THE BREAST

Comprehensive Management of Benign and Malignant Diseases

SECOND EDITION

Volume 2

Edited by

KIRBY I. BLAND, M.D.

J. Murray Beardsley Professor and Chairman
Department of Surgery
Professor of Medical Sciences
Brown University School of Medicine
Surgeon-in-Chief, Rhode Island Hospital
Executive Surgeon-in-Chief, Brown University Affiliated Hospitals
Brown University
Providence, Rhode Island

EDWARD M. COPELAND III, M.D.

The Edward R. Woodward Professor and Chairman
Department of Surgery
University of Florida College of Medicine
Director, University of Florida Shands Cancer Center
Gainesville, Florida

Illustrated by

Louis Clark and Jonathan Bland

W.B. SAUNDERS COMPANY
A Division of Harcourt Brace & Company
Philadelphia   London   Toronto   Montreal   Sydney   Tokyo

W.B. SAUNDERS COMPANY
A Division of Harcourt Brace & Company

The Curtis Center
Independence Square West
Philadelphia, Pennsylvania 19106

Library of Congress Cataloging-in-Publication Data

The breast: comprehensive management of benign and malignant diseases / [edited by] Kirby I. Bland, Edward M. Copeland III; illustrations by Louis Clark and Jonathan Bland.—2nd ed.

p.   cm.

Includes bibliographical references and index.

ISBN 0–7216–6656–6

1. Breast—Cancer—Treatment.   2. Breast—Diseases—Treatment.   I. Bland, K. I.   II. Copeland, Edward M.   [DNLM: 1. Breast Diseases—therapy. 2. Breast Neoplasms—therapy.   WF 900 B828 1998]

RC280.B8B674   1998   618.1′9—dc21

DNLM/DLC   97-135

THE BREAST: COMPREHENSIVE MANAGEMENT OF BENIGN
AND MALIGNANT DISEASES   ISBN 0–7216–6656–6

Printed in the United States of America.

Last digit is the print number: 9   8   7   6   5   4   3   2   1

CONTENTS

VOLUME 1

VOLUME 2

*Deceased

*Deceased

THE BREAST

SURGERY FOR BENIGN AND MALIGNANT DISEASES OF THE BREAST

CHAPTER 39

EVOLUTION OF SURGICAL PRINCIPLES AND TECHNIQUES FOR THE MANAGEMENT OF BREAST CANCER

Eric R. Frykberg, M.D. / Kirby I. Bland, M.D.

To understand a science it is necessary to know its history

Auguste Comte (1798–1857)

Let us not lightly cast aside things that belong to the past, for only with the past can we weave the fabric of the future.

Anatole France (1844–1924)

Those who cannot remember the past are condemned to repeat it.

George Santayana (1863–1952)

We see so far, because we stand on the shoulders of giants.

Sir Isaac Newton (1643–1727)

ANCIENT RECORDS

The ancient recordings of historical aspects of carcinoma of the breast document the development of thought regarding its biology and pathophysiology and the application of these concepts to rational treatment. Its description in the earliest medical literature indicates that this disease has always been the relatively common and virulent entity that we know today.

The Edwin Smith Papyrus, discovered at Thebes, Egypt, in 1862, the oldest known medical document, is thought to date from between 3000 B.C. and 2500 B.C. It contains the oldest known reference to tumors or ulcers of the breast.[29, 41, 176, 245] Believed to have been written by the first known physician, Imhotep, it describes "bulging tumors" of the breast that were cool, spreading, and hard; had no granulation; formed no fluid; and generated no secretion. These tumors were probably malignant lesions, and it was asserted that there was no treatment for them, even though cauterization with a fire drill was used for lesions thought to represent benign cysts or breast abscesses.[60, 176] Writings from India and Assyria that date from this same period also mention breast growths.[60] There is no evidence of the application of an operative procedure for breast carcinoma in these ancient records.

The earliest reference to breast carcinoma in the ancient Greek civilization was made by the historian Herodotus (ca. 484–425 B.C.). He credited the Persian physician Democedes (ca. 525 B.C.) with the successful treatment of a breast tumor that had already ulcerated and spread in Atossa, daughter of Cyrus and wife of Darius.[41, 60, 139, 176] This may be the first description of local and metastatic spread of cancer, although the fact that it was apparently cured raises doubt that it was a malignancy.[41, 317] The hindrance of early diagnosis by a woman's fear and cosmetic considerations, a problem that persists to the present day, is also demonstrated by this anecdote.[176]

Hippocrates, the Father of Medicine (ca. 460–370 B.C.), devoted little attention to breast Karkinoma in his vast collection of works. His diligent observations of disease processes did include two references to apparently advanced cases of breast malignancy[41, 56, 176]:

> The whole body becomes emaciated. . . . When they have gone as far as this, they do not recover, but die of this disease.

This probably also represents an early reference to metastatic breast carcinoma. Hippocrates was the first to distinguish benign from malignant breast neoplasms, applying the latter term to any growth that spread and caused death.[317] He advocated withholding any treatment for "hidden" or deep-seated breast tumors (presumably referring to those that did not yet involve the overlying skin) in view of his observations that medical therapy caused a "speedy death, but to omit treatment is to prolong life." Some have interpreted these hidden cancers to mean those occurring within the body (i.e., metastatic lesions), for which this caution is logical.[56] There is no evidence that surgery was then applied to this disease.

Aulus Cornelius Celsus (ca. 30 B.C.–38 A.D.) was a

Roman scholar and encyclopedist who, although not a physician, wrote one of the most extensive surveys of the practice of medicine of that era. This work, *De Medicina*, demonstrated remarkable insight into the natural history of cancer, particularly as it applied to the breast.[34, 176] He provided one of the first descriptions of the "dilated tortuous veins" that typically surround a tumor,[41] which later led Galen to liken the lesion to a crab and to apply the label of *cancer*.[60] Celsus described four stages in the clinical evolution of breast cancer, the first of which (*cacoethes*) represented either early malignancy or a benign premalignant lesion. He advised treatment only at this stage, first with caustics, followed by surgical excision and cauterization if symptoms improved. Like his Egyptian and Greek predecessors, he advised against any treatment for the three more advanced stages of malignancy, since any surgery seemed to "irritate" the process and hasten the demise of the patient. Despite this cautious approach, it is evident that extensive surgery was commonly carried out for breast carcinoma in this ancient Roman period. Celsus advised against removal of the pectoral muscles if breast amputation was done. He thus indicated the benefits of early detection and treatment and the dangers of surgery for locally advanced disease that were ultimately confirmed some 2000 years later.[41, 56, 176, 317]

Galen (ca. 131–203 A.D.) was a Greek physician whose abundant works on medicine centered around the humoral principle of disease first elaborated by Hippocrates. He asserted that cancer was a local manifestation of "melancholia" caused by an excess of black bile in the body. This was the rationale behind his recommendation that all treatment include purgatives, bleeding, proper nutrition, and restarting of menstruation (he noted that most cases of breast carcinoma occurred in postmenopausal females). Such a concept represents perhaps one of the earliest views of breast malignancy as a systemic disease that required systemic treatment and served to explain its poor prognosis at that time.[60, 97] After such treatment, Galen recommended surgical excision of the diseased breast if it was amenable to removal. In what may be the first description of an operation for cancer of any kind, he advised incising the breast through healthy, uninvolved tissue to widely encompass the whole tumor without leaving behind "a single root" that would allow recurrence. He also advised against the use of either ligatures or cautery, since free flow of blood was thought to maximize the drainage of black bile and thus minimize the chance of local recurrence and spread.[41, 56, 176]

The Greek physician and surgeon Leonides, who worked in the great school of Alexandria around 180 A.D., provided the first detailed factual description of a mastectomy as it was widely practiced at that time. He, like Galen, advocated wide excision of the tumor through normal tissues, but he used cautery to both stem the bleeding and eradicate the disease. The common association of enlarged axillary nodules with breast cancer was noted in his writings.[41, 60, 245] He was the first to describe nipple retraction as a clinical sign of breast cancer. He advised against surgical intervention in cases of locally advanced disease and also advocated systemic "detoxification of the body" in both the preoperative and postoperative phases of treatment.[56, 176, 234] His practice of performing mastectomy by alternate incision and cautery persisted largely unchanged for at least the next 1500 years.

Substantial progress was made in these ancient times toward understanding the pathophysiology of breast carcinoma and developing some of the basic surgical treatment principles that we still follow today. In the next several centuries further progress was scant, and some concepts were even forgotten.

MEDIEVAL AND RENAISSANCE PERIODS

The humoral theory of disease prevailed throughout the Dark Ages, and rigid adherence to Galen as the ultimate authority in medical matters prevented any further innovations in the treatment of breast carcinoma. A conservative and nihilistic view of this disease process was held by virtually all medical practitioners. The influence of the Church on all scholarly matters in this era is suggested by the fact that the Council of Tours in 1162 banned the "barbarous practice" of surgery for breast tumors.[41, 60] Cautery, purgatives, and caustic agents were the mainstays of treatment, as they largely were in the ancient Greek and Roman cultures. The treatises of the Spanish-Arabian surgeon Albucaisis (ca. 1013–1106) and the French surgeons Henri de Mondeville (ca. 1260–1320) and his pupil Guy de Chauliac (ca. 1300–1367) reflected Galen's approach to breast cancer in advocating only a limited role for surgery for tumors that could be completely removed.[200] De Chauliac emphasized the need for wide excision of these tumors to include all residual disease when surgery was indicated. Lanfranc (ca. 1296), the Father of French Surgery, practiced the same technique for mastectomy that Leonides had described 1100 years before and was largely responsible for this operation's becoming the standard treatment for breast cancer in the larger schools of medicine in Europe.[41, 176, 245]

As the Renaissance philosophy of enlightenment and learning spread throughout Europe in the fifteenth and sixteenth centuries, many of the principles that eventually led to the modern era of breast cancer treatment were developed or rediscovered. At the same time, however, several extreme and irrational modes of treatment persisted. The Spanish surgeon Francisco Araceo (1493–1571) cut directly into breast tumors to place a large ligature in an attempt to "dissolve" the disease. Some physicians applied frogs and bisected chickens or puppies to breast tumors. William Clowes (1560–1634), physician to Queen Elizabeth, advocated the laying on of hands by the monarch to cure this disease. Peter Lowe (ca. 1597) applied goat's dung, and James Cooke (1614–1688) advised bleeding from the basilic vein.[41, 60, 176] Incising into a diseased breast and through tumor in a piecemeal approach to removing the malignancy appears to have been commonly practiced during this period. The poor results of this practice, in terms of the rapid recurrence of ulcerating tumors, led Fabricius ab Aquapendente (1537–1619), the famed Italian surgeon and anatomist who was William Harvey's teacher, to condemn partial excision as worthless. He performed radical excisions of the entire breast, but only when the patient requested it.[41, 176, 322] This idea recalled the advice of Galen and Leonides that breast tumors be widely excised through normal tissue and represented an important conceptual basis for the ultimate evolution of the modern mastectomy.

One of the first scholars of this period to reject the entrenched doctrines of Galen and thus pave the way for a new era of medical progress was Andreas Vesalius (1514–1574), the Father of Modern Anatomy. He also advocated wide surgical excision of breast tumors but substituted ligatures for cautery to control hemorrhage. Ambrose Pare (1510–1590), the French military surgeon and Father of Modern Surgery, treated large and advanced breast malignancies with milk, vinegar, and ointments in the galenic tradition. He also widely excised smaller tumors, using sulfuric acid instead of hot cautery to control bleeding. He attempted a less mutilating procedure originally introduced by Lenard Fuchs (1501–1566) involving crushing the diseased breast between lead plates.[245] The observation of the probable relationship between breast carcinoma and swelling of the axillary glands was an important advance credited to Pare. His pupil, Bartholemy Cabrol, took a more radical approach to breast cancer by advocating mastectomy and removal of the underlying pectoral muscles, as did Jacques Guillemeau (1550–1601) and Michael Servetus (1509–1553). Servetus, a Spanish surgeon who was burned at the stake by Calvinists, was also perhaps the first to recommend that axillary lymph nodes be removed along with the radical excision of the breast in the treatment of breast carcinoma.[245, 322] This idea was also advanced by the Italian surgeon Marcus Aurelius Severinus (1580–1659), who was perhaps the first author since Hippocrates to emphasize the distinction between benign and malignant breast tumors. He also recommended excision of benign lesions to prevent their developing into cancers.[50, 60, 176]

The sixteenth and seventeenth centuries were marked by a variety of innovations in the technique of mastectomy for breast cancer that led to a more efficient, thorough, and swift operation in this preanesthetic era. Wilhelm Fabry von Hilden, also known as Fabricius Hildanus (1560–1624), a German surgeon taught by Vesalius, invented a surgical instrument that compressed the base of the breast to allow easy amputation with a knife. He emphasized the need for tumors to be mobile if the patient were to be a candidate for surgery and to avoid leaving behind "sprouts," asserting[12]:

But before everything we must carefully make out whether the tumour can be shifted and moved from one point to another, and whether it can be radically excised. For the operation will be fruitless if any part of the tumour, however minute—nay, even the membranes in which tumours of this sort are usually enveloped—be left behind. For the disease sprouts up again, and becomes more malignant than ever, while there is no hope that we can remove what remains behind by cauterising.

Fabry also removed axillary lymph nodes as a part of his procedure.[41, 69, 157, 245]

Johannes Scultetus (1595–1645) was another German surgeon whose method of treatment for breast carcinoma involved traction on the diseased breast with cords placed through the base with large needles, allowing complete amputation with a knife (see Figs. 1–7 and 1–8). Bidloo (1708) and Tabor (1721) described similar instruments and methods.[261] In all cases the large open wounds were cauterized, which generally led to a high incidence of infection and death.[56, 60]

The Reverend John Ward described in 1666 a mastectomy performed on a Mrs. Townsend, in which two surgeons bluntly separated a breast tumor from surrounding tissues by hand, after the skin incision. The skin was apparently closed back over the wound temporarily and in the succeeding 2 days reopened several times to allow further removal of more tumor. Several months later the patient died with malignancy still present in the breast, confirming the admonition against piecemeal removal of breast tumors given a century earlier by Fabricius ab Aquapendente.[56, 176, 234] Attempts at this more limited form of operation may have been initiated by a desire to be kinder to the patient by reducing the degree of mutilation and perhaps also to avoid the catastrophic complications from the large cauterized open wounds that took several months to heal, *if* the patient survived. The flaw in these attempts, as noted by Moore two centuries later, became obvious when these tumors quickly recurred and hastened the patient's death, presumably from residual tumor left behind.[41, 204] This observation had been made by Celsus 1800 years earlier. One of the first surgical attempts to allow healing by direct union of the incised skin edges following mastectomy was recorded by Van der Mullen in 1698. The fact that this patient also died contributed to the controversy over the safety of primary wound closure.[56]

THRESHOLD OF THE MODERN PERIOD

One of the greatest impediments to the advancement of knowledge of the treatment of breast carcinoma through these years was in the failure of physicians to keep comprehensive records of their results, the absence of scientific analysis of such results, and the poor communication among physicians. With the advent of the Age of Enlightenment in the eighteenth century, this situation began to change. The great hospitals of Paris and London became centers of scholarly study in both theoretical and practical aspects of medicine. Formal lectures in anatomy and surgery were instituted, prizes were awarded for scientific research, and in 1731 one of the first surgical societies was founded in France, the Academie de Chirurgie.[56] Its publication, *The Memoires*, was the first journal devoted entirely to surgery, and it pioneered the spread of surgical knowledge throughout Europe.

The systemic theory of origin of breast carcinoma persisted during this period, although derangements of the newly discovered and described lymphatic system replaced Galen's black bile as the stimulating agent.[60, 176, 317] John Hunter (1728–1793), a proponent of this idea, believed that cancer made its appearance wherever lymph coagulated. He also believed, however, that a local component of disease origin was important in the treatment of breast carcinoma, which required wide excision beyond the grossly visible disease if recurrences were to be avoided.[58] This typified the views of many surgeons of this period, and such views marked the beginning of a trend toward more aggressive and thorough local treatments that ultimately led to greatly improved results for women afflicted with breast cancer. The report of Guillaume de Houpeville in 1693, describing his removal of a breast with surrounding healthy tissue as well as the underlying pectoral muscle, indicated a revival of the radical operation first advocated 150 years before by Cabrol, Guillemeau, and Servetus.[245] Such an operation was not often performed at that time, but de Houpeville's report did illustrate the beginning of the idea that breast cancer may initially develop as localized disease.

One of the greatest contributions to this changing attitude was made by the French surgeon Henri Francois LeDran (1685–1770), who practiced at the Hôpital St. Come. He courageously repudiated the classic humoral theory of Galen, which was still firmly entrenched in the contemporary teachings of medical schools, by asserting in 1757 that breast cancer began in its earliest stages as a local process within the breast proper. As it grew, he believed it spread initially to the regional axillary lymphatics and then to distant sites through the general circulation.[172] He thus claimed, "we may hope for a perfect cure" by aggressive surgical ablation in its earliest stages. This presaged the benefits of early detection of this disease that were to be well demonstrated more than 200 years later,[262, 264, 285] as well as the benefits of a wide surgical resection of disease that were to be so famously demonstrated by Halsted 150 years later.[122] LeDran's operation included the dissection of enlarged axillary lymph nodes, as previously advocated by Servetus, Severinus, and Fabry. He also recognized the dismal prognostic implications of axillary lymph node involvement with the malignant process.[56, 176, 245, 317] The results of these

efforts can only be surmised by LeDran's vague statement, characteristic of this period, that he carried out "a great number" of such operations, "many" with success.

Jean Louis Petit (1674–1750), LeDran's contemporary, was a prominent French surgeon and the first Director of the Academie Francaise de Chirurgie (Fig. 39–1). He is credited by many as being the first to introduce an improved operation for breast carcinoma with the goal of curing rather than simply removing an inevitably fatal tumor.[41, 60, 176, 225, 234, 245] His book, *Traites des Operations*, was not published until 24 years after his death. In it, he recommended total removal of the breast and of any enlarged axillary lymph nodes as well as the pectoralis major muscle if it was involved by tumor. It is not clear whether the lymph nodes were removed in continuity, but he did begin the operation by removing them.[56] He discouraged the practice of partial or piecemeal removal of tumor and breast tissue that was so prevalent at the time and asserted, "the roots of a cancer (of the breast) were the enlarged lymphatic glands." This principle of wide excision without incising, or even viewing, the tumor itself recalls the original philosophy set forth by Galen.

Although Petit's operation may be considered the direct forerunner of the modern radical mastectomy in both principle and technique, it did differ principally in the amount of skin removed. He advised leaving the greater portion of overlying skin, and even the nipple, and dissecting breast tissue out from beneath it. His pupil and colleague, Rene Garangeot (1688–1760), was largely responsible for preserving

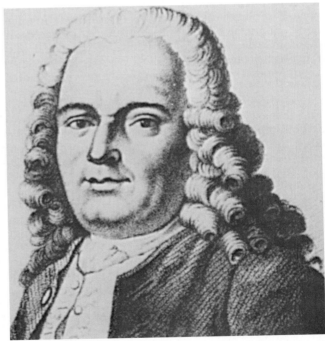

Figure 39–1 *Jean Louis Petit (1674–1750), the French surgeon who was the first to apply surgical intervention as a curative modality for breast carcinoma. (From Robinson JO: Am J Surg 151:317–333, 1986. Adapted with permission from American Journal of Surgery.)*

and spreading the teachings of this eminent surgeon who was so far ahead of his time. Garangeot explained the rationale for skin preservation in mastectomy in his own book, *Traite des Operations de Chirurgie* (1720):

> sewing up the lips of the wound immediately after operation, as was practiced by J. L. Petit, is not only the safest method of arresting hemorrhage but is also the quickest way of healing the wound and preventing the return of the cancer.

It probably also served to reduce the considerable number of infectious complications associated with the typically large and open wounds that most surgeons of that era left, although no definitive results were ever published.[234] Petit did recognize the necessity of removing any skin directly involved by the cancer, asserting[225]:

> Where the integuments are also affected and strictly joined to the cancer there is little hope to expect a perfect cure if they are not both cleanly extirpated together.

This further reinforced the principle of wide excision of all clinically evident malignancy. He also recognized the poor prognosis of cervical and supraclavicular lymph node involvement.[176, 245]

These principles of breast carcinoma beginning as a localized disease process and necessitating wide excision of the entire breast and surrounding tissues if cure was to be achieved gained momentum during this period. Lorenz Heister (1683–1758), a famous German surgeon, used a guillotine device to amputate the entire breast. He was also aware of the morbid implications of axillary lymph node involvement. Removal of axillary contents, the pectoralis major muscle, and even portions of the chest wall if necessary, for excision of the gross tumor were recommended by him in conjunction with mastectomy.[60, 136, 245] Bernard Peyrilhe (1735–1804) also embraced the concept that breast cancer began as a local disease in the breast and later spread by way of the lymphatics.[226] Like Heister and Petit, he advocated the total removal of a cancerous breast along with the axillary contents and pectoralis major muscle.[56, 60, 317]

Samuel Sharpe, an English surgeon, advocated a similarly aggressive approach in his *Treatise on the Operations of Surgery*, published in 1735. He recommended removing the entire breast through a longitudinal incision for small tumors, although an oval segment of skin was taken for larger tumors, to facilitate the dissection. He claimed that the breast should be cleaned away from the pectoral fascia and that this operation was impractical if the tumor involved the pectoral muscles. The necessity of removing any "knobs" in the armpit was also asserted by Sharpe, who wrote[12, 157, 245]:

> The possibility of extirpating these knobs without wounding the great vessels is very much questioned

by surgeons, but I have done it when they have not laid backwards and deep.

Benjamin Bell (1749–1806), surgeon to the Edinburgh Royal Infirmary, not only advocated a radical operation for all breast tumors but also emphasized the importance of early diagnosis.[54, 176, 234, 245] He echoed Petit's views in his book, *A System of Surgery* (1784), in which he wrote[18]:

> When practitioners have an opportunity of removing a cancerous breast early they should always embrace it, that as little skin as possible should be removed, and that the breast should be dissected off the pectoral muscle, which ought to be preserved. If any indurated glands be observed, they should be removed and particular care should be given to this part of the operation. For unless all the diseased glands be taken away, no advantage whatever will be derived from it.

These principles of treatment of breast carcinoma remained the standard in Scotland for the next century.

Henry Fearon (1750–1825), a British surgeon of this period, also recognized the importance of early treatment of breast carcinoma and the unlikely probability of achieving this goal. In 1784 he asserted[58]:

> The early period of the complaint is beyond all doubt the most favorable period for extirpating it, however patients can seldom be convinced that there is any necessity for an operation while the disease continues in a mild state.

In the latter years of the eighteenth century and the first half of the nineteenth century, a greater degree of conservatism and pessimism toward breast carcinoma pervaded the medical literature and the practice of many surgeons. This arose primarily from the poor results of the bold operations described above. William Hunter stated in 1778[12]:

> Amputation of the breast is an easy operation but a doubtful remedy. The little success attending it deters the patient, wherefore it ought not to be undertaken without great probability of cure, as we run the risque of a general prejudice against the operation, which may so affright others that they will not run the hazard, tho' their disease may be really curable.

Thus, although many agreed that the goal of surgery should be complete removal of the disease, the consensus was that no operation should be performed at all if this goal was not realistic.

The Dutch surgeon Hendrick Ulhoorn asserted in 1747 that even small breast cancers had already spread throughout the body, and there was thus no point in operating for this disease.[56] Such a belief was remarkably similar to the theories of breast carcinoma held more than 200 years later. His contemporary, Petrus Camper, commented on the reluctance of most surgeons at that time to perform mastectomy for breast carcinoma; he reported in 1757, "not six times a year a breast was amputated with reasonable chance of cure" in Amsterdam, which had a population of 200,000.[56, 59, 245]

The first efforts to record and analyze the results of treatment of breast carcinoma occurred during this period and reinforced these pessimistic attitudes. Most of the literature consisted of case reports of mastectomy. Alexander Monro Senior (1697–1767) reviewed the cases of 60 patients with this disease who had been treated by contemporary methods and found only four patients free of disease after 2 years.[201] He noted that the disease almost always returned, either locally or in distant sites, soon after operation. Operative mortality alone was reported to be as high as 20 percent, predominantly from sepsis.[60]

The Scottish surgeon James Syme (1799–1870) wrote in 1842 in his *Principles of Surgery* that palliative procedures for carcinoma of the breast should be abandoned when axillary glands are involved or the tumor is too extensive or fixed to allow complete removal.[176, 245, 283] He found that surgery is more likely to "excite greater activity" of the tumor left behind, echoing the observations of Celsus nearly 1900 years earlier.

A. Velpeau reviewed this subject in 1856 and listed several authors who had reported dismal results after treatment of breast carcinoma.[296] According to him, Boyer found four cases of cure out of 100 operations, and Mayo reported only a 5 percent cure rate.[56] MacFarlane had not seen a single cure after 118 operations. Although Velpeau did not attach great importance to these observations because they lacked scientific foundation, his own experience led him to believe that a true breast malignancy could not be cured.[54, 245]

Sir James Paget (1814–1899) wrote in 1856 that breast carcinoma was such a hopeless disease that he doubted the substantial mortality and morbidity of its treatment could be justified.[218] He found that women with "scirrhous" carcinoma of the breast actually lived longer without surgical intervention than those who underwent attempts at surgical excision.[56] In 235 cases he had an operative mortality of 10 percent and had never seen a cure or a case in which recurrence was delayed beyond 8 years.[176, 245]

Robert Liston (1794–1847) wrote in 1840 that only under the most favorable circumstances should a woman be subjected to operation for breast carcinoma and that it was rash and cruel to remove axillary lymph glands involved with tumor.[178, 245]

The first hospital ward for indigent cancer patients was opened in Middlesex Hospital in London in 1792.[56] The surgeon John Howard provided the major initiative in this effort by arguing that such a ward would not only benefit the patients themselves but would also provide an opportunity to study the natural history of this disease, which could lead to improvements in treatment. Private endowments eventually allowed this goal to be realized by contributing to its development into perhaps the first modern cancer institute. From this establishment came some of the most important advances in our knowledge and experience with carcinoma of the breast in the ensuing years.

By the middle of the nineteenth century, the basic principles of surgical treatment of breast carcinoma had been laid down. Several surgeons had already performed what would later be called the *standard radical mastectomy*; however, there was no consistency among various surgeons or between different geographic regions in the overall management of this disease or in the specific operations performed. This can be attributed to a less than optimal mechanism for widespread communication and dissemination of ideas, ignorance of the basic pathology and pathophysiology of the malignant process, and the poor results of treatment, evident in the few scientific analyses available. Advances in these areas were necessary for the evolution of a truly effective and widely accepted treatment for breast carcinoma.

THE MODERN ERA

Two major advances that paved the way for an effective operation for breast carcinoma were the discovery and development of general anesthesia and the dissemination of the germ theory of disease and principles of antisepsis.[56] These both occurred in the middle to late 1800s. One other series of scientific advances occurred during this same period that contributed to a basic understanding of tumor biology that many consider the most important contribution to the ultimate development of a rational treatment for breast carcinoma. The widespread use of the microscope led to the birth of cell pathology, and such scientists as Raspail (1826), Schleiden (1838), Schwann (1838), Muller (1838), and Remak (1852) established the cell as the basic structural and functional unit of normal tissue as well as of neoplasms.[176] The growth and behavior of malignancies were found by (among others) Virchow and Leydig to be caused primarily by cell division, thus removing cancer from the realm of body humors. Recamier first used the term *metastasis* in 1829 and described local tumor infiltration and venous invasion.[317] Rene Laennec (1781–1826) was the first to devise a classification of tumors based on scientific principles. Hannover (1843) and Lebert (1845) first described a *cancer cell*, which identified a malignancy and distinguished it from benign growths. Hannover also asserted that these cells could be found circulating in the blood and were responsible for distant metastases.[56, 317]

Virchow believed that these malignant cells originated from connective tissue. The meticulous and extensive studies of Thiersch (1822–1895) and Waldeyer (1872), however, established the epithelial origin of all carcinomas. These investigators also supported the mechanical theory of metastasis, asserting that emboli of cancer cells through the lymphatics and blood stream are responsible for the spread of disease.[317]

These scientific advances fostered an enlightened atmosphere in the second half of the nineteenth century, which led to the re-emergence of radical surgery for breast carcinoma. The increasing acceptance of the local theory of origin of this disease and the desire to eliminate its local recurrence further contributed to a decline in pessimistic and fatalistic attitudes and to the establishment of a more rational approach to management. Joseph Pancoast (1805–1882) was a professor of surgical anatomy at Jefferson Medical College in Philadelphia (Fig. 39–2). He revived the teachings of Petit and Bell, advocating routine removal of the entire breast for tumors of any size and removal of axillary lymph nodes if they were clinically involved. His assertion that the axillary contents should be removed in continuity with the breast represented the first description of an en bloc resection.[54, 56, 219, 234] This was not then a widely held view, as suggested by the fact that Pancoast's successor, Samuel D. Gross (1805–1884), felt, "the proper operation is amputation, not excision."[234] Gross taught that as much skin as possible should be preserved and that axillary lymph nodes should not be removed, in view of the hopelessness of cure if they were involved.

Thomas Bryant, an assistant surgeon at Guy's Hospital in London, echoed Pancoast's views in

1864.[234] He believed that local recurrence of breast carcinoma was caused by inadequate surgical resection and thus taught that the entire breast, along with a wide margin of overlying skin, should be removed in all cases of breast carcinoma.

A landmark paper by Charles Hewitt Moore (1821–1870) was presented before the Royal Medical and Surgical Society in London in 1867.[204] Moore was surgeon to the Middlesex Hospital, where he observed several breast cancer patients who had been subjected to the various operations then being practiced for this disease and who had subsequently developed local recurrences. He postulated that, since these recurrences virtually always occurred near the surgical scar, they probably represented direct extension of the primary disease rather than new foci of malignancy. Thus, they appeared to result from incomplete removal of the disease at the original operation rather than from a systemic predisposition, or diathesis. He advocated removal of the entire breast for any breast carcinoma, along with a wide margin of overlying skin, especially if there was any doubt about skin involvement by the tumor. Another principle set forth in this paper was to avoid cutting into the tumor or even seeing it in the course of resection—so as to prevent any of its cells from lodging in the wound. He also recommended removing diseased axillary glands en bloc with the breast, although he later stated that even normal-looking axillary lymph nodes can never be assumed to be healthy, suggesting that axillary dissection should be a routine part of the operation.[41, 56, 234, 245] He did not recommend removing the pectoral muscles. It is interesting to note that he reported the placement of a drainage tube through the armpit as early as 1858.[234] Moore gave new impetus to the theory of local origin of breast carcinoma with this report, and his remarkable clinical insight into the underlying pathophysiology of this disease served as the foundation on which a standard and widely accepted operation would later be based.

Richard Sweeting, a British surgeon from Stratford, advocated the same principles of wide excision but extended Moore's operation to include "the lower two thirds" of the pectoralis major muscle.[282] He did not mention removal of the axillary contents but articulated the concept of the local origin of disease:

> For if a purely localized cancer is to be cured by incisions, and is sure to return if not completely removed, then we are more likely to succeed in proportion as our incisions are as deep and as extensive as is consistent with the patient's safety.

He reported three patients who were "cured" by this operation on follow-up of 7 months, 25 months, and 31 months, respectively.

Joseph Lister (1827–1912) of Edinburgh, Scotland, revolutionized the surgical approach toward breast carcinoma with his introduction of antiseptic techniques; he also supported the principles laid down by

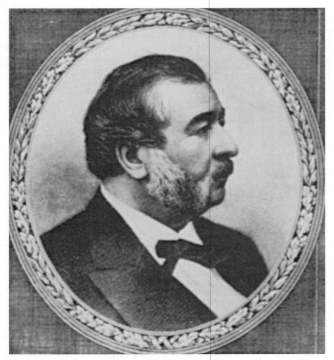

Figure 39–2   *Joseph Pancoast (1805–1882), the American surgeon who supported wide breast excision and first described en bloc axillary lymph node dissection. (From Robinson JO: Am J Surg 151:317–333, 1986. Adapted with permission from American Journal of Surgery.)*

Moore. In 1870 he reported removing the entire breast in continuity with the axillary glands and was the first to describe division of the origins of both pectoral muscles to facilitate the axillary dissection.[177]

In 1877 William Mitchell Banks, surgeon to the Liverpool Royal Infirmary, read a paper before the British Medical Association supporting the principles of Moore and emphasizing the merits of routine axillary dissection in continuity with wide excision of the entire breast.[11, 234] Banks' views were supported by his own clinical experience and that of his contemporaries in attempting to avoid the axillary recurrence that was often noted when the axillary nodes were left *in situ*. He reiterated Moore's observation that it was impossible clinically to judge axillary node involvement. Also described in his paper was the technique of first removing the breast until it was attached only to the axillary pedicle, which could then be meticulously dissected free of the axillary vein as far as the clavicle (thus recalling the advice of Sharpe more than a century before). He employed "undercutting" of the remaining skin to facilitate primary closure of the wound. He did not find it necessary to divide the pectoral muscles as Lister had but did subscribe to Lister's antiseptic techniques. By 1902, he had performed this operation 300 times and documented the course of 175 patients. In his last 80 consecutive cases he reported only one operative mortality and several ancedotal reports of cure. He also expressed an opinion, which was to be shared increasingly by others in subsequent years, concerning the desirability of achieving earlier detection of breast carcinoma in order to improve the chances for cure[12]:

> Have you ever imagined what the results would be if all cancers were thoroughly excised when they were no bigger than peas? But if this happy consummation is to be reached, it will not be by performing tremendous operations upon practically hopeless cases.

A German surgeon from Berlin, Ernst Küster (1839–1922), had practiced routine clearance of the axilla in conjunction with mastectomy since 1871.[166] A review of 95 recurrences in his series demonstrated only one in the axilla.[256] Halsted later credited Küster with being the first to advocate routine systematic axillary dissection.[60]

Theodor Billroth (1824–1887), the famous professor of surgery in Vienna, elevated the practice of surgery to a scientific discipline. He related the clinical manifestations of breast carcinoma to its underlying pathophysiology and in this way developed a rational mode of treatment. Although he generally removed the entire breast with the underlying pectoral fascia, he felt that wide local excision of smaller tumors might be just as effective. After removing the breast he lengthened the incision into the axilla, where he digitally removed any enlarged nodes and the axillary fat pad. He also removed a portion of the

pectoral muscle if it was involved by tumor.[20] The overall mortality of this operation was 15.7 percent, and it was 21.3 percent for cases with axillary dissection. With the introduction of antiseptic wound techniques, these rates were reduced to 5.8 percent and 10.5 percent, respectively. As was characteristic of most mastectomies of this period, 82 percent of Billroth's patients developed local recurrence, and only 4.7 percent had survived by the end of 3 years.[114]

Richard von Volkmann (1830–1889), a German professor of surgery from Halle, was among the first to apply histological observations to the treatment of breast carcinoma. He reported several cases in which the pectoral fascia was involved with tumor that was clinically evident, but microscopic foci were not. This led him routinely to supplement mastectomy and axillary dissection with removal of the pectoral fascia.[304] He also advocated removal of a wide margin of skin as well as a generous portion of underlying muscle if the tumor were fixed to it. In 38 cases of far advanced disease, he reported a 14 percent 3-year survival rate and no local recurrence.[176] It was Volkmann's belief that survival without disease for 3 years was a firm indication of cure, an idea that pervaded virtually all studies of that period.[56]

Lothar Heidenhain (1860–1940), an assistant to Küster, reported the histological observation of metastases in lymphatic channels running between the breast and pectoral muscle in two thirds of the cases of breast carcinoma.[135] He believed that contraction of the muscle was a major route of disease spread. Based on these observations, Heidenhain routinely extended the surgical treatment of this disease to include a superficial layer of the muscle for movable tumors and complete removal of the entire pectoralis major muscle and its underlying connective tissue when the tumor was fixed to it.

Samuel Weissel Gross (1837–1889) was a lecturer in clinical surgery at the Jefferson Medical College in Philadelphia, where his father, Samuel D. Gross, had succeeded Pancoast as professor of surgery. Unlike his father, he endorsed the tenets of Pancoast and Moore advocating total mastectomy, including all skin covering the breast, routine axillary dissection, and excision of the pectoral fascia. This became known as the *dinner plate operation* because of the shape of the wound it left.[176, 234, 245] In his report of 207 patients, he demonstrated a 19.4 percent 3-year survival rate and a 53 percent rate of local recurrence, with only a 4.6 percent operative mortality.[106] He also showed that 87.5 percent of all nonpalpable axillary lymph nodes were actually involved with tumor, reinforcing his belief in the necessity for routine axillary dissection.

Sir Henry Butlin provided figures at about this same period from his own experience with carcinoma of the breast that supported a conservative and more selective approach toward axillary dissection.[157, 245] He recommended this procedure only when enlarged axillary glands could be palpated. His operative mortality rate (20 percent) and 3-year survival rate (five percent) among 209 women whose axillas were opened were substantially worse than those rates (ten percent and 18 percent, respectively) among 101 women who did not undergo axillary dissection as part of their operation. He interpreted these figures as indicating that axillary dissection was dangerous, although in retrospect it can be seen that he was describing the more favorable prognosis associated with earlier lesions in which axillary lymph nodes would not be clinically evident. The high operative mortality was typical of that period and was attributable principally to infection.

Johannes Adrianus Korteweg (1851–1930) was a Dutch professor of surgery whose critical approach toward evaluating his operative experience was typical of European surgeons at the end of the nineteenth century.[161, 162] He reviewed the operative mortality and cure rates of surgery for breast carcinoma from several European clinics and made several observations. The widely differing operative procedures and degrees of adherence to antiseptic techniques between various surgeons made comparison difficult and largely explained the range of differences in their respective results.[41] Korteweg noted a lower level of local recurrence before the introduction of listerian antisepsis than after, presumably because of an increasing preference to preserve more skin for primary wound closure once infection became less of a threat. He postulated that some forms of breast carcinoma are more malignant than others, thus foreshadowing current knowledge of the individual differences in tumor biology and growth characteristics among patients with the disease. He noted the substantially higher 3-year survival rates in patients without axillary nodal involvement than in those *with* axillary involvement. He also shared a misconception common in the history of medicine, believing that no further improvement could be expected in the cure rates following treatment of this disease.

Development of the Standard Radical Mastectomy

The evolution of a standardized, effective, and widely accepted operation for the treatment of carcinoma of the breast culminated primarily with the efforts of William Stewart Halsted (1852–1922). Having completed his undergraduate education at Yale in 1874 and his medical education at Columbia in 1877, Halsted then spent 2 years (1878–1880) in Europe observing the practice of the noted surgeons of that era (Fig. 39–3). For much of this period he worked in Vienna under Billroth, whose experience he later reviewed along with that of many other European surgeons. He developed a working knowledge of the state of the art of surgical treatment of breast carcinoma, which predominantly involved Volkmann's operation. He returned to New York with a firm idea, based on his observations and analyses of the results of others, of what the appropriate surgical attack on this disease should encompass.[114] The high rates of local recurrence and low rates of survival of the oper-

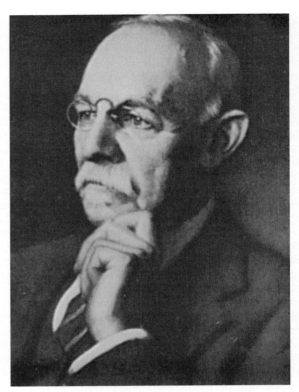

Figure 39–3 *William Stewart Halsted shortly before his death at age 70. (From Robinson JO: Am J Surg 151:317–333, 1986. Adapted with permission from American Journal of Surgery.)*

ations performed by the prominent European surgeons led him to extend the concept of wide excision, based on the theory of local origin of breast carcinoma. Halsted believed these poor results must be caused by an inadequate and inconsistent removal of tissue surrounding the tumor, thus failing to give the malignancy a wide enough berth to avoid leaving any cancer cells behind. He pronounced Volkmann's operation "a manifestly imperfect one."[120] Although Halsted's philosophy toward breast carcinoma was very much like that of Moore and Banks, he never referred to the work of these surgeons in his early reports. This was probably a result of the small circulation of the British journals in which they published.[234]

The major contribution that Halsted made in this area was his advocacy of the routine removal of the pectoralis major muscle (in addition to the entire breast) and meticulous clearing of the axillary tissue. He performed all of these maneuvers as an en bloc resection so as to avoid cutting across any cancer-involved tissues. He firmly believed that cancer spread entirely through the lymphatics and not through the blood stream, having been influenced by Heidenhain's studies that showed a high incidence of microscopic involvement of the pectoral muscles with tumor cells. He later asserted[119]:

From the careful microscopical examination of many very small cancers of the breast I am convinced that the pectoralis major muscle is usually at the time the operation involved in the new growth. Strange to say, no authority so far as I know suggests the advisability of always removing the pectoralis muscle or a portion of it in operations for the cure of cancer of the breast; and still stranger there are many surgeons of the first rank—surgeons in favor of methodically clearing out the axilla—who instead of recommending the excision of the muscle advise the removal of the fascia only from the pectoral muscle. . . . Surely it is absurd not to remove the muscle when its fascia is, even to the naked eye, diseased.

Halsted first performed his "complete operation" at Roosevelt Hospital in New York City in 1882. In 1883 he used it in "almost every case" of breast carcinoma, and it ultimately became known as the *radical mastectomy.*"[60, 114] His first 13 cases were summarized in an article he published on wound healing in 1891.[119] In 1894 he published his landmark study that described in detail both the operation he developed and the follow-up results from his first 50 patients.[120] There were no operative deaths in this series. The local recurrence rate of 6 percent (3 of 50 patients) and the 3-year survival (cure) rate of 45 percent stood in stark contrast to all of Halsted's contemporaries', which he meticulously analyzed in this same report (Table 39–1). He achieved his results in spite of his finding that 27 of the 50 patients had been labeled *hopeless* or *unfavorable* on presentation, that all had axillary node metastases, and that 10 percent had supraclavicular node metastases. By modern standards, his actual local recurrence rate was 18 percent. A follow-up study of this population by Lewis and Rienhoff in 1932[175] reported this local recurrence rate to have increased to 31.5 percent, which still represented a substantial improvement at that time. Another perspective was provided in 1980 by Henderson and Canellos,[60, 138] whose analysis of Halsted's data showed only 8 percent disease-free survival (DFS) at 4 years and no more than a 12 percent overall improvement in survival. Halsted

TABLE 39–1. RESULTS OF SURGICAL TREATMENT OF BREAST CARCINOMA UP TO 1894

Surgeon	Time	Cases (n)	Local Recurrence (%)	Three-Year Cure (%)
Banks	1877	46	——	20
Bergmann	1882–1887	114	51–60	20
Billroth	1867–1876	170	82	4.7
Czerny	1877–1886	102	62	18.8
Fischer	1871–1878	147	75	——
Gussenbauer	1878–1886	151	64	——
Konig	1875–1885	152	58–62	——
Küster	1871–1885	228	59.6	21.5
Lucke	1881–1890	110	66	16.2
Volkmann	1874–1878	131	60	11
Halsted	1889–1894	50	6	45

Compiled from Halsted WS: Johns Hopkins Hosp Rep 4:297–350, 1894–1895; and Cooper WA: Ann Med His 3:36–54, 1941.

himself continued to update his results, which he perceived as vindication of his original premise and reinforcing ement of the then prevalent concept of breast carcinoma as a disease that arises locally and spreads exclusively via the lymphatics.[121, 122]

Halsted's radical mastectomy involved wide excision of skin through a teardrop incision extending across the deltopectoral groove onto the arm, excision of the entire pectoralis major muscle, and simple division of the pectoralis minor muscle to expose the axillary contents for dissection (Fig. 39–4). By the time of his follow-up report in 1898, he had extended the operation routinely to include excision of the supraclavicular lymph nodes and pectoralis minor muscle and immediate skin graft of all wounds.[121] He learned this latter technique from Thiersch, in Germany, and was one of the few in the United States at that time to have mastered it. Halsted also described the dissection of mediastinal nodes by his house surgeon, Harvey Cushing, in three cases of recurrent breast carcinoma, prompting his prediction that this would probably be a routine part of the

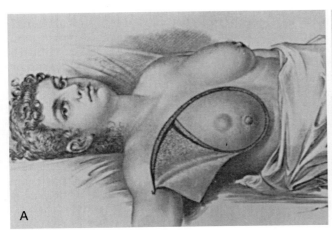 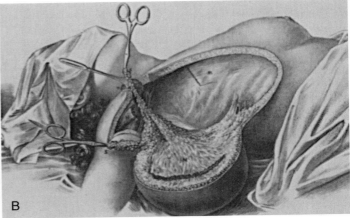

Figure 39–4 *A* and *B, Plates X and XI from Halsted's landmark 1894 paper (Johns Hopkins Hospital Reports, 4:297–350, 1894–1895) showing his incision and dissection for the radical mastectomy. (Courtesy of Johns Hopkins Hospital.)*

primary operation in the future. Halsted also favored stripping the fascial sheaths of the rectus, serratus anterior, subscapularis, and latissimus dorsi muscles in locally advanced cases and even indicated, "a part of the chest wall should, I believe, be excised in certain cases."[122]

In 1907 Halsted reported before the American Surgical Association an update of his results on 232 patients who underwent his complete operation at Johns Hopkins,[122] where he had served as professor of surgery since 1891. All patients in this series had been subjected to at least 3 years of follow-up. His operative mortality was 1.7 percent (4 patients), and only 18 patients had been lost to follow-up. No axillary lymph node metastasis was found in 64 of these 232 patients (27.6 percent), and this group had 70 percent overall cure rate (45 of 64 patients) and an 80 percent (51 of 64 patients) 3-year DFS rate. In 15 of these node-negative patients (23.4 percent), metastasis or local recurrence ultimately occurred: 6 developed such recurrence more than 3 years after treatment. This contrasted with the 24.5 percent cure rate for the 110 patients with axillary lymph node involvement but negative supraclavicular nodes, and the 7.5 percent cure rate in 40 patients with both axillary and supraclavicular lymph node involvement.

Halsted was pessimistic in this paper about the efficacy of routine supraclavicular node dissection and had abandoned this practice for cases with no clinical evidence of axillary or neck disease. He stated[122]:

> Before accepting the statement of anyone that he has cured a case of breast cancer with neck involvement, incontrovertible proof should be demanded. . . . We should demand as further proof of cure in these positive neck cases that the patient live at least five years after the operation. . . . With these stipulations fulfilled I should still be sceptical [sic] as to the cure.

This remarkable 1907 paper contained many of the fundamental precepts that are currently taken for granted. It was evident that the natural history of this disease was more protracted than was previously thought. The number of recurrences found more than 3 years after primary treatment led Halsted to first advance the idea that perhaps at least 5 years of survival was a more appropriate measure of "cure." His data also clearly demonstrated the importance of axillary lymph node involvement as a prognostic factor and that the prognosis for breast carcinoma is related to its stage or level of advancement at the time of diagnosis and treatment. This reinforced the findings of Butlin from several years before. The poor outcome of patients with supraclavicular node involvement, regardless of the extent of surgery, suggested systemic dissemination, which led Halsted eventually to abandon supraclavicular dissection. By 1910 Halsted had made his final modification to the operation, which was the elimination of the upper extension of the incision onto the arm. Instead, he carried his incision straight upward from the circular incision around the breast to the midclavicle.

All these observations emphasized the advantages of early detection of breast carcinoma, a principle strongly advocated by Halsted and one of the most vigorous thrusts of current research. Both the importance and the difficulty of such efforts were accurately described by Halsted[122]:

> But women are now presenting themselves more promptly for examination, realizing that a cure of breast cancer is not only possible, but, if operated upon early, quite probable. Hence the surgeon is seeing smaller and still smaller tumors, cancers which give not one of the cardinal signs . . . It would undoubtedly be possible for the expert to discover of the scirrhous growth earlier stages than he encounters, but unfortunately the tumor must first be recognized by the patient, and a scirrhous cancer large enough to attract her attention has quite surely already gone afield. Our problem, therefore, is to discover these tumors before the afflicted one can do so.

Halsted's operation resulted in the most significant improvement in survival and overall control of breast carcinoma that had occurred up to that time, which was reflected in its rapid and widespread adoption, by the turn of the century, as the standard treatment for this disease.[245] This was the first time in the long history of treatment of breast carcinoma that any single procedure was uniformly embraced. Halsted's 1907 paper, however, also contained the seeds of the eventual demise of the radical mastectomy some 70 years later. The fact that 23.4 percent of node-negative patients died of disseminated disease, despite having undergone the complete operation, provided the first indication that the theory of local origin does not adequately explain the underlying biology of this disease. Halsted was troubled by this observation but concluded simply that a more diligent and comprehensive surgical attack and an effort to diagnose the disease earlier would lead to an improved rate of cure in this group. Further studies in subsequent years were to confirm that metastasis must occur earlier than was originally thought (i.e., while the disease is still at a microscopic stage) and that more extensive local excision does not, in fact, improve the approximately 20 percent rate of relapse in stage I patients.[71, 78] This aspect of breast cancer biology led eventually to a diminished emphasis on ever wider and more extensive surgical excision in the initial treatment of primary disease.

The end of the nineteenth century provided an atmosphere of enlightenment and scientific approaches to disease that allowed the principles of breast cancer surgery to take root and flourish. In fact, in 1894 a professor of surgery at the New York Postgraduate Medical School, Willy Meyer (1858–1932), reported the details of an operation very simi-

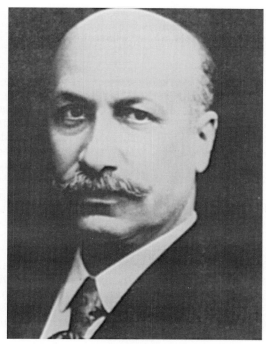

Figure 39–5   *Willy Meyer (1858–1932), German-born New York surgeon who conceived of and performed radical mastectomy independently of Halsted in 1894. (From Ravitch MM: A Century of Surgery, Vol 1. Philadelphia, JB Lippincott, 1980, p 471. Reprinted by permission.)*

2 months before and had performed only six other similar operations since 1891. The basis of Meyer's operation, like Halsted's, was removal en bloc of the entire breast, pectoralis muscles, and axillary contents. Meyer advocated routine removal of the pectoralis minor muscle, a modification later adopted by Halsted, and began his operation with the axillary dissection so as to minimize tumor manipulation and lymphatic dissemination.[121] Although he did not excise the supraclavicular lymph nodes at that time, he did add that to his procedure after reading Halsted's paper. He left more skin than Halsted did and sutured together as much of the skin as possible (Fig. 39–6). He grafted skin to any remaining defect only after 8 to 10 days to allow a bed of granulation tissue to develop. Drainage tubes were routinely placed in the axilla. Overall, he preferred his method to Halsted's since it seemed to be "more anatomical," although he recognized "Halsted's unprecedented percentage of cures." Meyer concluded[197]:

> That this kind of radical operation will be 'the' operation for the extirpation of carcinoma of the breast, there can be no doubt. . . . I venture to hope that, by absolutely and continuously working everywhere around the seat of disease, by never trespassing on the belly of the muscles, and always removing the latter completely, this extremely gratifying result might also be secured by others.
>
> Thus will then, at last, it is to be hoped, also this terrible foe of suffering mankind, this dread especially of the female sex, become oftener silenced and made more submissive to the surgeon's knife, provided the operation is done early, before remote parts of the system have become infected.

Here is still another independent recognition of the value of early detection and treatment of breast carcinoma.

lar to Halsted's radical mastectomy before the Section on Surgery of the New York Academy of Medicine.[197] Meyer (Fig. 39–5), born and educated in Germany, had independently conceived this operation based on the observations of Heidenhain and many of the other European surgeons who had also influenced Halsted.[2] Meyer's report was given only 10 days after the publication of Halsted's landmark paper on the "complete operation," although Meyer had performed his first fully developed operation only

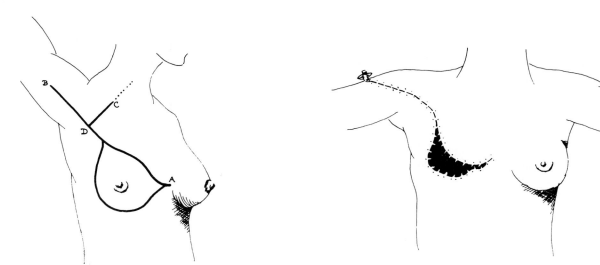

Figure 39–6   *Meyer's incision and closure for his radical mastectomy. (From Meyer W: JAMA 45:297–313, 1905. Copyright, 1905, American Medical Association. Reprinted by permission.)*

Meyer published an update of the results of his operation after 10 years[1] experience with 72 procedures in 70 patients.[198] His only modifications were supraclavicular dissection in cases of upper quadrant tumors and preservation of a portion of the pectoralis minor muscle to facilitate skin grafting. The operation took an average of 30 minutes to perform, one case being done in 12 minutes. He reported 1.4 percent operative mortality (one patient, who died of diabetic coma). Follow-up results were available for 67 patients, 30 (44.8 percent) of whom were alive at the time of his report. Twenty-four (35.8 percent) of these survivors were disease free, and six had developed local, regional, or distant recurrence. Of the 30 study patients with a 5- to 10-year follow-up, 8 (26.7 percent) were still alive, of whom 7 (23.3 percent) were disease free, and one had developed a regional recurrence 8 years after surgery. There was a 50 percent DFS (14 of 28 patients) among patients followed for 1 to 3 years. Thirty-five patients (52.3 percent) had died of their disease. Twenty-seven of those who died had distant metastases, accounting for 40.3 percent of all 67 traceable patients, while 4 died with regional recurrence, and the remaining 4 died with both local recurrence and distant metastasis. Meyer concluded this paper, as he did his original report, with an observation on the value of early detection[198]:

> I am convinced that final results could be further improved only, if we could get patients to come earlier for operation. The important task before us, therefore, is that of educating the public. . . . In view of the excellent results that can be obtained by radical operation . . . physicians, too, should advise early operation, not only in the plainly recognizable cases, but also in the doubtful ones, rather than keep such patients under observation until the disease has become manifest beyond question, and, perhaps, developed to a stage where it is beyond surgical reach.

Meyer was perhaps the first to believe in an immune-mediated basis for cancer, an idea that developed from his observation of the regression of a case of ulcerating breast carcinoma after the patient had developed and recovered from erysipelas.[2] He developed this thesis in his book, *Cancer*, published in 1931, and came to regard the disease as a systemic process, thus reviving a theory that had not been prevalent for more than 200 years.

An obscure report in *The Lancet* of February 4, 1893, is cited by Donegan[60] as evidence that other surgeons were performing similar radical breast excisions at the time of both Halsted's and Meyer's papers, perhaps even predating them. This report related a presentation by the British surgeon Arbuthnot Lane before the Clinical Society of London in 1893,[169] which described his operation as en bloc excision of the breast and underlying pectoral muscles and complete clearance of axillary contents:

> By these means not only were the primary growth and the cancerous glands removed, but, also, all the lymphatic channels along which infection had extended.

Halsted has nevertheless been accorded the primary credit for the radical mastectomy, in view of his meticulous and diligent correlation of the pathophysiology of breast carcinoma with an appropriate surgical attack as well as the esteem he engendered in his surgical pupils, who then became effective disciples of his technique.[56, 176, 245] Matas explained Halsted's prominence in this field by stating[191]:

> Though old the thought and oft expressed, 'tis his at last who says it best.

In the first decade of the twentieth century, several surgeons published their experiences with the radical mastectomy, indicating again how rapidly and widely it was accepted (Table 39–2). One of the most comprehensive such reports was published by J. Collins Warren of Boston in 1904,[312] describing the results of 100 consecutive cases of breast carcinoma accumulated during a 20-year period for which at least 3 years' follow-up was available. There was only 2 percent operative mortality among these patients, a 6 percent rate of local or regional recurrence, and a 30 percent rate of cure at 3 years. In following patients beyond 3 years, Warren found only a 12 percent rate of cure at 5 years and 5 percent at 10 years, leading him to assert, "the 3-year limit does not by any means constitute an infallible test of cure." He found that 56 percent of all locoregional recurrences that occurred did so within 5 years of surgery, and 37 percent occurred within 2 years. At the time of his report, nine patients treated for local recurrence were still alive and well; two of them lived 10 and 16 years, respectively, after resection for these recurrences. This was perhaps the first indication that

TABLE 39–2.   RESULTS OF RADICAL OPERATION FOR THE TREATMENT OF BREAST CARCINOMA SINCE 1904

Author	Date	No. Cases	Operative Mortality (%)	Locoregional Recurrence (%)	Five-Year Survival (%)
Warren[312]	1904	100	2	6	12
Meyer[198]	1905	72	1.4	9	26.7
Greenough[103]	1907	376	3.6	47.7	11.2
Halsted[122]	1907	232	1.7	19.5	30.9
Ochsner[214]	1907	98	3	——	18.4
Lee et al[173]	1924	75	——	——	15
White[316]	1927	157	——	22.6	36
Harrington[132]	1929	2083	0.76	——	34
Jessop[150]	1936	217	3.2	——	48
Rodman[246]	1943	132	——	2.2	46
Taylor and Wallace[288]	1950	2000	0.65	——	51
Haagensen and Stout[113]	1951	495	1.8	22.8	58.2

*Includes a mixture of cases, some of which were subjected to "complete" operations, others to lesser procedures.

local recurrence is not necessarily the inevitable death sentence that past authors had suggested. Skin involvement by the primary tumor had been noted in 17 percent of patients. Among 17 patients who had no axillary lymph node involvement, a 64 percent rate of cure was observed. An 8 percent rate of bilateral breast malignancy was also observed in this population. Another important observation made by Warren in this series was that the preoperative duration of symptoms did not appear to affect the prognosis.

Warren's first 50 cases had involved only total mastectomy with excision of the pectoral fascia and axillary lymph nodes, whereas his last 50 patients were subjected to the Halstedian operation. Interestingly, there was no difference in the overall survival for these two groups. In actuality, Warren's procedure more closely approximated that of Meyer, in that the axillary dissection was carried out first. He also added a hook-shaped lateral extension onto Halsted's classic racket-shaped (teardrop) incision (Fig. 39–7) and extended an incision onto the neck of several patients for supraclavicular node excision. He eventually abandoned this latter portion of the procedure, as Halsted did about this same time. Although Warren believed, as did Halsted, "any method which permits of an easy approximation of the edges of the wound is out of date," he was nevertheless able to close most of his wounds primarily by extensive mobilization of flaps and the opposite breast (Fig. 39–8). He thus made use of those same "plastic procedures" decried by Halsted, yet increasingly utilized by most other surgeons for primary wound closure.[122] A unique addition introduced by Warren was his insis-

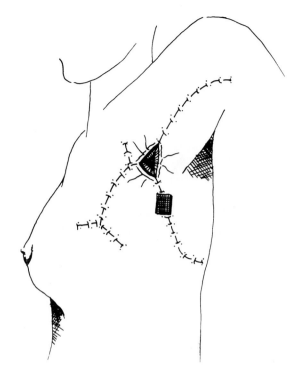

Figure 39–8 *Warren's closure following radical mastectomy. (From Warren JC: Ann Surg 40:805–833, 1904. Reprinted by permission.)*

tence that a pathologist be present in the operating room throughout the procedure to confirm that all margins were free of tumor before the dissection was completed.

In 1906 Jabez N. Jackson, of Kansas City, Missouri, published a detailed description of his own modification of the radical mastectomy, which he had performed on eight patients.[147] His operation involved a circular incision encompassing most of the breast skin and extending into the axilla and superiorly toward the supraclavicular area (Fig. 39–9). He also began his dissection at the axilla. This incision allowed ready mobilization of flaps for primary closure of the wound and eliminated dead space in the axilla (Fig. 39–10).

Albert J. Ochsner of Chicago in 1907 published the results of his surgical treatment of breast carcinoma in 98 patients who could be followed out of a total of 164 patients treated.[214] He reported 54 patients (55 percent) still alive at intervals of 1 to 13 years after surgery, 36 of these 54 patients having only a 5-year follow-up. Only 5 patients were alive 10 years or more after surgery. There was only 3 percent (5 of 164) operative mortality in this population. This paper typified the problems with many reports of this period in that it included patients with different stages of disease treated by different operative procedures. Ochsner's results dated back to 1887, and he did not perform his first radical mastectomy until 1896. Almost one third of his patients, therefore, underwent less extensive procedures, usually involving only total mastectomy and axillary dissection.

Robert B. Greenough, a Boston surgeon on the

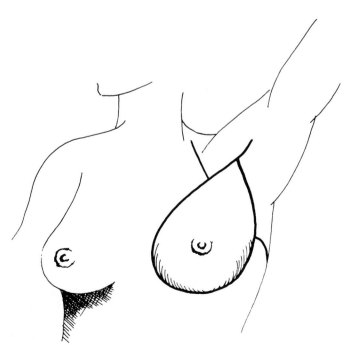

Figure 39–7 *Incision used by J. C. Warren of Boston for radical mastectomy. (From Warren JC: Ann Surg 40:805–833, 1904. Reprinted by permission.)*

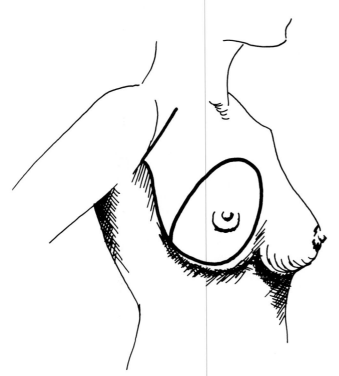

Figure 39–9 *Jabez Jackson's incision for radical mastectomy. (From Jackson JN: JAMA 46:627–633, 1906. Copyright 1906. American Medical Association. Reprinted by permission.)*

faculty of Harvard Medical School, presented "The Results of Operations for Cancer of the Breast at the Massachusetts General Hospital from 1894 to 1904" before the American Surgical Association in 1907.[104] There were 416 primary operations for breast cancer

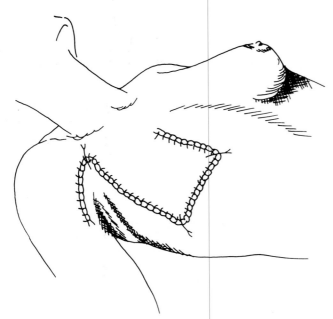

Figure 39–10 *Jackson's closure following radical mastectomy. (From Jackson JN: JAMA 46:627–633, 1906. Copyright 1906. American Medical Association. Reprinted by permission.)*

during this period, of which 376 patients (90 percent) could be adequately traced for long-term follow-up. These operations were performed by 20 different surgeons (one of them J. C. Warren). Only 160 patients had undergone a "complete operation"; a "semicomplete" procedure (differing only in that the pectoralis minor muscle was left in place) was performed in 75 patients. "Incomplete" procedures—those that lacked any one of the essential elements of a radical mastectomy—were performed in 85 patients, and 56 patients with hopelessly advanced disease underwent palliative procedures that probably left tumor behind. The 3-year survival rate in this last category was, predictably, only 7 percent. Paradoxically, though, a 25 percent 3-year DFS rate was found in the incomplete and semicomplete groups, while the complete group showed only a 16 percent rate. The authors attributed this difference to selection bias, again indicating the problem with failing to stratify a study population according to stage of disease. The overall operative mortality was 3.6 percent, dropping from 5.1 percent in the first 5 years to only 2 percent in the last 5 years. The overall DFS rate at 3 years, excluding the palliative group, was 21 percent and in the last 5 years of the study was 26 percent. Of the 64 patients alive and well 3 years or more after operation, 42 (65.6 percent) had survived 5 years or more, and 17 (26.6 percent) had survived 10 years or more. Almost 50 percent of the patients evaluable for recurrence (126 of 264) developed local chest wall recurrence, and the authors noted that local recurrence was least likely to occur in those who had the widest and most complete primary resections. Seventeen (19 percent) of the 88 patients free of disease at 3 years later developed recurrence; in four cases recurrence occurred more than 6 years after operation. This led to speculation that 3-year DFS probably was not an adequate measure of cure.

Greenough and coworkers' paper documented several clinical features associated with a poor prognosis, all of which were later recognized to be ominous signs.[111, 112] These included skin involvement, ulceration, axillary gland involvement, supraclavicular gland involvement (in which group there was not a single cure), bilateral cancer, and chest wall or axillary vein attachment. Also, like Warren, these authors found that preoperative duration of disease did not seem to affect prognosis.

In 1950 Taylor and Wallace updated this experience at the Massachusetts General Hospital.[288] They analyzed 2500 cases of primary breast carcinoma, 2000 of whom had been treated by radical mastectomy. A greater degree of uniformity was apparent in this study population, since patients with Greenough's unfavorable factors were eliminated from study. The operative mortality decreased to 0.65 percent. They reported a 51 percent overall 5-year "cure" rate. Those without axillary node involvement had a 77 percent rate of cure, whereas axillary involvement resulted in a 33 percent cure rate. Again, axillary node status was shown to be a significant prognostic factor. There was still a 76 percent cure rate when only one or two axillary nodes were involved.

These survival figures for breast cancer must be viewed in the context of what is known of the natural history of this disease. Bloom and associates in 1962 reviewed the clinical courses of 250 women with a confirmed diagnosis of breast carcinoma who had been admitted to the Middlesex Hospital Cancer Ward between 1805 and 1933 and were not treated.[26] He found a median survival of 2.7 years from onset of symptoms; 20 percent were alive at 5 years, 5 percent at 10 years, and approximately 1 percent were still alive at the end of 15 years (Fig. 39–11). Thus, in some series at the turn of this century radical mastectomy did not appear to affect survival at all.

Theories of Metastatic Dissemination

The perceived means by which carcinoma of the breast spreads throughout the body has, appropriately, always influenced its primary surgical treatment. The ancient belief that cancer is a systemic disease mediated through body humors persisted into the nineteenth century, when it was reinforced by Virchow's assertion that cancer was disseminated from the primary neoplasm by a toxic fluid.[97, 303] This

philosophy led to a pessimistic attitude toward local surgical ablation of breast carcinoma. In the late nineteenth century, Thiersch and Waldeyer demonstrated that metastasis occurred through seeding of distant organs with cells of the primary tumor, by way of embolization through the lymphatics and blood stream.[317] This formed the basis of the *mechanical theory* of tumor dissemination that was widely accepted at the beginning of the twentieth century.

William Sampson Handley (1872–1962) was a British surgeon at London's Middlesex Hospital who made a meticulous study of the pathological anatomy of the lymphatic circulation and cancer dissemination and applied his observations to the clinical management of carcinoma of the breast (Fig. 39–12). He extended the principle first espoused by his predecessor, Charles H. Moore, asserting that cancer cells spread centrifugally from the primary tumor, but more through continuous permeation of the lymph vessels than through episodic embolization. He believed that the lymphatics were the sole route by which this dissemination occurred, referring to earlier studies that indicated that blood-borne tumor cells are routinely destroyed because they stimulate a thrombotic process.[60, 157, 317] According to Handley's theory, regional lymph nodes act as filters for these permeating cancer cells, and only after the cells are able to grow beyond them are they capable of reach-

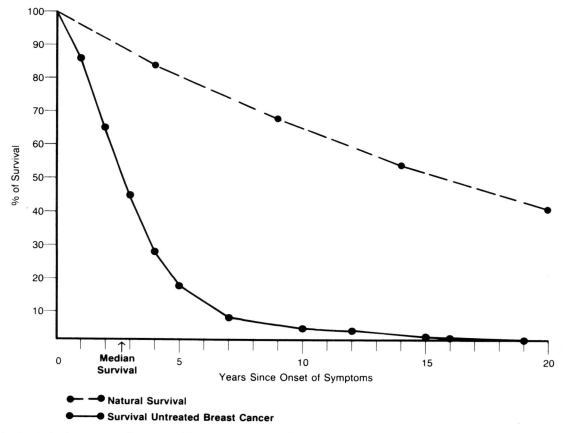

Figure 39–11 *Survival of women with untreated breast carcinoma. (Adapted from Bloom et al: Natural history of untreated breast cancer ([1805–1933]). BMJ 2:213–221, 1962.)*

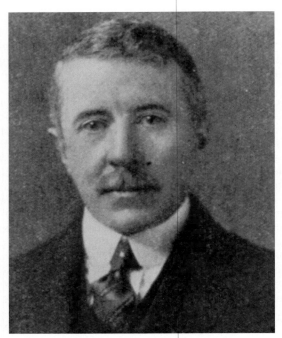

Figure 39–12   *William Sampson Handley (1872–1962), surgeon to Middlesex Hospital, whose permeation theory of breast cancer dissemination was embraced by Halsted. (Courtesy of Professor Irving Taylor, Department of Surgery, Middlesex Hospital, London, England.)*

ing the blood stream for embolic spread. These principles contributed to the idea that breast cancer begins as a local process in the breast proper and then spreads in an orderly, incremental fashion first to the regional lymphatics and then to distant sites. This formed the conceptual basis for radical mastectomy, because, according to this theory, complete ablation of all tissues through which the lymphatics travel provided the only chance of curing the disease as long as it had not already reached distant sites through the blood stream. It also supported the practice of excising all tissues in continuity, so as not to cut across and disperse the tumor-filled regional lymphatics. Not surprisingly, Halsted embraced and endorsed Handley's theory, and its publication in Handley's first book on breast cancer in 1906 was a significant contribution to the management of this disease that affected surgical practice throughout the world.[122, 129, 245] Handley recommended the modification of Halsted's operation to include smaller areas of skin and greater portions of the deep fascia, to more fully encompass the offending lymphatics.[41]

One of Halsted's major concerns, derived from the mechanical theory of tumor dissemination, was the danger of manipulating a breast tumor, especially for purposes of diagnosis. Moore had voiced these same concerns some 30 years earlier. Halsted asserted[121]:

Tumors should never be harpooned, nor should pieces even be excised from malignant tumors for diagnostic purposes. Think of the danger of rapid dissemi-

nation of the growth from . . . snipping off a piece of the tumor with scissors.

In studying the published histories of cases of malignant tumors, particularly sarcoma, I have been impressed with the great number of cases in which general dissemination of the neoplasm has seemed to follow swiftly upon exploratory incisions.

Breast tumors should not be incised on the operating table prior to their removal. The surgeon must learn to recognize malignant tumors not only with the microscope, but also with his naked eye and fingers.

. . . If the surgeon cannot, in a given case, make a diagnosis prior to operation . . . he should excise the breast or, at least, give the tumor a wide berth. If then, on incision, the tumor proved to be malignant, the complete operation should be performed immediately.

These concerns were supported by experimental evidence published in 1913 of tumor dissemination after manipulation of breast tumors in the Japanese waltzing mouse, although this was never corroborated in humans.[290]

The perceived necessity for a one-stage operation that encompassed both the diagnostic biopsy and a definitive procedure led to the development at Johns Hopkins of the frozen section examination. William H. Welch is credited with first using this technique in 1891 on a patient Halsted operated on for a benign breast tumor.[245] In 1895 a detailed description of this technique was published.[46] The one-stage procedure was to remain the standard approach to diagnosis and surgical management of primary breast carcinoma for the next 80 years.

Handley's permeation theory eventually was discredited in favor of the original theory of tumor cell embolization.[157] J. H. Gray showed in an extensive series of observations that cancer cells can be found only rarely along the entire course of a lymph channel, a well-known observation that Handley explained by postulating that an obliterative lymphangitis obscured cancer cells.[102, 130] He also found that the deep fascia was virtually devoid of lymphatics, contrary to Handley's assertion. Abundant evidence also accumulated of the existence of cancer cells in the circulating blood, which is now felt to be the primary route of metastatic dissemination.[8, 65] These changing attitudes toward the underlying biology of breast carcinoma were among many that in ensuing years led to a new appreciation of the extent of surgery necessary to control the disease.

Results and Modifications of Radical Mastectomy

Halsted made very little modification to his procedure during the 40 years that he performed it. Supraclavicular dissection, mediastinal dissection, and stripping of the fascia of the rectus and serratus muscles were all temporary additions that he eventually abandoned. In 1913 he published a fourth paper on breast cancer that summarized the technique and advantages of skin grafting in radical mastectomy, a part of the procedure to which he remained firmly committed.[114, 123] His last paper, published in 1921, dealt with lymphedema of the arm after radical mastectomy.[124] He emphasized the meticulous attention that must be paid to suturing the flaps and grafts without tension and to avoiding infection, both of which he believed to be major factors in the development of arm edema. As mentioned earlier, he had already abandoned extending his incision onto the arm in an effort to avoid arm edema.

Most of the modifications made by other surgeons to Halsted's procedure were relatively minor and unimportant but served to reinforce the essential principles he espoused, which remained widely accepted and practiced well after his death in 1922.[41] In fact, the operation done by most surgeons during the next several decades resembled Meyer's procedure more than Halsted's, especially in the sacrifice of smaller areas of skin to (usually) allow primary closure. F. T. Stewart introduced the transverse incision in 1915.[277]

In 1924 Burton J. Lee, a surgeon at the Cornell Medical School in New York, presented before the American Surgical Association the first survival curve for treated breast carcinoma.[238] Seventy-five of 87 cases were available for long-term follow-up, which showed a 15 percent 5-year recurrence-free survival. Like many other surgeons of this period, he advocated abandoning the 3-year standard for defining cure.

In 1929 Stuart W. Harrington of the Mayo Clinic updated the results of operation for primary breast carcinoma that had originally been reported by Judd and Sistrunk in 1914.[132, 151] From 2083 operations, he reported an operative mortality of only 0.76 percent. Axillary lymph node involvement was clearly demonstrated in this series to be "the most important factor in the prognosis" of breast carcinoma, a principle that has remained valid up to the present.[74, 280, 294] Those without lymphatic involvement had overall 3-year survival of 74.7 percent and 10-year survival of a 44.1 percent, while patients with regional lymph node involvement had 39 percent 3-year survival and a 13.4 percent 10-year survival. Harrington's skin incision was not uniform but was tailored to the extent of disease in each individual case. He made a vertical incision for upper or lower quadrant lesions (Fig. 39–13) and a transverse incision for lateral or medial lesions, approaching this part of the procedure with the following philosophy:

> I believe it important to make a wide excision of the skin, and, if the margins cannot be approximated, I graft skin. This, however, is not often necessary if the incision is properly planned, except in extensive cases.

Harrington observed gradual improvement in survival from this operation up to 1915, which he attributed to "improvement and standardization of technic and the gradual increase of the operative procedure." After 1915 these results reached a plateau, indicat-

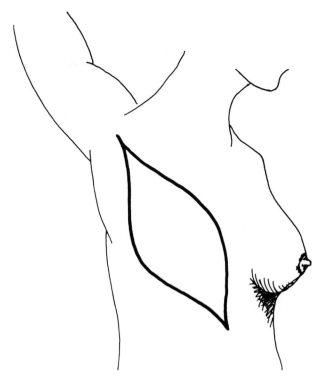

Figure 39–13 *The vertical skin incision of S. W. Harrington of the Mayo Clinic. (From Harrington SW: JAMA 92:208–213, 1929. Copyright 1929. American Medical Association. Reprinted by permission.)*

ing the limits of surgery for the disease. There was an 80 percent 3-year survival rate and 53 percent 10-year survival rate among those treated with primary radical operation who had no axillary node involvement. These were the best results obtained up to that time. He also observed the failure of various extensions to the operation—supraclavicular dissection, excision of the contralateral axillary nodes, and removal of the opposite breast—to improve results.

Harrington made several observations in this paper that were to become important issues in the future. Five patients who were pregnant at the time of operation had poor outcomes, leading him ultimately to the misguided conclusion that pregnancy is a poor prognostic factor. A group of 112 patients who had undergone inadequate forms of treatment before having a radical operation at the Mayo Clinic had substantially lower survival rates than those who underwent radical operation initially, demonstrating the validity of Moore's original thesis published more than 60 years earlier. For 51 patients with bilateral malignancy, the second malignancy did not have any additional adverse effect on survival. In 1092 cases, adding "roentgen ray" treatment to radical operation produced no demonstrable survival benefit which was to be expected with the state of knowledge at that time, as indicated by Harrington's statement:

> If the radical operation is performed, it should accomplish what the term implies, complete removal of

the diseased tissue, and should not depend on the roentgen ray to destroy remaining malignant tissue.... The best opportunity of eradicating the malignant disease is at the first operation and the magnitude of this operation must be sufficient to remove all of the diseased tissue. The prognosis depends on the possibility of accomplishing this.

Thus, Harrington understood that radiation therapy was strictly a modality for local control of disease and not a substitute for an incomplete or poorly executed operation. Since breast cancer is a systemic illness that ultimately kills, radiation treatment should have no effect on survival.

Harrington also emphasized the benefits of early detection of disease, which were evident in his statistics relating survival to lymph node involvement. He was concerned that the incidence of lymph node involvement had actually increased—from 59 percent before 1915 to 67 percent since then—suggesting that patients were presenting at later stages of disease. He stated:

> The results in these cases can be greatly improved if operation is performed early in the course of the disease. If operation is delayed until the signs of malignancy are obvious, it is too late to expect much more than a palliative result. There are few if any single tumors of the breast in which delay in the institution of treatment is safe for the patient, and few physicians care to assume the responsibility of determining the presence or absence of malignancy by the physical characteristics of the tumor.

He also supported Halsted's belief that, in doubtful cases a definite diagnosis must be made by wide excision of the tumor, microscopic examination, and immediate radical operation in one stage if the lesion is malignant.

J. Stewart Rodman of Philadelphia published in 1943 the results of 132 women who had undergone a modification of the Halsted radical mastectomy first proposed in 1908 by William L. Rodman.[246] This procedure combined wide removal of skin with the ability to close the wound in virtually every case and resulted in a negligible incidence of arm edema or limitation of arm function. Rodman reported a 2.2 percent incidence of local recurrence, among the lowest in the literature, and 46 percent 5-year DFS (63.5 percent in those without axillary metastasis).

In 1927 William Sampson Handley (see Fig. 39–12), still devoting his career at London's Middlesex Hospital to the investigation of breast carcinoma, published a report that revived an awareness of the internal mammary and mediastinal lymph node chains as a route of metastatic dissemination.[131] He observed that, despite the lower incidence of local recurrence (especially in the axilla) following radical mastectomy, involvement of axillary lymph nodes with tumor was still predictive of death from disseminated disease. Most of the recurrences in his patients occurred along the sternal border of the excised breast. He concluded that these lymph nodes must be seeded with microscopic deposits of tumor quite early in the course of the disease. The extent of surgical treatment would have no effect on outcome for these patients unless the nodes were also treated. Handley did not believe that surgical excision was appropriate, in view of the time and morbidity it added to the radical mastectomy, but he did advocate routine placement of radium tubes along the sternal border as an adjunct to mastectomy. This practice resulted in 56.5 percent DFS at 3 years, which he considered a significant improvement over the 47 percent 3-year survival for his patients not so treated. He also noted that local recurrences only rarely occurred in the sites where radium had been inserted.

After World War II, Handley's son Richard S. Handley (1909–1984) published the results of his practice of routine biopsy of the internal mammary lymph nodes in all cases of breast carcinoma.[125, 126] Among 119 patients, these nodes were involved with metastases in 34 percent of patients overall and in 48 percent of those with axillary lymph node metastasis. He felt this explained both the recurrence of disease when radical mastectomy is performed for early lesions and the fact that the lungs and pleura are the most common sites of distant metastasis; however, Handley seemed skeptical about the possibility of surgically eradicating these nodes, much as his father had been.[127]

The implications of Handley's observations that one third of all mastectomies are doomed to failure from the start led some surgeons to recommend treating breast carcinoma with an "extended" radical mastectomy, which included en bloc resection of the internal mammary lymph nodes. The first to do this routinely was the Italian surgeon Margottini in 1948, although Halsted had described this being done in three cases by his house surgeon, Harvey Cushing, in 1898.[60, 121, 186]

In 1952 Jerome Urban published his initial experience with radical mastectomy in continuity with en bloc internal mammary dissection at Memorial Hospital in New York.[292] He developed this procedure after observing that more than 70 percent of chest wall recurrences after radical mastectomy occurred in the medial parasternal area.[291] There was one operative death among 57 patients who underwent this procedure and no local recurrences, and 28 patients (49 percent) had internal mammary node metastasis. Like Handley, he found that medial quadrant lesions had the greatest risk of internal mammary involvement. Although the short follow-up period did not allow any assessment of survival, Urban postulated significant improvement and even considered the following:

> The next step to be considered is the further extension of this procedure to include en bloc dissection of the lymphatic-bearing tissues at the base of the neck.

Wangensteen and associates had already been performing a "super-radical" mastectomy, including supraclavicular, internal mammary, and mediastinal lymph node dissection.[310, 311] They found that 58 percent of their cases of operable breast carcinoma had internal mammary node involvement, but they were unable to demonstrate any significant improvement in survival with this procedure. Because of 12.5 percent operative mortality, they abandoned the procedure for treating breast carcinoma.

Dahl-Iversen published several reports from Denmark that detailed an operation that also combined radical mastectomy with supraclavicular and internal mammary dissection, although these extensions were not performed in continuity.[47–49] Prudente described upper extremity amputation en bloc with radical mastectomy for locally advanced disease.[237]

In 1964 E. D. Sugarbaker published a retrospective review of 156 extended radical mastectomies with internal mammary node dissection and compared them to 97 historical controls whose stage and demographic features were very comparable and who had undergone conventional radical mastectomies.[278] The 5-year survival rate in the former group was 70 percent, as compared with 57 percent in the latter group, prompting the conclusion that operable breast carcinoma should be treated by extended radical mastectomy. Other series, though, demonstrated either no difference in overall results between simple mastectomy plus postoperative irradiation and extended radical mastectomy or simply failure of internal mammary node dissection to improve survival.[152, 301] These extended procedures never became widely accepted because of the absence of any clear benefit despite the substantial added risk; however, they are still used selectively in some centers.[50]

During these same years the bilaterality of carcinoma of the breast became evident in a small percentage of cases, and victims of such disease were at greater risk of a second malignancy developing metachronously in the contralateral breast. In 1951 Pack advocated bilateral mastectomy for any unilateral breast malignancy, an idea that has continued to be sporadically advocated.[215] Several authors have suggested routine contralateral blind biopsy in conjunction with ipsilateral mastectomy and excision of the contralateral breast in those 10 percent to 20 percent of patients who show any microscopic findings of malignancy.[91, 159, 235, 263, 293, 309] Robbins and Berg demonstrated that the cumulative risk of developing clinically evident contralateral breast carcinoma following ipsilateral disease was less than 1 percent per year, which is less than the incidence of clinically occult carcinoma in the opposite breast detected by routine blind biopsy.[244] Metachronous contralateral breast carcinomas have been shown to have no adverse impact on ultimate survival over that of the original primary breast carcinoma, perhaps owing to the more aggressive mammographic surveillance of these women, which results in earlier detection of these second lesions.[84, 196, 231, 272] Although invasive lobular carcinomas have been associated with a greater risk of contralateral breast cancer than have invasive ductal carcinomas, most now agree that the their low incidence does not justify blind contralateral biopsy or prophylactic mastectomy in this setting.[19, 143, 173] Because of doubts about the clinical significance of occult contralateral malignancy that are raised by these considerations, most surgeons do not intervene in the opposite breast in the absence of standard clinical indications.[10, 84, 231, 274]

Biology and Detection of Early Breast Cancer

The potential improvement in survival through the detection of breast cancer in its earliest stages of development had been suggested by several investigators through the centuries, including Celsus, Severinus, LeDran, Fearon, Banks, Halsted, Meyer, and Harrington.* The first histologic studies of breast cancer in the late nineteenth century supported this concept by demonstrating that malignancy appeared to arise from normal epithelial cells.[42, 43, 243, 306, 307] Since Astley Cooper first reported an association between benign breast changes and carcinoma in 1845, numerous clinical investigators have provided evidence that certain benign breast lesions progress to malignancy.† These observations led to the "transition theory" of breast cancer development.[95, 98, 99] As originally postulated by MacCarty in 1913, it has since been firmly established that epithelial hyperplasia, especially atypical hyperplasia, is the benign change that leads to breast cancer, although this progression is nonobligate.‡

According to the transition theory, all cases of invasive breast carcinoma traverse a stage in which previously normal epithelial cells of the breast become malignant but have not yet invaded beyond their confining basement membranes.[248] Several authors of the late nineteenth and early twentieth centuries published illustrations of the histology of this "noninvasive" stage of breast malignancy.[42, 43, 67, 266, 307] MacCarty was probably the first to describe these lesions as preinvasive, suggesting the dynamic process of development of invasive cancer from normal cells.[180] Cheatle and Cutler asserted, "in these instances there is no doubt that these epithelial cells inside the normal boundaries are as histologically malignant as those that have transgressed them and are trespassing in the surrounding tissues."[35] In 1932, Broders first applied the term *in situ carcinoma* to this intermediate, noninvasive stage of cancer development, recognizing it as an independent entity, distinct from its benign precursors and invasive counterparts.[30] Broders also recognized the important opportunity for improved survival offered by detection of malignancy at this still localized stage.

---

*See references 12, 34, 41, 50, 56, 58, 60, 122, 132, 172, 176, 198, and 317.

†See references 40, 52, 53, 98, 103, 146, 153, 176, 306, and 313.

‡See references 7, 21, 37, 57, 63, 66, 83, 87, 95, 98, 108, 109, 153, 180, 193, 202, and 217.

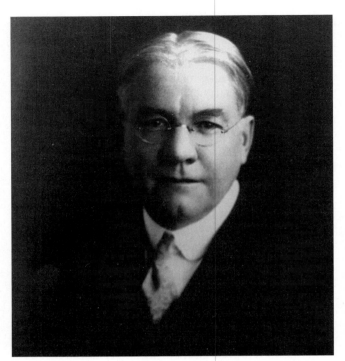

Figure 39–14 *Dr. Joseph Colt Bloodgood who made important observations on the biology of early breast malignancies.*

This opportunity would not be exploited to any significant extent for breast cancers for another 50 years.

Joseph Colt Bloodgood (Fig. 39–14) was a surgeon at Johns Hopkins Hospital in the early twentieth century who published several investigations of the biology and clinical behavior of the earliest forms of ductal carcinoma of the breast, which he termed "borderline breast tumors."[24, 25] His histologic illustrations are now recognized as typical examples of ductal carcinoma *in situ* of the breast. Bloodgood was the first to describe both the excellent prognosis for this lesion and the importance of public education for improving survival from breast cancer by detecting it in this earliest noninvasive stage.[23]

The most effective modality for the detection of breast carcinoma in its earliest forms, when treatment promises to be most successful, had its beginnings as early as 1913. Salomon then first applied radiography to the study of breasts.[253] By 1960, Egan demonstrated this new technique of mammography to be sufficiently effective and standardized to be clinically applicable to a large population.[64] Several prospective randomized trials over the next 30 years consistently demonstrated that routine mammographic screening detects breast carcinoma at an earlier stage and, consequently, leads to as much as a 46 percent reduction in mortality, as compared with standard physical examination.*

The increasing use of mammography in the United States during the 1980s resulted in substantial changes in the techniques used by surgeons to diagnose breast carcinoma. Standard open surgical biopsies could no longer be performed on the progressively smaller and nonpalpable lesions detected by mammography. Needle localization biopsy with specimen radiography evolved as the most common method to accurately localize and sample nonpalpable mammographically detected breast lesions (see Chapter 40).[14, 160, 289] The effectiveness of this technique at early diagnosis of breast cancer has been demonstrated in several published series that report an average yield of carcinoma *in situ* among all malignancies of over 43 percent, and fewer than 15 percent of invasive lesions that have axillary metastases (Table 39–3). These results are clearly superior to those of physical examination alone, which yields incidences of carcinoma *in situ* of less than 5 percent of all malignancies and of axillary metastases among invasive lesions of over 50 percent.[31, 212, 251]

Thanks largely to mammography, more than 80 percent of all breast carcinoma lesions in the United States are now smaller than 2 cm at the time of diagnosis. Early detection was therefore one of the most important factors that made possible the treatment of breast carcinoma with less extensive surgical procedures than were used in the first half of the twentieth century.

Emergence of Less Extensive Operative Procedures

Halsted's major contributions to the treatment of breast carcinoma include (1) substantial reduction in operative mortality rates through adherence to the surgical principles of sharp dissection, meticulous hemostasis, elimination of dead space, wound closure using skin grafts, and antiseptic techniques; (2) the demonstration of the importance of wide surgical excision in preventing locoregional recurrence of disease; and (3) the value of applying scientific principles of anatomy, physiology, and analysis of results to the development of a rational and effective treatment.

The basic flaw in the theory of local disease origin was quickly manifested by the fact that surgery alone did not consistently yield high rates of cure, regardless of how extensive the procedure or early the diagnosis. Although survival at 3 years appeared to show an improvement over that with earlier procedures, longer follow-up revealed steadily diminishing rates. The efforts of many surgeons to extend the scope of the radical mastectomy indicated their recognition of its inadequacy as the sole treatment for breast carcinoma. The abandonment of these extensive procedures by most surgeons, including Halsted himself, further testifies to the failure of surgery alone to eradicate most cases of this disease.

Rudolf Matas (1860–1957), of Tulane University, asserted in 1898 that Halsted's operation could never be considered complete because of all the lymph channels left behind.[190] Lane-Claypon published the first epidemiological analysis of the results of surgi-

---

*See references 94, 95, 179, 206, 262, 264, 285, 297, and 314.

TABLE 39–3. RESULTS OF BIOPSY OF NONPALPABLE MAMMOGRAPHICALLY DETECTED BREAST LESIONS—1986–1992

Investigator	No. Biopsies (n)	Malignancies (n)	Malignancies (%)	In Situ (n)	In Situ (%)*	Axillary Metastasis (n)	Axillary Metastasis (%)†
Bauer et al[13]	2077	286	14	82	29	29/251	12
Franceschi et al[92]	1144	269	24	98	36.5	31/171	18
Landercasper et al[168]	203	44	22	29	66	5/24	21
Marrujo et al[187]	237	64	27	23	36	7/54	13
Perdue et al[223]	536	96	18	48	50	4/41	10
Poole et al[232]	148	21	14	5	24	3/19	16
Shroff et al[267]	246	43	17.5	13	30	5/31	16
Silverstein et al[269]	653	147	22.5	88	60	6/127	5
Skinner et al[273]	179	41	23	9	22	7/30	23
Symmonds et al[284]	499	72	14	13	18	7/62	11
Wilhelm et al[318]	1464	264	18	178	67	18/78	23
Totals	7386	1347	18	586	43.5	122/888	13.7

*Percentage of all malignancies.
†Ratio (percentage) of cases of axillary metastasis to number of cases treated with axillary dissection.

cal treatment of breast carcinoma in 1924 and concluded in this and a follow-up report in 1928 that whatever improvement in survival may exist was primarily attributable to earlier diagnosis rather than to the radical mastectomy itself.[170, 171] In a retrospective review of 20,000 operations for breast carcinoma in the medical literature, she showed 43 percent 3-year survival and 33 percent 5-year survival for those subjected to radical mastectomy. Those treated with less extensive operations had 3-year survival of only 29 percent. Also shown was a twofold increase in survival in the absence of lymph node involvement.[56]

William Crawford White, a surgeon at New York's Roosevelt Hospital, reported survival data on 157 radical mastectomies in 1927.[316] He typified the tendency to extend the reporting interval to 5 years or more, showing 36 percent 5-year survival and only 24 percent survival at 10 years. This study also demonstrated the impact of disease stage, as determined by axillary node status, on prognosis.

The noted New York pathologist James Ewing was also pessimistic about the true value of radical mastectomy during this period, agreeing that the relatively good survival in most reports was more likely attributable to early detection than to the surgery. He was concerned that this operation was being performed too often for relatively harmless and sometimes benign lesions, while ultimately it seemed to make little difference to mortality for those with very aggressive and advanced lesions.[67, 245] In 1928 he stated[68]:

I have drawn the impression that in dealing with mammary cancer surgery meets with more peculiar difficulties and uncertainties than with almost any other form of the disease. The anatomical types are so numerous, the variations in clinical course so wide, the paths of dissemination so free and diverse, the difficulties of determining the actual conditions so complex, and the sacrifice of tissues so great, as to render impossible in the majority of cases a reasonably accurate adjustment of a means to an end.

The pessimistic extreme was represented by Park and Lees, who in 1950 published an extensive and elegant analysis of treatment results for breast carcinoma.[220] They cautioned that the variability of individual tumor growth rates may render survival rates meaningless and that the available forms of treatment were unlikely to alter mortality rates, since the rates were largely related to distant metastases. They concluded that there was no firm evidence that treatment had any effect whatsoever on survival.

The evident shortcomings of surgical treatment of breast carcinoma led some to consider using less extensive procedures in conjunction with other modalities, to spare patients unnecessary tissue loss. Radiation therapy was one of the first adjunctive modalities applied to breast carcinoma for this purpose, having first been used in this way by Emile Grubbe in Chicago within 2 months of the discovery of x-rays by Wilhelm Roentgen in 1895.[107] In 1917 Janeway described the use of interstitial irradiation instead of mastectomy for operable breast carcinoma, finding it an acceptable alternative for patients who refused surgery or for those tumors that were not amenable to surgical ablation.[149]

Geoffrey Keynes, a surgeon at St. Bartholomew's Hospital in London, began applying radium needles to the treatment of breast carcinoma in 1922 under the direction of his superior, George Gask.[157, 245] They treated only advanced, inoperable cases at first but extended the use of the procedure as their success became evident. Of their first 42 patients treated by radium implantation alone, without surgery, 13 (31 percent) were "apparently cured," six of those had been judged inoperable.[154] The follow-up in this series ranged from 8 months to 4 years, with only four patients having more than a 2-year follow-up. In 1932 Keynes reported similar results for 171 cases treated during a 7-year period, pointing out some of the harmful effects of this method on both patient and physician.[155] In this report he also first speculated that radium might be more efficacious if the bulk of the tumor were first surgically removed. Several patients had been subjected to this combination of surgery and radiotherapy by 1937, when Keynes published his results from 250 patients for whom at least a 3-year follow-up was available.[156] He stratified these patients according to disease stage, with 85 patients being clinically stage I. Pathological staging was not possible, since axillary dissections were not performed. There was a 71.4 percent 5-year survival rate for these patients, and 29 percent 5-year survival for those judged clinically to be stage II at presentation. This compared to 69 percent stage I and 30.5 percent stage II 5-year survivals among patients subjected to surgery alone as reported in a contemporary series by Jessop.[150] Assuming a 27 percent error rate in the clinical assessment of axillary nodes, Keynes speculated that the actual 5-year survival rate among his stage I patients might be as high as 86 percent. Since it is now known that such an error may be as high as 40 percent to 50 percent, Keyne's results appear to be remarkable.[3, 233] They demonstrated for the first time the possibility that extensive less surgical ablation of breast carcinoma may provide acceptable results.

George E. Pfahler, a Philadelphia radiologist, analyzed in 1932 a series of 1022 cases in which radiation therapy was applied to breast carcinoma.[227, 228] Patients given radiation after surgery, exhibited a 90 percent increase in 5-year survival as compared with surgery alone. By 1939, Keynes was also convinced of the necessity to routinely remove the gross bulk of tumor before irradiation because of an otherwise high local recurrence rate.[157, 245] This was the first assertion of the now widely accepted principle that surgery should be most effectively and appropriately applied to the removal of clinically evident disease, whereas radiation is best applied to ablation of the subclinical disease that is virtually always left behind after surgery. In other words, these modalities are complementary rather than competing forms of local treatment for breast carcinoma, though neither one can effectively treat the distant metastases that are largely responsible for death from the disease.

Haagensen and Stout in 1943 defined the clinical features of breast carcinoma that predicted a poor outcome after radical mastectomy in terms of a prohibitively high rate of local recurrence and poor overall survival (Table 39–4).[111, 112] Such cases were considered inoperable. This report recognizes the same limitations of surgery (especially for locally advanced disease) that such authorities as Banks, Moore, Petit, LeDran, and Hippocrates had espoused in centuries past.

In 1951 Haagensen and Stout reviewed, according to their strict and specific criteria of operability, a series of 495 radical mastectomies performed at Columbia Presbyterian Hospital in New York between 1935 and 1942.[113] They reported a 1.8 percent operative mortality, a relative 5-year survival rate of 58.2

TABLE 39–4.   GRAVE SIGNS OF INOPERABILITY IN PATIENTS WITH BREAST CARCINOMA

Skin edema
Skin ulceration
Chest wall fixation
Matted, enlarged, or fixed axillary nodes
Satellite skin nodules
Supraclavicular node enlargement
Arm edema
Inflammatory carcinoma

Data from Greenough et al: Surg Gynecol Obstet 3:39–50, 1907; and Haagensen CD, Stout AP: Ann Surg 118:859–876, 1032–1051, 1943.

percent and a relative 5-year clinical cure rate of 48.7 percent, which were among the best results ever achieved after radical mastectomy. These results represented a 10 percent to 75 percent improvement over earlier rates from that hospital, although the obvious contribution of selection bias to these results cannot be overlooked.[176]

Following World War II efforts to investigate the feasibility of less extensive operative procedures for breast carcinoma continued. High-voltage external-beam radiation was developed, allowing more effective and safer delivery of radiation to the breast with better cosmetic results. In 1948 Robert McWhirter, a surgeon at the Royal Infirmary in Edinburgh, Scotland, published the results of treatment of 1345 patients who presented with breast carcinoma between 1941 and 1945.[194] Simple mastectomy and radiotherapy were carried out in 757 patients whose disease appeared clinically to be localized to the breast. The surgery involved only limited skin excision and limited undermining of flaps, with no axillary dissection in the absence of clinically palpable nodes. Radiation was applied to the chest wall, axilla, and supraclavicular fields in a minimum dose of 3750 rad over 3 weeks. The 5-year survival rate for these patients was 62.1 percent, which was substantially better than that for women treated with radical mastectomy alone in most series.

McWhirter emphasized the validity of study techniques that are necessary to identify optimal treatment regimens. Exclusion of untreated patients (selection bias), use of historical or noncomparable controls, lack of comprehensive follow-up, short follow-up intervals, incomplete histological confirmation, and failure consistently to stratify cases according to stage of disease at presentation were all flaws in study design that he identified in many published series that contributed to confusion and misconceptions about appropriate treatment of breast carcinoma. He asserted that if these factors were taken into account and radical mastectomy was the only form of treatment available, then the 5-year survival rate for all patients with breast carcinoma was no more than 25 percent.[245] The overall survival rate for all 1345 cases of breast carcinoma referred to McWhirter's institution during the study period of 1941 to 1945 was 43.7 percent. For those 389 patients with only locally advanced but inoperable disease treated only with radiotherapy, 5-year survival was 29 percent. In those 1146 cases with no evidence of distant metastasis, the 5-year survival rate was 50.5 percent. These results were interpreted as demonstrating the efficacy of radiation as the sole treatment of the axilla, although future investigators, like Keynes in prior years, were not to find this true.[156] In 1964 McWhirter emphasized the need to address flaws in study design in order to determine scientifically the optimal treatment for breast carcinoma.[195] He advised that multicenter prospective clinical trials be organized for this purpose, something that was actually to occur in the near future.

Two surgeons from London's Middlesex Hospital, D. H. Patey (1889–1977) (Fig. 39–15) and W. H. Dyson, initiated a revolutionary change in the surgical management of breast carcinoma with the publication in 1948 of their technique of modified radical mastectomy.[222] There appeared to these authors to be no valid reason for routine removal of the pectoralis major muscle in conjunction with mastectomy, except in those rare cases when it was actually invaded by tumor. The work of Gray supported this contention by demonstrating the absence of lymphatics in the muscle and its fascia, which was contrary to the observations of Heidenhain in the nineteenth century.[102] The primary conceptual basis of Halsted's removal of the muscle was the belief that it served as a route of lymphatic dissemination of tumor. The steadily decreasing rates of survival following radical mastectomy with lengthening follow-up intervals also raised the question of the importance of the extent of local treatment. Mr. Patey did believe in the necessity for wide skin excision and thorough

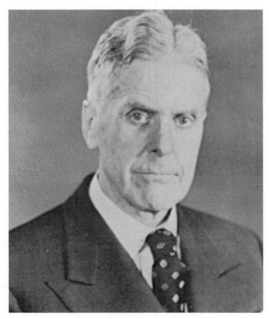

Figure 39–15   *D. H. Patey (1889–1977), surgeon at London's Middlesex Hospital, who demonstrated the benefits of the modified radical mastectomy in 1948 with complete dissection of Levels I to III nodes following removal of the pectoralis minor. (Courtesy of Professor Irving Taylor, Department of Surgery, Middlesex Hospital, London, England.)*

axillary dissection, the latter including excision of the pectoralis minor muscle to ensure completeness. He also emphasized preservation of the lateral pectoral nerve. The advantages of leaving the pectoralis major muscle included the improved cosmetic result, less operative blood loss, and "a more suitable bed for skin grafting than ribs and costal cartilages [would afford]." This plea to preserve the pectoralis major muscle echoed the advice given by Celsus almost 2000 years ago.

Patey had first performed this modified radical mastectomy in 1932 and began using it routinely in 1936. The results on his first 118 patients, stratified according to axillary lymph node involvement and types of operative procedures, showed equivalent outcomes between modified radical mastectomy and standard radical mastectomy (83 percent versus 78 percent 3-year survival in node-negative patients). The influence of postoperative irradiation could not be assessed, since it was applied inconsistently in both groups. This similarity of results, in terms of both survival and local recurrence rates, was confirmed in an updated review by Patey in 1967 of 146 patients, 69 of whom underwent modified radical mastectomy.[221] "Good" results were achieved in 38 patients, all with follow-up of at least 8 years.

In his 1948 report, Mr. Patey described 10 cases in which partial mastectomy and axillary dissection were performed. Interestingly enough, the survival rate for these patients did not appear to be significantly different from that for those who underwent total mastectomy, although the high rate of local recurrence led Patey to abandon this breast-sparing approach. Had he used radiation therapy on these patients, he could have been far ahead of his time in establishing an even more radical departure from the standard radical mastectomy.

Handley and Thackray, of the Middlesex Hospital, reported in 1969 their 10-year results on 143 patients who underwent Patey's modified radical mastectomy but received no adjuvant hormonal manipulation or chemotherapy.[128] They included in this procedure biopsy of the medial ends of the upper three intercostal spaces. Their adherence to Patey's philosophy of wide skin removal was reflected in the fact that 50 percent of their patients required skin grafting. Fifty-four percent of these patients were stage A of the Columbia Clinical Classification, and this group showed 61 percent 10-year survival and 16 percent local recurrence. In no case did the local recurrence arise from the pectoralis major muscle. This was felt to be equivalent to results after standard radical mastectomy.

Williams and colleagues published in 1953 a retrospective review of 1044 cases of breast carcinoma treated by various methods at St. Bartholomew's Hospital in London between 1930 and 1939 in an effort to identify possible differences in outcome according to treatment method.[319] The results indicated that there was no difference in 10-year survival rates among radical mastectomy, modified radical mastectomy, and simple mastectomy, and whether or not radiation therapy was used. Local recurrence rates appeared to be significantly reduced only in the radical mastectomy group and did not appear to be influenced by the use of radiation therapy. The conclusion of these authors was "that where efficient radiotherapy is available radical mastectomy should be abandoned in favor of conservative surgery." This supported the efforts of such contemporary investigators as McWhirter and Patey to explore the efficacy and safety of less extensive procedures and presaged the eventual widespread acceptance of these procedures.

Hugh Auchincloss, a surgeon at the Columbia Presbyterian Hospital, advanced the cause of the modified radical mastectomy using many of the same arguments as Patey did to conceptually justify its use.[9] He analyzed a series of 107 radical mastectomies for breast carcinoma associated with axillary metastases. Of 31 of these patients who were clinically free of disease 8 to 10 years after surgery, 27 had involvement of four or fewer nodes, all of which had been situated in the lower two axillary levels. This suggested that all disease could just as effectively have been removed by the modified procedure, with the same chance of cure. Auchincloss's procedure used a transverse elliptical incision but differed from that of Patey in leaving the pectoralis minor muscle in place and only dissecting the lower two thirds of the axilla to avoid the morbidity of arm edema. Postoperative irradiation to the chest wall and upper axilla was given only to those patients with axillary node involvement; this combined the best aspects of both radical surgery and radiation with the least morbidity.

John L. Madden of New York began in 1958 to perform modified radical mastectomy routinely on his patients with breast carcinoma, removing the chest wall musculature only when direct invasion occurred and using neither routine radiotherapy nor chemotherapy.[182] He used a vertical elliptical skin incision similar to that described by Harrington in 1929 and extensive subcutaneous dissection of the skin flaps that rarely required skin graft closure.[132] The pectoralis fascia was removed. The en bloc axillary dissection included all three levels, being more extensive than Auchincloss's procedure, and both pectoralis muscles were left *in situ*. Although, like Patey and Auchincloss, Madden made a point of removing the intermuscular nodes of Rotter, he did not believe these were clinically important because of their rare involvement by tumor. Drains were routinely placed under the skin flaps postoperatively. In subsequent reports, Madden's results were also compatible with those of the more extensive radical mastectomy. An important finding in his series was the absence of any local recurrences in the pectoral muscle at 10 years.[183]

Roses and coworkers reported in 1981 another variation of the modified radical mastectomy and advocated abandoning this term in favor of a more accurately descriptive name, since there are so many modifications of the radical mastectomy.[250] Their procedure involved a transverse or oblique skin incision and division of the humeral insertion of the pectoralis major muscle, with medial reflection of the sternal portion of this muscle to allow complete axillary dissection up to the apex. The pectoralis minor muscle is excised in continuity with the breast and axillary contents, preserving the lateral pectoral and long thoracic nerves, usually preserving the thoracodorsal nerve and sacrificing the intercostobrachial nerve and thoracodorsal vessels. The pectoralis major muscle is then resutured to its insertion on the humerus before skin closure and drain placement underneath the flaps. They called this procedure *total mastectomy with complete axillary lymph node dissection* and asserted that a similar procedure leaving the pectoralis minor muscle in place (i.e., that of Auchincloss or Madden) should be called *total mastectomy with lateral axillary dissection. Total mastectomy* is a term they reserved for procedures that only sample low-level axillary nodes. Roses' procedure is reminiscent of that originally described by Lister more than 110 years earlier.

The modified radical mastectomy is essentially the same operation described by Moore in 1867, although it was another century before this procedure became the standard surgical treatment for breast carcinoma. A report by the American College of Surgeons Commission on Cancer demonstrated a dramatic decline in the use of the radical mastectomy, from 47.9 percent of cases in 1972 to 3.4 percent in 1981 (Fig. 39–16). The modified radical mastectomy was increasingly utilized during this same period, making up 27.7 percent of cases in 1972 and 72.3 percent in 1981.[4, 50, 212] An NIH Consensus Development Conference in 1980 concluded that the modified radical mastectomy is a satisfactory alternative to the Halsted radical mastectomy for stage I or stage II breast carcinoma.[207] This was further supported by a randomized prospective clinical trial published in 1983 that showed no significant difference in DFS or overall survival or in local recurrence rates at 5 years between those of radical mastectomy and modified radical mastectomy.[184] The differences that existed in this study were attributable to a small number of stage III patients, indicating that locally advanced disease is not amenable to surgery alone and probably should not be included in these trials. The routine use of chemotherapy for patients with involved axillary lymph nodes also distinguished this trial from earlier studies.

As the validity of less extensive local treatments for breast cancer became established through the 1950s and 1960s, it seemed reasonable to postulate that tumor extirpation alone might be as effective as mastectomy. Keynes had approached this goal with the addition of radiotherapy, but Patey's small experience with a high local recurrence rate among patients undergoing only partial mastectomy lent a pessimistic outlook to this procedure.[157, 222] The reluctance of surgeons to attempt anything less than total mastectomy for this disease can be understood in the context of history, since such authorities as LeDran,

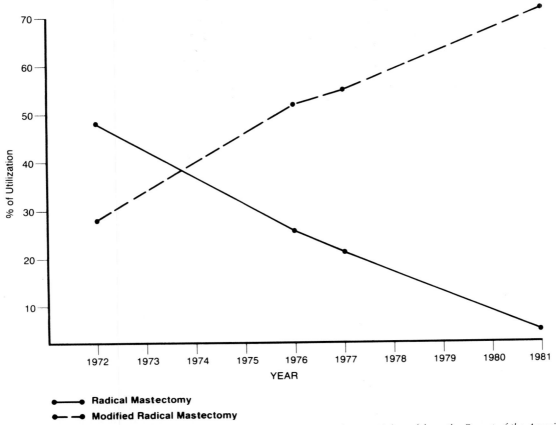

Figure 39–16 *Changing patterns of operation for breast carcinoma between 1972 and 1981. (Adapted from the Report of the American College of Surgeons Commission on Cancer, October 22, 1982.)*

Petit, Moore, and Halsted, among others, had all demonstrated the dangers of "inadequate operation," in terms of prohibitive rates of local recurrence and death from disease.[204] Of course the nature and extent of the disease being treated in the mid-twentieth century were quite different from the locally advanced disease most often treated by the earlier authorities, and the understanding of tumor biology and surgical principles had advanced to a remarkable degree during the intervening years.

Adair[1] in 1943 reported a small series of patients with breast carcinoma who had undergone local excision only; they actually had better 5-year survival (88 percent) than a larger group of patients who had undergone radical mastectomy, simple mastectomy, or local excision plus radiotherapy during the same time period.[1] The failure to stratify these patients according to variables, such as stage (known to influence survival) and the degree of selection bias, made these results inconclusive. Stimulated by these results, though, Crile and colleagues analyzed several series of patients during a 25-year period.[44, 45, 140] Their results suggested that partial mastectomy resulted in rates of local recurrence and overall survival that were statistically similar to those for radical mastectomy. This similarity was most prominent when partial mastectomy was applied to patients

with small tumors and no involvement of axillary lymph nodes and persisted up to 15 years of follow-up.[140] The retrospective and uncontrolled study design, the failure to confirm clear margins microscopically, and the selection bias in these studies, though, cast some uncertainty on these findings. Tagart in 1981 added to this uncertainty with his finding of a prohibitively high rate of local recurrence (37 percent) at only 3 years after wide local excision of operable (stage I or II) breast carcinoma in 44 patients, when a 2-cm margin of grossly normal tissue was obtained around all tumors.[286] Montgomery and colleagues followed a group of 31 patients with small (T1 or T2) breast carcinomas treated only with wide biopsy excision.[203] At 5 years, the overall locoregional recurrence rate was 33 percent. They stated the basic concerns that must be addressed in the treatment of breast carcinoma in the light of our current knowledge of tumor biology:

Treatment of breast cancer by radical surgery with or without radiotherapy has as its objective cure of the patient, or at least the prevention of distressing local recurrence. It is widely believed that recurrence in the operation area predisposes to early dissemination, and, since we now realize that the curative role of mastectomy is at least debatable, treatment is directed at preventing local tumor recurrence.

TABLE 39–5. RESULTS OF RETROSPECTIVE STUDIES OF PARTIAL MASTECTOMY AND POSTOPERATIVE BREAST IRRADIATION FOR OPERABLE STAGE I AND II BREAST CARCINOMAS

Author (Ref)	Patients (n)	Follow-up Interval (yr)	Local Recurrence (%)	Overall Survival (%)
Mustakallio[208]	127	10	26	71
Porritt[233]	263	10	——	70
Peters[224]	124	10	5	45
Wise et al[321]	49	10	8	62
Prosnitz et al[236]	49	5	2	97
Freeman et al[93]	115	5	16	80
Vilcoq et al[302]	314	5	10	84
Clark et al[38]	680	10	16	62
Romsdahl et al[247]	103	10	7	78
Leung et al[174]	493	10	10	68
Delouche et al[55]	410	10	10	63
DuBois et al[62]	392	10	16	78
Haffty et al[117]	278	10	20	67
Veronesi et al[300]	1232	10	8	78
Fowble et al[90]	697	10	18	83

*Stage I cases only.

Lagios and associates in 1983 prospectively studied 43 patients who underwent segmental mastectomy alone for primary operable breast carcinoma, comparing their outcomes with those of a similar group of patients who underwent total mastectomy.[167] A significantly greater incidence of local recurrence was found in the former group after an average follow-up of 24 months (28 percent versus 7.5 percent). A major factor related to this incidence of local recurrence was the unsuspected involvement of the resection margin by carcinoma in several cases. This emphasized the importance of ensuring an adequate resection of tumor, preferably by microscopic confirmation, if segmental mastectomy is to be at all successful. If the dangers of local recurrence are to be avoided, whether they be a persistent potential for distant dissemination or simply the morbidity associated with salvage mastectomy, these authors feel that any involvement of resection margins by tumor mandates either further surgery or postoperative radiotherapy. Subsequent studies have affirmed the importance of ensuring microscopically clear margins as a standard part of breast conservation therapy, to minimize local treatment failure.*

Several retrospective studies since the 1950s have confirmed the original observations of Keynes and McWhirter about the efficacy and safety of limited surgery followed by postoperative radiotherapy.† These studies demonstrate no differences in ultimate outcome of segmental mastectomy plus post-operative radiation as compared with more extensive surgery alone (Table 39–5). The addition of radiotherapy appears to control those multicentric or residual foci of subclinical disease in the breast that presumably

---

*See references 6, 110, 229, 255, 257, 275, and 320.
†See references 55, 62, 90, 93, 117, 133, 174, 208, 224, 233, 236, 247, 276, 300, 302, and 321.

give rise to the high rates of local recurrence observed following segmental mastectomy alone.

A small number of studies have explored the value of radiation therapy as the sole treatment for carcinoma of the breast. Although the results have been quite comparable with those of surgery at follow-up of 5 and 10 years, longer follow-up has revealed increased levels of local recurrence and distant metastases as well as severe late radiation damage to the treated breast. Radiation therapy is therefore generally applied as the sole form of treatment only to inoperable forms of breast carcinoma, in which its goal is strictly palliation rather than cure.[71, 142]

The appropriate roles of breast-sparing surgery and radiation therapy in the treatment of breast carcinoma appeared to be definitively established by the results of the National Surgical Adjuvant Breast and Bowel Project (NSABP) B-06 protocol.[73, 80, 81] This study improved on the design flaws of earlier ones in its prospective controlled design, its uniform assurance of complete tumor excision in segmental mastectomy through microscopic confirmation of clear margins, the use of pathological staging through the performance of axillary dissection in all patients, and treatment of all node-positive patients with chemotherapy. After 8 years' follow-up, this trial demonstrated no significant difference in S, DFS, or DDFS between women subjected to total mastectomy and those subjected to lumpectomy, with or without breast irradiation. Lumpectomy with breast irradiation resulted in a significantly lower rate of ipsilateral breast tumor recurrences (10 percent) than lumpectomy without breast irradiation (39 percent), although S and DDFS did not differ between these latter two groups. These results have been corroborated by several subsequent prospective randomized trials.[22, 115, 254, 295, 298, 320]

It thus seems that surgery is best applied to controlling grossly evident disease, and any extension of its application to attempt eradication of subclinical or microscopic disease increases its morbidity with no compensatory gain in survival. Conversely, it is this subclinical disease that is best controlled by radiation therapy, the morbidity of which becomes prohibitive when it is extended to the treatment of gross disease.[137] It has been demonstrated that a postoperative radiation dose of 5000 rad to a breast free of clinically detectable disease should provide control in 100 percent of cases.[88, 93]

It could be argued that segmental mastectomy alone is also justified by the results of the B-06 protocol if a predictably high rate of local recurrence is acceptable (i.e., approximately 40 percent, and perhaps higher for those lesions such as invasive lobular carcinoma or ductal carcinoma *in situ* known to be associated with high rates of multicentricity). The prognostic implications of local recurrence in the breast remain unresolved. Although many authors view local recurrence as a strong indicator, and perhaps instigator, of distant disease, many reports demonstrate that when it follows segmental mastectomy, it can be effectively treated by reexcision or salvage mastectomy without any apparent adverse effects on ultimate survival.* in the b-04 protocol of the NSABP, 88 percent of the local recurrences in the group undergoing radical mastectomy were ultimately associated with distant metastasis, while only 58 percent of local recurrences in the group treated with total mastectomy developed distant disease.[77, 79] Fisher has postulated from this observation that local recurrence following more radical surgical procedures may be caused by tumor cells that are already systemically disseminated lodging in the operative site; following lesser procedures, especially segmental mastectomy, it may result from residual or incompletely excised tumor in the absence of distant disease.[78] This may justify a less pessimistic attitude toward local recurrences after breast-sparing procedures and may explain their apparent lack of impact on survival in many series when treated appropriately.[242] Although invasive lobular carcinoma has been postulated to pose a higher risk of local treatment failure following breast conservation, in view of its high incidence of multicentricity, this has not been borne out in several studies.[165, 230, 259, 315] There is no evidence to support withholding breast conservation solely on the basis of invasive lobular histology.

Another perspective on this issue of local recurrence was provided by the results of the NSABP B-06 trial summarized previously.[73, 80, 81] In node-positive patients, local recurrence had no effect on survival. In node-negative patients, however, local recurrence was associated with a significant reduction in DFS ($p = .005$) and distant disease–free survival (DDFS; $p = .02$). This suggests that local recurrence should be vigorously prevented to optimize the chance of cure in those patients most capable of being cured and provides the strongest argument against treating breast carcinoma with segmental mastectomy alone, tending to vindicate the basic beliefs of Petit, Moore, and Banks. However, Fisher has offered a very different perspective on these observations. He asserts that the NSABP data do show a 3.4-fold increased risk of developing distant metastases among women who develop ipsilateral breast tumor recurrence but that this local recurrence should be viewed as a marker for poor prognosis rather than the cause of it.[72] This view is in accord with Fisher's alternative hypothesis, which asserts that the method of local treatment of breast carcinoma has no effect on a woman's ultimate survival. The answer to this dilemma awaits further data.

EVOLVING ISSUES

The one common thread found in virtually all recent studies on the surgical treatment of breast carcinoma is that the type and extent of local and regional treatment do not substantially affect survival. This concept represents a major change in thinking about the biology of breast carcinoma from the Halstedian beliefs that predominated at the turn of the twentieth century. This change resulted at least partially from scientific observations of the results of treatment that was predicated on the belief that the disease is local in origin. For several decades it has been apparent that breast carcinoma must in fact be a systemic disease at its earliest stages and that the development of distant metastases depends on a number of factors related to tumor cell kinetics, tumor growth rate, and complex host-tumor interactions, perhaps mediated through hormonal and immune mechanisms that are unique to each afflicted individual.[71, 72, 78, 137, 233]

Experimental studies have shown further that breast carcinoma does not evolve in the orderly, incremental fashion envisioned by Halsted and his contemporaries. Fisher and Fisher demonstrated that lymph nodes do not act as barriers to tumor cell dissemination and that there is extensive and complex intercommunication between the lymphatics and blood stream that contradicts the premise of the mechanical theory of tumor extension elaborated by Thiersch, Waldeyer, Handley, and Gray.[75, 76] These observations suggest that the status of regional lymph nodes in the patient with breast carcinoma should be viewed as a "marker" of the particular host-tumor relationship that exists, which is either conducive to (i.e., positive nodes) or not conducive to (i.e., negative nodes) the development of distant metastasis. This concept assumes that all patients have some potential for systemic dissemination from the earliest phases of disease development.[78]

The greatest promise for an effective cure must therefore lie in systemic treatment. Patey's understanding of this concept is reflected in the following assertion[222]:

> Until an effective general agent for the treatment of carcinoma of the breast is developed, a high proportion of cases are doomed to die of the disease whatever combination of local treatment by surgery and irradiation is used, because in such a high proportion of cases the disease has passed outside the field of local attack when the patient first comes for treatment.

The abundant experimental and clinical evidence that has emerged in support of this hypothesis has led to the current acceptance of a diminished emphasis on loco-regional treatment of this disease, as discussed in the previous section, while systemically oriented modalities have been increasingly emphasized. Hormone manipulation was the first systemic therapy applied to breast carcinoma when Sir George Beatson of Glasgow performed oophorectomy for an advanced case in 1896.[16] Since then, hormone therapies of various types have continued to be used, showing promising though less than optimal results.[116, 145, 181, 192, 209, 279] Cytotoxic chemotherapy became popular in the late 1950s and has since become

---

*See references 17, 36, 38, 93, 101, 163, 164, 203, 242, 258, 276, and 286.

a mainstay of adjuvant systemic therapy following surgical treatment and, as such, has demonstrated better survival than surgery alone.[27, 78, 105, 134] Advances in molecular biology have led to the discovery of oncogenes, which offer the opportunity of perhaps manipulating the process of malignancy to prevent it altogether.[213] Adoptive immunotherapy is another form of systemic treatment involving the application of the lymphokine interleukin 2 to activate "killer" lymphocytes with antitumor activity; this is currently being investigated for clinical use and may represent the next generation of treatment for breast carcinoma.[249]

The surgeon has thus become an integral part of a multidisciplinary team who manages patients with breast carcinoma. This team includes the diagnostic radiologist, radiation oncologist, medical oncologist, and pathologist. The surgeon's role has evolved to diagnosing and ensuring the removal of all clinically evident disease so as to maximize the efficacy of radiation and systemic therapy.[71] All members of this team must be committed to the total patient and to a thorough understanding of the disease process and of management options. Mastectomy is still a valid, and sometimes preferable, option for operable (stage I and II) breast carcinoma as well as all cases of locally advanced disease judged to be amenable to operation.

In the future, axillary dissection may assume diminished importance for treatment of breast carcinoma. Recent studies have demonstrated that there is no survival advantage to the routine removal of axillary lymph nodes and that the only therapeutic advantage of this practice is a substantial reduction in the rate of regional axillary recurrence.[3, 71, 77, 79, 82, 85] The clinical significance of axillary lymph node involvement, beyond its prognostic implications, has also been questioned.[85] In the past, the status of axillary lymph nodes has been the primary determinant of the need for systemic adjuvant chemotherapy; however, the National Cancer Institute now recommends routine systemic therapy, even in the absence of axillary metastases.[5] It would therefore seem reasonable, because of the absence of data to suggest any detriment to survival, to perform axillary dissection only in patients who present with palpable adenopathy or who develop such adenopathy after primary treatment.[32, 118, 270] This approach is currently practiced by some in the treatment of malignant melanoma; however, most investigators still advocate routine axillary dissection in the treatment of primary breast carcinoma, in view of some persistent uncertainty as to benefit.[51, 185, 241, 252, 320]

The therapeutic challenge posed by noninvasive breast carcinoma will be faced increasingly in the future because of more frequent detection of these lesions owing to the current emphasis on early detection of breast carcinoma and the use of mammography. *In situ* breast malignancies may be the one form of this disease that may still be governed by the precepts of the local origin theory, since by definition systemic dissemination should not yet have occurred

at this stage (see Chapter 52). Aggressive local treatment alone may thus be curative, as has been demonstrated in a number of studies.[94, 95, 262, 305] The evidence of the natural history of lobular carcinoma *in situ* currently available suggests that it may best be managed expectantly and may be more of a marker of increased risk for future development of invasive carcinoma than an actual precursor of it.[96] Ductal carcinoma *in situ* appears to be a more ominous lesion that requires definitive surgery, although breast-sparing procedures with postoperative irradiation result in survival rates comparable to those of total mastectomy, which, as would be predicted at this stage of disease, approach 100 percent.[86, 216, 239, 262] Further advances in hormone manipulation and molecular biology may halt the progression of these lesions to invasive carcinoma.

Although mammography has resulted in the detection of early malignancies that appear to be highly curable, 80 percent of biopsies of nonpalpable breast lesions are currently benign (see Table 29–3). This has led to an emphasis on a more selective approach to biopsy of mammographic lesions to improve the yield of malignancies without missing any.[15] Nonoperative observation of certain mammographic lesions that include smooth-bordered masses 1 cm or smaller, asymmetrical densities, and clustered microcalcifications that contain fewer than 10 flecks of calcium, has been shown to be safe when followed reliably for interval change.[268] This finding promises to reduce substantially the number of unnecessary surgical biopsies and improve the cost-effectiveness of diagnosis of breast carcinoma.

Fine-needle aspiration (FNA) biopsy, introduced in 1930 for cytologic tissue diagnosis, assumed an increasingly prominent role in the diagnosis of breast masses during the 1980s.[188] It is now the recommended diagnostic modality of choice for palpable breast masses, and has been applied successfully to the diagnosis of nonpalpable breast masses.[169, 189, 265, 308] Stereotactic devices have also been successfully applied to the diagnosis of nonpalpable breast lesions, using either FNAB or core biopsy techniques.[61, 70, 100, 205] The accuracy of these methods is entirely comparable to that of open surgical biopsy, and they also promise to reduce the need for diagnostic surgery of breast lesions that carry an intermediate risk for malignancy.[205]

Locally advanced carcinoma of the breast is no longer considered inoperable, as originally asserted by Haagensen and Stout.[111, 112] The introduction of multimodality treatment, including preoperative induction, or neoadjuvant, chemotherapy followed by mastectomy and postoperative chemotherapy and radiation therapy, has greatly improved the resectability of these complex breast tumors, their local control, and these patients' survival.[144, 281] Compelling evidence has also been reported that the substantial shrinking of these cancers afforded by neoadjuvant chemotherapy allows even breast conservation to be applied safely and successfully to them.*

---

*See references 28, 33, 148, 158, 260, 271, and 299.

Currently, radiation therapy is applied routinely in all cases of invasive breast carcinoma being treated conservatively because of the unacceptably high incidence of local recurrence following lumpectomy alone.[80, 320] Several recent studies have questioned the necessity for postlumpectomy radiation of small node-negative tumors of any tumor in an elderly woman.[141, 199, 211, 242] The only prospective randomized study of this issue concluded that local breast recurrence following lumpectomy alone remains prohibitively high, even in the most favorable-prognosis cases.[39] The current consensus, therefore, supports routine breast irradiation in this setting.[89, 240]

Despite the abundance of compelling data from numerous prospective randomized trials on the validity and safety of breast conservation treatment of breast carcinoma,[22, 80, 115, 254, 295, 298] only about 12 percent of all patients, and fewer than 30 percent of women with the most favorable T1 tumors, receive this treatment in the United States.[210, 287] This is due largely to the reluctance of surgeons to abandon mastectomy, as well as to unfounded fears of radiation therapy on the part of patients. Widespread education of both surgeons and patients is needed if breast conservation is to achieve its full potential.[287]

As we come to the end of the twentieth century, breast carcinoma is increasingly regarded as a systemic disease. This same concept was shared by Imhotep, Hippocrates, Galen, and Hunter at the crest of many other cycles of belief and practice. Although these swings in philosophy during the past several centuries may appear arbitrary, they have actually occurred in response to advances in clinical experience and scientific knowledge. It is likely that the remarkable rate of scientific advances currently being made in this field will result in further shifts in conceptual and practical approaches to breast carcinoma in the future. We can hope that this cycle will culminate in an ideal management regimen for this complex disease process. This sentiment was expressed by Lewison in 1953[176]:

> The soundest predication of future progress must come from a realistic view of the past. Only by carefully examining our present precepts and practice can we intelligently plan for the future. Our resolute purpose must always be to promote the best interest of each individual patient, and not those of surgery, radiotherapy or chemotherapy.

Bernard Fisher, among others, has much contributed to achieving this purpose by developing and establishing the clinical trial, as McWhirter had recommended.[195] Such trials become the primary tool for testing hypotheses and determining optimal treatment for breast carcinoma. He has asserted thus[78]:

> Therapeutic strategies for breast cancer have evolved over time in step-wise fashion and are the result of biological information, which has led to a better understanding of this disease. It is logical to anticipate that this course will continue and that future gains will occur as a result of the testing of new biological hypotheses. Breast cancer management has been, is, and will be related to science and not to populism!"

Interestingly enough, Fisher's sentiment on this issue closely echoes one of Virchow's many dictums, stated in 1896, as cited by DeMoulin[56]:

> Indeed, a great deal of industrious work is being done and the microscope is extensively used, but someone should have another bright idea!

This impatience with the status quo and commitment to shed light on the unknown will continue to advance the frontiers of our knowledge of breast carcinoma.

References

1. Adair FE: Role of surgery and irradiation in cancer of the breast. JAMA 121:553–558, 1943.
2. Anonymous: Dr. Willy Meyer. Am J Surg 17:287–292, 1932.
3. Anonymous: Cancer research campaign working party: Cancer research campaign (King's/Cambridge) trial for early breast cancer. Lancet 2:55–60, 1980.
4. Anonymous: Report by the American College of Surgeons Commission on Cancer. Chicago, October 22, 1982.
5. Anonymous: Clinical alert from the National Cancer Institute, Department of Health and Human Services. Bethesda, MD, May 16, 1988.
6. Anscher MS, Jones P, Prosnitz LR, et al: Local failure and margin status in early-stage breast carcinoma treated with conservation surgery and radiation therapy. Ann Surg 218:22–28, 1993.
7. Ashikari R, Huvos AG, Snyder RE, et al: A clinicopathologic study of atypical lesions of the breast. Cancer 33:310–317, 1974.
8. Ashworth TR: A case of cancer in which cells similar to those in the tumours were seen in the blood after death. Med J Aust 14:146–148, 1869.
9. Auchincloss H: Significance of location and number of axillary metastases in carcinoma of the breast: A justification for a conservative operation. Ann Surg 158:37–46, 1963.
10. Baker RR, Kuhajda FP: The clinical management of a normal contralateral breast in patients with lobular breast cancer. Ann Surg 210:444–448, 1989.
11. Banks WM: A plea for the more free removal of cancerous growths. Liverpool and Manchester Surgical Reports 192–206, 1878.
12. Banks WM: A brief history of the operations practised for cancer of the breast. Br Med J 1:5–10, 1902.
13. Bauer TL, Pandelidis SM, Rhoads JE, et al: Mammographically detected carcinoma of the breast. Surg Gynecol Obstet 173:482–486, 1991.
14. Bauermeister DE, Hall MH: Specimen radiography: A mandatory adjunct to mammography. Am J Clin Pathol 59:782–789, 1973.
15. Baute PB, Thibodeau M, Newstead G: Improving the yield of biopsy for nonpalpable lesions of the breast. Surg Gynecol Obstet 174:93–96, 1992.
16. Beatson GT: On the treatment of inoperable cases of carcinoma of the mamma: Suggestions for a new method of treatment, with illustrative cases. Lancet 2:104–107, 1896.
17. Bedwinek JM, Lee J, Fineberg B, Ocwieza M: Prognostic indicators in patients with isolated local-regional recurrence of breast cancer. Cancer 47:2232–2235, 1981.
18. Bell B: A System of Surgery, Vol 5. Edinburgh, Bell, Bradfute, 1791, pp 436–460.

19. Bernstein JL, Thompson WD, Risch N, et al: Risk factors predicting the incidence of second primary breast cancer among women diagnosed with a first primary breast cancer. Am J Epidemiol 136:925–936, 1992.
20. Billroth T: Die Krankheiten der brust Drusen. Stuttgart, F Enke, 1880.
21. Black MM, Barclay THC, Cutler SJ, et al: Association of atypical characteristics of benign breast lesions with subsequent risk of breast cancer. Cancer 29:338–343, 1972.
22. Blichert-Toft M, Brincker H, Andersen JA, et al: A Danish randomized trial comparing breast-preserving therapy with mastectomy in mammary carcinoma: Preliminary results. Acta Oncol 27:671–677, 1988.
23. Bloodgood JC: Cancer of the breast: Figures which show that education can increase the number of cures. JAMA 66:552–553, 1916.
24. Bloodgood JC: Borderline breast tumors. Ann Surg 93:235–249, 1931.
25. Bloodgood JC: Comedo-carcinoma (or comedo-adenoma) of the female breast. Am J Cancer 22:842–853, 1934.
26. Bloom HJG, Richardson WW, Harries EJ: Natural history of untreated breast cancer (1805–1933). Br Med J 2:213–221, 1962.
27. Bonadonna G, Valagussa P: Dose-response effect of adjuvant chemotherapy in breast cancer. N Engl J Med 304:10–15, 1981.
28. Bonadonna G, Veronesi U, Brambilla C, et al: Primary chemotherapy to avoid mastectomy in tumors with diameters of three centimeters or more. J Natl Cancer Inst 82:1539–1545, 1990.
29. Breasted JH: The Edwin Smith Surgical Papyrus, Vol 1. Chicago, University of Chicago Press, 1930, pp 363, 463.
30. Broders AC: Carcinoma in situ contrasted with benign penetrating epithelium. JAMA 99:1670–1674, 1932.
31. Brown PW, Silverman J, Owens E, et al: Intraductal "noninfiltrating" carcinoma of the breast. Arch Surg 111:1063–1067, 1976.
32. Cady B, Stone MD, Wayne J: New therapeutic possibilities in primary invasive breast cancer. Ann Surg 218:338–349, 1993.
33. Calais G, Berger C, Descamps P, et al: Conservative treatment feasibility with induction chemotherapy, surgery, and radiotherapy for patients with breast carcinoma larger than 3 cm. Cancer 74:1283–1288, 1994.
34. Celsus AM: De Medicina, Vol 2. Translated by Spencer WG. Cambridge, Harvard University Press, 1953, p 129.
35. Cheatle GL, Cutler M: Tumors of the Breast. Philadelphia, JB Lippincott, 1931.
36. Chu FCH, Lin F-J, Kim JH, et al: Locally recurrent carcinoma of the breast. Cancer 37:2677–2681, 1976.
37. Clagett OT, Plimpton NC, Root GT: Lesions of the breast: Relationship of benign lesions to carcinoma. Surgery 15:413–419, 1944.
38. Clark RM, Wilkinson RH, Mahoney LJ, Reid JG, MacDonald WD: Breast cancer: A 21 year experience with conservative surgery and radiation. Int J Radiol Oncol Biol Phys 8:967–975, 1982.
39. Clark RM, McCulloch PB, Levine MN, et al: Randomized clinical trial to assess the effectiveness of breast irradiation following lumpectomy and axillary dissection for node-negative breast cancer. J Natl Cancer Inst 84:683–689, 1992.
40. Cole WH, Rossiter LJ: Chronic cystic mastitis with particular reference to classification. Ann Surg 119:573–590, 1944.
41. Cooper WA: The history of the radical mastectomy. Ann Med Hist 3:36–54, 1941.
42. Cornil AV: Contributions a l'histoire du development histologique des tumeurs epitheliales (squirrhe, encephaloide, etc.). J Anat Physiol 2:266–276, 1865.
43. Cornil AV: Les Tumeurs du Sein. Paris, Libraire Germer Balliere, 1908.
44. Crile G: Treatment of breast cancer by local excision. Am J Surg 109:400–403, 1965.
45. Crile G, Hoerr SO: Results of treatment of carcinoma of the breast by local excision. Surg Gynecol Obstet 132:780–782, 1971.
46. Cullen TS: A rapid method of making permanent specimens from frozen sections by the use of formalin. Bull Johns Hopkins Hosp 6:67–73, 1895.
47. Dahl-Iversen E, Soerener B: Recherches sue les metastases microscopiques des ganglions lymphatiques parasterneaux dans le cancer du sein. J Int Chir 11:492–509, 1951.
48. Dahl-Iversen E, Tobiassen T: Radical mastectomy with parasternal and supraclavicular dissection for mammary carcinoma. Ann Surg 157:170–176, 1963.
49. Dahl-Iversen E, Tobiassen T: Radical mastectomy with parasternal and supraclavicular dissection for mammary carcinoma. Ann Surg 170:889–894, 1969.
50. Danforth DN, Lippman ME: Surgical treatment of breast cancer. In Lippman ME, Lichter AS, Danforth DN (eds): Diagnosis and Management of Breast Cancer. Philadelphia, WB Saunders, 1988, pp 95–154.
51. Danforth DN: The role of axillary lymph node dissection in the management of breast cancer. PPO Updates 6:1–16, 1992.
52. Davis HH, Simons M, Davis JB: Cystic disease of the breast: Relationship to carcinoma. Cancer 17:957–978, 1964.
53. Deaver JB: Malignant and benign diseases of the female breast. Trans South Surg Assoc 41:95–111, 1928.
54. Degenshein GA, Ceccarelli F: The history of breast cancer surgery, part 1: early beginnings to Halsted. Breast 3:28–36, 1977.
55. Delouche G, Bachelot F, Premont M, et al: Conservation treatment of early breast cancer: Long term results and complications. Int J Radiat Oncol Biol Phys 13:29–34, 1987.
56. De Moulin D: A Short History of Breast Cancer. Boston, Martinus Nijhoff, 1983.
57. DeOme K: Formal discussion of multiple factors in mouse mammary tumorigenesis. Cancer Res 25:1348–1351, 1965.
58. Dobson J: John Hunter's views on cancer. Ann R Coll Surg Engl 1:176–181, 1959.
59. Doets CJ: De Heelkunde van Petrus Camper 1722–1789. Thesis. Leiden, 1948, p 25.
60. Donegan WL: Introduction to the history of breast cancer. In Donegan WL, Spratt JS (eds): Cancer of the Breast, 3rd ed. Philadelphia, WB Saunders, 1988, pp 1–15.
61. Dowlatshahi K, Yaremko L, Kluskens LF, et al: Nonpalpable breast lesions: Findings of stereotaxic needle-core biopsy and fine-needle aspiration cytology. Radiology 181:745–750, 1991.
62. DuBois JB, Gary-Bobo J, Pourquier H, et al: Tumorectomy and radiotherapy in early breast cancer: A report on 392 patients. Int J Radiat Oncol Biol Phys 15:1275–1282, 1988.
63. Dupont WD, Page DL: Risk factors in women with proliferative breast disease. N Engl J Med 312:146–151, 1985.
64. Egan RL: Experience with mammography in a tumor institution: Evaluation of 1000 studies. Radiology 75:894–900, 1960.
65. Engell HC: Cancer cells in the circulating blood. Acta Chir Scand 201(suppl):1–70, 1955.
66. Ernster VL: The epidemiology of benign breast disease. Epidemiol Rev 3:184–202, 1981.
67. Ewing J: Neoplastic Diseases, 2nd ed. Philadelphia, WB Saunders, 1922.
68. Ewing J: Neoplastic Diseases, 3rd ed. Philadelphia, WB Saunders, 1928, p 582.
69. Fabry W: Observationum et curationum chirurgicarum centuriae, cent. II. Lugduni, IA Huguetan, 1641, pp 267–269.
70. Fajardo LL, Davis JR, Wiens JL, et al: Mammographically-guided stereotactic fine-needle aspiration cytology of nonpalpable breast lesions: Prospective comparisons with surgical biopsy results. AJR Am J Roentgenol 155:977–981, 1990.
71. Fisher B: A commentary on the role of the surgeon in primary breast cancer. Breast Cancer Res Treat 1:17–26, 1981.
72. Fisher B, Anderson S, Fisher ER, et al: Significance of ipsilateral breast tumour recurrence after lumpectomy. Lancet 338:327–331, 1991.
73. Fisher B, Bauer M, Margolese R, et al: Five year results of a randomized clinical trial: Comparing total mastectomy and segmental mastectomy with or without radiation in the treatment of breast cancer. N Engl J Med 312:665–673, 1985.
74. Fisher B, Bauer M, Wickerham DL, et al: Relationship of number of positive axillary nodes to the prognosis of patients with primary breast cancer—an NSABP update. Cancer 52:1551–1557, 1983.

75. Fisher B, Fisher ER: Transmigration of lymph nodes by tumor cells. Science 152:1397–1398, 1966.

76. Fisher B, Fisher ER: The interrelationship of hematogenous and lymphatic tumor cell dissemination. Surg Gynecol Obstet 122:791–798, 1966.

77. Fisher B, Montague ED, Redmond C, et al: Comparison of radical mastectomy with alternative treatments for primary breast cancer: A first report of results from a prospective randomized clinical trial. Cancer 39:2827–2839, 1977.

78. Fisher B, Redmond C, Fisher ER, et al: The contribution of recent NSABP clinical trials of primary breast cancer therapy to an understanding of tumor biology—an overview of findings. Cancer 46:1009–1025, 1980.

79. Fisher B, Redmond C, Fisher ER, et al: Ten-year results of a randomized clinical trial comparing radical mastectomy and total mastectomy with or without radiation. N Engl J Med 312:674–682, 1985.

80. Fisher B, Redmond C, Poisson R, et al: Eight-year results of a randomized clinical trial comparing total mastectomy and lumpectomy with or without irradiation in the treatment of breast cancer. N Engl J Med 320:822–828, 1989.

81. Fisher B, Redmond C: Lumpectomy for breast cancer: An update of the NSABP experience. J Natl Cancer Inst Monogr 11:7–13, 1992.

82. Fisher B, Wolmark N, Bauer M, et al: The accuracy of clinical nodal staging and of limited axillary dissection as a determinant of histological nodal status in carcinoma of the breast. Surg Gynecol Obstet 152:765–772, 1981.

83. Fisher ER: The impact of pathology on the biologic, diagnostic, prognostic and therapeutic considerations in breast cancer. Surg Clin North Am 64:1073–1093, 1984.

84. Fisher ER, Fisher B, Sass R, et al: Pathologic findings from the National Surgical Adjuvant Breast Project (Protocol No. 4) XI. Bilateral breast cancer. Cancer 54:3002–3011, 1984.

85. Fisher ER, Sass R, Fisher B: Biologic considerations regarding the one and two step procedures in the management of patients with invasive carcinoma of the breast. Surg Gynecol Obstet 161:245–249, 1985.

86. Fisher ER, Sass R, Fisher B, et al: Pathologic findings from the National Surgical Adjuvant Breast Project (protocol 6). I. Intraductal carcinoma (DCIS). Cancer 57:197–208, 1986.

87. Fisher ER, Shoemaker RH, Palekar AS: Identification of pre-malignant hyperplasia in methyl-cholanthrene–induced mammary tumorigenesis. Lab Invest 33:446–450, 1975.

88. Fletcher GH: Clinical dose-response curves of human malignant epithelial tumors. Br J Radiol 46:1–12, 1973.

89. Fowble B: Is there a subset of patients with early stage invasive breast cancer for whom irradiation may not be indicated after conservative surgery alone? Breast J 1:79–90, 1995.

90. Fowble BL, Solin LJ, Schultz DJ, et al: Ten-year results of conservative surgery and irradiation for Stage I and II breast cancer. Int J Radiat Oncol Biol Phys 21:269–277, 1991.

91. Fracchia AA, Robinson D, Legaspi A, et al: Survival in bilateral breast cancer. Cancer 55:1414–1421, 1985.

92. Franceschi D, Crowe JP, Lie S, et al: Not all nonpalpable breast cancers are alike. Arch Surg 126:967–971, 1991.

93. Freeman CR, Belliveau MD, Kim TH, Boivin J-F: Limited surgery with or without radiotherapy for early breast carcinoma. J Can Assoc Radiol 32:125–128, 1981.

94. Frykberg ER, Bland KI: In situ breast carcinoma. Adv Surg 26:29–72, 1993.

95. Frykberg ER, Bland KI, Copeland EM: The detection and treatment of early breast cancer. In Tompkins RK (ed): Advances in Surgery, Vol 23. Chicago, Year Book Medical Publishers, 1990, pp 119–194.

96. Frykberg ER, Santiago F, Betsill WL, O'Brien PH: Lobular carcinoma in situ of the breast. Surg Gynecol Obstet 164:285–301, 1987.

97. Galen: De tumoribus praeter naturam. In Kuhn CG (ed): Opera Omnia, Vol 7. Lipsiae, C Knobloch, 1821, pp 726–728.

98. Gallager HS, Martin JE: Early phases in the development of breast cancer. Cancer 24:1170–1178, 1969.

99. Gallager HS, Martin JE: An orientation to the concept of minimal breast cancer. Cancer 28:1505–1507, 1971.

100. Gent HJ, Sprenger E, Dowlatshahi K: Stereotaxic needle localization and cytologic diagnosis of occult breast lesions. Ann Surg 204:580–584, 1986.

101. Gilliland MD, Barton RM, Copeland EM: The implications of local recurrence of breast cancer as the first site of therapeutic failure. Ann Surg 197:284–287, 1983.

102. Gray JH: The relation of lymphatic vessels to the spread of cancer. Br J Surg 26:462–495, 1938.

103. Greenough RB: Early diagnosis of cancer of the breast. Ann Surg 102:233–238, 1935.

104. Greenough RB, Simmons CC, Barney JD: The results of operations for cancer of the breast at the Massachusetts General Hospital from 1894–1904. Surg Gynecol Obstet 3:39–50, 1907.

105. Greenspan EM, Fisher M, Lesnick G, Edelman S: Response of advanced breast carcinoma to the combination of the antimetabolic methotrexate and the alkylating agent Thio-Tepa. Mt Sinai J Med 33:1–26, 1963.

106. Gross SW: An analysis of two hundred and seven cases of carcinoma of the breast. Med News 51:613–617, 1887.

107. Grubbe EH: X-ray Treatment: Its Origin, Birth and Early History. St Paul, MN, Bruce Publishing, 1949.

108. Gullino PM: Natural history of breast cancer: Progression from hyperplasia to neoplasia as predicted by angiogenesis. Cancer 39:2697–2703, 1977.

109. Gump FE: Premalignant diseases of the breast. Surg Clin North Am 64:1051–1059, 1984.

110. Gwin JL, Eisenberg BL, Hoffman JP, et al: Incidence of gross and microscopic carcinoma in specimens from patients with breast cancer after re-excision lumpectomy. Ann Surg 218:729–734, 1993.

111. Haagensen CD, Stout AP: Carcinoma of the breast, I. Criteria of operability. Ann Surg 118:859–876, 1943.

112. Haagensen CD, Stout AP: Carcinoma of the breast, II. Criteria of operability. Ann Surg 118:1032–1051, 1943.

113. Haagensen CD, Stout AP: Carcinoma of the breast: Results of treatment 1935–1942. Ann Surg 134:151–172, 1951.

114. Haagensen CD: The history of the surgical treatment of breast carcinoma from 1863–1921. In Haagensen CD (ed): Diseases of the Breast, 3rd ed. Philadelphia, WB Saunders, 1986, pp 864–871.

115. Habibollahi F, Fentiman IS, Chaudary MA, et al: Conservation treatment of operable breast cancer (ABSTR). Proc Am Soc Clin Oncol 6:A231, 1987.

116. Haddow A, Watkinson JM, Paterson E: Influence of synthetic oestrogens upon advanced malignant disease. Br Med J 2:393–398, 1944.

117. Haffty BG, Goldberg NB, Rose M, et al: Conservative surgery with radiation therapy in clinical Stage I and II breast cancer: Results of a 20-year experience. Arch Surg 124:1266–1270, 1989.

118. Haffty BG, McKhann C, Beinfield M, et al: Breast conservation therapy without axillary dissection: A rational treatment strategy in selected patients. Arch Surg 128:1315–1319, 1993.

119. Halsted WS: The treatment of wounds with especial reference to the value of the blood clot in the management of dead spaces. Johns Hopkins Hosp Rep 2:255–314, 1890–1891.

120. Halsted WS: The results of operations for the cure of cancer of the breast performed at the Johns Hopkins Hospital from June 1889 to January 1894. Johns Hopkins Hosp Rep 4:297–350, 1894–1895.

121. Halsted WS: A clinical and histological study of certain adenocarcinomata of the breast: And a brief consideration of the supraclavicular operation and of the results of operations for cancer of the breast from 1889 to 1898 at the Johns Hopkins Hospital. Ann Surg 28:557–576, 1898.

122. Halsted WS: The results of radical operations for the cure of carcinoma of the breast. Ann Surg 46:1–19, 1907.

123. Halsted WS: Developments in the skin grafting operation for cancer of the breast. JAMA 60:416–435, 1913.

124. Halsted WS: The swelling of the arm after operations for cancer of the breast—elephantiasis chirurgica—its cause and prevention. Bull Johns Hopkins Hosp 32:309–313, 1921.

125. Handley RS, Thackray AC: Invasion of the internal mam-

mary lymph glands in carcinoma of the breast. Br J Cancer 1:15–20, 1947.

126. Handley RS, Thackray AC: Internal mammary lymph chain in carcinoma of the breast: Study of 50 cases. Lancet 2:276–278, 1949.

127. Handley RS: Further observations on the internal mammary lymph chain in carcinoma of the breast. Proc R Soc Med 45:565–566, 1952.

128. Handley RS, Thackray AC: Conservative radical mastectomy (Patey's operation). Ann Surg 170:880–882, 1969.

129. Handley WS: Cancer of the Breast, 2nd ed. New York, Paul B Hoeber, 1906.

130. Handley WS: Cancer of the Breast and Its Operative Treatment. London, John Murray, 1922.

131. Handley WS: Parasternal invasion of the thorax in breast cancer and its suppression by the use of radium tubes as an operative precaution. Surg Gynecol Obstet 45:721–728, 1927.

132. Harrington SW: Carcinoma of the breast: Surgical treatment and results. JAMA 92:208–213, 1929.

133. Harris JR, Connolly JL, Schnitt SJ, et al: The use of pathologic features in selecting the extent of surgical resection necessary for breast cancer patients treated by primary radiation therapy. Ann Surg 201:164–167, 1985.

134. Heidelberger C, Chaudhuri NK, Danneburg P, et al: Fluorinated pyrimidines, a new class of tumour—inhibitory compounds. Nature 179:663–666, 1957.

135. Heidenhain L: Ueber die ursachen der localen Krebsrecidive nach Amputation mammae. Arch Klin Chir 39:97–166, 1889.

136. Heister L: General System of Surgery, part II, section 4. London, Innys, 1745, p 13.

137. Hellman S, Harris JR: The appropriate breast cancer paradigm. Cancer Res 47:339–342, 1987.

138. Henderson IC, Canellos GP: Cancer of the breast: the past decade. N Engl J Med 302:17–20, 78,7–800, 1980.

139. Herodotus: The Histories. New York, Penguin, 1967.

140. Hermann RE, Esselstyn CB, Crile G, Cooperman AM, Antunez AR, Hoerr SO: Results of conservative operations for breast cancer. Arch Surg 120:746–751, 1985.

141. Hermann RE, Esselstyn CB, Grundfest-Broniatowski S, et al: Partial mastectomy without radiation is adequate treatment for patients with Stages 0 and 1 carcinoma of the breast. Surg Gynecol Obstet 177:247–253, 1993.

142. Hochman A, Robinson E: Eighty-two cases of mammary cancer treated exclusively with roentgen therapy. Cancer 15:670–673, 1960.

143. Horn PL, Thompson WD: Risk of contralateral breast cancer: Associations with histologic, clinical, and therapeutic factors. Cancer 62:412–424, 1988.

144. Hortobagyi GN, Ames FC, Buzdar AU, et al: Management of Stage III primary breast cancer with primary chemotherapy, surgery, and radiation therapy. Cancer 62:2507–2516, 1988.

145. Huggins C, Bergenstal DM: Inhibition of human mammary and prostatic cancers by adrenalectomy. Cancer Res 12:134–141, 1952.

146. Humphrey LJ, Swerdlow M: Relationship of benign breast disease to carcinoma of the breast. Surgery 52:841–846, 1962.

147. Jackson JN: A new technic for breast amputation. JAMA 46:627–633, 1906.

148. Jacquillat C, Weil M, Baillet F, et al: Results of neoadjuvant chemotherapy and radiation therapy in the breast-conserving treatment of 250 patients with all stages of infiltrative breast cancer. Cancer 66:119–129, 1990.

149. Janeway HH: Radium Therapy in Cancer at Memorial Hospital. New York, Hober, 1917, pp 184–190.

150. Jessop WHG: Results of operative treatment in carcinoma of the breast. Lancet 2:424–426, 1936.

151. Judd ES, Sistrunk WE: End-results in operation for cancer of the breast. Surg Gynecol Obstet 28:289–294, 1914.

152. Kaae S, Johansen H: Breast cancer: Five year results: Two random series of simple mastectomy with postoperative irradiation versus extended radical mastectomy. AJR 87:82–88, 1962.

153. Karpas CM, Leis HP, Oppenheim A, et al: Relationship of fibrocystic disease to carcinoma of the breast. Ann Surg 162:1–8, 1965.

154. Keynes G: Radium treatment of primary carcinoma of the breast. Lancet 2:108–111, 1928.

155. Keynes G: The radium treatment of carcinoma of the breast. Br J Surg 19:415–480, 1932.

156. Keynes G: Conservative treatment of cancer of the breast. Br Med J 2:643–647, 1937.

157. Keynes G: Carcinoma of the breast: A brief historical survey of the treatment. St. Bartholomew's Hosp J 56:462–466, 1952.

158. Khanna MM, Mark RJ, Silverstein MJ, et al: Breast conservation management of breast tumors 4 cm or larger. Arch Surg 127:1038–1043, 1992.

159. Kinne DW: Contralateral breast biopsy. Breast Dis 3:9–10, 1992.

160. Kopans DB, Meyer JE: Versatile spring hookwire breast lesion localizer. AJR 138:586–588, 1982.

161. Korteweg JA: Die statistischen Resultate der Amputation des Brustkrebses. Arch Klin Chir 38:679–685, 1889.

162. Korteweg JA: Carcinoom en statistiek. Ned Tijdschr Geneeskd 39:1054–1068, 1903.

163. Kurtz JM, Amalric R, Brandone H, Ayme Y, Spitalier J-M: Results of salvage surgery for mammary recurrence following breast-conserving therapy. Ann Surg 207:347–351, 1988.

164. Kurtz JM, Amalric R, Brandone H, Ayme Y, Spitalier J-M: Results of wide excision for mammary recurrence after breast-conserving therapy. Cancer 61:1969–1972, 1988.

165. Kurtz JM, Jacquemier J, Torhorst J, et al: Conservation therapy for breast cancers other than infiltrating ductal carcinoma. Cancer 63:1630–1635, 1989.

166. Küster E: Zur Behandlung des Brustkrebses. Arch Klin Chir 29:723–735, 1883.

167. Lagios MD, Richards VE, Rose MR, Yee E: Segmental mastectomy without radiotherapy: Short-term followup. Cancer 52:2173–2179, 1983.

168. Landercasper J, Gundersen SB, Gundersen AL, et al: Needle localization and biopsy of nonpalpable lesions of the breast. Surg Gynecol Obstet 164:399–403, 1987.

169. Lane WA: A case illustrating a more effectual method of removing a cancerous breast, lymphatics and glands. Trans Clin Soc London 26:85–87, 1893.

170. Lane-Claypon JE: Cancer of the breast and its surgical treatment. Reports on public health and medical subjects No. 28. London, Ministry of Health, 1924.

171. Lane-Claypon JE: Report on the late results of operation for cancer of the breast. Reports on public health and medical subjects No. 51. London, Ministry of Health, 1928.

172. LeDran F: Memoire avec une precis de plusiers observations sur le cancer. Mem Acad R Chir Paris 3:1–56, 1757.

173. Lee JSY, Grant CS, Donohue JH, et al: Arguments against routine contralateral mastectomy or undirected biopsy for invasive lobular breast cancer. Surgery 118:640–648, 1995.

174. Leung S, Otmezguine Y, Calitchi E, et al: Locoregional recurrences following radical external beam irradiation and interstitial implantation for operable breast cancer: A Twenty-three-year experience. Radiother Oncol 5:1–10, 1986.

175. Lewis D, Rienhoff WF: A study of the results of operations for the cure of cancer of the breast performed at the Johns Hopkins Hospital from 1889–1931. Ann Surg 95:336–400, 1932.

176. Lewison EF: The surgical treatment of breast cancer: An historical and collective review. Surgery 34:904–953, 1953.

177. Lister J: Collected Papers, Vol 2. Oxford, Clarendon Press, 1909.

178. Liston R: Practical Surgery. London, J Churchill, 1837.

179. Lung JA, Hart NE, Woodbury R: An overview and critical analysis of breast cancer screening. Arch Surg 123:833–838, 1988.

180. MacCarty WC: The histogenesis of cancer of the breast and its clinical significance. Surg Gynecol Obstet 17:441–446, 1913.

181. MacMahon CE, Cahill JL: The evolution of the concept of the use of surgical castration in the palliation of breast cancer in pre-menopausal females. Ann Surg 184:713–716, 1976.

182. Madden JL: Modified radical mastectomy. Surg Gynecol Obstet 121:1221–1230, 1965.

183. Madden JL, Kasndalaft S, Bourque R: Modified radical mastectomy. Ann Surg 175:624–633, 1972.
184. Maddox WA, Carpenter JT, Laws HL, et al: A randomized prospective trial of radical (Halsted) mastectomy versus modified radical mastectomy in 311 breast cancer patients. Ann Surg 198:207–212, 1983.
185. Margolis DS, McMillen MA, Hashmi H, et al: Aggressive axillary evaluation and adjuvant therapy for nonpalpable carcinoma of the breast. Surg Gynecol Obstet 174:109–113, 1992.
186. Margottini M: Recent developments in the surgical treatment of breast cancer. Acta Unio Int Contra Cancrum 8:176–190, 1952.
187. Marrujo G, Jolly PC, Hall MH: Nonpalpable breast cancer: Needle-localized biopsy for diagnosis. Am J Surg 151:599–602, 1986.
188. Martin H, Ellis E: Biopsy by needle puncture and aspiration. Ann Surg 92:169–181, 1930.
189. Masood S, Frykberg ER, McLellan GL, et al: Prospective evaluation of radiologically directed fine-needle aspiration biopsy of nonpalpable breast lesions. Cancer 66:1480–1487, 1990.
190. Matas R: In discussion of WS Halsted. Trans Am Surg Assoc 16:165–178, 1898.
191. Matas R: William Stewart Halsted, 1852–1922: An appreciation. Bull Johns Hopkins Hosp 36:2–7, 1925.
192. McGuire WL, DeLaGarza M: Similarity of the estrogen receptor in human and rat mammary carcinoma. J Clin Endocrinol Metab 36:548–552, 1973.
193. McLaughlin CW, Schenken JR, Tamisiea JX: A study of precancerous epithelial hyperplasia and non-invasive papillary carcinoma of the breast. Ann Surg 153:735–744, 1961.
194. McWhirter R: The value of simple mastectomy and radiotherapy in the treatment of cancer of the breast. Br J Radiol 21:599–610, 1948.
195. McWhirter R: Should more radical treatment be attempted in breast cancer? AJR Am J Roentgenol 92:3–13, 1964.
196. Mellink WAM, Holland R, Hendriks JHCL, et al: The contribution of routine follow-up mammography to an early detection of asynchronous contralateral breast cancer. Cancer 67:1844–1848, 1991.
197. Meyer W: An improved method of the radical operation for carcinoma of the breast. Med Rec 46:746–749, 1894.
198. Meyer W: Carcinoma of the breast: Ten years' experience with my method of radical operation. JAMA 45:297–313, 1905.
199. Moffat FL, Ketcham AS, Robinson DS, et al: Segmental mastectomy without radiotherapy for T_1 and small T_2 carcinomas. Arch Surg 125:364–369, 1990.
200. deMondeville H: Die Chirurgie des Heinrich deMondeville. Berlin, A. Hirschwald, 1892.
201. Monro A: Collections of blood in cancerous breasts. In The Works of Alexander Monro: Published by His Son Alexander Monro. Edinburgh, Ch. Elliot, 1781, pp 484–491.
202. Monson RR, Yen S, MacMahon B, et al: Chronic mastitis and carcinoma of the breast. Lancet 2:224–226, 1976.
203. Montgomery ACV, Greening WP, Levene AL: Clinical study of recurrence rate and survival time of patients with carcinoma of the breast treated by biopsy excision without any other therapy. J R Soc Med 71:339–342, 1978.
204. Moore CH: On the influence of inadequate operations on the theory of cancer. R Med Chir Soc London 1:244–280, 1867.
205. Morrow M, Schmidt R, Cregger B, et al: Preoperative evaluation of abnormal mammographic findings to avoid unnecessary breast biopsies. Arch Surg 129:1091–1096, 1994.
206. Moskowitz M, Gartside PS: Evidence of breast cancer mortality reduction: Aggressive screening in women under age 50. AJR 138:911–916, 1982.
207. Moxley JH, Allegra JC, Henney J, et al: Treatment of primary breast cancer: Summary of the National Institutes of Health Consensus Development Conference. JAMA 244:797–799, 1980.
208. Mustakallio S: Treatment of breast cancer by tumor extirpation and roentgen therapy instead of radical operation. J Fac Radiol 6:23–26, 1954.
209. Nathanson IT: The effect of stilbestrol on advanced cancer of the breast. Cancer Res 6:484, 1946. (Abstract)
210. Nattinger AB, Gottlieb MS, Veum J, et al: Geographic variation in the use of breast-conserving treatment for breast cancer. N Engl J Med 326:1102–1107, 1992.
211. Nemoto T, Patel JK, Rosner D, et al: Factors affecting recurrence in lumpectomy without irradiation for breast cancer. Cancer 67:2079–2082, 1991.
212. Nemoto T, Vana J, Bedwani RN, et al: Management and survival of female breast cancer: Results of a national survey by the American College of Surgeons. Cancer 45:2917–2924, 1980.
213. Nowell PC: Molecular events in tumor development. N Engl J Med 319:575–577, 1988.
214. Ochsner AJ: Final results in 164 cases of carcinoma of the breast operated upon during the past fourteen years at the Augustana Hospital. Ann Surg 46:28–42, 1907.
215. Pack GT: Argument for bilateral mastectomy. Surgery 29:929–931, 1951.
216. Page DL, Dupont WD, Rogers LW, et al: Intraductal carcinoma of the breast. Cancer 49:751–758, 1982.
217. Page DL, Dupont WD, Rogers LW, et al: Atypical hyperplastic lesions of the female breast: A long-term follow-up study. Cancer 55:2698–2708, 1985.
218. Paget J: On the average duration of life in patients with scirrhous cancer of the breast. Lancet 1:62–63, 1856.
219. Pancoast J: A treatise on operative surgery. Philadelphia, R Hart, 1852, pp 269–271.
220. Park WW, Lees JC: The absolute curability of cancer of the breast. Surg Gynecol Obstet 93:129–152, 1951.
221. Patey DH: A review of 146 cases of carcinoma of the breast operated on between 1930 and 1943. Br J Cancer 21:260–269, 1967.
222. Patey DH, Dyson WH: The prognosis of carcinoma of the breast in relation to the type of operation performed. Br J Cancer 2:7–13, 1948.
223. Perdue P, Page DL, Nellestein M, et al: Early detection of breast carcinoma: A comparison of palpable and nonpalpable lesions. Surgery 111:656–659, 1992.
224. Peters MV: Wedge resection and irradiation: An effective treatment in early breast cancer. JAMA 200:144–145, 1967.
225. Petit JL: Oeuvres Completes, section VII. Limoges, R Chapoulard, 1837, pp 438–445.
226. Peyrilhe B: Dissertatio Academia de Cancro. Paris, De Hansy Jeune, 1774.
227. Pfahler GE: Results of radiation therapy in 1,022 private cases of carcinoma of the breast from 1902 to 1928. AJR Am J Roentgenol 27:497–508, 1932.
228. Pfahler GE, Parry LD: Roentgen therapy in carcinoma of the breast: a statistical study of 977 private cases. Ann Surg 93:412–427, 1931.
229. Pittinger TP, Maronian NC, Poulter CA, et al: Importance of margin status in outcome of breast-conserving surgery for carcinoma. Surgery 116:605–609, 1994.
230. Poen JC, Tran L, Juillard G, et al: Conservation therapy for invasive lobular carcinoma of the breast. Cancer 69:2789–2795, 1992.
231. Pomerantz RA, Murad T, Hines JR: Bilateral breast cancer: Am Surg 55:441–444, 1989.
232. Poole GV, Choplin RH, Sterchi JM, et al: Occult lesions of the breast. Surg Gynecol Obstet 163:107–110, 1986.
233. Porritt A: Early carcinoma of the breast. Br J Surg 51:214–216, 1964.
234. Power D: The history of the amputation of the breast to 1904. Liverpool Med Chir J 42:29–56, 1934.
235. Pressman PI: Selective biopsy of the opposite breast. Cancer 57:577–580, 1986.
236. Prosnitz LR, Goldenberg IS, Packard RA, et al: Radiation therapy as initial treatment for early stage cancer of the breast without mastectomy. Cancer 39:917–923, 1977.
237. Prudente A: L'amputation inter-scapulo-mammothoracique (technique et resultants). J Chir 65:729–735, 1949.
238. Ravitch MM: A Century of Surgery, Vol I. Philadelphia, JB Lippincott, 1980, p 612.
239. Recht A, Danoff BS, Solin LJ, et al: Intraductal carcinoma

240. of the breast: Results of treatment with excisional biopsy and radiation. J Clin Oncol 3:1339–1343, 1985.

240. Recht A, Houlihan MJ: Conservative surgery without radiotherapy in the treatment of patients with early-stage invasive breast cancer: A review. Ann Surg 222:9–18, 1995.

241. Recht A, Houlihan MJ: Axillary lymph nodes and breast cancer: A review. Cancer 76:1491–1512, 1995.

242. Reed MWR, Morrison JM: Wide local excision as the sole primary treatment in elderly patients with carcinoma of the breast. Br J Surg 76:898–900, 1989.

243. Remak R: Ein Beitrag zur Entwickelungsgeschichte der krebshaften Geschuwulste. Deutsche Klin 6:170–174, 1854.

244. Robbins GF, Berg JW: Bilateral primary breast cancers: A prospective clinicopathological study. Cancer 17:1501–1527, 1964.

245. Robinson JO: Treatment of breast cancer through the ages. Am J Surg 151:317–333, 1986.

246. Rodman JS: Skin removal in radical breast amputation. Ann Surg 118:694–705, 1943.

247. Romsdahl MM, Montague ED, Ames FC, Richards PC, Schell SR: Conservation surgery and irradiation as treatment for early breast cancer. Arch Surg 118:521–528, 1983.

248. Rosen PP: Lobular carcinoma in situ and intraductal carcinoma of the breast. Monogr Pathol 25:59–105, 1984.

249. Rosenberg SA, Lotze MT, Muul LM, et al: Observations on the systemic administration of autologous lymphokine-activated killer cells and recombinant interleukin-2 to patients with metastatic cancer. N Engl J Med 313:1485–1492, 1985.

250. Roses DF, Harris MN, Potter DA, Gumport SL: Total mastectomy with complete axillary dissection. Ann Surg 194:4–8, 1981.

251. Rosner D, Bedwani RN, Vana J, et al: Noninvasive breast carcinoma: Results of a national survey by the American College of Surgeons. Ann Surg 192:139–147, 1980.

252. Ruffin WK, Stacey-Clear A, Younger J, et al: Rationale for routine axillary dissection in carcinoma of the breast. J Am Coll Surg 180:245–251, 1995.

253. Salomon A: Beitrage zur pathologie und klinik der mammacarcinome. Arch Klin Chir 101:573–668, 1913.

254. Sarrazin D, Le MG, Arriagada R, et al: Ten-year results of a randomized trial comparing a conservative treatment to mastectomy in early breast cancer. Radiother Oncol 14:177–184, 1989.

255. Sauter ER, Hoffman JP, Ottery FD, et al: Is frozen section analysis of reexcision lumpectomy margins worthwhile? Cancer 73:2607–2612, 1994.

256. Schmid H: Zur statisk der mammacarcinome und der heitung. Dtsch Z Chir 26:139–145, 1887.

257. Schnitt SJ, Abner A, Gelman R, et al: The relationship between microscopic margins of resection and the risk of local recurrence in patients with breast cancer treated with breast-conserving surgery and radiation therapy. Cancer 74:1746–1751, 1994.

258. Schnitt SJ, Connolly JL, Khettry V, et al: Pathologic findings on re-excision of the primary site in breast cancer patients considered for treatment by primary radiation therapy. Cancer 59:675–681, 1987.

259. Schnitt SJ, Connolly JL, Recht A, et al: Influence of infiltrating lobular histology on local tumor control in breast cancer patients treated with conservative surgery and radiotherapy. Cancer 64:448–454, 1989.

260. Schwartz GF, Birchansky CA, Komarnicky LT, et al: Induction chemotherapy followed by breast conservation for locally advanced carcinoma of the breast. Cancer 73:362–369, 1994.

261. Scultetus J: Armamentarium Chirurgicum. Ulm, B Kuhnen, 1653, pp 50–51.

262. Seidman H, Gelb SK, Silverberg E, et al: Survival experience in the Breast Cancer Detection Demonstration Project. CA 37:258–290, 1987.

263. Senofsky GM, Wanebo HJ, Wilhelm MC, et al: Has monitoring of the contralateral breast improved the prognosis in patients treated for primary breast cancer? Cancer 57:597–602, 1986.

264. Shapiro S, Venet W, Strax P, et al: Ten-to-fourteen year effect of screening on breast cancer mortality. J Natl Cancer Inst 69:349–355, 1982.

265. Sheikh FA, Tinkoff GH, Kline TS, et al: Final diagnosis by fine-needle aspiration biopsy for definitive operation in breast cancer. Am J Surg 154:470–475, 1987.

266. Shield AM: A Clinical Treatise on Diseases of the Breast. New York, MacMillan, 1898.

267. Shroff JH, Lloyd LR, Schroder DM: Open breast biopsy: A critical analysis. Am Surg 57:481–485, 1991.

268. Sickles EA: Periodic mammographic follow-up of probably benign lesions: Results in 3,184 consecutive cases. Radiology 179:463–468, 1991.

269. Silverstein MJ, Gamagami P, Rosser RJ, et al: Hooked-wire–directed breast biopsy and over penetrated mammography. Cancer 59:715–722, 1987.

270. Silverstein MJ, Gierson ED, Waisman JR, et al: Axillary lymph node dissection for T_{1a} breast carcinoma: Is it indicated? Cancer 73:664–667, 1994.

271. Singletary SE, McNeese MD, Hortobagyi GN: Feasibility of breast-conservation surgery after induction chemotherapy for locally advanced breast carcinoma. Cancer 69:2849–2852, 1992.

272. Singletary SE, Taylor SH, Guinee VF, et al: Occurrence and prognosis of contralateral carcinoma of the breast. J Am Coll Surg 178:390–396, 1994.

273. Skinner MA, Swain M, Simmons R, et al: Nonpalpable breast lesions at biopsy: A detailed analysis of radiographic features. Ann Surg 208:203–208, 1988.

274. Smith BL, Bertagnolli M, Klein BB, et al: Evaluation of the contralateral breast: The role of biopsy at the time of treatment of primary breast cancer. Ann Surg 216:17–21, 1992.

275. Smitt MC, Nowels KW, Zdeblick MJ, et al: The importance of the lumpectomy surgical margin status in long term results of breast conservation. Cancer 76:259–267, 1995.

276. Stehlin JS, Ipolyi PD, Greeff PJ, Gutierrez AE, Hardy RJ, Dahiya SL: A ten year study of partial mastectomy for carcinoma of the breast. Surg Gynecol Obstet 165:191–198, 1987.

277. Stewart FT: Amputation of the breast by a transverse incision. Ann Surg 62:250–251, 1915.

278. Sugarbaker ED: Extended radical mastectomy: Its superiority in the treatment of breast cancer. JAMA 187:96–99, 1964.

279. Suntzeff V, Burns EL, Moskop M, Loeb L: The effect of injections of estrin on the incidence of mammary cancer in various strains of mice. Am J Cancer 27:229–245, 1936.

280. Sutherland CM, Mather FJ: Long-term survival and prognostic factors in breast cancer patients with localized (no skin, muscle, or chest wall attachment) disease with and without positive lymph nodes. Cancer 57:622–629, 1986.

281. Swain SM, Sorace RA, Bagley CA, et al: Neoadjuvant chemotherapy in the combined modality approach of locally advanced non-metastatic breast cancer. Cancer Res 47:3889–3894, 1987.

282. Sweeting R: A new operation for cancer of the breast. Lancet 1:323, 1869.

283. Syme J: Principles of Surgery. London, H Balliere, 1842, p 73.

284. Symmonds RE, Roberts JW: Management of nonpalpable breast abnormalities. Ann Surg 205:520–528, 1987.

285. Tabar L, Fagerberg CJG, Gad A, et al: Reduction in mortality from breast cancer after mass screening with mammography. Lancet 1:829–832, 1985.

286. Tagart REB: Partial mastectomy for breast cancer. Br Med J 2:1268, 1978.

287. Tarbox BB, Rockwood JK, Abernathy CM: Are modified radical mastectomies done for T_1 breast cancers because of surgeon's advice or patient's choice? Am J Surg 164:417–422, 1992.

288. Taylor GW, Wallace RH: Carcinoma of the breast: Fifty years experience at the Massachusetts General Hospital. Ann Surg 132:833–843, 1950.

289. Threatt B, Appleman H, Dow R, et al: Percutaneous needle localization of clustered mammary microcalcifications prior to biopsy. AJR Am J Roentgenol 121:839–842, 1974.

290. Tyzzer EE: Factors in the production and growth of tumor metastases. J Med Res 28:309–333, 1913.

291. Urban JA: Radical excision of the chest wall for mammary cancer. Cancer 4:1263–1285, 1951.

292. Urban JA, Baker HW: Radical mastectomy in continuity with

en bloc resection of the internal mammary lymph-node chain: A new procedure for primary operable cancer of the breast. Cancer 5:992–1008, 1952.

293. Urban JA: Bilaterality of cancer of the breast. Cancer 20:1867–1870, 1967.

294. Valagussa P, Bonadonna G, Veronesi U: Patterns of relapse and survival following radical mastectomy. Cancer 41:1170–1178, 1978.

295. Van Dongen JA, Bartelink H, Fentiman IS, et al: Randomized clinical trial to assess the value of breast-conserving therapy in Stage I and II breast cancer, EORTC 10801 trial. J Natl Cancer Inst Monogr 11:15–18, 1992.

296. Velpeau A: A Treatise on the Diseases of the Breast and Mammary Regions. Translated by M Henry. London, The Sydenham Society, 1856.

297. Verbeek ALM, Hendriks JHCL, Holland R, et al: Reduction of breast cancer mortality through mass screening with modern mammography: First results of the Nijmegen project 1975–1979. Lancet i:1222–1225, 1984.

298. Veronesi U, Banfi A, Del Vecchio M, et al: Comparison of Halsted mastectomy with quadrantectomy, axillary dissection, and radiotherapy in early breast cancer: Long-term results. Eur J Cancer Clin Oncol 22:1085–1089, 1986.

299. Veronesi U, Bonadonna G, Zurrida S, et al: Conservation surgery after primary chemotherapy in large carcinomas of the breast. Ann Surg 222:612–618, 1995.

300. Veronesi U, Salvadori B, Luini A, et al: Conservative treatment of early breast cancer: Long term results of 1232 cases treated with quadrantectomy, axillary dissection, and radiotherapy. Ann Surg 211:250–259, 1990.

301. Veronesi U, Valagussa P: Inefficacy of internal mammary node dissection in breast cancer surgery. Cancer 47:170–178, 1981.

302. Vilcoq JR, Calle R, Stacey P, et al: The outcome of treatment by tumorectomy and radiotherapy of patients with operable breast cancer. Int J Radiat Oncol Biol Phys 7:1327–1332, 1981.

303. Virchow R: Cellular Pathology. Translated by R. Chance. Philadelphia, JB Lippincott, 1863.

304. Volkmann R: Beitrage zur Chirurgie. Leipzig, Breitkoff und Hartel, 1875, pp 329–338.

305. Von Rueden DG, Wilson RE: Intraductal carcinoma of the breast. Surg Gynecol Obstet 158:105–111, 1984.

306. Waldeyer W: Die Entwickelung der Carcinome. Arch Pathol Anat Phys Klin Med 41:470–523, 1867.

307. Waldeyer W: Die Entwickelung der Carcinome. Arch Pathol Anat Phys Klin Med 55:67–159, 1872.

308. Wanebo JH, Feldman PS, Wilhelm MC, et al: Fine needle aspiration cytology in lieu of open biopsy in management of primary breast cancer. Ann Surg 199:569–578, 1984.

309. Wanebo JH, Senofsky GM, Fechner RE, et al: Bilateral breast cancer: Risk reduction by contralateral biopsy. Ann Surg 201:667–677, 1985.

310. Wangensteen OH: Carcinoma of the breast. Ann Surg 132:833–843, 1950.

311. Wangensteen OH, Lewis FJ, Arhelger SW: The extended or super-radical mastectomy for carcinoma of the breast. Surg Clin North Am 36:1051–1062, 1956.

312. Warren JC: The operative treatment of cancer of the breast: With an analysis of a series of one hundred consecutive cases. Ann Surg 40:805–833, 1904.

313. Warren S: The relation of "chronic mastitis" to carcinoma of the breast. Surg Gynecol Obstet 71:257–273, 1940.

314. Wertheimer MD, Costanza ME, Dodson TF, et al: Increasing the effort toward breast cancer detection. JAMA 255:1311–1315, 1986.

315. White JR, Gustafson GS, Wimbish K, et al: Conservative surgery and radiation therapy for infiltrating lobular carcinoma of the breast. Cancer 74:640–647, 1994.

316. White WC: Late results of operations for carcinoma of the breast. Ann Surg 86:695–701, 1927.

317. Wilder RJ: The historical development of the concept of metastasis. J Mt Sinai Hosp 23:728–734, 1954.

318. Wilhelm MC, Edge SB, Cole DD, et al: Nonpalpable invasive breast cancer. Ann Surg 213:600–603, 1991.

319. Williams IG, Murley RS, Curwen MP: Carcinoma of the female breast: Conservative and radical surgery. Br Med J 2:787–796, 1953.

320. Winchester DP, Cox JD: Standards for breast-conservation treatment. CA Cancer J Clin 42:134–162, 1992.

321. Wise L, Mason AY, Ackerman LV: Local excision and irradiation: An alternative method for the treatment of early mammary cancer. Ann Surg 174:392–401, 1971.

322. Wolff J: Die Lehre von der Krebskrankenheit, Vol 1. Jena, G Fischer, 1907.

CHAPTER 40

INDICATIONS AND TECHNIQUES FOR BIOPSY

Wiley W. Souba, M.D., Sc.D. / Kirby I. Bland, M.D.

Breast biopsy is one of the most common surgical procedures performed today. Recently, however, there has been a shift away from open biopsy toward needle biopsy. Although a learning curve is associated with these newer techniques, accurate results can be obtained in the hands of an experienced operator. These newer techniques are safe, less expensive, and acceptable to patients.

Even though a presumptive diagnosis of breast cancer can be made from a patient's history and physical examination or from radiological studies, the actual removal of tissue from the breast or from a metastatic site, followed by microscopic examination, is essential to confirm the diagnosis. Unfortunately, most breast masses that appear benign have a real, although relatively small, probability of malignancy that cannot be ruled out until a biopsy is performed.[16, 63, 77] The morbidity and mortality associated with breast biopsy are acceptably low, primarily because of adherence to careful surgical technique and to the frequency with which local anesthesia can be utilized. A 1980 study on the cost effectiveness of breast cancer management demonstrated that screening costs are very high and that the most effective means of containing the economic cost of this illness is by targeted selection of high-risk patients for breast biopsy with local anesthesia.[13] Given the emotional impact of the possibility of a breast mass' being cancerous, however, and the traditional teaching that all breast masses in women older than 35 years should be removed, can the need for breast biopsy be questioned? Open biopsy of a breast mass under general or local anesthesia is associated with relatively low morbidity and essentially no mortality. Although most biopsies of "suspicious" breast lesions prove to be benign, certain clinical and mammographic features are associated with a high probability of malignancy.*

The history, physical examination, and preoperative staging each influence the timing and the type of breast biopsy performed. Should the patient have cancer confirmed by biopsy, the information gained from the specimen is crucial to staging, assessment of prognosis, and selection of the appropriate therapy. The biopsy findings, properly done, will be very useful in planning the work-up and definitive treatment of the patient. On the other hand, inconclusive data derived from insufficient tissue or a malpositioned biopsy incision can limit therapeutic options or render definitive treatment difficult or inconsequential.

The decision to perform breast biopsy requires thorough assessment of the individual patient and her radiographic and clinical presentation. Breast masses in adolescent and young adult women are often benign lesions that can be followed at specific intervals unless an indication for biopsy is apparent (e.g., positive family history or suspicious mammogram). Kopans and associates recently evaluated the positive predictive value (PPV) and its variation with age for 4778 women who underwent biopsy for an occult mammographic abnormality.[42] These authors did not detect abrupt changes in the PPV at any age for women aged 40 to 79 years, but diagnostic results increased steadily. This study affirms the existing evidence for the probability of disease at any age. The modeled PPV for cancer in these 4778 patients increased with age from approximately 12 percent at 40 years to 46 percent by 79 years.

For women older than 35 years, there are several clinical situations in which a biopsy is generally indicated without reservation. The first is the presence of a previously unrecognized three-dimensional mass that is anatomically distinct from the remainder of the breast tissue. Even though the mammogram is entirely normal, the presence of a new mass is usually an indication for biopsy. Criteria that should influence the surgeon's decision to perform the biopsy include mammographic findings that are suspicious for carcinoma,[24] a positive family history for breast cancer or previous personal history of breast cancer,[41] and physical findings (e.g., skin dimpling, *peau d'orange,* or clinically positive axillary nodes) indicative of neoplastic disease.[16] The second indication for breast biopsy is the presence of mammographic findings that are suggestive of, or compatible with, carcinoma.[6, 7, 24, 48, 50, 64–66] These radiographic features include architectural distortion of the surrounding breast tissue that may suggest carcinoma or clustered microcalcifications (see Chapter 35). In the absence of any physical abnormality, these findings are generally an indication for excisional biopsy of the nonpalpable lesion.

NONPALPABLE LESIONS

A "normal" breast may not present any physical signs of an underlying breast cancer but may harbor a neoplasm in the noninfiltrating (*in situ*) stage or, less often, as an occult infiltrating breast carcinoma.[32] Nonpalpable breast lesions are generally discovered on routine screening mammography, although incidental breast masses have been found on chest computed tomography (CT). In the past decade, the widespread application of high-quality film screen

---

* See references 17, 18, 31, 32, 48, 58, and 60.

mammography has resulted in the detection of increasing numbers of nonpalpable breast lesions.[48] The radiographic criteria on which the decision to perform biopsy is based include (1) a localized soft tissue mass within the breast parenchyma; (2) architectural distortion, including contracture of trabeculae producing stellate alterations, with severe asymmetrical periductal and lobular thickening; and (3) cluttered microcalcifications, with or without the aforementioned features.[16, 18, 24] However, the diagnosis of breast cancer in younger women (aged 30 to 40 years) by mammography is limited, with a sensitivity of approximately 75 percent.[4] Younger women should be informed that mammography and physical examination have limitations in diagnosis and that presentation and detection of their cancers is often delayed.

Preoperative Localization of Nonpalpable Breast Lesions

The widespread use of mammography has resulted in the detection of increasing numbers of suspicious but clinically occult, nonpalpable lesions of the breast.[24] Such lesions may represent up to as many as half of the detected cancers in screening clinics and account for a substantial proportion of breast tumors investigated by biopsy. Despite the frequency and simplicity of radiographic or mammographic identification of suspicious lesions, intraoperative localization with subsequent adequate excision presents challenging technical problems because the shape and position of the breast during compression mammography are often quite different from those seen by the surgeon in the operating room. This has led to the development of several methods for preoperative localization of nonpalpable lesions.* The aim of these methods is to facilitate complete removal of the tumor at the first attempt at excision while simultaneously minimizing the size of the resected specimen and shortening the duration of anesthesia. Radiologically guided, invasive, preoperative localization of nonpalpable breast lesions is a safe, simple, and established procedure that allows for accurate and expeditious biopsy that can often be performed under local anesthesia. It should be uniformly available wherever mammography and breast biopsy are performed. Since nonpalpable breast masses are often discovered as clustered microcalcifications or architectural distortions, they may remain nonpalpable, even on examination of the resected specimen. Thus, mammography is mandatory to document removal of the suspect area and to facilitate histological examination.†

Noninvasive Techniques

Noninvasive techniques for localization of mammographically suspicious breast lesions include visual estimation, external breast markers,[5] coordinates plotted on a diagram of the breast,[75] stereomammograms,[3] grid compression devices, and CT-directed biopsy. The latter technique may be of value for the 5 percent of mammographically suspicious lesions detectable in only one mammographic view (craniocaudal or mediolateral). More recently, magnetic resonance image (MRI)–guided techniques have been utilized.[21] Although superficial lesions of the breast or lesions adjacent to the nipple may be localized adequately preoperatively by visual estimation, deeper suspect areas cannot be accurately localized by noninvasive techniques.[5] Extrapolation of the depth and surface distances of the lesion obtained during compression mammography in the supine position introduces unacceptable error. External breast markers such as indelible ink or the needle scratch technique were introduced more than 25 years ago; Stevens and Jamplis were among the first investigators to describe preoperative localization of nonpalpable breast lesions with use of a "mammographic map" that established the relative position for the suspect area within the breast using coordinates.[75] With this localization technique, a wedge biopsy with adequate margins could be obtained. These authors emphasized the need for roentgenographic confirmation of removal of the suspect lesion. Following "bread loafing" of the specimen and repeat roentgenography, the exact site of the suspect lesion may be localized and submitted for pathological evaluation (Fig. 40–1). Although this technique for localization of nonpalpable lesions was an improvement over blind biopsy methods, it was fraught with error and sampling of the suspect breast lesion was inaccurate.

Invasive Techniques

Localization of occult breast masses has markedly improved with the use of small radiopaque needles

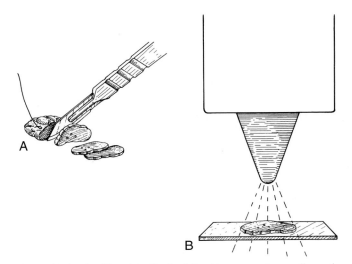

Figure 40–1 **A,** *"Bread loafing" of the biopsy specimen allows the exact site of the lesion to be determined and submitted for pathological evaluation.* **B,** *Following excision of the suspicious lesion, specimen radiography is completed to confirm the presence of the suspect lesion in the excised tissue.*

---

* See references 3, 5, 12, 28, 34–37, 46, 47, 65, 71, 74, and 75.
† See references 2, 40, 52, 61, 62, 71, 72, and 79.

that can be radiographically guided into the breast.[33, 36, 37, 46, 53] These needles are inserted by the radiologist in the radiology suite; subsequent mammography demonstrates the relationship of the needle to the suspect lesion. The success of breast localization procedures requires patient co-operation and communication between radiologist and surgeon; when specimen radiography is necessary, communication among radiologist, surgeon, and pathologist is of utmost importance. Failure of these three to communicate at preoperative planning of the procedure is a common cause of unsuccessful localization and excision of the nonpalpable breast lesion following needle localization.[5]

Injection (Spot) Localization

In 1972, Simon and colleagues first described the technique of spot localization of nonpalpable breast lesions using a percutaneously inserted needle.[69] The site for insertion of the localizing needle is selected by using co-ordinate measurements taken from the craniocaudal and mediolateral mammograms in relation to the nipple. Following local anesthesia of skin and subcutaneous tissues, the needle is inserted through the skin in the direction and to the depth determined by the biplanar radiographic measurements. Repeat craniocaudal and mediolateral radiographs are obtained with the needle in position, to confirm its relationship to the suspect lesion and to identify any necessary changes in needle position. Once the needle has been satisfactorily positioned, a 0.1-ml solution of equal parts of Evans blue dye and radiopaque contrast is injected. Thereafter, a small amount of air is flushed through the needle to ensure that all of the dye has been delivered into the breast. The needle is withdrawn, and repeat craniocaudal and mediolateral radiographic views are taken to determine the distance and direction of the lesion relative to the radiopaque contrast. This information is communicated to the surgeon, and the final set of radiographs are sent with the patient to the operating room. The surgeon performs the biopsy, using as a guide the dyed outline of breast tissue and its relation to the area of suspicion on the mammogram. The spot method of localization overcame the disadvantage of localization based on co-ordinates alone (i.e., the co-ordinates tended to shift substantially when the patient was placed in the supine position on the operating table). Unfortunately, this technique was limited by rapid absorption of the biodegradable dye from the vicinity of the tumor and the needle track and by dissemination of the dye well beyond the anatomical site of the tumor.

Needle Localization

Needle localization methods that utilized needles placed percutaneously in the vicinity of the suspect mass as a biopsy guide were first described by Dodd.[14] This technique, however, did not gain widespread acceptance until screening mammography achieved universal application. Variations of this technique have been reported by many radiologists[36, 37] and became popular and routinely accepted in the late 1970s. Thereafter, Libshitz and coworkers reported complete success in the removal of 83 suspicious breast lesions.[46] Unfortunately the authors did not state how often more than one biopsy was required to remove the suspicious area or the frequency of lesions that were palpable during the surgical procedure.

Common technical problems with this method of localization include (1) movement of the inflexible needle during the time between placement and operation, even when the needle hub is taped or secured in place; (2) compression of the breast during mammography and localization, creating tissue stress that may alter the position of the needle even when it is sutured in place; and (3) unavoidable dislodgement of the needle during the procedure, with operator manipulation often leading to inadequate tissue sampling (false-negative results) or inadvertent transection of the tumor with incomplete removal of the suspect mass.

Hasselgren and associates determined that the frequency of a malignancy in nonpalpable breast lesions is affected by various factors, including patient age and mammographic features.[29, 30] Utilizing these discriminants allows selective biopsy to enhance diagnostic accuracy and cost-effectiveness.

Self-Retaining Wire Localization

The two principal problems with needle localization of breast lesions are the inflexibility of the stainless steel needle and the unreliability of the position of the needle following breast compression, patient movement, and surgical manipulation.[28] These problems have been overcome, for the most part, by placing a flexible, hooked wire within the localizing needle, a technique first described by Frank and associates.[22] Ideally, the hook lodges within the suspicious breast lesion and prevents dislodgement from the specimen (Figs. 40–2 and 40–3). Local anesthesia is recommended,[9] and a small puncture wound is made in the skin that directly overlies the lesion using a no. 11 scalpel blade. The rigid introducer needle with the hooked wire within it is directed into the breast using biplanar mammographic guidance. The rigid needle is then removed, leaving the hooked wire in place. Because of its self-retaining feature, the wire is not easily withdrawn, advanced, or redirected. The operative approach is directed parallel and deep to the axis of the wire; the hooked tip of the wire is excised with contiguous tissues that surround the suspect lesion. Although wire localization has gained worldwide acceptance, several technical problems have been reported. The surgeon may have difficulty locating the flexible localization wire, especially if the lesion is approached via a circumareolar incision remote from the suspicious mass. To help eliminate this problem, Homer and colleagues advocate the placement of a postlocalization needle.[33]

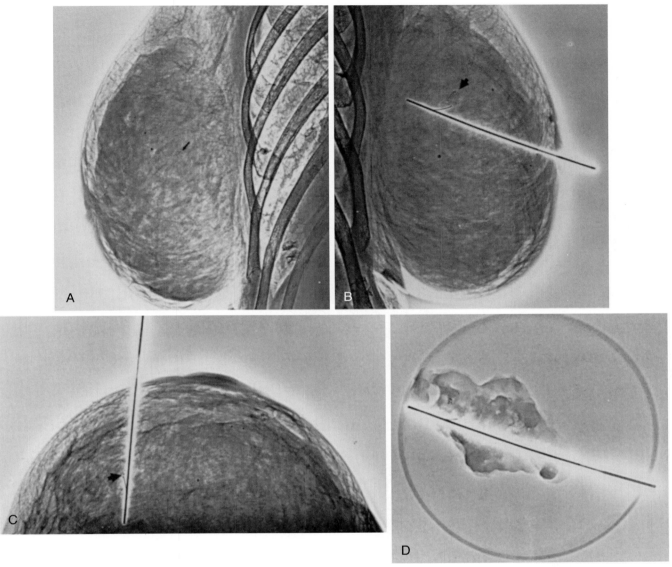

Figure 40–2 *Preoperative needle localization of a nonpalpable breast lesion* **(A)** *requires mediolateral* **(B)** *and craniocaudal* **(C)** *views of the breast. It is mandatory to obtain specimen mammography of the excised tissue* **(D),** preferably with the localization wire in place to confirm extirpation of the suspect lesion.

This needle is guided percutaneously by the surgeon over the flexible hooked wire, which was placed previously by the radiologist. The rigidity of the needle allows easy palpation of its course during the operative procedure.

Methods for preoperative localization represent a major contribution to the operative treatment of suspicious, occult (nonpalpable) lesions of the breast. As the therapeutic adequacy of tumor-free margins with this technique is unknown, repeat excision of the tumor bed (segmental or total mastectomy) is required to achieve margin-free eradication of the tumor.[1] Cox and coworkers estimate that more than 75 percent of patients who have diagnostic biopsy lesions (palpable or nonpalpable) harbor residual breast cancer.[10] The success and effectiveness of any invasive breast localization procedure to facilitate

specimen removal, decrease operating time and expense, and reduce biopsy size is enhanced by an experienced surgeon working in close co-operation with the radiologist. Obtaining a specimen radiograph after wire localization is strongly recommended to corroborate excision of the suspicious occult; however, Hasselgren and coworkers observed a false-positive specimen x-ray film rate of 7.8 percent and a false-negative rate of 55 percent.[29] Thus, a postoperative mammogram is essential, regardless of the specimen radiograph, to ensure excision of the suspicious lesion.

Stereotactic Needle-Core Biopsy of Nonpalpable Breast Lesions

Stereotactic mammographic devices and automated biopsy guns with core biopsy needles have radically

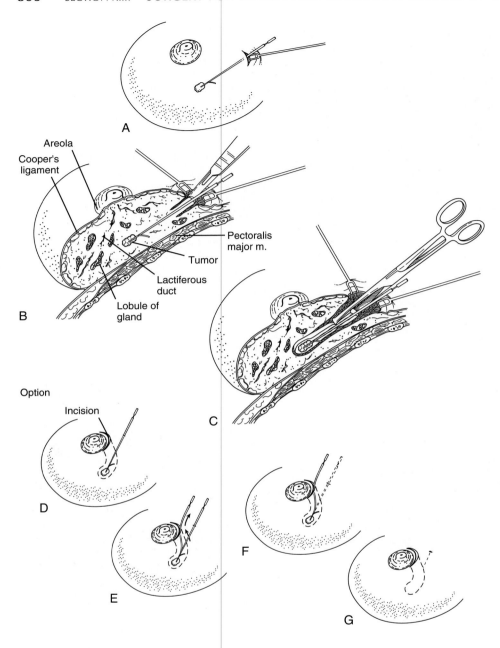

Figure 40–3 *Operative technique for needle localization biopsy: The suspicious lesion is "localized" on the mammogram immediately before surgery.* **A,** *At operation the needle serves as a guide for the surgeon to perform the biopsy.* **B,** *Development of tissue planes circumferential and parallel to the localization wire.* **C,** *Controlled dissection of the wire, which is purchased with tissues using an Allis clamp. The suspicious lesion is incorporated in the dissection, which includes tissue beyond the tip of the hooked wire. Specimen radiography confirms excision of the suspicious, nonpalpable mammographically identified lesion.* **Options.** **D,** *Deeply localized, suspicious lesion approached via circumareolar incision.* **E,** *Wire is repositioned from percutaneous localized position to exit via incision.* **F,** *Dissection completed circumferentially and parallel to wire via circumareolar incision.* **G,** *Completed dissection with breast defect.*

changed the methods by which nonpalpable, mammographically detected abnormalities are managed. In many cases, stereotactic needle-core breast biopsy (SNCB) obviates open biopsy and thus is associated with cost savings and greater patient satisfaction.[25, 49, 51, 56] The analysis by Wallace's group reiterated this view and further determined that SNCB is equivalent to needle-localized biopsy in the frequency of diagnosis of breast cancer.[78] Furthermore, these investigators determined that there was no statistical difference between the two biopsy techniques in diagnosis for women younger than and older than 50 years.

Stereotactic mammographic devices use the principle of triangulation, which allows precise location of the breast lesion to be determined in three dimensions.[57] Prone stereotactic devices are more expensive but more accurate, and patients generally find them more comfortable. A 14-gauge cutting needle that fits into an automated, spring-loaded biopsy gun is used. The device is somewhat similar to a hand-held Tru-Cut needle biopsy in that it consists of an inner tissue-sampling needle and an outer cutting needle. A core of tissue, measuring approximately 2 to 2.5 mm in diameter, is obtained during the procedure.

The procedure consists of placing the patient prone on the stereotactic core biopsy table with the breast dependent. The breast is compressed within the unit and a scout film is obtained and evaluated. The skin of the breast is sterilized with povidone iodine, and the region of the skin through which the biopsy needle will pass is anesthetized with lidocaine. A small (1- to 2-mm) puncture is made in the skin using a no. 11 knife blade. Using computed calculations, the center of the lesion is determined and the needle is advanced into the breast after passing through the skin puncture site (Fig. 40–4). The core biopsy needle is advanced to the leading edge of the lesion; its position is verified; and the biopsy gun is fired. After firing, repeat views are obtained to document that the needle traversed the lesion. The needle containing the tissue sample is then withdrawn. Additional cores can be obtained by targeting different areas within the index or other mammographic abnormalities. The cores are submitted for pathological evaluation. Following completion of the biopsy, pressure is held over the biopsy site for 5 to 10 minutes and a Band-Aid is placed over the puncture site.

The value of core biopsy of multiple synchronous ipsilateral lesions to identify neoplastic disease in more than one site in the breast has recently been confirmed by Liberman and colleagues at Memorial Sloan-Kettering Cancer Center.[45] Repeat biopsy of patients undergoing SNCB, with results that are not concordant with initial imaging and histopathology of the suspicious lesion, is emphasized by Dershaw's group.[11] This practice to ensure corroboration of SNCB results is necessary for the technique to be optimally effective. Further, pathological incidence of atypical duct hyperplasia diagnosed at SNCB requires open (needle-directed) biopsy to rule out intercurrent ductal *in situ* or invasive disease.[43]

Stereotactic core biopsy can also be done to evaluate suspicious microcalcifications. The extracted core of tissue should be examined by specimen mammography to confirm the presence of microcalcifications within the biopsy. For patients whose core biopsy documents the presence of carcinoma, a definitive surgical procedure should be planned. As noted above, when the core biopsy is unequivocal or shows atypia, needle-localized breast biopsy should be performed. Liberman and colleagues determined that 14-gauge SNCB achieved 99 percent diagnostic yield with five specimens obtained from masses.[44] Additional specimens may be essential to avoid false-negative results with the diagnosis of some calcified lesions.[20, 43, 55]

Patients who cannot lie prone or cannot tolerate breast compression are not candidates for stereotactic breast biopsy. In addition, if the breast compresses to less than 2 cm from the chest wall, biopsy is not recommended since the needle excursion is often slightly greater than 2 cm and violation of the chest wall, and possibly the pleura, can occur. Complications of stereotactic core breast biopsy include hematomas, infections, possible tumor seeding of the

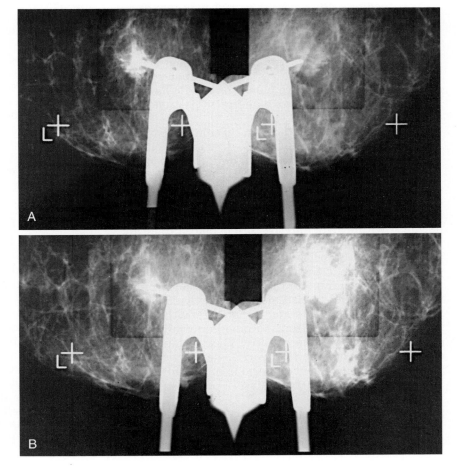

Figure 40–4 *Stereotactic image pair showing placement of the 14-gauge guide needle for stereotactic core biopsy.* **A,** *Prefire views with core needle in place in the center of the target lesion.* **B,** *Postfire views with the needle passing through the target, having sampled a core of the lesion.*

biopsy track, and some discomfort during the procedure itself. The complication rate is acceptably low.

In good hands, the procedure can be done in 30 minutes with a false-negative rate of less than 2 percent. Stereotactic core biopsies are associated with significant savings (possibly as much as $1000 per biopsy) as compared with needle-localized biopsy.[81] A comprehensive review of stereotactic biopsy technique is included in Chapter 36.

Ultrasound-Directed Percutaneous Fine Needle Biopsy of Mammographic Abnormalities

Ultrasound-guided fine needle aspiration (FNA) biopsy offers certain advantages over stereotactic core biopsy.[59, 64] In the hands of an experienced operator, the procedure is tolerated extremely well by patients, fluid (e.g., from a small cyst) can be aspirated, and noncystic lesions can be sampled with great accuracy.[55, 64] Samples obtained from FNA biopsy require evaluation by an expert cytopathologist and can be complicated by an inadequate specimen or by the inability to determine whether invasive carcinoma is present. Ultrasonography does not detect microcalcifications and is ineffective for solid masses smaller than 5 to 6 mm. Unlike for stereotactic core biopsy, a stereotactic device is not necessary since it involves the freehand technique. The operator who performs the technique can select any site of entry on the skin. As the needle is advanced or moved it is monitored in real time on the ultrasound monitor.

Complications of ultrasound-guided FNA include hematoma, infection, and failure to sample the abnormality in question. Inadequate cytologic smears require subsequent attempts that, if unsuccessful, should be followed by core biopsy or needle-localized breast biopsy. False-negative and false-positive rates are acceptably low.

Ultrasound-guided large-core needle biopsy can also be safely performed. New devices that include a firing mechanism provide a high-quality specimen with thinner (18-gauge) needles. Under ultrasonographic guidance the tip of the needle is directed toward the abnormality. When the biopsy needle is appropriately positioned, the mechanism is fired, the needle is withdrawn, and the core is placed in formalin. The procedure can be repeated several times through an introducer that is first inserted to the proximal surface of the lesion, permitting rapid reinsertion and avoiding reintroduction through breast tissue. Ultrasound-guided biopsy is particularly useful in pregnant patients and in patients with lesions that cannot be visualized mammographically. As a general rule, a negative result of needle biopsy or of core biopsy in the face of a worrisome physical finding or a mammographic abnormality should not delay definitive surgical removal.

PALPABLE LESIONS

Although nonpalpable breast lesions require needle localization before definitive biopsy, palpable lesions may be "biopsied" by one of several techniques. The choice of the biopsy technique is influenced by the physical characteristics and size of the breast mass, the site of the suspicious lesion in the breast, the use of local or general anesthesia, and the method of treatment that would be chosen should a malignancy be confirmed. For example, an incisional biopsy of a large breast tumor performed under local anesthesia in a woman who presents with bony metastases provides histological confirmation of the malignancy and adequate tissue for hormone receptor analysis before the initiation of preoperative chemotherapy. On the other hand, FNA biopsy of a suspicious mass done in an outpatient setting for a woman with clinical stage I breast cancer provides a diagnosis and allows surgeon and patient to discuss treatment strategies and options before the definitive surgical procedure. It is critical that the biopsy specimen be handled properly in both clinical situations, as failure or delay in transport to the surgical pathology laboratory can render a specimen invalid for histological or hormone receptor analysis (see Chapter 25).

Collection of Specimens for Cytologic Examination

Direct Smear

Specimens for exfoliative cytology in the patient with suspected Paget's disease of the breast may be obtained with direct smear of the weeping eczematoid lesion of the nipple. If the areola and surrounding skin is scaly and encrusted, a sterile glass slide can be used to scrape this area gently. The direct smear technique is simple and can be performed in the surgeon's office. Expert pathology consultation should be sought to differentiate invasive cancer from carcinoma *in situ* with this technique. The treatment of choice for Paget's disease is total (simple) mastectomy for carcinoma *in situ* and modified radical mastectomy for invasive disease. Comprehensive management of nipple cytology and secretions is reviewed in Chapter 4.

Fluid Aspiration

Fluid from breast cysts is simple to aspirate with a needle and syringe (Fig. 40–5). If the cyst is not palpable, ultrasound may confirm its presence and can be used as a guide to direct the depth and location of the biopsy needle. The return of greenish brown fluid virtually confirms the diagnosis of benign (nonproliferative) cystic disease and, unless otherwise indicated, should not be submitted for cytologic examination. Bloody cystic fluid, on the other hand, is more likely to be indicative of malignancy and therefore should always be examined histologically, either after direct smear or after centrifugation of the aspirated contents. Palpable breast cysts should no longer be detectable after aspiration of their contents since the walls of the cyst should subsequently collapse and conform to the configuration of contigu-

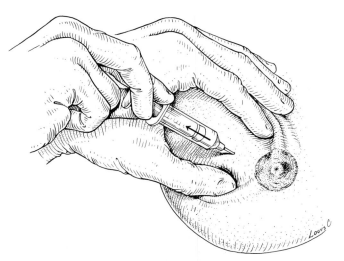

Figure 40–5 *Technique for aspiration of fluid from a breast cyst.*

ous breast tissues. Clinical and mammographic follow-up of patients who undergo fluid aspiration is mandatory, since excisional biopsy of the suspicious mass is indicated for most patients, should the mass recur within 6 weeks of aspiration.

Fine Needle Aspiration Biopsy

FNA biopsy of breast masses is a safe and reliable diagnostic technique that can be performed in the office using local anesthesia.[23] The skin overlying the palpable lesion is infiltrated with 1 percent plain lidocaine. The breast lump is held relatively immobile, using one hand to gently but firmly stabilize the quadrant containing the mass. Using a special cytology aspiration gun (Cameco, Enebyberg, Sweden) that activates the plunger of a disposable 10- or 20-ml syringe attached to a 22-gauge needle, the biopsy can effectively be performed using this technique (Fig. 40–6). The needle is inserted into the mass through the anesthetized skin, and maximum suction is applied to the syringe. By moving the needle into the suspect lesion at various angles over an area of no more than 1 cm, clumps of cells may be

dislodged from the tumor, aspirated into the syringe, and submitted for cytologic examination. FNA is quite safe, although the operator performing the procedure must be cognizant at all times of the relationship of the aspiration needle to the chest wall, as entry into the parietal pleura and iatrogenic pneumothorax is a potentially dangerous, although rare, complication. Following FNA biopsy of any breast mass, local pressure should be applied to the skin puncture site to prevent dispersion of cells and ecchymosis.

The diagnostic accuracy of FNA biopsy of breast masses approximates 80 percent.[39] False-positive results are unusual when the aspirated specimen is properly prepared and reviewed by a qualified cytopathologist. False-negative results are much more common, and it must be emphasized that the absence of malignant cells in the aspirate does not rule out the diagnosis of cancer. Thus, any clinically or mammographically suspicious breast mass investigated by FNA biopsy that does not yield a diagnosis of malignancy must be subjected to incisional or excisional biopsy. When patients undergo FNA of the breast to confirm the diagnosis of metastatic cancer before the institution of preoperative chemotherapy, quantitative hormone receptor (estrogen and progesterone) assays cannot be performed because the tissue sample is too small. Newer qualitative immunofluorescence monoclonal antibody techniques can be applied to the cytology specimen and may help eliminate the problem of insufficient tissue to provide accurate hormone receptor data.

Cutting Needle Biopsy

The technique of biopsy with a needle that incises a core of tissue from the breast is termed *cutting needle biopsy* or *large-core needle biopsy*. The standard Tru-Cut (Travenol, Deerfield, IL) needle (Fig. 40–7) is the cutting needle most often used for breast biopsy. The false-positive diagnostic rate is lower with tissue procured by cutting needles than by FNA biopsy, because more tissue is retained and can be submitted for analysis. Doyle and associates noted specificity of

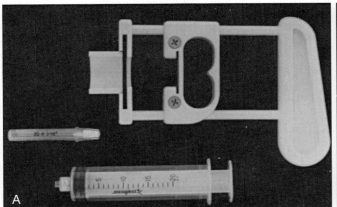
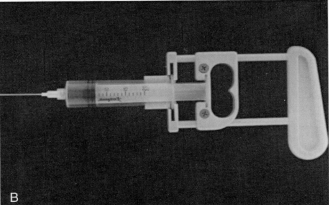

Figure 40–6 **A** *and* **B,** *Aspiration of a solid breast mass is best performed using a cytology fine needle "aspiration gun" (Cameco, Enebyberg, Sweden).*

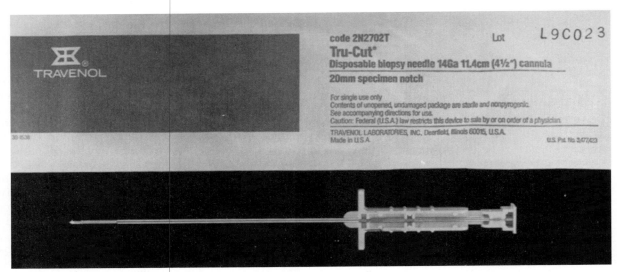

code 2N2702T   Lot   L9C023
Tru-Cut®
Disposable biopsy needle 14Ga 11.4cm (4½") cannula
20mm specimen notch

For single use only
Contents of unopened, undamaged package are sterile and nonpyrogenic.
See accompanying directions for use.
Caution: Federal (U.S.A.) law restricts this device to sale by or on order of a physician.

TRAVENOL LABORATORIES, INC., Deerfield, Illinois 60015, U.S.A.
Made in U.S.A.   U.S. Pat. No. 3,477,423

Figure 40–7   *The TruCut (Travenol) cutting needle is commonly utilized to obtain a core biopsy of solid, palpable breast masses.*

large-core needle biopsies to be 98 percent; sensitivity based on limited follow-up was 100 percent.[15] A core biopsy that yields no malignant cells cannot, however, conclusively be considered benign, since only a portion of the mass that did not contain cancer may have been sampled (sampling error). Thus, like FNA biopsy, the cutting needle biopsy is useful only when the results are positive for malignancy. Cutting needles are 12-gauge or larger and thus require local anesthesia. Since the biopsy yields a core of solid tissue rather than clumps of cells, the potential risk for hemorrhage and tissue disturbance is greater than with needle aspiration methods. Care must be taken to avoid advancing the cutting needle beyond the suspect mass, lest the contiguous normal breast or chest wall be implanted with malignant cells. Such complications can be reduced with operator experience. The site of the puncture and the biopsy track should always be planned so that these areas can be excised en bloc with the neoplasm at the time of the definitive surgical treatment.

Incisional Biopsy

Incisional biopsy of a suspicious breast mass involves removal of a portion of the lesion, which is then submitted for pathological examination. This type of biopsy is indicated for primary breast lesions larger than 4 cm that are to be treated by preoperative chemotherapy or radiotherapy. The incisional biopsy should excise only the amount of tissue necessary for histological confirmation of the diagnosis and for hormone receptor studies.

Technique. The biopsy site should be marked on the breast, typically in curvilinear fashion paralleling Langer's lines, to enable the surgeon to excise the entire scar and the primary neoplasm at the time of definitive surgical therapy (see Chapter 41). Meticulous attention to hemostasis is mandatory to avoid spreading potentially malignant cells. The technical aspects of incisional biopsy of breast masses are relatively simple and straightforward. Local anesthesia with 1 percent plain lidocaine is infiltrated into the dermis of the planned skin incision, directly over the tumor. The actual biopsy of tumor is best performed using a scalpel since electrocautery may distort the histological features of the tissue and possibly invalidate accurate tissue levels (expressed in mg of cytosol protein) of hormone receptors. Biopsy of a portion of the mass is followed by closure with absorbable 2-0 or 3-0 sutures.

Excisional Biopsy

As the terminology implies, excisional biopsy of a breast mass removes the entire lesion and generally includes a margin of normal breast tissue that surrounds it. It should be considered an error in surgical technique if the tumor is transected during excisional biopsy. Such technical errors virtually guarantee contamination of adjacent tissues with malignant cells. Occult suspicious breast lesions that are apparent only on mammograms should be removed by excisional biopsy using preoperative needle localization.[8] If the volume of tissue removed is smaller than 1 cm³, only permanent histological sections of the lesion should be planned, as the pathologist may not be able to distinguish between severe atypia and carcinoma on frozen section specimens. On rare occasion excisional biopsy of a large breast mass (e.g., giant fibroadenoma) is indicated to provide definitive therapy for breast disease.

Diagnostic excisional biopsy should *not* be considered a substitute for planned removal of malignant lesions. Tafra and coworkers determined that biopsy specimens with residual tumor had larger median tumor diameters than those that had no residual disease (2 cm versus 1 cm, $P < .01$), were more likely to be associated with positive axillary nodes ($P < .001$) and more likely to develop recurrence ($P < .025$).[76] The authors suggest that any procedure less extensive than the planned surgical operation is liable to leave behind malignant breast tissue.[76]

Lumpectomy (Segmental Mastectomy)

When the National Surgical Adjuvant Breast and Bowel Project (NSABP) was implemented in the 1950s, the standard surgical treatment for carcinoma of the breast was modified radical or radical mastectomy. Surgeons had essentially no familiarity with "breast conservation surgery" or terms such as *tylectomy, lumpectomy, segmental mastectomy*, and *quadrantectomy*. Through a series of workshops and other educational tools, the participating NSABP surgeons were instructed in the methods mandated by the protocol. Lumpectomy with axillary dissection (levels I and II) followed by radiation therapy to the breast is now an acceptable surgical treatment for certain carcinomas of the breast.

Some clinics currently advocate lumpectomy as the preferred technique for initial biopsy of suspicious breast masses.[54] Compared with traditional excisional biopsy, this technique more often provided adequate (clear) margins and decreased the number of subsequent procedures on the breast for conservation purposes. Lumpectomy as the initial biopsy method requires prolonged operation time to ensure clear surgical margins. We continue to prefer pathological studies of excision specimens with subsequent completion of lumpectomy after confirmation of the malignant diagnosis. A detailed review of the indications and techniques for conservation surgery advocated by Fisher and other investigators of the NSABP is provided in Chapter 46.

Curvilinear incisions are recommended for the majority of lumpectomies, regardless of the site of the primary breast lesion. Although radial incisions are preferred by some surgeons for lesions in the lower half of the breast, we use nonradial incisions in the majority of patients, as cosmetic results are equivalent or superior with curvilinear incisions that follow the breast contour parallel to Langer's lines. Chapter 40 reviews the placement of incisions for suspect breast masses in various quadrants of the breast. The surgeon must always be cognizant of the occasional necessity to convert a planned segmental mastectomy into a total mastectomy. Thus, placement of breast incisions that are readily incorporated into cosmetically acceptable incisions for total mastectomy is essential to planning the operative procedure.

It is helpful if the preoperative diagnosis of cancer has been established by needle aspiration biopsy or core biopsy. For breast lesions suggestive of carcinoma that require needle localization, the needle should be directed into the lesion perpendicular to the skin and as close as possible to the planned curvilinear incision, to avoid extensive flap elevation with subsequent wound hemorrhage and skin slough. The incision for lumpectomy should be placed directly over the lesion. Extensive tunneling through and elevation of contiguous breast tissue at an angle

is ill-advised and is *not recommended*, as tumor-free margins are invariably difficult to obtain.[38] In patients referred with biopsy-proven carcinoma, reexcision of the old scar and the entire biopsy site is essential to reducing the probability of tumor implantation and local recurrence in the scar and skin flaps.

It is imperative to excise a margin of healthy breast tissue contiguous with the suspect mass. Careful palpation of margins of the tumor by the operating surgeon during excision provides a three-dimensional perspective on the lesion that is essential to ensure that the tumor is not violated and is excised within the sphere of extirpated breast tissue. This technique does not necessitate removal of a predetermined volume of normal tissue; the goal of the operative procedure is to obtain margins that are grossly free of tumor. Skin edges need not be undermined, and the pectoralis major fascia is not included in the resected margin unless the lesion is contiguous with or is fixed to the fascia. The specimen should be oriented in all dimensions, using suture for tags. The designations *cranial-caudal, medial-lateral*, and *superficial-deep* allow the surgeon to identify clearly the margins of the excised specimen for the pathologist. Such margins may be dyed with indelible vital stains (e.g., India ink and various colored dyes) to verify and corroborate areas of concern and to ensure histological extirpation of the cancer. On occasion, the pathologist may complete frozen section tissue or cytologic analysis of the margins of all biopsy specimens (when indicated) to ensure histologically clear margins (see Chapters 39 and 41). The pathologist's role is essential: confirmation of histological diagnosis, establishing the presence of tumor-free margins, and submitting tissue for estrogen and progesterone receptor (ER/PR) analyses, and other prognostic determinants (e.g., oncogene biochemical markers, ploidy, S phase). The surgeon must be cognizant of tumor orientation with respect to the wound and the chest wall during resection of the breast mass. The presence of a positive margin requires re-excision of any area in which the frozen section was histologically positive. When lumpectomy cannot ensure tumor-free margins (e.g., multifocality, multicentricity, multiple histological types, diffuse microcalcifications), total mastectomy is performed.

Following confirmation of tumor-free margins by the pathologist, meticulous hemostasis is achieved and wound closure is begun. Special attention is paid to closure of the wound, since tissue defects created with lumpectomy may produce cosmetically unacceptable scars that may be further exaggerated after completion of breast irradiation. Care must be taken in closing the wound, as unacceptable cosmetic results occur when superficial or deep tissues are approximated under tension. Large defects are preferably closed in multiple layers with interrupted 2-0 or 3-0 absorbable chromic gut or synthetic sutures. Some surgeons make no attempt to obliterate dead space, and others make no effort to drain this space. Interrupted absorbable sutures are placed in the subcutaneous tissues, and the skin is closed using a running, subcuticular, absorbable 4-0 or 5-0 synthetic suture.

Surgical Biopsy of the Breast

Only by removing a sample of breast tissue sufficient for histological preparation can a diagnosis be made with ultimate confidence. The accuracy of pathological information obtained is limited only by the accuracy of sampling and the morphological interpretation. Because a negative biopsy result can be caused by sampling error, cancer cannot be excluded unless representative pathological tissue is removed and examined thoroughly. This principle is most important, as therapy for cancer can be predicated only on histological verification of its presence. Depending on histological and mammographic findings, bilateral biopsy may be indicated. Simkovich and colleagues determined that random contralateral breast biopsy is indicated with histological confirmation of infiltrating lobular carcinoma.[68] This treatment is considered debatable by many[70] and is reviewed comprehensively in Chapters 13, 14, and 39 through 47.

Breast biopsy is best performed in a surgical suite, under sterile conditions and with techniques of local or general anesthesia. This may be done on an outpatient basis, but the setting depends on patient and physician preference. It is essential that incisions be cosmetically designed, since approximately 70 percent of breast biopsies confirm benign (proliferative and nonproliferative) disease. Since the lines of tension in the skin of the breast (Langer's lines) are generally concentric with the nipple (Fig. 40–8), incisions that parallel these lines generally result in thin and cosmetically acceptable scars.[73] It is best to keep these incisions within the boundaries of potential incisions for future mastectomy or wide local excision, should those therapies be required for definitive treatment (Fig. 40–9).[19] Principles for planning breast biopsy are further reviewed in Chapters 41 and 59. The most cosmetically acceptable scars result from circumareolar (curvilinear) incisions. Most centrally located subareolar lesions can be approached in this manner.

Once the patient is positioned comfortably on the operating table, the thorax is slightly elevated ipsilaterally to the suspect lesion (using folded sheets), and the arm is placed in a relaxed position on an arm board. Incisions commonly used for all quadrants are depicted in Figure 40–6. In general, dermal tension is concentric with the nipple, becoming transverse over the sternum and diagonal toward the extreme upper lateral anterior chest. Periareolar and concentric lesions follow these lines of tension and therefore are optimally "aesthetic." The proposed incision is marked on the skin after the dimensions of the tumor are estimated, and local anesthesia (1 percent plain lidocaine) is infiltrated into the dermis (cutis vera). The surgeon is admonished to avoid lidocaine injections that contain epinephrine, lest it cause epidermolysis of the injection site with subsequent slough of the epidermis. It is not necessary to fill subcutaneous tissues with the local anesthetic, as this may make it difficult to palpate margins of the suspicious mass. This principle is most important when excisional biopsy is planned. Injection of the tumor with anesthetics is also contraindicated, as this adds nothing to patient comfort but risks dissemination of neoplastic cells into contiguous tissues. Preferably, biopsy should be performed with the scalpel rather than electrocautery, which can devitalize tissue and invalidate detectable hormone receptor values. We prefer to obtain ER and PR data from tissue removed at the initial biopsy rather than from residual tumor in the mastectomy specimen, particularly because warm ischemia time during mastectomy may alter the estrogen and progesterone content (see Chapter 25).

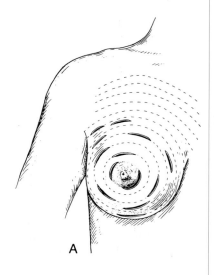

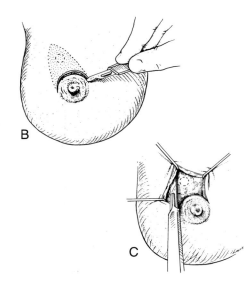

Figure 40–8 *Recommended locations of incisions for performing breast biopsy.* **A,** *The most cosmetically acceptable scars result from circumareolar incisions that follow the contour of Langer's lines.* **B** *and* **C,** *Technique for dissection of breast masses within 2 cm of the areolar margin. Thick skin flaps are advised to ensure cosmetically contoured and viable tissues about the areola.*

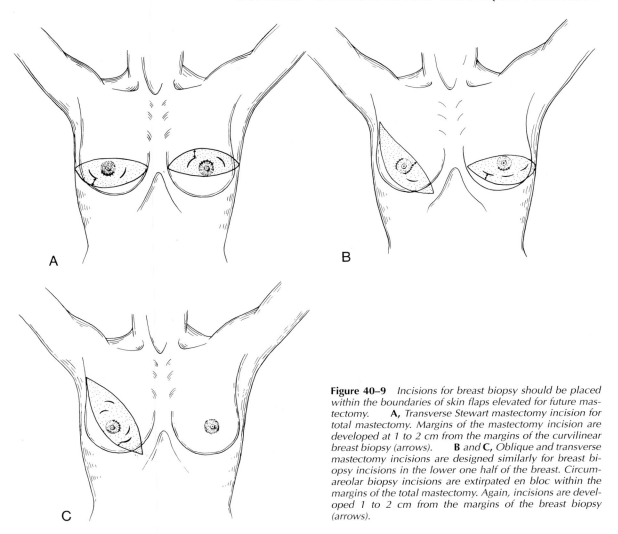

Figure 40–9 *Incisions for breast biopsy should be placed within the boundaries of skin flaps elevated for future mastectomy.* **A,** *Transverse Stewart mastectomy incision for total mastectomy. Margins of the mastectomy incision are developed at 1 to 2 cm from the margins of the curvilinear breast biopsy (arrows).* **B** and **C,** *Oblique and transverse mastectomy incisions are designed similarly for breast biopsy incisions in the lower one half of the breast. Circumareolar biopsy incisions are extirpated en bloc within the margins of the total mastectomy. Again, incisions are developed 1 to 2 cm from the margins of the breast biopsy (arrows).*

Following completion of the skin incision, dermal and subcutaneous bleeding is controlled and the incision is opened through the subcutaneous fat with sharp (scalpel) dissection to expose the tumor mass. Unless incisional biopsy is planned because of the size (larger than 4 cm) of the neoplasm, every effort is made to avoid incision into the tumor. Using sharp dissection guided by careful and gentle digital palpation, the operating surgeon excises the mass with a small rim of normal breast parenchyma. If the tumor is at least 4 cm, only incisional biopsy should be performed to confirm the diagnosis of cancer. If the diagnosis of cancer is not determined at histological review of permanent sections, the entire mass should be removed and the specimen placed immediately in a saline-soaked sponge for transport to the pathologist. Should prolonged transport of the tumor be anticipated (i.e., warm ischemia time longer than 20 minutes), the specimen should be packed on ice and delivered expeditiously to the pathology department.

During excisional biopsy, retractors can be utilized to facilitate exposure for dissection of the mass, but care must be taken not to violate the area to be removed. Once the specimen has been removed, attention to meticulous hemostasis with electrocautery or suture ligatures is mandatory. Catheter or Penrose drainage of the wound bed is unnecessary when adequate hemostasis is achieved. Further, drainage via suction methods had no impact on postoperative pain or long-term outcomes in the prospective analysis in the United Kingdom by Warren and coworkers.[80] Closure of the breast tissue defect is not mandatory, although we recommend closure with interrupted 2-0 or 3-0 absorbable chromic gut or synthetic sutures. The subcutaneous tissues are closed with 3-0 or 4-0 interrupted, absorbable sutures. A running subcuticular closure of the skin using 5-0 synthetic suture is performed, followed by Steri-Strip approximation of the skin edges. A light occlusive dressing is applied.

Goff and associates observed the long-term impact of previous breast biopsy on breast cancer screening modalities in a prospective analysis.[26] These investigators and others[67] concluded that excision at biopsy does not generally produce long-term changes that affect the interpretation of breast physical examination or mammography.

CHOICE OF ANESTHESIA FOR ONE- AND TWO-STAGE PROCEDURES

The choice of anesthesia (local or general) for breast biopsy depends on the following factors:

1. The presence of a lesion, palpable or nonpalpable
2. The age and general medical condition of the patient
3. The presumptive diagnosis
4. The necessity to procure adequate amounts of tissue for hormone receptor analysis before initiation of anticancer therapy
5. The type of biopsy (incisional, excisional, FNA) that the physician plans to perform
6. The location of the mass within the breast
7. The personal preference of the physician and the patient

In general, efforts should be made to avoid sequential general anesthesia when treating patients with a potentially malignant breast mass, although this is not always feasible or possible. For example, nonpalpable lesions that lie deep in the breast may be best excised under general anesthesia. In addition, an anxious patient who is apprehensive of the biopsy under local anesthesia may elect a general anesthetic if her medical condition is compatible with this technique.

Biopsy as a separate procedure under general anesthesia should be avoided when needle biopsy, cutting needle biopsy, or biopsy under local anesthesia can safely and comfortably be accomplished with supplemental anesthesia (intravenous sedation). The great majority of palpable and nonpalpable breast masses can be excised with local anesthesia and sedation, incurring minimal morbidity and no mortality with substantial cost reduction.[27] Local agents such as lidocaine are safe and effective and produce minimal discomfort after injection of the dermis and surrounding breast tissues. Contraindications to local anesthesia for breast biopsy generally include (1) a palpable or nonpalpable lesion deep within the breast parenchyma for which significant manipulation of tissue near the fascia is anticipated; (2) an anxious, apprehensive patient or one who prefers to have the biopsy done under general anesthesia; and (3) a patient with a breast mass suggestive of carcinoma who agrees to undergo biopsy, frozen section, and definite operative therapy, all during one procedure under general anesthesia. When it is anticipated that general anesthesia will be required for biopsy of a suspicious breast mass, a full work-up, including staging (see Chapter 21), with plans to implement comprehensive operative therapy, should be completed before the procedure, to avoid a second operation. Therefore, informed consent for definitive therapy should be obtained before any procedure in the patient with a suspicious breast mass. Additionally, the surgeon and operating room personnel must arrange preoperatively for specimen mammography to be performed (if needle localization is required) as soon as the biopsy is completed to allow analysis of the freshly procured tissue. Such arrangements with the radiologist and pathologist minimize the duration of the general anesthetic and its inherent morbidity.

For a highly suspect lesion, a two-stage procedure under general anesthesia is not recommended if frozen section evaluation at the time of the biopsy could provide the diagnosis and allow the surgeon to proceed with definitive therapy as a one-stage procedure. General anesthesia for biopsy should not be used solely because the clinic or hospital lacks the facilities for needle biopsy or frozen section analysis.

References

1. Acosta JA, Greenlee JA, Gubler KD, Goepfert CJ, Ragland JJ: Surgical margins after needle-localization breast biopsy. Am J Surg 170:643–645, 1995.
2. Bauermeister DE, Hall MH: Specimen radiography: Mandatory adjunct to mammography. Am J Clin Pathol 59:782–789, 1973.
3. Becker W: Stereotactic localization of breast lesions. Radiology 133:240–241, 1979.
4. Bennett IC, Freitas R Jr, Fentiman IS: Diagnosis of breast cancer in young women. Aust NZ J Surg 61:284–289, 1991.
5. Bigongiari LR, Fidler W, Skerker LB, Comstock C, Threatt B: Percutaneous localization of breast lesions prior to biopsy: Analysis of failures. Clin Radiol 28:419–425, 1977.
6. Block MA, Reynolds W: How vital is mammography in the diagnosis and management of breast carcinoma? Arch Surg 108:588–591, 1974.
7. Brobeil A, Bermann C, Clark R, Cox C, Reintgen D: Medical-legal pitfalls for the breast surgeon: Incomplete mammographic localization of suspicious lesions and the correlation between palpable and mammographic abnormalities. Am Surg 62:484–487, 1996.
8. Cady B: How to perform breast biopsies. Surg Oncol Clin North Am 4:47–66, 1995.
9. Cox G, Didlake R, Powers C, Scott-Conner C: Choice of anesthetic technique for needle localized breast biopsy. Am Surg 57:414–418, 1991.
10. Cox CE, Reintgen DS, Nicosia SV, Ku NN, Baekey P, Carey LC: Analysis of residual cancer after diagnostic breast biopsy: An argument for fine-needle aspiration cytology. Ann Surg Oncol 2:201–206, 1995. Comment.
11. Dershaw DD, Morris EA, Liberman L, Abramson AF: Nondiagnostic stereotaxic core breast biopsy: Results of rebiopsy Radiology 198:313–315, 1996. Comment
12. Dietler PC, Wineland RE, Marolo NM: Localization of nonpalpable breast lesions detected by xeromammography. Ann Surg 42:810–811, 1976.
13. Doberneck RC: Breast biopsy, a study of cost-effectiveness. Ann Surg 192:152–156, 1980.
14. Dodd GD: Pre-operative radiographic localization of non-palpable lesions. In Gallagher HS (ed): Early Breast Cancer; Detection and Treatment. New York, John Wiley & Sons, 1975, pp 151–152.
15. Doyle AJ, Murray KA, Nelson EW, Bragg DG: Selective use of image-guided large-core needle biopsy of the breast: Accuracy and cost-effectiveness. AJR Am J Roentgenol 165:281–284, 1995.
16. Egan RL: Breast biopsy priority: Cancer versus benign preoperative masses. Cancer 35:612–617, 1975.
17. Egan RL, McSweeney MB, Sewell CW: Intramammary calcifications without an associated mass in benign and malignant diseases. Radiology 137:1–7, 1980.
18. Egeli RA, Urban JA: Mammography in symptomatic women

50 years of age and under, and those over 50. Cancer 43:878–882, 1979.

19. Farley DR, Meland NB: Importance of breast biopsy incision in final outcome of breast reconstruction. Mayo Clin Proc 67:1050–1054, 1992.

20. Fine RE, Boyd BA: Stereotactic breast biopsy: A practical approach. Am Surg 62:96–102, 1996.

21. Fischer U, Vosshenrich R, Doler W, Hamadeh A, Oestmann JW, Grabbe E: MR imaging–guided breast intervention: Experience with two systems. Radiology 195:533–538, 1995.

22. Frank HA, Hall FM, Steer ML: Preoperative localization of non-palpable breast lesions demonstrated by mammography. N Engl J Med 295:259, 1976.

23. Frazier TG, Rowland CW, Murphy JT, Woolery CT, Ryan SM: The value of aspiration cytology in the evaluation of dysplastic breasts. Cancer 45:2878–2879, 1980.

24. Gallager HS: Breast specimen radiography: Obligatory, adjuvant and investigative. Am J Clin Pathol 64:749–755, 1975.

25. Gisvold JJ, Goellner JR, Grant CS, Donohue JH, Sykes MW, Karsell PR, Coffey SL, Jung SH: Breast biopsy: A comparative study of stereotaxically guided core and excisional techniques. AJR Am J Roentgenol 162:815–820, 1994.

26. Goff JM, Molloy M, Debbas MT, Hale DA, Jaques DP: Long-term impact of previous breast biopsy on breast cancer screening modalities. J Surg Oncol 59:18–20, 1995.

27. Grannan KJ, Lamping K: Impact of method of anesthesia on the accuracy of needle-localized breast biopsies. Am J Surg 165:218–220, 1993.

28. Hall FM, Frank HA: Preoperative localization of nonpalpable breast lesions. AJR Am J Roentgenol 132:101–105, 1979.

29. Hasselgren PO, Hummel RP, Fieler MA: Breast biopsy with needle localization: Influence of age and mammographic feature on the rate of malignancy in 350 nonpalpable breast lesions. Surgery 110:623–627, 1991.

30. Hasselgren PO, Hummel RP, Georgian-Smith D, Fieler M: Breast biopsy with needle localization: Accuracy of specimen x-ray and management of missed lesions. Surgery 114:836–840, 1993.

31. Hassler O: Microradiographic investigations of calcifications of the female breast. Cancer 23:1103–1109, 1969.

32. Hickey RC, Gallager HS, Dodd GD, Samuels BI, Paulus DD, Moore DI: The detection and diagnosis of early, occult and minimal breast cancer. Adv Surg 10:287–312, 1976.

33. Homer MJ, Fisher DM, Sugarman HJ: Post-localization needle for breast biopsy of nonpalpable lesions. Radiology 140:241–242, 1981.

34. Homer MJ, Rangel DM, Miller HH: Pre- and transoperative localization of nonpalpable breast lesions. Am J Surg 139:889–891, 1980.

35. Horns JW, Arndt RD: Percutaneous spot localization of non-palpable breast lesions. Am J Roentgenol 127:253–256, 1976.

36. Jensen SR, Luttenegger TJ: Wire localization of nonpalpable breast lesions. Radiology 132:484–485, 1979.

37. Kalisher L: An improved needle for localization of nonpalpable breast lesions. Radiology 128:815–817, 1978.

38. Khatri VP, Smith DH: Method of avoiding tunneling during needle-localized breast biopsy. J Surg Oncol 60:72–73, 1995.

39. Kline TS, Neal HS: Role of needle aspiration biopsy in diagnosis of carcinoma of the breast. Obstet Gynecol 46:89–92, 1975.

40. Koehl RH, Snyder RE, Hutter RVP: The use of specimen roentgenography to detect small carcinomas not found by routine pathologic examination. Cancer 21:2–10, 1971.

41. Kolbenstvedt A, Heldaas O: Value of radiography of the remaining breast following mastectomy for carcinoma. Acta Radiol Diagn 14:435–441, 1973.

42. Kopans DB, Moore RH, McCarthy KA, Hall DA, Hulka CA, Whitman GJ, Slanetz PJ, Halpern EF: Positive predictive value of *breast biopsy* performed as a result of mammography: There is no abrupt change at age 50 years. Radiology 200:357–360, 1996.

43. Liberman L, Cohen MA, Dershaw DD, Abramson AF, Hann LE, Rosen PP: Atypical ductal hyperplasia diagnosed at stereotaxic core biopsy of breast lesions: An indication for surgical biopsy. AJR Am J Roentgenol 164:1111–1113, 1995.

44. Liberman L, Dershaw DD, Rosen PP, Abramson AF, Deutch BM, Hann LE: Stereotaxic 14-gauge breast biopsy: How many core biopsy specimens are needed? Radiology 192:793–795, 1994.

45. Liberman L, Dershaw DD, Rosen PP, Morris EA, Cohen MA, Abramson AF: Core needle biopsy of synchronous ipsilateral breast lesions: Impact on treatment. AJR Am J Roentgenol 166:1429–1432, 1996.

46. Libshitz HI, Feig SA, Fetouh S: Needle localization of nonpalpable breast lesions. Radiology 121:557–560, 1976.

47. Loh CK, Perlman H, Harris JH, Rotz CT, Royal DR: An improved method for localization of nonpalpable breast lesions. Radiology 130:244–245, 1979.

48. McLelland R: Mammography in the detection, diagnosis and management of carcinoma of the breast. Surg Gynecol Obstet 146:735–740, 1978.

49. Meyer JE, Christina RL, Lester SC, Frenna TH, Denison CM, DiPiro PJ, Polger M: Evaluation of nonpalpable solid breast masses with stereotaxic large-needle core biopsy using a dedicated unit. AJR Am J Roentgenol 167:179–182, 1996.

50. Millis RR, McKinna JA, Hamlin IME, Greening WP: Biopsy of the impalpable breast lesion detected by mammography. Br J Surg 63:346–348, 1976.

51. Morrow M, Schmidt R, Cregger B, Hassett C, Cox S: Preoperative evaluation of abnormal mammographic findings to avoid unnecessary breast biopsies. Arch Surg 129:1091–1096, 1994.

52. Moss JP, Voyles RG: Operative localization of the suspicious lesion on mammography. J Ky Med Assoc 76:324–326, 1978.

53. Muhlow A: A device for precision needle biopsy of the breast at mammography. Am J Roentgenol Radium Ther Nucl Med 121:843–845, 1974.

54. Ngai JH, Zelles GW, Rumore GJ, Sawicki JE, Godfrey RS: Breast biopsy techniques and adequacy of margins. Arch Surg 126:1343–1347, 1991.

55. Parker SH, Burbank F: A practical approach to minimally invasive breast biopsy. Radiology 200:11–20, 1996.

56. Parker SH, Burbank F, Jackman RJ, et al: Percutaneous large-core breast biopsy: A multi-institutional study Radiology 193:359–364, 1994. Comment

57. Parker S, Burbank F, Tabar L, et al: Percutaneous large core breast biopsy: A multi-institutional experience. Radiology 193:359–364, 1994.

58. Pollei SR, Mettler FA, Bartow SA, Moradian G, Moskowitz M: Occult breast cancer: Prevalence and radiographic detectability. Radiology 163:459–462, 1987.

59. Price JG, Kortz AB, Clark DG: US-guided automated large-core breast biopsy. Radiology 187:507–511, 1993.

60. Rogers JV, Powell RW: Mammographic indications for biopsy of clinically normal breasts: Correlation with pathologic findings in 72 cases. Am J Roentgenol Radium Ther 115:794–800, 1972.

61. Rosen P, Snyder RE, Foote FW, Wallace T: Detection of occult carcinoma in the apparently benign breast biopsy through specimen radiography. Cancer 26:944–952, 1970.

62. Rosen PP, Snyder RE, Robbins G: Specimen radiography for nonpalpable breast lesions found by mammography: Procedures and results. Cancer 34:2028–2033, 1974.

63. Roses DF, Harris MN, Gorstein F, Gumport SL: Biopsy for microcalcification detected by mammography. Surgery 87:248–252, 1980.

64. Schmidt RA: Stereotactic breast biopsy. CA Cancer J Clin 144:172–191, 1994.

65. Schwartz AM, Siegelman S: A technique for biopsy of nonpalpable breast tumors. Surg Gynecol Obstet 23:1321–1322, 1966.

66. Seidman H, Gelb SK, Silverberg E, LaVerda N, Lubera JA: Survival experience in the breast cancer detection demonstration project. CA 37:258–290, 1987.

67. Sickles EA, Herzog KA: Mammography of the postsurgical breast. AJR Am J Roentgenol 136:585–588, 1981.

68. Simkovich AH, Sclafani LM, Masri M, Kinne DW: Role of contralateral breast biopsy in infiltrating lobular cancer. Surgery 114:555–557, 1993.

69. Simon N, Lesnick GJ, Lerer WN, Bachman AL: Roentgenographic localization of small lesions of the breast by the spot method. Surg Gynecol Obstet 134:572–574, 1972.

70. Smith BL, Bertagnolli M, Klein BB, Batter S, Chang M, Douville LM, Eberlein TJ: Evaluation of the contralateral breast. The role of biopsy at the time of treatment of primary breast cancer Ann Surg 216:17–21, 1992. Comment.

71. Snyder RE: Specimen radiography and preoperative localization of nonpalpable breast cancer. Cancer 46(4 suppl):950–956, 1980.

72. Snyder RE, Rosen P: Radiography of breast specimens. Cancer 28:1608–1611, 1971.

73. Spratt JS, Donegan WL: Surgical management. *In* Donegan WL, Spratt JS (eds): Cancer of the Breast. 3rd ed. Philadelphia, WB Saunders, 1988, pp 403–416.

74. Stephenson TF: Chiba needle–barbed wire technique for breast biopsy localization. AJR Am J Roentgenol 135:184–186, 1980.

75. Stevens GM, Jamplis RW: Mammographically directed biopsy of nonpalpable breast lesions. Arch Surg 102:292–295, 1971.

76. Tafra L, Guenther JM, Giuliano AE: Planned segmentectomy. A necessity for breast carcinoma. Arch Surg 128:1014–1018, 1993.

77. Urban JA: Biopsy of the "normal" breast in treating breast cancer. Surg Clin North Am 49:291–301, 1969.

78. Wallace JE, Sayler C, McDowell NG, Moseley HS. The role of stereotactic biopsy in assessment of nonpalpable breast lesions. Am J Surg 171:471–473, 1996.

79. Wallace TI: Radiographic identification of calcifications in breast specimens. Cancer 21(1):11–12, 1971.

80. Warren HW, Griffith CD, McLean L, Angerson WJ, Kaye B, McElroy M: Should breast biopsy cavities be drained? Ann R Coll Surg Engl 76:39–41, 1994.

81. Yim JH, Barton P, Weber B, Radford D, Levy J, Monsees B, Flanagan F, Norton JA, Doherty GM: Mammographically detected breast cancer. Benefits of stereotactic core versus wire localization biopsy. Ann Surg 223:688–697, 1996.

CHAPTER 41

GENERAL PRINCIPLES OF MASTECTOMY: EVALUATION AND THERAPEUTIC OPTIONS

Kirby I. Bland, M.D. / John B. McCraw, M.D. / Edward M. Copeland III, M.D.

"The treatment of a presumably surgically operable mammary carcinoma may be reinforced by two methods: radiation alone and combined radiation and operation. The outlook upon the adoption or otherwise of the reinforcing methods depends upon the experience and judgment of the surgeon."[10]

G. L. Cheatle and M. Cutler (1933)

With pathological confirmation of the diagnosis of breast cancer, a complete history, physical examination and accurate clinical staging evaluation are requisite to therapy of the primary invasive neoplasm. Mammary adenocarcinoma that is 5 cm or less in transverse diameter and limited to the central or lateral aspect of the breast with the absence of pectoral fascia, skin fixation, and axillary lymphadenopathy can usually be treated by surgery alone. Lesions that are smaller than 4 cm in diameter may be optionally treated by segmental mastectomy (partial mastectomy, lumpectomy, or tylectomy) and postoperative irradiation, with results comparable to radical surgical techniques; this is discussed in a subsequent section of this chapter. For cancers larger than 5 cm (T3) in transverse diameter (stage IIIA or IIIB), a combination of radical surgery and radiation therapy is often essential to achieve local and regional control of the breast, axilla, and chest wall (see Chapters 67, 68, and 69).

The significant contributions of investigators for breast cancer management in the twentieth century established the outcome results for conservation surgical techniques to be equivalent to those of radical approaches. Thus, the procedure to be completed and the anatomical site that should receive irradiation for stages 0, I, and II disease depend on the location of the primary neoplasm in the breast, the presence or absence of axillary metastases, and characteristics (phenotype) of the index cancer.[37]

Moreover, the increasing importance of the primary tumor characteristics and its phenotype relative to its natural history are emerging in clinical trials as important criteria for selection of the procedure. The integration of cellular, biochemical, immunohistochemical, and molecular biological features of the neoplasm will increasingly direct therapies of the next decade.

Lesions in the *lateral aspect of the breast* drain principally via axillary lymphatic channels (see Chapter 2). Disease in this location can be eradicated from the chest wall by employing the modified radical mastectomy. The latter procedure is defined as a total mastectomy with en bloc removal of the pectoralis minor muscle and Levels I to III axillary lymph nodes. These laterally placed neoplasms with axillary lymph node metastases may be associated with internal mammary or supraclavicular lymph node metastases in as much as 25 to 30 percent of patients; thus, irradiation therapy has been used to treat the peripheral lymphatic areas (internal mammary chain, supraclavicular sites).[12]

Centrally located lesions that are fixed to the pectoralis major fascia or high-lying (superiorly located) lesions that are fixed to this fascia may be treated by radical mastectomy or by a combination of radical mastectomy and peripheral lymphatic and chest wall irradiation when palpable axillary lymph node metastases smaller than 2 cm are evident. These centrally placed lesions commonly metastasize via lymphatics that parallel the course of the neurovascular bundle medial to the pectoralis minor muscle. This medial neurovascular bundle that contains the lateral pectoral nerve and innervates the pectoralis major muscle is preserved in the modified radical mastectomy to ensure function of the pectoralis major muscle after mastectomy. In the radical mastectomy procedure, this neurovascular bundle, associated lymphatics, and areolar tissue are resected en bloc with the specimen to accomplish adequate surgical extirpation of regional disease.

For *medially located neoplasms*, the principal lymphatic drainage is via routes that course to lymph nodes near the ipsilateral internal mammary vessels. These medial lesions may be associated with metastasis to the internal mammary lymphatics in 10 to 30 percent of patients, as previously confirmed by Handley.[34] The presence of pathologically positive axillary metastasis with an associated medial lesion escalates this incidence of internal mammary metastasis to as much as 50 percent. In the absence of clinically positive axillary metastases, medially located cancers may be adequately treated by segmental (partial) mastectomy or modified radical mastectomy and peripheral lymphatic irradiation.

Whether the surgeon chooses the conservation or radical approach depends on tumor size and characteristics, general medical status, patient choice, and desire for reconstruction. Regardless of the operative procedure selected, clearance of pathologically "free" margins about the neoplasm in three dimensions is paramount to enhancement of disease-free survival. Margins of the tumor resection that invade the costochondrium and periosteum of ribs or sternum or the intercostal musculature require full-thickness chest wall resection with immediate myocutaneous flap reconstruction. With "clear" margins pathologically, radiation may be administered concomitantly with the treatment regimen and depends on tumor characteristics and location, and the presence (number) of metastatic lymph nodes (see Chapters 60 and 61). Further, it is common to include chest wall irradiation when axillary metastases are identified pathologically in more than 20 percent of the removed axillary lymphatics. This principle was originally established because of the high incidence of skin flap recurrence evident with metastatic disease that courses to the axilla via the subdermal lymphatics from medially located primary lesions.

The principal determinant of actuarial survival of the patient following therapy of the primary breast lesion is the pathological stage of tumor. As established by the American Joint Committee on Cancer (AJCC), the staging system most used is the Tumor, Node, Metastasis (TNM) system. It is the responsibility of the surgeon and the radiation therapist to plan an operative procedure that encompasses, en bloc, the extent of the disease and provides the maximum probability for local and regional chest wall control of the tumor. It is also their responsibility to achieve this end result with minimal morbidity and mortality. These principles are best served by the avoidance of axillary irradiation following the Patey (complete) surgical dissection of Levels I to III axillary lymphatics; otherwise, the incidence of lymphedema of the ipsilaterally irradiated extremity will be increased approximately seven- to tenfold. Following radical resection of lymphatic channels with en bloc dissection of Levels I to III, the remaining lymphatics are destroyed by radiation therapy, thus increasing the incidence of lymphedema. In principle, operable breast cancer (stages I and II) treated by total mastectomy and axillary node removal with the radical or modified radical mastectomy should not require postoperative irradiation. In contradistinction, for the treatment of stage III disease with axillary metastases that clinically present with large, matted, or multiple nodes, the radiation therapist should plan the application of tangential fields to the apex of the axilla, including the peripheral lymphatics and chest wall after the extended simple (total) mastectomy is performed. This therapeutic regimen is essential, because Level III (apical) lymphatics remain intact after a resection that includes lymphatics lateral to the border of the pectoralis major and minor muscles. With the extended simple mastectomy performed for stage III breast cancer, the primary cancer or lymphatics, or both, that are larger than 1 cm in diameter are unlikely to be sterilized by irradiation and are thus surgically removed.

Extension of the primary neoplasm into the axillary space with invasion of the axillary artery, vein, or brachial plexus does not technically allow surgical removal and is best treated with ionizing irradiation to the area. Radiotherapy should be added to low or central axillary nodes that are determined pathologically to have *extranodal capsular extension*, because

local and regional control rates are enhanced with this modality, despite the increased risk of lymphedema in the ipsilateral arm. In the absence of clinically palpable nodes with primary neoplasms that exceed 5 cm in diameter, preoperative radiation therapy or combination chemotherapy may induce regression of the primary lesion. Thereafter, surgical treatment of the breast depends on the extent (volume) of regression of the primary tumor, the presence or absence of fixation to pectoralis major fascia, location, and the presence or absence of local grave signs (ulceration, skin edema and fixation, satellosis).[60]

Surgeons should plan the operation with the objective of achieving, at minimum, 1 to 2 cm skin margins with subcutaneous and parenchymal margins of 2 to 3 cm in all directions from the tumor, which can be accomplished with a radical, modified radical, or extended simple mastectomy. Patients presenting with distant metastases, including supraclavicular lymph node metastases, are best treated with systemic chemotherapy. Again, it is the responsibility of the surgeon and the radiotherapist to achieve local and regional control except when adequate surgical margins are unobtainable without regression of the tumor, thereby reducing the probability of radiotherapeutic responses. The choice of these operative procedures must be individualized for the patient following determination of the site, clinical stage, and histological type of the primary neoplasm. Similar principles guide the management of inflammatory breast cancers, which may be large, fixed, or ulcerated (see Chapters 67, 68, and 69).

As indicated in Chapters 13, 22, and 25, estrogen and progesterone receptor activity, ploidy and S-phase determination cytologic and nuclear grading indicators should be obtained on all pathological breast cancer specimens to aid the therapeutic planning of endocrine replacement and cytotoxic therapy should adverse prognostic indicators be evident. The prospective data available for analysis suggest that mean survival rates for patients receiving either chemotherapy or hormonal manipulation are high for patients who have positive estrogen/progesterone receptor activity and favorable biochemical and cellular growth phase indicators than for those who do not. Regardless of the pathological stage of the tumor or the receptor activity, the optimal chemotherapeutic regimen for patients with metastatic breast cancer is still evolving. Nonetheless, both the quantitative and qualitative values for receptor activity of the primary neoplasm and cellular/biochemical prognosticators are of significant value to the oncologist and should be obtained from the primary lesion and metastatic sites to prospectively guide subsequent therapy.

The proper technique for the processing of tissues that contain estrogen receptor (ER) and progesterone receptor (PR) activity is essential to the design and implementation of future chemotherapy protocols for specific patients; the surgeon's attention to the preservation and processing of biopsy tissues is mandatory. Despite the importance of the ER and PR activity and other cellular/biochemical and oncogene

TABLE 41–1. STEROID HORMONE RECEPTOR VERSUS ISCHEMIA TIME[17, 18]

Receptor (n = 11)	Ischemia Time (minutes)†				
	0	*30*	*60*	*90*	*150*
ER	100	79 ± 10‡	67 ± 11‡	54 ± 11‡	56 ± 13‡
PR	100	100 ± 21	101 ± 26	94 ± 14	84 ± 27
AR	100	57 ± 12‡	53 ± 15‡	28 ± 9†	42 ± 12‡

*Ischemia significantly decreased ER levels within the first 30 minutes ($p = 0.05$). ER values had sustained decrease throughout 150 minutes of ischemia. Similarly, AR levels were significantly lower by 30 minutes of ischemia ($p = 0.002$) and remained so throughout 150 minutes of ischemia. The largest decrease in ER and AR levels occurred within the first 30 minutes of ischemia. In contrast, PR levels were unchanged throughout 150 minutes of ischemia.
†Values are mean ± SEM, expressed as percent of control at baseline. AR = androgen receptor; ER = estrogen receptor; PR = progesterone receptor.
‡$p < 0.05$ compared with baseline by analysis of variance.

markers to guide future therapies, processing of neoplastic tissue for pathology, in all cases, must take *precedence* over determination of steroid receptor activity, and procurement of additional tissues to determine cellular, biochemical, and molecular prognostic characteristics that evaluate tumor phenotype (see Chapters 22, 24, and 25).

The surgeon should also be aware of the potential for the electrocautery to diminish steroid receptor activity. This has been confirmed by Ellis and associates[17, 18] and by Bland and colleagues[3] to be dependent on heat inactivation by the ambient temperature and by devascularization (Table 41–1). The procurement of primary breast cancer tissue for pathological diagnosis and for determination of quantitative and qualitative steroid receptor activity is best accomplished with the cold scalpel. This technique avoids the possibility of heat-induction artifact, tissue necrosis, cellular death, and temperature-dependent inactivation of steroid receptor activity in the procured tissues. Nonetheless, tumor excision with cautery can be used if the operator avoids direct contact of tumor specimen with the cautery blade. The indications and techniques for biopsy of suspicious breast masses are comprehensively reviewed in Chapter 40.

TOPOGRAPHICAL SURGICAL ANATOMY

Chapter 2 (Romrell and Bland, "Anatomy of the Breast, Axilla, Chest Wall, and Related Metastatic Sites") provides a detailed review of the anatomy of the breast, including discussions of regional vasculature, neurological structures, and lymphatics. Hollingshead[39] observed that the fibrous and fatty components of breast tissue occupied that interval between the second or third rib superiorly, with extension to the sixth or seventh ribs inferiorly. The breadth of extension includes the parasternal to the midaxillary lines. The glandular portion of the breast rests largely on the pectoral fascia and the serratus anterior musculature; however, mammary tissue extends typically into the anterior axillary fold (tail of Spence) and may be visible as a well-defined superolateral extension from the upper outer quadrant of breast tissue. Extent of the mammary tissue is ill-defined and varies considerably with patient habitus and lean muscle mass.

Parenchymal volume of the gland, with anterior and lateral projections, is variable and depends on lean body mass, habitus, age, and ovarian functional status. Because the ductal and lobular components are almost exclusively sensitive to the trophic effects of secretory estrogen and progestational compounds, the breast remains underdeveloped and rudimentary in the male. In men, short ducts with poorly developed acini are evident. Thus a deficiency of parenchymal fat and nipple-areola development are apparent and contribute to the nonspheroidal or flat appearance of the male breast.

Relative to the male breast, the nonparous breast is hemispheric and somewhat flattened above the nipple. The multiparous breast, on the other hand, is large and replaced in part with fat, which accounts for its lax, soft appearance; it rarely regains its initial configuration until menopause, when atrophy of glandular tissue is initiated. The breast is circumscribed anteriorly by a superficial layer and posteriorly by a deep layer of the superficial investing fascia of the chest wall. The superficial layer of the superficial fascia of the chest wall derives its anterior boundaries from the fibrous tissue of the tela subcutanea. Haagensen[31] observed the deep layer of the superficial fascia to be contiguous with the pectoral fascia.

Following loss of estrogen influence on breast parenchyma and ductal structures, the postmenopausal breast is consistently noted to lack parenchymal fat and active (proliferative) glandular components. Spratt and Donegan[61, 62] note the nonlactating breast to weigh between 150 g and 225 g, whereas the lactating organ may weigh as much as 500 g.

Neurological Innervation of the Pectoral Muscles

In major surgical texts, the surgical anatomy of the pectoral nerves and the innervation of the pectoral muscles has evoked only minimal interest. Major textbooks of surgical anatomy have long considered the names of the medial pectoral and lateral pectoral nerves on the basis of origin from the *brachial plexus*.

Therefore the names in classic anatomical teaching are *not* correlated with the anatomical position found at operation (Fig. 41–1). Moosman,[51] however, completed a detailed study of the pectoral nerves by dissection of 100 adult fixed and fresh cadaver pectoral regions (56 male and 44 female), and transposed the names of the medial and lateral pectoral nerves according to their anatomical relationship to the pectoral muscles and to the anterior chest wall. These nerves, sometimes referred to as the *anterior thoracic nerves*, originate cephalad and posterior to the axillary vein from an anastomotic nerve loop of variable size between the medial and lateral brachial plexus cords.

Moosman[51] noted in his anatomical dissections that the *lateral pectoral nerve* arises anatomically *medial* to the pectoralis minor and, in its course, to divide into two to four branches that pass downward and medial to supply the clavicular, manubrial, and

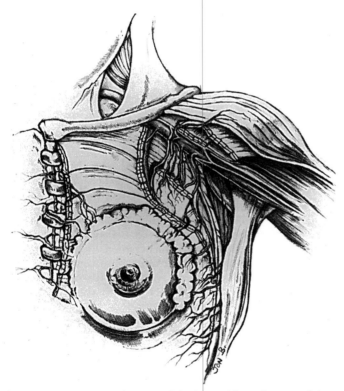

Figure 41–1 *Arteries and nerves of the breast. View of nerves of the axilla that provide innervation to the pectoral muscles and muscles of the chest wall and posterior axillary space. The long thoracic nerve is identified and protected at the juncture where the axillary vein passes over the second rib. Injury or division of this nerve will result in "winged scapula" due to paralysis of the serratus anterior. The thoracodorsal nerve is found in the posterior axillary space with origin medial to the thoracodorsal vessels. This nerve may accompany the thoracodorsal artery and vein en route to its innervation of the latissimus dorsi. Injury results in weakness of abduction; internal rotation of the shoulder will result. The medial (anterior thoracic) pectoral nerve is superficial to the axillary vein and lateral to the pectoralis minor muscle, which it variably penetrates en route to its innervation of the pectoralis major muscle. The lateral (anterior thoracic) pectoral nerve lies at the medial edge of the pectoralis minor muscle and superficial to the axillary vein. With origin from the lateral cord of the brachial plexus, this nerve supplies major motor innervation to the pectoralis major.*

sternal components of the pectoralis major muscle. Thereafter the nerve passes through the costocoracoid foramen with the thoracoacromial vessels and enters the interpectoral space to mix with tributaries of vascular origin to the muscle. Moosman observed that this nerve is larger than the medial pectoral nerve because of the greater volume of muscle it innervates.

The *medial pectoral nerve* is smaller (approximately 1 mm to 2 mm in diameter and 10 cm to 15 cm in length), with origin medial or posterior to the pectoralis minor. This nerve sends branches to the pectoralis minor and descends on its dorsal surface. Typically this nerve crosses the axillary vein and is accompanied by small tributaries from the axillary or thoracoacromial vessels. It enters the interpectoral space and supplies the lower third of the costoabdominal portion of the pectoralis major muscle. In this extensive review of the anatomy of the medial and pectoral nerve, Moosman[51] observed the relationship of the medial pectoral nerve to the pectoralis minor to be one of several variants: (1) descension as a single branch around the lateral border of the lower half of the muscle (38 percent); (2) division into two branches, with one branch passing *through* the muscle and the other *around* its lateral margin (32 percent); (3) descension as a single branch that passed *through* the muscle (22 percent); and (4) descension as two or three branches of varying size, each of which passed through the muscle often at different levels (8 percent). He observed motor branches to the pectoralis major coursing through the pectoralis minor in 62 percent of cases.

In rare circumstances, the medial pectoral nerve may pass through the medial muscular components of the pectoralis minor or, in other cases, may remain entirely on its medial surface. When numerous branches arise from the major trunks, a more diminutive size can be expected for branches that innervate the pectoralis major. The nerve is observed to remain relatively large when it is a single branch, while multiple branches passing through the muscle may be of thread size.[51]

Regardless of the anatomical nomenclature used, the surgeon must be cognizant of the potential for damage to the nerve supply to the pectoralis muscles at all levels of dissection. Manipulation, traction, electrocautery, or removal may destroy the lateral or medial pectoral nerves unless they are carefully separated from nerve branches of variable size.

For purposes of clarity and consistency, the editors have retained the classic anatomical description and nomenclature for the pectoral (anterior thoracic) nerves and the accompanying neurovascular bundles (see Section II, Chapter 2, Romrell and Bland, "Anatomy of the Breast, Axilla, and Chest Wall, and Related Metastatic Sites"). The name of the neurovascular bundle (lateral or medial) is synonymous with its course (position) in the axilla. Classic anatomy teaches that the pectoral nerves take the name of the brachial cord (medial or lateral) from which they originate. In the technical description of operative procedures within this chapter and in anatomical descriptions in other sections of this text, we have retained the classic nomenclature.

Vascular Distribution

Nutrient arterial supply to the skin and breast is via branches of the *lateral thoracic arteries*, the *acromiothoracic branch of the axillary artery*, and the *internal mammary artery*.[1] The venous drainage system includes the intercostal veins, which traverse the posterior aspect of the breast from the second or third through the sixth or seventh intercostal spaces to terminate and enter posteriorly into the vertebral veins. The intercostal veins may arborize centrally with the azygos system to terminate in the superior vena cava. The deep venous drainage of the breast in large part parallels the pectoral branches of the acromiothoracic artery and the lateral thoracic artery.

The large epithelial and mesenchymal surface area of the superior, central, and lateral aspects of the breast is drained by tributaries that enter the *axillary vein*. Venous supply from the pectoralis major and minor muscles also drain into tributaries that enter the axillary vein. Perforating veins of the *internal mammary venous system* drain the medial aspect of the breast and the pectoralis major muscle. This large venous plexus can be observed to traverse the intercostal musculature and terminate in the innominate vein, providing a direct embolic route to the venous capillary network of the lungs. Each plexus of veins in the lateral and medial aspects of the breast is observed to have multiple, racemose anastomotic connections.

Lymphatic Drainage and Routes for Metastases

The rich and elaborate lymphatic drainage generally parallels the arterial and venous supply of the breast. This lymphatic flow is primarily unidirectional except in subareolar and central aspects of the breast or in circumstances in which physiological lymphatic obstruction occurs as a consequence of neoplastic, inflammatory, or developmental processes that initiate a reversal of flow with bidirectional egress of lymph.[28] This bidirectional lymphatic flow (see Figs. 2–12 and 2–14) may account for metastatic proliferation in sites remote from the primary neoplasm (e.g., the opposite breast and axilla). The delicate lymph vessels of the corium are valveless and encircle the lobular parenchyma to enter each echelon of the regional lymphatic nodes in a progressive and orderly fashion (e.g., Level I → Level II → Level III). As indicated in Chapter 2 (see Figs. 2–14, 2–15, and 2–16), multiple lymphatic capillaries anastomose and fuse to form fewer lymph channels that subsequently terminate in the large left thoracic duct or the smaller right lymphatic duct (see Chapter 2, Figs. 2–6 and 2–16). As a consequence of the predominant unidirectional flow of lymph, two accessory drainage routes exist for lymph en route to nodes of the apex of the axilla and include the *transpectoral* and the *retropectoral* routes, as defined by Anson and McVay.[1] Lymphatics of the *transpectoral* or *interpectoral* routes that occupy the position between the pectoralis major and minor muscles were described by Rotter, a German pathologist, and bear his name: Rotter's nodes. Cody and coworkers[11] and Netter[53] observed Rotter's nodes to be present in up to 75 percent of individuals, with an average of two to three nodes per patient. Cody and colleagues[11] observed that 0.5 percent of node-negative patients and 8.2 percent of patients who were axillary node positive had evidence of Rotter lymph node metastases. This observation was rarely reported by Haagensen.[31] Therefore, although the Patey axillary dissection, included in the Halsted radical[32] and in the modified radical mastectomy, removes the interpectoral Rotter group en bloc, this nodal group plays only a diminutive role in the diagnosis and therapy of breast cancer. The retropectoral lymphatics, however, may play a more important physiological role in drainage of the breast, because they are exposed to the superior and internal portions of the mammary glands. These lymphatics arborize lateral and posterior to the surface of the pectoralis major muscle and terminate at the apex of the axilla. To achieve an adequate en bloc resection of major axillary nodal groups, a thorough conceptualization of breast lymphatic drainage is essential to the surgeon. Familiarization with the anatomy of this area is essential for staging and for curative resection.

Section II, Chapter 2, Romrell and Bland, "Anatomy of the Breast, Axilla, Chest Wall, and Related Metastatic Sites," deals with the *principal axillary nodal groups* as described by Anson and McVay.[1] Figure 41–2 topographically depicts anatomical Levels I to III of the axillary contents with the relations to the neurovascular bundle, the pectoralis minor, the latissimus dorsi, and the chest wall. The following principal axillary nodal groups are included in *Level I*:

1. The *external mammary group*, which parallels the course of the lateral thoracic artery from the sixth or seventh rib to the axillary vein. This group occupies the loose areolar tissue inferior and lateral to the pectoralis major muscle in the medial distal axillary space.

2. The *subscapular group*, which is contiguous with thoracodorsal branches of the subscapular vessels. This group extends from the ventral surface of the axillary vein to the lateral thoracic chest wall and includes loose areolar tissue on the serratus anterior and subscapularis musculature.

3. The *axillary vein group*, which is the most laterally placed nodal group of the axillary space. This group also contains the largest group of nodes in the axilla and is observed to be caudal and ventral to the surface of the axillary vein.

Level II, or the *central nodal group*, is immediately beneath the pectoralis minor muscle and is the most

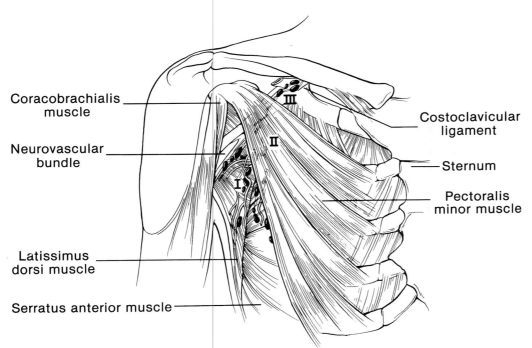

Coracobrachialis muscle

Neurovascular bundle

Latissimus dorsi muscle

Serratus anterior muscle

Costoclavicular ligament

Sternum

Pectoralis minor muscle

Figure 41–2 *Topographical anatomical depiction of Levels I, II, and III of the axillary contents with relation to the neurovascular bundle, pectoralis minor, latissimus dorsi, posterior axillary space, and chest wall. Level I comprises three principal axillary nodal groups, including the external mammary group, the subscapular group, and the axillary vein (lateral) group. Level II, the central nodal group, is centrally placed immediately beneath the pectoralis minor muscle. The subclavicular (apical) group is designated Level III nodes and is superomedial to the pectoralis minor muscle.*

centrally located of the axillary lymphatic groups. This nodal group is located between the anterior and posterior axillary fold and occupies a superficial position beneath the skin and fascia of the midaxilla. The highest and most medially placed of the lymph node groups is the *subclavicular (apical group)*, designated as *Level III*. This is the cephalomedial lymph node group that is located just proximal to the termination of the axillary vein at its confluence with the subclavian vein at the level of *Halsted's (costoclavicular) ligament* (condensation of the clavipectoral fascia). Figure 41–2 depicts the position of the nodes relative to the pectoralis minor muscle and the posterior axillary space. These nodal groups are described relative to topographical anatomical relationships with the pectoralis minor muscle and the medial, lateral, and posterior axillary space. These lymphatics may be different from the nodal groups described by pathologists to indicate the area of metastatic involvement within the axilla.

EVOLUTION OF SURGICAL TECHNIQUES FOR MASTECTOMY

In 1894, Halsted[32] and Meyer[49] simultaneously reported their operations for treatment of cancer of the breast. By demonstrating superior local and regional control rates using en bloc radical resection techniques, these eminent surgeons established the radical mastectomy as the "state-of-the-art" modality of that era to control cancer of the breast. Subsequently, many modifications of the original incision developed by Halsted have been reported and include those of Meyer, Kocher, Rodman, Stewart, Warren, Greenough, Orr, and MacFee, to mention only a few

variations of the incision.[19] Many of the original incisions were developed to permit multiple approaches for extirpation of the mamma and to allow access to the axillary contents.

The Halsted and Meyer radical mastectomies differed technically in the sequence in which the breast and nodes were removed. Halsted insisted on primary resection of the breast and pectoral muscles before dissection of the axillary contents. In contrast, the Meyer technique (modified Halsted incision) completed the axillary dissection first, which was followed in sequence by breast and pectoral muscle resections, respectively. As indicated in Figure 41–3, the result achieved and the final cosmetic appearance for the Halsted and Meyer mastectomies are similar. Both procedures use a vertical incision to facilitate detachment of the pectoralis major from the clavicle and humerus and removal of the pectoralis minor from the coracoid process of the scapula. The incisions that have been subsequently adopted by various European and American surgeons are indicated in Figure 41–3 and represent incision modifications for operable breast cancer that presents in each quadrant of the organ. It should be noted that Halsted[32] and Meyer[49] strongly advocated the necessity of en bloc resections for extirpation of the breast and the contents of the axilla but had little appreciation for clinical staging and the ultimate consequences of systemic disease. At that time, no modalities existed to provide effective cytoreduction of the advanced primary lesion; thus advanced stages of disease were extirpated with the use of wider skin margins and larger flaps. For this reason, incision modifications that incorporate breast resection and wound closure were developed.

Eminent breast surgeons of the late nineteenth

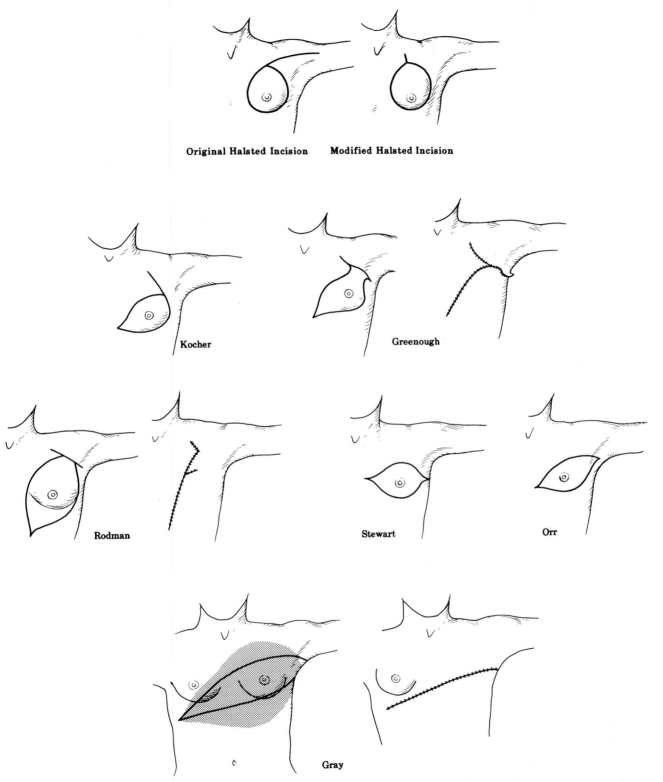

Figure 41–3 *Variants of the radical mastectomy incision used in the therapy of primary carcinoma of the breast by various surgeons. The original Halsted incision was revised to avoid encroachment on the cephalic vein, which was preserved in subsequent procedures.*

and early twentieth centuries appreciated early in the formulation of therapeutic principles that the total mastectomy incision should incorporate both the nipple and the biopsy site to reduce the possibility of tumor implantation in the wound. In original dissections of the axilla, both Halsted[32] and Meyer[49] advocated complete axillary dissection of three (all) nodal levels from the latissimus dorsi muscle laterally to the thoracic outlet medially. Both surgeons routinely sacrificed the long thoracic nerve and the thoracodorsal neurovascular bundle en bloc with the axillary contents. Therefore it is not surprising that much of the initial criticism leveled at the radical mastectomy in the treatment of breast carcinoma concerned itself with the limitation of motion in the shoulder and the ipsilateral lymphedema that followed the surgery. It may also be argued that the survival rates for these patients, especially those with advanced local and regional disease, were not increased in proportion to the resultant disabilities (e.g., the "winged scapula" and shoulder fixation) evident with the procedures. Subsequently, Haagensen[31] advocated preservation of the long thoracic nerve to avoid the winged scapula disability and motor apraxia evident with loss of innervation to the serratus anterior. Additionally, Haagensen[31] commonly advocated removal of the thoracodorsal neurovascular bundle (with neural innervation to the latissimus dorsi muscle) to allow clearance of the subscapular and external mammary lymphatics that may follow the course of this neurovascular structure. However, the majority of breast surgeons currently preserve *both* the long thoracic and the thoracodorsal nerves in the absence of gross invasion by the neoplasm or nodal fixation to these nerves. These principles are strictly enforced to ensure function of the scapula and to preserve viability and function of the latissimus dorsi such that myocutaneous breast reconstruction may be considered at a future date.

It should be noted that contemporary modifications of the Halsted or Meyer radical mastectomy, with preservation of the long thoracic nerve, can be performed with little or no increase in morbidity when compared with the simple mastectomy.[27, 28] Additionally, any argument based on the value of the simple versus the radical procedure should be concerned with the long-term survival of the patient, which is the ultimate goal of therapy. To deny the patient the benefit of an adequate operative procedure on the basis of difficulty in placing cosmetic incisions or difficulty with wound closure is tantamount to oblivious disregard of indisputable tenet that portends local or regional recurrence of disease.

The highly regarded and significant contributions of D. H. Patey[54, 55] of the Institute of Clinical Research, Middlesex Hospital, London, should be recognized. His careful clinical development and scientific demonstration of the worth of the "modified radical mastectomy" technique are quite laudable. In Britain in the 1930s, only a small minority of physicians questioned the absolute necessity of the radical mastectomy for carcinoma of lesser size with absence of

fixation to the pectoral muscles (stage I or II). Three major influences led Patey to consider alternatives and design the modified radical mastectomy technique. The first and most important consideration was the development and organization of radiation therapy. The second influence was the growing feeling of dissatisfaction with Sampson Handley's theory of "lymphatic permeation" as the primary process for the dissemination of carcinoma of the breast—a theory that, in its day, provided a logical pathological basis for some of the technical details of the radical mastectomy.[54] Lastly, with newer techniques for the study of lymphatic anatomy, Patey was able to refute the unproven postulates on which the original radical operations were based.[28, 61] Thereafter, Mr. Patey and his colleagues developed the technique for incontinuity removal of the breast and axillary contents with preservation of the pectoralis major muscle. This technique removed the pectoralis minor, like the standard radical operation, as an essential step to provide complete clearance of the axillary contents. Thereafter, objective demonstration of the efficacy for removal of axillary lymphatics with the technique was proven with lymphangiography by Kendall and associates[41] in 1963. Although this operation was performed by Patey for the first time in 1932, it was not adopted as a routine alternative to the standard radical mastectomy until late 1936.[61]

Although Patey is credited with the formulation and implementation of the modified radical mastectomy as a standard approach for operable breast cancer, Auchincloss[2] and Madden[48] also developed technical variants of the modified radical mastectomy. As described earlier, the Patey mastectomy differs from the Halsted mastectomy in that the pectoralis major muscle is preserved. Patey acknowledged the importance of the complete axillary dissection and appreciated the anatomical necessity for preservation of the medial and lateral pectoral (anterior thoracic) nerves, which may serve as dual innervation to the pectoralis major. In contrast, the Madden[48] and Auchincloss[2] modified radical mastectomies advocated preservation of *both* the pectoralis major and minor muscles. The similarities of the approaches were that these techniques required total mastectomy with at least partial axillary lymph node dissection. Because these approaches preserved the pectoralis minor, dissection of the apical (subclavicular, Level III) nodes was restricted, and in all cases, nodal recovery was less than with the Patey modified technique. The advantage of the Auchincloss[2] and Madden[48] procedures may be the higher probability for preservation of the medial pectoral nerve, which courses in the lateral neurovascular bundle of the axilla and may course through the pectoralis minor to supply the lateral border of the pectoralis major muscle. Expectantly, the Madden and Auchincloss techniques dissect only Levels I and II nodes and leave Level III lymphatics intact. Some surgeons advocate preservation of the pectoralis minor and simply detach the tendinous portion of the muscle from the coracoid process of the scapula to allow complete dissection of Level III nodes to Halsted's ligament. On completion of the nodal dissection, the tendon of the pectoralis minor was reapproximated to the coracoid with stainless steel wire or nonabsorbable suture.

Advanced students of breast surgery should recognize that incisions for the modified radical mastectomy are narrow, and wounds are commonly closed primarily. In contrast, radical procedures use wide incision margins, and skin is routinely grafted to wound defects. The application of modern radiobiological techniques and cytoreductive chemotherapy presently does not require primary incisions that totally ablate the skin of the breast (see Fig. 41–3). Before the application of modern adjuvant techniques, incisions for large tumors that were considered to be locally advanced (because of ulceration, edema, and other grave signs) were designed to encompass these lesions with wide margins.

All skin flaps should be designed so that the incision incorporates skin at least 1 cm from the periphery of the tumor in three dimensions. In principle, less skin is excised when lesions are located deep within the breast and are small in transverse diameter (T1 < 2 cm). As indicated in Chapter 2, viable breast tissue is anatomically distributed on the chest wall from the sternum to the axilla and from the clavicle to the aponeurosis of the rectus abdominis tendon. Haagensen[31] demonstrated that small foci of glandular tissue can be histologically identified in close proximity to the dermis just beneath the superficial fascia. Halsted[32] and Haagensen[31] each considered that wide skin excision of at least 5 cm in all directions from the tumor was essential because of the rich superficial lymphatic channels of the central subareolar tissue and subcutaneous dermal lymphatic plexuses of the breast. The rationale of the classic radical and modified radical mastectomies is increasingly being challenged because of the availability of adjuvant modalities that enhance local and regional control with potential lengthening of disease-free and overall survival rates. These tenets form the anatomical and pathological basis for the skin-sparing mastectomy, which is discussed subsequently in this chapter.

Issues continue to be debated with regard to the *thickness* of skin flaps that should be elevated in the planning of the total mastectomy as part of the radical or modified radical procedure. Krohn and colleagues[42] report a two-arm study to evaluate the necessity of the ultrathin skin flap and the autogenous skin graft as methods to enhance local wound control and 5- and 10-year survival. A similar group of women who underwent radical mastectomy with narrow margins of skin excision, with primary wound closure and without ultrathin flaps, had comparable 5- and 10-year survival and local recurrence rates. Wound complications, hospital stay, and subsequent lymphedema, however, were significantly greater in the patients with thinner skin flaps. Most surgeons acknowledge that superior cosmetic results are achievable with well-vascularized flaps and the

avoidance of split-thickness skin grafting. We maintain these basic tenets and avoid ultrathin flaps. Flaps developed at the plane of insertion of Cooper's ligament in the cutis with subcutaneous fat ensure extirpation of the underlying breast parenchyma. In general, flaps of 7- to 8-mm thickness usually ensure generous vascularity to the skin. As much subcutaneous fat is preserved as is consistent with complete breast resection. Although the deep layer of the superficial investing fascia that intervenes between the subcutaneous fat and the breast tissue is easily identified, the thickness of this well-vascularized flap varies considerably with the patient's habitus and lean body mass.

Total mastectomy for operable cancer that is not amenable to conservation surgical techniques has been previously addressed. In principle, advanced primary lesions (T2 or T3), with pectoralis major fixation, high-lying lesions, and perhaps some lesions with grave signs should be treated by radical or modified radical techniques. As previously discussed, the operations designed by Halsted, his predecessors, and his students reflect the necessity of designing wider flaps with large incisions for advanced primary cancers (T3A, T3B, T4) to encompass the primary lesion by at least 5 cm. When considering the advanced primary lesions that were treated in that era without adjuvant techniques, the necessity of larger resections can be rationalized, because surgery was the only option for treatment.

Design of incisions for removal of the entire mammary gland (total or simple mastectomy) must incorporate the nipple-areola complex with the primary tumor in a three-dimensional aspect such that margins are free of disease.[29] Donegan and coworkers[16] previously determined that incisions that resect skin and breast parenchyma at a distance of more than 4 cm from any margin of the palpable tumor achieve nothing therapeutically. At present, many surgeons consider a 1- to 2-cm margin adequate to achieve local control without tumor implantation. Intraoperative frozen section for marginal clearance is appropriate, especially margins 1 cm or less from the index neoplasm. As discussed previously in Chapter 40, incisions placed in the breast for suspicious masses must be planned with consideration for the subsequent need for total mastectomy. Incisions should incorporate the primary biopsy scar, which should be well planned at the time of biopsy to allow complete extirpation of the neoplasm with the definitive mastectomy. When the primary breast lesion has been totally removed with the original biopsy as an excisional technique, incisions at the time of total mastectomy should incorporate the skin and scar of the biopsy site by a 1-cm margin in all directions. We prefer incisions that are slightly oblique from the transverse line and that extend cephalad toward the axilla. Under no circumstances should the design of a cosmetic scar compromise the successful extirpation of the primary neoplasm in any way. Split-thickness skin grafting with T3 or T4 primary neoplasms becomes necessary when wider margins and larger flaps are required.

Figures 41–4 through 41–9 depict the various locations of breast primaries in which adequate therapy, with or without irradiation and chemotherapy, necessitates total mastectomy, which is completed with conventional technique in which reconstruction is not planned. For all mastectomy procedures, note that wide (radical) skin margin (> 5 cm) excisions are not considered essential for locoregional disease control. However, skin excisions of at least 1 to 2 cm distant are necessary to ensure pathology-free margins. Margins in excess of 2 cm are technically feasible for most total mastectomies in which reconstruction (early or delayed) will not be completed. Preoperative consideration should be given to the skin-sparing technique (see discussion later in this chapter) when reconstruction is desired.

DESIGN OF INCISIONS FOR MASTECTOMY IN THE TREATMENT OF BREAST CANCER

Central and Subareolar Primary Lesions

Figure 41–4 depicts the design of the classic Stewart elliptical skin incision (see Fig. 41–3) that is used for

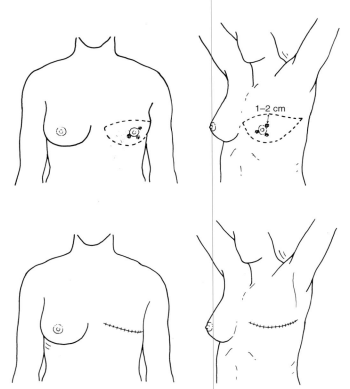

Figure 41–4   *Design of the classic Stewart elliptical incision for central and subareolar primary lesions of the breast. The medial extent of the incision ends at the margin of the sternum. The lateral extent of the skin incision should overlie the anterior margin of the latissimus dorsi. The design of the skin incision should incorporate the primary neoplasm en bloc with margins that are 1 to 2 cm from the cranial and caudal edges of the tumor.*

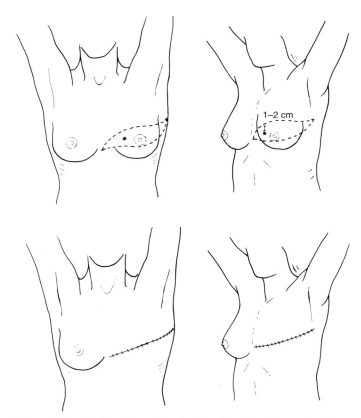

Figure 41–5   *Design of the obliquely placed modified Stewart incision for cancer of the inner quadrant of the breast. The medial extent of the incision often must incorporate skin to the midsternum to allow a 1- to 2-cm margin in all directions from the edge of the tumor. Lateral extent of the incision ends at the anterior margin of the latissimus.*

mastectomy of subareolar or central breast primaries. The original biopsy is preferably done via a periareolar incision for lesions in this location. The residual scan should have measurements for the cephalad and caudad extents of the incision to include at least a 1-cm margin. Availability of adequate skin to complete a primary closure is rarely difficult in the pendulous or large breast. For the majority of patients with small breasts, the Stewart incision will allow primary closure of skin except when more than 4 to 5 cm of skin are encompassed in the primary resection or if evidence of skin devascularization is apparent following completion of the procedure. Loss of skin secondary to ultrathin dissection planes or trauma to the flaps may necessitate even wider resections of skin margins.

Figure 41–5 shows an optional elliptical incision in the contour of the breast for an inner quadrant primary lesion. This incision would perhaps best be described as the *modified Stewart incision*, which has a predominant extension in a more oblique and cephalad direction toward the ipsilateral axilla. The Stewart incision is commonly preferred by plastic surgeons anticipating reconstruction with myocutaneous flaps, especially when a contralateral simple mastectomy is planned for treatment of benign or potentially malignant disease or as a prophylactic procedure.

Lesions of the Upper Outer or Lower Inner Quadrants

Figures 41–6 and 41–7 denote the incision design for operable breast cancer in the upper outer or lower inner quadrants. Minimal skin margins of 1 to 2 cm from the primary neoplasm are incorporated in a *modified Orr incision* that is slightly oblique from the transverse line with cephalad extension toward the axilla. Similar to the Orr and Stewart incisions, although somewhat more oblique, these incisions lend themselves to cosmetically satisfactory breast reconstruction using myocutaneous or subpectoral augmentation breast implants.

Lesions of the Upper Inner Quadrants

Lesions of the upper inner quadrants of the breast represent the most difficult to manage because of their anatomical location. The surgeon should recognize the inherent problems encountered with elevation of skin flaps that allow adequate surgical margins while providing cosmesis for wound closure and potential reconstruction. The surgeon is able to develop a 1- to 2-cm margin for lesions that are in

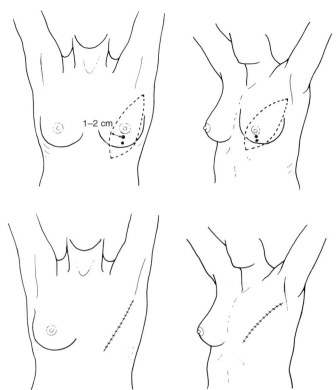

Figure 41–7 *Variation of the* Orr *incision for lower inner and vertically placed (6 o'clock) lesions of the breast. The design of the skin incision is identical to that of Figure 41–5, with attention directed to margins of 1 to 2 cm.*

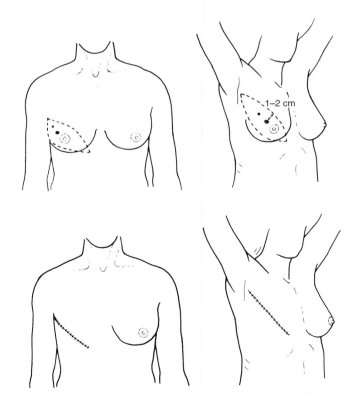

Figure 41–6 *Design of the classic* Orr *oblique incision for carcinoma of the upper outer quadrants of the breast. The skin incision is placed 1 to 2 cm from the margin of the tumor in an oblique plane that is directed cephalad toward the ipsilateral axilla. This incision is a variant of the original Greenough, Kocher, and Rodman techniques for flap development.*

this quadrant, providing the lesion is not cephalad (infraclavicular). These lesions may be operated via the modified Stewart incision. Commonly the surgeon encounters the dilemma of designing an elliptical incision that is widely based near the cephalomedial aspect of the breast to incorporate a 1- to 2-cm margin of the tumor with extension laterally and inferiorly such that the incision terminates at the anterior axillary line (Fig. 41–8). The surgeon should plan the cephalic portion of the incision for the superior flap such that adequate access to the pectoralis major and to the axillary contents is ensured.

Lesions of the Lower Outer Quadrants

Lesions of the lower outer quadrants of the breast should have an incision design similar to those of the upper inner quadrant, with margins of 1 to 2 cm around the primary lesion (Fig. 41–9) and with maximum extension of the cephalad margin to provide access to flaps for dissection of the pectoralis major and the axillary contents.

High-lying (Infraclavicular) Lesions

With large lesions (T2, T3, T4) that are high lying, infraclavicular, or fixed to the pectoralis major, incisions designed to provide a 1- to 2-cm margin will

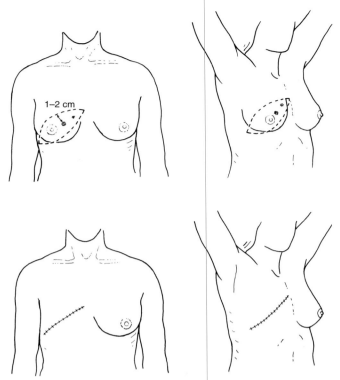

Figure 41–8 *Design of skin flaps for upper inner quadrant primary tumors of the breast. The cephalad margin of the flap must be designed to allow access for dissection of the axilla. With flap margins 1 to 2 cm from the tumor, variation in the medial extent of the incision is expectant and may extend beyond the edge of the sternum.*

On occasion, the modified Stewart incision can incorporate the tumor en bloc, provided that the cancer is not too high on the breast and craniad from the nipple-areola complex. All incision designs must be inclusive of the nipple-areola when total mastectomy is planned with primary therapy.

necessitate skin grafting of the defect. The original Halsted and Meyer incisions, with subsequent modifications by Greenough, Rodman, and Gray (see Fig. 41–3), are used for treatment of these primary lesions of T2, T3, and T4 size.[27] For T1 lesions in this

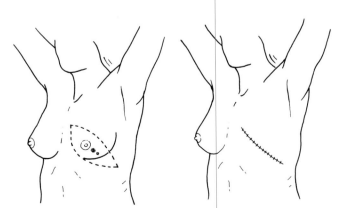

Figure 41–9 *Incisions for cancer of the lower outer quadrants of the breast. The surgeon should design incisions that achieve margins of 1 to 2 cm from the tumor with cephalad margins that allow access for dissection of the axilla. The medial extent is the margin of the sternum. Laterally, the inferior extent of the incision is the latissimus.*

position, design of an elliptical incision placed in a vertical dimension from the clavicle provides adequate access for axillary dissection and clearing of the pectoralis major muscle when indicated. Figure 41–10 depicts the design of the vertical, elliptical incision for these high-lying lesions and the vertical closure. Because these incisions are placed perpendicular to Langer's lines, cosmesis is minimized and the planes of cleavage for the medial breast are lost.

SKIN-SPARING MASTECTOMY

Mastectomy with Limited Skin Excision: Rationale and Technique of the "Skin-Sparing" Mastectomy

Wide skin excision is routinely employed with every radical and modified mastectomy. A mastectomy with wide skin excision is often inclusive of an excision that is in excess of 30 to 50 percent of the breast skin. This is removed as an ellipse, usually measured 10 cm (width) by 20 cm (length), and is closed primarily. The elliptical excision facilitates removing the dog-ears that are technically created by the wide skin removal and subsequent tension of excessive tissue at the terminal points of skin closure.

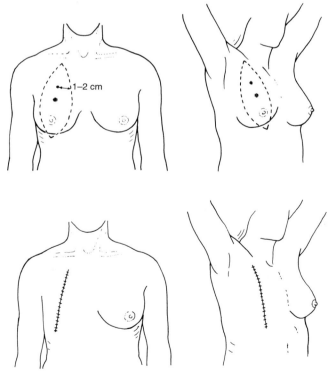

Figure 41–10 *Depiction of skin flaps for lesions of the breast that are high lying, infraclavicular, or fixed to the pectoralis major muscle. Fixation to the muscle and/or chest wall necessitates Halsted radical mastectomy with skin margins of a minimal 2 cm. Skin grafting is necessary when large margins of skin are resected for T3 and T4 cancers. Primary closure for T1 and some T2 tumors is often possible. General principles for skin-sparing techniques.*

Limited skin excision can be defined as excision of the nipple/areola complex, the skin around the biopsy site, and the skin within 2 to 3 cm of the tumor margin. This usually amounts to 5 to 10 percent of the breast skin and is either approximated primarily or closed with an autogenous myocutaneous flap that is used to replace the breast volume. Dog-ears do not occur with this technique, because the limited skin removal does not initiate skin contracture with closure.

Over the course of the twentieth century, the clinical guidelines for breast skin excision with mastectomy have developed anecdotally, and have been applied by convention. Further, the benefits of wide versus limited skin excision have not been subjected to prospective randomized trials. Because local-regional surgical control of breast cancer has improved over the last 60 years, the extent of the breast skin excision with mastectomy has decreased proportionally. Standards of practice have sequentially evolved from (1) total excision of the breast skin, to (2) wide excision without primary closure, to (3) wide excision with primary closure, and finally to (4) the "skin-sparing mastectomy." The indications and techniques for limited skin excision with mastectomy are reviewed here.

Factors Affecting Local Recurrence

With the increasing acceptance and application of breast conservation techniques for the therapy of ductal carcinoma *in situ* and invasive neoplasms of lobular and ductal origin, it is essential that the surgeon determine whether adequate excision margins are achieved to confer long-term local control. Gilliland and coworkers[26] and Johnson and associates[40] determined the necessity of total mastectomy with and without node dissection; with the exception of advanced disease (T3, T4 tumors), immediate breast reconstruction can be completed without any effect on the quality or duration of survival. As noted by Johnson and colleagues, local recurrence is usually a harbinger of systemic disease and, predictably, factors for local recurrence also represent prognostic indicators of survival. The 1992 report by Kurtz[44] reviewed common host and histological features that influence local failure following breast conservation and irradiation to the intact breast for clinical stage I and II disease. This author determined that the significant features that correlate with increased risk are young age at time of primary therapy and the presence of an extensive intraductal component within the invasive index (primary) neoplasm. Additionally, this clinical study determined that adequacy (volume) of the surgical excision, the use of systemic adjuvant therapy, and high-quality radiation therapy technique all contribute to a reduction in the risk of local-regional recurrence.

Biological Factors: Effect on Local Recurrence

Biological factors related to the tumor phenotype and cellular characteristics overshadow all other considerations in assessing various treatment modalities, including total excision of the breast. With the increasing acceptance and application of breast conservation techniques for treatment of both *in situ* and invasive neoplasms of lobular and ductal origin, it is essential that the surgeon determine whether adequate excisional margins are achieved to confer long-term local control. Many investigators* acknowledge the importance of patient selection to achieve optimal disease-free survival relative to local-regional recurrence within the ipsilateral mastectomy site. The large prospective analysis ($n = 1036$) by the German Breast Cancer Study Group for therapy of T1N0M0 disease concluded that the width of the margin of excision (in centimeters) had no impact on prognosis.[56] This analysis of patients who were randomized between breast preservation and mastectomy did establish conclusively, however, that poorer disease-free survival was associated with microscopically involved margins in the conservation technique when compared with the mastectomy study group (75 versus 90 percent at 3 years). Tumor size and tumor grade were also prognostic factors that accurately predicted recurrence. Age, ER/PR status, menopausal status, histological tumor type, and therapy (mastectomy versus breast preservation) were not significant predictive factors.

The full realization of the impact of contemporary developments in molecular and genetic markers as prognostic indicators of local and regional recurrences has not yet been assimilated into practice.[4] As these tests gain acceptance, our recognition of patients with unfavorable disease will be facilitated at the outset following cellular, biochemical, and molecular-genetic analysis of the primary neoplasm. Treatment can then be designed individually, rather than as done presently using one variant of the mastectomy for all patients. Moreover, the comprehensive prospective analysis of the National Surgical Adjuvant Breast and Bowel Project (NSABP) by Fisher and associates[22] suggests that the extent (type) of mastectomy and regional node excision are not associated with significant differences in survival from more radical procedures.

Tumor Volume (Size): Effect on Local Recurrence

For patients who are *not* treated with irradiation following breast conservation surgery, tumor size is an important determinant of risk for local recurrence, as reported in data from the NSABP by Fisher and co-investigators.[21, 24] Fowble et al,[25] Stotter et al,[63] and Kurtz et al[45] note that larger neoplasms (e.g., T3, T4) comprise the vast majority of these local failures. These findings are further amplified by the large, long-term study by Kurtz of operable T1 and T2 invasive breast cancers. Within the range of tumor diameter appropriate to breast conservation, this investigator[44] determined that the size of the

---

*See references 15, 30, 43, 44, 46, 56, 58, 59, 63, and 66.

TABLE 41–2.　CRUDE RATE OF LOCAL RECURRENCE IN THE BREAST FOR 1350 STAGE I AND II PATIENTS AS A FUNCTION OF CLINICAL BREAST TUMOR SIZE*

TNM Stage	Clinical Tumor Size (cm)	Local Recurrence (%)	P Value
T1a, T1b	<1	29/255 (11.4)	NS
T1c	1.1–2.0	45/438 (10.3)	NS
T2	2.1–3.0	40/392 (10.2)	NS
T2	3.1–4.0	21/179 (11.7)	NS
T2	4.1–5.0	21/86 (13.9)	NS

NS, Nonsignificant.

*Patients were treated at the Cancer Institute and associated clinics in Marseille between 1962 and 1981 (median follow-up 10 years).

Modified from Kurtz JM: Eur J Cancer 28:660–666, 1992, with kind permission from Elsevier Science Ltd, The Boulevard, Langford Lane, Kidlington OX5 16B, UK.

primary lesion had no apparent influence on the risk for local recurrence, provided that macroscopically complete resection was achieved (Table 41–2). Although the analysis by Kurtz includes radiation of the intact breast with the goal of preserving the organ, others[15, 43] have come to the same conclusions in patients undergoing mastectomy alone. Kroll and colleagues[43] and Dao and Nemoto[15] reiterate that this reduction in the local recurrence rate is evident when the adequacy of resection is confirmed.

Holland and coworkers[38] determined in serial subgross sectioning of mastectomy specimens that the percentage of breasts harboring residual foci 2 cm distal to the edge of the index tumor was similar for T1 (T1a, T1b, T1c) cancers 2 cm in diameter to those between 2 and 5 cm (T2) in transverse diameter. Data from virtually all large series designed to corroborate these findings determined that local failure is not more frequent in operable T2 than in T1 primary tumors. However, from a technical perspective, adequate local excision with macroscopically clear margins is more difficult to achieve in the T2 lesion, especially for patients with small breasts.

Breast Skin Excision: Effect on Local Recurrence

In 1963, Dao and Nemoto[15] confirmed that the risks associated with skin preservation in mastectomy are more theoretical than actual. In a series of 135 consecutive cases of breast cancer, these investigators observed that skin recurrence was evident in 27.5 percent of locally advanced tumors, but the incidence was only 2 percent for patients with nonadvanced disease. Kroll and associates[43] determined that a low recurrence rate (1.2 percent) can be achieved with conservation of the uninvolved breast skin. In this study, patients undergoing mastectomy with immediate autogenous breast reconstruction were treated by skin-sparing mastectomy. The limited breast skin excision included the nipple and areola, as well as a 1-cm margin around the previous biopsy scar. Of significance, this mixed group of T1, T2, T3 and Tx TNM-staged cancers did not demonstrate any addi-

tional risk for local recurrence when treated with a 1-cm skin margin around the biopsy scar and even narrower cutaneous margins for deep or small tumors. Both of these studies, therefore, relate local recurrences more to biological aspects of the tumor rather than extirpative (technical) differences of the procedure. Dao and Nemoto[15] concluded that "skin recurrence is nothing more than metastasis at an additional site in patients with widespread disease." These authors noted that "the frequency of skin recurrence is governed by the pathological stage of the disease, rather than by the amount of skin that is removed."

Evolution of Breast Skin Excision with Mastectomy

The Radical Mastectomy

The halstedian principles embodied an anatomical basis for cancer surgery, which presumed an improved survival with the more radical extirpative approach (see Chapter 42). Recurrences were usually interpreted as evidence of inadequate local-regional therapy, and therapy was rarely directed to systemic disease.[42] This premise dictated therapy of breast cancers managed in the halstedian era, because the majority were T3 and T4 neoplasms. Extremely wide excision of skin was established as an absolute dictum for the cancer cure, and this concept prevailed for 80 years, well into the twentieth century. Before World War II, mastectomies for cancer were designed to remove *all* breast tissue, and included the pectoralis major and minor muscles and the axillary lymph nodes. There was some variation, however, in the management of the volume and technique for breast skin excision (see Fig. 41–3).

Near-Total Excision of the Breast Skin Without Undermining to Develop Skin Flaps. In concurrent evolution of the technique of mastectomy, Halsted and Meyer advocated extremely wide skin excision because of the advanced presentation of disease at that time (T3, T4) for the majority of patients.[32, 33, 47, 49] Primary closure was rarely attempted, except by skin grafting. The wound was routinely allowed to granulate.

Wide Dissection of Skin Flaps with Extensive Skin Removal. Handley[36] popularized dissection of the breast skin away from the breast tissue as a thin skin flap. Because the skin removal was much less radical, primary closure of the skin flaps was occasionally attempted.

Wide Dissection of Thin Skin Flaps with Less-Extensive Skin Removal. Finney also developed thin skin flaps, but with less extensive skin removal.[7, 19] Primary closure of the skin flaps was usually attempted. The Finney modification of the Halsted-Meyer mastectomy evolved into the predominant method of radical mastectomy after World War II.

The Modified Radical Mastectomy

The technique for modified radical mastectomy was initially described by Patey and Dyson[55] in 1948 (see Chapter 44). Patey began using this method in 1932 and employed it routinely after 1936. This conservative approach was a revolutionary departure from the previous methods espoused by Halsted and Meyer and their surgical pupils, in that it preserved the pectoralis major muscle. Patey based his method on the belief that local-regional dissemination of the breast cancer did not commonly involve the pectoralis muscle, unless the tumor was attached to the fascia and/or the surface of this muscle. He did believe, however, that wide skin excision was essential to cancer control because of the histologic proximity of the ductal tissue and the breast skin and their lymphatic-venous connections. In 1969, Handley and Thackray,[35] also from the Middlesex Hospital in London, confirmed the effectiveness of Patey's modified mastectomy. Although the procedure preserved the pectoralis major muscle, all of these surgeons were firmly convinced of the necessity of wide skin excision, as evidenced by the fact that over 50 percent of their patients required skin grafting for closure. It was not until the 1960s that primary closure of the Patey mastectomy was routinely attempted. Auchincloss,[2] and later Madden,[48] preserved the pectoralis major and minor muscles, and advocated low axillary node dissection (levels I and II) with less extensive skin resection. Auchincloss used a horizontal skin closure, whereas Madden employed a vertical skin closure. The Auchincloss-Madden technique routinely allowed the surgeon to close the breast skin, with survival results that were comparable to the operations championed and advocated by Halsted, Meyer, and Patey. As noted by Bland and colleagues[6] (Chapter 39), the current modified radical mastectomy is essentially the same operation originally described by Moore[50] in 1867, a century before it became the worldwide standard of therapy.

Modified radical mastectomy remains the most common surgical therapy for both invasive and *in situ* carcinoma of the breast, despite the eligibility of many women for breast conservation techniques. Further, as of 1991, the majority of patients with ductal carcinoma *in situ* still had axillary node dissections, despite the low nodal positivity rate that approximates 1 to 2 percent (see Chapters 12, 52, and 53). Although the 1995 report of the Commission on Cancer of the American College of Surgeons[68] suggests increasing use of breast-conserving surgery for *in situ* disease from 20.9 percent in 1985 to 35.4 percent in 1991, modified radical mastectomy represented the principal therapy of the disease and remained constant at 42 percent. Moreover, the use of radiation for patients with ductal carcinoma *in situ* following partial mastectomy without node dissection ranged from 24.2 percent in 1990 to 37.7 percent in 1985. These contemporary trends suggest an enlightened awareness of the design of the technical procedure to accommodate patient desires, while achieving local-regional disease control equivalent to more radical approaches. However, similar reports emphasize the necessity of inculcation of various objective pathological and radiological criteria (e.g., cellular and biochemical variables, oncogenes, and mammograms) to integrate risk parameters of the tumor phenotype. These various factors allow the clinician to more accurately determine risk for local-regional recurrence. Future prospective clinical trials will determine the specter of limitations for breast conservation. Regardless, the necessity of total mastectomy with or without regional nodal dissection will maintain primacy as the desired therapeutic modality for various stages of presentation.

Skin Preservation Procedures

The breast conservation treatments of lumpectomy-radiation and quadrantectomy-radiation introduced the concept of minimal skin removal in the quadrant of the tumor and nipple/areolar complex preservation, if that site was clinically uninvolved.[23, 67] Lumpectomy-radiation was initially proposed by Mustakallio for patients who refused radical mastectomy.[52] This new treatment proved to be effective in providing disease-free survival, and evolved as a consequence of the interest and the advocacy of a number of clinical investigators.[8, 14] Fisher and his coworkers[23] first experimentally established a new concept of tumor cell dissemination that was not based solely on the mechanical and anatomical factors previously espoused by Halsted and others. Fisher's concepts of biological factors, hematogenous dissemination, and the ineffectiveness of regional lymphatic systems as tumor "filters" were truly revolutionary. Today, both lumpectomy and quadrantectomy are well-accepted variants of treatment because of the theories developed by Fisher and colleagues[20–24] and by Veronesi and coworkers,[67] respectively.

In the late 1970s, the mammographic diagnosis of *in situ* disease and minimal breast cancer (Tmic, T1a, T1b) produced a new subset of patients with early-stage disease. In 1983, Bland and associates[5] described a skin preservation technique in which the nipple is resected and augmentation is achieved with subpectoral prosthetic implants. Thereafter, in 1991, Toth and Lappert[65] described a total mastectomy without extensive skin resection as an appropriate treatment for patients with minimal breast cancer and *in situ* disease. These authors coined the term "skin-sparing mastectomy," which was employed primarily in patients with relatively favorable disease indicators. These patients had limited skin resection, which included the biopsy site, the nipple/areola complex, as well as any additional breast skin adjacent to the tumor needed to provide an adequate histologically free margin of tumor excision. Even though skin resection is limited, all ductal tissue is completely extirpated, as would be completed for any total glandular mastectomy. The technical dictum of complete parenchymal resection is scrupulously observed in this method, including the posterior margins and the axillary tail of Spence. The uninvolved breast skin can be preserved without compromise of oncological purpose of the procedure. The reconstruction and rehabilitation goal is to provide the patient with breast symmetry, form, and contour, which can be achieved without placement of incisions in medial and upper (infraclavicular) quadrants of the breasts.

The skin-sparing mastectomy has been used primarily for patients with AJCC-TNM stages 0, I and early II disease requiring mastectomy when eligible for immediate autogenous breast reconstruction.[9, 43, 57, 65] Most of the patients eligible for the technique of combined mastectomy-reconstruction were selected because they were *not* candidates for lumpectomy and postoperative radiation. The authors consider the following to be *indications for skin-sparing techniques*:

1. Multicentricity of disease (ductal *in situ,* any invasive histology),
2. Invasive carcinoma associated with an extensive intraductal component that is 25 percent or more of tumor volume,
3. T_2 tumors (2 to 5 cm), especially those with unfavorable features on radiographic or physical examination that defy confidence in follow-up,
4. A central tumor that would require removal of the nipple/areola complex.

None of the aforementioned indications necessitates wide skin removal to achieve adequate extirpation of the neoplasm. Additional patients have been selected for limited skin resection because of *relatively favorable indications,* and include

1. *In situ* cancers of lobular and ductal origin,
2. Multifocal, minimal breast cancer (Tmic, T1a, T1b),
3. All T1 and possibly T2a tumors deep within the breast parenchyma that, following neoadjuvant therapy, had significant cytoreduction of tumor volume,
4. A positive family history, together with worrisome histological features such as atypical lobular or ductal hyperplasia,
5. Patients with and without familial inheritable disease when physical or radiographic features, or both, defy confidence in follow-up, especially when multiple biopsies are indicated.

For these patients, extensive removal of breast skin *does not* enhance treatment by improving survival or decreasing local recurrences. Conversely, in cases with large tumors (e.g., 5 cm or greater, T3, T4), particularly with attachment to the overlying skin and subcutaneous tissues, with or without ulceration, extensive skin removal is clearly justified and advisable.

Finally, to achieve total glandular mastectomy, some clinics have advocated preservation of the areola by nipple-coring to enhance aesthetic appearance. Although this practice is acceptable, it may prove ill-advised for oncological procedures that attempt total extirpation of mammary ducts of the nipple/areola

complex, because this premise incorrectly assumes that the areola is devoid of mammary ductal tissue. Schnitt and associates[58] performed marginal excision of the nipple (nipple-coring) on eight consecutive mastectomy specimens, excised the areolas, and thereafter submitted all tissues for histological analysis. Mammary ducts in the areola were extensive and were identical to those of extralobular ducts in the breast parenchyma. Schnitt and colleagues concluded that mammary ducts represent a normal histological component of the areolar dermis and that nipple-coring alone does not result in complete removal of all mammary ductal tissue from the nipple/ areola complex. However, areolar preservation may be an insignificant risk parameter relative to local recurrence, because residual breast tissue is evident in all viable skin flaps following total glandular mastectomy.

Technical Aspects of Skin-Sparing Mastectomy

Unfortunately, total glandular mastectomy techniques with axillary lymph node dissection (e.g., modified radical mastectomy) and without axillary lymph node dissection (e.g., simple [total] mastectomy), followed by immediate reconstruction in which skin preservation is a prominent feature of the mastectomy, have received little attention in the general surgical or surgical oncology literature. Resection of the previous biopsy scar and wound cavity with skin overlying the neoplasm, the nipple or the nipple/areola complex, and the entire breast parenchymal contents are cardinal technical caveats of the skin-sparing mastectomy (Table 41–3). As indicated earlier, technical access to the axilla for lymph node dissection is essential; planning of cosmetically acceptable incisions that allow partial access as sampling (Levels I and II) or Patey dissection (Levels I, II, and III) are critical to the technical design. Further, Carlson[9] notes that breast symmetry with reconstruction will be enhanced with preservation of the native skin because of similar skin color and an improved shape.

The anatomy of the breast in regard to skin-sparing mastectomy has been properly outlined by Carlson.[9] The glandular tissue, including the nipple and areola, is removed en bloc. When the tumor is located within 3 cm or less from the surface, the overlying

TABLE 41–3. TECHNICAL FEATURES OF THE SKIN-SPARING MASTECTOMY

1. Skin excision (1-cm margins) of the previous biopsy site or scar overlying index neoplasm
2. Skin excision (marginal only) of nipple/areola complex
3. Total glandular mastectomy, which includes the index tumor or previous biopsy wound cavity en bloc with skin excisions #1 and #2
4. Skin incision design must ensure technical access to the axilla when lymph node dissection (sampling, Levels I/II; *Patey,* Levels I, II, III) is indicated

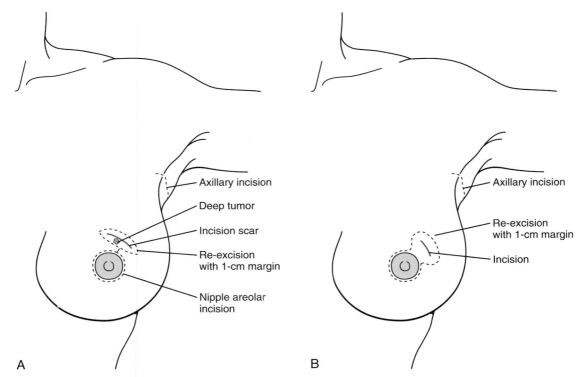

A   B

Figure 41-11   **A** and **B**, Breast incisions when the biopsy site is contiguous with the areola. Note: Axillary incision is remotely placed.

skin is removed with the specimen. A 1- to 2-cm margin of breast skin is removed around the biopsy scar, but the remaining breast skin is preserved.

Incision Design

Figures 41–11 through 41–25 depict the various therapeutic principles and their application that may exist for patients eligible for skin-sparing techniques. Figures 41–16, 41–18, 41–21, 41–23, and 41–25 show breast incision variants of skin-sparing mastectomy for all quadrants when the primary tumors and biopsy sites are located in a site *remote* from the nipple/areola complex. Essential to completion of the oncological aspects of this technique are removal of the nipple or the nipple/areola complex and a 1-cm margin of skin about the biopsy site. Lesions in juxtaposition to the areola may be excised with a single skin island flap (Figs. 41–26 to 41–36). Lesions with biopsy scars greater than 4 cm from the areola margin require *separate excisions* with attention to preservation of a well-vascularized intervening skin bridge. All excisions for both upper and lower hemispheres of the breast are excised via 1-cm margins placed elliptically as nonradial incisions that typically parallel Langer's lines.

Placement of superolateral (modified Orr) incisions (see Fig. 41–3) as an extension of the periareolar incision ensures comprehensive exposure for comple-

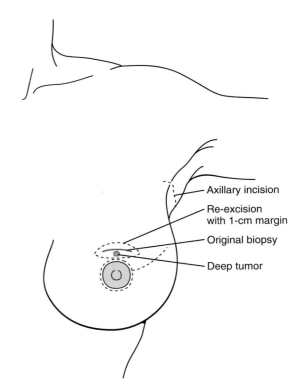

Figure 41-12   Lateral extension of the periareolar incision to enhance exposure for dissection. Remote axillary incision may not be essential if incision is extended toward axilla.

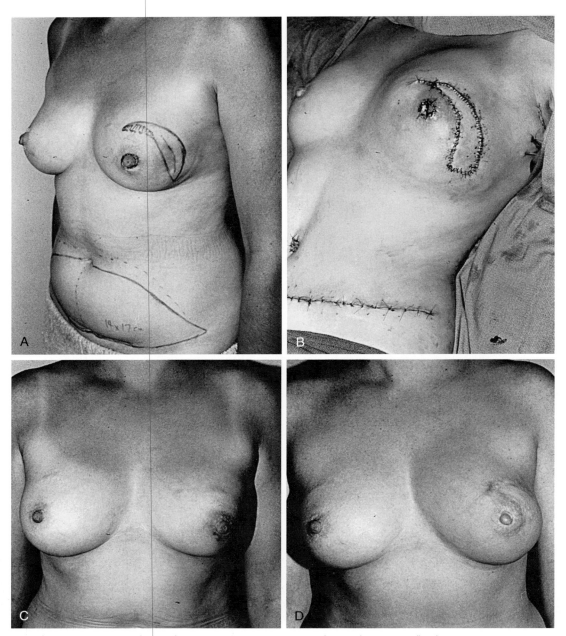

Figure 41–13 **A** *and* **B**, *Preoperative markings of a conservation mastectomy and immediate TRAM flap breast reconstruction. Intraoperative view of the skin replacement of the lateral breast in the area of the previous biopsy. The TRAM flap was used for volume, surface skin replacement, and immediate nipple reconstruction. Preoperative* **(C)** *and postoperative* **(D)** *views following completion of the left breast and nipple reconstruction. No procedure was completed in the right breast. Without the skin conservation mastectomy, it would not have been possible to match the normal right breast.*

Illustration continued on opposite page

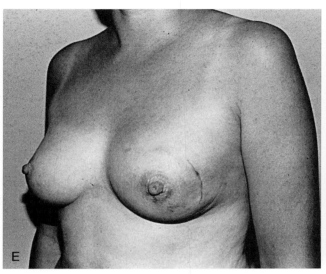
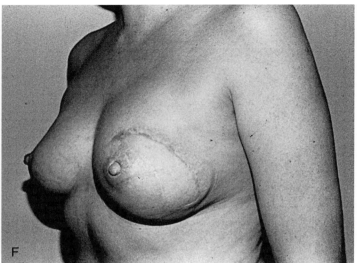

Figure 41–13 Continued *Oblique preoperative* (**E**) *and postoperative* (**F**) *views.*

tion of the total mastectomy and axillary lymph node dissection when limited exposure for flap elevation is evident following incision around 1-cm margins of the biopsy scar and marginal excision of the nipple/areola complex. The 1-cm skin margins that circumvent the biopsy site are resected en bloc with the breast parenchyma including the undisturbed (intact) tumor or the biopsy cavity of index neoplasm.

On occasion, separate axillary incisions designed

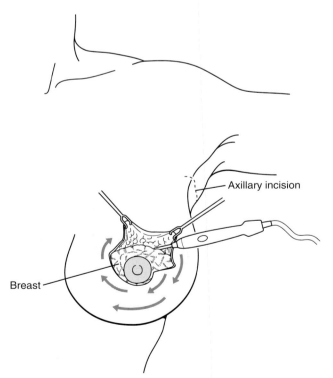

Figure 41–14 *Skin flap elevation is above the superficial fascia. Centripetal dissection enhances exposure. Flap contour with thickness of 7 to 8 mm ensures viability. Dissection should not enter breast parenchyma because margins are developed to chest wall en bloc.*

as indicated in Figure 41–37 for Level I and II nodal sampling or Patey dissection may be used to facilitate exposure with mastectomy. For all presentations of cancer in any quadrant or contiguous with the nipple/areola complex, the design of incisions is guided by oncologic principles with paramount concern for local-regional disease control. Incision planning jointly by oncologic and plastic surgeons ensures optimal appearance and functional outcome with mastectomy techniques that enhance these disease-control measures.

Exposure is gained through ample skin incisions, which are placed precisely parallel to the lines of skin tension. Incisions are placed below the level of the nipple, laterally and inferiorly, passing around the areola. The most satisfactory incisions, both from the standpoint of exposure and the quality of the final scar, extend from the areola at 2 to 3 o'clock and 6 to 8 o'clock. The lateral incision bends upward toward the axilla exactly in the lines of skin tension. If the incision is lengthened 10 to 12 cm lateral to the areola, the exposure of the axilla should be excellent. Alternatively, a separate 10-cm incision in the axillary hair-bearing skin can be used. The incision inferior to the nipple usually provides an excellent scar, even when it does not fall precisely in a skin tension line.

Flap Elevation

Skin flap mobilization is commenced following elevation of periareolar tissues centrally and those continuous with margins of the excised biopsy scar. Although flap thickness depends upon body habitus and fat content, typical thickness of the skin flap is 7 to 8 mm. Electrocautery scalpel using blended cut-coagulation mode may be used for flap elevation but with extreme caution. Uniform flap thickness that is well vascularized must be fastidiously sought and accomplished, or the sole remaining blood supply of

Text continued on page 848

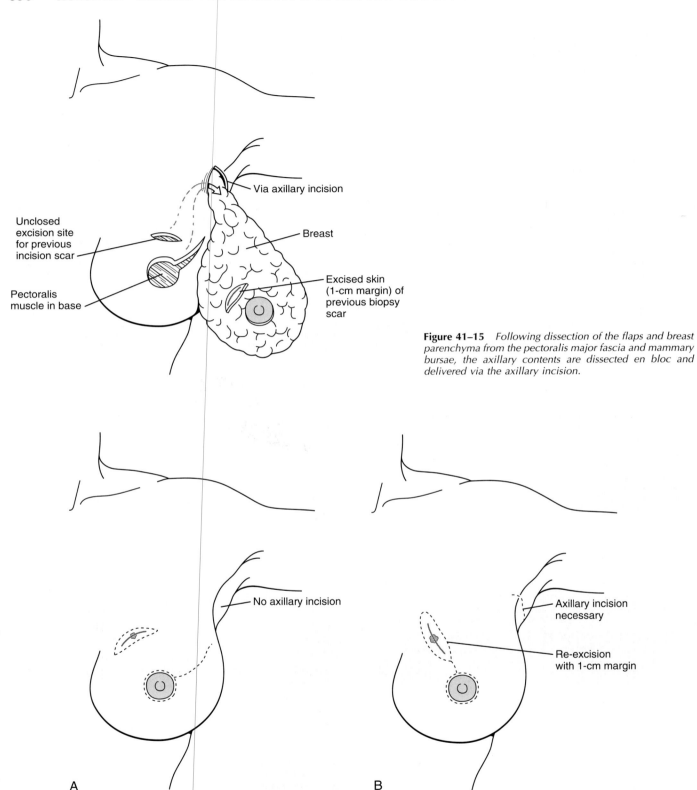

Figure 41–15 *Following dissection of the flaps and breast parenchyma from the pectoralis major fascia and mammary bursae, the axillary contents are dissected en bloc and delivered via the axillary incision.*

Figure 41–16 Upper-inner (medial) quadrant. *A, One-centimeter margin excision that is remote from periareolar incision with lateral extension of modified Orr incision. No axillary incision is necessary because exposure with this approach is adequate for lymph node sampling B, This figure depicts a primary tumor and biopsy site that are vertically placed and radial with 1-cm margins. Following incisions at margin of nipple/areola complex, continuous development of incision allows adequate breast parenchymal exposure. When axillary dissection is necessary, remote incision may be planned.*

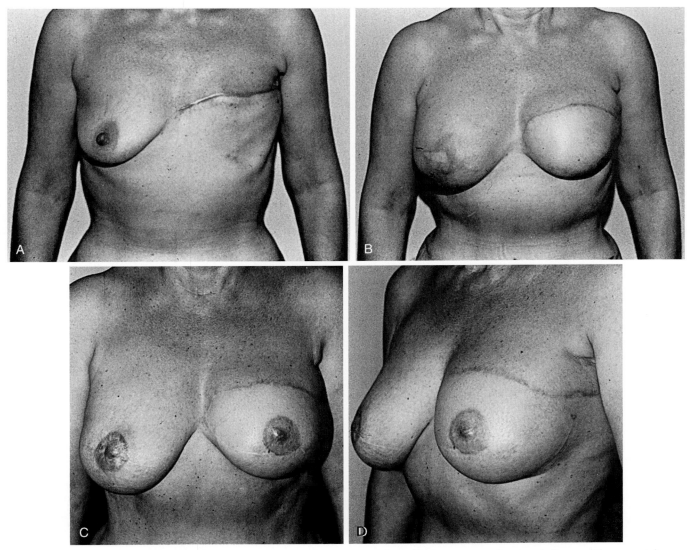

Figure 41–17   Upper-inner (medial) quadrant.   **A,** *Patient with a previous left modified mastectomy for stage I disease with no special reason for extensive skin removal.*   **B,** *Bilateral TRAM flap breast reconstruction done at the time of the right skin conservation mastectomy. Note the difficult skin replacement in the left breast. It was necessary to replace all of the missing skin below the mastectomy scar with a TRAM flap. In the right breast, all of the TRAM flap was buried, except for the part needed to form the nipple and areola.*   **C,** *One year following the completion of the breast and nipple reconstructions.*   **D,** *Achieving symmetry was difficult because of the radical skin excision of the left breast.*

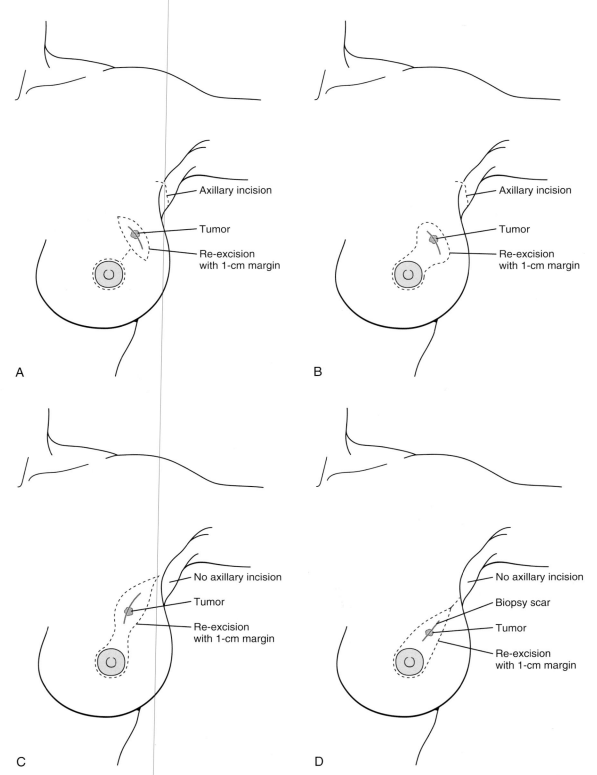

Figure 41–18 Upper-outer (lateral) quadrant. **A,** *Nonradial biopsy site excised with 1-cm margins; nipple/areola marginal incision becomes contiguous with biopsy site to give breast exposure for dissection. Remote axillary dissection incision may be essential for proper technical access to Level I and II nodes.* **B,** *Nonradial biopsy site excised with 1-cm margins at the most lateral extension of incision with resection of contiguous skin intervening between nipple-areola. Remote axillary incision is usually necessary for adequate sampling exposure.* **C,** *Vertically placed (radial) biopsy site necessitates modified Orr skin flaps inclusive of the 1-cm margins of the biopsy site. Axillary exposure is adequate without remote incision.* **D,** *Has similar radial biopsy site to C. Periareolar incision in continuity with 1-cm margin of biopsy site gives excellent exposure to breast and axilla.*

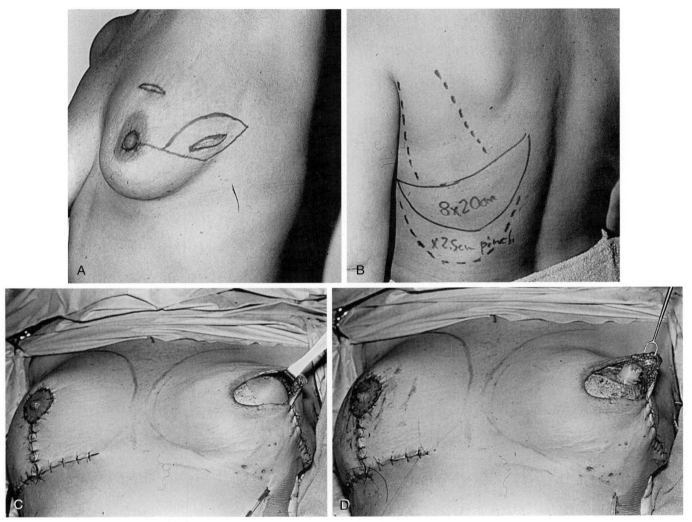

Figure 41–19   Upper-outer (lateral) and central. *Outline of two previous biopsies (upper central and lateral 3 o'clock) in a patient with stage I disease.*   **A,** *The skin excision in the skin conservation mastectomy encompasses the recent biopsy site, and the incision will be extended into the nipple.*   **B,** *Outline of the autogenous latissimus flap on the back. The dotted lines represent the margins of the fat which will be carried on the surface of the latissimus dorsi muscle.*   **C,** *Intraoperative view of the buried latissimus flap prior to de-epithelialization.*   **D,** *The nipple has been reconstructed from the central part of the skin paddle. A mastopexy was performed in the right breast for symmetry.*

Illustration continued on following page

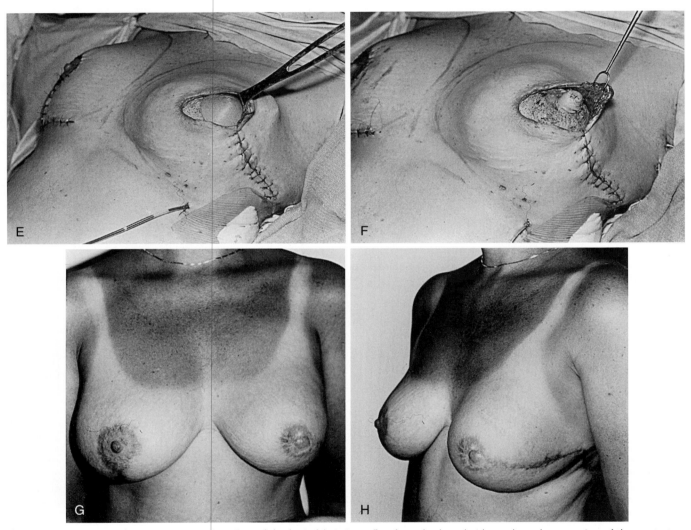

Figure 41–19 Continued   **E,** Intraoperative view of the buried latissimus flap from the lateral side to show the extension of the mastectomy incision.   **F,** Note the reconstructed nipple.   **G** and **H,** Five months following left mastectomy and reconstruction. No revision was done.

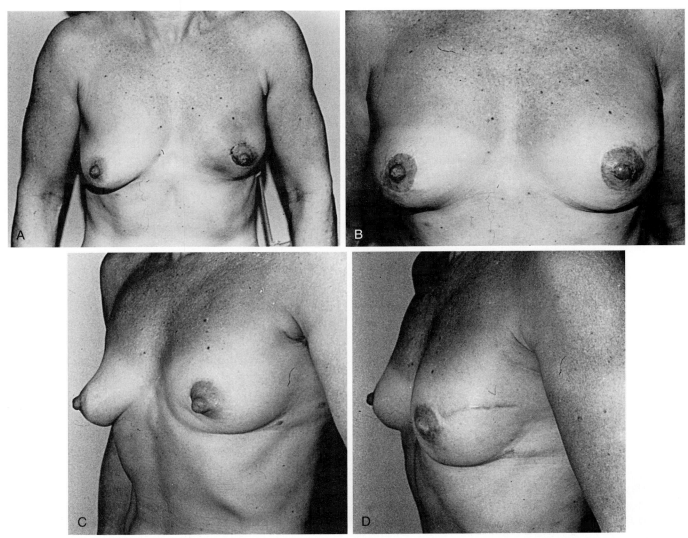

Figure 41–20   Upper-outer (lateral).   **A,** *Preoperative and,*   **B,** *postoperative views following left skin conservation mastectomy for stage I disease. At the time of mastectomy, an immediate free TRAM flap breast and nipple reconstruction were performed in a single stage, with a right mastopexy for symmetry.*   **C,** *Oblique preoperative and,*   **D,** *postoperative views at 1 year. No revision was needed. The areolar tattoo was performed in the office. Note the short lateral skin incision, which was used to encompass the previous biopsy sites.*

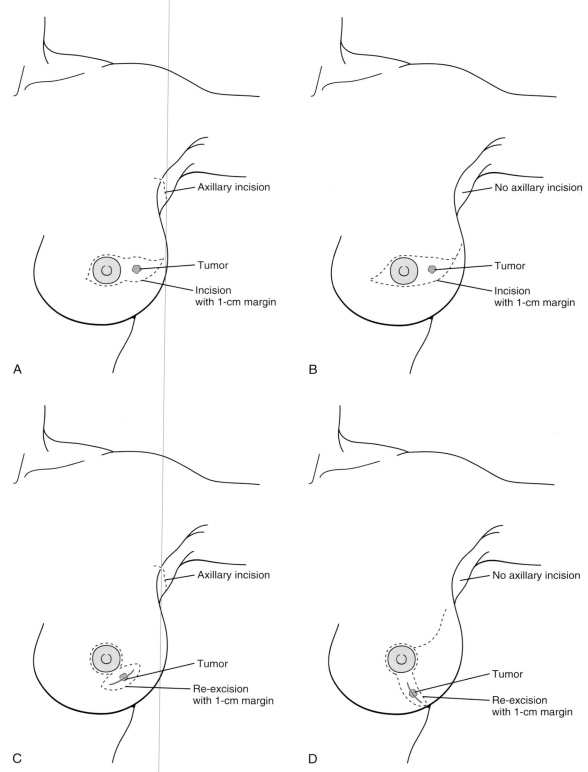

Figure 41–21   Lateral and lower-outer (lateral) quadrant.   *A, Incision around margin of areolar en bloc with 1-cm tumor margin completed as modified Stewart incision. Separate axillary incision may be required when nodal sampling is indicated.*   *B, Similar to A, tumor is noncontiguous with the areola. A modification of the transverse Stewart incision with superolateral extension provides excellent access to breast flap dissection and mastectomy. The axillary dissection can be readily completed with this approach with no need for a separate incision.*   *C, Nonradial biopsy incision contiguous with areolar margin allows adequate breast exposure. Remote axillary incision is necessary.*   *D, Radial biopsy incision contiguous with areolar. Superolateral extension is necessary to complete flap exposure to parenchyma of breast and axillary dissection.*

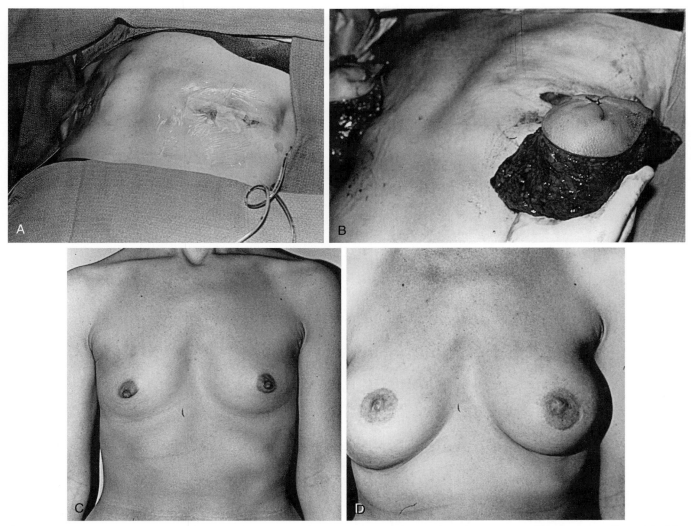

Figure 41–22   **A,** *Bilateral mastectomy for in situ disease using skin conservation technique through a 10-cm modified transverse (Stewart) incision.* **B,** *Bilateral latissimus flaps are brought out through the incisions before insetting in this immediate reconstruction.*   **C,** *Preoperative and,* **D,** *postoperative views following completion of nipple/areola reconstructions. Projection was enhanced with 100-ml implants.*

Illustration continued on following page

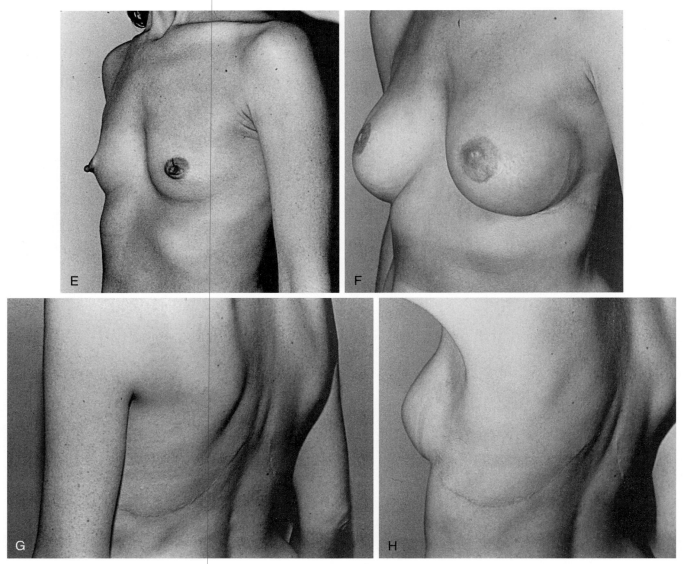

Figure 41–22 Continued   **E,** *Oblique preoperative and,*   **F,** *postoperative views. The excellent result is directly attributable to the skin conservation and the immediate reconstruction. This reconstruction was a prerequisite to the mastectomy in this patient, and there was no reason to delay the reconstruction. Radical skin excision would not have enhanced the extirpation.*   **G** and **H,** *Autogenous latissimus flap donor sites. The scar is usually inconspicuous if placed in the line of a posterolateral thoracotomy.*

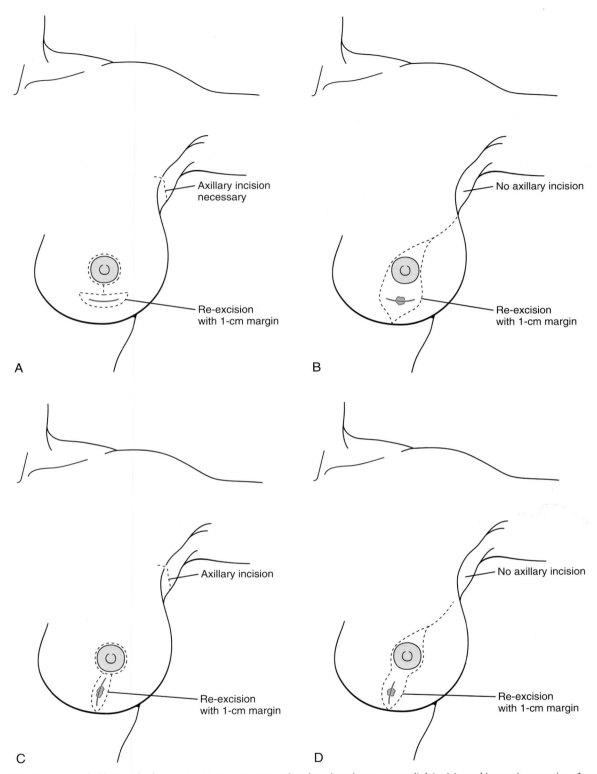

Figure 41–23 Lower one-half (6 o'clock).   *A, Biopsy site may often be placed as a nonradial incision; skin-sparing requires 1-cm marginal excision continuous with periareolar incision. Remote axillary incision is necessary for adequate exposure and dissection.   B, Biopsy site is nonradial in skin-fold contour. Similar to A, re-excision margins are 1 cm and contiguous with skin bridge cephalad toward areola. Superolateral extension of incision allows total mastectomy and axillary dissection (when indicated).   C, Biopsy site is radially placed. Excision of 1-cm biopsy site margin in continuity with areola allows proper breast exposure. Axillary access requires a separate incision.   D, Radial biopsy site excised with tumor inclusive of 1-cm skin-sparing margin. Superolateral extension provides adequate exposure for total mastectomy and axillary dissection.*

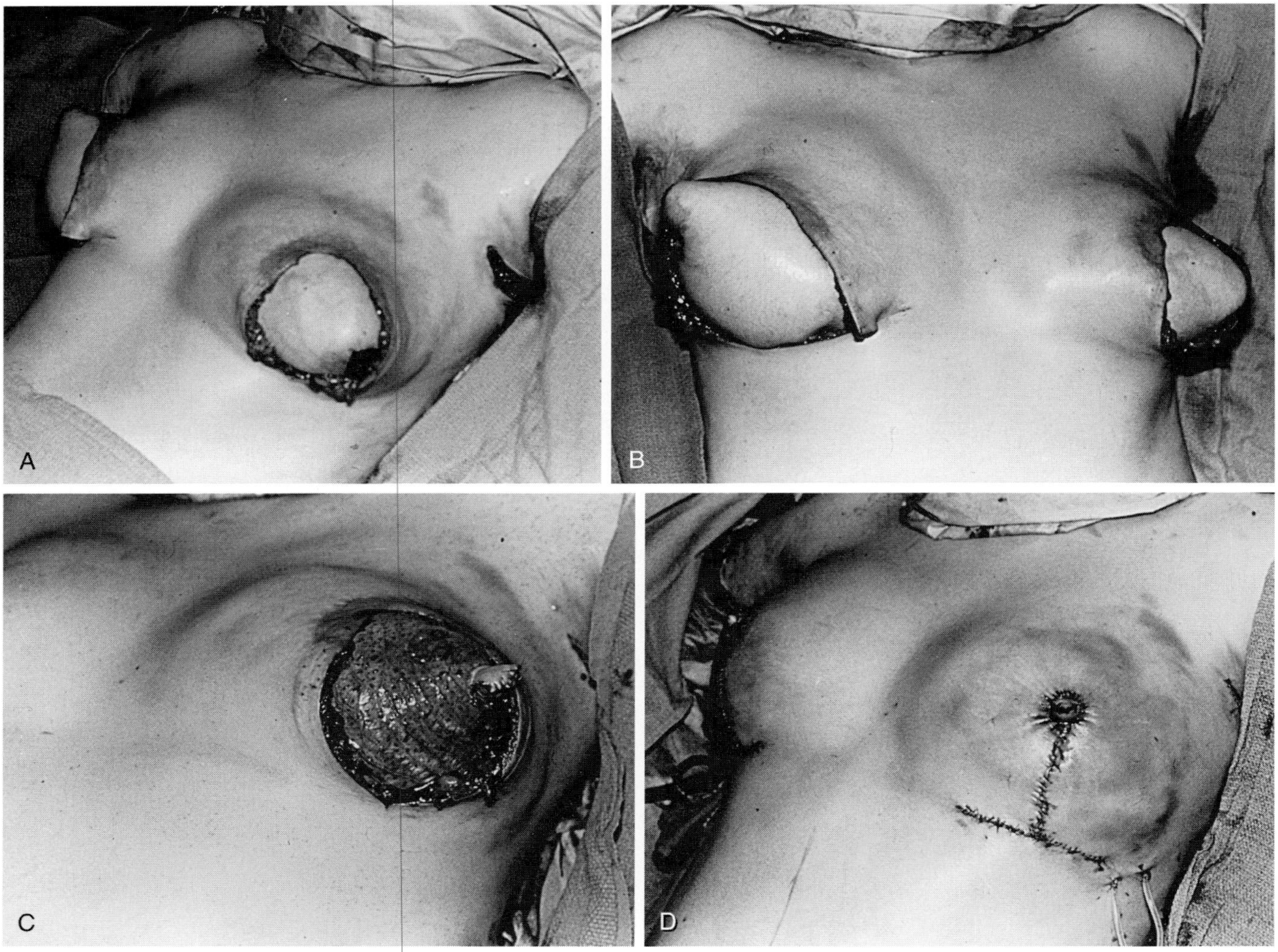

Figure 41–24 **A–B, Bilateral immediate TRAM flap** *reconstruction of skin conservation mastectomies for* in situ *disease. No breast skin was excised.* **C,** *View of the de-epithelialized TRAM flap with an immediate nipple reconstruction the surface of the flap.* **D,** *The mastectomy flaps were closed in the lines of a Wise reduction pattern to remove redundant skin.*

Illustration continued on opposite page

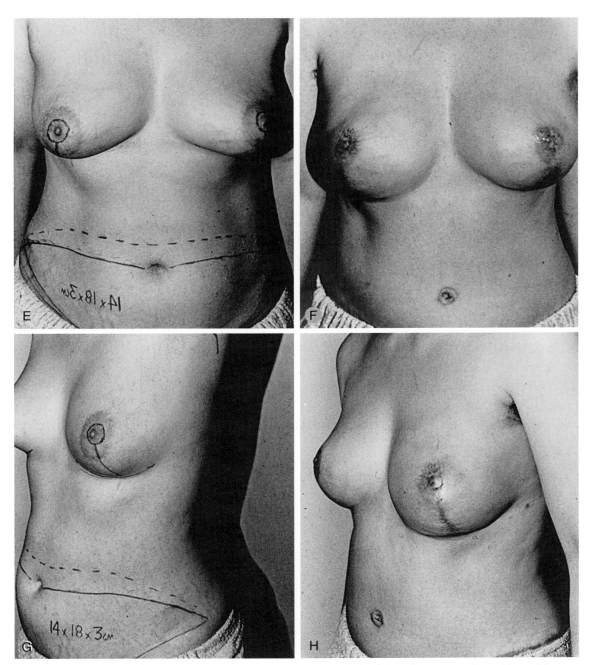

Figure 41–24 Continued   *E, Preoperative and,*   *F, postoperative views of the bilateral reconstructions. No revision was performed.*
G, Oblique views of the preoperative markings, and   *H, the postoperative results of breast and nipple reconstructions. The areolas and nipples*
were tattooed in an office procedure.

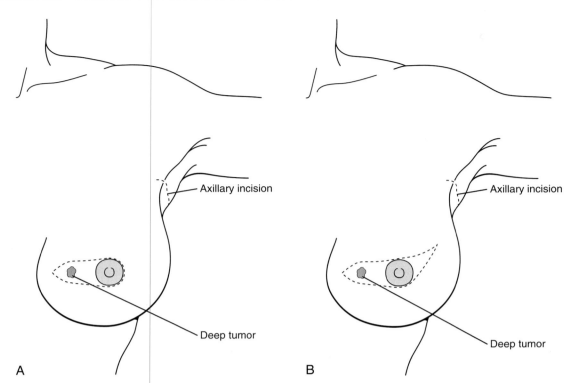

Figure 41–25 Inner (medial) quadrant.   *A, Contiguous 1-cm excision of superficial tumor with areolar margin. Remote incision for axillary dissection is always necessary if sampling of nodes is indicated.*   *B, Similar to A, a 1-cm margin around superficial tumor with lateral and superior extension of incision is essential for breast exposure. Remote axillary incision is necessary when dissection is indicated.*

the breast and skin—the subdermal plexus—will be injured. When the white undersurface of the dermis is exposed, the subdermal plexus will be injured, and flap viability may be harmed distal to the surgical injury. Variation in flap thickness in the process of thinning may devascularize the flap and initiate disastrous wound repair problems.

With completion of flap elevation in superior and medial boundaries, attention is focused to the inferiormost extent of the boundary dissection. Preoperative marking of the inframammary fold or fixation with 2–0 silk sutures allows the oncologic surgeon to determine readily the caudad extent of mammary parenchymal resection. The mammary bursa facilitates mobilization of the breast off the pectoralis major fascia. With axillary dissection, when nodal sampling of Levels I and II or Patey dissection (Levels I–III) is indicated (see Chapters 54, 55, and 56), preservation of the thoracodorsal neurovascular bundle and the long thoracic nerve are requisite to ensure intact motor innervation of the latissimus dorsi and serratus anterior muscles, respectively. Sensory innervation of the axilla and medial upper inner arm may be preserved when sacrifice of the traversing intercostobrachial nerves is avoided. However, transection of these sensory branches creates little long-term morbidity as innervation occurs usually within 8 to 10 months. Additionally, in the course of axillary lymph node dissection, avoidance of section of the medial pectoral neurovascular bundle ensures motor innervation and function of the pectoralis major and

minor muscles. Moreover, it is most important to protect the subscapular vascular pedicle and its thoracodorsal branch, which supplies the latissimus dorsi muscle. Injury of these vessels eliminates the vascular supply and survival of the latissimus myocutaneous flap, which is one of the primary reconstructive options. In addition, the subscapular pedicle is an important recipient vessel for free flaps, which may be needed some time in the future to reconstruct radiation injuries of the chest wall and axilla. It is also helpful, but not essential, to protect the serratus anterior branch of the subscapular pedicle, because this is the alternative vascular supply to the proximal latissimus dorsi muscle.

Once the autogenous flap is inset, the breast skin flaps are used to shape the breast replacement volume. It is at this juncture in the procedure that the breast skin is so important in obtaining a satisfactory shape of the reconstruction. The essential factor in breast reconstruction is symmetry between the normal and reconstructed breasts. This means that the reconstructed breast shape and color match must duplicate a normal shape. In practice, it is usually necessary to alter the normal breast with either a mastopexy or reduction mammoplasty to obtain symmetry. An important principle for the plastic surgeon to follow is to correct any deformity of the opposite breast rather than to shape the reconstructed breast to match an unattractive, ptotic breast.

Finally, the importance of the skin color provided by the skin-sparing mastectomy should be empha-

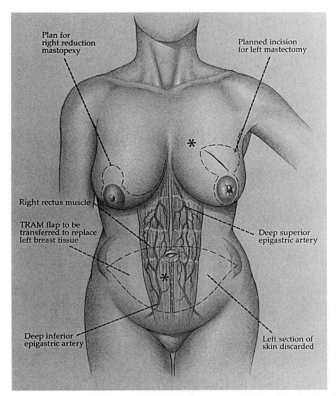

Figure 41–26 *The preoperative plan calls for a left modified radical mastectomy; reconstruction with a contralateral, single-pedicle, abdominal flap; and a matching mastopexy on the right. The asterisk indicates the position of the medial edge of the flap after its rotation and transfer to the chest. (From Copeland EM III, Yu LT: Skin-sparing mastectomy and immediate autologous flap reconstruction. Surg Illus 1993.)*

sized. The native breast skin gives the best possible color match, because it is identical to the opposite breast skin. A pale myocutaneous flap on the surface of the breast has the appearance of a "patch" and is remarkably detractive. Use of the autogenous flap on the surface to replace lost breast skin also diminishes the amount of flap that is available for shaping purposes. When implants are used, the breast skin is even more critical for coverage of the implant and subsequent shaping.

Discussion

Because of the availability of autogenous myocutaneous flaps, the majority of breast reconstructions are now completed at the time of mastectomy rather than at subsequent intervals. A byproduct of the preoperative planning in these cases by the surgical oncologist and the plastic surgeon has been a reconsideration of both the incisions and the absolute necessity for breast skin removal. There are two reasons to consider skin conservation in this setting: (1) when there is little justification to remove the usual 10- by 20-cm ellipse of breast skin around the nipple, and (2) preservation of the native breast skin dramatically enhances the quality of the reconstruction.

This skin conservation approach appears to be

justified in mastectomies when patients are ineligible for lumpectomy-radiation. Many of these factors have little to do with a need for wide skin excision (e.g., invasive T1, T2 with extensive intraductal component, a central tumor which would deform the breast, or multifocality). Favorable conditions for skin-sparing approaches include minimal cancers (T1a, T1b, ductal carcinoma *in situ*), diffuse microinvasive or multicentric cancers; or benign conditions, such as familial breast cancer or difficult diagnostic breasts; and small breast cancers that are deep in the breast and remote from the overlying skin. Even in large tumors (T2, T3, T4), the expected local recurrences virtually always represent systemic disease rather than inadequate local-regional excision. In no immediate reconstructive series has there been any increase in local recurrence that can be related to the autogenous reconstruction.[9, 43, 57, 65]

It is frequently said that the purpose of the skin-sparing mastectomy is to improve "cosmesis." To the

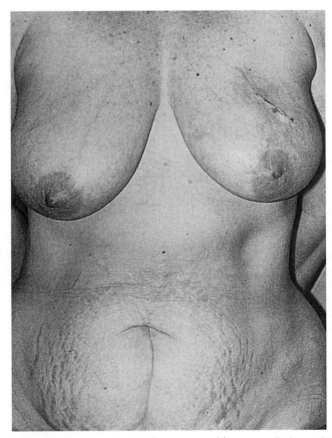

Figure 41–27 *The patient has been prepared for surgery. Perioperative antibiotics have been administered, and a corticosteroid and calcium channel blocker have been given to improve perfusion of the flap. Before anesthesia is induced and with the patient erect, her breast architecture is re-examined. The inframammary fold, midline, and breast width are noted, and after anesthesia, will be tattooed with methylene blue to facilitate reconstruction. The breast scar is from the incisional biopsy. A more radical incision in the upper-outer quadrant would have allowed preservation of maximal skin surface for the skin-sparing mastectomy. (From Copeland EM III, Yu LT: Skin-sparing mastectomy and immediate autologous flap reconstruction. Surg Illus 1993.)*

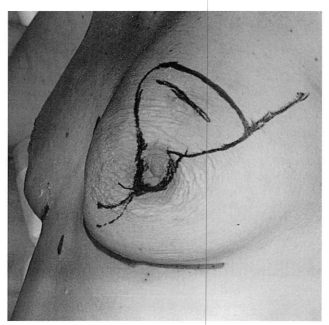

Figure 41–28   *General anesthesia has been induced, and the skin incision has been outlined on the left breast. (Nitrous oxide is not used for anesthesia, because it could distend the bowel and increase intra-abdominal pressure during closure.) The area to be resected includes the biopsy scar and the nipple. Both inframammary folds have been marked to guide the reconstruction and matching mastopexy. (From Copeland EM III, Yu LT: Skin-sparing mastectomy and immediate autologous flap reconstruction. Surg Illus 1993.)*

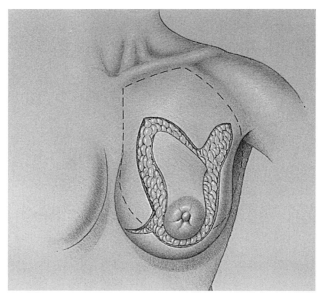

Figure 41–29   *The skin has been incised. Skin flaps are raised by electrocautery dissection, and breast tissue beneath the flaps is removed under direct vision. The subcutaneous margins of the flaps (shown by the dashed line) will extend superiorly to the medial half of the clavicle, superolaterally to the deltopectoral triangle and the cephalic vein, laterally to the anterior edge of the latissimus dorsi muscle, medially to the lateral border of the sternum, and inferiorly to the inframammary fold. (From Copeland EM III, Yu LT: Skin-sparing mastectomy and immediate autologous flap reconstruction. Surg Illus 1993.)*

reconstructive surgeon, the word cosmesis is a derogatory term that implies frivolous concern about minor differences of appearance. In actuality, the skin-sparing mastectomy does provide a major difference in the quality of every variant of the breast reconstructive procedure, particularly when implant augmentation is planned. Conversely, wide skin excision is the reason why the complex transverse rectus abdominis myocutaneous (TRAM) flap is usually employed in breast reconstruction; the skin deficit is so extensive that no other reconstruction method would be satisfactory. When limited skin excision has been planned and implemented, simpler variants of reconstruction, such as the autogenous latissimus flap and tissue expanders can be used because there will be no need for surface skin replacement. With increasing evidence that no deleterious outcome results from skin conservation in a broad range of mastectomy patients, this technique should gain general acceptance as the conventional approach. It can be expected in the future that wide skin excision will have limited indications, such as direct skin invasion or a massive tumor.

Incisions for Axillary Dissection

Figure 41–37 depicts the preferred incision and the optional incisions for axillary dissections performed synchronously with lumpectomy (segmental mastectomy, tylectomy). The surgeon is well-advised to complete incisions placed parallel with Langer's lines and designed in a curvilinear fashion just caudal to the axillary hairline. Preferably, axillary incisions are made separately from incisions of the segmental mastectomy. Optional incisions indicated in Figure 41–37 obliquely cross Langer's lines and are not positioned in axillary skin folds. It is perhaps for this latter reason that delay in primary healing and inferior cosmetic results are obtained. Adequate skin exposure should be provided so that dissection of

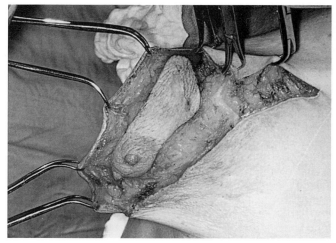

Figure 41–30   *For the skin-sparing mastectomy, the superior flap is elevated first by dissection in the plane between the subcutaneous tissue and the investing fascia of the breast. The skin edges are held with towel clips. (From Copeland EM III, Yu LT: Skin-sparing mastectomy and immediate autologous flap reconstruction. Surg Illus 1993.)*

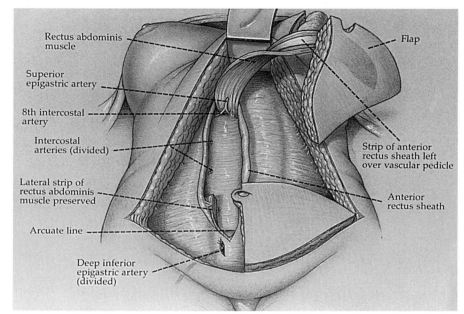

Figure 41–31 *Following skin-sparing modified radical mastectomy, formation of the TRAM flap and its pedicle is complete. The pedicle of rectus muscle includes sufficient deep epigastric vasculature to ensure the flap's viability. A narrower strip of anterior rectus sheath attached to the muscle helps protect the epigastric artery. A lateral segment of the muscle remains in place from the most inferior tendinous intersection to the arcuate line. (From Copeland EM III, Yu LT: Skin-sparing mastectomy and immediate autologous flap reconstruction. Surg Illus 1993.)*

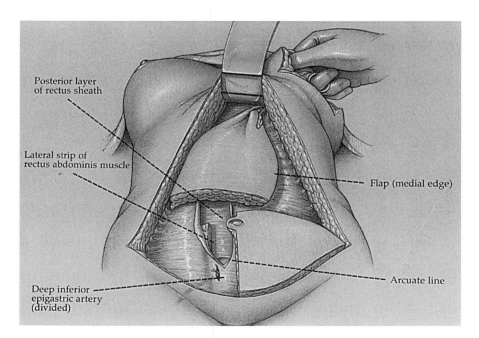

Figure 41–32 *The flap is passed through the tunnel into the mastectomy site. Counterclockwise rotation during passage ensures optimal drainage for the flap and avoids kinking of the pedicle. The pedicle is examined to ensure that it is not twisted. The flap will be allowed to perfuse while the abdomen is closed.*

The left wing of the skin flap is discarded. The right anterior rectus sheath is closed with a running 0 Prolene suture. An opening is left at the cephalad end of the closure to avoid constricting the muscular pedicle. The left sheath is imbricated to centralize the umbilicus. Two large Jackson Pratt drains are left anterior to the rectus sheath. (From Copeland EM III, Yu LT: Skin-sparing mastectomy and immediate autologous flap reconstruction. Surg Illus 1993.)

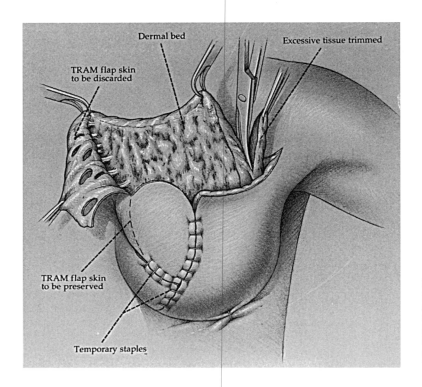

Dermal bed

Excessive tissue trimmed

TRAM flap skin
to be discarded

TRAM flap skin
to be preserved

Temporary staples

Figure 41–33 *Sections of poorly vascularized tissue have been excised from the TRAM flap, and the flap is temporarily stapled in place so that it can be trimmed and contoured. As the reconstruction proceeds, any excess skin is de-epithelialized, leaving a well-vascularized dermal bed, which will be buried. (From Copeland EM III, Yu LT: Skin-sparing mastectomy and immediate autologous flap reconstruction. Surg Illus 1993.)*

Figure 41–34 *To fill the infraclavicular hollow, the most superior edge of the flap is set onto the pectoralis major muscle. The buried, de-epithelialized portions of the flap are rolled and positioned to create an appropriate degree of projection and ptosis. A symmetrical inframammary fold is constructed by tacking the TRAM flap to the periosteum of a rib. (From Copeland EM III, Yu LT: Skin-sparing mastectomy and immediate autologous flap reconstruction. Surg Illus 1993.)*

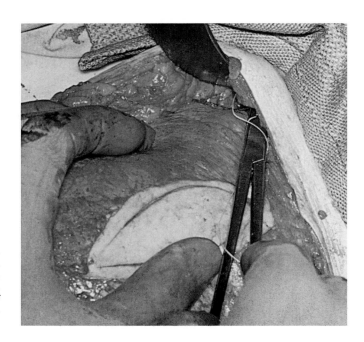

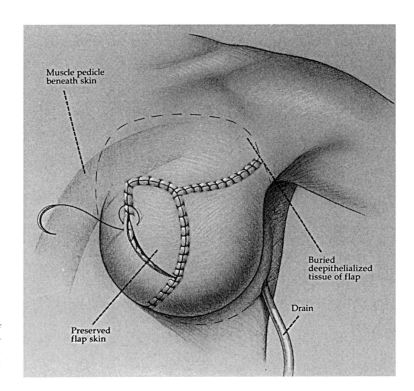

Figure 41–35   *The breast skin is closed with a single layer of continuous 5–0 Prolene suture. The axilla will be closed over a drain. (From Copeland EM III, Yu LT: Skin-sparing mastectomy and immediate autologous flap reconstruction. Surg Illus 1993.)*

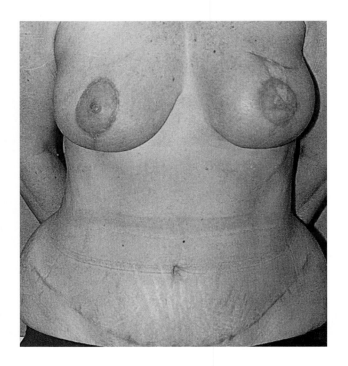

Figure 41–36.   *Nipple/areola reconstruction has completed the procedure. The left nipple/areola is tattooed for color symmetry. (From Copeland EM III, Yu LT: Skin-sparing mastectomy and immediate autologous flap reconstruction. Surg Illus 1993.)*

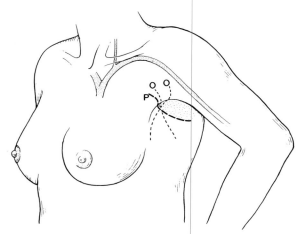

Figure 41–37   *Illustration of preferred (P) and optional (O) incisions used in axillary dissection. Ideally, incisions are placed in skin folds that parallel Langer's lines. Incisions are preferably curvilinear with placement just caudal to the hairline of the axilla.*

Optional incisions depicted are oblique or vertically placed with the chest wall. Because these optional incisions cross the lines of tension (Langer's lines), delay in wound repair and inferior cosmetic results may be observed.

Level I and Level II nodes beneath the pectoralis minor is possible without undue traction on the pectoralis major or minor muscles. This principle prevents damage to the medial and lateral (anterior thoracic) pectoral nerves located in the lateral and medial neurovascular bundles, respectively. Incisions placed in a curvilinear transverse, oblique, or vertical fashion all allow adequate access to the axillary vein, the medial border of the pectoralis minor muscle, and the lateral aspect of the latissimus dorsi muscle. This exposure should permit visualization of the long thoracic nerve to the serratus anterior and the thoracodorsal nerve to the latissimus dorsi.

References

1. Anson BJ, McVay CB: Breast or mammary region. *In* Anson BJ, McVay CB (eds): Thoracic Walls: Surgical Anatomy, vol 1. Philadelphia, WB Saunders, 1971, pp 339–356.
2. Auchincloss H: Significance of location and number of axillary metastases in carcinoma of the breast: a justification for a conservative operation. Ann Surg 158:37–46, 1963.
3. Bland KI, Freedman BE, Harris PL, Yun-Jo H, Wittliff JL: The effects of ischemia on estrogen and progesterone receptor profiles in the rodent uterus. J Surg Res 42(6):653–660, 1987.
4. Bland KI, Konstadoulakis MM, Vezeridis MP, Wanebo HJ: Oncogene protein co-expression: value of Ha-*ras*, c-*myc*, c-*fos*, and p53 as prognostic discriminants for breast cancer. Ann Surg 221:706–720, 1995.
5. Bland KI, O'Neal B, Weiner LJ, Tobin GR II: One-stage simple mastectomy with immediate reconstruction for high-risk patients: An improved technique: The biologic basis for ductal-glandular mastectomy. Arch Surg 121(2):221–225, 1986.
6. Bland KI, Copeland EM, Fisher B, Frykberg ER, Hundahl SA, Urban JA, Veronesi U: Primary therapy for breast cancer: Surgical principles and techniques. *In* Bland KI, Copeland EM (eds): The Breast: Comprehensive Management of Benign and Malignant Diseases. Philadelphia, WB Saunders, 1991, p 562.
7. Brooks B, Daniel RA Jr: Present status of the "radical operation" for carcinoma of the breast. Ann Surg 3:688, 1940.
8. Calle R, Pilleron JP, Schlienger P, Vilcoq JR, et al: Conserva-tive management of operable breast cancer: ten years' experience at the Foundation Curie. Cancer 42:2045–2053, 1978.
9. Carlson GW: Skin sparing mastectomy: anatomic and technical considerations. Am Surg 62:151–155, 1996.
10. Cheatle GL, Cutler M: Tumours of the Breast, 1st ed. Philadelphia, JB Lippincott Co, 1933, pp 314–315.
11. Cody HS, Egeli RA, Urban JA: Rotter's node metastases. Ann Surg 199:266–270, 1984.
12. Copeland EM III: Carcinoma of the breast. *In* Copeland EM III (ed): Surgical Oncology. New York, John Wiley & Sons, 1983, pp 43–58.
13. Copeland EM III, Yu LT: Skin-sparing mastectomy and immediate autologous flap reconstruction. Surg Illus 1993.
14. Crile G Jr: Treatment of breast cancer by local excision. Am J Surg 109:400, 1965.
15. Dao TL, Nemoto T: The clinical significance of skin recurrence after radical mastectomy in women with cancer of the breast. Surg Gynec Obstet 117:447–453, 1963.
16. Donegan WL, Perez-Mesa CM, Watson FR: A biostatistical study of locally recurrent breast carcinoma. Surg Gynecol Obstet 122:529–540, 1966.
17. Ellis LM, Wittliff JL, Bryant ML, Hogancamp WE, Sitren HS, Bland KI: Correlation of estrogen, progesterone, and androgen receptors in breast cancer; significance to the androgen receptor. Am J Surg 157(6):577–581, 1989.
18. Ellis LM, Wittliff JL, Bryant MS, Sitren HS, Hogancamp WE, Souba WW, Bland KI: Lability of steroid hormone receptors following devascularization of breast tumors. Arch Surg 124:39–42, 1989.
19. Finney JMT: Keen's Surgery. Philadelphia, WB Saunders, 1924, p 605.
20. Fisher B: Lumpectomy and axillary dissection. *In* Bland KI, Copeland EM (eds): The Breast: Comprehensive Management of Benign and Malignant Diseases. Philadelphia, WB Saunders, 1991, p 634–639.
21. Fisher B, Anderson S, Fisher ER, et al: Significance of ipsilateral breast tumour recurrence after lumpectomy. Lancet 338:327–331, 1991.
22. Fisher B, Redmond C, Fisher ER, Bauer M, Wolmark N, Wicherham L, Deutsch M, Montague E, Margolese R, Foster R: Ten-year results of a randomized trial comparing radical mastectomy and total mastectomy with or without radiation. N Engl J Med 312:674–681, 1985.
23. Fisher B, Redmond C, Poisson R, et al: Eight-year results of a randomized clinical trial comparing total mastectomy and lumpectomy with and without irradiation in the treatment of breast cancer. N Engl J Med 320:822–828, 1989.
24. Fisher ER, Sass R, Fisher B, et al: Pathologic findings from the National Surgical Adjuvant Breast Project (Protocol 6). II. Relation of local breast recurrence to multicentricity. Cancer 57:1717–1724, 1986.
25. Fowble B, Solin LJ, Schultz DJ, Rubenstein J, Goodman RL: Breast recurrence following conservative surgery and radiation: Patterns of failure, prognosis, and pathologic findings from mastectomy specimens with implications for treatment. Int J Radiat Oncol Biol Phys 19:833–842, 1990.
26. Gilliland MD, Barton RM, Copeland EM III: The implications of local recurrence of breast cancer as the first site of therapeutic failure. Ann Surg 197:284–287, 1983.
27. Gray DB: The radical mastectomy incision. Am Surg 35(10):750–755, 1969.
28. Gray JH: The relation of lymphatic vessels to the spread of cancer. Br J Surg 26:462–495, 1939.
29. Gray SW, Skandalakis JE: Atlas of Surgical Anatomy for General Surgeons. Baltimore, MD, Williams & Wilkins, 1985.
30. Greco RJ, Dascombe WH, Williams SL, Johnson RR, Kelley JL: Two-staged breast reconstruction in patients with symptomatic macromastia requiring mastectomy. Ann Plast Surg 32:572–579, 1994.
31. Haagensen CD: Anatomy of the mammary gland. *In* Haagensen CD (ed): Diseases of the Breast, 2nd ed. Philadelphia, WB Saunders, 1971, pp 1–28.
32. Halsted WS: Results of operation for cure of cancer of breast performed at Johns Hopkins Hospital from June 1889 to January 1894. Ann Surg 20:497–555, 1894.

33. Halsted WS: The results of radical operation for the cure of cancer of the breast. Trans Am Surg Assoc 25:61, 1907.

34. Handley RS: The conservative radical mastectomy of Patey: ten year results in 425 patients breasts. Dis Breast 2:16, 1976.

35. Handley RS, Thackray AC: Conservative radical mastectomy (Patey's operation). Ann Surg 170:880–882, 1969.

36. Handley WS: Cancer of the Breast and Its Treatment, 2nd ed. London, A. Murray, 1922.

37. Harris JR, Hellman S: Primary radiation therapy for early breast cancer. Cancer 52:2547–2552, 1983.

38. Holland R, Veling SHJ, Mravunac M, Hendriks JHCL: Histologic multifocality of Tis, T1-2 breast carcinomas. Implications for clinical trials of breast-conserving surgery. Cancer 56:979–990, 1985.

39. Hollingshead WH: The breast. *In* Hollingshead WH (ed): Anatomy for Surgeons, Vol 2. Thorax, Abdomen, and Pelvis, 2nd ed. New York, Harper & Row, 1971, pp 11–17.

40. Johnson CH, van Heerden JA, Donohue JH, Martin JK Jr, Jackson IT, Instrup DM: Oncological aspects of immediate breast reconstruction following mastectomy for malignancy. Arch Surg 124:819–824, 1989.

41. Kendall BE, Arthur JF, Patey DH: Lymphangiography in carcinoma of the breast: a comparison of clinical, radiological, and pathological findings in axillary lymph nodes. Cancer 16:1233–1242, 1963.

42. Krohn IT, Cooper DR, Bassett JG: Radical mastectomy. Arch Surg 227:760–763, 1982.

43. Kroll SS, Ames F, Singletary SE, Schusterman MA: The oncologic risks of skin preservation at mastectomy when combined with immediate reconstruction of the breast. Surg Gynecol Obstet 172:17–20, 1991.

44. Kurtz JM: Factors influencing the risk of local recurrence in the breast. Eur J Cancer 28:660–666, 1992.

45. Kurtz JM, Jacquemier J, Brandone H, et al: Inoperable recurrence after breast-conserving surgical treatment and radiotherapy. Surg Gynecol Obstet 172:357–361, 1991.

46. Lebovic GS, Laub DR, Berkowitz RL: Aesthetic approach to simple and modified radical mastectomy. Contemp Surg 45:15–19, 1994.

47. Lewis D, Rienhoff WF Jr: Study of the results of operation for cure of cancer of breast performed at Johns Hopkins Hospital 1889 to 1931. Ann Surg 95:336, 1932.

48. Madden JL: Modified radical mastectomy. Surg Gynecol Obstet 121:1221–1230, 1965.

49. Meyer W: An improved method of the radical operation for carcinoma of the breast. Med Rec NY 46:746–749, 1894.

50. Moore CH: On the influence of inadequate operation on the theory of cancer. J R Med Chir Soc London 1:244–280, 1867.

51. Moosman DA: Anatomy of the pectoral nerves and their preservation in modified mastectomy. Am J Surg 139:883–886, 1980.

52. Mustakallio S: Treatment of breast cancer by tumor extirpation and roentgen therapy instead of radical operation. J Fac Radiol 6:23, 1954.

53. Netter FH: CIBA collection of medical illustrations, 7:6, Summit NJ, CIBA Pharmaceutical, 1979.

54. Patey DH: A review of 146 cases of carcinoma of the breast operated upon between 1930–1943. Br J Cancer 21:260–269, 1967.

55. Patey DH, Dyson WH: Prognosis of carcinoma of the breast in relation to type of operation performed. Br J Cancer 2:7–13, 1948.

56. Sauer R, Schauer A, Rauschecker HF, Schumacher M, Gatzemeier W, Schmoor C, Dunst J, Seegenschmiedt MH, Marx D: Therapy of small breast cancer: a prospective study on 1036 patients with special emphasis on prognostic factors. Int J Rad Onc Biol Phys 23:907–914, 1992.

57. Sampaio Goes J: Mastectomy by periareolar approach with immediate breast reconstruction. Rev Loc Bras Cir Estet Reconstr 10:44–55, 1995.

58. Schnitt SJ, Goldwyn RM, Slavin SA: Mammary ducts in the areola: implications for patients undergoing reconstructive surgery of the breast. Plast Reconstr Surg 92:1290–1293, 1993.

59. Silverstein MJ, Gierson ED, Colburn WJ, Cope LM, Furmanski M, Senofsky GM, Gamagami P, Waisman JR: Can intraductal breast carcinoma be excised completely by local excision? Cancer 73:2985–2989, 1994.

60. Slavin SA, Love SM, Sadowsky NL: Reconstruction of the radiated partial mastectomy defect with autogenous tissues. Plast Reconstr Surg 90:854–865, 1992.

61. Spratt JS Jr, Donegan WL: Anatomy of the breast. *In* Donegan WL, Spratt JS Jr (eds): Cancer of the Breast, 3rd ed. Philadelphia, WB Saunders, 1979.

62. Spratt JS, Tobin GJ: Gross anatomy of the breast. *In* Donegan WL, Spratt JS (eds): Cancer of the Breast, 4th ed. Philadelphia, WB Saunders, 1995.

63. Stotter AT, McNeese MD, Ames FC, Oswald MJ, Ellerbroek NA: Predicting the rate and extent of locoregional failure after breast conservation therapy for early breast cancer. Cancer 64:2217–2225, 1989.

64. Toth BA, Glafkides MC: Immediate breast reconstruction with deepithelialized TRAM flaps: Techniques for improving breast reconstruction. Plast Reconstr Surg 85:967–970, 1990.

65. Toth BA, Lappert P: Modified skin incisions for mastectomy: the need for plastic surgical input in preoperative planning. Plast Reconstr Surg 87:1048–1053, 1991.

66. Verhoef LCG, Stalpers LJA, Verbeek ALM, Wobbes T, van Daal WAJ: Breast-conserving treatment or mastectomy in early breast cancer: A clinical decision analysis with special reference to the risk of local recurrence. Eur J Cancer 27:1132–1137, 1991.

67. Veronesi U, Volterrani F, Luini A, et al: Quandrantectomy versus lumpectomy for small size breast cancer. Eur J Cancer 26:671–673, 1990.

68. Winchester DP, Menck HR, Osteen RT, Kraybill W: Treatment trends for ductal carcinoma in situ of the breast. Ann Surg Onc 2:207–213, 1995.

CHAPTER 42

HALSTED RADICAL MASTECTOMY

Kirby I. Bland, M.D. / Edward M. Copeland III, M.D.

HISTORICAL ASPECTS FOR DEVELOPMENT OF RADICAL MASTECTOMY

The evolution of anatomical principles and the basic knowledge of cancer biology of the nineteenth century allowed renowned anatomists, physiologists, and surgeons to formulate what were considered "modern" biological and surgical therapies for cancer of the breast. The Halsted radical mastectomy, begun in 1882 by Halsted at the Roosevelt Hospital in New York City, was popularized and scientifically embraced at the Johns Hopkins Hospital in Baltimore. The operation embodied the concept of routine complete en bloc resection of the breast with the pectoralis major muscle and the regional lymphatics.[12, 13] The halstedian approach was largely directed at the proposition of preventing local or regional recurrences. Halsted's synthesis of the techniques of his predecessors in surgery and pathology allowed him to achieve local and regional recurrent rates of 6 percent and 22 percent, respectively.[5, 12, 13] The en bloc technique described by Halsted, although published simultaneously by Willy Meyer,[27] allowed a reduction in the local recurrence rate to 6 percent from rates of 51 percent to 82 percent for contemporary European surgeons. Table 42–1 compares the operations available to European surgeons during the halstedian era with the accompanying 3-year estimated cure rates for breast carcinoma.

Halsted was not the first surgeon to resect the pectoralis major muscle in the course of a radical mastectomy. Wolff[57] documents that Barthelemy Cabrol of Montpellier, France, reported in 1570 the cure of a mammary carcinoma in a 35-year-old woman in whom the pectoralis major muscle was excised and the wound sprinkled with vitriols.[5] The patient survived 12 years, only to succumb to cancer of the lower lip. Great European surgeons such as Petit, Billroth, Volkmann, and others of that period not infrequently removed portions of the pectoral muscles in resection of certain malignancies of the breast.[56] Joerss[19] has attributed the modern operation to Heidenhein. Nonetheless, it was Halsted who advocated routine resection of the pectoralis muscles en bloc with breast tissues and axillary nodes.

Halsted gave credit that substantiated the contributions of other renowned surgeons of this era in formulation and adoption of this procedure.[11]

TABLE 42–1. CHRONOLOGY OF THE MASTECTOMY FOR TREATMENT OF BREAST CANCER WITH EXPECTANT (AVERAGE) 3-YEAR "CURE RATES"

Type of Operation	Author	Year	No. of Cases	Percent 3-Year Cures
Simple mastectomy	Winiwarter (Billroth)[56]	1867–1875		4.7
Average				*4.7*
Complete mastectomy and axillary dissection in majority of cases	Oldekop[33]	1850–1878	229	11.7
	Dietrich (Lucke)[7]	1872–1890	148	16.2
	Horner[17]	1881–1893	144	19.4
	Poulsen[42]	1870–1888	110	20
	Banks[3]	1877	46	20
	Schmid (Kuster)[46]	1871–1885		21.5
Average				*18.1*
Complete (total) mastectomy, axillary dissection, removal of pectoral fascia and greater or lesser amounts of pectoral muscle	Sprengel (Volkmann)[49]	1874–1878	200	11
	Schmidt[47]	1877–1886	112	18.8
	Rotter[44]		30	20
	Mahler[24]	1887–1897	150	21
	Joerss[19]	1885–1893	98	28.5
Average				*19.9*
Modern radical mastectomy	Halsted[12]	1889–1894	76	45
	Halsted[13]	1907	232	38.3
	Hutchison's collected figures[18]	1910–1933		39.4
Average				*40.9*

Modified from Cooper WA: The history of the radical mastectomy. *In* Annals of Medical History. Vol 3. New York, Paul B. Hoeber, 1941, p 51.

In its final form, the technique of the radical mastectomy espoused by Halsted embodied the following principles:

1. Wide excision of the skin, covering the defect with Thiersch grafts.
2. Routine removal of *both* pectoral muscles.
3. Routine axillary dissection (Levels 1 to 3).
4. Removal of all tissues in one block, cutting as wide as possible on all sides of the growth.

The evolution of the modern radical mastectomy, which began with Cabrol in 1570 and ended with Halsted in 1890,[5] is one of discordant retrogressions. The wide acceptance of the incurability of carcinoma, the consequences of sepsis, and the necessity for anesthesia played prominent roles in the delay of the development for surgery of the breast. To attribute the development of the modern operation to a single individual would discredit the remarkable contributions of Halsted's predecessors. The early surgery and pathology pioneers extended the operation because of the clinical observations for the natural history of breast cancer. These leaders of medical science lacked the salient background in pathology, anatomy, and statistics that enabled Halsted to complete the evolution of the radical mastectomy in the late nineteenth century.

BREAST CANCER TREATMENT IN THE UNITED STATES

Trends and Patterns of Care, 1971–1984

Figures 39–16 and 42–1 confirm that the majority of surgeons used the modified radical mastectomy on patients reported in 1971, 1976, 1977, and 1981. In 1972, 48 percent of patients were reported to have had a Halsted-type radical mastectomy, whereas only 3 percent of patients underwent this procedure in 1981. Trends in the use of radiation therapy and chemotherapy also showed dramatic alterations in application from 1972 through 1981. The trends for the use of radiation therapy in these years are depicted in Figure 42–2. The proportion of patients at all stages reported to have received irradiation decreased from 33 percent in 1972 to 18 percent in 1981. This trend is most apparent for regional stage disease. In contrast, the introduction of effective adjuvant and systemic chemotherapy and the emerging principles of pharmacotherapeutics caused a dramatic increase in the application of chemotherapy. Chemotherapy increased from 7 percent of patients treated in 1972 to 22.7 percent in 1981. As depicted in Figure 42–3, this exponential increase in the use of chemotherapy was limited to patients with regional and distant stages of disease. Currently, the use of adjuvant chemotherapy for treatment of localized disease (stages 0 and I) has seen a renaissance. A discussion of the application of adjuvant chemotherapy and hormonal therapy for breast cancer is presented in Chapter 39.

The 1982 National Survey evaluated 5-year sur-

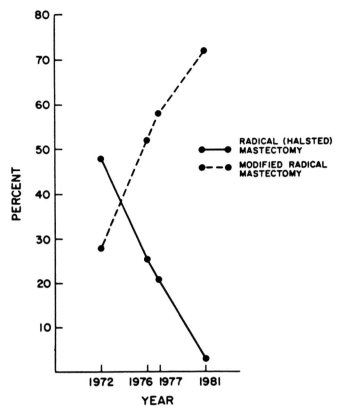

Figure 42–1   *Trends in the type of operation performed from 1972 to 1981 in the 1982 National Survey of Carcinoma of the Breast in the United States by the American College of Surgeons. (From Wilson RE, et al: Surg Gynecol Obstet 159:309–318, 1984.)*

vival rates by stage, type of treatment, and type of adjuvant therapy. Table 42–2 depicts survival rates for patients treated in 1976 by type of operation, with or without adjuvant irradiation and chemotherapy. Similar survival rates for patients with localized disease were observed for treatment by partial mastec-

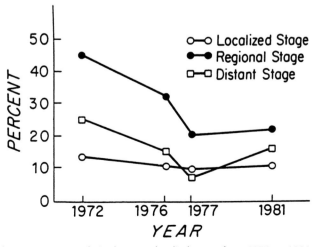

Figure 42–2   *Trends in the use of radiotherapy from 1972 to 1981 as reported in the 1982 National Survey of Carcinoma of the Breast in the United States by the American College of Surgeons. (From Wilson RE, et al: Surg Gynecol Obstet 159:309–318, 1984.)*

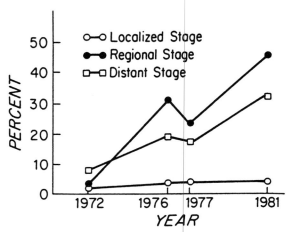

Figure 42–3   *Trends in the application of systemic chemotherapy from 1972 to 1981 as reported in the 1982 National Survey of Cancer of the Breast in the United States by the American College of Surgeons. (From Wilson RE, et al: Surg Gynecol Obstet 159:309–318, 1984.)*

tomy alone and by partial mastectomy plus irradiation to the breast, the axilla, or both. Additionally, 5-year survival rates for patients treated by the modified radical mastectomy technique were similar to 5-year survival rates for those treated by the Halsted radical mastectomy. Wilson and colleagues[54] noted that survival rates were also similar for those who received additional irradiation therapy or chemotherapy with one of the two surgical procedures.

It must be emphasized that these short- and long-term surveys are not prospective trials, and bias in treatment selection cannot be eliminated. In addition, follow-up studies are short, and data represent only trends. Nonetheless, there has been an important transition in curative surgical procedures used by American surgeons from the Halsted radical

to the modified radical mastectomy techniques.[52] This transition was apparent at the time of the 1977 survey reported by Nemoto and associates[28, 29] and the 1981 survey[29] confirmed that the vast majority of patients treated had had a modified radical rather than a radical mastectomy (77 percent versus 3 percent). The results of the short-term survey also confirmed an increase in the proportion of patients being treated by partial mastectomy, largely because of the convincing results of recent clinical trials conducted by Fisher and coworkers[8, 9] in association with the National Surgical Adjuvant Breast and Bowel Project (NSABP). Survival rates of patients treated by the various procedures are *not* comparable in the absence of more detailed data, because of confounding biological and patient-related factors that may affect prognosis.

The American College of Surgeons (ACS) conducted two surveys for the treatment of breast carcinoma in the United States: a long-term survey in 1976 and a short-term survey in 1982.[54] Table 42–3 shows that in the short-term survey, more than twice the percentage of patients were treated by partial mastectomy (7.2 percent) compared with the long-term survey, which reported that 2.8 percent of surgeons used this technique in the primary therapy of breast cancer ($p < 0.0001$). The most significant change in this survey was in the type of operations used for treatment of operable breast cancer. There is an increased use of modified radical mastectomy (55.6 percent in the long-term survey compared with 78.2 percent in the short-term survey) and a marked decline in the reported use of the Halsted radical mastectomy (27.5 percent of patients in the long-term survey compared with 3.4 percent in the 1981 data) (see Fig. 42–1). For each stage of disease, there was a greater reported use of the modified radical

TABLE 42–2.   FIVE-YEAR SURVIVAL RATE BY STAGE, TYPE OF OPERATION, AND TYPE OF ADJUVANT THERAPY

| | Type of Adjuvant Therapy by Stage | | | | | | | | |
| | Localized | | | Regional | | | Distant | | |
Type of Operation	None	Radiation	Chemotherapy	None	Radiation	Chemotherapy	None	Radiation	Chemotherapy
Partial mastectomy									
Five-year survival (%)	82.6	83.9	100.0	64.4	56.9	81.0	29.0	9.5	20.4
No. of patients	301	81	7	54	45	8	32	18	37
Total mastectomy only									
Five-year survival (%)	86.8	81.0	80.1	60.0	51.3	55.9	30.2	23.4	19.7
No. of patients	1034	154	37	183	116	32	72	44	43
Total mastectomy with low axillary dissection									
Five-year survival (%)	92.6	88.0	82.7	75.0	64.7	74.0	24.8	19.0	36.4
No. of patients	540	55	24	242	159	77	15	17	13
Modified radical mastectomy									
Five-year survival (%)	92.4	89.2	84.3	80.2	72.3	71.6	46.1	29.4	32.4
No. of patients	6537	630	280	2131	1292	1553	85	55	85
Radical (Halsted) mastectomy									
Five-year survival (%)	92.8	89.4	88.7	78.0	73.1	71.1	52.5	51.4	51.5
No. of patients	3058	335	104	1190	795	640	50	29	37

Adapted from Wilson RE, Donegan WL, Mettlin C, Natarajan N, Smart CR, Murphy GP: The 1982 national survey of carcinoma of the breast in the United States by the American College of Surgeons. Surg Gynecol Obstet 159:309–318, 1984.

TABLE 42–3. TYPE OF OPERATION AND STAGE DISTRIBUTION OF PATIENTS WITH CARCINOMA OF THE BREAST

| | Clinical Stage Regional To: | | | | | | | | | |
| Operation | Localized | | Axillary Nodes with or Without Adjacent Tissue | | Adjacent Tissue Only | | Distant | | Total | |
	No.	Percent	No.	Percent	No.	Percent	No.	Percent	No.	Percent
Long-term survey (1976)										
Partial mastectomy	408	3.0	74	0.8	58	8.1	153	14.3	693	2.8
Total mastectomy only	1,261	9.3	203	2.2	178	24.7	278	26.0	1,920	7.8
Total mastectomy with low axillary dissection	632	4.6	509	5.5	35	4.9	98	9.2	1,274	5.2
Modified radical mastectomy	7,584	55.7	5,481	59.1	295	41.0	361	33.7	13,721	55.6
Radical (Halsted) mastectomy	3,571	26.2	2,909	31.4	144	20.0	169	15.8	6,793	27.5
Extended radical mastectomy	152	1.1	99	1.1	9	1.2	11	1.0	271	1.1
Total	13,608	100.0	9,275	100.0	719	100.0	1,070	100.0	24,672	100.0
Short-term survey (1981)										
Partial mastectomy	819	8.5	236	3.4	58	12.1	170	22.1	1,283	7.2
Total mastectomy only	530	5.5	129	1.9	73	15.2	184	23.9	916	5.2
Total mastectomy with low axillary dissection	511	5.3	340	5.0	26	5.4	83	10.8	960	5.4
Modified radical mastectomy	7,436	77.1	5,777	85.0	302	62.9	312	40.6	13,827	78.2
Radical (Halsted) mastectomy	295	3.0	272	4.0	17	3.5	19	2.5	603	3.4
Extended radical mastectomy	57	0.6	41	0.6	4	0.8	1	0.1	103	0.6
Total	9,648	100.0	6,795	100.0	480	100.0	769	100.0	17,692	100.0

From Wilson RE, Donegan WL, Mettlin C, Natarajan N, Smart CR, Murphy GP: The 1982 national survey of carcinoma of the breast in the United States by the American College of Surgeons. Surg Gynecol Obstet 159:309–318, 1984.

procedure in the more recent short-term survey data compared with that for patients operated on 5 years earlier. Interestingly, no significant changes were observed in the other types of surgical procedures between 1976 and 1981.

When treatment modalities were evaluated according to clinical stage in the ACS survey, 95 percent of patients were treated in the long- and short-term surveys by surgical treatment alone or in combination with other modalities. Table 42–4 shows that in the long-term survey, 60.6 percent of patients were treated by operation alone, compared with 58.8 percent in the short-term analysis. Additionally, the use of surgical therapy plus irradiation (with or without chemotherapy) decreased from 19.8 percent to 16.6 percent, and the use of chemotherapy (with or without irradiation) with operation increased from 16.4 percent to 22.7 percent during this 5-year period. The change was limited to patients with regional and distant disease, and there was no significant change in the use of other treatment modalities between the long- and short-term surveys. For both analyses, 82 to 84 percent of patients in the localized disease stage were treated by surgery alone. For both surveys, the use of operative therapy as a sole modality decreased with advancing stage of disease, and the proportion of patients treated by operation alone was similar in both surveys (see Table 42-4). Further, operation plus irradiation was used more often than operation plus chemotherapy in treatment of patients having cancer diagnosed as localized or regional to adjacent tissue. For the long-term study, operation plus irradiation and operation plus chemotherapy were used equally (24.2 percent versus 24.1

percent) for treatment of patients with axillary node involvement. The short-term study confirmed that operation plus chemotherapy was 3.5 times more likely to be used than operation plus radiation (35 percent versus 10.4 percent) for treatment of patients with positive axillary nodes. Wilson and colleagues[54] noted that in both surveys, similar proportions of patients with regional disease underwent operation followed by radiation and chemotherapy. For patients with disease in the advanced stage, irradiation, chemotherapy, or hormone therapy, alone or in combination, were used more often (42.1 percent long-term and 38.7 percent short-term).

Trends and Patterns of Care, 1985–1995 National Cancer Data Base—American College of Surgeons' Commission on Cancer

The evolution of less-radical approaches for the therapy of breast cancer followed the convincing reports of the past two decades for the efficacy and equivalency for local/regional control with conservative approaches (see Chapter 46). The National Cancer Data Base (NCDB) of the Commission on Cancer of the ACS tracked therapy trends for breast cancer for the years 1985, 1988, and 1990. These data, illustrated in Tables 42–5 and 42–6, identify the high usage of breast conservation for early stage disease (T1, T2; stage 0.1) by U.S. Census Region in 1990.[55] The trends and patterns of care by board-certified Fellows of the ACS reflect decreasing usage of radical mastectomy in 1985, 1988, and 1990 (1.9 percent, 1.5 per-

TABLE 42–4.   TYPE OF TREATMENT AND STAGE DISTRIBUTION OF PATIENTS WITH CARCINOMA OF THE BREAST

	Clinical Stage Regional To:									
	Localized		Axillary Nodes with or Without Adjacent Tissue		Adjacent Tissue Only		Distant		Total	
Operation	No.	Percent	No.	Percent	No.	Percent	No.	Percent	No.	Percent
Long-term survey (1976)										
Surgical treatment only	11,592	84.4	3,395	35.8	454	53.9	261	14.1	15,702	60.6
Surgical treatment and radiation	1,275	9.3	2,289	24.2	148	17.6	165	8.9	3,877	15.0
Surgical treatment and chemotherapy	460	3.4	2,284	24.1	57	6.8	215	11.6	3,016	11.6
Surgical treatment and hormone therapy	75	0.5	132	1.4	12	1.4	103	5.6	322	1.2
Surgical treatment, radiation, and chemotherapy	154	1.1	911	9.6	34	4.0	142	7.7	1,241	4.8
Surgical treatment and others*	52	0.4	264	2.8	14	1.7	184	10.0	514	2.0
Others*	120	0.9	198	2.1	123	14.6	778	42.1	1,219	4.7
Total	13,728	100.0	9,473	100.0	842	100.0	1,848	100.0	25,891	100.0
Short-term survey (1981)										
Surgical treatment only	8,065	82.2	2,444	35.0	285	53.5	140	11.2	10,934	58.8
Surgical treatment and radiation	1,035	10.6	731	10.4	94	17.6	56	4.5	1,916	10.3
Surgical treatment and chemotherapy	355	3.6	2,444	35.0	44	8.3	209	16.7	3,052	16.4
Surgical treatment and hormone therapy	78	0.8	179	2.6	8	1.5	96	7.7	361	1.9
Surgical treatment, radiation, and chemotherapy	88	0.9	857	12.3	37	6.9	181	14.4	1,163	6.3
Surgical treatment and others*	27	0.3	140	2.0	12	2.3	87	6.9	266	1.4
Others*	162	1.6	192	2.7	53	9.9	485	38.7	892	4.8
Total	9,810	100.0	6,987	100.0	533	100.0	1,254	100.0	18,584	100.0

*Radiation, chemotherapy, or both, and radiation, hormone therapy, or both.
From Wilson RE, Donegan WL, Mettlin C, Natarajan N, Smart CR, Murphy GP: The 1982 national survey of carcinoma of the breast in the United States by the American College of Surgeons. Surg Gynecol Obstet 159:309–318, 1984.

cent, and 0.6 percent, respectively). A similar pattern was observed for modified radical mastectomy with 63.2 percent, 64.8 percent, and 59.7 percent of surgeons using the procedure in 1985, 1988, and 1990, respectively (see Table 42–6). The explanation for decreasing usage of the radical procedure is found in the shift to the segmental (partial) mastectomy, which represented 28.4 percent of mastectomies in 1990.

The most recent National Survey of Carcinoma of the Breast by the Commission on Cancer,[36] reported in 1994, indicates that patients diagnosed in recent years (1990) are being treated at an earlier stage of disease when compared with data from surveys published in 1978 and 1983. The 1994 survey suggested that this trend for diagnosis is most probably a result of the increasing use of mammography. Patient education and the increased access to diagnostic clinics have aided early diagnosis and downstaging

TABLE 42–5.   PERCENT OF BREAST CANCER CASES WITH PARTIAL (SEGMENTAL) MASTECTOMY BY U.S. CENSUS REGION, 1990, STAGES 0 AND I CASES

Region	1985	1988	1990
New England	39.9	44.0	52.6
Mid-Atlantic	16.4	33.6	48.9
South Atlantic	27.8	27.2	32.0
East North Central	19.6	25.9	40.7
East South Central	28.3	16.3	17.5
West North Central	14.1	20.1	24.2
West South Central	25.8	20.6	28.8
Mountain	14.5	25.0	40.1
Pacific	34.1	36.0	41.3
All regions	25.8	29.8	38.1
No. of cases	5,592	12,420	18,641

From Winchester DP: Standards of care in breast cancer diagnosis and treatment. Surg Oncol Clin North Am 3:85–99, 1994.

TABLE 42–6.   PERCENT OF BREAST CANCER CASES BY TYPE OF SURGERY BY YEAR OF DIAGNOSIS

Surgery	1985	1988	1990
Radical mastectomy	1.9	1.5	0.6
Modified radical mastectomy	63.2	64.8	59.7
Total mastectomy	3.4	3.8	2.8
Partial (segmental) mastectomy	18.4	22.2	28.4
Subcutaneous mastectomy	0.5	0.5	0.5
Surgery type unknown	3.5	1.0	1.1
No surgery	7.0	5.4	4.5
Unknown if surgery done	2.1	0.8	2.4
Total	100.0	100.0	100.0
No. of cases	14,509	26,465	39,869

Modified from Winchester DP: Standards of care in breast cancer diagnosis and treatment. Surg Oncol Clin North Am 3:85–99, 1994.

TABLE 42–7.   CHANGES IN DISTRIBUTION OF PATIENTS BY TYPE OF OPERATION BY YEAR OF DIAGNOSIS

	Percentage of Patients				
Type of Operation	*1972* (n = 15,132)	*1976* (n = 24,672)	*1981* (n = 17,692)	*1983* (n = 17,295)	*1990* (n = 24,356)
Partial (segmental) mastectomy	3.4	2.8	7.2	13.1	25.4*
Total mastectomy, no nodes	11.5	7.8	5.2	4.2	4.1†
Total mastectomy, nodes	32.6	55.6	78.2	75.2	65.8*
Radical mastectomy	45.3	27.5	3.4	1.7	0.4*
Extended radical	1.8	1.1	0.6	0.1	<0.1
None	5.4	5.2	5.4	4.6	4.2†

*The difference for the rates of these operations for 1985 and 1990 was statistically significant ($p < 0.0005$). For extended radical mastectomy, $p = 0.03$.
†Denotes $p > 0.05$ (not statistically significant). Data from 1972, 1976, and 1981 are included for comparison but were not analyzed statistically.
From Osteen RT, Cady B, Chmiel JS, Clive RE, Scotte Doggett RL, Friedman MA, Hussey DH, Kraybill WG, Urist MM, Winchester DP: 1991 National Survey of Carcinoma of the Breast by the Commission on Cancer. J Am Coll Surg 178:213–219, 1994.

of this neoplasm. Surgical therapy with breast conservation is being used with increasing frequency; partial (segmental) mastectomy use was 3.4 percent, 7.2 percent, and 25.4 percent in 1972, 1981, and 1990, respectively (Table 42–7). However, modified radical mastectomy remains the most frequently used surgical therapy for breast cancer by those surveyed. The most significant trend in usage was the decrease in radical mastectomy ($p < 0.0005$); the frequencies in 1972, 1981, and 1990 were 45.3 percent, 3.4 percent and 0.4 percent, respectively. Since 1972, the radical and extended radical procedures have been replaced by total mastectomy with or without axillary nodal sampling (see Table 42–7).

For the 1990 survey, the criteria on which the surgeon based his or her selection of the operative procedure are depicted in Tables 42–8 and 42–9. These data illustrate the stage distribution and age and geographic variations that affected the selection process. Radical and extended radical techniques are rarely used except in advanced local disease (stages IIIA or IIIB). Moreover, most U.S. surgeons have

replaced the radical procedure with the modified radical (Patey, Auchincloss-Madden) approach.[36, 37]

INDICATIONS FOR THE RADICAL MASTECTOMY

Although modern radiobiology and chemotherapy allow cytoreduction of the primary breast neoplasm, and these less-radical (modified radical and partial) mastectomies are increasingly used in clinics throughout the world, radical mastectomy is occasionally necessary to achieve local and regional control of disease in the breast, axilla, and chest wall. Breast cancer mortality rates before and after the introduction of the Halsted mastectomy attest to the effectiveness of this treatment as the most definitive step in the management of breast cancer.[1] Until the advent of adjuvant chemotherapy and modern irradiation, little improvement in survival data for patients with breast cancer was documented. A growing body of data confirms that the extent of the procedure

TABLE 42–8.   STAGE DISTRIBUTION OF PATIENTS BY SURGICAL PROCEDURES

			pAJCC Stage (%)							
Operation	Median Age (yr)	Stage Unknown (%)	*0*	*I*	*IIA*	*IIB*	*IIIA*	*IIIB*	*IV*	*No. of Patients*
<Total, no nodes	69.2	34.6	22.2	4.7	2.5	1.1	0.7	4.8	19.4	3,319
<Total, nodes	59.4	6.2	7.9	19.8	11.9	8.2	3.7	3.6	5.7	5,095
Subcutaneous	56.5	0.6	2.0	0.2	0.2	0.3	0.2	0.4	0.6	157
Total, no nodes	71.8	9.6	11.0	2.0	2.2	1.3	0.9	7.5	8.5	1,519
Total, nodes	63.0	21.2	52.4	71.0	81.1	87.6	90.3	75.5	39.5	28,960
Radical	60.8	0.8	0.4	0.5	0.9	1.0	2.2	3.1	1.8	392
Extended	55.0	0.0	0.1	0.0	0.0	0.0	0.2	0.3	0.2	17
Surgery type	62.4	26.1	3.8	1.3	0.9	0.5	1.5	4.4	22.5	1,863
Number of patients	—	3,980	2,484	13,600	10,614	5,871	1,786	1,527	1,773	—

pAJCC, Pathologic American Joint Committee on Cancer.
Each column represents the percentage of patients with that stage disease who had the operation listed in that row; that is, 22.2 percent of patients with stage 0 disease were treated by less than total mastectomy without a node dissection.
<Total = less than total mastectomy.
From Osteen RT, Cady B, Chmiel JS, Clive RE, Scotte Doggett RL, Friedman MA, Hussey DH, Kraybill WG, Urist MM, Winchester DP: 1991 National Survey of Carcinoma of the Breast by the Commission on Cancer. J Am Coll Surg 178:213–219, 1994.

TABLE 42–9. FREQUENCY OF SURGICAL PROCEDURES BY REGION

Operation	Canada + U.S. poss.	New England	Middle Atlantic	South Atlantic	E. North Central	E. South Central	W. North Central	W. South Central	Mountain	Pacific
<Total, no nodes	4.7	13.0	10.2	6.8	7.4	4.1	5.6	6.1	6.0	8.2
<Total, nodes	11.8	17.5	13.8	11.6	10.8	6.1	9.9	8.2	11.3	4.9
Subcutaneous	0.9	0.3	0.2	0.3	0.4	0.5	0.4	0.5	0.5	0.5
Total, no nodes	3.3	4.4	4.3	3.7	3.4	3.3	3.6	3.5	3.9	3.0
Total, nodes	66.0	58.0	64.6	72.4	72.2	79.0	74.5	75.5	72.9	68.3
Radical	5.2	0.7	1.0	0.9	0.7	2.5	1.2	1.4	1.3	0.4
Extended	—	—	—	0.1	0.1	—	—	—	—	—
Surgery type unknown	8.0	6.0	5.8	4.2	5.2	4.5	4.8	4.8	4.2	4.5
No. of patients	212	4,137	6,782	5,287	7,836	2,213	3,288	2,886	1,946	6,958

>Total = less than total mastectomy.
From Osteen RT, Cady B, Chmiel JS, Clive RE, Scotte Doggett RL, Friedman MA, Hussey DH, Kraybill WG, Urist MM, Winchester DP: 1991 National Survey of Carcinoma of the Breast by the Commission on Cancer. J Am Coll Surg 178:213–219, 1994.

can be lessened while maintaining survival rates equivalent to those of the radical approach for the treatment of breast cancer.*

The retrospective Italian study of 1995 by Scorpiglione and colleagues[48] reaffirms the importance of patient education to allow participation in therapeutic options; efforts to enhance awareness of alternative therapies appropriate for tumor stage should reduce unnecessary radical procedures.[25] The enlightening prospective report by Grilli and associates[10] suggests that the Halsted radical mastectomy was more likely to be inappropriately performed on less-educated patients and in institutions with low patient volume. Moreover, the 25-year prospective study by Staunton and coworkers[50] at St. Bartholomew's Hospital (London) further reaffirms the value of the Patey mastectomy with preservation of the pectoralis major muscle for patients with T1 and T2 tumors. The equivalent local/regional control rates of the Paley mastectomy (Chapter 44) and the Halsted mastectomy, account for the diminishing application of the radical procedure internationally.

The major consideration for operations less extensive than the classic Halsted mastectomy is based on tissue preservation to enhance the cosmetic and functional results. Table 42–10 depicts the relative indications for use of the Halsted radical mastectomy with presentation of advanced locoregional disease.

Major transitions from the halstedian era of breast cancer treatment have occurred as a result of the equivalent local/regional control evident with alternative breast conservation principles.[53] However, the increasing application of breast conservation surgery has more recently defined an indication for the Halsted procedure. With local recurrence, after conservation approaches, in the presence or absence of regional disease, the radical mastectomy is indicated when disease invades the pectoralis major muscle. This aggressive "salvage mastectomy" is necessary for large (bulky) recurrences, especially for posterior lesions that recur with fascial or muscle fixation. The

important study by Korzeniowski and associates[20] from the Skiodowska-Curie Institute in Poland has received little recognition. These investigators evaluated 10 years of data for survival and recurrence in 1068 breast cancer patients treated by Halsted radical mastectomy between 1952 and 1980. Univariate and multivariate analyses confirmed the prognostic significance of tumor size, histological type and grade (Bloom classification), and involvement of axillary nodes. In this large analysis, young age was a significant risk parameter for local/regional disease-free survival. For stage I T1 tumors, the prognosis was excellent regardless of histological grade (80 percent to 90 percent 10-year disease-free survival); for stage I, T2 tumors, survival was statistically dependent on histological grade and type. For stages II and III (node-positive) patients, evidence of increasing numbers of positive nodes and higher histological grade represented an *independent adverse* effect on survival and local/regional control. Hathaway and associates[15, 35] determined that radical surgical therapy and reconstruction is feasible in locally advanced and

TABLE 42–10. RELATIVE INDICATIONS FOR HALSTED RADICAL MASTECTOMY*

1. Advanced local/regional disease with fixation to pectoralis major muscle (T2, T3, T4a–c; stages IIIA, IIIB, IIIC), when refractory to induction chemotherapy and irradiation.
2. Advanced local/regional disease with skin ulceration (T4b; stage IIIB) unresponsive to radiochemotherapy.
3. Recurrent advanced, local/regional disease (T2, T3, T4) after partial (segmental) mastectomy with tumor fixation to pectoralis major muscle ("salvage" mastectomy).
4. For completion of the radical procedure with local/regional recurrence after modified/segmental mastectomy when tumor invades chest wall and is refractory to cytoinduction chemotherapy.
5. High-lying advanced peripheral lesions near clavicle/sternum with tumor fixation to muscle (stages IIA, IIB; stages IIIA, IIIB).

*All presentations of advanced local/regional disease should receive induction cytotoxic drug therapy, radiotherapy, or both before radical mastectomy. Staging to rule out systemic disease should precede induction therapy.

*See references 2, 6, 8, 9, 14, 22, 23, 28, 29, 39, and 40.

locally recurrent disease; the procedure was completed with low morbidity and mortality and provided excellent local control of disease. Radical surgical procedures may be the only available technique for local/regional control of locally advanced (fixed, ulcerated) disease, especially for patients who have previously received total breast irradiation and multidrug cytotoxic therapy.[21, 34, 51]

Indications for the extended radical mastectomy are reviewed in Chapter 43. Proponents of the extended procedure maintain that it has an advantage over the Halsted radical approach, especially for medial quadrant lesions.[4, 26, 30, 31]

TECHNIQUE OF RADICAL MASTECTOMY

After induction of general anesthesia, the patient is positioned supine on the operating table with a sheet roll that allows slight elevation of the ipsilateral shoulder and hemithorax. The ipsilateral hemithorax should be positioned at the margin of the operating table. The operator must be aware of the potential for subsequent subluxation and abduction of the shoulder on the arm board to prevent stretch of the brachial plexus with potential injury by motor denervation of the shoulder and arm. This complication is best avoided by padding the arm board to allow elevation of the forearm and hand in a relaxed position (Fig. 42–4). The operator should confirm that the ipsilateral arm and shoulder have free mobility for adduction across the chest wall; the elbow should be easily flexed and extended without tension.

The involved breast with the ipsilateral neck and hemithorax is prepped to the table margin inclusive of the shoulder, axilla, arm, and hand. Towels may

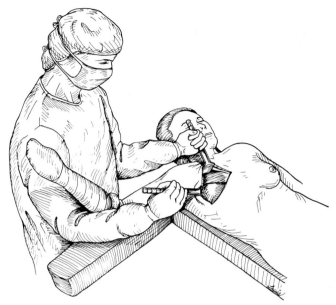

Figure 42–5 *Position of the first assistant for right radical mastectomy. The surgical assistant, positioned cephalad to the armboard and shoulder, is able to provide traction, control, and protection of the arm and shoulder. Undue traction of chest wall musculature with potential damage to the brachial plexus can be avoided by ensuring free mobility of the shoulder and elbow that is being controlled by the first assistant.*

be stapled or secured with towel clips to the skin with draping of the shoulder, lower neck, sternum, and upper rectus abdominus musculature within the planned operative field (see Fig. 42–4). The authors prefer to isolate the hand and forearm with an occlusive Stockinette (DeRoyal Industries, Powell, TN) cotton dressing and secure them with a Kerlex or Kling (Johnson and Johnson, New Brunswick, NJ) cotton roll that is carefully tied below the elbow. Thereafter, sterile sheets isolate the anesthesiologist from the operating site. We prefer to position the first assistant over the shoulder (cephalad to the arm board) on the ipsilateral side of the procedure (Fig. 42–5) so that the muscular retraction with extension and abduction of the arm and shoulder that is necessary for dissection of the axilla can be accomplished without undue stretch on the brachial plexus.

The operation is initiated with the ipsilateral arm in a relaxed, extended position on the arm board. Incisions are made according to the guidelines discussed in Chapters 39, 40, and 41. Incisions are made with a cold scalpel. Tissue dissection and flap elevation may be completed with electrocautery, cold scalpel, or neodymium:yttrium aluminum garnet (Nd:YAG) laser scalpel.[58]

The Halsted radical mastectomy is used for larger breast lesions (T2, T3, T4) that have gross involvement (fixation) of the skin or pectoralis major (see Fig. 42–6, inset) and for peripheral (high-lying) lesions near the clavicle in patients who are otherwise not candidates for radiation therapy. The skin flaps are designed to encompass wider margins than those for modified radical techniques. To obtain adequate

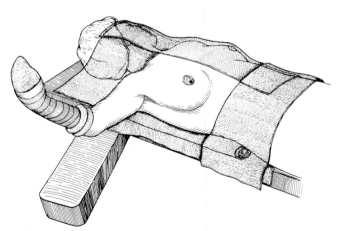

Figure 42–4 *Typical position for draping patient for operations of cancer of the right breast. The ipsilateral hemithorax is positioned at the margin of the operative table with a sheet roll that provides slight elevation to the ipsilateral shoulder and hemithorax. This position potentially prevents subluxation and abduction of the shoulder with stretch of the brachial plexus. Draping of the periphery of the breast is inclusive of the supraclavicular fossa and the entire shoulder to allow adequate mobility for adduction of the shoulder and arm across the chest wall. The elbow should be easily flexed and extended without undue tension.*

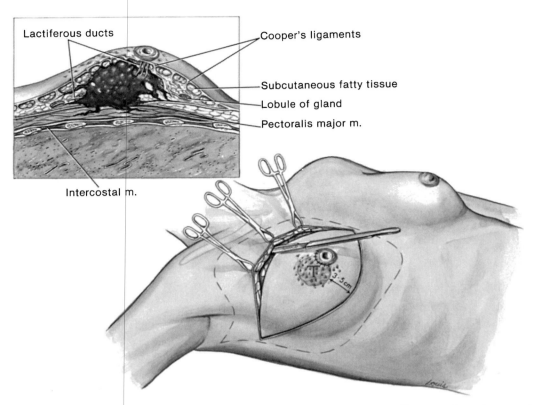

Figure 42–6   Inset, *Large breast lesions (T2, T3, T4) may present with gross fixation to the skin and/or pectoralis major musculature. The radical mastectomy is designed to encompass wider skin flaps than does the modified technique. The margins designed and developed should encompass normal skin and breast parenchyma 3 to 5 cm from the periphery of the tumor. The design of elevated flaps is inclusive of skin margins at the periphery of the breast on the chest wall. The broken line indicates the limits of the dissection and includes the following: superior, the inferior border of the clavicle at the subclavius muscle; lateral, the anterior margin of the latissimus dorsi muscle; medial, midline of the sternum; and inferior, the inframammary fold with extension of dissection to the cephalic extension of the aponeurosis of the rectus abdominis tendon.*

surgical margins that encompass the primary neoplasm and involved skin, the operator may need to elevate skin flaps at the periphery of the breast (see Fig. 42–6). This procedure necessitates an en bloc resection of the breast and the skin overlying the tumor as well as the pectoralis major and minor muscles with a complete axillary dissection of Levels 1 to 3 nodes. The limits of the dissection are delineated *superiorly* by the inferior border of the clavicle at the subclavius muscle, *laterally* by the anterior margin of the latissimus dorsi muscle, *medially* at the midline of the sternum, and *inferiorly* at the inframammary fold with extension to the aponeurosis of the rectus abdominis tendon, approximately 3 to 4 cm inferior to the caudal extent of the breast. As described previously, cutaneous flaps should be elevated with a thickness of 7 to 8 mm; however, flap thickness is invariably dependent on the patient's habitus and lean body mass. The interface for elevation of this flap is the plane deep to the cutaneous vasculature, which can be accentuated with tension on the flaps by towel clips placed in the margins of the incision or by retraction hooks. This technique of retraction is essential to allow exposure of the subcutaneous component of the flap as it overlies the breast parenchyma. Flap elevation may be accomplished with electrocautery or cold scalpel dissection.

Typically, exposure of the superolateral aspect of the wound allows identification of the humeral insertion of the pectoralis major muscle and then continuation of the dissection in a central and superomedial direction with muscular elevation to allow exposure of the pectoralis minor. The insertion of the pectoralis major on the humerus is transected and rotated medially. The operator must be aware of the anatomical position of the cephalic vein and its relationship to the deltopectoral triangle. The dissection begins medially with resection of the pectoralis major at its craniad clavicular attachments. This maneuver allows the surgeon direct access to the axilla; thereafter, the tendinous portion of the pectoralis minor muscle is divided at its insertion on the coracoid process of the scapula (Fig. 42–7). This muscle is likewise elevated from the axilla with careful ligature and division of perforating musculature branches from the thoracoacromial artery and vein. The *medial (anterior thoracic) pectoral nerve*, which commonly penetrates the pectoralis minor before innervation of the pectoralis major, is ligated and divided at its origin from the medial cord of the brachial plexus. As the surgeon continues the medial resection of the pectoralis major, the *lateral (anterior thoracic) pectoral nerve* (which originates from the lateral cord and runs in the medial neurovascular bundle) should be identified, ligated, and divided. We prefer to continue the dissection in the superomedial-most aspect of the elevated flap so that the pectoralis major is divided from its medial origin at the costo-sternal junction of ribs 2, 3, 4, 5, and 6 (Fig. 42–8). The resection of the pectoralis musculature invariably allows the operator to encounter multiple perforator vessels (lateral thoracic and anterior intercostal arteries) at its periphery that are end arteries to the pectoralis major and minor. Perforator branches from the intercostal muscles that take origin from the intercostal arteries and veins are also encountered. All divided tributaries should be individually clamped, ligated, and tied with nonabsorbable 2-0 or 3-0 suture. With division of the pectoral muscles and inferomedial traction of the specimen, the axillary contents are fully exposed, and origin of the pectoralis minor on ribs 2 to 5 can be visualized and divided at this level. With this maneuver, *Rotter's interpectoral nodes* are swept en bloc into the specimen to allow full visualization of the axillary vein to the level of Halsted's (costoclavicular) ligament, which is recognized as condensation of the clavipectoral fascia. *Level 3 (apical, subclavicular) nodes* can be dissected at this level.

Thereafter, we prefer to work lateral to medial to allow en bloc dissection of the axillary contents. (See Chapter 44 for figures that illustrate the techniques for axillary dissection.) The axillary vein is identified, and the investing deep layer of superficial fascia of the axillary space is incised sharply with the scalpel on the ventral and anterior surface of the vein, with dissection and exposure of all venous tributaries. It is inadvisable to dissect the axilla with electrocautery for fear of thermal damage to the axillary vein and electrostimulation of the brachial plexus or its motor branches. As the medial and lateral (anterior thoracic) pectoral nerves have previously been sacrificed with elevation of the pectoralis major and minor muscles, the entire extent of dissection along the anterior axillary vein allows ligation and division of venous tributaries coursing inferiorly and anteriorly without fear of neural injury.

All loose areolar tissues at the juncture of the axillary vein with the anterior margin of the latissimus dorsi are swept inferomedially to be inclusive of the *lateral (axillary) nodal group (Level 1)*. Care is taken to preserve the thoracodorsal artery and vein, and the operator should be aware of the origin of the *thoracodorsal nerve*, which is medial to this vascular structure. This nerve originates from the posterior cord and may run a variable course in the central axillary space as it courses inferolaterally to innervate the latissimus dorsi muscle. As dissection in the axilla commences, the major branch of the *intercostobrachial nerve*, which transverses the axillary spaces at right angles to the latissimus medial to lateral, will be identified. This nerve, which is sensory to the medial arm and axilla with fibers from lateral cutaneous branches of the second and third

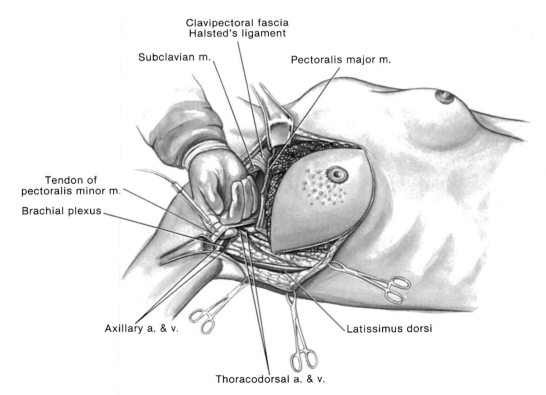

Figure 42–7 *Exposure of the superolateral aspect of the mastectomy wound following division of the humeral insertion of the pectoralis major muscle. The insertion of the pectoralis minor on the coracoid process of the scapula is transected and rotated medially with en bloc dissection of Rotter's interpectoral nodes. Technically, the dissection commences on the anterior and ventral aspects of the axillary vein to incorporate Levels 1 to 3 nodes. Division of the pectoralis major and minor tendons allows the surgeon direct access to the floor of the axilla.*

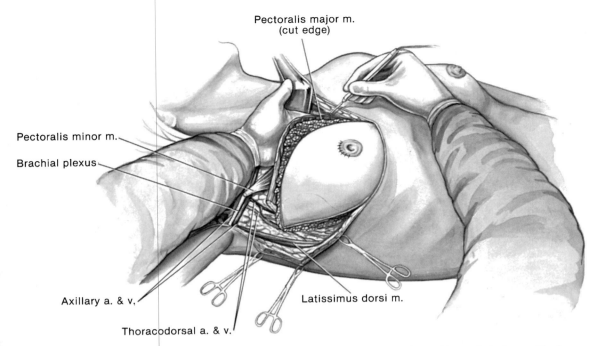

Figure 42–8 *Superomedial dissection of the elevated pectoralis minor and pectoralis major muscles en bloc with the breast. The breast parenchyma remains intact with the pectoralis major fascia. Illustrated is the medial extent of the dissection along the costoclavicular margin with division of insertion of the pectoralis major on ribs 2 through 6 and the pectoralis minor on ribs 2 through 5. Multiple perforator branches from the intercostal muscles are encountered at the origin of the intercostal arteries and veins. Following superomedial and inferomedial dissection, the axillary contents are fully exposed to allow completion of the Patey axillary dissection of Levels 1 to 3 nodes.*

intercostal nerves, is sacrificed without prolonged morbidity.

Typically, the *lateral (axillary) nodal group* is swept anteriorly or posteriorly around the thoracodorsal neurovascular bundle to be incorporated en bloc with the *subscapular group of nodes (Level 1),* which are medially placed between the thoracodorsal nerve and the lateral chest wall. With dissection of these two nodal groups and the investing areolar tissues, the posterior boundary of the axillary space with exposure of the teres major muscle is evident. Medial dissection with clearing of the ventral surface of the axillary vein allows direct visualization of the subscapularis muscle. Inferior dissection of the *external mammary nodes of Level 1* is deferred. Preferably, dissections of the *central nodal group (Level 2)* and the *apical or subclavicular (Level 3) nodes* are completed before removal of the external mammary level. We favor this technique with clearing of the superomedial areolar and nodal contents to the costoclavicular (Halsted's) ligament. Thereafter, the Level 3 group can be labeled with a metallic marker or suture to provide the pathologist precise identification of this nodal group, which may have therapeutic and prognostic value. These two nodal groups are subsequently retracted inferiorly with the partially dissected components of Level 1 groups. Nodal dissection begins with en bloc removal of the external mammary group that is medial and contiguous with the breast. The operator is reminded to dissect from a cephalad to caudad direction *parallel with* the thoracodorsal neurovascular bundle. This maneuver is important in dissection to prevent neural injury and allows direct access to venous tributaries posterior to the axillary vein. Thereafter, the surgeon will encounter the chest wall, and dissection is continued in a cephalocaudal direction to allow identification of the *long thoracic nerve (respiratory nerve of Bell)* that provides motor innervation to the serratus anterior muscle. After incision of the serratus fascia, this nerve is dissected throughout its course in the medial axillary space from its superior-most origin near the chest wall to the innervation of the serratus anterior.

On occasion, extranodal extension of metastatic disease with nodal involvement of the external mammary, subscapular, or lateral (axillary) nodal groups of Level 1 initiates tumor fixation and invasion of the thoracodorsal neurovascular bundle. When such pathology is encountered, the surgeon should sacrifice this neurovascular structure at the ventral surface of the axillary vein. Artery and vein should be ligated separately with nonabsorbable 2-0 sutures to avoid subsequent hematoma formation. Relatively little disability is evident with denervation of the latissimus dorsi muscle; however, myocutaneous flaps that use the latissimus dorsi must be excluded for reconstruction purposes. Every attempt should be made to preserve the long thoracic nerve for fear of permanent disability with the "winged scapula" and shoulder apraxia that follow denervation of the serratus anterior.

Thereafter, the axillary contents anterior and medial to the long thoracic nerve are swept inferomedially with the specimen, and the operator should ensure that division of the inferior-most boundaries of the axillary contents is deferred until preserved innervations of the long thoracic and thoracodorsal nerves are visualized. Any point of origin of the pectoralis major muscle from the second through the sixth rib left intact with the medial dissection is divided such that en bloc resection of the pectoralis major is accomplished over the retromammary bursa. The surgeon continues the dissection in this avascular plane to sweep the breast and axillary contents toward the aponeurosis of the rectus abdominis tendon to complete extirpation of the specimen as an en bloc procedure (Fig. 42–9).

The surgeon and assistants as well as the scrub nurse should reglove (and optionally regown). Clean instruments for flap closure are preferred to avoid the potential for wound implantation of tumor. Thereafter, the wound is copiously irrigated with distilled water or saline to evacuate residual tissue and clots. Points of bleeding from intercostal perforators are identified, clamped, and ligated to diminish hematoma and seroma accumulation. Closed-suction catheters (18–20 French) are placed via separate stab-type incisions that enter the inferior margin of the flap at approximately the anterior axillary line (see Fig. 42–9, inset). These Silastic catheters are positioned with the lateral catheter in the axillary space just medial to or on the surface of the latissimus dorsi to provide drainage of the axilla. The second, longer catheter is placed via the anterior-most

skin incision superomedially to evacuate serum and blood of the large surface area dissected from the chest wall. The drains are secured at skin level with 2-0 nonabsorbable sutures. Suction catheters should not be secured to the chest wall with sutures because of the potential for causing muscle injury and hemorrhage with removal.

Skin margins should be carefully inspected to evaluate devascularization that results from the trauma of dissection or tangential incisions that contribute to subsequent skin necrosis and wound dehiscence. We prefer closure with interrupted 2-0 absorbable synthetic sutures placed in the subcutaneous tissues without tension. The skin may be closed optionally with subcuticular 4-0 synthetic absorbable sutures or stainless-steel staples. Steri Strips are applied across (vertical to) the incision when subcuticular sutures are used in the closure. After irrigation, the closed-suction catheters are connected and maintained on continuous low to moderate suction with large reservoir vacuum bottles. Closure of dead space by suturing of skin flaps to underlying muscle combined with early removal of closed suction drains has been reported by O'Dwyer and colleagues[32] to diminish the incidence of seroma formation. Light, bulky dressings are applied to the entire area of dissection and are taped securely in place, although some surgeons prefer compression dressings over flaps inclusive of the margins of dissection. This practice may initiate central damage to the flap and po-

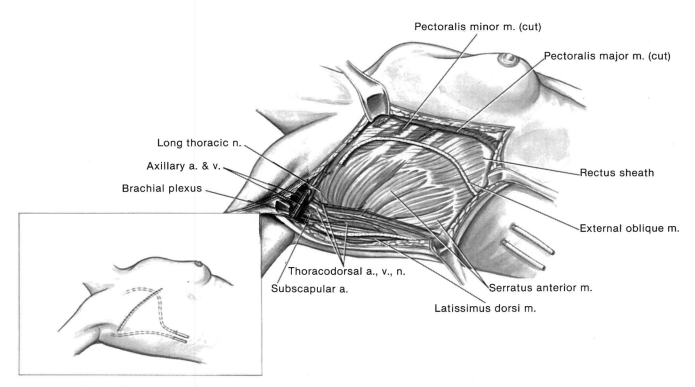

Figure 42–9 *The complete Halsted radical mastectomy with residual margins of the pectoralis major and minor muscles. Ideally, preservation of the long thoracic nerve ensures innervation of the serratus anterior. Innervation of the latissimus dorsi muscle is ensured with preservation of the thoracodorsal nerve that accompanies the neurovascular bundle of the posterior axillary space. Inset depicts position of closed-suction catheters (18–20 French) placed via separate stab wounds that enter the inferior margin of the flap at approximately the anterior axillary lines.*

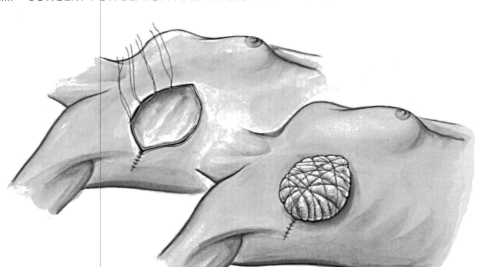

Figure 42–10 *Top, Large defect that is expectant with creation of large skin flaps inclusive of the periphery of the breast for T3 and T4 lesions with fixation to the pectoralis major. Such large defects must be grafted with split-thickness skin (0.018–0.020 in.) that is preferably obtained via a dermatome from skin of the anterior/lateral thigh or buttock. An additional option for closure is the myocutaneous latissimus dorsi flap. Bottom, The partial-thickness skin graft held in position with a compression stent created with cotton gauze mesh. These large skin defects do not require catheter drainage. Alternatively, compression foam-mesh as the stent may be applied over the split-thickness skin graft. Foam mesh may be stapled in place at the margin of the skin defect.*

tential skin necrosis if undue pressure is applied with taping. The dressing should remain intact until the third or fourth postoperative day. Typically, wound catheters may be removed when drainage becomes predominantly serous and has decreased to a maximum of 20 to 25 ml during a 24-hour interval. Shoulder exercises are initiated on the day after removal of the drainage catheters.

Often the defect created with the Halsted mastectomy is too great to allow primary wound closure. Thus, the defect must be grafted with split-thickness skin (0.018 to 0.020 in.) obtained with a dermatome from the anterolateral thigh or buttock (Fig. 42–10). To immobilize the skin graft and enhance the probability of adherence ("graft-take") to the chest wall, the partial-thickness skin is stented with bolsters (Fig. 42–10) or compression foam mesh. Catheters are not usually necessary when skin grafts are applied to the defect. The stents placed over the split-thickness skin grafts are not removed until the fifth or sixth postoperative day, unless undue drainage (serum, blood, or suppuration) from beneath the grafts is evident. This practice increases the probability of graft adherence, which is further enhanced with postoperative shoulder immobilization for large defects.

After development of protracted serosanguineous or serous drainage, the catheters may be shortened and the portable suction device secured in the most comfortable position for ambulation. This practice requires the patient to pay strict attention to hygienic care of the catheters and the sites of skin entry and necessitates frequent dressing changes. In addition, the patient should be instructed to temporarily limit the range of motion of the shoulder and arm to augment flap adherence to the chest wall. The physician should periodically inspect the volume and composition of fluid emanating from the catheter and should be aware of the potential for retrograde infection of the axillary space. Wound care and complications after mastectomy are reviewed more comprehensively in Chapter 50.

Patients should be offered immediate breast reconstruction after Halsted mastectomy; this alternative for cosmetic/functional enhancement of the patient is being applied more commonly internationally.[41, 43, 45] When the presence of adverse biological factors exist, the surgeon may defer reconstruction. However, the recent Wales prospective trial, conducted by Patel and colleagues[38] over 10 years, suggests that immediate reconstruction is widely applicable and technically feasible without long-term effect on the development of local recurrence or metastatic disease.

References

1. Anglem TJ, Leber RE: Characteristics of survivors after radical mastectomy. Am J Surg 121:363–367, 1971.
2. Baker RR, Montague ACW, Childs JN: A comparison of modified radical mastectomy to radical mastectomy in the treatment of operable breast cancer. Ann Surg 189(5):553–559, 1979.
3. Banks M: A plea for the more free removal of cancerous growths. *In* Liverpool and Manchester Surgical Reports. 1878, pp 192–206.
4. Cody HS III, Laughlin EH, Trillo C, Urban JA: Have changing treatment patterns affected outcome for operable breast can-

cer? Ten-year follow-up in 1288 patients, 1965 to 1978. Ann Surg 213:297–307, 1991.

5. Cooper WA: The history of the radical mastectomy. *In* Annals of Medical History. Vol 3. New York, Paul B. Hoeber, 1941, pp 36–54.

6. Dahl-Iversen E, Tobiassen T: Radical mastectomy with parasternal and supraclavicular dissection for mammary carcinoma. Am Surg 157:170–173, 1963.

7. Dietrich G (Lucke): Beitrag zur Statistik des Mammacarcinom. Duch Z F Chir 33:471–516, 1892.

8. Fisher B, Bauer M, Margolese R, Poisson R, Pilch Y, Redmond C, Fisher ER, Wolmark N, Deutsch M, Montague E, Saffer E, Wickerham L, Lerner H, Glass A, Shibata H, Deckers P, Ketcham A, Oishi R, Russell I: Five-year results of a randomized clinical trial comparing total mastectomy and segmental mastectomy with or without radiation in the treatment of breast cancer. N Engl J Med 312:665–673, 1985.

9. Fisher B, Redmond C, Poisson R, Margolese R, Wolmark N, Wickerham L, Fisher E, Deutsch M, Caplan R, Pilch Y, Glass A, Shibata H, Lerner H, Terz J, Sidorovich L: Eight-year results of a randomized clinical trial comparing total mastectomy and lumpectomy with or without irradiation in the treatment of breast cancer. N Engl J Med 320(13):822–828, 1989.

10. Grilli R, Mainini F, Penna A, Bertolini G, Scorpiglione N, Torri V, Liberati A: Inappropriate Halsted mastectomy and patient volume in Italian hospitals. Am J Public Health 83:1762–1764, 1993.

11. Halsted WS: Surgical Papers, 1852–1922. Vol 2. The Classics of Surgery Library. Baltimore, Johns Hopkins Press, 1984. Letter to Dr. William H. Welch of Baltimore, dated August 22, 1922.

12. Halsted WS: The results of operations for the cure of cancer of the breast performed at the Johns Hopkins Hospital from June, 1889, to January, 1894. Ann Surg 20:497–555, 1894.

13. Halsted WS: The results of radical operations for the cure cancer of the breast. Tr Am S A 25:61–79, 1907.

14. Handley RS: The conservative radical mastectomy of Patey: Ten year results in 425 patient's breasts. Dis Breast 2:16, 1976.

15. Hathaway CL, Rand RP, Moe R, Marchioro T: Salvage surgery for locally advanced and locally recurrent breast cancer. Arch Surg 129:582–587, 1994.

16. Havenga K, Welvaart K, Hermans J: Significance of local recurrence after mastectomy for breast cancer. Surg Oncol 1:363–369, 1992.

17. Horner F: Ueber die Endresultate von 172 operierten Fällen maligner Tumoren der weiblichen Brust. Beitr Z Klin Chir 12:619–703, 1894.

18. Hutchison RG: Radiation therapy in carcinoma of the breast. Surg Gynecol Obstet 62:653–664, 1936.

19. Joerss K: Ueber die beutige Prognose der Exstirpatio mammae carcinomatosae. Dtsch Z F Chir 44:101–130, 1897.

20. Korzeniowski S, Dyba T, Skolyszewski J: Classical prognostic factors for survival and loco-regional control in breast cancer patients treated with radical mastectomy alone. Acta Oncol 33:759–765, 1994.

21. Largiarder F: Surgical treatment of local recurrence after mastectomy (German). Helvetica Chir Acta 59:157–161, 1992.

22. Madden JL: Modified radical mastectomy. Surg Gynecol Obstet 121(6):1221–1230, 1965.

23. Maddox WA, Carpenter JT, Laws HL, Soong SJ, Cloud G, Urist MM, Balch CM: A randomized prospective trial of radical (Halsted) mastectomy vs modified radical mastectomy in 311 breast cancer patients. Ann Surg 198(2):207–212, 1983.

24. Mahler F: Ueber die in der Heidelberger Klinik 1887–1897 behandelten Fälle von Carcinoma Mammae. Beitr Z Klin Chir 26:681–714, 1900.

25. Marchant DJ: Invasive breast cancer: Surgical treatment alternatives. Obstet Gynecol Clin North Am 21:659–679, 1994. Review.

26. Meier P, Ferguson DJ, Karrison T: A controlled trial of extended radical versus radical mastectomy: Ten-year results. Cancer 63:188–195, 1989.

27. Meyer W: An improved method of the radical operation for carcinoma of the breast. Med Rec NY 46:746–749, 1894.

28. Nemoto T, Vana J, Bedwanni RN, Baker HW, McGregor FH, Murphy GP: Management and survival of female breast cancer; results of a national survey by the American College of Surgeons. Cancer 45:2917–2924, 1980.

29. Nemoto T, Vana J, Nararajan N, et al: Observations on short-term and long-term surveys of breast cancer by the American College of Surgeons. *In* Murphy GP (ed): International Advances in Surgical Oncology, Vol IV. New York, Alan R Liss, 1981, pp 209–239.

30. Noguchi M, Taniya T, Koyasaki N, Miyazaki I: A multivariate analysis of en bloc extended radical mastectomy versus conventional radical mastectomy in operable breast cancer. J Jpn Surg Soc 91:883–888, 1990. Japanese.

31. Noguchi M, Taniya T, Koyasaki N, Miyasaki I: A multivariate analysis of en bloc extended radical mastectomy versus conventional radical mastectomy in operable breast cancer. Int Surg 77:48–54, 1992.

32. O'Dwyer PJ, O'Higgins NJ, James AG: Effect of closing dead space on incidence of seroma after mastectomy. Surg Gynecol Obstet 172:55–56, 1991.

33. Oldekop J: Statistiche Zusammenstellung von 250 Fällen von Mamma-Carcinom. Arch F Klin Chir 24:536–581, 1879.

34. Osborne MP, Borgen PI, Wong GY, Rosen PP, McCormick B: Salvage mastectomy for local and regional recurrence after breast-conserving operation and radiation therapy. Surg Gynecol Obstet 174:189–194, 1992.

35. Osborne MP, Simmons RM: Salvage surgery for recurrence after breast conservation. World J Surg 18:93–97, 1994. Review.

36. Osteen RT, Cady B, Chmiel JS, Clive RE, Scotte Doggett RL, Friedman MA, Hussey DH, Kraybill WG, Urist MM, Winchester DP: 1991 National Survey of Carcinoma of the Breast by the Commission on Cancer. J Am Coll Surg 178:213–219, 1994.

37. Osteen RT, Steele GD Jr, Menck HR, Winchester DP: Regional differences in surgical management of breast cancer. CA Cancer Clin 42:39–43, 1992.

38. Patel RT, Webster DJ, Mansel RE, Hughes LE: Is immediate postmastectomy reconstruction safe in the long-term? Eur J Surg Oncol 19:372–375, 1993.

39. Patey DH: A review of 146 cases of carcinoma of the breast operated on between 1930 and 1943. Br J Cancer 21:260–269, 1967.

40. Patey DH, Dyson WH: Prognosis of carcinoma of the breast in relation to type of operation performed. Br J Cancer 2:7–13, 1948.

41. Patrizi I, Maffia L, Vitali CM, Boccoli G, La Rocca R: Immediate reconstruction after radical mastectomy for breast carcinoma with a Becker-type expander prosthesis. Minerva Chir 48:453–458, 1993. Italian.

42. Poulsen K: Die Geschwülste der Mamma. Arch F Klin Chir 42:593–644, 1891.

43. Pronin VI, Adamian AA, Smagin EN, Rozanov LUL, Akimov AA, Tkach AV, Kudaibergenova IO: A choice of reconstructive plastic surgery with endoprosthesis of the breast after radical mastectomy. Khirurgiia (Mosk) 3:37–9, 1994. Russian.

44. Rotter J: Günstigere Dauererfolge durch eine verbesserte operative Behandlung der Mammakarzinome. Berl Klin Wochenschr 33:69–72, 1896.

45. Russell IS, Collins JP, Holmes AD, Smith JA: The use of tissue expansion for immediate breast reconstruction after mastectomy. Med J Aust 152:632–635, 1990.

46. Schmid H (Kuster): Zur statistik der mammacarcinome und deren heilung. Dtsch Z F Chir 26:139, 1887.

47. Schmidt GB: Die Geschwülste der Brustdrüse. Beitr Z Klin Chir 4:40–136, 1889.

48. Scorpiglione N, Nicolucci A, Grilli R, Angiolini C, Belfiglio M, Carinci F, Cubasso D, Filardo G, Labbrozzi D, Mainini F, et al: Appropriateness and variation of surgical treatment of breast cancer in Italy: When excellence in clinical research does not match with generalized good quality care. J Clin Epidemiol 48:345–352, 1995.

49. Sprengel O (Volkmann): 131 Fälle von Brust-Carcinom. Arch F Klin Chir 27:805–892, 1882.

50. Staunton MD, Melville DM, Monterrosa A, Thomas JM: A 25-year prospective study of modified radical mastectomy (Patey) in 193 patients. J R Soc Med 86:381–384, 1993.
51. Sweetland HM, Karatsis P, Rogers K: Radical surgery for advanced and recurrent breast cancer. J R Coll Surg Edinb 40:88–92, 1995.
52. Vana J, Bedwani R, Nemoto T, Murphy GP: Long-term patient care evaluation study for carcinoma of the female breast. American College of Surgeons Commission on Cancer Final Report, Chicago, 1979.
53. Wickerham DL, Fisher B: Surgical treatment of primary breast cancer. Semin Surg Oncol 4:226–233, 1988. Review.
54. Wilson RE, Donegan WL, Mettlin C, Natarajan N, Smart CR, Murphy GP: The 1982 national survey of carcinoma of the breast in the United States by the American College of Surgeons. Surg Gynecol Obstet 159:309–318, 1984.
55. Winchester DP: Standards of care in breast cancer diagnosis and treatment. Surg Oncol Clin North Am 3:85–99, 1994.
56. Winiwarter V (Billroth): Beiträge zur statistik d. carcinome. Stuttgart, 1878.
57. Wolff J: Die Lehre von der Krebskrankheit. Vol 1. Jena, G Fischer, 1907, p 43.
58. Wyman A, Rogers K: Radical breast surgery with a contact Nd:YAG laser scalpel. Eur J Surg Oncol 18:322–326, 1992.

CHAPTER 43

EXTENDED RADICAL MASTECTOMY

Scott A. Hundahl, M.D. / Jerome A. Urban, M.D., D.Sci. (Hon)

RATIONALE FOR THE EXTENDED RADICAL MASTECTOMY

The internal mammary lymphatics constitute an important route of spread for breast cancers, particularly those located centrally or medially. Hidden beneath the medial chest wall, internal mammary nodes elude palpation and, unless specifically subjected to a biopsy, histological examination. Despite the independent prognostic significance of internal mammary metastases[28] (particularly if such metastases are not adequately treated[4]), staging systems have, until recently,[2] disregarded such involvement. The possibility that even carefully controlled, prospective, randomized trials of therapy have been confounded by failure to stratify for internal mammary metastases should not be dismissed.

Before succumbing to the popular neglect of the internal mammary lymphatics, the following conditions should be considered:

I. No internal mammary node metastases
II. Internal mammary node metastases
    A. With systemic dissemination
    B. Without systemic dissemination

Naturally, extended radical mastectomy cannot be expected to benefit category I patients without internal mammary metastases. Similarly, patients with internal mammary metastases and concurrent systemic disease (category IIA) will not enjoy survival benefit as a result of this or any other regional treatment. We should, however, carefully consider the fate of those patients in subgroup IIB, who have regional disease with internal mammary involvement but no associated systemic dissemination. What proportion of patients fits into this subgroup? Is it a significant proportion? Can such patients be reliably identified preoperatively? Can surgical extirpation of such regional disease generate long-term disease-free survival? If this or other treatment (e.g., radiotherapy) can eliminate such regional disease, which treatment is associated with the lowest treatment-related morbidity or mortality?

We believe that the subgroup of breast cancer patients at high risk for internal mammary metastases is identifiable and that such patients indeed do benefit from surgical removal of the internal mammary lymphatics by a properly performed extended radical mastectomy. This view has now been confirmed by both large retrospective studies and prospective randomized trials.

RISK FACTORS FOR INTERNAL MAMMARY METASTASES

Which patients harbor internal mammary metastases? In an effort to answer this question, R. S. Handley,[7] continuing the pioneering work of his father,[8] took biopsy specimens from the internal mammary nodes of 1000 patients with primary breast cancer. Handley reported his results according to location of the primary tumor and axillary nodal status. He found that patients with central or medial tumors, as well as patients with involved axillary nodes, exhibited internal mammary nodal metastases more frequently. Handley's data are presented in Table 43–1.

Handley's technique of sampling the internal mammary nodes through intercostal space incisions precluded a complete analysis of the internal mammary nodes, suggesting the possibility that internal mammary metastases were underestimated. In 1984, Li and Shen reported a large series of consecutive, unselected cases of primary breast cancer treated by extended radical mastectomy.[16] In this series, because all internal mammary lymph nodes were removed and available for histological analysis, sampling error was eliminated. Li and Shen's findings, shown in Table 43–2, are similar to Handley's; both centromedial location of the primary tumor and axillary metastases were associated with internal mammary metastases.

Other possible risk factors for internal mammary involvement, gleaned from a retrospective review of 1119 patients treated by extended radical mastectomy at the National Cancer Institute of Milan, are size of the primary tumor (diameter $\leq$ 2 cm, 16 percent; diameter $>$ 2 cm, 24 percent; $p = 0.007$) and age of the patient (age $\leq$ 40 years, 27.6 percent;

TABLE 43–1. RESULTS OF 1000 INTERNAL MAMMARY NODE BIOPSIES

Axillary Nodal Status	Location of Breast Cancer	
	Outer (% positive)	Central or Medial (% positive)
Negative (N = 465)	4	10
Positive (N = 535)	21	48
Total (N = 1000)	14	30

From Handley RS: Ann R Coll Surg Engl 57:59–66, 1975. Reprinted by permission.

TABLE 43–2. INTERNAL MAMMARY METASTASES IN 1242 CONSECUTIVE UNSELECTED CASES TREATED BY EXTENDED RADICAL MASTECTOMY

	Location of Breast Cancer	
Axillary Nodal Status	Outer (% positive)	Central or Medial (% positive)
Negative (N = 607)	2	9
Positive (N = 635)	25	35
Total (N = 1242)	14	22

From Li KY, Shen ZZ: Breast 10–19, 1984. Reprinted by permission.

age 41 to 50 years, 19.7 percent; age > 50 years, 15.6 percent; $p = 0.01$). Although this study confirmed axillary metastases as a risk factor (negative axillary nodes, 9.1 percent; positive axillary nodes, 29.1 percent; $p < 10^{-6}$), location of the primary tumor, in this study, failed to reach statistical significance as an independent risk factor ($p = 0.07$).[17]

In a 524-patient study of patients treated by partial mastectomy and radiation (i.e. no surgical treatment of internal mammary nodes), Ege and Clark have demonstrated that the survival of patients whose internal mammary lymph nodes appear abnormal on internal mammary lymphoscintigraphy appears much lower than that of patients with a normal study ($p < 0.0005$).[5] In another study by Noguchi and associates in Japan, internal mammary lymphoscintigraphy and parasternal ultrasonography accurately detected biopsy-proven internal mammary nodal metastases in 72 and 84 percent of cases, respectively.[22] First and second intercostal space lymph node biopsy detected 97% of those with disease.[22] Such detection techniques seem to offer a useful means of selecting those patients who might benefit from internal mammary nodal treatment.

Preoperative bone marrow aspiration with immunocytochemical analysis to detect breast cancer micrometastases might further refine patient selection by identifying those with systemic disease.[21, 23] Used in combination with internal mammary lymphoscintigraphy or parasternal ultrasonography, preoperative identification of those patients with internal mammary nodal metastases unassociated with systemic dissemination seems possible. Such an approach should probably be incorporated into entry criteria for future prospective, randomized studies of comparing various internal mammary nodal treatments (e.g., extended radical mastectomy versus internal mammary radiotherapy using modern techniques).

PROGNOSIS OF TREATED AND UNTREATED PATIENTS WITH INTERNAL MAMMARY METASTASES

Donegan[4] has reported on a series of 113 patients treated by radical mastectomy who underwent simultaneous internal mammary node biopsy. Twenty-five patients (22 percent) had histologically documented internal mammary metastases, and of these, 20 received no further treatment and five received adjuvant chest wall (but not internal mammary) irradiation. Only one of these 25 patients with untreated internal mammary metastases survived 10 years (4 percent 10-year survival), and even this patient subsequently died of disseminated cancer.[4]

In Table 43–3, Donegan's results with untreated internal mammary metastases are compared with results obtained when such metastases are treated by internal mammary radiotherapy[7] or by extended radical mastectomy.[3, 16, 27, 29] When only internal mammary metastases are present, 10-year survival rates for treated patients range from 40 to 61 percent. When both axillary and internal mammary metastases are present, 10-year survivals of 20 to 38 percent are obtained.

INTERNAL MAMMARY IRRADIATION VERSUS EXTENDED RADICAL MASTECTOMY

Comparison of Handley's results with those of investigators treating internal mammary metastases by

TABLE 43–3. REPORTED 10-YEAR SURVIVAL RATES ACCORDING TO STATUS OF AXILLARY AND INTERNAL MAMMARY NODES

Reference	Surgical Treatment	Adjuvant Radiotherapy	Adjuvant Chemotherapy	Ax− IM−	Ax+ IM−	Ax− IM+	Ax+ IM+
Donegan[4] (113 cases)	RM	5/113	—	40	21	0	6
Handley[7] (425 cases)	MRM	Yes	—	69	44	40	20
Veronesi and Valagussa[29] (342 cases)	ERM	—	—	79.5	Not given	45.8	20
Urban[27] (815 cases)	ERM	Yes	—	82	63	56	38
Li and Shen[16] (1242 cases)	ERM	—	—	84.5	44	61	27
Deemarksi and Seleznev[3] (325 cases)	ERM	—	Yes	77.4	57	45	39

Nodal Status (%)

Ax = Axillary nodes; ERM = extended radical mastectomy; IM = internal mammary nodes; MRM = modified radical mastectomy; RM = radical mastectomy; + = positive; − = negative.

extended radical mastectomy (see Table 43–3) suggests that surgical resection of the internal mammary nodes may be superior to internal mammary irradiation.

Ten-year survival of patients with both axillary and internal mammary metastases may be further improved if adjuvant treatment follows extended radical mastectomy. Urban and Egli's 38 percent 10-year survival rate for this subgroup, obtained when adjuvant base of neck and supraclavicular irradiation* was used,[27] is similar to the 39 percent 10-year survival reported by Deemarski and Seleznev when adjuvant chemotherapy was employed.[3] Combined adjuvant irradiation and adjuvant chemotherapy for patients with internal mammary metastases treated by extended radical mastectomy awaits investigation.

Ignoring, for the moment, the possible survival advantage associated with extended radical mastectomy, an additional argument against internal mammary irradiation relates to the increased incidence of myocardial infarction among patients receiving internal mammary irradiation. In a trial of postoperative radiotherapy conducted at the Norwegian Radium Hospital in Oslo, there was a significant increase in deaths from myocardial infarction in the group treated with cobalt 60 for internal mammary irradiation.[10] Older radiation therapy techniques appear to be associated with an increased risk of death from heart attack, and this risk parallels myocardial radiation dose.[24] The major consequence is that there is no increase in overall survival. A meta-analysis of postmastectomy radiotherapy incorporating studies using newer radiotherapeutic techniques that minimize myocardial dose, however, does suggest survival benefit for radiotherapy.[17] For patients with medial tumors and involved axillary nodes, internal mammary treatment appears to be associated with significantly diminished distant metastases and contralateral breast tumors.[15] Lymphoscintigraphy-guided treatment planning for internal mammary nodal irradiation can further improve radiotherapy.[11] Such advances invite speculation that postmastectomy radiotherapy might rival the efficacy of surgical internal mammary nodal treatment. At this point, however, available data suggest otherwise.

COMPARISON OF EXTENDED RADICAL MASTECTOMY WITH RADICAL MASTECTOMY IN HIGH-RISK PATIENTS

Clinical risk factors for internal mammary metastases that are identifiable preoperatively include central or medial location of the breast tumor,[7, 12, 16, 27] size > 2 cm,[28] presence of axillary lymph node metastases,[7, 12, 16, 27, 28] and age ≤ 40 years.[28] Although it is not possible to stratify the data from available stud-

ies according to all of these risk factors, detailed analysis of the patients with central or medial tumors is possible.

Ten and 20-year data from nonrandomized, large series comparing the survival of patients treated by extended radical mastectomy with that of concurrently treated patients who underwent radical mastectomy are available.[3, 16] Because extended radical mastectomy is likely to benefit only those patients with internal mammary metastases but no systemic dissemination, no study, except the extremely large series by Li and Shen,[16] has documented a statistically significant improvement in the overall survival of unselected patients undergoing extended radical mastectomy versus radical mastectomy. When analysis is restricted to the subgroup of patients with central or medial tumors larger than 2 cm, however, significant differences are apparent (Table 43–4). Data from Deemarski and Seleznev,[3] as well as from the trials summarized in Table 43–5, suggest that such differences are even more pronounced in the subgroup of patients who also have axillary metastases.

In the prospective randomized trials listed in Table 43–5, a similar analysis of the subgroup of patients with central or medial tumors confirms significant differences in survival following extended radical mastectomy versus radical mastectomy. If a subgroup of patients with all of the identified risk factors for internal mammary metastases could be compared, the results could be even more striking.

As stated earlier, future prospective, randomized trials will probably include selection criteria such as positive internal mammary lymphoscintigraphy, positive parasternal ultrasonography, and positive intercostal node biopsy.[22] Immunohistochemical screening of bone marrow aspirates to exclude those patients with systemic disease might further enhance patient selection.[21, 23] The efficacy of state-of-the-art radiotherapy versus extended radical mastectomy versus both for addressing those patients in the target subgroup (i.e., those with internal mammary nodal disease unassociated with systemic dissemination) seems worthy of prospective, randomized investigation.

RECOMMENDATIONS

Extended radical mastectomy, like any other treatment of breast cancer, should be selectively applied. Using the aforementioned internal mammary imaging techniques and possibly immunohistochemical screening of bone marrow, fairly precise patient selection seems possible. Unfortunately, these diagnostic methods are not widely available.

In countries with limited radiotherapy facilities but good surgical centers, extended radical mastectomy for those patients with central or medial tumors should certainly be considered, particularly when axillary adenopathy is detected.

In the United States, the widespread perception of

---

*Within this series, however, no statistically significant survival advantage for adjuvant radiotherapy was demonstrable.

TABLE 43–4. RESULTS OF NONRANDOMIZED STUDIES OF EXTENDED RADICAL MASTECTOMY VERSUS RADICAL MASTECTOMY IN PATIENTS WITH CENTRAL OR MEDIAL TUMORS

| Reference | Tumor Size or Stage | No. of Patients with Central or Medial Tumor | Adjuvant Treatment | | Axillary Node Status | Follow-up Interval (yrs) | Percent Survival | | p value* |
			Radiotherapy	Chemotherapy			ERM	RM	
Li and Shen[16]	Stage I	161	No	No	−	10	83.1	79.8	NS
						20	78.6	79.8	NS
	Stage II	354	No	No	±	10	66	51.8	<0.02
						20	63	46	<0.01
	Stage III	429	No	No	±	10	45	27	<0.001
						20	42	24	<0.001
Deemarski and Seleznev[3]	T1	119	For RM pts. only	Yes	±	10	72	62	NS
	T1 + T2 combined	311	For RM pts. only	Yes	−	10	77	60	0.001
		233	For RM pts. only	Yes	+	10	58	29	<0.001

*P values, not included in the original reports, were calculated by the chi-squared test.
ERM = Extended radical mastectomy; NS = not significant; RM = radical mastectomy; + positive; − = negative.

TABLE 43-5.   RESULTS OF PROSPECTIVE, RANDOMIZED TRIALS OF EXTENDED RADICAL MASTECTOMY VERSUS RADICAL MASTECTOMY IN PATIENTS WITH CENTRAL OR MEDIAL TUMORS

Trial	Tumor Size	No. of Patients with Central or Medial Tumor	Adjuvant Treatment		Axillary Node Status	Follow-up Interval (yrs)	Percent Survival		p Value
			Radiotherapy	Chemotherapy			ERM	RM	
Chicago Trial[6, 20]	T1–T2	70	No	Yes	±	10	86.0	60.0	0.025
International Cooperative Trial[12, 20]	T1–T2	192	No	No	+	5	71	52	0.01
						10	Subgroup not analyzed		
Milan[29]	T1–T3a	286	No	No	±	10	62	56	NS
Inst. Gustave Roussy[13]	T1–T2	70	No	No	+	15	53	28	0.05

*Data from centers participating in International Cooperative Trial.
ERM = Extended radical mastectomy; NS = not significant; RM = radical mastectomy; + = positive; − = negative.

poor cosmesis and excessive morbidity with surgical treatment of internal mammary nodes severely limit the use of extended radical mastectomy in the treatment of breast cancer. Proponents of radiotherapy for internal mammary disease largely ignore the treatment-related mortality rate associated with this technique, confident that modern radiotherapeutic techniques can eliminate this problem.

Given increasingly accurate internal mammary imaging techniques, better methods for detecting systemic disease, and improved reconstructive methods (see later), the stage is set for prospective, randomized assessment of various treatments for internal mammary disease: extended radical mastectomy, radiotherapy, or both.

OPERATIVE PROCEDURE

Histological confirmation of malignancy is mandatory before any surgical therapy. If immediate treatment is undertaken, gloves, instruments, and drapes should be changed following the biopsy.

A wide skin incision should be made extending at least 4 cm from the nearest palpable margin of the tumor and encompassing the areola. A transverse incision extending from just below the axillary hairline to the parasternal area is cosmetically more acceptable but less convenient than the more vertical incision indicated in Figure 43–1. Skin flaps are developed outside the superficial fascia, which separates the subcutaneous fat from the underlying breast parenchyma. This fascia is transected at the base of the flap, and the incision is beveled off to the underlying muscle fascia (Fig. 43–1). Flaps are

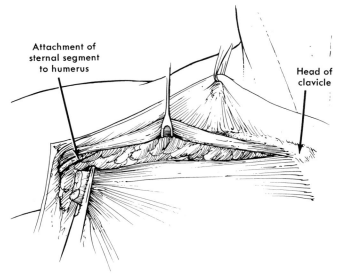

Figure 43–2   *Separation of the clavicular and sternal heads of the pectoralis major muscle.*

developed to the clavicle above, to the sternum medially, to the anterior margin of the latissimus laterally, and inferiorly to the sixth rib.

The fascia overlying the clavicular head of the pectoralis major muscle is dissected from this muscle downward to the plane that separates the sternal and clavicular heads. The pectoralis major muscle is separated in this plane (Fig. 43–2). Tissues overlying the first rib and the arch of the manubrium are dissected down to the bony structures and reflected inferiorly, exposing the lower margin of the first rib and the arch of the manubrium.

Inferiorly, the rectus sheath is cleared to the level of the sixth rib, where it is incised, or to the level of the fifth rib and reflected superiorly, exposing the lower portion of the fourth or fifth interspace (Fig. 43–3). The pectoralis muscle is freed from the underlying chest wall by inserting a finger beneath this muscle just lateral to the second costochondral junction and elevating the muscle from the level of the first interspace above to the fifth interspace below. Inferiorly, the pectoralis major muscle is transected at its attachment to the costochondral junction of the fifth rib, and the tunnel beneath the muscle is completed (Fig. 43–4).

The chest is entered through the first interspace just outside the costochondral junctions of the first and second ribs. The internal mammary artery, lying just beneath the first rib, can now be palpated from within the chest. The artery usually extends upward and laterally, whereas the vein extends upward and medially at this level. The base of the neck can be explored by palpation from within the chest, and the deeper mediastinal structures can also be examined before committing to resection of the internal mammary area. If no gross evidence of metastatic disease is noted in these areas, the procedure is continued.

The intercostal muscles of the first interspace are

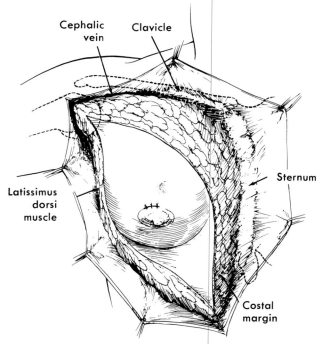

Figure 43–1   *Development of flaps.*

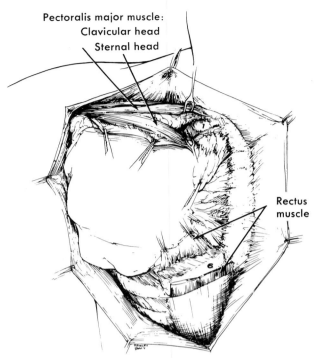

Pectoralis major muscle:
Clavicular head
Sternal head

Rectus muscle

Figure 43–3   *The first and fifth interspaces are exposed (label identifies the sixth rib).*

cut from the lower margin of the first rib and the arch of the manubrium, exposing the areolar tissue (between the parietal pleura and the intercostal muscle) that contains the internal mammary vessels and

nodes. This is reflected downward toward the operative specimen, the internal mammary vessels are doubly tied and cut, and the parietal pleura is transected just below the lower margin of the first rib.

In a similar fashion, dissection is carried through the lowermost portion of the fourth or fifth interspace, depending on the location of the primary tumor in the breast. With an upper inner quadrant lesion, dissection is usually carried down to the fourth interspace. If disease is found in the lower portion of the breast, dissection is usually carried down to the upper margin of the sixth rib to include this drainage area more thoroughly. Inferiorly, the internal mammary vessels lie between the intercostal muscles anteriorly and the anterior transverse thoracic muscle posteriorly. Dissection is carried through the entire thickness of the chest wall, and the vessels are isolated, tied off, and cut just above the lower rib.

The sternum is split vertically just inside its ipsilateral margin, developing a trap door in the chest wall (Fig. 43–5). This portion of the chest wall, which contains the internal mammary vessels and lymph nodes, is then resected from the chest wall by cutting through the ribs and soft parts at the level of the costochondral junctions of the second and third ribs with scissors. The chest wall area containing the internal mammary lymph node complex is now reflected laterally, still in continuity with the overlying breast and pectoralis major muscle (Fig. 43–6). The intercostal bleeders are tied off with 3-0 silk sutures,

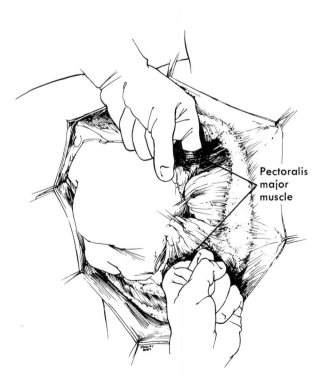

Pectoralis major muscle

Figure 43–4   *A tunnel is developed beneath the pectoralis major muscle.*

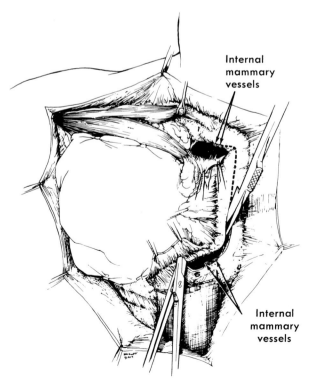

Internal mammary vessels

Internal mammary vessels

Figure 43–5   *Near the sternal margin, the sternum is split vertically with a Lebsche sternal knife.*

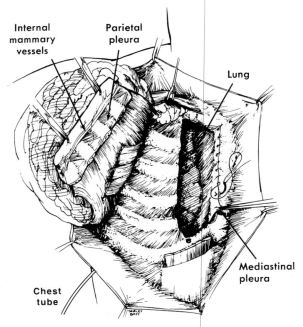

Figure 43–6   *A "trap door" excision of the parasternal chest wall, pleura, and internal mammary lymphatics is performed. The mediastinal pleura is sewn to the sternal periosteum. A chest tube is inserted.*

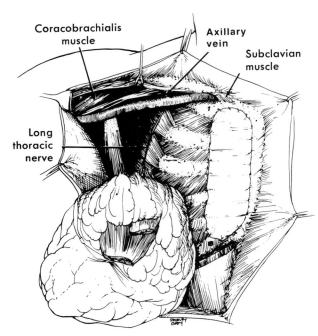

Figure 43–8   *The breast, pectoral muscles, and axillary contents are excised as indicated.*

and bone wax is used to control oozing from the sternal marrow cavity.

The pectoralis major and minor muscles are then reflected from the chest wall laterally. A No. 28 French chest tube, connected to water seal drainage, is inserted into the chest cavity through a separate inferolateral skin incision in the midaxillary line and secured with a stout dermal suture (see Fig. 43–6).

Reconstruction of the chest wall defect is then begun by suturing the free margin of the mediastinal pleura to the fascia overlying the sternum with a running suture of fine catgut. The cut rib margins are then approximated to the sternal margin with

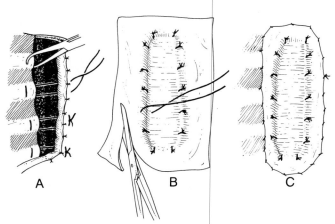

Figure 43–7   *"Traditional" reconstruction of chest wall defect. Use of a Marlex mesh–methylmethacrylate "sandwich" prosthesis is recommended, however (see text).*

four separate, parallel, heavy, stay sutures of No. 2 nylon (Fig. 43–7). These are applied through the anterior margin of the sternum first, carried across the space through the rib, over the rib, back through the rib, and back through the anterior margin of the sternum. The sutures are all put in place and then snubbed up tightly to minimize the chest wall defect and also to stabilize the chest wall. The defect in the chest wall is usually diminished by approximately one third by this maneuver, and the tense sutures serve as a stabilizing support (see Fig. 43–7). Finally, sterile ox fascia, autologous fascia lata, or synthetic Gore-Tex is applied over the stabilized chest wall and anchored under tension to the margins of the defect with interrupted double 0 nylon. Excess fascia is trimmed off, and the margins are approximated to the underlying chest wall with a running atraumatic 00 chronic catgut suture. This type of closure results in a flexible support of the chest wall that greatly prevents paradoxical motion.

An alternate means of chest wall reconstruction, appropriate to both small and large chest wall defects, appears superior to the traditional approach mentioned earlier, and has proven quite useful in those patients who require an associated chest wall resection for localized chest wall disease. A sandwich constructed of Marlex mesh and methylmethacrylate, constructed intraoperatively to conform to the dimensions of the excised tissue, may be simply sewn in place with full-thickness nonabsorbable monofilament sutures.[2, 18, 19] This construction provides a thin, rigid surface with a smooth contour and completely eliminates paradoxical motion. Patients may be extu-

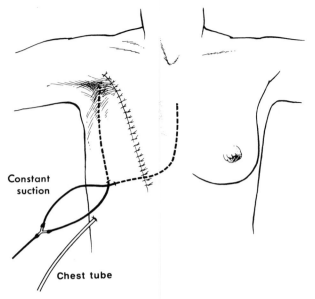

Figure 43–9 *Skin closure and placement of drains.*

bated as soon as they have sufficiently recovered from anesthesia. Particularly when combined with myocutaneous flap coverage, this technique seems to be superior to traditional reconstruction.

As shown in Figure 43–8, the excisional component of the procedure is completed by resecting remaining tissues as in a conventional radical mastectomy. We use closed-suction drains and a chest tube routinely (Fig. 43–9).

Immediate myocutaneous flap reconstruction improves both chest wall coverage and cosmesis. It should be considered in all cases, particularly if Marlex mesh methylmethacrylate is used (Fig. 43–10). In any previously irradiated patient, we consider myocutaneous coverage to be mandatory.

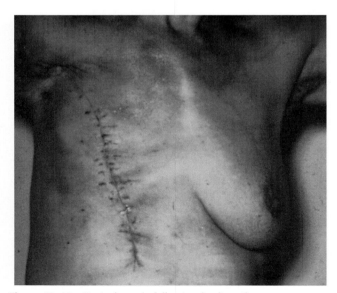

Figure 43–10 *Typical result following healing if no myocutaneous flap reconstruction is used (see text).*

POSTOPERATIVE CARE AND COMPLICATIONS

Patients undergoing the extended radical mastectomy are usually hospitalized for 8 days. The chest tube (usually left in place for 2 days) and the Relia-vac catheters (usually left in place for 5 to 7 days) are not removed until total drainage is less than 150 ml and 50 ml, respectively, for a 24-hour period.

One of the authors (JAU) has performed 1000 extended radical procedures with only three postoperative deaths within 1 month of surgery. One death occurred from a coronary infarction, another from a cerebrovascular accident, and a third from an uncontrolled perforated peptic ulcer. This minimal mortality rate is only possible through careful postoperative care of the patients, with particular attention to pulmonary ventilation and pleural drainage. The incidence of nonpulmonary postoperative complications is similar to that seen following radical mastectomy.

References

1. Beahrs O, Henson DE, Hutter RVP, Kennedy BJ: Manual For Staging of Cancer, 3rd ed. Philadelphia, JB Lippincott, 1988.
2. Boyd AB, Shaw WW, McCarthy JG: Immediate reconstruction of full-thickness wall defects. Ann Thorac Surg 32:337–346, 1981.
3. Deemarski LY, Seleznev IK: Extended radical operations on breast cancer of medial or central location. Surgery 96:73–77, 1984.
4. Donegan WL: The influence of untreated internal mammary metastases upon the course of mammary cancer. Cancer 39:533–538, 1977.
5. Ege GN, Clark RM: Internal mammary lymphoscintigraphy in the conservative management of breast carcinoma: An update and recommendations for new TNM staging. Clin Radiol 36:469–472, 1985.
6. Meier P, Ferguson DJ, Karrison T: A controlled trial of extended radical versus radical mastectomy. Ten-year results. Cancer 63:188–195, 1989.
7. Handley RS: Carcinoma of the breast. Ann Coll Surg Engl 57:59–66, 1975.
8. Handley RS: The conservative radical mastectomy of Patey: 10-year results in 425 patients. Breast 2(3):16–19, 1976.
9. Handley RS: Parasternal invasion of the thorax in breast cancer and its suppression by the use of radium tubes as an operative precaution. Surg Gynecol Obstet 45:721–782, 1927.
10. Host H, Brennhoud IO, Loeb M: Post-operative radiotherapy in the treatment of breast cancer—long-term results from the Oslo study. Int J Radiol Oncol Biol Phys 12:727–782, 1986.
11. Hunt MA, Shank B, McCormick B, Yahalom J, Graham M, Kutcher GJ: The use of lymphoscintigraphy in the treatment of primary breast cancer. Int J Radiat Oncol Biol Phys 17:597–606, 1989.
12. Lacour J, Bucalossi P, Caceres E, et al: Radical mastectomy versus radical mastectomy plus internal mammary dissection. Cancer 37:206–214, 1976.
13. Lacour J, Lé MG, Hill C, et al: Is it useful to remove internal mammary nodes in operable breast cancer? Eur J Surg Oncol 13:309–314, 1987.
14. Lacour J, Monique L, Caceres E, et al: Radical mastectomy versus radical mastectomy plus internal mammary dissection. Cancer 51:1941–1943, 1983.
15. Le MG, Arriagada R, Vathaire F, Dewar J, Fontaine F, Lacour J, Contesso G, Tubiana M: Can internal mammary chain treatment decrease the risk of death for patients with medial breast cancers and positive axillary nodes? Cancer 66:2313–2318, 1990.

16. Li KY, Shen ZZ: An analysis of 1,242 cases of extended radical mastectomy. Breast 10:10–19, 1984.

17. Lichter AS: Defining the role of post-mastectomy radiotherapy: The new evidence. Oncology 10:991–1002, 1996.

18. McCormack PM, Bains MS, Burt ME, Martini N, Chaglassian MD, Hidalgo DA: Local recurrent mammary carcinoma failing multimodal therapy—a solution. Arch Surg 124:158–161, 1989.

19. McCormack PM, Bains MS, Beattie ED Jr, et al: New trends in skeletal reconstruction after resection of chest wall tumors. Ann Thorac Surg. 31:45–52, 1981.

20. Meier P, Ferguson DJ, Karrison T: A controlled trial of extended radical mastectomy. Cancer 55:880–891, 1985.

21. Merkle E, Bahr J, Henke A, Buhner M, Martus P: Immunocytochemischer Nachweis von Tumorzellen im Knochenmark als Prognosefaktor beim Mammakarzinom. Geburtshilfe-Frauenheilkd 54:662–669, 1994.

22. Noguchi M, Michigishi T, Nakajima K, Koyasaki N, Taniya T, Ohta N, Miyazaki I: The diagnosis of internal mammary node metastases of breast cancer. Int Surg 78:171–175, 1993.

23. Osborne MP, Rosen PP: Detection and management of bone marrow micrometastases in breast cancer. Oncology 8:25–31, 1994.

24. Rutqvist LE, Lax I, Fornander T, Johansson H: Cardiovascular mortality in a randomized trial of adjuvant radiation therapy versus surgery alone in primary breast cancer. Int J Radiat Oncol Biol Phys 22:887–896, 1992.

25. Urban JA, Baker HW: Radical mastectomy in continuity with en bloc resection of the internal mammary lymph node chain. Cancer 5:992–1008, 1952.

26. Urban JA, Castro EB: Selecting variations in extent of surgical procedure for breast cancer. Cancer 28:1615–1623, 1971.

27. Urban JA, Egeli RA: Extended radical mastectomy. *In* Strombeck JO, Rosato FE (eds.): Surgery Of The Breast. New York, Thieme, 1986, pp 138–147.

28. Veronesi U, Cascinelli N, Greco M, et al: Prognosis of breast cancer patients after mastectomy and dissection of internal mammary nodes. Ann Surg 202:702–707, 1985.

29. Veronesi U, Valagussa P: Inefficacy of internal mammary node dissection in breast cancer surgery. Cancer 47:170–175, 1981.

CHAPTER 44

MODIFIED RADICAL MASTECTOMY AND TOTAL (SIMPLE) MASTECTOMY

Kirby I. Bland, M.D. / Helena R. Chang, M.D., Ph.D / Edward M. Copeland III, M.D.

> *Sometimes the tumor only is removed; sometimes the segment of the breast (where the tumor lies) is taken away . . . ; sometimes . . . the entire mamma. Mammary cancer requires the careful extirpation of the entire organ.*
>
> C. H. Moore (1867)

MODIFIED RADICAL MASTECTOMY

The rationale for the Halsted radical mastectomy was largely the prevention of local and regional recurrence on the chest wall and axilla. The synthesis of mastectomy techniques by Halsted's predecessors in surgery and pathology allowed him to achieve unprecedented success in obtaining this objective without the availability of irradiation and/or chemotherapy. From a historical perspective, C. H. Moore[58] was the first to introduce the concept of the modified radical mastectomy with *segmental resection* of the breast in which the tumor was located and *selective* axillary dissections for clinically positive nodal disease. He stated that "diseased axillary glands should be taken away by the same dissection as the breast itself, without dividing the intervening lymphatics."[58] Careful review of Moore's literature suggests that he performed axillary dissection *selectively* rather than as a routine procedure. In 1875, Volkmann[80] followed the postulates espoused by Moore but was opposed to the performance of partial amputation of breast tissue. Regardless of the small size of the primary breast tumor on initial evaluation, he advised total extirpation of the gland. He preserved the pectoralis major as the "floor" of the dissection, but stressed the necessity for resection of the pectoralis major fascia. When axillary lymphatics were observed to be "diseased," they were removed—a "cleaning of the axilla." Volkmann was also convinced of the inadvisability of supraclavicular node dissection when clinically involved and considered operation inappropriate with this presentation.

Like Volkmann, the American surgeon Samuel Gross,[32] in 1880, strongly advocated the principles and concepts developed by Moore.[58] Gross used total mastectomy and concomitant "cleaning out" of the axilla for the primary treatment of cancer in 19 of 48 patients (39.6 percent) treated for mammary carcinoma.[32] Gross allowed wounds to heal by secondary intention without skin grafting.

In 1882, Banks[4] reported a British series with use of the modified radical mastectomy in 46 patients. With regard to the axillary dissection, Banks stated: "As you cannot tell whether these glands are infected or not, remove them and dissipate the doubt." Banks indicated that Level 3 axillary lymphatics could be readily resected en bloc; he found no indication "for dividing the pectoral muscles." In this same year, Sprengel[71] of Germany reported the results of operations performed in 131 patients treated in the Volkmann Clinic between 1874 and 1878. He stressed the importance of the total mastectomy and "cleaned out" clinically involved axillary nodes as a staging and potentially therapeutic procedure. When disease was not palpable in the axilla, the "axilla was opened in order to ascertain the true diagnosis" (operative staging). Sprengel[71] treated 29 patients (22.1 percent) with total mastectomy, and the remaining 102 patients (77.9 percent) were treated with total mastectomy and concomitant dissection of varying levels of the axilla.

Soon after, in 1883, Küster[44] emphasized the importance of the total mastectomy performed in conjunction with routine dissection of the axillary nodes for the treatment of breast carcinoma. He advised axillary dissection despite node-negative clinical findings. Of 132 patients with carcinoma in Küster's series, 117 (88.6 percent) were so treated.[44] In the discussion of Küster's original presentation, Gussenbauer, von Langenbeck, and von Winiwater agreed that routine axillary dissection was an essential part of the therapy of breast carcinoma, despite the clinical negativity of the axilla with initial clinical staging.[44] Gussenbauer further advised the routine "extirpation of supraclavicular nodes . . . when the condition demanded it."[44]

In 1894, Halsted[33] and Meyer[56] independently reported their individual techniques for the successful therapy of breast carcinoma with radical mastectomy. The initial clinical experience by Halsted suggested that he removed only the pectoralis major concomitant with the axillary node dissection, which presumably included Levels 1 to 3 nodes. The pectoralis minor muscle was transected only for technical expediency in the conduct of the axillary dissection and was thereafter resutured to close the posterior superior axillary space. Soon after, Halsted advocated and was in complete agreement with Meyer's concept of the *routine* resection of *both* muscles. This concept, espoused by Meyer and Halsted, soon became the state-of-the-art operative procedure for cancer of the breast until challenged by American and British clinics on the basis of the worth of conservative methods for surgical management of the organ.

In 1912, J. B. Murphy[61] acknowledged that he had abandoned the Halsted radical mastectomy and did not remove either pectoral muscle. Murphy's practice for preservation of these muscles was based on the original report by Bryant of London, who acknowledged only one case of recurrent carcinoma of the breast in the pectoral muscles in patients followed during a 40-year clinical experience.[61] The recommendation by Grace,[30] in 1937, for use of the total (simple) mastectomy alone for the treatment of certain invasive carcinomas was unchallenged until the widely acclaimed report by McWhirter[55] in 1948 served to renew enthusiasm for the modified radical technique.

The notable and widely regarded contribution of D. H. Patey[64, 65] of the Middlesex Hospital, London, described modified radical mastectomy as an alternative to those more extended forms of mastectomy. Subsequently, a variant of modified radical mastectomy was introduced by J. L. Madden.[50, 51] A shift from radical to conservative surgery has been observed during the past three decades. In 1972, 30 percent of patients with breast cancer were treated with modified radical mastectomy and 50 percent with radical mastectomy. By 1981, only 3 percent received radical mastectomy as the primary modality of treatment, whereas 73 percent had modified radical mastectomy. The Consensus Development Conference on the treatment of breast cancer in 1979 stated that modified radical mastectomy was the standard of treatment for women with stages I and II breast cancer. Any other local/regional treatment developed thereafter must be compared with the results of modified radical mastectomy.*

In this chapter, we discuss the roles and outcomes of several retrospective and prospective studies that examined modified radical mastectomy in the treatment of breast cancer.

RETROSPECTIVE STUDIES OF MODIFIED RADICAL MASTECTOMY

Table 44–1 provides the results from various clinics and study groups for retrospective clinical trials conducted for the modified radical mastectomy. Inclusive are the absolute 5- and 10-year survival rates available from the various studies of these series between 1969 and 1986. In these series, completed in the United Kingdom, Canada, and the United States, it is evident that dramatic reductions in survival are expected with advancing stage of disease at operation. Handley and Thackray,[36] Baker and colleagues,[3] and Leis[47] used the classic Patey mastectomy with resection of the pectoralis minor and all three levels of axillary nodes. In contrast, the series reported by Madden and colleagues,[50, 51] Meyer and associates,[56, 57] DeLarue and associates,[12] Hermann and coworkers,[39, 40] and Robinson and colleagues[66] used the Auchincloss-Madden technique for the modified radical mastectomy with preservation of the pectoralis minor to complement regional control with the total mastectomy. Nemoto and colleagues,[62] in reporting the American College of Surgeons Survey of

*References 2, 6, 25, 66, 67, 77, 78.

TABLE 44–1. RESULTS OF RETROSPECTIVE CLINICAL TRIALS OF PATIENTS TREATED BY MODIFIED RADICAL MASTECTOMY ALONE*

Author and Year	Clinic or Study Group	Number of Patients	Disease Stage	Absolute-Survival (%)	
				5-yr	10-yr
Handley and Thackray, 1969[36]	United Kingdom	77	I	75	61
		58	II	57	25
DeLarue et al., 1969[12]‡	Toronto	75	I	61.8	—
		25	II	51.4	—
Madden et al., 1972[51]†	New York City	94	I	81.6	63
			II	32.4	17
Robinson et al., 1976[66]	Mayo Clinic	280	I	81	—
			II	54	—
Meyer et al., 1978[56]	Rockford, IL	175	I–III	74	43
Baker et al., 1979[3]‡	Johns Hopkins University	91	I	90	—
		22	II	72	—
		31	III	45	—
Leis, 1980[47]§	NY Medical College	397	I	—	72.2
		333	II	—	40.2
Nemoto et al., 1980[62]‡	American College of Surgeons	8906	I	65.1	—
		7832	II	35.1	—
Hermann et al., 1985[40]†	Cleveland Clinic	358	I	73	56
		211	II	55	28

*Includes some patients treated with radical mastectomy with equivalent therapy results.
†Manchester classification.
‡TNM classification.
§Columbia Clinical Classification.

1978, expectantly analyzed a mixed series of patients having both the Patey and Auchincloss-Madden techniques performed in this large series of stage I and II (TNM classification) patients. As a consequence of the various classifications for staging used in the series reported in Table 44–1, a variance in the absolute survivals at 5 and 10 years is evident.

Attempts to make comparisons with statistical and reproducible validity among retrospective series with varied reported stages are virtually impossible. Therefore, the series reported in Table 44–1 reflect a variance in the absolute survival at 5 years for stage I patients of 61.8 percent to 90 percent on the basis of these biological and anatomical differences in the tumor. However, the series clearly reflect the difference in survivorship at 5 and 10 years for stages I and II disease. Furthermore, with comparisons to Table 42–2 for the Halsted radical mastectomy and with consideration of stage classification, the results of the two procedures are comparable. With extensive analyses that allow comparisons of the Patey and the Auchincloss-Madden mastectomy techniques, the results of these two procedures would also appear to be similar with regard to survival. The retrospective analyses by Hermann and colleagues,[40] Robinson and colleagues,[66] DeLarue and associates,[12] and Madden and coworkers[51] suggest that no benefit in survival is obtained with completion of the axillary dissection inclusive of Level 3 nodes after removal of the pectoralis minor.

Table 44–2 further analyzes the 5- and 10-year survival rates as a function of the status of the axillary nodes at the time of modified radical mastectomy for operable cancer. In six series reported between 1969 and 1986, survivorship directly correlated with the presence or absence of nodes containing tumor metastasis. Table 44–2 also reflects a diminishing survival with any positive node and a decreasing survival rate with the number of positive nodes (1 to 3, ≥4) reported in the operative series. These six series confirm for node-negative patients a 5-year survival rate of 71.8 percent to 87 percent and a 10-year survival rate of 57 percent to 74 percent. The

presence of *any* positive node statistically diminished the probability of 5- and 10-year survival for all series. In this retrospective analysis, patients with any positive nodes had an expectant 5-year survival that varied from 32 percent to 61 percent and a 10-year survival of 17 percent to 56 percent. Robinson and colleagues,[66] Nemoto and associates,[62] Hermann and colleagues,[40] and Martin and colleagues[54] further confirm the statistically significant effect of reduction in 5-year survival as the number of nodes increases. Robinson and colleagues,[66] in the Mayo Clinic series of 339 patients, observed a 61 percent absolute (72 percent determinate) survival rate at 5 years for one to three nodes. Absolute 5-year survival data for four or more positive nodes was 37 percent (42 percent determinate). In the large series reported by Nemoto and associates[62] of the American College of Surgeons Survey of more than 24,000 patients, any positive node had the effect of reducing 5-year survivorship by greater than 30 percent. Vana and coworkers,[76] Nemoto and associates,[62] Hermann and colleagues,[40] and Martin and colleagues[54] further confirm that the number of the positive nodes has a reciprocal effect on 5- and 10-year survivorship.

The 5- and 10-year local and regional recurrence rates for chest wall, scar, operative field, and axilla are analyzed from six series in Table 44–3. The series by Madden and colleagues,[51] Handley and Thackray,[36] Leis,[47] and Crowe and colleagues[10] reported 10-year recurrence rates, whereas the series by DeLarue and associates[12] and Baker and colleagues[3] indicated 5-year relapse rates. Adjunctive irradiation was used in the series reported by Baker and colleagues[3] but was excluded for patients in the Leis, Handley and Thackray, DeLarue and associates, and Madden and colleagues analyses. Interestingly, DeLarue and associates[12] observed no recurrence at any site for stage I disease (n = 43) at 5-year follow-up. Leis[47] observed no recurrence in any site for stage 0 (minimally invasive ductal carcinoma ≤ 1 cm; *in situ* ductal and lobular carcinoma); for stage I disease, Leis noted a 5 percent recurrence rate at 10 years for chest wall, scar, and operative field, with a low axillary recur-

TABLE 44–2.   FIVE- AND 10-YEAR SURVIVAL RATES AS A FUNCTION OF AXILLARY NODAL STATUS AFTER MODIFIED RADICAL MASTECTOMY

| Author and Year | Clinic or Study Group | Number of Patients | Survival Rate for Patients with Negative Nodes | | Survival Rate by Number of Positive Nodes | | | | | |
| | | | | | Any | | 1–3 | | ≥4 | |
			5-yr	10-yr	5-yr	10-yr	5-yr	10-yr	5-yr	10-yr
Handley and Thackray, 1969[36]	United Kingdom	135	75	57	61	25	NA	NA	NA	NA
Madden et al., 1972[51]	New York City	94	82	63	32	17	NA	NA	NA	NA
Robinson et al., 1976[66]	Mayo Clinic	339	80† (93)		48† (55)		61† (72)		37† (42)	
Nemoto et al., 1980[62]	American College of Surgeons	24,136	71.8		40.4		63.1–58.8*		51.9–22.2*	
Hermann et al., 1985[40]	Cleveland Clinic	564	78	62	55	28	66	41	47	25
Martin et al., 1986[54]	Mayo Clinic	208	87	74	—	56	NA	NA	NA	NA

*Range inclusive of number of positive nodes.
† = Determinate survival.
NA = Not available.

TABLE 44–3.   LOCAL AND REGIONAL 5- AND 10-YEAR RECURRENCE RATES OF VARIOUS SITES IN RETROSPECTIVE STUDIES AFTER MODIFIED RADICAL MASTECTOMY

Author and Year	Clinic or Study Group	Number of Patients	Disease Stage	Site (%) Chest Wall, Scar, or Operative Field	Axilla
DeLarue et al., 1969[12]	Toronto General* (Canada)	43	I	0	0
		32	II	12.5	—
		25	III	15.0	—
Madden et al., 1972[51]	NYC†	94	I–III	10	0
Handley, 1976[35]	UK†	77	A‡	10.0	1.8
		58	B	22.6	0.1
		8	C	63.6	9.1
Baker et al., 1979[3]	Johns Hopkins*	91	I	13.2	1.1
		22	II	9.1	4.5
		31	III	22.6	22.6
Leis, 1980[47]	NY Medical College†	116	0	0	0
		397	I	5.0	0.08
		333	II	13.8	0.08
Crowe et al., 1991[10]	Case Western	917	LN−	6.5	2.7
		475	LN+	9.0	8.4

*5-year recurrence rates.
†10-year recurrence rates.
‡Columbia Clinical Classification.
Staging is TNM unless otherwise noted. LN − = lymph node negative; LN + = lymph node positive

rence rate of 0.8 percent when using the classic Patey mastectomy technique. This low axillary recurrence rate was similarly observed by Handley and Thackray[36] for Columbia Clinical Classification Stage A and B lesions of 1.8 percent and 0.1 percent, respectively.

Madden and colleagues[51] extol the virtues of the Auchincloss technique and stress the necessity to dissect completely the axillary contents. Auchincloss[1] originally questioned the value of removal of the apical (Level 3) nodes if they were invaded. In 38 patients who had metastases to apical nodes, only 4 (10.5 percent) remained free of disease in follow-up 8 to 10 years subsequently. Conversely, when apical nodes were clinically negative, Auchincloss considered completion of the axillary dissection unnecessary, because results equivalent to excision of the lower nodes (Levels 1 and 2) alone with removal of the breast and preservation of the pectoral muscles had control and survival rates identical to the more radical approaches. Furthermore, Crile[7–9] had previously presented inconclusive but intriguing data that supported the concept that node-negative cancer of the breast should have delayed axillary node dissection, performed only if nodal metastases became clinically evident. Crile[7–9] used experimental data to confirm the concept that excision of normal regional lymph nodes may remove a natural protective immunological barrier to the systemic dissemination of primary breast tumors.

In the series reported by Madden and colleagues,[51] the local recurrence rate using the Auchincloss-Madden technique was 10 percent. None of the patients in this series received prophylactic irradiation to the chest wall or peripheral lymphatics. Madden and colleagues considered removal of the pectoralis minor unnecessary on the basis of the experimental data

noted previously by Crile and the lack of evidence to suggest a reduction in survival or control rates when delayed metastases were evident. Furthermore, in this series of 93 patients, Madden[50] and Madden and colleagues[51] noted no involvement of Rotter's nodes and considered the clearance of this group of interpectoral lymphatics unnecessary. These authors considered preservation of both pectoral muscles to be equivalent to standard or extended radical procedures for the treatment of breast cancers when axillary nodes were clinically negative. The superior control rates for the axilla obtained by these authors justify this technique's application in the treatment of stage I patients.

Baker and colleagues[3] of Johns Hopkins University compared the results of modified radical mastectomy (n = 144) to radical mastectomy (n = 188) in the treatment of operable cancer of the breast. For 205 patients with stage I cancer, 60 with stage II disease, and 67 with stage III disease (TNM system), there were no statistically significant differences in 5-year survival when the results of the radical mastectomy were compared with those of the modified radical mastectomy. Furthermore, no statistically significant differences in incidence of local/regional recurrence were evident in patients with stage I and II disease when the results of the two surgical procedures were compared. In contrast, individuals with stage III disease treated by modified radical mastectomy had a statistically significant (p = 0.002) higher incidence of local recurrence (chest wall and axilla) when compared with patients treated with the radical mastectomy. Baker and colleagues[3] concluded that modified radical mastectomy is the treatment of choice in patients with TNM stage I and II disease. For patients with stage III disease, the radical mastectomy provided a greater probability of local/regional control of disease but did not enhance survival.

Crowe and colleagues[10] reported a 16-year experience of local-regional recurrence in a series of 1392 patients who were treated by modified radical mastectomy for operable breast cancer. They found that most local/regional recurrence occurred within the first 3 years of treatment. Among patients with local/regional recurrence, 64% had developed distant metastases. Large size of tumor and positive nodes were associated with rapid, local/regional recurrence. Furthermore, the incidence of developing distant failure was directly associated with the disease-free interval between the mastectomy and local/regional recurrence as well as to the size and nodal status of the initial tumor staging.

These and other observations support the conclusion that extirpation of the pectoralis major muscle is not essential to provide local/regional control of stage I and stage II disease (Columbia Clinical Classification A and B). It must be noted that either the modified radical mastectomy or the Halsted procedure *alone* would be inadequate for achieving local/regional control of TNM stage III and Columbia Clinical Classification C and D tumors (see discussion of stage III and IV disease, Chapters 68 and 69). In properly selected patients with stage I and II disease, these retrospective analyses for the modified radical procedure show survival and control rates comparable to the more radical procedure. Chapter 50 contains a comprehensive discussion of local, regional, and systemic complications that may ensue with the modified radical mastectomy.

PROSPECTIVE TRIALS FOR MODIFIED RADICAL MASTECTOMY

In contrast to the Halsted radical mastectomy, the modified radical mastectomy implies a total mastectomy with removal of the tumor, overlying skin, and axillary lymphatics with preservation of the pectoralis major muscle. Thus, the modified radical technique has the established precedent for preservation of the major muscle group, which preserves cosmesis of the chest wall. Retrospective analyses by Handley[35] and Dahl-Iversen and Tobiassen[11] confirm survival results similar to those of the classic radical mastectomy. Subsequently, Nemoto and Dao[63] reported that the modified radical mastectomy, which uses the Patey approach, can recover as many axillary lymphatic nodes as possible with the radical mastectomy. Similarly, the report by Fisher and associates[20] of the National Surgical Adjuvant Breast and Bowel Project (NSABP) confirmed the modified technique to be equivalent to the radical mastectomy in disease-free and overall survival in a carefully controlled, prospectively randomized trial.

Manchester Trial

Between 1969 and 1976, Turner and associates[74] in Manchester, England, prospectively randomized and treated T1 or T2 (N0 or N1) carcinomas of the breast with either Halsted radical mastectomy or modified radical mastectomy. Neither adjuvant chemotherapy nor irradiation were given after the operative procedure performed by six surgeons participating in the trial. In this series, Halsted radical mastectomy was performed in 278 patients, and modified radical mastectomy was performed in 256 patients.

At a median follow-up period of 5 years, Turner and associates[74] found no statistical differences with regard to disease-free or overall survival between the two surgical treatment groups. This was also true for local recurrence and distant metastases for stage I and stage II tumors (Figs. 44–1 to 44–4). Table 44–4 confirms that for clinical and pathological stage I and stage II patients, the 5-year local/regional recurrence rates for the chest wall, axilla, and skin were equivalent. Indeed, a trend favoring the modified radical technique was evident for all cases (25 percent local recurrence rate for radical versus 21 percent for modified radical). This clinical trial suggested that the modified radical mastectomy provided overall and disease-free survival rates similar to those of the Halsted radical technique, and the incidence of local recurrence and distant metastases was not significantly different between the two operations.

Investigators of the Manchester trial acknowledge the violation of protocol stipulations in eight patients who received surgical procedures other than those assigned to the study. In addition, the number of positive nodes recovered per patient is not reported,

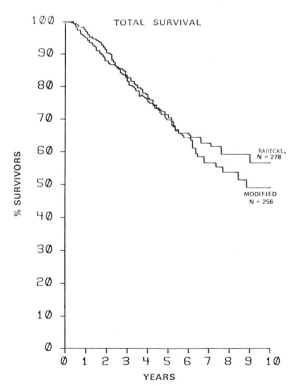

Figure 44–1   *Total survival rates for each of the two operations, including disease-free, locally recurrent disease, and metastatic disease. (From Turner L, et al: Ann R Coll Surg Engl 63:241, 1981. Reprinted by permission.)*

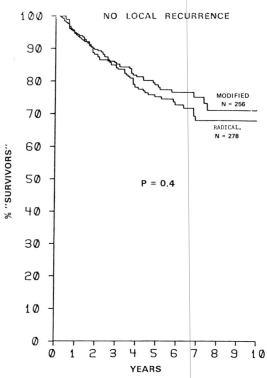

Figure 44–2 *Survival rates for patients free of either local recurrence or distant metastasis. (From Turner L, et al: Ann R Coll Surg Engl 63:241, 1981. Reprinted by permission.)*

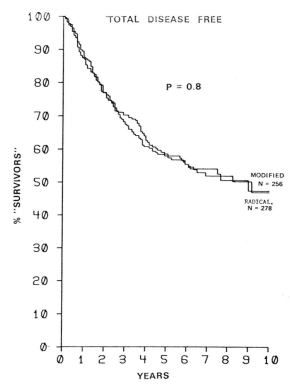

Figure 44–4 *Distant metastasis rates regardless of any other outcome. (From Turner L, et al: Ann R Coll Surg Engl 63:241, 1981. Reprinted by permission.)*

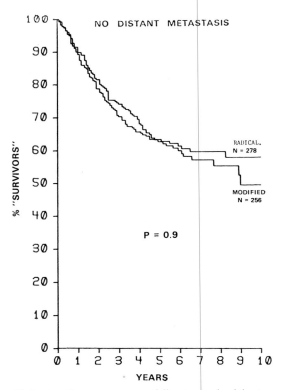

Figure 44–3 *Local recurrence rates following each of the two operations regardless of any other outcome. (From Turner L, et al: Ann R Coll Surg Engl 63:241, 1981. Reprinted by permission.)*

and the precise axillary dissection (Patey versus Auchincloss) methodology with which Levels 2 and 3 nodes were recovered is not specified for either surgical procedure. Despite these variances in reporting, staging classifications are equivalent. With regard to randomization, the only variance is that patients in the Halsted radical group were, on average, 3 years older than those in the modified radical group. Despite the minor infractions of protocol variation, the Manchester trial supports the comparability of the two surgical techniques with regard to overall survival, disease-free survival, and recurrence.

University of Alabama Trial, 1975–1978

In the absence of any clear consensus about the appropriate standard for surgical therapy of primary breast cancer, a controlled-network cancer demonstration project was initiated between 1975 and 1978 by Maddox and associates[52, 53] of the University of Alabama in Birmingham (UAB). This study was approved and supported by the Alabama Chapter of the American College of Surgeons (ACS) with the primary goal of establishing a prospective randomized trial to compare alternative forms of surgical therapy and adjuvant chemotherapy. Patients with operable breast cancer were randomized to receive either a Halsted radical mastectomy or a modified radical mastectomy. Three hundred and eleven patients with primary operable cancer were entered into this surgical and adjuvant chemotherapy trial. Although con-

TABLE 44–4.   MANCHESTER TRIAL RESULTS: OVERALL SURVIVAL, DISEASE-FREE SURVIVAL, AND LOCAL AND DISTANT DISEASE–FREE SURVIVAL RATES (%) FOR RADICAL AND MODIFIED RADICAL MASTECTOMY ACCORDING TO CLINICAL AND PATHOLOGICAL STAGE AT ENTRY

	No. of Patients Followed Up	Overall Survival, 5 yrs	Disease-Free Local Recurrence,* 5 yrs	Disease-Free of Distant Metastases,* 5 yrs	Overall Disease-Free Survival,* 5 yrs
All cases					
Radical	278	70	75	63	58
Modified	256	70	79	63	58
Clinical stage I					
Pathological stage I					
Radical	119	80	85	79	69
Modified	108	79	90	79	71
Pathological stage II					
Radical	52	57	57	52	39
Modified	49	62	74	62	57
Clinical stage II					
Pathological stage I					
Radical	41	85	91	79	79
Modified	38	78	88	71	70
Pathological stage II					
Radical	64	55	59	47	38
Modified	59	55	56	45	30

*Figures indicate the percentages of patients not experiencing each event regardless of any other outcome.
From Turner L, Swindell R, Bell WGT, Hartley RC, Tasker JH, Wilson WW, Alderson MR, Leck IM: Radical vs modified radical mastectomy for breast cancer. Ann R Coll Surg Engl 63:240–243, 1981. Reprinted by permission.

ducted and controlled by a single institution, 91 surgeons participated (all Diplomates of the American Board of Surgery and Fellows of the ACS). Patients with histologically positive metastatic axillary lymph nodes were randomized further to receive one of two forms of adjuvant chemotherapy (a combination of cyclophosphamide, methotrexate, and fluorouracil [CMF] or the single agent melphalan).

At the median follow-up of 5.5 years, Maddox and associates[52] found no statistically significant difference in disease-free survival between the two operative groups. However, at this early operative follow-up interval, a trend toward improvement in the 5-year survival rate was evident for the Halsted mastectomy group when compared with the modified radical group (84 percent versus 76 percent, respectively; $p = 0.14$). This trend became more evident when analysis was completed at 10 years[53] (Fig. 44–5). Figure 44–6 shows an improvement in survival rates for patients treated with the Halsted radical technique for T2 tumors with clinically positive axillary nodes or for T3 tumors. Maddox and associates[53] confirmed a statistically significant reduction in the local/regional recurrence rate ($p = 0.04$) after treatment with the radical mastectomy technique when compared with the modified technique (Fig. 44–7). Table 44–5 depicts the comparison of 5- and 10-year recurrence rates between the two techniques according to stage of disease. At the 5-year analysis, patients treated with the modified radical mastectomy technique (n = 175) had a local recurrence rate of 9.1 percent compared with 4.4 percent for 136 patients treated with Halsted mastectomy ($p = 0.09$). At 10-year follow-up, these investigators confirmed an increase in local recurrence rate for the

modified radical technique that was twice that of the radical mastectomy technique ($p = 0.04$). This increase in recurrence was evident with subset analysis of the more advanced stage lesions and, as expected, was greatest for stage III disease. This subset of patients with more advanced cancers (T2 and T3 with clinically positive axillary nodes) experienced significantly better survival at 10 years after the radical mastectomy compared with the modified radical mastectomy (59 percent versus 38 percent, respectively).

The results of this prospective randomized UAB study demonstrated no significant difference in the overall survival rates for the two techniques. However, there was a trend of increased survival rates for those having the radical mastectomy. These re-

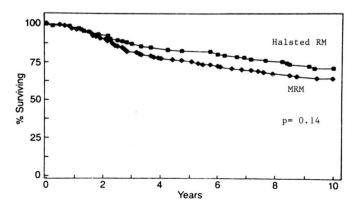

Figure 44–5 *Overall survival of patients who underwent radical (squares, n = 136) and modified radical (diamonds, n = 175) mastectomy (p = 0.14). (From Maddox WA, et al: Arch Surg 122:1319, 1987. Copyright 1987, American Medical Association.)*

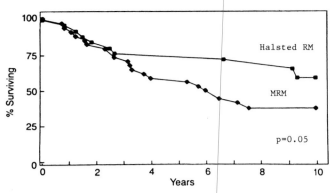

Figure 44–6 *Survival curves comparing radical (squares, n = 25) and modified radical (diamonds, n = 36) mastectomy for patients with T2 tumors with clinically positive axillary nodes or T3 tumors. There was significantly better survival after radical mastectomy (p = 0.05). (From Maddox WA, et al: Arch Surg 122:1319, 1987. Copyright 1987, American Medical Association.)*

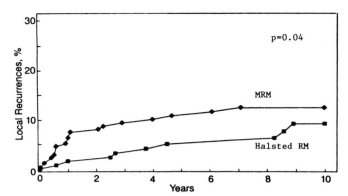

Figure 44–7 *Overall local recurrence rates in patients who underwent radical (squares, n = 136) and modified radical (diamonds, n = 175) mastectomy. Local recurrence rate was significantly higher after modified radical mastectomy (p = 0.04). (From Maddox WA, et al: Arch Surg 122:1319, 1987. Copyright 1987, American Medical Association.)*

sults are virtually identical to those reported by Turner and associates[74] in the Manchester trial (see Table 44–4 and Figs. 44–1 and 44–2) for overall survival between the two surgical treatment groups. However, disease-free survival was different at 10 years in the analysis by Maddox and associates.[53] Furthermore, this well-controlled and monitored study produced remarkable concurrence between the community pathologists and referees. Despite the large number of qualified surgeons who participated in the trial, recurrence rates among stages I and II patients were comparable at 5 years. The higher local/regional recurrence rate experienced using the lesser technique suggests that more advanced local disease (T2, T3 with clinically positive nodes) substantially benefited from the more comprehensive operation. This study further demonstrated the importance of conducting long-term follow-up analysis to confirm the results of a trial in which trends are evident in the earlier stages of the analysis. The

results of this study indicate that although overall survival was similar for patients treated with the two techniques, patients with more advanced disease had better ultimate survival when treated by the radical mastectomy.

University of Tokushima Trial, 1986–1989

A cooperative prospective study was carried out at the Shikoku District in Japan to compare modified radical mastectomy with extended radical mastectomy in treating stage II breast cancer. Ninety-six patients were randomized to each treatment group, with a median follow-up of 4.7 and 4.5 years for the modified and extended radical mastectomy groups, respectively. All patients received postoperative chemotherapy (mitomycin-C and fluorouracil) and tamoxifen. The 5-year disease-free survival rates were 87.2 percent for the modified radical mastectomy and

TABLE 44–5. UNIVERSITY OF ALABAMA PROSPECTIVE RANDOMIZED TRIAL TO COMPARE THE HALSTED RADICAL MASTECTOMY TO THE MODIFIED RADICAL MASTECTOMY: LOCAL RECURRENCE RATES OF THE TWO TECHNIQUES

	Modified Radical Mastectomy						Halsted Radical Mastectomy					
			Local Recurrence						Local Recurrence			
			5-year		10-year				5-year		10-year	
Disease Stage	No. of Patients	%	No.	%	No.	%	No. of Patients	%	No.	%	No.	%
I	43	13.8	4	9.3	NA	NA	37	11.9	2	5.4	NA	NA
II	112	36.0	8	7.1	NA	NA	83	26.7	3	3.6	NA	NA
III	20	6.4	4	20.0†	NA	NA	16	5.0	1	6.3†	NA	NA
Total	175	56.2	16	9.1*	20	11.4‡	136	43.7	6	4.4*	8	5.8‡

*p = 0.09.
†p = NS.
‡p = 0.04.
NA = Not available.
Modified from Maddox WA, Carpenter JT Jr, Laws HT, Soong S-J, Cloud G, Urist MM, Balch CM.: A randomized prospective trial of radical (Halsted) mastectomy versus modified radical mastectomy in 311 breast cancer patients. Ann Surg 198:207–212, 1983; and Maddox WA, Carpenter JT Jr, Laws HT, Soong S-J, Cloud G, Balch CM, Urist MM: Does radical mastectomy still have a place in the treatment of primary operable breast cancer? Arch Surg 122:1317–1320, 1987.

82.7 percent for the extended mastectomy group. The 5-year disease-free survival rates for patients with nodal metastases were 75.6 percent and 73.3 percent for the two groups, respectively. The 5-year overall survival rates for the two groups were also similar: 93.2 percent for the modified radical mastectomy group and 92.4 percent for the extended mastectomy group. Thus, the differences between the two treatment groups were not significant.

The presence of nodal metastasis adversely affected the 5-year overall survival rates in both groups. For the two groups receiving modified radical mastectomy or extended radical mastectomy, the rates of nodal metastasis were 84.4% and 87.8%, respectively. Not only were the survival rates indistinguishable between the two groups, but also the first recurrence sites were essentially the same in the two groups. Two patients of each group (2 percent) had recurrences in the operative field. The patterns of distant metastases were similar as well. Thus, the authors concluded that the more extended surgery did not improve the survival rates or reduce the incidence of relapse locally or distantly. Compared with the trials that did not include postoperative systemic adjuvant therapy, the 5-year survival rates appeared favorable for women with stage II breast cancer in this study.

St. Bartholomew's Hospital, 1993

A prospective 25-year follow-up in 193 patients with operable breast cancer who were treated with Patey's modified radical mastectomy was reported by Staunton and associates.[72] Of these patients, 66 percent were stage I, 24 percent were stage II, and 9 percent were stage III. Forty-two percent of patients received hormonal treatment and 9 percent received chemotherapy. Six percent of patients had radiation treatment as part of their initial treatment.

The 5-, 10-, and 15-year survival rates for clinical stage I breast cancer were 90 percent, 79 percent and 74 percent; for stage II, 81 percent, 64 percent, and 60 percent; and for stage III, 78 percent, 70 percent, and 0 percent. The 5-, 10-, and 15-year survival rates for patients without nodal metastases were 95 percent, 90 percent, and 84 percent; and for patients with positive nodes, 68 percent, 43 percent, and 40 percent. The isolated local recurrence rate was 5 percent. Symptomatic lymphedema occurred in 1 percent of patients, all of whom had had adjuvant radiation treatment. Given the excellent result in controlling the disease, rapidity in achieving the therapeutic and staging goals, and minimal morbidity, the authors concluded that modified radical mastectomy continued to be a good choice for treating patients with primary operable breast cancer.

TOTAL MASTECTOMY (WITH AND WITHOUT IRRADIATION)

The term *total mastectomy* should be considered synonymous with *simple mastectomy*. This technique represents a further modification of the modified and Halsted radical mastectomies in that the total mastectomy preserves *both* pectoral muscles and does not use any variant of the axillary dissection in the treatment of breast cancer. As discussed in a subsequent section of this chapter, the rationale for the procedure developed from the alternative hypothesis concept, which, in the most simplistic terms, considers breast cancer to be a biologically heterogeneous, systemic disease involving a complexity of host-tumor interrelationships. Furthermore, this alternative hypothesis suggests that variations in local/regional therapy are unlikely to substantially affect survival. Fisher and colleagues[23] of the NSABP have contributed significantly to this hypothesis.

It has previously been determined that regional lymph nodes have greater biological than anatomical importance and do not provide a barrier to tumor dissemination as considered by Halsted[33] Meyer,[57] and others during the late nineteenth and early twentieth centuries. These original concepts of the "orderliness" about tumor dissemination and the probability that clinically recognizable cancer was in many circumstances a local/regional disease have been essentially dispelled by the recognition of systemic disease in the presence of early stages of breast cancer. In that era, surgeons considered cancers of the breast to be more curable if the surgeon designed a more expansive operation to extirpate wider margins that encompassed the locally confined disease process. In this earlier era of breast cancer therapy, local/regional recurrences were considered to be the result of inadequate applications of surgical skill rather than a manifestation of systemic dissemination.

Fisher and associates[26] confirmed that biological rather than anatomical factors are responsible for metastatic dissemination. The findings of these investigators confirmed that hematogenously located tumor cells enter the lymph nodes and concluded that the hematopoietic and lymphatic systems are unified inasfar as tumor cell dissemination. Furthermore, there appeared to be no orderly pattern of tumor cell dissemination based on the primitive concepts of mechanical considerations and orderly permeation of lymphatics prior to systemic disease.[19] These investigators conducted important experiments in the 1950s to determine host factors for development of metastases and established that the tumor is not autonomous of its host.[18] Evidence for a "dormant" tumor cell was confirmed experimentally, and Fisher and Fisher[18] identified host perturbations that could produce lethal metastasis from these dormant cells. Other experiments support divergent hypotheses regarding the biology of breast cancer, with particular reference to the mechanism for tumor dissemination, and provide the major rationale for disagreement as to the surgical management for cancer of this organ. However, *these experiments support the concept that cancer of the breast is a systemic disease, perhaps from its inception.*[23] In contradistinction, this premise and its biological rationale do not suggest that every patient will develop overt metastasis (stage IV disease). It is this rationale that led Fisher and Fisher[21, 22] to formulate the thesis that the regional lymph node basin represents an *indicator* of the "existent host-tumor relationship." These and many other investigators consider the positive regional lymph node to be a reflection of the interrelationship that permits development of metastases rather than maintains the role as the instigator of distant disease. These principles and the evolution of scientific debate led to the establishment of the use of the total mastectomy alone or in combination with irradiation for the treatment of breast cancer. Data for the effectiveness of the total mastectomy with or without irradiation or chemotherapy for treatment of disease are derived from retrospective and prospective randomized trials.

Because the total (simple) mastectomy is designed to treat local disease or its recurrence, some authors have postulated that the addition of the regional node dissection should not influence survival. This premise maintains that the total mastectomy provides overall survival rates equivalent to those of the modified radical and radical mastectomy without incurring an additional operative risk or unnecessary cosmetic deformity. It has also been postulated that the intact axillary nodal basin may enhance immune competency and inherent tumoricidal activities. Should this be confirmed, we would expect a reduction in the local/regional recurrence rate reflected in an increased disease-free survival.

RETROSPECTIVE AND PROSPECTIVE STUDIES OF TOTAL MASTECTOMY

The previously cited data demonstrate the biological and anatomical considerations for use of the total mastectomy in the treatment of operable breast cancer. These data are derived from retrospective studies and prospective randomized clinical trials. These series make comparisons of the total mastectomy with and without radiation therapy; other studies make comparisons with radical surgical procedures.

Table 44–6 documents the survival results for nine retrospective clinical trials performed by seven institutions or study groups using total mastectomy with and without irradiation of the peripheral lymph nodes and chest wall. The Manchester and TNM classification systems were used in these trials, which varied in homogeneity and patient accrual size. The 3-, 5- and 10-year survival rates show an expected progressive attrition over time for patients who underwent irradiation of the peripheral lymphatics or for those in whom this modality was not used in postoperative therapy. Turnbull and colleagues[73] reported from Southampton (United Kingdom) the 3-year follow-up results of patients treated by simple mastectomy alone or by simple mastectomy with radical irradiation. There were no statistically significant differences in survival of patients in the two groups at 3 years, but local recurrence was significantly more frequent (28 percent) in the mastectomy-alone group. Early survival was not adversely affected by irradiation.

For these various trials, the 5-year survival rate for clinical TNM stage I tumors ranged from 51 percent to 78 percent; for clinical TNM stage II cancers, the range was 33.7 percent to 71 percent. Radical radiotherapy administered to the peripheral lymphatics in these nine series appears to have had little overall benefit in the groups compared by Williams and associates[81] at 5 years. However, at 10 years, absolute survival appeared to be improved in patients who had undergone radical irradiation of the

TABLE 44–6. SURVIVAL RESULTS OF RETROSPECTIVE CLINICAL TRIALS FOR TOTAL MASTECTOMY WITH OR WITHOUT RADIOTHERAPY (RT)

Author and Year	Clinic or Study Group	No. of Patients	Disease Stage	Absolute Survival (%) 5-year −RT	5-year +RT	10-year −RT	10-year +RT
Williams et al., 1953[81]	St. Bartholomew (U.K.)	110	I	77	67	33	40
		45	II	—	35	—	21
Smith and Meyer, 1959[70]	Rockford, IL	97	I & II	54	—	32	—
Shimkin et al., 1961[69]	Rockford, IL	103	I & II	51	—	31	—
Devitt, 1962[14]	Ottawa (Canada)	119	I	—	68	—	45
		30	II	—	56	—	47
Den Besten and Ziffren, 1965[13]	University of Iowa	133	I	55.7	—	—	—
		95	II	33.7	—	—	—
Kyle et al., 1976[45]	Cancer Research Campaign (U.K.)	1152	I*	78	79	—	—
		1116	II	71	76	—	—
Turnbull et al., 1978[73]	Southampton (U.K.)	96	I	84†	85†	—	—
		54	II	72†	81†	—	—
Meyer et al., 1978[56]	Rockford, IL	252	I & II	69	—	40	—
Hermann et al., 1985[40]	Cleveland Clinic	355	I	78	—	60	—
		47	II	53	—	37	—

*Manchester Staging Classification.
†3-year survival.

peripheral lymphatics. Hermann and associates[40] reported a 10-year absolute survival of 60 percent for stage 1 and 37 percent for stage II, respectively. No comparisons were made at 10 years for usage of radical irradiation in this series. These data must be viewed with the knowledge that these trials span three decades and use diverse techniques by varying physicians in retrospective reports. However, it seems evident that the survival rates achieved with total mastectomy (both with and without radiation therapy) are comparable to those obtained with radical mastectomy.

Table 44–7 catalogues local/regional recurrence rates after total mastectomy with and without irradiation in nine retrospective and prospective clinical trials conducted in the United Kingdom, South Africa, and the United States. The series by Williams and associates[81] of St. Bartholomew's-St. Albans Hospitals (U.K.) represents a 10-year study of patients with stage I, II, or III cancer. With comparable matching of patients in these stages, the authors used total mastectomy with and without irradiation or total mastectomy with radium implants. No differences were observed between the treatment groups using external beam irradiation or radium implants versus the surgery-only group. Recurrences at the chest wall, scar, or supraclavicular sites were not documented in this series.[81]

Crile[8] of the Cleveland Clinic treated operable stage I and II breast cancer with simple mastectomy alone (stage I) and occasionally used radical irradiation of the peripheral lymphatics for stage II disease. In 69 reported cases at this institution, 5 patients (7.2 percent) treated by simple mastectomy had local recurrence in the chest wall or the axilla; in a comparable group of 62 patients treated by radical operation, 5 (8.1 percent) had similar recurrence. Crile does not document recurrence rates in chest wall, scar, operative field, or supraclavicular sites.

Helman and associates[37] reported on a controlled trial to investigate the efficacy of simple mastectomy versus radical mastectomy in the treatment of TNM stage I and II operable breast cancer at the Groote Schuur Hospital in Capetown, South Africa. This interim study was rapidly terminated when follow-up analysis at the time of the report confirmed that 5 of 51 patients (9.8 percent) having simple mastectomy developed lymph node recurrence in the axilla, and 7 (13.7 percent) developed skin flap recurrence. Recurrence rates in the operative scar, chest wall, or supraclavicular sites were not reported. In contrast, Helman and associates[37] confirmed that of 44 patients undergoing radical mastectomy, only 1 (2.3 percent) developed skin flap recurrence, and none developed axillary nodal recurrence at the time of this brief follow-up of 2 to 5 years. This high rate of local/regional recurrence for the simple mastectomy persuaded the authors to recommend techniques that include axillary node dissection or postoperative irradiation therapy for treatment of operable breast cancer.

In the original report of the Cancer Research Campaign of the United Kingdom, Kyle and associates[45] compared the results of a radical therapeutic regimen (total mastectomy and radiotherapy) to those of a conservative policy (total mastectomy alone) in a prospective controlled clinical study. The study included 2268 patients to ensure that small but significant differences between the two treatments would be evident. Within a 5-year follow-up interval, there was no evidence that routine postoperative radiation therapy was detrimental to wound repair;

TABLE 44–7.   LOCAL AND REGIONAL RECURRENCE RATES AFTER TOTAL MASTECTOMY WITH OR WITHOUT RADIOTHERAPY

Author and Year	Clinic or Study Group	No. of Patients	Disease Stage	Follow-up (yrs)	Chest Wall	Scar	Operative Field	Supra-clavicular
Williams et al., 1953[81]	St. Bartholomew's	55*	I–III	10	—	—	16	—
	St. Albans (U.K.)	63†	I–III	10	—	—	14	—
		98§	I–III	10	—	—	13	—
Crile, 1964[9]	Cleveland Clinic*†	69	I + II	5	7.2	—	—	—
Helman et al., 1972[37]	Groote Schuur (Capetown)	51	I + II	2–5	—	—	13.7	—
Kyle et al., 1976[45]	Cancer Research Campaign (U.K.)	1152*	I + II	5	3.2	—	4.9	2.2
	King's College	1116†	I + II	5	0.8	—	1.5	0.7
Turnbull et al., 1978[73]	Holt Radium Inst.	76*	I + II	1–4	—	—	27.6	—
	Southampton (U.K.)	74†	I + II	1–4	—	—	10.8	—
Langlands et al., 1980[46]	Southeast Scotland	131†	I	12	—	—	8.4	3.1
		64†	II	12	—	—	12.5	6.3
		47†	III	12	—	—	12.8	4.3
Forrest et al., 1974, 1982[27, 28]	Edinburgh (Cardiff/St. Mary's)	75*	I	5	—	5.3	2.7	—
		49†	I	5	—	8.0	4.0	—
		39‡	II	10	25.6	—	—	—
Berstock et al., 1985[5]	Cancer Research Campaign (U.K.)	1121*	I + II	14	12.4	—	—	3.9
	King's College	1122	I + II	14	6.5	—	—	3.4
Fisher et al., 1985[20]	NSABP B-04*	365	I	10	5.2	1.6	0.8	3.0
	NSABP B-04†	352	I	10	0.9	0.3	0.0	0.3
	NSABP B-04†	294	II	10	0.7	0.3	0.7	0.0

*Total mastectomy alone.
†Total mastectomy with radical irradiation.
‡Total mastectomy with axillary irradiation only.
§Total mastectomy plus radium implant.

however, this modality also conferred no additional benefit as to survival or distant recurrence. Irradiation did, however, significantly reduce the incidence of local/regional recurrence, as indicated in Table 44–7. Almost a fourfold reduction in chest wall recurrence and a threefold reduction in supraclavicular recurrence was evident at 5-year follow-up with the addition of irradiation. Similar trends were observed in recurrence at the operative site. Berstock and associates[5] continued this trial, with follow-up ranging from 9 to 14 years (median, 11.4 years). Again, updated analyses showed no significant differences in survival and distant recurrence between the two treatment groups. Conversely, patients who received prophylactic irradiation postoperatively continued to have a reduced risk for development of local recurrence as the first sign of treatment failure ($p <$ 0.001). A twofold reduction was evident in chest wall recurrence at the median follow-up of 11.4 years. Specifics with regard to site and operative field recurrence were not reported. Interestingly, at the median follow-up of 11.4 years, prophylactic irradiation appeared to confer minimal benefit for control of the supraclavicular site.

Houghton and associates[42] reported a follow-up of the Cancer Research Campaign study recently. A total of 2800 patients with a median follow-up of 19 years were included in the recent analysis. Local recurrence after simple mastectomy was significantly reduced by the added radiation therapy (RR = 0.44 [0.39–0.51]). The reduction in risk continues, although to a lesser degree, even after 10 years (Table 44–8). The sites of local/regional failure are summarized in Table 44–9. The prognosis of patients with local recurrence is poor, with less than one third surviving for 5 years, and it is particularly bad in patients previously treated with radiation and in those who developed supraclavicular recurrence. The overall survival rates in the two treatment groups are similar; however, there are more non–breast cancer deaths observed in the irradiated patients (Fig.

TABLE 44–9. SITES OF FIRST LOCAL/REGIONAL FAILURE

Site	DXT	WP	Relative Risk	Log Rank p Value
Chest wall	69	135	0.50 (0.38–0.66)*	<0.001
Axilla	79	277	0.31 (0.25–0.38)	<0.001
Supraclavicular nodes	28	31	0.85 (0.51–1.42)	0.54
Internal mammary nodes	1	3	Inestimable†	
Multiple sites‡	53	96	0.53 (0.38–0.73)	<0.001
All sites§	230	542	0.42 (0.36–0.48)	<0.001

*The 95% confidence intervals are shown in parentheses
†Too few events have occurred to allow accurate estimation
‡Patients having recurrence simultaneously at more than one local site are included in this study
§Patients who did not have detailed site information available were excluded
From Houghton J, Baum M, Haybittle JL: Role of radiotherapy following total mastectomy in patients with early breast cancer. World J Surg 18:117–122, 1994.

44–8). These non–breast cancer deaths include increased cardiac causes of death and non–breast malignancies. Those patients with breast cancer on the left side in the group treated with radiation were particularly at increased risk for non–breast cancer deaths.

A prospective randomized trial was conducted by Turnbull and associates[73] in Southampton for treatment of early breast cancer with total mastectomy alone versus total mastectomy with radical radiotherapy. These investigators matched groups for age, menopausal status, duration of symptoms, size of tumor, and nodal involvement. In stage I and II patients (n = 76) treated with total mastectomy alone and followed for 1 to 4 years, operative field recurrence was 27.6 percent. Seventy-four patients with TNM stages I and II disease who were followed con-

TABLE 44–8. LOCAL RECURRENCE BY LENGTH OF FOLLOW-UP AFTER SIMPLE MASTECTOMY FOLLOWING RADIATION THERAPY

Follow-up Interval (yr)	No. of Patients	Relative Risk	Log Rank p Value
0–4.99	2800	0.40 (0.34–0.46)[a]	<0.001
5–9.99	1699	0.67 (0.51–0.88)	0.004
10–14.99	1152	0.61 (0.37–1.01)	0.06
15+	602	0.22 (0.06–0.82)	0.02
10+	1152	0.54 (0.34–0.87)	0.01
All	2800	0.44 (0.39–0.51)	<0.001

[a]The 95% confidence intervals are shown in parentheses.
From Houghton J, Baum M, Haybittle JL: Role of radiotherapy following total mastectomy in patients with early breast cancer. World J Surg 18:117–122, 1994.

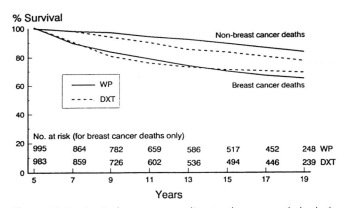

Figure 44–8 *Survival curves according to the cause of death for patients alive 5 years after randomization. When deaths from breast cancer only are considered as events: $\chi^2 = 0.76$, $p = 0.38$, RR = 0.93 (0.79 − 1.09); when only deaths from causes other than breast cancer were counted as events: $\chi^2 = 11.03$, $p < 0.001$, RR = 1.49 (1.18 − 1.89). The number at risk represents the number of patients alive in each group at 5 years and every 2 years thereafter. This number decreases during later years, because fewer patients have relevant trial times. From Houghton J, Baum M, Haybittle JL: Role of radiotherapy following total mastectomy in patients with early breast cancer. World J Surg 18:117–122, 1994.*

currently at the same interval but were treated with postoperative irradiation showed a reduction in operative field recurrence to 10.8 percent. Early survival was not affected by radiation therapy.

In the randomized trial conducted by Langlands and colleagues[46] in southeast Scotland, the overall survival rate with use of radical mastectomy was equivalent to that for patients treated by simple mastectomy and radical irradiation. At 12 years follow-up, these authors confirmed that survival in the radical mastectomy treatment group was significantly better ($p < 0.05$), but only for those with clinical stage I disease. The pattern of survival after recurrence was detected confirmed interesting differences between the two treatment modalities. Overall, there was a significantly prolonged survival after detection of recurrence in the radical mastectomy group ($p < 0.05$); this was greatest when local recurrence and distant metastases coincided ($p < 0.01$). Forrest and associates[27, 28] of the University Department of Clinical Surgery, Royal Infirmary, Edinburgh, confirmed scar recurrence rates of 5.3 percent and 8.0 percent for TNM stages I and II, respectively. Recurrence rates in the operative field were 2.7 percent and 4.0 percent at 5-year follow-up for stages I and II, respectively.

In NSABP B-04, Fisher and associates[20] conducted a randomized study to compare alternative local and regional treatments of breast cancer. Life table estimates were obtained for 1665 women enrolled for a mean of 126 months (see critique Total Mastectomy with/without Irradiation). For patients treated by total (simple) mastectomy without axillary irradiation but with regional irradiation versus those treated by total mastectomy alone, no differences were observed between patients with clinically positive nodes or clinically negative nodes with respect to recurrence-free survival, distant disease-free survival, or overall survival at 10 years follow-up. Ten-year survival was approximately 57 percent for node-negative patients and 38 percent for node-positive patients. These investigators concluded that variations of local and re-

gional treatment were not important in determining survival of patients with breast cancer. Results obtained at 5 years accurately predicted outcome at 10 years. Despite these similarities in survival, chest wall recurrence was significantly greater at 10-year follow-up for stage I patients treated with mastectomy alone (5.2 percent) versus patients treated with total mastectomy and radical irradiation (0.9 percent). Table 44–7 further documents the reduction in scar, operative field, and supraclavicular recurrence for stage I and stage II disease in patients treated with adjunctive radiotherapy.

The axillary recurrence rates for node-negative and node-positive patients treated with total mastectomy with and without radiation are depicted in Table 44–10. The series by Kyle and coworkers[45] and Berstock and associates[5] represent trials of the Cancer Research Campaign of the United Kingdom. The series reported by Langlands and colleagues[46] was updated at 10 years in the Cardiff-St. Mary's study by Forrest and associates.[27, 28] In the report by Crile[8] of 103 node-negative and 35 node-positive patients, the axillary recurrence rate for node-negative patients was 30.0 percent at 6-year follow-up. The recurrence rate for node-positive patients was not reported in this series.

In the Cancer Research Campaign of the UK initially reported by Kyle and coworkers,[45] with detailed follow-up at 14 years by Berstock and associates,[5] the benefit of radiotherapy was evident in the node-negative group. At 5 years, a reduction in axillary recurrence rate for stage I disease from 9.5 percent to 1.7 percent was attributed to the use of prophylactic radiotherapy. At 14 years follow-up, Berstock and associates[5] documented an axillary recurrence rate of 23.8 percent for stage I disease. A reduction of the relapse rate to 6.4 percent was evident in patients who had undergone radical radiotherapy to the chest wall and regional lymphatics. In the Scottish trial initially reported by Langlands and colleagues[46] with follow-up by Forrest and associates,[27, 28] 5-year axillary recurrence rate for node-negative and node-posi-

TABLE 44–10. AXILLARY RECURRENCE RATES FOR PATIENTS TREATED WITH TOTAL MASTECTOMY WITH OR WITHOUT RADIOTHERAPY

Author and Year	Clinic or Study Group	No. of Patients Neg./Pos.	Follow-up Interval (yr)	Recurrence Rates (%) Node-Negative	Node-Positive
Crile, 1964[9]	Cleveland Clinic	103/35	6	30.0	NA
Kyle et al., 1976[45]	Cancer Research Campaign (U.K.)‡	877/275	5	9.5*	—
		843/273	5	1.7†	—
Langlands et al., 1980[46]	Southeast Scotland	131/111	5	13.7	10.8+
Forrest et al., 1982[28]	Edinburgh (Cardiff)§	64/39	10	15.6	25.0+
Berstock et al., 1985[5]	Cancer Research Campaign (U.K.)‡	877/275	14	23.8*	—
		843/273	14	6.4†	—
Fisher et al., 1985[20]	NSABP B-04	365/294	10	1.1§	—
		352/294	10	3.1†	11.9†

*Overall axillary recurrence for node-positive and node-negative without radiation therapy.
†Overall axillary recurrence for node-positive and node-negative with radiation therapy.
‡No axillary node histology available at therapy.
§Treated with axillary radiotherapy if nodes positive clinically.
NA = Not available.

tive patients was 13.7 percent and 10.8 percent, respectively. The recurrence rate at 10 years was 15.6 percent for node-negative and 25 percent for node-positive patients. In the Cardiff-St. Mary's trial, patients were treated with axillary radiotherapy only if nodes were clinically positive.

In NSABP B-04, Fisher and associates[20] reported a 10-year axillary recurrence rate of 1.1 percent in stage I node-negative patients treated by total mastectomy alone, which was equivalent to the relapse rate for radical mastectomy (1.4 percent) for this site. The addition of irradiation therapy to the total mastectomy group conferred no benefit in this subset of patients with clinically negative nodes. However, in B-04, one third of the patients in the total mastectomy group had varying numbers of lymph nodes removed, ranging from 1 to 31 axillary lymph nodes as part of the total mastectomy specimen. Furthermore, 18 percent of patients with clinically negative axilla who were originally treated with total mastectomy developed clinically metastatic lymph nodes and required axillary dissection. The development of gross axillary metastases was not considered as axillary recurrence in B-04. The axillary recurrence rate after a delayed axillary dissection was 6.2 percent (4 of 65 patients) and was 1.1 percent in the entire group (4 of 365 patients). For patients with clinically positive nodes, the axillary recurrence rate was 11.9 percent in the group treated with irradiation and total mastectomy, which was significantly higher than that in the group treated by radical mastectomy alone (1.0 percent). These analyses note minimal enhancement of absolute survival at 5 and 10 years; some studies confirm that peripheral irradiation in the clinically node-positive group reduced local/regional relapse rates. These data further indicate the necessity of histological sampling of the axillary lymphatics for invasive ductal and lobular carcinoma to guide future therapy strategies. Unless axillary lymphatics are sampled at the time of total mastectomy, this information will not be available for the planning of peripheral irradiation and/or subsequent systemic chemotherapy. The advantages of adding systemic chemotherapy, hormonal therapy, or both to the premenopausal and postmenopausal patient are discussed in Chapters 66 and 73.

PROSPECTIVE TRIALS FOR TOTAL MASTECTOMY WITH AND WITHOUT IRRADIATION

A previous section in this chapter gave the history of the development of the Halsted radical mastectomy and its necessity in the absence of effective adjuvant therapy to control local and regional disease. This section has defined the rationale for the modified radical mastectomy as a more conservative approach than the Halsted procedure that can achieve similar local/regional and survival benefit. The evolution toward more conservative approaches with effective adjuvant therapy has led to prospective randomized

clinical trials for the treatment of breast cancer with total mastectomy with and without irradiation.

Groote Schuur Trial, 1968–1971

A prospective controlled trial was conducted in the breast clinic of the Groote Schuur Hospital in Capetown, South Africa, to evaluate the efficacy of simple mastectomy versus radical mastectomy in the treatment of stage I (T1N0, T2N0) and stage II (T1N1, T2N1) carcinoma of the breast. Helman and associates[37] in an interim report, believed that conservative approaches for the treatment of operable breast cancer should be investigated. The authors did not use routine postoperative radiotherapy or chemotherapy in the treatment of 51 patients undergoing simple mastectomy and 44 patients undergoing radical mastectomy. The median follow-up was not determined.

At the time of analysis, the authors confirmed that 5 of 51 patients (9.8 percent) having simple mastectomy developed lymph node recurrences in the axilla; 7 (13.7 percent) developed skin flap recurrence. In contrast, for the 44 patients undergoing radical mastectomy, only 1 (2.3 percent) developed skin flap recurrence, and none developed axillary node recurrence. After reviewing these results and the apparent discrepancy between the local recurrence rates after simple and radical mastectomy, the Groote Schuur Breast Clinic terminated the trial because of the high rate of axillary node recurrence in patients undergoing simple mastectomy.

Helman and associates[37] admitted that they had no justifiable predictions of prognosis for patients in the simple mastectomy trial. They concluded that simple mastectomy, in the absence of routine postoperative irradiation, should not be used for operable breast cancer. Because of the satisfactory survival data obtained with radical mastectomy, the authors suggest that this operation or any other form of mastectomy that includes axillary node dissection with postoperative irradiation is an effective therapy for breast cancer.

It is unfortunate that this trial was terminated after only 3.25 years. The small number of patients in each arm of the study and the short duration of the trial make ultimate conclusions difficult to formulate. Furthermore, the authors do not state in the study design regarding the mechanism for allocating patients to each of the randomization arms with regard to stage of disease. Without knowledge of the number of positive nodes and tumor size allocated into each arm, firm conclusions cannot be drawn. Despite these factors, the disturbingly high incidence of progression of disease in the axillary lymphatics (9.8 percent) of the simple mastectomy–only group is significant. The low local/regional recurrence rate (2.2 percent) and the absence of failure of the axilla in the Halsted radical group confirms the efficacy of the radical mastectomy to control axillary recurrence.

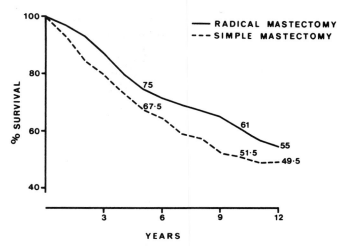

Figure 44–9 *Crude survival rates for 256 radical mastectomies and 242 simple mastectomies plus radiotherapy. Percentage survivals are indicated for 5, 10, and 12 years. (From Langlands AO, et al: Br J Surg 67:171, 1980. Reprinted by permission.)*

Copenhagen Trial, 1951–1957

Between 1951 and 1957, Johansen and coworkers conducted a study to compare the simple mastectomy with postoperative radiation to extended radical mastectomy in treating primary breast cancer.[43] A total of 666 patients were randomized, with 335 patients in the simple mastectomy group and 331 patients in the simple mastectomy plus radiation group. All the patients were followed for more than 25 years. The overall survival rates in the two groups were identical at 5 (60 percent), 10 (40 percent), and 25 (28 percent) years. When the stage IV disease patients were excluded, there was again no difference detected between the two treatment groups, and the survival rates were improved to 70 percent, 60 percent, and 40 percent at 5, 10, and 25 years, respectively. The disease-free survival rates were similar in the two treatment groups as well. Recurrence-free survival at 25 years (58 percent versus 45 percent) was slightly better in patients with clinical stage I

disease treated by the extended radical mastectomy; however, this is not statistically significant. In patients with extended radical mastectomy, one third were found to have histologically verified lymph node metastases. The 25-year survival rates for patients with and without lymph node metastasis were 20 percent and 60 percent, respectively. In conclusion, nodal status has a strong prognostic value. Although advances in adjuvant therapy necessitate removal of lymph nodes for accurate staging, locally, simple mastectomy plus irradiation is as effective as radical surgery for patients with primary operable breast cancer.

Edinburgh Trial, 1964–1971

Between 1964 and 1971, Hamilton and colleagues[34] and Langlands and colleagues[46] conducted a study for the treatment of operable cancer of the breast in the southeast region of Scotland. In this controlled clinical trial, 490 women aged 35 to 69 years were randomized to treatment by radical mastectomy (n = 256) or by simple mastectomy and postoperative radiotherapy (n = 242). Figure 44–9 confirms crude survival rates for the radical and simple mastectomy groups. Follow-up data for the first 12 years indicated that survival in the radical mastectomy group was significantly better ($p < 0.05$); however, the benefit accrued only to patients with clinical stage I disease (Fig. 44–10).

Table 44–11 demonstrates the pattern of survival once recurrence has been detected, confirming survival differences between the two treatment groups. Overall, there was a significant prolongation of survival after detection of recurrence in the radical mastectomy group ($p < 0.05$), which was greatest when local recurrence and distant metastases were observed ($p < 0.01$). At 12 years of study, Langlands[46] confirmed that duration of survival was independent of clinical stage of disease, tumor size, or menstrual status at diagnosis of recurrent disease. However, the duration of survival was observed to be directly

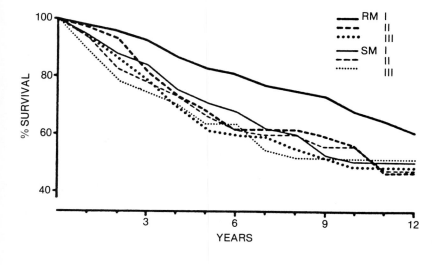

Figure 44–10 *Crude survival rates for cases according to international stage of the disease and treatment option (RM I = radical mastectomy for stage I, SM III = simple mastectomy plus radiotherapy for stage III, and so forth). (From Langlands AO, et al: Br J Surg 67:172, 1980. Reprinted by permission.)*

TABLE 44–11.   EDINBURGH TRIAL (1964–1971): SURVIVAL ACCORDING TO TYPE OF RECURRENCE

Type of Recurrence	Treatment	Observed No. of Patients	Expected No. of Deaths	No. of Deaths	X^2
Local only	RM	35	27	28.45	0.20
	SM	28	19	17.55	
Distant only	RM	58	45	51.26	1.56
	SM	69	62	55.74	
Local and distant	RM	12	9	13.88	7.32 ($p<0.01$)
	SM	10	10	5.12	
Combination	RM	105	81	93.59	4.09 ($p<0.05$)
	SM	107	91	78.41	
All recurrences without stratification	RM	105	81	96.43	5.90 ($p<0.05$)
	SM	107	91	75.57	

RM = Radical mastectomy; SM = simple mastectomy.
From Langlands AO, Prescott RJ, Hamilton T: A clinical trial in the management of operable cancer of the breast. Br J Surg 67:170–174, 1980. Reprinted by permission.

proportional to the duration of the disease-free interval ($p < 0.01$) (Fig. 44–11 and Table 44–12).

The enhanced survival determined in the Edinburgh trial is seen exclusively in the radical mastectomy group but is accounted for entirely by the use of this technique for the treatment of stage I disease. This well-controlled prospective study further demonstrated an excess number of deaths in the simple mastectomy plus irradiation group that were attributed to causes other than cancer. However, the difference in the pattern of local recurrence, which appears to be excessive in the simple mastectomy plus irradiation group, is almost entirely accounted for by recurrence in the axilla, which occurred in 12 percent of the simple mastectomy group compared with 3 percent in the radical mastectomy group. This recurrence appeared to be unaffected by stage of disease

at the time of presentation. Recurrence in skin flaps was more commonly observed in stage III disease; paradoxically, such recurrences were greater in the radical mastectomy group and are perhaps accounted for by the advantage of postoperative irradiation. Distant disease–free survival was equivalent for the two treatment groups.

Edinburgh Royal Infirmary–Cardiff Trial, 1967–1973

To determine if simple mastectomy combined with lower axillary node sampling (Level 1 and 2 node biopsy) was a safe therapeutic option for conservation of the breast, Forrest and associates[27, 28] of the Royal Infirmary in Edinburgh initiated the Cardiff trial. Two hundred patients were included in the study, all with tumors of TNM classification T1, T2, N0N1M0. Patients were randomized according to the site of tumor, clinical stage, and menopausal status and were randomly selected within subgroups for conservative (n = 103) or radical (n = 97) therapy. Patients treated by the conservative approach (simple mastectomy and axillary node sampling) received postoperative irradiation only if the node sample proved to be positive. Radiation therapy was restricted to the axilla and was given in ten fractions (40 Gy) over 3

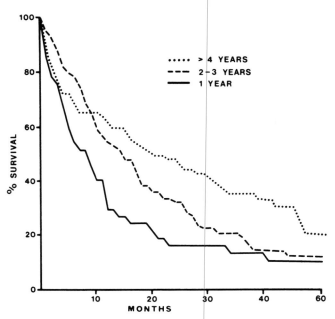

Figure 44–11 *Subsequent survival of patients according to the length of the disease-free interval. (From Langlands AO, et al: Br J Surg 67:174, 1980. Reprinted by permission.)*

TABLE 44–12.   EDINBURGH TRIAL (1964–1971): DISEASE-FREE INTERVAL ACCORDING TO TYPE OF RECURRENCE*

Stratum	RM Group	SM Group
Local recurrence only	33.5 (+ 4.8)	34.9 (+ 5.2)
Distant metastases only	45.8 (+ 4.4)	38.4 (+ 3.4)
Synchronous local and distant	41.4 (+ 7.4)	31.0 (+ 6.8)

*Mean times in months (+ standard errors) from initial treatment until the first detection of recurrent disease according to the three strata defined in the text.
RM = Radical mastectomy; SM = simple mastectomy.
From Langlands AO, Prescott RJ, Hamilton T: A clinical trial in the management of operable cancer of the breast. Br J Surg 67:170–174, 1980. Reprinted by permission.

TABLE 44–13.   EDINBURGH ROYAL INFIRMARY—CARDIFF TRIAL (1967–1973): AXILLARY RECURRENCE IN PATIENTS WITH NEGATIVE AND NONIDENTIFIED NODES TREATED BY SIMPLE AND RADICAL MASTECTOMY

	Number of Patients	
Treatment	Total	With Axillary Recurrent (%)
Mastectomy alone (simple mastectomy)	64	10 (15.6)
Mastectomy with axillary clearance (radical mastectomy)	66	1 (1.5)

From Forrest APM, Stewart HJ, Roberts MM, Steele RJC: Simple mastectomy and axillary node sampling (pectoral node biopsy) in the management of primary breast cancer. Ann Surg 196(3):371–378, 1982. Reprinted by permission.

weeks. The protocol also required that a biopsy sample be taken from the edge of the removed skin in proximity to the tumor; if biopsy results were positive, radiation therapy was also given to the chest wall. Patients randomized to the radical policy (Halsted radical mastectomy) also received irradiation when positive nodes were identified in the axillary specimen.

As of 1981 (14 years on study), the major revelation of this Scottish study was in the success of the two policies of treatment to achieve local control.[28] There was an increased incidence of recurrent disease affecting the axilla in patients who, on the basis of clinically negative nodes, were treated by simple mastectomy alone compared to those treated by radical mastectomy (Table 44–13). With simple mastectomy alone, axillary recurrence was noted in 10 of 64 patients (15.6 percent); only 1 of 66 patients (1.5 percent) treated with radical mastectomy had axillary recurrence. For patients having simple mastectomy and axillary radiotherapy for positive nodes, the observed chest wall recurrence rate was 25.6 percent (10 of 39 patients); only 2 of 31 patients (6.5 percent) with positive nodes having radical mastectomy and radical irradiation had chest wall recurrence (Table 44–14). Despite these differences in local/regional control and axillary recurrence rates,

TABLE 44–14.   EDINBURGH ROYAL INFIRMARY—CARDIFF TRIAL (1967–1973): CHEST WALL TUMOR RECURRENCE*

	Number of Patients	
Treatment	Total	With Chest Wall Recurrence (%)
Simple mastectomy and axillary radiotherapy	39	10 (25.6)
Radical mastectomy and radical radiotherapy	31	2 (6.5)

*Patients had positive nodes at the time of mastectomy.
From Forrest APM, Stewart HJ, Roberts MM, Steele RJC: Simple mastectomy and axillary node sampling (pectoral node biopsy) in the management of primary breast cancer. Ann Surg 196(3):371–378, 1982. Reprinted by permission.

the overall survival rates with the two therapies proved to be identical ($p = 0.4147$) (Fig. 44–12). Results from the Edinburgh trial shown in Table 44–15 suggest that radical irradiation may benefit patients with histologically negative or unidentified pectoral nodes recovered at mastectomy; this benefit is greater for patients with unidentified nodes (i.e., unstaged pathologically).

Although the previous Edinburgh trial showed that radiation after total mastectomy without any nodal removal reduced the local/regional recurrences from 41 percent to 19 percent, the recurrences were further reduced to 5 percent if histologically proved negative nodes were found in the mastectomy specimen. The question remains whether treatment with radiation in patients with histologically proved nodal metastases will be as effective as axillary clearance. Forrest and colleagues[29] conducted a randomized trial to study 417 patients who had mastectomy and node sampling or full axillary clearance. Those who had positive nodes by sampling received radiation. Patients with positive nodes received CMF or oophorectomy if they were premenopausal; tamoxifen was given to postmenopausal women and premenopausal women with negative nodes. The incidence of distant metastasis and the 12-year overall survival rate are the same in both groups. Although the radiation reduced chest wall recurrences in node-positive patients when compared with patients with axillary clearance, the latter group showed slightly less axillary recurrences (3 percent versus 5.4 percent). Adjuvant systemic treatment reduced local/regional recurrences in node-positive women of both groups.

Manchester Regional Breast Study, 1970–1975

Lythgoe and associates[48] and Lythgoe and Palmer[49] reported a prospective clinical trial for treatment of

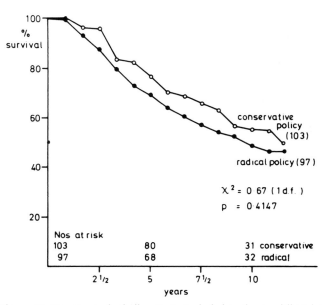

Figure 44–12 *Survival of all patients included in the Cardiff trial in April 1981. (From Forrest APM, et al: Ann Surg 196:371, 1982. Reprinted by permission.)*

TABLE 44–15.   EDINBURGH TRIAL: LOCAL/REGIONAL RECURRENCE ACCORDING TO WHETHER NODES WERE IDENTIFIED OR NONIDENTIFIED FOR HISTOLOGICAL EXAMINATION AT MASTECTOMY

Treatment	Number of Patients, Nodes Identified and Histologically Negative		Number of Patients, Nodes Not Identified	
	Total	With Recurrence (%)	Total	With Recurrence (%)
Mastectomy alone	114	18 (16)	59	24 (41)
Mastectomy with radiotherapy	112	6 (5)	57	11 (19)

From Forrest APM, Stewart HJ, Roberts MM, Steele RJC: Simple mastectomy and axillary node sampling (pectoral node biopsy) in the management of primary breast cancer. Ann Surg 196(3):371–378, 1982. Reprinted by permission.

operable breast cancer initiated by the Manchester Regional Association of Surgeons. Patients with TNM clinical stage I cancer (T1, T2, N0M0) were randomly allocated to be treated by total mastectomy and postoperative radiotherapy (TM + RT) or by total mastectomy (TM) alone. Patients with clinical stage II cancers (T1, T2, N1M0) were randomly allocated to treatment by TM + RT or by radical mastectomy (RM) alone.

Between March 1970 and October 1975, 1022 patients (714 stage I and 308 stage II) were admitted to this prospective trial. At a follow-up of 5 to 10 years, no statistically significant differences in overall survival were evident in clinical stage I cancers treated by TM + RT versus those treated by TM alone (Fig. 44–13). Local recurrence (defined as recurrence at the chest wall, axilla, or supraclavicular fossa) was observed twice as frequently in the group treated with TM alone, and this difference was statistically significant ($p < 0.0001$) (Fig. 44–14). Of clinical stage II breast cancers randomly allocated to either TM + RT or RM alone (n = 308), no statistically significant differences in survival or in the frequency of local/regional recurrence were observed between the two treatment groups. Table 44–16 depicts the primary control rates to the clinical stage of disease and the treatment allocated for the Manchester study. For clinical stage II disease, postoperative ir-

radiation therapy used with total mastectomy appears to have a 10-year survival rate equivalent to that of radical mastectomy. In addition, primary control rates of the chest wall, axilla, and supraclavicular fossa appear to be equivalent with the two modalities for this more advanced stage.

Cancer Research Campaign Clinical Trial, 1970–1975

Berstock and colleagues[5] of the King's College/Cambridge School of Medicine in the United Kingdom reported on the Cancer Research Campaign Multicenter Trial for the management of operable breast cancer. Patients were managed with two treatment policies: a total mastectomy alone ("watch policy") and a total mastectomy plus radiotherapy given as a four-field technique using a recommended dose of 1320 to 1510 ret (radiation equivalent therapy) during a 6-week period. Of 2800 patients randomized, 2243 were evaluated in the groups in which no formal axillary dissection was performed. Follow-up ranged from 9 to 14 years (median, 11.4 years). As seen in Figure 44–15, these data confirm no significant differences in terms of survival ($p = 0.37$) for the watch policy versus irradiated patients after total

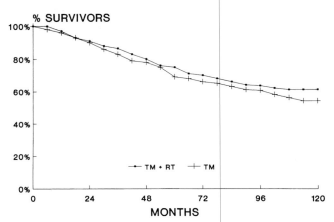

Figure 44–13 *Survival curves for all surgical cases entered as stage I. TM = Total (simple) mastectomy; TM + RT = total (simple) mastectomy and postoperative radiation therapy. (From Lythgoe JP, Palmer MK: Br J Surg 69:693, 1982. Reprinted by permission.)*

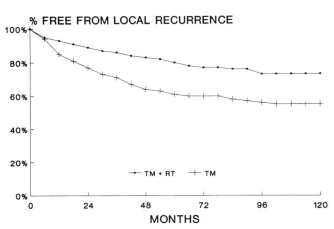

Figure 44–14 *Percentage of stage I patients free of local recurrence. TM + RT = Total mastectomy plus postoperative irradiation; TM = total mastectomy alone. The differences observed for local recurrence of the chest wall, axilla, and supraclavicular fossa were statistically significant (p < 0.0001). (From Lythgoe JP, Palmer MK: Br J Surg 69:693, 1982. Reprinted by permission.)*

TABLE 44–16.   MANCHESTER REGIONAL BREAST STUDY (1970–1975): PRIMARY CONTROL RELATED TO CLINICAL STAGE AND TREATMENT FOR STAGE I AND II DISEASE

Clinical Stage	Treatment	No. of Patients	Chest Wall		Axilla		Supraclavicular Fossa	
			5 yr	10 yr	5 yr	10 yr	5 yr	10 yr
I	Simple mastectomy	359	84	80	67	63	89	85
	Simple mastectomy + radiotherapy	355	94	91	84	81	92	89
			$p = 0.0002$		$p = 0.0001$		$p = 0.20$	
II	Radical mastectomy	149	66	64	76	71	80	77
	Simple mastectomy + radiotherapy	159	77	63	75	72	87	86
			$p = 0.22$		$p = 0.95$		$p = 0.15$	

% Free from Recurrence (column group header above Chest Wall, Axilla, Supraclavicular Fossa)

From Lythgoe JP, Palmer MK: Manchester regional breast study—5 and 10 year results. Br J Surg 69:693–696, 1982. Reprinted by permission.

mastectomy. However, the incidence of local recurrence in the two treatment groups (Fig. 44–16) shows a marked and significant difference favoring the radiotherapy group and represents a hazard ratio of observed-to-expected events in the "watch policy" group of 2.69 compared with the irradiated group ($p < 0.001$). The effect of radiotherapy on the distribution of local recurrence as reported by the authors of this trial is interesting, because irradiation tended to protect most effectively against axillary recurrence (hazard ratio = 3.95) and less effectively against chest wall recurrence (hazard ratio = 2.03). Furthermore, the use of irradiation appeared to have no protection whatsoever against supraclavicular recurrence, in spite of the supraclavicular field being included in the recommended protocol and used in 92 percent of the patients studied. The most significant variable that determined the future development of local recurrence was the histological grade of the primary tumor. As reported by Elston and associates,[17] high-grade tumors had a significantly higher incidence of local recurrence than did histologically

low-grade tumors (Fig. 44–17). The site of the primary tumor within the breast, dose of radiation therapy received, and menstrual status had little bearing on the subsequent development of local recurrence.

Of interest in the study is the finding that survival after development of local recurrence was different between the two treatment groups. Paradoxically, the radiotherapy arm did worse than the watch policy group ($p = 0.05$). The 5-year survival rate after any local/regional recurrence was 35.6 percent for the watch policy group and 30.6 percent for the total mastectomy plus irradiation group. Mean survival time was 3.3 years for the "watch policy" group and 2.7 years for the total mastectomy plus irradiation group (Table 44–17).

This study confirms that patients at high risk of local recurrence are those with high histological grade tumors, those with clinically or pathologically positive axillary nodes, and those with cancers that had diameters greater than 2 cm. Of patients who subsequently developed local/regional recurrence and died, 67 percent in the total mastectomy plus irradia-

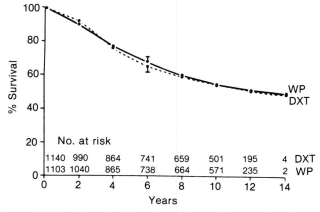

Figure 44–15   *All evaluable patients. Survival in watch policy and radiotherapy groups ($x^2 = 0.02$, p = 0.88, hazard ratio (HR) = 1.0). "No. at risk" represents the number of patients alive at entry and biennially thereafter. This number decreases in the later years, since there are fewer patients with relevant trial times. Vertical bars indicate the 95 percent confidence intervals. (From Berstock DA, et al: World J Surg 9:667, 1985. Reprinted by permission.)*

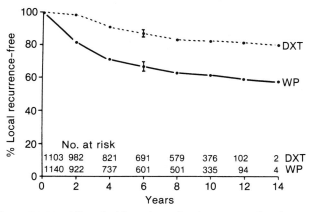

Figure 44–16   *All evaluable patients: local recurrence-free in watch policy and radiotherapy groups ($x^2 = 120.93$, p < 0.001, HR = 2.69). "No. at risk" represents the number of patients alive at entry and biennially thereafter. This number decreases in the later years, since there are fewer patients with relevant trial times. Vertical bars indicate the 95 percent confidence intervals. (From Berstock DA, et al: World J Surg 9:667, 1985. Reprinted by permission.)*

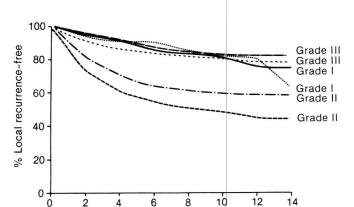

Figure 44–17 *Patients with histologically graded tumors subdivided by treatment policy: Grade I (n = 180) − x^2 = 0.01 ns, HR = 1.04; Grade II (n = 903)x^2 = 59.79, p < 0.001, HR = 2.98; Grade III (n = 456) − x^2 = 42.21, p < 0.001, HR = 3.28. (From Berstock DA, et al: World J Surg 9:667, 1985. Reprinted by permission.)*

tion group and 56 percent in the watch policy group did so with evidence of uncontrolled local/regional disease; the incidence of uncontrolled local disease at death was greater in the watch policy group (13.2 percent versus 6.8 percent, $p < 0.001$). Although much of the local/regional recurrence can be controlled by surgery, radiation therapy, chemotherapy, or adjunctive endocrine measures, this study indicated that the disease will remain uncontrolled in a percentage of patients until death. Importantly, this prospective study establishes the rationale for use of prophylactic irradiation for patients considered at high risk for recurrence to reduce the unfortunate sequelae of uncontrolled disease.

National Surgical Adjuvant Breast and Bowel Project (B-04), 1971–1974

In NSABP B-04, alternative local and regional treatments of breast cancer, all of which used breast removal, were compared in a prospectively randomized trial.[20] The findings are drawn from 1655 patients with primary operable breast cancer who were followed for 108 to 145 months (average, 126 months).

TABLE 44–17.   CANCER RESEARCH CAMPAIGN TRIAL (1970–1975): SURVIVAL AFTER THE DEVELOPMENT OF LOCAL RECURRENCE

Site	5-Yr Survival, % (± SE)		Median Survival (yr)	
	WP	DXT	WP	DXT
Chest wall	33.9 (4.2)	32.2 (5.9)	3.1	2.8
Axilla	33.7 (3.0)	26.7 (5.4)	3.2	2.6
Supraclavicular fossa	16.9 (5.8)	7.9 (4.4)	1.6	1.1
Overall	31.6 (2.5)	30.6 (3.9)	3.3	2.7

WP = Watch policy group; DXT = irradiated group.
From Berstock DA, Houghton B, Haybittle J, Baum M: The role of radiotherapy following total mastectomy for patients with early breast cancer. World J Surg 9:667–670, 1985. Reprinted by permission.

Among these, 100 patients (5.7 percent) were considered ineligible for analysis. Women who had clinically negative axillary nodes with T1 through T3 tumors were randomized to receive one of three distinctly different local/regional treatment regimens: a conventional radical mastectomy (RM); a total (simple) mastectomy followed by local/regional irradiation (TM + RT); or a total mastectomy alone (TM). Removal of axillary regional lymphatics was to be completed only when nodes became clinically positive. Similarly, clinically node-positive patients were treated with RM or TM + RT. No adjunctive chemotherapy was given to patients in any of the three randomization arms. Patients considered to have clinically negative nodes were randomly assigned so that one third were treated by RM, one third by TM + RT, and one third by TM alone. Patients with clinically positive axillary nodes were randomized so that one half were treated by RM and one half by TM + RT. A node biopsy was performed in patients with clinically negative axillary nodes who had undergone a total mastectomy without irradiation and subsequently had clinical evidence of axillary node involvement in the absence of other disease manifestations. When regional lymphatics were pathologically reported as positive, a delayed axillary dissection was completed. Patients whose disease progressed with positive axillary nodes after TM + RT were considered treatment failures.

Irradiation was administered using supervoltage techniques; radiation dosages of 4500 rad over 25 fractions were administered to the internal mammary and supraclavicular nodes at a depth of 3 cm. For patients with clinically negative axillary nodes, a dose of 5000 rad in 25 fractions was delivered to the midaxilla. Most of the dosage was delivered from the anterior supraclavicular portal, and the remainder, from the posterior axillary portal. Patients with clinically positive nodes received a boost of 1000 to 2000 rad via a direct appositional portal.[20]

Figure 44–18 shows that there was no significant difference ($p = 0.2$) in recurrence-free survival during the entire period of follow-up among groups of patients with *clinically negative nodes* treated by RM, TM + RT, or TM (panel A). When disease-free survival was evaluated in the first and second 5-year periods of follow-up, Fisher and colleagues observed no differences among groups within the first 5 years after surgery ($p = 0.08$) (panel B). Subsequently, an additional 15 percent of patients in all three groups had a treatment failure between the 5th and 10th year. There were no statistical differences in the probability of failure among the three groups during the second 5 years of follow-up ($p = 0.8$) (panel C). For each group, approximately 75 percent of patients who were free of disease at the end of 5 years remained so at the end of the 10th year. It is apparent that differences observed in the initial 5 years occurred secondary to the higher incidence of local/regional disease and occurred as the first evidence of disease in the total mastectomy group. The differences were not related to an increase in distant dis-

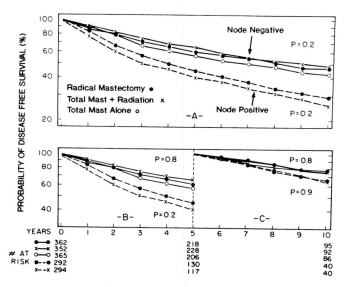

Figure 44–18 *Disease-free survival for patients treated by radical mastectomy (solid circle), total mastectomy plus radiation (x), or total mastectomy alone (open circle). There were no significant differences among the three groups of patients with clinically negative nodes (solid line) or between the two groups with clinically positive nodes (broken line). (From Fisher B, et al: N Engl J Med 312[11]:674, 1985. Reprinted by permission.)*

ease occurring as a first treatment failure (Fig. 44–19, upper panel). These investigators noted that patients undergoing TM + RT had a lower incidence of local and regional recurrence than did those in the other two groups.

This study showed no significant differences in disease-free survival among patients in the two groups (see Fig. 44–18) treated with RM or TM + RT who presented with *clinically positive nodes* ($p = 0.2$). These data held for the first and second 5-year intervals of follow-up. Almost two thirds of patients who were free of disease at the end of the 5th year remained so within the next 5-year interval of follow-up. Additionally, this NSABP study[20] observed little difference between the two groups with respect to the occurrence of distant, local, or regional disease (Fig. 44–19, lower panel).

Fisher and colleagues[20] observed no significant differences in the probability of survival free of any distant disease, whether occurring as a first treatment failure or after local or regional disease, among patients in the three randomized arms who had *clinically negative nodes* ($p = 0.6$) (Fig. 44–20, upper panel A). In addition, no significant differences were observed when groups were examined according to the first and second 5-year postoperative intervals for patterns of recurrence ($p = 0.3$ and 0.4, respectively) (Fig. 44–20, upper panels B and C).

A similar trend was also observed for patients with *clinically positive nodes*, with no significant differences in distant disease–free survival between those undergoing RM and those treated with TM + RT

($p = 0.8$) (Fig. 44–20, lower panel A). At 5 years follow-up, the distant disease–free survival for patients with clinically positive nodes was 53 ± 3.0 percent for patients treated by RM and 51 ± 3.0 percent for those treated by TM + RT ($p = 0.4$) (Fig. 44–20, upper panel B). At 10 years, the NSABP investigators noted the corresponding figures were 39 ± 3.1 percent and 40 ± 3.1 percent. Thus, the probability of distant disease occurring in the second 5-year interval was identical for the two treatment arms ($p = 0.4$) (Fig. 44–20, upper panel C). The occurrence of distant treatment failures reported by the NSABP suggests that the first evidence of recurrent disease does not differ significantly among node-negative (Fig. 44–19, upper panel) and node-positive (Fig. 44–19, lower panel) treatment subgroups.

It is no surprise that overall survival was not significantly different ($p = 0.5$) among the three *node-negative groups* (Fig. 44–20, lower panel A). Overall survival at mean follow-up of 126 months for the three arms was 58 ± 2.6 percent for the RM group, 59 ± 2.7 percent for the TM + RT group, and 54 ± 2.7 percent for the TM group. The probability of survival during the first and second 5-year follow-up intervals was not significantly different ($p = 0.9$ and

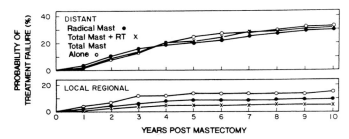

CLINICALLY NODE NEGATIVE

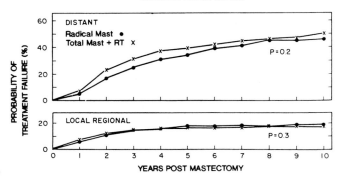

CLINICALLY NODE POSITIVE

Figure 44–19 *Local or regional and distant treatment failures as the first evidence of disease in patients with clinically negative and positive nodes who were treated by radical mastectomy (solid circle), total mastectomy and radiation (x), or total mastectomy alone (open circle). For node-negative patients there were no significant differences in distant disease occurring as a first treatment failure among the three groups, whereas local and regional disease was best controlled in the group receiving radiation. For node-positive patients there was no significant difference in distant or local and regional disease between the two groups. (From Fisher B, et al: N Engl J Med 312[11]:674, 1985. Reprinted by permission.)*

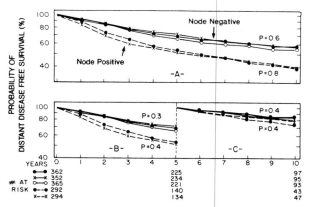

Survival Free of Distant Disease through 10 Years (A), during the First 5 Years (B), and during the Second 5 Years for Patients Free of Distant Disease at the End of the 5th Year (C).

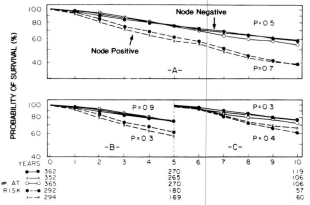

Survival through 10 Years (A), during the First 5 Years (B), and during the Second 5 Years for Patients Alive at the End of the 5th Year (C).

Figure 44–20 *Distant disease–free survival and overall survival for patients treated by radical mastectomy* (solid circle), *total mastectomy and radiation* (x), *or total mastectomy alone* (open circle). *There were no significant differences among the three groups of patients with clinically negative nodes* (solid line) *or between the two groups with positive nodes* (broken line). *(From Fisher B, et al: N Engl J Med 312[11]:674, 1985. Reprinted by permission.)*

0.3, respectively) (Fig. 44–20, lower panels B and C). Approximately 75 percent of patients with negative nodes who were alive in the first 5 years of follow-up remained alive at 10 years.

No statistical differences were observed in the *node positive group* with respect to survival at 10 years follow-up ($p = 0.7$) (Fig. 44–20, lower panel A). The probability of survival in the first 5 years and second 5 years of follow-up were not statistically different ($p = 0.3$ and 0.4, respectively) (Fig. 44–20, lower panels B and C). At the end of the 10th year of follow-up, only 38 ± 2.9 percent of the RM group and 39 ± 2.9 percent of the TM + RT group were alive. The authors observed that approximately 65 percent of patients with positive nodes who lived 5 years survived an additional 5 years.

Tumor Location and Survival

Figure 44–21 indicates the relationship of treatment to survival according to tumor location in the NSABP

study. Adjustments were made for intralymphatic extension, cell reaction, histological grade, and clinical tumor size.[20] For patients with clinically negative nodes and medial-central or laterally located tumors, no statistical differences ($p = 0.6$) were observed in outcome among the three treatment groups. For patients with clinically positive nodes, treatment was not observed to affect survival in those with lateral ($p = 0.8$) or medial-central tumors ($p = 0.3$).

Axillary Recurrence After Total Mastectomy

Among 365 patients with clinically negative axillary nodes who had total mastectomy without irradiation, Fisher and colleagues[20] observed that 17.8 percent subsequently developed histologically confirmed ipsilateral adenopathy. These patients were treated by delayed axillary dissection. Median time from TM to axillary dissection for recurrent disease was 14.7 months (range, 3 to 112.6 months). The majority of delayed axillary dissections (78.5 percent) were completed within 24 months of the original mastectomy. Only 4.6 percent of delayed dissections were completed in the second 5-year follow-up interval.

Summary

This well-controlled prospective study used patients who were meticulously analyzed for treatment results and follow-up. The findings indicate that location of the breast tumor does not influence prognosis and that irradiation of the internal mammary chain in patients with inner quadrant lesions does not improve survival. This clinical trial demonstrated that results obtained at 5 years accurately predict the outcome to be expected at 10 years. It would appear from this important study that variations of local and regional treatment parameters have less importance in determining survival of the patient with breast cancer than originally considered.

MODIFIED RADICAL MASTECTOMY TECHNIQUE

For the planning of mastectomy incisions, the reader is referred to Chapter 41, which describes the techniques for elevation of flaps for tumors of central-subareolar sites and each quadrant of the breast. The initial steps of the operation are conducted with the ipsilateral arm and shoulder in a relaxed, extended position on the arm board (see Fig. 44–23).

As indicated previously, the modified radical mastectomy, with removal of the pectoralis minor muscle (Patey dissection), allows access to Level 3 nodes so that all nodal levels can be extirpated. The Patey modified radical mastectomy is intended for lesions that cannot be extirpated with clear margins at the time of tylectomy and for lesions of so large a size (>T2, >5 cm) that cosmetic reconstruction and regional control cannot be accomplished with confidence. It is not intended for large tumors (T2, T3,

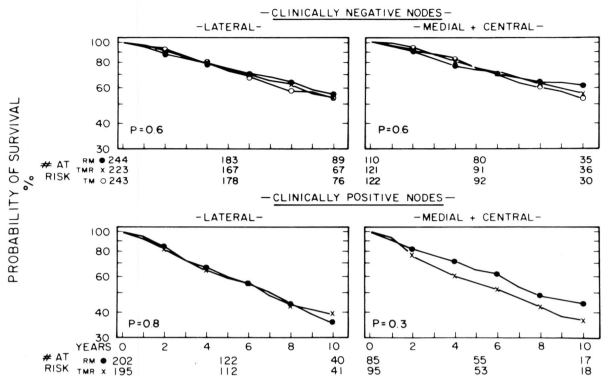

Figure 44–21 *Relation of treatment to survival according to tumor location. Patients were treated by radical mastectomy (solid circle), total mastectomy and radiation (x), or total mastectomy alone (open circle). The outcome for patients with clinically negative or positive nodes and lateral tumors or medial and central tumors was not affected by the treatment. (From Fisher B, et al: N Engl J Med 312[11]:674, 1985. Reprinted by permission.)*

T4) with evidence of skin or pectoralis major fixation for which major resection of this muscle is necessary to achieve adequate surgical margins. Therefore, patients with high-lying (peripheral) lesions near the clavicle are not considered candidates for the Patey,[64, 65] Auchincloss,[1] or Madden[50] techniques.

The modified radical mastectomy necessitates en bloc resection of the breast, the axillary lymphatics, and overlying skin near the tumor with a 3- to 5-cm margin to ensure marginal clearance of the tumor. The names *Auchincloss*[1] and *Madden*[50] (and occasionally *Handley*[35]) are used synonymously as modified radical techniques. The Patey mastectomy acknowledges the importance of the complete axillary dissection and the anatomical necessity for preservation of the medial and lateral pectoral (anterior thoracic) nerves, which may serve as dual innervation to the pectoralis major. The Madden and Auchincloss mastectomies advocate preservation of the pectoralis major and minor muscles, thus allowing adequate access to Level 2 lymphatics with incomplete dissection (or preservation) of Level 3. These approaches are similar in that both require total mastectomy with at least partial axillary lymph node dissection. With the limitation for dissection of the apical (subclavicular) nodal group, the Auchincloss[1] and Madden[50] procedures allow for higher probability of preservation of the *medial (anterior thoracic) pectoral nerve,* which courses in the *lateral neurovascular bundle* of the axilla and commonly penetrates the

pectoralis minor to supply the lateral border of the pectoralis major muscle.

The patient is positioned supine for induction with general anesthesia. A roll sheet allows modest elevation of the ipsilateral hemithorax and shoulder so that there is no limitation of range of motion of the shoulder and arm with abduction and adduction. The positioning of the patient at the margin of the operative table is important to allow the operator and assistant simple access without undue retraction on the major muscle groups or brachial plexus (Fig. 44–22). With positioning, the operator should be aware of potential subluxation and abduction of the shoulder. This complication is best prevented with padding of the armboard to avoid stretch of the brachial plexus and denervation of major muscle groups of the shoulder and arm. The surgeon must confirm adequate mobility of the ipsilateral arm for adduction and extension during operation.

The ipsilateral breast, neck, shoulder, and hemithorax are prepped with povidone iodine to the table margin and well beyond the midline (see Fig. 42–4). Additionally, the axilla, arm, and hand are fully prepped within the operative field. Towels are secured with clips or stainless steel staples to the skin within the operative field, which includes the shoulder, lower neck, sternum, and upper abdominal musculature. Alternative methods exist to include the arm and hand in the operative field. Our preference is to isolate the hand and forearm with an occlusive

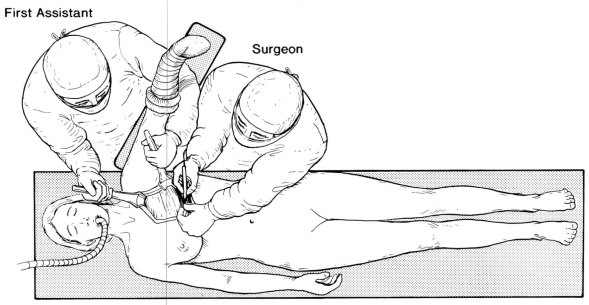

Figure 44–22   *Position of patient for left modified radical mastectomy at margin of operative table. The first assistant is cephalad to the armboard and shoulder of the patient to allow access to the axillary contents without undue traction on major muscle groups. Depicted is the preferential isolation of the hand and forearm with an occlusive Stockinette cotton dressing secured distal to the elbow. This technique allows free mobility of the elbow, arm, and shoulder to avoid undue stretch of the brachial plexus with muscle retraction.*

Stockinette (DeRoyal Industries, Powell, TN) cotton dressing that is further secured with Kling or Kerlex cotton roll (Johnson and Johnson, New Brunswick, NJ) distal to the elbow. Free mobility of the elbow, arm, and shoulder must be ensured with isolation of the forearm and hand. As in the Halsted radical mastectomy, we position the first assistant over the shoulder (craniad to the armboard) of the ipsilateral breast such that appropriate muscle retraction at the time of axillary dissection can be accomplished with free mobility of the shoulder to allow extension, abduction, and adduction without undue stretch of neurovascular structures of the axilla (see Fig. 42–5).

The limits of the modified radical mastectomy, regardless of the skin incisions used, are delineated *laterally* by the anterior margin of the latissimus dorsi muscle, *medially* by the midline of the sternum, *superiorly* by the subclavius muscle, and *inferiorly* by the caudal extension of the breast some 3 to 4 cm inferior to the inframammary fold (Fig. 44–23, inset).

The design of skin flaps is carefully planned with relation to the quadrant in which the primary neoplasm is located so that adequate margins can be ensured. In the majority of cases, primary closure should be possible unless undue tension or flap devascularization and the necessity of margin debridement are evident. Incisions and skin flaps should be developed perpendicular to the subcutaneous plane. Thereafter, retraction hooks or towel clips are placed on skin margins for appropriate elevation. Flaps are retracted with constant tension on the periphery of the elevated margin at right angles to the chest wall to expose the superficial and deep layers of superficial fascia. This maneuver allows the operator access to the anatomical boundaries described previously.

Flap thickness varies with patient habitus and proportional lean body mass. Ideally, flap thickness should be 7 to 8 mm, inclusive of skin and tela subcutanea. The interface for flap elevation is developed deep to the cutaneous vasculature, which is accentuated by flap traction as previously described. The surgeon must be aware of the necessity for flap elevation with consistent thickness to avoid creating devascularized subcutaneous tissue that contributes to wound seroma, skin necrosis, or flap retraction.

We prefer to elevate the cephalad skin flap with constant thickness to the level of the subclavius muscle. Dissection commences from lateral to medial with the optional use of the cold scalpel or electrocautery. Thereafter, the pectoralis major fascia is dissected from the pectoralis musculature in a plane that is parallel with the course of the muscle bundle from the origin of ribs two to six to its insertion on the humerus (Fig. 44–24). The operator places inferior traction (perpendicular to the clavicle) on the breast and fascia, this traction is maintained constantly with elevation of the fascia from the muscle. Multiple perforator vessels from the lateral thoracic or anterior intercostal arteries are invariably encountered in moving from lateral to medial with the dissection. These vessels represent end-arteries that supply the pectoralis major and minor and should be carefully identified, clamped, and ligated with 2-0 or 3-0 nonabsorbable suture. The breast and skin, inclusive of the elevated pectoralis fascia from the lateral humeral extension to the medial costochondral junction, are elevated en bloc to approximately the 5th or 6th rib, leaving the inferiormost portion of the breast intact. Depending on location of the lesion, if access to the central and lower aspect of the breast

Figure 44–23   Inset, *Limits of the modified radical mastectomy are delineated* superiorly *by the subclavius muscle,* laterally *by the anterior margin of the latissimus dorsi muscle,* medially *by the midline of the sternum, and* inferiorly *by the caudal extension of the breast approximately 3 to 4 cm inferior to the inframammary fold. Skin flaps for the modified radical technique are planned with relation to the quadrant in which the primary neoplasm is located. Adequate margins are ensured by developing skin edges 3 to 5 cm from the tumor margin. Incisions are planned so that they are developed perpendicular to the subcutaneous plane and are inclusive of skin and parenchymal tissue 3 to 5 cm around the neoplasm. Flap thickness is dependent on patient habitus and proportional lean body mass. Flaps should be 7 to 8 mm in thickness inclusive of the skin and tela subcutanea. Flap tension should be perpendicular to the chest wall with flap elevation deep to the cutaneous vasculature, which is accentuated by flap retraction.*

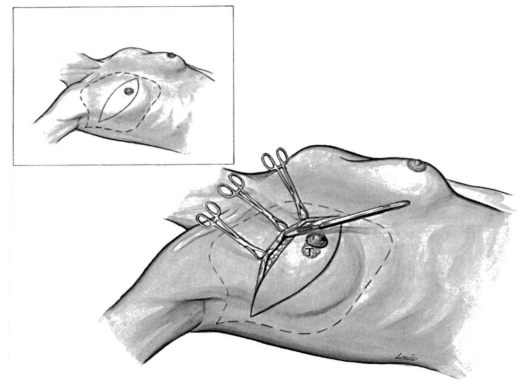

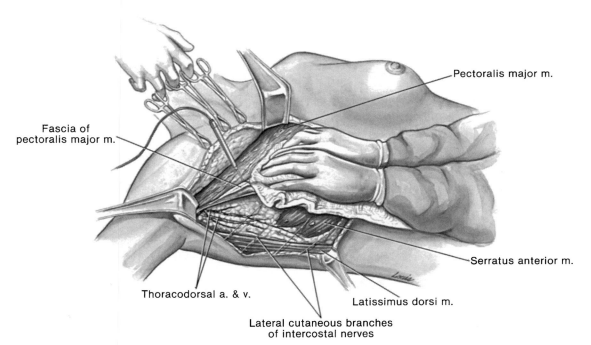

Pectoralis major m.

Fascia of
pectoralis major m.

Serratus anterior m.

Thoracodorsal a. & v.

Latissimus dorsi m.

Lateral cutaneous branches
of intercostal nerves

Figure 44–24   *Elevation of the superior flap to the level of the subclavius muscle at the superior-most extent of breast parenchyma. Skin flap thickness is constant at 7 to 8 mm from lateral to medial. Thereafter, dissection of the pectoralis major fascia from the pectoralis musculature may be completed with cold scalpel or electrocautery. Dissection commences lateral to medial in a plane that parallels the muscle bundles of the pectoralis major muscle from origin of ribs 2–6 to insertion on the humerus. Countertraction in a caudal direction allows tension on the fascia to facilitate its removal from the pectoralis major. Perforator vessels from the lateral thoracic or anterior intercostal arteries are encountered as end-arteries that supply the pectoralis major and minor muscles. Thereafter, the inferior flap is elevated medially in similar fashion to the midline, inferiorly to the aponeurosis of the rectus abdominis tendon, and laterally to the anterior margin of the latissimus. The inferior-most portion of the breast is left intact following clearing of the superolateral margin of the pectoralis major. This maneuver ensures an en bloc resection of the axillary contents with the breast, leaving the axillary tail of Spence intact.*

is not possible, the inferior flap should then be elevated as delineated previously. Preferably, the lateral margin of the flap is then elevated to the anterior margin of the latissimus dorsi with exposure from inferior to superior directions (Fig. 44–25). The loose areolar tissue of the lateral axillary space is elevated with identification of the lateral-most extent of the axillary vein in its course anterior and caudal to the brachial plexus and axillary artery. Dissection craniad to the axillary vein is inadvisable for fear of damage to the brachial plexus and the infrequent observation of nodal tissues cephalad to the vein. The axillary vein should be sharply exposed with cold scalpel dissection on its anterior and ventral surfaces after division of the investing deep layer of superficial fascia of the axillary space. Dissection with electrocautery may cause thermal damage to the surface of the anterior or inferior vein wall. Electrical stimulation with electrocautery of the brachial plexus or its motor branches to muscles of the arm and shoulder is an additional technical problem.

As the operator proceeds medially to complete dissection of the lateral-most margin of the pectoralis major, abduction of the shoulder and extension of the arm with finger dissection of the lateral and inferior margin of the pectoralis major allow visualization of the insertion of the pectoralis minor on the coracoid process of the scapula. The tendinous portion of the pectoralis minor is divided near its insertion on the coracoid process (Fig. 44–26, inset). The surgeon must be aware of the anatomical location of the lateral neurovascular bundle in which the medial pectoral nerve courses to its innervation of the pectoralis minor and major. If possible, this nerve should be preserved to abrogate the probability of atrophy of the lateral head of the pectoralis major. Should the entire nerve trunk penetrate the pectoralis minor, sacrifice may be necessary. It may also be necessary to sacrifice penetrating *branches* of the medial pectoral nerve with elevation and medial retraction of the pectoralis minor to its origin on ribs 2 through 5. With this maneuver, the *interpectoral nodes (Rotter's nodes)* are included en bloc with the operative specimen. Furthermore, resection of the pectoralis minor allows full visualization of the extent of the axillary vein in its course beneath the pectoralis minor and its entry into the chest wall at its confluence with the subclavian vein beneath the costoclavicular (Halsted's) ligament. With resection of the pectoralis minor muscle, exposure of Level 2 and 3 nodes is possible.

The operator should continue to work lateral to medial with complete visualization of the anterior and ventral surfaces of the axillary vein. The investing fascia of the axillary vein is dissected with elevation of the deep layer of superficial fascia and cold scalpel division after exposure, ligation, and division of all venous tributaries. With identification and retraction of the superomedial aspect of the pectoralis major, the lateral pectoral (anterior thoracic) nerve with origin from the lateral cord is exposed with the medial neurovascular bundle. This neuro-

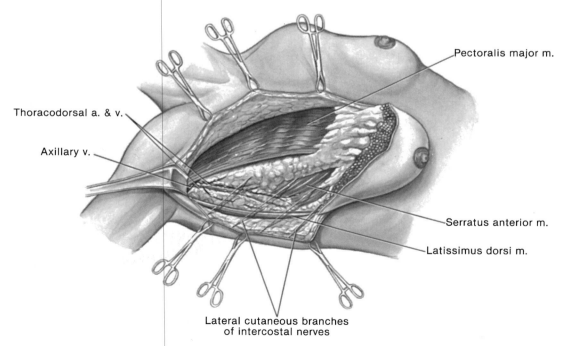

Pectoralis major m.

Thoracodorsal a. & v.

Axillary v.

Serratus anterior m.

Latissimus dorsi m.

Lateral cutaneous branches
of intercostal nerves

Figure 44–25 *The completed superior and inferior flap with breast parenchyma intact with the axillary tail of Spence and the axillary contents. The pectoralis major is completely cleared of its fascia en bloc with the breast parenchyma. At this juncture, the pectoralis minor has not been exposed to allow access to the axilla (Level 2 and 3 nodes). The latissimus dorsi muscle has been dissected on its anterior surface to delineate the lateral boundary of dissection. Illustrated in this view is the cutaneous innervation of skin of the lateral chest, axilla, and medial arm by intercostobrachial sensory nerves. These nerves are commonly divided in the course of dissection of the axilla and lateral skin flap following identification of the latissimus dorsi.*

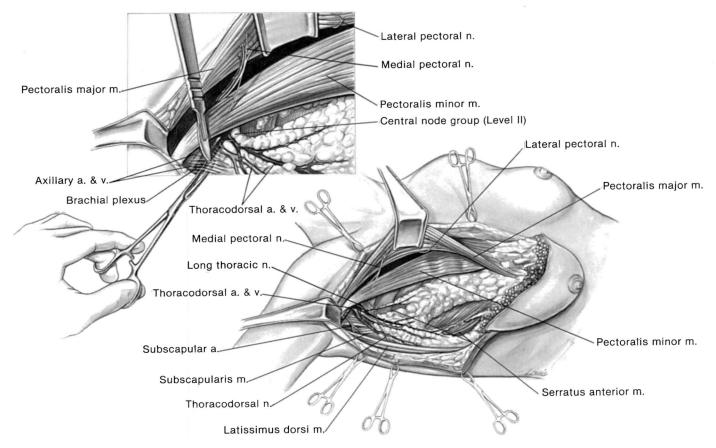

Figure 44–26   Inset, *Juncture of the latissimus (unexposed) with the ventral surface of the axillary vein. Sharp division with scalpel to incise the investing fascia of the axillary space. Following isolation of the tendinous portion of the pectoralis minor muscle with finger dissection, the insertion of this tendon on the coracoid process of the scapula can be readily identified. The surgeon must be cognizant of the anatomical location of the lateral neurovascular bundle and the laterally placed medial pectoral nerve, which takes origin from the medial cord. (See section entitled "General Principles of Mastectomy" for variance of this nerve.) Every attempt should be made to preserve the medial pectoral nerve, as sacrifice of the main trunk may allow atrophy of the lateral head of the pectoralis major. Further, the lateral pectoral nerve, which takes origin from the lateral cord and is medially placed, should also be preserved.*

vascular structure should likewise be protected to ensure innervation to the medial heads of the pectoralis major (Fig. 44–27). Dissection is continued medially on the anterior/ventral surface of the axillary vein to the costoclavicular ligament, which represents the condensation of the clavipectoral fascia.

Caudal to the vein, the loose areolar tissue at the juncture of the axillary vein with the anterior margin of the latissimus dorsi is swept inferomedially to include the *lateral (axillary) nodal group (Level 1).* The operator should take care to preserve the thoracodorsal artery and vein, which are deep in the axillary space and fully invested with loose areolar tissue and nodes of the lateral group. The operator should also be aware of the origin of the *thoracodorsal nerve* from the posterior cord, whose origin is medial to the thoracodorsal artery and vein. This nerve has a variable inferolateral course en route to its innervation of the latissimus dorsi muscle and must be visualized and protected throughout its course if subsequent reconstruction using myocutaneous flaps that incorporate the latissimus is planned. Thereafter, the lateral axillary nodal group is retracted inferomedi-

ally and anterior to the *thoracodorsal neurovascular bundle* to be dissected en bloc with the *subscapular group of nodes (Level 1),* which are medially located between the thoracodorsal nerve and the lateral chest wall. Dissection of the posterior contents of the axillary space and division of multiple tributaries from the thoracoacromial artery and vein allow free access to exposure of the posterior boundary of the axilla. With this dissection, the heads of the teres major laterally and the subscapularis muscle medially are visualized.

The dissection begins medially with extirpation of the *central nodal groups (Level 2)* and *apical (subclavicular) (Level 3) nodes.* The superomedial-most aspect of the dissection at the level of the costoclavicular ligament represents the point of termination of the dissection; this nodal group should be identified with a metallic marker or suture. This practice provides the pathologist the opportunity to examine for extension of nodal disease, which may have subsequent therapeutic and prognostic significance.

It is essential that the operator continue this dissection en bloc to avoid the separation of nodal

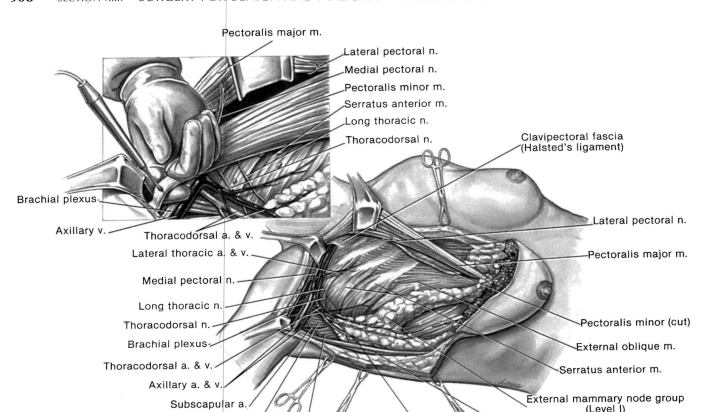

Pectoralis major m.

Lateral pectoral n.

Medial pectoral n.

Pectoralis minor m.

Serratus anterior m.

Long thoracic n.

Thoracodorsal n.

Clavipectoral fascia
(Halsted's ligament)

Brachial plexus

Axillary v.

Thoracodorsal a. & v.

Lateral thoracic a. & v.

Medial pectoral n.

Long thoracic n.

Thoracodorsal n.

Brachial plexus

Thoracodorsal a. & v.

Axillary a. & v.

Subscapular a.

Dissected lateral
axillary node group
(Level I)

Subscapularis m.

Subscapular node group
(Level I)

Lateral pectoral n.

Pectoralis major m.

Pectoralis minor (cut)

External oblique m.

Serratus anterior m.

External mammary node group
(Level I)

Latissimus dorsi m.

Figure 44–27   Inset, *Digital protection of the brachial plexus for division of the insertion of the pectoralis minor muscle on the coracoid process. All loose areolar and lymphatic tissues are swept en bloc with the axillary contents to ensure resection of the interpectoral (Rotter's) nodes.*

Dissection commences lateral to medial with complete visualization of the anterior and ventral aspects of the axillary vein. Dissection craniad to the axillary vein is inadvisable, for fear of damage to the brachial plexus and the infrequent observation of gross nodal tissue cephalic to the vein. Investing fascial dissection of the vein is best completed with the cold scalpel following exposure, ligation, and division of all venous tributaries on the anterior and ventral surfaces. Caudal to the vein, loose areolar tissue at the junction of the vein with the anterior margin of latissimus is swept inferomedially inclusive of the lateral (axillary) nodal group (Level 1). Care is taken to preserve the neurovascular thoracodorsal artery, vein, and nerve in the deep axillary space. The thoracodorsal nerve is traced to its innervation of the latissimus dorsi muscle laterally. Lateral axillary nodal groups are retracted inferomedially and anterior to this bundle for dissection en bloc with the subscapular (Level 1) nodal group. Preferentially, dissection commences superomedially before completion of dissection of the external mammary (Level 1) nodal group. Superomedial dissection over the axillary vein allows extirpation of the central nodal group (Level 2) and apical (subclavicular) Level 3 group. The superomedial-most extent of the dissection is the clavipectoral fascia (Halsted's ligament). This level of dissection with the Patey technique allows the surgeon to mark, with metallic clip or suture, the superior-most extent of dissection. All loose areolar tissue just inferior to the apical nodal group is swept off the chest wall, leaving the fascia of the serratus anterior intact. With dissection parallel to the long thoracic nerve (respiratory nerve of Bell), the deep investing serratus fascia is incised. This nerve is closely applied to the investing fascial compartment of the chest wall and must be dissected in its entirety, cephalic to caudal to ensure innervation of the serratus anterior and avoidance of the "winged scapula" disability.

groups and disruption of lymphatic vessels in the axilla. Inferomedial retraction of Level 2 and 3 nodes en bloc with the specimen, which is inclusive of the *external mammary group (Level 1)*, is conducted in a cephalad to caudad direction in parallel with the thoracodorsal neurovascular bundle. This dissection maneuver incorporates nodal groups en bloc and avoids neural injury while providing direct access and exposure of venous tributaries posterior to the axillary vein. With medial dissection, the operator encounters the chest wall deep in the medial axillary space and is able to identify the *long thoracic nerve (respiratory nerve of Bell)* applied in the deep investing (serratus) fascia of the axillary space. This

nerve is constant in its location anterior to the subscapularis muscle and is closely applied to the investing fascial compartment of the chest wall. Every effort should be made to preserve the long thoracic nerve; otherwise, permanent disability with a winged scapula and shoulder apraxia will follow denervation of the serratus anterior. This nerve is dissected throughout its course to innervation of the serratus anterior (see Figs. 44–26 and 44–27). The axillary contents anterior and medial to the nerve are swept inferomedially with this specimen, and the operator should ensure that innervations of the long thoracic and thoracodorsal nerves are visualized before division of the inferior-most extent of the axillary contents. Incompletely divided origins of the pectoralis minor from ribs 2 through 5 are resected with electrocautery, and the remaining portions of the muscle are swept en bloc with the axillary contents to be inclusive of Rotter's interpectoral and the retropectoral groups. The dissection continues in a caudal direction such that the entire breast and fascia are cleared medially and inferiorly from the aponeurosis of the rectus abdominis muscle (see Fig. 44–27). The specimen is immediately sent to the pathology department for examination of the fresh specimen and to procure steroid hormone receptors of the tumor if this procedure was not completed at the initial biopsy. It is essential that tissue be forwarded promptly to the laboratory for tissue preservation, because hormone receptor analyses are thermo- and ischemia-labile within the ambient temperature of the operating room environment.[15, 16]

Points of bleeding are inspected, clamped, and ligated individually with nonabsorbable 2-0 and 3-0 sutures. Before wound closure, the margins of the wound are carefully inspected for devascularization initiated by the trauma of flap retraction or by tissue dissection of thin, poorly vascularized skin. Obvious sites of devascularization are debrided back from the skin margin parallel with the original skin incision such that adequate closure without tension is possible. For equivocal areas of devascularized tissue, systemic intravenous injection of 4 to 5 cc of fluoroscein will allow the operator to visualize viable skin margins with a Wood's light.

The surgeon, all assistants, and the scrub nurse should reglove and, optionally, regown. Additionally, sterile instruments are used for wound closure to avoid the potential for implantation of exfoliated tumor cells in the wound. Thereafter, the wound may be closed after copious irrigation with distilled water or saline, which augments evacuation of residual tissue, clots, and serum. The wound is again inspected for bleeding sites, and if none are found, closed-suction Silastic catheters (18–20 French) are positioned via separate stab incisions that enter the inferior flap at approximately the anterior axillary line (Fig. 44–28).

The lateral Silastic catheter is positioned in the axillary space approximately 2 cm inferior to the

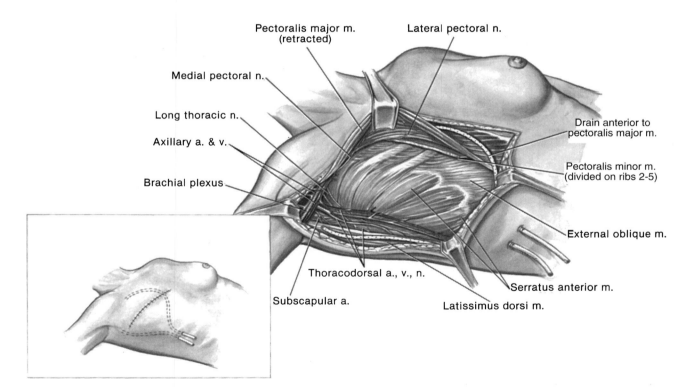

Figure 44–28 *The completed Patey axillary dissection variant of the modified radical technique. The dissection is inclusive of the pectoralis minor muscle from origin to insertion on ribs 2–5. Both medial and lateral pectoral nerves are preserved to ensure innervation of the lateral and medial heads, respectively, of the pectoralis major. With completion of the procedure, remaining portions of this muscle are swept en bloc with the axillary contents to be inclusive of Rotter's interpectoral and the retropectoral groups.*

Inset, Following copious irrigation with distilled water and saline, closed-suction Silastic catheters (18–20 French) are positioned via stab incisions placed in the inferior flap at the anterior axillary line. The lateral catheter is placed approximately 2 cm inferior to the axillary vein. The superior, longer catheter placed via the medial stab wound is positioned in the superomedial aspect of the defect anterior the pectoralis major muscle beneath the skin flap. The wound is closed in two layers with 2-0 absorbable synthetic sutures placed in subcutaneous planes. Undue tension on margins of the flap must be avoided; it may necessitate undermining of tissues to reduce mechanical forces. The skin is optionally closed with subcuticular 4-0 synthetic absorbable sutures or stainless steel staples

Following completion of wound closure, both catheters are irrigated copiously with saline to ensure patency and are connected and maintained on low to moderate continuous suction provided by reservoir portable vacuum bottles. Light, bulky dressings of gauze are placed over the dissection site and taped securely in place with occlusive dressings. The surgeon may elect to place the ipsilateral arm in a sling to provide immobilization.

axillary vein on the ventral surface area of the latissimus dorsi muscle to provide drainage of the axilla. A longer, second catheter placed via the medial stab incision is positioned in the superomedial aspect of the defect (see Fig. 44–28, inset) to provide continual evacuation of serum and blood that may accumulate within the large surface area of the dissected pectoralis major muscle. Both catheters are secured at skin level with a 2-0 nonabsorbable suture. We prefer not to secure the catheters to pectoral muscles or to the latissimus for fear of initiating bleeding at the time of catheter removal.

The flap margins are again inspected to evaluate sites of devascularization or "buttonhole" defects that result from tangential incisions or the trauma of dissection with flap elevation. The wound is closed in two layers with 2-0 absorbable synthetic sutures placed in the subcutaneous tissues. Undue tension on margins of the flap may necessitate extensive undermining of these tissues to reduce mechanical forces and maximize adherence to the underlying pectoralis major. The skin is optionally closed with subcuticular 4-0 synthetic absorbable sutures or stainless steel staples. Wounds closed with subcuticular sutures should have Steri-Strips applied perpendicular to the incision to enhance wound repair. Thereafter, both catheters are irrigated copiously with saline to ensure patency and are then connected and maintained on continuous low-to-moderate suction by large reservoir portable vacuum bottles. Light bulky dressings of cotton are applied to the dissection site and are taped securely in place. Optionally, the surgeon may immobilize the ipsilateral arm in an arm sling.

The dressings should remain intact on the operative wound until the third or fourth postoperative day, unless the surgeon is concerned about the viability of the dissected flap. Wound catheters should remain in the site of dissection until the drainage becomes predominantly serous and diminishes to 20 to 25 ml during a 24-hour interval. Most surgeons initiate shoulder and arm exercises on the day after removal of the drainage catheters.

We follow the same recommendations given in Chapter 42 for the Halsted radical mastectomy for patients with protracted serosanguinous or serous drainage. This is evident in approximately 20 percent of operative wounds and may be managed by continued suction using the lateral-most (dependent) Silastic drain. However, long-term catheter preservation requires the patient to be aware of hygienic care of the catheters and of the sites of skin entry and necessitates frequent changes of dressings. It is our practice to limit the range of motion of the arm and shoulder for patients with protracted drainage, because shoulder immobilization augments flap adherence to the chest wall. The surgeon must periodically inspect wound discharge from the catheters to evaluate the potential for retrograde bacterial infection of the axillary space, particularly when drainage catheters remain in place longer than 7 days.

References

1. Auchincloss H: Significance of location and number of axillary metastases in carcinoma of the breast. Ann Surg 158:37–46, 1963.
2. Bader J, Lippman ME, Swain SM: Preliminary report of the NCI early breast cancer (BC) study. A prospective randomized trial comparison of lumpectomy and radiation to mastectomy for Stage I and II BC. Int J Radiat Oncol Biol Phys 12 (suppl):160, 1987.
3. Baker RR, Montague ACW, Childs JN: A comparison of modified radical mastectomy to radical mastectomy in the treatment of operable breast cancer. Ann Surg 189(5):553–557, 1979.
4. Banks WM: On free removal of mammary cancer with extirpation of the axillary glands as a necessary accompaniment. Br Med J 2:1138, 1882.
5. Berstock DA, Houghton B, Haybittle J, Baum M: The role of radiotherapy following total mastectomy for patients with early breast cancer. World J Surg 9:667–670, 1985.
6. Blichert-Toft M: A Danish randomized trial comparing breast conservation with mastectomy in mammary carcinoma. Br J Cancer 62 (suppl 12):15, 1995.
7. Crile GC Jr: Results of simple mastectomy without irradiation in the treatment of operative stage I cancer of the breast. Ann Surg 168:330–336, 1968.
8. Crile GC Jr: Results of conservative treatment of breast cancer at ten and 15 years. Ann Surg 181:26–30, 1975.
9. Crile GC Jr: Results of simplified treatment of breast cancer. Surg Gynecol Obstet 118:517–523, 1964.
10. Crowe JP, Gordon NH, Antunez AR, Shenk R, Hubay CA, Shuck J: Local-regional breast cancer recurrence following mastectomy. Arch Surg 126:429–432, 1991.
11. Dahl-Iversen E, Tobiassen T: Radical mastectomy with peristernal and supraclavicular dissection for mammary carcinoma. Am J Surg 157:170–173, 1963.
12. DeLarue NC, Anderson WD, Starr J: Modified radical mastectomy in the individualized treatment of breast carcinoma. Surg Gynecol Obstet 129:79–88, 1969.
13. Den Besten L, Ziffren SE: Simple and radical mastectomy: A comparison of survival. Arch Surg 90:755–759, 1965.
14. Devitt JE: The influence of conservative and radical surgery on the survival of patients with breast cancer. Can Med Assoc J 87:906–910, 1962.
15. Ellis LM, Wittliff JL, Bryant MS, Sitren HS, Hogancamp WE, Souba WW, Bland KI: Effects of ischemia on breast tumor steroid hormone-receptor levels. Curr Surg 45(4):312–314, 1988.
16. Ellis LM, Wittliff JL, Bryant MS, Sitren HS, Hogancamp WE, Souba WW, Bland KI: Lability of steroid hormone receptors following devascularization of breast tumors. Arch Surg 124:39–42, 1989.
17. Elston CW, Gresham GA, Rao GS, Zebro T, Haybittle JL, Houghton J, Kerney G: The Cancer Research Campaign (King's/Cambridge) Trial for early breast cancer: Clinical pathological aspects. Br J Cancer 45:655, 1982.
18. Fisher B, Fisher ER: Experimental evidence in support of the dormant tumor cell. Science 130:918–919, 1959.
19. Fisher B, Fisher ER: Transmigration of lymph nodes by tumor cells. Science 152:1397–1398, 1966.
20. Fisher B, Redmond C, Fisher ER, Bauer M, Wolmark N, Wickerham L, Deutsch M, Montague E, Margolese R, Foster R: Ten-year results of a randomized clinical trial comparing radical mastectomy and total mastectomy with or without radiation. N Engl J Med 312(11):674–681, 1985.
21. Fisher ER, Fisher B: Host influence on tumor growth and dissemination. In Schwartz E (ed): The Biological Basis of Radiation Therapy. Philadelphia, JB Lippincott, 1966, pp 484–517.
22. Fisher B, Fisher ER: The interrelationship of hematogenous and lymphatic tumor cell dissemination. Surg Gynecol Obstet 122:791–798, 1966.
23. Fisher B, Redmond C, Fisher ER, et al: The contribution of recent NSABP clinical trials of primary breast cancer therapy

to an understanding of tumor biology—an overview of findings. Cancer 46 1009–1025, 1980.

24. Fisher B, Redmond C, Poisson R, Margolese R, Wolmark N, Wickerham L, Fisher E, Deutsch M, Caplan R, Pilch Y, Glass A, Shibata H, Lerner H, Terz J, Sidorovich L: Eight-year results of a randomized clinical trial comparing total mastectomy and lumpectomy with or without irradiation in the treatment of breast cancer. N Engl J Med 320(13):822–828, 1989.
25. Fisher B, Anderson S, Redmond CK, Wolmark N, Wickerham DL, Cronin WM: Reanalysis and results after 12 years follow-up in a randomized clinical trial comparing total mastectomy with lumpectomy with or without irradiation in the treatment of breast cancer. N Engl J Med 333:1456–1461, 1995.
26. Fisher B, Saffer EA, Fisher ER: Studies concerning the regional lymph node in cancer. VII. Thymidine uptake by cells from nodes of breast cancer patients relative to axillary location and histopathologic discriminants. Cancer 33:271–279, 1974.
27. Forrest APM, Roberts MM, Preece P, Henk JM, Campbell H, Hughes LE, Desai S, Hulbert M: The Cardiff-St. Mary's trial. Br J Surg 61:766–769, 1974.
28. Forrest APM, Stewart HJ, Roberts MM, Steele RJC: Simple mastectomy and axillary node sampling (pectoral node biopsy) in the management of primary breast cancer. Ann Surg 196(3):371–378, 1982.
29. Forrest APM, Everington D, McDonald CC, Steel RJC, Chetty U, Stewart HJ: The Edinburgh randomized trial of axillary sampling or clearance after mastectomy. Br J Surg 82:1504–1508, 1995.
30. Grace E: Simple mastectomy in cancer of the breast. Am J Surg 35:512, 1937.
31. Glastein E, Straus K, Lichner A: Results of the NCI early breast cancer trial. Proceedings of the National Institutes of Health Consensus Development Conference, June 18–21, 1990, p 32.
32. Gross SW: A Practical Treatment of Tumors of the Mammary Gland Embracing Their Histology, Pathology, Diagnosis and Treatment. New York. D Appleton & Co, 1880, pp 222–227.
33. Halsted WS: The results of operations for the cure of cancer of the breast performed at the Johns Hopkins Hospital from June 1889 to January 1894. Arch Surg 20:497–544, 1894.
34. Hamilton T, Langlands AO, Prescott RJ: The treatment of operable cancer of the breast. A clinical trial in the South-East region of Scotland. Br J Surg 61:758–761, 1974.
35. Handley RS: The conservative radical mastectomy of Patey: 10-year results in 425 patients' breasts. Dis Breast 2:16, 1976.
36. Handley RS, Thackray AC: Conservative radical mastectomy (Patey's operation). Ann Surg 170(6):880–882, 1969.
37. Helman P, Bennett MB, Louw JH, Wilkie W, Madden P, Silber W, Sealy R, Heselson J: Interim report on trial of treatment for operable breast cancer. South Afr Med J 46:1374–1375, 1972.
38. Henderson IC. Mourisden H, et al: Effects of adjuvant tamoxifen and of cytotoxic therapy on mortality in early breast cancer: An overview of 61 randomized trials among 28,896 women. N Engl J Med 319(26):1681–1692, 1988.
39. Hermann RE, Steiger E: Modified radical mastectomy. Surg Clin North Am 58(4):743–754, 1978.
40. Hermann RE, Esselstyn CB Jr, Crile G Jr, Cooperman AM, Antunez AR, Hoerr SO: Results of conservative operations for breast cancer. Arch Surg 120:746–751, 1985.
41. Hoffman GW, Elliott LF: The anatomy of the pectoral nerves and its significance to the general and plastic surgeon. Ann Surg 205(5):504–507, 1987.
42. Houghton J, Baum M, Haybittle JL: Role of radiotherapy following total mastectomy in patients with early breast cancer. World J Surg 18:117–122, 1994.
43. Johansen H, Kaae S, Schiødt T: Simple mastectomy with postoperative irradiation versus extended radical mastectomy in breast cancer: A twenty-five year follow-up of a randomized trial. Acta Oncol 29:709–715, 1990.
44. Küster E: Zur behandlung des brustkrebses verhandlungen der deutschen gesellschaft für Chirurgie. Leipsiz 12:288, 1883.
45. Kyle J, et al: Management of early cancer of the breast: Report on an international multicentre trial supported by the Cancer Research Campaign. Br Med J 1:1035–1038, 1976.

46. Langlands AO, Prescott RJ, Hamilton T: A clinical trial in the management of operable cancer of the breast. Br J Surg 67:170–174, 1980.
47. Leis HP Jr: Modified radical mastectomy: Definition and role in breast cancer surgery. Int Surg 65(3):211–217, 1980.
48. Lythgoe JP, Leck I, Swindell R: Manchester regional breast study: preliminary results. Lancet 1:744–747, 1978.
49. Lythgoe JP, Palmer MK: Manchester regional breast study—5 and 10 year results. Br J Surg 69:693–696, 1982.
50. Madden JL. Modified radical mastectomy. Surg Gynecol Obstet 121(6):1221–1230, 1965.
51. Madden JL, Kandalaft S, Bourque RA: Modified radical mastectomy. Ann Surg 175(5):624–634, 1972.
52. Maddox WA, Carpenter JT Jr, Laws HL, Soong SJ, Cloud G, Urist MM, Balch CM: A randomized prospective trial of radical (Halsted) mastectomy versus modified radical mastectomy in 311 breast cancer patients. Ann Surg 198(2):207–212, 1983.
53. Maddox WA, Carpenter JT Jr, Laws HT, Soong S-J, Cloud G, Balch CM, Urist MM: Does radical mastectomy still have a place in the treatment of primary operable breast cancer? Arch Surg 122:1317–1320, 1987.
54. Martin JK, van Heerden JA, Taylor WF, Gaffey A: Is modified radical mastectomy really equivalent to radical mastectomy in treatment of carcinoma of the breast? Cancer 57:510–518, 1986.
55. McWhirter R: The value of simple mastectomy and radiotherapy in the treatment of cancer of the breast. Br J Radiol 21:599–610, 1948.
56. Meyer AC, Smith SS, Potter M: Carcinoma of the breast: A clinical study. Arch Surg 113:364–367, 1978.
57. Meyer W: An improved method for the radical operation for carcinoma of the breast. Med Rec NY 46:746–749, 1894.
58. Moore CH: On the influence of inadequate operations on the theory of cancer. R Med Chir Soc London 1:244–280, 1867.
59. Morimoto T, Monden Y, Takashima S, Iton S, Kimura T, Yamamoto H, Kitamura M, Inui K, Tanaka N, Nagano T, Fujishima N, Yanada J, Tsurunom, Kamaki K: Five-year results of a randomized trial comparing modified radical mastectomy and extended radical mastectomy for Stage II breast cancer. Jpn J Surg 24:210–214, 1994.
60. Moxley JH III: Treatment of primary breast cancer: Summary of the NIH Consensus Development Conference. JAMA 244(8):797–800, 1980.
61. Murphy JB: Carcinoma of breast. Surg Clin 1(6):779, 1912.
62. Nemoto T, Vana J, Bedwani RN, Baker HW, McGregor FH, Murphy GP: Management and survival of female breast cancer: Results of a national survey by the American College of Surgeons. Cancer 45(12):2917–2924, 1980.
63. Nemoto T, Dao TL: Is modified mastectomy adequate for axillary lymph node dissection? Ann Surg 182:722–723, 1975.
64. Patey DH, Dyson WH: The prognosis of carcinoma of the breast in relation to the type of operation performed. Br J Cancer 2:7–13, 1948.
65. Patey DH: A review of 146 cases of carcinoma of the breast operated on between 1930 and 1943. Br J Cancer 21:260–269, 1967.
66. Robinson GN, Van Heerden JA, Payne WS, Taylor W, Gaffey TA: The primary surgical treatment of carcinoma of the breast: a changing trend toward modified radical mastectomy. Mayo Clin Proc 51:433–442, 1976.
67. Sarrazin D, Le MG, Fontaine MF, Arriagada R: Conservative treatment versus mastectomy in T1 or small T2 breast cancer. A randomized clinical trial. In Harris JR, Hellman S, Silen W (eds): Conservative Management of Breast Cancer. Philadelphia, JB Lippincott, 1983, pp 101–111.
68. Chevalier TL, Lacour J: Ten-year results of a randomized trial comparing a conservative treatment to mastectomy in early breast cancer. Radiother Oncol 14:177–184, 1989.
69. Shimkin MB, Koppel M, Connelly RR, Cutler SJ: Simple and radical mastectomy for breast cancer: a re-analysis of Smith and Meyer's report from Rockford, Illinois. J Natl Cancer Inst 27:1197–1215, 1961.
70. Smith SS, Meyer AC: Cancer of the breast in Rockford, Illinois. Am J Surg 98:653–656, 1959.
71. Sprengel O: Mittheilungen über die in den Jahren 1874 bis

1878 aur der Volkmann'schen Klinik operativ behandelten 131 Falle von Brust-carcinom. Archir F Klin Chir 27:805, 1882.

72. Staunton MD, Melville DM, Monterrosa A, Thomas JM: A 25-year prospective study of modified radical mastectomy; (Patey) in 192 patients. J Royal Soc Med 86:381–384, 1993.

73. Turnbull AR, Chant ADB, Buchanan RB, Turner DTL, Shepherd JM, Fraser JD: Treatment of early breast cancer. Lancet 2:7–9, 1978.

74. Turner L, Swindell R, Bell WGT, Hartley RC, Tasker JH, Wilson WW, Alderson MR, Leck IM: Radical vs modified radical mastectomy for breast cancer. Ann R Coll Surg Engl 63:239–243, 1981.

75. Urban JA: Treatment of primary breast cancer. Management of local disease. Minority report. JAMA 244(8):800–803, 1980.

76. Vana J, Bedwani R, Nemoto T, Murphy GP: American College of Surgeons Commission on Cancer Final Report on Long-Term Patient Care Evaluation Study for Carcinoma of the Female Breast. Chicago, American College of Surgeons, 1979.

77. Veronesi U, Valagussa P: Inefficacy of internal mammary nodes dissection in breast cancer surgery. Cancer 47:170–175, 1981.

78. Veronesi M, Banfi A, DelVecchio M, Saccozzi R: Comparison of Halsted mastectomy with quadrantectomy, axillary dissection, and radiotherapy in early breast cancer long term results. Eur J Cancer Clin Oncol 22:1085–1089, 1986.

79. Veronesi M, Luini A, Galimberti V, Zarrida S: Conservative approach for the management of stage I/II carcinoma of the breast. Milan Cancer Institute Trials. World J Surg 18:70–75, 1994.

80. Volkmann R: Geschwülste der mamma (36 Fälle) Beitrage zur Chirurgie. Leipsiz, 1895, pp 310–334.

81. Williams IG, Murley RS, Curwen MP: Carcinoma of the female breast: Conservative and radical surgery Br Med J 2:787–796, 1953.

82. Wilson RE, Donegan WL, Mettlin C, Smart CR, Murphy GP: The 1982 National Survey of Carcinoma of the Breast in the United States by the American College of Surgeons. Surg Gynecol Obstet 159:309–318, 1984.

CHAPTER 45
QUADRANTECTOMY

Umberto Veronesi, M.D.

GENERAL PRINCIPLES

A quadrantectomy is an operation that removes a significant portion of the quadrant of the breast where the primary carcinoma is located. For small tumors, the classic concepts of good oncological surgical practice (i.e., removal of an extensive portion of normal tissue around the primary, en bloc removal of overlying skin and underlying muscular fascia) may be maintained without performing a total mastectomy. This concept follows a similar evolution of thought in other fields of surgical oncology (e.g., lobectomy instead of total thyroidectomy, lung lobectomy or removal of a lung segment instead of pneumonectomy, partial resection of the bladder instead of a total cystectomy) when small tumors are found.

These concepts have evolved primarily because of the great change in the characteristics of the patient population that has occurred in the past 20 years. Better education, more extensive information, more refined diagnostic tools, and diffuse screening campaigns all contribute to earlier detection of cancer, particularly of breast carcinoma in women. It would be unwise to perform the classic surgical procedures that were introduced at the beginning of the century to treat patients with tumors that were totally different in character and more often than not were locally advanced. Many patients bear breast tumors of very limited dimensions, and sometimes these tumors are not even palpable. We have to consider that the feeling of women toward breast cancer and breast cancer surgery has also greatly changed; women today are aware that if the primary tumor is small, most of the breast may be spared with adequate surgical and radiotherapeutic procedures. This new optimistic view of breast cancer treatment has also stimulated women to participate more actively in detection programs and in breast self-examination, knowing that if a small cancer is found, treatment can preserve the breast rather than produce the scarring mutilation prevalent in previous eras.

Certainly, the quadrantectomy poses some cosmetic problems. In a breast of normal size, it produces acceptable results, but in small breasts, the cosmetic results may be unsatisfactory. Therefore in selected cases, the option of total mastectomy and immediate reconstruction may be considered. However, surgeons must be trained to reshape the breast after quadrantectomy, possibly with the help of a plastic surgeon, who may in the future become a component of the modern breast surgery team.

It must be emphasized that the quadrantectomy is a surgical procedure that may be defined as "radical," in the sense that it aims at removal of all the tumor cells of the primary carcinoma. Other procedures, such as the lumpectomy, tylectomy, or tumorectomy, are just "debulking" operations whose objective is to reduce the mass of cancer tissue in order to improve the efficacy of postsurgical radiotherapy.

Quadrantectomy followed by radiotherapy has had excellent results, not only in the overall survival but also in the incidence of local recurrences, with rates ranging from 3 to 5 percent, which is comparable to the rate of recurrence following the Halsted mastectomy and probably lower than the rate of local recurrence after modified radical mastectomy.[2, 4-6] Results of the QUART protocol (quadrantectomy, axillary dissection, radiotherapy) are reviewed comprehensively in Chapter 65.

SURGICAL TECHNIQUE

Biopsy

In principle, no definitive treatment for suspicious breast cancer should be adopted until the diagnosis is established by a satisfactory pathological examination. If a fine needle biopsy has previously unequivocally proved the diagnosis of malignancy and there are clear clinical and mammographic findings of invasive carcinoma, an open biopsy may be avoided and the quadrantectomy performed directly. Otherwise, an open biopsy is necessary.

Obtaining an adequate biopsy specimen has the following objectives:

1. To remove an adequate quantity of cancer tissue for an accurate pathological diagnosis and to allow an accurate measurement of the lesion.
2. To limit the disruption of the anatomical integrity of the breast to a minimum.
3. To avoid implantation of cancer cells.

As regards the last point, because cancer cells are easily transplantable, the surgeon must take special care not to implant them in the operative field. Therefore in the subsequent removal of the involved quadrant, the surgeon should avoid re-entering the biopsy site.

The incision must be made just over the site of the lesion in a radial direction. The tumor nodule must be carefully dissected and totally removed with a very limited margin of normal tissue in all directions. The surgeon should then cut the tumor in two parts and observe the cutting surface. In most cases the diagnosis is easy to assess with this macroscopic examination. If the mass is less than 2 to 3 cm in maximum diameter, the patient is considered to be a candidate for quadrantectomy. In the case of an extemporary biopsy, while the specimen is being processed in the pathology department to obtain the final histological diagnosis by frozen section examination, the mammary gland is carefully reconstructed with one layer of interrupted suture with 0 silk. Because the wound may contain free-floating cancer cells, it is filled with a gauze soaked in a solution (i.e., hypotonic saline or distilled water) apt to destroy free cancer cells. The skin is closed with a continuous or interrupted suture. This suture must be tight, and no fluid should spill from the wound. If this should happen, there is a risk of implantation of cancer cells during the subsequent quadrantectomy. If final surgery is delayed, some time (7 to 10 days) should elapse between the biopsy and the quadrantectomy, because this procedure is much more easily performed if the area of the biopsy has undergone a reparative fibrotic process.

Removal of the Quadrant

The quadrantectomy technique aims to remove a portion of a quadrant of the breast, including the skin and the superficial pectoralis fascia.[3] The objective is to obtain a radical removal of the primary tumor and its potential surrounding infiltrations through a wide excision. To perform such an operation, it is necessary that the primary cancer be of limited size; it is difficult to perform an appropriate quadrantectomy on tumors whose diameter is larger than 3 cm, unless the breast is large.

After the biopsy has been terminated and the malignant nature of the lesion confirmed, all the instruments, gloves, and drapes must be changed, and the skin resterilized.

The incision in the skin is first outlined with a sterile marking pencil. The shape of the incision is elliptical, with the major axis radial from the nipple. There must be a margin of at least 2 cm from the biopsy incision (Fig. 45–1).

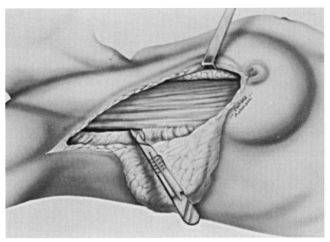

Figure 45–2 *Removal of the quadrant. Two to 3 cm of normal mammary tissue around the primary carcinoma is removed.*

Should the axillary dissection be performed in continuity, a peripheral extension of the incision is made to give adequate exposure of the axilla. The en bloc operation is generally performed when the primary tumor is situated in the upper external quadrants close to the axilla. In all other situations, the quadrantectomy must be carried out separately from the axillary dissection. The skin flaps are prepared with great accuracy to expose a portion of the mammary gland and allow an incision in the mammary gland at least 2 cm from the border of the tumor or the biopsy incision. The deep plane of the excision is the superficial fascia of the pectoralis major muscle (Fig. 45–2). This plane of dissection may be many centimeters from the primary cancer if the tumor is superficial, but when the cancer is deeply situated, only a few millimeters may separate the border of the tumor from the pectoralis muscle; thus the plane of dissection is very close to the edge of the tumor. In this case, the corresponding superficial portion of the pectoralis major muscle may be dissected en bloc with the breast quadrant.

Because a good cosmetic result is one of the major objectives of the quadrantectomy, it is important that the breast and the nipple be reconstructed with great care. This step requires time and often the collaboration of a plastic surgeon. The edges of the mammary gland must be sutured along one or two planes according to the thickness of the breast. However, the extent of reconstruction of the mammary tissue must be carefully evaluated in each case, because it is sometimes advisable to limit reconstruction to a minimum to avoid possible subsequent skin retraction or a bulky and excessively prominent breast.

Special care is needed for the good appearance of the nipple. One of the consequences of the quadrantectomy may be the excessive protrusion and sometimes distortion of the nipple. The protruded nipple tends in fact to bend in the direction of the removed quadrant. To avoid nipple distortion, it is advisable to free the nipple from the mammary gland through

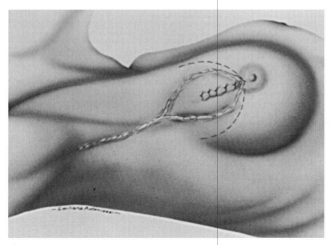

Figure 45–1 *Quadrantectomy and in-continuity axillary dissection lines of skin incision.*

an extensive dissection of the skin and by cutting the major ducts. If the breast resection has been extensive and results in the operated breast being much smaller than the opposite one, it may be reasonable to surgically reduce the contralateral breast during the same session. This bilateral simultaneous approach has the great advantage of granting to the surgeon the freedom to remove a very large portion of the involved breast, knowing that both breasts will be reshaped.

Axillary Dissection

The axillary dissection may sometimes be performed in continuity with the quadrantectomy. In the majority of cases, it is performed in discontinuity through a separate incision, preferably a posteroanterior one that crosses the axillary fossa in an upward direction. The incision follows the cutaneous lines of Langer, 3 to 4 cm down the axillary fold, and has a length of 12 to 15 cm. It gives excellent access to the axillary vein but should be retracted downward to obtain access to the thoracodorsal vessels and nodes (Fig. 45–3).

The first step of the axillary dissection, after the preparation of the skin flaps, is the exposure of the latissimus dorsi muscle. This muscle is a key part of the technique and, once identified, must be carefully followed upward to its white tendinous portion. After the latissimus dorsi muscle has been isolated, the axillary vein, which lies on the white tendon of the latissimus dorsi, is easily identified.

When the vein has been isolated in its lateral portion, the thoracodorsal vessels and nerve are exposed (Fig. 45–3). This may be achieved by cutting the deep pectoralis fascia. At this point, the surgeon should free the lateral margin of the pectoralis major muscle from its fascial connections. The muscle is then retracted upward to give access to the structures situated deep in the axilla. Great care must be taken not to injure the thoracoacromial vessels and the nerves

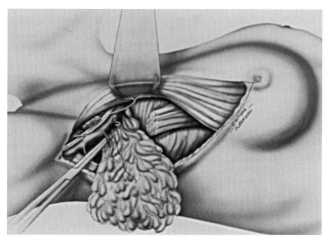

Figure 45–4 *The axillary dissection is completed.*

to the pectoralis major. The pectoralis minor muscle is then freed from its connections and isolated, keeping its nerves and vessels intact.

The next step is the dissection of the apex of the axilla, which may easily be obtained with the incision of the costocoracoid fascia at the point of its reflection into the chest wall. To improve the visibility of the apex of the axilla, the minor pectoralis muscle is retracted laterally. The fat and areolar tissues in the area between the chest wall and the medial aspect of the minor pectoralis muscle contain the highest axillary lymph nodes. To help the pathologist orient the specimen, it is advisable to put a metal disc on the tissue excised from the apex of the axilla.

Once the apex of the axilla has been cleared, the operation continues by dissecting the entire axillary vein and artery, with isolation and ligation of all their branches directed toward the breast. After the long thoracic nerve is identified and isolated, all of the axillary fatty and areolar tissues containing the axillary lymph nodes and vessels are set free and removed (Fig. 45–4). A suction drain is employed, and then the wound is closed (Fig. 45–5).

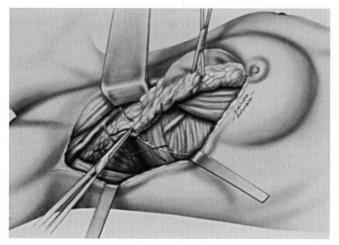

Figure 45–3 *Dissection of axillary nodes, with preservation of the pectoralis major muscle.*

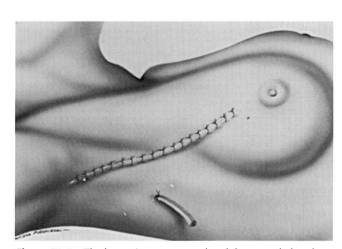

Figure 45–5 *The breast is reconstructed and the wound closed.*

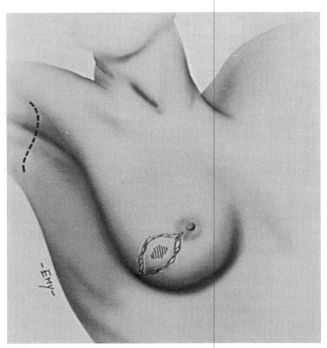

Figure 45–6 *Quadrantectomy and axillary dissection with separate incision.*

Figure 45–6 depicts quadrantectomy and axillary dissection with separate incisions developed for lesions in quadrants other than the upper outer quadrant.

SUMMARY

Quadrantectomy has as its objective the removal of all the cancer tissue in the breast. In principle, therefore, it might not need to be followed by radiotherapy; in Europe clinical trials on this issue are under evaluation.[4, 5] However, experience until now has been limited to the QUART protocol, which involves postquadrantectomy radiotherapy and axillary dissection. With this technique the results are equal, if not superior, to the Halsted mastectomy. The significance of the QUART protocol is its extremely low rate of local recurrence of disease, which approximates 3 to 5 percent in large series of cases.[1] A high rate of local recurrences often necessitates a second operation, which in many cases, is a mastectomy, thus frustrating the objectives of the conservative procedure and creating serious psychological distress for the patient.

References

1. Veronesi U: Rationale and indications for limited surgery in breast cancer: current data. World J Surg 11:493–498, 1987.
2. Veronesi U, Banfi A, Del Vecchio M, et al: Comparison of Halsted mastectomy with quadrantectomy, axillary dissection, and radiotherapy in early breast cancer: Long-term results. Eur J Cancer Clin Oncol 22:1085–1089, 1986.
3. Veronesi U, Costa A, Saccozzi R: Surgical technique of breast quadrantectomy and axillary dissection. *In* Stömbeck JO, Rosato FE (eds): Surgery of the Breast. Diagnosis and Treatment of Breast Disease. Stuttgart, Thieme Verlag, 1986, pp 127–131.
4. Veronesi U, Luini A, Del Vecchio M, Greco M, Galimberti V, Merson M, Rilke F, Sacchini V, Saccozzi R, Savio T, Zucali R, Zurrida S, Salvadori B: Radiotherapy after breast-preserving surgery in women with localized cancer of the breast. N Eng J Med 328:1587–1591, 1993.
5. Veronesi U, Saccozzi R, Del Vecchio M, et al: Comparing radical mastectomy with quadrantectomy, axillary dissection, and radiotherapy in patients with small cancers of the breast. N Engl J Med 305:6–11, 1981.
6. Veronesi U, Salvadori B, Luini A, Greco M, Saccozzi R, Del Vecchio M, Mariani L, Zurrida S and Rilke F: Breast conservation is a safe method in patients with small cancer of the breast. Long-term results of three randomised trials on 1,973 patients. Eur J Cancer 31:1574–1579, 1995.

CHAPTER 46
LUMPECTOMY (SEGMENTAL MASTECTOMY) AND AXILLARY DISSECTION

Bernard Fisher, M.D.

In less than two decades, revolutionary changes in the local and regional management of primary breast cancer have taken place. During that time, radical and extended radical mastectomy have become historic "milestones" against which progress can be measured. Total mastectomy (modified radical mastectomy) and axillary dissection can be considered the "radical" surgery of the present era. It is likely that, in the foreseeable future, these procedures will likewise be relegated to a position of historic significance. Breast-conserving procedures are being employed with ever increasing frequency. How strong is the justification for the changes that have occurred? Why have they come about? Has science played a role? Have these changes resulted because of anecdotal reporting of the experiences of a few who dared to tamper with tradition, or are there nebulous reasons, such as "consumer pressure," that some would suggest are the cause?

For more than a quarter of a century I have reported the results of laboratory and clinical investigations that have had an impact on the primary treatment of breast cancer, and I have repeatedly presented my perception of the reasons for the change in the surgical management of cancer.[12–17, 19, 20, 34, 41] The altered comprehension of cancer biology acquired over the past two decades is primarily responsible for the formulation of a new basis for cancer surgery, and any contribution from "nonscience" (anecdotage) has been entirely fortuitous.

On numerous occasions I have chronicled the pathway of change from Halsted's time to the present and have emphasized laboratory and clinical research conducted by my associates and me that led to the formulation of a hypothesis alternative to Halsted's. I have also repeatedly reported the results of clinical trials carried out to test the new paradigm. Space prohibits more than a brief presentation of the highlights of those efforts, and the reader is referred to the original publications and a complete bibliography for more details. This chapter provides information obtained from the only randomized trial in America carried out to determine the efficacy of breast conservation for the treatment of primary breast cancer. That study (protocol B-06) was begun in 1976 by the National Surgical Adjuvant Breast and Bowel Project (NSABP). This chapter presents findings through 12 years of follow-up and commentary on the major issues that have arisen as a result of the use of breast conservation and that have not been previously addressed in the literature. The original study reports used the term *segmental mastectomy* to identify the

operative procedure employed for breast preservation. The term was intended to indicate that the operation removed only enough breast tissue to ensure that margins of the resected surgical specimen were free of tumor. The term *segmental mastectomy*, however, failed to convey the image of the operation employed and was judged inappropriate since there are no true *segments* of breast, as there are in other anatomical structures (e.g., the lung). Consequently, we have resorted to the use of the term *lumpectomy*, which, although inelegant and equally imprecise, better conveys the intent of the operation. Other terms, such as *tylectomy*, *local excision*, and *tumorectomy*, are also imprecise and fail to indicate whether the primary tumor is completely or partially removed and whether an attempt is made to remove the tumor so that the specimen margins are tumor free.

FROM HALSTED'S RADICAL MASTECTOMY TO LUMPECTOMY: A HISTORICAL OVERVIEW

The Anecdotal Period

There must be a solid rationale for the surgical management of cancer. In tracing the evolution of cancer surgery, it is important to know how those who formulated and influenced treatment at a particular time in history conceived of the disease, for it was their conception of the disease process that provided the rationale for the therapy they employed.

The first true paradigm for cancer management was formulated in the late nineteenth century by William S. Halsted. To understand the rationale for the type of surgery he advocated, it is important to appreciate Halsted's concept of the biology of cancer, particularly the phenomenon of metastases. Halsted formulated a hypothesis based on a diverse group of findings that had been obtained by others around 1880. This hypothesis ultimately had its expression in the radical mastectomy. Of particular importance were the findings of Goldman and Schmidt that cancer cells in blood excited thrombosis and that the thrombosis destroyed or rendered cancer cells harmless.[50] The report by Handley that tumor cells spread along lymphatic pathways by direct extension rather than by embolization had a seminal effect on Halsted's thinking.[48] The investigations of Virchow indicating that regional lymph nodes were effective filters also influenced the evolution of Halstedian concepts.[83] Another precept in harmony with Halsted's hypothesis was that a growing tumor remains localized at its site of origin for a period of time, but that at some instant during its growth, tumor cell invasion of lymphatics and dissemination to regional nodes takes place. After another interval, during which the tumor is local or regional only, systemic dissemination occurs as the tumor increases in size.

As a consequence of these precepts and the understanding of the mechanism of cancer metastases at the time, there arose an "anatomical" basis for cancer surgery. The "proper" cancer operation consisted of removal of the primary tumor together with regional lymphatics and lymph nodes by en bloc dissection. Because there was deemed to be a certain orderliness about tumor spread and because clinically recognizable cancer was considered in many instances to be a local/regional disease, it was thought that tumors would be more curable if surgeons would only be more expansive in their interpretation of what constituted the *region* and, above all, if they utilized better technique so that they could eradicate every cancer cell. Local or regional recurrences were more often than not considered to be the result of inadequate application of surgical skill rather than a manifestation of systemic disease. There was hope that one more lymph node dissection would cure more cancers. Radical cancer surgery based on those anatomical considerations persisted for 75 years—and still endures to varying degrees. The Halstedian paradigm remained intact because few substantive challenges to it arose from the results of laboratory and clinical investigations. Findings from studies that were carried out could not be unified to produce a competing hypothesis.

The efficacy of performing the radical mastectomy to fulfill the tenets of the Halstedian hypothesis began to be seriously challenged during the 1950s and 1960s. The challenge was not to the principles on which the hypothesis was based but to whether the radical mastectomy adequately embodied those principles. If the removal of the entire lymphatic drainage area was of paramount importance, the radical operation for breast cancer was inadequate, since lymph nodes other than those in the axilla were frequently involved with tumor. A flurry of anecdotal reports by such leaders in surgery as Wangensteen, Margottini, Urban, Dahl-Iversen, Lacour, Veronesi, Caceres, and Sugarbaker appeared that recorded their personal experiences with *extended* radical mastectomy.[2, 4, 59, 64, 77, 78, 82, 85] In 1970, after an extensive evaluation of these reports, I concluded that the information presented by those investigators had not demonstrated that the extended radical procedure was more efficacious than the conventional radical mastectomy.[12] Despite the large number of patients in many of the studies, the evaluations were inadequate to test the worth of the extended radical operation. Nothing came from those reports that could provide a basis for challenging Halstedian principles, and nothing arose from them that added to comprehension of the disease.

At the same time that more extensive operations were being carried out, other investigators were reporting their experience with operations less extensive than the radical mastectomy. The deviation from radical mastectomy was not a result of the Halstedian hypothesis being displaced by new facts or concepts, but of a dissatisfaction with the results of the operation. The considerations of McWhirter, who in 1948 reported his results with simple mastectomy combined with postoperative radiotherapy, best exemplify that attitude.[65] McWhirter adopted his "new" therapeutic regimen because of his concern that radical operations were not radical enough because they failed to get rid of all tumor tissue in the operative area, and "at the time of operation tissues actually invaded by tumor must often be divided." It was McWhirter's opinion that, as a result of this trauma, malignant cells would have an increased tendency to disseminate to other sites. Although he appreciated the possibility that such cells could still be liberated from the area of operation when a simple mastectomy was performed, McWhirter was of the opinion that these cells would be trapped by the intact barrier of the axilla. Moreover, since wound healing was likely to take place more rapidly after simple rather than radical mastectomy, radiotherapy could be applied sooner, thus reducing the interval during which cells could be disseminated to distant sites. McWhirter's views were in keeping with the mechanistic approach to both tumor dissemination and eradication; they did not challenge the prevailing paradigm. As with extended radical mastectomy, aside from a demonstration of personal conviction, the data on operations less extensive than radical mastectomy were not definitive. The data failed to demonstrate unequivocally whether simple mastectomy should supplant the radical operation. While clinicians were debating the relative merits of radical, extended radical, and simple mastectomy, a few were reporting their experiences with modified radical mastectomy or local excision and radiation. The most ardent of the few supporters of the modified radical mastectomy (Patey's operation) was Handley.[49] Handley's rationale for that operation was based on his conviction that the radical mastectomy was inadequate because it left behind internal mammary nodes. It was his view that the use of radiation following modified radical mastectomy would be more beneficial, since the internal mammary nodes would be treated by employing this procedure.

The results of local excision of breast tumors followed by breast radiation were reported by Mustakallio in 1954 and by Porritt, Peters and Crile in the 1960s.[11, 67, 68, 73] While these studies failed clearly to determine the relative merits of that regimen, they did demonstrate that patients could survive free of disease for many years after such treatment. The more recent reports by Calle, Hellman, Prosnitz, Montague and their associates, and Pierquin continue to attest to that fact.[5, 55, 66, 72, 74] It is difficult to determine the rationale employed by the early advocates of breast conservation. What seems most certain is that no clear biological principle directed their approach. In many instances, as noted by Mustakallio, the procedure was initially performed because patients refused radical mastectomy.

Despite the fact that clinical efforts from 1950 to 1970 failed to determine with certainty the relative merits of the various methods for local or regional treatment of breast cancer, failed to evolve new biological principles, and failed to test the Halstedian hypothesis (allowing it to remain the paradigm for breast cancer management), operations of lesser extent were becoming accepted in clinical practice and in some places were considered standard. Thus, as previously mentioned, the retreat from radical mastectomy was more the result of frustration with its failure to support the tenets of the hypothesis than because new principles were attracting attention.

Laboratory and Clinical Research in the 1960s

During the time that anecdotal clinical information was accumulating, a series of laboratory and clinical investigations directed toward obtaining a better comprehension of the biology of metastases was being conducted by us and by other investigators. These studies (1958 to 1970) influenced our thinking about metastatic mechanisms and revealed that the blood and lymphatic vascular systems are so interrelated that it is impractical to consider them as independent routes of tumor cell dissemination.[32] The studies also revealed that the residence of a vast majority of tumor cells gaining access to an organ via the blood stream was transient.[30] As a consequence, we concluded that patterns of tumor spread are not dictated solely by anatomical considerations but are also influenced by intrinsic factors in tumor cells and in the organs to which they gain access. The thesis was accepted that there is no orderly pattern of tumor cell dissemination that could be based on mechanical and temporal factors.

Results from other experiments indicated that regional lymph nodes are not, as Virchow proposed, effective barriers to tumor spread.[8] Tumor cells traverse lymph nodes and gain access to the blood vascular system by lymphatic-venous communications in nodes. Additional studies indicated the biological importance of regional nodes, which were found to have a role in both initiation and maintenance of tumor immunity.[31] It was demonstrated that regional node cells are capable of destroying tumor cells; therefore, the presence of negative nodes may be a result of such a circumstance (because tumor cells traverse nodes) rather than the result of removal of a tumor prior to its dissemination.[38] Our findings indicated that biological rather than anatomical factors may be the reason that certain nodes contain metastases and others do not. Thus, we concluded that consideration of regional nodes as mechanical receptors for tumor cells and way stations for tumor dissemination is an anachronism. The findings also indicated that host factors are important in the de-

velopment of metastases and that a tumor is not autonomous of its host, as was believed in Halsted's time. The existence of dormant tumor cells was demonstrated for the first time, and it was shown that perturbation of a host by a variety of means could produce lethal metastases from those cells.[29] Our findings led us to consider that local reoccurrences following operation were apt to be the result of systemically disseminated cells lodging and growing at a site of trauma rather than because of inadequate surgical technique.[33] We proposed that a tumor is a systemic disease, probably from its inception. That premise does not imply that all patients will at some time develop overt metastases, nor that only patients with metastases have disseminated disease. We theorized in the 1960s that the regional node is an indicator of host-tumor relations. The lymph node that contains tumor cells reflects an interrelation between host and tumor that permits the development of metastases; it does not mean that the lymph node is an instigator of distant disease.

Concurrent with the laboratory studies, a series of clinical trials carried out by us provided new information that raised questions regarding concepts on which treatment was based. Tumor recurrence and survival of breast cancer patients were found to be independent of the number of axillary nodes removed and examined,[39] and tumor location failed to influence prognosis.[40]

Regardless of whether the results of all of the laboratory studies and clinical observations were interpreted correctly, whether they resulted from the methods and models employed rather than from biological circumstances, whether they could or could not be confirmed in every setting and in every detail, or whether they were obtained from simplistic experiments that did not really provide positive proof for any of our assumptions, they had in common the fact that they did not conform to the concepts that provided the principles for the Halstedian hypothesis. They provided a matrix within which an alternative thesis could be formulated. That hypothesis, synthesized by us in 1968, is biological rather than anatomical and mechanistic. Its components are completely antithetical to those in Halsted's hypothesis (Table 46–1).

Clinical Trials Testing the Alternative Hypothesis and Providing Justification for Evaluating Lumpectomy

During the time that laboratory investigations were reshaping thinking about the biology of metastases and anecdotal reporting was flourishing, one of the great advances of our time was taking place. The prospective, randomized, controlled trial was being introduced into clinical medicine as a means of testing hypotheses, obtaining natural history information, and evaluating the worth of a particular therapy. The use of that very sophisticated method instead of anecdotal reports represented a major step

TABLE 46–1. TWO DIVERGENT HYPOTHESES OF TUMOR BIOLOGY

Halstedian	Alternative
Tumors spread in an orderly defined manner based on mechanical considerations.	There is no orderly pattern of tumor cell dissemination.
Tumor cells traverse lymphatics to lymph nodes by direct extension, supporting en bloc dissection.	Tumor cells traverse lymphatics by embolization, challenging the merit of en bloc dissection.
The positive lymph node is an indicator of tumor spread and is the instigator of disease.	The positive lymph node is an indicator of a host-tumor relationship that permits development of metastases rather than the instigator of distant disease.
Regional lymph nodes are barriers to the passage of tumor cells.	Regional lymph nodes are ineffective as barriers to tumor cell spread.
Nodes are of anatomical importance.	Nodes are of biological importance.
The blood stream is of little significance as a route of tumor dissemination.	The blood stream is of considerable importance in tumor dissemination.
A tumor is autonomous of its host.	Complex host-tumor interrelationships affect every facet of the disease.
Operable breast cancer is a local/regional disease.	Operable breast cancer is a systemic disease.
The extent and nuances of operation are the dominant factors influencing patient outcome.	Variations in local-regional therapy are unlikely to substantially affect survival.
No consideration is given to tumor multicentricity.	Multicentric foci of tumor are not necessarily a precursor of clinically overt cancer.

toward transforming medicine from an art to a science.

In August 1971, a clinical trial (NSABP B-04) was begun, not only to test the validity of the principles on which our alternative hypothesis was based but also to simultaneously evaluate, in an unbiased fashion, different regimens of surgical management for primary breast cancer. The results of that trial, obtained from information on more than 1500 women,

indicate that, in patients with no clinical evidence of axillary node involvement (40 percent of whom had histologically positive nodes), three distinctly different treatment regimens—radical mastectomy, total (simple) mastectomy with local/regional irradiation, or total mastectomy and removal of nodes that later became clinically positive—yielded no significant difference in overall treatment failure, distant metastases (Fig. 46–1), or survival through more than 18

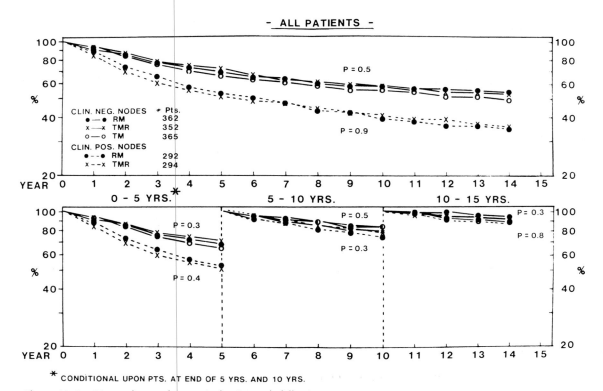

Figure 46–1 *Distant disease–free survival at intervals following mastectomy.*

years of follow-up.[37] (An update in progress indicates that the findings remain similar through 20 years of follow-up.) When patients free of disease at the end of 5 years were evaluated at between 5 and 10 years, not only was there no difference among the treatment groups, but the node-positive patients had results similar to patients with negative nodes. The same findings were observed between 10 and 18 years. Thus the 5-year results were indicative of future findings. In patients with clinical evidence of node involvement, there was no significant difference between the group treated by radical mastectomy and the group treated by total mastectomy and local/regional irradiation. The findings also indicated that radiation of internal mammary nodes in patients with inner quadrant lesions did not improve survival and that results obtained at 5 years accurately predicted the outcome through 10 years.

It was concluded that variations in local/regional treatment used in the study were not important in determining survival of breast cancer patients. The multiple findings from this study support and confirm the validity of the various components of the alternative hypothesis.

During the 1970s, other trials were unwittingly testing the alternative hypothesis. A major trial in the United Kingdom employed women with clinical stage I or stage II carcinoma of the breast.[7] A simple mastectomy was performed in all patients without surgical attention to the axillary nodes. Patients received either a course of regional radiotherapy or no further primary treatment (the "watch policy" group). Ten years later, no differences were found between the two groups, findings that supported the alternative hypothesis.

When early findings from the NSABP B-04 study indicated that patients treated by total mastectomy without axillary node dissection and pectoral muscle removal were at no higher risk for distant disease or death than those treated with Halsted radical mastectomy, we considered it clinically and scientifically justifiable to begin a new study (B-06) to evaluate breast conservation by local tumor excision, with or without radiation therapy. The rest of this chapter provides an overview of findings obtained from the NSABP study, which was the first and largest randomized trial in America to evaluate the worth of lumpectomy with and without breast irradiation.

DESIGN OF THE NSABP LUMPECTOMY TRIAL

In April 1973, a meeting was convened in Bethesda, Maryland, to plan and design the NSABP B-06 study. To ensure credibility of the findings from the NSABP lumpectomy trial, a sophisticated experimental design was needed (Fig. 46–2). Beginning in 1976, patients were randomly assigned to one of three treatment groups: total mastectomy, lumpectomy, or lumpectomy followed by breast irradiation. Women in all the treatment groups had axillary dissection,

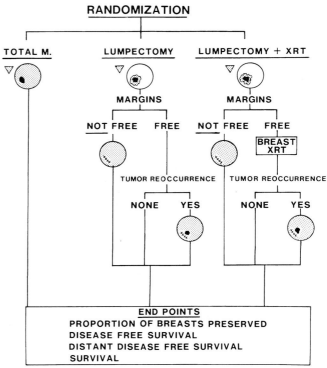

Figure 46–2 *Treatment strategy NSABP B-06.*

and those with positive nodes received chemotherapy. The lumpectomy operation completely abandoned conventional concepts of cancer surgery by removing only enough breast tissue to ensure that the margins of the resected surgical specimens were free of tumor. All resected lumpectomy specimens were examined pathologically to ensure that the margins were tumor free. The study was designed to determine (1) the effectiveness of lumpectomy for breast preservation, (2) whether radiation therapy reduces the incidence of tumor in the ipsilateral breast after lumpectomy, (3) whether breast conservation results in a higher risk of distant disease and death than does mastectomy, and (4) the clinical significance of multicentricity.

The protocol required that a subsequent mastectomy be performed if the margins of specimens removed by lumpectomy were not tumor free. It also mandated that a total mastectomy be carried out should tumor occur in the same breast subsequent to lumpectomy. Such a tumor occurring following a previous lumpectomy was designated a tumor "reoccurrence," not a "treatment failure" unless the tumor was so extensive that it could not be completely removed by mastectomy. However, because the breast was removed, the patient was regarded as having had a "cosmetic failure." It must also be emphasized that when determining disease-free survival (DFS), distant disease–free survival (DDFS), and survival (S) in the three treatment groups, it was necessary that all patients in each group be included, even those in the two lumpectomy groups who had margins involved and consequently had a mastectomy. Margin involvement was found to be associated with poorer patient prognosis than were tumors with free margins. Consequently, elimination of those patients from the lumpectomy groups would have created a bias, because patients with a similarly poor prognosis existed in the total mastectomy group. Elimination would have resulted in the appearance of a much more favorable outcome among lumpectomy patients.

Recurrences of tumor in the chest wall and operative scar, but not in the ipsilateral breast, were classified as local treatment failures. Tumors in the internal mammary, supraclavicular, or ipsilateral axillary nodes were classified as regional treatment failures. Tumors in all other locations were considered distant treatment failures. Patients classified as having any distant disease included those with a distant metastasis as a first treatment failure, a distant metastasis after a local or regional reoccurrence, or a second cancer (including tumor in the other breast). *Overall survival* refers to survival with or without recurrent disease.

OPERATIVE TECHNIQUE FOR LUMPECTOMY

When the NSABP study to evaluate the worth of local tumor excision was implemented in 1976, American surgeons had little familiarity with breast-conserving procedures. Through a series of workshops and other educational mechanisms, those NSABP surgeons participating in the trial were informed of the methods mandated by the protocol. With only minor variations, those procedures have been used in thousands of lumpectomies in patients entered into the initial and subsequent NSABP trials evaluating local/regional and systemic therapy for breast cancer. The following descriptions highlight the operative procedures employed; these are described in detail elsewhere.[43, 63]

Incisions and Skin Removal

Curvilinear incisions are employed by us, no matter where in the breast a lesion occurs (Fig. 46–3). Such incisions should be used even when tumors are in the upper outer quadrant of the breast, near the axilla. A separate incision for the axillary dissection is almost always made when a tumor is in that portion of the breast. To achieve the best cosmetic results, radial incisions are *not* recommended (Fig. 46–4). Some NSABP surgeons, however, prefer radial incisions for lesions at the "6 o'clock" position in the breast. Our own preference is for curvilinear incisions even for tumors in that site. To perform a satisfactory lumpectomy, it is essential that the incision be placed directly over the tumor (Fig. 46–5 [A]). A circumareolar incision is inappropriate for removal of a lesion that is not in proximity to the areola.

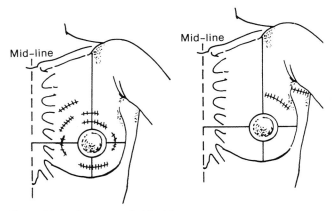

Figure 46–3 *Recommended incisions.*

Tunneling through breast tissue to remove a lesion that is not beneath the incision is to be condemned. Tumor-free specimen margins are difficult—and often impossible—to obtain when such an incision is made. Re-excision of the tumor site to obtain free margins is equally difficult. It should be determined before operation whether or not a patient is a candidate for lumpectomy. The decision about the location of the lumpectomy incision should be made independently of any consideration given to skin removal should a conventional mastectomy subsequently be performed. In those rare instances when it is found at operation that a planned lumpectomy cannot be carried out because of the inability to obtain tumor-free margins, the mastectomy incisions are tailored to accommodate the lumpectomy incision.

Because lumpectomy is not a Halstedian operation and patients with tumor involving the overlying skin are not apt to be candidates for the operation, skin removal is not a requisite of the operation. A small ellipse of skin may be removed with the underlying lesion to orient the pathologist to the anterior or superficial border of the specimen, but its removal does not enhance the effectiveness of the operation. We do not ordinarily remove any skin, because in our experience, the quality of cosmesis is inversely related to the amount of skin removed. If prior biopsy

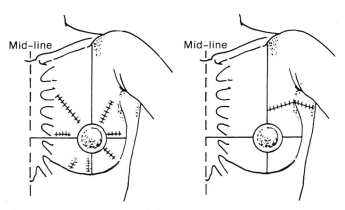

Figure 46–4 *Nonrecommended incisions.*

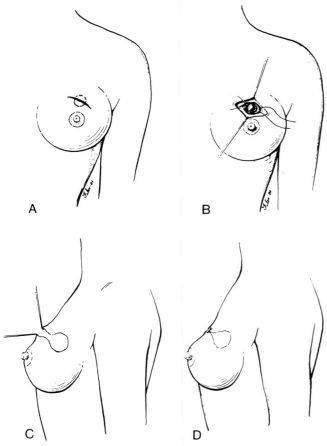

Figure 46–5   *Technique of lumpectomy.*

has been performed, skin encompassing the biopsy site is removed at lumpectomy.

Tumor Removal and Examination of Specimen Margins

The tumor is removed so that it is completely enveloped in normal fat or breast tissue. This does not necessitate removal of a predefined amount of normal tissue around the lesion. The aim is to remove an amount adequate to achieve specimen margins grossly free of tumor (Fig. 46–5B). A special point to be emphasized is that, when the excision is being carried out, skin edges are not undermined (i.e., thin skin flaps are not desirable) (Fig. 46–5C). Undermining of skin, like skin removal, results in an unfavorable cosmetic result. No special effort is made to include pectoral fascia in the specimen unless the lesion lies close to it.

Our practice is to tag the specimen before it leaves the operating field (see Fig. 46–5B). Any system for doing this may be employed. A long silk suture is used to mark the lateral surface, a short suture to identify the medial aspect of the specimen, and two short tags close together to identify the "top" of the specimen (i.e., the anterior or superficial margin). Additional tags may be placed to designate the supe-

rior, or cephalic, margin and the inferior, or caudal, border. The specimen is immediately delivered to the pathologist, or, ideally, he or she is present in the operating room to receive it. The pathologist's role is to confirm or establish the diagnosis of cancer, help the surgeon decide intraoperatively whether the specimen margins are *grossly* free of tumor, and to take an aliquot of tumor for estrogen and progesterone receptor analyses. Our procedure is to delay closure of the operative incision until the pathologist reports on the status of the specimen margins.

When the pathologist receives the specimen, he or she carefully orients it by means of the suture tags that the surgeon has placed (Fig. 46–6). After measurement, the uncut specimen is inspected for gross margin involvement. If there is evidence that the tumor has been transected, the surgeon is immediately apprised of the precise location of the margin involvement so that additional tissue can be removed from that area while the pathologist is completing inspection of the specimen. The pathologist then coats the entire surface of the specimen with India ink (Fig. 46–7A), blots it dry, and then bisects the tumor and specimen transversely. The anteroposterior and mediolateral diameters of the tumor are then measured, and the specimen is further examined to determine if the tumor is grossly "close" to any margin of the specimen. If there is concern about any border, the pathologist may do a frozen section to determine margin involvement. Our preference is to remove additional breast tissue in the area to obtain a new true margin any time that it is considered advisable that frozen section be done to check margin involvement. Rarely will there be a subsequent report of microscopic tumor at margins that have been reported to be grossly free. A multiplicity of frozen sections are *not* carried out to determine if the margins are free of tumor. Rarely is a frozen section done for that purpose. If tumor is found on gross examination to be "close" to a portion of the resected tissue margin, the resection in that area is extended by removing an additional rim of breast tissue and fat. The new true margin of the area that was considered to be "close" is identified for the pathologist

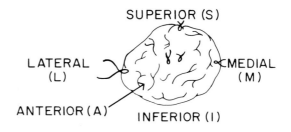

Figure 46–6   *Orientation of the lumpectomy specimen.*

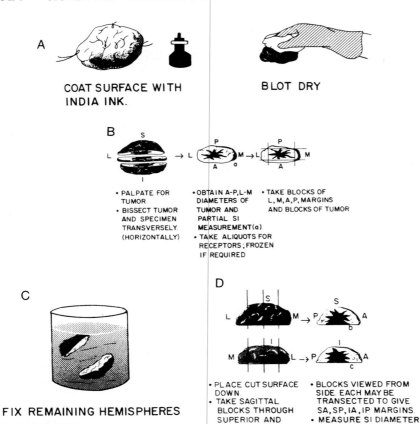

A, Application of India ink. **B,** Taking of blocks.

- PALPATE FOR TUMOR.
- BISSECT TUMOR AND SPECIMEN TRANSVERSELY. (HORIZONTALLY)

- OBTAIN A-P, L-M DIAMETERS OF TUMOR AND PARTIAL SI MEASUREMENT(a).
- TAKE ALIQUOTS FOR RECEPTORS; FROZEN IF REQUIRED

- TAKE BLOCKS OF L, M, A, P, MARGINS AND BLOCKS OF TUMOR.

FIX REMAINING HEMISPHERES 1-2 HOURS.

- PLACE CUT SURFACE DOWN.
- TAKE SAGITTAL BLOCKS THROUGH SUPERIOR AND INFERIOR PORTIONS.

- BLOCKS VIEWED FROM SIDE. EACH MAY BE TRANSECTED TO GIVE SA, SP, IA, IP MARGINS.
- MEASURE SI DIAMETER OF TUMOR: a+b+c

Figure 46–7 *Preparation of specimen for determination of margin involvement.* **A,** *Application of India ink.* **B,** *Taking of blocks.* **C,** *Fixing tissue for additional blocks.* **D,** *Taking further blocks.*

by placing methylene blue on the surface of the re-resected portion of tissue that is farthest from the initial resection site.

Aliquots of tumor are taken for receptor studies and for the preparation of blocks from which permanent sections are made (Fig. 46–7*B*). While the technique for examining the specimen for margin involvement may vary among pathologists, the following approach established by the NSABP project pathologist[45] is provided as a guideline that may be varied with circumstances. Blocks of the lateral, medial, anterior, and posterior margins are prepared from the original transverse block. The remaining hemispheres are fixed for 1 to 2 hours to facilitate subsequent blocking (Fig. 46–7*C*). These remnants are then blocked sagittally, with the cut surfaces placed down (Fig. 46–7*D*). This procedure provides for measurement of the superior-inferior diameter of the tumor and for the preparation of blocks that provide sections for additional examination of margins. At least 12 to 20 blocks are made from each specimen, depending on its size. Although there have been, and will continue to be, variations of this scheme by hospital pathologists, at least five lines of resection were available for review in patients having lumpectomy in the NSABP study.

Pathological assessment of lines of resection in a lumpectomy specimen is, admittedly, difficult because of the large surface area. This assessment is confounded by vague pathological criteria utilized for making a decision about whether tumor involves specimen margins. Many pathologists have the tendency to infer margin involvement by such subjective designations as tumor *too* or *very* close to it. When hospital pathologists resorted to these subjective criteria, there was residual cancer in only 12 percent of total mastectomy specimens removed because of presumed margin involvement. Thus, it is most appropriate to regard lines of resection as being involved only when cancer is transected.

Closure of the Lumpectomy Wound

After a decision has been made on the status of the specimen margins and meticulous hemostasis of the lumpectomy site has been achieved, the wound is closed (see Fig. 46–5*D*). Because lumpectomy is a cosmetic procedure, meticulous attention must be given to this part of the operation. Attempts at breast reconstruction by approximating breast tissue and deep fat can produce an unsatisfactory appearance, particularly following removal of tumors in the upper half of the breast. For optimal cosmesis, our approach is to make no attempt to obliterate the "dead space" in the breast by approximating breast tissue or fat, and no drain of any type is ever placed in the wound (Fig. 46–5*C*). In recent years we have found it desirable to use interrupted Dexon (5-0) sutures to approximate the subcutaneous fat. The skin is then carefully approximated with a continuous subcuticular suture of the same material (Fig. 46–5D).

Subareolar Tumors or Tumors Larger Than 4 cm

The aim of the NSABP lumpectomy protocol was to carry out the operation so that all patients would be left with a normal-appearing breast. Because subareolar tumors or those close to that position might require removal of the nipple and areola to ensure tumor-free specimen margins, with a resultant cosmetic defect, lesions in such a site were not considered to be amenable to lumpectomy. Patients with subareolar or periareolar lesions were considered candidates for lumpectomy when tumor-free margins could be obtained without removal of the nipple and areola and when a satisfactory cosmetic result could be achieved. This was particularly the case in women with large breasts and posteriorly located tumors. With increased experience, it was concluded that removal of subareolar lesions with the nipple and areola can be carried out with a satisfactory cosmetic result. The resulting breast mound is more normal than that achieved by breast reconstruction after total mastectomy.

After publication of the results of our trial, the erroneous impression was created that lumpectomy was appropriate for only those patients with very small tumors. This misconception occurred despite the fact that it had clearly been stated that women with tumors as large as 4 cm were eligible. That tumor size was originally selected because we had demonstrated that the incidence of multicentricity was apt to be greater in tumors larger than 4 cm. We later liberalized the tumor size requirement so that patients with tumors as large as 5 cm are eligible for our current protocols, providing they have a breast of ample size that would permit obtaining a favorable cosmetic result. Thus, patients with clinical stage I and II tumors are eligible for lumpectomy regardless of tumor location. It is our opinion that, when technically feasible, women with larger tumors and/or clinically positive nodes are better served by lumpectomy because they are at great risk for the development of distant metastases and death, regardless of what operation is performed.

AXILLARY DISSECTION

We do not recommend axillary sampling as a substitute for axillary dissection. The purpose of axillary dissection is to use the information about lymph node involvement with tumor (1) for determining patient prognosis, (2) for determining whether and what type of adjuvant chemotherapy should be employed, and (3) for local/regional disease control. Axillary dissection is not employed with the intent of enhancing curability, since it is our contention that regional lymph nodes serve as indicators rather than instigators of distant metastatic disease. Although we have

demonstrated that the qualitative status of axillary lymph node involvement (i.e., either positive or negative) may be accurately determined by examining relatively few nodes, a more complete dissection is required to accurately determine the number of nodes involved.[42] Because patient prognosis is significantly related to the number of positive nodes (i.e., 1–3, 4–9, ≥10), a sufficient number must be obtained to quantitate the prognosis more accurately.[27]

The incision used for axillary dissections is separate from that used for removal of the tumor in the breast. We prefer a curvilinear transverse incision just below the axillary hairline. Some surgeons favor a longitudinal incision placed along the posterolateral margin of the pectoralis major muscle; either incision is appropriate. In all NSABP breast protocols, axillary dissection includes all nodes from at least axillary levels I and II. The anatomical delineation of this dissection are the latissimus dorsi muscle laterally, the axillary vein superiorly, and the medial border of the pectoralis minor muscle medially. Removal of the pectoralis minor muscle is not required. The nerves to the serratus anterior and latissimus dorsi muscles should be identified and preserved. The axillary vein should be visualized and followed under the pectoralis minor muscle to the medial border. These are the minimal limits for the dissection. The average number of nodes removed compares favorably with the number obtained after a radical mastectomy or a modified radical mastectomy in previous NSABP trials. In all NSABP studies since 1971, the number of axillary nodes removed (a mean of 15) has remained remarkably constant. Although the surgical site in the breast is not drained, a suction drain is left in the axilla for several postoperative days.

When a lumpectomy is carried out for lesions in the upper outer quadrant of the breast, even when separate incisions are used for removal of the tumor and for the axillary dissection, the two cavities (i.e., those in the breast and in the axilla) may sometimes become confluent. In such a situation, we omit using any drain in the axilla or the breast. An axillary drain in such a circumstance prevents accumulation of serum at the lumpectomy site that would result in an unfavorable cosmesis. The omission of such a drain has produced no undesirable effect, and seroma of the axilla has not been observed.

A question asked with increasing frequency is whether all patients who have a lumpectomy require axillary dissection. The question arises most often with small tumors, i.e., those no larger than 1 cm, particularly patients whose lesions were detected by mammography and who have clinically negative axillary nodes. We demonstrated in a prior NSABP study (B-04) that patients who were treated by simple mastectomy and an axillary dissection when nodes became clinically positive had an outcome similar to that of patients who were treated by total mastectomy and an initial axillary dissection. Those findings indicate that such a dissection does not enhance curability. Moreover, if all node-negative and -positive patients are given the same systemic adjuvant therapy, there is no need to know the nodal status except for predicting prognosis. That is not yet entirely the case. Consequently, I currently recommend that all patients receiving lumpectomy have an axillary dissection. NSABP studies currently being carried out may provide reasons to alter that view.

RADIATION THERAPY AFTER LUMPECTOMY

In 1924, an English surgeon, Geoffrey Keynes, of St. Bartholomeus Hospital, London, began to treat breast carcinoma by implanting radium needles, often achieving good local control of cancer.[58] For the next half century, although a few surgeons such as Mustakallio of Finland; Porritt in England; and Adair, Crile, and Cope in the United States were attracting attention with their writings, much of the impetus for breast conservation in the management of mammary cancer came from radiation therapists. The French were particularly influential.[1, 3, 6, 10, 71, 84] Reports by Peters, Prosnitz, Montague, and Hellman and their respective colleagues are representative of the activities of American radiation therapists who were early advocates of breast preservation.* Some of these investigators promulgated the thesis of "primary treatment of breast cancer by radiation," a misleading description of therapy, because the radiation was administered after tumor excision. Essentially, it was only Baclesse, from the Institute Curie of Paris, who in 1965 reported his experience with the treatment of breast cancer exclusively by radiation.[3]

Reports in the 1960s were anecdotal and related to findings from heterogeneous groups of cases varying in stage of disease, operation employed, techniques of radiation, and other patient and tumor characteristics. While failing to provide definitive information on the worth of breast irradiation, these reports, together with evolving biological information, provided justification for evaluating breast irradiation in conjunction with breast conservation surgery by means of a proper clinical trial such as that conducted by the NSABP.

Radiation used by the NSABP in protocol B-06 was aimed at eliminating occult tumor foci remaining in the ipsilateral breast. The dose level used in the NSABP trial was a level that was considered to be tumoricidal and not likely to produce distortion and fibrosis of the breast or other undesirable sequelae. The dose used to meet those requirements was efficacious, as indicated by the findings from the study. The marked reduction in breast tumor recurrence following radiation, the failure to observe undesirable cosmetic sequelae, and the absence of complications such as rib fractures and pneumonitis that have been reported by others attest to the propriety of the

techniques and the amount of radiation administered.

The intent of the radiation therapy was to treat the skin, breast tissue, muscle, lymphatics, and entire scar of the breast. No attempt was made to include axillary, supraclavicular, interpectoral, or internal mammary lymph nodes. Because the internal mammary nodes, however, lie at the medial edge of the treatment field, they were sometimes either partially or wholly included. No special attempt was made to exclude them, because that would have interfered with irradiation of the entire breast. Our findings over the years indicate no advantage for axillary radiation when axillary dissection has been carried out, and radiation of the internal mammary nodes has resulted in no survival benefit in any of the NSABP trials.

When lumpectomy and axillary dissection were performed through separate incisions and the scar from the axillary dissection was extrinsic to the breast, no radiation was directed to that scar. If the axillary dissection scar was in continuity with that of the lumpectomy, no special attempt was made to irradiate the portion of the scar that was beyond the breast tissue.

Radiation therapy was initiated no later than 6 weeks after lumpectomy in patients with negative nodes and no later than 8 weeks after surgery in those with positive nodes. In patients with positive nodes, radiation therapy was delayed to permit completion of the first course of adjuvant chemotherapy. A minimum dose of 5000 rad was administered. This dose was calculated at a depth of two thirds the distance between the skin overlying the breast and the base of the tangential fields at mid-separation. This depth generally ranged from 3 to 7 cm. The maximum dose to the point of calculation did not exceed 5300 rad. The dose was given at a rate of 1000 rad per week (200 rad per day, 5 days per week), calculated at the minimum dose point. Both tangential fields were treated daily, with 100 rad and given to each. Dry desquamation with pigmentation or erythema at the end of treatment were considered desirable; limited patches of moist desquamation were acceptable. Extensive areas of moist desquamation were avoided.

Because proper administration of radiation is as important as surgical technique for obtaining a good cosmetic result and for preventing ipsilateral tumor recurrence, it is appropriate to present a detailed account of the method of irradiation employed for all lumpectomy patients entered into NSABP studies.

Patients lie supine, with the head straight (no pillows are used unless dorsal convexity is extreme), and the upper arm abducted 90°, with the forearm supported in an upright position by a vertical armboard. The breast (and the chest wall) are treated through opposing tangential fields to avoid direct irradiation of the lung.

The field boundaries employed are as follows: The medial border lies along the midsternal line and the lateral border along the midaxillary line. If the scar

---

*See references 51, 53, 54, 61, 66, 68–70, 74, and 86.

extends beyond this line, the lateral border may, within limits, be moved posteriorly to include the entire scar. The extent to which this line may be moved posteriorly should be guided by the amount of lung tissue that would be irradiated if this border is parallel-opposed to the medial border. If the irradiated slice of lung tissue exceeds a width of 5 cm, the lateral portal should be left along the midaxillary line and the end of the surgical scar treated by superficial irradiation. The inferior border of the tangential field is drawn horizontally across the hemithorax at a level about 2 cm below the inframammary fold. This line can be drawn by extension from the contralateral fold if the ipsilateral breast is distorted. The superior border is located along a horizontal line that bisects the sternomanubrial junction (angle of Louis). If necessary, this border may be moved superiorly to ensure that both the entire breast and the tail of the breast are included. If the scar extends above this boundary, the line should be moved superiorly to include the entire scar. The central axes of the medial and lateral fields lie on the same line. The angle of treatment ($\pm 180°$) can be determined with a rolling ball or an inclinometer bridge or by rotating the head of the machine until the back pointer and the front pointer lie on the lateral and medial field boundaries, respectively.

Cobalt 60 or a linear accelerator x-ray machine is employed. Superficial irradiation may be used only to treat or boost portions of the surgical scar as described. The use of a beam-blocking device ("breast gadget") greatly facilitates treatment of the breast. Because the lower half of the beam is blocked near its central axis, the tangential fields do not diverge into the lung.

The extent to which bolus should be used depends greatly on the details of the treatment situation at each institution. Bolus is added to reach the desired skin reaction (i.e., dry desquamation and erythema). Any accessories that enhance secondary electron scatter increase the dose to the skin and, thus, limit the need for buildup. Plastic blocking trays or shields may enhance the skin dose to the extent that the use of additional bolus is neither necessary nor desirable. In general, bolus may safely be used two to four times with each tangential field when no intervening tray is used.

The value of radiation therapy following lumpectomy has been demonstrated by our findings. Most important is the fact that those results were achieved with radiation therapy that did not include the use of radiation boosts or external beam or interstitial implants; radiation of regional nodes was not employed. Our incidence of breast tumor recurrence approximated that observed by proponents of such additive therapy, so it would seem that there is no need for a radiation boost to the excision site when proper attention is paid to specimen margins. A clinical trial to evaluate the effectiveness of radiation with and without boosts or to evaluate external-beam boosts versus boosts by interstitial implant would be nearly impossible to undertake because of the size of the patient population that would be required. Moreover, giving such a trial a high priority designation would be inappropriate. We are currently evaluating our data with respect to patient and tumor characteristics associated with tumor recurrence following radiation, in an attempt to identify which patients might benefit from a boost. Despite our findings indicating no need for a boost, if there are circumstances in which the radiation therapist feels more benefit would accrue from using a boost, an external-beam boost is more appropriate than interstitial implants because of the need for additional hospitalization, higher morbidity, imprecise radiation dose delivered, and the lack of data demonstrating the superiority of interstitial implants.

It is frequently asked whether all patients who have a lumpectomy need to have breast irradiation. For example, do women with tumors 1 cm or smaller and negative axillary nodes require such therapy? Data from the NSABP trial continue to indicate that, even in such patients, radiation reduces the incidence of ipsilateral breast tumor recurrence. Whether radiation is required for patients whose microinvasive tumors are treated by lumpectomy is unclear, particularly if these patients receive systemic therapy such as tamoxifen. There are no data to clarify this issue. The NSABP implemented a randomized trial (B-21) in 1989 to evaluate whether such patients require radiation therapy or tamoxifen. That study randomized patients, all of whom received lumpectomy, to receive radiation therapy, radiation therapy and tamoxifen, or tamoxifen alone. More than 700 patients were entered in the study. Although we currently advocate breast irradiation even for this subset of patients, rational empiricism may suggest that patients with negative nodes who have tumors no larger than 1 cm, particularly those whose tumors are estrogen receptor (ER)–positive and whose tumor specimen margins are tumor free, may be candidates for lumpectomy without breast irradiation, particularly if tamoxifen is being administered.

RESULTS FROM THE NSABP B-06 TRIAL EVALUATING LUMPECTOMY

Tumor Involvement of Specimen Margins

In our initial report we indicated that, of the 1257 patients treated initially by lumpectomy, 10 percent were found to have tumor at the margins of resected specimens and subsequently had a total mastectomy.[26] The incidence of positive specimen margins was related to certain patient and tumor characteristics. Evaluation according to patient age showed that about 10 percent of patients aged 49 years or younger and 10 percent of those 50 years and older had positive margins. A higher percentage of patients with positive nodes (15 percent) than with negative nodes (7 percent) had positive margins after lumpectomy, and the larger the number of positive axillary nodes was, the higher the incidence of positive specimen margins: 33 percent of patients with at least 10 positive nodes had margins containing tumor. Women with larger tumors (2.1 cm to 4 cm) had a higher percentage of positive margins (13 percent) than did those with tumors between 0 and 2 cm (7 percent). Women whose tumors were centrally located were most apt to have margin involvement.

Central review of material obtained from hospital pathologists relative to specimen margin involvement with tumor disclosed disparities in interpretation of the findings in some instances. This discrepancy was clearly related to hospital pathologists' statements indicating that tumor was "too" or "very" close to a line of resection, whereas it has been our practice to regard only transected invasive or noninvasive cancer as evidence of such involvement. Residual cancer was noted in 67 percent of the mastectomy specimens available for review when there was agreement on the line of involvement; however, it was noted in only 12 percent of the mastectomy specimens in which hospital, but not headquarters, pathologists had considered margins to be involved. This study did not allow for direct evaluation of the contribution of inadequate assessment of the lines of excision to the incidence of breast tumor recurrence, since total mastectomy was performed in most instances when involvement was considered to have been present.

When the specimen margin contains an amount of tumor that indicates that the tumor has been transected, there is little problem in deciding the future surgical management of the patient. Either re-excision (lumpectomy) of the area should be done to obtain free margins or a mastectomy should be performed if it is deemed that clear margins cannot be obtained with lumpectomy. If, however, the margin is involved with only a few cells, the question arises as to whether re-excision is necessary or whether radiation, perhaps with an external-beam boost plus systemic therapy will eliminate the minimal tumor that may or may not be present. No clear information exists to supply an answer, because, in our study, either re-excision or mastectomy was performed in such patients. Radiation with an external-beam boost may be adequate, particularly since all primary breast cancer patients receive systemic therapy that may, in conjunction with the radiation, be adequate for preventing breast tumor recurrence.

Tumor Recurrence

We have reported findings over an average of 12 years after randomization.[25] Radiation therapy resulted in a marked decrease in the rate of ipsilateral breast tumor recurrence. After 12 years' follow-up, the cumulative prevalence of tumor recurrence was 35 percent in the group treated by lumpectomy alone and 10 percent in those treated by lumpectomy and breast irradiation ($p<.001$; Fig. 46–8). (These values are lower than those previously reported because they estimate the probability of ipsilateral breast tumor reoccurrence in the presence of competing risks; that is, recurrences at other sites, and deaths.) In patients with node-negative cancer, the cumulative incidence was 32 percent and 12 percent, respectively ($p<.001$; Fig. 46–8). Among the patients with node-positive cancer, all of whom also received chemotherapy, the decrease in the likelihood of ipsilateral breast tumor recurrence was more evident after lumpectomy and breast irradiation than after lumpectomy alone (5 percent and 41 percent, respectively, $p<.001$; Fig. 46–8). This low incidence precludes considering positive axillary nodes as a contraindication to breast-conserving surgery.

Shortly after the initial report of our findings with lumpectomy, we provided information on our pathological experience with this procedure, particularly as it related to ipsilateral breast tumor recurrence.[45] Eighty-six percent of all breast tumor recurrences were noted within 4 years after lumpectomy, and 95 percent had occurred within 5 years. A review of the site of recurrences indicated that 95 percent involved the mammary parenchyma, and the remaining 5 percent involved the skin and/or nipple only. Ten percent of those in the breast parenchyma were noninvasive. The most common presentation of recurrence (86 percent) was a localized mass within or close to the quadrant of the cancer removed by lumpectomy. Fourteen percent of the recurrences within the breast were not only in the same quadrant as the primary cancer but also extended diffusely into other quadrants as well. Pathologically, intralymphatic exten-

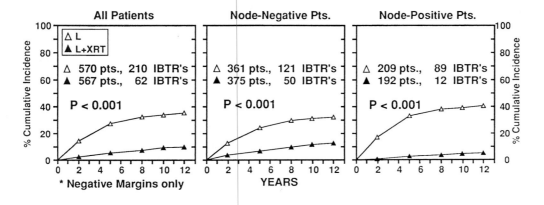

Figure 46–8 *Cumulative incidence of ipsilateral breast tumor recurrence (IBTR) following lumpectomy with and without breast irradiation, through 12 years of follow-up, according to nodal status.*

sion in this type was pronounced, being evident in remote quadrants, and not infrequently in overlying skin and/or nipple, as in so-called inflammatory or occult inflammatory breast cancer.[62] The extraparenchymal local breast tumor recurrences appeared to involve only the lymphatics (71 percent), the dermis of the skin or lymphatics, or the ducts or epidermis (Paget's disease) of the nipple. There were no significant differences in the time of appearance of the invasive and noninvasive breast tumor recurrences or those invasive forms that appeared locally or more diffusely in the breast. Too few examples of recurrences involving only the skin and/or nipple were available for this determination.

The histological types and grades of 93 recurrent, invasive cancers of breast parenchyma were identical to those of the original tumor in 86 percent of cancers, whereas in 14 percent the histological type differed from that of the initial lesion (Table 46–2); however, in eight (9 percent) of these, the recurrent cancer could have represented one portion of a combination-type tumor. The histological grades of these 13 cancers were similar to those of the initial cancer in seven, better-differentiated in four, and less-differentiated in only two.

When the probability of breast tumor recurrence was related to the pathological features of tumors (Table 46–3), there was a significantly greater ($p \leq .05$) incidence in patients whose tumors were 2 cm

TABLE 46–2. INCIDENCE OF HISTOLOGICAL TYPES OF INITIAL AND RECURRENT INVASIVE CANCERS INVOLVING BREAST PARENCHYMA ONLY

Same Types

Type	No.	%
NOS	40	50
Medullary	13	16
NOS + tubular	13	16
Papillary	6	8
Tubular	4	5
NOS + lobular invasive	4	5
Total	80	100

Different Types

Initial	Recurrence	No.
Mucoid	Mucoid + papillary*	1
Mucoid	NOS	2
NOS	NOS + tubular*	1
NOS	NOS + lobular invasive*	1
NOS	Lobular invasive + tubular	1
NOS + tubular	NOS*	2
NOS + tubular	Lobular invasive	1
NOS + lobular invasive	NOS*	1
NOS + lobular invasive	Lobular invasive*	1
Lobular invasive	NOS + lobular invasive*	1
Medullary	NOS + tubular	1
Total		13

*Could represent portion of combination tumor.
NOS = Not otherwise specified.

TABLE 46–3. PATHOLOGICAL FEATURES RELATED TO LOCAL BREAST TUMOR RECURRENCE

Feature	After All Lumpectomies		After Lumpectomy + Radiation	
	%	p	%	p
Tumor size ≥ 2 cm	12 vs 7*	0.02	5 vs 2	0.16
Nuclear grade		0.002		0.42
Grade 1	4		5	
Grade 2	8		3	
Grade 3	13		5	
Histological grade		0.01		0.11
Grade 1	2		0	
Grade 2	9		3	
Grade 3	12		6	
Intralymphatic extension		0.0004		0.07
Yes	41†		8	
No	12		3	

*12% of patients with tumors ≥ 2 cm had recurrence, whereas 7% with tumors <2 cm had recurrence.
†41% of patients with intralymphatic extension had recurrence, whereas 12% without intralymphatic extension had recurrence.

or larger, of high nuclear and histological grades, or revealed intralymphatic extension. Recurrences were less frequent with tubular-type primary cancers or with types 1 and 4 scar cancers. The majority of the latter cancers were tubular. Except for intralymphatic extension, the magnitude of difference noted with these discriminants was not great. For instance, 12 percent of patients with tumors of at least 2 cm and 7 percent with tumors of less than 2 cm had recurrences. Recurrences in the lumpectomy and irradiation group were related only to intralymphatic extension in the primary cancer ($p = .07$).

There was no relationship between recurrences in the breast and the level of estrogen and progesterone receptors in the primary cancer. The mean largest diameters of the initial and recurrent cancers were 2.5 ± 1.3 and 2.4 ± 1.4, respectively.

These findings indicate that the majority of breast tumor recurrences are a result of residual tumor. Whether the recurrences that exhibited a different histological appearance represent de novo cancers or are a portion of a combination tumor cannot be stated with certainty. Nevertheless, at the time of these analyses, the findings minimize the clinical significance of multicentric foci of cancer in the breast as a deterrent to performing lumpectomy.

This study has revealed three presentations of local tumor recurrence. In the most common presentation, the recurring lesion appears localized. In the second, more diffuse breast involvement is apparent, both clinically and pathologically. This presentation simulates inflammatory breast cancer or its occult form[62] and is often associated with skin and/or nipple involvement. The tumor is exceedingly multifocal or infiltrative or reflects the phenomenon of intramammary metastases. Intralymphatic extension is con-

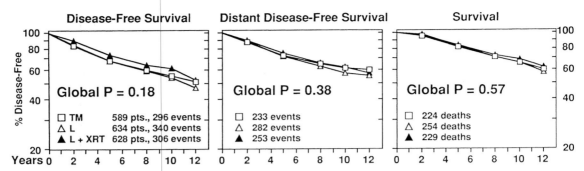

Figure 46–9   *Disease-free survival, distant disease-free survival, and survival through 12 years of follow-up according to treatment group.*

spicuous, not only locally but in other quadrants— and often in the skin of the breast as well. The third form of recurrence may represent a variant of the second and is characterized by intralymphatic extension to dermal or nipple lymphatics.

The second and third forms of recurrence appear to be local phenomena of highly aggressive cancers rather than an induced biological change attendant with lumpectomy. The failure to recognize any significant difference in the histological grades of all except two of the primary cancers and their local recurrences supports this view. In neither of these two with differing grades was the recurrence of the diffuse type. This information also suggests that, once established, it is highly unlikely that the histological grade vis-à-vis differentiation of breast cancer changes. This interpretation coincides with our previous assessment of the nuclear grades of primary breast cancer and their nodal metastases.[44]

Several pathological discriminants were recognized that appear to be statistically related to recurrence after lumpectomy. The magnitude of their significance, however, does not appear to be great. The only feature suggestively found to be related to recurrence in the group treated by lumpectomy and breast irradiation was intralymphatic extension. Our experience differs from that of Schnitt, Harris, Connolly and their associates[9, 52, 75] who related recurrence following biopsy and irradiation of breast cancer to anaplasia and a marked or moderate intraductal component of the initial cancer. One reason for the failure

to recognize the latter component as significant may well be the relatively frequent (44 percent) presence of an intraductal component at the periphery of all invasive breast cancers. The failure to discern any adverse effect of local recurrence on the ultimate survival of patients indicates to us that some of these events, particularly those mimicking occult inflammatory cancer, represent local manifestations of very aggressive cancers that would not be affected by any form of local control. This, as well as the relative infrequency of local breast tumor recurrence after lumpectomy and breast irradiation, indicates to us that there are no pathological discriminants that appear to contraindicate lumpectomy and breast irradiation.

Disease-Free Survival, Distant Disease–Free Survival, and Overall Survival

Recently, we reported findings through an average of 12 years after randomization.[25] There continues to be no significant difference in either disease-free survival (DFS) (global P = .18; Fig. 46–9) or distant disease–free survival (DDFS) (global P = .38; Fig. 46–9) among the three treatment groups. When the survival of patients in the three groups was examined overall or according to nodal status, no significant heterogeneity was found among the groups for all patients, for those with node-negative cancer, or for those with node-positive cancer (Fig. 46–10). De-

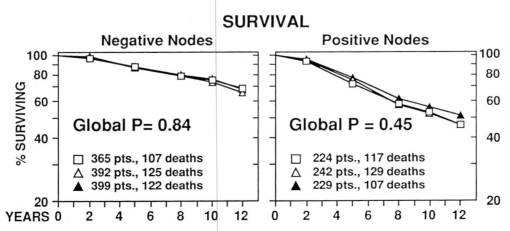

Figure 46–10 *Survival through 12 years of follow-up according to nodal status.*

tailed results on DFS and overall survival (S) appear in Table 46–4.

COMMENTS

The increasing use of lumpectomy has raised several issues that require attention. The following paragraphs present personal views on issues that I deem important.

Comparison of Lumpectomy and Quadrantectomy

A critical appraisal of the two very different methods—lumpectomy and quadrantectomy—for achieving breast preservation was presented in a recent editorial.[23] The difference between these two approaches relates to more than just how much "normal" breast tissue is removed. Not only are the surgical procedures considerably different, but they also seem to be conceptually unrelated. Lumpectomy was designed to remove, through a limited curvilinear incision, the tumor plus enough "normal" tissue to ensure that the margins of the resected specimen are tumor free (see Fig. 46–5).[43] The reason for insisting that specimen margins be tumor free is to better ensure that no gross tumor remains at the operative site. A tumor-free margin of 1 mm, or even less, is considered adequate. When lumpectomy is performed, en bloc dissections are not carried out, not even for upper outer quadrant lesions. No skin, fascia, or muscle is removed. Lumpectomy is used to treat patients of any age or axillary nodal status (positive or negative), regardless of the site or size of the tumor in the breast and regardless of any particular tumor characteristic. If there are two distinctly separate primary tumors in the breast (e.g., in different quadrants) and if it is possible to resect both so that clear, tumor-free specimen margins are obtained for each and a good cosmetic result can be obtained, both tumors can be removed through separate incisions.

In sharp contrast, a quadrantectomy, as originally described by the Milan group, uses a long radial incision through which tumors 2 cm or smaller (and, more recently, as large as 2.5 cm) are removed with a 2- to 3-cm cuff of normal tissue circumscribing the tumor.[80] Skin, pectoral fascia, and the pectoralis minor muscle are also removed. Moreover, dissection en bloc is employed for removal of at least 50 percent of lesions (i.e., those in the upper outer quadrant) in conjunction with total axillary nodal dissection. These requirements limit the feasibility of attaining a satisfactory cosmetic result and of removing even "small" tumors from "small" breasts. For example, for a tumor of 2 cm, the diameter of the resected specimen would be 6 to 8 cm. In a large percentage of such women, the anatomical site of the tumor may preclude removal of that much breast tissue in all directions.

Conceptually, quadrantectomy can be viewed as a next step in redefining the Halstedian paradigm, a step beyond Patey's operation (modified radical mastectomy) and simple mastectomy, all of which maintain attachments to the Halstedian paradigm. Lumpectomy, in contrast, has abandoned every vestige of Halstedian surgery and, in that regard, is conceptually and technically different from quadrantectomy.

In the editorial comparing lumpectomy with quadrantectomy, it was pointed out that the incidence of ipsilateral breast tumor recurrence after lumpectomy in the NSABP B-06 trial should be viewed as historical.[23] During that study, many American surgeons learned how to perform lumpectomy and numerous radiation oncologists learned the technique for breast irradiation. Also in the B-06 study, only node-positive patients received systemic therapy, whereas in more recent trials node-negative as well as node-positive patients received chemotherapy and/or tamoxifen therapy. Results from five recent NSABP studies in which patients received systemic therapy after lumpectomy and breast irradiation indicate that the incidence of ipsilateral breast tumor recurrence was probably at least as low as, and perhaps lower than, that after quadrantectomy (Table 46–5).

It must be emphasized that, despite any comparisons between Milan and NSABP data, physicians should not choose a breast-conserving operation on the basis of such comparisons, which are meaningless if for no other reason than that the patient populations are so different.[81] For example, in the Milan II trial, 89 percent of women had tumors no larger than 2 cm, and 71 percent were node negative. In contrast, 45 percent of NSABP patients had tumors larger than 2 cm, and nearly 40 percent were node positive.

In conclusion, we continue to believe that lumpectomy with tumor-free specimen margins, followed by breast irradiation and systemic adjuvant therapy, when indicated, is the appropriate therapy for most patients with stage I or II breast cancers. Because survival and ipsilateral breast tumor recurrence rates of NSABP lumpectomy-treated patients were similar to those of quadrantectomy-treated patients, despite the fact that the NSABP patients were at greater risk for failure, and because the cosmetic results after lumpectomy were superior, lumpectomy is preferable.

Reappraisal of Breast Biopsy

Paradoxically, just when the two-stage biopsy procedure has gained acceptance, not only is there a need to reassess the merits of that approach, but it is also necessary to reappraise and modify the entire method of breast cancer biopsy. With the increasing use of breast-conserving operations and evidence supporting their validity, there is a need to re-evaluate the surgical strategy employed in breast cancer management. I recently described how my experience with lumpectomy altered not only my views and policies on breast biopsy but also my entire approach to breast cancer surgery.[18] A detailed algorithm describ-

TABLE 46-4. ESTIMATES OF DISEASE-FREE SURVIVAL AND SURVIVAL FOR ALL TREATMENT GROUPS AFTER 12 YEARS OF FOLLOW-UP

Treatment Group	No. Pts. (n)	Disease-Free Survival						Survival					
		Events (n)	Censored*	Disease Free	DFS† %	Relative Odds of DFS (95% CI)‡	P Value	Dead	Censored*	Alive	Survival† (%)	Relative Odds of Survival (95% CI)‡	P Value
Total mastectomy	589	285	177	127	50	—		216	224	149	60	—	
Lumpectomy	634	331	192	111	47	0.94 (0.80–1.10)	0.43	242	247	145	58	0.96 (0.80–1.15)	0.66
Lumpectomy + radiation therapy	628	299	205	124	49	1.08 (0.91–1.27)	0.39	215	250	163	62	1.07 (0.89–1.29)	0.49

*Refers to patients who were free of events or who were alive at the most recent contact but who had been followed for <12 years.
†Life-table estimates were adjusted for the number of positive nodes (0, 1 to 3, 4 to 9, ≥10).
‡In all cases, the reference group is the group that underwent total mastectomy. CI denotes confidence interval.

TABLE 46–5.   CUMULATIVE INCIDENCE OF IPSILATERAL BREAST TUMOR RECURRENCE FOLLOWING LUMPECTOMY AND BREAST IRRADIATION FOR INVASIVE BREAST CANCER IN RECENT NSABP STUDIES

NSABP Protocols	Systemic Therapy	Pts. (n)	IBTR (n)	Follow-up (yrs.)*	Cumulative Incidence (%)	P†
Node–negative						
B-13	None	119	16	8	12.9	.001
	M→F	116	3	8	2.6	
B-19	M→F	196	11	5	5.8	.03
	CMF	194	3	5	1.5	
B-14	Placebo	532	78	10	11.6	<.0001
	Tamoxifen	530	23	10	3.3	
Node–positive						
B-15	AC	208	19	9	8.7	
	CMF	204	21	9	7.4	.67
	AC→CMF	212	23	9	9.5	
B-16	TAM	116	7	9	4.5	.31
	ACT	112	4	9	2.7	

*Years of follow-up in B-13, B-14, B-19; average years on study in B-15 and B-16.
†Based on comparison of average annual rates.

ing an optimal surgical strategy for the management of primary breast cancer was presented (Fig. 46–11). It was pointed out that, as a result of the increasing acceptance of lumpectomy, arguments for use of the two-stage procedure are in many, if not most, in-

stances nullified and obsolete. As in the Halstedian era (but now for different reasons), there is justification for performing more, rather than fewer, biopsies with general anesthesia and for more frequently carrying out biopsy and the definitive operation in

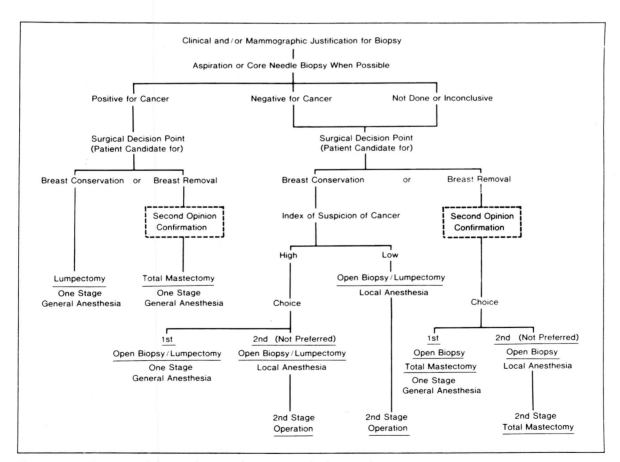

Figure 46–11 *Recommended surgical strategy for management of primary breast cancer.*

one stage. It is an absolute dictum that all open breast biopsies be carried out as if a lumpectomy were being performed. Attention must be given to ensuring that specimen margins are likely to be free of tumor, should a tumor be encountered. Today, biopsy done without attention to specimen margins is inappropriate. In all circumstances when breast conservation is feasible, the operation carried out to establish the definitive *diagnosis* of a breast lesion becomes the definitive *treatment*, along with axillary dissection.

Lumpectomy in Conjunction with Systemic Therapy

It is becoming increasingly meaningless to discuss the surgical management of breast cancer without considering how other therapeutic modalities might influence the surgeon's operative approach. It is highly likely that, with the use of more effective systemic therapy following operation, the incidence of breast tumor recurrence will be lower than that observed as a result of lumpectomy and breast irradiation alone. This finding is already evident in more recent NSABP studies. The NSABP B-06 study, which provided data for this chapter, was concerned almost entirely with assessing local/regional disease control by lumpectomy and radiation therapy without serious regard for how systemic therapy might affect patient outcome as influenced by the surgery. The study has, however, provided evidence to indicate the value of chemotherapy in enhancing the benefit from lumpectomy and radiation therapy. In the B-06 trial, only node-positive patients received systemic chemotherapy (melphalan + 5-fluorouracil), which had been demonstrated in a prior NSABP study to modestly improve DFS and S of node-positive patients following total mastectomy and axillary dissection. It has been observed that the incidence of ipsilateral breast tumor recurrence in the B-06 trial was lower in node-positive lumpectomy patients who received breast irradiation than in node-negative lumpectomy patients who received breast irradiation but no chemotherapy. The incidence of ipsilateral breast tumor recurrence after lumpectomy in the NSABP B-06 trial should be viewed as "historical."

In recent NSABP studies evaluating the use of adjuvant chemotherapy for node-negative breast cancer, evidence has indicated that effective systemic therapy reduces the incidence of breast tumor recurrence following lumpectomy and breast irradiation.[21, 22] In one trial (NSABP B-13), node-negative, ER-negative patients received methotrexate followed by 5-fluorouracil (M→F). After 8 years' follow-up, the incidence of ipsilateral breast tumor recurrence was 2.6 percent, as compared with an incidence of 12.9 percent in a control group treated by surgery alone. In another study (NSABP B-19) patients similar to those in B-13 received either cyclophosphamide, methotrexate, and 5-fluorouracil (CMF) or M→F. The incidence of ipsilateral breast tumor recurrence after 5 years was 1.5 percent in patients who received

CMF and 5.8 percent in those treated with M→F. When tamoxifen was administered to node-negative, ER-positive patients in NSABP B-14, only 2.1 percent demonstrated an ipsilateral breast tumor recurrence after 10 years' follow-up. In a trial (NSABP B-15) that evaluated the value of chemotherapy in node-positive patients with ER-negative tumors, the incidence of ipsilateral breast tumor recurrence, with a mean follow-up of 9 years, was similar whether Adriamycin-cyclophosphamide (AC) or CMF therapy was used (8.7 percent and 7.4 percent, respectively). Most notable was the low incidence of ipsilateral breast tumor recurrence in node-positive lumpectomy-treated patients (NSABP B-16) after either tamoxifen or tamoxifen and AC therapy (4.5 percent and 2.7 percent, respectively; mean follow-up 9 years).

Systemic therapy may also influence breast-conserving procedures when used before operation. Recently the NSABP judged that there is sufficient biological and clinical information available to justify the conduct of a randomized clinical trial to determine whether preoperative chemotherapy will more effectively prolong DFS and overall S of patients with stages I and II breast cancer than will the same therapy given postoperatively. That study (B-18) also evaluates the response of the primary tumor to preoperative chemotherapy and will correlate response with ultimate DFS and S. That study is particularly important to the surgeon in that it determines whether preoperative chemotherapy can shrink a large primary tumor sufficiently to permit a breast-conserving operation with a low incidence of ipsilateral breast tumor recurrence.

It is likely that a reduction in the extent of surgery may, indeed, result, since it has been demonstrated by other investigators that there was a 90 percent objective response following the use of primary chemotherapy for stage III disease.[76] A complete response was observed in 50 percent of these patients. Others have reported a similar experience with locally advanced disease.[57] Thus, it is reasonable to speculate that the present paradigm for the management of breast cancer—operation followed by systemic therapy—may be replaced by another that renders current management anachronistic. With the advent of increasingly better diagnostic procedures and the availability of better regimens of therapy, this outcome is almost inevitable.

Biological Significance and Clinical Management of Ipsilateral Breast Tumor Reoccurrence After Lumpectomy

Findings from NSABP B-06 indicated no significant difference in DDFS or S among women treated by lumpectomy alone and those treated by lumpectomy and ipsilateral breast irradiation, despite the fact that the former group had a much greater cumulative incidence of ipsilateral breast tumor recurrence than the latter group (35 percent vs. 10 percent, respectively, through 12 years). This led us to conclude that there is no causal relation between ipsilateral breast tumor recurrence and distant disease. A Cox regression model on fixed covariates—features such as tumor type or size at surgery, and on breast tumor recurrence, which is time dependent and not fixed—revealed that the risk of distant disease was 3.4 times greater after adjustment for covariates in patients who developed ipsilateral breast tumor recurrence.[87] We also provided data demonstrating that the earlier an ipsilateral breast tumor recurrence appeared, the less favorable was the DDFS.

We concluded that ipsilateral breast tumor recurrence is a powerful independent predictor of distant disease and that it is a marker of risk for, not a cause of, distant metastasis. Although mastectomy or breast irradiation following lumpectomy prevents expression of the marker, they do not lower the risk of distant disease. These findings further justify the use of lumpectomy.

Our findings, published in 1991, have been confirmed by several reports.[24] Whelan and colleagues also demonstrated from a randomized trial that local recurrence following lumpectomy was associated with increased risk of distant relapse and death, and that ipsilateral breast tumor recurrence within 1 year of surgery was associated with a higher risk of distant relapse and death.[87] Information from data collected retrospectively by Haffty's group also indicated that ipsilateral breast tumor recurrence early after lumpectomy and radiation therapy was a significant predictor of distant metastases.[47] Finally, Veronesi and colleagues concluded that the timing of ipsilateral breast tumor recurrence seems to be an important marker: the earlier the local recurrence after operation, the higher the risk of distant metastases.[79] Our report suggested that additional systemic therapy should be considered when ipsilateral breast tumor recurrence is diagnosed.[24]

The appropriate treatment for an ipsilateral breast tumor recurrence following lumpectomy is no longer as much of an issue as it was a decade ago. If patients treated by lumpectomy undergo regular clinical examinations and mammography at intervals consonant with those recommended for women in the general population, recurrences should be detected when they are amenable to excision with another lumpectomy. If satisfactory cosmesis and local disease control can be achieved by repeat lumpectomy, there is no reason for mastectomy. Radiation therapy to the area of re-excision may be considered, but no information exists to mandate its use.

Underutilization of Lumpectomy

Because many women in the United States, Europe, South America, and elsewhere are being treated by mastectomy, it is appropriate to comment on some of the reasons frequently given to justify underutilization of lumpectomy.[35, 60]

Patient Preference

The investigative and clinical findings on lumpectomy have provided physicians—and others who are interested in the breast cancer problem—with justification for offering breast preservation as an option for women, should they prefer it. It seems inappropriate to present breast preservation as an alternative to mastectomy, a procedure no longer supported by biological and clinical evidence. Giving breast cancer patients treatment options may be unfair—and perhaps deleterious to their outcome. If doctors offer options in a way that reflects their own biases, they are influencing the patient's choice, particularly since clinical guidance is what patients expect. It is invalid for physicians then to assert that they performed mastectomy instead of lumpectomy because the patient chose mastectomy. On the other hand, if options are presented to patients in an unbiased fashion, doctors become vendors who "dispense" whatever treatment patients choose, and, thus, play no role in the decision-making process.

Physicians must objectively communicate information that relates treatment to outcome. The patient's autonomy will not be compromised and paternalism will not be resurrected if physicians inform patients that, in almost all cases and based on current knowledge, mastectomy is no longer justifiable and lumpectomy followed by breast irradiation will not put them at greater risk of developing systemic disease or of dying than mastectomy would. The burden for implementing appropriate therapy still rests with the physician.

Patient Age

One of the reasons given for underutilization of lumpectomy in Europe and the United States stems from evidence that breast preservation is used less frequently as patient age increases.[46, 56, 60] This practice is likely related to male physicians' attitudes that cosmesis is less important to women as they get older. This bias is apt to be concealed in the recommendation that "it is more appropriate to remove the breast so you won't have to worry about the problem anymore." Information from our studies and from those of other investigators fails to confirm the thesis that lumpectomy carries increased risk that is age related.

Tumor Size, Nodal Status, and Tumor Location

Most women with either small or large tumors, tumors in any single location—including those that are subareolar—and women with either negative or positive axillary nodes are candidates for lumpectomy followed by breast irradiation. This conclusion is supported by findings from our current trials, which indicate that, with more effective systemic adjuvant therapy, the incidence of breast tumor recurrence following lumpectomy and radiation therapy is even lower in node-positive and node-negative patients than was originally reported in the study findings from the B-06 trial.

The idea that lumpectomy is feasible only for patients with tumors smaller than 2 cm, or for those with small, mammographically detected lesions, is erroneous. In all NSABP protocols, as previously noted, patients with tumors as large as 5 cm are eligible for lumpectomy. The main limitation to performing breast-preserving operations in patients with large tumors relates to the size of the woman's breast. If it is disproportionately small in relation to the size of the tumor so that an excellent cosmetic result cannot be achieved, lumpectomy may not be desirable. Similarly, the notion that lumpectomy is appropriate only for patients with negative nodes needs to be dispelled. Node-positive patients are particularly good candidates for lumpectomy. Since we first began to conduct trials to evaluate the value of lumpectomy, it has been judged that the rationale for performing the operation in patients with large tumors and/or positive nodes is equal to (and perhaps greater than) that for performing it in patients with small tumors and negative nodes. The justification for that thesis relates to the fact that women with large tumors and/or positive nodes are at increased risk for distant disease and death. To perform a radical or modified radical mastectomy, with its subsequent undesirable sequelae, on such patients, only to have them die of metastatic disease 6 months or a year later (as they often do), is not defensible. Finally, the presence of a tumor in the subareolar area is considered by some to preclude breast preservation. Lumpectomy with removal of the nipple-areolar complex can be achieved with an excellent cosmetic result and should be employed without consideration for tumor location.

Breast Irradiation After Lumpectomy

One reason for not performing lumpectomy relates to the need for postoperative breast irradiation. Many patients are terrified by the prospect of radiation therapy. Too often, their concerns are not adequately allayed by physicians who are, themselves, unfamiliar with the fact that the morbidity associated with breast irradiation is minor when radiation therapy is administered by experienced therapists using appropriate equipment. When balanced against the short-term inconvenience associated with its use, the advantage of radiation therapy far outweighs the psychological and physical damage that persists for a woman's lifetime after mastectomy.

Many physicians claim that they do not perform lumpectomy because of insufficient facilities for conveniently administering appropriate breast irradiation. If that excuse is valid, a disturbing contradiction exists that requires resolution. On the one hand, there is strong advocacy for mammography so that women can be treated by breast-preserving surgery if a clinically undetectable breast lesion is found. On the other hand, many women cannot gain full benefit from mammography because they appropriate radiation therapy is unavailable. If radiation therapy is not available, we could ask whether or not there are subgroups of patients in which the risk of an

ipsilateral breast tumor recurrence is sufficiently small to justify recommending that they may be treated by lumpectomy without breast irradiation, even though there may be some greater risk of an ipsilateral breast tumor recurrence. Although we previously reported observing a benefit from tamoxifen in patients with negative *or* positive nodes, regardless of tumor size, and recommended the use of radiation therapy after lumpectomy for all patients, regardless of tumor size, it has seemed appropriate to reassess that position to determine whether an argument can be made for performing lumpectomy even if radiation therapy cannot be administered.[36]

Such a reassessment seems germane because most patients, node-negative and node-positive alike, receive some form of systemic therapy after surgery and because it may be considered that such therapy alone will be sufficiently effective in reducing the incidence of ipsilateral breast tumor recurrence after lumpectomy so as to preclude radiation therapy. Unfortunately, to our knowledge, little or no information is available from randomized studies to either support or refute that thesis. Rational empiricism may suggest that patients with negative axillary nodes who have tumors no larger than 1 cm, particularly those whose tumors are ER positive and whose tumor specimen margins are tumor free, may be candidates for lumpectomy without breast irradiation, particularly if tamoxifen is being administered. The NSABP implemented a randomized trial (B-21) in 1989 to evaluate whether such patients require radiation therapy or tamoxifen. That study randomized patients, all of whom received lumpectomy, to receive radiation therapy, radiation therapy and tamoxifen, or tamoxifen alone. After more than 700 patients were entered into the study, it was suspended because of political intervention. The trial has since been reopened to enrollment, and there is hope that answers about the need for radiation therapy and/or tamoxifen in such patients will be forthcoming.

Lumpectomy for the Treatment of Intraductal Breast Cancer

Women with intraductal breast cancer (ductal carcinoma *in situ* or DCIS) have been treated in many different ways. Because there is little justification for mastectomy in the treatment of invasive breast cancer, that an operation for noninvasive breast cancer should be more radical than one for invasive disease seems counterintuitive. Uncertainty about the most appropriate treatment for women with these tumors prompted the NSABP to begin a randomized clinical trial in 1985 to test the hypothesis that, for women whose localized DCIS was thought to have been completely removed, local excision (lumpectomy) plus breast irradiation is more effective than local excision alone in preventing a second cancer in the ipsilateral breast.

The initial results from this trial (NSABP B-17) indicated that at 5 years' follow-up there was a significant reduction in the incidence of second ipsilat-

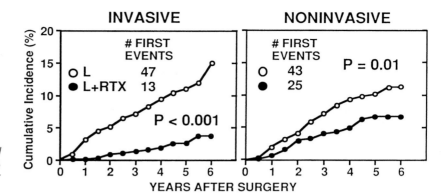

Figure 46–12 *Cumulative incidence of invasive and noninvasive second cancers in the ipsilateral breast, following lumpectomy with and without breast irradiation, through 6 years of follow-up.*

eral breast cancers with the use of breast irradiation after lumpectomy.[28] Not only was there a significant reduction in the incidence of second noninvasive breast cancers in the ipsilateral breast, but most important, there was a marked reduction in the incidence of invasive tumors as well. We concluded from these initial findings that, for women with localized DCIS that could be removed so that the margins of the resected specimen were tumor free, lumpectomy followed by breast irradiation was the treatment of choice. A current update of findings indicates that, through 6 years of follow-up of the group treated by lumpectomy alone, the cumulative incidence of noninvasive second cancers in the ipsilateral breast was reduced by 41 percent, from 11.3 percent to 6.7 percent ($p = .01$; Fig. 46–12). Even more impressive, the cumulative incidence of invasive second cancers was reduced by 75 percent, from 15.0 percent to 3.8 percent ($p < .001$).

Upon completion of accrual in the B-17 study, the NSABP implemented a new trial (B-24) to evaluate tamoxifen for the treatment of more extensive DCIS than that found in women in the B-17 trial. All too frequently, DCIS is not sufficiently localized as to be completely removed by local excision. Consequently, in the B-24 study, patients with mammographic findings of DCIS that cannot be removed completely so as to ensure tumor-free specimen margins and patients with persistent mammographic evidence of DCIS were randomized to two groups. Patients in both groups received radiation therapy after lumpectomy; one group then received placebo and the other tamoxifen. More than 12 patients have been randomized to this trial. The results should indicate whether there will be an even larger cohort of DCIS patients who can be spared the need for mastectomy.

SUMMARY

This chapter provides results obtained from patients who were entered into the NSABP clinical trial evaluating breast conservation. Twelve years after operation, the findings continue to justify the use of lumpectomy followed by breast irradiation for patients with stage I or II breast cancer no larger than 4 cm, provided that resected specimen margins are free of

tumor and that systemic adjuvant therapy is administered to those with pathologically positive axillary lymph nodes. The use of systemic therapy as well as breast irradiation markedly reduces the incidence of ipsilateral breast tumor recurrence after lumpectomy in patients with node-negative tumors. The findings continue to support the validity of the alternative paradigm for breast cancer management that I proposed in the 1960s.

ACKNOWLEDGMENTS

Most of the information presented was obtained as a result of support by a Public Health Service grant from the National Cancer Institute (NCI-U10-CA-12027) and by a grant from the American Cancer Society (ACS-RC-13).

References

1. Amalric R, Santamaria F, Robert F, Seigle J, Altshuler C, Pietra JC, Amalric F, Kurtz JM, Spitalier JM, Brandone H, Ayme Y, Pollet JF, Bressac C, Fondarai J: Conservative therapy in operable breast cancer—results at five, ten and fifteen years in 2216 consecutive cases. *In* Harris JR, Hellman S, Silen W (eds): Conservative Management of Breast Cancer. Philadelphia, JB Lippincott, 1983, pp 15–21.
2. Andreassen M, Dahl-Iversen E, Sorensen B: Extended exeresis of regional lymph nodes at operation for carcinoma of the breast and result of 5-year follow-up of first 98 cases with removal of axillary as well as supraclavicular gland. Acta Chir Scand 107:206–213, 1954.
3. Baclesse F: Five year results in 431 breast cancers treated solely by roentgentherapy. Ann Surg 161:103–104, 1965.
4. Caceres E: An evaluation of radical mastectomy and extended radical mastectomy for cancer of the breast. Surg Gynecol Obstet 125:337–341, 1967.
5. Calle R, Pilleron JP, Schlienger P, Vilcoq JR: Conservative management of operable breast cancer: Ten years experience at the Foundation Curie. Cancer 42:2045–2053, 1978.
6. Calle R, Vilcoq JR, Pilleron JP, Schlienger P, Durand JC: Conservative treatment of operable breast carcinoma by irradiation with or without limited surgery—ten-year results. *In* Harris JR, Hellman S, Silen W (eds): Conservative Management of Breast Cancer. Philadelphia, JB Lippincott, 1983, pp 3–9.
7. Cancer Research Campaign Working Party: Cancer research campaign (King's/Cambridge) trial for early breast cancer. Lancet 2:55–60, 1980.
8. Coman DR: Mechanisms responsible for the origin and distribution of blood-borne tumor metastases: A review. Cancer Res 13:397–404, 1953.

9. Connolly JL, Schnitt SJ, Harris JR, Hellman S, Cohen RB: Pathologic correlates of local tumor control following primary radiation therapy in patients with early breast cancer. *In* Harris JR, Hellman S, Silen W (eds): Conservative Management of Breast Cancer. Philadelphia, JB Lippincott, 1983, pp 123–136.

10. Cope O, Wang CA, Chu A, Wang CC, Schulz M, Castleman B, Long J, Sohier WD: Limited surgical excision as the basis of a comprehensive therapy for cancer of the breast. Am J Surg 131:400–406, 1976.

11. Crile G Jr: Treatment of breast cancer by local excision. Am J Surg 109:400, 1965.

12. Fisher B: The surgical dilemma in the primary therapy of invasive breast cancer: A critical appraisal. Curr Probl Surg October: 3–53, 1970.

13. Fisher B: Cancer: A Comprehensive Treatise, Vol 6. New York, Plenum, 1977, pp 401–421.

14. Fisher B: Breast cancer management: Alternatives to radical mastectomy. N Engl J Med 301:326–328, 1979.

15. Fisher B: Laboratory and clinical research in breast cancer—a personal adventure: The David A Karnofsky Memorial Lecture. Cancer Res 40:3863–3874, 1980.

16. Fisher B: The interdependence of laboratory and clinical research in the study of metastases. *In* Nicolson GL, Miles L (eds): Cancer Invasion and Metastasis: Biologic and Therapeutic Aspects. New York, Raven Press, 1984, pp 27–46.

17. Fisher B: The Role of Science in the Evolution of Breast Cancer Management. Austin, TX, University of Texas Press, 1984, pp 1–21.

18. Fisher B: Reappraisal of breast biopsy prompted by the use of lumpectomy. JAMA 253:3585–3588, 1985.

19. Fisher B: The revolution in breast cancer surgery: Science or anecdotalism? World J Surg 9:655–666, 1985.

20. Fisher B: Conservative surgery: The American experience. Semin Oncol 13:425–433, 1986.

21. Fisher B: Sequential methotrexate and 5-fluorouracil for the treatment of node negative breast cancer patients with estrogen receptor negative tumors: Results from NSABP protocol B-13. N Engl J Med 320:473–478, 1989.

22. Fisher B: Tamoxifen for the treatment of node negative breast cancer patients with estrogen receptor positive tumors: Results from NSABP protocol B-14. N Engl J Med 320:479–484, 1989.

23. Fisher B: Lumpectomy versus quadrantectomy for breast conservation: A critical appraisal. Eur J Cancer 31A:10:1567–1569, 1995.

24. Fisher B, Anderson S, Fisher ER, Redmond C, Wickerham DL, Wolmark N, Mamounas EP, Deutsch M, Margolese R: Significance of ipsilateral breast tumor recurrence after lumpectomy. Lancet 338:327–331, 1991.

25. Fisher B, Anderson S, Redmond CK, Wolmark N, Wickerham DL, Cronin WM: Reanalysis and results after 12 years of follow-up in a randomized clinical trial comparing total mastectomy with lumpectomy with or without irradiation in the treatment of breast cancer. N Engl J Med 333:1456–1461, 1995.

26. Fisher B, Bauer M, Margolese R, Poisson R, Pilch Y, Redmond C, Fisher ER, Wolmark N, Deutsch M, Montague E, Saffer E, Wickerham L, Lerner H, Glass A, Shibata H, Deckers P, Ketcham A, Oishi R, Russell I: Five-year results of a randomized clinical trial comparing total mastectomy and segmental mastectomy with or without radiation in the treatment of breast cancer. N Engl J Med 312:665–673, 1985.

27. Fisher B, Bauer M, Wickerham L, Redmond CK, Fisher ER: Relation of number of positive axillary nodes to the prognosis of patients with primary breast cancer—an NSABP update. (With the contribution of Cruz A, Foster R, Gardener B, Lerner H, Margolese R, Poisson R, Shibata H, Volk H, and other NSABP Investigators) Cancer 52:1551–1557, 1983.

28. Fisher B, Costantino J, Redmond C, Fisher E, Margolese R, Dimitrov N, Wolmark N, Wickerham DL, Deutsch M, Ore L, Mamounas E, Poller W, Kavanah M: Lumpectomy compared with lumpectomy and radiation therapy for the treatment of intraductal breast cancer. N Engl J Med 328:1581–1586, 1993.

29. Fisher B, Fisher ER: Experimental evidence in support of the dormant tumor cell. Science 130:918–919, 1959.

30. Fisher B, Fisher ER: The organ distribution of disseminated ^{51}Cr-labeled tumor cells. Cancer Res 27:412–420, 1967.

31. Fisher B, Fisher ER: Studies concerning the regional lymph node in cancer I. Initiation of immunity. Cancer 27:1001–1004, 1971.

32. Fisher B, Fisher ER: The interrelationship of hematogenous and lymphatic tumor cell dissemination. Surg Gynecol Obstet 122:791–798, 1966.

33. Fisher B, Fisher ER, Feduska N: Trauma and the localization of tumor cells. Cancer 20:23–30, 1967.

34. Fisher B, Gebhardt MC: The evolution of breast cancer surgery: Past, present and future. Semin Oncol 5:385–394, 1978.

35. Fisher B, Ore L: On the underutilization of breast-conserving surgery for the treatment of breast cancer. Ann Oncol 4:96–98, 1993.

36. Fisher B, Redmond C: Lumpectomy for breast cancer: An update of the NSABP experience. J Natl Cancer Inst Monogr 11:7–13, 1992.

37. Fisher B, Redmond C, Fisher ER, Bauer M, Wolmark N, Wickerham L, Deutsch M, Montague E, Margolese R, Foster R: Ten year results of a randomized clinical trial comparing radical mastectomy and total mastectomy with or without radiation. N Engl J Med 312:674–681, 1985.

38. Fisher B, Saffer E, Fisher ER: Studies concerning the regional lymph nodes in cancer. IV. Tumor inhibition by regional lymph node cells. Cancer 33:631–636, 1974.

39. Fisher B, Slack NH: Number of lymph nodes examined and the prognosis of breast carcinoma. Surg Gynecol Obstet 131:79–88, 1970.

40. Fisher B, Slack NH, Ausman RK, Bross IDJ: Location of breast carcinoma and prognosis. Surg Gynecol Obstet 129:705–716, 1969.

41. Fisher B, Wolmark N: New concepts in the management of primary breast cancer. Cancer 36:627–632, 1975.

42. Fisher B, Wolmark N, Bauer M, Redmond C, Gebhardt M: The accuracy of clinical nodal staging and of limited axillary dissection as a determinant of histologic nodal status in carcinoma of the breast. Surg Gynecol Obstet 152:765–772, 1981.

43. Fisher B, Wolmark N, Fisher ER, Deutsch M: Lumpectomy and axillary dissection for breast cancer: Surgical, pathological, and radiation considerations. World J Surg 9:692–698, 1985.

44. Fisher ER, Palekar AS, Sass R, Fisher B: Pathologic findings from the National Surgical Adjuvant Breast Project (protocol 4): IX. Scar cancers. Breast Cancer Res Treat 3:39–59, 1983.

45. Fisher ER, Sass R, Fisher B, Gregorio R, Brown R, Wickerham L, and collaborating NSABP investigators: Pathologic findings from the National Surgical Adjuvant Breast Project (protocol 6). II. Relation of local breast recurrence to multicentricity. Cancer 57:1717–1724, 1986.

46. Greenfield S, Blanco DM, Elashoff RM, Ganz PA: Patterns of care related to age of breast cancer patients. JAMA 257:2766–2770, 1987.

47. Haffty BG, Reiss M, Beinfield M, Fischer D, Ward B, McKhann C: Ipsilateral breast tumor recurrence as a predictor of distant disease: Implications for systemic therapy at the time of local relapse. J Clin Oncol 14:52–57, 1996.

48. Halsted WS: The results of radical operations for the cure of carcinoma of the breast. Ann Surg 46:1–19, 1907.

49. Handley RD: The technic and results of conservative radical mastectomy (Patey's operation). Prog Clin Cancer 1:462, 1965.

50. Handley WS: *In* Murray A (ed): Cancer of the Breast and Its Operative Treatment. London, Hoeber Publishing, 1922.

51. Harris JR, Botnick L, Bloomer WD, Chaffey JT, Hellman S: Primary radiation therapy for early breast cancer: The experience at the joint center for radiation therapy. Int J Radiat Oncol Biol Phys 7:1549–1552, 1981.

52. Harris JR, Connolly JL, Schnitt SJ, Cohen RB, Hellman S: Clinical pathologic study of early breast cancer treated by primary radiation therapy. J Clin Oncol 1:184–189, 1983.

53. Harris JR, Hellman S: Primary radiation therapy for early breast cancer. Cancer 52:2547–2552, 1983.

54. Harris JR, Levine MB, Hellman S: Results of treating stage I and II carcinoma of the breast with primary radiation therapy. Cancer Treat Rep 62:985–991, 1978.

55. Hellman S, Harris JR, Levene MB: Radiation therapy of early carcinoma of the breast without mastectomy. Cancer 46:988–994, 1980.
56. Interdisciplinary Group for Cancer Care Evaluation: Survey of treatment of primary breast cancer in Italy. Br J Cancer 57:630–634, 1988.
57. Jacquillat C, Baillet F, Blondon J, Auclerc G, Lefranc JP, Maylin CI, Weil M: Preliminary results of "neoadjuvant" chemotherapy in initial management of breast cancer (BC). Proc Am Soc Clin Oncol 2:C-437, 112, 1983.
58. Keynes G: Radium treatment of primary carcinoma of the breast. Lancet 2:108, 1928.
59. Lacour J: The place of the Halsted operation in treatment of breast cancer. Int Surg 47:282, 1967.
60. Lazovich DA, White E, Thomas DB, Moe RE: Underutilization of breast-conserving surgery and radiation therapy among women with stage I or II breast cancer. JAMA 266:3433–3438, 1991.
61. Levene MBF, Harris JR, Hellman S: Treatment of carcinoma of the breast by radiation therapy. Cancer 39:2840–2845, 1977.
62. Lucas FV, Perez-Mesa C: Inflammatory carcinoma of the breast. Cancer 41:1595–1605, 1978.
63. Margolese R, et al: The technique of segmental mastectomy (lumpectomy) and axillary dissection: A syllabus from the National Surgical Adjuvant Breast Project workshops. Surgery 102:828–834, 1987.
64. Margottini M, Bucalossi P: El metastasi lymphoghiandolari mammario interne nel cancro delia mammella. Boll Oncol 23:2, 1949.
65. McWhirter R: The value of simple mastectomy and radiotherapy in the treatment of cancer of the breast. Br J Radiol 21:599–610, 1948.
66. Montague ED, Gutierrez AE, Barker JL, Tapley N, Fletcher GH: Conservative surgery and irradiation for the treatment of favorable breast cancer. Cancer 43:1058–1061, 1979.
67. Mustakallio S: Treatment of breast cancer by tumor extirpation and roentgen therapy instead of radical operation. J Fac Radiol 6:23, 1954.
68. Peters MV: Wedge resection and irradiation, and effective treatment in early breast cancer. JAMA 200:134–135, 1967.
69. Peters MV: Cutting the "Gordian Knot" in early breast cancer. Ann R Coll Phys Surg Can 8:186–192, 1975.
70. Peters MV: Wedge resection with or without radiation in early breast cancer. Int J Radiat Oncol Biol Phys 2:1151–1156, 1977.
71. Pierquin B: Conservative treatment for carcinoma of the breast: Experience of Creteil—ten year results. In Harris JR, Hellman S, Silen W (eds): Conservative Management of Breast Cancer. Philadelphia, JB Lippincott, 1983, pp 11–14.
72. Pierquin B, et al: Radical radiation therapy of breast cancer. Int J Radiat Oncol Biol Phys 6:17, 1980.
73. Porritt A: Early carcinoma of the breast. Br J Surg 51:214, 1964.
74. Prosnitz LR, Goldenberg IS, Packard RA, Levene MB, Harris J, Hellman S, Wallner PE, Brady LW, Mansfield CM, Kramer S: Radiation therapy as initial treatment for early stage cancer of the breast without mastectomy. Cancer 39:917–923, 1977.
75. Schnitt SJ, Connolly JL, Harris JR, Hellman S, Cohen RB: Pathologic predictors of early local recurrence in stage I and II breast cancer treated by primary radiation therapy. Cancer 53:1049–1057, 1984.
76. Sorace RA, Bagley CS, Lichter AS, Danforth DN, Wesley MW, Young RC, Lippman ME: The management of nonmetastatic locally advanced breast cancer using primary induction chemotherapy with hormonal synchronization followed by radiation therapy with or without debulking surgery. World J Surg 9:775–785, 1985.
77. Sugarbaker ED: Extended radical mastectomy. Its superiority in the treatment of breast cancer. JAMA 187:96–99, 1964.
78. Urban JA: Discussion on radical mastectomy in breast cancer with supraclavicular and/or internal mammary node dissection. Proc Natl Cancer Conf 2:243, 1952.
79. Veronesi U, Marubini E, Del Vecchio M, Manzari A, Andreola S, Greco M, Luini A, Merson M, Saccozzi R, Rilke F: Local recurrences and distant metastases after conservative breast cancer treatments: Partly independent events. J Natl Cancer Inst 87:19–27, 1995.
80. Veronesi U, Saccozzi R, Del Vecchio M, Banfi A, Clemente C, De Lena M, Gallus G, Greco M, Luini A, Marubini E, Muscolino G, Rilke F, Salvadori B, Zecchini A, Zucali R: Comparing radical mastectomy with quadrantectomy, axillary dissection, and radiotherapy in patients with small cancers of the breast. N Engl J Med 305:6–11, 1981.
81. Veronesi U, Salvadori B, Luini A, Greco M, Saccozzi R, Del Vecchio M, Mariani L, Zurrida S, Rilke F: Breast conservation is a safe method in patients with small cancer of the breast. Long-term results of three randomised trials on 1,973 patients. Eur J Cancer 31A:1574–1579, 1995.
82. Veronesi U, Zingo L: Extended mastectomy for cancer of the breast. Cancer 20:677–680, 1967.
83. Virchow R: Cellular Pathology. Translated by Frank Chase. Philadelphia, JB Lippincott, 1863.
84. Volcoq JR, et al: The outcome of treatment of tumorectomy and radiotherapy of patients with operable breast cancer. Radiat Oncol Biol Phys 7:1327, 1981.
85. Wangensteen OH: Super-radical operation for breast cancer in the patient with lymph node involvement. Proc Natl Cancer Conf 2:230, 1952.
86. Weber E, Hellman S: Radiation as primary treatment for local control of breast carcinoma. A progress report. JAMA 234:608–611, 1975.
87. Whelan T, Clark R, Roberts R, Levine M, Foster G: Ipsilateral breast tumor recurrence postlumpectomy is predictive of subsequent mortality: Results from a randomized trial. Int J Radiat Oncol Biol Phys 30:11–16, 1994.

CHAPTER 47
EXTENDED SIMPLE MASTECTOMY

Edward M. Copeland III, M.D. / Kirby I. Bland, M.D.

The surgical definition of extended simple mastectomy is removal of the breast in continuity with Level I lymph nodes. In this procedure, the surgeon deliberately leaves intact Levels II and III lymph nodes of the axilla. The need for such an operation arises when radiation therapy to the apical axilla and supraclavicular region is indicated in conjunction with an axillary dissection or when an axillary lymph node sampling is required at the time of an indicated total mastectomy.

In 1972, Charles McBride[4] of the M.D. Anderson Hospital popularized the operation, although a look at the specimen photographed in Halsted's initial description of the radical mastectomy indicates the contents of the procedure may have been only the breast and Level I lymph nodes.[2] No chest wall muscles are visible.

Radiation therapy to the axilla should not be used in conjunction with complete surgical dissection (Patey operation) of the axilla. Major lymphatic channels are removed surgically, and collateral channels draining the arm are damaged by radiation therapy. The result is symptomatic lymphedema of the ipsilateral extremity. When the surgeon determines that all disease cannot be removed from the axilla by any surgical procedure and that radiation therapy to this area is inevitable, then only the bulky metastatic disease in Level I and Level II lymph nodes should be removed surgically. As a rule, moderate doses of radiation therapy sterilize lymph nodes 1 cm or smaller in size; therefore metastatic cancer in smaller, centrally located axillary lymph nodes (high Level II and Level III), often attached to or invasive of axillary structures and not adequately removed surgically, is sterilized by radiation therapy. By such a combination of therapeutic modalities, the entire axilla is treated with minimal overlap of radiation portals with the surgically dissected portion of the axilla. The entire axilla is irradiated with less chance of resultant symptomatic lymphedema.

The operation is ideally suited to the treatment of advanced stage III and inflammatory breast cancer. Preoperative chemotherapy reduces the size of axillary metastases and often reduces the size of the primary lesion, making operation possible. Even if a complete response to chemotherapy is obtained, extended simple mastectomy is still recommended, because the majority of patients will have microscopic residual breast cancer.[1, 3] Radiation therapy to the chest wall, apical axilla, and internal mammary and supraclavicular lymph nodes is used postoperatively to decrease the incidence of chest wall recurrence. Radiation therapy should start as soon as the wound has healed adequately. Consequently, thick skin flaps should be elevated, using the plane of the retinaculae cutis. All attempts to prevent skin slough should be employed. Because radiation therapy will be used, the skin incision to initiate the skin flaps can be relatively close to the tumor mass, because any residual disease remaining after the dissection will be in the radiation treatment field.

Extended simple mastectomy is also indicated when preoperative radiation therapy (with or without chemotherapy) is employed with treatment fields that cover the apical axilla or the supraclavicular region. A therapeutic dose of radiation should sterilize these areas. Surgical dissection of high Level II and Level III lymph nodes adds minimal therapeutic benefit and dramatically increases (seven- to tenfold) the incidence of symptomatic lymphedema of the ipsilateral arm.

Axillary lymph node dissection is usually not necessary when treating carcinoma *in situ* unless the disease is multifocal or has a large component of comedo carcinoma with necrosis. In both instances, multiple microscopic foci of invasive breast cancer may coexist with the *in situ* component and have the potential to metastasize to axillary lymph nodes. If total mastectomy is the treatment selected for the breast, the en bloc Level I axillary lymph node dissection adds minimum morbidity, gives adequate information as to the pathological status of the axilla, and allows easy access to the subpectoral area for breast reconstruction.

TECHNIQUE

The arm is draped free so that the elbow may be flexed or extended and the arm adducted across the chest wall. A roll is placed parallel to the thoracic spine beneath the ipsilateral scapula.

The orientation of the skin incision is somewhat dictated by the location of the tumor mass. To minimize bleeding of the inferior incision while the superior flap is developed, the superior flap is elevated first, before beginning the incision that outlines the inferior flap. Medially, the upper margin of the superior flap is the medial half of the clavicle; laterally, it is the deltopectoral triangle and cephalic vein. The lateral portion of the superior flap is developed until the anterior edge of the latissimus dorsi muscle is identified, at which point the superior flap is developed laterally and superiorly following the anterior edge of the latissimus dorsi muscle cephalad (Fig. 47–1). As the dissection continues toward the axilla, the major branch of the intercostobrachial nerve is identified and sacrificed if multiple clinically positive

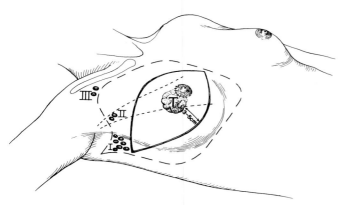

Figure 47–1 *Limits of dissection for the extended simple mastectomy (dotted line). The dissection is inclusive of tumor and overlying skin, with an adequate skin margin to allow primary wound closure. Only Level I and lower Level II nodes are dissected en bloc with the breast.*

lymph nodes are present. This nerve is composed of fibers from the lateral cutaneous branches of the second and third intercostal nerves and runs at right angles and anterior to the latissimus dorsi muscle. It should not be confused with either the thoracodorsal or long thoracic nerve. If the axilla is clinically negative, often the intercostobrachial nerve can be spared to reduce postoperative paresthesias on the medial side of the upper arm. The dissection is continued cephalad following the anterior border of the latissimus dorsi muscles until the white tendon of the latissimus dorsi muscle is identified. Immediately superior and anterior to this tendon, the axillary vein is identified and exposed.

Attention is then turned to dissection of the inferior flap, a portion of the operation that should proceed expeditiously, because the investing fascia of the breast is usually easy to identify inferiorly, and the position of the anterior border of the latissimus dorsi muscle is known laterally. In raising the skin flaps medially, the plane of penetration of the pectoralis major fascia by the perforating branches of the internal mammary vessel should be used as a guide for the medial extension of the dissection. Several of these branches often can be preserved, and the dissection need not extend to the middle of the sternum to remove all breast tissue.

The breast is dissected free from the pectoralis major muscle, beginning superomedially and progressing inferolaterally until the lateral border of the muscle is identified almost in its entirety (except for the superiormost portion, which crosses anterior and lateral to the latissimus dorsi muscle to insert on the humerus).

Allis clamps are placed on the lateral border of the pectoralis major muscle, and the muscle is retracted anteriorly and medially. Dissection is continued lateral and posterior to the pectoralis major muscle to identify the lateral border of the pectoralis minor muscle. The entire innervation of the pectoralis major and minor muscles can be preserved in this operation. The medial pectoral nerve is identified coursing lateral to (or penetrating) the pectoralis mi-

nor muscle at approximately the juncture between the superior one third and inferior two thirds of the pectoralis major muscle. Only rarely is the medially placed lateral pectoral nerve visualized in this procedure, because Level II and Level III nodes are incompletely exposed. The (lateral) neurovascular bundle that contains the medial pectoral nerve can be easily severed inadvertently. It represents an important landmark as it courses posterior to the pectoralis minor muscle with vascular and neural origin from the thoracoacromial trunk of the axillary artery, the axillary vein, and the medial cord of the brachial plexus.

The clavipectoral fascia lateral to the pectoralis minor muscle is opened, and the axillary vein is again identified.

Working laterally along the axillary vein, the venous tributaries coursing inferiorly are divided and ligated. Laterally, the neurovascular bundle to the latissimus dorsi muscle is identified; this bundle contains the thoracodorsal nerve and major branches of the subscapular artery and vein. The lateral thoracic artery is usually identified just medial to it and is removed with the specimen. The full extent of the thoracodorsal neurovascular bundle is often best demonstrated by dissecting the fibrofatty tissue from the anterior border of the latissimus dorsi muscle and retracting it laterally and inferiorly. At the site of confluence of the thoracodorsal neurovascular trunk with the latissimus dorsi muscle, a venous tributary courses medially to join the chest wall. At this site, with meticulous dissection in a plane parallel with the long axis of the patient, the long thoracic nerve to the serratus anterior muscle (respiratory nerve of Bell) is best identified. The long thoracic nerve is traced superiorly until it exits the operative field posterior to the axillary vein.

The axillary contents are removed from the serratus anterior muscle anterior and medial to the long thoracic nerve. The superior extent of the axillary dissection was defined previously by the axillary vein, and the medial extent of the dissection is represented by the lateral borders of the pectoralis major and minor muscles as well as the medial pectoral nerve and accompanying vascular structures. When operating on a patient with stage III AB or inflammatory breast cancer who is to receive postoperative radiation therapy, any lymph nodes that are clinically positive and larger than 1 cm in size should be removed from beneath the pectoralis minor muscle (within Level II lymph nodes). As the Level I axillary contents are removed from the serratus anterior muscle, the lateral cutaneous branches of the second and third intercostal nerves and accompanying vascular structures are identified. The specimen is removed from the operative field and the wound is irrigated copiously with warm saline.

When mastectomy is indicated for noninvasive or microinvasive breast cancer, the dissection can be performed with a skin-sparing incision that circumnavigates the nipple and extends radially for enough length to allow adequate visualization of the skin flaps to ensure that all visible breast tissue is removed from the flaps and that the axilla can be dissected safely. The skin-sparing incision allows the native skin and areola to be used during autologous tissue reconstruction simultaneous with the oncologic surgical procedure. Removal of all breast tissue to include the nipple and the recent biopsy scar (if one exists) in the specimen are imperative.

Instruments and gloves are discarded for clean ones. Two large-bore suction catheters are inserted, one anterior to the pectoralis major muscle and the other posterior to it within the dissected axilla. The drains are sutured in place at the skin entrance site. The wound is closed with interrupted absorbable sutures in the subcutaneous tissue, and the skin is closed with staples or optional subcuticular absorbable sutures. Continuous suction is maintained on the drains by attachment to a suction apparatus that generates approximately 60 cm of water-negative pressure, and a pressure dressing is applied to be removed within 48 hours. The drains are removed when their output falls below 20 ml per 24 hours. Following drain removal, shoulder exercises are begun.

References

1. Bonadonna G, Valagussa P, Zambetti M, Zucali R: Locally advanced breast cancer: 10-year results after combined treatment. Proc Am Soc Clin Oncol 7:9, 1988.
2. Halsted WS: The results of operations for the cure of cancer of the breast performed at the Johns Hopkins Hospital from June 1889, to January 1894. Ann Surg 20:497–555, 1894.
3. Manji M, Ragaz J, Worth A, Plenderleith IH, Harman J, Knowling M, Olivotto I, Basco V: Is mastectomy indicated in patients with stage III breast cancer treated with preoperative (neoadjuvant) therapy? Proc Am Soc Clin Oncol 7:36, 1988.
4. McBride CM: Extended simple mastectomy: anatomic definition and uses. South Med J 65:1427–1431, 1972.

CHAPTER 48

THERAPEUTIC VALUE OF AXILLARY LYMPH NODE DISSECTION FOR BREAST CANCER

Charu Taneja, M.D. / Bernard Gardner, M.D., F.A.C.S.

LYMPHATIC DRAINAGE OF THE BREAST

The breast is drained by a network of intercommunicating lymphatic channels from the walls of the lactiferous ducts and subcutaneous, subareolar, and deep plexus mainly into the axillary and the internal mammary groups of lymph nodes. Some lymphatic drainage also occurs to the contralateral breast via the lymphatics of the anterior abdominal wall and the diaphragm, but contralateral breast metastases are rarely seen clinically except in instances of widespread involvement. Studies show that both the axillary and internal mammary nodes receive lymph from all quadrants of the breast, with the axilla receiving 75 percent of the lymph and the internal mammary nodes receiving 25 percent. There is, however, a greater tendency for tumors in the medial quadrant to drain to the internal mammary nodes.[31]

The *axillary lymph nodes* receive approximately 75 percent of the drainage from the breast as well as drainage from the upper extremity and ipsilateral thorax. These lymph nodes are divided into six groups according to their position relative to the axillary vein and its tributaries.

1. *Axillary vein or lateral group of lymph nodes.* These are four to six nodes along the medial side of the axillary vein. They mainly receive lymphatic drainage from the upper extremity.

2. *External mammary group.* These are also known as the *anterior* or *pectoral* nodes. They are five to six nodes along the lower border of the pectoralis minor on the medial wall of the axilla, contiguous with the lateral thoracic vessels. They receive the majority of the lymph from the breast.

3. *Scapular or posterior group.* These are also known as the *subscapular* nodes. They are five to seven nodes along the posterior wall of the axilla along the subscapular vessels. They receive lymph from the axillary tail, lower back of the neck and shoulder, and the upper half of the trunk posteriorly.

4. *Central group of nodes.* These are three to four large nodes embedded in the fat in the center of the axilla, immediately posterior to the pectoralis minor. These receive lymph from the previously mentioned groups of nodes, as well as directly from the breast.

5. *Apical or subclavicular group of nodes.* These are nodes posterior and superior to the upper border of the pectoralis minor. They receive lymph from all the groups of axillary nodes and then drain via the subclavian trunk into the supraclavicular nodes and the thoracic and right lymphatic ducts. These nodes are not accessible without division of the pectoralis minor muscle.

6. *Interpectoral or Rotter's nodes.* These are one to four nodes between the pectoralis major and minor, along the branches of the thoracoacromial vessels and in direct line with the apical nodes of the axilla. They drain into the central and subclavicular nodes.

Surgeons also divide the axillary lymph nodes into three levels based on their relation to the pectoralis minor muscle:

- *Level 1:* Nodes below or lateral to the lower border of the pectoralis minor and medial to the latissimus dorsi muscle (including the axillary vein, external mammary, and scapular groups of nodes).
- *Level 2:* Nodes behind the pectoralis minor (central group of nodes).
- *Level 3:* Nodes above or medial to the upper border of the pectoralis minor and below the costoclavicular or Halsted's ligament (subclavicular group of nodes), including the apical nodes.

Level 1 nodes are the most numerous and Level 3 nodes the least. Approximately 60 percent of the axillary lymph nodes are present in Level 1, 20 percent in Level 2, and 20 percent in Level 3.[24]

The *internal mammary nodes* are few in number and lie along the internal mammary vessels deep to the plane of the costal cartilages. These nodes drain into the veins directly or via the major lymphatic ducts.

HISTORY OF NODE TREATMENT

The role of axillary dissection in the management of breast carcinoma was first advocated by the German surgeon Lorenz Heister, in the eighteenth century.[83] Over the next century, further progress was made in understanding the lymphatic drainage of the breast. In 1875 Richard von Volkmann advocated dissection of the axillary space after he observed the communication of the mammary lymphatics with the axillary nodes through the pectoral fascia.[118]

Charles Moore,[86] a surgeon at the Middlesex Hospital in London, believed that the cure of breast carcinoma was possible only when the "diseased glands" were removed along with the breast. Banks[8] supported Moore's view and, recognizing the occult involvement of the axillary nodes, said that the axillary nodes should be removed even when they were not clinically involved. In 1894 Meyer[84] and Halsted[51, 52] simultaneously described the radical mastectomy and demonstrated better regional control and survival rates with this procedure.

The radical mastectomy procedure subsequently underwent many modifications. In the 1930s Patey[91, 92] described his modification of preserving the pectoralis major muscles. Auchincloss[5] and Madden[76] preserved both the pectoralis major and minor muscles, with improved cosmesis but a resulting decrease in the number of lymph nodes removed as compared with the standard radical mastectomy.

Role of Extended Radical Dissection

In 1907 Halsted[53] reviewed his experience and recognized the fact that removal of the nodes might not affect survival when the nodes were demonstrably involved. Wangensteen[128] extended lymphatic dissection to include the supraclavicular, internal mammary, and mediastinal nodes. Dahl-Iverson[23] further refined internal mammary dissection to an extrapleural approach. However, these approaches were subsequently shown not to affect survival.[62, 63, 123]

Urban,[21, 120] in several publications, advocated the routine resection of internal mammary nodes for medial lesions. He treated moderate numbers of patients with 10-year survival rates of 58 percent when axillary nodes were negative and internal mammary nodes were positive and 53 percent when both groups of nodes were positive.[21] However, these were retrospective analyses. A randomized prospective study of internal mammary node resection versus simple mastectomy reported by Kaae and Johansen[62, 63] in 1962 demonstrated no survival advantage for the more radical resection.

Role of Radiation Therapy

Radiation to the breast was applied within months of the discovery of X rays by Roentgen in 1895. By the 1920s James Ewing was questioning the concept of radical operations on the breast. Sir Geoffrey Keynes[64] was the first to report that radiation was equivalent to mastectomy in terms of patient survival. By the 1940s radiation therapy was being used extensively for the treatment of breast cancer. In Edinburgh, McWhirter[81] introduced simple mastectomy with postoperative external-beam radiation to the axilla instead of surgical dissection, with results comparable to those of radical mastectomy.

ACCURATE STAGING

Comparison of Results When Different Studies Use Different Methods of Staging

The clinical assessment of axillary nodal status is unreliable in one third of patients with a low sensitivity and specificity.[33, 49, 74] Approximately 27 percent of axillae thought to be positive on clinical examination are found to be free of metastatic disease, whereas 38 percent of clinically uninvolved axillae have metastases on pathological examination.[106] The inaccuracy of clinical examination is increased further when done after fine needle aspiration cytology (FNAC) for the primary lesion, as this causes reactive lymph node hyperplasia. Imaging of the axilla with ultrasonography, scintigraphy, or positron emission tomography to detect the presence of lymph node metastases has not contributed significantly to the preoperative detection of axillary involvement.[22, 80, 117]

The pathological staging of the axilla is the most important prognostic factor, with survival rate being related to axillary node status rather than size of the tumor in one series.[2] In a 30-year follow-up of patients undergoing radical mastectomy at the Memorial Sloan-Kettering Cancer Center, patients with negative nodes had a 75 percent 30-year survival rate compared with 40 percent for patients with involvement of the lower axillary nodes. However, subsequent studies have shown that the number of nodes with metastases increases with the size of the primary lesion and that this is more important than the level of the nodes in determining prognosis.[9, 112]

Barth and coworkers[9] found that the number of involved nodes increased with the size of the primary tumor but that the number of nodes and the size of the tumor were independent prognostic variables. The number of involved nodes was divided into categories of zero, one to three, and four or more. Overall survival rates were 94 percent, 85 percent, and 58 percent, respectively, on a median follow-up period of 6.9 years. This difference was statistically significant. Disease-free survival for these groups was 83 percent, 73 percent, and 38 percent, respectively. These findings confirmed those of Smith and coworkers,[112] who also found that (1) there was a significant correlation between survival and the number of positive nodes and (2) the incidence of local recurrence was higher in patients with more than five positive nodes. When more than ten nodes are positive, and no adjuvant therapy is used, the 5-year survival rate is 39–55 percent, and at 10 to 15 years the survival rate is 12 percent.[126] With the use of systemic therapy, the reduction in mortality for patients with one to three positive nodes is 30 percent, whereas for those with less than ten positive nodes, the reduction in mortality is only 10 percent in short-term studies. Thus, although systemic therapy would be used for both these groups of patients, the estimated benefit in survival may not be significant in the group with more lymph node involvement.

The probability of all three levels of nodes being involved increases with the size of the primary tumor, being 11.3 percent with a T1 primary tumor and 32.1 percent with a T3 tumor. If a single node is the site of metastasis, the probability of the other levels being involved is low (8 percent), but this probability increases to 25 percent when two nodes are involved.[123]

Despite arguments about its therapeutic value, most clinicians agree as to the need for axillary staging.

Use of Adjuvant Treatment

Axillary lymph node dissection determines the need for adjuvant or systemic therapy in clinically node-negative patients and favorable-result primary biopsies. The number of positive nodes at the time of axillary dissection may determine the chemotherapy regimen used. In the axillary node-negative patient, recommendations for chemotherapy are modified to exclude the alkylating agents so as to avoid toxicity and the late development of other malignancies. The survival benefit is very small, 3 percent to 4 percent at best. Such patients should receive chemotherapy as part of a clinical trial unless there are other prognostic markers (S-phase function, nuclear grade, size of primary tumor, vascular invasion, and so forth) that indicate a poor prognosis.

For some investigators, the presence of matted nodes in the axilla is an indication for the use of preoperative induction chemotherapy followed by surgery with axillary dissection. The number of nodes in the axilla remaining positive after induction chemotherapy has prognostic significance. Patients with four or more positive nodes have a disease-free survival rate similar to that of patients with ten or more positive nodes.[126] Patients with more than ten positive nodes may be candidates for treatment with high-dose chemotherapy with autologous bone marrow transplantation with or without consolidation with high-dose intensification chemotherapy (cisplatin, etoposide, and cyclophosphamide).[126]

Tamoxifen is the standard of care in postmenopausal women regardless of lymph node status because of its low toxicity and evidence suggesting it might increase survival.[7] This is a subject under study at the time of this writing.

EXTENT OF LYMPHADENECTOMY NECESSARY FOR STAGING

Definition of Terms Used in Staging Procedures[65]

Table 48–1 presents the various terms used to describe the extent of axillary surgery.

Sampling. This is defined as the removal of nodes from the lower axilla without the definition of anatomical boundaries. *Pectoral node biopsy* is the term applied to the removal of the nodes around the axillary tail, probably some or all being Level 1.[41] It applies to the random, or blind, sampling of the nodes when no defined anatomical landmarks are used. Some studies use the term "sampling" when the procedure used is actually a low axillary dissection.[48] This use of terminology may bias the results obtained. However, most studies agree that a minimum of three to five nodes must be removed to stage the axilla adequately.[20, 48] When fewer than three nodes are studied, the number of false-negative results increases significantly. In the series of Steele and coworkers[113] 135 patients were randomized to either undergo a complete axillary dissection or receive no further therapy to the axilla after a sampling procedure. Steele and coworkers[113] observed that the axillary clearance did not add to the number of patients known to be node-positive. They concluded that the randomization of the patients is an important variable, because when the operating surgeon is aware that a complete axillary clearance is going to follow the sampling procedure, he or she might take less care to ensure that an adequate sampling is carried out.[66] Conversely, if no axillary dissection is to be carried out, the sampling procedure might be more extensive.

The advantage of sampling is that with modern screening techniques, and a decrease in the size of the primary lesion, approximately two thirds of all patients are node-negative. Sampling might also decrease the morbidity associated with complete axillary dissection (a strong advantage) or the practice of blindly giving radiotherapy to all patients. Furthermore, sampling could be used to determine nodal status and, followed by irradiation in node-positive patients, leave axillary dissection for the control of recurrences. However, when the primary sampling procedure is more extensive than planned, the use of radiotherapy may contribute to serious long-term morbidity in the arm.[48] Furthermore, radiotherapy is not effective when positive nodes are palpable.

The use of intraoperative imprint cytology or frozen sections to determine the need for further surgery to the axilla can increase the accuracy of the

TABLE 48–1.   STAGING TECHNIQUES FOR BREAST CANCER

Staging Technique	Advantages	Disadvantages	Error Rate in Missing Positive Axillae (%)
Sampling	Low morbidity; X-ray treatment still possible	Leaves disease behind	24
Low Axillary Dissection	Use for Level 1 nodes only; low morbidity; >90% accurate in identifying positive axillae	Leaves disease behind. Skip metastases in 5% of cases	5–10
Level 1 and 2 Dissection	99% accurate in identifying positive axillae	Moderate morbidity; X-ray treatment should not be used in axillae	1–2
Full Axillary Dissection	No recurrence in axillae; 100% accurate in identifying positive axillae	Arm edema in small percent of cases; X-ray treatment should not be used in axillae	0

sampling procedure from 86 percent to 90 percent[38] and can make it possible to proceed with axillary clearance at the same time. Nevertheless, a significant number of patients would still be left with positive nodes, and the procedure is time-consuming and not generally available.

The overall error of the sampling procedure has been reported as 24 percent owing to a failure to identify any nodal tissue in 10 percent of cases, and thus underestimating the number of positive nodes in 6 percent.[66] In four of 30 patients (13 percent) the sample was node-negative, but a complete axillary clearance demonstrated node-positivity. Therefore, the disadvantages of axillary sampling are (1) failure to identify node-positive patients who may benefit from axillary dissection and (2) failure to assess the total number of positive nodes, which may be an indication for more intensive chemotherapy and perhaps with bone marrow transplantation.

Low Axillary Dissection. This is defined as en bloc resection of Level 1 nodes of the axilla from the border of the latissimus dorsi to the lateral border of the pectoralis minor muscle medially and the axillary vein superiorly. It will identify 99 percent of all positive-node patients without incurring the higher rate of lymphedema associated with complete axillary dissection.[71] However, "skip metastases" occur in 3–5 percent of patients. Identification of the node-positive patient is not synonymous with removal of all nodal disease.

Level 1 and 2 Dissection. This is defined as en bloc resection of the low and middle portions of the axilla by relaxing and retracting the pectoralis minor muscle. Dissection extends from the latissimus dorsi to the medial border of the pectoralis minor muscle and the axillary vein cephalad. It is difficult to dissect behind the pectoralis minor if it is intact.

Full Axillary Dissection. This is a removal of the entire axillary contents, from the latissimus dorsi to the subclavius muscle (Halsted's ligament) medially with clearance of the axillary vein.

Effect of Technique of Axillary Dissection. The number of lymph nodes identified in the axillary dissection specimen depends on a number of factors, with the extent of the primary surgery being one of the major determinants. In the study of Veronesi and coworkers[123] the average number of nodes per patient was 20.5, but no significant difference was found between the Halsted and modified radical (Patey[91]) mastectomies as compared with quadrantectomy and axillary dissection in the number of nodes removed. In the series of Rosen and colleagues,[104] whereas the average number of nodes identified was similar (mean number of nodes was 21), there was a difference with the type of procedure performed: radical and extended mastectomies yielded more nodes than modified mastectomy. The mean number of nodes was 20 ± 8 for modified radical, 22 ± 7 for standard radical, and 23 ± 8 for extended radical. These differences were statistically significant. However, this was not a randomized study, and there was probably a bias on the part of the operating surgeon, with modified mastectomy being performed for stage I and II disease and standard radical mastectomy being performed for more advanced disease. Extended mastectomy was done only for patients with central and medial lesions.

Division of the pectoralis minor may not increase the number of nodes obtained,[82, 109, 123] but this issue has not been studied in a randomized fashion. In many patients the pectoralis minor tightly covers the axillary vein and makes it difficult to obtain the relaxation necessary to dissect behind or medial to it. The division of this muscle opens the axilla to direct vision and produces no noticeable disability for the patient.

In the NSABP-B04 trial, the average number of nodes identified varied from seven to 30 at various centers. This variation in the number of nodes may be due to a variation in the surgical technique or in the ability of the pathologist to identify the nodes in the surgical specimen. The diligence of the pathologist in finding axillary nodes is of paramount significance in all these studies. Surgical residents dissecting an axillary specimen while rotating on pathology routinely find 30 to 40 nodes in node-positive patients.

Pathological processing of the specimen has a major effect on the number of nodes found in the specimen. Chemical clearing of the specimen yields a greater number of nodes, but it is a laborious and expensive procedure. It is also doubtful whether the increased number of nodes thus identified will provide more accurate information about the presence of axillary metastases. The use of multiple sectioning also demonstrates the presence of micrometastases in 20 percent of otherwise uninvolved nodes, but this too is a very time-consuming and expensive process.[65]

At this time it is appropriate to discuss the characteristics of the surgical levels reported in many studies. When seen at the operating table, these levels may not correlate with the levels defined by the pathologist. With the breast lying on the axillary contents in the pathology laboratory, the nodes closest to the breast are actually Level 3. Therefore, studies reporting level involvement must rely on the surgeon carefully labeling the specimen before removing it from the patient. Because in the modified mastectomy the pectoralis minor is not removed, it is impossible for the pathologist to reconstruct the precise levels of involvement. Furthermore, Rotter's nodes, if they are removed at all, will always be submitted as a separate specimen as they cannot be removed in continuity with the axillary contents in a modified radical mastectomy. Consequently, only studies such as those reported by Rosen and coworkers,[104] where the surgeon labeled the specimen at operation, are valuable in demonstrating the orderly progression of lymph nodes and rarity of skip metastases.

The usefulness of sampling is questioned because

of the failure of the procedure to identify metastases in some cases[41] and the frequency of axillary failure when sampling is performed before a complete axillary dissection.[66, 105]

Less than complete axillary dissection fails to identify nodal metastases in 25–42 percent of patients who undergo axillary lymph node biopsy and in 14–30 percent of node-positive patients who undergo sampling. A Level 1 and 2 dissection is 95 percent accurate in identifying metastases but leaves behind micrometastases in the Level 3 nodes in 14–24 percent of patients and should be done only in clinically negative axillae.[41, 65, 66, 96]

One series showed that the failure to obtain nodes at the time of axillary sampling could be surgeon-dependent; when the surgeon is responsible for identifying at least four nodes in the specimen from the axillary sampling, nodes can be identified in 99.5 percent of cases.[113] This problem of failing to identify nodal metastases is further increased by the fact that different studies use different terms for the procedures of axillary biopsy and sampling. As these terms are inexact, they should not be used without defining the extent of dissection in anatomical terms of levels or in reference to landmarks within the axilla.

PRIMARY TUMOR CHARACTERISTICS IN RELATION TO AXILLARY METASTASES

The factor most strongly related to the presence or absence of axillary node involvement is the size of the primary tumor.* The reported incidence for a T1 tumor is 21–35 percent.[18] When the size of the primary tumor is 0–0.5 cm, the incidence of lymph node positivity is 3–20 percent,[15, 102, 119] and this incidence increases from 10–19 percent for all tumors less than 1 cm to 30–50 percent for larger tumors.[15, 18, 78, 79, 119, 127] Of all patients with positive nodes and a primary tumor less than 1 cm, 71 percent have only one to two positive nodes.[16, 115] Of those with positive nodes and a T1a, T1b, or T1c invasive tumor, 2 percent, 6 percent, and 9 percent, respectively, have more than three positive nodes.[15] The size of the invasive component is the predictor of lymph node metastasis rather than gross tumor size or volume. This fact is of great importance in cases of small tumors where the intraductal component could account for a sizeable portion of estimated tumor volume.[107]

A tubular histology of the primary tumor is associated with a low incidence of axillary node involvement.[16] The degree of tumor differentiation also affects nodal involvement. Incidence of node positivity is 14 percent for well-differentiated tumors as compared with 32 percent for moderately or poorly differentiated tumors.[6, 18, 25, 127] When the S-phase fraction is low, the incidence of lymph node positivity is 25 percent compared with 40 percent when it is high.[18, 97]

Lymphatic or vascular invasion from the primary tumor increases the incidence of nodal involvement from 20 percent to 64 percent and increases the number of nodes seen.[18, 72] Such invasion is also an independent prognostic variable associated with a significantly poorer prognosis in node-negative patients and a higher risk of death in node-positive patients.[73] Extracapsular metastases in the axillary node[28] are an important prognostic factor for survival in patients with one to three positive nodes. Extracapsular metastases do not influence locoregional recurrence in the axilla. The frequency of capsular invasion increases with the size of the metastases (none are found in patients with micrometastases).

Older patients are significantly more likely to have negative nodes, with nodal involvement present in 35 percent of patients younger than 60 years and in 21 percent of those older.[18, 73] Older patients are also more likely to have positive estrogen receptors, well-differentiated nuclear grade of the primary tumor, low S-phase fractions, and no lymphatic or vascular invasion.[18] Other studies have shown no effect of age on the incidence of axillary node involvement,[6] although younger patients have an overall poorer prognosis. Previous pregnancies also constitute an independent variable increasing the risk of axillary metastases.[73]

The *HER-2*/neu gene, a member of the *ERBB* oncogene family, is overexpressed in approximately 30–35 percent of patients with breast cancer. The amplification of this gene correlates with the number of positive nodes and is an independent prognostic variable in determining the overall survival and the time until relapse in node-positive patients.[85, 111] Newer modalities, such as the detection of altered glycosylation as a predictor of axillary involvement, need further validation.[12]

In a series of 263 patients with T1 tumors, Chadha and coworkers[18] found that size of tumor, histological subtype, nuclear grade, DNA ploidy, S-phase fraction, and presence of lymphatic or vascular invasion all correlated with the presence of axillary involvement. However, multivariate analysis showed that only the size of the primary tumor and the presence of lymphatic or vascular invasion from the primary tumor were independent variables affecting the presence of axillary metastases. In the presence of a tumor larger than 1 cm with lymphatic or vascular invasion, 68 percent of patients had axillary involvement, compared with 9 percent when the tumor was less than 1 cm with no lymphatic or vascular involvement.

SENTINEL LYMPH NODE DISSECTION

There has been increasing interest in the identification and significance of the "sentinel" node in breast carcinoma ever since Morton and researchers[88, 89] demonstrated the accuracy of sentinel lymphadenectomy in detecting metastasis in melanoma. In brief, the technique consists of injecting 3–5 ml of a vital

---

*See references 6, 18, 19, 28, 67, 73, 107.

dye into the breast lesion, or into its cavity if the lesion has already been excised, and 5 minutes later identifying the blue-staining lymphatic channels in the axilla through a transverse incision. These lymphatics are then followed to the first lymph node draining the primary site (the sentinel node). If the sentinel node is negative, then theoretically the rest of the nodes in the lymphatic basin should also be negative.

In the series of Giuliano and coworkers,[47] the sentinel lymph node could be accurately identified in 65.5 percent of 174 patients, and in 38 percent of patients with clinically negative but pathologically positive axillae, the sentinel node was the only positive node found. When it could be identified, the sentinel node was 95.6 percent accurate in predicting axillary nodal status. False-negative rate was 4.3 percent (five patients), with all these cases occurring earlier in the series. On retrospective review with the use of immunohistochemical techniques, the tissue was found to have been wrongly identified as nodal tissue in three patients (60 percent) as the amount of lymphoid tissue was less than 2 mm. One of the remaining two patients was found to be positive for metastatic disease with immunohistochemical techniques, and the other was found to be negative. The location of the sentinel node within the lymphatic basin was variable. On analysis, in 23.7 percent of cases the sentinel node was in Level 2 (skip metastasis) and would probably have been missed by random sampling.

A later series examined the role of immunohistochemical staining and multiple sectioning of the sentinel node to facilitate the pathological staging of the axilla in patients with breast carcinoma.[46] A prospective randomized study was performed comparing the use of these techniques in the sentinel node with the current gold standard—axillary dissection of Level 1 to 2 nodes and some Level 3 nodes. To overcome the problem of wrong identification of blue-stained fatty tissue as the sentinel lymph node, the tissue was subjected to frozen section examination in this study.[46] There was a significantly higher incidence of axillary metastases in the group undergoing sentinel lymphadenectomy followed by axillary lymphadenectomy (SLND) as compared with the axillary lymphadenectomy group (ALND)—42 percent versus 29.1 percent. There was also a significantly higher incidence of micrometastases (less than 2 mm) in the node-positive SLND group (38.2 percent versus 10.3 percent in the ALND group). Of these, 42.3 percent of the micrometastases in the SLND group were identified only on immunohistochemical staining for cytokeratin in the sentinel lymph node.

A major criticism of this study is that the sentinel node underwent serial sectioning while the other nodes underwent single-section sampling during the process of looking for metastases. In many of these patients the "positive" axilla actually consisted of the sentinel node itself. It is therefore not possible to fully evaluate this technique.

In a study by Krag and coworkers,[68] preoperative lymphoscintigraphy was used to identify the sentinel node with similar results. The combined use of preoperative lymphoscintigraphy using a hand-held gamma probe with the injection of a vital dye intracutaneously in patients with melanoma facilitated the identification of the sentinel node.[121] This approach decreases the technical expertise required to identify and follow the lymphatics to the sentinel node, as it is possible to localize the sentinel node preoperatively with the gamma probe and then incise right on top of it. This method may have an application in treating breast carcinoma as well.

The use of immunohistochemical methods and multiple sectioning facilitates the detection of axillary metastases and micrometastases. However, these methods are too expensive and time-consuming to apply to all the nodes in the ALND specimen. Identification of the sentinel node, the node most likely to bear metastatic disease, makes the application of these techniques more practical. This finding also suggests that only patients with metastatic disease in the sentinel node undergo further treatment of the axilla to minimize the morbidity associated with unnecessary radiation therapy or ALND. A further advantage of this procedure is that it can be done under local anesthesia. The false-negative rate of 3–4 percent in the study of Giuliano is the same as the incidence of Level 3 metastasis that most surgeons will miss with a routine Level 1 and 2 dissection. The probability of excising positive nodes in a clinically node-negative patient with the use of lymphatic mapping and sentinel lymphadenectomy was 61.9 percent compared with 17.5 percent by random sampling in the series of Giuliano and associates.[47]

A major disadvantage of the procedure is that in approximately 20 percent of patients it is not possible to correctly identify the sentinel node. There is a definite learning curve for this procedure, with the accuracy of detection of the sentinel lymph node increasing from 58.6 percent in the initial 87 cases to 78.6 percent in the last 50 cases in the series of Giuliano and coworkers.[47] The internal mammary nodes may account for some of the missed sentinel nodes, and the use of preoperative scintigraphy would possibly decrease this number. This study demonstrates that it may be possible to determine with minimal morbidity the extent of treatment required to treat a clinically negative axilla. However, while the new approach has an advantage over random sampling in the staging of a clinically negative axilla, it needs to be tested more extensively in prospective studies. There is a significant possibility of leaving positive nodes behind. At this time it is clear that the technique should not be recommended for clinical use.

CURE OF BREAST CANCER

The cure rate for all patients with breast cancer is 18 percent. The cure rate is 30 percent for patients with stage II disease and approximately 20–30 percent for patients with positive axillary nodes.[45, 61, 65] Studies show that the predicted survival from the date of locoregional recurrence is less for patients who experienced failure than for those who did not.[74] The maximum number of deaths resulting from breast cancer occur in the first decade after diagnosis, and then the rate declines.[90] Late deaths resulting from breast cancer continue to be seen after several decades.[6] Overall survival of these patients never equals that of age-matched controls.

Some women achieve a personal cure (die of another cause before succumbing to breast cancer). Statistics are further confounded by the fact that these patients are at a higher risk of developing a second malignancy such as cancers of the colon, lung, uterus, ovary, bladder, thyroid, or opposite breast. There is also an increased rate of cardiac deaths owing to the long-term effects of irradiation on the heart.

If all women with cancer developing in the contralateral breast are excluded, the survival rate at 20 years for stage I and II cancers smaller than 2 cm is 70–80 percent.[102] The relative survival is 1.0: (observed rate = expected rate at 15–25 years).[61] In one study the 30-year survival was 80 percent for postsurgical stage I patients (node-negative patients with tumors less than 2 cm) and 41 percent for stage II patients. These patients were all treated with locoregional therapy only. No late deaths occurred as a result of breast cancer on follow-up of 23 years in this study.[55]

Short-term data also suggest that the 5-year and 10-year survival rates for patients with breast cancer diagnosed in the 1980s are better than the survival rates for most patients in the 30-year follow-up studies who were diagnosed in the 1940s to 1970s. This may, in part, be due to the smaller size of the cancers detected during the 1980s because of more aggressive screening measures.[15]

In an analysis of 1024 patients, Gardner and Feldman[45] reported that after 7 years, regional (positive-node) patients had the same survival rate as negative-node patients. Thirty percent of the regional patients were alive at 10 years, which is remarkably similar to data from the Surveillance, Epidemiology and End Results (SEER) program and other studies. Furthermore, SEER data demonstrating conditional relative survival for 18,220 women supported this finding (Table 48–2). "Conditional relative survival" is the survival expectation relative to the general population after the patient has survived a given number of years. After 10 years, 30 percent of patients with regional disease were still alive in the SEER study. Moreover, the probability of a patient who had regional disease, surviving 10 years and living another 5 years (80 percent) was the same as for a patient who had survived, surviving to 20 years (82 percent) (Table 48–3).

DO POSITIVE NODES INDICATE DISSEMINATED DISEASE?

Clinical evidence suggests that breast cancer is a very heterogeneous disease, with some patients dying as a result of metastatic disease despite negative axillary nodes (25 percent), and another subset of patients surviving for a long time despite positive axillary nodes at initial presentation (35 percent of patients)[11] (Figure 48–1). The argument has been made that once positive lymph nodes have been demonstrated, the disease has disseminated, and local and regional treatment will not affect survival. Patients with untreated breast cancer have less than a 5 percent survival rate at 10 years.[10] Patients with known stage IV disease rarely survive 5 years. Yet, there is a distinct correlation between the survival of operable breast cancer patients and the number of positive nodes. How can one explain this correlation and the long survival of 30 percent of node-positive patients (overall), as well as the survival advantage of patients with micrometastases versus macrometastases unless the cancer has progressed from one group of nodes to the next *prior to systemic spread.*

TABLE 48–2. PROBABILITY DENSITIES FOR FIRST 10 YEARS AFTER DIAGNOSIS OF LOCAL OR REGIONAL BREAST CANCER

| Year | Localized Disease = 330 | | Regional Disease = 433 | |
	Probability of Death (%)	*95% C.I.*	*Probability of Death (%)*	*95% C.I.*
1	.058	.032–.084	.134	.103–.168
2	.067	.039–.095	.162	.126–.198
3	.048	.024–.072	.106	.076–.136
4	.076	.046–.106	.058	.036–.180
5	.030	.012–.048	.102	.072–.132
6	.033	.013–.053	.055	.032–.077
7	.055	.029–.081	.044	.024–.064
8	.018	.004–.032	.016	.004–.028
9	.024	.008–.040	.030	.014–.046
10	.023	.008–.038	.015	.001–.031

C.I. = confidence interval.
Gardner B, Ann Surg 218(3):270–278, 1993.

TABLE 48–3.   CONDITIONAL 5-YEAR RELATIVE SURVIVAL RATES FOR PATIENTS WHO SURVIVED THE INDICATED COMPLETE NUMBER OF YEARS AFTER SURGERY FOR BREAST CANCER (WHITE FEMALES DIAGNOSED 1950–1959)

Completed Years of Survival	Localized Disease		Regional Disease	
	No. of Cases	*Conditional Relative Survival Rate (%)*	*No. of Cases*	*Conditional Relative Survival Rate (%)*
0	6526	85	6531	55
1	6210	83	5775	55
2	5853	84	4892	59
5	4791	86	3167	68
10	3469	91	1847	80
15	2525	90	1219	82

From Surveillance, Epidemiology and End Results (SEER).

Therefore, in this chapter we have shunned the nihilistic attitude that no node-positive patients are ever cured in favor of the view that patients with nodal disease may be cured by nodal treatment along with treatment of the primary tumor.[45]

Negative Nodes

With the use of immunocytochemical techniques, tumor cells can be identified in the bone marrow aspirates of 23 percent of patients who have operable breast cancer and negative nodes. These immunocytochemical methods employ epithelial-specific monoclonal antibodies to detect low concentrations of malignant cells in the aspirate.[11] The subgroup of patients in whom these malignant cells are found may suffer recurrent disease despite having negative nodes. Also, in 80 percent of patients who have breast cancer and negative nodes, cancer cells are found in the blood if large enough samples are taken.[17] The significance of this is unknown in relation to whether these cells will produce metastases.

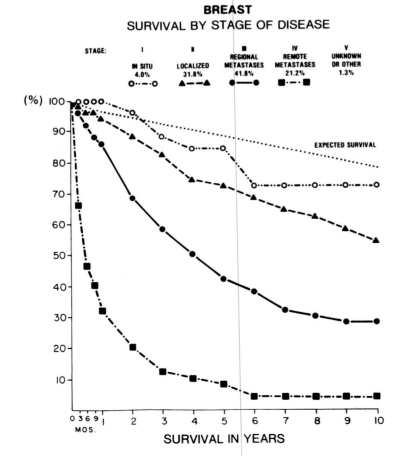

Figure 48–1   *The stages are defined as indicated and not according to the staging system of the American Joint Committee.*

Treatment of node-negative disease yields a 70 percent cure rate after locoregional treatment.[98] The length of time for 10 percent of patients to relapse is inversely related to the size of the primary tumor,[98] the size being the strongest predictor of outcome. The use of adjuvant chemotherapy in node-negative patients has been shown to improve the short-term 5-year disease-free survival rate from 67 percent to 75 percent, with only an 8 percent absolute improvement in survival.[98]

EXTENT OF TREATMENT REQUIRED FOR THE AXILLA: PARTIAL VERSUS COMPLETE DISSECTION

The function of sampling is to obtain with minimal morbidity, sufficient nodes to identify the node-negative patient. There is no doubt that the first level of the axilla is quite accurate for the staging of a clinically negative axilla. However, when one or more positive nodes are found in this level, the question of residual disease in the axilla has to be addressed. The probability of residual disease depends on the number of positive nodes found and on the size of the primary tumor. When Level 1 and 2 are positive for nodal metastases, the chances of the third level being involved varies from 22 percent to 42 percent.[65, 123] These nodes will then require further treatment. Consequently, a decision has to be made on what to do for the axillary disease, because the Level 2 and 3 nodes are difficult to assess by physical examination and the axillary metastases will become manifest only when they reach a certain size. Required treatment involves either an axillary re-exploration or radiation to the axilla. If only a Level 1 dissection is done, the risk of incorrect assessment of nodal status is 19.6 percent, and higher in patients with larger tumors. If a Level 1 and 2 dissection is done, 3.9 percent of patients are incorrectly assessed.

Advantages of Complete Axillary Dissection

Advantages of complete axillary dissection are as follows:

1. There is no risk of understaging the disease because of fewer than ten nodes being identified if a complete dissection is performed. When Level 1 and 2 dissections are done, the risk of understaging the disease is at least 2.6 percent,[109] with the same morbidity as for a complete dissection.

2. No additional treatment is required if the axilla is pathologically positive. This benefit is important when there are features in the primary tumor suggestive of extensive nodal involvement. In the series of Senofsky and coworkers,[109] if only Levels 1 and 2 had been removed, nodal metastases would have been left behind in 10.4 percent (29 of 278) of axillae, or 31.5 percent of all node-positive axillae. Prophylac-

tic radiotherapy to the axilla is unnecessary and harmful.

3. Complete dissection minimizes the risk of local recurrence. There was no local recurrence on 50-month follow-up after total lymphadenectomy in one series.[27] In the NSABP-B04 trial, the risk of axillary recurrence was inversely proportional to the number of nodes removed, and the risk was higher when nodal metastases were present. The NSABP-B04 trial reported a 1.4 percent rate of axillary recurrence at 10-year follow-up in patients treated with radical mastectomy, 3.1 percent in patients treated with total mastectomy and postoperative radiotherapy, and 17.8 percent in patients who had axillary recurrence when the axilla was not treated, with 78 percent of these recurrences being in the first 2 years after mastectomy.[38] However, the dose of axillary irradiation in the NSABP-B04 trial was 60 Gy, and this dose increases the complications seen in the axilla. Lin and coworkers[75] report an improvement in axillary control with a complete ALND as compared with irradiation with 45 Gy to the axilla.

In a series of 259 women treated with a Level 1–2 dissection of the axilla, two had recurrences in the axilla within 2 years of surgery.[112] Some series report a 20 percent axillary recurrence when only axillary sampling is used and there is no further treatment to the axilla. Greenall and Davidson[48] reported a 2 percent recurrence after axillary sampling and radiotherapy for positive-node patients and four relapses in node-negative patients who did not receive radiotherapy. The estimated probability for axillary recurrence is 19 percent when no nodes are examined, 10 percent when there are one to two negative nodes, 5 percent when there are three to four negative nodes, and 3 percent when there are more than five negative nodes.[6]

4. Randomization of treatment to determine the effectiveness of nodal resection to improve survival has failed to resolve this issue because, at the time of this writing, no study has the statistical power to provide an answer. Comparing different treatments fails to consider that only a small percentage of patients (those with only regional disease) are at risk for such a study. Any group of patients with operable breast cancer includes some with disease that has already metastasized (the overall recurrence rate after mastectomy is 50 percent). Among those with purely local disease, 40 percent is the minimal cure rate after lumpectomy. Therefore, a small number of patients with only local and regional disease would be at risk for a study involving the importance of axillary node treatment (roughly 10 percent). Harris and Osteen[55] estimated that a survival rate difference of 7 percent would require 1000 patients in each arm of such a study. Gardner[45] reported that if a 10 percent difference in survival at 10 years were to be significant at $p < .05$, then 3900 patients would be required in each arm. In this scenario, even if a modified radical mastectomy had a significant advantage over total mastectomy (no nodes removed), the actual overall survival rates of the groups (90 percent

of patients not at risk for the study) would be reported as 52 percent for modified radical mastectomy and 48 percent for total mastectomy, well comparable to those of the Fisher NSABP-B04 study[38] (Figs. 48–2 and 48–3). *All current randomized studies of nodal treatment therefore conclude that the treatments are equivalent.*

This most widely quoted study (B04) had some additional problems in that 35 percent of the patients randomized to receive no treatment to the axilla actually had a partial lymph node dissection. In addition, patients who failed in the axilla as part of systemic recurrence were not counted as axillary failures.

DO METASTASES METASTASIZE?

Studies have demonstrated that metastatic sites can produce generalized cancer.[13] In a series of experiments using parabiotic mice, cells spread to a second animal from lung metastases in the first animal after the primary tumor had been removed.[58] Similar results were reported for B16 melanoma.[56]

The question of whether metastases metastasize is important because it reflects on the significance of recurrent disease for survival. When cancer recurs in the ipsilateral breast, the prognosis for survival decreases markedly.[116] In randomized studies, ipsilateral recurrence was associated with an increased risk of distant metastases and death.[40, 129] Therefore, serious consideration must be paid to the risk of axillary recurrence as well, although equivalent studies are not available on this manifestation of the disease.

ORDERLY PROGRESSION OF METASTASES (SKIP METASTASIS)

In an era when minimally invasive surgery is the norm, and procedures such as sampling and low axillary dissection are gaining popularity for detecting the presence of axillary metastases, it becomes important to understand the patterns of lymphatic drainage of the breast. It is widely accepted that involvement of the axillary nodes occurs in a progressive fashion from the lower to the higher levels of the axilla.

Veronesi and coworkers,[123] in an analysis of 539 patients with carcinoma of the breast and positive nodes, demonstrated that Level 1 nodes were the only site of nodal involvement in 58.2 percent of cases. In 21.7 percent of cases, both Level 1 and 2 were involved, and in 16.3 percent, all three levels of the axilla were involved. This orderly progression of metastases occurred in 96.2 percent of cases. In 1.5 percent of cases, the first level was skipped by metastases. In 0.4 percent, both the first and second levels were skipped, and in 2.6 percent, the second level was skipped.

These data concur with those of Rosen and colleagues,[104] who, in a study of 1228 patients undergoing modified, radical, and extended mastectomy, found that the incidence of axillary positivity was 46 percent in patients with an invasive tumor. Metastases were limited to Level 1 in 54 percent of these cases, with Level 1 and 2 being involved in 10 percent. Level 3 was the highest level of involvement in 11 percent. Metastases were found more often at Level 2 or 3 after radical or extended mastectomies

Theoretical study of Total Mastectomy (TM) vs. Modified Radical Mastectomy (MRM) in breast cancer patients.

L = Local Disease   LM = Local disease actually metastatic

R = Regional Disease   RM = Regional disease actually metastatic

1,000 patients entered. Those with local disease clinically have 20% LM and those with clinical regional disease have 60% RM.

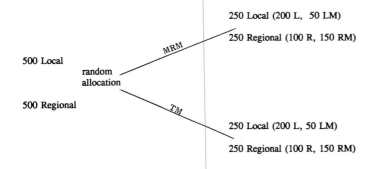

250 Local (200 L, 50 LM)

250 Regional (100 R, 150 RM)

500 Local

random allocation

MRM

500 Regional

TM

250 Local (200 L, 50 LM)

250 Regional (100 R, 150 RM)

Figure 48–2 *Distribution of cases in a theoretical study in which a perfect randomization for patients with local or regional disease is obtained. (After Gardner B, Feldman J: Ann Surg 218:270–278, 1993.)*

Results of our theoretical study of Total vs. Modified Radical Mastectomy:

SCENARIO I

10 Year Survival

Sample size needed to have a 95% chance of detecting the difference with an alpha = .05

All R in MRM survive
and no R in TM survive

$$MRM = \frac{200+100}{500} = 60\%$$

800

$$TM = \frac{200}{500} = 40\%$$

SCENARIO II

80% R in MRM survive
40% R in TM survive

$$MRM = \frac{200+80}{500} = 56\%$$

2,400

$$TM = \frac{200+40}{500} = 48\%$$

SCENARIO III

60% R in MRM survive
40% R in TM survive

$$MRM = \frac{200+60}{500} = 52\%$$

7,800

$$TM = \frac{200+40}{500} = 48\%$$

Figure 48–3 *Results of the theoretical study proposed in Figure 2. Three scenarios are depicted. Note the large number of patients required to produce results significant at P = 0.05 (after Gardner B, Feldman J: Ann Surg 218:270–278, 1993.)*

than after the modified mastectomy. Skip metastases were found in 1.6 percent of all cases and in 3 percent of all node-positive cases. Most of the primary tumors associated with skip metastases were present in the outer quadrants of the breast, although the difference was not statistically significant from the rest of the series. It is important for the surgeon to tag the specimen at the time of operation, as it is otherwise impossible to identify the levels of the axillary nodes in a modified radical mastectomy specimen.

Rotter's nodes are involved in up to 10 percent of patients with breast cancer but are not always looked for and removed at the time of axillary clearance. In a study evaluating the presence and involvement of the interpectoral nodes,[27] these nodes were identified in 15 of 73 patients (20 percent) and were positive in 10 of these patients (14 percent). Three patients had positive Rotter's nodes in the absence of any axillary involvement (7.5 percent of all node-positive patients in this series), and these patients were significantly younger, with larger tumors. All patients with involved interpectoral nodes had tumors involving the upper half of the breast. Rotter's nodes were the only involved nodes in 0.1 percent of all women with invasive tumors in this series.[104] The higher incidence of Rotter's node involvement could be related to (1) the larger tumor size, (2) the multiple sections being taken from each node, and (3) the routine division of the pectoralis minor muscle.

In the series of Senofsky and associates,[109] Rotter's nodes were involved in 5 percent of all cases and in 15.2 percent of all node-positive cases. This study found metastases in the apical or Rotter's nodes without involvement of the Level 1 or 2 nodes in 2.6 percent of cases (5.5 percent of node-positive patients). This study also found that 18.2 percent of cases with only micrometastases in Levels 1 or 2 had involvement of the apical or Rotter's nodes. Failure to remove the interpectoral nodes could contribute to the recurrence seen after complete axillary clearance. The removal of these nodes is a simple procedure and adds little to the operative time. Rotter's nodes should be looked for in all patients undergoing a complete axillary dissection; if palpable, they should definitely be removed.

As the number of involved nodes increases, so does the involvement of the Level 3 nodes; i.e., the involvement of the axillary nodes shows an orderly progression, with higher levels being involved at a later stage of the disease. This fact is related to the worse prognosis of patients with positive Level 3 nodes.[104, 123] When the nodes in the first level are positive, the chances of the higher levels being positive varies from 22 percent to 42.9 percent, and this incidence increases from 28.4 percent in patients with T1 tumors to 67.9 percent in those with T3 tumors.

No satisfactory explanation can be found for the presence of skip metastases, although it has been postulated that the intervening nodes might harbor micrometastases.[104]

These data confound the hypothesis that once the nodes are involved, the disease has spread systemically.

MEDIASTINAL NODES RESECTION?

The internal mammary nodes are involved in 0–22 percent of invasive breast cancers when an extended radical mastectomy is performed.[74, 87, 100] This involvement is influenced by the size and position of the primary tumor as well as by the presence of positive axillary nodes. However, in only 4 percent of patients is this node involvement clinically detected following a radical mastectomy. On the basis of the low incidence of clinically detected involvement, it has been proposed that treatment for these nodes is not required. Some studies show no survival benefit or decrease in parasternal recurrence when only a radical mastectomy is done.[26, 37, 70, 125] Other studies have demonstrated a survival benefit when the internal mammary nodes are treated, especially in patients with medial lesions and positive axillary nodes.[4, 100] Yet the survival benefit and local control achieved is the same for irradiation and surgery, and in patients with laterally situated primary tumors, no such benefit is seen.

The greatest proponent of mediastinal node resection was Urban.[21, 120] A review of his data reveals a 10-year disease-free survival of 42 percent in patients with positive axillary and mediastinal nodes and an overall survival of 53 percent at 10 years. Most of Urban's studies were nonrandomized. The randomized studies showed no survival advantage to internal mammary node resection.[62] In 5–10 percent of patients, the internal mammary nodes are involved in the absence of axillary involvement but usually only when the primary is medially placed.[87] Other studies have shown that the internal mammary nodes were not the site of first relapse in any patients.[26] Current thought is that there is no role for resection or irradiation if the patient is going to receive systemic therapy. Urban[21] himself postulated that the therapeutic dilemma posed by the internal mammary nodes remains unsolved and the benefit of extended mastectomy unproven.

ROLE OF RADIOTHERAPY

Almost all the complications of radiotherapy as the primary treatment of breast cancer are related to the irradiation of the nodal fields. Surgery is better at preventing local recurrence than radiotherapy.[26, 38, 74, 75] Also, approximately one fifth of all mammary cancers are radioresistant.[122] Radiotherapy to the breast after lumpectomy and axillary dissection decreases the risk of ipsilateral breast tumor recurrence as well as the incidence of nodal recurrence but does not affect long-term survival.[26, 36] Radiotherapy should be reserved for nonpalpable disease as it has a high failure rate when positive axillary nodes are palpable.

In patients with T1–2 tumors treated with lumpectomy and irradiation to the breast and axilla, without any surgery to the axilla, the 5-year survival was 87 percent and 10-year survival was 71 percent. The incidence of axillary recurrence was 2.4 percent, and the incidence of lymphedema was also very low.[50, 69] Radiation can induce brachial plexus neuropathy and radiation pneumonitis. The risk of brachial plexus neuropathy is 1.3 percent with axillary radiation of less than 50 Gy; but with an increase in the dose to greater than 50 Gy, the risk increases to 5.6 percent.[99] This risk is related to technique, fraction size, and the use of overlapping fields. A rare complication is radiation-induced sarcoma, which has a significant mortality rate and may require forequarter amputation for local control. Radiotherapy has no role in treating patients with clinically positive disease, as the dose of radiation required to treat positive nodes is much higher and is associated with a significantly higher complication rate. The rate of axillary failure with inadequate radiation is 13–19 percent.[101]

Regional nodal failure was the first site of failure in 2.3 percent of 1624 patients with stage I–II disease. The conclusion was that regional nodal failure is uncommon in patients with radiation to the breast with an adequate axillary dissection when the nodes are negative or when one to three nodes are positive. Regional nodal failure is also uncommon in patients with clinically uninvolved axillae treated with nodal radiotherapy without axillary dissection. Of these patients, 2.3 percent had regional nodal failure, and 32 percent had distant metastases simultaneously.

COMPLICATIONS OF AXILLARY DISSECTION

Lymphedema

Lymphedema is a "permanent disability requiring daily attention."[93] It is associated with patient discomfort and recurrent episodes of cellulitis. The incidence of lymphedema following axillary surgery is 2–32 percent,* varying according to the enthusiasm with which it is looked for, the method of measuring it, and the interval after surgery at which it is assessed.

The most commonly used method for measuring the presence of lymphedema is the circumference of the arm and forearm and the presence of pitting edema on the dorsum of the hand.[51, 95] There is a discrepancy of 20 percent in the measurement of the two arms in a control population. This discrepancy is

---

*See references 32, 57, 77, 95, 100, 109, 124.

related to the greater muscle mass of the dominant arm. A difference of 2–2.5 cm or greater is usually taken as being indicative of lymphedema.

The use of volume displacement by the arm (greater than 150 cc between two arms being significant) is a more accurate indicator of lymphedema than is arm circumference,[57, 106] but this measurement is more cumbersome to perform. The clinical criteria of Senofsky and colleagues[109] use the extent of treatment required for lymphedema, with grade 1 (minimal or mild lymphedema) requiring no intervention or only elevation on one to two pillows at night, grade 2 requiring an external compression stocking for satisfactory control, grade 3 requiring the use of a lymphedema pump and stocking for control, and grade 4 being poorly controlled lymphedema or lymphedema complicated by recurrent lymphangitis. The lower incidence of lymphedema in the series reported by Senofsky and colleagues[109] may be due to this method of measuring lymphedema.

Lymphedema appearing late (2 or more years after nodal dissection) is often associated with recurrent disease and probably represents disease involving the next level of lymph nodes or lymphatics. It is often associated with other evidence of dissemination within 6 months of its appearance.

The pathogenesis of lymphedema has been related to lymphatic stasis and decreased venous return as well as to the efficiency of the lymphogenous anastomosis in the arm. Patients without lymphedema have had rapid transfer of injected radiolabeled serum albumin from the lymphatic to the venous system, whereas patients with lymphedema have not; thus the absence of adequate anastomoses may play a role in the development of lymphedema.[1, 95] Studies have also shown greater arterial inflow following axillary surgery with or without radiation. This increased inflow is maximum in patients with clinical lymphedema and has been attributed to a loss of sympathetic tone in these patients.[100]

Increased patient age has been associated with an increase in lymphedema incidence (25 percent versus 7 percent in patients older and younger than 60 years, respectively).[95] Other studies, however, have shown no effect of patient age.[100, 106] Obesity has been associated with a significantly higher risk of developing lymphedema.[106] Whether or not the arm was used immediately postoperatively, and whether or not the surgery was on the dominant side had no effect.[93, 106] In 89 percent of patients with a history of multiple infections in the ipsilateral arm, lymphedema developed in one series.[106] The presence of postoperative wound infections increased the incidence of lymphedema to 10 percent in another series.[95]

There is an equal incidence of lymphedema when the axilla is treated by surgery or radiotherapy alone,[14, 93] but this incidence increases threefold to sevenfold when the two modalities are used in combination,[57, 93, 106, 109] and the extent of lymphedema is usually greater.

The presence of lymphedema correlates with the extent of surgery in most cases. Veronesi and coworkers[124] reported a 6.6 percent incidence in patients after radical mastectomy compared with 3.1 percent in those undergoing conservative treatment—that is, lumpectomy with axillary clearance. This incidence was not related to the number of nodes removed but was significantly higher in patients with gross rather than microscopic metastases to the axillary nodes.[109] No such association was found in other studies.[57]

The incidence of lymphedema varies from zero to 3 percent when the axilla is not treated or when only axillary sampling is done versus 2.7–9.4 percent when a Level 1 and 2 dissection is done.[57, 95, 109] When complete axillary clearance is performed, the incidence varies from 4.8 percent to 16 percent. The technique of lymphadenectomy also affects the incidence of lymphedema. Skeletonizing the axillary vein, or dividing the pectoralis minor muscle increases the incidence of lymphedema.[82, 109] The use of an oblique incision compared with a transverse or vertical incision also increases the risk of lymphedema.

Radiation may cause obstruction of the small lymphatic vessels directly or by scarring and is considered by some to be the most important factor in the development of arm edema.[14, 32, 43] There is some controversy about the importance of this factor, as variations in the dosage of external radiation have not always been accounted for. This is especially true for earlier studies, in which the dose and technique of radiotherapy sometimes varied greatly. The only important factor is the direct radiation of the axilla, as the radiation of the breast or supraclavicular and parasternal nodes does not affect the incidence of lymphedema.[95, 106] In two studies the incidence of lymphedema was 4 percent when only radiation was given to the axilla, and this percentage increased to 5–6 percent when axillary radiation was combined with a Level 1 and 2 dissection. Durand and associates[29] found that adding 55 Gy radiation to the axilla of patients undergoing axillary lymphadenectomy and radiotherapy to the breast increased the incidence of lymphedema from 1 percent to 9 percent.

Despite the high incidence of measurable lymphedema in some studies, the presence of clinically severe edema remains low; i.e., 2–3 percent,[32, 75] and is rarely encountered in the practice of many surgical oncologists.

It is extremely important for the surgeon and radiotherapist to agree that no axillary radiation will be given if a complete axillary dissection has been done.

Care of the hand after axillary dissection should include

- Avoiding blood pressure monitoring or intravenous or intramuscular injections in the affected hand.
- Avoiding cuts, scrapes, or puncture wounds on hands.
- Using protective gloves or mittens while gardening or cooking.

- Treating all minor wounds with care.
- Using lotions to soften skin and prevent it from drying and cracking.

Seroma

The presence of seroma in the axilla is related to the division of the lymphatics at the time of surgery and perhaps could more accurately be called "lymphoma." Its importance lies in the fact that the excessive accumulation of fluid causes patient discomfort, impairs wound healing, and may predispose to infection.[94] The seroma usually accumulates in the first 2 weeks following surgery, stays stable over the next 2–3 weeks, and then starts to resorb.[60] The incidence of seromas varies from 4.2 percent of "clinically detectable and bothersome to the patient" seromas[108] to 92 percent of seromas discovered on ultrasonography.[60] However, 8–72 percent of these seromas required aspiration of an average of 100 cc of fluid for patient comfort in some series.[60, 108, 109]

There was no relationship between the amount or duration of the drainage to the degree of arm mobilization after surgery[59, 93] or of the use of single or multiple drains in the axilla.[94] Closing the dead space at the time of surgery did decrease seroma formation, but the time required for this procedure and the restriction in arm movement of the patient that it causes prevent it from being widely accepted.[93]

Seroma formation increases significantly with the presence of positive nodes.[93] The division of the pectoralis minor at the time of surgery was found to be a significant variable in older patients in one series[109] but had no effect in another.[82] Other modalities to decrease seroma formation have included the use of lasers, sclerotherapy with tetracycline, and the use of fibrin glue, all with little success.[93] The only surgeon-controlled variable is the extent of surgery, which should be dictated by the characteristics of the malignancy and of the patient, as only 0.2–2 percent of all patients with seromas require drainage and antibiotics.[108, 109]

Over the years one of the authors has used the following techniques to avoid the development of seromas: (1) closed suction with two catheters and (2) large retention sutures over soft dental packs, tied so as to compress the flaps, particularly in the axilla. This author no longer sutures the flaps or restricts the motion of the patient's shoulder (e.g., by using a sling and swathe). Clinical seromas develop in fewer than 2 percent of patients and are rarely clinically significant. Shoulder exercises are begun on the 8th to 10th postoperative day, after suture removal. The packs are removed on day 5 or 6. Patients are usually discharged from the hospital on day 2 or 3.

Wound Infection

The incidence of wound infection after axillary dissection varies from 5.6 percent to 14.2 percent.[3, 93] The predisposing factors are decreased blood supply, advanced age, prolonged catheter drainage of the wound, skin necrosis, malnutrition, and associated medical diseases such as diabetes mellitus. Administration of prophylactic antibiotics in patients undergoing axillary surgery has been shown to decrease the incidence of wound infection.[93] The authors never use postoperative antibiotics and yet see very little wound infection (less than 0.5 percent). Necrosis of the flaps can be prevented by fashioning flaps with appropriate backcuts and flap rotation to release tension. In some instances closure may require skin grafting to avoid creating tension.

Frozen Shoulder/Decreased Range of Motion

Frozen shoulder is a rare but disabling complication that is avoided by early mobilization and, occasionally, physical therapy. The incidence of decreased range of motion varies from zero to 10 percent.[32, 43, 109] In one series there was a 19 percent incidence of reduction in one of the shoulder movements (abduction, adduction, rotation, or flexion) of 20 degrees at 1 year follow-up as compared with preoperative function.[59] Another series showed that at 1 year follow-up, 17 percent of patients had a 15-degree or less reduction in shoulder motion and only 4 percent had a reduction of 15 to 30 degrees in the range of motion. In general, it was found that in patients undergoing radiation the range of motion decreases as the dose of radiation increases.[32] As indicated earlier, abandonment of all shoulder-restrictive dressings has eliminated this complication, particularly if the patient is well motivated to exercise.

Chronic Pain Syndrome/Neuropathies

Chronic pain syndrome is described as a chronic stable pain of long duration starting soon after surgery. The syndrome occurs in 4–22 percent of patients after axillary surgery[32, 43, 75, 93, 114] and is thought to occur because of injury to the intercostobrachial nerve during axillary dissection. This pain is a distinctive neuropathic or deafferentation one, starting soon after surgery and localized to the axilla in 84 percent of patients, the medial upper arm in 74 percent, and the anterior chest wall of the same side in 58 percent.[114] It is described as paroxysms of lancinating pain against a background of burning aching and constricting pain in the axilla.

In most patients the pain is exacerbated by movement and does not decrease with time. Nevertheless, only 25 percent of these patients require mild analgesics. The major consequence of their pain is an interference with their daily activities, and because the pain is increased by movement, they tend to immobilize their arms. This immobilization in turn may contribute to a higher incidence of frozen shoulder in patients without adequate pain relief. This study suggests that chronic pain syndrome tends to be undertreated, as tricyclic antidepressants, which have been shown to be of benefit in neuropathic pain, are seldom tried for chronic or postmastectomy pain syndromes.[114] The incidence of this syndrome is *decreased with the preservation of the nerve during surgery*. It is sometimes possible to identify a single point on the axilla that is extremely painful because of a neuroma in the stump of the nerve. The neuroma may then be treated with excision or injection or both. One series showed that the incidence of chronic pain was higher in patients with lymphedema.[93] Approximately 70–81 percent of all patients undergoing axillary dissection have a subjective or objective loss of sensation in the distribution of the intercostobrachial nerve following surgery unless the nerve is preserved.[32, 75]

Brachial plexus neuropathy is seen only in patients treated with external radiation with or without surgery and is unheard of when surgery is the only modality of treatment to the axilla.[32, 99] The risk of brachial plexus neuropathy is 1.3 percent with axillary radiation of less than 50 Gy, but with an increase in the dose to greater than 50 Gy, the risk increases to 5.6 percent.[99] The incidence of this complication increases from 0.3 percent to 3.4 percent with the concurrent use of chemotherapy.[99]

Painful Lymphatic Occlusion

Painful lymphatic occlusions are reported as extreme pain on movement of the shoulder or elbow,[77] with palpable tender bands in the axilla that limit shoulder movement after axillary node biopsy or clearance. They may occur 4–6 weeks following the primary surgery and are treated, with good results, by biopsy and division of the bands during general anesthesia, followed by physiotherapy. The biopsy shows lymphatic occlusion without any involvement by tumor. This may be in part due to the lymph stasis following axillary surgery but appears to be distinct from lymphedema. The incision must be planned so that it does not enter the axillary fold when sutured.

Other Complications

Other complications of axillary surgery include axillary vein thrombophlebitis and superficial vein phlebitis. These are minor complications with an incidence of zero to 3 percent of all patients.[108, 109] The incidence increases when the axillary vein is not visualized at the time of surgery.

In summary, the overall complication rate for patients treated by experienced breast surgeons is very low. Although measurable edema may be present, the incidence of visible edema is less than 1 percent. Pain over the chest wall is usually due to the mastectomy rather than the axillary dissection, and a full range of motion and return to normal activity is to be expected. Exercises are started after the 8th postoperative day, and the patient can be reassured that full range of motion will be back by 6 weeks.

EVALUATION OF PATIENTS FOR ALND

In-situ *Invasive*. Incidence of lymph node positivity is 0–2 percent in patients with DCIS.[7, 30, 44, 78, 102, 110]

Positive axillary nodes from a patient with DCIS are rare even when a palpable lesion is present unless invasion is also present or suspected because of the large area involved. The incidence is approximately zero percent when the lesion is detected mammographically.

Invasive (Size versus Axillary Nodes). In regard to screen-detected cancer, the size of the primary tumor has been related to the incidence of axillary metastases in various studies. This incidence varies from 10 percent to 32 percent for a T1 lesion.[102] The number of nodes also increases as the size of the primary tumor increases.[74]

ALND is indicated only for a T1b lesion or greater—i.e., an invasive lesion larger than 6 mm in size.[110] The incidence of axillary lymph node involvement in patients with small cancers is as follows: DCIS, 0 percent; T1a, 3 percent; T1b, 17 percent; T1c, 32 percent; T2, 32 percent; and T3, 60 percent. These incidences are directly related to the size of the invasive component. So if 100 dissections were done in patients with T1a lesions, only three patients are likely to have metastases and thus derive a potential benefit. The survival rate for patients with T1a lesions undergoing axillary dissection is 90 percent at 10 years, but it is not known whether survival would have been the same if ALND had not been done.

ALND is therapeutic in patients with palpable nodes and in most centers is done only for those patients. The procedure is performed less often for patients with clinically negative nodes, resulting in an understaging of disease in those patients. Only 27 percent of patients with small primary tumors get any form of axillary dissection.

No Treatment to the Axilla. Observation of clinically node-negative axillae in patients with T1 or T2 tumors results in an 8–37 percent incidence of axillary recurrence,[18, 38, 39, 42] whereas 45–60 percent of these patients should have had positive nodes on histopathology. This approach of observation alone may be an option for older or postmenopausal women who would be treated with tamoxifen regardless of axillary nodal status and are less likely to benefit from polychemotherapy.[16, 34, 35, 36] The most widely quoted study in favor of this approach is the NSABP-B04 trial, which demonstrated no effect on survival when there was a delay in treating the clinically negative axilla, but no prospective studies exist to prove this. The NSABP-B06 trial also demonstrated a survival benefit for node-negative patients receiving chemotherapy.[36] As ipsilateral breast recurrence is associated with decreased survival, one would expect similar findings with ipsilateral axillary recurrence.

The histological status of the axillary nodes is the most important prognostic feature in breast cancer. The information gained from other factors, such as the size of the primary tumor, the presence of vascular invasion, the estrogen and progesterone receptor status, the histological grade, and the S-phase fraction, can make a major contribution to assessing the prognosis in individual patients, but these factors are less accurate than formulae that include the nodal status of the patient.

Patients with a small primary tumor who do not undergo an axillary dissection may be misdiagnosed as stage I when they are actually node-positive; i.e., stage II. These patients would then contribute to a higher rate of relapse in this group. The argument against this conclusion is that with a tumor less than 1 cm, the 20-year mortality is about 10 percent.[16, 103] In a series of 130 lumpectomy patients treated without surgery or irradiation to the breast, followed by mammography and clinical examination, 9 percent developed nodal failure, which failure was associated with local recurrence or distant metastases in all cases. When the breast was irradiated, the rate of recurrence in the axilla decreased, possibly because the radiation field usually includes the lower half of the axilla.

Markers for Axillary Involvement (Histological). Favorable features of the primary tumor in patients with negative nodes are papillary, medullary, colloid, or tubular histology, especially when tumors are less than 1 cm diameter, for which the associated disease-free survival rate is 88 percent at 18 years follow-up.[11, 115] Patients who have markers indicating aggressive disease with poor prognosis require more aggressive operative treatment. These markers include poor nuclear grade, vascular or lymphatic invasion, high S-phase fraction, extensive intraductal disease, and large primary tumors. Some surgeons favor more aggressive surgery in younger patients. The nodal resection may be indicated regardless of the treatment of the primary breast cancer.

SUMMARY

Breast cancer is a heterogeneous disease for which a wide range of treatment options are available. Radiation to or surgical excision of the axillary nodes in conjunction with the treatment of the primary tumor is recommended to avoid local recurrence with an associated decrease in survival. Radiation cannot provide adequate staging and is not effective when palpable disease is present.

Current randomization studies do not have the statistical power to answer questions relating to the efficacy of nodal excision.

The authors strongly recommend complete axillary node resection with treatment of the primary breast cancer in patients with invasive cancer over 1 cm in size or with prognostic markers indicating aggressive disease in order to

1. Provide accurate staging.
2. Provide a survival advantage (unproved).
3. Prevent axillary recurrence.

The importance of local treatment to the survival of breast cancer patients has been demonstrated in two recently published studies, which appeared after this chapter was completed. They add emphasis to the importance of complete nodal treatment as a first line of defense against recurrence.

1. Ragaz J, Jackson SM, Le N, et al: Adjuvant radiotherapy and chemotherapy in node positive premenopausal women with breast cancer. N Engl J Med 337:956–962.
2. Overgaard M, Hansen PS, Overgaard J, et al: Post operative radiotherapy in high risk premenopausal women with breast cancer who receive adjuvant chemotherapy. N Engl J Med 337:949–955.

References

1. Aboul-Enein A, Eshmawy I, Arafa S, Abboud A: The role of lymphogenous communication in the development of postmastectomy lymphedema. Surgery 95:562–565, 1984.
2. Adair F, Berg J, Joubert L, et al: A long-term follow-up of breast cancer patients: The thirty-year report. Cancer 33:1145–1150, 1974.
3. Aitken DR, Minton JP: Complications associated with mastectomy. Surg Clin North Am 63:1331–1352, 1983.
4. Arriagada R, Le MG, Mouriesse H, et al: Long-term effects of internal mammary chain treatment. Results of a multivariate analysis of 1195 patients with operable breast cancer and positive axillary nodes. Radiother Oncol 11(3):213–222, 1988.
5. Auchincloss H: Significance of location and number of axillary metastasis in carcinoma of the breast. Ann Surg 158:37–46, 1963.
6. Axelsson CK, Mouridsen HT, Zelder K: Axillary dissection of level 1 and 2 lymph nodes is important in breast cancer classification. Eur J Cancer 28A(8/9):1415–1418, 1992.
7. Balch CM, Singletary SE, Bland KI: Clinical decision-making in early breast cancer. Ann Surg 217(3):207–225, 1993.
8. Banks WM: On free removal of mammary cancer with extirpation of the axillary glands as a necessary accompaniment. BMJ 2:1138–1141, 1882.
9. Barth RJ, Danforth DN, Venzon DJ, et al: Level of axillary involvement by lymph node metastases from breast cancer is not an independent predictor of survival. Arch Surg 126:574–577, 1991.
10. Bloom HJG: Survival of women with untreated breast cancer—Past and present in prognostic factors in breast cancer. *In* Forrest APM and Kunkler PB (eds): Prognostic Factors in Breast Cancer. Baltimore, Williams and Wilkins Co., 1968, pp 3–19.
11. Brady MS, Osborne MP: The biological basis of breast cancer treatment. Surgical Rounds pp. 27–33, 1993.
12. Brooks S, Leathem AJC: Prediction of lymph node involvement by detection of altered glycosylation in the primary tumor. Lancet 338:71–74, 1991.
13. Bross IDJ, Blumenson LE: Metastatic sites that produce generalized cancer: Identification and kinetics of generalizing sites. *In* Weis, L (ed): Fundamental Aspects of Metastasis. Amsterdam, North-Holland Publishing Co., 1976, pp. 359–375.
14. Cabanes PA, Salmon RJ, Vilcoq JR, et al: Value of axillary dissection in addition to lumpectomy and radiotherapy in early breast cancer. Lancet 339:1245–1248, 1992.
15. Cady B: The need to re-examine axillary lymph node dissection in invasive breast cancer. Cancer 73(3):505–508, 1994.
16. Cady B, Stone MD, Wayne J: New therapeutic possibilities in primary invasive breast carcinoma. Ann Surg 218(3):338–349, 1993.
17. Candar Z, Ritchie AC, Hopkirk JF, Long RC: The prognostic value of circulating tumor cells in patients with breast cancer. Surg Gynec Obstet 113:291–294, 1962.
18. Chadha M, Chabon AB, Friedman P, Vikram B: Predictors of axillary lymph node metastases in patients with T1 breast cancer: A multivariate analysis. Cancer 73:350–353, 1994.

19. Chevinsky AH, Ferrara J, James AG, et al: Prospective evaluation of clinical and pathological detection of axillary metastases in patients with carcinoma of the breast. Surgery 108:612–618, 1990.
20. Christensen SB, Jansson C: Axillary biopsy compared with dissection in the staging of lymph nodes in operable breast cancer: A randomized trial. Eur J Surg 159:159–162, 1993.
21. Cody HS III and Urban JA: Internal mammary node status: A major prognosticator in axillary node–negative breast cancer. Ann Surg Oncol 2(1):32–37, 1995.
22. Crowe JP, Lee MD, Adler MD, et al: Positron emission tomography and breast masses: Comparison with clinical, mammographic, and pathological findings. Ann Surg Oncol 1:132–140, 1994.
23. Dahl-Iverson E, Tobiassen T: Radical mastectomy with parasternal and supraclavicular dissection for mammary carcinoma. Ann Surg 170:889–891, 1969.
24. Danforth DN, Findlay PA, McDonald HD, et al: Complete axillary lymph node dissection for stage 1-2 carcinoma of the breast. J Clin Oncol 4:655–662, 1986.
25. Davis BW, Gelber RD, Goldhirsch A, et al: Prognostic significance of tumor grade in clinical trials of adjuvant therapy for breast cancer with lymph node metastasis. Cancer 58:2662–2670, 1986.
26. Deutsch M: Radiotherapy after breast conservation therapy: How much is enough. Semin Surg Oncol 8:140–146, 1992.
27. Dixon JM, Dobie V, Chetty U: The importance of interpectoral nodes in breast cancer. Eur J Cancer 29A(3):334–336, 1993.
28. Donegan WL, Stine SB, Samter TG: Implications of extracapsular nodal metastases for treatment and prognosis of breast cancer. Cancer 72:778–782, 1993.
29. Durand JC, Poljicak M, Lefranc JP, Pilleeron JP: Wide excision of the tumor, axillary dissection and postoperative radiotherapy as treatment of small breast cancers. Cancer 53:2439–2443, 1984.
30. Eberlein TJ: Current management of carcinoma of the breast. Ann Surg 220(2):121–136, 1994.
31. Ellis H, Colburn GL, Skandalakis JE: Surgical embryology and anatomy of the breast and its related anatomic structures. Surg Clin North Am 73;2:611–632, 1993.
32. Falk SJ: Radiotherapy and the management of the axilla in early breast cancer. Br J Surg 81:1277–1281, 1994.
33. Fentiman IS, Chetty U: Axillary dissection in breast cancer—Is there still a debate? Eur J Cancer 28A(6/7):1013–1014, 1992.
34. Fentiman IS, Mansel RE: Axillary dissection in breast cancer. Lancet 337:682, 1991.
35. Fentman IS, Mansel RE: The axilla—not a no-go zone. Lancet 337:221–223, 1991.
36. Fisher B, Anderson S: Conservative surgery for the management of invasive and noninvasive cancer of the breast: NSABP trials. World J Surg 18:63–69, 1994.
37. Fisher B, Boyle S, Burke M, Price AB: Intraoperative assessment of nodal status in the selection of patients with breast cancer for axillary clearance. Br J Surg 80(4):457, 1993.
38. Fisher B, Redmond C, Fisher ER, et al: Ten-year results of a randomized trial comparing radical mastectomy and total mastectomy with or without radiation. N Eng J Med 312:674–681, 1985.
40. Fisher B, Wolmark N, Bauer M, et al: The accuracy of clinical nodal staging and of limited axillary dissection as a determinant of histological nodal status in carcinoma of the breast. Surg Gynecol Obstet 152:765–772, 1981.
41. Forrest A, Roberts M, Cant E, Shivas A: Simple mastectomy and pectoral node biopsy. Br J Surg 63:569–575, 1976.
42. Fowble B, Solin L, Schultz D, Goodman R: Frequency, sites of relapse and outcome of regional nodal failures following conservative surgery and radiation for early breast cancer. Int J Radiat Oncol Biol Phys 13:475–481, 1987.
43. Fowble BL, Solin LJ, Schultz DJ, Goodman RL: Ten-year results of conservative surgery and irradiation for stage 1 and 2 breast cancer. Int Radiat Oncol Biol Phys 21:269–277, 1991.
44. Frazier TG, Copeland EM, Gallaher HS, et al: Prognosis and treatment in minimal breast cancer. Am J Surg 133:697–701, 1977.
45. Gardner B, Feldman J: Are positive axillary nodes in breast cancer markers for incurable disease? Ann Surg 218(3):270–278, 1993.
46. Giuliano AE, Dale PS, Turner RR, Morton DL, et al: Improved axillary staging of breast cancer with sentinel lymphadenectomy. Ann Surg 222(3):394–401, 1995.
47. Giuliano AE, Kirgan DM, Guenther JM, Morton DL: Lymphatic mapping and sentinel lymphadenectomy for breast cancer. Ann Surg 220(3):391–401, 1994.
48. Greenall MJ, Davidson T: How should the axilla be treated in breast cancer? Eur J Surg Oncol 21:2–7, 1995.
49. Haagensen CD: Diseases of the Breast. 3rd ed. Philadelphia: WB Saunders, 1986, 658–663.
50. Haffty BG, McKhann C, Beinfield M, Fischer D, Fischer JJ: Breast conservation without axillary dissection: A rational treatment in selected patients. Arch Surg 128:1315–1319, 1993.
51. Halsted WS: The results of operations for the cure of cancer of the breast performed at the Johns Hopkins from June 1889 to January 1894. Arch Surg 20:497–455, 1894.
52. Halsted WS: A clinical and histological study of certain adenocarcinoma of the breast. Ann Surg 28:557–576, 1898.
53. Halsted WS: The results of radical operations for the cure of carcinoma of the breast. Ann Surg 46:1–19, 1907.
54. Handley RS, Thackray AC: Invasion of the internal mammary lymph glands in carcinoma of the breast. Cancer 1:15–20, 1947.
55. Harris JR, Osteen RT: Patients with early breast cancer benefit from effective axillary treatment. Breast Cancer Res Treat 5:17–21, 1985.
56. Hart IR, Fidler IJ: Role of organ selectivity in the determination of metastatic patterns of B16 melanoma. Cancer Res 40:2281–2287, 1980.
57. Hoe AL, Iven D, Royle GT, Taylor I: Incidence of arm swelling following axillary clearance for breast cancer. Br J Surg 79:261–262, 1992.
58. Hoover HC, Ketcham AS: Metastasis of metastases. Am J Surg 130:405–411, 1975.
59. Jansen RFM, van Geel AN, de Groot HGW, et al: Immediate versus delayed shoulder exercises after axillary lymph node dissection. Am J Surg 160:481–484, 1990.
60. Jeffrey SS, Goodson WH, Ikeda DM, et al: Axillary lymphadenectomy for breast cancer without axillary drainage. Arch Surg 130:909–913, 1995.
61. Joensuu H, Toikkanen S: Cured of breast cancer? J Clin Oncol 13:62–69, 1995.
62. Kaae S, Johansen H: Five-year results: Two random series of simple mastectomy with postoperative irradiation versus extended radical mastectomy. Am J Roetgen 87:82–88, 1962.
63. Kaae S, Johansen H: Simple mastectomy plus postoperative irradiation by the method of McWhirter for mammary carcinoma. Ann Surg 170:895–899, 1969.
64. Keynes G: Radium treatment of primary carcinoma of the breast. Lancet 2:108–111, 1928.
65. Kinne DW: Controversies in primary breast cancer management. Am J Surg 166:502–508, 1993.
66. Kissin MW, Thompson EM, Price AB, et al: The inadequacy of axillary sampling in breast cancer. Lancet 1:1210–1212, 1982.
67. Koscielny S, Tubiana M, Le MG, et al: Breast cancer: Relationship between the size of the primary tumor and the probability of metastatic dissemination. Br J Cancer 49(6):709–715, 1984.
68. Krag DN, Weaver DL, Alex JC, Faitbank JT: Surgical resection and radiolocalization of the sentinel lymph node in breast cancer using a gamma probe. Surg Oncol 2(6):335–339, 1993.
69. Kurtz JM: Radiation therapy and breast conservation: Past achievements, current results, and future prospects. Semin Surg Oncol 8:147–152, 1992.
70. Lacour J, Le MG, Hill C, et al: Is it useful to remove the internal mammary nodes in operable breast cancer? Eur J Surg Oncol 13(4):309–314, 1987.

71. Larson D, Weinstein M, Goldberg I, et al: Edema of the arm as a function of the extent of axillary surgery in patients with stage 1-2 carcinoma of the breast treated with primary radiotherapy. Int J Radiat Oncol Biol Phys 12:1572–1582, 1986.

72. Lauria R, Perrone F, Carlomagno C, et al: The prognostic value of lymphatic and blood vessel invasion in operable breast cancer. Cancer 76:1772–1778, 1995.

73. Lehrer S, Garey J, Shank B: Nomograms for determing the probability of axillary nodal involvement in women with breast cancer. J Cancer Res Clin Oncol 121:123–125, 1995.

74. Levitt SH: The importance of locoregional control in the treatment of breast cancer and its impact on survival. Cancer 74:1840–1846, 1994.

75. Lin PP, Allison DC, Wainstock J, et al: Impact of axillary lymph node dissection on the therapy of breast cancer patients. J Clin Oncol 11(8):1536–1544, 1993.

76. Madden JL: Modified radical mastectomy. Surg Gynecol Obstet 121:1221–1230, 1965.

77. Marcus RT, Pawade J, Vella EJ: Painful lymphatic occlusion following axillary lymph node surgery. Br J Surg 77:683, 1990.

78. Margolis DS, McMillen MA, Hashmi H, Wasson DW, MacArthur JD: Aggressive axillary evaluation and adjuvant therapy for nonpalpable carcinoma of the breast. Surg Gynecol Obstet 174:109–113, 1992.

79. Marujo G, Jolly P, Hall M: Nonpalpable breast cancer: Needle-localized biopsy for diagnosis and considerations for treatment. Am J Surg 151:599–602, 1986.

80. McLean RG, Ege GN: Prognostic value of axillary lymphoscintigraphy in breast cancer patients. J Nucl Med 27:1116, 1986.

81. McWhirter R: The value of simple mastectomy and radiotherapy in the treatment of cancer of the breast. Br J Radiol 21:599–610, 1948.

82. Merson M, Pirovano C, Balzarini A, et al: The preservation of the minor pectoralis muscle in axillary dissection for breast cancer: Functional and cosmetic evaluation. Eur J Surg Oncol 18:215–218, 1992.

83. Meyer KK, Beck WC: Mastectomy performed by Lorenz Heister in the eighteenth century. Surg Gynecol Obstet 159:391–394, 1984.

84. Meyer W: An improved method of the radical operation for carcinoma of the breast. Medical Record pp. 746–748, 1894.

85. Mittra I, Redkar AA, Badwe RA: Prognosis of breast cancer: Evidence for interaction between c-erb-b2 overexpression and number of involved axillary lymph nodes. J Surg Oncol 60:106–111, 1995.

86. Moore C: On the influence of inadequate operations on the theory of cancer. R Med Chir Soc, London 1:244–280, 1867.

87. Morrow M, Foster R: Staging of breast cancer: A new rationale for internal mammary node biopsy. Arch Surg 116:748–751, 1981.

88. Morton DL, Wen DR, Cochran A: Management of early-stage melanoma by intraoperative lymphatic mapping and selective lymphadenectomy: An alternative to routine elective lymphadenectomy or "watch and wait." Surg Oncol Clin North Am 1:246–259, 1992.

89. Morton DL, Wen DR, Wong JH, et al: Technical details of intraoperative lymphatic mapping for early-stage melanoma. Arch Surg 127:392–399, 1992.

90. Osborne MP: The biologic basis for breast cancer treatment options. Am Coll Surg Bulletin 71(9):4–14, 1986.

91. Patey DH: A review of 146 cases of carcinoma of the breast operated on between 1930 and 1943. Br J Cancer 21:260–269, 1967.

92. Patey DH, Dyson WH: The prognosis of carcinoma of the breast in relation to the type of operation performed. Br J Cancer 2:7–13, 1948.

93. Petrek JA, Blackwood MM: Axillary dissection: Current practice and technique. Curr Probl Surg Vol 32(4), 1995.

94. Petrek JA, Peters MM, Cirrincione C, Thaler HT: A prospective randomized trial of single versus multiple drains in the axilla after lymphadectomy. Surg Gynecol Obstet 175:405–409, 1992.

95. Pezner RD, Patterson MP, Hill LR, et al: Arm lymphedema in patients treated conservatively for breast cancer: Relationship to patient age and axillary node dissection technique. Int J Rad Oncol Biol Phys 12(12):2079–2083, 1986.

96. Pigott J, Nichols R, Maddox WA, Balch CM: Metastasis to the upper levels of the axillary nodes in carcinoma of the breast and its implications for nodal sampling procedures. Surg Gynecol Obstet 158:255–259, 1984.

97. Pisansky TM, Ingle JN, Schaid DJ, Hass AC, et al: Patterns of tumor relapse following mastectomy and adjuvant systemic therapy in patients with axillary lymph node-positive breast cancer: Impact of clinical, histopathological, and flow cytometric factors. Cancer 72:1247–1260, 1993.

98. Quiet C, Ferguson DJ, Weichselbaum RR, Hellman S: Natural history of node-negative breast cancer: A study of 826 patients with a long-term follow-up. J Clin Oncol 13:1144–1151, 1995.

99. Recht A: Radiotherapy and the management of the axilla in early breast cancer. Br J Surg 82:421–422, 1995.

100. Recht A, Houlihan MJ: Axillary lymph nodes and breast cancer. Cancer 76:1491–1512, 1995.

101. Recht A, Pierce SM, Abner A, et al: Regional nodal failure after conservative surgery and radiotherapy for early-stage breast carcinoma. J Clin Oncol 9(6):988–996, 1991.

102. Robinson DS, Senofsky GM, Ketcham AS: Role and extent of lymphadenectomy in early breast cancer. Semin Surg Oncol 8:78–82, 1992.

103. Rosen PP, Groshen S, Saigo PE, et al: A long-term follow-up study of survival in stage 1 (T1N0M0) and stage 2 (T1N1M0) breast carcinoma. J Clin Oncol 7:355–366, 1989.

104. Rosen PP, Lesser ML, Kinne DW, Beattie EJ: Discontinuous or "skip" metastases in breast carcinoma. Ann Surg 197:276–283, 1983.

105. Salvadori B, Rovini D, Squicciarini P, et al: Surgery for local recurrence following deficient radical mastectomy for breast cancer: A selected series of 39 cases. Eur J Surg Oncol 18:438–441, 1992.

106. Segerstrom K, Bjerle P, Graffman S, Nystrom A: Factors that influence the incidence of brachial edema after treatment of breast cancer. Scand J Plast Reconstr Surg Hand Surg 26:223–227, 1992.

107. Seidman JS, Schnaper LA, Aisner SC: Relationship of the size of the invasive component of the primary breast carcinoma to axillary lymph node metastases. Cancer 75:65–71, 1995.

108. Seigel BM, Mayzel KA, Love SM: Level 1 and 2 axillary dissection in the treatment of early breast cancer. Arch Surg 125:1144–1147, 1990.

109. Senofsky GM, Moffat FL, Davis K, et al: Total axillary lymphadenectomy in the management of breast cancer. Arch Surg 126:1336–1342, 1991.

110. Silverstein M: Axillary dissection for T1a breast cancer—Is it indicated? Cancer 73:664–667, 1994.

111. Slamon DJ, Clark GM, Wong SG, et al: Human breast cancer: Correlation of relapse and survival with the amplification of the HER-2 neu oncogene. Science 235:177–182, 1987.

112. Smith JA, Gamez-Araujo LL, Gallager HS, et al: Carcinoma of the breast. Analysis of total lymph node involvement versus level of metastasis. Cancer 39:527–532, 1977.

113. Steele RJC, Forrest APM, Gibson T, Stewart HJ, Chetty U: Sampling in obtaining lymph node status in breast cancer: A controlled randomized trial. Br J Surg 72:368–369, 1985.

114. Stevens PE, Dibble SL, Miaskowski C: Prevalence, characteristics, and impact of postmastectomy pain syndrome: An investigation of women's experiences. Pain 61:61–68, 1995.

115. Strierer M, Rosen HR, Weber R, et al: Long-term analysis of factors influencing the outcome in carcinoma of the breast smaller than one centimeter. Surg Gynecol Obstet 175:151–160, 1992.

116. Strotter A, Atkinson EN, Fairston BA, et al: Survival following locoregional recurrence after breast conservation therapy for cancer. Ann Surg 212:166–172, 1990.

117. Tate J, Lewis V, Archer T, et al: Ultrasonographic detection of axillary lymph node metastases in breast cancer. Eur J Surg Oncol 15:139–142, 1989.

118. Thorek M: Surgery of the breast. *In* Modern Surgical Technic. 2nd ed. Philadelphia, JB Lippincott, 1949.

119. Tinnemans J, Wobbes T, Hollan R, et al: Treatment and survival of female patients with nonpalpable breast carcinoma. Ann Surg 209:249–253, 1989.

120. Urban JA: Radical mastectomy in continuity with en bloc resection of internal mammary lymph node chain: New procedure for primary operable cancer of the breast. Cancer 5:992–1006, 1952.

121. van der Veen H, Hoekstra OS, Paul MA, et al: Gamma probe guided sentinel node biopsy to select patients with melanoma for lymphadenectomy. Br J Surg 81:1769–1770, 1994.

122. Veronesi U, Luini A, Galimberti V, Zurrida S: Conservation approaches for the management of stage 1–2 carcinoma of the breast: Milan Cancer Institute trials. World J Surg 18:70–75, 1994.

123. Veronesi U, Rilke F, Luine A, et al: Distribution of axillary metastases by level of invasion. Cancer 59:682–687, 1987.

124. Veronesi U, Saccoozzi R, Del Vecchio M, et al: Comparing radical mastectomy with quadrantectomy, axillary dissection, and radiotherapy in patients with small cancers of the breast. N Eng J Med 305:6–11, 1981.

125. Veronesi U, Valagussa P: Inefficiency of internal mammary node dissection in breast cancer surgery. Cancer 47:170–175, 1981.

126. Walker MJ, Osborne MD, Young DC, et al: The natural history of breast cancer with more than ten positive nodes. Am J Surg 169:575–579, 1995.

127. Walls J, Boggis CRM, Wilson M, et al: Treatment of the axilla in patients with screen-detected breast cancer. Br J Surg 80:436–438, 1993.

128. Wangensteen OH: Super radical operation for breast cancer in the patient with lymph node involvement. Proc Natl Cancer Conf 2:230, 1952.

129. Whelan T, Clark R, Roberts R, et al: Ipsilateral breast tumor recurrence post-lumpectomy is predictive of subsequent mortality: Results from a randomized trial. Int J Radiat Oncol Biol Phys 30:11–16, 1994.

CHAPTER 49
BREAST RECONSTRUCTION FOLLOWING MASTECTOMY

John B. McCraw, M.D. / Christoph Papp, M.D. / Anne Cramer, M.D. /
Virginia Huang, M.D. / Abdullah Bandek, M.D. / Ann McMellin, C.S.T.

THE ROLE OF RECONSTRUCTION IN BREAST CANCER TREATMENT

In its broadest sense, breast reconstruction is a replacement of lost breast tissue and lost breast skin. The reasons for the loss of breast tissue, except for congenital deformities, include partial and complete mastectomies, radiation damage, infection, and trauma. By definition, the deformity that is caused by the breast injury produces an anatomically abnormal state.

Breast reconstruction is always performed to correct anatomical abnormalities, and for this reason, it is always a functional procedure. Breast reconstruction has nothing to do with the word cosmesis, which implies an improvement of normal. It is expected that any reconstructive breast procedure would improve the appearance compared with a mastectomy or a radiation injury but not when compared with normal anatomy.[13, 35, 118]

Until recently, breast cancer patients were not routinely considered for reconstruction at the time of mastectomy. Although there were good reasons for this in the past, such as large tumors and less than adequate methods of reconstruction, both of these concerns are infrequent considerations. Most mastectomies today are now performed for totally curable lesions, such as *in situ,* multifocal, and minimal breast cancers. Routine consideration of breast reconstruction at the time of mastectomy can now be defended for patients with stages 0, I, and IIa disease, and this subset of patients describes the vast majority of the patients who presently undergo mastectomy. (See Section XIII, Chapter 41.) In fact, there is no scientific basis for denying this group of patients immediate reconstruction.* Immediate reconstruction is usually ignored more than it is denied, out of deference to past convention.

Women are no different from men in their desire to correct a physical deformity, yet the only cancer patients who are not routinely considered for some form of reconstruction are breast cancer patients.

Breast reconstruction is considered cosmetic or unessential by some because the replacement breast apparently does not add to bodily function. Many procedures in men are performed purely to improve form rather than function, including excision of gynecomastia, placement of a scrotal prosthesis, or removal of an unsightly skin graft of the arm. Until the advent of managed care rationing, none of the male procedures were scrutinized as to whether they were cosmetic or not. Breast reconstruction in women should require no justification if a mastectomy is either planned or completed. When the extirpation causes a physical deformity, reconstruction should be routinely considered by the treating doctors, and this choice should not be arbitrarily denied solely for economic reasons by insurance reviewers. Breast reconstruction serves as one aspect of the overall process of cancer rehabilitation, which is conducted to restore the patient physically, emotionally, and spiritually.[36, 57, 72, 113]

In addition to postmastectomy reconstruction, autogenous flap reconstructions are essential for treatment of radiation injuries of the breast and chest wall. It is now recognized that both postmastectomy radiation and lumpectomy radiation cause a vasculitis that progressively destroys skin and muscle over a period of time.[15] Higher radiation dosages, particularly when concentrated in a localized area, eventually cause fibrosis of the pectoralis muscle, and ischemic necrosis of the costal cartilages and sternum with breakdown of the overlying skin. These radiation injuries were much more common with the older techniques, yet they remain as an inherent part of radiation therapy. This is an important consideration in younger women, because the progressive vasculitis may cause problems 20 or 30 years after treatment. No matter how carefully it is performed, radiation therapy eventually produces a certain number of radiation ulcers, lumpectomy-radiation failures, and other problem wounds that can only be corrected by the introduction of well-vascularized tissue to replace the radiated tissue.[70, 102] Particularly when resection of the chest wall is needed, myocutaneous flaps are absolutely necessary for a safe closure of the wound.[3]

---

*See references 27, 67, 69, 72, 97, 118, and 139.

DEFINITION OF THE MASTECTOMY DEFORMITY

The Ideal Total Mastectomy

From the standpoint of the reconstructive surgeon, the ideal total mastectomy should preserve the pectoralis major muscle and all of the skin that is not essential to the tumor resection. When this approach is used, the functional considerations of mobility of the shoulder and soft tissue coverage of the ribs will be achieved (Fig. 49–1A and B). Extensive skin excision, which results in a tight skin closure, has *not* been shown to enhance survival, but it does make reconstruction much more difficult. Tissue expanders cannot overcome a large skin deficit, and the need for the more complex autogenous flaps is ensured by a mastectomy with radical skin excision. The difference between skin laxity and skin tightness is usually a difference of an added 2 cm of skin with each mastectomy flap. The addition of 4 to 6 cm of skin to the closure is tremendously helpful to any type of reconstruction and usually is the determining factor as to whether a myocutaneous flap will be required to correct the deformity.

In addition to crossing tension, the placement of the incision is the other important factor that determines whether mastectomy scars will be good or bad. In this regard, the foremost consideration is to place the incision in the appropriate lines of skin tension. It is easy to identify the exact direction of the skin tension lines by pinching the skin to accentuate the wrinkles. When incisions follow these lines precisely, this offers the best chance of favorable healing, and usually avoids prolonged redness and hypertrophic scarring. Rather than using the standard transverse ellipse, an incision is chosen in the lower or lateral breast, which provides adequate access for any mastectomy. A low and oblique closure is preferred because it is better hidden and offers much better shoulder and chest mobility than a higher incision. The worst choice for a closure in a patient who will eventually have a breast reconstruction is the transverse Patey incision. It is inelastic and unexpandable, and gives the least attractive scars (Figs. 49–2 and 49–3).

Partial Mastectomy

It is still not generally recognized that any partial breast deformity is preferable to any complete breast deformity. By far the easiest reconstruction is replacement of up to 50 percent of the breast volume without skin replacement.[77, 102, 130] This can be accomplished with an autogenous latissimus flap in a single stage, under local (tumescent) anesthesia with deep sedation. The usual skin defects of the modified mastectomy, which is approximately 7 cm by 15 cm, can also be accomplished with the latissimus flap.[85, 87] The favorable nature of the partial mastectomy defect is the reason that a central tumor should never be the sole justification for choosing a complete mastectomy instead of lumpectomy and radiation. When the lumpectomy deforms the breast, and even when it is necessary to remove the nipple, conservation therapy is still a good option. Although a partial central mastectomy does deform the breast, the deformity of a complete mastectomy is always worse than this partial deformity (Figs. 49–4 and 49–5). The loss of the central breast and nipple are simple problems to correct and can be achieved either before or after radiation.[15, 100]

The skin-conservation, or skin-sparing, mastectomy limits the skin excision to the skin needed for

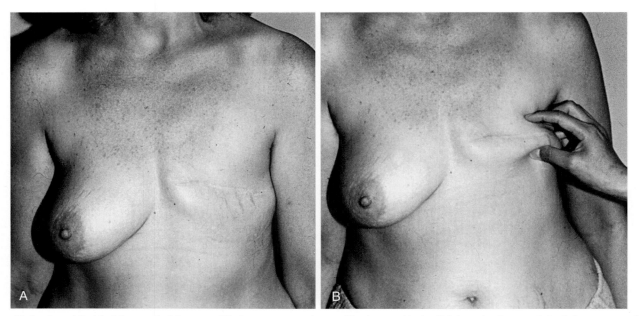

Figure 49–1 **A** *and* **B,** *Ideal low and oblique modified mastectomy closure. The breast skin is slightly redundant, and the inframammary fold is still present.*

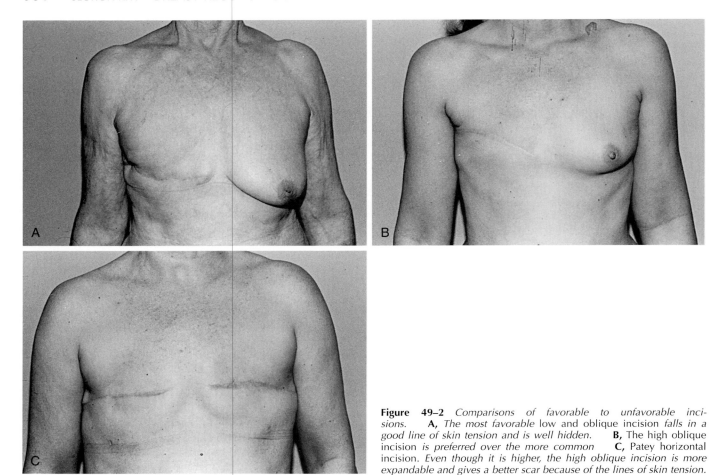

Figure 49–2 *Comparisons of favorable to unfavorable incisions.*   **A,** *The most favorable low and oblique incision falls in a good line of skin tension and is well hidden.*   **B,** *The high oblique incision is preferred over the more common*   **C,** *Patey horizontal incision. Even though it is higher, the high oblique incision is more expandable and gives a better scar because of the lines of skin tension.*

adequate tumor removal, which includes the nipple, the biopsy site, and any breast skin that is within 1 to 2 cm of the tumor. (See Section XIII, Chapter 41.) In most patients with stages I and IIa tumors, this is a reasonable approach because tumors are more often deep than they are close to the skin. Even when

the tumor lies beneath the nipple, a wide skin ellipse is usually unnecessarily radical. At the periphery of the ellipse, the margin of tumor excision is 10 to 15 cm, which is far in excess of any treatment protocol. A circular excision of the nipple/areola complex usually provides satisfactory margins and exposure with

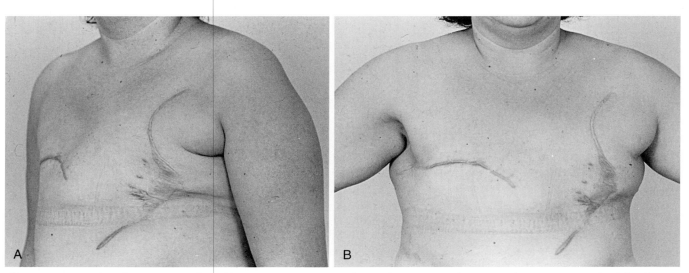

Figure 49–3   **A** *and* **B,** *The two most unfavorable incisions: transverse and vertical. Asymmetrical incisions always accentuate the deformity.*

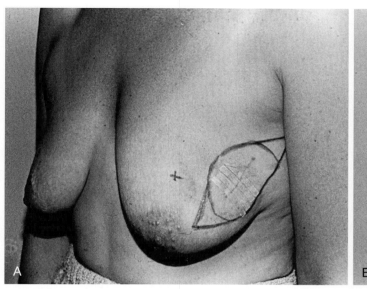
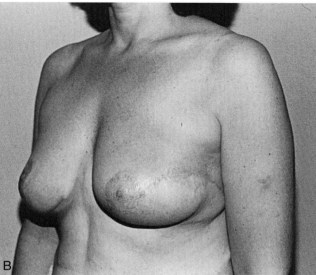

Figure 49–4 **A,** *Outline of quadrantectomy to be followed by radiation without boost to the area of the tumor.*   **B,** *Postoperative view at 1 year following an autogenous latissimus reconstruction to replace the 50 percent loss of breast volume. No implant was used. The quadrantectomy skin removal was closed through a lateral incision and used to correct breast ptosis.*

far less harm to the breast. It should be remembered that the primary purpose of the elliptical closure, compared with a circular closure, is to avoid dogears. Skin conservation facilitates reconstruction with tissue expanders alone, and greatly improves the result that can be achieved with autogenous flaps. Even in cases in which reconstruction will never be performed, in the vast majority of patients there is no reason to excise the skin widely and cause functional deformities. It should not be just the reconstructive surgeon who encourages skin conservation (Figs. 49–6 to 49–8). It should be in everyone's interest

to avoid unnecessarily radical skin excision when glandular removal and limited skin excision provides the same margin of safety.*

Modified Mastectomy with Extensive Skin Excision

By convention, the amount of skin excision is just as radical with a modified radical mastectomy as it is with a standard radical mastectomy in present-day

*See references 39, 40, 47, 63, 67, 69, 72, 129, and 132.

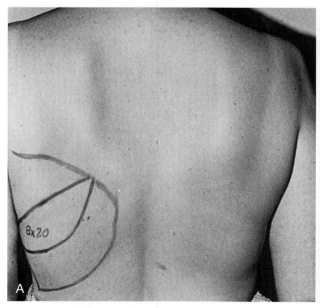
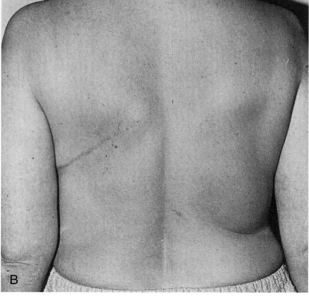

Figure 49–5 **A,** *Outline of the autogenous latissimus flap on the back. The skin "paddle" is drawn as an ellipse. The circular outline depicts the area of fat that will be carried on the surface of the latissimus muscle.*   **B,** *Postoperative view of the back donor site at one year. This gives a good scar when the closure follows the skin tension lines.*

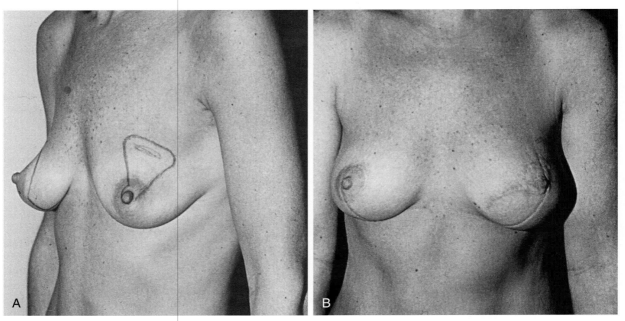

Figure 49–6   A, *Outline of limited skin removal, including the biopsy site, in a patient with DCIS and minimal breast cancer. A free TRAM flap is planned for breast volume replacement because of the thin build of the patient.*   **B,** *Two months following skin conservation mastectomy with a buried TRAM flap and first stage of nipple reconstruction. A mastopexy was performed in the normal breast.*

practice. Extensive skin excision has been the cornerstone of mastectomy for breast cancer since Handley promoted the permeation theory of centrifugal tumor spread in 1915.[55] Today's modified mastectomy is patterned after Patey's method of radical skin excision with the primary closure, which was popularized by Auchincloss and Madden.[4, 74, 101] It is very similar to the original description of Moore in 1867.[94] It was

Patey's belief that removal of the pectoralis major muscle contributed little to the cure of breast cancer because the tumor seldom invaded the muscle unless it was in close proximity. Instead, skin permeation with tumor was Patey's primary concern in tumor extirpation, so that he attempted primary closure in only about half of his cases. When compared with the radical mastectomy, the Patey mastectomy is less

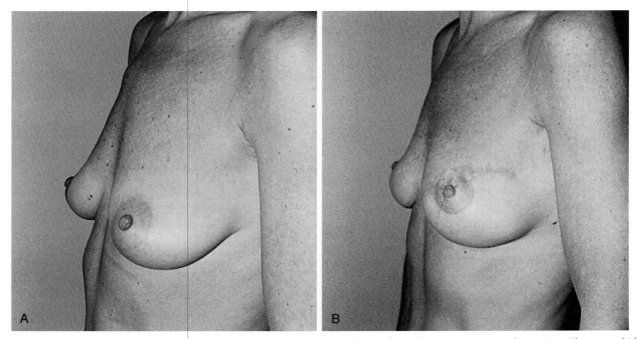

Figure 49–7   A, *Preoperative view.*   **B,** *Postoperative view following completion of nipple reconstruction and tattooing. The tattoo hides the central third of the oblique scar.*

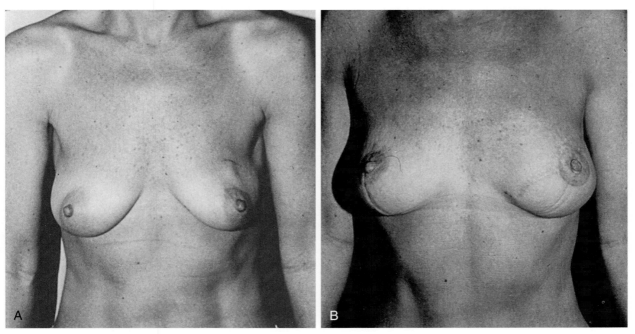

Figure 49–8   **A** *and* **B,** *Preoperative and postoperative views at 6 months. Note the perfect symmetry that is made possible by three factors:* skin conservation, autogenous tissue, and immediate reconstruction. *Removing additional skin, as in a traditional modified mastectomy, would not have contributed anything to the extirpation in this patient, but it would have prevented an excellent reconstructive result.*

radical in regard to the pectoralis major muscle but just as radical in regard to skin removal.[54]

In the normal breast, there is no tightness of either the skin or pectoralis major muscle and 180 degrees of shoulder abduction is the full range of motion. By comparison, the skin closure of the standard modified mastectomy usually causes skin tightness at 90 degrees of shoulder abduction, as well as some limitation of shoulder motion, beginning at 130 degrees of abduction (Figs. 49–9 and 49–10). In practice, the elliptical skin excision usually measures 10 by 17

cm, which is more than enough to cause a skin contracture across the chest. A horizontal skin ellipse has the most detrimental effect on shoulder motion compared with any other incision because of the tethering of the extensile skin between the inframammary fold and the axilla. The usual transverse skin closure is also the most unfavorable scar for breast reconstruction, because it crosses the skin tension lines perpendicularly, which results in scar hypertrophy and stiffness. The low and oblique scar is much more extensible, and even a vertical closure gives a

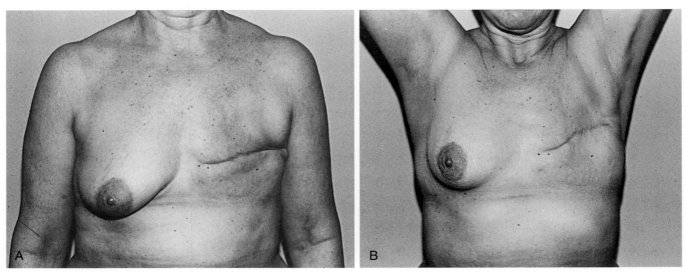

Figure 49–9   **A** *and* **B,** *Typical modified mastectomy with extensive skin resection. The skin tightness is noticed at 90 degrees and limits shoulder motion beginning at 130 degrees. Because of the scarring, the skin between the incision and the inframammary fold cannot be used in the breast reconstruction and must be replaced by an autogenous flap.*

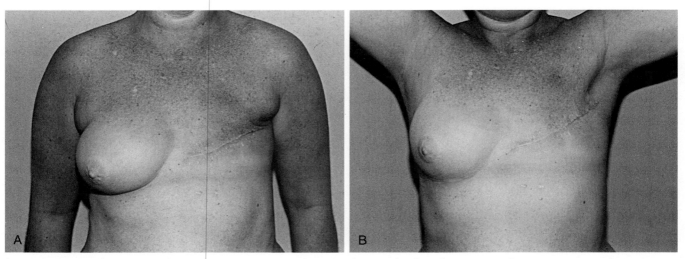

Figure 49–10 **A** and **B,** *Massive skin resection in a patient with stage I disease. The skin ellipse measured 10 cm × 22 cm. Skin expansion is precluded by the skin deformity.*

better scar than the transverse closure (Figs. 49–11 and 49–12).

Reconstruction in a patient who has had a modified mastectomy with extensive skin excision can be just as difficult as reconstruction of the radical mastectomy deformity.[36] Reconstruction cannot usually be accomplished with an implant or a tissue expander alone because the surrounding skin has already been "recruited" for closure of the mastectomy defect.[8] Autogenous skin flaps are usually required to replace the breast skin because tissue expanders cannot overcome the tightness of the skin closure.[14, 59, 73, 80]

Radical Mastectomy

In the radical mastectomy, the skin resection is always extensive and produces chest wall tightness, visible ribs, and some compromise of shoulder mobility.[50] Radical mastectomies are still performed, and patients still present with these massive deformities

from years before (Fig. 49–13). Because of the inadequate soft tissue cover, it is usually impossible for patients to wear an external prosthesis. Reconstruction of this deformity is never possible with an implant or tissue expander alone, and always requires the addition of a myocutaneous flap. Even under ideal circumstances, it is almost impossible to achieve an excellent result of radical mastectomy reconstruction.[37, 84, 90]

Mastectomy and Radiation

When the treatment includes postoperative radiation, functional deformities caused by extensive skin excision are magnified.[15] Radiation causes scarring between the skin and pectoralis major muscle, and shrinkage of both the skin and muscle, and may also have a direct effect on stiffness of the shoulder joint. Adding radiation to a modified mastectomy converts the functional deficit to that of a radical mastectomy

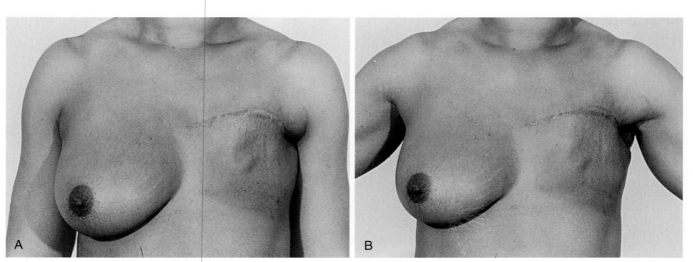

Figure 49–11 **A** and **B,** *Massive skin resection with a high transverse closure in a patient with stage I disease. A satisfactory reconstruction cannot be achieved without autogenous tissue replacement.*

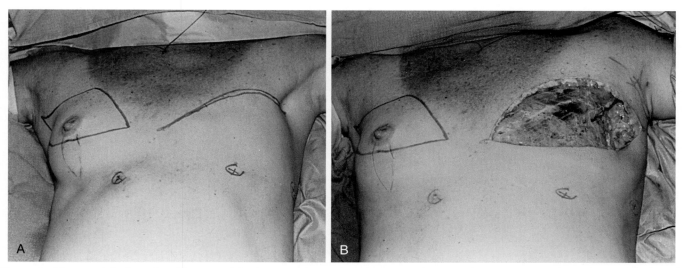

Figure 49–12 **A** *and* **B,** *Extensive skin removal in the upper breast done for stage I disease with a 1-cm tumor above the nipple. The right mastectomy was done for DCIS, but the incisions were identical to the left breast. A skin conservation mastectomy could have been performed in both breasts.*

or worse.[112] Because radiation causes a perivascular inflammation, which continues to damage the tissue forever, the mastectomy flaps must be presumed to have poor vascularization. For this reason, much of the radiated breast skin must be discarded and replaced with autogenous tissue.[18, 102] It is imperative to remove as much of the pigment-altered irradiated skin as possible because this is a sign of very advanced radiation damage. This skin may survive a re-elevation, but it frequently develops ischemic necrosis many years later. Radiation precludes an implant reconstruction in almost every instance, because the radiated skin lacks pliability and extensibility, and is subject to late skin ulcerations from the underlying implant.[18] Patients who have had augmentation can be considered for conservation therapy, which preserves the implant, but the value

of this has been questioned.[53] These implants usually become firm because of the irradiation, and mammographic follow-up is impaired by both silicone and saline implants. Even with a perfect implant, this would probably not be an acceptable combination (Figs. 49–14 to 49–16).

RECONSTRUCTIVE SURGICAL METHODS

Historical Developments

The history of reconstructive breast surgery has several identifiable periods, and the developments of each period have had a dramatic effect on the course of breast cancer surgery in general. From antiquity

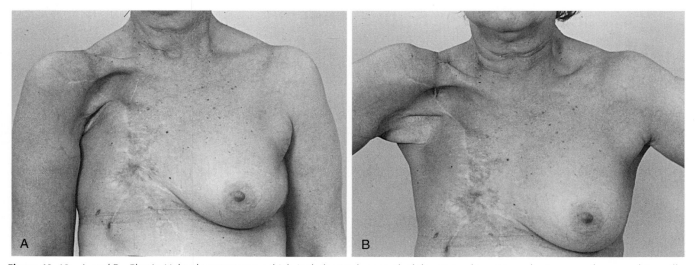

Figure 49–13 **A** *and* **B,** *Classic Halsted mastectomy, which includes total removal of the pectoralis major and minor muscles, complete axillary dissection, and skin closure by secondary healing. This procedure was used into the 1980s because surgeons believed that it would prolong survival in patients with advanced disease.*

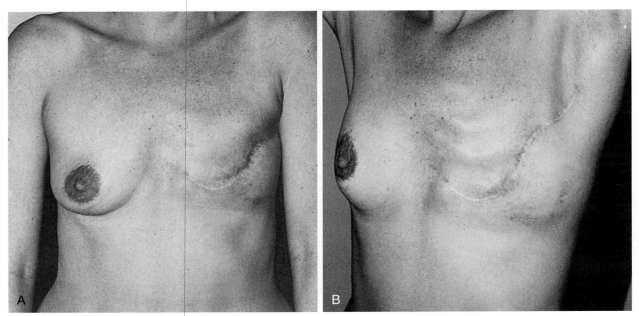

Figure 49–14   A and **B,** *Thirty-seven-year-old patient treated for stage IIa disease with removal of the pectoralis major muscle, extensive skin excision, and postoperative radiation. Reconstruction must be performed with autogenous tissue that carries its own permanent blood supply and replaces most of the irradiated breast skin. Because of the massive defect, reconstruction can only be accomplished with either a double-muscle or free TRAM.*

until very recent times, healing of the mastectomy wound was the primary reconstructive concern in undertaking any extensive mastectomy procedure. Until skin grafting became available, radical mastectomies were all allowed to heal by secondary epithelialization.[52] Small skin grafts were described in the 1870s but were not applied to the mastectomy deformity until the turn of the century.[31, 99, 110, 127, 138] Sheet skin grafting was developed in the late 1920s but was only available in a few major medical centers until after World War II.[12, 31, 51] By 1950, only a few hundred surgeons were trained in sheet skin grafting, a technique that was not generally used until the Brown motorized dermatome became available.[22, 100] Elevation of breast skin flaps with primary closure of the mastectomy first appeared during the 1940s, but it was not accepted as a routine part of the mastectomy until the 1960s.[4, 54, 74] Breast reduction and nipple reconstruction were introduced in the late 1940s but did not become popular until the 1970s.*

*See references 1, 2, 5, 75, 76, 103, 109, 121, 128, and 137.

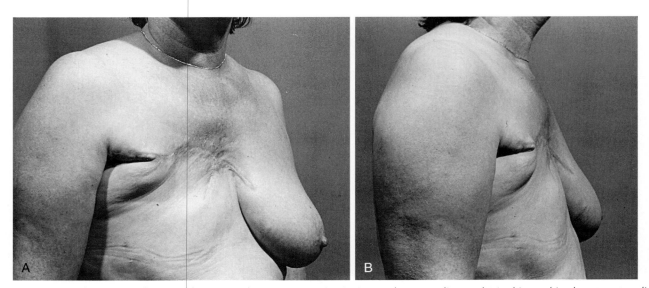

Figure 49–15   A and **B,** *Forty-eight-year-old patient with a 2-cm tumor impinging on the pectoralis muscle. In this combined treatment, radiation compounds the problem of the tight skin closure. Without radiation, this would be an extremely difficult reconstruction. With radiation, it is nearly impossible.*

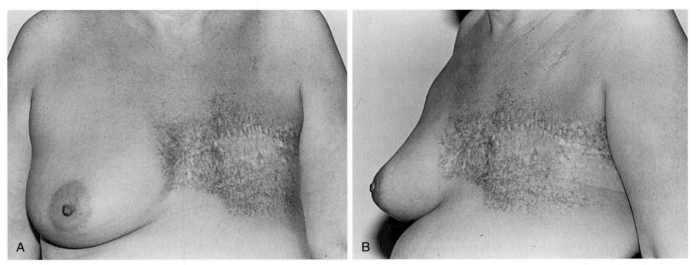

Figure 49–16 *A* and **B**, *Fibrotic destruction of the breast skin by radiation. This progressive injury took 15 years to develop and made even an autogenous reconstruction almost impossible.*

The first breast reconstructions were performed using tubed skin flaps or silicone implants beginning in the early 1960s.[20, 44, 45, 89, 135] In Europe, the Tansini latissimus dorsi myocutaneous flap was commonly used for the closure of radical mastectomies between 1900 and 1925, but myocutaneous flap procedures were abandoned until 1975.[78, 122, 123] Campbell first reported on the use of the latissimus dorsi muscle flap for chest wall reconstruction in 1950, but his method went unnoticed for another generation.[25] By 1975, myocutaneous flaps were used for delayed breast and chest wall reconstructions, but myocutaneous flaps were seldom used for immediate reconstruction before 1990.[81–83, 86] Today it would be difficult to imagine extirpative breast surgery without primary closure, skin grafts, or myocutaneous flaps.

Primary Closure

Extensive skin excision has always been a hallmark of both radical, modified, and even simple mastectomies (Fig. 49–17). In each procedure, as much breast skin was removed as possible, in hope that this would improve the effectiveness of the mastectomy. This practice was so well accepted that it was continued for 60 years before it was subjected to scientific study. The various mastectomies are still differentiated by factors other than skin excision. For example, the modified mastectomy is a radical mastectomy in which the pectoralis major muscle is preserved, and the simple mastectomy is a modified mastectomy without an axillary dissection. Patey's mastectomy is still considered less radical than the Halsted mastectomy because the pectoralis major muscle is preserved, but Patey believed in extremely wide skin excision, in which only half of his mastectomies were primarily closed. Since the reports of Madden and Auchincloss in the early 1960s, primary closure has not been considered harmful and has been accepted as the prevailing method. Today, extensive skin exci-

sion is still the standard of practice in mastectomy, because of the lingering suspicion that limited skin excision might be less effective in curing the cancer, even though this belief has never been tested by prospective and randomized scientific studies. Fifty years from now, students will be just as puzzled about our current practices of extensive skin excision as they are about the total breast skin excision at the turn of the century.

Primary closure is a relatively recent development in mastectomy surgery. The Halsted mastectomy, like other radical mastectomies in the early part of the century, was rarely closed primarily.[51] This procedure included resection of skin and breast tissue in a three-dimensional block (Fig. 49–18). This near-total removal of the breast skin was routinely used until the 1940s, because elevation of breast skin flaps was believed to interfere with the tumor resection by either spreading the breast cancer or leaving it within the substance of the breast skin. At the time, it was presumed that the breast cancer permeated the entire breast skin, not just the part of the skin that was adjacent to the tumor. When total excision of the breast skin was eventually abandoned, it was replaced with such extreme resections of the skin in the modified radical mastectomy that primary closure was the exception until the late 1960s.[54]

Skin Grafting

Primary healing of the radical mastectomy was rarely considered until sheet skin grafts became available in the 1920s.[22] Until that time, very small, postage stamp grafts were used. Beginning in 1870, small split-thickness grafts and full-thickness grafts were used on the face.[99, 110, 127, 138] Most of these grafts were postage stamp–sized grafts only because knives had not been developed for harvesting larger grafts. In the 1920s, John Staige Davis popularized pinch grafts, which were harvested by shaving a "divot" of

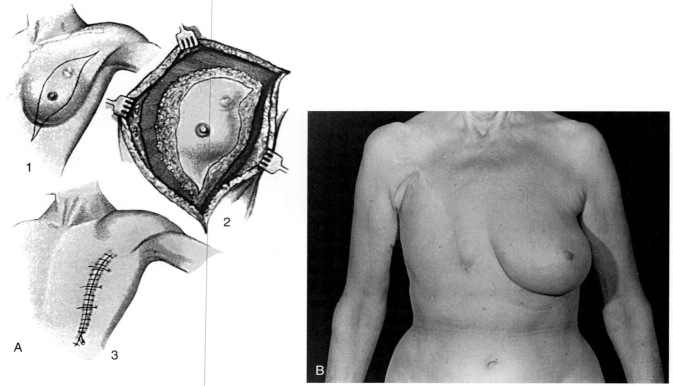

Figure 49–17 **A,** *Illustration from Geschickter's* Diseases of the Breast *(1943), published by J.B. Lippincott. Note the extent of the proposed skin excision in this* simple mastectomy, *in which primary closure is obviously a challenge.* **B,** *A 1979 clinical example of this mastectomy with a vertical closure demonstrates the same principles of wide skin excision, performed nearly 40 years later.*

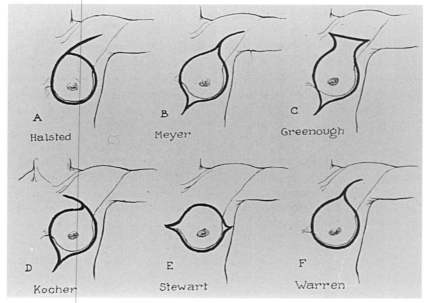

Figure 49–18 *Illustration from Geschickter's* Diseases of the Breast *(1943), published by J.B. Lippincott. Note that in each design for radical mastectomy incisions virtually all of the breast skin was excised in the shape of a circle. The differences were in the extensions, which facilitated exposure. Primary closure would be impossible for most of these designs.*

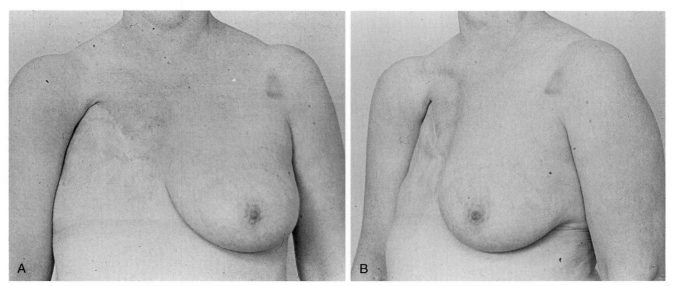

Figure 49–19 **A** *and* **B,** *Example of a skin-grafted radical mastectomy done in 1978. The sheet skin graft was a major advance in healing the mastectomy wound.*

skin with a flat knife.[31] This graft was a full-thickness graft in the center and a partial-thickness in the periphery to enhance the take of the graft. Even though these small grafts were available, most mastectomies were allowed to heal secondarily by scar epithelium. Beginning in the late 1920s, Blair and Brown in the United States and Humby and Braithwaite in England popularized sheet skin grafts, which were taken with large hand-held knives. These knives were variations of the straight razor of the day and required such exquisite dexterity that less than a hundred surgeons were trained in these techniques by the start of World War II. Most of these surgeons were general surgeons who took additional training in plastic surgery. In the late 1930s, calibrated dermatomes, such as the Padgett and Reese dermatomes, were introduced.[100, 109] The motorized Brown dermatome was not developed until after World War II, when it was conceived by Dr. Brown during his war time imprisonment in Bataan.[22] Even as late as 1950, only a few hundred surgeons in the world attempted skin grafting procedures, and very few of these procedures were performed on mastectomy patients (Fig. 49–19).

Early Flaps

In 1896, the latissimus dorsi flap was described by Iginio Tansini, a professor of surgery at the University of Pavia in Italy.[122, 123] In the early part of the century, the breast was removed without elevation of skin flaps, which left a large circular defect that took a number of months to heal. The Tansini method used the same extirpative technique as the Halsted radical mastectomy, but the latissimus dorsi myocutaneous flap was transposed anteriorly for wound closure (Figs. 49–20 to 49–23). The purpose of the

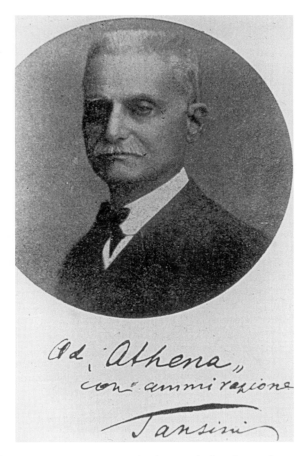

Figure 49–20 *Iginio Tansini, the distinguished professor of surgery at the University of Pavia at the turn of the century. The Tansini method of mastectomy used the latissimus dorsi myocutaneous flap to close the radical mastectomy. His primary closure predated sheet skin graft closure by some 20 years. (From Maxwell, GP: Iginio Tansini and the origin of the latissimus dorsi musculocutaneous flap. Plast Reconstr Surg 65:686–693, 1980.)*

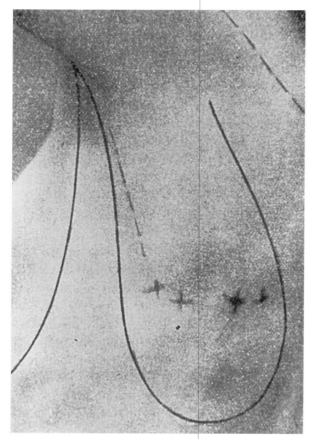

Figure 49–21 *Outline of the latissimus myocutaneous flap in the lateral view. Skin was carried on the anterior surface of the latissimus muscle in this proximally based flap. (From Maxwell GP: Iginio Tansini and the origin of the latissimus dorsi musculocutaneous flap. Plast Reconstr Surg 65:686–693, 1980.)*

latissimus myocutaneous flap was to replace the pectoralis major and provide skin from the back to heal the breast wound primarily. Tansini's description of the latissimus dorsi myocutaneous flap is virtually identical to that described independently by Olivari,[98] McCraw,[83] and Muhlbauer,[95] in 1974. The Tansini method was the prevailing technique of mastectomy in Europe until about 1920, when Halsted made a grand tour of the European medical centers. Halsted said: "Beware of the man with the plastic operation . . ." because he thought that the latissimus flap was both "unnecessary and hazardous."[78] At a time when intravenous fluids, transfusions, and anesthetics were in a stage of rudimentary development, Halsted's statement was probably reasonable. Nevertheless, it set back the legitimate uses of myocutaneous flaps for breast or chest wall reconstruction for another 50 years. Between 1920 and 1974, the Tansini procedure was completely abandoned, and myocutaneous flaps were not used for immediate reconstruction of the breast until after 1980.

Because of the notable success of Sir Harold Gillies in repairing World War I maxillofacial injuries, the tubed skin flap became the dominant method of flap reconstruction until myocutaneous flaps were re-

introduced in the mid-1970s.[44, 45] Tubed flaps were not applicable to immediate breast reconstruction, because the transfer of the tube of skin from the abdomen to the breast consumed a period of at least a year and more than a dozen operations. Tubed flaps were also impractical to use for radiation injuries because they did not carry a permanent blood supply to the ischemic area. Until the advent of myocutaneous flaps, flap resurfacing of an irradiation ulcer was seldom attempted because of the high morbidity and the frequent recurrence of radiation ulcers in the skin surrounding the flap. As late as the 1970s, tubed flaps were used for elective breast reconstruction (Figs. 49–24 to 49–27).

Silicone Breast Implants

Silicone breast implants were first introduced by Cronin and Gerow[29] in 1964 and popularized by a number of surgeons over the next 20 years.[32, 62, 105, 106, 108, 126] This pioneering surgical work was conducted in collaboration with the Dow Chemical Company using polymers constructed from silicone. Silicone is an elemental metal adjacent to carbon on the periodic table and was chosen as an implant material because of its nonreactive potential and its availability as both a solid and a gel. These physiochemical characteristics allow a broad range of design capabilities

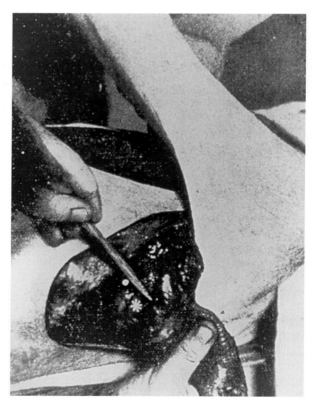

Figure 49–22 *Elevation of the latissimus flap with the patient in the supine position. The radical mastectomy defect is seen anteriorly. Note that Professor Tansini is operating without gloves. (From Maxwell GP: Iginio Tansini and the origin of the latissimus dorsi musculocutaneous flap. Plast Reconstr Surg 65:686–693, 1980.)*

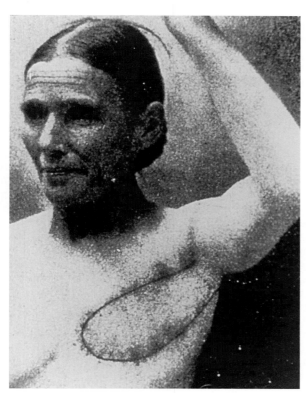

Figure 49–23 *Transposed latissimus flap into the left radical mastectomy defect. Instead of taking months to heal the wound, the latissimus flap provided immediate closure. Halsted called this myocutaneous flap procedure "Unnecessary and hazardous . . . ," even though it was the predominant method of mastectomy closure in Europe at the time. (From Maxwell GP: Iginio Tansini and the origin of the latissimus dorsi musculocutaneous flap. Plast Reconstr Surg 65:686–693, 1980.)*

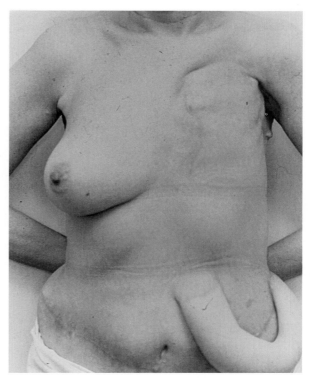

Figure 49–24 *Correction of a radical mastectomy defect with a tube flap created from the abdominal pannus.*

that can be achieved by manipulating the molecular weight of the polymer. Linear, short-chain lightweight silicone polymers form lubricants and oils. With increasing molecular weight, the viscosity of silicone increases. Use of a catalyst and heating cause the polymers to branch into chains and form gels. With side branching of the linear chains, the oils are vulcanized into elastomers that can be used as adhesives, sealants, and rubbers. The first silicone implant design, a silicone gel contained within a thin, solid silicone envelope sealed with silicone adhesive, is basically unchanged to the present time.

Compared with the previously available human breast implants, which were made of polyurethane foam, paraffin, or allogenic implants, all of which were capable of disastrous complications, the silicone gel implants represented a historic medical breakthrough.[21, 62, 76, 104] This development also initiated a completely new group of medical products from silicone, including silicone tubes, lubricants, and linings, which were relatively inert in a biological setting. By the late 1960s, silicone gel implants were sporadically used for breast reconstruction. The early experience with these implants was not good because of the fibrous encapsulation of the implant that occurred beneath the thin mastectomy skin flaps. The better soft tissue cover of subpectoral placement of the im-

plants improved the results, just as the even better cover of autogenous flaps improved it further. Over time, it became apparent that silicone implants were not as nonreactive as had been expected, and many local wound problems—such as scarring, low-grade infection, and implant intolerance—were cause for concern. Eventually, many of the early implant breast reconstructions failed because distortion of the shape produced an appearance known as the "half

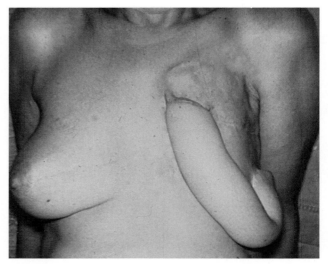

Figure 49–25 *Intermediate inset of the tube flap following separation from its abdominal blood supply. This process of "waltzing" a tube flap from the abdomen to the chest was used by Halsted and Billroth.*

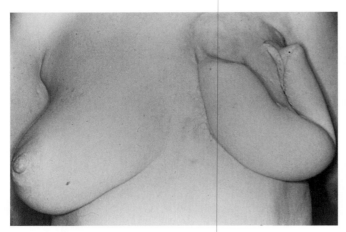

Figure 49–26 *Final inset into the sternum before shaping.*

grapefruit" shape which accurately described the elevated, rounded, and firm implant (Fig. 49–28).

In 1992, the federal Food and Drug Administration (FDA) restricted the availability of silicone gel implants, in deference to a class action legal suit involving hundreds of thousands of claims. Saline-filled silicone breast implants, which were not implicated as causing any autoimmune symptoms, were still allowed under the new FDA regulations. After several years of study, no association was found between silicone implants and atypical autoimmune diseases. Statistical association did not prove causation. One unanticipated benefit of the FDA changes was the acceleration of the search for implant filler materials that are more biologically compatible, that is, inert and harmless when leaked.[41] Besides good performance characteristics, the new implants are expected to offer no interference with mammograms. The only material that appears to have satisfied most of these basic criteria is the triglyceride implant.[68] Made from soybean oil, the triglyceride implant has the same radiolucency as breast tissue, so that microcalcifica-

tions can be viewed through the implant material. To date, at least one breast cancer has been diagnosed mammographically with the triglyceride implant in place. Several other new filler materials can be expected in the next few years, and silicone gel will eventually be replaced completely.

Tissue Expansion

In the early 1980s, tissue expanders were developed as an alternative to simple silicone implant breast reconstruction.[8, 17, 107] These inflatable implants were used to stretch the remaining breast skin and create an oversized pocket in an effort to decrease encapsulation of the silicone implant. Unfortunately, this method was initially applied to unfavorable candidates, such as those who had undergone the Patey mastectomy with extensive skin excision, and it was the poor mastectomies that gave the method an initial bad reputation (Fig. 49–29). As experience has been gained, the tissue expander has become the predominant means of breast reconstruction in patients who have not had extensive skin removal. The device is useful at the time of mastectomy to preserve the space and prevent shrinkage of the mastectomy flaps.[34, 117] Over a period of 10 to 14 days, the device is gradually expanded, which should not cause any problems with wound healing. The most ideal circumstance for tissue expansion is when a skin-sparing mastectomy has been performed and neither expansion nor recruitment is required. At a second stage, a permanent implant is placed, or an autogenous myocutaneous flap can be buried to replace the lost breast. If the new permanent implants are significantly better than our present implants and more skin-sparing mastectomies are performed, the method of tissue expansion will gain even wider acceptance.

Myocutaneous Flaps

The subpectoral reconstruction was expected to solve the problem of periprosthetic scarring by protecting

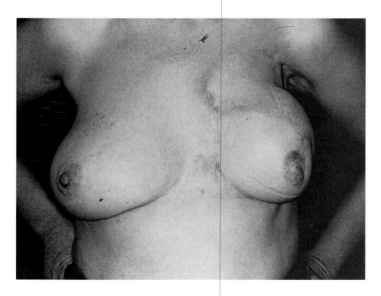

Figure 49–27 *The lateral half of the tube flap was then detached laterally and inset into the upper sternum to create the breast shape. This type of reconstruction usually took over a year to complete with more than a dozen procedures.*

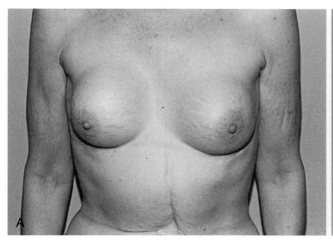
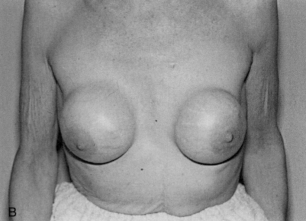

Figure 49–28 **A** *and* **B,** *Silicone implant reconstruction of a subcutaneous mastectomy, a procedure that was popular in the 1970s. The fibrous capsule around the silicone implant eventually constricts the shape to cause firmness, roundness, and elevation of the implant.*

the implant beneath the pectoralis major muscle.[65] This reduced the incidence of symptomatic capsular contracture from nearly 100 percent to less than 30 percent in the first 2 years because of a reduction in scarring around the implant.[23, 24] In retrospect, this was the first evidence of the protective effect of muscle in the prevention of periprosthetic scarring and firmness (Fig. 49–30). Unfortunately, the skin defect of the modified mastectomy was too extensive to correct with a simple implant, whether it occurred beneath the pectoralis muscle or not.

The latissimus dorsi breast reconstruction was introduced in 1977 by Schneider, Hill, and Brown[114] and popularized by Bostwick[14] and others.[79, 80, 89, 90] The latissimus dorsi breast reconstruction offered several breakthroughs with immediate replacement of the lost breast skin, replacement of the pectoralis muscle with the latissimus dorsi muscle, and complete muscle coverage of the silicone implant.[16, 28] Replacement of the pectoralis major muscle, the anterior axillary fold, and at least part of the missing

skin revolutionized the reconstruction of the radical mastectomy defect (Fig. 49–31). The muscular coverage of the implant was expected to reduce the rate of capsular contracture to a minimal level, which it did for a period of 1 to 2 years. McCraw and Maxwell reported the first 5-year results, which were disappointing because of either firmness or contour deformities in 39 percent of the patients with modified mastectomies and 75 percent of the patients with radical mastectomies.[84] Nevertheless, the latissimus dorsi myocutaneous flap gave the first acceptable results with breast reconstruction following radical mastectomy. From the time of its description in 1977 to the height of its popularity in 1982, the latissimus breast reconstruction was recognized as the standard by which all of the methods of breast reconstruction should be measured. By 1985, the standard latissimus reconstruction was all but abandoned in favor of either tissue expander or the transverse rectus abdominis myocutaneous (TRAM) flap reconstruction because of the problems of shape and softness caused

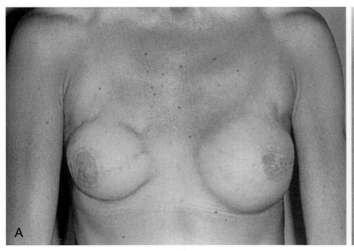
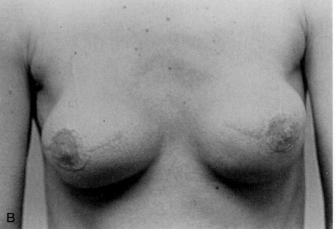

Figure 49–29 **A** *and* **B,** *Encapsulated silicone implant reconstruction corrected with tissue expansion. The capsule is first excised, and the tissue expander is used to create an oversized pocket for the implant.*

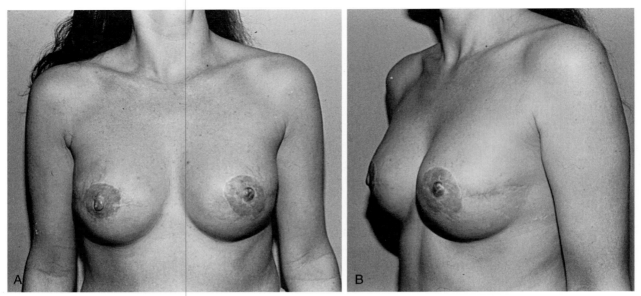

Figure 49–30 **A** and **B**, *Placement of silicone implants beneath the pectoralis major muscle at the time of a skin conservation mastectomy. Reasonably good results can be expected with subpectoral simple implant reconstructions when the skin removal is limited.*

by the silicone implant. If the new implant designs solve the problems of capsular contracture, the latissimus myocutaneous flap reconstruction may regain its previous popularity.

Autogenous Myocutaneous Flaps

Beginning in 1982, the era of autogenous myocutaneous flaps was introduced with the description of Hartrampf's TRAM flap.[60] This was the first breast reconstruction using only living tissue, and it achieved the first uniformly good results with any type of mastectomy. Over the period of a decade this procedure reached a level of perfection which would have been unthinkable only a decade before. In the

late 1980s, the autogenous latissimus flap was developed as an alternative procedure to the TRAM flap.[10, 85, 87] In the 1990s, microvascular transfer of the TRAM flap expanded the indications for the breast reconstruction to "high-risk" patients who were not acceptable candidates for the pedicle TRAM flap.[11, 36, 49, 130] This included patients with diabetes, smoking, obesity, and radiation injuries. In the future, these complex and expensive procedures will assuredly be rationed by the managed care system, and they may be lost for a generation, just as myocutaneous flaps disappeared between 1925 and 1975.

The autogenous latissimus breast reconstruction carries fat on the surface of the latissimus muscle to replace the breast tissue removed at mastectomy.[57, 87]

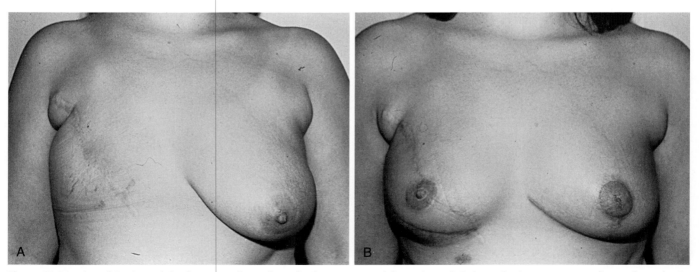

Figure 49–31 **A** and **B**, *One of the first corrections of a radical mastectomy defect using a latissimus dorsi myocutaneous flap and a reduction mammoplasty of the normal breast. The latissimus flap provided immediate expansion of the breast skin and complete coverage of the silicone implant. This created a "teardrop" shape and symmetry for the first time in radical mastectomy reconstruction.*

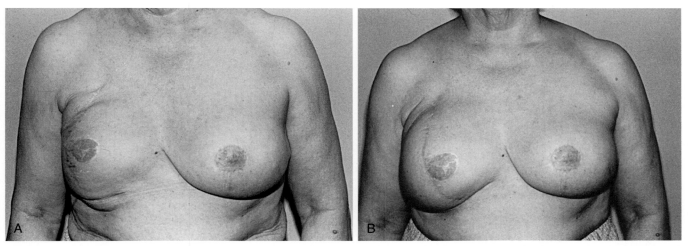

Figure 49–32 **A** *and* **B,** *Failed implant reconstruction of the right breast following a modified mastectomy with very extensive skin excision. The implant was removed and replaced with 1600 gm of fat from the autogenous latissimus flap.*

In an average-sized person, a 2-cm layer of fat on the surface of the latissimus dorsi muscle provides 800 gm of fat, and the skin paddle will carry an additional 500 to 700 gm of fat. This total of 1300 to 1500 gm is usually enough to replace the entire volume of breast tissue (Figs. 49–32 to 49–34). When additional volume is needed, a small implant can be used. The autogenous latissimus dorsi flap can be raised at the time of the mastectomy, and an immediate reconstruction can be performed with only a moderate increase in operative time. With a skin-sparing mastectomy, most reconstructions can be completed in a single stage. Delayed reconstruction, on the other hand, requires a second, longer operation and has a less satisfactory outcome than an immediate reconstruction. The autogenous latissimus dorsi reconstruction is particularly well suited for the modified mastectomy defect (Figs. 49–35 and 49–36). The autogenous latissimus dorsi flap is also the procedure of choice for partial mastectomy defects rather than the more complex TRAM flap. If less than 50 percent of the breast volume is removed, the autogenous latissimus flap can give a perfect correction for lumpectomy-irradiation failures, which require mastectomy. Because of the excellent blood supply, the autogenous latissimus dorsi flap is particularly useful in high-risk patients who have a history of smoking, diabetes, or marked obesity. Like the posterior lateral thoracotomy scar, the donor site scar is usually very good. The functional loss of the latissimus muscle is unnoticed except in the most vigorous athlete. It is certainly possible to play golf and tennis and even climb ropes in the absence of latissimus dorsi muscular function.

The TRAM flap is the gold standard of breast reconstruction. Since its description by Hartrampf in 1982, this procedure has gained worldwide acceptance as the procedure of choice for difficult recon-

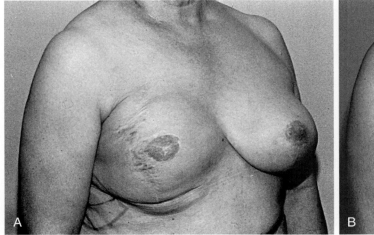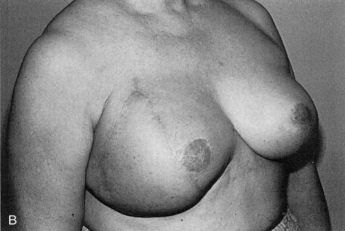

Figure 49–33 **A** *and* **B,** *Note the replacement of the vertical skin deficit lateral to the nipple. Fat from the back on the surface of the latissimus muscle is usually similar in volume to the normal breast in most patients.*

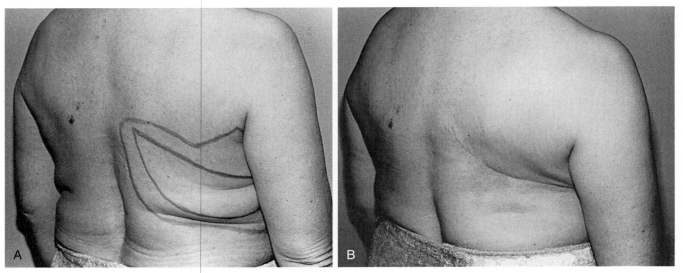

Figure 49–34   *Preoperative outline of the skin paddle* (**A**) *and postoperative view of the healed donor site* (**B**).

structions, particularly the mastectomy with extensive skin removal.* In experienced hands, the TRAM flap is extremely reliable and gives very predictable results (Figs. 49–37 and 49–38). Although it is a long operative procedure, patients recovery quickly and can usually be discharged by the fourth postoperative day. Management of the abdominal closure with the TRAM flap is critically important, because fascial bulges occur in 3 percent of the patients.[59] The rectus muscle can usually be raised with only a small strip of fascia, for example, 2 to 3 cm in width, which can be easily closed primarily. Bilateral flaps are more difficult to close, and Prolene mesh is occasionally

*See references 6, 7, 10, 19, 48, 56, 61, 96, 111, 119, 124, 125, 130, and 131.

used as an overlay patch in order to relieve the tension on the fascial closure. End-to-end patches of Gortex or Marlex are never used because of the high incidence of hernia formation because of graft failure. If patients are selected properly, true hernia formation should be rare, with an incidence of 0.3 percent in 400 consecutive patients treated by Hartrampf.[58, 92] The functional loss of a single rectus abdominis muscle is seldom noticed, and 95 percent of Hartrampf's patients believe that their work performance and sports activities were unchanged following surgery.[93] Overall, the TRAM flap reconstruction is very well accepted by patients. When Hartrampf surveyed his first 300 patients, he asked two questions: "was the operation worth the time and effort you have invested in it" and "would you recommend this method

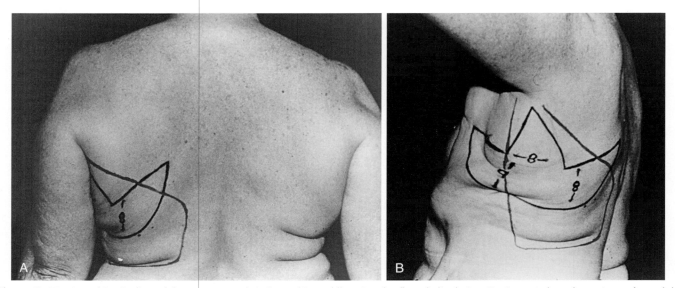

Figure 49–35   **A** *and* **B**, *Outline of the autogenous latissimus skin paddle using the fleur-de-lis design. Fat is carried on the entire surface of the latissimus muscle.*

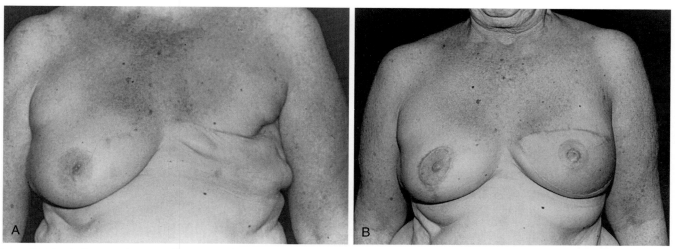

Figure 49–36   A, *Preoperative view of a 67-year-old patient following a modified mastectomy.*   **B,** *Postoperative view following a left autogenous latissimus reconstruction without an implant. A reduction mammoplasty was required in the opposite breast for symmetry.*

of breast reconstruction to other patients"? Both questions were answered affirmatively by 98 percent of the patients.[59]

Free Tissue Transfers

Free tissue transfers to the breast have gained acceptance for immediate reconstruction, extensive defects, and high-risk patients (Figures 49–39 and 49–40).* If the free-TRAM flap is done with the double team approach, the operative time is very similar to that required for the pedicle TRAM flap, and the free-TRAM reconstruction is actually associated with fewer complications and revisions.[36, 37] Other free flap donor sites are available but are used only in cases in which the TRAM or latissimus dorsi flaps cannot be used. These alternative flaps include the gluteus maximus myocutaneous flap and the Rubens flap,

---

*See references 42, 49, 56, 64, 71, 115, 116, 133, and 134.

but not the tensor fascia lata and the gracilis myocutaneous flaps, which have been largely abandoned. The expense of these complex operations will probably limit their use to very special situations in the future.

CLINICAL INDICATIONS FOR RECONSTRUCTIVE PROCEDURES

Myocutaneous Flaps

Problem surface wounds provide the most frequent indication for myocutaneous flaps, including replacement of the skin grafts, unstable scars, and radiation ulcers (Figs. 49–41 and 49–42). Before the development of myocutaneous flaps, most of these problems went untreated. Local skin flaps could not be transposed because tight mastectomy closure left no surrounding laxity for donor site tissue. Tubed flaps

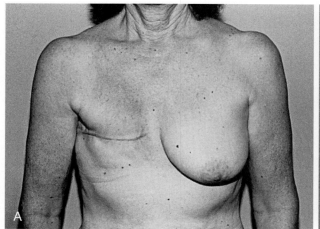
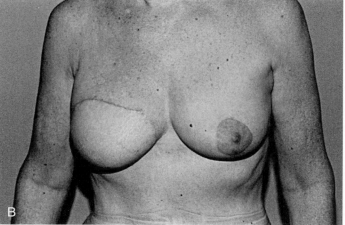

Figure 49–37   A *and* **B,** *Delayed reconstruction following a modified mastectomy with extensive skin excision in a patient with stage I disease. As was done in this patient, it is usually necessary to replace all of the skin between the mastectomy scar and the inframammary fold.*

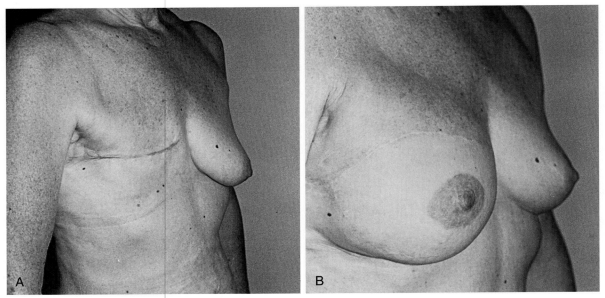

Figure 49–38 **A** and **B,** *Preoperative and postoperative views. Note the extensive skin replacement. Reconstruction of the nipple was done with small local flaps. The areola and nipple were tattooed.*

were cumbersome procedures and did not contribute a new permanent blood supply to the injured area. Myocutaneous flaps can be taken from the back, abdomen, buttocks, and thighs, depending on the type of tissue needed.

Reconstruction of full-thickness chest wall defects may be required for tumor invasion or, more often, for radiation defects. Severely irradiated skin undergoes a progressive vascular injury, which eventually results in painful skin ulceration or necrosis of the costal cartilages, sternum, and ribs. Full-thickness chest wall resection was first performed in 1950 by Campbell using a latissimus muscle flap.[25] The team approach encompassing both thoracic and plastic surgeons was first developed in the mid-1970s by Arnold and Pairolero at the Mayo Clinic.[3] The latissi-

mus and serratus muscles are still the most commonly used muscle flaps for chest wall problems, but the TRAM flap is used when massive skin replacement is needed.

Tumor recurrence following lumpectomy and radiation requires a mastectomy with wide skin excision, which makes primary skin closure difficult or impossible.[15, 102, 112, 118] Myocutaneous flaps are needed to obtain a healed wound because skin grafts are unreliable in radiated beds. This mastectomy usually requires extensive removal of the surrounding unstable irradiated skin and release of axillary contractures caused by radiation fibrosis. The TRAM flap is preferred over the autogenous latissimus dorsi flaps for large skin defects or when a total autogenous reconstruction (without an implant) is needed.

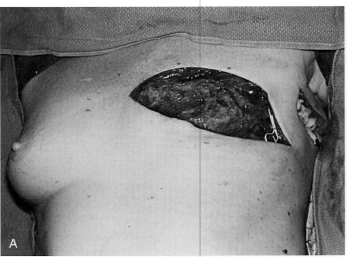
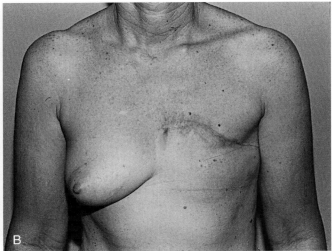

Figure 49–39 **A** and **B,** *Example of a modified mastectomy with extensive skin removal and a very high closure. Note the massive intraoperative skin defect, which can only be reconstructed with a TRAM flap.*

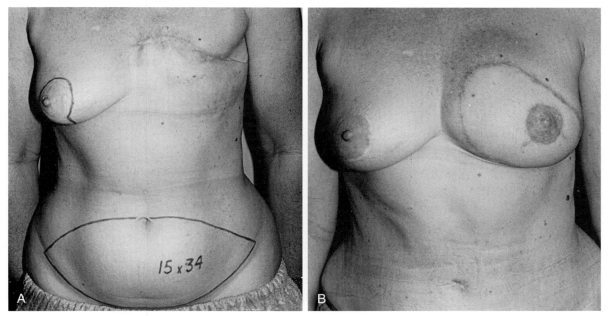

Figure 49–40   **A** *and* **B,** *Preoperative and postoperative views following the left free TRAM breast reconstruction. Skin replacement included all of the skin between the mastectomy scar and the inframammary fold. The nipple reconstruction and the opposite mastopexy were done at a separate procedure.*

Partial mastectomy defects offer the best chance of a reconstruction with predictably excellent results.[87] Quadrantectomy or quadrantectomy followed by irradiation can be repaired by a latissimus muscle flap with or without skin replacement (see Fig. 49–4). This avoids a contracted and deformed breast, and has little or no effect on the mammographic diagnosis of future breast cancer recurrences. It is an uncommon procedure only because quadrantectomy is uncommon. Reconstruction of partial defects is always preferred to any larger reconstruction of a total mastectomy defect. The failure of logic in excluding central tumors from lumpectomy-radiation treatment is the justification that the excision would deform the breast, which is nonsensical. Although that is par-

tially true, the deformity is easy to reconstruct compared with a total mastectomy. A central tumor should never be used as the sole justification for a complete mastectomy, any more than a tumor anywhere else in the breast should be.

The skin-sparing mastectomy removes all of the breast tissue, the nipple/areola complex, and the previous biopsy site (see Figs. 49–6 to 49–8). In the future, this technique should be the mastectomy of choice for patients with stage T0, T1, and T2 disease.[26, 47, 48, 118] Limited skin excision does not affect the rate of recurrence or survival in this group of patients and should be considered as a routine approach rather than as a special procedure. The skin-sparing mastectomy simplifies the reconstructive

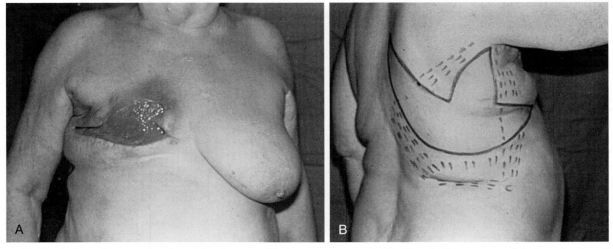

Figure 49–41   **A,** *Loss of mastectomy flaps following a modified mastectomy.*   **B,** *The fleur-de-lis autogenous latissimus flap is outlined.*

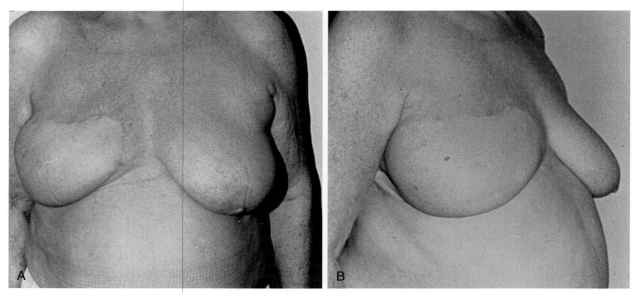

Figure 49–42 *A* and **B,** *Single-stage reconstruction of the right breast defect. The autogenous latissimus flap is the procedure of choice for full-thickness chest wall defects.*

procedure and improves the quality of the result of both autogenous flaps and tissue expanders in immediate reconstructions.

Modified and radical mastectomies create two obstacles to breast reconstruction: skin deficiency and a transverse scar. Both factors make reconstruction difficult and create a need for a myocutaneous flap.[118] The Patey mastectomy with its extensive transverse skin excision prevents tissue expansion in most cases because of the skin deficiency of the lower breast. A low-oblique scar that parallels the skin lines is the best choice for breast reconstruction, and even a vertical closure is better than the Patey closure.

Implant and Tissue Expander Reconstructions

The pectoralis major muscle will cover the upper half of the tissue expander, but complete coverage of the implant requires a rotation of the latissimus muscle. When skin removal is limited, a good reconstruction can be obtained. When skin removal is very extensive and the closure is transverse, which is usually the case, tissue expansion may not be possible. Skin-sparing mastectomies can be reconstructed with any method, and the best results are obtained when this is done as an immediate reconstruction when the tissues are malleable and unscarred. Tissue expanders are helpful in delayed reconstructions, when there is a tight skin closure. The transverse closure of the Patey mastectomy is the most unfavorable line of closure on the breast for purposes of expansion, because it is unyielding and stiff. Tissue expanders can be used at the time of mastectomy as a staging procedure to maintain a space for a later myocutaneous flap placement. This maintains the skin surface area and can be performed without any harmful effect on healing. The tissue expander is left unin-

flated until the mastectomy wound is healed, then it is gradually inflated over a period of weeks. At a second stage, the tissue expander is replaced with an implant or myocutaneous flap.

Opposite Breast Considerations

Reduction Mammaplasty

Reduction mammaplasty involves removal of 400 to 2000 gm of breast tissue as well as a skin tightening procedure, or mastopexy.[30, 66] Reduction mammaplasty removes a wedge of breast tissue from the inferior pole of the breast. Mastopexy corrects the breast ptosis by tightening the skin without removing any breast tissue. Both of these procedures can be performed without having an adverse effect on palpation or mammographic diagnosis of future breast masses. Reduction mammaplasty may be the only procedure indicated in mastectomy patients who do not want a reconstruction. A unilaterally large breast frequently causes more neck and back pain than bilateral enlargement because of the marked asymmetry in weights. In patients who have breast reconstruction, reduction mammaplasty or mastopexy procedures are essential for symmetry, which is the whole reason for the reconstruction.

Augmentation Mammaplasty

Augmentation of the normal breast is generally discouraged because saline and silicone implants are densely radiolucent, which obscures mammographic diagnosis of breast cancer. The new triglyceride implant has the same radiodensity of breast tissue, so that tiny calcifications can be visualized through the implant. Subpectoral augmentation is always preferred over prepectoral augmentation, which has a higher incidence of firmness and interferes with mammographic examination.

Prophylactic Mastectomy

Prophylactic mastectomy is rarely indicated in the treatment of breast cancer, except when bilateral prophylactic mastectomies are performed for special reasons. When an opposite prophylactic mastectomy is performed, either immediately or later, this makes a quantum difference in the complexity of the reconstruction. For instance, thin patients may have adequate tissue for a single breast reconstruction but not nearly enough soft tissue for a bilateral reconstruction. To achieve adequate volume, implants must be used and second flaps should be considered. On the other hand, it is important for the reconstructive surgeon to know that an opposite mastectomy might be considered in the future. If there is a good chance that it will be performed at a future time, the TRAM flap should be reserved, because it is only available once.

Nipple Reconstruction

Nipple/areola reconstruction is a very important part of breast reconstruction. Without the nipple, the breast does not look like a breast. This alone makes the breast look asymmetric, and our eyes are highly critical of asymmetry, whether it is a mole on the cheek or the absence of a nipple. A successful nipple/areola reconstruction restores the shape of the nipple, the shape of the areola, and the color of both entities. The shape of the areola is the foundation for the nipple and is created by a constricted circular closure of the autogenous flap. The nipple is formed

by local bilobed or trilobed flaps. The arms of these flaps are wrapped around themselves to form a standing cone. The color of the nipple and areola are provided by imbedding pigments with a tattoo machine. The color of the nipple is usually darker than the areola, which provides additional spatial differentiation. Nipple reconstruction can be performed at the time of an immediate reconstruction, but it is usually performed at a later time, when the shape of the reconstructed breast is definitive.

Delayed Reconstruction

Clearly not all patients treated for cancer survive, but that is not an indication to withhold reconstruction from the vast majority of patients (Figs. 49–43 to 49–45). The existing treatment protocols use the severity of the disease as the primary gauge of whether and when reconstruction should be performed. For example, most patients with ductal carcinoma *in situ* or minimal breast cancer are considered for immediate reconstruction, whereas only 5 percent of patients with invasive breast cancer undergo immediate reconstruction. Most patients are advised to wait at least until chemotherapy is completed to consider breast reconstruction. After 6 months of trauma from the mastectomy and chemotherapy, many patients are completely exhausted and have no interest in a second surgical procedure. The most common reason patients give for refusing delayed breast reconstruction is the fear of the second operation.

The commonly expressed goals of the patient seeking delayed reconstruction include

1. *Relief from negative feelings:* Mastectomy patients may accept the mastectomy and the cancer

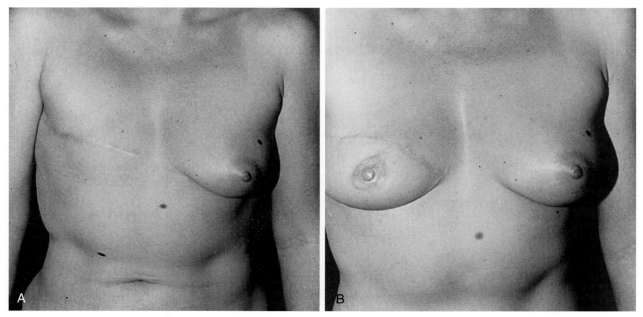

Figure 49–43   **A** *and* **B,** *Preoperative and postoperative views of a delayed reconstruction of a Patey mastectomy using a free TRAM flap. The right breast shape and nipple-areola reconstruction achieve nearly perfect symmetry with the normal breast.*

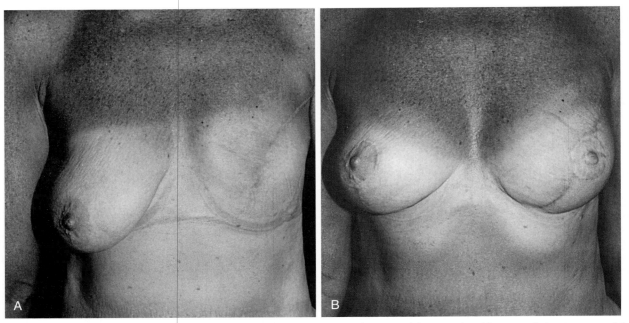

Figure 49–44   **A** *and* **B,** *Difficult reconstruction of a vertical modified mastectomy because of the extensive skin removal. A mastopexy of the right breast is essential so that the reconstructed breast can be shaped to match a normal shape rather than a ptotic shape.*

without question, but at some point, they tire of the physical and emotional loss they have sustained. Feelings of "weariness" with the mastectomy deformity and the stigma of being considered abnormal or different from other women are common. This post-mastectomy stigma is reinforced by well-intentioned friends and family ascribing great strength and character to the mere survival of a mastectomy. These stigmatized patients seek a time when they can

think, feel, and express themselves as they did before the mastectomy. Whether the problem is perceived as an anatomical deformity, asymmetry of the breast, or something that can be translated into a loss of femininity, the mirror is a constant reminder that they are not a "whole" person.

2. *Symmetry:* Symmetry with the opposite breast is always the goal of any mastectomy patient, whether this factor is stated or not. This goal is

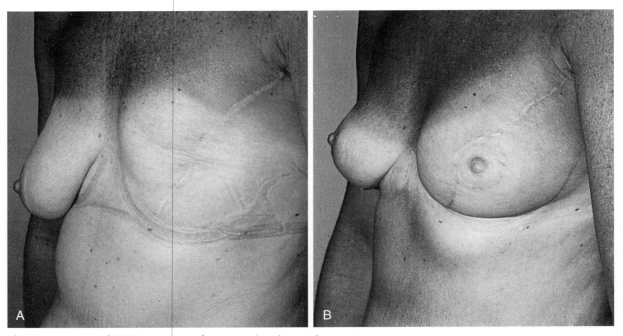

Figure 49–45   **A** *and* **B,** *Preoperative and postoperative views at 2 years.*

seldom obtainable without an autogenous reconstruction, which must be consciously chosen by the patient.

3. *Lasting result:* The desire for a lasting result is a desire for completion. At some point, the patient wants to feel that the reconstruction is finished and no more revisions will be required. The reason that implant reconstructions are not acceptable to some patients is because implants are more likely to need revision in later years.

4. *Forgetting about the mastectomy:* This is the "ultimate" goal of any breast reconstruction. In reality, most patients do not have limited expectations, such as being able to dress in normal clothes. Most patients want to return to their condition before the mastectomy. They want to forget the trauma of the mastectomy and completely recover physically and emotionally. For this to happen, the symmetry must be good enough that the patient can walk by a mirror and not think anything, good or bad, about the way they look. This type of sophisticated reconstruction requires autogenous flaps, an excellent nipple/areola reconstruction, and usually a mastopexy or reduction of the opposite breast. If a large amount of skin was removed with the mastectomy, or the mastectomy was followed by radiation, it is even more difficult to achieve and may necessitate prior tissue expansion, permanent implants, and later revisions of either the autogenous flaps or the implant.

5. *Emotional recovery:* The psychological aspects of the recovery process are not well understood by most doctors, because the emotional healing has been traditionally left to outside groups such as Reach to Recovery that function independent of surgeons and physicians. These groups are effective primarily because their members have actually suffered both physically and emotionally with the disease. Psychiatrists and psychologists, no matter how well intentioned, have learned these feelings second hand and usually are not as effective in counseling mastectomy patients as are women who have experienced the pain of losing a breast. Generally, breast reconstruction is an appropriate addition to the late recovery process, at a time when self-esteem is high and life is viewed as worth living. At this point, doing something for yourself is seen as healthy rather than as a way of denying unpleasant truths. It is clearly a mistake to proceed with plans for a breast reconstruction before these issues have been resolved with the patient and her family.

Both physicians and surgeons should be concerned about undertaking a reconstruction in patients who are poor candidates. It is always a disservice to undertake a complex reconstruction when a patient is still emotionally unstable, has unrealistic expectations, or is in poor health and informed consent cannot be properly obtained. The surgeon accepts the patient at the urging of a personal physician who recommends reconstruction as a rehabilitative measure to restore breast contour, form, and function. However, this patient often has a nonexistent sup-

port group and there is usually a long history of continuing medical care for a litany of minor symptoms. Prozac is typical of medications used by a patient in this emotional state. Under such negative conditions complications are poorly tolerated, and lawsuits are common because the surgeon and the referring physicians are obvious outlets for the patient's anger. It is better to delay reconstruction than to have the reconstruction negatively impact the patient's life.

Immediate Reconstruction

Treatment of the breast cancer and reconstruction of the lost breast have traditionally been conceptualized as separate and unrelated issues—one necessary, the other optional. Unlike that for any other cancer patient, treatment is completed before reconstruction is considered. In virtually all other cancer patients, the reconstruction is completed at the time of the extirpation. Although reconstruction may not be reasonable in a patient with a life span limited to 1 to 2 years, it is a reasonable consideration in any patient who is being treated for a cure of the cancer (Figs. 49–46 to 49–48).[27, 34, 134] Even in patients with advanced disease, immediate autogenous reconstruction is reasonable and does not interfere with subsequent treatment or follow-up.[46, 47, 97]

There are understandable historical reasons for the separation of treatment and reconstruction: (1) Treatment protocols were developed before reconstructive procedures were available. (2) Extensive skin resection has always been a hallmark of both radical and modified mastectomies. (3) Autogenous flap reconstructions have only become refined during the past 10 years. (4) The mastectomy and reconstructive procedures are done by two different specialties of surgery.

If autogenous flaps had developed within the specialty of surgery instead of plastic surgery, they would be used in a more routine fashion at the time of mastectomy. Extensive skin resection would have been the exception rather than the rule, and reconstruction would not be viewed as incompatible with adjuvant therapy.

For the foreseeable future, mastectomies will not be totally replaced by other forms of treatment. Specifically, there are several conditions that are not accommodated by the lumpectomy and irradiation paradigm, including

- Familial breast cancer
- *In situ,* minimal, and multifocal breast cancers
- Central breast cancer that requires sacrifice of the nipple
- Cancers that are too large for lumpectomy
- Recurrent breast cancer following lumpectomy-radiation
- Patients who cannot accept radiation

Routine consideration of breast reconstruction at the time of mastectomy can now be scientifically de-

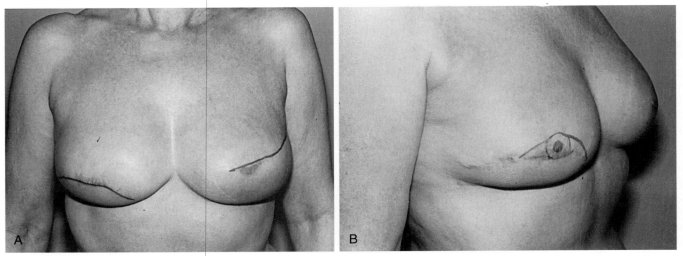

Figure 49–46   **A** *and* **B,** *Six weeks following bilateral skin conservation mastectomies and free TRAM flap breast reconstructions in a patient with stage I disease. The low and oblique closures facilitated the reconstruction. The nipple flaps are outlined in* B.

fended for patients with stages 0, 1/2, I, and II-A. This subset of patients describes more than 70 percent of the patients who are undergoing mastectomy, at present. As the safety of breast reconstruction has been demonstrated in careful studies, there is no more reason to deny breast cancer patients reconstruction than there is to deny any other cancer patients reconstruction.

There is no data to suggest that immediate reconstruction interferes with surgical treatment by either spreading the cancer, hiding a local recurrence, or adversely affecting the survival. It is now recognized that essentially all local recurrences are harbingers of systemic disease, and that recurrences can only exist within breast tissue. The only remaining breast tissue following a mastectomy is either in the breast skin or in breast tissue that was not removed with the mastectomy. After a reconstruction, what would

have been a chest wall recurrence becomes a skin recurrence, only because the skin is physically separated from the chest wall by the reconstruction. Recurrences are never seen within the substance of an autogenous flap, because the fat and muscle of the flap are inhospitable to the transplantation of the breast cancer (Figs. 49–49 to 49–51).

There are a number of recent reports in which the safety of immediate reconstruction is documented for the first time. Wang and colleagues reviewed survival data in 172 immediate breast reconstructions performed between 1970 and 1990, and compared them with a control group of similar patients who had had only a mastectomy.[134] In these groups, the flap reconstruction did not interfere with either diagnosis or treatment of the recurrence. There was no difference in a 5- and 10-year disease-free survival, and there was no difference between reconstructions per-

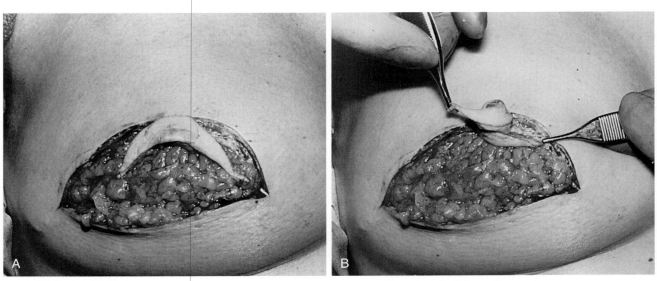

Figure 49–47   **A** *and* **B,** *Nipple reconstruction done as an office procedure, using fishtail bilobed flaps of breast skin.*

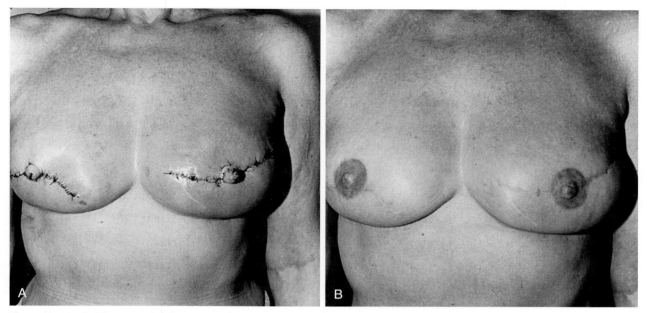

Figure 49–48   **A,** *View 1 week following nipple reconstruction and,* **B,** *1 year following completion of the reconstruction.*

formed with implants versus autogenous flaps or immediate versus delayed reconstructions. Slaven, Love, and Goldwyn reported on 161 immediate breast reconstructions, including 41 salvage mastectomies using myocutaneous flaps.[118] Local recurrences that developed were consistent with the stage of the disease, and 76 percent of these local recurrences represented systemic disease. All local recurrences were found within the native breast skin rather than in relation to the flap. There were no cases of a delay

in diagnosis or compromise of the cancer treatment. Godfrey and associates reviewed patients having immediate reconstruction with advanced disease and confirmed the findings of Slavin that the reconstruction itself had no effect on the outcome of the cancer treatment.[46] Noone and coworkers reported on 306 patients who had undergone implant reconstruction with long-term follow-up.[97] The local and distant recurrences in this group of patients were similar to those expected in patients with similar disease. Kroll

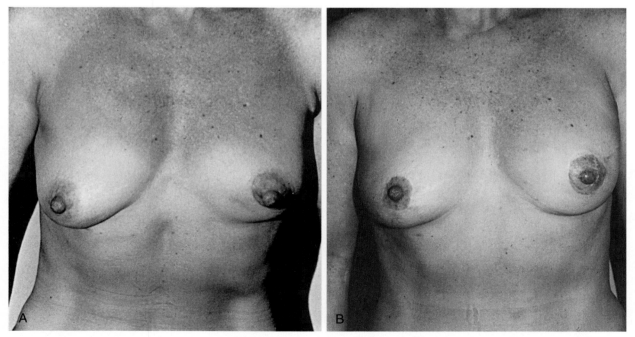

Figure 49–49   **A,** *Preoperative view of the patient following a biopsy of a 1-cm invasive breast cancer in the left breast.*   **B,** *Postoperative view 5 years following skin conservation mastectomy, immediate free TRAM breast reconstruction, and nipple-areola reconstruction as a one-stage procedure.*

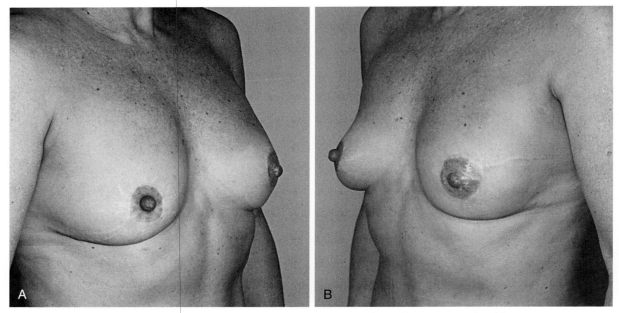

Figure 49–50   A and **B,** *Oblique view at 5 years. A mastopexy was done in the right breast for symmetry. The oblique mastectomy scar is partially covered by the nipple-areola reconstruction. The original nipple was removed with the mastectomy and replaced with skin from the TRAM flap. The reconstruction, including the nipple, was completed in a single stage at the time of mastectomy and without any subsequent revisions.*

and colleagues collected 131 patients who had undergone immediate reconstruction, of which 104 had skin-sparing mastectomy. When compared with matched patients, these authors concluded that the skin-sparing mastectomy with immediate reconstruction had no effect on the outcome in this 5-year follow-up.[69]

Although the potential harmful effects on local recurrence or survival have not materialized, there should be concern about the effect of breast reconstruction on adjuvant therapy. It is important biologically to begin chemotherapy within 28 to 40 days of extirpative therapy, so the reconstruction must be primarily healed during the first month. Chemotherapy can be started while there is still a surface

wound that has not yet epithelialized, but it cannot be started in the face of necrotic tissue, seromas, or infection. When it is known in advance that the patient will undergo chemotherapy, the choices of reconstructions should include only flaps that are well vascularized and known to heal primarily as the first choice. Implants can be used, but if the implants have problems with seroma or infections, it may be necessary to remove the implant to correct the healing problem and allow the chemotherapy to progress. When radiation is planned, tissue expander and implant reconstruction should not be used, because unsatisfactory firmness is inevitable when implants are radiated. Only autogenous flaps offer satisfactory solutions in these patients, and it is preferable to com-

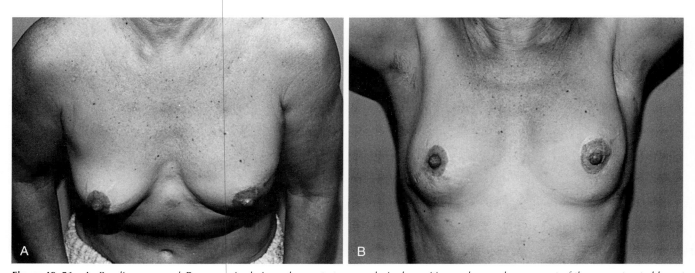

Figure 49–51   A, *Bending-over and,* **B,** *arms-raised views demonstrate normal nipple position and normal movement of the reconstructed breast.*

plete the reconstruction at the time of mastectomy. Radiation is usually performed because the margin of tumor resection at the chest wall is suspect or because the tumor is large and aggressive. In either case, the reason for tumor recurrence or poor patient survival is the stage of the disease, not the reconstruction. Should a flap hide a recurrence at a questionable chest wall margin, this would only delay the diagnosis of systemic disease, but it is so rare as to be a reportable event. Whether immediate reconstruction should be performed at all in stages IIb and III is more of a social decision than a medical decision. The survival in these patients will not be as good as in most patients, but it will not be affected by an autogenous reconstruction. If it is known that the patient wants a reconstruction at some point, the time to do it is immediately. For the few hours added to the mastectomy, the reconstruction can be completed, and the patient does not have to face a second major surgical procedure following chemotherapy. If the flap is constructed immediately, the radiation may shrink the flap volume, but delayed reconstruction is much more problematical from the standpoint of healing.

CONCLUSIONS

We have just now reached the point at which our understanding of breast cancer treatment allows new combinations of chemotherapy, reconstruction, and radiation that could not have been considered a generation ago. Early in this century, the surgeon was alone in taking responsibility for breast cancer treatment, when the only treatment was the radical mastectomy. Today, there is support from several disciplines, and the surgical oncologist should be the leader of this coordinated effort. Helping the patient choose among these sophisticated treatment options requires the efforts of both the surgical oncologist and the reconstructive surgeon.

References

1. Adams WM: Free composite grafts of the nipples in mammaplasty. South Surg 13:615–623, 1947.
2. Adams WM: Labial transplant for correction of loss of the nipple. Plast Reconstr Surg 4:295–304, 1949.
3. Arnold, PG and Pairolero, PC: Chest wall reconstruction: Experience with 100 consecutive patients. Ann Surg 199:725–741, 1984.
4. Auchincloss H: Significance of location and number of axillary metastases in carcinoma of the breast: A justification for a conservative operation. Ann Surg 158:37–46, 1963.
5. Aufricht G: Mammaplasty for pendulous breasts: Empiric and geometric planning. Plast Reconstr Surg 4:13–22, 1949.
6. Baldwin BJ, Schusterman MA, Miller MJ, Kroll SS: Bilateral breast reconstruction. Conventional versus free TRAM. Plast Reconstr Surg 93:1410–1417, 1994.
7. Beasley ME: The pedicled TRAM as preference for immediate autogenous tissue breast reconstruction. Clin Plast Surg 21:191–205, 1994.
8. Becker H: Breast reconstruction using an inflatable with detachable reservoir. Plast Reconstr Surg 73:678–683, 1984.
9. Becker H: Breast augmentation using the expander mammary prosthesis. Plast Reconstr Surg 79:192–199, 1987.
10. Berrino P, Campora E, Leone S, Zappi L, Nicosia F, Santi P: The transverse rectus abdominis musculocutaneous flap for breast reconstruction in obese patients. Ann Plast Surg 27:221–231, 1991.
11. Berrino P, Santi P: Applications of the "recharged" TRAM flap. Clin Plast Surg 21:233–245, 1994.
12. Blair VP, Brown JB: Use and uses of large split skin grafts of intermediate thickness. Surg Gynecol Obstet 49:82–85, 1929.
13. Bostwick J 3rd: Breast reconstruction following mastectomy. Contemp Surg 27:15–23, 1985.
14. Bostwick J III, Vasconez LO, Jurkiewicz MJ: Breast reconstruction after a radical mastectomy. Plast Reconstr Surg 61:682–693, 1978.
15. Bostwick J III: Breast reconstruction after radiation therapy and conservative treatment. Contemp Surg 30:13–22, 1987.
16. Bostwick J III: Latissimus dorsi flap Current applications. Ann Plast Surg 9:377–380, 1982.
17. Bostwick J III: Breast reconstruction using modified tissue expansion for matching a small opposite breast. Perspect Plast Surg 1:79–92, 1987.
18. Bostwick J III, Paletta C, Hartrampf CR Jr: Conservative treatment for breast cancer: Complications requiring reconstructive surgery. Ann Surg 203:481–490, 1986.
19. Boyd JB, Taylor GI, Corlett R: The vascular territories of the superior epigastric systems. Plast Reconstr Surg 73:1–16, 1984.
20. Braithwaite F: Preliminary observations on the vascular channels in tubed pedicles. Br J Plast Surg 3:40, 1950.
21. Broadbent TR, Woolf RM: Augmentation mammoplasty. Plast Reconstr Surg 40:517–523, 1967.
22. Brown JB, Mc Dowell F: Skin Grafting. 3rd ed. Philadelphia, JB Lippincott, 1958.
23. Burkhardt BR: Capsular contracture: Hard breasts, soft data. Clin Plast Surg 15:521–532, 1988.
24. Burkhardt BR: Comparing contracture rates: Probability theory and the unilateral contracture. Plast Reconstr Surg 74:527–529, 1984.
25. Campbell DA: Reconstruction of the anterior chest wall. J Thorac Surg 19:456–477, 1950.
26. Carlson G: Skin sparing mastectomy: Anatomical and technical considerations. Am Surg 62:151–155, 1996.
27. Clough KB, Bourgeois D, Falcou MC, Renolleau C, Durand JC: Immediate breast reconstruction by prosthesis: A safe technique for extensive intraductal and microinvasive carcinomas. Ann Surg Oncol 3:212–218, 1996.
28. Cohen BE, Cronin ED: Breast reconstruction with the latissimus dorsi musculocutaneous flap. Clin Plast Surg 11:287–302, 1984.
29. Cronin TD, Gerow F: Augmentation mammoplasty: A new Anatural feel prosthesis. *In* Blocker T (ed): Transactions of the Third International Congress of Plastic Surgeons. Amsterdam, Excerpta Medica, 1964.
30. Courtiss EH, Goldwyn RM: Reduction mammaplasty by the inferior pedicle technique: An alternative to free nipple and areolar grafting for severe macromastia or extreme ptosis. Plast Reconstr Surg 59:500–517, 1977.
31. Davis JS: Small deep skin grafts. Surg Gynecol Obstet 19:554, 1907.
32. Dempsey WC, Latham WD: Subpectoral implants in augmentation mammaplasty. Plast Reconstr Surg 42:515–521, 1968.
33. Dick GO, Brown SA: Breast reconstruction using modified tissue expansion. Plast Reconstr Surg 77:613–620, 1986.
34. DiMartino L, Murenu G, Demontis B, Licheri S: Reconstructive surgery in operable breast cancer. Ann NY Acad Sci 698:227–245, 1993.
35. Dowden RV, Horton CE, Rosato FE, McCraw JB: Reconstruction of the breast after mastectomy for cancer. Surg Gynecol Obstet 149:109–115, 1978.
36. Elliott LF, Eskenazi L, Beegle PH, Podres PE, Drazan L: Immediate TRAM flap breast reconstruction: 128 consecutive cases. Plast Reconstr Surg 92:217–227, 1992.
37. Feller AM, Horl HW, Biemer E: The transverse rectus abdominis musculocutaneous free flap: A reliable alternative for delayed autologous tissue breast reconstruction. Ann Plast Surg 25:425–434, 1990.

38. Fisher B, Fisher ER: Transmigration of lymph nodes by node tumor cells. Science 152:1397–1398, 1966.
39. Fisher B, Fisher ER: The interrelationship of hematogenous and lymphatic tumor cell dissemination. Surg Gynecol Obstet 122:791–798, 1966.
40. Fisher B, Redmond C, Fisher ER: The contribution of recent NSABP clinical trials of primary breast cancer therapy to an understanding of tumor biology—an overview of findings. Cancer 46:1009–1025, 1980.
41. Friedman R, Gyimesi I, Robinson J, Rohrich R: Saline made viscous with polyethylene glycol: A new alternate breast implant filler material. Plast Reconstr Surg 98:1208–1213, 1996.
42. Fugino T, Harashina T, Aoyagi F: Reconstruction for aplasia of the breast and pectoral region by microvascular transfer of a free flap from the buttock. Plast Reconstr Surg 56:178–181, 1975.
43. Furey PC, MacGillivray DC, Castione CL, Allen L: Wound complications in patients receiving adjuvant chemotherapy after mastectomy and immediate reconstruction for breast cancer. J Surg Oncol 55:194–197, 1994.
44. Gillies HD: The tubed pedicle in plastic surgery. NY J Med 111:1–13, 1920.
45. Gillies HD: Surgical replacement of the breast. Proc R Soc Med 52:597–602, 1959.
46. Godfrey PM, Godfrey NV, Romita MC: Immediate autogenous breast reconstruction in clinically advanced disease. Plast Reconstr Surg 95:1039–1043, 1995.
47. Goes JCS: Mastectomy by periareolar approach with immediate breast reconstruction. Rev Soc Bras Cir Plast 10:44–55, 1995.
48. Goes JCS: Periareolar mammaplasty: double skin technique. Rev Soc Bras Cir Plast 4:55–63, 1989.
49. Grotting JC, Urist MM, Maddox WA, Vasconez LO: Conventional TRAM flap versus free microsurgical TRAM flap for immediate breast reconstruction. Plast Reconstr Surg 83:828–844, 1989.
50. Halsted WS: Results of operation for cure of cancer of the breast performed at the Johns Hopkins Hospital from June 1889 to January 1894. Ann Surg 20:497–516, 1894.
51. Halsted WS: Skin grafts. Trans Am Surg Assoc 30:287–290, 1912.
52. Halsted WS: The results of operations for the cure of cancer of the breast performed at the Johns Hopkins Hospital from June 1889 to January 1894. Johns Hopkins Hosp Rev 4:297–350–70, 1895.
53. Handel N, Lewinsky B, Jensen A, Silverstein M: Breast conservation therapy after augmentation: Is it appropriate? Plast Reconstr Surg 98:1216–1224, 1996.
54. Handley RS, Thackray AC: Conservative radical mastectomy. Ann Surg 170:880–882, 1969.
55. Handley WS: Cancer of the Breast and Its Treatment. 2nd ed. London, A. Murray, 1922.
56. Harashina T, Sone K, Inoue T, Fukuzumi S, Enomoto K: Augmentation of circulation of pedicled transverse rectus abdominis musculocutaneous flaps by microvascular surgery. Br J Plast Surg 40:367–370, 1987.
57. Hartrampf CR Jr: Breast Reconstruction with Living Tissue. New York, Raven Press, 1990.
58. Hartrampf CR Jr: Abdominal wall competence in transverse abdominal island flap operations. Ann Plast Surg 12:139–146, 1984.
59. Hartrampf CR Jr, Bennett GK: Autogenous tissue reconstruction in the mastectomy patient: A critical review of 300 patients. Ann Surg 105:508–519, 1987.
60. Hartrampf CR Jr, Scheflan M, Black PW: Breast reconstruction with a transverse abdominal island flap. Plast Reconstr Surg 69:216–225, 1982.
61. Hartrampf CR Jr: Transverse Abdominal Island Flap Technique for Breast Reconstruction after Mastectomy. Baltimore, University Park Press, 1984.
62. Hester TR: The polyurethane-covered mammary prosthesis: Facts and fiction. Perspect Plast Surg 2:135, 1988.
63. Hinton CP, Doyle PJ, Blamey RW, Davies CJ, Holliday HW, Elston CW: Subcutaneous mastectomy for primary operable breast cancer. Br J Surg 71:469–472, 1984.
64. Holmstrom H: The free abdominoplasty flap and its use in breast reconstruction. Scand Plast Reconstr Surg: 13:423–427, 1979.
65. Horton CE, Adamson JE, Mladick RA, Carraway JC: Simple mastectomy with immediate reconstruction. Plast Reconstr Surg 53:42–47, 1974.
66. Hugo NE, McClellan RM: Reduction mammaplasty with a single superiorly based pedicle. Plast Reconstr Surg 63:230–244, 1979.
67. Johnson CH, Van Heerden JA, Raine TJ: Oncological aspects of immediate breast reconstruction following mastectomy for malignancy. Arch Surg 124:819–827, 1989.
68. Knapp T: A new triglyceride breast implant. Presented at Breast Surgery in the 90's Symposium. Santa Fe, NM, August, 1996.
69. Kroll S, Ames F, Singletary SE, Schusterman MA: The oncologic risks of skin preservation at mastectomy when combined with immediate reconstruction of the breast. Surg Gynecol Obstet 172:17–20, 1991.
70. Kroll SS, Shusterman MA, Reese GP, Miller MJ, Smith B: Breast reconstruction with myocutaneous flaps in previously irradiated patients. Plast Reconstr Surg 93:460–469, 1994.
71. Kroll S, Schusterman M, Tadjalli H, Singletary E, Ames F: Risk of recurrence after treatment of breast cancer with skin-sparing mastectomy. Submitted for publication Plast Reconstr Surg 1996.
72. Lejour M, De May A, Mattheim W: Local recurrences and metastases of breast cancer after 194 operations. Chir Plast 7:131–134, 1983.
73. Lejour M, Alemanno P, De May A: Analysis of 56 breast reconstructions using the latissimus dorsi flap. Ann Chir Plast Esthet 30:7, 1985.
74. Madden JL: Modified radical mastectomy. Surg Gynecol Obstet 121:1221–1230, 1965.
75. Maliniac JW: Arterial blood supply of the breast. Arch Surg 47:329–344, 1943.
76. Maliniac JW: Breasts and Their Repair. New York. Grune & Stratton, Inc., 1950.
77. Marshall DR, Anstee EJ, Stapleton MJ: Immediate reconstruction of the breast following modified radical mastectomy for carcinoma. Br J Plast Surg 35:438–442, 1982.
78. Maxwell GP: Iginio Tansini and the origin of the latissimus dorsi musculocutaneous flap. Plast Reconstr Surg 65:686–693, 1980.
79. Maxwell GP: Latissimus dorsi breast reconstruction: An aesthetic assessment. Clin Plast Surg 8:373–387, 1981.
80. Maxwell GP, Horton CE, McCraw JB: Cancer trends: Breast reconstruction after mastectomy. Va Med Q 108:328–337, 1981.
81. McCraw JB, Bostwick J III, Horton CE: Methods of soft tissue coverage for the mastectomy defect. Clin Plast Surg 6:57–69, 1979.
82. McCraw JB, Dibbell DG: Experimental definition of independent myocutaneous vascular territories. Plast Reconstr Surg 60:212–227, 1977.
83. McCraw JB, Dibbell DG, Carraway JH: Clinical definition of independent myocutaneous vascular territories. Plast Reconstr Surg 60:341–352, 1977.
84. McCraw JB, Maxwell GP: Early and late capsular deformation as a cause of unsatisfactory results in the latissimus dorsi breast reconstruction. Clin Plast Surg 15:717–726, 1988.
85. McCraw JB, Papp C, Zanon E: Breast volume replacement using the de-epithelialized latissimus dorsi myocutaneous flap. Eur J Plast Surg 11:120–125, 1988.
86. McCraw JB, Massey FM, Shanklin KD, Horton CE: Vaginal reconstruction with gracilis myocutaneous flaps. Plast Reconstr Surg 58:176–183, 1976.
87. McCraw JB, Papp C, Edwards A, McMellin A: The autogenous latissimus breast reconstruction. Clin Plast Surg 21:279–288, 1994.
88. McKissock PK: Reduction mammaplasty with a vertical dermal flap. Plast Reconstr Surg 49:245–264, 1972.
89. Millard DR Jr: Breast reconstruction after radical mastectomy. Plast Reconstr Surg 58:283–291, 1976.

90. Millard DR Jr: Breast aesthetics when reconstruction with the latissimus dorsi musculocutaneous flap. Plast Reconstr Surg 70:161–172, 1982.

91. Milloy FG, Anson BJ, McAfee DK: The rectus abdominis muscle and the epigastric arteries. Surg Gynecol Obstet 110:293–302, 1960.

92. Mizgala CL, Hartrampf CR Jr, Bennett GK: Abdominal function after pedical TRAM flap. Clin Plast Surg 21:255–272, 1994.

93. Mizgala CL, Hartrampf CR Jr, Bennett GK: Assessment of the abdominal wall after pedicle TRAM flap surgery: Five-to-seven year follow-up of 150 consecutive patients. Plast Reconstr Surg 93:988–1002, 1994.

94. Moore CH: On the influence of inadequate operation on the theory of cancer. J R Med Cir Soc London 1:244–280, 1867.

95. Muhlbauer W, Olbrisch R: The latissimus dorsi myocutaneous flap for breast reconstruction. Chir Plast 4:27, 1977.

96. Mukagerjee R, Gottlieb B, Hacker LC: Experience with the ipselateral upper TRAM flap for postmastectomy breast reconstruction. Ann Plast Surg 23:187–196, 1989.

97. Noone RB, Frazier TG, Noone GC, Blanchet NP, Murphy JB, Rose D: Recurrence of breast carcinoma following immediate reconstruction: A 13-year review. Plast Reconstr Surg 93:96–106, 1994.

98. Olivari N: The latissimus flap. Br J Plast Surg 29:126–128, 1976.

98a. Olivari N: Use of thirty latissimus dorsi flaps. Plast Reconstr Surg 64:654–661, 1979.

99. Ollier L: Greffes cutanees ou autoplastiques: Bull Acad Med (Paris) 1:243–247, 1872.

100. Padgett EC: Calibrated intermediate skin grafts. Surg Gynecol Obstet 69:799–807, 1939.

101. Patey DH, Dyson WH: The prognosis of carcinoma of the breast in relation to the type of operation performed. Br J Cancer 2:7–13, 1948.

102. Pearl RM, Wisnicki J: Breast reconstruction following lumpectomy and irradiation. Plast Reconstr Surg 76:83–86, 1985.

103. Penn J: Reduction mammaplasty. Br J Plast Surg 7:357–371, 1955.

104. Peters W, Smith D: Ivalon breast prostheses: Evaluation 19 years after implantation. Plast Reconstr Surg 67:514–518, 1981.

105. Pickrell KL, Puckett CL, Given KS: Subpectoral augmentation mammoplasty. Plast Reconstr Surg 60:325–336, 1977.

106. Pollock H: Polyurethane-covered breast implant. Plast Reconstr Surg 74:729–730, 1984.

107. Radovan C: Tissue expansion in soft tissue reconstruction. Plast Reconstr Surg 74:282–292, 1984.

108. Rees T, Guy C, Coburn J: The use of inflatable breast implants. Plast Reconstr Surg 52:609–615, 1973.

109. Reese JD: Dermatape: A new method for management of split skin grafts. Plast Reconstr Surg 1:98–105, 1946.

110. Reverdin JL: Epidermal skin grafts. Boston Med Surg J 6:196–211, 1870.

111. Robbins TH: Rectus abdominis flap for breast reconstruction. Aust NZ Surg 49:527–530, 1979.

112. Rouanet P, Fabre JM, Tica V, Anaf V, Jozwick M, Pojol H: Chest wall reconstruction for radionecrosis after breast carcinoma therapy. Ann Plast Surg 34:465–470, 1995.

113. Schain WS, Wellisch DK, Pasnau RO: The sooner the better: A study of psychological factors in women undergoing immediate versus delayed breast reconstruction. Am J Psychol 40:142–150, 1985.

114. Schneider WJ, Hill LH Jr, Brown RG: Latissimus dorsi myocutaneous flap for breast reconstruction. Br J Plast Surg 30:277–281, 1977.

115. Schusterman MA, Kroll SS, Weldon ME: Immediate breast reconstruction: Why the free TRAM over the conventional TRAM? Plast Reconstr Surg 90:255–261, 1992.

116. Shaw WW: Breast reconstruction by superior gluteal microvascular free flaps without silicone implants. Plast Reconstr Surg 72:490–501, 1983.

117. Slavin SA: Improving the latissimus dorsi myocutaneous flap with tissue expansion. Plast Reconstr Surg 93:811–824, 1994.

118. Slavin SA, Love SM, Goldwyn RM: Recurrent breast cancer following immediate reconstruction with myocutaneous flaps. Plast Reconstr Surg 93:1191–1204, 1994.

119. Slavin SA, Goldwyn RM: The mid-abdominal rectus abdominis myocutaneous flap: Review of 236 flaps. Plast Reconstr Surg 81:189–199, 1988.

120. Snyderman RK, Guthrie RH: Reconstruction of the female breast following radical mastectomy. Plast Reconstr Surg 47:565–567, 1971.

121. Strombeck JO: Mammaplasty: Report of a new technique based on the two pedicle procedure. Br J Plast Surg 13:79–89, 1960.

122. Tansini I: Nuovo processo per l= amputazione della mammaella per cancre. Reforma Medica 12:3–19, 1896.

123. Tansini I: Sopra il mio nuovo processo di amputazione della mammaella. Reforma Medica 12:757–772, 1906.

124. Taylor GI, Corlett RJ, Boyd JB: The extended deep inferior epigastric flap: A clinical technique. Plast Reconstr Surg 72:751–765, 1983.

125. Taylor JI, Caddy CM, Watterson PA, Crock JG: The venous territories (venosomes) of the human body: Experimental study and clinical implications. Plast Reconstr Surg 86:185–198, 1990.

126. Tebbetts JB: Transaxillary subpectoral augmentation mammaplasty. Plast Reconstr Surg 74:636–647, 1984.

127. Thiersch J: Skin grafts. Verh Dtsch Ges Chir 69–78, 1874.

128. Thorek M: Plastic reconstruction of the breast and free transplantation of the nipple. J Int Coll Surg 9:194–202, 1946.

129. Toth B, Lappert P: Modified skin incision for mastectomy: The need for plastic surgical input in preoperative planning. Plast Reconstr Surg 87:1048–1053, 1991.

130. Trabulsy PP, Anthony JP, Mathes SJ: Changing trends in post mastectomy breast reconstruction: A 13-year experience. Plast Reconstr Surg 93:1418–1427, 1994.

131. Vasconez HC, Holley DT: Use of the TRAM and latissimus dorsi flaps in autogenous breast reconstruction. Clin Plast Surg 22:153–166, 1995.

132. Veronesi U, Banfi A, Del Vecchio M: Comparison of Halsted mastectomy with quadrantectomy, axillary dissection, and radiotherapy in early breast cancer: Long-term results. Eur J Cancer Clin Oncol 22:1085–1089, 1986.

133. Wagner DS, Michelow BJ, Hartrampf CR Jr: Double-pedicle TRAM flap for unilateral breast reconstruction. Plast Reconstr Surg 88:987–997, 1991.

134. Wang B, Chang B, Dooley W, Chang L, Hamad G, Vander-Kolk C, Manson P: Breast cancer recurrence following mastectomy with reconstruction. Submitted for publication Arch Surg 1996.

135. Webster JP: Thoraco-epigastric tubed pedicles. Surg Clin North Am 17:145–161, 1937.

136. Weiner DL, Aiache AE, Silver L, Tittiranonda T: A single dermal pedicle for nipple transposition in subcutaneous mastectomy, reduction mammaplasty, and mastopexy. Plast Reconstr Surg 51:115–127, 1973.

137. Wise RJ: A preliminary report on a method of planning the mastopexy. Plast Reconstr Surg 17:367–379, 1956.

138. Wolfe JR: A new method for performing plastic operations. Br Med J 2:360–368, 1875.

139. Woods JE, Irons GB, Arnold PG: The case for submuscular implantation of prostheses in reconstructive breast surgery. Ann Plast Surg 5:115–122, 1980.

CHAPTER 50
WOUND CARE AND COMPLICATIONS OF MASTECTOMY

Kirby I. Bland, M.D. / Michael C. Coburn, M.D.

Rehabilitation of the postmastectomy patient produces problems of varying complexity. This chapter reviews commonly used approaches for the care of the postmastectomy wound and addresses the complications encountered in these patients.

WOUND CARE

The various operative techniques used in the treatment for breast carcinoma are described in detail in Chapters 39 to 47 and 49. The surgeon should recognize that the essential parts of optimal wound repair are the application of meticulous technique, hemostasis, and wound closure at operation. We prefer closed-suction catheter drainage of the mastectomy wound, commercially available as Relavac 400, CWS 400, Davol (Davol-Bard, Cranston, RI), or Jackson-Pratt tubing (Baxter Healthcare, Deerfield, IL), and each system should be appropriately placed at operation to allow superomedial and inferolateral positioning of these apparati to ensure thorough, dependent aspiration. After the wound is closed, the tubing is connected to ensure removal of all wound contents (e.g., clots, serum). An optional technique includes wound irrigation with saline via the closed flaps to flush the drainage system and provide patency of the suction catheters. Thereafter, the skin margins may be covered with strips of nonadherent, nonporous dressing (Telfa [Kendall Healthcare, Mansfield, MA]) or a porous dressing (Adaptic [Johnson & Johnson Medical Inc., Arlington, TX]). In addition, surgeons may apply fluffs of 4 × 4 dressings of cotton gauze, over the entire operative site, to provide uniform gentle compression within the limits of flap dissection. These compression dressings are then taped with Elastoplast or an equivalent elastic adherent dressing that is further secured by the application of benzoine over the periphery of the dissected operative sites. This technique affords optimal coverage of the axilla with uniform gentle compression, yet leaves the upper arm and forearm free of dressing application.

Other surgeons criticize the application of pressure dressings over the dissected skin flaps and prefer occlusive dressings alone (e.g., light dressing, Opsite). This technique is inadvisable for drainage methods that do not use active suction, because flap adherence is reduced, with subsequent seroma formation. The application of the operative dressing is an essential part of the operative procedure and should not be delegated to surgical assistants or nurses unfamiliar with this detail.

Suction catheter drainage, as a rule, is necessary for 4 to 7 days postoperatively. Premature removal of the catheters is only allowed when the function of this closed-system technique is compromised. Routinely, catheters are removed only when less than 20 ml of serous or serosanguinous drainage is evident during a 24-hour interval. Thereafter, the wound is carefully inspected with regard to flap adherence, and the patient is encouraged to begin graded, active range of motion of the ipsilateral arm and shoulder.

The patient usually experiences moderate pain in the operative site, shoulder, and arm in the immediate postoperative period. Because of the necessity of extensive flap development, the patient may note hypesthesia and paresthesia as well as occasional "phantom" hyperesthesia. Hypesthesia is a common postmastectomy complaint and results from denervation of one or more of the intercostobrachial nerves traversing the axillary space that are sectioned in the conduct of the axillary dissection. These sensations disappear gradually with wound healing.[33] The patient should be assured that abnormal sensations will usually subside within 3 to 8 months postoperatively. However, normal sensation may never return to the denervated axilla, medial arm, and hemithorax.

In the immediate postoperative period, the patient is encouraged to resume activity on the evening after her operative procedure. We regularly prescribe fluids by mouth within 2 to 4 hours postoperatively, and often the patient is able to eat a normal or light meal before retiring. Early ambulation is encouraged. Use of portable suction units allows the patient to be up and about her room early postoperatively. We routinely encourage the patient to continue immobilization of the ipsilateral shoulder and upper arm, although mobility is permitted below the elbow in the forearm and hand. Application of closed-suction catheter techniques ensures wound evacuation in this circumstance. Isometric exercises, such as squeezing a ball, are not encouraged because they increase blood and lymph volume without facilitating lymph flow. Initial exercises following drain removal should include graded, active shoulder exercises.

Although a moderate degree of bacterial contamination can be demonstrated in mastectomy procedures, we do not routinely administer preoperative, perioperative, or postoperative antibiotics unless mandated by other medical conditions (e.g., cardiac valvular disease, prosthetic appliances, or skin ulceration). If postoperative erythema and cellulitis are evident, treatment with topical antibacterial creams such as Silvadene are of particular value to prevent progressive epidermolysis and invasive soft tissue infections. Early debridement of obviously devascularized tissue is an important prophylactic adjunct to prevent progressive invasive infection.

Skin grafting after radical mastectomy as originally proposed by Halsted[13] occasionally is required in the management of the mastectomy wound. Stents applied over split-thickness skin grafts, which are necessary for large tissue defects, should be removed on the 5th or 6th postoperative day. Early and periodic wound care, including debridement with wet-to-dry saline dressings, affords optimal wound management to ensure adequate "take" of the graft application.

COMPLICATIONS OF MASTECTOMY

The operative therapy of breast carcinoma can produce a variety of physical problems with regard to patient care. Rehabilitation for the postmastectomy patient has been greatly facilitated by the Reach to Recovery programs sponsored by the American Cancer Society and similar patient/family rehabilitation agencies (see Chapters 87, 90, and 91). In most circumstances, the breast cancer patient is allowed to begin the gradual resumption of presurgical activities within 2 weeks after surgery. Younger women usually regain full range of motion of the arm and the shoulder soon after drain removal, whereas older patients may require intense (supervised) exercise for several months before attaining their former levels of activity. Visits from volunteers of the American Cancer Society or the Visiting Nurse Association are of particular value for psychosocial and physical recovery of the postmastectomy patient.

Lymphedema

The pathogenesis of ipsilateral arm lymphedema after radical, modified, and segmental mastectomy is reviewed in Chapter 51. Lymphedema occurs as a consequence of the en bloc ablation of lymphatic routes (nodes and channels) within the field of resection of the primary mammary tumor. The subsequent increase in plasma hydrostatic pressure that results with removal of these conduits may follow the surgical procedure, irradiation, or uncontrolled progression of neoplasm. Injury, capillary disruption, infection, obstruction to lymphatic or venous outflow, hyperthermia, or exercise will accelerate protein leakage into these tissues. In addition, venous Doppler ultrasound studies of edematous arms after axillary dissection have demonstrated abnormalities in 70 percent of cases.[37]

Previous attempts to evaluate the degree of arm lymphedema have been classified by Stillwell[36] according to the percentage of volume increase. This methodology has been subsequently investigated and further refined.[28] We grade an increase of less than 10 percent in arm volume as insignificant, whereas an increase of greater than 80 percent is classified as severe.

Lymphedema affects some 50 percent to 70 percent of all radical mastectomy patients but is severe and incapacitating in only approximately 10 percent.[10, 34] The incidence of lymphedema after modified radical mastectomy has been found to be significant, but considerably less (12.5 percent).[3] Factors that have been identified as independent risks for the development or progression of lymphedema include the extent of axillary dissection, the use of axillary radiotherapy, pathological nodal status, and obesity.[4, 19] Gilchrist[12] stresses the importance of free and complete active range of motion of the arm and shoulder in the early postoperative period. Patient education emphasizing the avoidance of excessive sun exposure, injections, infections, or other potentially active or passive injury to the ipsilateral extremity is paramount to avoid lymphedema. Further, early recognition of incipient edema by the patient and immediate therapy with compression massage of the area by the patient or nursing personnel may abrogate the ensuing morbidity of lymphedema. Early application of compression massage with the thumb, including stroking of the edematous extremity, will often alleviate and augment the prophylaxis of further edema.

When lymphedema is severe, hospitalization for mechanical expression of tissue fluid, with application of an intermittent pneumatic compression device (Jobst pump), may be of value. The Jobst compression pump (Jobst, Toledo, OH) allows sequential, uniform, and progressive compression of the involved extremity in a proximal direction, thus allowing egress to the obstructed flow of lymph. The physician may wish to prescribe antibiotics, especially if there is evidence of supervening cellulitis. Additionally, it is advisable to prescribe diuretic therapy concomitant with a low-salt diet. An elastic Ace bandage is applied when the patient is not treating herself with the pump, and the arm should be elevated above heart level when the patient is inactive.

We recommend daily measurements at a fixed point on the extremity before and after Jobst therapy is initiated. The arm circumference is measured daily at positions above and below the elbow. These measurements should be recorded before and after therapy. This method is completed in a cycle when progressive resolution of the edema is evident. When optimal improvement is apparent, the patient is measured for a Jobst Venous Pressure sleeve, which is custom-tailored with specific circumferential compression pressure (30 to 40 mm Hg). Daily application of compression treatments is necessary until the sleeve is received and the results of therapy are realized. A more thorough discussion of medical, mechanical, and surgical treatment of chronic lymphedema is provided in Chapter 51.

Wound Infection

Although wound infection occurs infrequently, infection and cellulitis of the mastectomy wound or ipsilateral arm may represent serious morbidity in the postoperative patient (see Chapter 5). The majority of reported wound infections occur as a result of the primary tissue ischemia resulting from extensive tissue dissection that creates thin, devascularized skin flaps. Thereafter, progressive tissue necrosis provides a medium that supports bacterial proliferation with invasive tissue infection.

The 18.9 percent infection rate reported for radical mastectomy by the National Research Council is exorbitantly high for a clean operation. In contrast, wound infection rates after modified radical mastectomy range from 2.8 percent to 15 percent.[39, 40] These reported rates for modified radical mastectomy may be lower because the operation is of lesser magnitude, but more likely it is less because of the efficient evacuation of hematoma and serum with closed wound suction drainage. A wound infection rate of less than 10 percent after radical mastectomy can be achieved when suction drains are routinely used.[1]

Except in patients with pre-existing medical diseases (e.g., prosthetic devices, cardiac valvular disease, or ulcerative carcinoma), we do not administer prophylactic antibiotics routinely; however, irrigation of the wound with antibiotics at operation is desirable for reduction of bacterial flora.

Wound infection or cellulitis produces an immediate disability that may progress to late postoperative lymphedema of the arm. The compromised lymphatic flow, with resultant stasis produced by the standard technique of developing thin skin flaps, predisposes the wound to resultant infection. Early attempts should be made to culture the wound for aerobic and anaerobic organisms with immediate Gram stain of identifiable strains to document the bacterial contaminant. In the absence of lymphedema, wound cellulitis uniformly responds to appropriate antibiotic therapy and elevation of the extremity.

Seroma

Seromas occur in the axillary dead space beneath the elevated skin flaps and represent the most frequent complication of mastectomy, developing in approximately 30 percent of cases.[39, 40] In a retrospective analysis of 87 axillary regional lymph node (Patey) dissections performed as isolated procedures discrete from en bloc breast resections, Bland and associates[6] observed seromas in 26 percent of patients.

With surgical ablation of the breast, the intervening lymphatics and fatty tissues are resected en bloc; thus, the vasculature and lymphatics of the gland are transected. Thereafter, transudation of lymph and the accumulation of blood in the operative field are expected. Further, extensive dissection of the mastectomy flaps results in a large potential dead space beneath the flaps, as does the irregularity of the chest wall, especially in the deep axillary fossa. Continual chest wall respiratory excursions and motion in the shoulder initiate shearing forces that further delay flap adherence and wound repair. Operative technique should minimize lymphatic spillage and transudation of serum to allow rapid adherence of the skin flaps to deep structures without compromise of blood flow to skin flaps or the axilla. Various techniques for flap fixation and wound drainage have been used to enhance primary wound repair and to minimize seroma accumulation.

Two types of external suture fixation have been advocated. In the study by Orr,[31] tension sutures tied over a rubber tubing bolster to fixate the flaps to underlying intercostal muscles and the latissimus dorsi muscle were used. In the report by Keyes and colleagues,[18] through-and-through flap sutures were tied directly to the skin surface to secure the breast flap to the chest wall. Penrose drains were used to drain excessive accumulation of lymph and blood. Thereafter, Larsen and Hugan[21] recommended the application of buried fixation sutures of silk or absorbable material to secure the flaps. These authors secured skin flaps with 30 to 50 subcutaneous cotton sutures and avoided the insertion of any type of drain when possible. With few exceptions, these flap fixation techniques using bolsters and through-and-through sutures from the flap to the underlying chest wall have fallen into disfavor, because of the emergence of simple and improved suctioning devices.[30]

Removal of serum accumulation was first accomplished by the use of static drains, such as Paul's tubing, and the insertion of various soft Penrose drains. Both Paul's tubing and Penrose drains required bulky gauze dressings and multiple dressing changes for the continuous serous soilage expected with wound discharge. Murphy in 1947[29] and Morris in 1973[27] proposed continuous closed-suction drainage methods to prevent serum collection beneath extensive flaps. Presently, the majority of surgeons use this technique of closed-suction drainage to aspirate excessive collections of serum, lymph, and blood from the mastectomy wound.

In the classic report by Maitland and Mathieson in 1970,[23] 1193 wounds were drained during a 5-year period. Of 153 mastectomies, 72 underwent traditional drainage (i.e., wicks, Penrose), whereas 81 had suction drainage. For operations at various sites, including the genitourinary, alimentary, and biliary tract and soft tissue areas (e.g., breast, thyroid), significant differences were not evident for the two techniques. However, in evaluation of the breast as a subset of the overall analysis, the incidence of wound infection with suction drainage (4.9 percent) versus traditional drainage (12.50 percent) was 1.7 times less frequent ($p = 0.045$). For this subset of the patient population, the authors noted a diminished wound infection rate and increased primary healing with the application of closed-suction drainage techniques.

These results were confirmed by Morris[27] after a controlled clinical trial performed to compare the effectiveness of suction drainage with that of static drainage. For radical mastectomy wounds, this trial established that the rate of wound repair was superior with suction drainage technique. Furthermore, the volume of aspirated drainage was greater with the closed-suction method, which also afforded a reduction in the infection, tissue necrosis, and wound disruption frequency.

Thereafter, Bourke and associates[7] conducted a randomized, prospective trial of closed-suction wound drainage compared with corrugated wound drainage after simple mastectomy for early breast cancer (lesion confined to the breast and without skin ulceration). In 51 patients admitted to the study, there were no statistically significant differences between the two groups with respect to local complications such as infection, serum collection beneath the flaps, skin necrosis, and wound repair. However, as shown in Table 50–1, the number of dressing changes required were significantly reduced with suction catheters as opposed to corrugated drainage, and suction drains could be removed significantly sooner than corrugated drains. In today's cost-conscious medical environment, the reduction in dressing changes per day and the morbidity related to prolonged *in situ* drainage clearly favors the use of closed-suction drainage methods. Moreover, with the exception of one small prospective randomized study, suction drainage has been found to be superior to siphon drains.[41]

The extent of surgery also influences local complication rates. Aitken and coworkers[1] evaluated 204 consecutive mastectomies in which the techniques used for flap closure and wound management were identical. All potential dead space was obliterated with absorbable sutures that incorporated the pectoralis major, serratus anterior, and latissimus dorsi muscles as well as the subdermal skin of the axillary flap. Two closed-suction Hemovac drains, one placed in the axillary apex along the lateral part of the chest wall and the other placed over the anterior portion of the chest, were inserted via a separate lower flap stab incision. The average initial volume and total volume of the fluid aspirated from the wounds were similar in both radical and modified radical mastectomy groups (91.1 ml versus 91.7 ml).

Table 50–2 summarizes the wound complications observed in this series. Postoperative fluid accumulation occurred in 9.31 percent, with greater frequency in the radical mastectomy group. Infected seroma was identified only in the radical mastectomy group, with an overall frequency of 0.98 percent. The magnitude of the radical mastectomy procedure perhaps also accounted for the frequency of superficial wound infections, which were more than four times as frequent in this group as in the modified radical mastectomy group. Aitken and Minton[2] identified a decreased incidence of seroma accumulation in these less-extensive operations on the breast (simple mastectomy had less incidence than modified radical, which in turn had less incidence than radical mastectomy). These results agree with the results of other reports, in which the incidence of seroma was higher for modified radical mastectomy compared with lumpectomy and axillary dissection.[40]

Tadych and Donegan[38] determined the daily wound drainage and total hospital drainage (THD) for 49 consecutive patients undergoing mastectomy to evaluate the frequency of seroma and lymphedema formation. No patient received preoperative or postoperative radiation. Of this series of patients undergoing modified radical mastectomies and who did not receive irradiation, all had wound closure with suction drainage and none had flap necrosis or infection. The THD varied from 227 to 3607 ml and did not correlate with body weight. Twenty-six patients had wound seromas requiring drainage for periods of as much as 7 months, most often requiring repeated aspirations and, more infrequently ($n = 4$), open drainage. Ipsilateral edema of the arm directly correlated with THD. No patient with less than 500 ml of THD had edema, whereas the frequency rate was 75 percent in patients with THD that exceeded 900 ml. These authors concluded that THD likely reflects the magnitude of lymphatic interruption after mastectomy and thus the probability of lymphatic insufficiency and the development of lymphedema. Of clinical and practical significance, no patient with less than 20 ml of drainage in the 24 hours before catheter removal developed a seroma.

The use of closed-system suction catheter drainage during the past decade has greatly facilitated the reduction in protracted serum collections. Seromas of the axillary dead space and the anterior chest wall are manifested in the first week postoperatively. Therapy consists of retention of the suction apparatus until drainage diminishes to less than 20 ml per day. Thereafter, compression dressings are applied after catheter removal in anticipation of protracted wound discharge.

McCarthy and associates[24] reported on attempts at management of the chronic serous discharge from

TABLE 50–1.   FREQUENCY OF DRESSINGS, LENGTH OF DRAINAGE, AND TIME OF SUTURE REMOVAL

	Suction Drains ($n = 24$)	Corrugated Drains ($n = 27$)	t	p
Number of dressings/day	0.071 ± 0.19	1.02 ± 0.30	3.88	0.001
Drains *in situ* (days)	4.79 ± 1.66	6.55 ± 1.33	4.18	0.001
Sutures removed (days)	9.91 ± 0.65	10.28 ± 0.93	1.15	NS

NS = Not significant.
From Bourke JB, Balfour TW, Hardcastle JD, Wilkins JL: A comparison between suction and corrugated drainage after simple mastectomy: A report of a controlled trial. Br J Surg 63:67–69, 1976. Reprinted by permission.

TABLE 50–2. SUMMARY OF WOUND COMPLICATIONS

| Complication | Type of Mastectomy | | | |
	Radical (n = 72)	Modified Radical (n = 117)	Simple (n = 15)	Total (n = 204)
Hematoma or seroma	14 (19.44)	5 (4.27)	—	19 (9.31)
Infected seroma	2 (2.78)	—	—	2 (0.98)
Superficial wound infection	5 (6.94)	2 (1.71)	—	7 (3.43)

Numbers in parentheses are percentages.
From Aitken DR, Hunsaker R, James AG: Prevention of seromas following mastectomy and axillary dissection. Surg Gynecol Obstet 158:327–350, 1984. Reprinted by permission.

mastectomy wounds that were observed in approximately 25 percent of their patients. In this prospective, randomized controlled trial, the effect of tetracycline as a sclerotherapy agent for flap adherence was evaluated. Six patients in the control group and eight patients in the treated group were evaluated. One patient in the control group developed a seroma after drain removal. In contrast, half of the patients treated with tetracycline therapy developed seromas after removal of drains. Because of the severe pain associated with tetracycline sclerotherapy treatment and the lack of demonstrable benefit to those treated, the study was aborted by the investigators.

In addition, postoperative oral administration of the antifibrinolytic tranexamic acid has been investigated as a means of decreasing seroma formation.[11] The results are encouraging but far from conclusive. Although a beneficial effect was observed in a rat model, intraoperative application of fibrin glue before flap closure has not been shown to be of any benefit in preventing seroma formation.[14, 15]

The effect of shoulder mobility restriction in diminishing serous wound discharge after radical mastectomy was evaluated in a randomized prospective clinical trial by Flew.[9] Of 64 consecutive patients nursed in the wards of the Guy's Breast Unit in London, shoulder movement restriction reduced the mean volume of drainage by 40 percent in those who had immobility for the first 7 postoperative days when compared with the group in whom early arm exercises were encouraged (Table 50–3). This study confirmed a reduction in drainage duration (days) by 29 percent. Both the number of patients requiring operation and the need for multiple aspirations were reduced in the shoulder-restricted group; however, differences were not statistically significant between the two subgroups in duration of hospital stay. Shoulder mobilization did not result in increased shoulder stiffness, although the author confirmed an increased incidence of mild, but transient, lymphedema of the arm when the technique was used. It may be concluded from this study that active shoulder movement immediately after mastectomy is not advisable.

Furthermore, there is evidence that immobilization significantly decreased drainage in volume ($p < 0.01$) and duration ($p < 0.05$) without affecting eventual shoulder mobility, as shown in Table 50–3. It

appears that the liability of lymphedema is enhanced with use of the restriction technique but can be limited in extent when the complication is recognized.

Similar conclusions were reached in a prospective randomized study performed at the National Cancer Institute of early versus delayed shoulder motion following axillary dissection.[22] Patients randomized to early motion demonstrated significantly greater total wound drainage, days of drainage, and days of hospitalization, without any differences in functional range of motion. Also, wound infection and flap necrosis were observed more frequently in the early motion group. In another study, the incidence of

TABLE 50–3. WOUND DRAINAGE AFTER MODIFIED RADICAL MASTECTOMY: EFFECT OF RESTRICTION OF SHOULDER MOVEMENT

	Fixed (n = 29)		Free (n = 35)	
Drainage volume (ml, mean ± S.E.)		725.4 ± 77.3		1203.1 ± 137.7†
Total drainage time* in days (range and mean)	4-21	11.69 ± 0.93	6-60	16.40 ± 1.79‡
Time until removal of all drains (range and mean)	4-21	11.17 ± 0.92	6-31	13.66 ± 0.93§
Aspirations				
No. patients		2		7§
No. aspirations		4		33‖
Hospital stay (days, mean ± S.E.)		14.66 ± 0.66		16.03 ± 0.75§

*Including aspirations.
†$t = 2.862; p < 0.01$.
‡$t = 2.195; p < 0.05$.
§N.S.
‖$t = 1.791; p < 0.1$.

| Group | Shoulder Abduction at 4 Months | |
	Limitation > 30° (No. of Patients)	Mean Limitation (Degrees ± S.E.)
Fixed (n = 29)	8	19.8 ± 3.3
Free (n = 34)	13	21.2 ± 3.6

The differences are not significant.
From Flew TJ: Wound drainage following radical mastectomy: The effect of restriction of shoulder movement. Br J Surg 66:302–205, 1979. Reprinted by permission.

seroma formation postmastectomy was tenfold less when shoulder immobilization was used compared with when active range of motion was allowed.[20]

Pneumothorax

Pneumothorax, a rare complication, develops when the surgeon perforates the parietal pleura with extended tissue dissection or with attempts at hemostasis for perforators of the intercostal musculature. Pneumothorax is more commonly seen in patients undergoing a radical mastectomy after removal of the pectoralis major musculature. Respiratory distress is recognized in the operative or the immediate postoperative periods, and pneumothorax is confirmed by chest roentgenogram. Immediate therapy with closed thoracostomy drainage of the pleural space is essential as soon as pneumothorax is verified.

Tissue Necrosis

A commonly recognized complication of breast surgery is necrosis of the developed skin flaps or skin margins. Budd and colleagues[8] observed major skin necrosis in 8 percent of their patients, a rate similar to that found in other series. Bland and colleagues[5, 6] observed an incidence of 21 percent for minor and major necrosis of skin flaps with associated wound infection for this operative site.

Local debridement is usually not necessary in minor areas of necrosis (i.e., ≤ 2 cm^2 area). Larger areas of partial or full-thickness skin loss require debridement and, on occasion, the application of split-thickness skin grafts. Rotational composite skin flaps and subcutaneous skin tissue can be used from the lateral chest wall or the contralateral breast to cover the defect.

Hemorrhage

Although not specifically designed to detect bleeding, the use of closed-suction catheter drainage allows early recognition of hemorrhage, an infrequent complication of mastectomy. Hemorrhage is reported as a postoperative complication in 1 to 4 percent of patients and is manifested by undue swelling of flaps of the operative site.[3, 4, 35] Early recognition of this complication is imperative. Hemorrhage may be treated by aspiration of the liquefied hematoma and the establishment of patency of the suction catheters. The application of a light compression dressing reinforced with Elastoplast tape should diminish the recurrence of this adverse event. Moderate to severe hemorrhage in the immediate postoperative course is rare and is best managed with wound re-exploration. Early, severe hemorrhage is most often related to arterial perforators of the thoracoacromial vessels or internal mammary arteries. Direct suture ligation is advisable. Thereafter, closed drainage systems are replaced, and tubing patency is ensured before wound closure.

Surgeons hold varying opinions as to the best technique to elevate skin flaps for performance of total mastectomy. Electrocautery, cold scalpel, Shaw hot knife, and, more recently, the laser, have been used to create skin flaps for modified radical and radical mastectomies. The cold scalpel has the advantage of minimal tissue injury but may present formidable bleeding problems unless used concomitantly with direct suture ligation or electrocoagulation. Excessive bleeding may obscure the operative field with blood, and the extensive dissection may leave the hematologically compromised patient anemic at termination of the procedure. In contrast, electrocoagulation minimizes blood loss.[2, 16] However, the experimental studies by Keenan and colleagues[17] suggest that the tissue damage initiated with cautery injury may diminish the host response to infection.

In the prospective, nonrandomized study of 60 patients undergoing total mastectomy by Osborne and colleagues,[32] no statistical differences for infection rate, operating time, wound discharge, or hospital stay were noted with use of the cold scalpel compared with the electrocautery. These authors determined that use of the electrocautery allowed significantly greater blood loss, estimating that blood loss was 440 ml versus 651 ml for the scalpel and electrocautery, respectively. Kakos and James[16] completed a similar prospective analysis for comparison of blood loss with the electrocautery versus the scalpel in 50 mastectomy patients. Average blood loss in this series was 960 ml in the scalpel group versus 160 ml in the electrocautery group. Twenty-four of 25 scalpel patients (96 percent) received transfusions, compared with only 6 of 25 (24 percent) in the electrocautery group. Wound necrosis was not different in the two groups.

Miller and associates[25] conducted a randomized prospective study to investigate differences in blood loss and postoperative complications in patients undergoing modified radical mastectomy with use of the electrocautery and scalpel. Table 50–4 demonstrates the demographic features identifiable with use of electrocoagulation versus the scalpel in mastectomies. Twenty-four patients had skin flaps created with the cold scalpel, and 25 had skin flaps created with the electrocautery. The two groups were similar with respect to age, stage of disease, size of tumor, and body weight. Use of the electrocautery allowed patients to have significantly reduced operative blood loss when compared with scalpel patients (352 versus 507 ml, respectively; $p < 0.05$). No electrocautery patient required transfusion. The primary advantage of the electrocautery was the reduction in blood loss; surprisingly, operating time was not significantly shortened with use of the electrocautery technique. These authors acknowledge that the axillary dissection is the time-limiting factor of the procedure, and, because of neurological injury induced with use of electrocoagulation, axillary dissection techniques used by the surgeons were identical in both subgroups. Total postoperative Hemovac drainage and hospital stay were not significantly different between

TABLE 50–4. BLOOD LOSS, HEMATOCRIT CHANGE, TRANSFUSION, LENGTH OF OPERATION, DRAINAGE, STAY, AND INFECTIONS IN SCALPEL AND ELECTROCAUTERY MASTECTOMY PATIENTS

	Scalpel Patients	Electrocautery Patients	p Value
Estimated blood loss (ml)	507 ± 122	352 ± 106	<0.05
Decrease in hematocrit	8.2 ± 2.2	5.9 ± 1.6	<0.05
Number transfused	3	0	<0.005
Length of operation (minutes)	120 ± 19	117 ± 20	NS
Postoperative drainage (ml)	208 ± 56	256 ± 66	NS
Stay (days)	5.8 ± 0.1	5.9 ± 0.6	NS
Number fever days	6	9	NS
Wound complications	3	6	NS
Cellulitis	2	5	NS
Flap necrosis	1	1	NS

NS = Not significant.
From Miller E, Paull DE, Morrissey K, Cortese A, Novak E: Scalpel versus electrocautery in modified radical mastectomy. Am Surg 54:284–286, 1988. Reprinted by permission.

the two groups. Although the number of fever days and wound complications were slightly higher in the electrocoagulation group, this difference was not statistically significant. Miller and associates[25] concluded that use of the electrocautery for development of skin flaps in the performance of a mastectomy reduces blood loss without incurring a greater incidence of wound complications.

Cautery appears to be the most suitable surgical instrument for tissue plane dissection in the procedure. However, it has the expectant limitation of neurostimulation and heat injury with dissection around motor nerves, such as the brachial plexus, and of motor innervation to muscles of the axillary space, including the medial/lateral pectoral, long thoracic, and thoracodorsal nerves to the pectoralis major/minor, serratus anterior, and latissimus dorsi muscles, respectively. For these reasons, a combination of both techniques is used by the majority of surgeons.

As indicated by Miller and associates,[26] the known risk for blood transfusions include hepatitis (0.26 to 1 percent), transfusion allergic reactions (1 to 19 percent), and a lower, but fatal, risk for acquisition of AIDS. Each of these transfusion-related complications necessitates constant reexamination of the indications for transfusion, with deliberate attempts to reduce transfusion requirements at mastectomy in the nonanemic patient.

Injury to Neurovascular Structures of the Axilla

Injury to the brachial plexus is also a rare complication of mastectomy. This is most commonly avoided by meticulous (cold scalpel) sharp dissection in and about the neurovascular bundle and by development of tissue planes that parallel the neurilemma and the wall of the axillary vein to allow en bloc resection of lymphatic structures and fatty tissues.

More common are injuries to the thoracodorsal nerve and the long thoracic nerve (respiratory) of Bell in the postoperative period. The thoracodorsal, or subscapular, nerve innervates the latissimus dorsi muscle in its course with the thoracodorsal (subscapular) vessels and is commonly sacrificed when lymphatics are discovered to be involved with metastases at axillary dissection. Sacrifice of this nerve results in minimal physical disability; the patient observes weakness of internal rotation and abduction of the shoulder after denervation and paralysis of the latissimus dorsi muscle.

Conversely, injury or transection of the long thoracic nerve of Bell, which innervates the serratus anterior muscle, produces instability and unsightly prominence of the scapula ("winged scapula"). The patient sustaining such an injury will often complain of shoulder pain at rest and with motion for many months after the procedure. All attempts should be made to preserve this nerve, yet its involvement with invasive neoplasm or nodal extension may require that it be sacrificed to ensure adequate en bloc resection.

The lateral and medial pectoral nerves to the pectoralis major muscles and the motor innervation to the pectoralis minor exit the brachial plexus to enter the posterior aspects of these muscles in the proximal axilla. Preservation of the pectoralis major and its function is the objective of the modified radical mastectomy. Thus, maintenance of the integrity of the medial and lateral pectoral nerves is paramount to ensure subsequent function of the pectoralis major. Section of the medial pectoral nerve with motor denervation of the pectoralis musculature allows progressive atrophy of these muscle groups with resultant cosmetic and neurological morbidity.

Technical precision must be exercised in dissection of the axillary vein and its tributaries. The surgeon should dissect in a plane that is parallel, anterior, and ventral to the vein surface with inclusion of perivascular fat and lymphatics (see Chapter 39). The rare complication of injury to the vein with dissection is immediately controlled by use of compression and vascular clamps and by suture repair with fine cardiovascular nylon suture. Tumor invasion of the axillary vein is best managed by vein resection and subsequent ligation of the proximal and distal ends. Ligation of the axillary vein for pre-existing venous tumor invasion has not been associated with an increased incidence of postoperative edema of the extremity.[42]

Injuries to the axillary artery likewise must be carefully repaired with cardiovascular suture; however, such injuries are less likely to occur than are venous injuries, because the axillary artery is located posterior and superior to the axillary vein. The interior aspect of the axillary vein must be "skeletonized" when performing the axillary dissection, but there is no need to dissect the axillary artery. Lymphatics around the axillary artery serve an important physiological purpose in preventing postoperative arm edema. These perivascular lymphatics are involved with metastatic disease only in advanced stages of regional disease in which locally invasive tumor or extranodal involvement extends into the axilla space.

References

1. Aitken DR, Hunsaker R, James AG: Prevention of seromas following mastectomy and axillary dissection. Surg Gynecol Obstet 158:327–330, 1984.
2. Aitken DR, Minton JP: Complications associated with mastectomy. Surg Clin North Am 63:1331–1351, 1983.
3. Axelrod DM, Osborne MP: The swollen extremity. In Wittes RE (ed): Manual of Oncologic Therapeutics. Philadelphia; JB Lippincott, 1989.
4. Bertelli G, Venturini M, Forno G, Macchiavello F, Dini D: An analysis of prognostic factors in response to conservative treatment of postmastectomy lymphedema. Surg Gynecol Obstet 175:455–460, 1992.
5. Bland KI, Heuser LS, Spratt JS Jr, Polk HC Jr: The postmastectomy patient: Wound care, complications, and follow-up. In Strombeck JO, Rosato FE (eds): Surgery of the Breast. Stuttgart, Thieme Verlag, 1986, pp 158–163.
6. Bland KI, Klamer TW, Polk HC Jr, Knutson CO: Isolated regional lymph node dissection: Morbidity, mortality, and economic considerations. Ann Surg 193:372–376, 1981.
7. Bourke JB, Balfour TW, Hardcastle JD, Wilkins JL: A comparison between suction and corrugated drainage after simple mastectomy: A report of a controlled trial. Br J Surg 63:67–69, 1976.
8. Budd DC, Cochran RC, Sturtz DL, Fouty WJ Jr: Surgical morbidity after mastectomy operations. Am J Surg 135:218–220, 1978.
9. Flew TJ: Wound drainage following radical mastectomy: The effect of restriction of shoulder movement. Br J Surg 66:302–305, 1979.
10. Flippetti M, Santoro E, Graziano F, Petric M, Rinaldi G: Modern therapeutic approaches to postmastectomy brachial lymphedema. Microsurgery 15: 604–610, 1994.
11. Gertli D, Laffer U, Haberthuer F, Kreuter U, Harder F: Preoperative and postoperative tranexamic acid reduces the local wound complication rate after surgery for breast cancer. Br J Surg 81:856–859, 1994.
12. Gilchrist RK: The postmastectomy massive arm: A usually preventable catastrophe. Am J Surg 122:363, 1971.
13. Halsted WS: Developments in the skin-grafting operation for cancer of the breast. JAMA 60:416–418, 1913.
14. Harada RN, Pressler VM, McNamara JJ: Fibrin glue reduces seroma formation in the rat after mastectomy. Surg Gynecol Obstet 175:450–454, 1992.
15. Jonk A, van Dongen JA, Kroon BBR: Prevention of seroma following axillary lymph node dissection or radical mastectomy: Ineffectiveness of fibrin glue sealing technique. Neth J Surg 39:135, 1987.
16. Kakos GS, James AG: The use of cautery in "bloodless" radical mastectomy. Cancer 26:666–668, 1970.
17. Keenan KM, Rodeheaver GT, Kenney JG, Edlich RF: Surgical cautery revisited. Am J Surg 147:818–821, 1984.
18. Keyes IW, Hawk BO, Sherwin CS: Basting the axillary flap for wounds of radical mastectomy. Arch Surg 66:446–451, 1953.
19. Kissin MW, della Rovere GQ, Easton D, Westbury G: Risk of lymphoedema following the treatment of breast cancer. Br J Surg 73:580–584, 1986.
20. Knight CD Jr, Griffen FD, Knight CD: Prevention of seromas in mastectomy wounds: The effect of shoulder immobilization. Arch Surg 130:99–101, 1995.
21. Larsen BB, Hugan C: Fixation of skin flaps in radical mastectomy by subcutaneous sutures. Arch Surg 71:419–423, 1955.
22. Lotze MT, Duncan MA, Gerber LH, Woltering EA, Rosenberg SA: Early versus delayed shoulder motion following axillary dissection: A randomized prospective study. Ann Surg 193:288–295, 1981.
23. Maitland IL, Mathieson AJM: Suction drainage: A study in wound healing. Br J Surg 57:193–197, 1970.
24. McCarthy PM, Martin JK, Wells DC, Welch JS, Ilstrup DM: An aborted, prospective, randomized trial of sclerotherapy for prolonged drainage after mastectomy. Surg Gynecol Obstet 162:418–420, 1986.
25. Miller E, Paull DE, Morrissey K, Cortese A, Novak E: Scalpel versus electrocautery in modified radical mastectomy. Am Surg 54:284–286, 1988.
26. Miller PJ, O'Connell J, Leipold A, Wenzel RP: Potential liability for transfusion associated AIDS. JAMA 253:3419–3423, 1985.
27. Morris AM: A controlled trial of closed wound suction drainage in radical mastectomy. Br J Surg 60:357–359, 1973.
28. Mridha M, Odman S: Fluid translocation measurement: A method to study pneumatic compression treatment of postmastectomy lymphedema. Scand J Rehab Med 21:63–69, 1989.
29. Murphy DR: The use of atmospheric pressure in obliterating axillary dead space following radical mastectomy. South Surg 13:372–375, 1947.
30. O'Dwyer PJ, O'Higgins NJ, James AG: Effect of closing dead space on incidence of seroma after mastectomy. Surg Gynecol Obstet 172:55–56, 1991.
31. Orr TG: An incision and method of wound closure for radical mastectomy. Ann Surg 133:565–566, 1951.
32. Osborne MP, Andrakis C, Rankin RA: The thermal scalpel: A comparative study with conventional scalpel and electrocautery. Contemp Surg 29:51–54, 1986.
33. Paredes JP, Puente JL, Potel J: Variations in sensitivity after sectioning the intercostobrachial nerve. Am J Surg 160:525–528, 1990.
34. Schottenfeld D, Robbins GF: Quality of survival among patients who have had radical mastectomy. Cancer 26:650, 1970.
35. Somers RG, Jablon LK, Kaplan MJ, Sandler GL, Rosenblatt NK: The use of closed suction drainage after lumpectomy and axillary node dissection for breast cancer. Ann Surg 215:146–149, 1992.
36. Stillwell GK: Treatment of postmastectomy lymphedema. Mod Treat 6:396–412, 1969.
37. Svensson WE, Mortimer PS, Tohno E, Cosgrove DO: Colour Doppler demonstrates venous flow abnormalities in breast cancer patients with chronic arm swelling. Eur J Cancer 30A:657–660, 1994.
38. Tadych K, Donegan WL: Postmastectomy seromas and wound drainage. Surg Gynecol Obstet 165:483–487, 1987.
39. Tejler G, Aspegren K: Complications and hospital stay after surgery for breast cancer: A prospective study of 385 patients. Br J Surg 72:542–544, 1985.
40. Vinton AL, Traverso LW, Jolly PC: Wound complications after modified radical mastectomy compared with tylectomy with axillary lymph node dissection. Am J Surg 161:584–588, 1991.
41. Whitfield PC, Rainsburg RM: Suction versus siphon drainage after axillary surgery for breast cancer: A prospective randomized trial. Br J Surg 81:546–547, 1994.
42. Zintel HA, Nay HR: Postoperative complications of radical mastectomy. Surg Clin North Am 44:313, 1964.

CHAPTER 51

LYMPHEDEMA IN THE POSTMASTECTOMY PATIENT: PATHOPHYSIOLOGY, PREVENTION, AND MANAGEMENT

Douglas S. Reintgen, M.D. / Charles E. Cox, M.D. / Christopher A. Puleo, PA-C

In the postmastectomy patient, chronic lymphedema has the potential to become a permanent, progressive condition. Once the condition is allowed to progress, it can become extremely treatment-resistant, and in most cases cannot be completely relieved by either medical or surgical means. Short-term complications, such as increased fullness of soft tissue and heaviness of the extremity, make the patient susceptible to long-term complications of decreased functional ability and range of motion. The lymphedema in turn may lead to subsequent fibrosis of the tissues as a result of deposition of protein-rich fluids in the interstitial tissues. This protein-rich fluid becomes an excellent growth medium for bacteria and fungi, causing an increase in recurrent infections of the affected extremity. With each infection, the lymphedema condition becomes worse.

The surgical management of the patient with chronic lymphedema is usually reserved for those with massive lymphedema and severe skin breakdown. These procedures have a potentially high morbidity, with a success rate of only 30 percent, and with a large number of patients returning to their presurgical girth within 3 to 4 years. For these reasons, a surgical approach is usually not recommended.

Medical management of chronic lymphedema, when instituted early in the postoperative period, has been shown to decrease overall limb volume and girth. These therapies usually allow the patient to prophylactically and later intermittently receive treatment for this potentially disabling condition.

HISTORY

Anatomical dissections around the year 1622 described the detection of mesenteric lacteals by Gasparo Aselli of Italy. In well-fed dogs, these vessels contained a milky white fluid that drained into a large mesenteric node.[13] Later, the French anatomist Jean Pecquet recognized the thoracic duct and its importance in the understanding of the lymphatic system. In 1953, the Scandinavians Rudbeck and Bartholin were the first to use the term *lymphatics*, but the function of the lymphatics remained a mystery.[13]

In the 18th century, those in William Hunter's School of Anatomy in London worked on the anatomy and physiology of the lymphatic system. The work, as summarized by Hunter, showed that "the lymphatic vessels are the absorbing vessels all over the body . . . and constitute one great and general system."[10]

Virchow[52] in 1806 was one of the first to recognize the importance of the lymphatic system in cancer, believing that the lymph nodes acted as a barrier to cancer spread. The radical surgical procedures developed shortly thereafter, including radical mastectomy, radical neck dissection, and abdominal perineal resection, were based on the concept that there was a stepwise progression of cancer spread from the lymph nodes to systemic areas. In fact, Sir Berkeley Moynihan (1865–1936) wrote "The surgery of malignant disease is not the surgery of organs, it is the anatomy of the lymph node system."[15]

One of the first articles to describe chronic lymphedema as a complication was written by Matas[28] in 1913, and was expounded upon later by Halsted[16] with his article concerning "elephantiasis chirurgica." Matas stated: "By elephantiasis we mean a progressive histopathologic state or condition which is characterized by a chronic inflammatory fibromatosis or hypertrophy of the hypodermal and dermal connective tissue which is preceded by and associated with lymphatic and venous stasis, and may be caused by any obstruction or mechanical interference with the return flow of the lymphatic and venous currents. . . ."

Surgical treatment for lymphatic problems evolved and advanced with Leriche stating in 1940 that "the treatment of lymphedema will only improve if radiography of lymphatic vessels has demonstrated the pathophysiology.[11, 42] In 1938, Veal performed venography in the arm of a patient with postmastectomy lymphedema and attributed swelling to axillary vein obstruction. However, his belief could not be confirmed, and in 1955, Kinmouth and colleagues[23] published conclusive evidence of lymphatic obstruction without axillary vein compromise to show that this was the true mechanism of postmastectomy lymphedema. Axillary vein obstruction has been documented with postmastectomy lymphedema in only about 20% of cases.

DEFINITION

Lymphedema is the accumulation of protein-rich fluid in soft tissues as a result of interruption of lymphatic flow. It occurs most frequently in the extremities, but it can also be found in the head, neck, abdomen, lungs, and genital regions. If the lymphatic system is damaged or blocked, edema accumulates over a period of time, with subsequent thickening of the tissues. This thickening is caused by fibrosis of the interstitial soft tissues.

Lymphedema is divided into two forms. Primary lymphedema, associated with developmental abnormalities of the lymphatic system, may be manifested in neonates (congenital), adolescents (praecox), or in patients older than age 35 years (tarda).

The most common form of lymphedema is secondary lymphedema. This usually occurs after oncological surgery or radiation therapy. The condition occurs as a result of damage by metastatic disease to the lymphatic system, postradiation changes to the underlying skin structures, or surgical removal of the lymphatic nodal basin(s).[12] After the onset of secondary lymphedema, the accumulation of lymphatic fluid in the subcutaneous tissue spaces and skin leads to a cosmetically displeasing and mechanically cumbersome enlargement of the extremity. Overall limb heaviness and fullness limit the daily life activities of the patient with chronic extremity lymphedema and a corresponding complaint of vague aches and pain. Recurrent infection also tends to make the lymphedematous limb worsen over time. The incidence of acute edema of the upper extremity after mastectomy is approximately 40 percent and is usually resolved with conservative measures. The incidence of chronic lymphedema (more than 6 months) is markedly varied in studies completed during the last 20 years. The incidence can be as low as 5.5 percent[14] to as high as 80 percent,[26] depending on the definition of chronic lymphedema. However, with the use of more conservative surgical modalities in the treatment of breast cancers, i.e., lumpectomy versus radical mastectomy (including perhaps only Levels 1 and 2 nodal dissections), the average incidence may be as low as 3 percent. Studies by Smith and associates[44, 45] demonstrated the incidence of postoperative upper extremity lymphedema to be 3 percent after surgical removal of the axillary regional lymph node basins at risk in patients with malignant melanoma. These numbers have been found applicable to breast cancer patients.

Fibrosis of the axilla is a universal phenomenon after mastectomy and is implicated as a cause of lymphedema. This fibrosis may compress main lymphatic trunks and act as a barrier to the regeneration of lymphatic vessels. Many authors agree that radiation therapy to the axilla after axillary node dissection greatly increases the incidence of lymphedema, and the incidence can be as high as 52 percent, compared with 3 to 25 percent incidence in those who did not receive postoperative radiation therapy. Radiation therapy causes fibrosis of the lymph nodes and channels. Infection in the extremity will cause the lymphedema to worsen and may be an important contributor to secondary lymphedema, once dermal lymphatic collaterals develop. Recurrent breast cancer rarely worsens the lymphedema; this is usually

easily detected because of the presence of a mass or recurrent adenopathy. However, the most common cause of lymphedema remains the interference and obstruction of the lymph flow from the arm by division and removal of the lymphatic channels and lymph nodes of the axilla by the surgical procedure.

CONTRIBUTING FACTORS

Segerstrom and associates[41] identified six contributing factors that influenced the incidence of brachial edema after treatment for breast cancer: radiation therapy, obesity, age, operative site, incision type, and history of infection.[1] With postoperative weight gain, a decrease in effectiveness of conservative therapy was evident in 10.3 percent.[3] Adding radiation therapy has been shown to increase the incidence of lymphedema from 20 to 52 percent.[18, 40] Lymphedema is lessened if transverse rather than oblique incisions are used.[41] Others have suggested that the extent of axillary dissection is an important contributing factor. Limiting the axillary dissection to Levels 1 and 2 and preserving the Level 3 nodes and lymphatic collateral channels around the shoulder may decrease the incidence of the acute and chronic lymphedema. In addition, some believe that the dissection of Levels 1 and 2 nodes is an adequate sampling of the axilla for staging purposes.[9] Recent technology has introduced the concept of lymphatic mapping and sentinel lymph node (SLN) biopsy for women with invasive breast cancer. With the hypothesis that the histology of the SLN reflects the histology of the remaining nodes in the basin, full nodal staging information can be garnered with a simple lymph node biopsy of 1 or 2 nodes. This approach may limit the possibility of lymphedema to only those women with histological evidence of metastatic disease in the axilla, e.g., only those women with a positive SLN who would then go on to have a complete axillary node dissection.[38]

PATHOPHYSIOLOGY

The lymphatic system develops during the embryological phase as part of the vascular system. The components of the lymphatic fluid include endothelial cells, protein, water, tissue products and other foreign particles. It is believed that the mammalian lymphatic system evolves from the fusion of clefts in the perivenous mesoderm layers.

The lymph capillaries form a network more extensive than that of blood capillaries. In some tissues, such as the skin, gastrointestinal tract, and lung, the lymphatics can be quite extensive. Other organs, such as the bone marrow, brain, and muscle do not contain any lymphatics. In the breast, the lymphatics may penetrate the pectoralis fascia when coursing to the axilla. The lymph capillaries, which begin as closed saccules, consist of a single layer of endothelium without gaps. Unlike blood vessels, the lymphatic vessels have an absent or poorly developed basement membrane. This facilitates intracellular movement of plasma proteins and lipids that are too large for venous absorption. Lymphatics reabsorb the fluid exuded by the blood capillaries, but they are also capable of taking up material that is quite large to drain into the collecting lymph vessels.[13] Normally, the pressure in the lymphatic vessels is negative or 0 mm H_2O. After an axillary dissection, intralymphatic pressure becomes positive, and lymphatic flow can be 10 times slower than normal.

The collecting lymph vessels are thin-walled structures with valves every 2 to 3 mm. The smaller collecting vessels have an inner coat of elastic longitudinal fibers and endothelial cells and an outer layer of connective tissue. The larger vessels have an additional middle smooth muscle coat, which aids transport of the fluid. These larger vessels coalesce and travel parallel with the veins to the draining lymph nodes.[13]

In the fetus, the lymph nodes form after the various plexuses develop. Foci of lymphocytes begin to accumulate within a network of lymphatic capillaries and eventually form lymph nodes. The afferent lymphatic enters the outside of the node into the marginal sinus. This structure surrounds the node and has a delicate retinaculum that will trap particulate material, including metastatic cells. Thus, the marginal sinus is the first site for metastases to be found. The efferent lymphatic vessel leaves the hilum of the node.[13]

The basic function of the lymphatic system is to circulate interstitial proteins and lipids back into the vascular system through lymphatic capillaries. As mentioned, these capillaries are valveless, intradermal vessels that drain into unidirectional valved lymphatic vessels located at the junction between the dermis and the subcutaneous tissue. These unidirectional vessels then drain into afferent lymphatics. The lymph is propelled by muscular movement and contraction of the larger lymphatic vessels, with the flow controlled by valves located at 1 to 2-mm intervals. The lymphatic fluid is subsequently filtered by regional lymph nodes that eventually empty into larger vessels in the venous system, primarily at the thoracic duct. The lymphatic system is a regional drainage system unlike the blood circulatory system. However, there are communicating lymph vessels between various regions, which allows for the successful use of complex physical therapy in the treatment of lymphedema.[51]

Application of the Starling equation suggests that edema represents an imbalance between net capillary filtration and lymphatic drainage. Capillary fluid filtration is promoted by capillary hydrostatic pressure and the colloid osmotic pressure of the interstitial fluid; it is impeded by interstitial hydrostatic pressure and the osmotic pressure of plasma proteins. Under normal conditions, the capillary wall is permeable to water and electrolytes, and filtration exceeds resorption, resulting in a net fluid flow from the capillaries to the interstitial spaces. This fluid is removed from the tissues by the lymphatic vessels. Abnormal interstitial fluid accumulation, or edema, occurs when there is a disequilibrium in the balanced fluid exchange. This can be classified by the principal causes leading to lymphedema development.

Fibrosis of the axilla usually develops after mastectomy, as reported by Hughes and Patel in 1966.[19] This, in turn, may cause venous and lymphatic obstruction. The postmastectomy fibrous tissue causes compression of the main lymphatic and venous structures of the axilla. It also acts by sclerosing the attempted regeneration of lymphatic and venous collateral channels, influencing the tributaries found in the superficial system over the anterior shoulder and chest, along with the subscapular and cephalic veins and their abilities to form a collateral system of drainage.

Some recent studies have shown increased arterial inflow[49] and venous outflow[48] to the extremity of the affected side. Svenson and colleagues, using color Doppler ultrasound, noted that the mean percentage of blood flow was 32 percent higher in the arm from the side of the mastectomy, compared with the contralateral arm. If the arm on the side of the mastectomy had lymphedema, then blood flow was 68 percent higher, compared with contralateral normal arms. This study showed an identifiable increase in arterial flow to the treatment-side arms that was worse in those arms already edematous. This was believed to be caused by a neurological deficit with loss of sympathetic vasoconstrictor control. Svenson and colleagues noted that more than half of their patients showed evidence of venous outflow obstruction, with venous congestion present in 14 percent of them.

DIAGNOSIS AND SYMPTOMS

There is no uniform agreement on the criteria for lymphedema, probably accounting for the wide variation in the reported incidence of the condition. Diagnosis can be established on the basis of an accurate history and a thorough physical examination. Assessment of the progression of edema is hallmark in the postoperative care of the patient. Several methods have been attempted. Each alone may have its inherent shortcomings, but when used in combination, they can give the practitioner an adequate means of following a patient's progression or response to therapy.

Photography at pre-operative and postoperative visits can be very useful in determining the onset and progression of lymphedema.[31] It is important that the photographs be taken from the same focal distance and time of day. Lymphedema is time- and activity-dependent. Therefore, views taken in the morning generally show an overall decreased edema in the patients. For this reason, afternoon photographs depict a more accurate assessment of the patient's progression and level of disability.

Circumferential measurements using reference

points to bony landmarks may also be a practical and simple way to follow a patient's lymphedema.[3] In severe cases, the bony landmarks may be obscured. In postmastectomy patients, the ulnar styloid and the tip of the olecranon are the best landmarks. Differences in circumferential measurement between two opposing limbs are noted at multiple landmarks. These measurements are totaled for each limb and compared. If there is a difference of greater than 10 cm, lymphedema exists.[3]

A third type of measurement, *water displacement*, may also be used.[31] It is accomplished by measuring the volume of fluid displaced after the affected extremity is placed in a tank of water. This is the most accurate method of documenting changes in edema. Kissen and colleagues[24] found that a water displacement measurement of 15 cm above the epicondyle was the most sensitive index. A value of 200 ml included 96.4 percent of patients with subjective lymphedema. This would appear to be the best objective criterion with which to judge lymphedema and response to therapy. However, these techniques are time-consuming and are limited to facilities that have the equipment to perform the study.

Symptoms of chronic lymphedema are usually elicited by taking an accurate history of the patient. The patients complain of an overall increase or "fullness" of the extremity, with a corresponding "heaviness" and decreased functional ability of the extremity. In chronic cases after mastectomy, there may be considerable decreased range of motion and function caused by interstitial fibrosis along the tendon and ligamentous structures, resulting from the increased deposition of the protein-rich lymphatic fluids in the tissues.

TREATMENT OPTIONS

Prevention

The radical mastectomy of the past has been replaced with more conservative procedures that have the potential for decreasing the incidence of this complication. Decreasing rates of lymphedema have been reported with the development of the modified radical mastectomy, lumpectomy, and confining the axillary dissection to the Level 1 and 2 nodal groups. The new technique of lymphatic mapping and SLN biopsy[38] promises to provide full nodal staging information with a simple lymph node biopsy. Lymphedema should be nonexistent after this procedure.

Primary healing creates less fibrosis than does scarring by secondary intention. Attention to detail and good surgical techniques of sharp dissection, adequate hemostasis, suction drainage, and closure without tension should lessen the chance of postoperative lymphedema. Wound infection and sepsis should be avoided, suggesting a role for perioperative antibiotics.

Radiation therapy after lumpectomy should not include the axilla, unless the chance of recurrence in the axilla is overwhelming, such as in those women with 4 or more positive nodes or with extranodal extension. If axillas are included in the radiation field, the incidence of lymphedema may be as high as 52 percent.

Surgical Treatment

Surgical treatment should be instituted in those patients who have either failed previous medical modalities or have had long-term complications. The earliest form of surgical intervention dates back to Lis Franc in 1841 and mostly consisted of excision of the swollen tissue.

In the last century, a number of surgical treatment plans have been attempted on the basis of reconstruction of the lymphatic channels. The initial trials were attempted by Handley[17] in 1908 involving the burying of silk and other synthetic materials in the soft tissues to mimic lymphatic channels. High rates of infection, extrusion of the suture, and very limited transient improvement caused this technique to be abandoned. Emmanuel Kondoleon (1879–1939) devised the "Kondoleon operation" for elephantiasis of the lower extremity in which long, elliptical incisions on the lateral aspect of the extremity were made, starting from the iliac crest and ending above the external malleolus. Subcutaneous tissue and fascia were excised corresponding to the skin incision. Heavy continuous catgut was used to close the incision, and a tightly applied wrap was used over the extremity during the postoperative period.[43]

A modern approach involves the removal of the subcutaneous fat along with the placement of a dermal flap within the muscle to encourage superficial-to-deep lymphatic anastomoses. A retrospective review of the surgical techniques available was completed by Chilvers and Kinmonth.[8] This review showed that only 30 percent of patients undergoing a surgical repair had good sustained results. Not only was the overall success rate found to be low, but they also found that many of the successful patients regressed to their pretreatment girth measurements within 3 to 4 years after the original reduction surgery. They also noted a surgical morbidity of 23 percent in the patients, consisting of major skin necrosis resulting in extended hospitalization.[22]

In patients who have massive lymphedema with overlying skin breakdown, the Charles procedure may be implemented. In this technique, the skin and subcutaneous tissue are removed to the level of the underlying fascia, and the extremity is covered with split-thickness skin grafts. Although the cosmetic appearance of the limb is not favorable, this procedure can allow an incapacitated patient to return to normal activity. A moderate hospital stay is required, and wound healing problems can occur in the skin-grafted areas. The risk/benefit evaluation is favorable because these patients are homebound and or bedridden if left untreated.

In those patients who have shown no further improvement or failure after conservative management, a staged approach to excision of the skin and subcutaneous tissue may be attempted. The initial procedure addresses the inner aspect of the extremity. In the second stage, an excision is carried out on the lateral aspect. The technique can be performed with a low morbidity and short hospitalization time. To maintain the improvement that is obtained surgically, long-term compression therapy is necessary. At this point, more conservative medical therapies may again be attempted. However, neither surgery nor conservative modalities will produce long-term results without lifetime diligence in follow-up care.

There are new microsurgical techniques that are currently being attempted using either lymphatic venous shunts (LVS) or lymphatic venous anastomosis (LVA).[11, 23] These procedures allow a lymphatic egress of fluid into the venous circulation. These procedures are done in conjunction with multiple limb fasciotomies and can improve lymphatic drainage through muscles and the deep lymphatic circulation. Complications include thrombophlebitis and lymphangitis. These patients must be carefully evaluated before surgery. In those with diffuse interstitial fibrosis, the more traditional option of total superficial lymphangiectomy (Servelle's) or partial superficial lymphangiectomy (Kondoleon's) is recommended.

An alternative microsurgical technique described by Campisi and colleagues[5] involves performing interposition autologous lymphatic-venous-lymphatic anastomoses (LVL). This procedure represents an alternative to direct lymphatic-venous shunting and is based on the abundance of large-caliber venous tributaries. The lymphatic collectors can be placed at both ends of the venous graft sites. The LVL anastomoses consist of inserting suitably large and lengthy autologous venous grafts between lymphatic collectors above and below the site of obstruction to the lymphatic flow. Contraindications to this procedure include lymph node hyperplasia or aplasia and extensive obliteration of superficial and deep lymphatic collectors.

Medical Treatment

The initial treatment of chronic secondary lymphedema should be managed by nonsurgical measures. Adequate patient education with respect to activity levels and infection prophylaxis play an important role in the patient's long-term care. Physical therapy in conjunction with the application of compression garments or the use of sequential gradient compression–type pumps has been added recently to the overall care of the patient with chronic lymphedema. A multidiscipline and multimodal approach to the treatment of chronic lymphedema has been shown to reduce overall limb volume by at least half in 72 percent of patients treated.[4]

Infection prophylaxis is an important component in the care of patients with chronic extremity lymphedema who are prone to repeated infections because the accumulation of protein-rich fluid creates a rich culture medium for bacterial growth. The more

lymphedematous the tissues, the more susceptible they are to infections. Simple injuries may lead to generalized infections, lymphangitis, and cellulitis, which can cause further lymphatic destruction and blockage of remaining channels.[1] The need for extensive patient education in skin care such as the immediate care of any open wound and proper nail care is a simple but important necessity in lymphedema treatment. There is ample evidence in the literature to suggest that the more severe the lymphedema, the greater the risk of cellulitis and extremity infection. Each subsequent episode of infection increases the risk of bacteremia and systemic toxicity to the patient and worsens the lymphedematous condition in the arm.

Extremity elevation (periodic elevation, of the affected extremity) is the simplest form of self-care that a patient can do to reduce chronic lymphedema. Instruction should be given as to proper height and elevation of the affected extremity for the most satisfactory results. Night-time elevation of the extremity has been shown to have the most dramatic effect.

Although not all forms of exercise are beneficial to patients with extremity edema, those that help the affected extremity to increase circulation are recommended. Some examples include swimming, biking, and isometric exercises. Activities that involve heavy lifting or repetitive motion, such as aerobics and jogging, should be avoided because they have been shown to cause pooling of the lymph fluid.

Medical management should involve a multidisciplinary approach in the long-term care of the patient. This includes patient education, instruction in home physical therapy exercises, maintaining normal range of motion and strength in the affected extremity, and preservation of existing motion. The overall treatment plan may include education and instruction in elevation of the affected extremity, skin care precautions, massage techniques, pumping exercises, and appropriate active-assistive and active and/or resistive exercises. The physical therapist may be asked to train the patient in the fitting and use of compression garments and in the monitoring during the use of gradient sequential compression–type pumps. Therapy used in conjunction with garments and pumps as well as patient education, skin maintenance, and eradication of bacterial and fungal skin infections can reduce extremity girth and lymphatic volume (Table 51–1).

Physiologically, because of communication of the lymphatic vessels between various body regions, *complex physical therapy (CPT)* can be used to help shunt fluid out of the compromised extremity. The CPT can be performed either in a hospital setting or through home-based physical therapy in treating the chronic lymphedema patient. Physical therapy is offered in two phases. Phase I lasts for a period of 4 weeks and can be divided into four segments. The first is skin care, which improves and maintains the normal skin integrity while decreasing the risks of infection. The second segment involves *manual lymphatic drainage*. This is a daily therapy designed to remove ex-

TABLE 51–1.   LYMPHEDEMA CHECKLIST GUIDELINES

Do's
Do keep skin clean.
Do moisturize skin.
Do elevate limb while sleeping and traveling.
Do wash with hypoallergenic soaps and cleaners.
Do use electric not straight razors to remove hair.
Do use mild detergents for clothes.
Do keep temperature in house constant.
Do eat a balanced nutritional diet.
Do treat infections early and thoroughly with antibiotics
    prescribed by your doctor.
Do exercise: walk, swim, prescribed isometrics.
Do wear prescribed garments and or bandages.
Do avoid cuts, burns, and insect bites.
Do avoid sunburn—use sunblock.
Do wear loose-fitting clothing.
Don't's
NO PROCEDURES SHOULD BE PERFORMED ON THE
    AFFECTED EXTREMITY!
No blood drawing.
No injections.
No intravenous dye x-rays.
No acupuncture.
No liposuction.
No blood pressure testing.
No heavy, traumatic or repetitive exercises.
No picking up heavy objects.

cess lymphatic fluid and open collateral lymphatics, allowing the nonsurgical or unaffected regions to aid the compromised regions in draining excess lymphatic fluid. The third segment deals with compression bandaging to maintain and increase compartment pressure and prevent retrograde flow of lymphatic fluid. The fourth segment involves specialized physical therapy exercises followed by lymphatic massage. Massage therapy is based on first emptying the lymphatics of the trunk. The Foldi technique[4, 32] of massage is then applied to areas adjacent to the compromised extremity. The therapist can then concentrate on the central portions of the limb, gradually working toward the distal portion of the extremity. This forces the excess lymphatic fluids into watershed regions of the body, which allows the fluid access to the nonaffected lymphatic collateral circulation.

Phase II consists of fitting the patient with specially measured compression garments. The use of elastic sleeve therapy alone has been shown to decrease limb girth by 15 percent.[3] Maintenance of the overall benefits from therapy depends largely on whether the patients continue their exercises and have intermittent CPT. Studies from Australia have shown that these techniques reduce extremity size by 65 percent.[54] However, they require skilled personnel and a strong daily commitment to complete.

Few drugs are being studied for treatment of chronic lymphedema.[36] Benzopyrones can decrease the overall volume of high-protein-concentrate edema by stimulating proteolysis.[7] They directly increase the number of macrophages at the site of high-protein lymphedema, which increases the normal proteolysis by the cells.[6] By increasing proteolysis and the number of macrophages, excess plasma protein is removed and overall edema decreases. Venalot, a benzopyrene, is a drug that breaks down large protein molecules, facilitating the absorption of the proteins into the vascular system at the level of the capillaries. This drug is currently not available in the United States.

Diuretics are of minimal aid in the treatment of chronic lymphedema resulting from oncological surgery or metastatic spread of the disease. This type of therapy should be reserved for early treatment of primary lymphedema patients, although its effects are transient at best.

Compression pumps are rapidly becoming a major factor in medical management of the patient with chronic lymphedema.[2, 30, 37, 55, 56] As previously stated, massage can be a very effective therapy in the long-term treatment of the chronic, lymphedematous extremity. However, the lack of experienced personnel limits the availability of this treatment. Researchers have recently focused attention on recreating the beneficial effects of massage by mechanical or compression means, leading to the development of compression devices.[35, 39] These compression machines are based on two basic principles. The first is the single-cell compartment system providing absolute pressure. The intermittent, single-chamber, nonsegmental compression pumps are the oldest devices available. They are characterized by equal pressure throughout the extremity. With these devices, no direction is offered for the fluid to be transported, which causes some backflow of the lymphatic fluid. This retrograde flow may cause an overall increase in lymphatic fluid to the tissues in the distal extremity. The second-generation devices are multicell systems based on sequential compression of the extremity. These sequential compression machines use compressed air forced into an arm or leg sleeve fitted over the affected extremity. The multicell systems can be subdivided into standard sequential systems and gradient sequential systems. The standard sequential compression system without calibrated gradient pressure is a multichamber pump. It delivers the compression at the same pressure in each garment section from distal to proximal. However, this does not imitate the normal muscular and vascular activities of an extremity. Because of muscle and tissue mass within the extremities and the varying diameters of the circulatory vessels, the underlying venous pressures vary within each extremity compartment. On the other hand, peristaltic sequential gradient compression systems more closely mimic normal extremity pressure changes. The pressures delivered by the gradient sequential systems average to an approximate 10 mm Hg difference between each chamber. The higher pressures are delivered to the distal chamber, with each chamber having around 10 mm Hg less pressure than the one preceding it (Fig. 51–1).[47]

For increased efficiency, the delivery of lymphedema therapy must be physiologically compatible with the lymph system and strong enough to imitate

MULTICOM 500- FIVE CHAMBER PERISTALTIC GRADIENT SEQUENTIAL PRESSURES

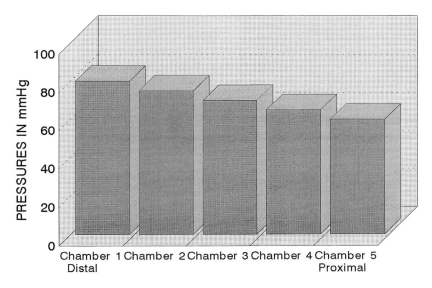

Figure 51–1 *Graph of pressures delivered by a gradient sequential compression pump more closely mimics the physiology of the lymph system.*

Maximum pressures per chamber during peristaltic cycle with adjustment at 80 mmHg

the rhythmic motion of the skeletal muscles to transfer the excess lymphatic fluid in a distal-to-proximal fashion. Placing an extremity in the horizontal or flat position decreases the pressure within the veins, because the fluids do not have to travel against gravity. Therefore, with a patient in a reclined position, a peristaltic sequential gradient system resembles what occurs in an unencumbered extremity. Good results occur in those patients who are lying down for treatment of the legs or placing the upper extremities on elevated pillows. The best results are seen in patients who use a pump on an intermittent daily basis. For this type of therapy to be effective, the treatment should be maintained for a minimum of 1 hour each session. Lower pressures for longer periods of time are more effective than higher pressures for shorter periods of time. Patients should be reminded to wear their fitted compression garments and to elevate the extremity whenever possible. The greatest advantage of this therapy is that it may be self-administered by the patient in the comfort of a home setting (Fig. 51–2).

Contraindications to the use of gradient sequential compression devices include the following:

1. Massive edema of the extremity secondary to congestive heart failure.
2. Concurrent neurological symptoms.
3. Severe arteriosclerosis.
4. Deformity of the extremity.
5. Skin changes (i.e., dermatitis, gangrene, recent skin grafts, cellulitis, deep venous thrombosis).

LYMPHANGIOSARCOMA

One of the rare complications of chronic extremity lymphedema is the development of lymphangiosar-

coma. This tumor is a rare form of soft tissue neoplasms. Lownestein first commented on this condition in 1906[27] with respect to post-traumatic chronic lymphedema of the upper extremity. Stewart and Treves were the first to associate the condition with post-mastectomy edema in 1948.[46, 50] The incidence ranges from 0.07 to 0.45 percent.[21]

Histologically, the tumor consists of vascular cavities lined with spindle-shaped endothelial cells with large nuclei and a prominent nucleoli.

The median time between mastectomy and development of this tumor is 10 years.[53] The primary le-

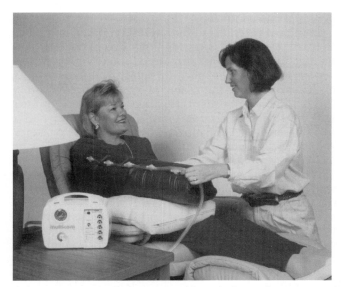

Figure 51–2 *Home therapy is possible with the gradient sequential compression devices. Arm should be treated in the elevated position for 1 hour on a daily basis.*

sion tends to form multiple satellites that may spread further or enlarge and ulcerate. Involvement of the underlying muscle is a late finding and is usually rare. Metastasis usually occurs early in the disease and is generally to the lungs.[20] Development can be divided into three phases[29]: prolonged lymphedema, angiomatosis, and angiosarcoma. Treatment includes local excision, wide excision, amputation, radiation therapy, chemotherapy, and combination therapy. Median survival of patients is 19 months after diagnosis.[53] The disease has a predictable course with rapid progression and a fatal outcome.

SUMMARY

Postmastectomy patients and their caregivers are often faced with the problematic management of upper-extremity chronic lymphedema. Until recent years, this condition was neglected because of poor understanding of the cause and abnormal physiology behind the condition. Consequently, most patients were completely untreated or undertreated. This resulted in a lifelong struggle for many patients with a condition that eventually led to crippling disability. In the past patients were told that this condition was something that they had to live with.

An accurate knowledge of the physiology and pathophysiology of lymphedema is necessary to understand the rationale of treatment techniques available. An accurate assessment of the degree of impairment should be established before initiating either short-term or long-term care. Although surgical intervention and treatment have been tried in the past, the standard of care now is a conservative medical management.[25, 33] The basis behind conservative therapy is to reduce existing edema while controlling formation of new edema. Observation techniques, including photography, circumferential measurement, and water displacement, aid in the long-term monitoring of the condition.

Standard methods of managing lymphedema, such as rest, elevation, wearing heavy constrictive garments, diuretics, and dietary changes, may fail to arrest the progress of this debilitating disease. A multidisciplinary approach is needed to maximize the available treatment regimes. Surgeons, nurses, and physical and occupational therapists play active roles in the care of chronic lymphedema patients. Appropriate patient education and instruction in self-care are paramount in the long-term care of the patient, because repeated infections would only worsen the lymphedema. Patient education should include instruction in exercise, what activities to avoid, extremity elevation, and infection prophylaxis.[34] With the recent advancements in external compression therapies that use peristaltic sequential gradient compression devices, patients have an effective, available treatment option that is safe, comfortable, and in many instances the least costly for long-term care. It may be administered on an intermittent basis, in the comfort of a home setting and on an as-

needed basis throughout the course of the illness. A realistic approach to the long-term care of this condition coupled with therapeutic and emotional support can ensure a productive and less debilitating lifestyle to the patient with chronic extremity lymphedema.

References

1. Aitken D, Minton JP: Complications associated with mastectomy. Surg Clin North Am 63:1331–1352, 1983.
2. Bastien MR, Goldstein BG, Lesher JL, et al: Treatment of lymphedema with a multicompartmental pneumatic compression device. J Am Acad Dermatol 20:853–854, 1989.
3. Bertelli G, Venturini M, Forno G, Macchiavello F, Dini D: An analysis of prognostic factors in response to conservative treatment of postmastectomy lymphedema. Surg Gynecol Obstet 175:455–460, 1992.
4. Bunce I, Mirolo B, Hennessy J, Ward L, Jones L: Post-mastectomy lymphoedema treatment and measurement. Med J Aust 161:125–128, 1994.
5. Campisi C, Boccardo F, Tacchella M: Reconstructive microsurgery of lymph vessels: The personal method of lymphatic-venous-lymphatic (LVL) interpositioned grafted shunt. Microsurgery 16:161–166, 1995.
6. Casley-Smith J: Modern treatment of lymphoedema: II. The benzopyrones. Australas J Dermatol 33:69–74, 1992.
7. Casley-Smith J, Morgan R, Piller N: Treatment of lymphedema of the arms and legs with 5,6-benzo-[alpha]-pyrone. N Engl J Med 329:1158–1163, 1993.
8. Chilvers AS, Kinmonth JD: Operations for lymphedema for the lower limbs. J Cardiovasc Surg 16:115–119, 1975.
9. Copeland EM: Carcinoma of the breast. Fifth Annual General Surgery Forum, Telluride, CO. Abstract.
10. Cruikshank WC: The Anatomy of the Absorbing Vessels of the Human Body. London, G. Nicol, 1786.
11. Filippetti M, Santoro E, Graziano F, Petric M, Rinaldi G: Modern therapeutic approaches to postmastectomy brachial lymphedema. Microsurgery 15:604–610, 1994.
12. Fitts WT, Keunelian, JG, Ravdin IS, Schor S: Swelling of the arm after radical mastectomy. Surgery 35:460, 1954.
13. Foster RS: General anatomy of the lymphatic system. Surg Clin North Am 5:1–13, 1996.
14. Golematis BC, Delikaris PG, Balarutsos C, Karamanakos PP: Lymphedema of the upper limb after surgery for breast cancer. Am J Surg 129:286–288, 1975.
15. Haagensen CD, Feind CR, Herter FP, et al: The Lymphatic in Cancer. Philadelphia, WB Saunders, 1972.
16. Halsted W: The swelling of the arm after operations for cancer of the breast—elephantiasis chirurgica—its cause and prevention. Bull John Hopkins Hosp 32:309–313, 1921.
17. Handley WS: Lymphangioplasty: A new method for the relief of the brawn arm of breast cancer and for similar conditions of lymphatic edema—preliminary note. Lancet 1:1783, 1908.
18. Hoe A, Iven D, Royle G, Taylor I: Incidence of arm swelling following axillary clearance for breast cancer. Br J Surg 79:261–262, 1992.
19. Hughes J, Patel A: Swelling of the arm following mastectomy. Br J Surg 53:4–14, 1966.
20. Janse A, Coevorden F, Peterse H, Keus R, Van Dongen J: Lymphedema induced lymphangiosarcoma. Eur J Surg Oncol 21:155–158, 1995.
21. Kaufmann T, Chu F, Kaufman R: Post-mastectomy lymphangiosarcoma (Stewart-Treves syndrome): Report of two long-term survivals. Br J Radiol 64:857–860, 1991.
22. Kinmonth JB, Patrick JH, Chilvers AS: Comments on operations for lower limb lymphedema. Lymphology 8:56–59, 1975.
23. Kinmonth J, Harper R, Taylor G: Lymphangiography: A technique for its clinical use in the lower limb. Br Med J 1:940–942, 1955.
24. Kissin M, Querci Della Rovere G, Easton D, Westbury G: Risk of lymphedema following the treatment of breast cancer. Br J Surg 73:580–584, 1986.
25. Lerner R, Requena R: Upper extremity lymphedema second-

ary to mammary cancer treatment. Am J Clin Oncol 481–487, 1986.

26. Loeb AW, Harkins HN: Postmastectomy swelling of the arm. West J Surg 57:550–557, 1949.

27. Lowenstein S: Der Aetiologische Zusammengang zwischen akutem und malignem Trauma und Sarko. Beitr Klin Chir 48:708–724, 1906.

28. Matas R: Surgical treatment of elephantiasis and elephantoid states dependent upon chronic obstruction of lymphatic and venous channels. Am J Trop Dis 1:60–85, 1913.

29. McConnell E, Haslam P: Angiosarcoma in postmastectomy lymphedema: A report of five cases and review of the literature. Br J Surg 46:322–332, 1959.

30. McLeod A, Brooks D, Hale J, et al: A clinical report on the use of three external pneumatic compression devices in the management of lymphedema in a pediatric population. Physiother Can 43:28–31, 1991.

31. Miller TA, Das SK: Classification and treatment of lymphedema. In Rutherford R (ed): Vascular Surgery, 4th ed. Philadelphia, WB Saunders, pp 232–240.

32. Mirolo B: Lymphoedema Treatment Programme. 2nd ed. Brisbane, Wesley Clinic for Haematology and Oncology, 1991.

33. Nava V, Lawrence W: Liposuction in a lymphedematous arm. Ann Plast Surg 21:366–368, 1988.

34. O'Donnell TF: The management of primary lymphedema. In Ernst CB, Stanley CJ (eds): Current Therapy in Vascular Surgery. 2nd ed. Philadelphia, BC Decker, 1991, pp 1022–1029.

35. Pappas CJ, O'Donnell TF: Long-term results of compression treatment for lymphedema. J Vasc Surg 16:555–562, 1992.

36. Piller NB: Conservative treatment of acute and chronic lymphedema with benzopyrones. Lymphology 9:132, 1976.

37. Raines JK, O'Donnell TF, Kalisher L, et al: Selection of patients with lymphedema for compression therapy. Am J Surg 133:430–437, 1977.

38. Reintgen DS, Cruse CW, Wells K, et al: The orderly progression of melanoma nodal metastases. Ann Surg 220:759–767, 1991.

39. Richmond DM, O'Donnell TF, Zelikovski A: Sequential pneumatic compression for lymphedema: A controlled trial. Arch Surg 120:1116–1120, 1985.

40. Sauter E, Eisenberg B, Hoffman J, Ottery F, Boraas M, Goldstein L, Solin L: Postmastectomy morbidity after combination preoperative irradiation and chemotherapy for locally advanced breast cancer. World J Surg 17:237–242, 1993.

41. Segerstrom K, Bjerle P, Graffman S, Nystrom A: Factors that influence the incidence of brachial oedema after treatment of breast cancer: Scand J Plast Reconstr Hand Surg 26:223–227, 1992.

42. Servelle M: Surgical treatment of lymphedema: A report on 652 cases. Surgery 101:485–495, 1987.

43. Skandalakis JE: I wish I had been there: Highlights in the history of the lymphatics. Am Surg 61:799–802, 1995.

44. Smith TJ, Balch CM, Bartolucci AA, Urist MM, Karakousis CP, Ross MI: Current results of the intergroup surgical trial in intermediate thickness melanoma. Houston, Concurrent Symposium, M D Anderson, 1995. Abstract.

45. Smith TJ, Balch C, Bartolucci A, Karakousis C, Ross M, Urist M, Tampa, FL: Risks and complications of elective inguinal node dissection. SSO, 1995. Abstract.

46. Stewart F, Treves N: Lymphangiosarcoma in postmastectomy lymphedema: A report of six cases on elephantiasis chirurgica. Cancer 1:64–81, 1948.

47. Stillwell GK: Physiatric management of postmastectomy lymphedema. Med Clin North Am 46:1051–1063, 1962.

48. Svensson W, Mortimer P, Tohno E, Cosgrove D: Colour Doppler demonstrates venous flow abnormalities in breast cancer patients with chronic arm swelling. Eur J Cancer 30A:657–660, 1994.

49. Svensson W, Mortimer P, Tohno E, Cosgrove D: Increased arterial inflow demonstrated by Doppler ultrasound in arm swelling following breast cancer treatment. Eur J Cancer 30A:661–664, 1994.

50. Tomita K, Yokogawa A, Oda Y, Terhata S: Lymphangiosarcoma in post-mastectomy Stewart-Treves syndrome. J Surg Oncol 38:275–228, 1988.

51. Vasudevan SV, Melvin JL: Upper extremity edema control: Rationale of the techniques. Am J Occup Ther 33:520–523, 1979.

52. Virchow R: Die Krankhaften Geshwulste. 3rd lesson, Nov 22, 1806. Berlin, A Hirschwald, 1963.

53. Woodward A, Ivins J, Soule E: Lymphangiosarcoma arising in chronic lymphedematous extremities. Cancer 30:562–572, 1972.

54. Zeissler RH, Rose GB, Nelson PA: Postmastectomy lymphedema: Late results of treatment in 385 patients. Arch Phys Med Rehabil 53:159–166, 1972.

55. Zelikovski A, Melamed I, Kott M, et al: The "Lympha-Press": A new pneumatic device for the treatment of lymphedema—clinical trials and results. Folia Angiol 28:165–169, 1980.

56. Zelikovski A, Manoach M, Giler S, et al: Lympha Press, a new pneumatic device for the treatment of lymphedema of the limbs. Lymphology 13:68–73, 1980.

CURRENT CONCEPTS AND MANAGEMENT OF EARLY BREAST CARCINOMA (Tis, Tmic, T1)

CHAPTER 52

CURRENT CONCEPTS ON THE BIOLOGY AND MANAGEMENT OF *IN SITU* (Tis, STAGE 0) BREAST CARCINOMA

Eric R. Frykberg, M.D. / Kirby I. Bland, M.D.

Ever since the first histological investigations of cancer were undertaken in the nineteenth century, it has been accepted that carcinoma of the breast evolves from normal epithelial cells through several progressive stages.* This transition theory has been supported by several studies that demonstrate that the benign proliferative changes of hyperplasia and cellular atypia ultimately give rise to invasive carcinoma.† As a corollary to this concept, it was logical to postulate that the detection and treatment of breast carcinoma in its earliest stages of development, before it could spread, should provide the best chance of cure or favorable outcome.[64, 67, 145] As long ago as the eighteenth century, the British surgeon Henry Fearon asserted, regarding breast tumors, that "the early period of the complaint is beyond all doubt the most favorable period for extirpating it."[84] Several studies of mammographic screening over the past few decades have confirmed this belief by clearly documenting the diagnosis of malignancy in its earliest phases results in as much as a 46% reduction in mortality from breast carcinoma.‡

These efforts led to the increasingly frequent diagnosis of borderline forms of breast carcinoma in which the epithelial cells have undergone malignant transformation yet remain confined within their natural basement membrane boundaries. Most authorities agree that all invasive breast carcinomas pass through this intraepithelial phase in the course of their development from normal tissue, but it is not clear that all such noninvasive carcinomas evolve into invasive lesions nor how long this stage lasts.[122, 131–133, 287] In 1932, Broders[52] labeled this stage *in situ* carcinoma, the term that is most commonly applied to what may be considered the earliest and most favorable form of breast malignancy.

The actual point at which benign tissue becomes malignant and those criteria that most accurately define malignancy have long been debated. It is understandable that increasing attention has been focused on the *in situ* phase of breast disease, in view of the opportunity it may provide to alter the natural history of, and perhaps prevent, invasive carcinoma.[124, 127, 156, 290, 306] On the other hand, there may be reason to question the clinical implications of carcinoma *in situ* (CIS) of the breast, whether it is a true malignancy, whether it merits our extensive and costly efforts to detect, whether treatment actually affects ultimate outcome, and what treatment, if any, is most appropriate.[118, 170, 175, 177, 296, 395] Both the complexity and the promise of this unique form of breast carcinoma warrant an analysis of its history, epidemiology, pathology, and biology in order to understand its appropriate diagnosis and treatment.

HISTORICAL OVERVIEW

Studies of the origin of breast carcinoma published in the late nineteenth century demonstrated that this malignancy arises from epithelial cells.[278, 357] Cornil[72, 73] and Waldeyer[368, 369] both documented the histological progression of breast epithelium into invasive carcinoma. Several of their drawings clearly show malignant cells still confined within the basement membranes of breast lobules and the morphological similarity of these cells to those that have invaded into the surrounding stroma in cases of fully developed invasive carcinoma.[287] An 1898 textbook by Shield[321] contains a histological drawing of intraepithelial carcinoma arising within a breast lobule, which he described as "the earliest change usually observable by the microscope in carcinoma of the mamma." James Ewing published typical illustrations of noninvasive breast carcinoma arising from both lobules and major lactiferous ducts in every edition of his textbook, referring to these lesions as precancerous to suggest that they represent one stage in the evolution of invasive carcinoma. Ewing asserted that these lesions are slow to involve the lymph nodes, and eventually break through the base-

---

*See references 64, 72, 212, 213, 278, 287, 368, and 369.
†See references 23, 82, 87, 108, 148, 253, and 254.
‡See references 100, 141, 194, 199, 210, 316, 319, 353, 365, and 379.

ment membrane to infiltrate surrounding tissues.[91, 92] Like some of his contemporaries,[145] he did not believe these lesions to be malignant.

MacCarty was probably the first to apply the term "preinvasive" to this phase of breast carcinoma to indicate a dynamic process of evolution, and published illustrations of the transition of noninvasive lesions into invasive carcinoma.[212, 213] As early as 1911, he explained the nature of this concept by stating[211]:

> Is it necessary to wait for the penetration of the basement membrane before making a diagnosis of carcinoma? . . . If the pathologist considers the penetration of the basement membrane the essential characteristic of carcinoma, then it must be admitted that the cells in adenoma are often as irregular as in carcinoma.

The difficulty of distinguishing this preinvasive stage from benign hyperplasia was described by Stout in 1932.[350] The pathologist Dawson also understood the concept of preinvasive carcinoma and believed that most breast malignancies arise from the terminal duct–lobular apparatus.[80] In 1931, Cheatle and Cutler[66] illustrated a classic example of an intraepithelial carcinoma of the breast lobules surrounded by cytologically identical invasive lobular carcinoma. In fact, the British surgeon John Birkett is credited with the first use of the term lobular carcinoma in 1850 to describe the earliest stage of breast malignancy.[40, 286]

The introduction of the term carcinoma *in situ* by Broders represented a recognition of this lesion as an entity distinct from its benign precursors and invasive counterparts, although another 50 years would pass before it became widely studied and accepted. His definition still holds true today[52]:

> Carcinoma in situ is a condition in which malignant epithelial cells and their progeny are found in or near positions occupied by their ancestors before the ancestors underwent malignant transformation . . . At least they have not migrated beyond the juncture of the epithelium and connective tissue of the so-called basement membrane.

Broders also appreciated the unique opportunity offered by this lesion in the possibility of altering its natural history and potentially preventing the development of invasive carcinoma:

> If carcinoma in situ appears alone, its recognition is necessary, for failure to recognize it may constitute an error of omission fraught with grave danger to the patient; if it goes unrecognized, carcinoma is allowed to masquerade as a benign or not more than a precarcinomatous process, with the possibility of its becoming too far advanced to be amenable to treatment.

Foote and Stewart published the landmark histologic and biologic description of the entity alluded to by all the aforementioned investigators, calling it lobular carcinoma *in situ* (LCIS). This term is still the most widely applied label.* This disease was believed to

arise from the terminal duct–lobular apparatus of the breast. Although these authors viewed LCIS as a "rare form of mammary carcinoma", agreeing with Broders, Cheatle and Cutler, and MacCarty that it is malignant, it has since become evident that it occurs more frequently than was originally suspected.[124, 125, 129, 150, 316] Muir also published a study of this lesion in that same year,[239] calling it intra-acinous carcinoma. However, the term LCIS has persisted as the standard label, in view of the assertion of Dawson[80] that the acinus is a functional rather than an anatomical unit of the breast and should refer only to the secretory lobules of pregnancy.[287]

Warren of Boston was perhaps the first to describe the noninvasive stage of ductal carcinoma of the breast, the most common histological type of breast malignancy believed to arise from the major lactiferous ducts. He called this lesion abnormal involution, noting that[377]:

> The transition stage is observed when the epithelium no longer confines itself to the cyst cavity, but breaks through the limiting membrane and infiltrates the adjacent structures.

Cheatle and Cutler published several photomicrographs from whole organ sections early in the twentieth century, which depict the evolution of breast carcinoma from benign tissue, many of which can be recognized today as noninvasive, or ductal carcinoma *in situ* (DCIS).[64–66] In 1935, Muir and Aitkenhead probably first applied the term intraduct carcinoma to this entity, noting that the proliferating ductal epithelial cells "have acquired the essential characters of malignant neoplasia, and they acquire this character before they transgress the normal boundaries."[240]

Joseph Colt Bloodgood (see Chapter 39) was a surgeon at Johns Hopkins Hospital in the early twentieth century who developed much of our current knowledge of the clinical behavior and pathological characteristics of this early stage of ductal carcinoma of the breast, which he termed borderline breast tumors.[44] He found these tumors to be very favorable in their prognosis, and called them "comedocarcinoma" on the basis of a gross appearance of extruding grayish-white cylinders from their surface.[45] He distinguished comedocarcinoma associated with fully developed breast cancer from pure comedotumor, or comedoadenoma, and his photomicrographs of this latter lesion are now recognized as typical DCIS. Bloodgood believed this to be a benign but precancerous tumor and did not emphasize the distinction between invasive and noninvasive forms, indicating the imprecision of the term comedocarcinoma as a diagnostic label.[115, 124, 128] He believed that comedoadenomas could be treated by a procedure that is less invasive than mastectomy and also mentioned the possibility of treatment by radiation, modalities that took another 50 years to apply successfully to this lesion.

Lewis and Geschickter[200] confirmed Bloodgood's impression of the favorable prognosis of comedocarci-

---

*See references 116, 117, 129, 140, 223, 283, 287, and 290.

noma, but considered it as a fully malignant tumor. Although they emphasized the importance of distinguishing histologic invasion, as did Muir,[239] their results clearly indicate that both invasive and noninvasive disease was included in this study.[124, 287] Radical mastectomy was recommended as the appropriate treatment.

Foote and Stewart were the first to establish the noninvasive form of ductal carcinoma of the breast as a distinct pathologic entity, [117] just as they had for LCIS.[116] In 1950, Stewart appears to have first applied the term DCIS to this lesion,[348] as did Gillis and colleagues in 1960,[137] who believed this to be a true malignancy requiring treatment by radical mastectomy. Although Haagensen included lesions with as much as 50 percent of their mass involved with invasive disease in his definition of DCIS,[153] and several authors have continued to include microinvasive disease in studies of DCIS,* McDivitt and associates clearly established in 1968 that DCIS is the purely noninvasive form of ductal breast carcinoma.[223, 331]

The concept of minimal breast cancer developed in the late 1960s from studies of whole organ sectioning of the breast, which affirmed the tenets of the transition theory.[122, 131–133, 159, 265, 373] Minimal breast cancer included LCIS, DCIS, and minimally invasive breast carcinoma less than 0.5 cm in size. However, it became evident that these are all very different biological entities that demand very different management approaches.[105, 391, 398] The evolution of breast carcinoma from proliferative epithelium appears to be a

---

*See references 104, 262, 298, 299, 322, 327, 331, and 392.

complex process involving several reversible stages that are not necessarily inevitable or obligate precursors to invasive malignancy (Fig. 52–1).[82, 87, 144, 177, 344] Our knowledge of CIS is still relatively young, with many outstanding issues still to be resolved by further investigation.

EPIDEMIOLOGY

Until the 1980s, physical examination was the predominant means of detecting breast abnormalities, and CIS was considered as only a clinical oddity. This disease comprised only 1.4 percent of all breast biopsies and only approximately 5 percent of all breast malignancies before 1980, and was treated routinely by mastectomy.[16, 22, 43, 288, 298, 386] As CIS became more widely recognized and accepted by pathologists over the past 50 years, and as mammography has led to earlier detection of breast carcinoma, the diagnosis of this disease has dramatically increased.[196, 296, 306, 316, 333, 334] In earlier years, CIS was under diagnosed in as many as 50% of cases.[36, 115, 177, 298, 337]

Data from the National Cancer Institute document a fivefold increase in the overall incidence of CIS in the United States between 1973 and 1987, with the major portion of this increase occurring in women over 50 years of age (Fig. 52–2).[296] The average age-adjusted incidence of CIS in the United States rose from 3 per 100,000 in 1973 to 11 per 100,000 in 1987, a fourfold greater rate of increase than for any other form of breast malignancy.[70] There was a 2.5-fold increase in the total number of cases of CIS reported

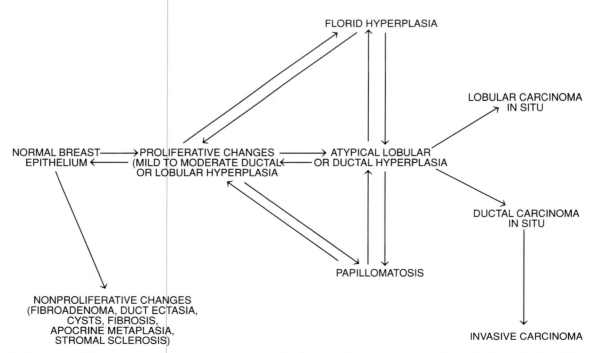

Figure 52–1   *Depiction of the current consensus as to the path of development of breast carcinoma. (From Frykberg ER, Bland KI: In situ breast carcinoma. Adv Surg 26:29–72, 1993.)*

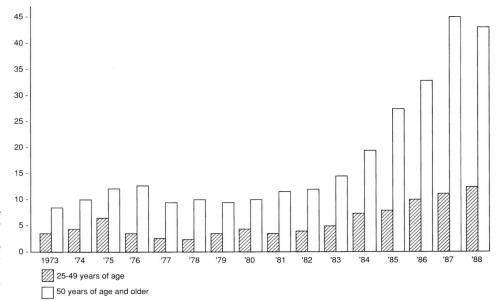

Figure 52–2   *The increased frequency of diagnosis of carcinoma in situ, expressed as number of cases per 100,000 U.S. women, stratified according to year and age group, from data from the National Cancer Institute. (From Frykberg ER, Bland KI: In situ breast carcinoma. Adv Surg 26:29–72, 1993.)*

in the state of Connecticut from 1984 to 1988, whereas the number of invasive breast cancers rose by only 30%.[374] Although CIS occurs most commonly in young white women, the greatest increase in this diagnosis in Detroit between 1973 and 1988 occurred in elderly black women.[333, 334]

Mammographic screening, which became widely established in the United States during this same time period, was largely responsible for this increased frequency of diagnosis.[115, 194, 196, 319, 353] Initially, mammography was applied only to the diagnosis of breasts with abnormal physical findings in the 1960s and 1970s, which resulted in a yield of CIS of 6 percent to 12 percent of all breast malignancies.* This was clearly an improvement over the yields from physical examination alone. The yield of CIS was further improved in the 1980s with routine mammographic screening of asymptomatic women, during which time most breast lesions that were biopsied were nonpalpable.[141, 194, 210, 288, 379] The ten-year results of the Breast Cancer Detection Demonstration Project documented that 16 percent of all breast malignancies detected by mammography were CIS.[316]

The combined results of 21 clinical series, all published since 1989, which report a total of 13,125 biopsies of nonpalpable mammographically detected breast lesions document a 39 percent overall incidence of CIS among all breast malignancies (range 19 to 67 percent) and a 7.5 percent overall incidence of CIS among all breast biopsies (Table 52–1). Some earlier series have shown CIS to comprise as much as 78 percent of all nonpalpable breast malignancies.[294] Mammography has also led to a predominance of DCIS among all *in situ* lesions, averaging 5:1 and ranging up to 17:1, over LCIS.[5, 124, 127, 288, 297, 351] The overall frequency of CIS has been estimated as up to

nine cases per 100,000 woman-years, and the cumulative lifetime risk of developing CIS is 0.53 percent.[42, 43, 279] The average age of women with this disease is approximately ten years younger than that of women with invasive breast carcinoma. One study[351] found that 69 percent of all cases occurred in premenopausal women. This is consistent with the transition theory tenet that CIS is a preinvasive stage of breast malignancy.*

Lobular Carcinoma *In Situ*

This form of noninvasive breast carcinoma occurs almost exclusively in females, although a small number of anecdotal cases occur in males, most commonly those exposed to estrogen or with genetic abnormalities.[226] The absence of lobular breast elements in males, from which LCIS is believed to arise, explains this.[381] Women with this disease average 44 to 47 years of age, which is ten to 15 years younger than those who typically develop invasive breast carcinoma. The coexistence LCIS with invasive disease occurs at an intermediate average age of 54 years.[24, 61, 77, 78, 287, 351]

As many as 90 percent of cases of LCIS occur in premenopausal women, compared with only 30 percent of cases of invasive breast carcinoma.† Further evidence that hormonal influence is an important factor in LCIS is that its cells manifest a greater incidence of estrogen receptor activity than do those of invasive ductal carcinoma.[14, 18, 55, 79, 291]

The true incidence of LCIS in the general population cannot be reliably determined, because it has no clinical or radiographic manifestations. This lesion is always a random and incidental microscopic finding. Its incidence directly correlates with the frequency

---

*See references 5, 15, 42, 43, 100, 123, 279, and 319.

*See references 43, 60, 122, 129, 167, 194, and 380.
†See references 93, 155, 156, 193, 286, 287, 290, 292, and 351.

TABLE 52–1. RESULTS OF BIOPSY OF MAMMOGRAPHICALLY DETECTED NONPALPABLE BREAST LESIONS SINCE 1989

Author	Reference Number	Number of Biopsies	Number Malignant (%)	Number of *In Situ* Cancers		
				Lobular	Ductal	Total (%)*
Petrovich et al	266	106	13 (12.3)	3	2	5 (38.5)
Rusnak et al	300	200	48 (24)	2	8	10 (21)
Silverstein et al	325	1162	238 (20.5)	—	—	131 (55)
Franceschi et al	121	825	203 (24.6)	0	54	54 (26.6)
Griffen and Welling	146	266	38 (14.3)	1	15	16 (42)
Meyer et al	224	1261	275 (19)	38	85	123 (52)
Papatestas et al	259	475	149 (31.4)	8	52	60 (40)
Bauer et al	34	2077	284 (13.7)	15	67	82 (29)
Hasselgren et al	160	350	66 (19)	0	23	23 (35)
McCreery et al	221	358	95 (26.5)	0	20	20 (21)
Roses et al	297	183	97 (53)	2	35	37 (37)
Wilhelm et al	383, 384	1464	264 (18)	—	—	178 (67)
Goedde et al	141	330	38 (11.5)	8	12	20 (53)
Miller et al	229	530	90 (17)	5	27	32 (35.6)
Perdue et al	264	536	96 (18)	14	35	49 (50)
Bowers et al	49	207	49 (23.7)	0	11	11 (22.5)
Opie et al	246	332	48 (14.5)	1	8	9 (18.8)
Patton et al	263	98	18 (18.4)	1	8	9 (50)
Sailors et al	301	559	92 (16.5)	2	21	23 (25)
Acosta et al	4	890	152 (17)	2	43	45 (30)
Letton et al	199	916	143 (16)	12	31	43 (30)
Total		**13,125**	**2496 (19)**	**114**	**557**	**980 (39)**

*Percentage of all malignancies.

of breast biopsy and is probably underestimated.[14, 129, 149, 287] LCIS occurs 12 times more frequently in white females than in black females, although blacks with this disease have a tenfold higher recurrence rate, all of which probably relates more to socioeconomic differences in access to early detection programs than to any biologic differences in racial predilection.[129, 371] The results of 19 published series that report a total of 10,149 biopsies of nonpalpable breast lesions (see Table 52–1) show that LCIS comprises 1.1 percent of all biopsy specimens and 5.7 percent of all 1994 evaluable mammographically detected breast malignancies.

Ductal Carcinoma *In Situ*

This most common histologic form of noninvasive breast carcinoma occurs predominantly in females, but also comprises approximately 5 percent of male breast carcinomas because the male breast contains the ductal elements from which this lesion arises.[57, 161] The average age of women with DCIS is approximately 54 years, which lies between the age of women with LCIS and those with invasive breast carcinoma.* Two studies have found no statistically significant difference between the ages of women with DCIS and those with invasive disease,[307, 380] suggesting that this is a more ominous disease than LCIS, having a closer relationship with invasive malignancy.

Those older series in which physical examination was the primary diagnostic modality, report the inci-

dence of DCIS to average less than 1 percent (range 0.3 to 3 percent) of all breast biopsies (Table 52–2) and only up to 6 percent of all breast malignancies.[16, 117, 288, 337, 374] The fact that some autopsy series documented a greater incidence of DCIS in asymptomatic women than most clinical series suggests either the possibility that DCIS is underdiagnosed by physical examination (244) or that many cases are not clinically significant (306). Although LCIS predominated over DCIS by as much as 3:1 in these early years,[16, 21, 61, 93, 94, 288, 298] DCIS came to predominate among all cases of CIS with the later use of mammography (Table 52–3). This latter observation is most likely attributable to the characteristic mammographic manifestations of DCIS[144, 307, 367, 374] and to its presen-

TABLE 52–2. INCIDENCE OF DUCTAL CARCINOMA IN SITU (DCIS) IN BREAST BIOPSY SPECIMENS BEFORE 1985

Author	Reference Number	Number of Breast Biopsies	Incidence of DCIS	
			No.	%
Brown et al	54	1,300	40	3.0
Foote and Stewart	117	500	3	0.6
Gillis et al	137	603	36	6.0
Kramer and Rush	181*	140	4	2.9
Nielsen et al	244*	83	9	13.3
Page et al	256	2,404	52	2.2
Rosen et al	288	10,000	30	0.3
Rosner et al	298	23,972	202	0.8
Total		**39,002**	**376**	**0.96**

*See references 21, 54, 190, 230, 256, 287, 298, 367, and 391.

*Autopsy series.

TABLE 52–3.   PROPORTIONS OF DCIS AND LCIS AMONG ALL IN SITU BREAST CARCINOMAS 1977–1992

Author	Reference Number	No. *In Situ* Carcinomas	No. DCIS (%)	No. LCIS (%)
Albert et al	5	404	286 (71)	118 (29)
Blichert-Toft et al	43	78	48 (61.5)	30 (38.5)
Frazier et al	122	155	138 (89)	17 (11)
Howard et al	167	59	55 (93)	4 (7)
Kinne et al	179	128	85 (66)	43 (34)
Pagana et al	252	20	18 (90)	2 (10)
Ringberg et al	279	167	134 (80)	33 (20)
Rosen et al	293	122	64 (52.5)	58 (47.5)
Rosner et al	298	323	202 (62.5)	121 (37.5)
Schwartz et al	310	101	81 (80)	20 (20)
Sunshine et al	351	106	70 (66)	36 (34)
Ward et al	374	319	220 (69)	99 (31)
Total		**1982**	**1401 (71)**	**581 (29)**

tation as a palpable mass in as many as 65 percent of cases even in recent years.*

A review of 19 published series of mammographically detected breast lesions (see Table 52–1) shows that DCIS occurs in 5.3 percent of all 10,499 evaluable nonpalpable breast biopsy specimens and 28 percent of all 1944 evaluable nonpalpable breast malignancies. DCIS also predominates over LCIS by an average ratio of 5:1 (556:114 total cases), ranging from 2:1 to 17:1.

PATHOLOGY

The essential pathological feature of CIS is still the same as originally defined by Broders,[52] being the malignant transformation of epithelial cells without evidence of invasion into the surrounding stroma. The basement membrane that confines these cells, its interaction with the surrounding stroma, and the outer layer of myoepithelial cells that invest the ductal and lobular breast elements, are all critical factors in determining the presence or absence of invasion.[17] Histological studies of the mammary basement membrane, and ultrastructural studies of the basal lamina, using a variety of immunocytochemical assays for type IV collagen and laminin, generally demonstrate a correlation between the integrity of this structure and the degree of malignant degeneration[306] with benign and *in situ* lesions having intact basement membranes, microinvasive lesions showing focal disruption with myoepithelial cells still present, and frankly invasive lesions having no detectable membrane or myoepithelial cells.[11, 31, 249, 251, 361] The degree of basement membrane disruption also tends to correlate directly with nuclear grade and histological type of CIS.[273] Electron microscopy has shown extrusion of malignant cells through gaps in the basal lamina of CIS not seen by light microscopy, which may explain the small incidence of axillary metastasis, recurrence, and mortality that occurs in women with this lesion.[200, 298]

Enough variability exists in these techniques to render them unreliable in consistently distinguishing between *in situ* and invasive disease.[62, 250, 273] Most pathologists rely only on light microscopy to diagnose CIS and exclude invasion, which indicates how subjective and arbitrary this diagnosis may be.[109, 115, 137, 156, 223, 307, 340]

The cellular and extracellular components of the stroma surrounding foci of CIS appear to play a critical role in the behavior of mammary epithelial cells and their invasive potential.[14, 16, 98, 251] Alterations in the biology of stromal fibroblasts and basement membrane proteins such as fibronectin correlate with the development of invasive disease. Angiogenesis is an essential process for the development of breast malignancy and may serve as a reliable marker of invasive potential in cases of CIS.[17, 51, 148, 184, 346] The mechanism by which the confined neoplastic cells escape through the basement membrane to initiate invasion has been postulated as a pressure necrosis on the myoepithelial cells or an enzymatic degeneration of the basement membrane.[116, 251, 360] The expression of the proteinase stromelysin 3 by fibroblasts has been implicated as a mechanism of invasion and thus a marker of poor prognosis.[335, 390]

The field of molecular biology promises to clarify our understanding of CIS, and supports the transition theory of evolution of breast carcinoma. The *HER2* (*c-erbB-2*) oncongene shows a greater frequency of amplification and overexpression in CIS than in invasive carcinoma, suggesting that alterations of this locus are among the earliest genetic disturbances leading to invasive breast carcinoma.[206] Estrogen receptor activity of specimens of CIS closely correlate with that of adjacent areas of invasive disease and also with the degree of histological differentiation.[30, 55, 63, 214] The tumor-associated antigen DF3 is expressed more strongly in specimens of atypical hyperplasia, CIS, and invasive carcinoma than in nonproliferative lesions or proliferative lesions without atypia.[245]

---

*See references 21, 54, 101, 115, 137, 150, 200, 230, 252, 298, 307, 332, 340, 367, and 380.

The many histological and cytologic factors involved in the pathological diagnosis of CIS and its distinction from benign and invasive disease have been thoroughly discussed in Section IV, Chapter 8, Section VI, Chapters 12 and 13 and Section XI, Chapter 37. Both LCIS and DCIS have distinct histopathological features that clearly differentiate them in most cases.[335] Several aspects of the pathology of these entities require emphasis, however, because they significantly impact on biological behavior and appropriate diagnosis and management.

Lobular Carcinoma *In Situ*

The unique histological appearance of this disease, once described as the "busy bosom"[201], is well established and easily recognized by pathologists.* It is believed to arise from the terminal duct–lobular apparatus of the breast, which explains its diffuse involvement of all breast tissue and the consistent absence of any clinical manifestations. Most authorities agree that LCIS should be assumed to be present throughout both breasts whenever detected in a biopsy specimen, because extensive tissue and whole organ sectioning have shown rates of ipsilateral multicentricity and contralateral bilaterality approaching 100 percent.† Its homogeneous appearance, slow growth, and low nuclear grade[228] explain the absence of calcium deposition in foci of LCIS and thus its lack of radiographic manifestations.[109, 130, 171, 173, 311, 351] LCIS most often falls into the microfocal growth pattern of benign-appearing cellular morphology and histological architecture with little surrounding stromal reaction.[13, 15]

There are several potential difficulties in the pathological diagnosis of LCIS. Most agree that at least 75 percent of a lobule must be involved with these proliferating neoplastic cells in order for this diagnosis to be made, although the true significance of lesser degrees of involvement is uncertain.[117, 156, 193, 257, 287] The well-differentiated appearance of LCIS can pose some difficulty in its distinction from benign lobular hyperplasia.[169, 171, 201, 223, 381] On the other hand, it also may resemble DCIS or invasive carcinoma, especially when these lesions coexist in the same duct-lobule unit.[283, 285, 287] The cells of LCIS may spread outside the lobules into major lactiferous ducts, and ductal forms of breast carcinoma likewise may involve lobules (cancerization of lobules), all of which may obscure the proper diagnosis.[9, 95, 96, 223]

Several studies have documented that LCIS typically has a high rate of estrogen receptor activity, low nuclear grade, low proliferative rate, and diploid DNA morphology.[55, 209, 225, 335] The tumor-suppressor gene nm 23 is strongly expressed in specimens of LCIS, whether or not it is associated with invasive disease, correlating with a low metastatic potential

and improved survival.[30, 335, 347] The *HER2* oncogene has shown no overexpression or amplification in most specimens of LCIS.[269] Genetic instability and chromosomal aberrations occur to a lesser degree and on different chromosomes in LCIS than in DCIS although both lesions show more genetic instability than benign proliferative breast tissue.[74, 366] These molecular characteristics are consistent with a relatively benign and indolent biologic behavior, and with a low likelihood of progression to invasive disease.[124, 125, 149]

Ductal Carcinoma *In Situ*

The well-established histopathological features of DCIS, described in detail in Section VI, Chapter 12, are usually distinct from LCIS, and are recognized easily by pathologists.[21, 117, 137, 223, 287] The aforementioned gross features of palpable tumors containing DCIS, which originally led Bloodgood[45] to label this entity comedocarcinoma are actually nonspecific and may be found also in cases of mastitis, hyperplasia, and stasis.[287] Most cases of DCIS are diagnosed by mammographic screening and are small, nonpalpable lesions, a trend with important diagnostic, prognostic, and therapeutic implications.* It must be emphasized that microscopic examination by a pathologist is the only reliable method of making this diagnosis, of ensuring its distinction from benign hyperplasia, and of excluding microinvasion.

Four histological patterns of DCIS are recognized by pathologists, which may represent successive stages in an evolution toward invasive carcinoma.[186, 287, 352] All are characterized by the essential elements of malignant cells confined within the basement membranes of major lactiferous ducts. Papillary and micropapillary DCIS involve well-differentiated cells that proliferate as papillary ingrowths into the ductal lumen and may be difficult to distinguish from ductal hyperplasia.[108] The cribriform pattern of DCIS, a term attributed to Schultz-Brauns,[239, 287, 308] occurs when cellular proliferation largely fills the duct except for scattered rounded spaces and the cells show increasing levels of atypia, hyperchromasia, and loss of polarity. Solid DCIS results when cellular proliferation obliterates all spaces, distending the duct with anaplastic cells and mitotic figures. As this process continues, the cells in the center of the lumen become necrotic, presumably from outgrowing their blood supply,[219] resulting in the characteristic microscopic appearance of the comedo pattern. This pattern is the most common form of DCIS,[37, 178, 262, 315, 332, 336] and may be confused with benign inflammatory processes.[176] Necrosis may also occur in cases of benign ductal hyperplasia,[124] emphasizing how nonspecific this feature is. Calcium is usually deposited in areas of rapid growth and necrosis, which accounts for the most common mammographic manifestation of DCIS.[89, 121, 141, 230, 383, 384] Individual cases of this disease typically show a large

---

*See references 9, 12, 117, 133, 156, 169, 171, 193, 222, 223, 239, 287, and 376.

†See references 10, 16, 94, 124, 125, 129, 155, 156, 280, 287, 289, and 361.

---

*See references 141, 150, 189, 190, 310, 332, and 358.

degree of histological heterogeneity.[195, 197, 262, 335] The more advanced patterns tend to be located centrally, with earlier patterns located peripherally, suggesting a radial growth process.[197]

These histological categories have significant prognostic implications.[71] Comedo-DCIS, in particular, has been associated with larger tumor size, higher nuclear grade, and greater risks of multicentricity, microinvasion, lymph node metastasis, and recurrence than noncomedo patterns, suggesting a more aggressive biological behavior.* This has been corroborated by studies of various tumor markers that show, in comedo-DCIS, a high incidence of aneuploid DNA and chromosome abnormalities,† rapid proliferative rates,[53, 225, 238] increased p53 expression,[195, 268, 354] extensive amplification of the *c-erbB-2* (*HER2/neu*) oncogene,‡ increased levels of transforming growth factor-β[370] reduced levels of the tumor-suppressor gene nm 23,[29] and lower levels of estrogen receptor activity[53, 55, 63, 214] when compared with noncomedo-DCIS, LCIS, or benign hyperplasia. Comedo-DCIS that is associated with concomitant invasive breast carcinoma exhibits more aggressive tumor characteristics and biological behavior than pure DCIS or noncomedo DCIS with invasion, and the level of these indicators of poor prognosis is directly proportional to the amount of synchronous invasion present.[53, 59, 218, 234, 322, 366] Therefore, the comedo architectural pattern appears to represent the noninvasive stage of evolution that is "closest" to invasive disease, or perhaps even an early indolent form of invasive carcinoma.

Investigators have focused on the need to standardize the definitions and classification of these architectural features in order to correlate more accurately with biological behavior and prognosis, and to allow valid comparisons among different studies.[37, 186-188] In the past, the presence of necrosis has been the central determinant of the comedo variant of DCIS.§ Some authors have failed to define their histological criteria for comedo-DCIS,[27] and others have failed to stratify their data according to histological subtype, assuming that all cases of DCIS are the same.[25, 58, 104, 113, 115, 258] Several studies and reviews have suggested that high nuclear grade is the independent factor that most closely correlates with poor prognosis in DCIS (i.e., greatest risk of recurrence and synchronous invasion) and therefore should be the major histological determinant of the comedo subtype regardless of architectural pattern or the presence of necrosis.¶ Although DCIS with high nuclear grade is very commonly associated with necrosis[262, 315, 336] and this combination is associated with the most aggressive biological characteristics,[187]

some now believe that necrosis is the least important factor in the designation of comedo-DCIS.[37, 234] The widespread inconsistency in definition of what exactly constitutes the comedo form of DCIS is perhaps a good reason to abolish this term as a diagnostic label in favor of a precise pathological description of the size, grade, presence and extent of necrosis, and margin status. This would allow a more accurate assessment of risk and therefore of the most appropriate form of management of each individual case.[118, 328, 329]

Noninvasive ductal carcinoma of the breast has been termed "intraductal" carcinoma in the past by many authors, denoting the essential histological feature of containment of malignant cells within the ductal elements of the breast.[115, 137, 234, 307] Comedocarcinoma, the term originated by Bloodgood[45] to describe typical gross and histological features of early breast carcinoma, has also been applied to DCIS. Many authors, however, have included both invasive and noninvasive lesions under these terms or have failed to make this critical distinction, resulting in confusion in the proper interpretation of the biology of true DCIS.[44, 45, 117, 200, 287, 306] This explains the surprisingly low 5-year survival rate reported in some studies of DCIS,[200, 298] as compared with those series that include only noninvasive lesions.[48, 316, 343]

The presence of any stromal invasion clearly denotes an entirely different biological entity from noninvasive breast carcinoma, with distinct prognostic and therapeutic implications. Any invasion signifies a potential for systemic metastasis and death that is not theoretically possible with *in situ* lesions, which suggests the need for more aggressive therapy.[117, 179, 187, 311, 337] Some retrospective studies have suggested that DCIS with microinvasion has a long-term survival similar to that of DCIS alone, apparently having no impact on outcome.[299, 392] Several recent published studies of DCIS have continued to include cases of microinvasion,[104, 262, 327, 331, 332, 336] and some authors have actually defined DCIS as including certain proportions of invasive disease.[153, 322] A prognostic distinction has been conjectured between microinvasion, defined as nests of malignant cells that have invaded within only 0.1 mm beyond a duct, and focal invasion, which involves classic invasion into the stroma with a significant risk of systemic disease.[99, 352] However, this theoretical distinction has never been supported by hard evidence. In fact, most available evidence confirms that even the earliest and smallest invasive breast carcinomas have a definite potential for metastatic spread and death.[19, 179, 234, 252, 337, 341]

It has been recommended that these imprecise terms and potentially misleading definitions no longer be applied to DCIS, because they tend to confuse the interpretation of its biological behavior.[115] At present, it is agreed widely that DCIS is the most appropriate diagnostic label for noninvasive ductal carcinoma of the breast and that this term must only be applied to lesions that have undergone extensive sectioning and special staining with histological markers to exclude any evidence of invasion.[179, 187, 223,]

---

*See references 27, 113, 147, 178, 189, 190, 233, 267, 306, 312, 315, and 336.

†See references 1, 53, 59, 71, 74, 114, 178, 195, 207, 243, and 366.

‡See references 6, 29, 33, 47, 152, 269, 354, and 363.

§See references 101, 111, 158, 223, 230, 247, 262, 312, and 331.

¶See references 1, 37, 164, 165, 178, 186, 187, 189, 197, 234, 258, and 343.

TABLE 52–4.   SALIENT CHARACTERISTICS OF LCIS AND DCIS

Characteristic	LCIS	DCIS
Average age (years)	44–47	54–58
Incidence*		
% Breast biopsies	1	5–6
% Breast cancers	5–6	25–35
Clinical findings	None	Mass, nipple discharge
Mammographic signs	None	Calcifications
Premenopausal (%)	70–90	30–35
Incidence synchronous IBC (%)†	5	2–46‡
Multicentricity (%)	60–90	25–40
Bilaterality (%)	50–90	10–20
Axillary metastasis (%)	<1	1–2‡
Subsequent carcinomas		
Average incidence (%)	18	36
Laterality	Bilateral	Ipsilateral
Interval to diagnosis (years)	15–20	5–10
Predominant histology	Ductal	Ductal
Cellular Characteristics		
DNA ploidy	Diploid	Aneuploid
Proliferative rates	Low	High
Hormone receptor activity	High	Moderate to Low
nm23 expression	High	Low
Oncogene expression	Low	High
Nuclear grade	Low	High
Necrosis	Absent	Present

* Among all nonpalpable mammographically detected breast biopsies and breast malignancies.
† DCIS = ductal carcinoma *in situ*, IBC = invasive breast carcinoma, LCIS = lobular carcinoma *in situ*.
‡ Higher in high-risk lesions (i.e., large size, high nuclear grade, necrosis).

[287, 293, 306] Some have advocated even abolishing the term DCIS altogether because of the confusion caused by the term carcinoma and to develop nomenclature that provides an appropriate assessment of risk. Blanket terminology denoting simple benign or malignant paradigms have been outdated by the complexities of DCIS pathology and the diversity of risk based on this pathology.[118]

NATURAL HISTORY AND PROGNOSIS

Until the 1980s, many investigators viewed CIS as one entity because of its uncommon occurrence and uniform treatment with mastectomy.[61, 94, 122, 265] The concept of minimal breast cancer fostered this perspective by blurring the distinctions between its components.[131–133, 373] Surprisingly, this view has persisted in some recent reports,[5, 159, 167, 279, 351, 356] although it is now generally accepted that LCIS and DCIS are distinct in their biological behavior and diagnostic and therapeutic implications (Table 52–4).*

Lobular Carcinoma *In Situ*

The diagnosis of LCIS from a breast biopsy specimen imparts one of the greatest risks currently known for the subsequent development of invasive carcinoma.[129, 149] Long-term follow-up studies of untreated women with LCIS have documented the ultimate development of invasive breast malignancy in up to 37 percent of cases,[290] with this risk ranging as high as 18 times that of the general population of women (Table 52–5).[13, 138, 179] Relative risk figures are a more accurate and informative method of expression of risk for LCIS than a single percentage, in view of the cumulative nature of this risk that is spread over a lifetime, as well as differences in length of follow-up, selection bias, and treatment regimens found in individual studies.[129, 149, 154, 270] These figures suggest a rate of development of subsequent ipsilateral invasive carcinoma of approximately 1 percent per year,* which is equivalent to the risk of contralateral malignancy following mastectomy for invasive carcinoma.[281] Several distinctive aspects of the pattern of risk associated with LCIS help clarify the appropriate management.

Studies have suggested that the hazard rate for LCIS, or the risk of development of subsequent invasive breast carcinoma, actually increases with time, with over half of these future malignancies occurring more than 15 years after diagnosis of LCIS, and 38 percent occurring after more than 20 years.[127, 129, 156, 171, 287, 290] This risk pattern is different from that observed in all other forms of breast carcinoma, in which most recurrences develop within 5 years and then taper with time.[39, 95, 115, 298] Surveillance strategies for women with LCIS must take this into account. Page and colleagues have reported contrasting results, in which two thirds of invasive carcinomas following LCIS in women with a 19-year mean follow-

---

*See references 50, 129, 150, 177, 179, 364, 371, 374, and 391.

*See references 12, 156, 222, 290, 302, 364, and 382.

TABLE 52–5.   INCIDENCE OF INVASIVE BREAST CARCINOMA FOLLOWING A BIOPSY DIAGNOSIS OF LCIS

| Author | Reference Number | No. Patients | No. Lost to Follow-up | Years of Follow-up | | No. Subsequent Cancers (%) | Relative Risk* |
				Mean	*Range*		
Andersen et al	12	52	0	15	2–28	15 (29)	12
Carson et al	60	51	0	7	1–20	3 (6)	—
Curletti and Giordano	75	19	0	11.7	7–21	2 (11)	—
Haagensen et al	156	285	2	16.3	1–47	53 (18.5)	7
Hutter and Foote	172	52	3	—	4–27	14 (29)	—
McDivitt et al	222	42	8	—	2–23	9 (22.5)	10
Ottesen et al	248	69	0	5†	2–8	8 (11.6)	11
Page et al	257	39	0	19	—	10 (25.6)	8
Ringberg et al	279	11	0	8†	4–13	1 (9)	—
Rosen et al	290	99	15	24	1–35	31 (37)	9.6
Wheeler et al	382	35	0	16	1–24	6 (17)	18
Zurrida et al	398	120	1	5	—	8 (6.7)	10.3
Total		**874**	**29**			**160 (18)**	

* Compared with women from Denmark (Andersen, Ottesen), Connecticut (Haagensen, McDivitt, Rosen), Atlanta (Page), Lombardy, Italy (Zurrida), and historical controls from the literature (Wheeler).
† Median follow-up.

up occurred within 15 years.[257] The actual risk beyond 15 years must be considered uncertain in view of the scant data available, although these observations suggest that standard surveillance regimens should be maintained throughout the life of the patient.

Another unique feature of LCIS is that the risk of subsequent malignancy applies equally to all breast tissue in both breasts, regardless of which breast contains the diagnosed focus of disease.* A review of 554 women reported in the literature who were subjected to a long-term follow-up of LCIS confirms this equal bilateral risk (Table 52–6). The only studies that have failed to find this are those with the shortest follow-up intervals.[60, 248, 302] This risk pattern is consistent with the extensive involvement of all breast tissue known to occur in women with LCIS,[60] and the therapeutic implication of this risk is that all breast tissue must be viewed as one organ and treated equally when LCIS is found.[270]

The risk of synchronous invasive carcinoma in either breast in women with a biopsy diagnosis of LCIS ranges from 4 to 13 percent[61, 287, 318, 361, 362] but is most commonly reported as occurring in 5 percent of patients.[171, 289, 293] This stresses the importance of a diligent and extensive review of several tissue sections by the pathologist to ensure the correct diagnosis. Ward and associates[374] have demonstrated a 6-percent incidence of unrelated nonbreast carcinomas in women with LCIS. The incidence of axillary nodal metastasis in mastectomy specimens from women with LCIS is generally less than 1 percent[61, 284] and is presumably a result of either overlooked or regressed foci of occult invasive disease.

Most invasive carcinomas that follow a diagnosis of LCIS (50 to 65 percent) are of the ductal histological type.* This is not consistent with the transition theory, which would predict an overwhelming predominance of invasive lobular carcinoma if LCIS were truly a direct precursor of these future breast malignancies. Although invasive lobular carcinoma does occur in this setting at 18 times its expected

*See references 12, 156, 171, 172, 222, 257, and 290.

*See references 77, 78, 109, 156, 222, 287, 290, 302, and 381.

TABLE 52–6.   LATERALITY OF RISK AND MORTALITY OF INVASIVE BREAST CARCINOMA FOLLOWING A BIOPSY DIAGNOSIS OF LCIS

| Author | Reference Number | Years of Follow-up | | Number of Ipsilateral Breasts/Carcinoma | Number of Contralateral Breasts/Carcinoma | Number of Cancer-Related Deaths |
		Mean	*Range*			
Andersen et al	12	15	2–28	46/9	52/9	6
Haagensen et al	156	16.3	1–47	281/33	286/37	11
Hutter and Foote	172	—	4–27	40/10	49/7	2
Page et al	257	19	—	35/6	39/4	3
Rosen et al	290	24	1–35	83/18*	83/17*	16
Wheeler et al	382	15.7	1–24	25/1	34/5	2
Total (N = 554)				**510/77 (15%)**	**543/79 (14.5%)†**	**40 (7.2%)**

* One patient excluded, side not known.
† Eleven percent if prior carcinoma excluded.
LCIS = Lobular carcinoma *in situ*.
Data from Haagensen CD: Diseases of the Breast, 3rd ed. Philadelphia, W.B. Saunders, 1986, p 209.

rate,[382] and it is reasonable to presume that it does develop from LCIS, these observations raise some doubt as to the validity of the transition theory, and suggest a more complex mechanism governing the development of invasive carcinoma.[124] It has been postulated that LCIS may transform into a ductal histological type as it becomes invasive,[14, 16, 156] or that the original diagnosis may have confused a ductal lesion with LCIS. Page and coworkers[257] support this latter suggestion in their finding that 70 percent of invasive breast carcinomas following LCIS were of lobular histology. Another explanation for the high rate of ductal carcinoma following LCIS involves the frequent coexistence of DCIS and LCIS in the same breast[109, 129, 248, 285, 290] and the fact that DCIS typically develops into invasive carcinoma more frequently and sooner than LCIS.[39, 256, 380] One study that supports this contention demonstrates a significantly greater incidence of lobular histology among all noninvasive breast carcinomas than among invasive carcinomas.[317] This differential in growth rates would lead to the initial appearance of invasive ductal carcinomas, which in the past generally have been treated by mastectomy, thus precluding any subsequent appearance of the slower developing and more indolent invasive lobular lesions. The current trend toward breast conservation for invasive breast carcinoma may lead to a change in this pattern.[127]

The behavior and prognosis of those invasive carcinomas that follow a diagnosis of LCIS are perhaps more important than their frequency.[381] Although a minority of authors have found these subsequent malignancies to have a poor prognosis,[286, 290] most have documented them to have a favorable prognosis.[12, 75, 155, 193, 381] Those studies of the longest follow-up intervals of women with LCIS who have developed invasive breast carcinoma report an overall cancer-related mortality of only 7.2 percent (see Table 52–6), which is substantially lower than that generally reported for invasive breast carcinoma.[337] More recent studies have shown even lower mortality rates in these women,[257] with many now reporting no cancer-related deaths over long follow-up periods.* The favorable prognosis of these subsequent malignancies is more likely a result of the increased surveillance of these women, owing to their known high risk, than of any biological differences stemming from the temporal relationship. This surveillance allows detection of subsequent carcinomas at an early stage, which is associated with good outcome following treatment.[127, 129] This has been supported by studies that document a smaller average tumor size among those malignancies that follow LCIS when compared with the overall size of all breast carcinomas.[248]

The determination of which women with a diagnosis of LCIS ultimately will develop invasive carcinoma is certainly desirable, because it would allow the selective application of aggressive treatment while avoiding unnecessary treatment of most of these women. Factors that have shown promise in

this regard in having demonstrated a correlation with high risk include young age at diagnosis, high nuclear grade, and extensive involvement of a large number of lobules.[248, 257] Notably absent of risk in these women is a family history of breast carcinoma and a history of exogenous hormone administration.[257] Page and colleagues have suggested that much of our uncertainty and the wide variation in magnitude of risk of LCIS reported in the literature stems from imprecise diagnosis and the inclusion of many cases of atypical lobular hyperplasia in studies of this disease.[257]

These unique biological features of LCIS, in terms of its bilaterality of risk of predominantly ductal invasive carcinoma in only a minority of afflicted women; the increasing level of risk over long periods of time; and its diffuse involvement of all breast tissue without any clinical manifestations has led to the prevailing consensus that LCIS is more a marker of increased risk than a true premalignant lesion.* LCIS may be viewed in the same way as other known risk factors such as family history or atypical hyperplasia, both of which are also bilateral in their risk and associated with no clinical manifestations. A small number of studies continue to suggest that LCIS may be a true precursor of invasive malignancy that requires surgical ablation,[248, 257, 371] indicating the persistent uncertainties as to its biology and how much more there is to learn about this disease.

Haagensen has labeled this disease process lobular neoplasia in order to emphasize its clinically benign behavior and to discourage physicians from inappropriately aggressive treatment that may be prompted by the term carcinoma.[149, 154–156, 193] Others apply this term to the spectrum of borderline lesions that include both benign hyperplasia and noninvasive lobular carcinoma of the breast.[257, 282] However, the original term of LCIS prevails to describe only noninvasive lesions because of its anatomical accuracy in terms of the malignant morphology of its cells.† Also, the term neoplasia has no precise pathological meaning. *CIS* does not necessarily imply an inevitable progression to invasion, as evidenced by the fact that most women with this diagnosis never develop invasive carcinoma.[16, 75, 283, 381] Finally, a knowledge of the biology of this lesion indicates that the term LCIS refers to certain histological and biological features that are distinct from lesions arising from major lactiferous ducts, and cytological morphology is not necessarily the sole diagnostic criterion.[117, 223, 287]

Ductal Carcinoma *In Situ*

Less published evidence is available of the natural history of DCIS than of LCIS, because DCIS has been recognized as a distinct entity for a shorter

---

*See references 60, 156, 179, 193, 248, 279, 302, and 398.

*See references 3, 60, 129, 149, 156, 171, 177, 193, 270, 302, 381, and 398.
†See references 14, 16, 24, 116, 117, 222, 223, 241, 242, 283, 288, and 381.

period of time, has been relatively rare, and has been treated more frequently by mastectomy. Only recently, with its increased incidence of diagnosis, have the uncertainties of its biological implications and appropriate management been clarified.[126, 128, 186, 287, 306, 391] The few published long-term follow-up studies of DCIS after biopsy only document an overall incidence of subsequent invasive breast carcinoma of over 36 percent (Table 52–7), which is twice the average rate of women with LCIS (see Table 52–5). Although most of these subsequent malignancies occur within ten years, as many as one third have been found to develop after 15 years.[39, 255] Page and colleagues[255, 256] calculated a 9.1-fold increased risk of invasive breast carcinoma among women with DCIS over that expected in the general population. Unfortunately, the validity of these observations is uncertain because these studies are flawed by small numbers, retrospective design, selection bias, the inclusion of invasive lesions, and failure to stratify for those variables now known to affect prognosis.[153, 186, 187, 200]

All of these subsequent breast malignancies in women with DCIS are of ductal histology and most commonly occur not only in the same breast but also in the same quadrant as the initial DCIS.[39, 150, 153, 287, 307, 389] Studies in past years[298] have reported substantially lower 5-year survival rates in women with DCIS (64 percent) than in those with LCIS (84 percent).

These characteristics indicate that DCIS is more ominous than LCIS in its biological implications (see Table 52–4). The twofold greater risk of subsequent invasive carcinoma of ductal histology occurring within ten years in the original biopsy site are consistent with the tenets of the transition theory and strongly suggest that DCIS is a true anatomical precursor of invasive carcinoma.[150, 190, 306] Earlier studies have viewed this entity as an aggressive disease process with rapid progression to invasion, because of its rare occurrence as a purely noninvasive lesion, and its frequent association with invasive disease.[117, 137, 200, 298, 344] Other studies have emphasized the long

duration of symptoms before diagnosis, the relatively young age distribution and the large size that some cases attain to support a more indolent and slow-growing entity with a long preinvasive phase.[380]

In recent years, the prognostic importance of several variables has been documented, which allows a more rational assessment of treatment options and a more appropriate evaluation of the published results of treatment than was possible in earlier years.[328, 329] Tumor size is among the strongest correlates with the prognosis of DCIS.[150, 167, 189, 190, 286, 332] Most studies have shown that large and palpable forms of this disease (>1 to 2 cm) are associated with as much as a 46 percent rate of synchronous occult invasion,[190] and significantly higher rates of multicentricity, local recurrence, axillary lymph node metastasis, and cancer-related mortality than smaller, nonpalpable and microscopic forms.[115, 137, 166, 186, 200, 298] This was first noted by Bloodgood in the 1930s.[44, 45] Although the B-17 trial of the National Surgical Adjuvant Breast and Bowel Project (NSABP) found no such relationship of size with prognosis, only a small percentage of its cases of DCIS (32/573) were larger than 1.0 cm.[111, 258] High nuclear grade has also been associated with a poor prognosis,[37, 137, 178, 187, 189, 230] as has comedo histology and the presence and degree of necrosis,[71, 187, 189, 247, 336, 343] as mentioned in the previous section of this chapter on pathology. Young age has been suggested as a poor prognostic factor that increases the risk of local breast recurrence following breast conservation therapy of DCIS.[150] Unlike LCIS, most cases of DCIS are associated with the poor prognostic features of high nuclear grade and comedonecrosis.[336]

The accuracy of risk assessment in patients with DCIS is affected and may be distorted substantially by the characteristics of individual lesions as well as by the specific form of management. Studies of mastectomy specimens from patients who had a biopsy diagnosis of DCIS have shown residual DCIS in the biopsy site in up to 77 percent of cases,[61, 293, 326, 389] suggesting that more complete excision of the primary lesion may reduce the risk of recurrence.[115, 164–166] Conversely, removal of the more common non-

TABLE 52–7.   INCIDENCE OF INVASIVE BREAST CARCINOMA FOLLOWING A BIOPSY DIAGNOSIS OF DCIS

| Author | Reference Number | Number Patients | Years of Follow-up | | No. Subsequent Cancers (%) | Years to Subsequent Cancer | |
			Mean	(Range)		Mean	(Range)
Betsill et al	39	10	21.6	(7–30)	7 (70)	9.7	(0.8–24)
Farrow	94	25	—	—	5 (20)	—	(1–8)
Haagensen	153	11*	13.5	—	8 (73)	4.7	—
Lagios et al	190	20	7.25	—	3 (15)	1.5	(0.75–3.0)
Lewis et al	200	8*	—	(1–11)	6 (75)	1.6	(1–4)
Millis and Thynne	230	8	—	(5–20)	2 (25)	3.8	(0.5–7.0)
Page et al	255, 256	28†	24‡	(8–29)	9 (32)	8	(3–31)
Total		**110**			**40 (36.4)**		

* Invasive lesions are included.
† All cases of low-grade forms.
‡ Median follow-up of all women in whom invasive carcinoma did not develop.
DCIS = ductal carcinoma *in situ*.

TABLE 52–8. INCIDENCE OF MULTIPLE SITES OF INVASIVE AND NONINVASIVE CARCINOMA IN BREASTS WITH A PRIMARY FOCUS OF CARCINOMA *IN SITU*

Author	Reference Number	DCIS		LCIS	
		Number of Patients	Number of Malignant Foci (%)	Number of Patients	Number of Malignant Foci (%)
Carter and Smith	61	38	25 (66)	49	34 (69)
Fisher et al	115	28	15 (54)	—	—
Gump et al	151	42	34 (81)	—	—
Rosen et al	293	50	34 (68)	50	30 (60)
Schwartz et al	310	42	17 (40.5)	6	4 (67)
Shah et al	318	45	29 (64)	40	28 (70)
Wobbes et al	389	30	23 (77)	—	—
TOTAL		**275**	**177 (64)**	**145**	**96 (66)**

DCIS = Ductal carcinoma *in situ*, LCIS = lobular carcinoma *in situ*.

palpable specimens of DCIS for diagnosis may completely ablate its risk and obscure its true natural history on follow-up.[17, 252] Also, some long-term follow-up studies of DCIS involved only low-grade lesions that had initially been confused with atypical hyperplasia.[39, 255, 256] These considerations may explain why all cases of DCIS do not appear to develop into invasive carcinoma, as would be expected if this were truly an obligate precursor, and suggest that the prognostic implications of DCIS are being underestimated by our current study techniques.[124]

These findings explain the pessimistic attitude toward DCIS that is evident in older series, which almost exclusively included larger palpable forms of this disease and did not reliably exclude invasive lesions.[21, 137, 153, 200, 344, 380] A more optimistic perspective presently prevails toward DCIS, because most cases are now small nonpalpable lesions detected only by mammography.* This view must be tempered, however, by the consensus that DCIS is a premalignant lesion that will develop into invasive carcinoma in a substantial portion of cases (perhaps all) if not aggressively treated. The aforementioned pathological features are the most accurate predictors of the biological behavior of a given lesion.[312, 315] The wide variation in the presentation and natural history of DCIS is most likely due to its histological and biological heterogeneity, as well as to differences in each individual's host resistance.[108]

MULTICENTRICITY AND BILATERALITY

The tendency of CIS to involve multiple sites within both breasts is an important factor to consider in assessing its natural history and appropriate treatment. An abundance of evidence indicates that breast carcinoma is a diffuse disease process and that malignant breast tumors arise from a coalescence of multiple sites of origin within the breast.† This concept is supported by the histological heterogeneity of

specimens of both CIS and invasive breast carcinoma, as well as the substantial incidence of multiple foci of occult malignancy in breasts with a primary focus of CIS (Table 52–8).* These occult foci of disease consist largely of the same *in situ* carcinoma as the primary lesion.[61, 108, 293, 318] The fact that the size of the primary tumor has been shown to correlate with the frequency and extent of these multiple occult foci of malignancy and that the frequency of these foci diminish with increasing distance from the tumor have led to the theory that this phenomenon represents a spread of tumor cells outward from the primary tumor, probably through the ductal system.[65, 150, 151, 166, 190]

The variations in the reported frequency of multiple sites of malignancy in breasts with CIS can be attributed to differences among published series in whether invasive or noninvasive lesions are included, the extent of histological sectioning and microscopic examination, and the location in the breast being examined.[359] It has been well demonstrated that the more diligently these occult foci are sought by the pathologist, the more will be found,[88] which is why those series in which a small number of histological sections are examined typically report the lowest yields.[115, 293, 324] Imprecise definitions also obscure this issue. Multicentricity is defined as invasive or noninvasive malignant foci found outside the quadrant of the primary breast tumor, whereas multifocality and residual disease are defined as malignant foci within the same quadrant as the primary tumor.[108, 115] Often these terms are used interchangeably in published studies, which makes comparisons and valid conclusions difficult.[19, 54, 61, 359] It is generally agreed that LCIS has a substantially higher rate of true multicentricity than DCIS, which approaches 100 percent when most diligently sought, supporting the consensus that LCIS should be presumed to be present throughout all breast tissue whenever it is detected.† Analysis of those studies of DCIS that carefully adhere to the true definition of multicentricity shows

---

*See references 124, 162, 267, 309, 310, 312, 315, and 336.
†See references 122, 131, 132, 140, 151, 272, 287, and 313.

*See references 53, 64, 108, 132, 197, 257, 315, 318, and 335.
†See references 10, 14, 58, 94, 129, 287, and 376.

that this phenomenon occurs in approximately one third of these women (Table 52–9)[119, 352] and predominantly consists of other microscopic foci of DCIS. Lagios and associates[185, 187, 189, 190] and others[7, 37, 58, 164, 277] have documented a direct correlation of multicentricity of DCIS with extent and size of the primary focus in that small nonpalpable cases of DCIS that were detected only by mammography, or were less than 25 mm in size, were multicentric in only 12 to 17 percent of cases, compared with an incidence of 47 percent when larger than 25 mm.[397] Nipple involvement with DCIS is also a risk factor for multicentricity, with an incidence of 12 percent in its absence and 37.5 percent in its presence.[191] Young age has also been shown to correlate with a risk of multicentricity.[7] As previously stated in this chapter, multifocality is found in up to 80 percent of cases of DCIS and is usually considered to represent residual disease from inadequate excision of the primary lesion.[88, 101, 293, 326, 389]

Theoretically, multicentricity and multifocality may influence the outcome of breast conservation treatment of DCIS by possibly increasing the incidence of ipsilateral breast tumor recurrence (IBTR). Studies have shown a higher incidence of multicentricity in breasts with CIS than in those with invasive carcinoma, which supports the theory that breast carcinoma develops from a coalescence of multiple sites of origin.* Because the studies that have validated breast conservation therapy have largely involved only invasive carcinoma,[106] these results and thus the safety of breast conservation should not automatically be extrapolated to DCIS without further cautious study.

The phenomenon of bilaterality of CIS probably stems from the same underlying biologic etiology as multicentricity and also may have a significant impact on therapeutic decisions.[7, 168, 198, 287] A 22-percent incidence of bilaterality was reported in one series of patients with all forms of breast carcinoma, and 74 percent of these tumors also demonstrated multicentricity in the ipsilateral breast.[318] As much as a 67-percent rate of bilaterality has been reported for CIS in general.[351] The rate of synchronous bilaterality of CIS, like multicentricity, is dependent on how extensively it is sought through tissue sampling and histological sectioning, suggesting that most published rates underestimate its true incidence.[166, 287] Like multicentricity, the frequency of contralateral breast malignancy varies significantly with the histological type of CIS. LCIS has shown a statistically significant rate of bilaterality,[378] which has been reported as high as 90 percent.* One study suggested that LCIS associated with invasive lobular carcinoma does not reliably predict contralateral disease,[28] again supporting the theory that this phenomenon regresses with progression to invasive disease. On the other hand, DCIS is associated with only a 10 to 15 percent average incidence of bilaterality, ranging as high as 30 percent,[122, 351] which is similar to that found in invasive ductal carcinoma.† As is also true of multicentricity, a substantial portion of these occult contralateral malignancies are *in situ* lesions.[280, 293, 307] The reader is referred to Section XXII, Chapter 78 for further discussion of bilateral breast carcinoma.

The true clinical significance of occult multicentric or contralateral breast malignancies in the setting of a primary focus of CIS should be questioned. Many studies of this issue provide conflicting data and fail to address such variables as how diligently these lesions were sought, what risk factors these patients had in terms of tumor size, grade and necrosis, and how these lesions related to patient outcome in terms of recurrence and mortality.[313, 318] The reported rates of subsequent ipsilateral or contralateral clinically evident breast carcinoma falls short of the published rates of occult multicentricity and bilaterality[281, 290, 378] and autopsy studies show higher rates of occult CIS than clinically evident breast malignancy.[181, 244] Those cases of subsequent breast carcinoma that do develop

---

*See references 7, 32, 151, 275, 293, 313, 314, and 336.

*See references 28, 155, 156, 241, 242, 280, 287, and 361.
†See references 21, 54, 101, 280, 307, 367, 378, and 380.

TABLE 52–9.   INCIDENCE OF TRUE MULTICENTRICITY* IN THE BREASTS OF PATIENTS WITH A PRIMARY FOCUS OF DCIS

Author	Reference Number	Number of Patients	Number with Multicentricity (%)
Bellamy et al	37	88	21 (24)
Brown et al	54	40	13 (32.5)
Cutuli et al	76	34	12 (35)
Lagios et al	190	53	17 (32)
Nielsen et al	244†	11	4 (36)
Rosen et al	293	53	10 (19)
Schuh et al	307	51	9 (18)
Schwartz et al	311, 315	50	18 (36)
Silverstein et al	324	98	15 (15)
Simpson et al	336	36	28 (78)
Von Rueden and Wilson	367	47	18 (38)
Total		**561**	**165 (29.4)**

* Malignant foci outside the quadrant of the primary lesion.
† Autopsy series.
DCIS = Ductal carcinoma *in situ*.

most commonly occur within 5 years, suggesting that they were probably present synchronously in a smaller, less easily detectable form.[361] Many studies do not distinguish whether metachronous carcinomas occurred in the region of the original biopsy site, which, especially for DCIS, would implicate incomplete excision of the primary tumor rather than a new malignancy arising from multicentric foci.[110] Despite the high rate of multicentricity and multifocality in breasts with CIS (see Table 52–8), it is rare to have two or more clinically detectable malignancies occur synchronously either in the same breast (approximately 0.1 percent)[112] or contralaterally (approximately 2 percent).[28] Despite the high rates of multicentricity and multifocality associated with DCIS, the only prospective randomized trial of breast conservation therapy for DCIS[104] documents rates of IBTR at 5 years that are no different than those found for invasive carcinoma treated in this way.[106] In fact, most recent studies have reported rates of multicentricity in DCIS that are similar to those associated with invasive breast carcinoma (see Table 52–9).[198, 318] Fisher and colleagues have published evidence that contralateral breast malignancy has no added impact on outcome beyond that of the primary ipsilateral tumor.[110] Because most cases of IBTR following DCIS occur in the biopsy site, multifocality and residual disease is probably a more important concern with regard to therapeutic implications than is multicentricity or bilaterality.[119] The ultimate clinical implications of multicentricity can only be defined by studies that follow these patients for over 20 years.[19]

DIAGNOSIS

The principles and techniques of diagnosis of breast carcinoma have been reviewed comprehensively in Section XI, Chapters 35 and 37, and Section XIII, Chapter 40. However, there are several considerations and issues unique to the detection and characterization of CIS which warrant emphasis.

Lobular Carcinoma *In Situ*

The pathologist carries the ultimate responsibility for diagnosis of LCIS, according to the histological criteria discussed earlier in this chapter, and as comprehensively discussed in Section IV, Chapter 8, Section VI, Chapters 12 and 13, and Section XI, Chapter 37. Any finding of lobular hyperplasia in a breast biopsy specimen with or without atypia, especially in women with a history of breast carcinoma, should mandate further sectioning in order to exclude any foci of LCIS or invasive lobular carcinoma.[8, 138, 169, 287] It has been recommended that as many as 40 blocks of tissue should be examined in order to reliably exclude LCIS.[10, 133, 201] If LCIS is found, further sectioning is necessary to exclude invasion in view of the significant change in prognosis and therapy this finding would entail.[171] Many pathologists have as-

serted the necessity of identifying synchronous foci of LCIS in order to accurately diagnose invasive lobular carcinoma,[8, 155, 228, 242] although others do not believe this is necessary.[97, 109] The histological appearance of LCIS may be confused with DCIS, because they often coexist and may be similar in their cytological and architectural morphology.[181, 262, 285, 287, 335, 366] Although frozen section examination has been advocated for the diagnosis of LCIS,[223] virtually all now agree that this is unreliable and unnecessary for this entity.* The need for extensive sectioning and deliberate examination of several permanent sections to detect LCIS and to exclude invasive disease far outweighs any need for rapid diagnosis.[283, 293] Fine needle aspiration cytology cannot be relied on to diagnose LCIS in view of the well-differentiated morphology of this lesion and the inability to examine the histological architecture in order to exclude invasion.[135, 143, 279, 372]

LCIS is unique in its diagnostic implications in that it is not associated with any clinical or radiographic manifestations. Its detection is always an incidental finding, most commonly in breast biopsy specimens of otherwise benign disease.† In past years, the most common indication for a breast biopsy that led to a diagnosis of LCIS was a palpable mass,[79, 202, 222, 378] but more recently it has been reported as nonpalpable mammographic masses or microcalcifications.[121, 173, 215, 339, 345, 383] However, in all cases, the microscopic foci of LCIS are outside these areas of abnormality.[60, 235, 287, 295, 345, 351] This so-called neighborhood calcification pattern is best explained by the absence of necrosis and extracellular secretions by the cells of LCIS, which fails to provide any stimulus for calcium deposition in the involved lobule. However, the neoplastic proliferation of these cells tends to plug up neighboring normal lobules, causing them to involute and calcify.[129, 130, 149, 173] Clearly, the increased frequency of diagnosis of LCIS in recent years (see Table 52–1) is related to increased mammographic screening, but this is presumably an indirect consequence of the increased rate of biopsy of high-risk mammographic findings.[141, 194, 288, 311]

Ductal Carcinoma *In Situ*

Unlike LCIS, DCIS most commonly presents as a clinically evident lesion, either as a palpable mass or as a nonpalpable mammographic finding. As stated earlier in this chapter, those cases of DCIS that are small and nonpalpable have the best prognosis, and fortunately are also the most commonly detected forms of this entity (see Table 52–1). Therefore, it is important to understand the typical radiographic features of DCIS.

Clustered microcalcifications represent the most common mammographic finding that warrants biopsy, being associated with carcinoma in up to 34

---

*See references 38, 77, 93, 94, 109, 171, 202, 351, and 381.

†See references 46, 109, 129, 149, 171, 179, 201, 202, 288, and 376.

percent of cases.[121, 311, 383] As many as 95 percent of all cases of CIS detected by mammography are associated with microcalcifications. Up to 90 percent of all carcinomas that manifest mammographic microcalcifications are CIS, and 80 percent of these are DCIS.[14, 310, 317, 358] Moreover, a linear and branching pattern of calcifications is most commonly associated with the most aggressive high-grade variants of DCIS.[187] The aforementioned pathological characteristics of DCIS, especially of the high-grade forms, explains its predominance in this setting, because rapidly dividing cells and necrosis stimulate calcium deposition.[89, 230]

An interval change in a mammographic lesion is another indication for biopsy and is associated with an 18-percent rate of malignancy, most of which is also CIS.[141, 192, 383] Nonpalpable mammographic masses, which are associated with a 20- to 25-percent rate of predominantly invasive malignancies, and asymmetrical densities, which are malignant in less than 10 percent of cases, have a minimal impact on the diagnosis of DCIS.[192, 313, 315, 317]

As a general rule, all nonpalpable clustered microcalcifications and interval progression of densities should undergo biopsy in view of their substantial risk of being early malignancies such as DCIS. Needle localization breast biopsy under local anesthesia is the most common technique used to sample nonpalpable, mammographically suspicious tissue that may harbor DCIS for examination by the pathologist and is a safe, accurate, and cost-effective modality.[180, 194, 210] The addition of specimen radiography improves the accuracy of this technique by confirming removal of the suspicious lesion and aiding the pathologist as to the specific location in the specimen where sectioning should be carried out (Fig. 52–3).[35, 294, 295]

Fine needle aspiration biopsy (FNAB) is an increasingly common modality being applied to the cytological diagnosis of both palpable and nonpalpable breast lesions that may contain DCIS, using ultrasound or stereotactic guidance for localization of nonpalpable lesions. Its overall accuracy in these settings compares favorably with any other diagnostic procedure,[135, 231, 232, 320, 385] although CIS in general and DCIS in particular have been documented as the most common causes of false-negative results.[143, 216, 231] As is true of LCIS, this is due to the inability to examine the histological architecture in cytological specimens in order to accurately distinguish between the benign precursors and invasive counterparts of DCIS. Although recent studies have suggested cytologic features that may improve the accuracy of diagnosing DCIS by FNAB,[2, 205] most pathologists now agree that cytologic aspirates of low-grade DCIS cannot be distinguished reliably from hyperplasia. High-grade DCIS usually is reported as malignant in cytologic specimens but still cannot be distinguished as yet from invasive disease. Therefore, FNAB should not be relied on to specifically diagnose DCIS.

In recent years, core needle biopsies have been applied increasingly to the diagnosis of palpable breast masses, as well as to nonpalpable breast le-

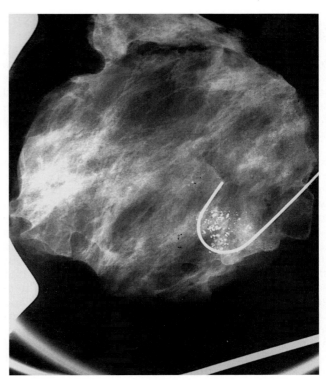

Figure 52–3 *Specimen radiograph of clustered microcalcifications removed from the breast of a 55-year-old female by wire localization, which was a 0.9-cm ductal carcinoma* in situ, *comedo type, without evidence of invasion. Margins were clear, and breast conservation was carried out with adjuvant radiation therapy. Axillary dissection was not performed.*

sions under ultrasound or stereotactic guidance, in an attempt to resolve the inherent inaccuracy of FNAB for the diagnosis of CIS.[236] However, this inaccuracy of FNAB has not shown any improvement with the use of core needle biopsies for the diagnosis of nonpalpable DCIS, despite the histological examination that this modality allows. In 839 patients reported in seven published series of stereotactic core needle biopsy of nonpalpable breast lesions (SCNBB), only 66 percent of all cases of DCIS were successfully diagnosed, overall sensitivity was as low as 71 percent, and in as many as 17 percent of cases, samples were insufficient for diagnosis.* A selection bias was also evident in these studies against the application of SCNBB to mammographic calcifications, in which DCIS is most commonly found.[236] Other studies have documented a 50- to 60-percent false-negative rate in cases diagnosed by SCNBB as atypical ductal hyperplasia, with most of the missed malignancies being DCIS, but as many as 35 percent being invasive carcinoma.[83, 86, 174, 203] Additionally, 20 percent of cases diagnosed as DCIS by SCNBB were demonstrated to contain invasive carcinoma by standard surgical excision.[204] Apparently even multiple cores of tissue do not permit the degree of examination required following standard excisional biopsy for the most ac-

---

*See references 85, 86, 90, 139, 227, 260, and 261.

curate diagnosis of DCIS, indicating that SCNBB should not be applied as yet to this purpose.[86]

Another problem posed by SCNBB is that small lesions may be completely removed by zealous core sampling. The consequent difficulty of definitive wide local excision for malignant lesions has been reported to lead to mastectomy in women otherwise eligible for breast conservation, simply owing to the inability to localize the site for margin clearance.[227, 236]

Several difficulties and limitations exist in the histological diagnosis of DCIS by pathologists, which overlap with those already discussed for LCIS. Deliberate analysis of several tissue sections is necessary whenever atypical hyperplasia or DCIS is found in order to exclude a more advanced stage of malignancy.[144, 306] Careful attention is also required in those cases of close coexistence of DCIS and LCIS to prevent confusion of these two entities.* One recent study demonstrated the great variability and subjectivity that exists among experienced pathologists in distinguishing between hyperplasia and DCIS in that there was not a single case of unanimous agreement.[282] Another study reported disagreement in the distinction between CIS and atypical hyperplasia among three pathologists in 20 percent of cases.[356] This has led to some doubt as to the need to make such rigorous histological distinctions, which may be somewhat artificial, especially when major therapeutic decisions are made on this basis.[247, 309] It has been suggested that a new diagnostic category of minimal intraepithelial neoplasia should be applied to all borderline lesions.[282] Others have postulated that these difficult diagnostic distinctions can be rendered more consistently objective and reproducible through the standardization of histological and architectural criteria,[305] or through the application of a numerical grading system based on specific cytologic criteria.[216, 217] Interobserver reliability in the determination of histological grade of DCIS approaches 100 percent when specific diagnostic criteria are followed.[188] The application of emerging techniques in immunocytochemical staining, ultrastructural analysis, and flow cytometry also promises to improve the critical distinctions between DCIS and benign or invasive variants of breast disease.[74] As is true of LCIS, frozen section is unreliable and unnecessary in the diagnostic evaluation of DCIS.[293, 306, 364] In the case of small, mammographically detected cases, frozen section may waste tissue that could otherwise be evaluated with a variety of tumor markers considered necessary for prognostic assessment.[125, 186]

TREATMENT OF LOBULAR CARCINOMA *IN SITU*

Ipsilateral radical or modified radical mastectomy was the standard recommended treatment for LCIS until the late 1970s, because this entity was viewed as simply an interesting and uncommon variant of invasive breast carcinoma.* In support of this view were observations of its high rate of multicentricity and bilaterality, a substantial incidence of subsequent invasive carcinoma, and an approximately 5-percent incidence of associated synchronous invasive carcinoma, suggesting that any compromise in treatment would jeopardize the patient's life.[171, 293]

By the 1970s, with its increasing rate of diagnosis, evidence accumulated as to the relatively benign course of LCIS, its predominance among young females, the predominance of ductal histology in subsequent invasive carcinomas, the bilaterality of its relatively low risk, and its unique pattern of increased hazard rate after 15 years. These observations indicating that LCIS is more a marker of risk than a premalignant lesion led Haagensen and coworkers to be the first to advocate nonoperative lifelong surveillance.[154–156] This has become the standard management approach toward LCIS.† Some authors no longer even consider LCIS a malignancy.[121, 143, 151] In support of this approach are long-term follow-up studies showing that the rate of clinically apparent invasive carcinomas which follow a diagnosis of LCIS falls well below the rate of associated occult multicentric and bilateral malignant foci, casting doubt on their clinical significance (see Table 52–5). Tulusan and associates[361] found a 16-percent rate of microscopic occult invasive carcinoma in subcutaneous mastectomy specimens from women with a recent (i.e., within 2 years) diagnosis of LCIS. This represents substantially more than 50 percent of the rate of clinically evident carcinoma expected over intervals of up to 30 years in these women,[257, 290] indicating either that most of these occult lesions never become clinically evident or that they are very indolent in their growth and behavior.

Nonoperative observation of LCIS certainly is not a risk-free management option, because overall mortality rates of approximately 7 percent have been reported (see Table 52–6). Up to 37 percent of these women ultimately develop invasive carcinoma, with mortality rates of up to 16 percent.[290] A meta-analysis of 13 combined series of LCIS[50] showed that treatment with biopsy only was associated with a 2.8-percent overall mortality rate and 4-percent recurrence rate over 10.9 years of mean follow-up, which is significantly greater than the 0.9-percent mortality rate and 2.7-percent recurrence rate following mastectomy. Although nonoperative observation has a higher recurrence rate, initial mastectomy did not significantly improve the ultimate cancer-related mortality rate following LCIS. These results still compare favorably with those following invasive breast carcinoma,[196, 337] although the diligence with which invasive disease was excluded in many older series is suspect. The goal of nonoperative observation with lifelong mammographic surveillance of both breasts is to detect any subsequent malignancy,

---

*See references 9, 95, 96, 248, 262, 285, and 287.

*See references 93, 94, 116, 140, 172, 222, 228, and 241.
†See references 8, 14, 60, 125, 129, 138, 149, 150, 171, 193, 257, 270, 302, 381, 382, 394, and 398.

which may develop in a minority of these women, at an early enough stage to have a high likelihood of cure and thus a negligible impact on overall survival. The feasibility of this goal is supported by the results of mammographic screening trials,[316, 319, 353] as well as the absence of mortality in several recent studies of this management for LCIS.[60, 156, 193, 302, 398] Although wide local excision of the biopsy site following a diagnosis of LCIS has been recommended in order to obtain clear margins,[235] no benefit of such a practice has ever been demonstrated, nor should it be expected, because this disease is known to involve all breast tissue when it occurs.[149, 286, 290]

The rationale and demonstrated success of nonoperative observation of LCIS emphasizes the intriguing question as to the validity of the rigid distinction between atypical lobular hyperplasia and LCIS that is maintained.[3, 23, 156, 171, 223, 382] Both entities carry approximately the same bilateral risk for the development of invasive carcinoma,[23] both are most appropriately viewed as risk factors rather than anatomical precursors of malignancy, and both are so morphologically similar that a histological or cytologic distinction by the most experienced pathologists is frequently subjective and arbitrary.[169, 201, 223, 257, 282, 381] Some have recommended abolishing the *in situ* concept based on these considerations in favor of categorizing these transitional lesions collectively as precancerous mastopathy[41, 145] or as minimal intraepithelial neoplasia.[282]

Routine mastectomy appears to be an overly radical treatment for LCIS in view of the low level of risk the lesion poses.[12, 129] Ipsilateral mastectomy and blind contralateral biopsy has been recommended on the basis of some evidence that the risk of subsequent carcinoma is higher in the breast in which LCIS is found and that a normal contralateral biopsy may indicate a lower risk of contralateral malignancy.[154, 222, 287–290, 351, 362] Surprisingly, it is apparent that a substantial minority of surgeons still treat LCIS with ipsilateral mastectomy, although this number is declining.[149, 371] Most authors now agree that, in women with LCIS, routine contralateral breast biopsy is not justified in the absence of standard clinical or mammographic indications, because the likelihood of finding a lesion requiring treatment (i.e., invasive carcinoma or DCIS) is very small, the clinical significance of such lesions may be negligible, and a normal biopsy has never clearly been shown to reduce risk to any degree.[28, 338]

Bilateral mastectomy is the most rational therapeutic option for those cases of LCIS in which surgical treatment is deemed necessary or is chosen by the patient in view of the well-established bilaterality of risk, which is not addressed by unilateral mastectomy. Although few recommend this approach as primary management,[38, 351] it may be considered in cases of exceptionally high risk. The association of LCIS with invasive carcinoma in either breast poses a fourfold greater risk of subsequent carcinoma than does either entity alone and may be an indication for bilateral mastectomy.[78, 97] The current sophistication

of breast reconstruction techniques may make this an acceptable option to some women. This procedure can be considered a prophylactic mastectomy, and issues such as indications and patient preferences, discussed in Section VI, Chapter 12, and Section IX, Chapter 23 and Section VI, Chapter 14, should apply.

Subcutaneous mastectomy with preservation of the nipple/areola complex has been advocated as an appropriate surgical option for LCIS.[38, 79, 361] However, available evidence does not support this option because of the substantial amount of breast tissue left behind compared with total mastectomy and the numerous reports of invasive carcinoma developing in breasts subjected to this procedure.[142, 171, 271] There is also no evidence to suggest that any significant reduction in risk results from reducing the amount of breast tissue short of a total mastectomy.[129] Therefore, any surgical procedure less than a bilateral total mastectomy cannot be considered an acceptable surgical option for LCIS.

The incidence of axillary node metastasis in women with LCIS is generally less than 1 percent, and these instances indicate the presence of occult invasion in the breast. Therefore, axillary dissection is not justified in cases of LCIS in the absence of palpable axillary adenopathy. In the event mastectomy is performed, a low-level I node sampling adds virtually no time or morbidity and may provide important information.[109, 171, 287, 293, 302, 351]

Clinical trials sponsored by the European Organization for the Research and Treatment of Cancer and by the NSABP are in progress to evaluate the prophylactic efficacy of tamoxifen in women with LCIS,[364] although several years of follow-up will be required before results are available. There is no evidence that radiation therapy or cytotoxic chemotherapy holds any therapeutic benefit for this disease.

TREATMENT OF DUCTAL CARCINOMA *IN SITU*

Mastectomy

Mastectomy has been the standard treatment of DCIS through the first 4 decades of its recognition as a distinct entity because of the same perceived hazards of extensive multicentricity and substantial incidence of synchronous and metachronous invasive carcinoma that characterized the initial observations of LCIS.* In earlier years, the application of mastectomy to DCIS can be understood in the light of the rarity of its diagnosis (most commonly achieved only by physical examination); the fact that mastectomy was the only treatment for any form of breast carcinoma; the typical presentation of DCIS as large, palpable tumors that were characterized by aggressive pathological features and biological behavior; and the

---

*See references 3, 21, 137, 200, 230, 287, 288, 293, 307, 313, 336, 367, and 380.

consequent view that DCIS represented simply an interesting variant of invasive breast carcinoma, in which microscopic invasion could not be excluded reliably.[44, 45, 54, 117, 137, 230]

The results of mastectomy in this setting are therefore abundant and well established, comparing very favorably with the results of mastectomy for invasive breast carcinoma, as should be expected for such an early stage of disease.[105, 106, 112, 337] A meta-analysis of 12 published reports of the treatment of 585 patients with DCIS by mastectomy shows an overall recurrence rate of 3.2 percent and cancer-related mortality of only 1.7 percent after an average follow-up of 8.6 years.[50] A compilation of 1575 patients with DCIS reported in 20 published series reveals overall locoregional recurrence and cancer-related mortality rates of only 1.1 and 1.3 percent, respectively, following mastectomy, after as much as an 18-year average follow-up (Table 52–10). The documentation of microinvasion in up to 21 percent of patients in three of these series (accounting for less than 1.9 percent of total patients) had no adverse impact on these excellent results,[101, 190, 336] which corroborates other recent studies.[299, 392] These data show that a risk of recurrence and death, although small, still exists even at this early and theoretically nonmetastatic stage of disease, most likely owing to the inability to completely exclude some degree of occult microinvasion. In fact, the results in Table 52–10 probably overestimate the true levels of recurrence and mortality from this treatment because of the inclusion of older studies[21, 54, 61, 94, 101, 298] in which the exclusion of invasive disease was not as stringently ensured as in more recent studies. Also, mastectomy tends to be applied to the most aggressive lesions.[329] Despite anecdotal reports of chest wall recurrence of DCIS following mastectomy for DCIS,[107] virtually all local recurrences in this setting, although rare, are invasive, thus marking the poor prognosis of the original lesion.[37, 94, 115, 190, 329] Contralateral mastectomy or biopsy is not necessary in this setting in the absence of standard clinical indications because of the low incidence of synchronous occult contralateral malignancy (10 to 15 percent), which approximates that of invasive breast carcinoma. Breast reconstruction should be offered to these women on either an immediate or delayed basis following mastectomy.[136] These observations indicate that mastectomy is clearly the gold standard against which all other forms of treatment for DCIS must be measured,[119, 134, 167, 233, 306, 356] although its nearly 100 percent efficacy suggests that it is probably overtreatment for this disease.[175]

Breast Conservation: Wide Local Excision Alone

The widespread application of mammography during the 1980s led to a substantial increase in the diagnosis of DCIS (see Fig. 52–2), as well as to a substantial reduction in its average size. This led to an increased application of breast conservation to DCIS in view of the excellent results achieved in patients with invasive breast carcinoma with this therapy.[106] Bloodgood[45] and Foote and Stewart[117] were the first to suggest that less extensive procedures than mastectomy may be valid for DCIS. Rosner and colleagues[298]

TABLE 52–10.   RESULTS OF TREATMENT OF DCIS WITH MASTECTOMY

Author	Reference Number	Number of Patients	Mean Follow-up (Years)	No. Locoregional Recurrence	Number of Cancer-Related Deaths
Arnesson et al	20	28	6.5	0	0
Ashikari et al	21	110	<10	2	1
Bellamy et al	37	94	5*	3	1
Brown et al	54	40	5	0	0
Carter and Smith	61	38	—	1	3
Farrow	94	181	—	2	3
Fentiman et al	101	82†	4.7*	1	1
Fisher et al	115	27	3.2	1	1
Griffin and Frazee	147	60	5	1	0
Kinne et al	179	101	11.5*	1	1
Lagios et al	190	53†	<15	2	1
Millis and Thynne	230	18	—	0	0
Rosner et al	298	182	5	—	4
Schuh et al	307	52	5.5	0	1
Silverstein et al	323	167	6.5*	2	0
Simpson et al	336	36†	17.7	0	0
Sunshine et al	351	68	>10	0	3
Temple et al	355	116	7.5	0	0
Von Rueden and Wilson	367	47	—	0	0
Warneke et al	375	75	4	1	0
Total		**1575**		**17 (1.1%)**	**20 (1.3%)**

* Median years of follow-up.
† Includes cases of microinvasion.
DCIS = Ductal carcinoma *in situ*.

TABLE 52–11. RESULTS OF TREATMENT OF DCIS WITH WIDE LOCAL EXCISION ALONE

| Author | Reference Number | Number of Patients | Mean Follow-up (Months) | Number of Recurrences (%) | | Number of Cancer-Related Deaths (%) |
				Total	Invasive	
Arnesson et al	20	38	60*	5 (13)	2	0
Baird et al	27	30	39	4 (13)	1	0
Bellamy et al	37	31	60*	10 (32)	5	0
Carpenter et al	58	28	38	5 (18)	1	0
Fisher et al	104†	391	43	64 (16.4)	32	0
Fisher et al	115†	22	39	5 (23)	3	0
Gallagher et al	134	13	100	5 (38)	3	3
Griffin and Frazee	147	13	30	0	—	0
Lagios et al	186, 189, 190	79	68*	10 (12.6)	5	0
Ottesen et al	247	112	53*	25 (22)	5	1
Page et al	255	28	360	10 (36)	9	3
Price et al	271	35	108	22 (63)	12	1
Schwartz et al	309, 312	72	49	11 (15)	3	0
Temple et al	356	17	72	2 (12)	2	1
Warneke et al	375	28	89	3 (11)	1	0
Total		**937**		**181 (19.3)**	**84 (46.4)‡**	**9 (0.96%)**

* Median follow-up.
† Prospective randomized trial.
‡ Percentage of all recurrences.
DCIS = Ductal carcinoma *in situ*.

were the first to document an equivalent survival rate between wedge resection of DCIS and mastectomy, although the unusually low survival rates reported for DCIS in that study tend to invalidate the results because invasive lesions were probably included. More recently, simple wide local excision of DCIS has been shown to be associated with substantial rates of IBTR, although with a relatively low mortality rate.[50] A combined total of 937 patients with DCIS treated by wide local excision alone, reported in 15 published series since 1986, documents an overall IBTR rate of over 19 percent (ranging up to 63 percent), and a cancer-related mortality rate of less than 1 percent over follow-up intervals ranging up to 30 years (Table 52–11). These are considered prohibitive levels of IBTR, especially because they consistently continue to increase over time.[104, 134, 258, 336] Because a substantial portion of IBTR occurs more than 5 years after the original diagnosis of DCIS,[119, 258, 271] it is important to be cautious in the interpretation of results from the large number of studies with relatively short follow-up intervals. This consideration also applies to the cancer-related mortality rate, which ranges as high as 23 percent in those studies with the longest follow-up.[134, 258, 356] Some authors have recommended that young women with DCIS should undergo mastectomy routinely because of the longer life span over which recurrences may develop, as well as the more aggressive behavior of breast carcinoma in younger women.[150, 182]

The consensus is that wide local excision alone should be applied cautiously to DCIS, and only in those carefully selected women with a low probability of recurrence according to presently accepted prognostic factors and who agree to it with a full understanding of its risks and uncertainties. Under such conditions, some promising results have been achieved.[186, 189, 190] Recent data suggest that this option may be applied most appropriately to cases of incidental DCIS, in which very small (<0.5 cm) and isolated microscopic foci are detected in specimens of predominantly benign breast tissue with no clinical or even mammographic manifestations of their presence[262, 312, 315, 328, 329] and in which no evidence of further disease is found after re-excision of the biopsy site.[126, 128, 309] Schwartz and coworkers[309, 312] found that in this setting, there were no recurrences among those cases qualifying as incidental over follow-up intervals ranging up to 168 months.

These observations led to the increasingly relevant suggestion that low-risk variants of DCIS that are small, low-grade, and without necrosis may be viewed as markers of risk rather than true anatomical precursors of malignancy in the same way that LCIS is viewed, because the subsequent risks are equivalent to those of LCIS. Consequently, these low-risk forms of DCIS may be treated most appropriately by observation after excision.* This viewpoint must be tempered by a substantial risk of long-term recurrence and mortality rates that have been demonstrated even in cases of low-grade DCIS.[39, 255, 256] These considerations further emphasize the necessity to stratify all DCIS according to prognostic factors that correlate with risk in order to apply the appropriate treatment rationally.

Breast Conservation: Wide Local Excision and Radiation Therapy

The addition of breast irradiation following wide local excision has been increasingly applied to DCIS in

_____
*See references 98, 162, 175, 187, 188, 267, and 328.

view of its established efficacy for invasive breast carcinoma.[106] Bloodgood was the first to report the successful use of excision and radiation therapy on three women with so-called pure comedo-tumor in 1934,[45] and the first studies of this treatment option for DCIS were published in the mid-1980s.[102, 277] The predominantly retrospective studies of this treatment that have been published since 1985 have documented recurrence rates significantly lower than those from wide local excision alone and similarly low cancer-related mortality rates over relatively short follow-up periods.[50] Fifteen published studies of this treatment applied to 1186 cases of DCIS document an overall rate of IBTR of 9 percent, 42 percent of which were invasive lesions, and a cancer-related mortality of 1.1 percent, over follow-up intervals of from 3 to almost 8 years (Table 52–12). Most cases of IBTR occur in the original biopsy site, suggesting inadequate excision as the cause rather than the intrinsic biological behavior of DCIS.[58, 111, 255, 258, 323]

The only complete prospective randomized trial to date of the efficacy of wide local excision and radiation therapy for DCIS, which compares this approach with wide local excision alone, is the B-17 protocol of the NSABP.[104, 111] Although the NSABP B-06 trial included 78 randomized cases of DCIS,[115] it had not been designed to evaluate this specific disease. The results of the B-17 trial showed a significant reduction in IBTR from 16.4 to 7 percent with the addition of breast irradiation following wide local excision of DCIS, and also a reduction in the percentage of IBTR that was invasive (50 to 28 percent), after 43 months of mean follow-up. This represented a reduction in the average annual incidence of IBTR by 58.8 percent and a reduction in the average annual rate of ipsilateral recurrence of invasive carcinoma by 77 percent,

with the use of radiation therapy. There were only three cancer-related deaths and an overall incidence of invasive recurrence of only 2.9 percent in the entire study population.

Evaluation of Study Results

An analysis of the results of the NSABP B-06 and B-17 trials, as well as those of many other studies of DCIS therapy (see Tables 52–10 to 52–12), provides several interesting insights into the biology and therapeutic implications of DCIS. The IBTR following wide local excision with or without breast irradiation is entirely equivalent to that following the same treatment of invasive breast carcinoma over the same follow-up periods,[106] despite the increased rates of multicentricity known to be associated with DCIS. This suggests that occult multicentricity has negligible clinical significance and should not influence the treatment decision. The lower IBTR following wide local excision alone of DCIS in the B-17 trial compared with that of the B-06 trial (16.4 versus 23 percent) can be attributed to the smaller average tumor size in B-17 (1.3 cm versus 2.2 cm), as well as the more thorough attention given in B-17 to excluding occult microinvasion and involvement of tumor margins.[111] This indicates that attention to minimizing those factors related to poor prognosis can reduce IBTR to more acceptable levels even without breast irradiation. The addition of breast irradiation appeared to negate the impact of these factors, because there was no difference in the low levels of IBTR between the B-06 and B-17 trials in this study arm (see Table 52–12).

Although the results of the NSABP B-17 trial appear to minimize prior uncertainties[389] as to the true

TABLE 52–12.   RESULTS OF TREATMENT OF DCIS WITH WIDE LOCAL EXCISION AND BREAST IRRADIATION

Author	Reference Number	Number of Patients	Median Follow-up (Months)	Number of Recurrences (%)		Number of Cancer-Related Deaths (%)
				Total	Invasive	
Baird et al	27	8	39*	2 (25)	1	0
Bornstein et al	48	38	81	8 (21)	5	0
Cutuli et al	76	34	56	3 (9)	1	0
Fisher et al	104, 111†	399	43*	28 (7)	8	3
Fisher et al	113, 115†	29	83*	2 (7)	1	0
Haffty et al	157	60	43	4 (7)	1	0
Kurtz et al	183	43	61	3 (7)	3	1
McCormick et al	220	54	36	10 (18)	3	0
Ray et al	274	56	67*	5 (9)	1	0
Recht et al	277	40	44	4 (10)	2	0
Silverstein et al	323	133	94	16 (12)	8	2
Solin et al	340, 343	172	84	16 (9)	7	4
Stotter et al	349	44	92	4 (9)	4	2
Warneke et al	375	21	37*	0	0	0
Zafrani et al	396	55	55	3 (5.5)	1	1
Total		**1186**		**108 (9)**	**46 (42.6)‡**	**13 (1.1)**

* Mean follow-up.
† Prospective randomized trial.
‡ Percentage of all recurrences.
DCIS = Ductal carcinoma *in situ*.

benefit of radiation therapy in the conservation treatment of DCIS, several doubts persist regarding the validity of that study and the role of this modality. Mastectomy remains substantially superior to any other form of treatment in its low risk of both IBTR and mortality (see Tables 52–10 to 52–12). Silverstein and associates[324] have documented a significantly reduced 7-year actuarial disease-free survival after excision and radiation therapy for DCIS when compared with mastectomy. The failure of the B-17 trial to stratify its patients according to the aforementioned prognostic variables of size, margin status, nuclear grade, occult microinvasion, extent of tumor involvement, and presence of necrosis make treatment comparisons difficult, and prevent any conclusions regarding those low-risk populations that may avoid radiation therapy with safety.[187, 258] Some specialists have asserted that longer follow-up of irradiated patients seems to show a progressive decline in the rate of disease-free survival, suggesting that the impressive short-term results of radiation therapy may simply represent a postponement of the appearance of IBTR rather than a true reduction in its incidence. Therefore, this modality may not affect long-term outcome at all.[187] The benefits of radiation therapy on local control of DCIS in the B-17 trial corroborate the findings of others[81, 119, 303] in refuting earlier suggestions that an extensive component of DCIS associated with invasive breast carcinoma (extensive intraductal carcinoma [EIC]) increases the risk of IBTR.[163, 304]

An important and unique perspective on breast conservation treatment of DCIS is the fact that approximately 50 percent of all cases of IBTR are invasive (see Tables 52–11 and 52–12).[71] This imparts a theoretical potential for systemic metastasis and death from a lesion that should be curable by simple local excision. Unlike IBTR following breast conservation treatment of invasive carcinoma, which has shown no clear causative impact on outcome,[103] an invasive recurrence after a noninvasive primary lesion represents a worsening of the stage and conceivably could increase the risk of death.[26, 68, 271] Therefore, poor local control of DCIS may be equated with reduced survival time. This possibility is supported by studies showing rates of cancer-related mortality among women with DCIS who develop IBTR as high as 43 percent,[256, 288] as well as a 14-fold higher rate of distant metastasis among women with IBTR than in those women who do not develop IBTR following DCIS.[342] Most deaths and distant metastases that follow this diagnosis afflict those women with invasive recurrences.[271, 343, 349] On the other hand, breast irradiation has resulted in significantly improved local control and a reduction of invasive recurrences to less than 3 percent of all women with DCIS.[104, 120] This low incidence is unlikely to have any significant impact on the overall outcome of breast conservation treatment of DCIS,[104, 111] as is supported by the absence of any clear adverse impact of the specific procedure used for local treatment on ultimate mortality (see Tables 52–10, 52–11, and 52–12).[50, 375] However,

any such differences that may exist in outcome likely will require more than 20 years of follow-up to demonstrate.[237] Regardless of its impact on survival, local control is still important in terms of avoiding subsequent salvage mastectomy, which defeats a major purpose of breast conservation and subjects these women to a second operative procedure. The ultimate long-term effect of breast conservation on the survival of women with DCIS has yet to be ascertained, and therefore caution is warranted in the application of this treatment.

Treatment Recommendations for Ductal Carcinoma *In Situ*

The aforementioned observations indicate that the same treatment options are available for DCIS as for invasive breast carcinoma, with some exceptions. The safety and efficacy of breast conservation is not as certain for DCIS, in view of the unknown impact of invasive IBTR on survival. Also, wide local excision alone without adjuvant breast irradiation appears to have a valid role in the management of low-risk variants of DCIS, whereas this method has yet to be accepted for any form of invasive breast carcinoma.[69, 387] The wide variations in treatment found in published studies reflect the lack of consensus that derives from incomplete biological information on the natural history of this disease.[70] It is clear that DCIS is a highly diverse and heterogeneous disease process that should not be viewed any longer as a single entity, nor be encompassed by one single form of management. A rational approach to treatment must depend on an evaluation of all characteristics of each individual case of DCIS that are known to affect prognosis, and an integration of this information with the desires of each patient (Table 52–13).[162, 267]

Available evidence indicates that mastectomy is the safest and most effective treatment for DCIS and is associated with the lowest risks of IBTR and death (see Table 52–10).[50, 323, 324] This is entirely consistent with the noninvasive stage of this disease. Some have asserted that routine mastectomy is difficult to justify in this setting when lesser procedures are accepted widely for the treatment of more advanced invasive breast carcinoma.* However, this is an overly simplistic argument, because DCIS and invasive breast carcinoma are not completely comparable disease processes[332] and there is still a clear role for mastectomy in certain high-risk cases of invasive carcinoma. Also, the noninvasive stage of disease offers the only opportunity for aggressive local treatment to alter the biological progression to invasive disease and thereby favorably affect survival, because the potential for systemic spread is not yet present.[150] On the other hand, most cases of DCIS are now small, nonpalpable lesions that typically are detected only as mammographic calcifications,[104, 111, 332] for which mastectomy clearly appears to be

---

*See references 101, 115, 149, 177, 267, 276, 306, and 391.

TABLE 52–13. TREATMENT OPTIONS FOR IN SITU BREAST CARCINOMA*

	LCIS		DCIS	
	High Risk†	*Low Risk*	*High Risk†*	*Low Risk*
OBS	Yes	Yes	No	Yes‡
WLE‡	No	No	No	Yes
WLE + RT‡	No	No	Yes	No
MASTX§	No	No	Possibly‖	No
BIL MASTX§¶	Possibly	Possibly	No	No

* Axillary lymph node dissection is indicated in cases of ipsilateral palpable adenopathy, invasive local breast recurrences, mastectomy, or possibly high-risk variants.

† Cases with high nuclear grade, large size (DCIS only), necrosis, or molecular markers of poor prognosis.

‡ Requires microscopically clear margins of at least 0.5 cm.

§ Total mastectomy with breast reconstruction should always be recommended. No indication for blind contralateral breast biopsy.

‖ Should only be considered for (1) inability to perform breast conservation or (2) salvage of local breast recurrences

¶ Should be considered only in women with multiple additonal risk factors or those who insist on surgical ablation after comprehensive genetic and psychological counseling. This is the only valid surgical option for LCIS.

BIL MASTX = bilateral mastectomy with reconstruction, DCIS = ductal carcinoma *in situ*, LCIS = lobular carcinoma in situ, MASTX = ipsilateral mastectomy, OBS = nonoperative observation with lifelong mammographic surveillance, WLE = wide local excision alone, WLE + RT = wide local excision and breast irradiation.

overtreatment. At present, the most appropriate indication for mastectomy for DCIS is the inability to completely excise the lesion with pathologically clear margins and with documentation of complete removal of the mammographic abnormality while maintaining an acceptable cosmetic result (i.e., the inability to perform breast conservation). Large palpable tumors or extensive nonpalpable multicentric disease in small breasts represent the most common settings in which mastectomy is the best treatment

option, and fortunately these presentations are increasingly uncommon (Fig. 52–4).[164, 352] Salvage mastectomy is also indicated for invasive local breast recurrences following breast conservation treatment of DCIS.

Since 1980, there has been a gradually increasing trend in the application of breast conservation therapy to DCIS in the United States, although a substantial number of cases still are being treated by mastectomy.[68, 70, 388] Certainly breast conservation should be offered to that majority of women with small, nonpalpable DCIS who are eligible, as long as the uncertainties, risks, and limitations discussed earlier are elaborated fully and understood. It is not clear that a high risk of IBTR (i.e., high nuclear grade, presence of microscopic necrosis, size larger than 2 cm) alone should lead to mastectomy and thus deprive a woman of the opportunity to conserve her breast, because no adverse impact of IBTR on survival has been proven conclusively as yet. Also, there are effective means of reducing these risks to improve local control. Adjuvant breast irradiation should be applied to all high-risk cases of DCIS that are amenable to breast conservation so as to minimize the incidence of IBTR as well as the percentage of invasive recurrences, at least over the short term. Achieving a complete local excision of the primary focus of DCIS is another means of minimizing risks and maximizing local control. The high levels of multifocality and residual disease following local excision of high-risk forms of DCIS,[58, 389] the fact that residual disease is found in up to 43 percent of cases in which even clear margins were microscopically ensured,[326] and the fact that most cases of IBTR following DCIS occur in the original biopsy site[27, 48, 58, 76, 111, 255] emphasize the importance of complete

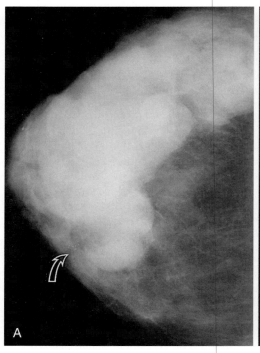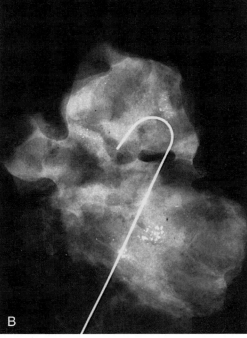

Figure 52–4 *A, Left breast of a 50-year-old female with a suspicious focal cluster of microcalcifications in the lower inner quadrant (arrow).* **B,** *Specimen radiograph demonstrates unsuspected multicentric foci of calcifications, which were comedo ductal carcinomas in situ on histological examination. Clear margins could not be obtained owing to widespread microscopic disease, and therefore, total mastectomy was performed. Extensive residual disease without evidence of invasion remained in breast specimen, and a low axillary sampling showed no nodal metastases. No adjuvant therapy was given. The patient remains free of disease 3 years later.*

excision with generous margins.[164] Microscopic margins of 1 cm or more are desirable, though probably 0.5 cm is the most realistic goal in view of the realities of surgical technique and breast cosmesis, and the uncertainties of the differences in risk between differing margin widths.[187, 329] Surgical excision appears to be the most effective means of reducing the risks of residual disease, and radiation therapy probably should not be relied on to substitute for inadequate margin clearance.

Low-risk DCIS (size less than 1 cm, no necrosis, low nuclear grade, wide clear margins) should be considered amenable to observation with no further treatment. Rigorous mammographic surveillance of women with these lesions should allow detection of any subsequent invasive recurrences at an early enough stage to maintain the risk of death at the same level as that following mastectomy. This low level of estimated risk is comparable to that following LCIS, a strong family history of breast carcinoma, and atypical hyperplasia, all of which are managed by observation alone.[162, 187, 188, 267, 328, 329] Re-excision of any lesion with involved or unknown margins is an essential component of this management because of the prognostic significance of histologically proven clear margins.[329]

Axillary lymph node dissection generally is considered unnecessary in the treatment of DCIS, in view of the very low yield of positive results (1 to 2 percent).[56, 115, 277, 327, 330, 356] Despite this fact, recent reports document that a surprisingly large number of women with DCIS are undergoing routine axillary node dissection.[70, 388] This procedure may be indicated in cases that are associated with palpable axillary adenopathy, when there is a reasonable suspicion of the possibility of occult invasion (i.e., comedo-type, high-grade, histological necrosis, large size) or in cases of invasive local recurrence.[150, 315] A low level I axillary sampling can be carried out with minimal added time or morbidity in conjunction with a mastectomy and may provide the only evidence of occult invasion.[393]

At present, there is no role or proven benefit for the use of cytotoxic chemotherapy or hormonal manipulation in the management of DCIS. The ongoing NSABP B-24 trial is designed to evaluate the benefit of tamoxifen for this disease.[162]

The persistent uncertainties regarding the appropriate treatment of DCIS are clarified only through further clinical and laboratory investigations. Available studies of the management of DCIS (see Tables 52–10 to 52–12) are somewhat inaccurate and limited in their implications because they tend to approach DCIS as a single disease entity and ignore its diverse manifestations and biology. A consensus must be reached on an appropriate system of pathological classification of DCIS.[165, 187, 188] The increasingly relevant question as to the validity and safety of breast conservation for DCIS will be resolved only by a prospective randomized comparison with mastectomy, in which DCIS is stratified according to known prognostic variables.[70]

POST-TREATMENT SURVEILLANCE

All women who have been treated for CIS require lifelong follow-up to facilitate early detection of any subsequent malignancy. This represents the complete management recommended for women with LCIS, who should be encouraged to follow the standard screening guidelines of monthly self-breast examination, yearly physician examination, and yearly mammography. This same regimen applies to all women with DCIS, although physical examination may be carried out more often during the first 5 years in high-risk cases. Women with DCIS who have undergone breast conservation treatment should have a mammogram of the treated breast following wide local excision to confirm complete removal of the suspicious lesion and to serve as a baseline study. Mammography of the treated breast also should be performed 6 months after completion of radiation therapy to serve as a baseline for radiation-induced changes. Bilateral mammography, or contralateral mammography following mastectomy, should be performed yearly thereafter. There is no indication for mammography of a reconstructed breast following mastectomy.[208, 276] Local breast recurrences may be re-excised according to the same strict guidelines for tumor margin clearance as required for the primary lesion. Radiation therapy may be added if not given originally. Salvage mastectomy is otherwise indicated and provides a good chance of long-term survival.[119, 343] The prognostic implications and most appropriate management of recurrent disease is still uncertain and requires further study.

SUMMARY

In situ breast carcinoma represents an early localized stage in the development of invasive breast carcinoma that has an excellent prognosis with appropriate management. Its increased frequency of diagnosis in recent years is a tribute to the success of early detection efforts through mammographic screening. The two histological forms of this disease are distinct in their pathological and behavioral characteristics, as well as in their therapeutic implications. LCIS may be viewed as a marker of high risk for subsequent carcinoma and is generally managed with nonoperative observation. DCIS behaves more as a direct precursor to invasive breast malignancy and should be treated according to the same therapeutic options as are available for invasive breast carcinoma, with some exceptions. Low-risk forms of DCIS are probably amenable to nonoperative observation following wide local excision and documentation of clear margins. Most high-risk forms of DCIS should be treated with radiation therapy of the involved breast following wide local excision. Mastectomy is reserved only for those high-risk cases of DCIS that are not amenable to adequate local excision, most commonly due to larger tumor size or extensive multicentricity. Axillary dissection is not generally necessary for *in situ* carcinoma of the breast. There are still many outstanding issues in the biology and management of this intriguing disease to be resolved by further investigation. Physicians involved in the management of breast disease must have a thorough understanding of the established principles and controversies relating to *in situ* carcinoma of the breast in order to establish a rational plan of treatment and to achieve optimal results.

References

1. Aasmundstad TA, Haugen OA: DNA ploidy in intraductal breast carcinomas. Eur J Cancer 26:956–959, 1990.
2. Abendroth CS, Wang HH, Ducatman BS: Comparative features of carcinoma in situ and atypical ductal hyperplasia of the breast on fine-needle aspiration biopsy specimens. Am J Clin Pathol 96:654–659, 1991.
3. Ackerman LV, Katzenstein AL: The concept of minimal breast cancer and the pathologist's role in the diagnosis of early carcinoma. Cancer 39:2755–2763, 1977.
4. Acosta JA, Greenlee JA, Gubler KD, et al: Surgical margins after needle-localization breast biopsy. Am J Surg 170:643–646, 1995.
5. Albert S, Belle S, Eckert D, et al: Current surgical management of in situ cancer of the female breast. J Surg Oncol 20:99–104, 1982.
6. Allred C, Clark GM, Molina R, et al: Overexpression of HER-2/neu and its relationship with other prognostic factors change during the progression of in situ to invasive breast cancer. Hum Pathol 23:974–979, 1992.
7. Anastassiades O, Iakovou E, Stavridou N, et al: Multicentricity in breast cancer: A study of 366 cases. Am J Clin Pathol 99:238–243, 1993.
8. Andersen JA: Lobular carcinoma in situ: A long-term follow-up of 52 cases. Acta Pathol Microbiol Scand 82:519–533, 1974.
9. Andersen JA: Lobular carcinoma in situ of the breast with ductal involvement: Frequency and possible influence on prognosis. Acta Pathol Microbiol Scand 82:655–662, 1974.
10. Andersen JA: Multicentric and bilateral appearance of lobular carcinoma in situ of the breast. Acta Pathol Microbiol Scand 82:730–734, 1974.
11. Andersen JA: The basement membrane and lobular carcinoma in situ of the breast: A light microscopic study. Acta Pathol Microbiol Scand 83:245–250, 1975.
12. Andersen JA: Lobular carcinoma in situ of the breast: An approach to rational treatment. Cancer 39:2597–2602, 1977.
13. Andersen JA, Blichert-Toft M, Dyreburg U: In situ carcinomas of the breast: Types, growth patterns, diagnosis, and treatment. Eur J Surg Oncol 13:105–111, 1987.
14. Andersen JA, Fechner RE, Lattes R, et al: Lobular carcinoma in situ: Lobular neoplasia of the breast (a symposium). Pathol Ann 15:193–223, 1980.
15. Andersen JA, Nielsen M, Blichert-Toft M: The growth pattern of in situ carcinoma in the female breast. Acta Oncol 27:739–743, 1988.
16. Andersen JA, Schiodt T: On the concept of carcinoma in situ of the breast. Pathol Res Pract 166:407–414, 1980.
17. Anonymous: Intraduct carcinoma of the breast (editorial). Lancet 2:24, 1984.
18. Antoniades K, Spector H: Correlation of estrogen receptor levels with histology and cytomorphology in human mammary cancer. Am J Clin Pathol 71:497–501, 1979.
19. Arbutina DR, Cruz BK, Harding CT, et al: Multifocality in the earliest detectable breast carcinomas. Arch Surg 127:421–423, 1992.
20. Arnesson LG, Smeds S, Fagerberg G, et al: Follow-up of two treatment modalities for ductal cancer in situ of the breast. Br J Surg 76:672–675, 1989.
21. Ashikari R, Hajdu SI, Robbins GF: Intraductal carcinoma of the breast (1960–1969). Cancer 28:1182–1187, 1971.
22. Ashikari R, Huvos AG, Snyder RE: Prospective study of non-infiltrating carcinoma of the breast. Cancer 39:435–439, 1977.
23. Ashikari R, Huvos AG, Snyder RE, et al: A clinicopathologic study of atypical lesions of the breast. Cancer 33:310–317, 1974.
24. Ashikari R, Huvos AG, Urban JA, et al: Infiltrating lobular carcinoma of the breast. Cancer 31:110–116, 1973.
25. Azzopardi JG: Problems in Breast Pathology. Philadelphia, WB Saunders, 1979, p 466.
26. Bahnsen J, Warneke B, Frishbier JH, et al: The intraductal carcinoma of the breast. Geburtshilfe Frauenheilkd 45:488–493, 1985.
27. Baird RM, Worth A, Hislop G: Recurrence after lumpectomy for comedo-type intraductal carcinoma of the breast. Am J Surg 159:479–481, 1990.
28. Baker RR, Kuhajda FP: The clinical management of a normal contralateral breast in patients with lobular breast cancer. Ann Surg 210:444–448, 1989.
29. Barnes DM: C-erb B-2 amplification in mammary carcinoma. J Cell Biochem 176:132–138, 1993.
30. Barnes R, Masood S: Potential value of hormone receptor assay in carcinoma in situ of the breast. Am J Clin Pathol 94:533–538, 1990.
31. Barsky SH, Siegal GP, Janotta F, et al: Loss of basement membrane components by invasive tumors but not by their benign counterparts. Lab Invest 49:140–147, 1983.
32. Bartelink H, Borger JH, Van Dongen JA, et al: The impact of tumor size and histology on local control after breast cancer: Conservative therapy. Radiother Oncol 4:297–303, 1988.
33. Bartkova J, Barnes DM, Millis RR, et al: Immunohistochemical demonstration of c-erb B-2 protein in mammary ductal carcinoma in situ. Hum Pathol 21:1164–1167, 1990.
34. Bauer TL, Pandelidis SM, Rhoads JE, et al: Mammographically detected carcinoma of the breast. Surg Gynecol Obstet 173:482–486, 1991.
35. Bauermeister DE, Hall MH: Specimen radiography: A mandatory adjunct to mammography. Am J Clin Pathol 59:782–789, 1973.
36. Beahrs OH, Shapiro S, Smart CR: Report of the working group to review the National Cancer Institute/American Cancer Society breast cancer detection demonstration projects. J Natl Cancer Inst 62:639–710, 1979.
37. Bellamy COC, McDonald C, Salter DM, et al: Noninvasive ductal carcinoma of the breast: The relevance of histologic categorization. Hum Pathol 24:16–23, 1993.
38. Benfield JR, Fingerhut AG, Warner NE: Lobular carcinoma of the breast 1969: A therapeutic proposal. Arch Surg 99:129–131, 1969.
39. Betsill WL, Rosen PP, Lieberman PH, et al: Intraductal carcinoma: Long-term follow-up after treatment by biopsy alone. JAMA 239:1863–1867, 1978.
40. Birkett J: The Diseases of the Breast and Their Treatment. London, Longman, Brown, Green and Longman, 1850.
41. Black MM, Barclay THC, Cutler SJ, et al: Association of atypical characteristics of benign breast lesions with subsequent risk of breast cancer. Cancer 29:338–343, 1972.
42. Blichert-Toft M, Andersen JA, Dyreborg U: In situ carcinomas of the female breast: Diagnostic and therapeutic aspects with special reference to histological growth patterns: Clinical review. Acta Chir Scand 156:113–119, 1990.
43. Blichert-Toft M, Graversen HP, Andersen JA, et al: In situ breast carcinomas: A population-based study on frequency, growth pattern, and clinical aspects. World J Surg 12:845–851, 1988.
44. Bloodgood JC: Border-line breast tumors. Ann Surg 93:235–249, 1931.
45. Bloodgood JC: Comedo carcinoma (or comedo-adenoma) of the female breast. Am J Cancer 22:842–853, 1934.
46. Borden AG, Gershon-Cohen J: Mammography of lobular carcinoma. Radiology 81:17–23, 1963.
47. Borg A, Linell F, Idvall I, et al: HER2/neu amplification and comedo type breast carcinoma. Lancet 2:1268–1269, 1989.
48. Bornstein BA, Recht A, Connolly JL, et al: Results of treating ductal carcinoma in situ of the breast with conservative surgery and radiation therapy. Cancer 67:7–13, 1991.

49. Bowers GJ, Getz JB, Roettger RH, et al: Nonpalpable breast lesions: Association of mammographic abnormalities with diagnosis after needle-directed biopsy. South Med J 86:748–752, 1993.
50. Bradley SJ, Weaver EW, Bowman DL: Alternatives in the surgical management of in situ breast cancer: A meta-analysis of outcome. Am Surg 56:428–432, 1990.
51. Brem S, Jensen H, Gullino P: Angiogenesis as a marker of pre-neoplastic lesions of the human breast. Cancer 41:239–244, 1978.
52. Broders AC: Carcinoma in situ contrasted with benign penetrating epithelium. JAMA 99:1670–1674, 1932.
53. Brower ST, Ahmed S, Tartter PI, et al: Prognostic variables in invasive breast cancer: Contribution of comedo versus noncomedo in situ component. Ann Surg Oncol 2:440–444, 1995.
54. Brown PW, Silverman J, Owens E, et al: Intraductal "noninfiltrating" carcinoma of the breast. Arch Surg 111:1063–1067, 1976.
55. Bur ME, Zimarowski MJ, Schnitt SJ, et al: Estrogen receptor immunohistochemicstry in carcinoma in situ of the breast. Cancer 69:1174–1181, 1992.
56. Cady B: Duct carcinoma in situ. Surg Oncol Clin North Am 2:75–89, 1993.
57. Camus MG, Joshi MG, Mackarem G, et al: Ductal carcinoma in situ of the male breast. Cancer 74:1289–1293, 1994.
58. Carpenter R, Boulter PS, Cooke T, et al: Management of screen detected ductal carcinoma in situ of the female breast. Br J Surg 76:564–567, 1989.
59. Carpenter R, Gibbs N, Matthews J, et al: Importance of cellular DNA content in pre-malignant breast disease and pre-invasive carcinoma of the female breast. Br J Surg 74:905–906, 1987.
60. Carson W, Sanchez-Forgach E, Stomper P, et al: Lobular carcinoma in situ: Observation without surgery as an appropriate therapy. Ann Surg Oncol 1:141–146, 1994.
61. Carter D, Smith RRL: Carcinoma in situ of the breast. Cancer 40:1189–1193, 1977.
62. Carter D, Yardley JH, Shelley WM: Lobular carcinoma of the breast: An ultrastructural comparison with certain duct carcinomas and benign lesions. Johns Hopkins Med J 125:25–43, 1969.
63. Chaudhuri B, Crist KA, Mucci S, et al: Distribution of estrogen receptor in ductal carcinoma in situ of the breast. Surgery 113:134–137, 1993.
64. Cheatle GL: Early recognition of cancer of the breast. BMJ 1:1205–1210, 1906.
65. Cheatle GL: Cysts, and primary cancer in cysts of the breast. Br J Surg 8:149–166, 1920–1921.
66. Cheatle GL, Cutler M: Tumors of the Breast. Philadelphia, JB Lippincott, 1931.
67. Christopherson WM: The changing concepts of early cancer. J Med Assoc Ala 35:261–266, 1965.
68. Ciatto S, Grazzini G, Iossa A, et al: In situ ductal carcinoma of the breast analysis of clinical presentation and outcome in 156 consecutive cases. Eur J Surg Oncol 16:220–224, 1990.
69. Clark RM, McCulloch PB, Levine MN, et al: Randomized clinical trial to assess the effectiveness of breast irradiation following lumpectomy and axillary dissection for node-negative breast cancer. J Natl Cancer Inst 84:683–688, 1992.
70. Coleman EA, Kessler LG, Wun L-M, et al: Trends in the surgical treatment of ductal carcinoma in situ of the breast. Am J Surg 164:74–76, 1992.
71. Cooke TG: Ductal carcinoma in situ: A new clinical problem. Br J Surg 76:660–662, 1989.
72. Cornil A-V: Contributions a l'histoire du developpement histologique des tumeurs epitheliales (squirrhe, encephaloide, etc.). J Anat Physiol 2:266–276, 1865.
73. Cornil A-V: Les Tumeurs du Sein. Paris, Libraire Germer Bailliere and Co, 1908.
74. Crissman JD, Visscher DW, Kubus J: Image cytophotometric analysis of atypical hyperplasias and intraductal carcinomas of the breast. Arch Pathol Lab Med 114:1249–1253, 1990.
75. Curletti E, Giordano J: In situ lobular carcinoma of the breast. Arch Surg 116:309–310, 1981.
76. Cutuli B, Teissier E, Piat J-M, et al: Radical surgery and conservative treatment of ductal carcinoma in situ of the breast. Eur J Cancer 28:649–654, 1992.
77. Dall'Olmo CA, Ponka JL, Horn RC, et al: Lobular carcinoma of the breast in situ: Are we too radical in its treatment? Arch Surg 110:537–542, 1975.
78. Davis N, Baird RM: Breast cancer in association with lobular carcinoma in situ: Clinicopathologic review and treatment recommendation. Am J Surg 147:641–645, 1984.
79. Davis RP, Nora PF, Kooy RG, et al: Experience with lobular carcinoma of the breast: Emphasis on recent aspects of management. Arch Surg 114:485–488, 1979.
80. Dawson EK: Carcinoma of the mammary lobule and its origin. Edinb Med J 40:57–85, 1933.
81. Delouche G, Bachelot F, Premont M, et al: Conservation treatment of early breast cancer: Long-term results and complications. Int J Radiat Oncol Biol Phys 13:29–34, 1987.
82. DeOme K: Formal discussion of multiple factors in mouse mammary tumorigenesis. Cancer Res 25:1348–1351, 1965.
83. Dershaw DD, Caravella BA, Liberman L: Limitations and complications in the utilization of stereotaxic core breast biopsy. Breast J 2:13–17, 1996.
84. Dobson J: John Hunter's views on cancer. Ann R Coll Surg 1:176–181, 1959.
85. Dowlatshahi K, Yaremko L, Kluskeus LF, et al: Nonpalpable breast lesions: Findings of stereotaxic needle-core biopsy and fine-needle aspiration cytology. Radiology 181:745–750, 1991.
86. Dronkers DJ: Stereotaxic core biopsy of breast lesions. Radiology 183:631–634, 1992.
87. Dupont WD, Page DL: Risk factors in women with proliferative breast disease. N Engl J Med 312:146–151, 1985.
88. Egan RL: Multicentric breast carcinoma: Clinical-radiographic-pathologic whole organ studies and 10-year survival. Cancer 49:1123–1130, 1982.
89. Egan RL, McSweeney MB, Sewell CW: Intramammary calcifications without an associated mass in benign and malignant diseases. Radiology 137:1–7, 1980.
90. Elvecrog EL, Lechner MC, Nelson MT: Nonpalpable breast lesions: Correlation of stereotaxic large-core needle biopsy and surgical biopsy results. Radiology 188:453–455, 1993.
91. Ewing J: Neoplastic Diseases: A Textbook on Tumors. Philadelphia, WB Saunders, 1919, pp 473, 494, 495.
92. Ewing J: Neoplastic Diseases: A Treatise on Tumors. Philadelphia, WB Saunders, 1940, p 568.
93. Farrow JH: Clinical considerations and treatment of in situ lobular breast cancer. Am J Roent Rad Ther Nucl Med 102:652–656, 1968.
94. Farrow JH: Current concepts in the detection and treatment of the earliest of early breast cancers. Cancer 25:468–477, 1970.
95. Fechner RE: Ductal carcinoma involving the lobule of the breast: A source of confusion with lobular carcinoma in situ. Cancer 28:274–281, 1971.
96. Fechner RE: Epithelial alterations in extralobular ducts of breasts with lobular carcinoma. Arch Pathol 93:164–171, 1972.
97. Fechner RE: Infiltrating lobular carcinoma without lobular carcinoma in situ. Cancer 29:1539–1545, 1972.
98. Fechner RE: One century of mammary carcinoma in situ: What have we learned? Am J Clin Pathol 100:654–661, 1993.
99. Fechner RE, Mills SE: Ductal carcinoma in situ. *In* Breast Pathology: Benign Proliferations, Atypias, and In Situ Carcinomas. Chicago, ASCP Press, 1990, pp 107–145.
100. Feig SA, Schwartz GF, Nerlinger R, et al: Prognostic factors of breast neoplasms detected on screening by mammography and physical examination. Radiology 133:577–582, 1979.
101. Fentiman IS, Fagg N, Millis RR, et al: In situ ductal carcinoma of the breast: Implications of disease pattern and treatment. Eur J Surg Oncol 12:261–266, 1986.
102. Findlay P, Goodman R: Radiation therapy for treatment of intraductal carcinoma of the breast. Am J Clin Oncol 6:281–285, 1983.
103. Fisher B, Anderson S, Fisher ER, et al: Significance of ipsilateral breast tumor recurrence after lumpectomy. Lancet 338:327–331, 1991.

104. Fisher B, Costantino J, Redmond C, et al: Lumpectomy compared with lumpectomy and radiation therapy for the treatment of intraductal breast cancer. N Engl J Med 328:1581–1586, 1993.

105. Fisher B, Redmond C, Fisher ER, et al: The contribution of recent NSABP clinical trials of primary breast cancer therapy to an understanding of tumor biology—an overview of findings. Cancer 46:1009–1025, 1980.

106. Fisher B, Redmond C, Poisson R, et al: Eight-year results of a randomized clinical trial comparing total mastectomy and lumpectomy with or without irradiation in the treatment of breast cancer. N Engl J Med 320:822–828, 1989.

107. Fisher DE, Schnitt SJ, Christian R, et al: Chest wall recurrence of ductal carcinoma in situ of the breast after mastectomy. Cancer 71:3025–3028, 1993.

108. Fisher ER: The impact of pathology on the biologic, diagnostic, prognostic and therapeutic considerations in breast cancer. Surg Clin North Am 64:1073–1093, 1984.

109. Fisher ER, Fisher B: Lobular carcinoma of the breast: An overview. Ann Surg 195:377–385, 1977.

110. Fisher ER, Fisher B, Sass R, et al: Pathologic findings from the National Surgical Adjuvant Breast Project (protocol no. 4): XI. Bilateral breast cancer. Cancer 54:3002–3011, 1984.

111. Fisher ER, Costantino J, Fisher B, et al: Pathologic findings from the National Surgical Adjuvant Breast Project (NSABP) Protocol B-17: Intraductal carcinoma (ductal carcinoma in situ). Cancer 75:1310–1319, 1995.

112. Fisher ER, Gregorio R, Fisher B: The pathology of invasive cancer: A syllabus derived from the findings of the National Surgical Adjuvant Breast Project (protocol 4). Cancer 36:1–85, 1975.

113. Fisher ER, Leeming R, Anderson S, et al: Conservative management of intraductal carcinoma (DCIS) of the breast. J Surg Oncol 47:139–147, 1991.

114. Fisher ER, Paulson JD: Karyotypic abnormalities in precursor lesions of human cancer of the breast. Am J Clin Pathol 69:284–288, 1978.

115. Fisher ER, Sass R, Fisher B, et al: Pathologic finding from The National Surgical Adjuvant Breast Project (Protocol 6). I. Intraductal carcinoma (DCIS). Cancer 57:197–208, 1986.

116. Foote FW, Stewart FW: Lobular carcinoma in situ: A rare form of mammary carcinoma. Am J Pathol 17:491–495, 1941.

117. Foote FW, Stewart FW: A histological classification of carcinoma of the breast. Surgery 19:74–99, 1946.

118. Foucar E: Carcinoma-in-situ of the breast: Have pathologists run amok? Lancet 347:707–708, 1996.

119. Fowble B: Intraductal noninvasive breast cancer: A comparison of three local treatments. Oncology 3:51–58, 1989.

120. Fowble B: The role of radiotherapy in the treatment of ductal carcinoma in situ—the challenge of the 1990s. Breast J 2:45–51, 1996.

121. Franceschi D, Crowe J, Zollinger R, et al: Biopsy of the breast for mammographically detected lesions. Surg Gynecol Obstet 171:449–455, 1990.

122. Frazier TG, Copeland EM, Gallager HS, et al: Prognosis and treatment in minimal breast cancer. Am J Surg 133:697–701, 1977.

123. Frisell J, Glas U, Hellstrom L, et al: Randomized mammographic screening for breast cancer in Stockholm. Breast Cancer Res treatment 8:45–54, 1986.

124. Frykberg ER, Bland KI: In situ breast carcinoma. Adv Surg 26:29–72, 1993.

125. Frykberg ER, Bland KI: Management of in situ and minimally invasive breast carcinoma. World J Surg 18:45–57, 1994.

126. Frykberg ER, Bland KI: Overview of the biology and management of ductal carcinoma in situ of the breast. Cancer 74:350–361, 1994.

127. Frykberg ER, Bland KI, Copeland EM: The detection and treatment of early breast cancer. Adv Surg 23:119–194, 1990.

128. Frykberg ER, Masood S, Copeland EM, et al: Ductal carcinoma in situ of the breast. Surg Gynecol Obstet 177:425–440, 1993.

129. Frykberg ER, Santiago F, Betsill WL, et al: Lobular carcinoma in situ of the breast. Surg Gynecol Obstet 164:285–301, 1987.

130. Gad A, Azzopardi AG: Lobular carcinoma of the breast: A special variant of mucin-secreting carcinoma. J Clin Pathol 28:711–716, 1975.

131. Gallager HS, Martin JE: The study of mammary carcinoma by mammography and whole organ sectioning. Cancer 23:855–873, 1969.

132. Gallager HS, Martin JE: Early phases in the development of breast cancer. Cancer 24:1170–1178, 1969.

133. Gallager HS, Martin JE: An orientation to the concept of minimal breast cancer. Cancer 28:1505–1507, 1971.

134. Gallagher WJ, Koerner FC, Wood WC: Treatment of intraductal carcinoma with limited surgery: Long-term follow-up. J Clin Oncol 7:376–380, 1989.

135. Gent HJ, Sprenger E, Dowlatshahi K: Stereotaxic needle localization and cytological diagnosis of occult breast lesions. Ann Surg 204:580–584, 1986.

136. Gilliland MD, Larson DL, Copeland EM: Appropriate timing for breast reconstruction. Plast Reconstr Surg 72:335–339, 1983.

137. Gillis DA, Dockerty MB, Clagett OT: Preinvasive intraductal carcinoma of the breast. Surg Gynecol Obstet 110:555–562, 1960.

138. Giordano JM, Klopp CT: Lobular carcinoma in situ: Incidence and treatment. Cancer 31:105–109, 1973.

139. Gisvold JJ, Goellner JR, Grant CS, et al: Breast biopsy: A comparative study of stereotaxically guided core and excisional techniques. AJR Am J Roentgenol 162:815–820, 1994.

140. Godwin JT: Chronology of lobular carcinoma of the breast: Report of a case. Cancer 5:229–266, 1952.

141. Goedde TA, Frykberg ER, Crump JM, et al: The impact of mammography on breast biopsy. Am Surg 58:661–666, 1992.

142. Goodnight JE, Quagliana JM, Morton DL: Failure of subcutaneous mastectomy to prevent the development of breast cancer. J Surg Oncol 26:198–201, 1984.

143. Goodson WH, Mailman R, Miller TR: Three year follow-up of benign fine-needle aspiration biopsies of the breast. Am J Surg 154:58–61, 1987.

144. Graversen HP, Blichert-Toft M, Dyerborg U, et al: In situ carcinomas of the female breast: Incidence, clinical findings, and DBCG proposals for management. Acta Oncol 27:679–682, 1988.

145. Greenough RB: Early diagnosis of cancer of the breast. Ann Surg 102:233–238, 1935.

146. Griffen MM, Welling RE: Needle-localized biopsy of the breast. Surg Gynecol Obstet 170:145–148, 1990.

147. Griffin A, Frazee RC: Treatment of intraductal breast cancer—noncomedo type. Am Surg 59:106–109, 1993.

148. Gullino PM: Natural history of breast cancer: Progression from hyperplasia to neoplasia as predicted by angiogenesis. Cancer 39:2697–2703, 1977.

149. Gump FE: Lobular carcinoma in situ: Pathology and treatment. Surg Clin North Am 70:873–883, 1990.

150. Gump FE, Jicha DL, Ozzello L: Ductal carcinoma in situ (DCIS): A revised concept. Surgery 102:790–795, 1987.

151. Gump FE, Shikora S, Habif DV, et al: The extent and distribution of cancer in breasts with palpable primary tumors. Ann Surg 204:384–390, 1986.

152. Gusterson BA, Machin LG, Gullick WJ, et al: Immunohistochemical distribution of c-erbB-2 in infiltrating and in situ breast cancer. Int J Cancer 42:842–845, 1988.

153. Haagensen CD: Diseases of the breast, 2nd ed, Philadelphia, WB Saunders, 1971, pp 586–590.

154. Haagensen CD: Diseases of the breast, 3rd ed. Philadelphia, WB Saunders, 1986.

155. Haagensen CD, Lane N, Lattes R: Neoplastic proliferation of the epithelium of the mammary lobules: Adenosis, lobular neoplasia, and small cell carcinoma. Surg Clin North Am 52:497–524, 1972.

156. Haagensen CD, Lane N, Lattes R, et al: Lobular neoplasia (so-called lobular carcinoma in situ) of the breast. Cancer 42:737–769, 1978.

157. Haffty BG, Peschel RE, Papadopoulos D, et al: Radiation therapy for ductal carcinoma in situ of the breast. Conn Med 54:482–484, 1990.

158. Hardman PDJ, Worth A, Lee U: The risk of occult invasive

breast cancer after excisional biopsy showing in-situ ductal carcinoma of comedo pattern. Can J Surg 32:56–60, 1989.

159. Hartmann WJ: Minimal breast cancer: An update. Cancer 53:681–684, 1984.

160. Hasselgren P-O, Hummel RP, Fieler MA: Breast biopsy with needle localization: Influence of age and mammographic feature on the rate of malignancy in 350 nonpalpable breast lesions. Surgery 110:623–628, 1991.

161. Heller KS, Rosen PP, Schottenfeld D, et al: Male breast cancer: A clinicopathologic study of 97 cases. Ann Surg 188:60–68, 1978.

162. Heteledikis S, Schnitt SJ, Morrow M, et al: Management of ductal carcinoma in situ. CA Cancer J Clin 45:244–253, 1995.

163. Holland R, Connolly JL, Gelman R, et al: The presence of an extensive intraductal component following a limited excision correlates with prominent residual disease in the remainder of the breast. J Clin Oncol 8:113–118, 1990.

164. Holland R, Hendriks JHCL, Verbeek ALM, et al: Extent, distribution, and mammographic/histological correlations of breast ductal carcinoma in situ. Lancet 335:519–522, 1990.

165. Holland R, Peterse JL, Millis RR, et al: Ductal carcinoma in situ: A proposal for a new classification. Sem Diagn Pathol 11:167–180, 1994.

166. Holland R, Veling SHJ, Mravunac M, et al: Histologic multifocality of T_{is} T_{1-2} breast carcinoma. Cancer 56:979–990, 1985.

167. Howard PW, Locker AP, Dowle CS, et al: In situ carcinoma of the breast. Eur J Surg Oncol 15:328–332, 1989.

168. Hutler RV, Kim DV: The problem of multiple lesions of the breast. Cancer 28:1591–1607, 1971.

169. Hutter RVP: The pathologist's role in minimal breast cancer. Cancer 28:1527–1536, 1971.

170. Hutter RVP: Is cured early cancer truly cancer? Cancer 47:1215–1220, 1981.

171. Hutter RVP: The management of patients with lobular carcinoma in situ of the breast. Cancer 53:798–802, 1984.

172. Hutter RVP, Foote FW: Lobular carcinoma in situ. Cancer 24:1081–1085, 1969.

173. Hutter RVP, Snyder RE, Lucas JC, et al: Clinical and pathologic correlation with mammographic findings in lobular carcinoma in situ. Cancer 23:826–839, 1969.

174. Jackman RJ, Nowels KW, Shepard MJ, et al: Stereotaxic large-core needle biopsy of 450 nonpalpable breast lesions with surgical correlation in lesions with cancer or atypical hyperplasia. Radiology 193:91–95, 1994.

175. Jatoi I, Baum M: Mammographically detected ductal carcinoma in situ: Are we overdiagnosing breast cancer? Surgery 118:118–120, 1995.

176. Jones EL, Codling BW, Oates GD: Necrotic intraduct breast carcinomas simulating inflammatory lesions. J Pathol 110:101–103, 1973.

177. Ketcham AS, Moffat FL: Vexed surgeons, perplexed patients, and breast cancers which may not be cancer. Cancer 65:387–393, 1990.

178. Killeen JL, Namiki H: DNA analysis of ductal carcinoma in situ of the breast: A comparison with histologic features. Cancer 68:2602–2607, 1991.

179. Kinne DW, Petrek JA, Osborne MP, et al: Breast carcinoma in situ. Arch Surg 124:33–36, 1989.

180. Kopans DB, Meyer JE: Versatile spring hook-wire breast lesion localizer. AJR Am J Roentgenol 138:586–588, 1982.

181. Kramer WM, Rush BF: Mammary duct proliferation in the elderly. Cancer 31:130–137, 1973.

182. Kurtz JM, Jacquemier J, Amalric R, et al: Why are local recurrences after breast-conserving therapy more frequent in younger patients? J Clin Oncol 8:591–598, 1990.

183. Kurtz JM, Jacquemier J, Torhorst J, et al: Conservation therapy for breast cancers other than infiltrating ductal carcinoma. Cancer 63:1630–1635, 1989.

184. Labat-Robert J, Birembaut P, Adnett JJ, et al: Loss of fibronectin in human breast cancer. Cell Biol Int Rep 4:609–616, 1980.

185. Lagios MD: Multicentricity of breast carcinoma demonstrated by routine correlated serial subgross and radiographic examination. Cancer 40:1726–1734, 1977.

186. Lagios MD: Duct carcinoma in situ: Pathology and treatment. Surg Clin North Am 70:853–871, 1990.

187. Lagios MD: Ductal carcinoma in situ: Controversies in diagnosis, biology and treatment. Breast J 1:68–78, 1995.

188. Lagios MD: Ductal carcinoma in situ: Biological and therapeutic implications of classification. Breast J 2:32–34, 1996.

189. Lagios MD, Margolin FR, Westdahl PR, et al: Mammographically detected duct carcinoma situ: Frequency of local recurrence following tylectomy and prognostic effect of nuclear grade on local recurrence. Cancer 63:618–624, 1989.

190. Lagios MD, Westdahl PR, Margolin FR, et al: Duct carcinoma in situ: Relationship of extent of noninvasive disease to the frequency of occult invasion, multicentricity, lymph node metastases, and short-term treatment failures. Cancer 50:1309–1314, 1982.

191. Lagios MD, Westdahl PR, Rose MR: The concept and implications of multicentricity in breast carcinoma. Pathol Ann 16:83–102, 1981.

192. Lang NP, Talbert GE, Shewmake KB, et al: The current evaluation of nonpalpable breast lesions. Arch Surg 122:1389–1391, 1987.

193. Lattes R: Lobular neoplasia (lobular carcinoma in situ) of the breast: A histological entity of controversial clinical significance. Pathol Res Pract 166:415–429, 1980.

194. Lay SF, Crump JM, Frykberg ER, et al: Breast biopsy: Changing patterns during a five-year period. Am Surg 56:79–85, 1990.

195. Leal CB, Schmitt FC, Bento MJ, et al: Ductal carcinoma in situ of the breast: Histologic categorization and its relationship to ploidy and immunohistochemical expression of hormone receptors, p53, and c-erb B-2 protein. Cancer 75:2123–2131, 1995.

196. Lenhard RE: Cancer statistics: A measure of progress. CA 46:3–27, 1996.

197. Lennington WJ, Jensen RA, Dalton LW, et al: Ductal carcinoma in situ of the breast: Heterogeneity of individual lesions. Cancer 73:118–124, 1994.

198. Lesser ML, Rosen PP, Kinne DW: Multicentricity and bilaterality in invasive breast carcinoma. Surgery 91:234–240, 1982.

199. Letton AH, Mason EM, Ramshaw BJ: Twenty-year review of a breast cancer screening project: Ninety-five percent survival of patients with nonpalpable cancers. Cancer 77:104–106, 1996.

200. Lewis D, Geschickter CF: Comedo carcinoma of the breast. Arch Surg 36:225–244, 1938.

201. Lewison EF: Lobular carcinoma in situ of the breast. Am Surg 31:787–789, 1965.

202. Lewison EF, Finney GG: Lobular carcinoma in situ of the breast. Surg Gynecol Obstet 126:1280–1286, 1968.

203. Liberman L, Cohen MA, Dershaw DD, et al: Atypical ductal hyperplasia diagnosed at stereotaxic core biopsy of breast lesions: An indication for surgical biopsy. AJR Am J Roentgenol 164:1111–1113, 1995.

204. Liberman L, Dershaw DD, Rosen PP, et al: Stereotaxic core biopsy of breast carcinoma: Accuracy at predicting invasion. Radiology 194:379–381, 1995.

205. Lilleng R, Hagmar BM, Farrants G: Low-grade cribriform ductal carcinoma in situ of the breast: Fine-needle aspiration cytology in three cases. Acta Cytol 36:48–54, 1992.

206. Liu E, Thor A, He M, et al: The HER2 (c-erb B-2) oncogene is frequently amplified in in situ carcinomas of the breast. Oncogene 7:1027–1032, 1992.

207. Locker AP, Horrocks C, Gilmour AS, et al: Flow cytometric and histological analysis of ductal carcinoma in situ of the breast. Br J Surg 77:564–567, 1990.

208. Loomer L, Brockschmidt JK, Muss HB, et al: Postoperative follow-up of patients with early breast cancer: Patterns of care among clinical oncologists and a review of the literature. Cancer 67:55–60, 1991.

209. Ludwig AS, Okagaki T, Richart RM, et al: Nuclear DNA content of lobular carcinoma in situ of the breast. Cancer 31:1553–1560, 1973.

210. Lung JA, Hart NE, Woodbury R: An overview and critical analysis of breast cancer screening. Arch Surg 128:833–838, 1988.

211. MacCarty WC: Carcinoma of the breast. Trans South Surg Assoc 23:262–270, 1911.

212. MacCarty WC: The histogenesis of cancer of the breast and its clinical significance. Surg Gynecol Obstet 17:441–446, 1913.

213. MacCarty WC: Clinical suggestions based upon a study of primary, secondary (carcinoma?) and tertiary or migratory (carcinoma) epithelial hyperplasia in the breast. Trans South Surg Assoc 26:208–213, 1913.

214. Malafa M, Chaudhuri B, Thomford NR, et al: Estrogen receptors in ductal carcinoma in situ of the breast. Am Surg 56:436–439, 1990.

215. Martin JE, Gallager HS: Mammographic diagnosis of minimal breast cancer. Cancer 28:1519–1526, 1971.

216. Masood S, Frykberg ER, McLellan GL, et al: Prospective evaluation of radiologically directed fine-needle aspiration biopsy of nonpalpable breast lesions. Cancer 66:1480–1487, 1990.

217. Masood S, Frykberg ER, McLellan GL, et al: Cytologic differentiation between proliferative and nonproliferative breast disease in mammographically guided fine-needle aspirates. Diag Cytopathol 7:581–585, 1991.

218. Matsukuma A, Enjoli M, Toyoshma S: Ductal carcinoma of the breast: An analysis of proportions of intraductal and invasive components. Pathol Res Pract 187:62–67, 1991.

219. Mayr NA, Staples JJ, Robinson RA, et al: Morphometric studies in intraductal breast carcinoma using computerized image analysis. Cancer 67:2805–2812, 1991.

220. McCormick B, Rosen PP, Kinne DW, et al: Duct carcinoma in situ of the breast: Does conservation surgery and radiotherapy provide acceptable local control? (Abstract.) Int Radiat Oncol Biol Phys 19:17, 1990.

221. McCreery BR, Frank LG, Frost DB, et al: An analysis of the results of mammographically guided biopsies of the breast. Surg Gynecol Obstet 172:223–226, 1991.

222. McDivitt RW, Hutter RVP, Foote FW, et al: In situ lobular carcinoma: Prospective follow-up study indicating cumulative patient risks. JAMA 201:96–100, 1967.

223. McDivitt RW, Stewart FW, Berg JW: Tumors of the breast. Washington, D.C., Armed Forces Institute of Pathology, 1968, pp. 63–85.

224. Meyer JE, Eberlein TJ, Stomper PC, et al: Biopsy of occult breast lesions: Analysis of 1261 abnormalities. JAMA 263:2341–2343, 1990.

225. Meyer JS: Cell kinetics of histologic variants of in situ breast cancer. Breast Cancer Res Treat 7:171–180, 1986.

226. Michaels BM, Nunn CR, Roses DF: Lobular carcinoma of the male breast. Surgery 115:402–405, 1994.

227. Mikhail RA, Nathan RC, Weiss M, et al: Stereotactic core needle biopsy of mammographic breast lesions as a viable alternative to surgical biopsy. Ann Surg Oncol 18:353–367, 1994.

228. Miller HW, Kay S: Infiltrating lobular carcinoma of the female mammary gland. Surg Gynecol Obstet 102:661–667, 1956.

229. Miller RS, Aderman RW, Espinosa MH, et al: The early detection of nonpalpable breast carcinoma with needle localization: Experience with 500 patients in a community hospital. Am Surg 58:193–198, 1992.

230. Millis RR, Thynne GSJ: In situ intraduct carcinoma of the breast: A long-term follow-up study. Br J Surg 62:957–962, 1975.

231. Mitnick JS, Vazquez MF, Pressman PI, et al: Stereotactic fine-needle aspiration biopsy for the evaluation of nonpalpable breast lesions: Report of an experience based on 2,988 cases. Ann Surg Oncol 3:185–191, 1996.

232. Mitnick JS, Vazquez MF, Roses DF, et al: Stereotactic localization for fine-needle aspiration breast biopsy: Initial experience with 300 patients. Arch Surg 126:1137–1140, 1991.

233. Moore MM: Treatment of ductal carcinoma in situ of the breast. Semin Surg Oncol 7:267–270, 1991.

234. Moriya T, Silverberg SG: Intraductal carcinoma (ductal carcinoma in situ) of the breast: A comparison of pure noninvasive tumors with those including different proportions of infiltrating carcinoma. Cancer 74:2972–2978, 1994.

235. Morris DM, Walker AP, Coker DC: Lack of efficacy of xeromammography in preoperatively detecting lobular carcinoma

in situ of the breast. Breast Cancer Res Treat 1:365–367, 1982.

236. Morrow M: Clinical applications of stereotactic biopsy. Breast J 1:326–329, 1995.

237. Morrow M: The natural history of ductal carcinoma in situ: Implications for clinical decision making. Cancer 76:1113–1115, 1995.

238. Mourad WA, Setrakian S, Hales ML, et al: The argyrophilic nucleolar organizer regions in ductal carcinoma in situ of the breast. Cancer 74:1739–1745, 1994.

239. Muir R: Evolution of carcinoma of the mamma. J Pathol Bacteriol 52:155–172, 1941.

240. Muir R, Aitkenhead AC: The healing of intra-duct carcinoma of the mamma. J Pathol Bacteriol 38:117–127, 1935.

241. Newman W: In situ lobular carcinoma of the breast: Report of 26 women with 32 cancers. Ann Surg 157:591–600, 1963.

242. Newman W: Lobular carcinoma in situ of the female breast: Report of 73 cases. Ann Surg 164:305–314, 1966.

243. Nielsen KV, Blichert-Toft M, Andersen JA: Chromosome analysis of in situ breast cancer. Acta Oncol 28:919–922, 1989.

244. Nielsen M, Jensen J, Andersen JA: Precancerous and cancerous breast lesions during lifetime and autopsy. Cancer 54:612–615, 1984.

245. Ohuchi N, Page DL, Merino MJ, et al: Expression of tumor-associated antigen (DF3) in atypical hyperplasias and in situ carcinomas of the human breast. J Natl Cancer Inst 79:109–117, 1987.

246. Opie H, Estes NC, Jewell WR, et al: Breast biopsy for nonpalpable lesions: A worthwhile endeavor? Am Surg 59:490–494, 1993.

247. Ottesen GL, Graversen HP, Blichert-Toft M, et al: Ductal carcinoma in situ of the female breast: Short-term results of a prospective nationwide study. Am J Surg Pathol 16:1183–1196, 1992.

248. Ottesen GL, Graversen HP, Blichert-Toft M, et al: Lobular carcinoma in situ of the female breast: Short-term results of a prospective nationwide study. Am J Surg Pathol 17:14–21, 1993.

249. Ozzello L: The behavior of basement membranes in intraductal carcinoma of the breast. Am J Pathol 35:887–899, 1959.

250. Ozzello L: Ultrastructure of intraepithelial carcinomas of the breast. Cancer 28:1508–1515, 1971.

251. Ozzello L, Sanpitar P: Epithelial—stromal junction of intraductal carcinoma of the breast. Cancer 26:1186–1198, 1970.

252. Pagana TJ, Lubbe WJ, Schwartz SM, et al: A comparison of palpable and nonpalpable breast cancers. Arch Surg 124:26–28, 1989.

253. Page DL: Cancer risk assessment in benign breast biopsies. Hum Pathol 9:871–874, 1986.

254. Page DL, DuPont WD, Rogers LW, et al: Atypical hyperplastic lesions of the female breast: A long-term follow-up study. Cancer 55:2698–2708, 1985.

255. Page DL, DuPont WD, Rogers LW, et al: Continued local recurrence of carcinoma 15–25 years after a diagnosis of low grade ductal carcinoma in situ of the breast treated only by biopsy. Cancer 76:1197–1200, 1995.

256. Page DL, DuPont WD, Rogers LW, et al: Intraductal carcinoma of the breast: Follow-up after biopsy only. Cancer 49:751–758, 1982.

257. Page DL, Kidd TE, DuPont WD, et al: Lobular neoplasia of the breast: Higher risk for subsequent invasive cancer predicted by more extensive disease. Hum Pathol 22:1232–1239, 1991.

258. Page DL, Lagios MD: Pathologic analysis of the National Surgical Adjuvant Breast Project (NSABP) B-17 trial: Unanswered questions remaining unanswered considering current concepts of ductal carcinoma in situ. Cancer 75:1219–1222, 1995.

259. Papatestas AE, Hermann D, Hermann G, et al: Surgery for nonpalpable breast lesions. Arch Surg 124:399–402, 1990.

260. Parker SH, Lovin JD, Jobe WE, et al: Stereotactic breast biopsy with a biopsy gun. Radiology 176:741–747, 1990.

261. Parker SH, Lovin JD, Jobe WE, et al: Nonpalpable breast lesions: Stereotactic automated large-core biopsies. Radiology 180:403–407, 1991.

262. Patchefsky AS, Schwartz GF, Finkelstein SD, et al: Heterogeneity of intraductal carcinoma of the breast. Cancer 63:731–741, 1989.

263. Patton ML, Haith LR, Goldman WT: An improved technique for needle localized biopsy of occult lesions of the breast. Surg Gynecol Obstet 176:25–29, 1993.

264. Perdue P, Page D, Nellestein M, et al: Early detection of breast carcinoma: A comparison of palpable and nonpalpable lesions. Surgery 111:656–659, 1992.

265. Peters TG, Donegan WL, Burg EA: Minimal breast cancer: A clinical appraisal. Ann Surg 186:704–710, 1977.

266. Petrovich JA, Ross DS, Sullivan JW, et al: Mammographic wire localization in diagnosis and treatment of occult carcinoma of breast. Surg Gynecol Obstet 168:239–243, 1989.

267. Pierce SM, Schnitt SJ, Harris JR: What to do about mammographically detected ductal carcinoma in situ? Cancer 70:2576–2578, 1992.

268. Poller DN, Roberts JA, Bell RA, et al: p53 Protein expression in mammary ductal carcinoma in situ: Relationship to immunohistochemical expression of estrogen receptor and c-erb B2 protein. Hum Pathol 24:463–468, 1993.

269. Porter PL, Garcia R, Moe R, et al: C-erb B-2 oncogene protein in in situ and invasive lobular breast neoplasia. Cancer 68:331–334, 1991.

270. Powers RW, O'Brien PA, Kreutner A: Lobular carcinoma in situ. J Surg Oncol 13:269–273, 1980.

271. Price P, Sinnett HD, Gusterson B, et al: Duct carcinoma in situ: Predictors of local recurrence and progression in patients treated by surgery alone. Br J Cancer 61:869–872, 1990.

272. Qualheim RE, Gall EA: Breast carcinoma with multiple sites of origin. Cancer 10:460–468, 1957.

273. Rajan PB, Perry RH: A quantitative study of patterns of basement membrane in ductal carcinoma in situ (DCIS) of the breast. Breast J 1:315–321, 1995.

274. Ray GR, Adelson J, Hayhurst E, et al: Ductal carcinoma in situ of the breast: Results of treatment by conservative surgery and definitive irradiation. Int J Radiat Oncol Biol Phys 28:105–111, 1994.

275. Recht A, Connolly JL, Schnitt SJ, et al: Conservative surgery and radiation therapy for early breast cancer: Results, controversies and unsolved problems. Semin Oncol 13:434–449, 1986.

276. Recht A, Connolly JL, Schnitt SJ, et al: Therapy of in situ cancer. Hematol Oncol Clinics North Am 3:691–708, 1989.

277. Recht A, Danoff BS, Solin LJ, et al: Intraductal carcinoma of the breast: Results of treatment with excisional biopsy and irradiation. J Clin Oncol 3:1339–1343, 1985.

278. Remak R: Ein beitrag zur entwickelungsgeschichte der krebshaften geschuwulste. Deutsche Klin 6:170–174, 1854.

279. Ringberg A, Andersson I, Aspegren K, et al: Breast carcinoma in situ in 167 women—incidence, mode of presentation, therapy, and follow-up. Eur J Surg Oncol 17:466–476, 1991.

280. Ringberg A, Palmer B, Linell F: The contralateral breast at reconstructive surgery after breast cancer operation—a histological study. Breast Cancer Res Treat 2:151–161, 1982.

281. Robbins GF, Berg JW: Bilateral primary breast cancers: A prospective clinicopathologic study. Cancer 17:1501–1527, 1964.

282. Rosai J: Borderline epithelial lesions of the breast. Am J Surg Pathol 15:209–221, 1991.

283. Rosen PP: Lobular carcinoma in situ: Recent clincopathologic studies at Memorial Hospital. Pathol Res Pract 166:430–455, 1980.

284. Rosen PP: Axillary lymph node metastases in patients with occult noninvasive breast carcinoma. Cancer 46:1298–1306, 1980.

285. Rosen PP: Coexistent lobular carcinoma in situ and intraductal carcinoma in a single lobular-duct unit. Am J Surg Pathol 4:241–246, 1980.

286. Rosen PP: Clinical implications of preinvasive and small invasive breast carcinomas. Pathol Ann 16:337–356, 1981.

287. Rosen PP: Lobular carcinoma in situ and intraductal carcinoma of the breast. Monogr Pathol 25:59–105, 1984.

288. Rosen PP, Braun DW, Kinne DE: The clinical significance of pre-invasive breast carcinoma. Cancer 46:919–925, 1980.

289. Rosen PP, Braun DW, Lyngholm B, et al: Lobular carcinoma in situ of the breast: Preliminary results of treatment by ipsilateral mastectomy and contralateral breast biopsy. Cancer 47:813–819, 1981.

290. Rosen PP, Lieberman PH, Braun DW, et al: Lobular carcinoma in situ of the breast: Detailed analysis of 99 patients with average follow-up of 24 years. Am J Surg Pathol 3:225–251, 1978.

291. Rosen PP, Menedez-Botet CJ, Nisselbaum JS, et al: Pathological review of breast lesions analyzed for estrogen receptor protein. Cancer Res 35:3187–3193, 1975.

292. Rosen PP, Senie RT, Farr GH, et al: Epidemiology of breast carcinoma: Age, menstrual status, and exogenous hormone usage in patients with lobular carcinoma in situ. Surgery 85:219–224, 1979.

293. Rosen PP, Senie RT, Schottenfeld D, et al: Noninvasive breast carcinoma: Frequency of unsuspected invasion and implications for treatment. Ann Surg 189:377–382, 1979.

294. Rosen PP, Snyder RE: Non-palpable breast lesions detected by mammography and confirmed by specimen radiography. Breast 3:13–16, 1977.

295. Rosen PP, Snyder RE, Robbins GF: Specimen radiography for non-palpable breast lesions found by mammography: Procedures and results. Cancer 34:2028–2033, 1974.

296. Rosenthal E: Quandary created by gain in detecting breast cancer. New York Times, July 21, 1990, pp 1, 11 section 1.

297. Roses DF, Mitnick J, Harris MN, et al: The risk of carcinoma in wire localization biopsies for mammographically detected clustered microcalcifications. Surgery 110:877–886, 1991.

298. Rosner D, Bedwani RN, Vana J, et al: Noninvasive breast carcinoma: Results of a national survey by the American College of Surgeons. Ann Surg 192:139–147, 1980.

299. Rosner D, Lane WW, Penetrante R: Ductal carcinoma in situ with microinvasion: A curable entity using surgery alone without need for adjuvant therapy. Cancer 67:1498–1503, 1991.

300. Rusnak CH, Pengelly DB, Hosie RT, et al: Preoperative needle localization to detect early breast cancer. Am J Surg 157:505–507, 1989.

301. Sailors DM, Crabtree JD, Land RL, et al: Needle localization for nonpalpable breast lesions. Am Surg 60:186–189, 1994.

302. Salvadori B, Bartoli C, Zurrida S, et al: Risk of invasive cancer in women with lobular carcinoma in situ of the breast. Eur J Cancer 27:35–37, 1991.

303. Schnitt SJ, Abner A, Gelman R, et al: The relationship between microscopic margins of resection and the risk of local recurrence in patients with breast cancer treated with breast-conserving surgery and radiation therapy. Cancer 74:1746–1751, 1994.

304. Schnitt SJ, Connolly JL, Khettry U, et al: Pathologic findings on re-excision of the primary site in breast cancer patients considered for treatment by primary radiation therapy. Cancer 59:675–681, 1987.

305. Schnitt SJ, Connolly JL, Tavassoli FA, et al: Interobserver reproducibility in the diagnosis of ductal proliferative breast lesions using standardized criteria. Am J Surg Pathol 16:1133–1143, 1992.

306. Schnitt SJ, Silen W, Sadowsky NL, et al: Ductal carcinoma in situ (intraductal carcinoma) of the breast. N Engl J Med 318:898–903, 1988.

307. Schuh ME, Nemoto T, Penetrante RB, et al: Intraductal carcinoma: Analysis of presentation, pathologic findings, and outcome of disease. Arch Surg 121:1303–1307, 1986.

308. Schultz-Brauns O: Die geschwulste der brustdruse. *In* Henke L, Lubarsch G (eds): Handbuch der speziellen pathologischen. Berlin, 1993.

309. Schwartz GF: Sub-clinical ductal carcinoma in situ of the breast: Selection for treatment by local excision and surveillance alone. Breast J 2:41–44, 1996.

310. Schwartz GF, Feig SA, Patchefsky AS: Significance and staging of nonpalpable carcinomas of the breast. Surg Gynecol Obstet 166:6–10, 1988.

311. Schwartz GF, Feig SA, Rosenberg AL, et al: Staging and treatment of clinically occult breast cancer. Cancer 53:1379–1384, 1984.

312. Schwartz GF, Finkel GC, Garcia JC, et al: Subclinical ductal carcinoma in situ of the breast: Treatment by local excision and surveillance alone. Cancer 70:2468–2474, 1992.

313. Schwartz GF, Patchefsky AS, Feig SA, et al: Clinically occult breast cancer: Multicentricity and implications for treatment. Ann Surg 191:8–12, 1980.

314. Schwartz GF, Patchefsky AS, Feig SA, et al: Multicentricity of non-palpable breast cancer. Cancer 45:2913–2916, 1980.

315. Schwartz GF, Patchefsky AS, Finklestein SD, et al: Nonpalpable in situ ductal carcinoma of the breast: Predictors of multicentricity and microinvasion and implications for treatment. Arch Surg 124:29–32, 1989.

316. Seidman H, Gelb SK, Silverberg E, et al: Survival experience in the breast cancer detection demonstration project. CA Cancer J Clin 37:258–290, 1987.

317. Sener SF, Candella FC, Paige ML, et al: Limitations of mammography in the identification of noninfiltrating carcinoma of the breast. Surg Gynecol Obstet 167:135–140, 1988.

318. Shah JP, Rosen PP, Robbins GF: Pitfalls of local excision in the treatment of carcinoma of the breast. Surg Gynecol Obstet 136:721–725, 1973.

319. Shapiro S, Venet W, Strax P, et al: Ten-to-fourteen year effect of screening on breast cancer mortality. J Natl Cancer Inst 46:1298–1303, 1982.

320. Sheikh FA, Tinkoff GH, Kline TS, et al: Final diagnosis by fine-needle aspiration biopsy for definitive operation in breast cancer. Am J Surg 154:470–475, 1987.

321. Shield AM: A Clinical Treatise on Diseases of the Breast. New York, MacMillan, 1898.

322. Silverberg SG, Chitale AR: Assessment of significance of proportions of intraductal and infiltrating tumor growth in ductal carcinoma of the breast. Cancer 32:830–837, 1973.

323. Silverstein MJ, Barth A, Poller DN, et al: Ten-year results comparing mastectomy to excision and radiation therapy for ductal carcinoma in situ of the breast. Eur J Cancer 37:1425–1427, 1995.

324. Silverstein MJ, Cohlan BF, Gierson ED, et al: Duct carcinoma in situ: 227 cases without microinvasion. Eur J Cancer 28:630–634, 1992.

325. Silverstein MJ, Gamagami P, Gierson ED, et al: 238 consecutive nonpalpable breast carcinomas (abstract): Proc Am Soc Clin Oncol 8:27, 1989.

326. Silverstein MJ, Gierson ED, Colburn WJ, et al: Can intraductal breast carcinoma be excised completely by local excision? Cancer 73:2985–2989, 1994.

327. Silverstein MJ, Gierson ED, Colburn WJ, et al: Axillary lymphadenectomy for intraductal carcinoma of the breast. Surg Gynecol Obstet 172:211–214, 1991.

328. Silverstein MJ, Lagios MD, Craig PH, et al: The Van Nuys prognostic index for ductal carcinoma in situ. Breast J 2:38–40, 1996.

329. Silverstein MJ, Poller DN, Waisman JR, et al: Prognostic classification of breast ductal carcinoma-in-situ. Lancet 345:1154–1157, 1995.

330. Silverstein MJ, Rosser RJ, Gierson ED, et al: Axillary lymph node dissection for intraductal breast carcinoma—Is it indicated? Cancer 59:1819–1824, 1987.

331. Silverstein MJ, Waisman JR, Gamagami P, et al: Intraductal carcinoma of the breast (208 cases): Clinical factors influencing treatment choice. Cancer 66:102–108, 1990.

332. Silverstein MJ, Waisman JR, Gierson ED, et al: Radiation therapy for intraductal carcinoma: Is it an equal alternative? Arch Surg 126:424–428, 1991.

333. Simon MS, Lemanne D, Schwartz AG, et al: Recent trends in the incidence of in situ and invasive breast cancer in the Detroit Metropolitan area (1975–1988). Cancer 71:769–774, 1993.

334. Simon MS, Schwartz AG, Martino S, et al: Trends in the diagnosis of in situ breast cancer in the Detroit Metropolitan area, 1973 to 1987. Cancer 69:466–469, 1992.

335. Simpson JF, O'Malley F, DuPont WD, et al: Heterogeneous expression of nm 23 gene product in noninvasive breast carcinoma. Cancer 73:2352–2358, 1994.

336. Simpson T, Thirlby RC, Dail DH: Surgical treatment of ductal carcinoma in situ of the breast: 10-to-20-year follow-up. Arch Surg 127:468–472, 1992.

337. Smart CR, Myers MH, Gloeckler LA: Implications from SEER data on breast cancer management. Cancer 41:787–789, 1978.

338. Smith BL, Bertagnolli M, Klein BB, et al: Evaluation of the contralateral breast: The role of biopsy at the time of treatment of primary cancer. Ann Surg 216:17–23, 1992.

339. Snyder RE: Mammography and lobular carcinoma in situ. Surg Gynecol Obstet 122:255–260, 1966.

340. Solin LJ, Fowble BL, Schultz DJ, et al: Definitive irradiation of intraductal carcinoma of the breast. Int J Radiat Oncol Biol Phys 19:843–850, 1990.

341. Solin LJ, Fowble BL, Yeh I-T, et al: Microinvasive ductal carcinoma of the breast treated with breast-conserving surgery and definitive irradiation. Int J Rad Oncol Biol Phys 23:961–968, 1992.

342. Solin LJ, Recht A, Fourquet A, et al: Ten-year results of breast-conserving surgery and definitive irradiation for intraductal carcinoma (ductal carcinoma in situ) of the breast. Cancer 68:2337–2344, 1991.

343. Solin LJ, Yeh I-T, Kurtz J, et al: Ductal carcinoma in situ (intraductal carcinoma) of the breast treated with breast-conserving surgery and definitive irradiation: Correlation of pathologic parameters with outcome of treatment. Cancer 71:2532–2542, 1993.

344. Somers SC: Histologic changes in incipient carcinoma of the breast. Cancer 23:822–825, 1969.

345. Sonnenfeld MR, Frenna TH, Weidner N, et al: Lobular carcinoma in situ: Mammographic-pathologic correlation of results of needle-directed biopsy. Radiology 181:363–367, 1991.

346. Stampfer MR, Viddavsky I, Smith HS, et al: Fibronectin production by human mammary cells. J Natl Cancer Inst 67:253–261, 1981.

347. Steeg PS, Bevilacqua G, Kopper L, et al: Evidence for a novel gene associated with low tumor metastatic potential. J Natl Cancer Inst 80:200–204, 1988.

348. Stewart FW: Tumors of the breast. In Atlas of Tumor Pathology, Fascicle 34, Washington, D.C., Armed Forces Institute of Pathology, 1950.

349. Stotter AT, McNeese M, Oswald MJ, et al: The role of limited surgery with irradiation in primary treatment of ductal in situ breast cancer. Int J Radiat Oncol Biol Phys 18:283–287, 1990.

350. Stout AP: Human Cancer: Etiological Factors, Precancerous Lesions, Growth, Spread, Symptoms, Diagnosis, Prognosis, Principles of Treatment. Philadelphia, Lea & Febiger, 1932, p 282.

351. Sunshine JA, Moseley HS, Fletcher WS, et al: Breast carcinoma in situ: A retrospective review of 112 cases with a minimum 10 year follow-up. Am J Surg 150:44–51, 1985.

352. Swain SW: Ductal carcinoma in situ. Cancer Invest 10:443–454, 1992.

353. Tabar L, Fagerberg CJG, Gad A, et al: Reduction in mortality from breast cancer after mass screening with mammography. Lancet 1:829–832, 1985.

354. Tavassoli FA, Man Y: Morphofunctional features of intraductal hyperplasia, atypical intraductal hyperplasia, and various grades of intraductal carcinoma. Breast J 1:155–162, 1995.

355. Temple WJ, Jenkins M, Alexander F, et al: In situ breast cancer in Alberta 1951–1984. (Abstract.) Am J Clin Oncol 9:109–110, 1986.

356. Temple WJ, Jenkins M, Alexander F, et al: Natural history of in situ breast cancer in a defined population. Ann Surg 210:653–657, 1989.

357. Thiersch C: Der Epithelial Krebs, Namentlich Der Haut: Eine Anatomischer-Klinische Untersuchung. Leipzig, Engelmann, 1865.

358. Tinnemans JGM, Wobbes T, Holland R, et al: Mammographic and histopathologic correlation of nonpalpable lesions of the breast and the reliability of frozen section diagnosis. Surg Gynecol Obstet 165:523–529, 1987.

359. Tinnemans JGM, Wobbes T, Van Der Sluis RF, et al: Multicentricity in nonpalpable breast carcinoma and its implications for treatment. Am J Surg 151:334–338, 1986.

360. Tobon H, Price HM: Lobular carcinoma in situ: Some ultrastructural observations. Cancer 30:1082–1091, 1972.

361. Tulusan AH, Egger H, Schneider ML, et al: A contribution to the natural history of breast cancer, IV. Lobular carcinoma in situ and its relation to breast cancer. Arch Gynecol 231:219–226, 1982.

362. Urban JA: Biopsy of the "Normal" breast in treating breast cancer. Surg Clin North Am 49:291–301, 1969.

363. Van DeVijver MJ, Peterse JL, Mooi WJ, et al: Neu-protein overexpression in breast cancer: Association with comedo-type ductal carcinoma in situ and limited prognostic value in stage II breast cancer. N Engl J Med 319:1239–1245, 1988.

364. Van Dongen JA, Harris JR, Peterse JL, et al: In situ breast cancer: The EORTC consensus meeting. Lancet 2:25–27, 1989.

365. Verbeek ALM, Hendricks JHCL, Holland R, et al: Reduction of breast cancer mortality through mass screening with modern mammography: First results of the Nijmegen project, 1975–1981. Lancet 1:1222–1224, 1984.

366. Visscher DW, Wallis TL, Crissman JD: Evaluation of chromosome aneuploidy in tissue sections of preinvasive breast carcinomas using interphase cytogenetics. Cancer 77:315–320, 1996.

367. Von Rueden DG, Wilson RE: Intraductal carcinoma of the breast. Surg Cynecol Obstet 158:105–111, 1984.

368. Waldeyer W: Die entwickelung der carcinome. Arch Pathol Anat Phys Klin Med 41:470–523, 1867.

369. Waldeyer W: Die entwickelung der carcinome. Arch Pathol Anat Phys Klin Med 55:67–159, 1872.

370. Walker RA, Dearing SJ: Transforming growth factor beta, in ductal carcinoma in situ and invasive carcinomas of the breast. Eur J Cancer 28:641–644, 1992.

371. Walt AJ, Simon M, Swanson GM: The continuing dilemma of lobular carcinoma in situ. Arch Surg 127:904–909, 1992.

372. Wanebo HJ, Feldman PS, Wilhelm MC, et al: Fine needle aspiration cytology in lieu of open biopsy in management of primary breast cancer. Ann Surg 199:569–578, 1984.

373. Wanebo HJ, Huvos HG, Urban JA: Treatment of minimal breast cancer. Cancer 33:349–357, 1974.

374. Ward BA, McKhann CF, Ravikumar TS: Ten-year follow-up of breast carcinoma in situ in Connecticut. Arch Surg 127:1392–1395, 1992.

375. Warneke J, Grossklaus D, Davis J, et al: Influence of local treatment on the recurrence rate of ductal carcinoma in situ. J Am Coll Surg 180:683–688, 1995.

376. Warner NE: Lobular carcinoma of the breast. Cancer 23:840–846, 1969.

377. Warren JC: Abnormal involution of the mammary gland with its treatment by operation. Am J Med Sci 134:521–535, 1907.

378. Webber BL, Heise H, Neifeld JP, et al: Risk of subsequent contralateral breast carcinoma in a population of patients with in situ breast carcinoma. Cancer 47:2928–2932, 1981.

379. Wertheimer MD, Costanza ME, Dodson TF, et al: Increasing the effort toward breast cancer detection. JAMA 255:1311–1315, 1986.

380. Westbrook KC, Gallager HS: Intraductal carcinoma of the breast: A comparative study. Am J Surg 130:667–670, 1975.

381. Wheeler JE, Enterline HT: Lobular carcinoma of the breast in situ and infiltrating. Pathol Annu 11:161–188, 1976.

382. Wheeler JE, Enterline HT, Roseman JM, et al: Lobular carcinoma in situ of the breast: Long-term follow-up. Cancer 34:554–563, 1974.

383. Wilhelm MC, DeParedes ES, Pope T, et al: The changing mammogram: A primary indication for needle localization biopsy. Arch Surg 121:1311–1314, 1986.

384. Wilhelm MC, Edge SB, Cole DD, et al: Nonpalpable invasive breast cancer. Ann Surg 213:600–605, 1991.

385. Wilkinson EJ, Scheuttke CM, Ferrier CM, et al: Fine-needle aspiration of breast masses: An analysis of 207 aspirates. Acta Cytol 33:613–619, 1989.

386. Wilson RE, Donegan WL, Mettlin C, et al: The 1982 national survey of carcinoma of the breast in the United States by the American College of Surgeons. Surg Gynecol Obstet 159:309–318, 1984.

387. Winchester DP, Cox JD: Standards for breast conservation treatment. CA Cancer J Clin 42:134–147, 1992.

388. Winchester DP, Menck HR, Osteen RT, et al: Treatment trends for ductal carcinoma in situ of the breast. Ann Surg Oncol 2:207–213, 1995.

389. Wobbes T, Tinnemans JGM, van der Sluis RF: Residual tumor after biopsy for non-palpable ductal carcinoma in situ of the breast. Br J Surg 76:185–186, 1989.

390. Wolf C, Rouyer N, Lutz Y, et al: Stromelysin 3 belongs to a subgroup of proteinases expressed in breast carcinoma fibroblastic cells and possibly implicated in tumor progression. Proc Natl Acad Sci USA 90:1843–1847, 1993.

391. Wolmark N: Minimal breast cancer: Advance or anachronism? Can J Surg 28:252–255, 1985.

392. Wong JH, Kopald KH, Morton DL: The impact of microinvasion on axillary node metastases and survival in patients with intraductal breast cancer. Arch Surg 125:1298–1302, 1990.

393. Wood WC: Should axillary dissection be performed in patients with DCIS? Ann Surg Oncol 2:193–194, 1995.

394. Wood WC: In situ carcinoma of the breast: Ductal and lobular cell origin. *In* Cameron JL (ed): Current Surgical Therapy, 5th ed. St. Louis, Mosby–Year Book, Inc., 1995, pp 560–565.

395. Wright CJ: Breast cancer screening: A different look at the evidence. Surgery 100:594–598, 1986.

396. Zafrani B, Fourquet A, Vilcoq JR, et al: Conservative management of intraductal breast carcinoma with tumorectomy and radiation therapy. Cancer 57:1299–1301, 1986.

397. Zavotsky J, Gardner B: Postexcisional recurrence of carcinoma of the breast. J Am Coll Surg 182:71–77, 1996.

398. Zurrida S, Bartoli C, Galimberti V, et al: Interpretation of the risk associated with the unexpected finding of lobular carcinoma in situ. Ann Surg Oncol 3:57–61, 1996.

CHAPTER 53

DUCTAL CARCINOMA *IN SITU*: CONTROVERSIAL ISSUES

Melvin J. Silverstein, M.D. / Pamela H. Craig, M.D., Ph.D.

Her agony came from the fact that mastectomy would be curative and it was hard to turn that down. A lesser procedure, while preserving her breast and her femininity, offered her somewhat less chance for a complete cure—but exactly how much less was unknown. Perhaps only a small amount less. It didn't seem worth losing her breast for a few percentage points. Yet, maybe it was. It was the most difficult decision of her life. But medicine had failed her. The data upon which to base her judgment was weak, and we had shifted the burden of that judgment to her.[95]

The preceding quote was written in 1991 about a woman with ductal carcinoma *in situ* (DCIS) of the breast and her difficult journey through the medical system as she searched for the "right" treatment. There were a number of "right" treatments then for her particular form of DCIS, but each was flawed in some way, confounding her thoughts, making her decision more difficult. But that was 1991. Today, we know a great deal more about DCIS. But the decision-making process is no easier.

The long-awaited results of National Surgical Adjuvant Breast and Bowel Project (NSABP) Protocol B-17 were published in 1993[30] and updated in 1995 and 1997.[35, 62a] This prospectively randomized study was designed to solve, once and for all, the complex treatment controversy. More than 800 patients with DCIS excised with clear surgical margins were randomized into two groups: excision only and excision plus radiation therapy. At 5 and 8 years, there were statistically significant decreases in local recurrence of DCIS and invasive breast cancer in patients treated with radiation therapy. These data led the NSABP to recommend postexcision radiation therapy for *all* patients with DCIS who chose to save their breasts, a recommendation that some consider too broad.[57, 76] The study was criticized for a number of reasons, including the NSAPB's definition of clear margins (which will be discussed in a later section of this chapter), the lack of size measurements for more than 40 percent of cases, and perhaps most importantly, a lack of pathological subset analysis.[57, 76]

Consider the following two patients, both of whom merit radiation therapy according to NSABP recommendations. Patient no. 1 is a woman with a 7-mm low-grade papillary DCIS widely excised with a minimum of 12-mm margins in all directions. Compare her with patient no. 2, a woman with a 35-mm high-grade comedo-lesion with DCIS approaching to within 0.1 mm of the inked margin but not involving it. According to the NSABP, both of these patients should be treated with radiation therapy. At our facil-

ity, based on data that will be presented later, the first patient would receive no additional therapy. She would be carefully followed with physical examination and mammography every 6 months. The second patient would undergo a wide re-excision before making a final treatment decision. Significant residual disease approaching the new margins would earn a recommendation for mastectomy and immediate reconstruction; widely clear new margins with little or no residual DCIS would earn a recommendation for radiation therapy. In spite of the results of NSABP protocol B-17, there continues to be much debate regarding the DCIS decision-making process, which is not much clearer now than it was in 1991.

There are numerous clinical, pathological, and laboratory factors that might aid clinicians and patients wrestling with the difficult treatment decision-making process. Our research has shown that nuclear grade, the presence of comedo-type necrosis (coagulative necrosis), tumor size, and margin width are all key factors in predicting local recurrence in patients with DCIS.[101, 102] By using a combination of these factors, it is possible to select subgroups of patients who do not require irradiation, if breast conservation is elected, or to select patients whose recurrence rate is potentially so high, even with breast irradiation, that mastectomy is preferable.

DCIS: A CHANGING DISEASE

As discussed in Chapter 12, DCIS is a biologically and histologically heterogeneous group of lesions.[59, 77] With the appreciation and acceptance of this heterogeneity, DCIS has become confusing for both patients and physicians. Currently, it is not uncommon for DCIS patients to seek second, third, and even fourth opinions and to receive a diverse spectrum of advice ranging from biopsy only, to wide excision, segmental resection, quadrant resection, mastectomy, or even bilateral mastectomy. With all treatments other than mastectomy, radiation therapy may or may not be advised, and there are physicians willing to support most of these options.[38, 95, 118] The second-opinion givers are usually oncologists, specializing in medicine, surgery, or radiation therapy. Some patients, however, seek this advice from gynecologists, internists, or family practitioners. Many women also seek advice from family, friends, and other women who have had breast cancer.

Table 53–1 shows the changing nature of DCIS during the last decade. Before mammography was

TABLE 53–1. DCIS: A CHANGING DISEASE

	Before 1985	After 1985
Frequency	Unusual	Common
Presentation	Palpable	Nonpalpable
Classification	Architectural	Biological
Treatment	Mastectomy	Breast conservation
Reconstruction	None/delayed	Immediate
Confusion	None	Great

Adapted from Silverstein MJ, Lagios MD: Oncology 10(11):393–410, 1997.

common, DCIS was rare, representing less than 1 percent of all breast cancer.[68, 69] Today, DCIS is common, representing at least 12 to 15 percent[88] of all newly diagnosed cases and as many as 20 to 40 percent of cases diagnosed by mammography.[56, 97] In 1997, there were more than 36,000 new cases of DCIS[128] in the United States.

Previously, most patients with DCIS were first seen with clinical symptoms, such as a breast mass, bloody or serous nipple discharge, or Paget's disease.[6, 10, 68, 115] Today, most lesions are nonpalpable, clinically unapparent, and detected by mammography alone.

Until recently, the treatment for most patients was mastectomy. Today, many patients are being treated with breast preservation. Fifteen years ago, when mastectomy was common, reconstruction was uncommon and if performed, it was generally done as a delayed procedure with implants. Today, reconstruction for patients with DCIS treated by mastectomy is common and when performed, it is generally done immediately, at the time of mastectomy and often with autologous tissue. In the past, when a mastectomy was performed, large amounts of skin were discarded. Today, it is considered safe to perform a skin-sparing mastectomy for DCIS.[48, 49, 51, 90] In the past, there was no confusion. All breast cancers were considered the same and mastectomy was the only treatment. Today, all breast cancers are different. There are many treatments and there is great confusion.

These changes were brought about by numerous factors, the most important of which were increased mammographic utilization, the improvement in mammographic technique, and the acceptance of breast-conservation therapy for invasive breast cancer.

The acceptance of mammography not only changed the way we detect DCIS, it changed the nature of the disease we detected by allowing us to enter the neoplastic continuum at an earlier time. Screening mammography and its impact on breast cancer diagnosis has been covered in detail in Chapter 33, but it is interesting to note the impact that mammography has had on our facility, The Breast Center in Van Nuys, California,[92] in terms of the number and type of DCIS cases.

From 1979 to 1981, our group treated a total of only 15 patients with DCIS, an average of 5 per year.

Only two lesions (13 percent) were nonpalpable. We added two new mammography machines and a full-time experienced mammographer in 1982, and immediately the number of new DCIS cases increased to more than 30 per year, most of them nonpalpable. With the addition of a third mammography machine in 1987, we began diagnosing almost 40 new cases per year. In 1994, we added a fourth machine and a stereotactic biopsy unit. Analysis of our series through 1995 (484 patients) reveals that 388 lesions (80 percent) were nonpalpable. If we look at only those lesions diagnosed after 1990, 87 percent were nonpalpable.

The second factor that affected how we think about DCIS was the acceptance of breast-conservation therapy (lumpectomy, axillary node dissection, and radiation therapy) for patients with invasive breast cancer. Until 1980, the treatment for most patients with any form of breast cancer was mastectomy. Since that time, numerous prospective randomized trials have revealed an equivalent survival for selected patients with invasive breast cancer treated with lumpectomy and radiation therapy.* Based on these results, it was difficult to continue treating less aggressive DCIS with mastectomy while treating more aggressive invasive breast cancer with breast preservation.

Patients often ask the question "You mean if I waited until my cancer was invasive, I could have saved my breast?" The answer of course is not simple. Although most authorities agree that there is a relationship between DCIS and invasive breast cancer, the nature of this relationship is unclear (the two entities clearly represent two different heterogeneous groups of diseases). The invasive breast cancers that are best treated by lumpectomy and radiation therapy are small invasive lesions (≤ 4 cm) with little or no intraductal component.

Nevertheless, current data suggest that many patients with DCIS can be successfully treated with breast preservation, with or without radiation therapy. In this chapter, we will show how easily available data can be used to help in the complex treatment selection process.

The majority of this chapter will be surgical in its orientation. The incidence, biology, natural history, mammography, and pathology of DCIS are discussed in Chapters 12, 17, and 27. They will be discussed in this chapter only to the extent necessary to develop the concepts that apply to the special and specific problems encountered in detecting, recognizing, classifying, and treating DCIS. Although we will review the work of others, our opinions are based largely on our own experiences. Our personal data come from a 16-year experience at The Breast Center in Van Nuys, the first free-standing breast center in the United States,[92] and includes 482 patients with DCIS treated through 1995.

---

*See references 13, 14, 29, 32, 60, and 122–124.

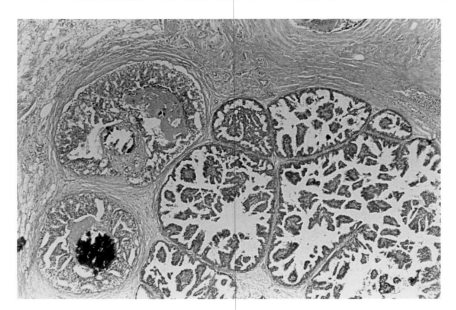

Figure 53–1 *Right side of the field reveals a low-grade micropapillary DCIS without comedo-type necrosis. The left side of the field shows two foci of an intermediate grade cribriforming DCIS with comedo-type necrosis and microcalcifications (× 20). (From Silverstein MJ, Lagios MD: Oncology 10(11):393–410, 1997.)*

CLASSIFICATION

In Chapter 12, Lagios and Page point out that there is no single universally accepted histopathological classification for DCIS. Pathologists divide DCIS into five architectural subtypes—papillary, micropapillary, cribriform, solid, and comedo—often grouping the first four together as noncomedo and comparing them with comedo.[56, 74, 120] Comedo DCIS is frequently associated with high nuclear grade,[56, 74, 83, 120] aneuploidy,[1] a higher proliferation rate,[65] *HER2* (*ERBB2*) gene amplification or protein overexpression,[2, 9, 11, 15, 62, 121] and clinically more aggressive behavior.[55, 87, 96, 111] Noncomedo lesions tend to be the opposite. However, such a division by architecture, comedo versus noncomedo, is an oversimplification and is not applicable in all cases.

Although the convention is as stated above, any architectural subtype may present with any nuclear grade with or without comedo-type necrosis. It is not uncommon for high–nuclear grade noncomedo lesions to express markers similar to high-grade comedo lesions and, as discussed later in this chapter, such lesions may require more aggressive treatment. Furthermore, mixtures of various architectural subtypes within a single biopsy specimen are common. In our series, 73 percent of all lesions had significant amounts of two or more architectural subtypes (Fig. 53–1).

Adding to the confusion, there is no uniform agreement among pathologists of exactly how much comedo DCIS needs to be present to consider the lesion a comedo DCIS. Lagios and colleagues,[54] in their original work, did not specify a specific amount. Lagios has confirmed that his earlier work was qualitative rather than quantitative and that any amount of comedo DCIS (10 or 20 percent) was sufficient to earn the label "comedo." Tavassoli[120] and Page and Anderson[74] also confirm that if any amount of comedo DCIS is present, the lesion should be considered a comedo lesion. Our group considered a lesion comedo if it was predominantly comedo, that is, 50 percent or more. Moriya and Silverberg[66, 67] required 70 percent. Poller and associates[78] used comedo-type necrosis to divide DCIS in three groups. Lesions containing at least 75 percent comedo DCIS were called pure comedo. Lesions with a lesser amount of comedo DCIS, but at least 5 percent, were called non–pure-comedo DCIS, and those with less than 5 percent or no comedonecrosis were called noncomedo DCIS. Using this

TABLE 53–2. VARYING DEFINITIONS OF COMEDO DCIS

	Percent Comedo-Necrosis Required	Nuclear Grade	Growth
Fisher et al[33, 35]	33 percent = moderate to marked	Not Applicable	Independent feature, not histological subtype
Lagios et al[54]	Any	3	Solid
Lennington et al[59]	Extensive	3	Solid, cribriform, micropapillary
Moriya and Silverberg[66]	70 percent	3	Solid
Page and Anderson[74]	Any	3	Solid or perforated
Patchefsky et al[77]	Abundant	Usually 3	Solid, cribriform, micropapillary
Poller et al[78] (pure comedo)	75 percent	3	Solid
Poller et al[78] (non–pure comedo)	5 to 74 percent	1, 2, 3	Any
Silverstein et al[96, 97]	50 percent	2, 3	Solid, cribriform, micropapillary
Tavassoli[120]	Any	3	Any

classification, they were able to correlate a variety of markers (*ERBB2*, S-phase) and outcome, as measured by local recurrence.

To complicate matters further, before a lesion is called comedo DCIS, most pathologists require the cells to be high–nuclear grade (grade 3) and their growth pattern to be solid. However, some pathologists will allow nuclear grade 2 lesions with significant comedo necrosis to be labeled comedo DCIS, and some may even allow nuclear grade 1 lesions to be called comedo DCIS. Others will allow a cribriform or micropapillary architectural pattern with significant comedo necrosis to be called comedo DCIS.

Moriya and Silverberg[67] required 70 percent of the lesion be high grade with solid growth and comedo-type necrosis before considering the lesion a comedo DCIS. Hence, only 8 percent of their DCIS cases met this criteria. Our group used a much less strict definition. We allowed nuclear grade 2 and 3 lesions to be considered comedo DCIS; we did not require uniform solid growth; and as mentioned, only 50 percent of the lesion had to be of this type. This resulted in 46 percent of our DCIS lesions being considered comedo DCIS. To add more confusion to the comedo/noncomedo classification scheme, Fisher and colleagues[33, 35] do not recognize comedo DCIS as a specific histological architectural subtype. Rather, they consider comedo-necrosis as an independent feature of DCIS, recognizing three main architectural subtypes: solid, papillary (including micropapillary), and cribriform.

Our point is clear. Architecture, without a strict set of universally agreed on criteria (which currently do not exist), is a poor way to classify DCIS. Table 53–2 points out some of the different comedo definitions in clinical use today. Current classification systems should be based on factors that reflect the biological potential of each individual lesion. Because of this, we will not present any of our data analyzed by histological architecture.

Nuclear grade is a more dependable biological indicator than architecture and has emerged as a key histopathological factor for identifying more probable aggressive behavior.* In an analysis of our own series, using only DCIS patients treated with excision plus radiation therapy, nuclear grade was the only significant factor, by multivariate analysis, that predicted for local recurrence of both DCIS and invasive breast cancer.[102]

This result led us to a more detailed analysis,[101, 105] using all breast-preservation patients in our series (excision only and excision plus radiation therapy). We analyzed 16 prognostic factors by univariate analysis (log rank test). All statistically significant predictors of local recurrence by univariate analysis were then evaluated using a Cox multivariate regression analysis with backward elimination. Nine factors were not significant predictors of local recurrence by univariate analysis: estrogen receptor (ER), progesterone receptor (PR), S-phase, ploidy, p53, mi-

crocalcifications, palpability, year of diagnosis, and age. Six factors, listed in Table 53–3, were significant predictors of local recurrence by univariate analysis; only three (nuclear grade, tumor size, and margin width) were significant predictors of local recurrence by multivariate analysis. The presence of comedo-type necrosis also approached multivariate significance ($p = 0.09$). With this in mind, in May 1995, our group introduced a new pathological DCIS classification[103] (the Van Nuys classification) based on two statistically important predictors of local recurrence: the presence or absence of high nuclear grade and comedo-type necrosis. Both factors are thought to be indicators of tumor biology. Our classification has been described and compared with other classifications in Chapter 12.

To use the Van Nuys pathological classification (Fig. 53–2), all high-grade lesions, regardless of the presence or absence of comedo-type necrosis, are placed into the worst prognostic group (Group 3). The remaining non–high-nuclear-grade lesions (nuclear grades 1 or 2) are then divided by the presence (Group 2) or absence (Group 1) of any amount of

TABLE 53–3. UNIVARIATE AND MULTIVARIATE P VALUES OF SIX PROGNOSTIC FACTORS FOUND TO BE SIGNIFICANT PREDICTORS OF LOCAL BREAST RECURRENCE

	Univariate *p* Value	Multivariate *p* Value
Nuclear grade	0.0002	0.001
Margin width	0.004	0.01
Tumor size	0.005	0.01
Presence of necrosis	0.009	0.09
Comedo architecture	0.01	NS
HER2neu (*ERBB2*)	0.02	NS

NS = not significant.

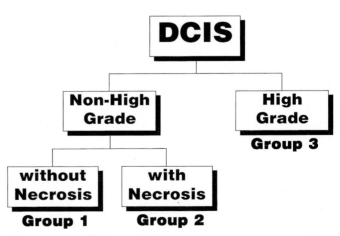

Figure 53–2 *Pathologic classification. DCIS patients are sorted into high nuclear grade and non–high nuclear grade. Non–high nuclear grade cases are then sorted by the presence or absence of comedo-type necrosis. Lesions in Group 3 (high nuclear grade) may or may not show comedo-type necrosis. (From Silverstein MJ, Poller DN, Waisman JR, Colburn WJ, Barth A, Gierson ED, Lewinsky B, Gamagami B, Slamon DJ: Lancet 345:1154–1157, 1995. © by The Lancet Ltd, 1995.)*

---

*See references 47, 53, 55, 68, 74, 103, 111, and 120.

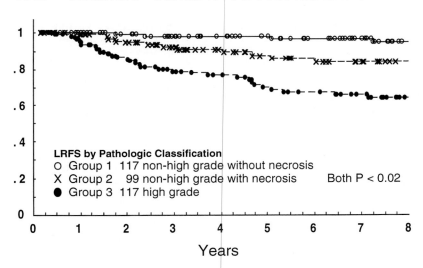

Figure 53–3 *Probability of local recurrence-free survival using Van Nuys DCIS pathological classification. (From Silverstein MJ, Lagios MD, Craig PH, Waisman JR, Lewinsky BS, Colburn WJ, Poller DM: Cancer 77:2267–2274, 1996. Copyright © (1996) American Cancer Society. Reprinted by permission of Wiley-Liss, Inc., a subsidiary of John Wiley & Sons, Inc.)*

comedo-type necrosis. This results in three easily identifiable groups with significantly different outcomes as measured by local tumor recurrence (Fig. 53–3).

High nuclear grade was chosen as the most important factor in the Van Nuys classification because of the results of our multivariate analysis (see Table 53–3) and because there is general agreement that patients with high–nuclear grade lesions are more likely to recur at a higher rate after breast conservation than patients with low–nuclear grade lesions.* Comedo-type necrosis was chosen because its presence also suggests a poor prognosis[12, 56, 78, 87, 96, 111] and it is easy to recognize.[108]

In our pathological classification, no requirement is made for a minimum or specific amount of high–nuclear grade DCIS, nor is there any requirement for a minimum or specific amount of comedo-type necrosis. Occasional desquamated or individually necrotic cells are ignored and are not scored as comedo-type necrosis.

The most difficult part of nuclear grading is the intermediate grade lesion. The subtleties of the intermediate grade lesion are not important to our classification; only nuclear Grade 3 needs to be recognized. This is fairly straightforward for most pathologists.[103] The cells must be large and pleomorphic, lack architectural differentiation and polarity, have prominent nucleoli and coarse clumped chromatin, and generally show mitoses.[56, 74, 78, 120] This pathological classification, when combined with tumor size and margin width, is an integral part of the Van Nuys prognostic index, a system that will be explained in detail later in this chapter.

DIAGNOSTIC AND SURGICAL PRETREATMENT ISSUES

Mammography

The importance of high-quality mammography cannot be overstated. During the last 5 years, 85 percent

of our DCIS patients had nonpalpable lesions. A few percent were detected as random findings during biopsy for a breast thickening or some other benign fibrocystic change; most lesions, however, were detected by mammography. The most common mammographic finding was microcalcifications, frequently clustered and generally without an associated soft tissue abnormality. Seventy-five percent of our DCIS patients exhibited microcalcifications on preoperative mammography: 61 percent of patients with nuclear Grade 1 lesions, 72 percent with Grade 2 lesions, and 84 percent with Grade 3 lesions. Because lower grade lesions are less likely to have mammographic calcifications, they are more difficult to find initially and more difficult to follow mammographically, if treated conservatively.

A major problem confronting surgeons relates to the fact that calcifications do not always map out the entire extent of the DCIS lesion, particularly in those lesions without comedo-type necrosis. Even though all the calcifications are removed, the surgeon may be leaving some DCIS behind. Sometimes, the majority of the calcifications are benign. In other words, the DCIS lesion may be smaller, larger, or the same size as the calcifications that lead to its identification. Calcifications more accurately approximate the size of high-grade than low-grade DCIS.[26, 45, 46]

In the years before mammography was common and of good quality, most DCIS presented as clinically apparent gross disease, diagnosed by palpation or inspection. Gump and associates[41] divided DCIS by the method of diagnosis into gross and microscopic disease. Similarly, Schwartz and coworkers[86] divided DCIS into clinical and subclinical disease. Both groups believed that patients with palpable masses, nipple discharge, or Paget's disease of the nipple (clinical or gross disease) required more aggressive treatment. Schwartz and coworkers believed that palpable DCIS should be treated as though it were an invasive lesion, suggesting that the pathologist simply has not found the area of invasion because of sampling error.[87] Although it is perfectly logical to believe that the change from nonpalpable to palpable

---

*See references 47, 54, 55, 68, 103, 122, and 124.

disease is a poor prognostic sign, an analysis of our data does not demonstrate a higher local recurrence rate or mortality rate for palpable DCIS when equivalent patients (by size and margin status) with palpable and nonpalpable DCIS are compared.

When a mammographic abnormality (microcalcifications, a nonpalpable mass, a subtle architectural distortion, etc.) is found, further mammographic work-up is indicated. This may include cone-down compression mammography, magnification views, or ultrasonography.[119] After this, the radiologist should render an opinion as to whether the lesion should be biopsied or followed. Although mammographic follow-up in 3 to 6 months may be medically correct for many benign-appearing lesions, it is often anxiety-provoking. If there is any question about the neoplastic nature of a lesion, we prefer that a diagnosis, benign or malignant, be made reasonably soon.

Biopsy

If a biopsy is required, there are three types: fine needle aspiration (FNA), stereotactic core, and dye or wire-directed open surgical biopsy. Fine needle aspiration is generally of little help for nonpalpable DCIS. By using mammography to localize the lesion, it is possible, with FNA, to obtain cancer cells; but because there is no tissue, there is no architecture. So although the cytopathologist can say that malignant cells are present, the cytopathologist cannot say whether the lesion is invasive. In addition, FNA of a nonpalpable lesion is difficult to do. Because the lesion cannot be felt, the FNA must be done under mammographic or stereotactic control.

Stereotactic core biopsy is relatively new, but its importance is increasing rapidly. Dedicated tables with digital attachments (Lorad and Fischer Imaging) make this a precise tool in experienced hands. For DCIS, stereotactic core biopsy, although far better than FNA, continues to present some problems. Because the biopsy sample is small, the possibility of invasion, in an area of the lesion that was not sampled, cannot be ruled out. Decisions that require a knowledge of whether invasion is present, such as axillary node dissection, may need to be based on excision of the entire lesion rather than on core biopsy. If multiple core biopsies have been performed and the lesion is subsequently removed surgically, the area of the core biopsies (performed with a large 14-gauge needle) may be disrupted, making it occasionally difficult to tell whether there is true invasion. Nevertheless, stereotactic core biopsy is extremely useful for patients with DCIS.[98]

Open surgical-directed breast biopsy makes use of an aid, such as a hooked wire or a dye-like methylene blue, to direct the surgeon to the nonpalpable mammographic abnormality. Because the wire is solid and can be palpated by the surgeon, we think that it is more reliable than dye. We have no problem with dye being used in conjunction with a wire. But by itself, without a wire, dye has disadvantages, the most important of which is that the abnormality may be

difficult to find, which in turn makes complete excision less likely. For DCIS, a single wire is better than dye without a wire, but this may not be adequate for many cases.

What remains is probably the best tool for DCIS: multiple wire–directed breast biopsy. When excising a lesion that is probably DCIS, the surgeon faces two opposing goals: clear margins versus good cosmesis. Oncologically, the largest specimen possible should be removed to achieve the widest possible margins. Cosmetically, a much smaller amount of tissue should be removed, disturbing the breast as little as possible. Because 80 percent of currently diagnosed DCIS cases are both nonpalpable and nonvisualizable, the surgeon must essentially operate blindly. Multiple wires, to a major extent, solve this problem.

The first attempt to remove a cancerous lesion is the most important. The first excision is the best chance to remove the entire lesion in one piece and to achieve the best possible cosmetic result. If involved margins force re-excision, the chances of achieving excellent cosmesis decrease. If the specimen is removed in multiple pieces, rather than a single piece, there is less likelihood of accessing margins and size accurately.

Currently, we use two (Fig. 53–4A and B) to four wires (Fig. 53–5A to D) to bracket all DCIS lesions.[94, 95] We never remove a possible DCIS using a single wire, because it may result in incomplete removal of the abnormality, calcifications at the edge of the specimen (Fig. 53–6A to C), positive histological margins, and the need to re-excise the biopsy cavity. The bracketing wire technique, although not guaranteeing complete removal during the initial biopsy, makes it more likely. Incomplete excisions are more likely to result when the mammographic abnormality does not correspond to the entire extent of the lesion.[71]

Handling of the Biopsy Specimen/Tissue Processing

Needle localization, intraoperative specimen radiography, and correlation with the preoperative mammogram should be performed in every nonpalpable case. Margins should be inked or dyed (Fig. 53–7), and specimens should be serially sectioned at 2- to 3-mm intervals (Fig. 53–8). The tissue sections should be arranged and processed sequentially. Pathological reporting should include a determination of nuclear grade, an assessment of the presence or absence of comedo-type necrosis, the measured size or extent of the lesion, the margin status with measurement of the closest margin, and a description of all architectural subtypes and the relative amounts of each.

Tumor size should be determined by direct measurement or ocular micrometry from stained slides for smaller lesions. For larger lesions, a combination of direct measurement and estimation, based on the distribution of the lesion in a sequential series of slides, should be used. The proximity of DCIS to an

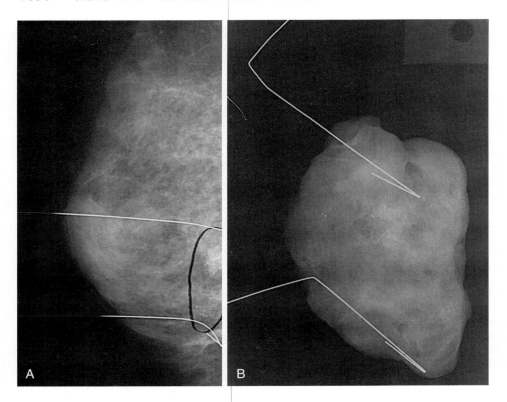

Figure 53–4 A, *Mediolateral mammogram taken after insertion of two bracketing wires around an area of microcalcifications in the extreme posterior aspect of the right breast.* **B,** *Magnification specimen radiograph of two-wire–directed breast biopsy showing a cluster of microcalcifications with mammographically clear margins (same patient as* **A***).*

inked margin should be determined by direct measurement or ocular micrometry. The closest single distance between any involved duct containing DCIS and an inked margin should be reported.

The Coordinated Biopsy Team

Removal of nonpalpable lesions is best performed with an integrated and coordinated team, consisting of a surgeon, a radiologist, and a pathologist. To obtain the most reliable results, the radiologist who places the wires must be experienced, as must the surgeon who removes the lesion and the pathologist who processes the tissue.

At the Breast Center, we were fortunate to be able to develop an optimal system for wire-directed breast biopsy. A pathologist is always present in the operating room to receive the specimen and to be oriented as to its exact position in the patient. Our pathologist then takes the specimen to our radiology department, only 100 feet away and on the same floor, where specimen radiology is carried out under the direction of the radiologist who placed the wires. We believe it is a mistake for the pathologist to perform the specimen radiology in the pathology department, particularly if the mammographic abnormality is a subtle mass or an architectural distortion. The pathologist should not be responsible for determining whether the surgeon has properly removed an area that was initially identified by another physician, the radiologist.

Ideally, the radiologist who identified the lesion

initially should place the wires, read the specimen radiogram, and inform the surgeon and the pathologist that the proper area has been removed and that the margins appear adequate by specimen radiography. When multiple radiologists are involved, passing the case from one to another, there is a greater risk of error.

Once our radiologist confirms that the proper area has been removed, our pathologist returns to the pathology laboratory, which is housed within our operating suite, and dyes the specimen, using a different color for each surface (see Fig. 53–6). Should the red surface show involved margins on final histopathological evaluation, we know it is the superior surface of the biopsy specimen and it will be relatively easy to re-excise. The entire specimen should be serially sectioned and submitted for histological evaluation (see Fig. 53–7). No tissue should be discarded.

Frozen sections should not be performed on nonpalpable lesions because of the loss of tissue caused by the frozen section process. In addition, because much of the specimen is fat (which does not freeze well), they are technically difficult to perform, often inaccurate, and may be extremely difficult to interpret. Most important, definitive treatment should not be decided on until permanent sections have been thoroughly evaluated. If questionable margins are visible to the pathologist, they can be evaluated by cytologic touch preparations. Hormone receptors, DNA analysis, *HER2*, etc., can be determined on paraffin-fixed tissue.

Once the surgeon has been told that the proper

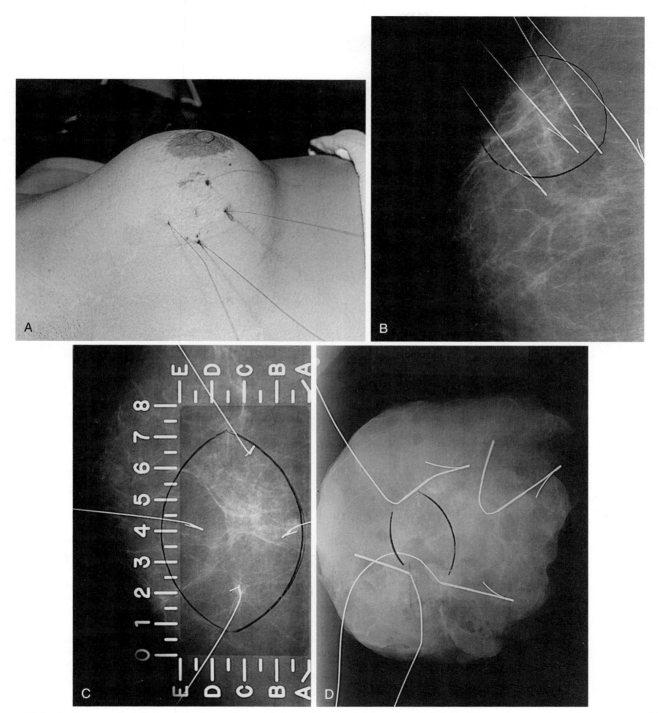

Figure 53–5   **A**, *Preoperative photograph of a patient with four wires in place.*   **B**, *Mediolateral mammogram taken after insertion of four bracketing wires around an area of architectural distortion and microcalcifications.*   **C**, *Craniocaudal mammogram taken after insertion of four bracketing wires around an area of architectural distortion and microcalcifications (same patient as* **B***).*   **D**, *Magnification specimen radiograph of four-wire–directed breast biopsy showing a cluster of microcalcifications and the architectural distortion excised with mammographically clear margins (same patient as* **B***).*

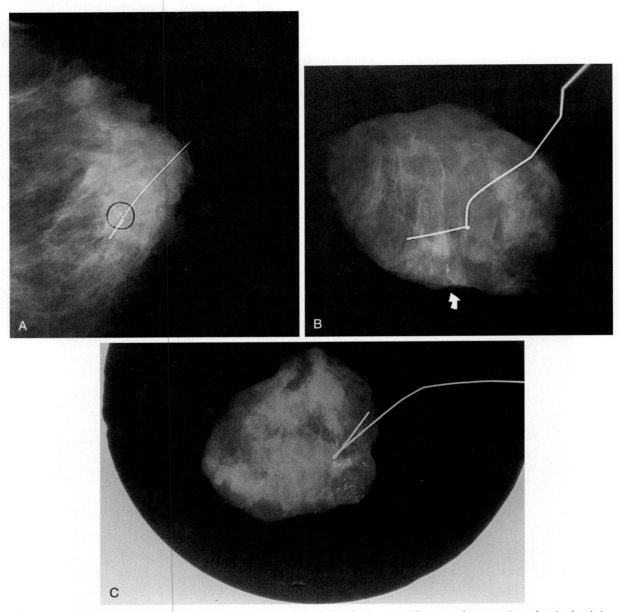

Figure 53–6   **A**, *Mediolateral mammogram taken after insertion of a single bracketing wire. The wire placement is perfect in that it is extremely close to the microcalcifications and goes 1 cm beyond them.*   **B**, *Magnification specimen radiograph of single-wire–directed breast biopsy showing a cluster of microcalcifications at the edge of the biopsy specimen (arrow) in spite of perfect wire placement (same patient as **A**).* **C**, *Specimen radiograph of another patient with a perfectly placed single wire in which the microcalcifications extend to the edge of the specimen and have been incompletely removed.*

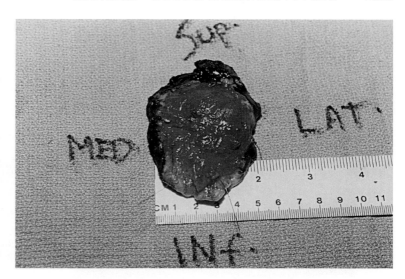

Figure 53–7   *The color-coded excision specimen with multiple wires in place oriented for the pathologist.*

area has been removed, the biopsy cavity should be marked with metallic clips (Fig. 53–9). This will identify the area of the biopsy if radiation therapy is elected or if there is a local recurrence. The surgeon should then perform a cosmetic closure. When a large amount of tissue has been removed, a flap advancement is sometimes required. At the conclusion of the procedure, we wrap the patient with a 30-foot bias pressure dressing (Fig. 53–10) over Steri-strips and fluff gauze. Using meticulous hemostasis and the bias pressure wrap, we have had to drain only four hematomas in more than 6,000 biopsies. Even ecchymoses are unusual if this wrap is applied properly.

If the lesion is large and the diagnosis unproven, we would suggest either FNA or stereotactic core biopsy as a first step to prove that malignant cells are present. If the patient is motivated for breast conservation, a multiple-wire–directed excision can be planned. This will give the patient her best chance at clear margins and good cosmesis. Our best chance at completely removing a large lesion is with a large initial excision. Our best chance at good cosmesis is

with a small initial excision. It is the surgeon's job to optimize these opposing goals. A large quadrant resection should not be performed unless there is cytologic or histological proof of malignancy or an extremely suspicious (unequivocal) mammogram. This type of resection may lead to varying degrees of breast deformity, and should the diagnosis prove to be benign, the patient will be quite unhappy. Our guidelines for excision and tissue processing of a suspected DCIS are summarized in Table 53–4.

Histological Excision Margins

We have previously mentioned how tissues should be processed and the importance of marking all margins. When this has been done properly and the pathologist reports the margins to be free of disease, what does that mean? Does it really mean that the entire lesion has been excised? First, we must define what is meant by clear margins. An initial problem is that there is no consensus on what constitutes a clear margin because different researchers use differ-

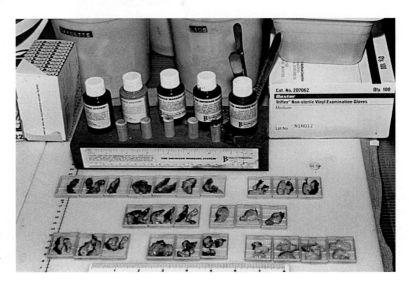

Figure 53–8   *The specimen has been color coded with dyes and serially sectioned, and will be sequentially submitted. (From Silverstein MJ: Obstet Gynecol Clin North Am 21:639–658, 1994.)*

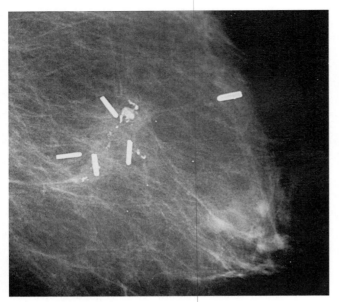

Figure 53–9 *Postoperative mediolateral mammogram. Metal clips mark biopsy cavity.*

ent criteria. Our group has used 1 mm in all directions. Shortly, we will show that 1 mm is probably inadequate.

Solin and colleagues have used 2 mm.[111] The NSABP[33] requires that the tumor has not been transected; only a few adipose cells between the tumor and the inked margin are needed to call the margin clear. Holland and associates[44] require normal breast structures between the tumor and the inked margin. Recently, the Nottingham group has required 10 mm in all directions.[89] The work of Faverly and colleagues[26] suggests that 10 mm would be an excellent

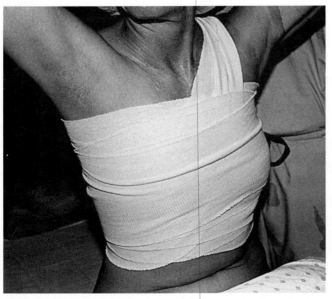

Figure 53–10 *A bias wrap, approximately 20–25 feet long, has been used to apply pressure to the biopsy site. This wrap is left in place for 48 hours.*

TABLE 53–4. GUIDELINES FOR EXCISION OF SUSPECTED DCIS

Team approach (surgeon, radiologist, pathologist)
Initial diagnosis using stereotactic core biopsy or FNA
Use multiple hooked-wires to mark extent of lesion
Remove tissue in one piece
Multiple wire placement and magnification specimen radiography by the same radiologist
Pathologist and radiologist communicate adequacy of gross excision to surgeon
No frozen sections
Mark margins with ink or colored dyes
Process all tissue sequentially
Prognostic markers, if indicated, on paraffin fixed tissue

choice for clear margins. Using serial subgross technique, they showed that only 8 percent of DCIS lesions have gaps (skip lesions) greater than 10 mm.

We have looked at the importance of margins in our series. Figure 53–11 compares the actuarial local recurrence rates when 1 mm or more is used as the definition of a clear margin. Conservatively treated tumors with a margin of 1 mm or more had a 20 percent local recurrence rate at 10 years. Those with less than 1 mm experienced a 52 percent local recurrence rate at 10 years. When the margin is 10 mm, there is a dramatic lessening of the local recurrence rate. Conservatively treated tumors with a margin of 10 mm or more had only a 4 percent local recurrence rate at 10 years. Those with less than 10 mm had a 28 percent local recurrence rate at 10 years (Fig. 53–12). As mentioned above, the three-dimensional work of Faverly and associates[26] suggests that skip areas are generally less then 10 mm in length and that 10-mm margins may be the gold standard. Our results and the low rate of local recurrence reported by the Nottingham Group[89] support this conclusion.

However, 10-mm margins in every direction may be difficult to achieve in some cases while obtaining good cosmesis. In the operating room, the surgeon is faced with a difficult problem: a lesion that generally can neither be seen nor felt. The best chance for a complete excision with widely clear margins comes with the placement of multiple hooked-wires around a lesion whose extent is well delineated by microcalcifications. If the lesion extends significantly beyond the calcifications, complete excision is far less likely and will only occur if the surgeon is not only competent but lucky.

TREATMENT

For most patients, there will be no single correct treatment approach. There will generally be a choice, and the choices, although seemingly simple, are not. As the treatment alternatives increase and become more complicated, frustration will increase for both patient and physician.[95]

Counseling the Patient with Biopsy-Proven DCIS

There is no easy way to tell a patient that she has breast cancer. But is DCIS really breast cancer?

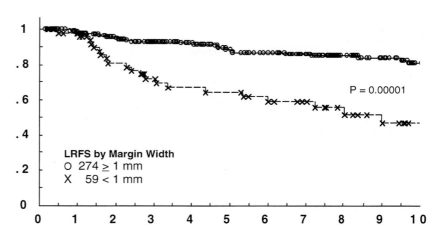

Figure 53–11 *Probability of local recurrence-free survival comparing margins 1 mm or more with margins 1 mm or less for 333 breast conservation patients.*

When we think of cancer, we think of a disease, that if untreated, runs an unrelenting course toward death. That is certainly not the case with DCIS. The cancer phenotype consists of at least five factors: unlimited growth, genomic elasticity (resistance to treatment), angiogenesis, invasion, and metastasis.[23, 61] DCIS lacks the latter two. In all likelihood, when we understand why some DCIS lesions develop the ability to invade and metastasize and why others do not, we will have opened the door to far greater understanding of the neoplastic process.

When counseling a patient with DCIS, it must be emphasized that she has a borderline cancerous lesion, a "preinvasive" lesion, which, at this time, is not a threat to her life. In our series of 482 patients with DCIS, the absolute mortality rate is less than 0.6 percent (there have been only three breast cancer–related deaths). The 10-year actuarial mortality rate is 1 percent for all patients and 2 percent for breast-preservation patients. Numerous other DCIS series* confirm an extremely low mortality rate (Table 53–5).

One of the most frequent concerns expressed by patients once a diagnosis of cancer has been made is the fear that the cancer has "spread." The patient with DCIS can be assured that no invasion was seen

---

*See references 4–6, 20, 22, 25, 27, 30, 56, and 102.

microscopically and that the likelihood of systemic spread is minimal.

The patient needs to be educated that the term *breast cancer* encompasses a wide variety of lesions with a wide range of aggressiveness and lethal potential. The patient with DCIS must be, and needs to be, reassured that she has a minimal lesion and that she may need some additional treatment, which might include further surgery, radiation therapy, or both. She needs to know that she will not need chemotherapy, that her hair will not fall out, and that it is highly unlikely that she will die of this lesion. She will, of course, also need careful clinical follow-up.

Mastectomy

Until the 1980s, just about all breast cancer, including the occasional rare case of DCIS, was treated with mastectomy. Although clinicians began using breast conservation (excision of the tumor, axillary dissection, and whole-breast irradiation) for small invasive lesions, the treatment of DCIS did not keep pace. Surgeons continued to perform mastectomies for less aggressive DCIS while recommending breast conservation for more aggressive invasive lesions. Because of this, there is a large amount of data available regarding outcome after mastectomy for DCIS. Most mastectomy studies, however, reflect le-

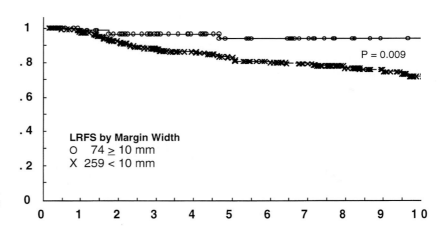

Figure 53–12 *Probability of local recurrence-free survival comparing margins 10 mm or more with margins less than 10 mm for 333 breast conservation patients.*

TABLE 53–5.   LOCAL RECURRENCE AND DEATH FROM BREAST CANCER AFTER MASTECTOMY FOR DCIS

Author	No. of Patients	Follow-up (yr)	Local Recurrence	No. Dead of Breast Cancer
Archer et al[4]	52	11.1	0	0
Arnesson et al[5]	28	6.4	0	0
Ashikari et al[6]	110	1–10	2	1
Brown et al[18]	39	1–15	0	0
Carter and Smith[20]	38	6.2	0	1
Ciatto et al[22]	210	5.5	3	1
Farrow[25]	181	2–20	2	4
Fentiman et al[27]	76	4.8	1	1
Fisher et al[34]	28	7.1	0	1
Kinne et al[50]	101	11.5	1	1
Lagios et al[54]	53	3.7	2	1
Rosner et al[84]	182	5	—	3
Schuh et al[85]	51	5.5	0	1
Silverstein et al[102]	221	6.1	2	0
Simpson et al[107]	34	17.7	0	0
Sunshine et al[117]	68	10	0	3
Von Reuden and Wilson[125]	47	1–22	0	0
Westbrook and Gallager[126]	60	5–25	1	0
Total	**1579**	**7.7 (mean)**	**14 (0.09 percent)**	**18 (1.1 percent)**

sions that were palpable and generally larger than those routinely discovered today.

Table 53–5 lists 18 studies with a total of 1579 patients, in which mastectomy was used as the treatment for DCIS. The local recurrence rate was 0.9 percent; the mortality rate was 1.1 percent. In our series at the Breast Center through 1995,[102] there were 221 patients treated with mastectomy; 2 of whom (1 percent) have recurred, neither of whom (0 percent) has died of breast cancer. Mastectomy clearly works for DCIS. But for many patients, it represents overtreatment. Mastectomy is physically deforming and may be psychologically mutilating even with optimal breast reconstruction. Our challenge is to select for mastectomy only those patients who require it because a lesser procedure would lead to an unacceptably high local recurrence rate.

Mastectomy is indicated for large diffuse lesions, for patients with documented multicentric disease (biopsy proof of DCIS in multiple quadrants), for patients unwilling to take even the slightest increased risk of death from an invasive local recurrence, for patients who have no interest in breast conservation or who are medically unsuited for breast conservation, and for patients who are unwilling or unable to undergo careful long-term clinical follow-up.

When mastectomy is required and reconstruction is desired, we generally perform a procedure that we call glandular replacement therapy (GRT).[48, 49] Glandular replacement therapy consists of the combination of a skin-sparing mastectomy and an autologous tissue reconstruction. Because DCIS does not invade the skin, there is no reason to discard large amounts of skin as when mastectomy is performed for a large invasive breast cancer close to or involving overlying skin. Figure 53–13 shows the skin incision for GRT compared with standard mastectomy. By saving most of the skin, the original skin envelope is preserved. When this is filled with autologous tissue,

it generally yields a breast of similar size, shape, and consistency when compared with the remaining contralateral breast (Fig. 53–14). Our usual choice for autologous tissue is generally a free TRAM (transrectus abdominus myocutaneous) flap, although pedicle TRAM flaps are used occasionally.

Breast Conservation for DCIS

Currently, breast conservation for small invasive tumors is being used with increasing frequency. Because of this, it is extremely difficult to justify the continued use of mastectomy for less aggressive noninvasive disease.

Breast conservation for DCIS is performed differently from breast conservation for invasive breast cancer. An invasive lesion requires excision of the primary tumor with clear margins, axillary node dissection, whole breast irradiation, a possible radiation

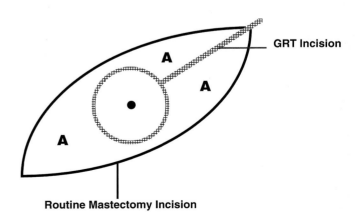

Figure 53–13   *Skin incision for glandular replacement therapy (skin-sparing mastectomy and immediate reconstruction). The area marked by the letter A (about 70 cm² in the average patient) represents the additional skin that would have been removed with a standard mastectomy.*

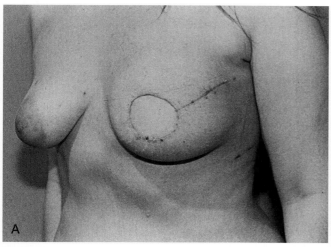
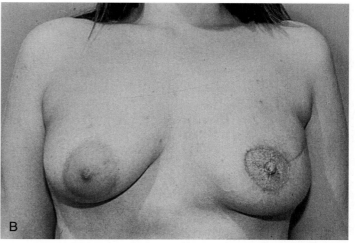

Figure 53–14 *Cosmetic results of glandular replacement therapy.* **A,** *A reconstructed breast after skin-sparing mastectomy and TRAM flap reconstruction (GRT). The island of skin that has been replaced is circular and exactly the same size as the nipple/areolar complex that has been removed.* **B,** *The nipple/areolar complex has been reconstructed.*

boost to the area of the tumor, and chemotherapy, if nodes are positive or if the primary tumor has poor prognostic features.

Breast conservation for DCIS is different. It requires, at a minimum, excision of the primary tumor, preferably with clear histological margins. Radiation therapy may or may not be added. Neither chemotherapy nor axillary dissection is indicated.

The serial subgross studies of Holland and associates[45] in which they found that 81 of 82 DCIS lesions were unifocal (not multifocal) suggests that, at least theoretically, many DCIS lesions can be completely excised surgically. Unfortunately, 23 percent of the lesions studied by Holland and associates occupied more than a full quadrant of the breast. Nevertheless, in a large percentage of cases, it is potentially possible to excise the entire lesion while achieving acceptable cosmesis. High-quality mammography and an aggressive biopsy policy using stereotactic cores and multiple hooked wires will yield a higher percentage of smaller lesions that can be completely excised with excellent cosmetic results.

Why Is Local Recurrence Important?

If all local recurrences were noninvasive (DCIS), there would be little danger and, therefore, little indication for mastectomy as the initial procedure for patients with DCIS. In our own series,[102] as in most other reported series,[21, 24, 56, 58, 111, 114] approximately half of all local recurrences were invasive (Tables 53–6 and 53–7). Local recurrences are, therefore, extremely important. When they occur in patients who have struggled to save their breasts, they are both demoralizing and theoretically, a threat to life. By avoiding mastectomy, we gain psychological and physical advantages, but when there is an invasive recurrence, we have permitted an almost totally curable noninvasive lesion to advance to a potentially less curable form. An invasive recurrence represents

TABLE 53–6.   RECURRENCE AFTER LOCAL EXCISION ONLY

Author	No. of Patients	Follow-up (yr)	No. of Recurrences	
			Total	Invasive
Arnesson et al[5]	38	5	5	2
Baird et al[7]	30	3.3	4	1
Carpenter et al[19]	28	3.2	5	1
Cataliotti et al[21]	46	7.8	5	5
Eusebi et al[24]	80	17.5	16	11
Fisher et al[30]	391	3.6	64	32
Fisher et al[34]	21	7.1	9	5
Gallagher et al[40]	13	8.3	5	3
Laigos et al[58]	79	10	13	6
Price et al[79]	35	9	22	12
Schwartz et al[86, 87]	72	4	11	3
Silverstein*	122	3.1	18	6
Total	**955**	**5.8 (mean)**	**177 (18 percent)**	**87 (49 percent)**

*Unpublished data.

TABLE 53–7.   RECURRENCE AFTER EXCISION PLUS RADIATION THERAPY

Author	No. of Patients	Follow-up (yr)	No. of Recurrences Total	Invasive
Archer et al[4]	21	11.1	3	3
Baird et al[7]	8	3.3	2	1
Fisher et al[30]	399	3.6	28	8
Fisher et al[34]	27	7.1	2	1
Fourquet et al[37]	67	8.7	7	5
Haffty et al[42]	60	3.6	4	1
Hiramatsu et al[43]	76	6.2	7	4
Kurtz et al[52]	43	5.1	3	3
Kuske et al[53]	70	4.0	3	3
McCormick et al[64]	54	3.0	10	3
Ray et al[80]	58	5.1	5	1
Silverstein et al[102]	139	7.8	23	12
Sneige et al[109]	49	7.2	5	3
Solin et al[114]	270	10.3	45	24
Stotter et al[116]	42	7.7	4	4
White et al[127]	53	5.7	3	1
Zafrani et al[129]	55	4.6	3	1
Total	**1489**	**6.3 (mean)**	**157 (11 percent)**	**77 (49 percent)**

a biological worsening of the stage of disease that may, in turn, ultimately translate into higher mortality for patients initially treated conservatively.

Local breast recurrence is usually treated with mastectomy. Solin and associates[110–114] reported 45 local recurrences occurring in 270 breasts treated with excision and radiation therapy. The median time to local recurrence was 5.2 years; 53 percent of the local recurrences were invasive; and 42 patients were treated with salvage mastectomy. The breast cancer–specific survival rate at 5 years for those who recurred was 84 percent.

In our own series, the median time to local failure in radiated patients was 4.8 years, similar to Solin and associates. The median time to local failure for nonradiated patients treated with excision was only 1.8 years. Radiation therapy may prevent some local recurrences and merely delay others.

Excision Alone

For more than a decade, Lagios and associates[54–56] have promoted breast conservation without radiation therapy. They began, in the 1970s, by treating selected patients with DCIS with excision only. Their strict criteria for eligibility required that all lesions be nonpalpable, discovered mammographically, 25 mm or less in maximum size, and free of microcalcifications on postoperative mammography. Recently, Lagios reported a 12 percent actuarial local recurrence rate at 5 years and 16 percent at 10 years.[58] There were no breast cancer–related deaths and no patients have developed distant metastases.

A number of other investigators[30, 72, 87] have reported similar but slightly higher rates of local recurrence for DCIS treated by excision only. The NSABP (whose prospective randomized trial will be discussed shortly) has reported an actuarial local recurrence rate of 20.9 percent at 5 years.[30] Schwartz[87] has reported a 15.3 percent (absolute rate) at 4 years. On an actuarial basis, this is likely to be about 20 percent at 5 years, similar to the NSABP.

At our facility, we have treated 122 DCIS patients with excision only. There were 18 local recurrences, 6 of which were invasive, and no breast cancer–related deaths through 1995. The 5-year actuarial local recurrence rate was 21 percent.

The average size of the tumors in Lagios' series was 7 mm. In addition, Lagios used the strictest criteria for inclusion in his protocol, explaining why his local recurrence rates are lower than other reported studies, in spite of longer follow-up.

Table 53–6 lists 12 studies with a total of 955 patients, in which excision alone was used as the treatment for DCIS. The raw local recurrence rate was 18 percent; 49 percent of all local recurrences were invasive. The mean follow-up was only 5.8 years. With longer follow-up, the local recurrence rate is likely to climb to as much as 30 percent.

We did not include the "biopsy only" series of Rosen and colleagues[82] and Page and associates[73, 75] in Table 53–6 because in these studies, the diagnosis of DCIS was initially missed and therefore no attempt was made to obtain clear surgical margins. All cases in both series were low- to intermediate-grade DCIS without comedonecrosis (generally micropapillary and cribriform architecture). Page's recent update[75] revealed a 22 percent breast cancer–specific mortality and a 42 percent local recurrence rate with a median follow-up of 24 years. Because these patients were essentially untreated, they offer insight into the natural history of low- to intermediate-grade DCIS.

These findings and the fact that autopsy studies[70] reveal an occult incidence of DCIS as high as 14 percent suggest that many DCIS lesions are not clinically significant and are unlikely to progress to invasive breast cancer.[3, 67]

Excision with Radiation Therapy

Numerous retrospective analyses of patients with DCIS treated with breast-conserving surgery and radiation therapy have been published.[16, 42, 53, 64, 110, 111] Table 53–7 lists 17 studies with a total of 1489 patients, in which excision followed by radiation therapy was used as the treatment for DCIS. The local recurrence rate was 11 percent. Again, 49 percent of the recurrences were invasive. The mean follow-up is relatively short (6.3 years).

The largest of the retrospective radiation analyses is that of Solin and associates.[110–114] They combined the data of nine institutions in the United States and Europe. A total of 270 DCIS lesions were treated with excision plus breast irradiation. The 15-year actuarial local recurrence rate was 19 percent. Half the recurrences were DCIS and half were invasive. The 15-year breast cancer–specific survival rate was 96 percent.[113, 114]

At our facility, we have treated a total of 139 DCIS patients with excision plus radiation therapy. There were 23 local recurrences, 12 of which were invasive. There have been 3 breast cancer–related deaths. The 5- and 10-year actuarial local recurrence rates for DCIS patients treated with excision plus radiation therapy were 12 percent and 22 percent respectively.

In 1985, the NSABP began a prospective randomized trial to evaluate the worth of postoperative breast irradiation after excision of the DCIS lesion. After lesionectomy with clear margins (remember that the NSABP defines clear margins as tumor not transected), patients were randomized to receive ipsilateral breast irradiation or no further therapy. Axillary node dissection was required until June 1987. Thereafter, it was optional, at the surgeon's discretion. If an axillary dissection was performed, the nodes had to be negative.

In May 1993, the first NSABP report was published.[30] A total of 790 patients were evaluable: 391 treated by excision only and 399 treated by excision plus breast irradiation. The 5-year actuarial local recurrence rate was 10.4 percent for excision plus irradiation and 20.9 percent for excision only. The difference was significant. There were 64 recurrences in the excision-only group, exactly half of which were invasive. There were 28 recurrences in the excision plus irradiation group, only 8 of which were invasive (29 percent). The NSABP concluded that excision plus breast irradiation was more appropriate than excision alone for patients with localized DCIS, and if there were a local recurrence, radiation statistically decreased the likelihood that it would be invasive. After years of retrospective analyses, this was the first prospective randomized clinical trial for patients with DCIS, and it is of profound importance.

The NSABP recommended lesionectomy and irradiation for all conservatively treated patients with localized DCIS and clear margins (by their definition), regardless of histological architectural subtype, nuclear grade, or size of the DCIS lesion. In other words, they concluded that excision alone for DCIS was inappropriate. Although we give great credit to the NSABP for organizing and conducting an outstanding study, it is difficult for clinicians to use global recommendations in an age of sophisticated consumer medicine. NSABP B-17 was designed in the mid 1980s. By the mid 1990s, physicians and patients had become more sophisticated and required significantly more data than were available from NSABP B-17.

The NSABP gave no recurrence analysis by subset. The NSABP reported that almost 50 percent of patients had comedonecrosis, more than 85 percent of patients had lesions 20 mm or smaller, and 81 percent of lesions were nonpalpable. But there was no analysis of how any of these parameters affected outcome. The initial report stated that more than 40 percent of lesions measured less than 1 mm. This was later corrected in a letter to the editor of *The New England Journal of Medicine*[31] in which it was stated that no size had been listed on the pathology report and that these tumors should have been listed as "size unknown."

The NSABP reported that radiation-treated patients had a 5-year actuarial local recurrence rate of 10.4 percent, and nonirradiated patients had a 20.9 percent actuarial local recurrence rate. They stated how many recurrences were invasive and how many were noninvasive in each group. But because there was no subset analysis, there was no way for the reader to see whether the local recurrence rate was different for a 6-mm low-grade micropapillary lesion with widely clear margins compared with a 30-mm high-grade comedo DCIS with minimally (0.2 mm) clear margins. The NSABP did not state whether patients with palpable DCIS recurred at a higher rate than patients with nonpalpable lesions. Because of these shortcomings, the paper was criticized[57, 76] and vigorous debate followed.[36]

In 1995, the NSABP published a second report, detailing the pathological findings from NSABP protocol B-17.[35] Microscopic slides were available for 573 of the original 790 patients. After central pathology review, all met the criteria for the diagnosis of DCIS. In this analysis, both comedo-type necrosis and margin status (close or involved) were found to be significant predictors of an increased likelihood of local recurrence. Some patients, originally thought to have clear margins, were found to have involved margins at review. The NSABP, however, did not change its recommendation that all patients with DCIS electing breast conservation receive radiation therapy in addition to excision with clear margins. In fact, at the 1995 St. Gallen Adjuvant Therapy of Breast Cancer Meeting,[63] Fisher and Margolese independently reiterated the NSABP position that all conservatively treated patients with DCIS should receive postoperative radiation therapy.

Detailed pathology, as described here, with careful measurements of margins, size, and nuclear grade, may be impractical for many pathologists during an era of increasing cost-consciousness. Therefore, the NSABP's recommendation of radiation therapy for all patients with DCIS who wish conservative treatment may be the safest approach, in the absence of meticulous pathological assessment.

We find, however, that we cannot agree with this position. Detailed subset analysis has allowed clinicians to select which patients with infections need antibiotics and which patients with invasive breast cancer might benefit from chemotherapy. Similarly, subset analysis should allow us to select which patients with DCIS might benefit from radiation therapy and which might not. Although we agree with the national need to economize, we do not believe that incomplete pathology is the answer to our financial troubles.

The Van Nuys Prognostic Index

Should all conservatively treated patients with DCIS receive postoperative radiation therapy? It is clear that breast irradiation reduces the local recurrence rate by about 50 percent at 5 years (from around 20 percent to around 10 percent). Series with longer follow-up,[42, 110] however, suggest that as time passes, recurrences will continue to accrue in the patients treated with radiation therapy. This raises speculation that at least in some patients, radiation merely delays, rather than prevents, an inevitable recurrence. There is now sufficient, easily available information that can aid clinicians in differentiating patients who require radiation therapy after excision from those who do not. These same data can point out patients who are better served by mastectomy because recurrence rates with breast conservation are unacceptably high with or without radiation therapy.

Our research[101–103] and the research of others* has shown that various combinations of nuclear grade, the presence of comedo-type necrosis, tumor size, and margin status are all important factors that can be used in predicting local recurrence in conservatively treated patients with DCIS (see Table 53–3). It may be possible, by using a combination of these factors, to select subgroups of patients who do not require radiation therapy in addition to complete excision or to select patients whose recurrence rate is theoretically so high, even with breast irradiation, that mastectomy is preferable.

We used the first two of these prognostic factors (nuclear grade and necrosis) to develop the Van Nuys DCIS pathological classification[103] described earlier in this chapter (henceforth, called pathological classification). Nuclear grade and comedo-type necrosis reflect the biology of the lesion, but neither are adequate as the sole guidelines in the treatment decision-making process. Tumor size and margin width reflect the extent of disease, the adequacy of surgical treatment, and the likelihood of residual disease and are, therefore, extremely important. The results of the multivariate analysis confirm the critical importance of these variables.

*See references 12, 35, 54, 55, 56, 58, 72, 78, 87, 111, and 130.

Therefore, the Van Nuys prognostic index (VNPI)[104–106] was devised by combining these three statistically significant predictors of local tumor recurrence in patients with DCIS: tumor size, margin width, and pathological classification. A score, ranging from 1 for lesions with the best prognosis to 3 for lesions with the worst prognosis, was given for each of the three predictors. The objective with all three predictors was to create three statistically different subgroups for each, using local recurrence as the marker of treatment failure. Cutoff points (for example, what size or margin width constitutes low, intermediate or high risk of local recurrence) were determined statistically using the log rank test with an optimum p-value approach.

Size Score. A score of 1 was given for small tumors 15 mm or less, 2 was given for intermediate sized tumors 16 to 40 mm, and 3 was given for large tumors 41 mm or more in diameter.

Margin Score. A score of 1 was given for widely clear tumor-free margins of 10 mm or more. This was most commonly achieved by re-excision with the finding of no residual DCIS or only focal residual DCIS in the biopsy cavity. A score of 2 was given for intermediate margins of 1 to 9 mm and a score of 3 for margins less than 1 mm (involved or close margins).

Pathological Classification Score[103]. A score of 3 was given for tumors classified as Group 3 (all high-grade lesions), 2 for tumors classified as Group 2 (non–high-grade lesion with comedo-type necrosis), and a score of 1 for tumors classified as Group 1 (non–high-grade lesion without comedo-type necrosis).

Calculating the Van Nuys Prognostic Index. The initial VNPI formula was determined by using the beta values, obtained from the multivariate analysis (Table 53–8), which show the relative contribution of each factor in the estimation of the likelihood of local recurrence.[102]

$$VNPI = 0.869 \text{ pathological classification score} + 0.864 \text{ margin score} + 0.749 \text{ size score}$$

Using this relatively user-unfriendly formula, 27 groups of patients were generated, with scores ranging from the lowest possible value of 2.482 to the highest possible value of 7.446. The 27 groups natu-

TABLE 53–8. RESULTS OF COX REGRESSION ANALYSIS

	Beta	Standard Error	t-Value	p Value
Tumor size	.749	.200	3.737	<0.001
Margin width	.865	.243	3.564	<0.001
Pathological classification	.869	.201	4.313	<0.0001

TABLE 53–9.   THE VAN NUYS PROGNOSTIC INDEX (VNPI)*

Score	1	2	3
Size (mm)	≤15	16–40	≥41
Margins (mm)	≥10	1–9	<1
Pathological classification	Non–high-grade without necrosis	Non–high-grade with necrosis	High-grade with or without necrosis

* One to three points are awarded for each of three different predictors of local breast recurrence (size, margins, and pathological classification). Scores for each of the predictors are totaled to yield a VNPI score ranging from a low of 3 to a high of 9. From Silverstein MJ, Lagios MD, Craig PH, Waisman JR, Lewinsky BS, Colburn WJ, Poller DM: Cancer 77:2267–2274, 1996.

rally divided into three prognostic subgroups: one with a low risk of recurrence, one with an intermediate risk of recurrence, and one with a high risk of local recurrence. Additional analyses revealed that the formula could be simplified, without compromising validity, by omitting the beta weighting, suggested by the multivariate analysis, and by readjusting the numerical range for each of the three subgroups. The final formula became:

$$\text{VNPI} = \text{pathological classification score} \\ + \text{margin score} + \text{size score.}$$

This formula yielded seven groups with whole number scores ranging from 3 to 9. The best possible VNPI score was 3, resulting from a score of 1 for each predictor, e.g., a 5-mm low-grade lesion with widely clear margins (≥ 10 mm) would earn a score of 3. The worst possible score was 9, a score of 3 for each predictor, e.g., a 50-mm high-grade lesion with close or involved margins (< 1 mm) would earn a score of 9. Table 53–9 summarizes the scoring for the VNPI. When patients were subdivided into groups with scores of 3 or 4; 5, 6, or 7; and 8 or 9, the results were identical when compared with the more complicated beta-weighted version, and the VNPI was much easier to use.

Results of Analysis Using the VNPI

The VNPI was initially tested on 254 breast-conservation patients from The Breast Center. After this,

it was independently validated by analyzing Lagios' series of 79 patients.[106] Both groups use similar tissue processing and have consulted each another for more than 10 years. The local recurrence-free survival (LRFS) curves for comparable patients in each group were almost identical, with no statistical differences found in any subgroup tested (Fig. 53–15). The two groups of patients were therefore combined to yield 333 patients with DCIS treated with breast preservation.

The LRFS for all 333 patients is shown by tumor size in Figure 53–16, by margin width in Figure 53–17, and by pathological classification in Figure 53–3. The differences between every survival curve for each of the three predictors that make up the VNPI are statistically significant.

Figure 53–18 shows the disease-free survival for each of the 7 VNPI groups, 3 through 9. Figure 53–19 groups patients with low (VNPI = 3 or 4), intermediate (VNPI = 5, 6, or 7), or high (VNPI = 8 or 9) recurrence rates together. Each of these three groups are statistically different from one another.

Patients with low VNPI scores of 3 or 4 do not show a decrease in local recurrence from breast irradiation (Fig. 53–20) ($p = 0.43$). Patients with intermediate VNPI scores of 5, 6, or 7 benefit from irradiation (Fig. 53–21). There is a statistically significant average 14 percent decrease in the local recurrence rate in irradiated breasts compared with those treated by excision alone ($p = 0.017$). Patients with high VNPI scores of 8 or 9 benefit most by the addition of radiation therapy to their treatment regimen (Fig. 53–22).

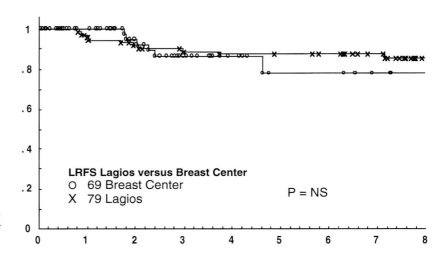

Figure 53–15 *Probability of local recurrence-free survival comparing equivalent patients (by tumor size and margin width) from The Breast Center and the series of Lagios and colleagues.*[54, 58]

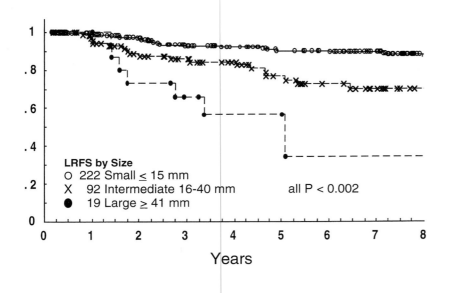

LRFS by Size
O 222 Small ≤ 15 mm
X 92 Intermediate 16-40 mm   all P < 0.002
● 19 Large ≥ 41 mm

Figure 53–16 *Probability of local recurrence-free survival by tumor size for 333 breast-conservation patients. (From Silverstein MJ, Lagios MD, Craig PH, Waisman JR, Lewinsky BS, Colburn WJ, Poller DM: Cancer 77:2267–2274, 1996. Copyright © (1996) American Cancer Society. Reprinted by permission of Wiley-Liss, Inc., a subsidiary of John Wiley & Sons, Inc.)*

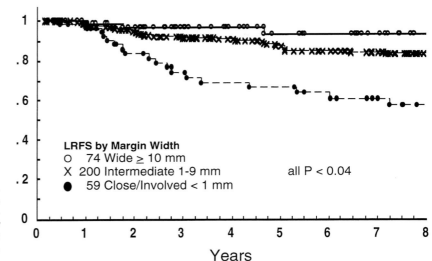

LRFS by Margin Width
O 74 Wide ≥ 10 mm
X 200 Intermediate 1-9 mm   all P < 0.04
● 59 Close/Involved < 1 mm

Figure 53–17 *Probability of local recurrence-free survival by margin width for 333 breast-conservation patients. (From Silverstein MJ, Lagios MD, Craig PH, Waisman JR, Lewinsky BS, Colburn WJ, Poller DM: Cancer 77:2267–2274, 1996. Copyright © (1996) American Cancer Society. Reprinted by permission of Wiley-Liss, Inc., a subsidiary of John Wiley & Sons, Inc.)*

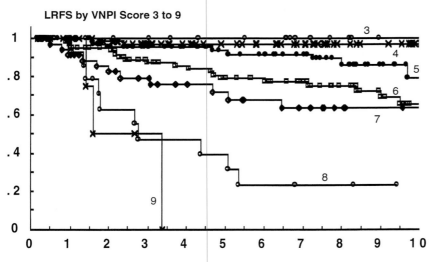

LRFS by VNPI Score 3 to 9

Figure 53–18 *Probability of local recurrence-free survival by Van Nuys Prognostic Index (VNPI) score 3 to 9.*

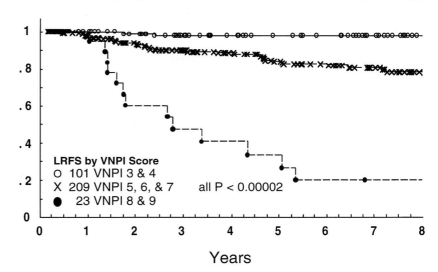

Figure 53–19 *Probability of local recurrence-free survival grouped by VNPI score for 333 breast-conservation patients. (From Silverstein MJ, Lagios MD, Craig PH, Waisman JR, Lewinsky BS, Colburn WJ, Poller DM: Cancer 77:2267–2274, 1996. Copyright © (1996) American Cancer Society. Reprinted by permission of Wiley-Liss, Inc., a subsidiary of John Wiley & Sons, Inc.)*

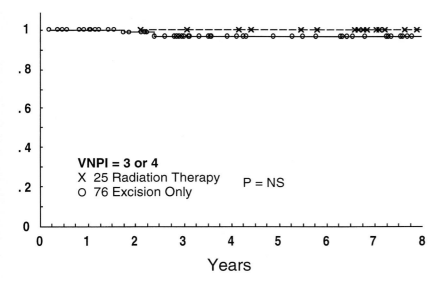

Figure 53–20 *Probability of local recurrence-free survival by treatment for 101 breast-conservation patients with VNPI scores of 3 or 4. (From Silverstein MJ, Lagios MD, Craig PH, Waisman JR, Lewinsky BS, Colburn WJ, Poller DM: Cancer 77:2267–2274, 1996. Copyright © (1996) American Cancer Society. Reprinted by permission of Wiley-Liss, Inc., a subsidiary of John Wiley & Sons, Inc.)*

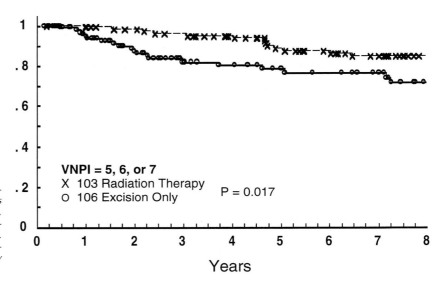

Figure 53–21 *Probability of local recurrence-free survival by treatment for 209 breast-conservation patients with VNPI scores of 5, 6 or 7. (From Silverstein MJ, Lagios MD, Craig PH, Waisman JR, Lewinsky BS, Colburn WJ, Poller DM: Cancer 77:2267–2274, 1996. Copyright © (1996) American Cancer Society. Reprinted by permission of Wiley-Liss, Inc., a subsidiary of John Wiley & Sons, Inc.)*

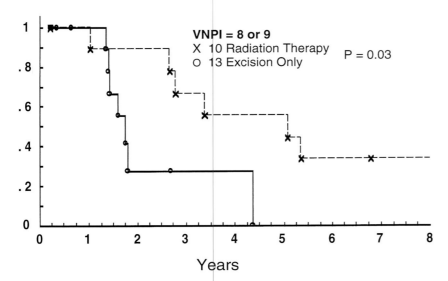

Figure 53–22 *Probability of local recurrence-free survival by treatment for 23 breast-conservation patients with VNPI scores of 8 or 9. (From Silverstein MJ, Lagios MD, Craig PH, Waisman JR, Lewinsky BS, Colburn WJ, Poller DM: Cancer 77:2267–2274, 1996. Copyright © (1996) American Cancer Society. Reprinted by permission of Wiley-Liss, Inc., a subsidiary of John Wiley & Sons, Inc.)*

However, even though the difference between the two groups is significant ($p = 0.026$), patients with a VNPI of 8 or 9 recur at an extremely high rate with or without radiation therapy.

Although mastectomy is curative for approximately 98 to 99 percent of patients with DCIS,* mastectomy represents overtreatment for most cases detected by current methods. When breast conservation is elected, radiation therapy statistically decreases the likelihood of local recurrence when compared with excision alone[30, 35]; but radiation therapy, like mastectomy, may also represent overtreatment for a significant number of patients who elect breast preservation.

Subsets of patients who are not likely to receive any significant benefit from radiation therapy can be identified, e.g., those with VNPI scores of 3 or 4 in the series presented here, low-grade lesions in the series of Lagios and colleagues,[55, 58] small noncomedo lesions with uninvolved margins in the series of Schwartz,[87] or the well-differentiated lesions of Zafrani and associates.[130] Such patients may account for 30 to 40 percent of all currently diagnosed DCIS patients.[55, 58, 87, 103, 130]

The recommendation by the NSABP that radiation therapy is appropriate for all patients with DCIS who are treated with breast preservation does not allow for the heterogeneity of DCIS nor the significant differences in subsets demonstrated by our data,[102, 103] the data of others,† and more recently, their own data.[35]

With radiation therapy, as with all treatments, there are side effects. It changes the texture of the breast and may make subsequent mammography more difficult to interpret. Perhaps most important, its use precludes additional radiation therapy and breast conservation should invasive breast cancer develop at a later date. The risks and benefits of radiation therapy must be carefully weighed and compared before making a recommendation. Radiation therapy should then be encouraged only for those patients likely to obtain a benefit.

Patients in this series with VNPI scores of 8 or 9 present a special problem. Although these patients show the greatest relative benefit from postexcisional radiation therapy, their local recurrence rate continues to be unacceptably high, more than 60 percent at 5 years, and a recommendation for mastectomy should be considered.

Treatment recommendations for the intermediate group (patients with VNPI scores of 5, 6, or 7) are the most difficult. For patients with intermediate VNPI scores and margin scores of 2 or 3, re-excision may decrease the risk of local recurrence by downscoring their VNPI score. If the score remains intermediate after re-excision, radiation therapy should be considered. However, some patients with scores of 7 may be better treated with mastectomy (for example, a patient with a large nuclear grade 2 lesion without necrosis with involved margins after re-excision). Some patients with scores of 5 may elect no further treatment (for example, a patient with widely clear margins, small tumor size, but high nuclear grade). These are independent judgments that must be made by the patient and physician. We are hopeful that the VNPI will be a helpful adjunct as these difficult decisions are discussed. If the VNPI, or some similar system, is not used, there are little data in the literature to aid clinicians in the complex DCIS treatment selection process.

There is a strong selection or treatment bias among the patients used to develop the VNPI. The treatment for all patients was selected by the patient and physician, not by random assignment. But treatment selection does not bias the results because the VNPI compares patients with different scores, not different treatments. Although the patient and the clinician control treatment selection, neither can control final margins, tumor size, or pathological classification. The fact that some patients opted for suboptimal treatments that were not recommended (for

---

*See references 4–6, 17, 25, 27, 34, 50, 84, and 102.
†See references 12, 35, 54, 55, 56, 58, 72, 78, 87, 111, and 130.

TABLE 53–10. TREATMENT GUIDELINES VAN NUYS PROGNOSTIC INDEX (VNPI)

VNPI Score	Recommended Treatment
3 or 4	Excision only
5, 6, or 7	Excision + radiation
8 or 9	Mastectomy

example, 23 patients with VNPI scores of 8 or 9 who selected breast conservation were all advised to undergo mastectomy) was helpful in developing and evaluating the VNPI.

Counseling patients with DCIS in a rational manner can be extremely difficult when the range of treatment options is extreme. The VNPI allows a scientifically based discussion with the patient, using the parameters of the lesion obtained after an initial excision. Thus, in some cases, a patient can choose re-excision, in an effort to downscore her lesion. Successful downscoring of a patient with a VNPI of 8 or 9 could result in substantial reduction in the risk of local recurrence, perhaps changing a recommendation from mastectomy to radiation therapy. Similarly, patients with close or involved margins, with VNPI scores of 5 or 6 after initial excision, could opt for re-excision. Successful downscoring by achieving widely clear margins could result in a final VNPI score of 3 or 4 and a recommendation for careful clinical follow-up without radiation therapy.

Downscoring can only be accomplished by re-excision in patients with margins scores of 2 or 3. Re-excision will not lower the pathological classification score nor will it reduce the size of the tumor. In some cases, re-excision will upscore the tumor, increasing the VNPI score by revealing a larger tumor size, a higher nuclear grade, the presence of previously undetected comedonecrosis, or an involved margin.

The VNPI is the first attempt to quantify known important prognostic factors in DCIS, making them clinically useful in the treatment decision-making process. It may be useful to clinicians because it

divides DCIS into three groups with different risks for local recurrence after breast-conservation therapy. Although there is an obvious treatment choice for each group (Table 53–10), the VNPI is offered only as a guideline, a starting place in the discussions with patients. Clearly, the validity of the VNPI must be independently confirmed by other groups with large series of DCIS patients and sufficient data to complete the subset analysis as outlined here. Prospective confirmation, however, would be better.

In the future, other factors, such as molecular markers, may be integrated into the VNPI or other prognostic indices when they are shown to statistically influence the likelihood of local recurrence after breast-conservation therapy.

Case Presentations Using the VNPI to Aid in Treatment Selection

Case 1—Downscoring (VNPI 6 to 4). The patient was a 49-year-old woman with mammographically detected microcalcifications. Wire-directed excision yielded a 12-mm non–high-grade cribriform DCIS with comedo-type necrosis. The lesion abutted the margin. VNPI score = 6 (size score = 1, pathological classification score = 2, and margin score = 3). Re-excision was performed, and a 2-mm focus of residual DCIS was found on the biopsy cavity wall. The re-excision margins were judged to be clear by more than 10 mm in all directions. This procedure downscored the lesion by converting the margin score to 1. The pathological classification score and size score remained unchanged. The patient now has a VNPI of 4 and can be considered for no further therapy. The potential benefit of downscoring is seen in Figure 53–23.

Case 2—Upscoring (VNPI 6 to 8). The patient was a 55-year-old woman with mammographically detected microcalcifications. Wire-directed biopsy reveals an 8-mm, solid DCIS of intermediate grade with focal comedo-type necrosis. The margins appear transected. VNPI score = 6 (size score = 1, patholog-

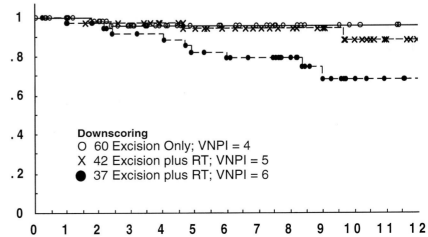

Figure 53–23 *The potential benefit of downscoring is illustrated. Thirty-seven patients with a VNPI = 6 treated with excision plus radiation therapy have a probability of local recurrence-free survival at 12 years of 69%. The probability of local recurrence-free survival for 42 patients with VNPI = 5 treated with excision plus radiation therapy is 89%. The probability of local recurrence-free survival for 60 patients with VNPI = 4 treated with excision alone is 96%. Re-excision of the patient illustrated in case 1 changed the VNPI from 6 to 4, eliminating the need for additional radiation therapy while yielding a 27% local recurrence-free survival benefit. If re-excision had achieved clear margins of only 3 to 4 mm rather than more than 10 mm, the patient would have been downscored to VNPI = 5. The benefit in local recurrence-free survival with the additional of radiation therapy would be 20%.*

ical classification score = 2, and margin score = 3). Re-excision revealed extensive residual disease measuring 45 mm. In addition, four foci of high-grade DCIS were found. The margins, however, were clear. The closest margin was now 4 mm. Final VNPI score = 8 (size score = 3, pathological classification score = 3, and margin score = 2). This procedure upscored her size score to 3 and her pathological classification score to 3. It downscored her margin score to 2. The patient now has a VNPI of 8 and would be best treated with mastectomy. An alternative would be to let the area heal for 3 to 6 months and then re-excise one more time in the hope of obtaining widely clear margins. If this were to happen, her margin score would become 1 and her VNPI would equal 7, at that point, radiation therapy would be an alternative. However, in this case, we would clearly prefer a mastectomy.

Case 3—A Random Finding. A 7-mm low-grade micropapillary DCIS without necrosis was found inadvertently within a breast reduction specimen in a 52-year-old woman. Because this was a reduction, margins were not marked and tissue was not serially sectioned and sequentially processed. Microscopically, the margins appear widely clear but the pathologist could not be certain. Prereduction mammography was negative. VNPI score = 3 or 4 (size score = 1, pathological classification score = 1, and margin score = 1 or 2). The pathologist cut in the remaining tissue and no additional foci of DCIS was found. The patient has a final VNPI of 3 or 4. We would not treat her with radiation therapy. Reduction mammoplasty causes significant postoperative mammographic scarring. Radiation therapy added to this would make future mammography even more difficult. Additionally, this DCIS was found inadvertently without mammographic signs. Under the best of circumstances, mammographic follow-up will be difficult. This patient should be fully apprised that this is a less-than-optimal circumstance in that margins could not really be evaluated. However, Schwartz and colleagues[86] have reported no local recurrences in 12 patients with incidental DCIS treated with excision only.

Case 4—A VNPI Score of 5 That Does Not Require Radiation Therapy. The patient was an 81-year-old woman with a screen-detected 11-mm area of microcalcifications. Wire-directed breast biopsy revealed a 10-mm high-grade comedo DCIS. The margins were widely clear (> 10 mm in all directions). VNPI score = 5 (size score = 1, pathological classification score = 3, and margin score = 1). Patients in the intermediate group (5, 6, or 7) generally require more thought and discussion. Some patients with scores of 5 may be better served by omitting radiation. Some patients with scores of 7 may be better served by mastectomy. In this particular case, we would not irradiate for the following reasons. The lesion was well marked by calcifications. It measured 11 mm on mammography and 10 mm on the micro-

scopic slide. Postoperative mammography showed no residual calcifications. The margins were widely clear. Although we prefer to omit radiation therapy in a patient of this age whenever possible, we would have no quarrel with the physician who elected to give radiation to this patient. If this patient were 54 years old, we would be much more likely to treat her with radiation therapy.

Case 5—Downscoring (VNPI 6 to 5). The patient was a 57-year-old woman with a screen-detected 22-mm area of microcalcifications. Wire-directed breast biopsy revealed a 25-mm intermediate grade DCIS with comedonecrosis. The closest margin measured 3 mm. VNPI score = 6 (size score = 2, pathological classification score = 2, and margin score = 2). This patient could be treated with radiation therapy. However, we would prefer to re-excise first. If widely clear margins were obtained, she would be downscored to a VNPI = 5. Radiation therapy would still be indicated, but the probability of local recurrence would be less than in a patient with a VNPI of 6.

Case 6—VNPI Score of 7 That Is Better Treated with Mastectomy. The patient was a 51-year-old woman with a vaguely palpable upper outer quadrant thickening. Mammography showed a nondiagnostic architectural distortion. Fine needle aspiration revealed moderately atypical cells, and biopsy was suggested. Core biopsy revealed a low-grade DCIS without necrosis (micropapillary architecture). The patient was strongly motivated for breast conservation. A four-wire–bracketed upper outer quadrant segmental resection was done. A 70-mm DCIS identical to the core biopsy, extending tenuously close to three margins, was found. VNPI = 7 (size score = 3, pathological classification score = 1, and margin score = 3). In this particular case, a skin-sparing mastectomy with immediate TRAM reconstruction would be our preference. We would choose this because the lesion is large and extends to multiple margins. Because it is not marked by microcalcifications, it is more difficult to completely excise and it will be more difficult to follow postoperatively, if this patient elects breast preservation. If she refused mastectomy, we would allow the wound to heal for 3 to 6 months and a formal quadrantectomy could be performed. With a low-grade micropapillary lesion, there is little risk in delaying definitive treatment for 6 months. If margins were then clear, consideration should be given to adding radiation therapy; however, data are weak regarding the benefits of radiation therapy for low-grade lesions.

Case 7—The First Excision Is the Best Chance to Get Clear Margins and Good Cosmesis. The patient was a 52-year-old woman with microcalcifications measuring 48 mm on mammography. Core biopsy showed high-grade DCIS with comedonecrosis. She had a large breast and was strongly motivated for breast preservation if possible. A four-wire–directed segmental resection revealed a 52-mm high-grade DCIS with widely clear margins (> 11 mm in all directions). VNPI = 7 (size score = 3, pathological classification score = 3, and margin score = 1). She is a candidate for breast preservation with radiation therapy.

At another facility not using stereotactic core biopsy or multiple wires, the case might have been handled somewhat differently. The scenario might have gone like this. A single-wire–directed biopsy would be performed. A 36-mm high-grade DCIS with involved margins would be found. VNPI = 8 (size score = 2, pathological classification score = 3, and margin score = 3). Postoperative mammography would reveal residual microcalcifications. The patient would continue to be strongly motivated for breast preservation and a quadrant type re-excision would be done. Residual DCIS would be found, but the margins would be clear by more than 10 mm in all directions. VNPI = 7 (size score = 3, pathological classification score = 3, and margin score = 1). The same score as the first scenario would be obtained, but in two operations. A formal quadrantectomy would not result in quite as good a cosmetic result. Another possibility also exists. With a VNPI = 8 and residual microcalcifications on postoperative mammography, many surgeons would prefer to proceed directly to mastectomy and reconstruction rather than re-excision.

Case 8—A Young Woman with a VNPI Score of 6 and a Family History of Breast Cancer. The patient was a 32-year-old woman whose mother and maternal grandmother had both had premenopausal breast cancer. The patient's mother died of breast cancer 5 years after diagnosis. Because of her family history, this patient had her first screening mammogram 2 years earlier at age 30. No abnormalities were seen. But her breasts were dense and difficult to evaluate by physical examination and mammography. This was her second screening mammogram, and it revealed worrisome microcalcifications measuring 26 mm in diameter in the upper outer quadrant of her left breast. Stereotactic core biopsy revealed a high-grade lesion with comedonecrosis. No invasion was seen. Because high-grade comedo-type lesions are generally well marked by microcalcifications, the surgeon believed that by using multiple wires, the entire lesion could be completely excised. If this had happened, the VNPI would have equaled 6 (size score = 2, pathological classification score = 3, and margin score = 1), and the patient could have been treated with radiation therapy.

She sought numerous additional opinions while wrestling with an extremely difficult decision. Because she was so young, she desperately wanted to save her breast. But because she had so much more time to live, she believed that a future invasive recurrence was highly likely. She was concerned that careful clinical and mammographic follow-up would be difficult because she had a mammographically dense breast, and radiation therapy would make mammography even more difficult. Most of all, she was affected by her mother's premature death, which occurred when the patient was still a teenager. This patient decided to undergo a unilateral mastectomy and immediate reconstruction. She planned to undergo a contralateral prophylactic mastectomy 5 years later regardless of whether any abnormalities developed.

Not all patients would have made this choice. Some might have opted for immediate bilateral mastectomies with or without reconstruction, whereas others might have chosen breast preservation with careful follow-up. The choices for this patient would have been clearer had genetic testing been available.

Axillary Lymph Node Dissection

In 1986, our group suggested that axillary lymph node dissection be abandoned for DCIS.[91, 93] In 1987, the NSABP made axillary node dissection for patients with DCIS entered into protocol B-17, optional, at the discretion of the surgeon. Since that time, we have published a series of papers that continue to show that axillary node dissection is not indicated for patients with DCIS.[96, 99–102] Through 1995, our group had performed a total of 293 node dissections (230 Level 1 and 2 dissections and 63 samplings), one of which contained two positive nodes. Frykberg and associates[39] compiled the data of nine studies with 754 patients. The incidence of axillary lymph node metastasis for patients with DCIS was 1.7 percent. In spite of these numbers, some authors continue to advocate removal of the axillary nodes in patients with palpable or extensive DCIS because of their belief that these patients have a higher risk of occult invasion.[8, 41, 87]

Our current policy is as follows. In any patient with DCIS (regardless of size of the DCIS, palpability, etc.) who is undergoing breast preservation, we do not remove any axillary nodes. In patients being treated with mastectomy, a thorough dissection of the axillary tail often yields 1 to 10 nodes.[28] In addition, most of our current patients who undergo mastectomy have breast reconstruction with a free TRAM flap. This procedure requires dissection of the subscapular vessels. It is not uncommon to remove a few nodes during the dissection as the vessels are exposed.

Most patients with DCIS who elect mastectomy have larger tumors and, therefore, a greater possibility that occult invasion was missed during routine histological evaluation.[81] In light of this, most patients are generally happy to have a few lower axillary nodes examined pathologically. A few negative nodes rewards many patients with additional peace of mind.

CONCLUSIONS

Ductal carcinoma *in situ* is relatively common and its frequency is increasing. Most of this is the result of better mammographic detection. We are not sure whether there is a true increase in incidence.

Not all microscopic DCIS will progress to clinical cancer, but if a patient has DCIS and is not treated, she is more likely to develop an ipsilateral invasive breast cancer than a woman without DCIS.

The separation of DCIS into two groups by architecture (comedo versus noncomedo) is an oversimplification and does not reflect the biological potential of the lesion as well as separation by nuclear grade and comedo-type necrosis.

High-grade DCIS is more aggressive and malignant in its histological appearance and is more likely to be associated with subsequent invasive cancer than non–high-grade DCIS. High-grade DCIS is more likely to have a high S-phase, overexpress *HER2* (*ERBB2*), and show increased thymidine labeling as compared with non–high-grade DCIS. High-grade DCIS treated conservatively is also more likely to recur locally than non–high-grade DCIS.

Most DCIS detected today will be nonpalpable. It will be detected by mammography with microcalcifications as the most common finding. It is not uncommon for DCIS to be larger than expected by mammography, to involve more than a quadrant of the breast, and to be unifocal in its distribution.

Preoperative evaluation should include film-screen mammography with compression magnification. The surgeon and the radiologist should plan the excision procedure carefully. The first attempt at excision is the best chance to get a complete excision with a good cosmetic result. Re-excisions are more likely to yield poor cosmetic results. In patients with suspicious mammographic lesions, consideration should be given to stereotactic core biopsy to make a definitive diagnosis.

After the establishment of the diagnosis, the patient can be apprised of all alternative procedures, their risks and advantages. If she is motivated for breast conservation, the surgeon and radiologist should plan the procedure carefully, using multiple wires to map out the extent of the lesion. Once the multiple-wire–directed excisional biopsy has been done, two factors can be evaluated: cosmesis and histopathology. If the cosmetic result is acceptable and the margins are clear, the patient can proceed with breast conservation. If she has a VNPI score of 3 or 4, no further therapy can be considered. If her score is 5, 6, or 7, re-excision may be a possibility. If re-excision is not possible or if her score remains in the mid-range, breast irradiation should be considered. Occasional patients with VNPI scores of 5 may be treated with excision alone, whereas some patients with VNPI scores of 7 may be better served with mastectomy. Individual judgment is required for all patients with intermediate scores. For patients with VNPI scores of 8 or 9, a mastectomy with immediate reconstruction is usually recommended.

If the initial margins are involved, consideration can be given to a re-excision procedure, but it may yield a poor cosmetic result and margins may continue to be involved. At this point, mastectomy with or without immediate reconstruction should be considered. Reconstruction can be accomplished with a variety of techniques, including expander, implant, TRAM flap, etc. In general, immediate reconstruction in combination with a skin-sparing mastectomy is to be preferred. It eliminates at least one surgical procedure in the future and usually results in a happier patient with a better cosmetic result.

For women with larger lesions (relative to breast size) that cannot be totally excised, mastectomy remains the treatment of choice. However, the NSABP is doing a prospective study (protocol B-24) that randomizes patients into two groups: excision plus breast irradiation with or without tamoxifen. In this study, positive margins and residual calcifications are allowed. The results of this study are eagerly awaited. However, judging from the results of B-17, the recurrence rates in B-24 are likely to be even higher.

THE FUTURE

Our knowledge of DCIS genetics and molecular biology is increasing at a remarkably rapid rate. Future studies are likely to identify markers that will allow us to differentiate DCIS with an aggressive potential from DCIS that is merely a microscopic finding. Once this happens, the treatment selection process will become much simpler.

Acknowledgments

The authors wish to thank Michael D. Lagios, M.D., for his counsel and the use of his patient data base.

References

1. Aasmundstad TA, Haugen OA: DNA ploidy in intraductal breast carcinomas. Eur J Cancer 26:956–959, 1992.
2. Allred DC, Clark GM, Molin R, et al: Overexpression of progression of in situ to invasive breast cancer. Hum Pathol 23:974–979, 1992.
3. Alpers C, Wellings S: The prevalence of carcinoma in situ in normal and cancer-associated breast. Hum Pathol 16:796–807, 1985.
4. Archer SG, Kemp BL, Gadd M, Shallenberger R, Ames FC, Singletary SE: Ductal carcinoma in situ of the breast: Comedo versus noncomedo subtype nonpredictive of recurrence of contralateral new breast primary. Breast Dis 7:353–360, 1994.
5. Arnesson LG, Smeed S, Fagerberg G, Grontoff O: Follow-up of two treatment modalities for ductal carcinoma in situ of the breast. Br J Surg 76:672–675, 1989.
6. Ashikari R, Hadju SI, Robbins GF: Intraductal carcinoma of the breast. Cancer 28:1182–1187, 1971.
7. Baird RM, Worth A, Hislop G: Recurrence after lumpectomy for comedo-type intraductal carcinoma of the breast. Am J Surg 159:479–481, 1990.
8. Balch CM, Singletary ES, Bland KI: Clinical decision-making in early breast cancer. Ann Surg 217:207–222, 1993.
9. Barnes DM, Meyer JS, Gonzalez JG, Gullick WJ, Millis RR: Relationship between c-erbB-2 immunoreactivity and thymidine labelling index in breast carcinoma in situ. Breast Cancer Res Treat 18:11–17, 1991.
10. Barth A, Brenner J, Giuliano AE: Current management of ductal carcinoma in situ. West J Med 163:360–366, 1995.

11. Bartkova J, Barnes DM, Millis RR, Gullick WJ: Immunohistochemical demonstration of c-erbB-2 protein in mammary ductal carcinoma in situ. Hum Pathol 21:1164–1167, 1990.
12. Bellamy COC, McDonald C, Salter DM, Chetty U, Anderson TJ: Noninvasive ductal carcinoma of the breast: The relevance of histologic categorization. Hum Pathol 24:16–23, 1993.
13. Blichert-Toft M, Brincker H, Andersen J, et al: A Danish randomized trial comparing breast preserving therapy with mastectomy in mammary carcinoma. Acta Oncol 27:671, 1988.
14. Blichert-Toft M, Rose C, Andersen J, et al: Danish randomized trial comparing breast conservative treatment with mastectomy: Six years of life table analysis. J Natl Cancer Inst Monogr 11:19, 1992.
15. Bobrow LG, Happerfield LC, Gregory WM, Springall RD, Millis RR: The classification of ductal carcinoma in situ and its association with biological markers. Semin Diagn Pathol 11:199–207, 1994.
16. Bornstein BA, Recht A, Connolly JL, et al: Results of treating ductal carcinoma in situ of the breast with conservative surgery and radiation therapy. Cancer 67:7–13, 1991.
17. Bradley SJ, Weaver DW, Bouwman DL: Alternatives in the surgical management of in situ breast cancer. Am Surg 56:428–432, 1990.
18. Brown PW, Silverman J, Owens P, et al: Intraductal "noninfiltrating" carcinoma of the breast. Arch Surg 111:1063–1067, 1976.
19. Carpenter R, Boulter PS, Cooke T, Gibbs NM: Management of screen detected ductal carcinoma in situ of the female breast. Br J Surg 76:564–567, 1989.
20. Carter D, Smith RRL: Carcinoma in situ of the breast. Cancer 40:1189–1193, 1977.
21. Cataliotti L, Distante V, Ciatto S, et al: Intraductal breast cancer: Review of 183 consecutive cases. Eur J Cancer 28A:917–920, 1992.
22. Ciatto S, Bonardi R, Cataliotti L, Cardona G: Intraductal breast carcinoma: Review of a multicenter series of 350 cases. Tumori 76:552–554, 1990.
23. Dickson RB, Lippman ME: Growth factors in breast cancer. Endocrine Rev 16:559–589, 1995.
24. Eusebi V, Feudale E, Foschini MP, et al: Long-term follow-up of in situ carcinoma of the breast. Semin Diag Pathol 11:223–235, 1994.
25. Farrow JH: Current concepts in the detection and treatment of the earliest of the breast cancers. Cancer 25:468–477, 1970.
26. Faverly DRG, Burgers L, Bult P, Holland R: Three dimensional imaging of mammary ductal carcinoma in situ: Clinical implications. Semin Diag Pathol 11:193–198, 1995.
27. Fentiman IS, Fagg N, Millis RR, Haywood JL: In situ ductal carcinoma of the breast: Implications of disease pattern and treatment. Eur J Surg Oncol 12:261–266, 1986.
28. Fisher B, Montague E, Redmond C, et al: Comparison of radical mastectomy with alternative treatments for primary breast cancer. Cancer 39:2827–2839, 1977.
29. Fisher B, Redmond C, Poisson R, et al: Eight-year results of a randomized clinical trial comparing total mastectomy and lumpectomy with or without irradiation in the treatment of breast cancer. N Engl J Med 320:822–828, 1989.
30. Fisher B, Costantino J, Redmond C, Fisher E, Margolese R, Dimitrov N, et al: Lumpectomy compared with lumpectomy and radiation therapy for the treatment of intraductal breast cancer. N Engl J Med 328:1581–1586, 1993.
31. Fisher B, Redmond CK, Fisher ER: Radiation therapy for in situ or localized breast cancer: The authors reply. N Engl J Med 329:1578, 1993.
32. Fisher B, Anderson S, Redmond CK, et al: Reanalysis and results after 12 years of follow-up in a randomized clinical trial comparing total mastectomy with lumpectomy with or without irradiation in the treatment of breast cancer. N Engl J Med 333:1456–1461, 1995.
33. Fisher ER, Sass R, Fisher B, et al: Pathologic findings from the National Surgical Adjuvant Breast Project (Protocol 6) 1. Intraductal carcinoma (DCIS). Cancer 57:197–208, 1986.
34. Fisher ER, Leiming ER, Anderson S, et al: Conservative management of intraductal carcinoma (DCIS) of the breast. J Surg Oncol 47:139–147, 1991.
35. Fisher ER, Constantino J, Fisher B, et al: Pathologic findings from the National Surgical Adjuvant Breast Project (NSABP) Protocol B-17. Cancer 75:1310–1319, 1995.
36. Fisher ER, Costantino J, Fisher B, Palekar AS, Mamounas E: Response: Blunting the counterpoint. Cancer 75:1223–1227, 1995.
37. Fourquet A, Zafrani B, Campana F, Durand JC, Vilcoq JR: Breast-conserving treatment of ductal carcinoma in situ. Semin Radiat Oncol 2:116–124, 1992.
38. Fowble B: Intraductal noninvasive breast cancer: A comparison of three local treatments. Oncology 3:51–58, 1989.
39. Frykberg ER, Masood S, Copeland EM, Bland KI: Duct carcinoma in situ of the breast. Surg Gynecol Obstet 177:425–440, 1993.
40. Gallagher WJ, Koemer FC, Wood WC: Treatment of intraductal carcinoma with limited surgery: Long term follow-up. J Clin Oncol 7:376–380, 1989.
41. Gump FR, Jicha DL, Ozzello L: Ductal carcinoma in situ (DCIS): A revised concept. Surgery 102:190–195, 1987.
42. Haffty BG, Peschel RE, Papadopoulos D, Pathare P: Radiation therapy for ductal carcinoma in situ of the breast. Conn Med 54:482–484, 1990.
43. Hiramatsu H, Bornstein BA, Recht A, et al: Local recurrence after conservative surgery and radiation therapy for ductal carcinoma in situ: Possible importance of family history. Cancer J Sci Am 1:55–61, 1995.
44. Holland R, Veling SHJ, Mravunac M, Hendriks JHCL: Histologic multifocality of Tis, T1-2 breast carcinomas: Implications for clinical trials of breast conserving surgery. Cancer 56:979–990, 1985.
45. Holland R, Hendriks JHCL, Verbeek ALM, Mravunac M, Schuurmans SJH: Extent, distribution, and mammographic/histological correlations of breast ductal carcinoma in situ. Lancet 335:519–522, 1990.
46. Holland R, Hendriks JHCL: Microcalcifications associated with ductal carcinoma in situ: Mammographic-pathologic correlation. Semin Diag Pathol 11:181–192, 1994.
47. Holland R, Peterse JL, Millis R, et al: Ductal carcinoma in situ: A proposal for a new classification. Semin Diag Pathol 11:167–180, 1994.
48. Jensen JA, Handel N, Silverstein MJ: Glandular replacement therapy (GRT) for intraductal breast carcinoma (DCIS). Proc Am Soc Clin Oncol 14:138, 1995.
49. Jensen JA, Handel N, Silverstein MJ: Glandular replacement therapy: An argument for a combined surgical approach in the treatment of noninvasive breast cancer. Breast J 2:121–123, 1996.
50. Kinne DW, Petrek JA, Osborne MP, et al: Breast carcinoma in situ. Arch Surg 124:33–36, 1989.
51. Kroll SS, Ames F, Singletary SE, et al: The oncologic risks of skin preservation at mastectomy when combined with immediate reconstruction of the breast. Surg Gynecol Obstet 172:17–20, 1991.
52. Kurtz JM, Jacquemier J, Torhorst J, et al: Conservation therapy for breast cancers other than infiltrating ductal carcinoma. Cancer 63:1630–1635, 1989.
53. Kuske RR, Bean JM, Garcia DM, et al: Breast conservation therapy for intraductal carcinoma of the breast. Int J Radiat Oncol Biol Phys 26:391–396, 1993.
54. Lagios MD, Westdahl PR, Margolin FR, Rose MR: Duct carcinoma in situ: Relationship of extent of noninvasive disease to the frequency of occult invasion, multicentricity, lymph node metastases, and short-term treatment failures. Cancer 50:1309–1314, 1982.
55. Lagios NM, Margolin FR, Westdahl PR, Rose NM: Mammographically detected duct carcinoma in situ: Frequency of local recurrence following tylectomy and prognostic effect of nuclear grade on local recurrence. Cancer 63:619–624, 1989.
56. Lagios MD: Duct carcinoma in situ: Pathology and treatment. Surg Clin North Am 70:853–871, 1990.
57. Lagios MD, Page DL: Radiation therapy for in situ or localized breast cancer. N Engl J Med 21:1577–1578, 1993. Letter.

58. Lagios MD: Ductal carcinoma in situ: Controversies in diagnosis, biology, and treatment. Breast J 1:68–78, 1995.
59. Lennington WJ, Jensen RA, Dalton LW, Page DL: Ductal carcinoma in situ of the breast: Heterogeneity of individual lesions. Cancer 73:118–124, 1994.
60. Lichter A, Lippman M, Danforth D, et al: Mastectomy versus breast conserving therapy in the treatment of stage I and II carcinoma of the breast: A randomized trial at The National Cancer Institute. J Clin Oncol 10:976, 1992.
61. Lippman ME: The rational development of biological therapies for breast cancer. Science 259:631–632, 1993.
62. Liu E, Thor A, He M, Barcos M, Ljung BM, Benz C: The HER2 (c-erbB-2) oncogene is frequently amplified in in situ carcinomas of the breast. Oncogene 7:1027–1032, 1992.
62a. Mamounas E, Fisher B, Dignam J, et al: Effect of breast irradiation following lumpectomy in intraductal breast cancer (DCIS); updated results from NSABP B-17. (Abstract.) Proc Soc Surg Oncol 50:7, 1997.
63. Margolese R: Ductal carcinoma in situ. Rec Results Cancer Res 140:131–138, 1995.
64. McCormick B, Rosen PP, Kinne D, Cox L, Yahalom J: Duct carcinoma in situ of the breast: An analysis of local control after conservation surgery and radiotherapy. Int J Radiat Oncol Biol Phys 21:289–292, 1991.
65. Meyer J: Cell kinetics of histologic variants of in situ breast carcinoma. Breast Cancer Res Treat 7:171–180, 1986.
66. Moriya T, Silverberg SG: Intraductal carcinoma (ductal carcinoma in situ) of the breast: A comparison of pure noninvasive tumors with those including different proportions of infiltrating carcinoma. Cancer 74:2972–2978, 1994.
67. Moriya T, Silverberg SG: Intraductal carcinoma (ductal carcinoma in situ) of the breast: Analysis of pathologic findings of 85 pure intraductal carcinomas. Int J Surg Pathol 3:83–92, 1995.
68. Morrow M, Schnitt SJ, Harris JR: Ductal carcinoma in situ. In Harris JR, Lippman MC, Morrow M, Hellman S (eds): Diseases of the Breast. Philadelphia, Lippencott-Raven, 1995, pp 355–368.
69. Nemoto T, Vana J, Bedwani RN, Baker HW, McGregor FH, Murphy GP: Management and survival of female breast cancer: Results of a national survey by The American College of Surgeons. Cancer 45:2917–2924, 1980.
70. Nielson M, Thomsen JL, Primdahl S, Dreyborg U, Anderson JA: Breast cancer and atypia among young and middle-aged women: A study of 110 medicolegal autopsies. Br J Cancer 56:814–819, 1987.
71. Noguchi S, Aihara T, Koyama H, Motomura K, Inaji H, Imaoka S: Discrimination between multicentric and multifocal carcinomas of breast through clonal analysis. Cancer 74:872–877, 1994.
72. Ottesen GL, Graversen HP, Blichert-Toft M, Zedeler K, Andersen JA: Ductal carcinoma in situ of the female breast: Short-term results of a prospective nationwide study. Am J Surg Pathol 16:1183–1196, 1992.
73. Page DL, Dupont WD, Roger LW, Landenberger M: Intraductal carcinoma of the breast: Follow-up after biopsy only. Cancer 49:751–758, 1982.
74. Page DL, Anderson TJ: Intraductal carcinoma. In Page DL, Anderson TJ (eds): Diagnostic Histopathology of the Breast. New York, Churchill Livingstone, 1987, pp 157–174.
75. Page DL, Dupont WD, Rogers LW, Jensen RA, Schuyler PA: Continued local recurrence of carcinoma 15-25 years after a diagnosis of low grade ductal carcinoma in situ of the breast treated only by biopsy. Cancer 76:1197–1200, 1995.
76. Page DL, Lagios MD: Pathologic analysis of the NSABP-B17 Trial: Unanswered questions remaining unanswered considering current concepts of ductal carcinoma in situ. Cancer 75:1219–1222, 1995.
77. Patchefsky AS, Schwartz GF, Finkelstein SD, et al: Heterogeneity of intraductal carcinoma of the breast. Cancer 63:731–741, 1989.
78. Poller DN, Silverstein MJ, Galea M, et al: Ductal carcinoma in situ of the breast: A proposal for a new simplified histological classification association between cellular proliferation and c-erbB-2 protein expression. Mod Pathol 7:257–262, 1994.
79. Price P, Sinnett HD, Gusterson B, et al: Duct carcinoma in situ: Predictors of local recurrence and progression in patients treated by surgery alone. Cancer 61:869–872, 1990.
80. Ray GR, Adelson L, Hayhurst E, et al: Ductal carcinoma in situ of the breast: Results of treatment by conservative surgery and definitive irradiation. Int J Radiat Oncol 28:105–111, 1994.
81. Rosen PP, Senie R, Schottenfeld D, Ashikari R: Noninvasive breast carcinoma: Frequency of unsuspected invasion and implications for treatment. Ann Surg 189:377–382, 1979.
82. Rosen PP, Braun DW, Kinne DE: The clinical significance of pre-invasive breast carcinoma. Cancer 46:919–925, 1980.
83. Rosen PP, Oberman HA: Intraepithelial (preinvasive or in situ) carcinoma. In Rosen PP, Oberman HA (eds): Atlas of Tumor Pathology: Tumors of the Mammary Gland. Washington, DC, Armed Forces Institute of Pathology, 1993, pp 119–156.
84. Rosner D, Bedwani RN, Vana J, Baker HW, Murphy GP: Noninvasive breast carcinoma: Results of a national survey of The American College of Surgeons. Ann Surg 192:139–147, 1980.
85. Schuh ME, Nemoto T, Penetrante RB, Rosner D, Dao TL: Intraductal carcinoma: Analysis of presentation, pathologic findings, and outcome of disease. Arch Surg 121:1303–1307, 1986.
86. Schwartz GF, Finkel GC, Garcia JC, Patchefsky AS: Subclinical ductal carcinoma in situ of the breast. Cancer 70:2468–2474, 1992.
87. Schwartz GF: The role of excision and surveillance alone in subclinical DCIS of the breast. Oncology 8:21–26, 1994.
88. SEER Cancer Statistics Review: 1973–1990. National Cancer Institute. NIH Pub no. 93-2789, 1993.
89. Sibbering DN, Robertson JSR, Blamey RW, et al: With a clear margin of excision radiation therapy may be unnecessary after local excision of DCIS. Proc Br Assoc Surg Oncol Nov 1994. Abstract.
90. Singletary ES: Skin-sparing mastectomy with immediate breast reconstruction: Is it safe? Breast Dis 6:259–260, 1995.
91. Silverstein MJ, Rosser RJ, Gierson ED, Gamagami P, Colburn WJ, Handel N, et al: Axillary lymph node dissection for intraductal carcinoma: Is it indicated? (Abstract.) Proc Am Soc Clin Oncol 5:265, 1986.
92. Silverstein MJ, Handel N, Hoffman RS, et al: The breast center: A multidisciplinary model. In Paterson AHG, Lees AW (eds): Fundamental Problems in Breast Cancer. Boston, Martinus Nijhoff, 1987, pp 47–58.
93. Silverstein MJ, Rosser RJ, Gierson ED, et al: Axillary lymph node dissection for intraductal carcinoma: Is it indicated? Cancer 59:1819–1824, 1987.
94. Silverstein MJ, Gamagami P, Colburn WJ, et al: Nonpalpable breast lesions: Diagnosis with slightly overpenetrated screen-film mammography and hook wire-directed breast biopsy in 1014 cases. Radiology 171:633–638, 1989.
95. Silverstein MJ: Intraductal breast carcinoma: Two decades of progress? Am J Clin Oncol 14:534–537, 1991.
96. Silverstein MJ, Waisman JR, Gierson ED, et al: Radiation therapy for intraductal carcinoma: Is it an equal alternative? Arch Surg 126:424–428, 1991.
97. Silverstein MJ, Cohlan B, Gierson ED, et al: Duct carcinoma in situ: 227 cases without microinvasion. Eur J Cancer 28:630–634, 1992.
98. Silverstein MJ, Waisman JR, Colburn WJ, et al: Intraductal breast carcinoma with and without microinvasion: Is there a difference in outcome? Proc Am Soc Clin Oncol 12:56, 1993.
99. Silverstein MJ: Noninvasive breast cancer: The dilemma of the 1990s. Obstet Gynecol Clin North Am 21:639–658, 1994.
100. Silverstein MJ, Gierson ED, Colburn WJ, et al: Can intraductal breast carcinoma be excised completely by local excision? Clinical and pathologic predictors. Cancer 73:2985–2989, 1994.
101. Silverstein MJ, Barth A, Waisman JR, et al: Predicting local recurrence in patients with intraductal breast carcinoma (DCIS). Proc Am Soc Clin Oncol 14:117, 1995.
102. Silverstein MJ, Barth A, Poller DN, et al: Ten-year results comparing mastectomy to excision and radiation therapy for

ductal carcinoma in situ of the breast. Eur J Cancer 31:1425–1427, 1995.

103. Silverstein MJ, Poller DN, Waisman JR: Prognostic classification of breast ductal carcinoma in situ. Lancet 345:1154–1157, 1995.

104. Silverstein MJ, Lagios MD, Craig PH, et al: The Van Nuys Prognostic Index for Ductal Carcinoma in Situ. Breast J 2:38–40, 1996.

105. Silverstein MJ, Poller DN, Craig PH, et al: A prognostic index for breast ductal carcinoma in situ. Breast Cancer Res Treat 37(suppl):34, 1996. Abstract.

106. Silverstein MJ, Poller DN, Craig PH, et al: A prognostic index for ductal carcinoma in situ of the breast. Cancer 77:2267–2274, 1996.

107. Simpson T, Thirlby RC, Dail DH: Surgical treatment of ductal carcinoma in situ of the breast: 10 to 20 year follow-up. Arch Surg 127:468–472, 1992.

108. Sloane JP, Ellman R, Anderson TJ, Brown CL, Coyne J, Dallimore NS, et al: Consistency of histopathological reporting of breast lesions detected by breast screening: Findings of the UK national external quality assessment (EQA) scheme. Eur J Cancer 30:1414–1419, 1994.

109. Sneige N, McNeese MD, Atkinson EN, Ames FC, Kemp B, Sahin A, Ayala AG: Ductal carcinoma in situ treated with lumpectomy and irradiation: Histopathological analysis of 49 specimens with emphasis on risk factors and long term results. Hum Pathol 26:642–649, 1995.

110. Solin LJ, Recht A, Fourquet A, Kurtz J, Kuske R, McNeese M, et al: Ten-year results of breast-conserving surgery and definitive irradiation for intraductal carcinoma of the breast. Cancer 68:2337–2344, 1991.

111. Solin LJ, Yet I-T, Kurtz J, et al: Ductal carcinoma in situ (intraductal carcinoma) of the breast treated with breast-conserving surgery and definitive irradiation: Correlation of pathologic parameters with outcome of treatment. Cancer 71:2532–2542, 1993.

112. Solin LJ, Fourquet A, McCormick B, et al: Salvage treatment for local recurrence following breast-conserving surgery and definitive irradiation for ductal carcinoma in situ (intraductal carcinoma) of the breast. Int J Radiat Oncol Biol Phys 30:3–9, 1994.

113. Solin L, Kurtz J, Fourquet A, et al: Fifteen year outcome for conservative surgery and radiotherapy for ductal carcinoma in situ (DCIS). Proc Am Soc Clin Oncol 14:107, 1995.

114. Solin L, Kurtz J, Fourquet A, et al: Fifteen year results of breast conserving surgery and definitive breast irradiation for the treatment of ductal carcinoma in situ (intraductal carcinoma) of the breast. J Clin Oncol 14:754–763, 1996.

115. Stockdale AD, Brierley JD, Whire WF, Folkes A, Rostom AY: Radiotherapy for Paget's disease of the nipple: A conservative alternative. Lancet 8664:664–666, 1989.

116. Stotter AT, McNeese M, Oswald MJ, et al: The role of limited surgery with irradiation in primary treatment of ductal carcinoma in situ breast cancer. Int J Radiat Oncol Bio Phys 18:283, 1990.

117. Sunshine JA, Moseley HS, Fletcher WS, Kripphaene WW: Breast carcinoma in situ: A retrospective review of 112 cases with a minimum 10 years follow-up. Am J Surg 150:44–51, 1985.

118. Swain SM: Ductal carcinoma in situ: Incidence, presentation and guidelines to treatment. Oncology 3:25–42, 1989.

119. Tabar L, Dean PB: Basic principles of mammographic diagnosis. Diagn Imag Clin Med 54:146–157, 1985.

120. Tavassoli FA: Intraductal carcinoma. *In* Tavassoli FA (ed): Pathology of the Breast. 261. Norwalk, CT, Appleton & Lange, 1992, pp 229–261.

121. Van de Vijver MJ, Peterse JL, Mooi WJ, Wisman P, Lomans J, Dalesio O, Nusse R. Neu-protein overexpression in breast cancer: Association with comedo-type ductal carcinoma in situ and limited prognostic value in stage II breast cancer. N Engl J Med 319:1239–1245, 1988.

122. Van Dongen JA, Bartelink H, Fentiman IS, et al: Randomized clinical trial to assess the value of breast-conserving therapy in stage I and II breast cancer: EORTC 10801 trial. Monogr Natl Cancer Inst 11:15–18, 1992.

123. Veronesi U, Saccozzi R, Del Vecchio M, et al: Comparing radical mastectomy with quadrantectomy, axillary dissection and radiotherapy in patients with small cancers of the breast. N Engl J Med 305:6, 1981.

124. Veronesi U, Banfi A, Salvadori B, et al: Breast conservation is the treatment of choice in small breast cancer: Long-term results of a randomized trial. Eur J Cancer 26:668–670, 1990.

125. Von Reuden DG, Wilson WE: Intraductal carcinoma of the breast. Surg Gynecol Obstet 158:105–111, 1984.

126. Westbrook KC, Gallager HS: Intraductal carcinoma of the breast: A comparative study. Am J Surg 130:667–670, 1975.

127. White J, Gustafson G, Levine A, et al: Outcome and prognostic factors for local recurrence in mammographically detected ductal carcinoma in-situ of the breast treated with conservative surgery and radiation therapy. Int J Radiat Oncol Bio Phys 27:145, 1993. Abstract.

128. Wingo PA, Tong T, Bolden S, Parker SL: Cancer statistics, 1995. CA Cancer J Clin 47:5–27, 1997.

129. Zafrani B, Fourquet A, Vilcoq JR, et al: Conservative management of intraductal breast carcinoma with tumorectomy and radiation therapy. Cancer 57:1299, 1986.

130. Zafrani B, Leroyer A, Fourquet A, et al: Mammographically detected ductal carcinoma in situ of the breast analysed with a new classification: A study of 127 cases: Correlation with estrogen and progesterone receptors, p53 and c-erbB-2 proteins and proliferative activity. Semin Diagn Pathol 11:208–213, 1994.

CHAPTER 54

SMALL INVASIVE CARCINOMAS: THE ROLE OF AXILLARY LYMPH NODE DISSECTION

Pamela H. Craig, M.D., Ph.D. / Melvin J. Silverstein, M.D.

The optimal management of the axilla for the surgical treatment of invasive breast cancer is an area of active debate and evolution.* Tumor size and node positivity are acknowledged by a large body of evidence to be the two most powerful long-term and independent predictors of outcome in invasive breast cancer.† Because clinical detection of axillary node involvement is unreliable,[54, 66, 247, 248] traditionally the only method of obtaining information about the axillary lymph nodes has been through the pathological examination of the axillary nodes obtained from a surgical dissection. But currently, there are those who advocate elimination of axillary dissection in selected patients‡ and those who routinely advocate total axillary clearance in all patients.§ As more patients are diagnosed with small breast cancers,[91, 158] and as more patients are treated with breast conservation, the role of axillary dissection will come under even more scrutiny as we try to define which subsets of patients may not need axillary surgery because there is no effect on outcome or because chemotherapy is given to all regardless of nodal status.

The goals of this chapter are to examine the current views of the role of axillary dissection of the breast, review the definitions and types of axillary dissection, explore in depth the rationale between different types of surgical axillary dissections and pathological axillary dissections, analyze the information available concerning other ways to predict axillary nodal status besides surgical dissection, and discuss the role of axillary dissection in minimally invasive breast cancer.

ROLE OF AXILLARY LYMPH NODE DISSECTION

Axillary dissection can be thought of as a tool that provides prognostic information and therapy. The therapy may be the prevention of either local or distant recurrence. The microscopic status of the axillary lymph nodes is generally regarded as the most powerful predictor of the natural history of breast cancer.¶ However, there is no universal consensus regarding how extensive an axillary dissection is

needed to achieve accuracy of nodal prognostic status. Because of the significant difference in overall survival between node-negative and node-positive patients, this information has been useful in determining the necessity of chemotherapy. However, chemotherapy, hormonal therapy, or both is now also offered to many node-negative patients.[69, 96, 150, 151, 267] The axillary lymph node status may therefore not be crucial in all patients for the selection of adjuvant therapy. Wood[267] and others[98] have stated that lymph node status is important, even in tumors 1 cm or less. Even though the benefit of chemotherapy in terms of relative reduction of risk of recurrence and death is fairly constant, the absolute risk is closely related to the presence and number of nodal metastases; therefore, the absolute percentage difference between treated and untreated patient populations is markedly related to nodal status.[115, 267] However, more than 70 percent of patients with T1 invasive carcinomas are node-negative.[4, 30, 34] With a well-functioning screening mammography program resulting in the detection of smaller cancers, there will be an even greater shift toward more node-negative cancers.[30, 238] There is an increasing tendency to give systemic therapy to nearly all patients with invasive breast cancer larger than 1 cm, regardless of nodal status, and to all patients with node-positive breast cancer, regardless of tumor size.[96, 98, 191] Although it has been stated that women with lesions smaller than 1 cm generally should not receive systemic chemotherapy because of their overall excellent prognosis,[115] a recent International Consensus Panel on the treatment of primary breast cancer still considered adjuvant chemotherapy or hormonal therapy appropriate for node-positive patients with invasive carcinomas 1 cm or less in diameter.[98] In addition, there are subsets of patients with small node-negative carcinomas with a significantly poor recurrence-free survival in whom consideration of adjuvant systemic therapy is warranted.[137]

The therapeutic role of axillary dissection is to achieve regional control by preventing axillary recurrences as well as to theoretically prevent distant recurrence. How much of the axilla needs to be removed to prevent axillary recurrences? What is an appropriate axillary dissection that adequately and safely treats the axilla while minimizing recurrences? Why not perform a delayed axillary dissection in those patients who develop positive nodes? The theoretical therapeutic role of axillary dissection to improve survival by preventing axillary recurrences is debatable. What is the evidence that initial

---

*See references 12, 31, 32, 40, 62, 63, 100, 108, 135, 145, 160, 177, 192, 209, and 263.
†See references 34, 35, 36, 43, 47, 50, 64, 67, 74, 76, 90, 92, 128, 199, 200, 205, 237, 238, 251, and 262.
‡See references 4, 31, 32, 181, 223, 224, and 225.
§See references 15, 51, 52, 63, 160, 195, and 219.
¶See references 65, 66, 76, 77, 97, 174, 200, and 251.

removal of the axillary nodes at the time of primary surgery affects breast cancer–specific survival? Do unresected positive lymph nodes serve as a nidus for the development of metastatic disease?

IS AXILLARY DISSECTION NECESSARY FOR PROGNOSTIC INFORMATION?

The status of the axillary nodes, along with tumor size, is currently the most important prognostic factor for prediction of breast carcinoma outcome because it is thought that the presence of regional metastatic disease functions as a marker for tumors capable of causing systemic metastatic disease.[70, 75] The role of the lymph nodes as the pivotal predictor, however, is being questioned because it is far from being consistently predictive.[87, 155, 188] Nodal status is not a sharp, binomial, yes-or-no prognostic factor that bifurcates patients into two distinct groups. For example, long-term survival occurs in about 30 percent of node-positive patients, whereas 15 to 30 percent of all node-negative patients relapse, and 24 percent of node-negative patients die within the first 10 years after local-regional therapy.[150] Twelve percent of axillary node–negative patients with lesions 1 cm or less in diameter develop metastases within 20 years of diagnosis, and almost 30 percent of node-negative T1c patients relapse within 20 years.[200, 203] In addition, specific subgroups of node-negative patients with small carcinomas 10 cm or less have been shown to have only a 44 to 67 percent distant disease-free survival.[1, 137] If you look at very long-term survival, an excess breast cancer mortality is observed for at least 40 years even in node-negative patients.[24, 208] We know little about assessing the virulence of lymph node metastases in addition to their mere presence. But there are clearly factors other than node-positivity impacting breast cancer survival. The disease may never be truly localized even though the nodes are negative.

According to halstedian thinking, breast cancer progressed centrifugally and contiguously from the primary lesion by direct extension to the draining lymph nodes, which acted as a barrier/filter, and then to distant metastatic sites. The Fisher hypothesis of the biology of breast cancer is that it is a systemic disease involving complex host-tumor interactions and that variations in the local-regional treatment do not substantially alter survival. This hypothesis suggests that the presence of positive axillary nodes means that the cancer is more aggressive, that it has a greater tendency to metastasize, or that it has already metastasized elsewhere. Thus, lymph node metastases are thought to be "indicators" but not "governors" of survival,[28] and "indicators" not "instigators" of distant disease.[66] The lymph nodes may not be the sole indicators, however, nor even the best indicators.[87, 90, 155] Other histological factors of the primary tumor or biological predictors and clinical characteristics are being examined as correlates with the risk of nodal involvement to better predict

risk of nodal positivity or, indeed, to better predict long-term outcome and therefore to define subgroups that may or may not need node dissections.

Evidence suggests that tumorigenesis, and by extension, metastagenesis, results from an accumulation of genetic abnormalities.[140] It is logical, therefore, to investigate other markers to attempt to predict more aggressive phenotypes even more accurately than axillary nodal status to replace axillary dissection altogether. Thus, there are two ways to address the problem: use prognostic factors to predict nodal status or use prognostic factors other than axillary lymph node status to produce models predictive of clinical outcome that are equal to or better than axillary node staging.

Perhaps our understanding of the natural history of invasive breast cancer may lie somewhere in between the halstedian and fisherian views, as in the spectrum hypothesis proposed by Hellman.[112, 113] He proposes that breast cancer is a heterogeneous disease that has a spectrum of proclivities, ranging from a disease that remains local throughout its course to one that is systemic when first detected. Persistent disease, either locally in the axillary nodes or in the breast, can serve as the source of distant disease. One of the unanswered questions relevant to this hypothesis is the issue of whether lymph node positivity occurs only as a function of time.[159] As shown in Figure 54–1, the smaller the tumor, the less the likelihood of positive lymph nodes.[97, 109] Is it because as tumors get larger, they simply have more opportunity to metastasize?[132] Or is it because as tumors increase in size, the likelihood of metastases increases because there is a critical volume for each tumor that must be reached before metastases occur?[111] Or is it because lymph node positivity is a function of the inherent aggressiveness of the primary tumor and not necessarily only a function of the chronological age as inferred by size? The relationship among tumor size, lymph node status, and survival is shown in Figure 54–2. Although the presence of positive lymph nodes and size of tumor are correlated, they also appear to be independent prognostic variables.[50, 64, 92] This suggests that lymph node positivity can be a function of the inherent aggressiveness of the primary tumor. But node-positive breast cancer may not just be a late manifestation of node-negative disease.[163] Although size is correlated with survival and the number of axillary metastases, examination of the subset of patients with invasive carcinomas 1 cm or less indicates that tumor size and lymph node status may lose their roles as prognostic indicators of overall survival. Other biological factors such as histological grade, particularly nuclear grade,[235] or lymphovascular invasion[1, 137] assume statistically significant roles.[113, 199, 200, 205, 207, 238] Tubiana and Koscielny analyzed a large series of patients at the Institute Gustave-Roussy to determine the relationship between the size of the primary tumor and the probability of distant metastatic spread. Even in tumors smaller than 1 cm, there is a calculated 4 percent probability of occult distant metasta-

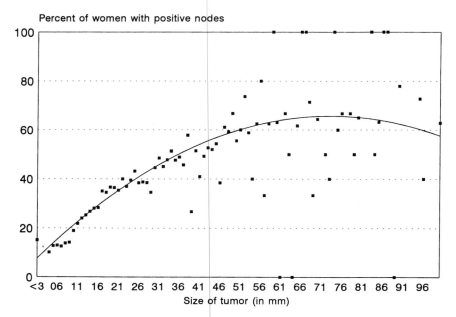

Figure 54–1 *Invasive female breast cancer showing percent of women with positive axillary lymph nodes by tumor size, excluding cases with further extension or distant metastases, SEER data 1983–1987. (From Gloeckler-Ries LA, Henson DE, Harras A: Survival from breast cancer according to tumor size and nodal status. Surg Oncol Clin North Am 3:35–53, 1994.)*

ses.[244] There is also enormous variation in growth rates of breast cancer and survivability.[114, 230] If one examines the median survival of breast cancer patients after first recurrence as a function of initial nodal status within a given tumor size (<2 cm), the presence of positive axillary nodes at initial diagnosis identifies a more aggressive phenotype that continues to affect outcome even after first recurrence.[125]

Regarding the question of axillary lymph node status being prognostic in small invasive carcinomas less than 11 mm, one key issue is whether there is a size limit below which an axillary dissection can be safely avoided because no additional meaningful prognostic information will be provided beyond the characteristics of the primary tumor. If so, how does

one set the threshold of probability of axillary lymph node metastases? A 3, 5, or 10 percent risk of nodal positivity? Long-term survival of patients with carcinomas 1 cm or less shows a significant impact of positive nodes. Review of our data on 345 small carcinomas less than 11 mm in diameter indicates a breast cancer–specific survival at 10 years of 95 percent in node-negative patients versus 83 percent for this same subset of patients with positive nodes. Hellman suggested that T1a or T1b invasive cancers are precisely one clinical situation in which there could be involved nodes but no distant disease, and therefore prompt initial treatment of the regional lymph nodes in this group is especially important.[113] Consequently, elimination of the prognostic role of

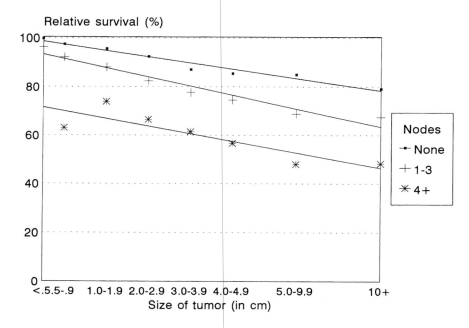

Figure 54–2 *Invasive breast cancer. 5-year relative survival rates by tumor size and number of positive regional lymph nodes, excluding cases with further extension or distant metastases, SEER 1977–1982. (From Gloeckler-Ries LA, Henson DE, Harras A: Survival from breast cancer according to tumor size and nodal status. Surg Oncol Clin North Am 3:35–53, 1994.)*

axillary lymph node dissection may not negate the therapeutic role in these small cancers.

IS AXILLARY NODE DISSECTION NECESSARY FOR THERAPY?

The results of the National Surgical Adjuvant Breast and Bowel Project (NSABP) protocol B-04[68] provided strong evidence against the halstedian concept of centrifugal breast cancer spread. After its publication, the necessity of axillary dissection as a therapeutic procedure became seriously debated, and attempts were made to define those patients in whom axillary dissection could be omitted because it may represent overtreatment.* The therapeutic goals of axillary lymph node dissection are to prevent axillary recurrence and theoretically to improve overall survival. We shall examine each goal separately.

Prevention of Axillary Recurrence

In NSABP B-04, patients with clinically negative axillas were randomized to one of three treatment arms: radical mastectomy, total mastectomy and postoperative radiation to the chest wall and axilla, or total mastectomy alone.[68] Careful scrutiny by Harris and Osteen[107] indicates that at a mean follow-up of 94 months, of the 236 patients who had a total mastectomy and no nodes removed, 21.2 percent went on to develop clinical axillary disease that was histologically confirmed. Of the remaining 142 patients treated with total mastectomy who had 5 or fewer nodes removed as part of the mastectomy procedure, 12 percent subsequently had axillary recurrence and required an axillary dissection. Of those patients who had more than 5 nodes removed as part of the total mastectomy specimen, none required a subsequent axillary dissection. Thus, the axillary relapse rate clearly depends on the number of nodes removed. The Danish Breast Cancer Group, in a series of more than 3000 axillary dissections, found a 21 percent rate of axillary recurrence if no nodes were removed, but no axillary recurrences if 5 or more axillary nodes were removed.[99] Based on the assumption that approximately 40 percent of patients who had no nodes removed in NSABP B-04 were actually node positive (based on the incidence of nodal positivity in the radical mastectomy arm of the B-04 trial), approximately half of those who actually had positive nodes required an axillary dissection, suggesting that unremoved, involved axillary nodes do not invariably develop into clinically significant adenopathy.[129] Alternatively, about half of the patients with untreated, pathologically involved axillary nodes will develop clinically evident disease in the axilla.

In addition to NSABP B-04, other studies that look at the incidence of subsequent axillary nodal failure in patients who initially had simple mastectomies

and no surgical or radiotherapeutic treatment of the axilla are the King's Cambridge Cancer Research Campaign trial,[33] the Manchester series,[142] the Cardiff–St. Mary's trials,[78] and the Danish series.[99] These studies show highly variable axillary recurrence rates of 7 to 37 percent at 10 years, partly because these are not truly comparable groups. The Cardiff–St. Mary's trial, for example, performed total mastectomies, but careful attention was paid to isolate several nodes either in the specimen in the tail of the breast or with the pectoral nodal sampling.[79] If any positive nodes were found, postoperative radiotherapy was given to the axilla. The recent 20-year update of the Cardiff local therapy trial[234] comparing mastectomy and axillary clearance with mastectomy and axillary node sampling shows that patients treated with node sampling (with an average of less than eight nodes removed) had a significantly worse distant disease-free survival and axillary recurrence rate (16 percent) compared with patients treated with axillary clearance. Thus, these trials confirm that not treating or undertreating the axilla will result in significant axillary recurrence.

Does Treatment of the Axilla Affect Survival?

A delayed axillary dissection could be performed in those 50 percent of patients with clinically negative, but pathologically positive, axillary lymph nodes who do not undergo an axillary dissection and who eventually develop axillary disease. The critical question, however, is whether untreated nodes contribute to a decrease in overall survival. Examination of NSABP B-04 data at 10 years[68] shows no statistically significant effect on survival between the total mastectomy group (42 percent) and the radical mastectomy group (47 percent). Harris and Osteen[107] question whether enough patients were entered into NSABP B-04 to actually prove that there is no effect on overall survival, because axillary dissection cannot be expected to improve survival in axillary node–negative patients (approximately 60 percent of the 236 patients who had no nodes removed). Furthermore, to prove a small, but statistically significant, survival benefit, at least 2000 patients would be required.[90] Sample size is critical in proving statistical significance when the magnitude of difference is 10 percent or less. The Manchester trial[142] included 1022 clinically node-negative patients randomly allocated to simple mastectomy alone versus simple mastectomy plus irradiation to the axilla. Notably, at 10 years, there was a survival advantage of 7 percent for the surgically axillary-treated group, although this too was not statistically significant. The Danish Breast Cancer Group examined overall survival in 3128 patients as a function of number of nodes removed and found an overall survival benefit of 8 percent at 10 years in those patients who had more than five nodes removed compared to no nodes removed.[99] The King's/Cambridge trial showed no difference in overall survival in the untreated axilla group.[33] The update of

---

*See references 4, 32, 55, 193, 206, 209, and 223.

the Southeast Scottish trial in which patients who had a "simple" mastectomy with excision of one or more lymph nodes lying close to the top of the axillary tail of the breast or in the adjacent axillary fat were randomized to either immediate radical radiotherapy or managed by a watch policy. At 15 years, of the 118 patients in whom no nodes were found, there was an approximately 10 percent difference in distant disease-free survival in favor of those from whom nodes were proved to be negative compared with the group who had no axillary nodes identified in the specimen.[233] These mature studies all suggest a small (4 to 10 percent) but consistent survival benefit in those patients who had some initial treatment to the axilla. A retrospective review of 1126 patients with invasive carcinomas 1 cm or less in overall tumor diameter was performed by White and associates.[263] Of this large series of small carcinomas, 969 patients had an axillary dissection as part of breast conservation treatment or a modified radical mastectomy, and 157 patients did not have an axillary dissection. At 5 years, there was a statistically significant difference in overall, disease-free, and breast cancer–specific survival. The majority of patients in whom an axillary recurrence is the first site of recurrent disease usually die of their disease.[55, 99] In the NSABP B-04 study, the 21 percent of patients who had no axillary dissection and developed axillary disease had a poor overall prognosis.[107] Thus, there is a small but significant survival value of initial treatment of the regional nodes with surgery or radiotherapy.

BREAST CONSERVATION AND AXILLARY DISSECTION

There are no trials comparing wide excision plus breast irradiation and axillary dissection to wide excision plus breast irradiation without axillary dissection. Furthermore, with proper irradiation techniques to the breast alone, it is probable that the lower axilla is radiated in the tangential fields and thus may be therapeutically "equivalent" to a lower axillary dissection alone.[192] But an analysis of the effect of irradiating only the breast on the rate of axillary recurrences has not been thoroughly evaluated. The Guy's Hospital trial[110] compared wide excision alone to radical mastectomy. Although the radiotherapy given to the conservatively treated group was far less than optimal for breast conservation therapy, at 10 years there was no statistically significant advantage in the incidence of distant metastases for the group who had axillary dissections. There was a small (6 percent) beneficial difference in overall survival at 10 years for those clinically node-negative patients who had an axillary dissection. Hoskin and colleagues[119] treated 94 patients with clinically negative axillas with wide excision alone and standard breast irradiation. There were five axillary relapses in this group (5.3 percent) at a short follow-up of 35 months. At 51 months median follow-up, Halverson and associates[104] found no axillary relapses in a small series of 21 patients treated with radiotherapy given only to the conservatively treated breast. In this study, the majority of the primary tumors (17) were 10 mm or less in diameter. Cabanes and coworkers[27] prospectively compared axillary dissection in the conservatively treated breast to no axillary dissection. However, all patients received radiation to the breast, axillary, and internal mammary nodes as well. There were 332 patients in the group that received no axillary dissection and 326 in group with axillary dissection. At a 54-month mean follow-up, the survival difference was 4 percent (92.6 percent without axillary dissection versus 96.6 percent with axillary dissection; $p = 0.014$). At this short follow-up, a survival advantage is suggested for those patients who had axillary dissection, but such a conclusion has been criticized because all the patients received axillary radiation, and those patients who had axillary dissection and were found to have positive nodes received chemotherapy.

As more patients with small cancers are being treated with conservative surgery and breast irradiation, the question of performing only excision of the tumor in those patients with clinically negative axillas, followed by breast and axillary radiation without axillary dissection, has been raised. Haffty and colleagues,[102] in 242 clinical stage I patients treated by lumpectomy alone without axillary dissection followed by radiation therapy to the intact breast and regional lymph nodes, found a 3 percent 5-year actuarial nodal recurrence rate. Other studies confirm an axillary recurrence rate of 1 to 3 percent in patients with clinically negative axillas treated with breast conservation without axillary dissection who receive axillary radiotherapy specifically directed to the axilla, and that axillary-directed radiation is not necessary after a surgical axillary dissection in the conservatively treated breast.* Whether axillary irradiation is used as an alternative method of treating the axilla to replace axillary dissection in the conservatively treated breast has been reviewed by Recht and Houlihanm[192] and will not be discussed here.

Axillary recurrences after either appropriate axillary surgery or axillary radiation are low, generally 1 to 3 percent whether the nodes are positive or not, and in the absence of any treatment to the axilla, there will be a significantly higher axillary relapse rate (7 to 37 percent). As noted above, if there is no treatment to the axilla, approximately half of the clinically negative, but histologically undetected positive axillas, will develop clinically significant axillary nodal disease within approximately 10 years. These patients will require axillary treatment. It appears that the effect of delayed treatment on overall survival is low, but such axillary relapses are demoralizing and can be very difficult to treat. When lymph node failure occurs, successful regional control is achieved in less than half of patients.[93, 190] From the standpoint of ability to prevent axillary relapse, the

---

*See references 13, 45, 56, 58, 138, 175, 190, 194, and 258.

high efficacy of axillary treatment in prevention of such relapse argues for surgical or radiotherapeutic treatment in patients who are at significant risk for having positive nodes. Which patient subsets are at such a low risk of involvement that any axillary treatment is of so little value that it should be eliminated, remains to be defined. We shall discuss such subsets in the section on selective axillary node dissection.

EXTENT OF AXILLARY DISSECTION

Levels of the Axilla

The axillary contents are divided into three anatomical levels that are defined by their relationship to the pectoralis minor muscle.[9, 52] These levels are summarized in Table 54–1.

Types of Axillary Node Dissections

There is great variation among surgeons in what is meant by an "axillary dissection." The following terminology currently is used to define the types of axillary dissections.

1. *Axillary sampling:* Removal of an axillary node or nodes from the lower axilla. Precise anatomical boundaries are not clear, but it includes the nodes in the tail of the breast as well as a low level 1 dissection. This technique is widely practiced in the United Kingdom and provides an average of four[130] to seven nodes.[38]

2. *Low Level 1 dissection:* Nodes removed from the latissimus dorsi muscle laterally and to the pectoralis major muscle medially, but the dissection stops superiorly at the level of the major intercostobrachial nerve, thus sparing the nerve and not dissecting the axillary vein.

3. *Level 1 dissection:* An en bloc excision of Level 1 of the axilla, from the latissimus dorsi muscle laterally to the lateral border of the pectoralis minor muscle medially and the axillary vein superiorly. Provides a mean number of ten nodes in this level.[52, 253]

4. *Level 1 and 2 dissection:* A procedure similar to that described above, but this also includes removal of axillary tissue beneath the pectoralis minor muscle and interpectoral (Rotter's) nodes. Facilitated by elevation of the pectoralis minor muscle and mobilization of the ipsilateral arm to relax the pectoralis major muscle. This dissection proceeds from the latissimus dorsi muscle laterally to the medial border of the pectoralis minor muscle medially. Provides a mean number of 11 to 17 nodes.[52, 253]

5. *Level 1, 2, or 3, total axillary lymphadenectomy, or radical axillary dissection:* Radical axillary dissection (total axillary dissection; total axillary lymphadenectomy; total axillary clearance) involves removal of the entire axillary contents, from the latissimus dorsi muscle laterally to the subclavius muscle (Halsted's ligament) medially, clearing the axillary vein, with preservation or excision of the pectoralis minor muscle (removing nodes below and lateral to pectoralis minor muscle). Provides a mean number of 20 nodes.[52, 54, 253]

ANALYSIS OF THE SURGICAL EXTENT OF AXILLARY DISSECTION

The range of axillary dissections varies among surgeons, ranging from axillary sampling to total axillary clearance. There are proponents of either extreme, and there is much debate regarding the best method of assessing the axilla. The arguments for a complete or total axillary dissection are similar to the arguments for performing any axillary dissection at all; namely, that it is therapeutic by reducing the risk of axillary recurrence to less than 5 percent and prognostic, by allowing even more accurate determination of nodal metastases.* But are these arguments valid? What constitutes an "adequate" axillary dissection?

Investigative approaches to answer this question include what are the minimum number of axillary nodes needed to accurately predict node positivity, and how often do skip metastases occur, that is, involvement of nodes in the higher axillary levels (2 and/or 3) with negative nodes in Level 1? Is there a difference in rates of local recurrence in patients who have different surgical extents of axillary dissection? The small, but consistent, difference in overall survival between those who have an axillary dissection and those who do not (4 to 10 percent) was thoroughly discussed in a previous section. As we have come to appreciate the heterogeneity of breast cancer, we are also recognizing the feasibility of tailoring the extent of axillary dissection to each patient (see section on selective axillary dissection). Another consideration is how often are positive axillary nodes missed by the pathologist, despite extensive surgical dissection, and what effect may this have on the survival of patients who are understaged? Thus, the more extensive the surgery, the more nodes will be removed, and the more diligently the pathologist searches, the more nodes, both positive and negative,

TABLE 54–1.   SURGICAL AXILLARY LEVEL DEFINITIONS

LEVEL 1: Also called *low axilla.* Refers to those nodes between the latissimus dorsi muscle, the lateral border of the axilla, and the lateral border of the pectoralis minor muscle.

LEVEL 2: The midaxilla. Refers to the axillary tissue behind or deep to the minor muscle (between the lateral and medial borders of the pectoralis minor muscle and inferior to the muscle) and the interpectoral (Rotter's) nodes.

LEVEL 3: Apex of the axilla. Refers to those nodes medial to the medial border of the pectoralis minor, extending to Halsted's ligament (costoclavicular ligament). Medial to this structure, the axillary vein enters the thorax.

---

*See references 15, 19, 51, 52, 53, 63, 160, 195, 219, and 253.

will be found. The issue is whether this makes any prognostic or therapeutic difference to the patient.

There are several studies examining the distribution of lymph nodes in the axilla and the distribution of positive lymph nodes in the axilla.* The more lymph nodes examined, the more positive lymph nodes will be found.[12] Danforth[52] tabulated the results of seven series analyzing the distribution of lymph nodes according to each level. Although there is much variation in these studies because of the natural imprecision in defining the levels, clearly 80 to 90 percent of axillary lymph nodes are found in Levels 1 and 2. Although a total axillary dissection (Levels 1, 2, and 3) in all cases is recommended by some,[42, 63, 160, 249, 254, 264] others concur that a Level 1 and 2 dissection is adequate in the absence of gross disease.† Pigott and colleagues[184] and Veronesi and associates[249] conclude from their extensive studies of axillary levels that metastatic invasion of the axillary nodes in patients with carcinoma of the breast follows a regular, progressive pattern, and as a rule, the nodes of the first level are first involved and then the second and the third level are seeded in successive steps. Most‡ but not all[184] have found a low incidence of skip metastases (1 to 3 percent) to Level 3, low potential understaging of 3 or less, and a low risk of regional recurrence if a Level 3 dissection is not performed.[160, 198, 220] There are also those who contend that a Level 1 dissection is adequate for staging purposes in the majority of cases because it is an accurate predictor of the entire axilla in 95 to 96 percent of patients.[23, 129, 249] Veronesi and associates[249] and Kjaergaard and colleagues[131] have shown that Level 1 nodes were positive in 96 percent of all patients who had positive nodes. Therefore, if axillary dissection is viewed solely as a prognostic tool, that information is theoretically available from a Level 1 dissection.

The therapeutic role of a Level 1 or 2 axillary dissection can be viewed with the following example. In patients with T1c carcinomas who have positive Level 1 nodes, there is a significant (28 percent) risk of metastases at Level 2 or 3.[249] By having only a Level 1 dissection, and assuming fewer than ten but more than five nodes are removed, this patient would have a 10 to 15 percent risk of progressing to clinically positive axillary disease and subsequently requiring an axillary dissection.[68] Although we do not know the incidence of positive lymph nodes by level in small carcinomas 1 cm or less, the overall incidence of positive lymph nodes in these small lesions may be significant (see Table 54–5).

The incidence of skip metastases to Level 2 (that is, negative nodes in Level 1 with positive nodes in Level 2) is extremely low: 1.2 percent in Veronesi and colleagues, series (6 of 539),[249] 5 percent (6 of 120) in the series by Chevinsky and associates,[42] 2.5 percent in the series of 200 patients by Boova and

colleagues,[23] and 4.7 percent (23 of 492) in a series by Gaglia and colleagues.[85] Rosen and coworkers[198] found skip metastases to Level 2 in only 7 of 1228 patients. However, two studies found skip metastases to Level 2 in 22 percent and 27 percent of cases.[51, 248] Lesser procedures, such as axillary sampling,[80, 81, 231, 232] or what amounts to a low Level 1 dissection,[53] are generally discouraged because of the small number of nodes retrieved and the potential understaging in up to 45 percent of cases.[54, 130] Proponents of sampling indicate that a mean of seven nodes are removed, and there is a low axillary failure rate.[38, 231] Others[100, 106] contend that it should not be performed because it is not anatomically precise, is not considered to denote a precise surgical procedure, and does not adequately stage the axilla.

Another approach to the problem of determining the optimal extent of axillary dissection is to determine the minimum number of axillary nodes that should be resected to predict nodal positivity. Although Mouridsen and associates[162] found that even in node-negative patients, the number of nodes examined alone served as a prognostic indicator, Mathiesen and colleagues demonstrated that removing a minimum of ten nodes would accurately stage the axilla.[148] In this study, the axillary nodal status of 960 consecutive patients was analyzed according to the number of nodes removed, and the incidence of node positivity in each subgroup was calculated. They found the probability of finding at least one metastatic node increased continuously up to about ten removed nodes. This minimum number was similarly confirmed by Wilking and associates.[264] In addition, recurrence-free survival by nodal status in a subgroup of patients who had one to three positive nodes was statistically poorer for patients who had fewer than five nodes removed, compared with patients who had five to nine nodes removed or ten or more nodes removed. However, there was no difference in recurrence-free survival in node-negative patients as a function of number of nodes removed. Kissin and associates[130] initially performed a lower axillary dissection, removing an average of four lymph nodes; thereafter, in the same session, a total mastectomy and radical axillary dissection were performed on 50 patients. In patients who had an average of four lymph nodes removed, a false negative axillary status occurred in 17 percent of the cases, whereas a positive axillary status was underdiagnosed in about 30 percent of cases. Davies[54] calculated that a lower axillary dissection with the removal of an average of six lymph nodes would have entailed a false negative nodal status in 10 percent of the cases and underdiagnosed a positive axillary status in 15 percent.

The rate of axillary recurrence as a function of the number of nodes that should be removed to provide an acceptably low rate of axillary recurrences has also been studied. Recht and coworkers demonstrated an increased rate of axillary recurrence in node-negative patients as a function of number of nodes removed.[190] Graversen and colleagues[99] also

---

*See references 20, 23, 51, 52, 141, 249, and 253.
†See references 66, 67, 68, 198, 206, 215, and 220.
‡See references 23, 29, 51, 85, 144, 198, and 249.

examined axillary recurrences in patients as a function of the number of nodes removed in an axillary dissection. In a series of 3128 women followed for a mean of 6.5 years, the probability of axillary recurrence was 2 percent if ten or more nodes were removed, and 5 percent if fewer than five nodes were removed. Kjaergaard and coworkers also found a significant risk of axillary relapse if fewer than three nodes were examined.[131] Dewar found an axillary relapse rate of 1.2 percent at 5 years with a minimum of seven nodes removed in node-positive patients and a much lower relapse rate of 0.7 percent in node-negative patients.[58] In NSABP B-04 there were no axillary recurrences in the group of patients who had at least five nodes removed as part of the total mastectomy group.[68]

In summary, performing a defined Level 1 and 2 dissection with removal of at least ten nodes will not significantly underestimate the metastatic involvement of the axilla, will provide accurate prognostic information, and will result in a very low axillary recurrence rate. Furthermore, the advantage of performing an anatomically defined Level 1 and 2 dissection is that if fewer than ten nodes are recovered, the surgeon knows that the entire contents of Levels 1 and 2 were removed, so the low count represents a variation in normal anatomy or a less-than-thorough pathological evaluation rather than inadequate removal of axillary tissue. Such a dissection will also minimize the risk of lymphedema.[5, 27, 181, 220]

ANALYSIS OF THE ANATOMICAL EXTENT OF PATHOLOGICAL AXILLARY DISSECTION

Because lymph node status is pivotal in the assessment of prognosis, careful study of the methods of pathological examination has been made to further refine and expand the information obtained from the lymph nodes removed by the surgeon.[73, 127, 265] These studies include how the nodes are first detected in the axillary specimen, how the nodes are then processed for slides, and how metastases are found in the lymph nodes.

In most laboratories, the axillary fat is examined for lymph nodes by visual and tactile inspection. The numbers of lymph nodes detected varies by individual, the extent of the surgical dissection, and by the diligence of the pathologist's search. The gross examination process was thoroughly reviewed by Fisher and Slack.[65] Pickren[183] was the first to show that clearance of axillary fat in cedar oil and more thorough sectioning increases the yield of positive nodes, but Morrow and colleagues[161] and Kingsley and associates[127] reported that clearing of the axillary fat may yield more nodes but does not change the clinical staging when compared with routine examination of the axillary fat.

If, however, more careful analysis changes the pathological staging, the discovery of additional nodes might be relevant. Therefore, the issue of how the nodes are sectioned has also been studied. Rosen and associates[196] and others[11, 74, 122] maintain that a single slice dividing the node into two halves, preferably at the hilum of the node,[109] providing a gross single section, is adequate for histopathological examination of the nodes. However, serial sub-gross step sectioning, cutting each node into approximately 1.5- to 2.0-mm thick slices, is performed by some groups.[58, 84, 147] Such macroscopic sectioning reveals an additional 17 to 24 percent positive nodes and alters the stage in 8.8 percent of cases.[72, 265] Although Kinne[129] states that microscopic serial lymph node sectioning is tedious and costly, serial sub-gross step sectioning is less time-consuming than serial microscopic sectioning of the paraffin blocks at 10- to 12-μ intervals. Serial sub-gross lymph node sectioning results in the detection of more micrometastases, and the prognostic significance of micrometastases has been investigated.

The term *micrometastasis* has evolved since Pickren[183] originally referred to micrometastases as occult metastases or those that escaped routine hematoxylin and eosin (H&E)–stained pathological examination. Attiyeh and coworkers,[11] Rosen and colleagues,[197] and Huvos and associates[122] define micrometastases as being less than 2 mm in largest diameter. Fisher and colleagues[73] have defined micrometastases as 1.3 mm in diameter or less. Others define micrometastasis as less than 0.5 mm.[147] The American Joint Committee on Cancer defines micrometastasis as 0.2 cm or less for purposes of staging.[9] Pickren[183] and Fisher and associates[72] found that on microscopic step sectioning, not sub-gross macroscopic step sectioning, of the paraffin blocks, 22 to 24 percent of the patients with so-called negative lymph nodes indeed had occult metastases, but the survival in this group was no different than those with negative nodes. Review of the NSABP B-04 data showed no difference in overall survival in patients who had negative nodes versus those who had a micrometastasis less than 2.0 mm.[73] There was a difference in disease-free survival, however, at 4 years, with 60 percent disease-free survival in patients with micrometastases less than 2 mm versus 90 percent disease-free survival in patients with no nodal metastases. Because the number of patients with micrometastases was only 21, the number was too small for statistical purposes. But the presence of micrometastases may indicate an aggressive breast cancer phenotype, and the size of the primary breast carcinoma may be of importance in interpreting the significance of micrometastases. For example, Rosen and colleagues[197] found that patients with smaller tumors and micrometastases do worse: during the first 6 years of follow-up, patients with T1 breast carcinoma with negative lymph nodes and those with a single micrometastasis less than 2 mm had similar survival curves; however, at 12 years, the survival of those T1 patients with micrometastases or macrometastases was nearly identical to those T1 patients with macrometastases, and both were significantly worse than those with negative nodes. But T2 tumors with negative nodes or a single micrometastasis had survival curves that did not differ throughout the long follow-up. Clayton and Hopkins[46] also noted an unfavorable relationship between small carcinomas and micrometastases. At a median follow-up of 10 years, patients with small primary carcinomas (<1.8 cm in diameter) showed a statistically significant worse overall survival if a micrometastasis less than 2 mm was present compared with patients with negative nodes (78 versus 89 percent).

The importance of detecting axillary node micrometastases has been examined by the International (Ludwig) Breast Cancer Study Group. Microscopic serial sectioning of lymph nodes at six different levels from 921 patients initially thought to be node-negative resulted in 83 patients (9 percent) who had missed nodal micrometastases.[21, 168] In their series of 921 patients, 122 had tumors 1 cm or less in diameter. Of these 122, 8 (6.6 percent) had micrometastases. In addition, in a much larger series of 633 small carcinomas less than 11 mm, in which meticulous sub-gross lymph node sectioning was performed, a 6.4 percent incidence of axillary micrometastases was similarly noted (Trojani M: Personal communication, 1995).

There is no consensus on the prognostic significance of micrometastases. In the Ludwig series, at 6 years of median follow-up there was a definite outcome disadvantage for those who converted to the node-positive classification after detection of micrometastases. The 6-year overall survival was 70 percent for those who converted versus 86 percent for those in whom no micrometastases were found ($p = 0.0009$).[21, 168] At 10 years, this survival disadvantage remains unaltered (Gelber RD and associates: Personal communication, 1995). The 10-year disease-free survival for the 8 patients with small carcinomas (≤ 1 cm) with axillary micrometastases in the Ludwig series was 63 percent compared with 73 percent for the 114 patients with small tumors without micrometastasis. Although this difference is not statistically significant because of the small numbers, the concept that micrometastases in small tumors portend an aggressive tumor must be considered. The Bordeaux series,[147, 243] in which micrometastases were found by serial sub-gross macroscopic sectioning, noted a significant difference in disease-free survival, but not in overall survival at 10 and 15 years between those patients with a micrometastasis of less than 0.5 mm versus those with no metastases. These authors and others[84] who routinely perform this technique claim that the serial gross step sectioning technique is not overly tedious or time-consuming. But Sacks and associates[209] believe that its value over and above finding new tumor markers awaits confirmation.

Others have analyzed the importance of serial sub-gross sectioning of lymph nodes and studied the incidence of occult lymph node metastases. These were previously undiagnosed or missed metastases but not necessarily micrometastases. In a series of 525 cases, occult metastases were found in 17 percent of patients, but there was no difference in overall survival between patients with negative nodes and those with occult nodes at 15 years.[265] Nasser and associates[166] also reported a 17 percent incidence of occult lymph node metastases by H & E stain after serial microscopic section, but no difference in disease-free survival at 14 years.

Overall, there is an approximately 9 to 17 percent incidence of occult or missed metastases by the pathologist and a similar incidence of micrometastases. Although there is some suggestive evidence, it is not clear whether the presence of micrometastases in small carcinomas 1 cm or less portends a particularly virulent tumor. Although more than routine single-section axillary node examination may be required, further research is needed to ascertain the most appropriate methods of diagnostic return.[167]

Other methods for examination of the lymph nodes, in addition to relying on H & E stains and the diligence of the pathologist, include immunohistochemical staining and polymerase chain reaction (PCR) in homogenized or sectioned lymph nodes. Ten published studies of immunohistochemical analyses of axillary lymph nodes in breast cancer (Table 54–2) show a 9 to 30 percent incidence of metastases detected by immunohistochemical methods. But only two of these ten studies show that these immunometastases affect prognosis. Using several monoclonal antibodies directed against epithelial cell antigens, Trojani and de Mascarel and associates[147, 242] detected immunohistochemical metastases in 14 percent of 150 node-negative patients. They found that the presence of immunometastases predicts only disease recurrence and not overall survival. Hainsworth and colleagues[103] reported on 343 apparently node-negative patients who were assessed with antimucin monoclonal antibodies. Twelve percent of these patients were found to have metastases by this method. With a median follow-up of 79 months, these patients also had a statistically significant decreased disease-free survival but no decrease in overall survival. However, there was a significant decrease in overall survival if two or more nodes were found to contain immunometastases. A report by Giuliano and co-workers has shown that careful processing of the blue-stained sentinel node in the axilla, obtained after injection of the breast tissue in proximity to the primary tumor with a blue vital dye, significantly increases the yield of both micrometastases detected by H & E and by immunohistochemistry.[95] In this study, no patients who had routine axillary lymph node dissection were found to have immunometastases, but 6.8 percent of the patients who had targeted processing of the sentinel node by serial microscopic sectioning were found to have immunometastases. Although the yield may be increased, the impact on survival remains to be established. Certainly, careful processing of only the axillary sentinel node or nodes for micrometastases by either H & E staining or immunohistochemical staining or both would be more time and cost efficient.

Recently, PCR has been used to determine if the

TABLE 54–2. LYMPH NODE METASTASIS BY IMMUNOHISTOCHEMISTRY

Author	No. of Pts IHC-Positive/Total	Percent IHC-Positive	DFS	OS
Sedmark et al[217]	45	20	Not examined	48% decrease at 10 years
Wells et al[261]	12/57	21	Not examined	Not examined
Trojani et al[242]	21/150	14	28% decrease—10 yr*	25% decrease—10 yr*
Nasser et al[166]	159	31	No effect	No effect
Hainsworth et al[103]	41/343	12	16% decrease—5 yr	No effect
Galea[86]	9/98	9	No effect	No effect
de Mascarel et al[147]	166	30	20% decrease—15 years	No effect
Bussolati et al[26]	12/50	24	No effect	No effect
Chen et al[41]	23/80	29	16% decrease	
Raymond and Leong[189]	7/30	23	Not examined	Not examined

* Significant difference seen in infiltrating ductal carcinoma only.
OS = overall survival; DFS = disease-free survival; IHC = immunohistochemistry; Pts = patients.

detection rate of micrometastases could be improved. Schoenfeld and associates[213] and Noguchi and associates[172] have demonstrated that measurement of a marker gene by amplifying the mRNA product with a reverse transcriptase-PCR will dramatically improve the detection of micrometastases in axillary lymph nodes (perhaps 1 abnormal cell in 10^7 lymphocytes) in patients with breast cancer. This preliminary work must be correlated with patient outcome, and further refinements in the specificities of the markers used are necessary.

OTHER PREDICTORS OF AXILLARY LYMPH NODE METASTASES

Surgical axillary dissection to determine the status of axillary nodes remains the standard of care in the management of breast cancer. But with the acknowledgment of the small therapeutic benefit of axillary node dissection, increasing use of chemotherapy in node-negative breast cancer, and breast-conserving treatment, efforts have focused on the development of other prognostic factors for breast cancer to replace the role of axillary node dissection and to improve the patient selection strategies for chemotherapy or hormonal therapy. Current therapeutic approaches rely on the pathological TNM grouping as well as histopathological features of the primary tumor, including histological and nuclear grade, but many other prognostic parameters have been evaluated alone and in combination to refine our ability to predict patient outcome in node-negative patients.[16, 92, 152, 236, 268] These markers generally include (1) measures of proliferation and steroid or estrogen-related markers (e.g., DNA flow cytometry and hormone receptors) and (2) multiple other prognostic factors such as oncogenes and their protein products (e.g., P53, HRAS, MYC) enzymes (cathepsin D), growth factors and receptors, and angiogenesis.* If the axillary lymph node status of patients with breast cancer could be accurately predicted from characteristics of the primary tumor, from other prognostic markers,

or from some combination of these parameters, then the current standard of TNM staging might be replaced.

Primary tumor size with the pathological characteristics of histological grade, nuclear grade, and the presence of lymphovascular invasion was examined in a group of T1 tumors with regard to predicting axillary nodal positivity. Chadha and colleagues[37] reviewed 263 patients with T1 cancers and clinically negative axillas who had a Level 2 axillary dissection and found that only tumor size and the presence of lymphovascular invasion were statistically significant predictors of axillary involvement. On multivariate analysis, nuclear grade did not predict nodal involvement.

Worsening histological tumor grade as a predictor of nodal positivity has also been demonstrated.[12, 256] A review of 11,173 patients showed that those patients with tumors showing a histological grade of 1 had 37 percent positive nodes, whereas those patients with grade 3 carcinomas had 56 percent positive nodes.[12] In this study of 1474 tumors 10 mm or less, only 10 percent of these were grade 3. Our data of 322 tumors 10 mm or less revealed a 13 percent incidence of histological grade 3. Other factors such as hormone receptors, S-phase fraction, and ploidy fail to improve the predictive value of tumor size alone,[4, 83] but recently the estrogen-related protein PS2 was shown by Nichols and colleagues[170] to correlate with nodal positivity, although this work needs verification. The data on the relationship between the oncogene P53 and nodal positivity is conflicting,[146, 173, 255] and simultaneous expression of P53 with cathepsin D does appear to correlate with positive nodal metastases. More work on the standardization of these prognostic factors and the definition of a limited set of markers that are independently predictive is necessary.[143]

By combining multiple factors, various attempts have been made to construct a predictive model of axillary node positivity.[156, 188] From a large data base of 6,356 patients, Ravdin and associates[188] examined multiple parameters, including tumor size, number of positive nodes, patient age, quantitative estrogen

*See references 22, 44, 134, 140, 143, 259, and 260.

and progesterone receptor levels, ploidy, and S-phase fraction. Tumor size was still identified as the strongest predictor on multivariate analysis. Groups with a probability of less than 10 percent or greater than 75 percent of having positive nodes can be identified using these models, but subsets could not be identified with more certainty. Another study using a large data base from the American College of Surgeons survey found that the percentage of cases in which the probability of positive nodes could be accurately predicted was very small.[89] Friedman and Friedman[83] also examined readily available prognostic factors in 110 patients to see if there were any correlation with axillary node status. Multiple regression analysis, followed by repeated univariate analyses, revealed that DNA ploidy, percent S-phase fraction, and hormone receptors failed to improve the predictive value of tumor size alone in determining the likelihood of having positive nodes. We reviewed our data on axillary lymph node metastases, which focuses on small carcinomas only, in 918 patients with T1 breast lesions who had a Level 1 or 2 axillary lymph node dissection.[225] To assess the ability to predict axillary lymph node metastases, we examined a total of eleven prognostic factors, including pathological tumor size, lymphatic/vascular invasion, nuclear grade, S-phase fraction, ploidy, palpability, age, estrogen and progesterone receptor status, HER2/NEU overexpression, and histological type. These factors were analyzed by univariate analysis and, when significant, by multivariate analysis. Of these 11 factors, only tumor size, lymphatic/vascular invasion, nuclear grade, and method of detection (nonpalpable versus palpable) remained statistically significant (Table 54–3). Using this information, among 117 patients with nonpalpable, non–high nuclear grade carcinomas less than 1 cm without lymphatic or vascular invasion, the incidence of positive lymph nodes was only 3.4 percent (4 of 117). Such an approach, based on readily available prognostic factors, may help develop those subsets of patients who have a very low

probability, which we would define as 5 percent or less, of positive lymph nodes and justify avoiding an axillary dissection.

Another method to define groups of patients in whom axillary dissection can be eliminated is to analyze whether prognostic factors can be used to produce models predictive of clinical outcome in lieu of axillary node status. Can we predict overall survival better than axillary nodal status? Menard and coworkers,[155] for example, have developed a prognostic score based on histological grade, tumor size, *CERBB2* oncogene overexpression, and laminin receptor overexpression. Overall survival of 463 patients with clinically negative axillas, all of whom had axillary node dissection as part of a radical or modified radical mastectomy, were studied. None of the patients received chemotherapy. The overall survival of the patients in the four different score groups was compared with the overall survival in node-positive and node-negative patients. The use of this scoring system resulted in a refinement of prognosis by allowing a more accurate grouping of overall patient survival compared with pathological nodal status. Further studies are needed to confirm this work. Querzoli and coworkers[185] compared the biological profile of 907 invasive carcinomas using several biological prognostic markers, such as hormone receptors, proliferative index, and *CERBB2* expression, and compared these with standard histological markers. Such studies may lead to the integration of and eventual substitution for the current TNM staging system. Such an approach and the development of a scoring system based on readily available characteristics of the primary tumor might be more universally applicable.

The status and utility of bone marrow micrometastases in breast cancer has been reviewed.[49, 176] Although this technique may identify a group of patients with an increased probability of relapse, further studies are necessary to address basic issues such as standardizing the criteria for defining micrometastases and the methodology. Although immunohistochemical methods are effective in identifying occult micrometastases in the bone marrow of patients with operable breast cancer, these methods are laborious, time-consuming, and require a high degree of expertise to perform and interpret. There appears to be little correlation between the presence of bone marrow micrometastases and positive axillary lymph nodes. Recently, Diel and colleagues[59] examined bilateral iliac crest bone marrow biopsies from 727 patients. Of the 19 patients with T1 breast cancers, 14 had tumor cells detected in their bone marrow aspirates, but only 8 of the 14 had positive axillary nodes. With improvements in technology, examination of the bone marrow may replace axillary node dissection.

OTHER METHODS OF AXILLARY STAGING

Several stepwise approaches to axillary staging are used to minimize the extent of axillary dissection. At

TABLE 54–3.   PREDICTIVE FACTORS OF AXILLARY LYMPH NODE METASTASIS IN 922 PATIENTS WITH T1 INVASIVE CARCINOMA

Variable	Percent Lymph Node Positive	Univariate p Value	Multivariate p Value
Tumor size			
T1a	4		
T1b	17	<0.0001	<0.01
T1c	28		
Tumor palpable			
Yes	28	<0.0001	<0.0004
No	10		
Lymph/vasc invasion			
Yes	46	<0.0001	<0.0000001
No	19		
Nuclear grade			
1	9		
2	21	<0.0001	<0.0004
3	34		

the Institute Gustave-Roussy,[58] a Level 1 axillary dissection is performed and the specimen is examined at the time of surgery by a pathologist. If a minimum of seven nodes are free of tumor, no further axillary surgery is performed. If any node is positive, the surgeon proceeds to perform an axillary clearance. Alternatively, an intraoperative touch-prep cytologic method has been described, in which four nodes are initially identified by palpation in the axillary fat pad alongside the pectoralis muscle. A contact cytologic smear of these sliced nodes is then made and examined, and if any nodes are positive, a total axillary dissection is performed.[71, 101] Such an imprint cytology method failed to identify only 1 of 51 positive nodes.

The concept of lymphatic mapping or identification of the sentinel node, the first node or nodes draining the primary tumor in the affected lymph node basin, has been examined by Giuliano and colleagues[94] (see Chapter 56). A blue vital dye was injected into the breast, followed by an axillary dissection to remove the blue-stained sentinel node. This technique accurately predicted axillary lymph node metastasis in 95.6 percent of cases. Multiple sectioning of the sentinel node for more extensive pathological analysis markedly increased the yield of micrometastases and immunometastases.[95]

Other methods of staging the axilla in lieu of surgical dissection have been investigated. Mammography, ultrasonography,[25, 123, 164] lymphangiography,[165] and computed tomography[144] of the axilla have not proved useful in determining positive axillary lymph nodes. Preliminary results with newer imaging techniques, such as positron emission tomography[3, 171] and magnetic resonance imaging[8] have been reported and may prove useful in the future.

Lymphoscintigraphy using an intraoperative gamma probe[6, 154, 239, 246] is under investigation as a method for identification of the sentinel node.[7, 133] Immunoscintigraphy, the detection of involved nodes with radioactively lableled monoclonal antibodies, is also an area of active research interest.[57, 120, 136, 179, 211, 241]

MINIMALLY INVASIVE BREAST CANCER AND THE ROLE OF AXILLARY DISSECTION

What Is Minimal Breast Cancer?

When Gallager and Martin first introduced the term *minimal breast cancer*,[88] it was intended to delineate a group of patients with a highly favorable prognosis and an extremely low risk of axillary metastasis. The original definition was applied to lobular carcinoma *in situ*, ductal carcinoma *in situ* (DCIS), and small invasive carcinomas no larger than 0.5 cm.[88, 121] The term was broadened and variously applied to tumors 1 cm or less in diameter, *in situ* and microinvasive carcinomas,[2, 169, 245] invasive cancers less than 0.5 cm with negative axillary nodes, clinically occult (nonpalpable) cancer,[157, 182, 214, 216] and special histological

entities such as cystosarcoma phyllodes, intracystic cancers, or low-grade infiltrating carcinomas, including medullary and colloid carcinoma.[82, 121, 258] Currently, there is no justification[250] for maintaining the original category of minimal breast cancer, because the biological behavior and natural history of these entities are so divergent. Although *minimal breast cancer* has been redefined to mean only invasive carcinomas 1 cm or less, the use of the term has been discouraged.[214] As discussed in a previous section, small breast cancers that are detected are not necessarily *early* or uniformly favorable. *Early-stage* cancer has been used to refer to carcinomas of any size not associated with lymph node metastases, according to the American Joint Committee on Cancer.[9] Small invasive cancers 1 cm in diameter represent approximately 1 billion cells and may contain a metastasizing phenotype. Knowledge of doubling times also indicates that these are not necessarily biologically early.[75, 244] And as noted above, some small, invasive, node-negative breast cancers demonstrate metastatic potential. Twelve percent of node-negative T1a and T1b palpable breast cancers detected in the premammographic era will recur within 20 years.[203] This is, however, substantially less than the 28 percent relapse rate of T1c carcinomas.[201] Approximately half of all invasive carcinomas 1 cm or less are of intermediate or high histological grade.[12, 235] Our own data on 322 invasive carcinomas 10 mm or less indicate that 81 percent of these lesions are of intermediate or high histological grade. However, examination of nuclear grade indicated only 21 percent of these small carcinomas demonstrate high nuclear grade.

To avoid confusion, the terms *minimal breast cancer, early breast cancer,* and *minimally invasive breast cancer* should be avoided. The T category or tumor classification system of the American Joint Committee's *Manual for Staging of Cancer* should be used instead.[216, 250] Thus, T1a cancers are equal to or less than 5 mm in diameter, and T1b cancers are greater than 5 mm but equal to or less than 1 cm in diameter.

To obtain accurate information regarding the risk of positive axillary nodes and tumor size, consistency, clarity, and precision of the measurement of the size of the invasive lesion are essential. Unfortunately, the method of determining the size has not always been reported. Furthermore, in some cases it is difficult to compare reports of incidence of positive lymph nodes as a function of tumor size because the size reported may refer to the clinical or palpable size,[61, 204] which usually overestimates tumor size measurements by 50 to 100 percent[50, 178] or is determined from the mammogram, correcting for magnification[60, 214] or gross pathological measurement.[82] These measurements do not always correlate.[178, 258] Precise histological measurements of the size of the tumor or of the invasive component within the tumor are also not always possible,[50, 214] especially if there has been a previous biopsy with partial tumor removal. In addition, when a macroscopic measurement of the tumor is made after cutting the specimen, microscopic tumor extensions may not be measured.[254]

Furthermore, there is still the tendency to group noninvasive DCIS, DCIS with microinvasion, and small "minimally" invasive T1a breast carcinomas together.[157, 182] For example, 17 percent of the series of small breast cancers less than 10 mm reviewed by Arnesson and associates[10] included "microinvasive DCIS." The American Joint Committee on Cancer/TNM Committee of the International Union Against Cancer system for staging states that the pathological T-stage of the lesion should be based on the extent of the invasive component, not the intraductal component.[9] Hence, a 30-mm DCIS with a 6-mm invasive component is a T1b invasive carcinoma with an extensive intraductal component (EIC). Seidman and colleagues[221] have discussed the importance of precise size measurement, noting that the most common method of obtaining this measurement from the gross pathological report may be suboptimal for small tumors. He cites a number of papers in which the method of measurement was either not stated or is vague. Furthermore, in invasive ductal carcinomas with an intraductal component, the invasive and intraductal components are often admixed. If one measures the total tumor size to include the intraductal component, as initially noted by Silverberg and Chitale,[221] the dimension will be larger than that obtained if one measures only the invasive component. This is especially true in cases of an EIC, because in cases where the predominant "tumor" is DCIS and microinvasion is noted, these tumors may not be correctly sized.[61]

Ductal carcinoma *in situ* with microinvasion and "microinvasive carcinoma" also must be scrutinized because currently there is no uniformly accepted definition of microinvasive breast carcinoma. Our group allows as many as 3 foci of up to 1 mm of invasion. The guidelines for pathologists prepared by a U.K. Royal College of Pathologists Working Group for the National Health Service Breast Screening Program also define microinvasive carcinoma as a tumor in which the dominant lesion is noninvasive but in which there are 1 or more foci of infiltration, none of which measures more than 1 mm.[229] Rosen and Oberman discuss the importance of microinvasion without precisely defining the lesion.[202] Rosen, however, has stated that *microinvasion* is a term he applies to unequivocal invasion less than 1 mm in size (Rosen PP: Personal communication, 1994). Rosen allows up to 2 or 3 foci of microinvasion. If there are more, he assigns the case as a T1a lesion, adding the microinvasive foci together and reporting an aggregate size. Leitner and colleagues define a tumor as *microinvasive* if the infiltrative component is 1 mm or less in maximum dimension.[137] Hutter recommends that all areas of microinvasive foci should be measured with a calibrated ocular lens, and if there are several areas of microinvasion, these should be measured, noted in the pathology report, and added together for the appropriate T classification (Hutter RVP: Personal communication, 1994). The difficulties

pathologists face in agreeing on what constitutes microinvasion will not be addressed in this chapter.

Incidence of Small Breast Cancers

There has been a well-documented increase in the incidence of T1a and T1b breast cancers. Surveillance Epidemiology and End Results Program (SEER) data demonstrate that the proportion of all invasive breast cancers less than 1 cm has quadrupled in a 7-year period (from about 9 in 100,000 in 1982 to 36 in 100,000 in 1989), which reflects improved detection with mammographic screening.[158] Others have noted a decrease in the mean and median diameters of invasive cancers.[30] There has been a 61 percent increase in the incidence of primary tumors 1 cm or smaller when analyzing data from the Seattle-Puget Sound registry for the periods of 1983 to 1985 and 1986 to 1987.[262] With the increased use of mammographic screening, smaller cancers are being detected. Tabar and colleagues[238] and Cady and associates[30] report that approximately 13 to 15 percent of all cancers detected in a screening program are 1 cm or less. Recent series show that invasive breast cancers smaller than 1 cm represent 15 to 35 percent of all operable invasive breast cancers,* although Veronesi has reported an incidence rate as high as 45 percent.[251]

Prognosis of Small Breast Cancers

Long-term prognosis of tumors less than 1 cm is very favorable. Table 54–4 tabulates studies with long-term follow-up of node-negative small invasive breast cancers. Rosen and associates found that 171 node-negative palpable invasive breast cancers 1 cm or less show an 88 percent disease-free survival at 20 years.[203] Arnesson and colleagues[10] noted a 96.8 percent overall survival at 7 years in 254 node-negative small carcinomas and a significant impact of positive nodes on overall survival at 12 years in cancers less than 10 mm (98.7 percent versus 79.3 percent). In node-negative tumors less than 1.5 cm, Tabar reported a 98 percent 5-year survival.[238] In addition, analysis of patients with small node-positive lesions 1 cm or less shows a marked difference in 10-year disease-free survival if one node is positive (95 percent versus two to three nodes positive (73 percent).[186]

Because smaller breast cancers are being diagnosed, along with increased utilization of breast conservation treatment and the preferability of breast conservation for small invasive cancers,[252] the question has been asked whether axillary dissection is indicated for small invasive carcinomas.†

Incidence of Positive Nodes in Small Breast Cancer

If positive axillary nodes are a reflection of "metastatic potential" or more virulent carcinomas, the

---

*See references 34, 97, 105, 203, 205, 207, 224, and 225.
†See references 4, 30, 32, 39, 55, 207, 223, and 240.

TABLE 54–4.   LONG-TERM SURVIVAL WITH NODE-NEGATIVE BREAST CANCER 1 CM OR LESS

Author	No. of Pts	Percent DFS	Percent CSS	Percent OS	Follow-up (yr)
Arnesson et al[10]	254			96.8	7
Rosen et al[203]	171	88			20
Silverstein (personal communication)	300	84	95	86	10
Abner et al[1]	57	80			10
Rosner and Lane[204]	91	91		96	7
Russo et al[207]	188	80	94	92	10
Fisher et al[76]	24	96		75	15

Pts = patients; DFS = disease-free survival; CSS = cause-specific survival; OS = overall survival.

current available data on the incidence of positive nodes in T1a and T1b cancers are relevant. As shown in Figure 54–1, as size increases so does the probability of having positive nodes. Table 54–5 summarizes recent studies, showing the percentage of patients with positive nodes in those studies in which T1a and T1b lesions were analyzed separately. The problem is that there are very few studies in which careful microscopic measurement, especially crucial in invasive carcinomas less than 1 cm, was obtained. In T1a lesions, for example, the published range of node positivity ranges from 0 to 28.5 percent; for T1b lesions, the range is 7 to 25 percent. There is concordance that the incidence of nodal positivity in carefully measured invasive carcinomas less than 5 mm is 5 percent or less in the reports of Sinn and colleagues,[228] Silverstein and associates,[224] and Seidman and coworkers.[218] Also, the studies of Sinn and Silverstein provided similar incidences of positive nodes in T1b lesions of 12 to 15 percent, but Seidman's carefully measured, but much smaller, series noted a 22 percent incidence of positive nodes in T1b lesions.[218] Thus, it is clearly difficult to be certain of the probability of finding positive nodes in a given patient with a T1a or T1b tumor until more carefully measured larger analyses are published.

Other factors may refine the ability to predict posi-

tive nodes, in addition to the pathologically measured size. Occult T1 tumors detected mammographically may differ biologically from palpable T1 tumors.[224] As shown in Figure 54–3, there is a higher incidence of node positivity in palpable invasive T1 cancers compared to nonpalpable occult, mammographically detected T1 lesions. Although it has been shown that there is no pathological difference between palpable and nonpalpable invasive carcinomas,[153] such mammographically detected lesions may have a different natural history than those palpable at the time of diagnosis.[48] In one series,[10] 324 patients with tumors 10 mm or less in diameter were analyzed, of which 77 percent were detected mammographically. In this study, positive lymph nodes were significantly more common in those cases detected clinically. Holland and associates[116] have also noted that the incidence of axillary nodal metastases in tumors 10 mm or less is higher (30 percent) in mammographically detected carcinomas at the first incidence screening compared with those same-sized small tumors detected at the interval screen (5 percent). The impact of method of detection on the incidence of positive nodes, particularly in these small lesions, needs further study and confirmation. Others,[187, 227] but not all,[108] have shown a lower incidence of positive nodes in mammographically detected carcinomas.

TABLE 54–5.   INCIDENCE OF AXILLARY NODE INVOLVEMENT IN INVASIVE BREAST CANCER 1 CM OR LESS

Author	How Measured	No. of Pts	Percent Positive Nodes	
			T1A	T1B
Silverstein et al[224]	Gross/micro measurement of invasive component	336	5	15
Reger et al[193]	Not stated	178	3	10
Winchester et al[266]	Cancer data base	317, 272	23.0	23.6
Carter et al[34]	SEER data	339	20	20.5
Ciatto et al[43]	Not stated	163	0	6.9
Tinnemans et al[240]	Pathological diameter	47	7.7	12.5
Seidman et al[218]	Gross/micro measurement of invasive component	37	0	22
Schnabel and Estabrook[210]	Not stated	621	9	20
Halverson et al[105]	Microscopic measurement	168	0	14.7
Lin et al[139]	Not stated	60	6	7
Dowlatshahi et al[60]	Pathological measurement	92	5	10
Ravdin et al[188]	Not stated	712	Not stated	19.7
Rosen and Groshen[201]	Gross measurement	171	11	15
White et al[263]	Not stated	969	9.8	18.2
Sinn et al[228]	Pathological measurement	157	3.8	12

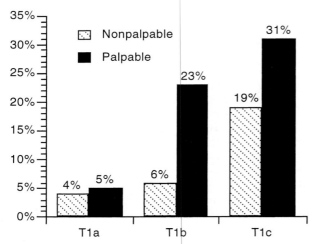

Figure 54–3 *Incidence of positive axillary nodes by T category and palpability in 922 patients with invasive breast cancer. The difference in positive nodes between palpable and nonpalpable T1b and T1c lesions are significant (p values < 0.002).*

The presence of associated intraductal carcinoma or EIC appears to increase the incidence of positive nodes in small invasive carcinomas. Thus, Sinn and colleagues[228] found no positive nodes in 73 T1b lesions with no associated intraductal carcinoma, but there was an 11 percent incidence of node positivity in 84 patients with T1b lesions if there was an associated intraductal component. Recurrences in the axilla after initial nodal dissection were also higher for invasive carcinomas less than 1 cm that were EIC positive (9.3 percent versus 4.2 percent).

Age may also affect the incidence of positive nodes within a given tumor size. For example, Holmberg and colleagues[117] examined the probability of axillary metastases given a certain tumor size as a function of age. The effect of age on node-positive risk was found to be nonlinear and peaked in the group 50 to 59 years, with the lowest effect in patients older than 70 years. A study by the Danish Breast Cancer Cooperative Group, which looked at median tumor diameters as a function of age and node positivity, found no difference between patients younger or older than 60 years.[12] In our series of 345 small breast cancers, we have not found that age (<50 years versus >50 years) is a significant predictor of positive nodes,[225] nor have we noted any difference between those patients younger than 60 years (12 percent) versus those older than 60 years (15.5 percent). But Chadha and colleagues[37] did find a statistically significant difference in positive nodes in 116 T1 carcinomas in women younger than 60 years versus those older than 60 years (35 percent versus 21 percent). Rosner and Lane have reported that women older than 50 years with T1a and T1b tumors had a 99 percent 10-year disease-free recurrence compared with women younger than 50 years, (91 percent), although this was not statistically significant.[205]

Very few studies have examined the relationship between histological grade and nodal positivity with specific reference to small carcinomas. Although

there is a trend for worsening histological grade as tumors increase in size, approximately half of all invasive carcinomas 1 cm or less are high or intermediate grade.[12] Although the NSABP B-04 trial noted a relationship at 10 years between histological grade and nuclear grade and prognosis,[74] at 15 years these factors did not show any independent influence on recurrence or survival.[76] It must be noted that there were only 24 patients in NSABP B-04 with lesions 1 cm or less. Halverson and associates[105] studied the incidence of positive nodes in tumors 1 cm or less. In 102 patients with these small carcinomas for whom histological grade was known and an axillary dissection performed, only 8 percent of those patients with positive nodes had well-differentiated tumors.[105] These authors found the incidence of nodal involvement in patients with histological grade 1, 2, or 3 tumors to be 7 percent, 8 percent, and 38 percent, respectively.

Although nuclear grade in tumors 1 cm or less has not been examined specifically with regard to the incidence of positive nodes, nuclear grade is highly significant in predicting poor recurrence-free survival and poor overall survival in these small tumors.[137, 235] Rosen and Greshen's series does not show a significant correlation between histological and nuclear grade and nodal positivity.[201] Multivariate analysis of 11 prognostic parameters in 922 T1 invasive carcinomas shows that only nuclear grade, the presence or absence of lymphatic/vascular invasion, and method of detection predict node positivity[225] (see Table 54–3).

Lymphatic/vascular invasion in lesions 1 cm or less indicates a more aggressive phenotype.[1] The presence or absence of lymphatic/vascular invasion was also found by Chadha and colleagues to be the only significant predictor of positive lymph nodes after multivariate analysis of five variables in T1 tumors.[37] Leitner and associates[137] found that the combination of poor nuclear grade and lymphatic/vascular invasion identified a subset of node-negative small carcinomas less than 11 mm with a significantly poorer recurrence-free survival (67 percent at 7 years). Rosen and coworkers also noted that the presence of vascular invasion was only significant in tumors less than 11 mm in diameter, not larger tumors, for predicting survival and recurrence at 10 and 20 years.[200] Others have reported the significance of lymphatic/vascular invasion in predicting the presence of micrometastases,[122, 124] and data from NSABP B-04 demonstrated that the presence of lymphatic/vascular invasion also predicted positive nodes.[74]

The presence of angiogenesis has been shown to correlate with risk of nodal involvement. Vascular counts were highly correlated with tumor size (<2 cm versus >2 cm) and histological grade.[118] There is no published information in this context for tumors 1 cm or less in diameter, although the authors note in the text that tumors 1 cm or less all showed normal vascular counts.

Examination of specific histological subtypes by Winchester and associates[266] from a large current data base of 317,272 patients and correlation with positive axillary lymph nodes reveals that the incidence of positive lymph nodes in predominantly tubular (3505 patients) and colloid (6007 patients) carcinomas less than 10 mm in size exhibits less than a 10 percent incidence of positive nodes. Using 10 percent as an arbitrary risk cutoff, Winchester and associates concluded that axillary dissection is not necessary in T1a and T1b lesions of these subtypes. McDivitt and colleagues reported positive lymph nodes in only 1 percent (1 of 71) of tubular carcinomas less than 1 cm in size.[149]

Selective Axillary Node Dissection

The concept of selective axillary lymph node dissection has been proposed.[4, 10, 30, 39, 181] Although size alone should not be the only criterion in the decision-making process, at the Breast Center we do not routinely perform axillary node dissection in patients with DCIS without microinvasion treated with breast conservation.[222] This approach is also advocated by others.[268] In Chapter 53, the role of axillary node dissection in DCIS is discussed. We do not perform axillary node dissections in patients with T1a carcinomas because of the very low probability of positive nodes (≤ 5 percent).[223] Because our data show positive nodes in 23 percent of palpable T1b lesions, we currently routinely perform axillary dissections in this group of patients. In nonpalpable T1b pure invasive lesions, without any associated DCIS, attention is paid to the presence or absence of lymphatic vascular invasion and the nuclear, not histological, grade of the lesion. If either of these unfavorable factors are present, we would perform a Level 1 or 2 axillary dissection. In favorable T1b lesions, it is reasonable to omit axillary dissection in patients who have nonpalpable, non–high nuclear grade lesions without lymphatic or vascular invasion; in our experience, the incidence of positive nodes in this subset is 3.4 percent.[225] In T1a or T1b lesions showing special histology, including tubular and colloid (mucinous) carcinoma, we agree with others[266] that an axillary lymph node dissection can be omitted because the incidence of positive axillary nodes is 5 percent or less. However, when making the decision to omit an axillary dissection, the surgeon must be absolutely clear that the pathologist has meticulously measured the size of the invasive lesion and that this is noted on the pathology report. Additional relevant tumor characteristics, such as nuclear grade, histological grade, the presence or absence of DCIS, and lymphatic/vascular invasion must also be carefully documented.[126, 212]

Others have explored the concept of selective axillary dissection. Elderly or infirm patients who elect breast conservation, who have a high anesthesia risk, and in whom tamoxifen will be used regardless of the results of the dissection do not require axillary dissection.[18, 181, 206, 258] Patients with predominantly tubular carcinomas 1 cm or less (T1a and T1b) may forego axillary dissections[14, 180] or undergo only a Level 1 axillary dissection.[216] Chang and Bland[39] also concur that it is reasonable to perform only a Level 1 dissection in patients with tumors 1 cm or less in diameter with well-differentiated histological grade and low nuclear grade.

Without question, as we continue to detect smaller breast cancers and as more women are treated with breast conservation, the need for performing an axillary dissection at the time of the excision of the breast primary tumor will be questioned. As the methods of measurement of these small carcinomas are refined, and as further studies confirm a consistent 5 percent or less incidence of positive axillary nodes in certain subsets of patients with lesions 10 mm or less, it may be appropriate to eliminate axillary dissection in these patients. Although not universally accepted,[115] current therapeutic recommendations are to give adjuvant therapy to node-positive patients with tumors 1 cm or less.[98] Thus, knowledge of nodal status is still therapeutically important in most of these cases. As noted, there are aggressive small carcinomas with unfavorable long-term outcome.[1, 10] The presence of positive lymph nodes in these small carcinomas does have a significant detrimental impact on recurrence and survival. A step approach to an axillary dissection, using intraoperative pathological analysis before proceeding further or identification of the sentinel node, is a reasonable alternative, but requires careful coordination with the pathologist. Until lymph node status is supplanted with another system for determining adjuvant therapy that is universally accepted, we think it is appropriate to perform a limited (Level 1 or 2) dissection with the exception of the above-noted subsets.

References

1. Abner A, Recht A, Connolly J, et al: Prognosis of pathologic T1 infiltrating cancer of the breast. Int J Radiat Oncol Biol Phys 27(Suppl 1):148, 1993.
2. Ackerman LV, Katzenstein AL: The concept of minimal breast cancer and the pathologist's role in the diagnosis of "early carcinoma." Cancer 39:2755–2763, 1977.
3. Adler LP, Crowe JP, Al-Kaisi NK, et al: Evaluation of breast masses and axillary lymph nodes with (F-18) 2-deoxy-2-fluoro-D-glucose PET. Radiology 187:743–750, 1993.
4. Ahlgren J, Stal O, Westman G, et al: Prediction of axillary lymph node metastases in a screened breast cancer population. Acta Oncol 33:603–608, 1994.
5. Aitken D, Minton J: Complications associated with mastectomy. Surg Clin North Am 63:1331–1352, 1983.
6. Alazraki N: Lymphoscintigraphy and the intraoperative gamma probe. J Nucl Med 36:1780–1783, 1995.
7. Albertini J, Cox C, Yeatman T, et al: Lymphatic mapping and sentinel node biopsy in the breast cancer patient. Proc Am Soc Clin Oncol 14:100, 1995.
8. Allan SM, McVicar D, Sacks NPM: Prospects for axillary staging in breast cancer by magnetic resonance imaging. Radiology 66(suppl):15–16, 1993.
9. Beahrs OH, Henson DE, Hutter RVP, Kennedy BJ (eds): Handbook for Staging of Cancer. 4th ed. Philadelphia, JB Lippincott, 1993.
10. Arnesson LG, Smeds S, Fagerberg G: Recurrence-free survival in patients with small breast cancers: An analysis of cancers 10 mm or less detected clinically by screening. Eur J Surg 160:271–276, 1994.

11. Attiyeh FF, Jensen M, Huvos AG, et al: Axillary micrometastasis and macrometastasis in carcinoma of the breast. Surg Gynecol Obstet 144:839–842, 1977.
12. Axelsson CK, Mouidsen HT, Zedeler K, et al: Axillary dissection of level I and II lymph nodes is important in breast cancer classification. Eur J Cancer 28A:1415–1418, 1992.
13. Baeza M, Sole J, Leon A, et al: Conservative treatment of early breast cancer. Int J Radiol Oncol Biol Phys 14:669–676, 1988.
14. Baker RR: Unusual lesions and their management. Surg Clin North Am 70:963–975, 1990.
15. Ball ABS, Waters R, Fish S, et al: Radical axillary dissection in the staging and treatment of breast cancer. Ann Coll Surg Engl 74:126–129, 1992.
16. Balslev I, Axelsson CK, Zedeler K, et al: The Nottingham prognostic index applied to 9,149 patients from the studies of the Danish Breast Cancer Cooperative Group (DBCG). Breast Cancer Res Treat 32:281–290, 1994.
17. Barth RJ, Danforth Jr MD, Venzon DJ, et al: Level of axillary involvement by lymph node metastases from breast cancer is not an independent predictor of survival. Arch Surg 126:574–577, 1991.
18. Bates T, Riley DL, Houghton J, et al: Breast cancer in elderly women: A cancer research campaign trial comparing treatment with tamoxifen and optimal surgery with tamoxifen alone. Br J Surg 78:591–594, 1995.
19. Benson EA, Thorogood EA: The effect of surgical technique on local recurrence rates following mastectomy. Eur J Surg Oncol 12:267–271, 1986.
20. Berg JW: The significance of axillary node levels in the study of breast carcinoma. Cancer 8:776–778, 1955.
21. Bettelheim R, Price KN, Gelber RD, et al: Prognostic importance of occult axillary lymph node micrometastases from breast cancers. Lancet 335:1565–1568, 1990.
22. Bland KI: The emerging importance of molecular biology in the therapy of breast carcinoma. Breast J 1:125–127, 1995.
23. Boova RS, Boananni R, Rosato FE: Patterns of axillary nodal involvement in breast cancer: Predictability of level one dissection. Ann Surg 196:642–644, 1982.
24. Brinkley D, Haybittle JL. Long-term survival of women with breast cancer. Lancet 1:1118, 1984.
25. Bruneton JN, Caramella E, Hery M, et al: Axillary lymph node metastases in breast cancer: Preoperative detection with US. Radiology 158:325–326, 1986.
26. Bussolati G, Gugliotta P, Morra I, et al: The immunohistochemical detection of lymph node metastases from infiltrating lobular carcinoma of the breast. Br J Cancer 54:631–636, 1986.
27. Cabanes PA, Salmon RJ, Vilcoq JR, et al: Value of axillary dissection in addition to lumpectomy and radiotherapy in early breast cancer. Lancet 339:1245–1248, 1992.
28. Cady B: Lymph node metastases: Indicators, but not governors of survival. Arch Surg 119:1067–1072, 1984.
29. Cady B, Sears HF: Usefulness and technique of axillary dissection in primary breast cancer. J Clin Oncol 4:623–624, 1986.
30. Cady B, Stone MD, Wayne J: New therapeutic possibilities in primary invasive breast cancer. Ann Surg 218:338–349, 1993.
31. Cady B: The need to reexamine axillary lymph node dissection in invasive breast cancer. Cancer 73:505–508, 1994.
32. Cady B: Dilemmas in breast disease. Breast J 1:121–124, 1995.
33. Cancer Research Campaign Working Party: Cancer research campaign (King's/Cambridge) trial for early breast cancer. Lancet July 12:55–60, 1980.
34. Carter CL, Allen C, Hendson DE: Relation of tumor size, lymph node status, and survival in 24,740 breast cancer cases. Cancer 63:181–187, 1989.
35. Cascinelli N, Greco M, Bufalino R, et al: Prognosis of breast cancer with axillary node metastases after surgical treatment only. Eur J Cancer Clin Oncol 23:793–799, 1987.
36. Cascinelli N, Anderson MD: Long-term survival and prognostic factors for 2,170 breast cancer patients treated at two cancer centers (Milan and Houston). Tumori 75:123–131, 1989.
37. Chadha M, Chabon AB, Friedmann P, et al: Predictors of axillary lymph node metastases in patients with T1 breast cancer: A multivariate analysis. Cancer 73:350–353, 1994.
38. Chan HY, Behen S, Greenall MJ: Adequacy of axillary node sampling for evaluation of the axilla and control of axillary disease in breast cancer. Eur J Surg Oncol 19:213–214, 1993.
39. Chang HR, Bland KI: An overview of breast-conserving surgery in breast cancer treatment. Breast J 1:91–95, 1995.
40. Chaudary MA: Radical axillary dissection in the staging and treatment of breast cancer. Ann R Coll Surg Engl 74:126–129, 1992.
41. Chen ZL, Wen DR, Coulson WF, et al: Occult metastases in the axillary lymph nodes of patients with breast cancer node negative by clinical and histologic examination and conventional histology. Dis Markers 9:239–248, 1991.
42. Chevinsky AH, Ferrara J, James AG, et al: Prospective evaluation of clinical and pathologic detection of axillary metastases in patients with carcinoma of the breast. Surgery 108:612–618, 1990.
43. Ciatto S, Cecchini S, Lossa A, et al: T category and operable breast cancer prognosis. Tumori 75:18–22, 1989.
44. Clark GM: Prognostic and predictive factors. In Harris J et al (eds): Diseases of the Breast. Philadelphia, Lippincott-Raven, 1996.
45. Clark RM: Breast cancer: Experiences with conservation therapy. Am J Clin Oncol 10:461–468, 1987.
46. Clayton F, Hopkins CL: Pathologic correlates of prognosis in lymph node-positive breast carcinomas. Cancer 71:1780–1790, 1993.
47. Collan YU, Eskelinen MJ, Nordling SA, et al: Prognostic studies in breast cancer: Multivariate combination of nodal status, proliferation index, tumor size, and DNA ploidy. Acta Oncol 33:873–878, 1994.
48. Consensus Panel: National Institute of Health Consensus Panel Consensus statement: Treatment of early-stage breast cancer. Natl Cancer Inst Monogr 11:1–5, 1992.
49. Cote RJ, Taylor C, Neville AM: Review: Detection of occult metastases. Cancer 8:49–51, 1995.
50. Crowe JP, Gordon NH, Shenk RR, et al: Primary tumor size: Relevance to breast cancer survival. Arch Surg 127:910–916, 1992.
51. Danforth DN Jr, Findlay PA, McDonald HD, et al: Complete axillary lymph node dissection for stage I–II carcinoma of the breast. J Clin Oncol 4:655–662, 1986.
52. Danforth DN Jr: The role of axillary lymph node dissection in the management of breast cancer. PPO Updates 6:1–16, 1992.
53. Davidson T: Why I favour axillary node clearance in the management of breast cancer. Eur J Surg Oncol 21:5–7, 1995.
54. Davies GC: Assessment of axillary lymph node status. Ann Surg 192:148–151, 1980.
55. Deckers P: Axillary dissection in breast cancer: When, why, how much, and for how long? Another operation soon to be extinct? J Surg Oncol 48:217–219, 1991.
56. Delouche G, Bachelot F, Premont M, et al: Conservative treatment of early breast cancer: Long term results and complications. Int J Radiat Oncol Biol Phys 13:29–34, 1987.
57. Dessureault S, Koven I, Couture J, et al: Pre-operative assessment of axillary lymph node status in patients with breast adenocarcinoma using intravenous technetium-99M Mab-1770. Breast Cancer Res Treat 37(Suppl A):133, 1955.
58. Dewar JA, Sarraxin D, Benhamou E, et al: Management of the axilla in conservatively treated breast cancer: 592 patients treated at Institute Gustave-Roussy. Int J Radiat Oncol Biol Phys 13:475–481, 1987.
59. Diel IJ, Kaufman M, Solomayer EF, et al: Micrometastatic tumor cells in bone marrow versus nodal status in breast cancer: Impact on prognosis in patients with primary breast cancer. Proc Am Soc Clin Oncol 14:110, 1995.
60. Dowlatshahi K, Snider Jr HC, Kim R: Axillary node status in nonpalpable breast cancer. Ann Surg Oncol 2:424–428, 1995.
61. Eberlein TJ, Connolly JL, Schnitt SJ, et al: Predictors of local recurrence following conservative breast surgery and radiation therapy: The influence of tumor size. Arch Surg 125:771–777, 1990.

62. Epstein RJ: Routine or delayed axillary dissection for primary breast cancer? Eur J Cancer 31A:1570–1573, 1995.
63. Fentiman IS, Mansel RE: The axilla: Not a no-go zone. Lancet 337:221–223, 1991.
64. Fisher B, Slack NH, Bross IDJ, et al: Cancer of the breast: Size and neoplasm and prognosis. Cancer 24:1071–1080, 1969.
65. Fisher B, Slack NH: Number of lymph nodes examined and the prognosis of breast carcinoma. Surg Gynecol Obstet 131:79–88, 1970.
66. Fisher B, Wolmark N, Bauer M, et al: The accuracy of clinical nodal staging and of limited axillary dissection as a determinant of histologic nodal status in carcinoma of the breast. Surg Gynecol Obstet 152:765–772, 1981.
67. Fisher B, Bauer M, Wickerham L, et al: Relation of number of positive axillary nodes to the prognosis of patients with primary breast cancer: An NSABP update. Cancer 52:1551–1557, 1983.
68. Fisher B, Redmond C, Fisher ER, et al: Ten-year results of a randomized clinical trial comparing radical mastectomy and total mastectomy with or without radiation. N Engl J Med 312:674–681, 1985.
69. Fisher B, Redmond C, Wickerham DL, et al: Systemic therapy in patients with node-negative breast cancer: A commentary based on two NSABP clinical trials. Ann Intern Med 111:703–712, 1989.
70. Fisher B: The evolution of paradigms for the management of breast cancer: A personal perspective. Cancer Res 52:2371–2383, 1992.
71. Fisher CJ, Boyle S, Burke M, et al: Intraoperative assessment of nodal status in the selection of patients with breast cancer for axillary clearance. Br J Surg 80:457–458, 1993.
72. Fisher ER, Swamidoss S, Lee CH, et al: Detection and significance of occult axillary node metastases in patients with invasive breast cancer. Cancer 42:2025–2031, 1978.
73. Fisher ER, Palekar A, Rockette H, et al: Pathologic findings from the NSABP (Protocol No. 4) V: Significance of axillary nodal micro- and macrometastases. Cancer 42:2032–2038, 1978.
74. Fisher ER, Sass R, Fisher B, et al: Pathologic findings from the NSABP (protocol No. 4) X: Discriminants for tenth year treatment failure. Cancer 53:712–723, 1984.
75. Fisher ER: The impact of pathology on the biologic, diagnostic, prognostic, and therapeutic considerations in breast cancer. Surg Clin North Am 64:1073–1093, 1984.
76. Fisher ER, Constantino J, Fisher B, et al: Pathologic findings from the NSABP Protocol 4. Discriminants for 15-year survival. Cancer 71:2141–2150, 1993.
77. Fisher ER, Anderson S, Redmond C, et al: Pathologic findings from the NSABP Protocol B-06: 10-year pathologic and clinical prognostic discriminants. Cancer 71:2507–2514, 1993.
78. Forrest APM, Roberts MM, Preece P, et al: The Cardiff-St. Mary's trial. Br J Surg 61:766–769, 1974.
79. Forrest APM, Roberts MM, Cant ELM, et al: Simple mastectomy and pectoral node biopsy. Br J Surg 63:569–575, 1976.
80. Forrest APM, Roberts MM, Cant ELM, et al: Simple mastectomy and pectoral node biopsy: The Cardiff-St. Mary's trial. World J Surg 1:320–323, 1977.
81. Forrest APM, Stewart HJ, Roberts MM, et al: Simple mastectomy and axillary node sampling (pectoral node biopsy) in the management of primary breast cancer. Ann Surg 196:371–378, 1982.
82. Frazier TG, Copeland EM, Gallager HS, et al: Prognosis and treatment in minimal breast cancer. Am J Surg 133:697–701, 1977.
83. Friedman NS, Friedman MD: Correlation of DNA flow cytometry and hormone receptors with axillary lymph node status in patients with carcinoma of the breast. Proc Am Soc Clin Oncol 13:83, 1994.
84. Friedman S, Bertin F, Mouriesse H, et al: Importance of tumor cells in axillary node sinus margins ('clandestine' metastases) discovered by serial sectioning in operable breast carcinoma. Acta Oncol 27:483–487, 1988.
85. Gaglia P, Bussone R, Caldarola B, et al: The correlation between the spread of metastases by level in the axillary nodes and disease-free survival in breast cancer: A multifactoral analysis. Eur J Cancer 23:849–854, 1987.
86. Galea MH: Occult regional lymph node metastases from breast carcinoma: Immunohistological detection with antibodies CAM 5.2 and NCRC-11. J Pathol 165:221–227, 1991.
87. Galea MH, Blamey RW, Elston CE, et al: The Nottingham prognostic index in primary breast cancer. Breast Cancer Res Treat 22:207–219, 1992.
88. Gallager HS, Martin JE: An orientation to the concept of minimal breast cancer. Cancer 28:1505–1507, 1971.
89. Gann PH, Colilla SA, Gapstur SM, et al: Factors associated with axillary node metastasis in breast cancer. Breast Cancer Res Treat 37:51, 1995.
90. Gardner B, Feldman J: Are positive axillary nodes in breast cancer markers for incurable disease? Ann Surg 218:270–278, 1993.
91. Garfinkel L, Boring CC, Hearth Jr CW: Changing trends: An overview of breast cancer incidence and mortality. Cancer 743:222–227, 1994.
92. Gasparini G, Weidner N, Bevilacqua P, et al: Tumor microvessel density, p53 expression, tumor size, and peritumoral lymphatic vessel invasion are relevant prognostic markers in node-negative breast carcinoma. J Clin Oncol 12:454–466, 1994.
93. Gateley CA, Mansel RE, Owen J, et al: Treatment of the axilla in operable breast cancer. Br J Surg 78:750, 1991. Abstract.
94. Giuliano AE, Kirgan DM, Guenther JM, et al: Lymphatic mapping and sentinel lymphadenectomy for breast cancer. Ann Surg 220:391–401, 1994.
95. Giuliano AE, Dale PS, Turner RR, et al: Improved axillary staging of breast cancer with sentinel lymphadenectomy. Ann Surg 222:394–401, 1995.
96. Glick J, Gelber RD, Goldhirsch A, et al: Meeting highlights: Adjuvant therapy for primary breast cancer. J Natl Cancer Inst 84:1479–1485, 1992.
97. Gloeckler Ries LA, Henson DE, Harras A: Survival from breast cancer according to tumor size and nodal status. Surg Oncol Clin North Am 3:35–53, 1994.
98. Goldhirsch A, Wood WC, Senn HJ, et al: Meeting highlights: International consensus panel on the treatment of primary breast cancer. J Natl Cancer Inst 87:1441–1445, 1995.
99. Graversen HP, Blichert-Toft M, Anderson JA, et al: Breast cancer: Risk of axillary recurrence in node-negative patients following partial dissection of the axilla. Eur J Surg Oncol 14:407–412, 1988.
100. Greenall MJ: Current controversies in the surgical management of breast cancer. Ann Oncol 5(suppl 4):S39–S43, 1994.
101. Hadjimas DJ, Burke M: Intraoperative assessment of nodal status in the selection of patients with breast cancer for axillary clearance. Br J Surg 81:1615–1616, 1994.
102. Haffty BG, McKhann D, Beinfield M, et al: Breast conservation without axillary dissection: A rational treatment strategy in selected patients. Arch Surg 128:1315–1319, 1993.
103. Hainsworth PJ, Tjandra JJ, Stillwell RG, et al: Detection and significance of occult metastases in node-negative breast cancer. Br J Surg 80:459–463, 1993.
104. Halverson KJ, Taylor ME, Perez CA, et al: Regional nodal management and patterns of failure following conservative surgery and radiation therapy for stage I and II breast cancer. Int J Radiat Oncol Biol Phys 26:593–599, 1993.
105. Halverson KJ, Perez CA, Myerson R, et al: Management of the axilla in patients with breast cancers one centimeter or smaller. Am J Clin Oncol 17:461–466, 1994.
106. Harris JR, Hellman S, Kinne DW: Limited surgery and radiotherapy for early breast cancer. N Engl J Med 313:1365–1368, 1985.
107. Harris JR, Osteen RT: Patients with early breast cancer benefit from effective axillary treatment. Breast Cancer Res Treat 5:17–21, 1985.
108. Harris JR, Morrow M: Treatment of early-stage breast cancer. In Harris J et al (eds): Diseases of the Breast. Philadelphia, Lippincott-Raven, 1996.
109. Hartveit F: Axillary metastasis in breast cancer: When, how, and why? Semin Surg Oncol 5:126–136, 1989.

110. Hayward JL: The Guy's trial of treatments in "early" breast cancer. World J Surg 1:314–316, 1977.

111. Hellman S, Harris JR: The appropriate breast cancer paradigm. Cancer Res 47:339–342, 1987.

112. Hellman S: Dogma and inquisition in medicine. Cancer 71:2430–2433, 1993.

113. Hellman S: Natural history of small breast cancer. J Clin Oncol 12:2229–2234, 1994.

114. Henderson IC: Biologic variations of tumors. Cancer 69:1888–1895, 1992.

115. Henderson IC: Adjuvant systemic therapy for early breast cancer. Cancer 74:401–409, 1994.

116. Holland PA, Walls J, Boggis C, et al: Incidental screen detected breast cancers require axillary node clearance. Eur J Cancer 30A(suppl):S30, 1994.

117. Holmberg L, Lindgren A, Norden T, et al: Age as a discriminant of axillary node involvement in invasive breast cancer. Acta Oncol 31:533–538, 1992.

118. Horak ER, Leek R, Klenk N, et al: Angiogenesis, assessed by platelet/endothelial cell adhesion molecule antibodies, as indicator of node metastases and survival in breast cancer. Lancet 340:1120–1124, 1992.

119. Hoskin PJ, Rahan B, Ebbs S, et al: Selective avoidance of lymphatic radiotherapy in the conservative management of early breast cancer. Radiother Oncol 25:83–88, 1992.

120. Hughes K, Nabi H, Barron A, et al: Radioimmunodetection (RAID) of operable breast cancer with 99mTc-labeled anti-CEA Fab fragment. Proc Am Soc Clin Oncol 14:101, 1995.

121. Hutter RVP: The pathologist's role in minimal breast cancer. Cancer 28:1527–1536, 1971.

122. Huvos AG, Hutter RVP, Berg JW: The significance of axillary macrometastases and micrometastases in mammary cancer. Ann Surg 173:44–46, 1971.

123. Ilkhaniipour ZS, Harris KM, Staiger MJ, et al: Characteristics of axillary adenopathy as a predictor of malignancy at mammography and sonography. Radiology 189:244, 1993.

124. International (Ludwig) Breast Cancer Study Group: Prognostic importance of occult axillary lymph node micrometastases from breast cancers. Lancet 335:1565–1568, 1990.

125. Jatoi I, Clark GM, de Moor C, et al: Axillary lymph node metastasis in primary breast cancer: An indicator of tumor chronology or biology? (Abstract.) Proc Am Soc Clin Oncol 14:100, 1995.

126. Kamel OW, Hendrickson MR, Kempson RL: Breast biopsies: The content of the surgical pathology report. Path: State of the Art Reviews 1:161–180, 1992.

127. Kingsley WB, Peters GN, Cheek H: What constitutes adequate study of axillary lymph nodes in breast cancer? Ann Surg 201:311–314, 1985.

128. Kinne DW: Surgical management of stage I and stage II breast cancer. Cancer 66:1373–1377, 1990.

129. Kinne DW: Controversies in primary breast cancer management. Am J Surg 166:502–508, 1993.

130. Kissin MW, Price AB, Thompson EM, et al: The inadequacy of axillary sampling in breast cancer. Lancet May 29:1210–1212, 1982.

131. Kjaergaard M, Blicher-Toft JA, Anderson JA, et al: Probability of false negative nodal staging in conjunction with partial axillary dissection in breast cancer. Br J Surg 72:365–367, 1985.

132. Koscielny S, Tubiana M, Le MG, et al: Breast cancer: Relationship between size of the primary tumour and the probability of metastatic dissemination. Br J Cancer 49:709–715, 1984.

133. Krag DN, Weaver DL, Alex JC, et al: Surgical resection and radiolocalization of the sentinel lymph node in breast cancer using a gamma probe. Surg Oncol 2:335–339, 1993.

134. Krontiris TG: Molecular medicine. N Engl J Med 333:303–306, 1995.

135. Kuznetsova M, Graybill JC, Zusag TW, et al: Omission of axillary lymph node dissection in early-stage breast cancer: Effect on treatment outcome. Radiology 197:507–510, 1995.

136. Lamki LM, Buzdar AU, Singletary E, et al: Indium-111-labeled B72.3 monoclonal antibody in the detection and staging of breast cancer: A phase I study. J Nucl Med 32:1326–1332, 1991.

137. Leitner SP, Swern AS, Weinberger D, et al: Predictors of recurrence for patients with small (one centimeter or less) localized breast cancer (T1a,b N0 M0). Cancer 76:2266–2274, 1995.

138. Leung S, Otmezguine Y, Calitchi E, et al: Locoregional recurrences following radical external beam irradiation and interstitial implantation for operable breast cancer—A twenty three year experience. Radiother Oncol 5:1–10, 1986.

139. Lin PP, Allison DC, Wainstock J, et al: Impact of axillary lymph node dissection on the therapy of breast cancer patients. J Clin Oncol 11:1536–1544, 1993.

140. Lippman ME: The development of biological therapies for breast cancer. Science 259:631–632, 1993.

141. Lloyd LR, Waits Jr RK, Shroder D, et al: Axillary dissection for breast carcinoma: The myth of skip metastasis. Am Surg 55:381–384, 1989.

142. Lythgoe JP, Palmer MK: Manchester regional breast study: 5 and 10 year results. Br J Surg 69:693–696, 1982.

143. Mansour EG, Ravdin PM, Dressler L: Prognostic factors in early breast cancer. Cancer 74:381–400, 1994.

144. March DE, Wechsler RJ, Kurtz AB, et al: CT-pathologic correlation of axillary lymph nodes in breast carcinoma. J Comput Assist Tomogr 15:440–444, 1991.

145. Margolese RG: Axillary surgery in breast cancer: There still is a debate. Eur J Cancer 29A:801, 1993.

146. Marsigiliante S, Leo G, Mottaghi A, et al: p53 associated with cathepsin D in primary breast cancer. Int J Clin Lab Res 23:102–108, 1993.

147. de Mascarel I, Bonichon F, Coindre JM, et al: Prognostic significance of breast cancer axillary lymph node micrometastases assessed by two special techniques: Reevaluation with longer follow-up. Br J Cancer 66:523–527, 1992.

148. Mathiesen O, Carl J, Bonderup O, et al: Axillary sampling and the risk of erroneous staging of breast cancer: An analysis of 960 consecutive patients. Acta Oncol 29:721–725, 1990.

149. McDivitt RW, Boyce W, Gersell D: Tubular carcinoma of the breast: Clinical and pathological observations concerning 135 cases. Am J Surg Pathol 6:401–411, 1982.

150. McGuire WL, Abeloff MD, Fisher B, et al: Adjuvant therapy in node-negative breast cancer. Breast Cancer Res Treat 13:97–115, 1989.

151. McGuire WL: Adjuvant therapy of node negative breast cancer. N Engl J Med 320:525–527, 1989. Editorial.

152. McGuire WL, Atul TK, Allred DC, et al: How to use prognostic factors in axillary node-negative breast cancer patients. J Natl Cancer Inst 82:1006–1015, 1990.

153. McKinney CD, Frierson Jr HF, Fechener RE, et al: Pathologic findings in nonpalpable invasive breast cancer. Am J Surg Pathol 16:33–36, 1992.

154. McLean RG, Ege GN: Prognostic value of axillary lymphoscintigraphy in breast carcinoma patients. J Nucl Med 27:1116–1124, 1986.

155. Menard S, Bufalino R, Rilke F, et al: Prognosis based on primary breast carcinoma instead of pathological nodal status. Br J Cancer 70:709–712, 1994.

156. Menard S, Cascinelli N, Rilke F, et al: Prediction of axillary lymph node status in breast cancer patients by use of prognostic indicators. J Natl Cancer Inst 87:607, 1995.

157. Meterissian S, Fornage BD, Singletary SE: Clinically occult breast carcinoma: Diagnostic approaches and role of axillary node dissection. Ann Surg Oncol 2:314–318, 1995.

158. Miller BA, Feuer EJ, Hankey BF: Recent incidence trends for breast cancer in women and the relevance of early detection: An update. CA Cancer J Clin 43:27–41, 1993.

159. Mittra I, MacRae KD: A meta-analysis of reported correlations between prognostic factors in breast cancer: Does axillary lymph node metastasis represent biology or chronology? Eur J Cancer 27:1574–1583, 1991.

160. Moffat FL, Senofsky GM, Davis K, et al: Axillary node dissection for early breast cancer: Some is good, but all is better. J Surg Oncol 51:8–13, 1992.

161. Morrow M, Evans J, Rosen PP, et al: Does clearing of axillary lymph nodes contribute to accurate staging of breast carcinoma? Cancer 53:1329–1332, 1984.

162. Mouridsen HT, Andersen J, Andersen KW, et al: Classical

prognostic factors in node-negative breast cancer: The DBCG experience. J Natl Cancer Inst 11:163–166, 1992.

163. Mueller CB: Stage II breast cancer is not necessarily a progression of stage I disease. *In* Wise L, Johnson H (eds): Breast Cancer: Controversies in Management. Armonk, NY, Futura, 1994.

164. Mustonen P, Farin P, Kosunen O: Ultrasonographic detection of metastatic axillary lymph nodes in breast cancer. Ann Chir Gynaecol 79:15–18, 1990.

165. Musumeci R, Tesoro-Tess JD, Costa A, et al: Indirect lymphography of the breast with iotasul: A vanishing hope? Lymphology 17:118–123, 1984.

166. Nasser IA, Lee AKC, Bosari S, et al: Occult axillary lymph node metastases in "node-negative" breast carcinoma. Hum Pathol 24:950–957, 1993.

167. Neville AM: Are breast cancer axillary node micrometastases worth detecting? J Pathol 161:283–284, 1990.

168. Neville AM, Price KN, Gelber RD, et al: Axillary node micrometastases and breast cancer. Lancet 337:1110, 1991.

169. Nevin JE, Pinzon G, Morgan TJ, et al: Minimal breast carcinoma. Am J Surg 139:357–359, 1980.

170. Nichols PH, Ibrahim NBN, Padfield JH, et al: Correlation of pS2 expression of involved lymph nodes in relation to primary breast carcinoma. Eur J Surg Oncol 21:151–154, 1995.

171. Nieweg O, Kim E, Wong WH, et al: Positron emission tomography with fluorine-18-deoxyglucose in the detection and staging of breast cancer. Cancer 71:3920–3925, 1993.

172. Noguchi M, Kitagawa H, Kinoshita K, et al: The relationship of p53 protein and lymph node metastases in invasive breast cancer. Jpn J Surg 24:512–517, 1994.

173. Noguchi M, Ohta N, Thomas M, et al: Clinical and biological prediction of axillary and internal mammary lymph node metastases in cancer. Surg Oncol 2:51–58, 1993.

174. Noguchi S, Aihara T, Nakamori S, et al: The detection of breast carcinoma micrometastases in axillary lymph nodes by means of reverse transcriptase-polymerase chain reaction. Cancer 74:1595–1600, 1994.

175. Osborne MP, Ormiston N, Harmer CL, et al: Breast conversation in the treatment of early breast cancer: A 20-year follow-up. Cancer 53:349–355, 1984.

176. Osborne MP, Rosen PP: Detection and management of bone marrow micrometastases in breast cancer. Oncology 8:25–42, 1994.

177. Pack MS, Thomas RS: Axillary lymph node dissection: Does it have a role in primary breast cancer? Am Surg 62:159–161, 1996.

178. Pain JA, Ebbs RPA, Hern A, et al: Assessment of breast cancer size: A comparison of methods. Eur J Surg Oncol 18:44–48, 1992.

179. Pecking AP, Bertrand FG, Lokiec FM, et al: Preoperative staging of lymph node status in breast cancer using radiolabeled monoclonal antibodies. Eur J Cancer 30A(suppl 2):S32, 1995.

180. Peters GN, Wolff M, Haagensen CD: Tubular carcinoma of the breast: Clinical pathologic correlations based on 100 cases. Ann Surg 193:138–149, 1981.

181. Petrek JA, Blackwood MM: Axillary dissection: Current practice and technique. Curr Probl Surg 32:259–323, 1995.

182. Petrovich JA, Ross DS, Sullivan JW, et al: Mammographic wire localization in diagnosis and treatment of occult carcinoma of the breast. Surg Gynecol Obstet 168:239–243, 1989.

183. Pickren JW: Significance of occult metastases: A study of breast cancer. Cancer 14:1266–1271, 1961.

184. Pigott J, Nichols R, Maddox WA, et al: Metastases to the upper levels of the axillary nodes in carcinoma of the breast and its implications for nodal sampling procedures. Surg Gynecol Obstet 158:255–259, 1984.

185. Querzoli R, Ferretti S, Albonico G, et al: Application of quantitative analysis to biologic profile evaluation in breast cancer. Cancer 76:2510–2517, 1995.

186. Quiet C, Ferguson D, Hellman S: The natural history of node positive breast cancer: Predictors of outcome with 40 year follow-up. Proc Am Soc Clin Oncol 13:79, 1994.

187. Ranaboldo CJ, Mitchel A, Royle GT, et al: Axillary nodal status in women with screen-detected breast cancer. Eur J Surg Oncol 19:130–133, 1993.

188. Ravdin PM, DeLaurentiis M, Vendely T, et al: Prediction of axillary lymph node status in breast cancer patients by use of prognostic indicators. J Natl Cancer Inst 86:1771–1775, 1994.

189. Raymond WA, Leong AS-Y: Immunoperoxidase staining in the detection of lymph node metastases in stage I breast cancer. Pathology 21:11–15, 1989.

190. Recht A, Pierce SM, Abner A, et al: Regional nodal failure after conservative surgery and radiotherapy for early-stage breast carcinoma. J Clin Oncol 9:988–996, 1991.

191. Recht A: Nodal treatment for patients with early stage breast cancer: Guilty or innocent? Radiother Oncol 25:79–82, 1992.

192. Recht A, Houlihan MJ: Axillary nodes and breast cancer: A review. Cancer 76:1491–1512, 1995.

193. Reger V, Beito G, Jolly PC: Factors affecting the incidence of lymph node metastases in small cancers of the breast. Am J Surg 157:501–502, 1989.

194. Ribeiro GG: The Christie Hospital Breast Conservation Trial: An update at 8 years from inception. Clin Oncol 5:278–283, 1993.

195. Robinson DS, Senofsky GM, Ketcham AS: Role and extent of lymphadenectomy for early breast cancer. Semin Surg Oncol 8:78–82, 1992.

196. Rosen PP, Saigo PE, Braun DW, et al: Prognosis in Stage II (T1N1M0) breast cancer. Ann Surg 194:576–584, 1981.

197. Rosen PP, Saigo PE, Braun DW, et al: Axillary micro- and macrometastases in breast cancer: Prognostic significance of tumor size. Ann Surg 194:585–591, 1981.

198. Rosen PP, Lesser ML, Kinne DW, et al: Discontinuous or "skip" metastases in breast carcinoma: Analysis of 1228 axillary dissections. Ann Surg 197:276–283, 1983.

199. Rosen PP, Groshen S, Saigo PE, et al: A long-term follow-up study of survival in stage I (T1N0M0) and stage II (T1N1M0) breast carcinoma. J Clin Oncol 7:355–366, 1989.

200. Rosen PP, Groshen S, Saigo PE, et al: Pathological prognostic factors in stage I and stage II breast carcinoma: A study of 644 patients with median follow up of 18 years. J Clin Oncol 7:1239–1251, 1989.

201. Rosen PP, Groshen S: Factors influencing survival and prognosis in early breast carcinoma. (T1N0M0-T1N1M0): Assessment of 644 patients with median follow up of 18 years. Surg Clin North Am 70:937–962, 1990.

202. Rosen PP, Oberman HA: Tumors of the Mammary Gland. Armed Forces Institute of Pathology, fascicle 1993.

203. Rosen PP, Groshen S, Kinne DW, et al: Factors influencing prognosis in node-negative breast carcinoma: Analysis of 767 T1N0M0/T2N0M0 patients with long-term follow-up. J Clin Oncol 11:2090–2100, 1993.

204. Rosner D, Lane WW: Node-negative minimal invasive breast cancer patients are not candidates for routine systemic adjuvant therapy. Cancer 66:199–205, 1990.

205. Rosner D, Lane WW: Predicting recurrence in axillary-node negative breast cancer patients. Breast Cancer Res Treat 25:127–139, 1993.

206. Ruffin WK, Stacey-Clear A, Younger J, et al: Rationale for routine axillary dissection in carcinoma of the breast. J Am Coll Surg 180:245–251, 1995.

207. Russo SA, Fowble B, Fox K, et al: The identification of a subset of patients with axillary node-negative minimally invasive breast cancer who may benefit from systemic adjuvant therapy. Breast J 1:163–172, 1995.

208. Rutqvist LE, Wallgren A: Long-term survival of 458 young breast cancer patients. Cancer 55:658–665, 1985.

209. Sacks NPM, Barr LC, Allan SM, et al: The role of axillary dissection in operable breast cancer. Breast 1:41–49, 1992.

210. Schnabel FR, Estabrook A: Results of axillary lymph node dissection in early breast cancer. Breast Cancer Res Treat 32(suppl):40, 1994.

211. Schneebaum S, Stadler J, Yaniv D, et al: Gamma probe-guided sentinel node biopsy optimal timing for injection. Breast Cancer Res Treat 37(suppl A):137, 1995.

212. Schnitt SJ, Connolly JL: Processing and evaluation of breast excision specimens. Am J Clin Pathol 98:125–137, 1992.

213. Schoenfeld A, Luqmani Y, Smith D, et al: Detection of breast cancer micrometastases in axillary lymph nodes by using polymerase chain reaction. Cancer Res 54:2986–2990, 1994.

214. Schwartz GF, Feig SA, Rosenberg AL, et al: Staging and treatment of clinically occult breast cancer. Cancer 53:1379–1384, 1984.
215. Schwartz GF: Extent of axillary dissection preceding irradiation for carcinoma of the breast. Arch Surg 121:1395–1398, 1986.
216. Schwartz GF, Carter DL, Conant EF, et al: Mammographically detected breast cancer: Nonpalpable is not a synonym for inconsequential. Cancer 73:1660–1665, 1994.
217. Sedmark DD, Meineke TA, Knechtges DS, et al: Prognostic significance of cytokeratin-positive breast cancer metastases. Mod Pathol 2:516–520, 1989.
218. Seidman JD, Schnaper LA, Aisner SC: Relationship of the size of the invasive component of the primary breast carcinoma to axillary lymph node metastases. Cancer 75:65–71, 1995.
219. Senofsky GM, Moffat FL, Davis K, et al: Total axillary lymphadenectomy in the management of breast cancer. Arch Surg 126:1336–1342, 1991.
220. Siegel BM, Mayzel KA, Love SM: Level I and II axillary dissection in the treatment of early-stage breast cancer: An analysis of 259 consecutive patients. Arch Surg 125:144–1147, 1990.
221. Silverberg SG, Chitale AR: Assessment of significance of proportions of intraductal and infiltrating tumor growth in ductal carcinoma of the breast. Cancer 32:830–837, 1973.
222. Silverstein MJ, Rosser RJ, Gierson ED, et al: Axillary lymph node dissection for intraductal carcinoma: Is it indicated? Cancer 59:1819–1824, 1987.
223. Silverstein MJ, Gierson ED, Waisman JR, et al: Axillary lymph node dissection for T1a breast carcinoma: Is is indicated? Cancer 73:664–667, 1994.
224. Silverstein MJ, Gierson ED, Waisman JR, et al: Predicting axillary node positivity in patients with invasive carcinoma of the breast by using a combination of T category and palpability. J Am Coll Surg 180:700–704, 1995.
225. Barth A, Craig PH, Silverstein MJ: Predictors of axillary lymph node metastases in patients with T1 breast carcinomas. Cancer 79:1918–1922, 1997.
226. Simon MS, Lemanne D, Schwartz AG, et al: Recent trends in the incidence of in situ and invasive breast cancer in the Detroit metropolitan area (1975–1988). Cancer 71:769–774, 1993.
227. Singhal H, O'Malley PP, Stitt L, et al: Management of the axilla in screen detected breast cancer. Breast Cancer Res Treat 37:50, 1995.
228. Sinn HP, Oelmann A, Anton HW, et al: Metastatic potential of small and minimally invasive breast carcinoma. Virchows Arch 425:237–241, 1994.
229. Sloan JP, Ellman R, Anderson T, et al: Consistency of histopathological reporting of breast lesions detected by breast screening: Findings of the UK National External Quality (EQA) Scheme. Eur J Cancer 30:1414–1419, 1994.
230. Spratt JA, von Fourmoer D, Spratt JS, et al: Mammographic assessment of human breast cancer growth and duration. Cancer 71:2020–2026, 1993.
231. Steele RJC, Forrest APM, Gibson T, et al: The efficacy of lower axillary sampling in obtaining lymph node status in breast cancer: A controlled randomized trial. Br J Surg 72:368–369, 1985.
232. Steele RJC: Lower-axillary-node sampling in conjunction with local excision for breast cancer. N Engl J Med 315:1358, 1986.
233. Stewart HJ: South-east Scottish trial of local therapy in node negative breast cancer. Breast 3:31–39, 1994.
234. Stewart HJ, Everington D, Forrest APM: The Cardiff local therapy trial: Results at 20 years. Breast 3:40–45, 1994.
235. Stierer M, Rosen HR, Weber R, et al: Long term analysis of factors influencing the outcome in carcinoma of the breast smaller than one centimeter. Surg Gynecol Obstet 175:151–160, 1992.
236. Sunderland MC, McGuire WL: Prognostic indicators in invasive breast cancer. Surg Clin North Am 70:989–1004, 1990.
237. Sutherland CM, Mather J: Long-term survival and prognostic factors in breast cancer patients with localized (no skin,

238. Tabar L, Fagerberg G, Day NE, et al: Breast cancer treatment and natural history: New insights from results of screening. Lancet 339:412–414, 1992.
239. Thompson CH, Stacker SA, Salehi N, et al: Immunoscintigraphy for detection of lymph node metastases from breast cancer. Lancet December 1:1245–1247, 1984.
240. Tinnemans JGM, Wobbes T, Holland R, et al: Treatment and survival of female patients with nonpalpable breast carcinoma. Ann Surg 209:249–253, 1989.
241. Tjandra JJ, Russell IS, Collins JP, et al: Immunolymphoscintigraphy for the detection of lymph node metastases from breast cancer. Cancer Res 49:1600–1608, 1989.
242. Trojani M, de Mascarel I, Bonichon F, et al: Micrometastases to axillary lymph nodes from carcinoma of the breast: Detection of immunohistochemistry and prognostic significance. Br J Cancer 55:303–306, 1987.
243. Trojani M: Detection and significance of occult metastases in node-negative breast cancer. Br J Surg 81:1241, 1994.
244. Tubiana M, Koscielny S: The natural history of breast cancer: Implications for a screening strategy. Int J Radiat Oncol Biol Phys 19:1117–1120, 1990.
245. Unzeitig GW, Frankl G, Ackerman M, et al: Analysis of the prognosis of minimal and occult breast cancers. Arch Surg 118:1403–1404, 1983.
246. Uren RF, Howman-Giles RB, Thompson JF, et al: Mammary lymphoscintigraphy in breast care. J Nucl Med 36:1775–1780, 1995.
247. Van Lancker M, Goor C, Sacre R, et al: Patterns of axillary lymph node meastasis in breast cancer. Am J Clin Oncol 18:267–272, 1995.
248. Veronesi U, Saccozzi R, Del Vecchio M, et al: Comparing radical mastectomy with quadrantectomy, axillary dissection, and radiotherapy in patients with small cancers of the breast. N Engl J Med 305:6–11, 1981.
249. Veronesi U, Rilke F, Luini A, et al: Distribution of axillary node metastases by level of invasion: An analysis of 530 cases. Cancer 59:682–687, 1987.
250. Veronesi U: Clinical management of minimal breast cancer. Semin Surg Oncol 5:145–150, 1989.
251. Veronesi U, Salvadori B, Luini A, et al: Conservative treatment of early breast cancer: Long term results of 1232 cases treated with quadrantectomy, axillary dissection, and radiotherapy. Ann Surg 211:250–259, 1990.
252. Veronesi U, Banfi A, Salvadori B, et al: Breast conservation is the treatment of choice in small breast cancer: Long term results of a randomized trial. Eur J Cancer 26:668–670, 1990.
253. Veronesi U, Luini A, Galimberti S, et al: Extent of metastatic axillary involvement in 1446 cases of breast cancer. Eur J Surg Oncol 16:127–133, 1990.
254. Voogd E, Peterse JL, Rutgers EJ, et al: T-staging of breast cancer: What is the correct T size? Eur J Surg Oncol 20:257–258, 1994.
255. Walker RA, Dearing SJ, Lane DP, et al: Expression of p53 protein in infiltrating and in situ breast carcinomas. J Pathol 165:203–206, 1991.
256. Walls J, Boggis CRM, Wilson M, et al: Treatment of the axilla in patients with screen detected breast cancer. Br J Surg 80:436–438, 1993.
257. Wanebo HJ, Huvos AG, Urban JA: Treatment of minimal breast cancer. Cancer 33:349–357, 1974.
258. Wazer DE, Erban JK, Robert JK, et al: Breast conservation in elderly women for clinically negative axillary lymph nodes without axillary dissection. Cancer 74:878–883, 1994.
259. Weidner N, Folkman J, Pozza F, et al: Tumor angiogenesis: A new significant and independent prognostic indicator in early-stage breast carcinoma. J Natl Cancer Inst 84:1875–1887, 1992.
260. Weidner N: Tumor angiogenesis: A review of current applications in tumor prognostication. Semin Diag Pathol 10:302–313, 1993.
261. Wells CA, Heryet A, Brochier J, et al: The immunocytochemical detection of axillary micrometastases in breast cancer. Br J Cancer 50:193–197, 1984.

262. White E, Lee CY, Kristal AR: Evaluation of the increase in breast cancer incidence in relation to mammography use. J Natl Cancer Inst 82:1546–1552, 1990.

263. White RE, Vezeridis MP, Konstadoulakis M, et al: Therapeutic options and results for the management of minimally invasive breast cancer: Influence of axillary dissection for the treatment of T1a and T1b lesions. J Am Coll Surg 183:575–582, 1996.

264. Wilking N, Rutquist J, Carstensen J, et al: Prognostic significance of axillary nodal status in primary breast cancer in relation to the number of resected nodes. Acta Oncol 31:29–35. 1992.

265. Wilkinson EJ, Hause LL, Hoffman RG, et al: Occult axillary lymph node metastases in invasive breast carcinoma: Characteristics of the primary tumor and significance of the metastases. Pathol Annu 17:67–91, 1982.

266. Winchester DJ, Menck HR, Fremgen AM, et al: Selection criteria for axillary dissection in breast cancer. Soc Surg Oncol 1995. Abstract no. 82.

267. Wood WC: Integration of risk factors to allow patient selection for adjuvant systemic therapy in lymph node-negative breast cancer patients. World J Surg 18:39–44, 1994.

268. Wood WC: Should axillary dissection be performed in patients with DCIS? Ann Surg Oncol 2:193–194, 1995.

CHAPTER 55

SELECTIVE MANAGEMENT OF AXILLA IN MINIMALLY INVASIVE AND EARLY INVASIVE DUCTAL CARCINOMA

Blake Cady, M.D.

Controversy has long existed in the biological implication and technical surgical treatment of regional lymph node metastases in invasive breast cancer. Currently, there is renewed interest in the issue of axillary nodal dissection. Several factors have led to this renewed interest. First is the continuing biological controversy, now more securely understood because of large clinical trials,[20] that axillary lymph node metastases are "indicators but not governors"[6] of outcome in breast cancer. Indeed, in all human solid cancers, this biological concept has been proved repeatedly,* and in every study addressing this issue,* lymph node metastases have proved to be indicators only. Greater cure rates have never been achieved simply by performing more radical lymph node dissections.

The second factor is the markedly decreasing size of invasive breast cancer under the impact of mammographic screening, which has, as a result, markedly decreased the incidence of axillary nodal metastases.[9, 54] Over recent years, the mean and median diameters of invasive breast cancers have decreased to 2.1 cm and 1.5 cm, respectively, in studies we recently published from the Deaconess Hospital (Boston) and Mt. Auburn Hospital (Cambridge, MA).[9] Between 1989 and 1993, almost 30 percent of all patients with invasive breast cancer had primary cancers 1 cm or less in diameter. Furthermore, mammographic screening programs are becoming more widespread since a significant reduction in death rates has been demonstrated.[54] If the entire population of appropriately aged women were screened with mammography, the median maximum diameter of all invasive breast cancers would be only 1 cm, and 20 to 40 percent of all patients might have noninvasive ductal carcinoma in situ (DCIS). This rapid change in breast cancer presentation is being reported from all parts of the United States and the world where mammographic screening is common. This declining size in the presentation of invasive breast cancer has resulted in an accompanying significant decline in regional lymph node metastases.[25, 37, 54] In many reports about mammographically discovered invasive breast cancer, the incidence of lymph node metastases ranges between 5 and 15 percent.[16, 49] This is in stark contrast to the findings of previous decades and to the incidence of lymph node metastases in larger or palpable invasive breast cancer. Because of the declining overall incidence of axillary regional node metastases and the increasing proportion of micrometastases (< 2 mm in diameter) that comprise the lymph node metastases in small, mammographically discovered breast cancers,[25, 51] other features of the primary invasive breast cancer[36, 46] will be regarded as indicators for prognostication and selection of adjuvant therapy.

The third factor is the increasing number of primary tumor features[26, 36, 41, 46] that have statistically significant correlations with outcome and that serve as prognostic markers and adjuvant therapy selectors, roles previously played almost entirely by detection of axillary metastases. All that is missing is a consensus of important features that can be reliably reproduced in pathology laboratories. It is probable that a combination of these prognostic variables will act as the surrogate test for nodal metastases. When a consensus can be achieved, axillary lymph node analysis will no longer be required for prognostication or selection of adjuvant therapy. Increasingly, these features are being used to advocate adjuvant therapy in the presence of negative axillary dissections.[38]

The fourth factor that will probably eliminate the need for axillary dissection is the technical advance of a "sentinel" lymph node biopsy.[24, 34, 50] Reports have shown that blue dye[24] or radioactive sulfur colloid[34] can be used to reliably detect (> 90 percent) the sentinel lymph node in the lymphatic drainage pathways of the breast. One or two sentinel lymph nodes can be removed under local anesthesia, and these have been proved to be highly accurate in determining the status of the entire axillary lymph node basin. This physiological demonstration of the first or sentinel lymph node may be better than axillary dissection because it permits detection of "skip" nodes or internal mammary sentinel lymph node metastases, which have been ignored in recent decades since the decline of routine internal lymph node dissection in medial breast cancers. Recent reports[25] show that with experience there is at least a 90 percent rate of detecting a sentinel lymph node and a 98 percent accuracy in the prediction of regional node metastases by the status of the indicator or sentinel lymph node. If this concept becomes firmly established, regional lymph node dissection and its attendant requirements of general anesthesia, hospitalization,

---

*See references 7, 12, 15, 35, 47, 53, 55, and 57.

1094

significant recovery period, and risk of arm edema will be unnecessary.

The last factor that further reduces the role of axillary dissection is the usefulness of induction (neoadjuvant) multidrug chemotherapy in the initial treatment of patients with advanced primary breast cancer.[52] Patients who fail to respond to induction chemotherapy, which may indicate an extremely poor prognosis, may benefit by prompt, aggressive, local and regional therapy through combinations of mastectomy, axillary dissection, and radiotherapy to attempt local control. In contrast, patients who respond to induction chemotherapy have a reasonable chance for continual freedom from systemic metastases and local disease recurrence, enabling breast preservation in a majority of patients.[52] If the primary cancer or palpable axillary metastases are removed before induction chemotherapy, the chance to obtain evidence of clinical response is lost, and the prognostic category cannot be defined because chemotherapy can no longer demonstrate clinical shrinkage. In these patients, the prime indicator of prognosis is the substantial clinical response of the regional axillary metastases and of the primary cancer to induction chemotherapy. Therefore, these patients should avoid axillary dissection before induction chemotherapy. Only after the prognostic category has been established can further therapeutic decisions be made, including the possibility of breast conservation therapy. If palpable axillary lymph node metastases remain after the local resection of the residual primary cancer and radiotherapy, removal of enlarged axillary lymph nodes for palliation should be considered, although survival will not be altered. In patients who do not undergo axillary dissection because of complete axillary response to chemotherapy and radiotherapy, the infrequent later recurrence in the axilla can be managed by axillary dissection.[48] Prophylactic axillary dissection will not improve survival, and palliation should be the goal of removing later axillary node recurrence. Such a passive surgical attitude toward regional lymph node metastases is practical and function preserving, because regional lymph node metastases only serve as indicators. There is no absolute indication to remove nonpalpable axillary lymph nodes to prepare for systemic therapy, because this has already occurred by induction chemotherapy.

We are entering an era in which we must reconsider the entire role of axillary lymph node dissection as an adjunct to breast cancer treatment. We must be extremely selective when choosing patients for traditional regional lymph node dissection.

IMPLICATION OF LYMPH NODE METASTASES

The history of lymph node dissection puts the current controversy in perspective. In the late 1800s, Halsted postulated that lymph node drainage from the primary cancer in the breast was the paramount route of the cancer cell spread that caused later metastatic disease.[28] He viewed the cancer cell exit as occurring exclusively through lymphatic routes, and he hypothesized that if lymph channels and lymph nodes could be resected en bloc with the primary cancer, then increased cure rates and better local and regional control would result. The concept of lymphatic and lymph node drainage was so dominant that it was postulated that direct lymphatic channels ran from the breast cancer across the diaphragm into the liver as the primary source of liver metastases! Other disseminated metastases also were fit into such a conceptual framework, such as brain metastases via paravertebral lymphatics. It was believed that only after the lymphatic system was filled would cells then enter the hematogenous system for further dissemination.

Halsted's en bloc radical axillary dissection and mastectomy technique was acclaimed as a major advance at the time and led to significant reductions in local recurrence on the chest wall.[28] Unfortunately, in retrospect it did not produce major improvements in survival because of the advanced nature of the disease. In fact, long-term survival results in Halsted's reports were extremely modest (less than 10 percent).

After World War II, with the development of safer general anesthesia and improved understanding of wound healing and surgical recovery, the field of radical oncological surgery developed. Super-radical operations evolved that included concomitant supraclavicular and internal mammary lymph node resections as a routine extension of radical mastectomy.[13] Wide sacrifices of skin overlying the breast and routine skin graft applications were also performed. The blunting of this movement toward super-radical breast cancer surgery occurred when randomized prospective clinical trials revealed that neither supraclavicular nor internal mammary lymph node dissection led to improved survival, compared with regional lymph node dissections confined to the axilla.[35, 55] Even in early studies of local excision of breast cancer in Finland[33] and England,[30] axillary nodal dissections continued to be part of the basic surgical approach. The first randomized trial at Guy's Hospital in London[30] compared radical mastectomy to wide excision only in breast cancer, and surprisingly both resulted in equivalent cure rates. These patients received a low dose of radiation therapy either to the bed of the radical mastectomy or to the breast, including the axilla in the wide-excision-only patients. These startling results led to suspicions that perhaps lymph node metastases did not play a vital role in survival from breast cancer and that the extent of the surgical treatment of the primary disease perhaps also was immaterial to long-term survival. This concept was tested in an early National Surgical Adjuvant Breast and Bowel Project Program (NSABP) study in which patients with clinically negative axillas were randomly assigned to radical mastectomy, total mastectomy and radiation therapy to the axilla, or total mastectomy without treatment of the axilla (Protocol B-04).[20] In the latter group, about 30 percent actually had a few lymph nodes removed without formal axillary dissection. In patients with clinically positive axillas, radical mastectomy was compared with total mastectomy with radiation therapy to the axilla as part of the same trial. After a 14-year follow-up, patients with clinically negative or clinically positive axillas had identical survival despite the wide variations in treatment of the axillary lymph nodes.[20] These studies along with supporting animal experiments led to the conceptual shift from a lymphatic-dominant dissemination pattern as proposed by Halsted to the hypothesis that lymphatic and vascular dissemination occurred simultaneously and uniformly. Therefore, lymph node metastases performed as an indicator rather than as a controlling factor in survival.[21] Many studies have since confirmed this concept not only in breast cancer but across the whole spectrum of human solid cancers.*

With the advent of multidrug adjuvant chemotherapy, however, the need rapidly emerged for accurate staging to select patients with poor prognoses for toxic systemic adjuvant treatment designed to improve survival by killing micrometastatic disease. The prime prognostic factor, after size of the primary cancer itself, was the status of the axillary lymph nodes. Many studies demonstrated the direct linear relationship between the increasing number of axillary lymph node metastases and worsening prognosis, so that patients with ten or more lymph node metastases were found to have only 25 percent 10-year survival.[56] Patients with a single micrometastasis, however, did not have any significant decrement in survival.[51] Looked at another way, among 5-year survivors with invasive breast cancer, Harvey and Auchincloss[29] found that 70 percent of patients surviving for 5 years had negative lymph nodes, 13 percent had one lymph node metastasis, 7 percent had two lymph node metastases, 5 percent had 3 node metastases, and less than 5 percent of patients had more than three lymph node metastases. For decades, axillary lymph node status was the only reliable indicator used in prognostication and selection of adjuvant systemic chemotherapy or administration of tamoxifen.[14, 23] Negative nodes, one to three positive nodes, four to ten positive nodes, and more than ten positive nodes became established as the general prognostic categories. It has recently been suggested that patients with more than five or ten positive nodes, with an unusually poor prognosis, might be selected for extremely aggressive experimental chemotherapy programs. For clinical trials, the exact number of lymph node metastases became important in selecting patients for highly morbid and sometimes lethal, aggressive systemic chemotherapy trials that eventually culminated in the tactic of bone marrow transplantation after super-lethal chemotherapy in an attempt to improve survival by escalating the drug dose.[40] No randomized trial has demonstrated that bone marrow transplantation results in better survival than standard chemotherapy.[11]

Because of the presumed reliability of many new primary tumor prognostic indicators (histochemical, biochemical, and genetic), patients, even with negative axillary lymph nodes, are being treated with adjuvant chemotherapy because of their high statistical risk of metastases.[10] However, a large meta-analysis demonstrated that because 75 percent of patients with breast cancer are postmenopausal, they do not benefit significantly from systemic adjuvant chemotherapy.[18] Statistically significant but small reductions in recurrence rates (12 to 15 percent) were demonstrated by the use of tamoxifen, but survival was only slightly improved.[18] Patients who receive adjuvant systemic therapy (chemotherapy or antiestrogen therapy) because of primary tumor features even in the presence of negative axillary lymph nodes, will not benefit from removal of axillary lymph nodes.[58]

Within 5 years, axillary lymph node removal will probably not be a regular component of the primary treatment of invasive breast cancer, but will instead be confined to research institutions conducting randomized prospective controlled trials. Axillary dissection will be confined to patients with recurrent or persistent palpable axillary metastases after initial therapy.

ANATOMY AND FUNCTION OF THE LYMPHATIC SYSTEM

The new tactical thinking regarding lymph node metastases and the need to determine their presence is also based on the biology of the lymphatic system, lymph nodes, and lymph node metastases. A brief analysis of the anatomy, physiology, biological function, and metastatic specificity of the lymphatic system will add to our understanding of changing attitudes toward surgical regional lymph node dissection.

The lymphatic system was first described by Asellius in Pavia in 1622. While performing an animal dissection to display the nerve supply, he accidentally incised an abdominal structure that spilled white fluid.[2] Shortly afterward, he published a color atlas of the newly discovered lymphatic vessels (the first colored anatomical atlas). He did not, however, understand how lymph nodes related to his lymphatic vessels. This relationship was not completely described until 1863 when His[32] linked the lymph nodes with the lymphatic system and described the anatomy and structure of both in such detail that no significant more recent description has been added.

The lymphatic system serves four purposes[17, 27]: (1) return of interstitial fluids and proteins to the blood and conduction of absorbed fats from the intestinal tract to the vascular system by way of intestinal lacteals and the thoracic duct; (2) production and dissemination of small T lymphocytes; (3) production of large lymphocytes and plasma cells that produce humeral antibodies; and (4) exposure of foreign antigens to lymph node lymphocytes that serve as anti-

*See references 6, 7, 12, 15, 35, 47, 53, 55, and 57.

gen recognition points for the production of circulating antibodies, the humeral component of the immunological system of the organism.

Circulating lymphocytes arrive in the lymph node through the artery and not through lymphatic channels. The specificity of lymphocytes in embryological development and normal physiology is extraordinary; Peyer's patch lymphocytes do not lodge in other lymph nodes, and conversely, other lymph node lymphocytes do not lodge in Peyer's patches.[1, 42]

Lymph nodes have four basic anatomical components[39]: lymphoid tissue, lymphatic capillaries, arterial and venous vessels, and the supportive structure of fibrous and connective tissue. The lymphatic vessels connect to and surround the lymph nodes in different patterns.[19, 39] One pattern involves afferent lymphatic channels that bypass lymph nodes completely or partially. In other patterns, lymphaticovenous anastomoses are noted in the prenodal afferent or postnodal efferent lymphatic channels. Such lymphaticovenous and bypass lymphatic channels allow fluids, foreign antigens, and metastatic cells direct access to the hematogenous system without traversing lymph nodes at all. In the predominant pattern, however, lymph flow goes from the afferent lymphatics directly to the pericapsular sinus of the regional lymph node, where the lymph flow successively moves to the central portion of the lymph node for the immunological function that maximally exposes interstitial foreign antigens to lymphocytes for the induction of humeral antibodies. After this, lymph exits the lymph node via efferent lymphatics.

Studies in animals show that metastatic cancer cells arriving at the lymph node by afferent lymphatics may bypass the node entirely through lymphatic channels or lymphaticovenous anastomoses, or, they may flow into the lymph node through the pericapsular sinus, then via centrally directed lymph channels where lymph flows sluggishly through varied routes exposed to lymphocytes, and then out the efferent lymphatic channel.[31, 43] Metastatic cancer cells following this path may lodge in the lymph node and remain, without progressive growth or with destruction by physiological processes that occur in the lymph node itself. Other cells may lodge and grow progressively.

Anatomically, lymph flows progressively and sequentially through regional lymph node groups. Recent surgical reports defined the concept of a sentinel lymph node and demonstrated lymph flow sequentially through successive lymph nodes.[25, 34, 50] Using blue dye[25] or radioactive sulfur colloid injection,[34, 50] it has been shown in melanoma and breast cancer that there are usually one or two lymph nodes in the regional lymphatics that can be reliably identified as the initial entrance point of lymphatic fluid (and presumably metastatic cells) traversing the regional lymph nodes. In these physiological studies, bypassing lymphatic channels that go to a different lymph node than what would be anatomically expected are similarly detected with staining or radioactive labeling as a sentinel node. Thus, anatomical and physiological variations of the lymphatic flow via lymph vessels out of the breast may lead to the detection of a sentinel lymph node. This sentinel node is usually in the low axilla, but it also may be in the upper axilla, internal mammary node, or supraclavicular space. The finding of an aberrant sentinel lymph node will undoubtedly explain the occasional "skip" nodal metastases. In studies reported thus far, sentinel lymph nodes are the reliable surrogate of the regional lymph node basin; multiple studies confirm that positive lymph nodes seldom remain after sampling of the negative sentinel lymph node.[25, 34, 50] There seems to be a coherent flow of lymph through lymph node basins with at least one, two, or three nodes at the initial entrance of lymphatic flow. These physiological studies are rational and intuitively sensible, because we know from past anatomical studies that patients with only one or two nodal metastases almost always display them in close proximity to the primary cancer. Thus, the distribution of lymph, metastatic cells, and nodal metastases is not a random event, but highly structured and sequential.

To understand lymph node function in human solid tumors, extensive research work is being conducted on metastatic cancer cell organ specificity that is crucial to explain the indicator rather than governing function of lymph node metastases in patient survival.[44] Cancer cells, selected by sequential harvesting of specific organ site metastases and injected intravenously in animals, display an inability to lodge and grow in organs other than their source in liver, lung, or lymph node from which they were obtained. Thus, despite obvious wide circulation of metastatic cancer cells in these animal models, only in the liver, lungs, or lymph node will specific metastatic cells lodge or display progressive growth. Unknown as yet are the exact physiological mechanisms that permit or prevent lodging and progressive growth of organ-specific metastatic cells, but they may be related to cytokine function, electrical charge, structural aspects of their surface, or other tissue features in the receptor organ.[3, 4, 45]

Brodt and colleagues[5] demonstrated the lymph node specificity of human lymphatic metastatic cells grown in nude mice and offer the probable physiological explanation for why lymph node metastases act as indicators but not governors of survival and why patients who have lymph node metastases may survive for long periods otherwise disease free. Such breast cancers may shed only lymph node–specific metastatic cells that, despite wide circulation, cannot grow in other organ sites. Their presence would demonstrate the statistical likelihood of dissemination of other clones of cells from the primary breast cancer that in turn may have their own organ specificity for lodging and growth in other organs such as bone, brain, lung, and liver. It has been postulated that only the lymph node–specific metastatic cells would lodge and grow in the regional lymph node site without threat to the life of the host. However, the resultant visceral organ metastatic distribution of cells has the capability of progressive growth, causing subsequent dysfunction of the recipient organ. Many human models of such organ specificity of metastatic cells occur, such as hepatic-only metastases in colorectal carcinomas that can be cured by hepatic resection,[8] or lung-only metastatic sarcomas that can also be resected for cure.[22] Other human cancers, such as low-risk differentiated thyroid cancer, have extensive lymph node metastases in as many as 75 or 80 percent of patients, yet they rarely have systemic metastatic disease. Such patients are cured in more than 98 percent of cases, whether or not the lymph nodes are removed.[7] Such lymph node metastases may be quiescent for many years, without apparent progressive growth or other dissemination that would pose a threat to host survival, because of the apparent lymph node–specific capacity of such cells.

COST-BENEFIT ANALYSIS

Another element to the re-evaluation of axillary lymph node metastases is the cost-benefit ratio. When invasive ductal cancers are small (≤ 1 cm), the positive lymph node rate will be 10 percent or perhaps 15 percent[9]; the routine use of axillary dissection in this situation increases survival of these patients by only 1 percent at ten years, at the cost of $1 million per 100 patients. Thus, if 100 axillary dissections (approximately $10,000 each) are performed (cost = $1 million) to define ten patients who have a positive node and those ten patients receive systemic chemotherapy, the resultant 33 percent reduction[18] in mortality (from 30 to 20 percent), would save only one life, because the seven of ten positive node survivors would increase to eight. The majority of breast cancer patients are postmenopausal, however, in whom the demonstrated effectiveness of tamoxifen is only one-half that of premenopausal multidrug chemotherapy[18]; the cost-benefit ratio in these patients would be even less justified. If there is an average of 20 years of life lost in women who die of breast cancer, then the $1 to $2 million cost of axillary dissections to save one life would equal $50,000 to $100,000 per year of life saved; this figure far exceeds current health estimates of justifiable and sustainable costs.

From these assumptions, one can see the immediate cost and morbidity advantage of performing a sentinel lymph node biopsy under local anesthesia to determine the status of the regional lymph node basin in patients without adverse primary tumor features who would benefit from adjuvant therapy.

SUMMARY

There are many reasons to avoid axillary lymph node dissection in the modern management of invasive breast cancer. (1) There is a lack of correlation between the management of the regional lymph node basin and survival. (2) It is desirable to avoid the complications and morbidity of surgery and general anesthesia resulting from axillary dissection. (3) There is a need to reflect in practical, functional terms on the lack of impact on survival by lymph node removal. This apparently counter-intuitive concept is given physiological explanation by experimental and clinical data that demonstrate highly organ-specific metastatic lodging and growth of circulating cells disseminated from primary cancers and that describe why lymph node metastases are indicators but not governors of survival. (4) The cost-benefit ratio of performing axillary dissection in the increasingly large proportions of very small invasive cancers indicates that the cost of lives saved exceeds $50,000 per year of life, far above sustainable costs. Increasingly, axillary lymph metastases detection will be irrelevant because of the dependence on primary tumor features for prognosis through routine pathological reports of size, grade, and lymph vessel involvement and through sophisticated analysis of genetic make-up, histochemical features, or biological markers in the primary cancer. (5) The new technology of sentinel node biopsy under local anesthesia produces a reliable surrogate for the status of the regional nodal basin and obviates the need to do regional nodal resection. (6) By deliberately not dissecting palpable lymph nodes in patients with advanced primary cancer in order to observe the clinical response to induction chemotherapy, axillary dissection would be detrimental to their overall management.

References

1. Abernathy NJ, Hay JB: The recirculation of lymphocytes from blood to lymph: Physiological considerations and molecular mechanisms. Lymphology 25(1):1–30, 1992.
2. Asellius G: De Lactibus sine Lacteis Venis. Mediolani, apud Io B Bdellium, 1627.
3. Brodt P: Adhesion mechanisms in lymphatic metastasis. Cancer Metastasis Rev 10(1):23–32, 1991.
4. Brodt P, Reich R, Moroz LA, et al: Differences in the repertoires of basement membrane degrading enzymes in two carcinoma sublines with distinct patterns of site-selective metastasis. Biochim Biophys Acta 1139(1–2):77–83, 1992.
5. Brodt P, Fallavollita L, Sawka RJ, et al: Tumor cell adhesion to frozen lymph node sections: A correlate of lymphatic metastasis in breast carcinoma models of human and rat origin. Breast Cancer Res Treat 17(2):109–120, 1990.
6. Cady B: Lymph node metastases: Indicators, but not governors of survival. Arch Surg 119:1067–1072, 1984.
7. Cady B, Rossi R: An expanded view of risk group definition in differentiated thyroid carcinoma. Surgery 104:947–953, 1988.
8. Cady B, Stone MD, Steele GD, et al: Technical and biological factors in disease-free survival after hepatic resection for colorectal cancer metastases. Arch Surg 127:561–568, 1992.
9. Cady B, Stone MD, Schuler J, et al: The new era in breast cancer: Invasion, size, and nodal involvement dramatically decreasing as a result of mammographic screening. Arch Surg 131:301–308, 1996.
10. Clark GM, Wenger CR, Beardslee S, et al: How to integrate steroid hormone receptor, flow cytometric, and other prognostic information in regard to primary breast cancer. Cancer 71(Suppl 6):2157–2162, 1993.
11. Cote RJ, Rosen PP, Lessser ML, et al: Prediction of early relapse in patients with operable breast cancer by detection of occult bone marrow micrometastases. J Clin Oncol 9(10):1749–1756, 1991.
12. Cuschieri A, Fayers P, Fielding J, Craven J, Bancewicz J,

Joypaul V, Cook P: Surgical treatment of gastric cancer postoperative morbidity and mortality after D1 and D2 resections for gastric cancer: Preliminary results of the MRC randomized controlled surgical trials. Lancet 347:995–999, 1996.

13. Dahl-Iversen E: Recherche sur les metastases microscopique des ganglions lymphatiques parasternaux dans le cancer du sein. Int J Chir 11:492, 1951.

14. Danforth DN: The role and necessity of axillary lymph node dissection in management of stage I or II breast cancer. Breast J 2:116–120, 1995.

15. Dent DM, Madden MV, Price SK: Controlled trials and the R1/R2 controversy in the management of gastric carcinoma. Surg Oncol Clin N Am 2:433–441, 1993.

16. Dowlatshahi K, Snider HC, Kim R: Axillary node status in nonpalpable breast cancer. Ann Surg Oncol 2(5):424–428, 1995.

17. Drinker CK, Yoffey JM: Lymphatics, Lymph and Lymphoid Tissue: Their Physiological and Clinical Significance. Cambridge, MA, Harvard University Press, 1944.

18. Early Breast Cancer Trialists' Collaborative Group: Systemic treatment of early breast cancer by hormonal, cytotox, or immune therapy. Lancet 339:1–15, 1992.

19. Edwards IM, Kinmonth JB: Lymphovenous shunts in man. Br Med J 4:579, 1959.

20. Fisher B, Redmond C, Fisher ER, et al: Ten-year results of a randomized clinical trial comparing radical mastectomy and total mastectomy with or without radiation. N Engl J Med 312:674–681, 1985.

21. Fisher ER, Anderson S, Redmond C, et al: Pathologic findings from the National Surgical Adjuvant Breast Project Protocol B-06: 10-year pathologic and clinical prognostic discriminants. Cancer 71:2507–2514, 1993.

22. Frost DB: Pulmonary metastasectomy for soft tissue sarcomas: Is it justified? J Surg Oncol 59(2):110–115, 1995.

23. Gardner B, Feldman J: Are positive axillary nodes in breast cancer markers for incurable disease? Ann Surg 218:270–275, 1993.

24. Giuliano AE, Kirgan DM, Guenther JM, Morton DL: Lymphatic mapping and sentinel lymphadenectomy for breast cancer. Ann Surg 220:391–398, 1994.

25. Giuliano AR, Dale PS, Turner RR, Morton DL, et al: Improved axillary staging of breast cancer with sentinel lymphadenectomy. Ann Surg 222:394–399, 1995.

26. Gotteland M, May E, May-Levin F, et al. Estrogen receptors (ER) in human breast cancer: The significance of a new prognostic factor based on both ER protein and ER mRNA contents. Cancer 74:864–871, 1994.

27. Guyton AC, Taylor AE, Granger HJ: Circulatory Physiology II: Dynamics and Control of the Body Fluids. Philadelphia, WB Saunders, 1975.

28. Halsted WS: The result of operations for the cure of cancer of the breast performed at the Johns Hopkins Hospital from June, 1889 to January, 1894. Johns Hopkins Hosp Bull 4:297, 1894–1895.

29. Harvey HD, Auchincloss H: Metastases to lymph nodes from carcinomas that were arrested. Cancer 21:684–691, 1968.

30. Hayward JL: The Guy's Hospital trial of treatment of "early" breast cancer. World J Surg 1:314–316, 1977.

31. Heys SD, Eremin O: The relevance of tumor draining lymph nodes in cancer. Surg Gynecol Obstet 174:533–540, 1992.

32. His W: Uber das Epithel der Lymphagefasswwrzeln und über die von Recklinghausen's schen Saftcanalchen. Z Wiss Zool 13:455, 1863.

33. Joensuu H, Taikkanen S: Cured of breast cancer? J Clin Oncol 13:62–69, 1995.

34. Krag DN, Weaver DL, Alex JC, Fairbank JT: Surgical resection and radio localization of the sentinel lymph node in breast cancer using a gamma probe. Surg Oncol 2:335–339, 1993.

35. Lacour J, Le MG, Kramar A, et al: Is it useful to remove internal mammary nodes in operable breast cancer? Eur J Surg Oncol 13:309–314, 1987.

36. Leitner SP, Swern AS, Weinberger D, Duncan LJ, Hutter

RVP: Predictors of recurrence for patients with small (one centimeter or less) localized breast cancer (T1a,b N0 M0). Cancer 76:2266–2274, 1995.

37. Letton AH, Mason EM, Ramshaw BJ: Twenty-year review of a breast cancer screening project: Ninety-five percent survival of patients with nonpalpable cancers. Cancer 77:104–106, 1996.

38. Loprinzi CL, Ravdin PM, DeLaurentiis M, et al: Do American oncologists know how to use prognostic variables for patients with newly diagnosed primary breast cancer? J Clin Oncol 12(7):1422–1426, 1994.

39. Ludwig J: General anatomy of the lymphatic system: Five types of arrangements of afferent and efferent lymphatics of lymph nodes. Pathol Microbiol 25:329, 1962.

40. Mansi JL, Easton D, Berger U, et al: Bone marrow micrometastases in primary breast cancer: Prognostic significance after 6 years' follow-up. Eur J Cancer 27:1552–1555, 1991.

41. Marks JR, Humphrey PA, Wu K, et al: Over expression of p53 and HER-2/neu proteins and prognostic markers in early stage breast cancer. Ann Surg 219:332–341, 1994.

42. Miura S, Asakura H, Tsuchiya M: Dynamic analysis of lymphocyte migration into Peyer's patches of rat small intestine. Lymphology 20:252–256, 1987.

43. Morris B, Salami M: The blood and lymphatic capillaries of lymph nodes in the sheep foetus and their involvement in cell traffic. Lymphology 20:244–251, 1987.

44. Nicolson GL, Dulski KM: Organ specificity of metastatic tumor colonization is related to organ-selective growth properties of malignant cells. Int J Cancer 38:289–294, 1986.

45. Nip J, Shibata H, Loskutoff DJ, et al: Human melanoma cells derived from lymphatic metastases use integrim A^vB^3 to adhere to lymph node vitronectin. J Clin Invest 90:1406–1413, 1992.

46. Osborne CK: Prognostic factors for breast cancer: Have they met their promises? J Clin Oncol 10:679–682, 1992.

47. Pezim ME, Nicholls RJ, Chir E: Survival after high or low ligation of the inferior mesenteric artery during curative surgery for rectal cancer. Ann Surg 200:729–733, 1984.

48. Recht A, Pierce SM, Abner A, et al: Regional nodal failure after conservation surgery and radiotherapy for early-stage breast carcinoma. J Clin Oncol 9:988–996, 1991.

49. Reger V, Beito G, Jolly PC: Factors affecting the incidence of lymph node metastases in small cancers of the breast. Am J Surg 157:501–502, 1989.

50. Reintgen D, Cruse CW, Wells K, Berman C, et al: The orderly progression of melanoma nodal metastases. Ann Surg 220:759–767, 1994.

51. Rosen PP, Saigo PE, Braun DW, et al: Axillary micro-and macro metastases in breast cancer: Prognostic significance of tumor size. Ann Surg 194:585–591, 1981.

52. Schwartz GF, Birchansky CA, Komarnicky LT, et al: Induction chemotherapy followed by breast conservation for locally advanced carcinoma of the breast. Cancer 73:362–369, 1994.

53. Slingluff CL, Stidham KR, Ricci WM, et al: Surgical management of regional lymph nodes in patients with melanoma: Experience with 4682 patients. Ann Surg 219:120–130, 1994.

54. Tabar L, Fagerberg G, Chen HH, Phil M, Duffy SW, Smart CR, Gad A, Smith RA: Efficacy of breast cancer screening by age: New results from the Swedish two-county trial. CA Cancer J Clin 75:2507–2517, 1995.

55. Veronesi U, Valagussa P: Inefficacy of internal mammary nodes dissection in breast cancer surgery. Cancer 47:170–175, 1981.

56. Walker MJ, Osborne MD, Young DC, et al: The natural history of breast cancer with more than 10 positive nodes. Am J Surg 169:575–579, 1995.

57. Weisenburger TH: Effects of postoperative mediastinal radiation on completely resected stage II and stage III epidermoid cancer of the lung. Chest 106(Suppl 6):297S–301S, 1994.

58. Wood WC: Integration of risk factors to allow patient selection for adjuvant systemic therapy in lymph node-negative breast cancer patients. World J Surg 18(1):39–44, 1994.

CHAPTER 56
LYMPHATIC MAPPING AND SENTINEL LYMPHADENECTOMY FOR BREAST CANCER

Mark C. Kelley, M.D. / Armando E. Giuliano, M.D.

THE ROLE OF AXILLARY DISSECTION IN STAGING AND TREATMENT

Axillary lymph node status is the single strongest predictor of survival in women with breast cancer. For decades it has played a critical role in determining adjuvant treatment and prognosis, and accurate pathological staging of the axilla has therefore been considered an integral part of the management of invasive breast cancer. The National Institutes of Health (NIH) consensus conference on early-stage breast cancer therapy recommended routine Level 1 and 2 axillary dissection to achieve this goal.[1] Although this approach has a low false-negative rate, it does result in significant morbidity. Permanent lymphedema has been documented in 7 to 37 percent of breast cancer patients undergoing axillary dissection, and the frequency and severity of lymphedema increases with the extent of axillary surgery and addition of radiation therapy.[3–5] Other side effects or complications such as wound infection, seroma, arm weakness, decreased shoulder range of motion, and neurological changes also occur frequently. These sequelae are a major source of emotional distress and functional impairment for women with breast cancer and significantly increase the monetary cost of treating the disease.[2–7] This is particularly relevant for the 60 to 70 percent of patients who do not have axillary node metastases, and therefore will not have a change in adjuvant therapy based on the results of the procedure.[8] Because many patients now receive adjuvant therapy regardless of nodal status, the benefit of axillary dissection has recently been challenged.[9–13]

Before examining the role of lymphatic mapping and sentinel lymphadenectomy in breast cancer, we should consider the therapeutic benefit of axillary dissection more closely. It is generally accepted that regional disease control is higher in patients undergoing axillary dissection than in those having no axillary treatment. Radiation therapy also enhances regional control, but axillary dissection is equivalent or superior in this regard.[9–17] Table 56–1 summarizes four randomized trials comparing axillary dissection to radiation therapy or observation alone. In each study the regional failure rate for axillary dissection was 1 percent, whereas observation and technically inadequate radiotherapy were associated with axillary relapse rates of 13 to 19 percent.[14–17] A recent prospective trial of breast-conserving therapy without axillary dissection documented a 28 percent nodal recurrence rate at 10 years, confirming poor long-term regional control in the absence of effective axillary treatment.[12, 18] The issue of regional control is often omitted from discussions about the role of axillary dissection in breast cancer therapy, but its importance cannot be overemphasized. The patient who unfortunately develops uncontrollable axillary disease, experiences tremendous pain and suffering. Axillary dissection therefore provides significant benefit by allowing accurate staging and appropriate selection of adjuvant therapy as well as reducing the morbidity of axillary recurrence in patients with lymph node metastases.[9–12]

It is less clear if axillary dissection directly affects patient survival. The results of several randomized trials addressing this issue are reviewed in Table 56–2.[8–13] Approximately 30 percent of women with lymph node metastases treated with mastectomy, axillary dissection, and no adjuvant therapy survive 10 years without recurrence. This suggests that a subset of patients with regional disease are cured by axillary dissection.[19] This hypothesis is supported by a prospective, randomized trial comparing lumpectomy with axillary dissection to lumpectomy with axillary irradiation that found improved survival in the group

TABLE 56–1. AXILLARY DISSECTION AND REGIONAL RECURRENCE OF BREAST CANCER

Study	No. of Patients	Dissection (%)	Radiation (%)	Observation (%)	Comments
Institut Curie[14]	658	1	2	—	
Edinburgh[15]	275	1†	14	—	Inadequate radiotherapy
Guy's Hospital II[16]	258	1†	13	—	Inadequate radiotherapy
NSABP B-04[17]	1079	1*	3*	19	

* = $p<0.05$ compared to observation.
† = $p<0.05$ compared to radiation.
Adapted from Recht A, Houlihan MJ: Axillary lymph nodes and breast cancer: A review. Cancer 76:1491–1512, 1995.

TABLE 56–2. AXILLARY DISSECTION AND SURVIVAL IN BREAST CANCER

Study	No. of Patients	Dissection (%)	Radiation (%)	Observation (%)	Measure (Overall Survival)	Comments
Institut Curie[14]	658	89*	87	—	5 yr	
Edinburgh[15]	275	62*	50	—	12 yr	Inadequate radiation
Guy's Hospital II[16]	258	71*	53	—	10 yr	Inadequate radiation
NSABP B-04[17]	1079	58	57	54	10 yr	

*$p<0.05$ compared to radiation.
Adapted from Recht A, Houlihan MJ: Axillary lymph nodes and breast cancer: A review. Cancer 76:1491–1512, 1995.

undergoing axillary dissection.[14] However, only patients with histologically proven lymph node metastases received adjuvant chemotherapy. Thus, the observed difference in survival may be the result of adjuvant therapy dictated by the procedure rather than the procedure itself. In either case, the combination of the procedure and the resultant alteration in therapy led to improved survival. A recent retrospective study also indicated that patients treated with lumpectomy alone had lower survival rates than those undergoing lumpectomy and axillary dissection or modified radical mastectomy.[20] This finding persisted after correction for other confounding variables, including age and tumor size, but not adjuvant therapy. The authors concluded that performance of an axillary dissection was associated with improved survival, but that it was unclear if this was related to the procedure itself. The positive impact of axillary dissection on survival is also supported by two randomized studies from Great Britain showing greater survival in patients undergoing axillary dissection compared with those receiving inadequate axillary radiation therapy.[15, 16]

In contrast, the National Surgical Adjuvant Breast and Bowel Project (NSABP) protocol B-04 trial showed no survival advantage to axillary dissection.[17] This study randomized patients to receive radical mastectomy, total mastectomy with chest wall and axillary radiation therapy, or total mastectomy alone. Although the rate of regional recurrence was higher in patients undergoing mastectomy alone, there was no difference in survival after 10 years of follow-up (see Tables 56–1 and 56–2). However, many patients in the mastectomy alone arm had a significant number of axillary nodes removed, which could have biased survival data for this group favorably. The number of patients included in the trial may also be insufficient to detect as much as a 10 percent difference in survival resulting from axillary dissection.[12] These considerations dictate caution when using this study as support for the contention that axillary dissection does not directly affect survival.[12] This question will only be answered unequivocally by a large, well-designed randomized study that controls for variations in adjuvant therapy based on the results of axillary dissection.

Because axillary dissection has significant morbidity and its survival benefit remains controversial, a debate has arisen over the appropriate method for axillary staging.[9–13] Recommendations have ranged from routine Level 1, 2, and 3 (total) axillary dissection[21] to no axillary staging.[13, 22, 23] It has recently become apparent that the average primary tumor size and incidence of axillary lymph node metastases are decreasing.[13, 23] The trend toward less extensive surgery for the breast primary has continued, and increasing emphasis is now placed on outpatient therapy and cost effectiveness. This has led some to suggest that routine axillary dissection should be abandoned in certain patients with invasive breast cancer.[13, 22, 23] Others have sought to develop less-invasive methods to accurately detect lymph node metastases. This chapter reviews the proposed noninvasive methods of predicting axillary node status and describes the development of a minimally invasive lymphatic mapping and sentinel lymphadenectomy technique for breast cancer. Results of several clinical trials of this technique performed at the John Wayne Cancer Institute and perspectives for its future clinical application are discussed.

NONINVASIVE METHODS OF PREDICTING AXILLARY LYMPH NODE METASTASES

Several noninvasive methods have been described to identify lymph node metastases in patients with breast cancer. Clinical examination is the oldest and simplest, but its accuracy is limited. Ten to 50 percent of clinically positive axillas do not contain tumor by hematoxylin and eosin (H&E) staining, whereas 15 to 40 percent of clinically negative axillas harbor metastases.[9–11, 24] Radiographic techniques such as mammography, ultrasound, magnetic resonance imaging (MRI), lymphoscintigraphy, and radiolabeled monoclonal antibody scanning may detect axillary node metastases, but lack the sensitivity or specificity required to have significant clinical utility.[10, 25–29] Nieweg and colleagues described the use of positron emission tomography (PET) scanning to identify axillary lymph node metastases in patients with breast cancer.[30] However, only metastases greater than 0.8 cm in diameter were detected with this technique, limiting its usefulness.

Patient age, tumor size, nuclear and histological grades, lymphatic and vascular invasion, angiogenesis, hormone receptor status, DNA ploidy, S-phase fraction, *ERBB2* (*HER2*/neu), cathepsin D, and integrin expression in the primary tumor have all been correlated with axillary metastases.[10, 31–44] Among these clinical and pathological factors, the best predictor of nodal status is tumor size. This is demonstrated by the review of 24,740 breast cancer cases in the Surveillance Epidemiology and End Results (SEER) Program study.[31] A linear relationship was found between tumor size and the incidence of axillary metastases. Tumor diameter and nodal status were independent and additive prognostic factors for survival, suggesting that both should be considered when making treatment decisions. Fisher and colleagues[32] also confirmed the strong correlation between tumor size and axillary metastases in a review of the pathological findings from 614 patients in the radical mastectomy arm of NSABP protocol B-04. Univariate analysis also identified 13 other factors associated with nodal status including clinical stage; nuclear and histological grades; and lymphatic, vascular, and perineural invasion.

The incidence of axillary metastasis in patients with T1 breast cancers has been evaluated extensively in an effort to define a subgroup of patients with a low enough risk of nodal metastasis that axillary dissection may be omitted.[13] Table 56–3 summarizes the results from several studies examining this issue. Review of more than 8000 T1 tumors in the SEER data base showed that the incidence of axillary metastases was 20 percent for tumors less than 0.5 cm (T1a), 21 percent for tumors 0.5 to 0.9 cm (T1b), and 33 percent for tumors 1.0 to 1.9 cm (T1c).[31] Approximately one third of the patients with nodal metastases in each T stage had four or more positive nodes. Rosen and colleagues reported a pathological analysis of 644 patients with T1 invasive carcinomas followed at Memorial Sloan-Kettering Cancer Center for 18 years.[33] The incidence of axillary metastasis was 11 percent for patients with T1a tumors, 15 percent for T1b lesions, 25 percent for 1.1- to 1.3-cm lesions, 34 percent for 1.4- to 1.6-cm lesions, and 43 percent for 1.7- to 2.0-cm lesions. White and associates evaluated 931 patients from the Rhode Island Tumor Registry and found axillary node metastases associated with 10 percent of T1a and 19 percent of T1b tumors.[20] These studies emphasize the high incidence of lymph node metastases in patients with T1 primary breast cancers and strongly support the use of routine axillary staging in these patients.

In contrast, a study by Reger and colleagues detected axillary metastases in only 3 percent of patients with T1a tumors, 10 percent with T1b tumors, 21 percent with 1.1- to 1.5-cm lesions, and 35 percent with 1.6- to 2.0-cm lesions.[34] Silverstein and associates also reported a 3 percent incidence of axillary metastasis in patients with T1a invasive carcinomas, which rose to 17 percent with T1b lesions and 32 percent with T1c tumors.[35] The authors concluded that axillary dissection could be omitted for patients with T1a tumors but should be performed routinely in patients with T1b or larger lesions. However, it is important to recognize that these studies included patients with *in situ* and microinvasive carcinomas (foci of invasion ≤ 2 mm in size), which are rarely associated with nodal metastases. Cady and colleagues noted a 13 percent incidence of axillary metastases in patients with T1a and T1b tumors and a 34 percent incidence with T1c primary lesions.[13] Based on the "low" frequency of nodal metastases in this group and only modest survival advantage for women with positive nodes treated with adjuvant therapy, they did not favor routine axillary dissection in patients with T1 breast cancers.

A recent review of 256 patients with T1 invasive breast carcinoma at our institution showed that 10 percent of patients with T1a, 12 percent of those with T1b, and 27 percent of patients with T1c tumors had axillary metastases detected by H&E staining.[36] When immunohistochemistry was performed on sentinel nodes removed from the subgroup of 50 patients who underwent lymphatic mapping, the incidence of axillary metastases rose to 15 percent for both T1a and T1b lesions. This highlights the importance of focused histopathological analysis of the sentinel lymph node, which will be discussed in greater detail later in this chapter. Although there is significant variation among studies, these data suggest that the risk of axillary metastases is approximately 10 to 15 percent in patients with T1a and T1b tumors. Avoiding lymph node evaluation would understage at least 10 percent of these patients, which most would consider an unacceptably high percentage.

Because tumor size cannot independently predict lymph node status, several authors combined multiple clinical and pathological factors into prognostic risk models.[37–39] Chada and associates[37] studied the prognostic factors related to axillary lymph node status in 263 patients with T1 breast carcinoma. The

TABLE 56–3. INCIDENCE OF AXILLARY NODE METASTASIS IN T1 BREAST CARCINOMA

Author	No. of Patients	T1a (%)	T1b (%)	T1c	Comments
Carter et al[31]	8319	20	21	33	30–40% with >3 nodes in each T
Rosen et al[33]	644	11	15	25–43	
White et al[20]	931	10	19	N/A	
Reger et al[34]	626	3	10	21–35	Included noninvasive tumors
Silverstein et al[35]	609	3	17	32	Included DCIS with microinvasion
Giuliano et al[36]	256	15	15	27	IHC used in 50 SLND patients

DCIS = Ductal carcinoma *in situ;* IHC = immunohistochemistry; SLND = sentinel lymphadenectomy; N/A = not evaluated.

overall incidence of axillary metastasis was 15 percent in T1a and T1b tumors and 35 percent in T1c lesions. Tumor size greater than 1 cm, intermediate or high nuclear grade, lymphatic or vascular invasion (LVI), and age younger than 60 years were all associated with axillary lymph node metastases by univariate analysis. Only tumor size and LVI were significant by multivariate analysis. These factors were then combined to stratify the population into high-risk (tumor >1 cm, LVI) and low-risk (tumor < 1 cm, no LVI) subgroups that had a 68 percent and 9 percent incidence of axillary metastases, respectively. This model has not been verified in a separate population of patients, and even the "low" risk group had a 9 percent incidence of axillary metastases.

Menard and associates also studied the factors associated with axillary metastasis in a group of 463 clinically node-negative breast cancer patients with T1 and T2 tumors.[38] They identified tumor size greater than 2 cm, histological grade III, laminin receptor and *ERBB*2 overexpression as predictors of axillary metastasis in multivariate analysis. The overall survival rate was higher in patients with a low score (none of the 4 factors) and lower in patients with a high score (3 or 4 factors) when the population used to generate the model was evaluated. However, when this model was validated in a separate group of 260 clinically node-positive patients, there was no significant difference in survival between the low and high score groups. Data regarding the ability of the model to predict pathological node status in the validation group were not presented. Both authors concluded that axillary dissection could be avoided in a subset of patients based on prognostic factors obtained from the primary tumor. This conclusion seems unjustifiable based on the data presented in their studies.

A larger study conducted by Ravdin and colleagues evaluated 11,964 patients from the Breast Cancer Tissue Resource Database.[39] Prognostic factors related to axillary metastases were studied in 5963 of these patients. Tumor size, age, progesterone receptor status, and S-phase fraction were found to be independent predictors of nodal status. Multiple models were then generated using these variables and tested in a separate group of 6001 patients from the data base. No patient subsets had more than a 95 percent chance of being node negative or node positive. The authors concluded that predictive models could not replace axillary dissection in situations where nodal status would affect therapeutic decisions.

Because more patients now have nonpalpable, mammographically detected breast carcinoma, several studies have addressed the incidence of axillary metastasis in palpable and nonpalpable tumors. A 13 percent incidence of axillary metastasis was reported in a recent series of patients with nonpalpable, clinically occult breast carcinomas.[45] Arnesson and colleagues identified axillary metastases in 9 percent of nonpalpable T1a and T1b tumors compared with 20 percent of those that were palpable.[46]

Silverstein and associates found the probability of nodal involvement was significantly higher for palpable tumors in the T1b, T1c, and T2 categories.[47] However, the average tumor diameter was also significantly larger for palpable lesions within each T category, and multivariate analysis was not performed to determine if palpability was an independent predictor of node status. We also noted a significantly higher frequency of axillary metastases in palpable (29 percent) than nonpalpable (17 percent) T1 tumors in our recent study.[36] In contrast, Halverson and colleagues found no difference in the incidence of axillary metastases in palpable and nonpalpable T1 tumors.[48] Although several studies suggest that the incidence of axillary node involvement may be lower in nonpalpable T1 carcinomas than in those that are palpable, 9 to 17 percent of nonpalpable T1 tumors are associated with axillary metastases. This supports the continued use of routine axillary staging in this subgroup.

The benefit of axillary dissection in elderly patients with estrogen receptor (ER)–positive tumors and clinically negative axillary nodes has also been questioned.[8–11] In most cases, these patients will receive tamoxifen postoperatively regardless of axillary lymph node status. They also frequently have comorbid medical illnesses, increasing the risk of complications and death from intercurrent disease.[8–10] Martelli and colleagues treated a group of 321 elderly patients with conservative surgery under local anesthesia without axillary dissection.[49] Patients received tamoxifen postoperatively for an indefinite period of time regardless of hormone receptor status. No adjuvant radiotherapy was given. At 72 months, relapse-free survival was 76 percent, with a regional recurrence rate of 4.3 percent. Local recurrence and distant metastases were more frequent in patients with ER-negative tumors, but there was no difference in overall survival between the ER-positive and ER-negative patients. A smaller prospective trial of tumor excision, axillary irradiation, and adjuvant tamoxifen documented a 100 percent regional control rate and 94 percent breast cancer–free survival at 8 years.[50] Although these studies suggest that this approach may provide acceptable survival and local control rates in selected elderly patients, a randomized trial is needed to confirm this.

AXILLARY BIOPSY AND SAMPLING TECHNIQUES

Surgical procedures of lesser extent than Level 1 and 2 dissection have been suggested as alternate methods to achieve axillary staging.[8–11] These include nonanatomical axillary node biopsy, axillary "sampling," and low (Level 1) axillary dissection. Forrest and associates described the technique of simple mastectomy and pectoral node biopsy.[51] This procedure initially involved excision of several Level 1 nodes adjacent to the axillary tail of the breast (pectoral nodes) along with simple mastectomy (including the lymph nodes within the axillary tail). The Cardiff–St. Mary's trial randomized patients to simple mastectomy and pectoral node biopsy versus radical mastectomy, with 40 Gy radiotherapy to the axilla for node-positive cases.[52] Lymph nodes were identified in only 83 percent of patients in the simple mastectomy arm, yet there was no difference in the overall incidence of positive nodes or survival between the two groups. The axillary relapse rate was 16 percent, and the chest wall recurrence rate was 25 percent in the simple mastectomy and pectoral node biopsy group. All axillary relapses occurred in patients with "negative" pectoral node biopsies or in those who had no lymph nodes identified. The authors then modified their technique to include palpation of the axilla and four-node axillary sampling. The modified technique was evaluated in the second Edinburgh study, which randomized 417 patients to total mastectomy and axillary clearance (Level 1 to 3 dissection) versus total mastectomy and axillary sampling.[53] Patients in the axillary sampling group received 40 Gy radiotherapy to the chest wall and axilla if positive nodes were identified. The incidence of involved lymph nodes was similar in both groups, and there was no significant difference in local or regional recurrence or survival. However, the authors concluded that axillary dissection was preferable to axillary sampling to avoid the cost and morbidity of radiotherapy.

The staging accuracy of axillary sampling was evaluated by Davies and coworkers who performed pectoral node biopsy and dissection of the axillary tail lymph nodes before radical mastectomy.[54] The false-negative rate was 42 percent for pectoral node biopsy and 14 percent for low axillary dissection. Fisher and colleagues evaluated Forrest's four-node axillary sampling procedure before axillary dissection and found a 10 percent false-negative rate.[55] There is also no definite evidence that any of these procedures result in less morbidity than Level 1 and 2 axillary dissection.

In summary, none of these less-invasive methods can predict the status of axillary lymph nodes with sufficient accuracy to replace routine axillary dissection. However, current data suggest that intraoperative lymphatic mapping and sentinel lymphadenectomy may fulfill this role.[23, 36, 56–58]

LYMPHATIC MAPPING AND SENTINEL LYMPHADENECTOMY

The sentinel node concept assumes that a malignancy that metastasizes by the lymphatic route will initially travel to one or a few lymph node(s), which are designated the sentinel node(s) (Fig. 56–1). Although a tumor may disseminate to other nodes, it will remain in the sentinel node, and therefore the status of the entire basin is predicted by the sentinel node. This allows patients with negative sentinel nodes to be spared the morbidity of complete node dissection, while those with positive sentinel nodes may undergo complete lymphadenectomy for staging and therapy.

Morton and colleagues confirmed the transit of intradermally injected dye to the sentinel lymph node in a feline model, and then applied the technique to a group of patients with melanoma undergoing wide excision and elective lymphadenectomy.[59, 60] Despite a significant learning curve, these investigators found that the sentinel node could be identified in more than 80 percent of their initial patients and that it predicted the pathological status of the lymph node basin in 97 percent of cases.[60] With further experience and refinement of the technique, the sentinel node was identified in 95 percent of patients, with false-positive and false-negative rates of 0 percent and 1 percent, respectively.[61] The procedure has been evaluated as a staging tool for melanoma at several centers with similar results, and is currently the subject of an international multicenter randomized trial.[62–64]

In October 1991, our group began to study the feasibility of lymphatic mapping and sentinel lym-

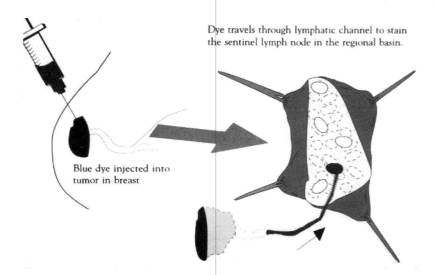

Dye travels through lymphatic channel to stain the sentinel lymph node in the regional basin.

Blue dye injected into tumor in breast

Figure 56–1 *Schematic diagram of transit of blue dye from primary breast cancer to sentinel lymph node.*

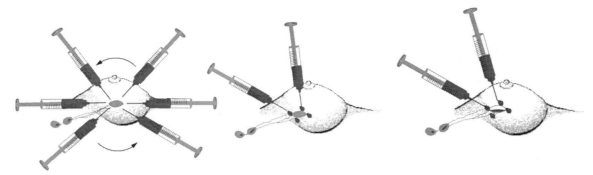

Figure 56–2 *Injection technique for lymphatic mapping and sentinel lymphadenectomy. Dye is injected in a circumferential pattern* (left). *When the tumor is palpable, dye is injected into the breast parenchyma around the tumor* (middle). *If the tumor has been previously removed, dye is injected into the wall of the biopsy cavity* (right).

phadenectomy in breast cancer.[57] With no prior experience with the technique in this disease, a learning period was required to define the technical aspects of the procedure. Several factors were identified that determine its success. These include patient selection, injection technique, dissection technique, and histopathological evaluation of the sentinel node.[65]

Patient Selection

For the technique to be successful, the lymphatic drainage pattern of the primary tumor must be followed by the dye. Several factors may interfere with this process and decrease the chance of correctly identifying the sentinel node. Injection of large biopsy cavities or segmental mastectomy defects may not accurately predict the lymphatic drainage pattern of the excised primary tumor. Similarly, large (>5 cm) or multifocal carcinomas can have complex lymphatic drainage patterns that make correct identification of the sentinel node difficult. Prior axillary surgery, trauma, or infection may also alter the lymphatic drainage of the primary tumor. Previous breast surgery does not appear to interfere with this process, and we have successfully identified the sentinel node in women with prior breast biopsy, reduction, or augmentation mammaplasty. The effects of pregnancy or lactation on the procedure and safety of isosulfan blue dye in this setting are unknown. We therefore consider large biopsy cavities, large or multifocal carcinomas, prior axillary surgery, trauma or infection, and pregnancy or lactation to be contraindications to lymphatic mapping and sentinel lymphadenectomy. Routine Level 1 and 2 axillary dissection is recommended for axillary staging in these patients.[65]

Injection Technique

With the patient under local or general anesthesia and positioned for axillary dissection, 3 to 5 cc of 1 percent isosulfan blue (Lymphazurin) is injected into the breast at the site of the primary tumor. For palpable lesions, dye is injected into the breast parenchyma around the periphery of the tumor. Mam-

mographically or ultrasonographically detected lesions are injected through needles placed with mammographic or ultrasound guidance. For tumors previously removed by excisional biopsy, dye is injected into the wall of the biopsy cavity, but not in the cavity itself (Fig. 56–2). Dye injected into biopsy cavities or directly into the tumor will not gain access to the afferent lymphatics and therefore will not identify the sentinel node.[65]

Dissection Technique

A 3- to 10-minute interval between dye injection and axillary incision is used to allow adequate visualization of the lymphatics. Too short a delay between injection and incision may prevent identification of the afferent lymphatics and location of the sentinel node. Too long a delay can result in dye transit to multiple nonsentinel nodes, which inhibits accurate identification of the sentinel node. The time required for dye transit to the axilla is related to the location of the primary lesion within the breast. Lesions in the axillary tail closer to the lymph node basin have shorter transit times, and those in the lower inner quadrant have longer transit times. We therefore typically allow 3 to 4 minutes and 7 to 10 minutes, respectively, for lesions in these locations. Breast size, postbiopsy edema and ecchymosis, and proximity of the tumor to the skin or chest wall do not appear to be related to transit time.[65]

A 2 to 3 cm transverse incision is made in the axillary fossa in the area used for Level 1 and 2 dissection. Care is taken to extend the incision only through the skin to avoid transection of the afferent lymphatics. The lymphatic channels are located with careful blunt dissection and followed to the sentinel node (Fig. 56–3). Any blue-stained lymphatics are traced proximally and distally to locate other possible sentinel nodes and lymphatic channels. After all sentinel nodes are identified, they are excised and forwarded for pathologic evaluation.[65] It is critical to initially search for the afferent lymphatics and not the lymph node. Lymphatic channels are then used as a "road map" to locate the node. Patience and meticulous dissection technique are essential during

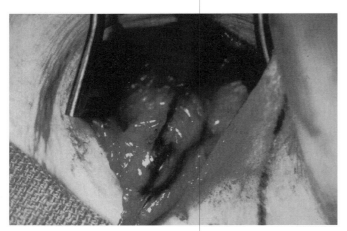

Figure 56–3 *Lymphatic channel leading to sentinel node.*

this part of the procedure to reliably and accurately identify the sentinel node.

Pathological Evaluation

All sentinel nodes are evaluated by intraoperative frozen section examination. This was initially done to confirm that nodal tissue had been removed, because misidentification of blue-stained fat as a sentinel node was a cause of false-negative results early in our experience.[57] More recently, frozen section has been used to identify the presence of axillary metastasis in the sentinel node, in which case the patients undergo standard Level 1 and 2 axillary dissection. If axillary metastases are not identified, no further axillary surgery is performed.[66] While awaiting frozen section results, the definitive procedure for the primary tumor (segmental or total mastectomy) is completed.

Frozen-section negative sentinel nodes are subsequently studied by permanent H&E staining. The nodes are bivalved, and the two sections are examined for the presence of metastases. If none are found, cytokeratin immunohistochemical staining is performed using the MAK-6 antibody cocktail to low and intermediate molecular weight cytokeratin. Six sections of the sentinel node are examined with immunohistochemistry to detect occult metastases.[58] A portion of the lymph node is also processed for multiple marker reverse transcriptase-polymerase chain reaction (RT-PCR) analysis. This technique identifies occult lymph node metastases not detected by immunohistochemistry.[67–69] We are currently prospectively evaluating this technique to determine the incidence and prognostic significance of metastases detected in this manner.

Results of Clinical Trials

In our initial study, we reported the results of our first 174 sentinel node procedures[57]; 172 patients were included, with 2 patients having synchronous bilateral breast cancer. All patients underwent lym-

phatic mapping and sentinel lymphadenectomy followed by Level 1 and 2 axillary dissection and surgical treatment of the primary lesion. Sentinel nodes were identified in 114 (66 percent) of procedures overall, but this rate improved to 78 percent in the final 50 cases. Axillary lymph node status was correctly predicted by sentinel node pathology in 109 of 114 (96 percent) of cases. The 5 false-negative results occurred in the first 87 procedures, and 2 were in the first 10 procedures. Three of these 5 patients had dye-stained axillary fat misidentified as a sentinel node. This prompted the routine use of frozen section to confirm lymph node recovery. Another patient was subsequently found to have micrometastases in the sentinel node after re-examination using anticytokeratin immunohistochemisty. We have used routine immunohistochemistry to detect occult metastases since that time. Only 1 of these 5 false-negative sentinel nodes was a 'true' false-negative, indicating the presence of metastases in other axillary nodes but not the sentinel node. With all 5 cases considered as false-negatives, the technique predicted axillary node status with 88 percent sensitivity and 100 percent specificity.[57] If only the single "true" false-negative result is considered, sensitivity increases to 97 percent.

The axillary dissection specimens of patients with histologically positive nodes were examined to determine if the sentinel node could have predicted their status simply by chance. Thirty-four patients had a total of 751 lymph nodes removed, of which 63 (8 percent) were sentinel nodes and 688 (92 percent) were nonsentinel nodes. Thirty-nine of 63 (62 percent) of the sentinel nodes contained tumor, whereas only 93 of 688 (14 percent) of nonsentinel nodes were involved ($p<0.0001$).[57] This confirmed the hypothesis that breast cancer metastases occur through a non-random pathway that can be identified by lymphatic mapping. It also suggests that random axillary biopsy or sampling could not recreate these results through chance alone.

The second report of this technique evaluated the first 162 patients undergoing successful lymphatic mapping and sentinel lymphadenectomy followed by completion axillary dissection (SLND group) and compared them with 134 patients undergoing axillary dissection without sentinel lymphadenectomy (ALND group).[58] Although the groups were not randomized, they were contemporaneous, and all procedures were performed at the same institution by a single surgeon. The sentinel nodes were evaluated by H&E and anticytokeratin staining, whereas other nodes were evaluated by H&E alone. Both groups had comparable clinical characteristics and a similar total number of axillary nodes excised. The SLND group had a 42 percent incidence of axillary metastases compared with 24 percent in the ALND group ($p<0.05$). This was primarily because of a dramatic increase in the detection of micrometastases in the SLND group. Sixteen percent of SLND patients had metastases less than 2 mm in diameter compared with 3 percent of the ALND group. Detection of micrometastases by both H&E (9 percent versus 3 percent) and immunohistochemistry (7 percent versus 0 percent) was increased with SLND. We concluded that the technique not only accurately predicts the status of the axillary nodes, but actually improves axillary staging compared to standard axillary dissection. This results from a focused histopathological evaluation of the sentinel lymph node, which increases the detection of micrometastases.

The significance of axillary micrometastases in breast cancer has been questioned.[70–72] Earlier studies using serial sectioning and H&E staining reported no significant difference in survival between patients with negative nodes and those with occult metastases.[70–72] However, axillary micrometastases were associated with decreased survival in certain subgroups, including those with T1 tumors[71] or tumors larger than 1.3 mm in diameter.[72] A more recent evaluation of 921 patients in the Ludwig study indicated that axillary micrometastases detected by serial sectioning were associated with a lower disease free survival (58 percent versus 78 percent) and lower overall survival (79 percent versus 88 percent).[73] Trojani and associates also reported lower overall and disease-free survival at 12 years in patients with ductal carcinoma and micrometastases detected by immunohistochemistry compared with those with no lymph node metastases.[74] Based on these studies, there is increasing agreement that patients with micrometastases have a high risk of recurrence and mortality. Most currently receive adjuvant therapy, although the efficacy of adjuvant therapy in this subgroup has not been addressed in a prospective, randomized trial.

In the last 100 patients undergoing lymphatic mapping and sentinel lymphadenectomy followed by axillary dissection, we identified the sentinel node in 94 percent of patients. There were no false-negative results, indicating a sensitivity and specificity of 100 percent.[66] We attribute our increased success to refinement of the technical details and extensive experience with the technique (approximately 400 cases in the last 5 years). Based on these results, we began a trial to investigate lymphatic mapping and sentinel lymphadenectomy alone in patients with negative sentinel nodes in October 1995.[66] Those with histologically positive sentinel nodes or in whom a sentinel node cannot be identified still undergo Level 1 and 2 axillary dissection. This approach allows women without axillary metastases to be spared the expense and morbidity of a complete axillary dissection. Those with metastases benefit from the local control and potential survival advantage of axillary dissection. The number of involved nodes is accurately identified, allowing selection of the appropriate adjuvant therapy.[8, 75]

UNANSWERED QUESTIONS AND FUTURE PERSPECTIVES

Although we have established the feasibility and accuracy of sentinel lymphadenectomy as a staging procedure in selected women with breast cancer, several important questions remain. The first issue relates to the use of lymphoscintigraphy. This study has been used for two decades to identify the lymphatic drainage pattern of primary melanoma.[76] It has become a routine part of the lymphatic mapping procedure for melanoma, in which it allows identification of aberrant drainage patterns and marking of the location of the sentinel node on the patient's skin to facilitate its location in the operating room.[60–64] In breast cancer, we noted early in our experience that we were able to identify a sentinel node less frequently in patients with medial primary lesions than in those with lateral lesions. This led to the hypothesis that medial quadrant tumors may have primary drainage to a sentinel node in the internal mammary chain, which precludes identification of an axillary sentinel node. We therefore began to evaluate all women with medial lesions with lymphoscintigraphy before lymphatic mapping and sentinel lymphadenectomy. Preliminary data indicate that approximately 25 percent of women with medial quadrant lesions have primary or exclusive drainage to the internal mammary nodes (A.E. Giuliano and E. Glass, unpublished data).

The management of this small subgroup of patients is quite difficult. Several studies indicate that patients with internal mammary node metastases have a high risk of recurrence and mortality, even in the absence of axillary node metastases.[77–80] We suspect that patients with primary lymphatic drainage to the internal mammary chain have a relatively high incidence of metastases in this location. If this is the case, a negative axillary sentinel node may not be a reliable indicator of the risk of recurrence and mortality in this group. However, routine internal mammary node dissection has significant morbidity and does not improve survival.[78–80] It has therefore been abandoned as a staging procedure. To define the incidence of primary internal mammary node drainage and role of lymphoscintigraphy in lymphatic mapping of breast cancer, we continue to perform the study in all women with medial tumors entered in our trial. Although we are reluctant to perform internal mammary node dissection on those with primary internal mammary drainage, we are investigating lymphatic mapping and internal mammary sentinel lymphadenectomy in selected patients to identify those who may benefit from more aggressive adjuvant therapy.

The other related issue is that of gamma-probe–guided resection of radiolabeled axillary lymph nodes. Isosulfan blue has been an effective agent for lymphatic mapping and sentinel lymphadenectomy for breast cancer and melanoma at our institution, but some surgeons have been unable to routinely identify the sentinel node with this technique.[81–83] Others who observed or performed the procedure in a supervised fashion have not experienced this problem and have been able to reproduce results similar to ours at other institutions (A.E. Giuliano and M. Guenther, unpublished data). Because of the perceived difficulties with the dye technique, routine lymphoscintigraphy and gamma-probe–guided resection of radiolabeled lymph nodes have been suggested as an alternate method of lymph node staging for melanoma and breast cancer.[81–83]

There are several potential problems with this approach in breast cancer. Most importantly, it has not been documented that radiolabeled nodes identified with this technique predict the status of the axilla based on complete node dissection in a large number of patients. The single study by Krag and associates reporting this technique included only 22 patients.[83] It is unclear if nodes removed with this procedure represent sentinel nodes, nonsentinel nodes, or a combination of both. Our experience has shown that the number of nodes identified by lymphatic mapping using radiolabeled colloids or blue dye is time dependent. If the timing is not precise, multiple nonsentinel nodes may be removed. Krag and associates reported an interval between injection and node identification of 1 to 4 hours,[83] raising concern that multiple nonsentinel nodes may have been excised. This could compromise the principle of selective node dissection by removing more nodes than required to determine the pathological status of the axilla. Evaluation of this question is hampered by the lack of data regarding the total number of nodes removed using this procedure.[83] The approach also requires the use of radioactive material and a gamma probe, making it more cumbersome and expensive than our routine technique using isosulfan blue dye alone.

If the gamma-probe technique detects true sentinel nodes not identified with blue dye, without removing an excessive number of nonsentinel nodes, it is a complementary procedure. This appears to be the case in melanoma, where an additional 5 to 10 percent more positive sentinel nodes are detected using the gamma probe and blue dye compared with dye alone.[81, 84] It seems likely that this procedure will add significantly to the blue dye technique in breast cancer, where it currently identifies the sentinel node in 93 percent of cases and predicts axillary node status with 100 percent accuracy.[30] To clarify this issue, we are beginning a prospective study of routine lymphoscintigraphy and intraoperative gamma-probe–guided resection of radiolabeled nodes to determine if they can complement our standard technique.

A major reason given for investigating the use of lymphoscintigraphy and gamma-probe–guided resection of radiolabeled nodes is the perceived difficulty of identifying lymphatics and locating the sentinel node using blue dye. As in melanoma,[60] there is a substantial learning curve to master before the technique becomes reliable. This is particularly apparent when the technical details of the procedure have not been defined, as seen in our early experience.[57] Success is achieved more rapidly when the established technique is taught by an experienced surgeon. This is evidenced by the ability of surgical oncology fellows at John Wayne Cancer Institute to identify the sentinel node in 75 to 80 percent of

patients after as few as ten cases (A.E. Giuliano, unpublished data). One of the critical issues regarding lymphatic mapping and sentinel lymphadenectomy in breast cancer is quality control. It will be important to evaluate the accuracy of this procedure at each institution before recommending it as a substitute for routine axillary dissection. Standardization of the technical details, educational process, and quality control will be integral parts of any multicenter trial of sentinel lymphadenectomy.

It appears that lymphatic mapping and sentinel lymphadenectomy result in much less morbidity than complete axillary dissection. The incision is smaller, and there is less pain, less limitation of motion, and fewer neurological sequelae. Lymphedema and seroma rates appear to be lower in patients having sentinel lymphadenectomy alone. However, these are subjective impressions that await confirmation by an ongoing prospective study of morbidity and complication rates in patients undergoing sentinel lymphadenectomy. An essential part of this study is evaluation of patient quality of life using objective scales such as the Functional Assessment of Cancer Therapy Scales—Breast Version (FACT—B) and Profile of Mood States (POMS).[85, 86] Because this procedure may be performed on an outpatient basis and may limit costly complications related to axillary dissection (e.g., infection, lymphedema), it should be more cost effective than routine axillary dissection. A prospective analysis of cost effectiveness is also underway to confirm this hypothesis.

In summary, the lymphatic mapping and sentinel lymphadenectomy procedure is a highly accurate method of axillary staging in breast cancer. Focused histopathological evaluation of the sentinel node improves axillary staging by increasing the detection of micrometastases. The procedure can be performed as an outpatient procedure with local anesthesia and may have less morbidity, fewer complications, and be more cost effective than routine axillary dissection. Refinements of the technical aspects of the procedure allow identification of the sentinel node in more than 90 percent of patients, with 100 percent diagnostic accuracy in our most recent series. This has led us to abandon routine axillary dissection in selected patients with invasive breast cancer, reserving this procedure only for those with histologically positive sentinel nodes or in whom the sentinel node cannot be identified. Several issues such as the role of lymphoscintigraphy and gamma-probe–guided resection of radiolabeled nodes remain to be defined. Because no other method accurately predicts axillary node status without complete axillary dissection, this technique merits further evaluation at other institutions to determine if it may become the standard method of axillary staging for breast cancer in the twenty-first century.[23, 87]

References

1. NIH consensus conference on the treatment of early-stage breast cancer. JAMA 265:391–395, 1991.

2. Ivens D, Hoe AL, Podd TJ, Hamilton CR, Taylor I, Royle GT: Assessment of arm morbidity from complete axillary dissection. Br J Cancer 66:136–138, 1992.
3. Kissin MW, Querci della Rovere G, Easton D, Westbury G: Risk of lymphoedema following the treatment of breast cancer. Br J Surg 73:580–584, 1986.
4. Larson D, Weinstein M, Goldberg I, Silver B, Recht A, Cady B, Silen W, Harris JR: Edema of the arm as a function of the extent of axillary surgery in patients with stage I-II carcinoma of the breast treated with primary radiotherapy. Int J Radiat Oncol Biol Phys 12:1575–1582, 1986.
5. Penzer RD, Patterson MP, Hill LR: Arm edema in patients treated conservatively for breast cancer: Relationship to patient age and axillary node dissection technique. Int J Radiol Oncol Biol Phys 12:2079–2083, 1986.
6. Tobin MB, Lacey HJ, Meyer L, Mortimer PS: The psychological morbidity of breast cancer-related arm swelling: Psychological morbidity of lymphoedema. Cancer 72:3248–3252, 1993.
7. Vecht CJ, Van de Brand HJ, Wajer OJM: Post-axillary dissection pain in breast cancer due to a lesion of the intercostobrachial nerve. Pain 38:171–176, 1989.
8. Lin PC, Allison DC, Wainstock J, Miller KD, Dooley WC, Friedman N, Baker RR: Impact of axillary dissection on the therapy of breast cancer patients. J Clin Oncol 11:1356–1544, 1993.
9. Ruffin WK, Stacey-Clear A, Younger J, Hoover HC: Rationale for routine axillary dissection in carcinoma of the breast. J Am Coll Surg 180:245–251, 1995.
10. Recht A, Houlihan MJ: Axillary lymph nodes and breast cancer: A review. Cancer 76:1491–1512,1995.
11. Kinne DW: Controversies in primary breast cancer management. Am J Surg 166:502–508, 1993.
12. Harris JR, Osteen RT: Patients with early breast cancer benefit from effective axillary treatment. Breast Cancer Res Treat 5:17–21, 1985.
13. Cady B, Stone MD, Wayne J: New therapeutic possibilities in primary invasive breast cancer. Ann Surg 218:338–349, 1993.
14. Cabanes PA, Salmon RJ, Vilcoq JR, Durand JC, Fourquet A, Gautier C, Asselain B: Value of axillary dissection in addition to lumpectomy and radiotherapy in early breast cancer. Lancet 339:1245–1248, 1992.
15. Langlands AO, Prescott RJ, Hamilton T: A clinical trial in the management of operable cancer of the breast. Br J Surg 67:170–174, 1980.
16. Hayward JL, Caleffi M: The significance of local control in the primary treatment of breast cancer. Arch Surg 122:1244–1247, 1987.
17. Fisher B, Redmond C, Fisher ER, Bauer M, Wolmark N, Wickersham L, Deutsch M, Montague E, Margolese R, Foster R: Ten year results of a randomized clinical trial comparing radical mastectomy and total mastectomy with or without radiation. N Engl J Med 312:674–681, 1985.
18. Baxter N, McCready D, Chapman JA, Fish E, Kahn H, Hanna W, Trudeau M, Lickley HL: Clinical behavior of untreated axillary nodes after local treatment for primary breast cancer. Ann Surg Oncol 3:335–340, 1996.
19. Gardner B, Feldman J: Are positive axillary nodes in breast cancer markers for incurable disease? Ann Surg 218:270–278, 1993.
20. White RE, Vezeridis MP, Konstadoulakis M, Cole BF, Wanebo HJ, Bland KI: Therapeutic options and results for the management of minimally invasive carcinoma of the breast: Influence of axillary dissection for the treatment of T1a and T1b lesions. J Am Coll Surg 183:575–582, 1996.
21. Senofsky GM, Moffat FL, Davis K, Masri MM, Clark KC, Robinson DS, Sabates B, Ketcham AS: Total axillary lymphadenectomy in the management of breast cancer. Arch Surg 126:1336–1342,1991.
22. Haffty BG, McKhann C, Beinfield M, Fischer D, Fischer JJ: Breast conservation therapy without axillary dissection: A rational treatment in selected patients. Arch Surg 128:1315–1319, 1993.
23. Cady B, Stone MD, Schuler JG, Thakur R, Wanner M, Lavin PT: The new era in breast cancer. Arch Surg 131:301–307, 1996.
24. Fisher B, Wolmark N, Bauer M, Redmond C, Gebhardt M: The accuracy of clinical nodal staging and of limited axillary dissection as a determinant of histologic nodal status in carcinoma of the breast. Surg Gynecol Obstet 152:765–772, 1981.
25. Dershaw DD, Panicek DM, Osborne MP: Significance of lymph nodes visualized by the mammographic axillary view. Breast Dis 4:271–280, 1991.
26. Bruneton JN, Caramella E, Hery M, Aubanel D, Manzino J, Picard JL: Axillary lymph node metastases in breast cancer: Preoperative detection with ultrasound. Radiology 158:325–326, 1986.
27. Allan SM, McVicar D, Sacks NPM: Prospects for axillary staging in breast cancer by magnetic resonance imaging. Br J Radiol 66(suppl):15, 1993. Abstract.
28. Black RG, Taylor TV, Merrick MV, Forrest APM: Prediction of axillary metastases in breast cancer by lymphoscintigraphy. Lancet 2:15–17, 1980.
29. Tjandra JJ, Sacks NPM, Thompson CH, Leyden MJ, Stacker SA, Lichtenstein M, Russell IS, Collins JP, Andrews JT, Pietersz GA, McKenzie IFC: The detection of axillary lymph node metastases from breast cancer by radiolabelled monoclonal antibodies: A prospective study. Br J Cancer 59:296–302, 1989.
30. Nieweg OE, Kim EE, Wong WH, Broussard WF, Singletary SE, Hortobagyi GN, Tilbury RS: Positron emission tomography with fluorine-18-deoxyglucose in the detection and staging of breast cancer. Cancer 71:3920–3925, 1993.
31. Carter CL, Allen C, Henson DE: Relation of tumor size, lymph node status, and survival in 24,740 breast cancer cases. Cancer 63:181–187, 1989.
32. Fisher ER, Sass R, Fisher B: Pathologic findings from the National Surgical Adjuvant Project for Breast Cancers (Protocol no. 4). Cancer 53:712–723, 1984.
33. Rosen PP, Groshen S, Saigo PE, Kinne DW, Hellman S. Pathological prognostic factors in stage I (T1N0M0) and stage II (T1N1M0) breast carcinoma: A study of 644 patients with a median follow-up of 18 years. J Clin Oncol 7:1239–1251, 1989.
34. Reger V, Beito G, Jolly PC: Factors affecting the incidence of lymph node metastases in small cancers of the breast. Am J Surg 157:501–502, 1989.
35. Silverstein MJ, Gierson ED, Waisman JR, Senofsky GM, Colburn WJ, Gamagami P: Axillary lymph node dissection for T1a breast carcinoma: Is it indicated? Cancer 73:664–667, 1994.
36. Giuliano AE, Barth AM, Spivack B, Beitsch PD, Evans SW: Incidence and predictors of axillary metastasis in T1 carcinoma of the breast. J Am Coll Surg 183:185–189, 1996.
37. Chada M, Chabon AD, Friedmann P, Vikram B: Predictors of axillary lymph node metastases in patients with T1 breast cancer. Cancer 73:350–353, 1994.
38. Menard S, Bufalino R, Rilke F, Cascinelli N, Veronesi U, Colnaghi MI: Prognosis based on primary breast carcinoma instead of pathological nodal status. Br J Cancer 70:709–712, 1994.
39. Ravdin PM, De Laurentiis M, Vendley T, Clark GM: Prediction of axillary lymph node status in breast cancer patients by use of prognostic indicators. J Natl Cancer Inst 86:1771–1775, 1994.
40. Weigand RA, Isenberg WM, Russo J, Brennan MJ, Rich MJ: Blood vessel invasion and axillary lymph node involvement as prognostic indicators for human breast cancer. Cancer 50:962–969, 1982.
41. Horak ER, Leek R, Klenk N, LeJeune S, Smith K, Stuart N, Greenall M, Stepniewska K, Harris AL: Angiogenesis, assessed by platelet endothelial cell adhesion molecule antibodies as an indicator of node metastases and survival in breast cancer. Lancet 340:1120–1124, 1992.
42. Noguchi M, Naohiro K, Ohta N, Kitagawa H, Earashi M, Thomas M, Miyazaki I, Mizukami Y: Internal mammary nodal status is a more reliable prognostic factor than DNA ploidy and c-erbB2 expression in patients with breast cancer. Arch Surg 128:242–246, 1993.
43. Winstanley JH, Leinster SJ, Cooke TG, Westley BR, Platt-Higgins AM, Rudland PS: Prognostic significance of Cathepsin-D in patients with breast cancer. Br J Cancer 67:767–772, 1993.

44. Gui GPH, Wells CA, Browne PD, Yeomans P, Jordan P, Puddlefoot JR, Vinson GP, Carpenter R: Integrin expression in primary breast cancer and its relation to axillary nodal status. Surgery 117:102–108, 1995.
45. Meterissian S, Fornage BD, Singletary SE: Clinically occult breast carcinoma: Diagnostic approaches and role of axillary node dissection. Ann Surg Oncol 2:314–318, 1995.
46. Arnesson L-G, Smeds S, Fagerberg G: Recurrence-free survival in patients with small breast cancers. Eur J Surg 160:271–276, 1994.
47. Silverstein MJ, Gierson ED, Waisman JR, Colburn WJ, Gamagami P: Predicting axillary node positivity in patients with invasive carcinoma of the breast by using a combination of T category and palpability. J Am Coll Surg 180:700–704, 1995.
48. Halverson KJ, Taylor ME, Perez CA, Garcia DM, Myerson R, Philpott G, et al: Management of the axilla in patients with breast cancers one centimeter or smaller. Am J Clin Oncol 17:461–466, 1994.
49. Martelli G, DePalo G, Rossi N, Coradini D, Boracchi P, Galante E, Vetrella G: Long-term follow-up of elderly patients with operable breast cancer treated with surgery without axillary dissection plus adjuvant tamoxifen. Br J Cancer 72:1251–1255, 1995.
50. Wazer DE, Erban JK, Robert NJ, Smith TJ, Marchant DJ, Schmid C, DiPetrillo T, Schmidt-Ullrich R: Breast conservation in elderly women for clinically negative axillary lymph nodes without axillary dissection. Cancer 74:878–883, 1994.
51. Forrest APM, Roberts MM, Cant E, Shivas AA: Simple mastectomy and pectoral node biopsy. Br J Surg 63:569–575, 1976.
52. Forrest APM, Stewart HJ, Roberts MM, Steele RCJ: Simple mastectomy and axillary node sampling (pectoral node biopsy) in the management of primary breast cancer. Ann Surg 196:371–377, 1982.
53. Forrest APM, Everington D, McDonald CC, Steele RCJ, Chetty U, Stewart HJ: The Edinburgh randomized trial of axillary sampling or clearance after mastectomy. Br J Surg 82:1504–1508, 1995.
54. Davies GC, Millis RR, Hayward JL: Assessment of axillary lymph node status. Ann Surg 192:148–151, 1980.
55. Fisher CJ, Boyle S, Burke M, Price AB: Intraoperative assessment of nodal status in the selection of patients with breast cancer for axillary clearance. Br J Surg 80:457–458, 1993.
56. Coburn MC, Bland KI: Surgery for early and minimally invasive breast cancer. Curr Opin Oncol 7:506–510, 1995.
57. Giuliano AE, Kirgan DM, Guenther JM, Morton DL: Lymphatic mapping and sentinel lymphadenectomy for breast cancer. Ann Surg 220:391–401, 1994.
58. Giuliano AE, Dale PS, Turner RR, Morton DL, Evans SW, Krasne DL: Improved axillary staging of breast cancer with sentinel lymphadenectomy. Ann Surg 222:394–401, 1995.
59. Wong JH, Cagle LA, Morton DL: Lymphatic drainage of the skin to a sentinel lymph node in a feline model. Ann Surg 214:637–641, 1991.
60. Morton DL, Wen D-R, Wong JH, Economou J, Foshag LJ, Cochran AJ: Technical details of intraoperative lymphatic mapping for early stage melanoma. Arch Surg 127:192–399, 1992.
61. Morton DL, Wen D-R, Cochran AJ: Management of early stage melanoma by intraoperative lymphatic mapping and selective lymphadenectomy: An alternative to routine elective lymphadenectomy or "watch and wait." Surg Oncol Clin North Am 1:247–259, 1992.
62. Ross MI, Reintgen D, Balch CM: Selective lymphadenectomy: Emerging role for lymphatic mapping and sentinel node biopsy in the management of early stage melanoma. Semin Surg Oncol 9:219–223, 1993.
63. Reintgen D, Cruse CW, Wells K, Berman C, Fenske N, Glass F, Schroer K, Heller R, Ross M, Lyman G, Cox C, Rappaport D, Seigler HF, Balch C: The orderly progression of melanoma nodal metastases. Ann Surg 220:759–767, 1994.
64. Thompson JF, McCarthy WH, Bosch CM, O'Brien CJ, Quinn MJ, Paramaesvaran S, Crotty K, McCarthy SW, Uren RF, Howman-Giles R: Sentinel lymph node status as an indicator of the presence of metastatic melanoma in regional lymph nodes. Melanoma Res 5:255–260, 1995.
65. Jones RC, Statman RC, Cabot M, Giuliano AE: Technical details of sentinel lymphadenectomy for breast cancer staging. Presented at the 48th Annual Cancer Symposium, Society of Surgical Oncology, 1995.
66. Statman RC, Jones RC, Cabot MC, Giuliano AE: Sentinel lymphadenectomy: A technique to eliminate axillary dissection in node-negative breast cancer. Proc Am Soc Clin Oncol 15:125, 1996.
67. Hoon DSB, Sarantou T, Doi F, Chi DDJ, Kuo C, Conrad AJ, Schmid P, Turner R, Giuliano A: Detection of metastatic breast cancer by β-HCG polymerase chain reaction. Int J Cancer 69:1–6, 1996.
68. Nogchi S, Tomohiko A, Nakamori S, Kazuyushi M, Inagi H, Imaoka S, Koyama H: The detection of breast carcinoma micrometastases in axillary lymph nodes by means of a reverse transcriptase-polymerase chain reaction. Cancer 74:1595–1600, 1994.
69. Mori M, Mimori K, Inoue H, Barnard GF, Tsuji K, Nanbara S, Ueo H, Akiyashi T: Detection of cancer micrometastases in lymph nodes by reverse transcriptase-polymerase chain reaction. Cancer Res 55: 2417–2420, 1995.
70. Wilkinson EJ, Hause LL, Hoffman RG, et al: Occult axillary lymph node metastases in invasive breast carcinoma: Characteristics of the primary tumor and significance of the metastases. Pathol Annu 17:67–91, 1982.
71. Rosen PP, Saigo PE, Braun DW, Weathers E, Fracchia AA, Kinne DW: Axillary micro and macrometastases in breast cancer. Ann Surg 194:585–591, 1981.
72. Fisher ER, Palekar A, Rockette H, Redmond C, Fisher B: Pathological findings from the National Surgical Adjuvant Breast Project (Protocol No. 4): Significance of axillary nodal micro and macrometastases. Cancer 45:2025–2031, 1978.
73. International (Ludwig) Breast Cancer Study Group: Prognostic importance of occult axillary lymph node micrometastases from breast cancers. Lancet 335:1565–1568, 1990.
74. Trojani M, DeMarscel I, Coindre JM, Bonichon F: Micrometastases to axillary lymph nodes from carcinoma of the breast: Detection by immunohistochemistry and prognostic significance. Br J Cancer 565:303–306, 1987.
75. Bonadonna G, Zambetti M, Valagussa P: Sequential or alternating doxorubicin and CMF regimens in breast cancer with more than three positive nodes. JAMA 273:524–547, 1995.
76. Robinson DS, Sample WF, Fee HJ, Morton DL: Regional lymphatic drainage in primary malignant melanoma of the trunk determined by colloidal gold scanning. Surg Forum 28:147–148, 1977.
77. Cody HS, Urban JA: Internal mammary node status: A major prognosticator in node-negative breast cancer. Ann Surg Oncol 2:32–37, 1995.
78. Handley RS: Carcinoma of the breast: The Bradshaw Lecture. Ann R Coll Surg Engl 57:59–66, 1975.
79. Lacour J, Bucalossi P, Caceres E, et al: Radical mastectomy versus radical mastectomy plus internal mammary node dissection: Five year results of an international cooperative study. Cancer 37:206–214, 1976.
80. Veronesi U, Valagussa P: Inefficacy of internal mammary node dissection in breast cancer surgery. Cancer 47:170–175, 1981.
81. Albertini JJ, Cruse CW, Rappaport D, Wells K, Ross M, DeConti R, Berman CG, Jared K, Messina J, Lyman G, Glass F, Fenske N, Reintgen D: Intraoperative radiolymphoscintigraphy improves sentinel node identification for patients with melanoma. Ann Surg 223:217–224, 1996.
82. Krag DN, Meijer SJ, Weaver DL, Loggie BW, Harlow SP, Tanabe KK, Laughlin EH, Alex JC: Minimal-access surgery for the staging of malignant melanoma. Arch Surg 130:654–658, 1995.
83. Krag DN, Weaver DL, Alex JC, Fairbank JT: Surgical resection and radiolocalization of the sentinel node in breast cancer using a gamma probe. Surg Oncol 2:335–340, 1993.
84. Essner R, Foshag LJ, Morton DL: Intraoperative radiolymphoscintigraphy: A useful adjunct to intraoperative lymphatic mapping and selective lymphadenectomy in patients with clinical stage I melanoma. Presented at the Society of Surgical Oncology, 1994.
85. Cella DF, Tulsky DS, Gray G, Sarafian B, Linn E, Bonomi A,

Silberman M, Yellen SB, Winicour P, Brannon J, Eckberg K, Lloyd S, Purl S, Blendowski C, Goodman M, Barnicle M, Stewart I, McHale M, Bonomi P, Kaplan E, Taylor S IV, Thomas CR Jr, Harris J: Functional assessment of cancer therapy scale: Development and validation of the general measure. J Clin Oncol 11:570–579, 1993.

86. McNair DM, Lorr M, Doppleman LF: Profile of mood states instrument. *In* McNair DM, Lorr M, Doppleman LF (eds): Manual for the Profile of Mood States. San Diego, Educational and Industrial Testing Service, 1971.

87. Bland KI: Enhancing the accuracy for predictors of axillary nodal metastasis in T1 carcinoma of the breast: Role of selective biopsy with lymphatic mapping. J Am Coll Surg 183:262–264, 1996.

CHAPTER 57

INTRAOPERATIVE CYTOLOGIC EVALUATION OF SURGICAL MARGINS IN BREAST CANCER

Soheila Korourian, M.D. / V. Suzanne Klimberg, M.D.

Intraoperative pathological consultation for breast biopsy is among the most frequent (16 to 62 percent) and the most difficult.[1-5] The National Institutes of Health 1991 Consensus Conference on Breast Cancer stated that breast-conserving surgery followed by radiation is the preferred method of treatment for stage I and II breast cancer.[6] It follows that the performance of the primary excisional biopsy as well as its pathological evaluation is a very important component in the implementation of breast conservation, both cosmetically and medically. Cosmetically, because the best cosmetic results are obtained at the time of the original operation and with a single excision. Medically, because several recent well-controlled retrospective studies have shown a significantly elevated recurrence rate when focally positive margins were not re-excised.[7, 8] Thus, with the increasing utilization of breast-conserving techniques, a methodology for reliable intraoperative pathological diagnosis and evaluation of margins is necessary.

IMPACT OF MARGIN STATUS ON BREAST CANCER RECURRENCE

Despite the recommendation that conservative surgery (lumpectomy and radiation with or without axillary lymph node dissection) is the preferred procedure for stage I and II breast cancer, the 1991 Consensus Conference could not agree on the necessity for negative margins.[6] Table 57–1 shows a summary of the largest available retrospective studies examining the necessity of negative margins. Eight of the studies clearly show a statistically significant higher recurrence rate in patients with focally positive margins. In two of the "negative" studies, the recurrence rate is higher, although it does not reach statistical significance because of the limited size of the studies. The most recent study in Table 57–1 is that of Spivack and colleagues, which was one of the best controlled studies in terms of conformity of surgery and radiation therapy.[8] This group showed a recurrence rate of 18.2 percent ($n = 44$) if focally positive margins were not re-excised but only 3.7 percent ($n = 214$) if negative margins were obtained ($p < 0.0001$). Similarly, Schnitt and colleagues showed that patients with focally positive margins had a relative ratio of 14.9 of developing recurrence compared with patients with negative margins ($p < 0.0001$).[7] Although all the studies are relatively small and by necessity retrospective, the bulk of the presently available evidence favors obtaining negative margins whenever possible. Despite this evidence, many centers report between 20 percent and 55 percent positive margins on the initial diagnostic biopsy.[9-11] A report from Japan indicates the positive margin rate was 95 percent when serial sections were performed on the lumpectomy site in mastectomy specimens.[12] In part, this is because of the lack of technology for intraoperative diagnosis and assessment of margins.

Few studies have attempted to determine the factors in a primary tumor that consistently influence incomplete microscopic excision and resection margin involvement.[13-15] Presence of microcalcifications in the original mass makes the resected margin twice

TABLE 57–1. MARGIN STATUS AND LOCAL RECURRENCE AFTER BREAST-CONSERVING SURGERY

	Surgery	Radiotherapy (Gy)	Boosts (Gy)	Follow-up (yr)	Recurrence (% Positive versus Negative)
Clarke et al[10]	+/−	45	15	10	10/4
Bartelink et al[32]	1 cm	50	0–25	6	9/2
Schmidt-Ullrich[16]	2–5 mm	50–70	0–20	5	0
Solin et al[33]	0–2 mm	45–50	10–15	5	0/2.7
Spivack et al[8]	1 cm	45–50	9–16	4	18.2/3.7
Schnitt et al[7]	1 mm	60	+	5	21/0
Pezner et al[34]	nmd*	45–50	10	4	14/0
Ryoo et al[35]	>5 mm	50	16–20	8	13/5
Fourquet et al[36]	+/−	57	7 if +	8.6	29/7.6
Hallahan et al[37]	nmd*	46	14–16	3	8.5/4.7
Kurtz et al[38]	1 cm	50	20–25	7.5	66.7/31.3
Anscher et al[39]	+/−	43–50	0–15	3.5	9/1.5

*nmd = No margin defined.

as likely to be involved, but assessment of the margin by intraoperative two-dimensional specimen radiography is of no value. Schmidt-Ullrich and associates evaluated 108 women with stage I and II invasive carcinoma for adequacy of histopathology margins.[16] Inadequate margins were found in the initial lumpectomy specimen in 32 percent of the T1 carcinomas and 49 percent of the T2 carcinomas. For patients with tumors larger than 2 cm in diameter in which re-excision was required, 71 percent had residual carcinoma.[16] Cox and colleagues suggest that knowing (via fine needle aspiration) that a mass is cancer before diagnostic biopsy decreases the chance of positive margins from greater than 50 percent to 5 percent.[17] The problem of focally positive margins is being addressed at many centers with the use of a radiation therapy boost to the primary site, but no randomized prospective studies validate this concept.

DIFFICULTIES IN THE ASSESSMENT OF MARGINS WITH TRADITIONAL TECHNOLOGY

The problem arises in how best to evaluate margins when it most matters, that is, at the time of the original operation. Pathologically, there is no standardized sampling method. The "orange peel" technique suggested by Carter allows evaluation of the entire resection margin (tangential margins), but is tedious and time consuming and is not feasible intraoperatively.[18] The technique of sectioning the lumpectomy specimen in several different planes to topographically localize tumor cells in representative margins (radial margins) is likewise tedious without truly sampling all the margins. It has been suggested that it would take 3000 sections, 6 μ thick, to fully evaluate the margins of a 2-cm breast biopsy.[18]

Regardless of the method of sectioning, margin evaluation via frozen section presents its own set of difficulties. These include technical problems secondary to freezing adipose tissue, tissue artifacts of freezing, cost, loss of tissue in smaller specimens for permanent section diagnosis, and sampling error in large specimens. In addition, frozen section is too time consuming to use for intraoperative evaluation of the multiple specimens required for margin evaluation. With the increased utilization of mammography and the prevalence of *in situ* and small carcinomas (<1 cm), frozen section is not advisable for diagnosis because it can actually compromise the final diagnosis by loss of a small lesion.

Touch preparation (TP) allows simple, safe, quick, and full evaluation of all margins. In the hands of an experienced pathologist with extensive knowledge of cytology, TP may actually be more accurate than permanent section. This statement is based on sampling error for margins in permanent section, problems associated with ink running, and the arboreal nature of the ductal system of the breast.

DEVELOPMENT AND USE OF TOUCH PREPARATION TECHNOLOGY

History and Methodology

Most noncytologic methods assess only 10 to 15 percent of the surface of a relatively rounded breast lesion.[18] Wet-film cytology, which was first perfected by Shaw[19] in 1910 and later introduced as a method of pathological investigation by Dudgeon and Patrick[20] in 1927, theoretically can assess all the margins. This technique has been published under many names, including imprint cytology,[21] TP,[22, 23] scrape cytology,[24] cytologic smears,[25] and Scrimp technique.[26] Despite many publications demonstrating the diagnostic accuracy and capability to predict margins intraoperatively,[23] the full potential of the TP technique has not been realized for a number of reasons: acceptance of breast-conserving therapy as the preferred treatment for stage I and II breast cancer, lack of cytologic skills by general pathologists now more commonly available, and the wider usage of screening mammography, which has led to smaller lesions and increased frequency of diagnosis of ductal carcinoma *in situ*, both of which are difficult to detect with frozen section.

The TP method consists of simply touching the specimen onto a glass slide, similar to pressing a rubber stamp onto paper. The principle is that tumor cells, if present, will adhere to the slide. On a given specimen, careful gross examination is performed and margins assessed by taking imprints of all six margins. Subsequently, the margins are inked and the specimen is serially sectioned at 0.5-cm intervals. Diagnosis of the lesion then is made separately again by careful gross examination of the specimen, identification of any masses, and scraping of the lesion(s) with a blade. Smears of the scraped material can then be air dried or fixed in 95 percent methanol. A number of staining methods can then be used, but usually hematoxylin and eosin suffice. Cytologic features of malignancy include loosely cohesive and individually scattered malignant cells, malignant epithelial cells arranged in three-dimensional clusters, syncytial grouping and acinar pattern, tumor diathesis, and nonpolar naked nuclei.[27] Diagnostic categories used in reporting cytologic findings include negative, suspicious, malignant, or indeterminate. Suspicious and malignant categories are used by the surgeon as an indication to obtain additional tissue from the indicated margins.

Comparison of TP Technology and Frozen Section

Frozen section has been the gold standard for intraoperative diagnosis of breast lesions. Table 57–2 demonstrates that TP compares favorably in older studies with frozen section in terms of percent of false positives and negatives. Advances and availability of screening technology in recent years have led to an increased diagnosis of *in situ* and small

TABLE 57–2. DIAGNOSIS OF BREAST LESIONS: COMPARISON OF TP AND FROZEN SECTION

		TP		Frozen Section	
	Number	FP (%)	FN (%)	FP (%)	FN (%)
Tribe[21]	311	0.65	5.15	0	1.6
Sakai and Lanslanti[40]	196*	0	0	0	0.1
Helpap and Tschubel[41]	700	NS	NS	NS	NS
Suen et al.[42]	473*	0	10	NS	NS
Esteban et al.[25]	140	1	2	1.1	0.7
Ku/Cox et al.[22, 23]	90	2.2	0	0	4.4

FN = False negative; FP = false positive.
*>5 percent of deferred cases; NS > 95% agreement but FP/FN not specified.

invasive carcinomas. Studies evaluating frozen section alone in the intraoperative diagnosis of nonpalpable lesions demonstrate positive predictive values ranging from 68 percent to 97.7 percent, with greater than 5 percent of cases being deferred in every series.[28, 29] In Fessia and associates' report of more than 4436 consecutive breast biopsies, there were no false positives, 1.7 percent false negatives, and there were 1.8 percent deferred diagnoses.[30] However, with minimally invasive cancers, the false-negative rate was 8.8 percent and the deferral rate, 11 percent. With

noninvasive cancers, the false-negative and deferral rates were 76.8 percent and 12.2 percent, respectively. Particular problems for frozen section in intraoperative diagnosis include sclerosing adenosis, proliferating or lactating fibroadenomas, papillomas *in situ*, and small (<1 cm) invasive carcinomas, especially well-differentiated carcinomas such as tubular carcinomas. TP compares favorably with frozen section in diagnosing small and *in situ* lesions and in distinguishing sclerosing adenosis from malignancy.

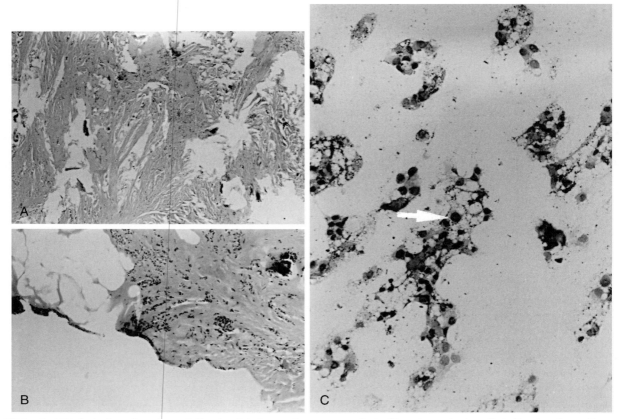

Figure 57–1 **A**, *Histological section shows infiltrating lobular carcinoma; note single files of neoplastic cells infiltrating dense fibrous stroma. Original power of magnification: 40 ×.* **B**, *Histological section shows infiltrating lobular carcinoma present at ink margin of resection marked by an arrow. Original power of magnification: 200 ×.* **C**, *Touch preparation of the surgical margin shows neoplastic cells as single cells and in clusters; note the uniform cell population and absence of bipolar myoepithelial cells. Original power of magnification: 400 ×.*

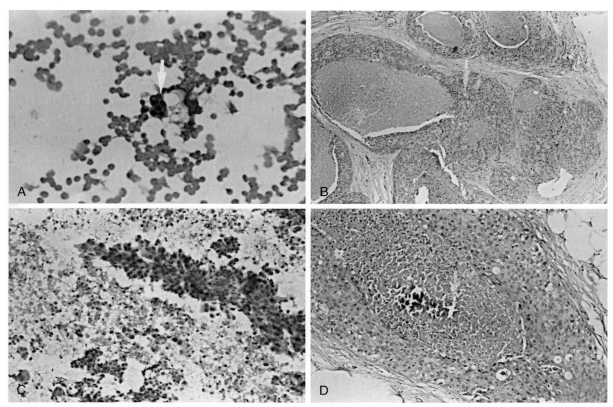

Figure 57–2   A, *Histological section shows ductal carcinoma* in situ, *comedo type. Original power of magnification: 100 ×.*   **B,** *Histological section shows ductal carcinoma* in situ, *comedo type; note presence of central necrosis, marked by an arrow. Original power of magnification: 400 ×.*   **C,** *Touch preparation of the margin of resection shows rare neoplastic cells. Original power of magnification: 400 ×.*   **D,** *Scrape preparation of the mass shows a large number of neoplastic cells arranged in clusters and as single cells in a background of extensive necrosis. These features are consistent with the diagnosis of comedocarcinoma* in situ. *Original power of magnification: 200 ×.*

Intraoperative Evaluation of Breast Lesions

Cox and colleagues and Ku and colleagues compared TP and frozen section in a similar group of patients (114 and 90 patients, respectively) in which patients already diagnosed with cancer underwent segmentectomy for margins.[22, 23] Two false-positive TPs in each study were associated with lesions <1 mm from the margin. Careful pathological re-evaluation of these margins suggested the margins may have truly been positive.[17] Klimberg and associates evaluated the TP technique prospectively on 428 consecutive patients undergoing breast biopsy for undiagnosed breast masses during a 2-year period. Of these 428 patients, approximately 20 percent underwent preoperative needle localization for a nonpalpable breast mass. Tumor size averaged 2.2 cm, of which 26.5 percent were *in situ*. The pathological diagnosis by TP was correct as compared with permanent section in 99.3 percent of the lesions (0.7 percent false negatives and 0 percent false positives). Diagnostic sensitivity was 96.4 percent, and specificity and positive predictive value were 100 percent. Indeterminate or deferred diagnosis represented less than 1 percent of the lesions. There were three missed diagnoses, two of which were focal ductal and one, focal lobular

carcinoma *in situ*. These three misses were thought to be sampling error, and all three had negative margins. Margin evaluation was correct in 100 percent of the lesions and was used to re-excise the margins when initial TP results were positive. Initial positive margins were diagnosed intraoperatively in 7.2 percent of the cases. TP evaluation was particularly useful in reassuring a patient that a mastectomy was her only choice when the surgeon was unable to obtain margins after multiple attempts at the time of initial biopsy. Figures 57–1 to 57–3 demonstrate the ability of TP to show positive margins in a number of histological types, including infiltrating lobular, ductal carcinoma *in situ*, and infiltrating ductal carcinoma.

POTENTIAL IMPACT OF INTRAOPERATIVE MARGIN EVALUATION

Assessment on the Outcome of Breast Cancer Surgery

The best cosmetic results with conservative breast surgery are obtained at the time of initial excisional biopsy. TP may aid in cosmesis because it circum-

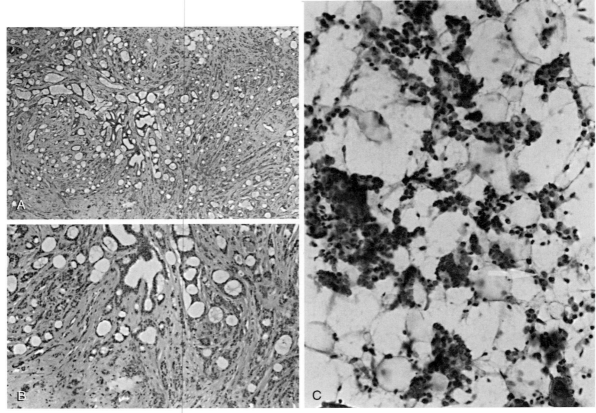

Figure 57–3 **A**, *Histological section shows an infiltrating ductal carcinoma. Original power of magnification: 40 ×.* **B**, *Histological section shows a grade I infiltrating ductal carcinoma. Original magnification power: 200 ×.* **C**, *Scrape preparation of the mass shows a large number of neoplastic cells organized in a cluster or in the form of acini. Individual neoplastic cells are also present. Original power of magnification: 200 ×.*

vents the need for a separate operative procedure for involved margins. Touch prep provides rapid, reliable, topographically accurate evaluation of the entire resection margin. Cox recently compared results among a group of patients in which 701 margins were evaluated by TP and 193 were not.[31] Local recurrence was lower with TP (2.3 percent) than in those patients diagnosed with conventional histology (13.5 percent). Cox suggests that TP evaluation of margins is more thorough, rapid, and accurate than standard histological techniques. Touch prep has the advantage of being a simple, quick (2 to 3 minutes), safe (no loss of diagnostic material), and accurate method for diagnosis and estimation of tumor margins at the time of the original surgery. It overcomes frozen sampling errors and artifacts related to fat and calcifications. It is feasible for large specimens with little diagnostic material such as seen in needle localization breast biopsies for nonpalpable lesions. TP is also cost effective because it requires fewer frozen sections, fewer re-excisions, possibly fewer salvage mastectomies, and minimal equipment, supply, maintenance, and personnel costs. The evidence suggests that cytologic evaluation of lumpectomy margins via TP may have a future role in improving cosmesis and reducing local recurrence after conservation therapy.

References

1. Holaday WJ, Assor D: Ten thousand consecutive frozen section: A retrospective study focusing on accuracy and quality control. Am J Clin Pathol 61:769–777, 1974.
2. Lessells AM, Simpson JG: A retrospective analysis of the accuracy of immediate frozen section diagnosis in surgical pathology. Br J Surg 63:327–329, 1976.
3. Nakazawa H, Rosen P, Lane N, Lattes R: Frozen section experience in 3,000 cases: Accuracy, limitations and value in residency training. Am J Clin Pathol 49:41–51, 1968.
4. Rosai J, Ackerman LV: The pathology of tumors. Part II: Diagnostic techniques. CA Cancer J Clin 29:22–39, 1979.
5. Shidham VB, Dravid NV, Grover S, Kher AV: Role of scrape cytology in rapid intraoperative diagnosis: Value and limitations. Acta Cytol 28:477–482, 1984.
6. National Institutes of Health Consensus Conference: Treatment of early-stage breast cancer. JAMA 265:391–395, 1991.
7. Schnitt SJ, Abner A, Gelman R, Connolly JL, Recht A, Duda RB, Eberlein TJ, et al: The relationship between microscopic margins of resection and the risk of local recurrence in patients with breast cancer treated with breast-conserving surgery and radiation therapy. Cancer 74:1746–1751, 1994.
8. Spivack B, Khanna MM, Tafra L, Juillard G, Giuliano AE: Margin status and local recurrence after breast-conserving surgery. Arch Surg 129:952–957, 1994.
9. Mokbel K, Ahmed M, Nash A, Sacks N: Re-excision operations in nonpalpable breast cancer. J Surg Oncol 58:225–228, 1995.
10. Clarke K, Le MG, Sarrazin D, Lacombe MJ, Fontaine F, Travagli JP, May-Levine F: Analysis of local-regional relapses in patients with early breast cancers treated by excision and radiotherapy: Experience of the Institute Gustave-Roussy. Int J Radiat Oncol Biol Phys 11:137–145, 1985.

11. Hustreich DJ, Dunn JM, Armstrong JS, et al: Diagnostic and therapeutic aspects of fine wire localization biopsy for impalpable breast cancer. Br J Surg 79:1038–1041, 1992.
12. Haga S, Makita M, Shimizu T, Watanabe O, Imamura H, Kajiwara R, Fujibayashi M: Histopathological study of local residual carcinoma after simulated lumpectomy. Surg Today 25:329–333, 1995.
13. Walls J, Knox F, Baildam AD, Asbury DL, Mansel RE, Bundred NJ: Can preoperative factors predict for residual malignancy after breast biopsy for invasive cancer? Ann R Coll Surg Engl 77:248–251, 1995.
14. Aitken RJ, Going JJ, Chetty U: Assessment of surgical excision during breast conservation surgery by intraoperative two-dimensional specimen radiology. Br J Surg 77:322–323, 1990.
15. Hall FM, Houlihan MJ, Baum JK: Efficacy of specimen radiography in evaluating the surgical margins of impalpable breast carcinoma. AJR 162:33–36, 1993.
16. Schmidt-Ullrich R, Wazer D, Tercilla O, Safaii HS, Marchant DJ, Smith TJ, Robert NJ: Tumor margin assessment as a guide to optimal conservation surgery and irradiation in early-stage breast carcinoma. Int J Radiat Oncol Biol Phys 17:733–738, 1989.
17. Cox CE, Reintgen DS, Nicosia SV, Ku NN, Baekey P, Carey LC: Analysis of residual cancer after diagnostic breast biopsy: An argument for fine-needle aspiration cytology. Ann Surg Oncol 2:201–206, 1995.
18. Carter D: Margins of "Lumpectomy" for breast cancer. Hum Pathol 17:330–332, 1986.
19. Shaw EH: The immediate microscopic diagnosis of tumours at the time of operation. Lancet Sept 4, 1910.
20. Dudgeon LS, Patrick CV: A new method for the rapid microscopical diagnosis of tumours. Br J Surg 15:250–261, 1927.
21. Tribe CR: A comparison of rapid methods including imprint cytodiagnosis for the diagnosis of breast tumours. J Clin Pathol 26:273–277, 1973.
22. Cox CE, Ku NK, Reintgen DS, Greenberg HM, Nicosia SV, Wangensteen S: Touch preparation cytology of breast lumpectomy margins with histologic correlation. Arch Surg 126:490–493, 1991.
23. Ku NK, Cox CE, Reintgen DS, Greenberg HM, Nicosia SV: Cytology of lumpectomy specimens. Acta Cytol 35:417–421, 1991.
24. Gal R: Scrape cytology assessment of margins of lumpectomy specimens in breast cancer. Acta Cytol 32:838–839, 1988.
25. Esteban JM, Zaloudek C, Silverberg SG: Intraoperative diagnosis of breast lesions: Comparison of cytologic with frozen section technics. Am J Clin Pathol 88:681–688, 1987.
26. Abrahams C: The "Scrimp" technique: A method for the rapid diagnosis of surgical pathology specimens. Histopathology 2:255–266, 1978.
27. Silverman JF: Breast. In Bibbo M (ed): Comprehensive Cytopathology. Philadelphia, WB Saunders, 1991.
28. Tinnemans JGM, Wobbes T, Holland R, Hendriks JHCL, van der Sluis RF, Lubbers E-J C, de Boer HHM: Mammographic and histopathologic correlation of nonpalpable lesions of the breast and the reliability of frozen section diagnosis. Surg Gynecol Obstet 165:523–529, 1987.
29. Ferreiro JA, Gisvold JJ, Bostwick DG: Accuracy of frozen-section diagnosis of mammographically directed breast biopsies: Results of 1,490 consecutive cases. Am J Surg Pathol 19:1267–1271, 1995.
30. Fessia L, Ghiringhello B, Arisio R, Botta G, Aimone V: Accuracy of frozen section diagnosis in breast cancer detection: A review of 4436 biopsies and comparison with cytodiagnosis. Pathol Res Pract 179:61–66, 1984.
31. Cox CE: Techniques to achieve a pathologic free margin during lumpectomy: Cytologic imprint. 49th Annual Cancer Symposium, Plenary Session. Presented at Society of Surgical Oncology, Atlanta, March 21 to 24, 1996.
32. Bartelink H, Borger JH, van Dongen JA, Peters JL: The impact of tumor size and histology on local control after breast-conserving therapy. Radiother Oncol 11:297–303, 1988.
33. Solin LJ, Fowble BL, Schultz DJ, Goodman RL: The significance of the pathology margins of the tumor excision on the outcome of patients treated with definitive irradiation for early-stage breast cancer. Int J Radiat Oncol Biol Phys 21:279–287, 1991.
34. Pezner RD, Lipsett JA, Desai K, Vora N, Terz J, Hill LR, Luk KH: To boost or not to boost: Decreasing radiation therapy in conservative breast cancer treatment when "inked" tumor resection margins are pathologically free of cancer. Int J Radiat Oncol Biol Phys 14:873–877, 1988.
35. Ryoo MC, Kagan AR, Woolin M, Tome MA, Tedeschi MA, Rao AR, Hintz BL, et al: Prognostic factors for recurrence and cosmesis in 393 patients after radiation therapy for early mammary carcinoma. Radiology 172:555–559, 1989.
36. Fourquet A, Campana F, Zafrani B, Messeri V, Vileh P, Durand JC, Vilcoq JR: Prognostic factors of breast recurrence in the conservative management of early breast cancer: A 25-year follow-up. Int J Radiat Oncol Biol Phys 17:719–725, 1989.
37. Hallahan DE, Michel AG, Halpern HJ, Awan AM, Desser R, Bitran J, Recant W, et al: Breast-conserving surgery and definitive irradiation for early-stage breast cancer. Int J Radiat Oncol Biol Phys 17:1211–1216, 1989.
38. Kurtz JN, Jacquemier J, Amalric K, et al: Why are local recurrences after breast-conserving surgery more frequent in young patients? J Clin Oncol 8:591–598, 1990.
39. Anscher MS, Jones P, Prosnitz LR, et al: Local failure and margin status in early-stage breast carcinoma treated with conservation surgery and radiation therapy. Ann Surg 218:22–28, 1993.
40. Sakai Y, Lanslanti K: Comparison and analysis of the results of cytodiagnosis and frozen sections during operation. Acta Cytol 13:359–368, 1969.
41. Helpap B, Tschubel K: The significance of imprint cytology in breast biopsy diagnosis. Acta Cytol 22:133–137, 1978.
42. Suen K, Wood W, Syed A, Quenville N, Clement P: Role of imprint cytology in intraoperative diagnosis: Value and limitations. J Clin Pathol 31:328–337, 1978.

CHAPTER 58

INTRAOPERATIVE IMPRINT CYTOLOGY

Charles E. Cox, M.D. / Ni Ni K. Ku, M.D. / Emmanuella Joseph, M.D. /
Douglas S. Reintgen, M.D. / Harvey Greenberg, M.D. /
Santo V. Nicosia, M.D., M.S.

IMPRINT CYTOLOGY FOR LUMPECTOMY MARGIN EVALUATION

The advent of breast conservation therapy has brought about the need for more precise, timely, and cost-effective ways of evaluating tumor margins. Such evaluation is critical to a successful disease-free outcome in patients with stage I or II breast cancer treated by lumpectomy and radiation therapy.* Surgical margins have been evaluated histologically, but a number of technical and diagnostic pitfalls may arise when trying to evaluate the entire resected surface by this approach.[3, 15, 27, 31, 36, 37] At the Moffitt Cancer Center (MCC), use of imprint cytology has unified the roles of the pathologist, surgeon, and radiation oncologist in the multidisciplinary treatment of the breast cancer patient. Imprint cytology has also reduced local recurrence in those patients receiving breast preservation and has avoided multiple re-excisions, therefore reducing the number of procedures required to obtain negative margins.[27-29]

History

A wide acceptance of breast conservation surgery has raised issues in the assessment and definition of negative margins. In the original study assessing lumpectomy as an alternative to mastectomy, Fisher and colleagues[12] described a method of evaluation of margins and defined as negative any margin that did not show tumor at the inked surface of the resected specimen.[12] These authors also recommended sectioning inked lumpectomy specimens in several different planes to topographically localize tumor cells in representative margins.[12] Likewise, the National Surgical Adjuvant Breast and Bowel Project (NSABP) protocols required tumor extension to an inked surgical margin before a margin could be called positive.[10, 11] Additional methods have also been used to evaluate surgical margins in breast conservation therapy. In 1986, Carter[4] proposed parallel sectioning of the entire outer surface of lumpectomy specimens for complete histological examination. Others have tried applying frozen section techniques to lumpectomy margins, but fat is notoriously difficult to freeze and section, and pathologists have difficulty using this technique.† Subsequently, Gal[15] applied the scraping technique of Shidham and associates[44] for

rapid cytologic evaluation. Investigators at MCC were the first to use imprint cytology to evaluate the margins of breast cancer specimens during breast-conserving surgery.[5, 28] In addition, the efficacy of imprint cytology has recently been validated by Klimberg and colleagues[24] as an ideal method to evaluate lumpectomy margins.

Technique

The general principles for specimen handling during the evaluation of tumor margins by imprint cytology are few but important. The lumpectomy specimen is marked by the surgeon to orient the specimen for the pathologist. The specimen must be fresh, wrapped in a saline-moistened Telfa pad; placed inside a clean, capped container; and submitted immediately to the pathology laboratory. Upon receipt of the specimen, its margins are oriented as anterior, superior, medial, lateral, inferior, or deep (Fig. 58–1). The IZI Corporation manufactures prelabeled orientation marker clips that are routinely used by us for orientation.[21] Immediately after excision, imprint smears are prepared from the freshly cut surfaces of the lumpectomy specimen using previously labeled glass slides by gentle but firm pressure over each margin. Four or five imprints can be made on each margin, using the same slide. Slides are then air-dried and stained with Diff-Quik followed by intraoperative evaluation under a light microscope (Table 58–1). After the imprints are made, the lumpectomy specimen is inked using different colors for each margin and sectioned for histopathological examination. If tumor is still

TABLE 58–1. DIFF-QUIK STAIN PROCEDURE

A	Thoroughly air dry slides.
B	Stain with Diff-Quik solution as follows.
Step 1	Fix for 15–20 seconds in solution I. Drain excess solution onto a paper towel.
Step 2	Dip slides repeatedly for 15–20 seconds in solution II until slides are uniformly coated and turn red-pink. Drain excess stain.
Step 3	Dip slides repeatedly for 10–15 seconds into solution III. Rinse in tap water.
Step 4	Drain excess water. Examine slide smears for quality of stain (purple). If the stain is too pale or too intense (deep blue), it may be destained by repeated immersion in solution I for 20–30 seconds.
Step 5	Intraoperative/stat reading may be performed on uncoverslipped wet slides. Mount in resin and coverslip slides when dry.

---

*See references 14, 36, 38, 39, 41, 47, 48, 49, and 50.
†See references 4, 5, 8, 9, 24, 40, and 45.

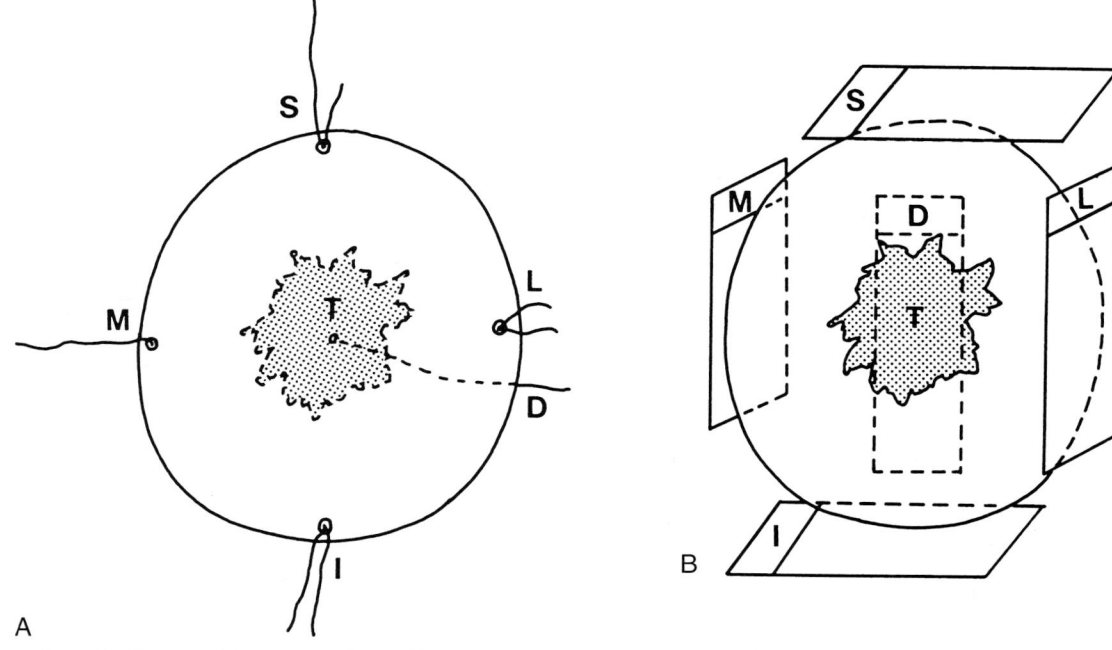

Figure 58–1 *Schematic diagram of imprint cytology of lumpectomy specimens.*   **A,** *Lumpectomy margins are first oriented by various sutures.* **B,** *Margins are then sampled by imprint cytology. S = superior, M = medial, D = deep, I = inferior, L = lateral, T = tumor. (From Ku NNK, Cox CE, Reingten DS, et al: Cytology of lumpectomy specimens. Acta Cytologica 35:417–421, 1991.)*

present, this is also imprinted to serve as a positive control for margin assessment.

Diagnostic Reporting

Cytologic evaluation and final reports on tumor margins can be rendered within 15 minutes, using the diagnostic criteria of negative, atypical, suspicious, or malignant. If the tumor is found at a given margin, the cytopathologist notifies the surgeon so that additional tissue can be resected until no tumor cells are identified. After lumpectomy, the tumor cavity is examined by the surgeon for residual disease by visual inspection and palpation. Intraoperative application of a triple diagnostic approach (specimen gross

appearance, along with radiographic assessment of calcifications and cytologic findings) plays an important role for accurate diagnosis. Familiarity with cytologic features of breast lesions is important for speed and accuracy of diagnosis (Figs. 58–2 to 58–4). The general cytologic criteria for benign or malignant lesions are similar to that of aspiration biopsy cytology (Table 58–2).[25, 31, 46]

Comparison to Frozen Section

At MCC, we routinely use imprint cytology of lumpectomy margins as an alternative to conventional frozen section. After more than 8 years since the implementation of this technique, more than 800 lumpectomies have been evaluated. Based on the follow-up of these patients, imprint cytology identifies microscopic disease not always detectable grossly or by frozen section (Table 58–3).[29] Our study as well as those of Veneti and colleagues[55] and Klimberg and associates[24] thus show that imprint cytology is superior to frozen section in the intraoperative assessment of tumor margins.[5, 8, 24, 29, 40, 55]

Limitations

Imprint cytology is not without technical limitations. Errors may be related to specimen surface irregularity, cauterization, and dryness as well as diagnostic misinterpretation. Another limitation is the possibility of a false positive report resulting from an overinterpretation of atypical or reactive cells. False positives are not considered a liability because most surgeons would remove another 1 cm of breast tissue

TABLE 58–2.   USEFUL GENERAL CYTOLOGIC CRITERIA IN EVALUATION OF BREAST LESIONS

Parameter	Benign Lesions	Malignant Lesions
Cellularity	+	+ / + + +
Dyshesion	– / +	+ + +
Monomorphism	–	+ + +
Crowding overlapping	+ / –	+ + +
Myoepithelial cells	+	– / +
Irregular chromatinic rim	– / +	+ +
Anisonucleosis	+ / +	+ +
Macronucleoli	– / +	+ +
Cytoplasmic diameter (μm)	<12	>10 <15
Nuclear diameter	<10	>9 <13
N/C ratio > 90%	<10%	50–90%

Modified from Kline TS, Kline IK: Breast. *In* Guide to Clinical Aspirator Biopsy. New York, Igaku-Shoin, 1989, pp 1–7.

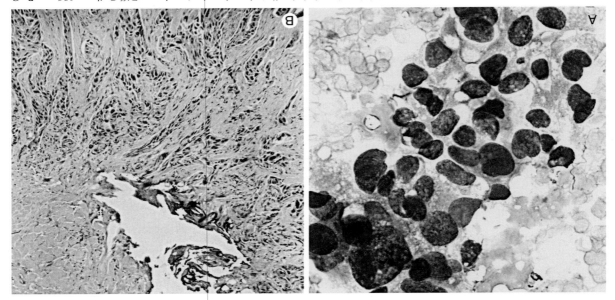

Figure 58–3 Infiltrating ductal carcinoma. **A,** Abnormal ductal epithelial cells in loosely cohesive cluster. Diff-Quik, × 630. **B,** Corresponding histology of the lumpectomy margin. H & E, × 100. (From Ku NNK, Cox CE, Reintgen DS, et al: Cytology of lumpectomy specimens. Acta Cytologica 35:417–421, 1991.)

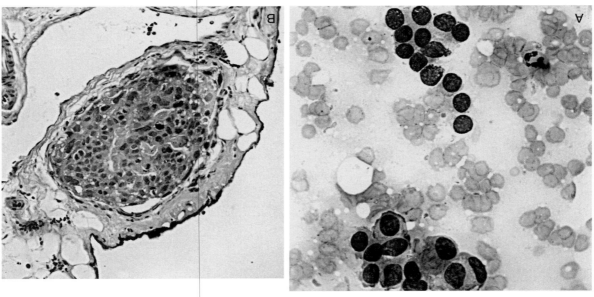

Figure 58–2 Intraductal carcinoma. **A,** Cohesive clusters of abnormal ductal epithelial cells. Diff-Quik, × 630. **B,** Corresponding histology of the lumpectomy margin. H & E, × 400. (From Ku NNK, Cox CE, Reintgen DS, et al: Cytology of lumpectomy specimens. Acta Cytologica 35:417–421, 1991.)

Local Recurrence

Numerous studies indicate that margin involvement is a significant predictor for local recurrence (Table 58-4). The use of standard or modified histological techniques has yielded local recurrence rates of 2 percent to 24 percent (mean, 15.8 percent) after breast conservation.[14, 19, 38, 43, 48, 53] At the MCC, we have studied the local recurrence rate after breast

conservation surgery using imprint cytology. From 1984 to 1996, 849 women were treated with breast conservation and radiation therapy (XRT) consisting of 4600 cGy and a 1400 cGy electron boost to the lumpectomy site. All patients with outside breast biopsies had their pathology reviewed before treatment to verify diagnosis and assess margins, and each radiation treatment was given under the direction of a radiation oncologist (H.G.) after margins were deemed negative. A standard linear accelerator with tangential fields was used. All patients were then followed prospectively and evaluated for recurrence at 6-month intervals with physical exams and concomitant mammography. Recurrence was evaluated by fine-needle aspiration biopsy (FNAB) of palpable masses or needle-localized breast biopsy of suspicious nonpalpable masses. Seven hundred and one patients had lumpectomy margins evaluated by imprint cytology, and the remaining 193 were evaluated by conventional histology. In both groups, margins were declared negative before proceeding with XRT. The mean age was comparable between the two groups (imprint cytology, 57.3 ± 13.0 yr versus conventional histology, 55.2 ± 12.3 yr). The tumor size and histology were similar with the exception of the patients with in situ lesions evaluated by imprint cytology (Table 58-5). Early in the series, the evaluation of the lumpectomy margins for patients with ductal carcinoma in situ (DCIS), comedocarcinoma variant, was greatly aided by imprint cytology, allowing us to offer breast conservation rather than mastectomy to more patients. The overall recurrence rate for all patient groups was 16 of 701 (2.27 percent) by imprint cytology versus 26 of 193 (13.5 percent) by conventional histology. The histological subgroup analysis demonstrated a significant increase in recurrence rates when lumpectomy margins were

in the direction of the positive margin, and this usually does not have a significant effect on cosmesis. False negative diagnoses are associated with lesions demonstrating extensive desmoplasia or bland cytologic features (lobular, colloid, papillary and monomorphic ductal carcinomas). An experienced cytopathologist is critical in these circumstances, and concurrent frozen sections may be invaluable to verify uncertain findings. These limitations notwithstanding, the need for routine frozen sections has been greatly reduced by imprint cytology.

TABLE 58-3. CORRELATION BETWEEN GROSS, FROZEN SECTION, PERMANENT HISTOLOGICAL, AND IMPRINT CYTOLOGY EXAMINATION OF LUMPECTOMY MARGINS OF 347 CASES

Margins	Type of Examination			
	Gross	Cytologic	Frozen Section*	Permanent
True positive	23	60	39	64
True negative	214	275	169	283
False positive	25	8	0	—
False negative	85	4	19	—

*Frozen section was not performed in 120 (34 percent) cases. Cytology alone was used for margin evaluation.

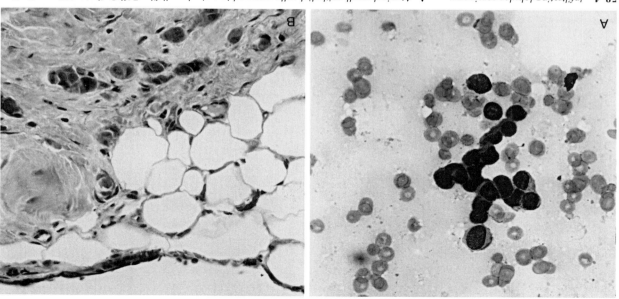

Figure 58-4 Infiltrating lobular carcinoma. **A,** Atypical small epithelial cells arranged in a single cell-file. Diff-Quik, × 400. **B,** Corresponding histology of the lumpectomy margin. H & E, × 400. (From Ku NNK, Cox CE, Reintgen DS, et al: Cytology of lumpectomy specimens. Acta Cytologica 35:417–421, 1991.)

TABLE 58–4.   LOCAL RECURRENCE RATES IN RELATION TO STATUS OF MICROSCOPIC MARGINS OF RESECTION AFTER BREAST CONSERVATION

| Author | Follow-up (mo) | n | Status of Microscopic Margin | | | | p Value |
			Positive (%)	Negative (%)	Close (%)	Unknown (%)	
Solin et al[49]	60	697	2	7	11	9	.53
Zanfrani et al[59]	103	433	24	8.3	—	—	<.0001
Van Dongen[54]	96	431	20	9	—	—	.1
Ansher et al[3]	44	164	9	1.5	—	—	.014
Schnitt et al[41]	60	133	21	0	4	—	.02
Spivack et al[50]	48	258	18	3.7	—	7.1	.0001
Veronesi et al[56]	60	289	17.4	8.6	—	8.9	—

evaluated by conventional histology in all categories, with the exception of those patients with infiltrating lobular carcinoma. The cells of this tumor are monomorphic, small, and quite bland on imprint cytology, rendering their identification from normal cellular component difficult (Table 58–6).[7, 58]

IMPRINT CYTOLOGY FOR DIAGNOSTIC EVALUATION

Intraoperative cytology for the diagnosis of breast cancer in needle-localized breast lesions has selective advantages[1, 6, 9] over excisional biopsy with frozen section. In specimens where small microcalcifications are present, diagnosis can be rendered without loss of tissue that may occur during cryosectioning. The technique allows for ancillary studies, including estrogen and progesterone receptor determination, and careful histological assessment of extremely small tumors while providing immediate determination of the malignant or nonmalignant status of the lesion.[34] Emphasis can then be placed on the definitive histopathologic characterization of these lesions. Another advantage of the technique is that rapid diagnosis with margin assessment can be achieved. Therefore, multiple surgeries may be avoided and a better cosmetic appearance obtained if diagnostic intraoperative cytology is used in conjunction with imprint cytology of margins when a decision is made to perform a lumpectomy at the time of excisional biopsy. Of course, all is dependent on the diagnostic experience of the cytopathologist.

History

The use of imprint cytology in the diagnosis of breast lesions was described in 1965 by Tribe and in 1968 by Pilar and sporadically evaluated in the past ten years.[35, 53] At the MCC we have used intraoperative imprint cytology for the diagnosis of nonpalpable breast lesions since 1987.[43]

Technique for Needle-Localized Breast Lesions

Lesions are radiographically localized with a needle by the radiologist in the standard fashion before the specimen is sent to the pathology laboratory. The specimens are mounted on a specboard with graduated X and Y coordinates, along with the preoperative mammogram and specimen radiograph.[1, 9, 17] The needle-localized area(s) are assigned coordinates and surfaces are marked with ink. Different ink colors may be used for each coordinate, and India ink covers the remainder of the specimen. The needle is then gently removed from the specimen, which is then bisected or serially sectioned at 3- to 5-mm intervals. The flat surface of the freshly cut lesion is firmly touched once or twice with a clean, prelabeled glass slide. The lesional surface may also be scraped gently, three or four times in the same direction, using the edge of a second glass slide or a dry scalpel blade if the lesion is found to be sclerotic or fibrotic.[44] The material is then smeared evenly on the other half of the glass slide. Gentle scraping is necessary because vigorous pressure may result in cellular dis-

TABLE 58–5.   TUMOR RECURRENCE VERSUS TUMOR SIZE

| Tumor Size | Imprint Cytology | | | Histology | | |
	Number of Patients	Number Recurred	Percent Recurred	Number of Patients	Number Recurred	Percent Recurred
T_0	144	2	1.3%	29	4	13.8%
T_1	434	9	2.0%	115	13	11.3%
T_2	117	5	4.3%	19	4	21%
T_3	6	0	0.0%	3	1	33.0%
T_x	—	—	—	27	4	14.8%
Totals	701	16	2.3%	193	26	13.5%

TABLE 58–6. TUMOR RECURRENCE BY HISTOLOGICAL SUBGROUP

Histologic Type	Imprint Cytology (%)	Histology (%)
DCIS	6/297 (3.0)	5/57 (15.8)
Infiltrating ductal and DCIS	3/297 (3.0)	4/57 (3.0)
Infiltrating ductal	5/356 (1.4)	17/136 (12.5)
Infiltrating lobular	2/48 (4.1)	—
Totals	16/701 (2.3)	26 (13.5)

TABLE 58–7. PAPANICOLAOU STAIN

95% ethyl alcohol	10 dips (×2)
70% ethyl alcohol	10 dips
Tap water	10 dips
Hematoxylin	20 seconds
Tap water	30 dips
Bluing reagent	10 dips
Tap water	30 dips
70% ethyl alcohol	10 dips
95% ethyl alcohol	10 dips
Cytostain	3 minutes
Tap water	30 dips
95% ethyl alcohol	10 dips (×3)
100% ethyl alcohol	10 dips (×3)
Xylene	10 dips (×3)

tortion and difficult or erroneous cytodiagnoses. The slides may be stained with Diff-Quik (see Table 58–1) or Papanicolaou stain (Table 58–7).

Diagnostic Evaluation

The diagnostic approach to imprint cytology is in general similar to that of aspiration biopsy cytology with the exception of cellularity, which may be artificially higher in cytological material obtained by scraping and not imprinting.[23, 24, 32, 54] General cytologic criteria for the evaluation of breast specimens rely on pattern recognition (best studied at 4 times magnification) and cytologic, nuclear, and cytoplasmic features (best evaluated at 25 to 63 times magnification) (see Table 58–2).[25] We also prefer the combined use of Diff-Quik (see Table 58–1) and Papanicolaou (see Table 58–7) stains for optimal recognition of cytoplasmic and extracellular material and nuclear details, respectively. Evaluation of nuclear and cytoplasmic features should be applied in a panel fashion because no single criterion is diagnostic of benignity or malignancy. Recognition of a combination of cytologic features will, however, assist in accurate cytodiagnosis on identification of specific benign or malignant histopathological subtypes (i.e., isolated small cells with targetoid mucin vacuoles in lobular carcinoma, large pleomorphic nuclei with very little surrounding cytoplasm and overlapping lymphocytes in medullary carcinoma, small monomorphic cells with extracellular mucin lakes, and occasional arborizing vascular networks in colloid carcinoma). Familiarity with these and with cytologic features of other entities is of fundamental importance (Figs. 58–5 to 58–11). Assessment of nuclear grading can also be attempted in most instances by accurately recognizing a number of features, including nuclear size, anisonucleosis, chromatin irregularities, and frequency of nucleoli and mitoses.

Comparison to Frozen Section

With increasing experience, intraoperative cytology has been shown to have rare false negative rates, with a diagnostic accuracy ranging from 98.3 percent to 100 percent.[5, 43] These data are comparable to frozen section results reported in other series.[16, 32] Using this technique, we have achieved a diagnostic accuracy of approximately 98 percent while retaining the entire specimen for permanent histological diagnosis and determination of prognostic factors.[5, 6, 43] Imprint cytology can clearly detect microscopic disease not

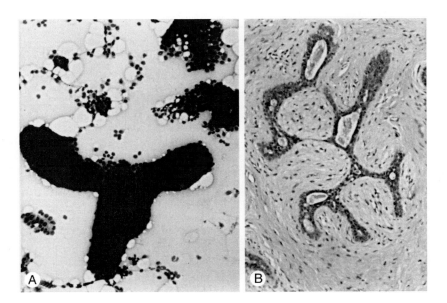

Figure 58–5 *Fibroadenoma. Note the pattern of cohesive and branching tissue fragments with scattered bare stromal nuclei* (**A**), *which is similar to that on the corresponding histological study* (**B**).   **A**, *Diff-Quik,* × *30;*   **B**, *(H & E),* × *110.*

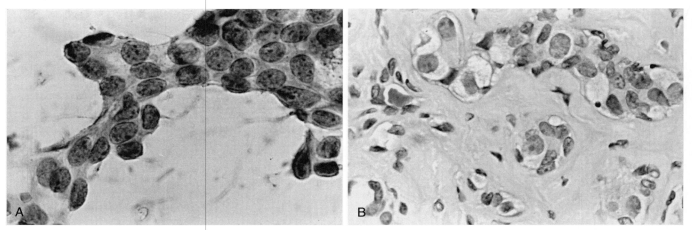

Figure 58–6 *Sclerosing adenosis.* **A,** *Cohesive fragment of enlarged and focally atypical ductal epithelial cells. Papanicolaou stain, ×* *1050.* **B,** *Noting the presence of myoepithelial cells in such fragments and the usually scant cellularity may reduce the incidence of overdiagnosing this benign proliferative lesion. H & E, × 670.*

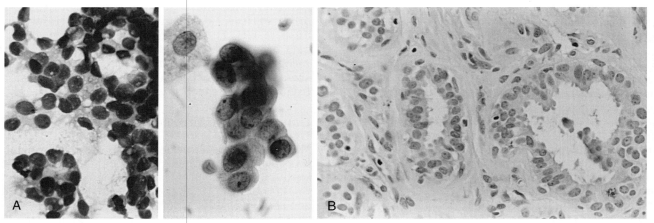

Figure 58–7 *Ductal hyperplasia with atypia.* **A,** *Note dyshesive ductal epithelial cells (left panel) and small epithelial fragments with enlarged nuclei (right panel). Papanicolaou stain: left panel, × 670; right panel, × 1050.* **B,** *An atypical mammary duct is shown in the corresponding biopsy. H & E, × 420.*

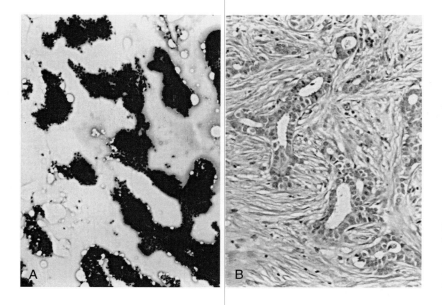

Figure 58–8 *Tubular carcinoma. Acute angle branching and cohesive fragments of neoplastic ductal epithelium without interspersed bare stromal cells differentiate from fibroadenoma the low-power cytological (**A**) and histological (**B**) pattern of this well-differentiated carcinoma.* **A,** *Diff-Quik, × 30.* **B,** *H & E, × 110.*

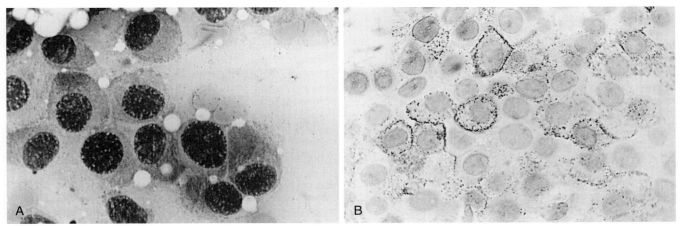

Figure 58–9 *Argyrophilic tumor.* **A,** *The aspirate of this variant of ductal carcinoma contains several dyshesive and monomorphic cells with intense and diffuse cytoplasmic granularity best observed in air-dried, Diff-Quik preparations. Diff-Quik, × 1050.* **B,** *The neuroendocrine nature of these granules is supported by intensive argyrophilia and chromogranin immunoreactivity. Grimelius stain, × 1050.*

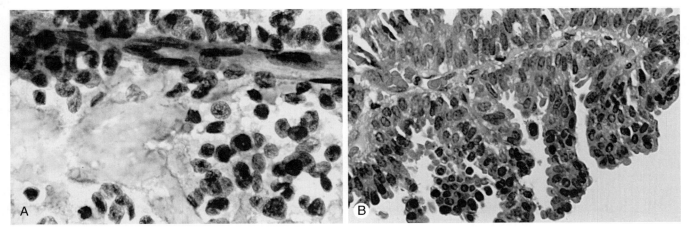

Figure 58–10 *Papillary carcinoma. Note pattern of abnormal epithelial cells singly or attached to microvessels* **(A)**, *which is similar to the corresponding histological study* **(B)**. **A,** *Papanicolaou, × 420;* **B,** *H & E, × 270.*

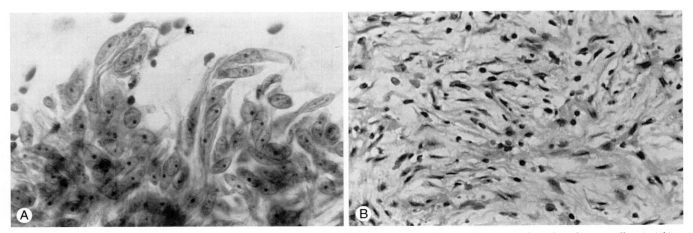

Figure 58–11 *Metaplastic carcinoma with sarcomatoid features.* **A,** *The aspirate contains spindly and moderately cohesive cells mimicking a soft tissue neoplasm. Papanicolaou stain, × 670.* **B,** *A similar pattern is noted in the corresponding histological study. A positive cytokeratin immunoreactivity is needed to confirm the epithelial nature of this neoplasm. H & E, × 420.*

visible by gross evaluation or frozen section of selective margins. Problems associated with frozen section such as potential tissue loss, sampling errors, and freezing artifacts are also overcome. It is our experience that false negative evaluations were rendered by gross examination in 13 percent of cases, by frozen section analysis in 4 percent of cases, and by imprint cytology 0 percent of cases.[27–29, 43] Another advantage of imprint cytology over frozen section is that it does not require the use of significant laboratory space and expensive equipment. In cases of borderline lesions[2] or infiltrating lobular carcinoma,[7, 58] where imprint cytology has a higher likelihood of false negativity, the technique may be complemented by frozen section.

LYMPHATIC MAPPING

The most powerful and predictive prognostic factor for breast cancer is the status of the regional nodes. Histological examination after routine complete axillary clearance is at present the only reliable method for assessing axillary node status. However, this exposes a large number of patients to perioperative and long-term morbidity with axillary seromas and lymphedema. Lymphatic mapping and sentinel node biopsy were first introduced by Morton and coworkers[30] for melanoma and Giuliano and associates[18] for breast cancer as a way to sample the axilla. The initial report with this technique from the John Wayne Cancer Institute showed a success rate of 71 percent with identification of the first node in the chain (the sentinel node, SLN) in 200 patients.[18, 26] At the MCC, we have introduced a lymphatic mapping technique to improve the staging and to decrease the morbidity in patients with all types of invasive breast cancers. We have used lymphatic mapping of patients with invasive breast cancer with preoperative lymphoscintigraphy followed by intraoperative injection with 3 cc of lymphazurin blue dye and 40 mCU of 99m Tc-radiolabeled sulfur colloid. In our ongoing prospective study, 174 patients with 178 nodal basins underwent radioguided surgery.[22] The technique was successful in identifying a SLN in 92 percent or 165 of 178 nodal basins. Of the 14 putative failures, 9 of 14 (64 percent) of the tumors were located in the inner quadrant of the breast and may have exclusive drainage to the internal mammary chain and thus may not need any axillary nodal staging procedure. The remaining 5 of 14 (36 percent) were the result of technical errors. After the identification of the SLN, lumpectomy or mastectomy was performed. When possible, the diagnosis of breast cancer was made with either FNAB of palpable lesions or stereotactic biopsies of mammographic abnormalities. After successful localization of 316 SLN, 50 of 316 (16.5 percent) of nodes found in 37 of 165 (23 percent) of the 164 patients exhibited metastatic disease. One hundred and thirty-six of the 164 patients went on to have complete axillary lymph node dissections. Only 1 patient had a false negative result of lymphatic mapping with a skip metastasis defined as a negative SLN and a positive higher node found after a complete axillary dissection. However, an error in identification of the true SLN may have also occurred, because this patient had undergone excisional biopsy before lymphatic mapping with disruption of breast lymphatic flow from the primary tumor. After complete axillary dissection, 23 of 37 (67 percent) of patients had positive nodes in addition to the SLN. A true positive complete node dissection (positive SLN and positive complete node dissection) was found in 22 patients and true negative SLNs (negative SLN and negative complete dissection) in 100 patients, for a negative predictive value of 99 percent.[22] Therefore, lymphatic mapping and SLN biopsy, using a combination of mapping techniques, provide accurate nodal staging of women with invasive breast cancer, sparing 77 percent of women without evidence of micrometastasis in their SLN the morbidity and expense of a complete node dissection.

Fisher and colleagues[13] studied preliminary axillary node sampling with intraoperative reporting of imprint cytology to detect positive nodes in 50 consecutive patients with T1 and T2 breast cancer. Patients undergoing axillary clearance had histologically positive nodes in 21 (42 percent) of cases.[13] This study showed that a sample of four axillary lymph nodes examined by imprint cytology detected nodal metastases. Imprint cytology failed to identify only 1 of 51 positive nodes, with 84 percent of sampled nodes containing tumor in node-positive patients. False negative results occurred in 1 of 10 and 1 of 17 positive nodes. In Fisher's study,[13] imprint cytology detected tumor cells that could not be shown by any other method, including immunostaining for epithelial cell membranes and cytokeratin. In addition, operative time for their procedure was limited to 10 minutes, and random cytological sampling of the axillary nodes but no lymphatic mapping was used. We suggest that if our lymphatic mapping techniques, including preoperative lymphoscintigraphy and a combination of intraoperative injection of a vital blue dye and radiocolloid, are used in a complementary style with imprint cytology, there would be an even higher rate of diagnostic accuracy. In addition, SLNs may be examined later and in more detail with serial sectioning, immunohistochemical staining, and perhaps reverse transcriptase–polymerase chain reaction analysis with keratin markers.[32, 55] Inevitably, this will upstage some breast cancer patients that heretofore had been deemed histological node negative to the pathologist and provide a more accurate staging for prognosis and treatment decisions.

Based on our study and those of Fisher and associates[13] and Quill and associates,[37] imprint cytologic examination is unaffected by lymphazurin blue dye or other mapping agents and is able to detect minimal disease. Lymphatic mapping selectively samples the axilla in women with breast cancers, providing accurate nodal staging and at the same time decreasing the morbidity for the patient and the expense for the health care system.[13, 22, 26] Clearly, the wave of the future is to perform in the same operative setting intraoperative imprint cytology for the diagnosis and evaluation of the margins of lumpectomy specimens as well as a limited axillary lymph node sampling with imprint cytology of the node.

DISCUSSION

Management Recommendations Based on Cytology Reports

The diagnostic categories used in reporting intraoperative cytologic diagnosis are unsatisfactory, negative, atypical, suspicious, or malignant. From a surgical management point of view, atypical diagnoses are considered as benign, whereas suspicious diagnoses are malignant. Thus, margin(s) with suspicious or malignant findings require additional intraoperative resection until a negative report is obtained.

The clinical management of breast masses should first include mammographic evaluation. Fine-needle aspiration biopsy should be performed for all palpable masses. Benign lesions or cysts can be followed. Even in the presence of negative or atypical cytologic findings, clinically suspicious lesions should undergo excisional biopsy with intraoperative imprint cytology. An unsatisfactory report should prompt the physician to repeat FNAB or perform excisional biopsy with intraoperative imprint cytology if clinically indicated. Those lesions reported as malignant by FNAB or imprint cytology can undergo definitive lumpectomy or mastectomy. This scheme allows FNAB and imprint cytology to be used in a complementary fashion. In addition, by obtaining a diagnosis of breast cancer with FNAB in palpable lesions or stereotactic biopsy for mammographic abnormalities, efferent lymphatic flow from the primary breast cancer is preserved. Lymphatic mapping and SLN biopsy techniques that sample the axilla can then be accepted as much more reliable and accurate.

Role in Breast Conservation Therapy

Cosmesis and cytologic negative margins are essential for successful breast conservation therapy. Breast conservation is offered in most cancer centers; however, management of the primary lesion and the axillary lymph nodes differs. Variations begin with initial biopsy or FNAB for diagnosis, followed by lumpectomy with re-excision for positive margins. The axilla may be managed with lymphatic mapping for node sampling or full dissection based on protocols. Where imprint cytology is offered, the diagnosis and treatment of stage I and II breast cancers can be completed in one operation.

The extent of radiation to be given is often determined by tumor characteristics and the number of nodes involved.[3, 16, 20, 34] Additional boost radiation to the affected quadrant is routinely used unless it is determined to be clinically unnecessary based on tumor histology or size. Definite knowledge of a nega-tive tumor bed in low-grade lesions may spare some patients from toxic boost doses.[20] Complications of radiation include edema, retraction, and pain to the breast. Radiation in some patients may significantly change the appearance and consistency of the breast so that it is difficult to assess for local recurrence. Imprint cytology of the margins can thus be used to guide radiation therapy recommendations.[3, 20, 34]

Examination of cytological imprints from lymph nodes has been shown to be useful for intraoperative staging in patients with breast cancer.[13, 51] Combined axillary node sampling with intraoperative reporting of cytological imprints from nodes can spare the node-negative patient from unnecessary complete lymphadenectomy. The imprint cytology technique is also an excellent adjunct to lumpectomy with lymphatic mapping, because it eliminates possible radiation contamination of equipment produced during frozen section.

SUMMARY

Intraoperative imprint cytology provides a rapid, reliable, and topographically accurate evaluation of lumpectomy margins. It overcomes sampling errors and artifacts of frozen section. The evaluation is more thorough, rapid, and accurate than frozen section and conventional histological techniques. False positive results may be encountered with imprint cytology, but these are usually "false-false" positive results caused by multifocal cancer not detected by frozen or permanent histological section of selected margins.[6, 28] However, imprint cytology may be complemented by frozen sections, especially with infiltrating lobular cancers.[58] Overall, when imprint cytology is used, local recurrence is lower (2.27 percent) than with conventional histology (13.5 percent). This becomes important because the goal of any lumpectomy program is to effectively treat cancer while preserving the breast. Local recurrences after lumpectomy and radiation therapy are best handled by salvage mastectomy. In addition, imprint cytology is exquisitely sensitive for evaluation of the comedocarcinoma DCIS in lumpectomy margins without necessity for frozen section. Imprint cytology is also an excellent tool for the diagnosis of needle-localized breast biopsies.

The cytological examination of the SLN in radioguided lymphatic specimens may avoid reoperation and radiation contamination. The cost effectiveness of imprint cytology is proved by fewer frozen sections, fewer re-excisions, fewer salvage mastectomies, minimal equipment and supplies, and fewer personnel. These significant advantages should be considered in the current and future management of breast conservation.

References

1. Acosta JA, Greenlee JA, Gubler KD: Surgical margins after needle-localization breast biopsy. Am J Surg 170:643–646, 1995.

2. Al-Kaisi N: The spectrum of the "gray zone" in breast cytology: A review of 186 cases of atypical and suspicious cytology. Acta Cytol 38:898–908, 1994.

3. Anscher MS, Jones P, Prosnitz LR, Blackstock W, et al: Local failure and margin status in early stage breast carcinoma treated with conservation surgery and radiation therapy. Ann Surgery 218:22–28, 1993.

4. Carter D: Margins of lumpectomy for breast cancer. Hum Pathol 17:330–332, 1986.

5. Cox CE, Ku NN, Reintgen DS, et al: Touch preparation cytology of breast lumpectomy margins with histologic correlation. Arch Surg 126:490–493, 1991.

6. Cox CE, Greenberg H, Fleisher D, et al: Natural history and clinical evaluation of the lumpectomy scar. Am Surg 59:55–59, 1993.

7. De las Morenas A, Clips POP, Moroz K, Donnelly MM: Cytologic diagnosis of ductal versus lobular carcinoma of the breast. Acta Cytol 39:865–876, 1994.

8. DeRosa G, Boschi IT, Boscaino A, Petrella O, Vetrani A, Palombim L, Pettinato O. Intraoperative cytology in breast cancer diagnosis, comparison between cytologic and frozen section techniques. Diagn Cytopathol 9:623–631, 1993.

9. Dixon JM, Ravi Sekar O, Walsh J, et al: Specimen oriented radiography helps define excision margins of malignant lesions detected by breast cancer screening. Br J Surg 80:1001–1002, 1993.

10. Fischer ER, Constantino, Fisher B: Pathologic findings from the national surgical adjuvant breast project. Cancer 71:2141–2150, 1993.

11. Fisher B, Wickerham DL, Deutsch M, et al: Breast tumor recurrence following lumpectomy with and without breast irradiation: An overview of recent NSABP findings. Semin Surg Oncol 8:153–160, 1992.

12. Fisher B, Redmond C, Poisson IT, et al: Eight year results of a randomized clinical trial comparing total mastectomy and lumpectomy with or without irradiation in the treatment of breast cancer. N Engl J Med 320:822–828, 1989.

13. Fisher CJ, Boyle S, Burke M, Price AB: Intraoperative assessment of nodal status in the selection of patients with breast cancer for axillary clearance. Br J Surg 80:457–448, 1993.

14. Frazier TG, Wong WYR, Rose D: Implications of accurate pathologic margins in the treatment of primary breast cancer. Arch Surg 124:37–38, 1989.

15. Gal R: Scrape cytology assessment of margins of lumpectomy specimens in breast cancer. Acta Cytol 36:838–839, 1992.

16. Ghossein NA, Alpert S, Barba J, Pressman P: Breast cancer: Importance of adequate surgical excision prior to radiotherapy in the local control of breast cancer in patients treated conservatively. Arch Surg 127:411–415, 1992.

17. Graham RA, Homer MJ, Sigler CJ, et al: The efficacy of specimen radiography in evaluating the surgical margins of impalpable breast carcinoma. AJR 162:33–36, 1994.

18. Giuliano AE, Kirgan DM, Guenther MD, et al: Lymphatic mapping and sentinel lymphadenectomy for breast cancer. Ann Surg 220:391–401, 1994.

19. Harris JR, Connolly JL, Schnitt SJ, Cady B, Love S, Osteen RT, Panerson WB, Shirley IT, Heliran S, Cohen IT, Silen W: The use of pathologic features in selecting the extent of surgical resection necessary for breast cancer patients by primary radiation. Ann Surg 201:164–169, 1985.

20. Hartsell WF, Kelly CA, Greim KL, et al: Breast-conserving therapy: A boost of radiation therapy is not necessary when negative margins of excision are achieved. Breast Cancer Treat Res 27:190, 1993.

21. IZI Corporation, Suite 334 1498-M Reistertown Road, Baltimore, Maryland 21208.

22. Reintgen DS, Joseph E, Lyman GH: The role of selective lymphenectomy in breast cancer. Cancer Control Journal 4:112–125, 1997.

23. KI Ukie TS, et al: Appraisal of cytomorphologic analysis of common carcinomas of the breast. Diagn Cytopathol 1:188–193, 1985.

24. Klimberg VS, Westbrook KC, Korourian SR: Use of touch preps for diagnosis and surgical margins in breast cancer. Proceedings from Annual Cancer Symposia, Society of Surgical Oncology. March 1996.

25. Kline TS, Kline IK: Breast. *In* Guide to Clinical Aspiration Biopsy. New York, Igaku-Shoin, 1989, pp 1–7.

26. Krag DN, Weaver DL, Alex JC, et al: Surgical resection and radiolocalization of the sentinel node in breast cancer using a gamma probe. Surg Oncol 2:335–340, 1993.

27. Ku NNK, Nicosia SY: Role of cytopathology in the management of breast cancer. Cancer Control 1:402–408, 1994.

28. Ku NNK, Cox CE, Reingten DS, et al. Cytology of lumpectomy specimens. Acta Cytol 35:417–421, 1991.

29. Ku NNK, Cox CE, Reintgen DS, Greenberg IN, Nicosia SV: Local recurrence after cytological evaluation of lumpectomy margins: A follow-up of 520 breast cancers. Lab Invest 70:17a, 1994.

30. Morton DL, Wen DR, Wong JH, et al: Technical details of intraoperative lymphatic mapping for early stage melanoma. Arch Surg 127:392–399, 1992.

31. Nicosia SV, Williams JA, Horowitz SA, et al: Fine needle aspiration biopsy of palpable breast lesions: Review and statistical analysis of 1875 cases. Surg Oncol 2:145–160, 1993.

32. Noguchi M, Masahide M, Mitsuharu E, et al: Intraoperative histologic assessment of surgical margins and lymph node metastasis in breast-conserving surgery. J Surg Oncol 60:185–190, 1995.

33. Pelosi G, Bresaola E, Rodella S, et al: Expression of proliferating cell nuclear antigen, Ki-67 antigen, estrogen receptor protein, and tumor suppressor P53 gene in cytologic scrapings of breast cancer: An immunocytochemical study with clinical, pathobiological and histological correlations. Cytopathol 11:131–140, 1994.

34. Pezner RD, Wagman LD, Ben-Ezra J, Odom-Maryon T: Breast conservation therapy: Local tumor control in patients with pathologically clear margins who receive 5000 cGy breast irradiation without local boost. Breast Cancer Treat Res 32:261–267, 1994.

35. Pilar P, Rubenstone A: A correlation of breast imprints (stained by the methods of papanicolaou) and tissue sections. Acta Cytol 12:462–472, 1968.

36. Pittinger TP, Marionian NC, Poulter CA, Peacock JL: Importance of margin status in outcome of breast-conserving surgery for carcinoma. Surgery 116:605–609, 1994.

37. Quill R, Leahy A, Lawler R, Finney R: Lymph node imprint cytology for the rapid assessment of axillary node metastases in breast cancer. Br J Surg 69:282, 1984.

38. Renton SC, Gazet JC, Ford HT, Corbishley C, Sutcliffe R: The importance of the resection margin in conservative surgery for breast cancer. Eur J Surg Oncol 22:17–22, 1996.

39. Rubin P, O'Hanlon D, Browell D, Callanan K, et al: Tumor bed biopsy detects the presence of multifocal disease in patients undergoing breast conservation therapy for primary breast carcinoma. Eur J Surg Oncol 22:23–26, 1996.

40. Sauter ER, Hoffman JP, Ottery FD, Kowalyshyn MJ, Litwin S, Eisenberg BL: Is frozen section analysis of reexcision lumpectomy margins worthwhile? Cancer 73:2607–2612, 1994.

41. Schnitt SJ, Abner A, Gelman R, et al: The relationship between microscopic margins of resection and the risk of local recurrence in patients with breast cancer treated with breast-conserving surgery and radiation therapy. Cancer 74:1746–1751, 1994.

42. Schnitt SJ, Connolly JL: Processing and evaluation of breast excision specimens: A clinically oriented approach. Am J Clin Pathol 98:125–137, 1992.

43. Shabaik AS, Cox CE, Clark RA, Reintgen DS: Imprint cytology of needle-localized breast lesions. Acta Cytol: 36:11–14, 1992.

44. Shidham VB, Nandkumar DV, Grover S, Kher AV: Role of scrape cytology in rapid intraoperative diagnosis. Acta Cytol 23:477–482, 1983.

45. Silva EG, Kraemer BB: The examination of margins of resection by frozen section: Part I. Surg Pathol 1:303-306, 1988.

46. Silverman IF: Breast. *In* Bibbo M (ed): Comprehensive Cytopathology. Philadelphia, WB Saunders, 1991, pp 703–710.

47. Smitt MC, Jeffrey S, Carlson RC, et al: The importance of the lumpectomy surgical margin status in breast conservation. Breast Cancer Treat Res 32:30, 1995.

48. Smitt MC, Nowels KW, Zbedlick MJ, Jeffrey S, et al: The importance of the lumpectomy surgical margin status in long term results of breast conservation. Cancer 76:259–267, 1995.

49. Solin LJ, Fowble B, Martz K, et al: Results of reexcisional biopsy of the primary tumor in preparation for definitive irradation of patients with early stage breast cancer. Int J Radiat Oncol Biol Phys 12:721–725, 1986.

50. Spivak B, Khanna MM, Tafra L, Juillard G, Giuliano AE: Margin status and local recurrence after breast-conserving surgery. Arch Surg 129:952–957, 1994.

51. Suen K, Wood W, Syed A, Quenville N, Clement P: Role of imprint cytology in intraoperative diagnosis: Value and limitations. J Clin Pathol 3:328–337, 1978.

52. Tribe C: Cytological diagnosis of breast tumors by imprint method. J Clin Pathol 18:31, 1965.

53. Tribe C: A comparison of rapid methods including imprint diagnosis for the diagnosis of breast tumors. J Clin Pathol 26:273–277, 1973.

54. Van Dogen JA, Bartelink H, Fentiman IS, et al: Factors influencing local relapse and survival and results of salvage treatment after breast-conserving therapy in operable breast cancer: EORTC Trial 10801. Breast conservation compared with mastectomy in TNM stage I and II breast cancer. Eur J Cancer 28A:801–805, 1992.

55. Veneti S, Oannl ou-Mouzaka L, Toufexi H, Xenitides J, Anastasiadis P: Imprint cytology: A rapid, reliable method of diagnosing breast malignancy. Acta Cytol 40:649–652, 1996.

56. Veronesi U, Liuni A, Galimberti V, et al: Conservation approaches for the management of stage I/II carcinoma of the breast: Milan Cancer Institute trials. World J Surg 18:70–78, 1994.

57. Wells C, Heyet A, Brochier J, Gatter KC, Mason D: The immunocytochemical detection of axillary micrometastases in breast cancer. Br J Cancer 50:193–197, 1984.

58. Yeatman TJ, Cantor AB, Smith TJ, et al: The tumor biology of infiltrating lobular carcinoma: Implications for management. Ann Surg 222:549–561, 1995.

59. Zanfrani B, Vielh P, Fourquet A, et al: Conservative treatment of early breast cancer: Prognostic value of the ductal in situ component and other pathological variables on local control and survival. Eur J Cancer Clin Oncol 25:1645–1650, 1989.

CHAPTER 59
CHOICE OF OPERATIONS FOR EARLY BREAST CANCER: AN EXPANDING ROLE FOR BREAST CONSERVATION INSTEAD OF MASTECTOMY

Blake Cady, M.D.

SELECTION OF THERAPY IN EARLY BREAST CANCER

The definition of early breast cancer has been controversial and is not completely agreed upon[82]; for this chapter it will include breast cancers that could be expected to have a better than 75 percent disease-free survival rate at 10 years. This would include noninvasive cancers (T0) and T1 N0 M0 and T1 N1 M0 invasive cancers (Table 59–1).[3] This arbitrary definition is chosen deliberately to highlight the surgeon's role in treating the current preponderance of breast cancer patients, and to emphasize the choice of operations, adjuvant treatment selection, the decision process regarding the management of the breast cancer itself, the breast as the host organ, and the patient with breast cancer. The roles of adjuvant chemotherapy and hormone therapy are presented in other chapters.

Primary breast cancer management is becoming increasingly complex, with rapid changes in management policy based on maturing clinical trials, new data, rapid improvement in clinical presentation resulting from mammographic screening, the development of cellular prognostic indicators that may enable more specific treatment selection, and an increased biological understanding. Because of this management complexity, patient involvement in decision making is critical. Surgeons must accept that patient involvement requires a great deal of time in presentation and explanation of data as well as empathy and understanding about the complexity of decision-making responsibility and the anxiety patients face. When surgeons are well informed and willing to address their patients as individuals and include them in management decisions, and when adequate pathology sophistication and radiotherapy units are available, modern breast cancer management can be conducted in any setting. Most patients today are informed through the public media and personal contacts about varying opinions and options in breast cancer management, and surgeons who do

not explicitly recognize this management complexity when talking to their patients invite a loss of confidence and a search for second opinions and other consultations. Dogmatic approaches to the management of early primary breast cancer ought to be avoided, and surgeons who recommend only local excision are as unlikely to be believed as those that suggest only mastectomy. Because the details of local breast cancer removal and management of the tissue specimen are critical to the conduct of contemporary breast cancer therapy, it is urged that surgeons develop special skill in and knowledge of breast-preserving therapy. The purposes of breast-preservation therapy are cosmetic appearance, maintenance of femininity, and comfortable sexual relations. It is vital that the details of the local breast cancer removal be well thought out and as precise as possible. Eventual results of breast-preserving surgery, cosmetic and clinical, are more critically related to technical surgical factors than results of mastectomy.

Careful handling of the tissue specimen is important to outcome, as is a good professional relationship with the patient. A collegial relationship with the pathologist is essential to acquire complete data for decision making, and there is increasing need for sophisticated analysis of the pathology because of decreasing size of the mass at diagnosis and the development of new prognostic markers. At present, there are no standards of pathological analysis of regional lymph nodes, and increasingly detailed ad hoc study of them has thrown the implication of what a "positive" lymph node is into confusion, when it is only a micrometastasis detected by histochemical staining. A pathology report containing a check list of every important feature is the best method of communication between pathologist and surgeon.

The contemporary approach to therapy selection in breast cancer, when true surgical options exist, involves the patient who must make the ultimate decision about breast preservation and, consequently, assume some of the associated risks and responsibilities of the decisions made. A thoughtful, open, and empathetic approach to patients yields enormous

TABLE 59–1. TNM BREAST CANCER CLASSIFICATION SYSTEM

Primary Tumor

TX		Primary tumor cannot be assessed
T0		No evidence of primary tumor
Tis		Carcinoma *in situ:* intraductal carcinoma, lobular carcinoma *in situ,* or Paget's disease of the nipple with no tumor
T1		Tumor 2 cm or less in greatest dimension
	T1a	0.5 cm or less in greatest dimension
	T1b	More than 0.5 cm but not more than 1 cm in greatest dimension
	T1c	More than 1 cm but not more than 2 cm in greatest dimension
T2		Tumor more than 2 cm but not more than 5 cm in greatest dimension
T3		Tumor more than 5 cm in greatest dimension
T4		Tumor of any size with direct extension to chest wall or skin
	T4a	Extension to chest wall
	T4b	Edema (including peau d'orange) or ulceration of the skin of the breast or satellite skin nodules confined to the same breast
	T4c	Both (T4a and T4b)
	T4d	Inflammatory carcinoma

Regional Lymph Node

NX	Regional lymph nodes cannot be assessed (e.g., previously removed)
N0	No regional lymph node metastasis
N1	Metastasis to moveable ipsilateral axillary lymph nodes
N2	Metastasis to ipsilateral axillary lymph nodes fixed to one another or to other structures
N3	Metastasis to ipsilateral internal mammary lymph nodes

Pathological Classification (pN)

pNX		Regional lymph nodes cannot be assessed (e.g., previously removed or not removed for pathological study)
pN0		No regional lymph node metastasis
pN1		Metastasis to moveable ipsilateral axillary lymph nodes
	pN1a	Only micrometastasis (none larger than 0.2 cm)
	pN1b	Metastasis to lymph nodes, any larger than 0.2 cm
	pN1bi	Metastasis in 1 to 3 lymph nodes, any more than 0.2 cm, and all less than 2 cm in greatest dimension
	pN1bii	Metastasis to 4 or more lymph nodes, any more than 0.2 cm, and all less than 2 cm in greatest dimension
	pN1biii	Extension of tumor beyond the capsule of a lymph node metastasis less than 2 cm in greatest dimension
	pN1biv	Metastasis to a lymph node 2 cm or more in greatest dimension
pN2		Metastasis to ipsilateral axillary lymph nodes that are fixed to one another or to other structures
pN3		Metastasis to ipsilateral internal mammary lymph nodes

Distant Metastasis

MX	Presence of distant metastasis cannot be assessed
M0	No distant metastasis
M1	Distant metastasis (includes metastasis to ipsilateral supraclavicular lymph nodes)

Stage Grouping

Stage 0	Tis	N0	M0
Stage I	T1	N0	M0
Stage IIA	T0	N1*	M0
	T1	N1	M0
	T2	N0	M0
Stage IIB	T2	N1	M0
	T3	N0	M0
Stage IIIA	T0	N2	M0
	T1	N2	M0
	T2	N2	M0
	T3	N1, N2	M0
Stage IIIB	T4	Any N	M0
	Any T	N3	M0
Stage IV	Any T	Any N	M1

*Note: The prognosis of patients with N1a is similar to that of patients with pN0.
Used with the permission of the American Joint Committee on Cancer (AJCC®), Chicago, Illinois. The original source for this material is the AJCC Manual for Staging of Cancer, 4th edition (1992) published by JB Lippincott, Philadelphia.

benefits in their satisfaction and positive attitudes about outcome, and also in our professional gratification of guiding women through a difficult experience, with implicit threats of mortality, physical disfigurement, and perceived loss of sexual appeal. This patient involvement should continue throughout the entire therapeutic process; patients frequently will want guidance from their surgeon regarding radia-

tion therapy or adjuvant systemic therapy. The surgeon, then, should be knowledgeable enough to be involved in these decisions and in the careful, detailed follow-up so important to patients selecting breast preservation. Few nonsurgeons are comfortable with or skilled in examining patients after breast preservation, particularly if the patients have also had radiation therapy. Therefore, continued follow-up by the original operating surgeon is extremely important for sophisticated cancer management and is very comforting to patients. Such careful follow-up is in danger of being refused by insurance company plans that are too focused on their gatekeeper function. Cancer specialists are usually more cost effective because they can confidently avoid expensive technology.

NONINVASIVE AND MARKER LESIONS

There is an increasing incidence of benign breast pathology that defines a risk of later invasive breast cancer but by itself carries no connotations of reduced survival. This has occurred because of widespread screening mammography. Four such histological entities must be addressed: ductal carcinoma *in situ* (DCIS), lobular carcinoma *in situ* (LCIS), atypical ductal hyperplasia (ADH), and atypical lobular hyperplasia (ALH). Other lesions, such as sclerosing adenosis, have some implication of increased risk of later breast cancer, but of a lower order of magnitude. Although they are not dealt with here, general principles of risk apply.

Ductal Carcinoma *In Situ*

Ductal carcinoma *in situ* is being encountered with increasing frequency as a result of the expanding use of screening mammography.[12, 89] In the premammography era, these lesions made up only 1 to 2 percent of palpable breast cancers.[5, 81] In recent studies, DCIS may make up to 20 percent of all breast cancers, and in some reports, more than 40 percent of all breast cancers detected only by mammography.[12, 51, 64, 86, 89, 94] With continued rapid expansion of mammographic screening programs, cases of DCIS may be diagnosed more frequently; patients will view DCIS as cancer with accompanying concerns about death, but the surgeons will recognize it as a lesion that carries a virtually 100 percent cure. Before mammography, the DCIS diagnosed was a large palpable comedocarcinoma or a tiny lesion discovered accidentally in the process of biopsy for other reasons.[81] The vast majority were not only palpable but frequently several centimeters in diameter. Even at that relatively advanced extent of intraductal carcinoma, if no invasive component was found, the prognosis for the patient undergoing mastectomy approached 100 percent freedom from disease.[44] Now that small, nonpalpable DCIS lesions are frequently found by mammography, a re-evaluation of our traditional approach of mastectomy for noninvasive ductal carcinoma has been accepted. At a time when mastectomy is not routinely required for invasive breast cancers, it is increasingly illogical to routinely perform mastectomy for noninvasive cancers.[102]

Important work has been done on the pathology, biological behavior, and outcome of breast-preserving surgery of DCIS by Lagios and colleagues[51] and many others.[28, 44, 55, 69, 89] In a series of papers culminating

in a summary report in 1989,[55] Lagios empirically divided DCIS into lesions 25 mm or less and 26 mm or more in diameter, after extensive pathological analysis involving meticulous whole organ sectioning of mastectomies for DCIS. The median diameter of the small lesions was 8 mm (akin to mammographically discovered DCIS), whereas the median diameter of the larger lesions was 50 mm (consistent with premammographic, large, palpable DCIS). In 115 patients undergoing mastectomy after a biopsy diagnosis of DCIS, the breasts were carefully studied by whole organ sections. There were no areas of microinvasion in the small lesions, but there was a 29 percent incidence of microinvasion in the larger lesions. Only two patients had positive axillary lymph nodes in these mastectomy specimens. They had occult invasion and DCIS more than 68 mm in diameter, and both patients had micrometastases in one lymph node. Almost half of the larger DCIS lesions had multifocal disease, whereas only an occasional smaller lesion was thus classified. Lagios and colleagues[52] subsequently treated a series of 79 patients[37, 103] with local excision only for DCIS lesions 25 mm or smaller that were detected mammographically by microcalcifications; there were 11 recurrences (14 percent). Six (55 percent) were DCIS only and occurred a median of 13 months (range, 9 to 25 months) after the local excision; none exceeded 23 mm in diameter. All these patients were living, and only one patient selected a mastectomy for treatment of the recurrent DCIS. Five patients (45 percent) had an invasive carcinoma as the recurrence a median of 36 months (range, 18 to 87 months) after the initial DCIS excision; all these lesions were 13 mm or less in diameter. These patients for the most part underwent mastectomy, although repeat local excision would certainly have been possible, and all were living free of disease at the time of the report.

Among the initial 20 patients in this series who were followed for a minimum of 80 months and a median of 118 months, there have been four recurrences (20 percent), whereas for the last 59 patients, there have been seven recurrences (12 percent) during a median 4-year follow-up (range 1 to 80 months). Thus, based on this initial therapeutic trial, it would

TABLE 59–2. STUDIES OF DUCTAL CARCINOMA *IN SITU* TREATED WITH WIDE EXCISION ALONE

Reference	No. of Patients	Mean Follow-up (months)	Recurrence No. (%)	Invasive (%)
Arnesson et al	38	60	5 (13)	40
Carpenter et al	28	38	5 (18)	20
Lagios et al	79	124	13 (16)	46
Schwartz et al	72	49	11 (15)	27
Silverstein et al	26	56	2 (8)	50
Fisher et al (B-06)	21	83	9 (43)	56
Fisher et al (B-17)	391	43	64 (16)	50

From Hetelekidis S, Schnitt SJ, Morrow M, Harris JR: Management of ductal carcinoma in situ. CA Cancer J Clin 45:244–253, 1995.

TABLE 59–3. STUDIES OF DUCTAL CARCINOMA *IN SITU* TREATED WITH EXCISION AND RADIATION THERAPY

Reference	No. of Patients	Mean Follow-up (months)	Recurrence No. (percent)	Invasive (percent)
Hiramatsu et al.	76	74	7 (9)	57
McCormick et al.	54	36	10 (18)	30
Ray et al.	56	67	5 (9)	20
Silverstein et al.	103	56	10 (10)	50
Solin et al.	172	84	16 (9)	44
Stotter et al.	42	92	4 (9)	100
Fisher et al. (B-06)	27	83	2 (7)	50
Fisher et al. (B-17)	399	43	28 (7)	40

From Hetelekidis S, Schnitt SJ, Morrow M, Harris JR: Management of ductal carcinoma in situ. CA Cancer J Clin 45:244–253, 1995.

appear that the local recurrence rate in the breasts of women treated by local excision only for small DCIS may not exceed 20 percent even in long-term follow-up.[52] The later 59 patients constituted the first long-term prospective study of DCIS deliberately selected for local excision only of nonpalpable, mammographically detected lesions.

There are several retrospective reports of local excision for palpable lesions before the use of mammography in which the lesions were discovered by retrospective histological reclassification to be DCIS. These reports indicate higher recurrence rates, ranging from 20 percent to more than 50 percent,[23, 32, 69, 77] but because these lesions were not known to be DCIS, margins were uncertain and adequacy of excision was not known. Several retrospective studies report local recurrence rates from 12 percent to 30 percent for DCIS excision alone, but after better margin analysis and control.[52, 85, 89, 93] In other retrospective surveys, it appears that radiation therapy of locally excised, clinically manifest DCIS may reduce the recurrence rate considerably, perhaps by half.[15, 28, 30, 73, 104] Tables 59–2 and 59–3 summarize the published literature for DCIS treated by local excision with or without radiation therapy. These reports demonstrate higher recurrence rates with longer follow-up periods. The National Surgical Adjuvant Breast and Bowel Project (NSABP) protocol B-17[28] prospectively evaluated radiation to observation after lumpectomy for DCIS and concluded that all DCIS cases should receive radiotherapy. This trial was seriously flawed, however, with misassignment of cases by size and without recognition of separate pathological subcategories of DCIS. Overall, in-breast recurrence was reduced by 40 percent by radiotherapy with statistically significant prevention of invasive ductal carcinoma recurrence, whereas recurrent DCIS was not significantly reduced.

Several recent reports by Silverstein[89] and Lagios and Silverstein,[54] although neither prospective nor randomized, nevertheless demonstrate convincingly that the best contemporary characterization of DCIS can be achieved by assignment by nuclear grade, size, and surgical resection margin (Table 59–4). In a 10-year follow-up report, they demonstrated that high-grade DCIS, which made up 28 percent of cases, has a high rate of local recurrence (up to 80 percent) after breast preservation. This high recurrence rate could be reduced by about 50 percent by using radiation therapy to the preserved breast, but recurrence rates remained too high in some cases to be acceptable. In contrast, non–high-grade DCIS without necrosis made up 34 percent of cases and had a local recurrence rate of only 10 percent, and non–high-grade DCIS with necrosis made up 38 percent of all cases and had a local in-breast recurrence rate of about 20 percent. Both groups of patients with non–high-grade DCIS (without or with necrosis) undergoing breast preservation had no reduction in local recurrence rate by the addition of breast radiation. Thus, almost 75 percent of patients with DCIS had a low risk of in-breast recurrence after breast preservation and did not benefit from the addition of adjuvant breast radiotherapy. Silverstein's cases all had negative histological specimen margins and were less than 4 cm in diameter. His chapter in this book (Chapter 53) is an extensive study of DCIS, and the Van Nuys Prognostic Scoring System (VNPSS) (Table 59–4) is the best contemporary analysis of treatment and results that are to be achieved in DCIS.

Other reports also addressed the issue of local recurrence after breast-preserving therapy for DCIS and conclude that little is gained by the addition of adjunctive radiotherapy.[45, 54] One report indicated that the only factor increasing local recurrence after local excision alone of DCIS was the presence of a positive surgical margin of the excision specimen.[45] This report demonstrated only a 10 percent local in-breast recurrence rate in very carefully selected patients, all discovered by mammography.

TABLE 59–4. THE VAN NUYS PROGNOSTIC INDEX SCORING SYSTEM

Score	1	2	3
Size (mm)	≤15	16–40	≥41
Margin width (mm)	≥10	1–9	<1
Pathological classification	Non–high-grade without necrosis	Non–high-grade with necrosis	High grade with or without necrosis

One to three points are awarded for each of three different predictors of local breast recurrence (size, margin width, and pathological classification). Scores for each of the predictors are totaled to yield a Van Nuys Prognostic Index score ranging from a low of 3 to a high of 9.

From Silverstein MJ, Lagios MD, Craig PH, Waisman JR, Lewinsky BS, et al: A prognostic index for ductal carcinoma in situ of the breast. Cancer 77:2267–2274, 1996. Copyright © (1996) American Cancer Society. Reprinted by permission of Wiley-Liss, Inc., a subsidiary of John Wiley & Sons, Inc.

TABLE 59–5. GUIDELINES FOR THE EVALUATION OF PATIENTS BEING CONSIDERED FOR BREAST-CONSERVING TREATMENT WITH MAMMOGRAPHICALLY DETECTED NONPALPABLE LESIONS WITH MICROCALCIFICATIONS

1. Careful mammographic evaluation of the breast before biopsy, including magnification views, to delineate the extent of the microcalcifications.
2. Needle localization of the biopsy.
3. Specimen radiography, preferably with magnification views as well as contact views, to confirm that the lesion has been excised and to direct pathological sampling.
4. Careful gross description of the excised specimen by the pathologist.
5. Inking of the specimen margins by the pathologist before sectioning to facilitate evaluation of margins of permanent sections.
6. On microscopic examination, description of the relation of the calcifications to the lesion and the distance of the tumor from the inked margins of resection.
7. Postbiopsy mammography with magnification views to confirm that all suspicious microcalcifications have been removed.
8. Repeat excision of the primary site if residual microcalcifications are seen on postbiopsy mammography or if tumor involves margins of resection microscopically.

From Schnitt SJ, Silen W, Sadowsky NL, Connolly JL, Harris JR: Ductal carcinoma in situ (intraductal carcinoma) of the breast. N Engl J Med 318:898–903, 1988. Reprinted by permission.

Thus, for women who want to preserve their breasts, it seems reasonable and safe to treat small, mammographically discovered DCIS by local excision only, particularly if it is non–high grade, of small size, and with an adequate surgical margin.[54, 89] However, the patient must understand the risks of recurrence, and the criteria suggested by Schnitt and associates[84] should be followed. These criteria are presented in Table 59–5 and indicate a rational approach to the breast-conservation management of small mammographically discovered DCIS lesions. Of utmost importance are adequate margins in the inked specimen (>10 mm), complete removal of microcalcifications as demonstrated by a postexcision mammogram, patient desire, and careful follow-up. An important element of such breast-preserving surgery is explanation to the patient of all the risks, benefits, and potential problems. Discussions with patients and families require presentation of data, consideration of alternatives, an empathetic attitude, and a great deal of time.[20, 48] Repeated discussion sessions may be required. A rapid resolution of the clinical situation is not important, because the lesions are noninvasive, very small, and not life-threatening, because these are almost exclusively discovered by mammography. It is more important that the patient make a considered, thoughtful decision than adhere to some arbitrary time schedule. Roughly, the same number of patients will have an intact breast and be free of cancer at 10 years regardless of whether radiation therapy is used, even in those with small high-grade DCIS (Table 59–6). This apparent anomaly occurs because even if the local recurrence rate may be higher without adjunctive radiation, two

thirds of patients that do have recurrence can be treated again with lumpectomy and breast preservation, and if necessary, radiotherapy. Patients initially treated with radiotherapy, even if they have a lower recurrence rate, usually require mastectomy for the recurrence.

When the DCIS is of intermediate size, between 15 mm and 40 mm, separate decision making is required because risks of multifocal or multicentric disease may be higher, high-grade lesions are more common, negative surgical margins may be more difficult to achieve, and cosmetic results might be less satisfactory because of the larger tissue volume required for complete removal. Negative surgical margins, at least 1 cm in width, and a postexcision mammogram without residual calcification are essential, as are the other criteria suggested by Schnitt.[84] If these intermediate lesions are non–high grade, the addition of radiotherapy will probably not further reduce the low recurrence rate. However, if the lesion is high grade or a comedo type DCIS, recurrence rates may be high but are only reduced by half by adding radiation therapy to the preserved breast; thus, the patient may still have a substantial recurrence rate of 10 to 15 percent. Such patients will require careful counseling, and considered judgments, balancing the desire to preserve the breast against the recurrence rate, still emphasizing that the risk of death is very small, although not zero.

For DCIS lesions of larger size (>40 mm in diameter) or when adequate negative surgical margins cannot be achieved, mastectomy should be recommended with or without reconstruction. The recommendations generated by the VNPSS are the best current guidelines to therapy, although they seem to be too liberal with recommendations for radiotherapy.[54]

The incidence of lymph node metastases in such patients is no more than 2 or 3 percent and, if present, are usually only micrometastases. Thus, when mastectomy is required for DCIS, or because of patient desire, axillary dissection should not be performed, although a few low axillary nodes adjacent to the breast are frequently removed with the breast without a formal axillary dissection.

TABLE 59–6. BREAST CANCER RADIATION THERAPY AFTER BREAST CONSERVATION

		%	Intact Breast
No RT	100 patients: 30% local recurrence		
	15% new primary cancer		
	No further breast surgery	55	
	Recurrence or new primary	45	85%
	67% breast preservation	30	
Initial RT	100 patients: 15% local recurrence		
	10% new primary cancer		
	No further breast surgery	75	
	Recurrence or new primary	25	83%
	33% breast preservation	8	

Cost: Benefit; DCIS < 25 mm; comedo; adequate excision; management.

Particular prognostic or histological features associated with recurrence and with the more aggressive high-grade or progressive forms of DCIS have been reported. *NEU* oncogene overexpression has been described by a group from the Netherlands[99] as being exclusively associated with comedo-type DCIS, which, by implication, is more likely to have microinvasion,[55] to recur after local excision,[89] to exhibit progressive growth, and to be of high grade. Another report[91] confirms that high-grade histology is associated with a high rate of recurrence, even with adjunctive radiotherapy. Such specific prognostic indicators are important in understanding the genetics, biology, and progress of DCIS, particularly when of limited extent and in selecting therapy. It seems clear that the larger DCIS lesions of high grade or comedo-type are slated to progress (i.e., develop the clinical course to invasive ductal carcinoma) if not removed surgically. However, many of the small non–high-grade DCIS lesions currently detected by mammography, and of low VNPSS, may well be pathological curiosities, or be of very indolent growth pattern with little potential progression to invasive disease even if not removed, because they are found with considerable frequency in routine autopsy studies of patients dying of other causes.[65] Because these DCIS lesions are all categorized as breast cancer in tumor registries, the detection by mammography of large numbers of such DCIS lesions may alter reported incidence and survival rates of carcinoma of the breast; such biases may not be accurately assessed without a sophisticated analysis of cancer registry data. As in other hormone organ cancers, microscopic foci of noninvasive carcinoma are frequent and in many cases may be of no biological significance. However, it has been impossible up to the present to accurately predict which tiny DCIS lesions might have the potential for progressive growth and which are clinically unimportant, a situation similar to that in prostate[5] or thyroid[10] cancer. Because all these DCIS lesions are discovered only by excision, the debate may be academic, but the possible impact on cancer statistics must be appreciated.

One result of the large number of DCIS and small invasive cancers detected by mammography has been to produce highly speculative estimations of breast cancer incidence in American women. The media publicity estimating that one of eight women will develop breast cancer was based on two questionable statistical assumptions: that the sharp increase in incidence[62] (now shown to be a temporary artifact produced by mammographic screening)[66, 84, 103] would continue unabated into the future and that all women would live to be 100 years old. In addition, the speculation was estimated for the cohort of women born in 1990, and therefore would only apply in the mid to late twenty-first century! These incidence assumptions are unquestionably erroneous because the incidence of breast cancer peaked between 1987 and 1989 and is now declining sharply.[62] What the eventual incidence will be is unknown, but it certainly will be markedly lower than one in eight.

The most important principle to support the concept of local excision of small DCIS lesions has been to address the biological issue of whether extensive (large) DCIS is the result of a multifocal origin within the breast or is the result of progressive intraductal growth from a single focus that does not breach the basement membrane. The model of Paget's disease with progressive intraductal spread of cells even onto the surface of the nipple may be illustrative of this particular biological growth pattern of a significant proportion of DCIS. A recent exhaustive anatomical study from Japan of three-dimensional reconstructions of the ductal extent of DCIS accompanying invasive cancers offers a fascinating demonstration of the complex intraductal spread of noninvasive cancer throughout an anatomical unit of the breast.[67] These authors clearly demonstrated occasional extension to adjacent anatomical units of the breast through crossing or bridging lactiferous ducts to gain intraductal entrance to adjacent major lactiferous ducts. The conclusion of this study was that extensive ductal spread from a solitary initial focus is the most likely method of progressive growth of much, if not all, DCIS. Such an implication is substantiated by the relatively low recurrence rate of DCIS after only local excision. If multifocal or multicentric origin were common, a very high rate of new or recurrent DCIS would be expected in the breast surrounding the initial lumpectomy or in other regions of the breast.

Long-term follow-up results from the series reported by Lagios and Silverstein[54] and Silverstein and associates[89] reaffirm the absence or low likelihood of "multifocal" or "multicentric" DCIS in the breasts of women treated by local excision only and support the concept that DCIS arises as a single intraductal focus and spreads only intraductally initially in the majority of cases. If DCIS were truly a multifocal or multicentric lesion, the low recurrence rates reported by Lagios and Silverstein[54] and Silverstein and associates[89] over long-term follow-up would not be maintained, and recurrences would be multifocal and in other parts of the same breast (multicentric). This hypothesis of ductal spread from a single focus was first explicitly proposed by Gump and colleagues[37] and has subsequently been reiterated by others.[54, 89] Clearly, the most interesting biological information that will result from future trials of local excision of DCIS will be to solidify this assumption about the origin of extensive DCIS lesions, both high grade and non–high grade, particularly as screening mammography progressively cleans out the pool of patients with slowly evolving focal DCIS (prevalence screening).

Follow-up data are consistent with the assumption that high-grade DCIS is a true precursor or preinvasive lesion in most if not all cases; when later invasive disease occurs, it appears in the same breast and in the same quadrant. The risk of later invasive cancer occurring in the ipsilateral breast after local excision can be estimated and is presented in Table 59–7.[89] This continuing risk is probably at least 2

TABLE 59–7.   ESTIMATED OUTCOME IN PATIENTS WITH HIGH-RISK, NONINVASIVE BREAST PATHOLOGY TREATED BY LOCAL EXCISION

Histology	Family History	Incidence of Invasive Cancer (%)		Maximum Estimated 20-Year Mortality if Breast Preserved (%)
		Annually	*At 20 Years*	
ADH ⎫	No	0.5	10	1
ALH ⎭	Yes	1	20	2
LCIS	No	1	20	2
	Yes	2	40	4
DCIS	No	2	40	4
	Yes	(4)	(60 at 15 yrs)	(6)

( ) = no data available—author's estimate.

percent per year for high-grade DCIS, although it may abate after a decade. This risk is increased and probably doubled by the presence of a family history of premenopausal breast cancer. The specific high-grade pathological subtype adds to the predictability of invasive cancer recurrence, as suggested by the data of Lagios and associates,[55] van de Vijver and associates,[99] and Silverstein and colleagues.[89]

However, of most concern and importance is not the risk of later noninvasive or invasive breast cancer, but the risk of ever dying from a later cancer that would not have occurred if the breast had been sacrificed initially. Clearly, risk of death is only a small fraction of the recurrent invasive cancer incidence if patients are followed carefully and subjected to regular screening mammography.[86] Estimates of eventual death risk are extrapolated from survival rates achieved by screening programs such as Breast Cancer Detection Demonstration Project (BCDDP),[86] Health Insurance Plan of Greater New York (HIP),[87] and more contemporary trials of mammographic screening[95, 96] and are probably less than 5 percent of *the cancers discovered by screening*.[86] In addition, it is assumed that 10 percent of new breast cancers would not be detected by screening programs and that these "interval cancers" may well carry a worse prognosis (50 percent survival).[40] Thus, at most, 5 percent of patients having cancers detected by screening will die, as will one half of the 10 percent not detected (5 percent), so that total risk of death will be no more than 10 percent (and may well be less) of the patients who actually develop invasive cancer recurrence after breast preservation. Table 59–6 gives the authors' estimate of the risk of developing invasive cancer and the risk of dying that would not have occurred if a mastectomy had been performed for DCIS, and the other lesions that communicate increased risk of developing breast cancer.

Lobular Carcinoma *In Situ*

Another noninvasive breast lesion of importance is LCIS. From reports in the literature[38, 79] and a collective review,[31] it seems clear that LCIS is a marker lesion for patients at high risk of developing breast cancer and not an explicit precursor lesion for the later local development of invasive carcinoma. This

can be appreciated by the fact that later-appearing breast cancers are as likely to be in the contralateral breast as in the ipsilateral breast, and in the ipsilateral breast, they are more likely to be in a different quadrant than the original biopsy that revealed LCIS. Table 59–8 summarizes data from Haagensen and associates[38] illustrating this generalized risk. He preferred the term *lobular neoplasia* to LCIS to emphasize its risk effects rather than its precursor status.[39] This is in marked contrast to the data reported in DCIS, where recurrences appear in large measure in the ipsilateral breast and in the same quadrant of the ipsilateral breast as the original biopsy when local excision only is performed. The risk of later invasive carcinoma developing in patients with LCIS treated by local excision seems to be roughly 1 percent per year (see Tables 59–7 and 59–8). This risk is probably doubled if there is an associated family history of a first-degree relative with premenopausal breast cancer or a previous personal breast cancer.[31] Thus, patients with LCIS need careful analysis of other risk factors, including family history, before making decisions regarding treatment.

Two aspects of LCIS that re-emphasize the concept of a marker, rather than a precursor lesion, are the pathological types of invasive cancers that later develop and the age range at which LCIS occurs. In follow-up of patients with LCIS, invasive lobular carcinoma is not the predominant later cancer. Invasive ductal carcinoma is by far the most common subse-

TABLE 59–8.   INCIDENCE OF INVASIVE CANCER WHEN ORIGINAL LCIS WAS TREATED BY BIOPSY

Years After LCIS Diagnosis	No. at Risk	Cumulative Probability of Ipsilateral Breast Cancer (%)	Cumulative Probability of Contralateral Breast Cancer (%)
5	236	4	5
10	224	7	8
15	135	11	9
20	94	18	12
25	42	21	15

From Haagensen CD, et al (eds): Breast Carcinoma Risk and Detection. Philadelphia, WB Saunders, 1981, p 267. Reprinted by permission.

quent cancer, suggesting that the LCIS is not itself developing invasion and is not a precursor lesion. Furthermore, LCIS is found predominantly in premenopausal women. The incidence of LCIS in biopsies from postmenopausal women is not as high as in biopsies from premenopausal women.[31] Autopsy studies also indicate a declining incidence of LCIS with age.[65] Thus, the implication of the high risk associated with LCIS is manifest even after the apparent regression of the LCIS lesion itself, probably because of the influence of declining estrogen levels. More specific prognostic aspects of LCIS have not been reported, but clearly *BRCA* gene expression, DNA ploidy, histological variation, and other disease patterns need to be analyzed so that more specific individual prognostication can be made for patients with LCIS.

It seems illogical on the basis of the reports published thus far to treat LCIS by ipsilateral mastectomy, because risk is distributed throughout all breast tissue. The most logical therapeutic options are bilateral mastectomy, a prevention strategy to remove the vast majority of breast tissue at risk, or local excision only with meticulous follow-up. Surgical margins are irrelevant. Patients who have a diagnosis of LCIS with a strong family history, particularly of a premenopausal breast cancer in a first-degree relative, may opt for bilateral mastectomy (with or without reconstruction) with the assumption that the marker lesion of LCIS indicates a genetic pattern with a high probability of later invasive breast cancer. Whether genetic analysis of the *BRCA1* or *BRCA2* gene will add a dimension to advising such patients is currently not known but may be clinically available in the near future.

Whether multifocal LCIS or recurrent LCIS portends a still higher risk of later development of invasive carcinoma in the absence of a strong family history or other risk factors is unknown. It is apparent that if local excision only is performed for LCIS, the follow-up of such patients should be continued until age 75 years or so. Although data have only been reported for 20 years of follow-up,[31, 38] the risk may continue unabated at similar rates. Thus, with the 40-year life expectancy of a woman who first underwent biopsy in her forties, it would appear that the risk of later invasive cancer might approach 40 percent in the absence of a family history and be even higher if a positive family history is present. Such rates of invasive cancer are remarkably similar to *BRCA1* gene carriers in family clusters of breast cancer estimated to have an 80 percent chance of developing breast cancer by the age of 80.[90] The data presented indicate the need to discuss at length with patients the available therapeutic options and the risks involved when LCIS is treated by excision only. The long-term management of patients with LCIS treated by biopsy and observation clearly requires involvement by the patient and implies that the patient understands and assumes the risks involved and will adhere to careful follow-up screening. This should include annual mammography and physical examination to detect abnormalities. We must keep in mind, however, that although the risk of developing invasive cancer after LCIS may be high, the risk to a patient's life will be no more and probably considerably less than 10 percent of the cancer risk, given the assumption made for LDCIS previously. Table 59–7 indicates my interpretation of the risk of later invasive breast cancer and the probable maximum risk of dying of the breast cancers developing that would not have occurred if bilateral mastectomy had initially been elected for LCIS, and is based on the assumptions previously mentioned.

Atypical Ductal Hyperplasia and Atypical Lobular Hyperplasia

Atypical ductal hyperplasia and atypical lobular hyperplasia have been shown by Page and coworkers[70] and Dupont and Page[18] to also be indicators of risk for the later development of invasive carcinoma of the breast. This risk is apparently doubled by the addition of a first-degree relative with breast cancer; however, the details of the family history were not recorded in their articles, and thus the contrasting risks of premenopausal or postmenopausal first degree relatives were not distinguished. Interpretation of these articles and data indicates that the level of risk after biopsy only of ADH or ALH is roughly 10 percent at 20 years, or 0.5 percent per year cumulative risk, and roughly 20 percent at 20 years, or 1 percent per year cumulative, if there is a family history of breast cancer (see Table 59–7). The location of the later carcinomas that develop in such patients is ipsilateral in 56 percent of ADH patients and 69 percent of ALH patients, somewhat at variance from expectations based on DCIS and LCIS. Thus, whether ADH and ALH represent precursor lesions or marker lesions is not fully understood at the present time; however, there is clearly a substantial risk in the contralateral breast. Again, the fraction of patients who develop invasive cancer and who will actually die of it is very small, at most only 10 percent and probably only 5 percent of the cancers developing given the current effectiveness of screening (see Table 59–7). Although ADH and ALH make up less than 5 percent of benign breast lesions,[18, 70] they may mark a significant proportion of patients at risk for later development of invasive breast cancer. Ductal hyperplasia without atypia and stromal changes or nonproliferative ductal lesions is not associated with increased risks of invasive breast cancer during the 20-year follow-up period in the reports by Page and coworkers[70] and Dupont and Page[18] when treated by biopsy only. These studies cannot be overemphasized, because they now provide clearcut evidence that certain well-defined benign lesions serve as indicators for patients at higher risk of later invasive breast cancer but also point out that the great majority of benign breast lesions have no measurable impact on risk of later cancer. Patients with ADH or ALH will benefit from repeated screening, including yearly mammography and physical examination. Although these reports have not yet been confirmed by others, their comprehensive data seem to secure this viewpoint and interpretation. A previous review by Love and associates[59] pointed out the lack of risk generally associated with "fibrocystic disease" and brought into focus the epithelial component of breast changes that are associated with increased breast cancer risk. These assumptions of increased risk are logical also when it is appreciated that ADH is a precursor for DCIS. Indeed, the border between ADH and DCIS is controversial and not always reproducible.[57] The progression from ductal proliferation to ADH to DCIS is most likely a continuum, and at transition areas of this continuum, significant disagreements among pathologists occur that may lead to confusion in diagnosis and management recommendations. Pathological consultation is extremely useful in cases of ADH, ALH, LCIS, or DCIS, because alterations of diagnosis on review may considerably change therapeutic decisions. When consensus of diagnosis is not achieved, clinical evaluation and patient participation in decisions will need to be recognized. Just as not all DCIS proceeds on to invasive cancer, not all ADH or ALH proceeds on to DCIS or LCIS. Genetic aspects of these transitions are only beginning to be described.[90]

Therapeutic recommendations in ADH and ALH consist of local excision and careful follow-up, because mastectomy or bilateral mastectomy would be completely unjustified. In patients with a strong family history and other features such as cancer phobia, the marker lesions of ADH and ALH may in the future lead to further genetic studies. Whether the lesions of ADH and ALH that are multifocal, recurrent, or bilateral in nature alters the increased risk is yet to be elucidated. Attainment of negative surgical margins probably is not essential, but it must be realized that areas of DCIS may lie in or near areas of ADH. Therefore, if mammographic calcification remains or margins are extensively involved, wider excision should be considered. The majority of subsequent cancers are ductal; only 3 of 16 cancers (19 percent) occurring after ALH were lobular carcinomas.

Table 59–7 summarizes my interpretation of the risks involved for later development of invasive carcinoma in DCIS, LCIS, ADH, and ALH if treated by breast preservation. In discussion with patients, it is important to emphasize that the mere occurrence of invasive cancer after local excision for these lesions is not the critically important risk feature by which to evaluate decisions for breast-conservation therapy. The slight risk of death from cancer after breast preservation in contrast to the negligible risk after sacrifice of the breast should be the criterion for risk or acceptability of the limited surgical approach to these lesions and the basis on which discussion with patients should be undertaken.

Again, it should be emphasized that the woman's desire for breast preservation contrasted to the small extra risks of death in the distant future is the balance to be considered. If the surgeon is fearful of the risks of ipsilateral breast recurrence, the patient will be too; if the surgeon views these risks with equanimity as a reasonable price to pay for keeping the breasts intact, the patient very likely will not be alarmed either and will be able to make a less emotional, more considered, and more thoughtful decision.[20] Patients vary widely in their willingness to accept or avoid risk, as do surgeons. Many patients, and surgeons, seek out risky avocational interests such as skydiving, whereas others try to preserve the illusion of living a risk-free life. It should also be mentioned when discussing options with patients that unilateral or bilateral mastectomy used to treat LCIS or DCIS lesions and to prevent later invasive carcinoma is not uniformly successful and is itself not free of risk; cases of breast cancer developing after "preventive" mastectomy do occur; every bit of breast tissue cannot be removed even by radical mastectomy.

In summary, management recommendations to patients regarding ADH, ALH, LCIS, and DCIS should balance risks and benefits estimated from published data and as perceived by the patient; the surgeon should help by providing data, objectivity, empathy, and maturity of judgment. Surgical therapy can be selected by addressing particular attention to the details of the histology of the lesion removed, the family history and other risk factors of the patient (i.e., previous invasive or noninvasive breast cancer), the patient's desire to retain the breast, and the patient's comprehension of and willingness to assume risks associated with breast conservation. Careful detailed follow-up by the responsible surgeon with a willingness to perform a biopsy on any suspicious lesion that develops in breast tissue is required for such a program.

INVASIVE BREAST CANCER OF LIMITED EXTENT

The most recent criteria for carcinoma of the breast adopted by the American Joint Committee on Cancer (AJCC) emphasizes the importance of size in analysis of very early breast cancer (see Table 59–1). T1 lesions are separated into those 5 mm or less in diameter (T1a), those more than 5 mm but not over 10 mm in diameter (T1b), and those more than 10 mm but not more than 20 mm in diameter (T1c). Because size is the most important prognostic indicator in breast cancer, it is vital that all studies be sophisticated in analyzing cancer by size to be able to address new therapeutic issues such as suitability for local excision only without radiotherapy and the likely incidence of lymph node metastases. These small primary cancers are significantly increasing in incidence, with a progressively declining incidence of positive nodes since widespread adoption of breast mammography. The use of mammogram screening has not only reduced the proportion of advanced-stage cases by 25 to 50 percent but has also markedly increased the number of small invasive breast cancers.[11, 40, 58, 95] In the BCDDP study,[58, 86] 27 percent of patients had invasive breast cancers less than 1 cm in diameter. In a randomized clinical study, 36 percent of repeatedly screened patients had cancers of 1 cm or less in diameter, in contrast to only 10 percent of the control group.[40] Our recent reports[11, 12] indicate that the median maximum diameter of all invasive breast cancers seen between 1989 and 1993 was only 1.5 cm, and 29 percent were T1a or T1b. If the statistically significant slope of decreasing size (Fig. 59–1) continues with more widespread use of screening mammography, it can be predicted that within a decade, the median maximum diameter of all invasive breast cancer will be only 1 centimeter, a remarkable achievement for a public health initiative.

In the not too distant future, it can be expected that more than 50 percent of breast cancers will be a very early stage, either noninvasive (DCIS) or invasive and 1 cm or less in diameter (T1a and T1b). In addition, most of the remaining breast cancers will be between 1 cm and 2 cm in diameter with either negative nodes or with only a few axillary nodes involved. Sixty-nine percent of all patients with invasive breast cancer between 1989 and 1993 in our report had negative axillary lymph nodes, and only 10 percent of patients had more than three positive nodes.[11] Controlled trials of mammography screening in Sweden[95] and the Netherlands[14] have indicated a similar reduction in the stage of presentation (i.e., smaller size and fewer lymph node metastases) of breast cancers that were detected. Between 1981 and 1985, in one report, 75 percent of all patients with cancers detected by repeated screening were stage I.[40] All these trends indicate that the vast majority of patients in the future will be classified as having early breast cancer. Treatment guidelines for management of these patients must remain flexible during this time of rapidly changing stage of disease presentation, attitudes, and procedures, when so many patients will have long-term survival expectations of more than 90 or even 95 percent.

One of the most informative analyses of results that might be achieved in patients with early breast cancer was published by Rosen and associates in 1989.[78] These patients originally had palpable T1 primary cancers and either N0 or N1 axillas and have been followed for almost 20 years. Patients with cancers 1 cm or less in diameter (T1a and T1b) have a better than 80 percent disease-free survival rate at 20 years, and patients with cancers between 1 and 2 cm in diameter survive disease free in 70 percent of cases. It is wise to keep in mind that these patients were first treated in the years 1964 to 1976, before mammography, and thus represent historical analysis of patients from a different era, all with palpable cancers. Another analysis of premammographic T1N0 breast cancers is contained in a detailed report from Finland,[46] where disease-specific 10-year survival is 96 percent and 20-year survival is 85 percent. It could certainly be expected that patients encountered in the late 1990s will have far earlier breast cancers and better results stage for stage, because even within overall stage categories there will be a shift toward earlier and smaller cancers as a result of early detection techniques. The analysis by Rosen and associates[78] and the Finnish data[46] included *no* patients who were detected by mammographic screening; however, in recent years, the number of cancer patients detected by mammography has significantly increased, and these patients have a far earlier presentation. Of all patients encountered in one series between 1977 and 1987, lymph node metastasis was present in only 5 percent if the invasive cancer was less than 0.5 cm in diameter and in only 10 percent if the invasive cancer was 1 cm in diameter or less.[76] Several other reports[17, 61] demonstrate similar low rates of axillary nodal metastases. Some reports[68] demonstrate a higher nodal metastatic rate, particularly if the lymph nodes are examined by more sophisticated techniques,[33] with multiple sections or histochemical staining, and include a high

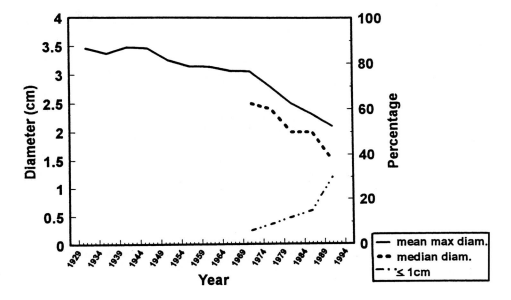

Figure 59–1   *Size of Invasive Breast Cancer—New England Deaconess Hospital.*

proportion of micrometastases. As an indication of the continued improvement in clinical presentation, Rosen's patients treated in the late 1960s had an overall node-positive rate of 27 percent in all T1 lesions,[78] whereas the report by Reger and colleagues[76] of patients seen from 1977 to 1987 indicated a 23 percent overall incidence of positive nodes in T1 cancers. Our recent report[11] indicates only a 31-percent overall rate of nodal metastases in the years 1989 to 1993 for all cases and only a 10-percent rate for T1a and T1b cancers. Silverstein demonstrated a node-positive rate of 6 percent and 13 percent in nonpalpable T1b and T1c invasive cancers, but 22 percent and 33 percent in palpable T1b and T1c cancers, respectively.[88] Thus, for similarly staged cancers, clinical and pathological presentations will continue to improve, and the incidence of lymph node metastases within each T category will decrease because of the decreasing median diameter within each T category resulting from early detection by mammography.

There will be differences in outcome based on the detection method even within limited cancer stage categories. In BCDDP patients,[58, 86] 36 percent of cancers were detected by mammogram only; such mammogram-only detected T1 node negative primary cancers had a 10-year survival rate of 92 percent. For Rosen's T1N0 patients,[78] who were detected only by physical examination, survival at the end of 10 years was 86 percent. T1N0 cases from Finland in the premammographic era from 1945 to 1969 revealed a disease-specific 10-year survival of 96 percent.[46] In a recent report, 7-year disease-free survival was more than 90 percent for T1a and T1b N0 cases and more than 95 percent for the 90 percent of patients without the two adverse prognostic features analyzed.[56] Thus, we can expect that therapeutic results will be even better than these older reports and may continue to improve with the increasing use of mammography screening to match the more recent reports.[56]

It has been amply demonstrated in a variety of studies throughout the world that the survival results comparing lumpectomy plus radiation therapy to mastectomy after prolonged follow-up are essentially identical.[13, 20, 29, 100] These results can be achieved regardless of the histological subtype.[50] In addition, patients who are at risk of failure after breast-preserving therapy have been so well defined that treatment selection can be relatively accurate.[49, 83, 72] Thus, patients younger than 35 years have a high risk of local recurrence regardless of whether they have negative margins or an extensive intraductal component (EIC) (Fig. 59–2). The most thorough study of local recurrence after breast conservation and radiotherapy analyzes recurrence by presence or absence of EIC and the histological assessment of lumpectomy margins[83] (Table 59–9). This report indicates that 83 percent of patients have less than a 5 percent risk of in-breast recurrence. The 17 percent of patients at high risk of local recurrence (28 percent) are defined by more than a focally positive margin, particularly if an EIC is present (42 percent

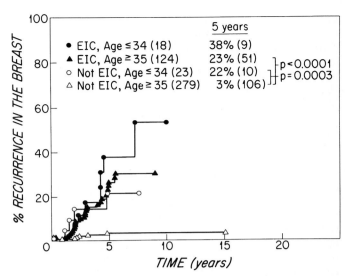

Figure 59–2 *Breast cancer recurrence as a function of age at diagnosis and presence of an extensive intraductal component (EIC). (Excisional biopsy and dose to primary site ≥ 60 Gy, infiltrating ductal histology, with evaluable specimen.) (From Recht A, et al: Int J Radiat Oncol Biol Phys 14:3, 1988. Reprinted by permission.)*

local recurrence). Accurate margin analysis is aided immeasurably by the use of multicolored inks.[6]

Breast conservation can be done in the future with increasing confidence and relatively accurate prediction of recurrence risks as seen by the increasing proportion of patients with cancer detected by mammography; the decreasing size of the primary inva-

TABLE 59–9.   LOCAL RECURRENCE AFTER CONSERVATIVE SURGERY AND RADIATION THERAPY FOR INVASIVE BREAST CANCER IN 290 PATIENTS BEFORE 1986

Margin Status	Patients No.	Patients %	Local Recurrence No.	Local Recurrence %	Distant Metastases No.	Distant Metastases %
Margin −	161	56	4	2.5	28	17
Margin +	79	27	7	9	15	19
Margin + +	50	17	14	28	15	30
Total	290	100	25	9	58	20
Low Risk	240/290	83	11/240	4.5	43/240	18

| | Recurrence | | | | | |
| | EIC Negative | | | EIC Positive | | |
Margins	No.	Local (%)	Distant (%)	No.	Local (%)	Distant (%)
Negative	137	1.5	20	24	8	4
Positive						
Focally	65	9	20	14	7	14
> Focally	31	19	39	19	42	16
Total	233 (80%)			57 (20%)		

From Schnitt SJ, Abner A, Gelman R, Connolly JL, Recht A, Duda RB, Eberline TJ, Mayzel K, Silver B, Harris JR: The relationship between microscopic margins of resection and the risk of local recurrence in patients with breast cancer treated with breast-conserving surgery and radiation therapy. Cancer 74:1746–1751, 1994. Copyright © (1994) American Cancer Society. Reprinted by Wiley-Liss, Inc., a subsidiary of John Wiley & Sons, Inc.

sive cancer; the greater attention to specimen margin analysis; the development of more precise prognostic studies such as flow cytometry, S-phase study, and oncogene analysis; and the improving overall prognosis. Thus, patients and surgeons are able to make decisions more comfortably regarding the selection of mastectomy or breast preservation and adjuvant therapy based on likelihood of local recurrence.

Several overall comments can be made regarding treatment selection for patients with early primary breast cancer. The essential decision in the selection of therapy for early breast cancer is the patient's desire for preservation of her breast. Although breast preservation in the large majority of women has been found to be extremely satisfactory,[20, 22, 48] there are many women who, for a variety of reasons, wish to have mastectomy (age, marital status, community beliefs, availability of radiotherapy, fear of recurrence, desire to minimize risks, etc.). This number of women may decrease in the future as breast preservation becomes increasingly publicized, more widely known, and safer; has more predictable results; and is extensively accepted by the public and physicians, particularly as the cancers become smaller and standards of margin analysis and resection become widely adopted. Nevertheless, elderly patients who do not wish to travel extensively and repeatedly for radiation therapy and for whom the breast is of less cosmetic, sexual, and functional importance may well choose mastectomy as the most expeditious therapy. In addition, of course, women who have an EIC within and around the primary invasive cancer may select mastectomy because of the extremely high local failure rate in the radiated breast despite extensive lumpectomy if pathologically positive margins are present in the inked lumpectomy specimen.[83] When patients are educated to recognize that a local in-breast recurrence does not alter survival, they may well appreciate that a 20 percent breast recurrence means an 80 percent chance of keeping the breast with no penalty of reduced survival. Therefore, although the surgeon may be concerned about a high local recurrence risk, the patient, if properly advised, may accept a more than modest risk of recurrence as part of an overall plan to preserve the breast if at all possible. Clearly, how the data are presented to the patient by the surgeon has an enormous impact on the patient's decision.[20, 21, 48]

Women desiring breast preservation by local excision and radiation therapy who have cancers that are large in proportion to the breast size or who have two or more widely separated primary lesions in the same breast will have a worse cosmetic outcome, a high likelihood of breast recurrence because of the need to radiate the entire breast at a high dose, and a poor chance of retaining the breast.

Lumpectomy without radiation therapy may be suitable for a proportion of patients with early breast cancer.[11, 43, 63, 71, 98] The NSABP protocol B-06 at 10 years[6] demonstrated no statistically significant reduction in survival (distant disease-free or overall) in patients who had local excision only compared with those who had local excision plus radiation therapy for all cancers 4 cm or less in diameter. In protocol B-06, patients whose cancers are 1 cm or less in diameter, there was only a 9 percent reduction in risk of local excision by the addition of radiotherapy to breast conservation at 6 years. Several other trials have demonstrated similar results: only modest decreases in local recurrence and identical long-term survival. Because the entire trend of breast cancer management during the recent decades has been toward more conservative treatment overall and more restrictive use of radiation therapy based on risk:gain analysis (i.e., elimination of supraclavicular, axillary, internal mammary node basin radiation, and avoidance of cardiac and pulmonary exposure) and more liberal use of systemic adjuvant treatment, one can expect that the subset of patients suitable for treatment by local excision and careful follow-up without radiation therapy will certainly increase.[11, 43, 63, 71, 98] This will result from earlier detection, smaller size,[12] a higher proportion of well-differentiated histology,[95] better definition of the risk of local recurrence in the breast,[83] comprehension of the lack of a survival penalty, more widespread use of careful pathologic margin analysis,[83] and the use of adjuvant tamoxifen, which may reduce the incidence of local recurrence and new primary cancers in other breast tissue (both ipsilateral and contralateral). It is difficult to predict what the standards of therapy will be for early breast cancer 10 or even 5 years in the future, however, because expanded therapy selections will evolve from sophisticated subset analyses of patients in current trials, more careful individualization of therapy based on patient wishes, wider public education and publicity, improved stage of disease resulting from wider usage of mammography, use of more sophisticated and individual prognostic indicators in the primary breast cancer, and the knowledge of excellent salvage that can occur even if locally excised breast cancers recur in the ipsilateral breast without a reduction in survival.

Therapy Selection

Therapy selection for patients with early invasive breast cancer can best be achieved by establishing the diagnosis, defining the details of the pathology, obtaining a sophisticated analysis of the margins of the lumpectomy specimen, evaluating the cosmetic appearance, and defining the risk of in-breast recurrence and systemic metastatic disease. Prolonged discussions to determine patient attitudes toward breast preservation and treatment aggressiveness and to describe the risk:benefit ratios are required. It is more important for the patient to make thoughtful, considered decisions than to adhere to any arbitrary time schedule for therapy once the primary cancer has been removed. Emphasis must be placed on patient participation in decisions for which true options for therapy exist; indeed, in situations with equivalent options, the patient *should* make the ultimate decision regarding breast preservation.[48] Obviously,

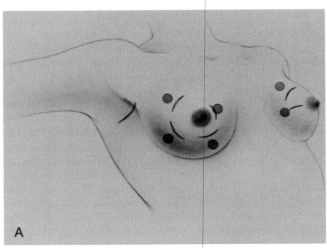 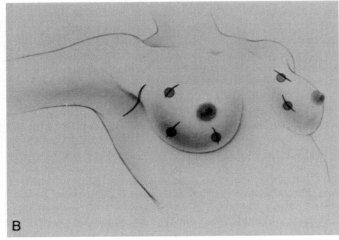

Figure 59–3 **A,** *The preferred incisions: circular, except in the extreme medial aspect, and more centrally placed. The extent of peripheral dissection to excise the primary lesion should not be excessive, and circumareolar incisions are generally avoided.* **B,** *Commonly advocated incisions that are less suitable. Radial incisions inferiorly cross Langer's lines of skin tension. Incisions placed directly over peripheral cancers are cosmetically more difficult to hide under clothing and mandate more difficult mastectomy incisions. Radial incisions in the upper medial area are to be condemned, because they are difficult to conceal or incorporate within mastectomy incisions.*

when the surgeon believes that options are not reasonable because of the clinical or pathological data and ensuing risks, he or she must assume responsibility for recommending a specific course of action.

Mammographically Detected Invasive Breast Cancer

For those patients whose primary invasive cancer is detected by mammography as part of a screening program, the therapeutic selection process begins with wire localization or stereotactic biopsy of the mammographically identified calcification or mass and adequate local excision. Stereotactic biopsy of

mammographically discovered lesions is being performed more frequently, but if a mammographic lesion is likely to be cancer, based on radiological characterics (> 20 percent risk of cancer), lumpectomy as the initial procedure (not just stereotactic biopsy) seems more rational because it completely excises the lesion for sophisticated pathological analysis, avoids an extra diagnostic step, and eliminates concern about future mammograms. Careful discussion and a close working relationship with the radiologist who performs the mammography, wire localization, or stereotactic biopsy are essential to achieve the best results. Increasingly, stereotactic biopsies will be performed by surgeons who will provide overall

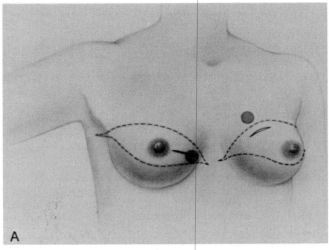 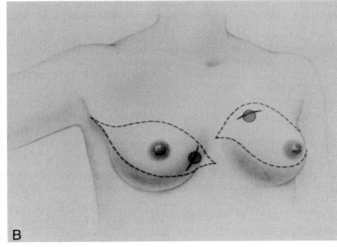

Figure 59–4 **A,** *Mastectomy, if required, can be performed with minimal skin sacrifice if biopsy incisions are more centrally placed and if medial incisions are radial.* **B,** *With the biopsy incision placed directly over peripheral cancers, the later mastectomy incision may have to be contorted to achieve inclusion within the skin ellipse. If medial biopsies are circular, wide skin sacrifice is required in a location where excess skin is not available. Because 30 percent of patients may require mastectomy, careful biopsy incision placement is critical. Furthermore, with immediate reconstruction, minimal skin sacrifice is desirable.*

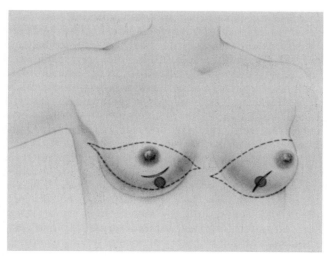

Figure 59–5   *Appropriate (left breast) and inappropriate (right breast) biopsy incision placements are demonstrated with the resulting mastectomy incisions.*

case management, which may integrate steps in management better, but selective use of stereotactic biopsy should be the rule.

Localization, stereotactic biopsy, and the subsequent open biopsy/lumpectomy can essentially always be performed under local anesthesia. The incisions for removing mammographically detected breast cancer should be circular except for a horizontal radial incision in the very medial breast so that later mastectomy incisions can be more easily placed if required (Fig. 59–3). Breast biopsy incisions placed along Langer's lines give superior cosmetic results and allow adequate excision of the breast lesions; they should be placed as centrally as possible, however, to allow subsequent mastectomy (if required) to be achieved without unusual distortion or arrangement of skin flaps or difficulty in approxima-

tion of the postmastectomy skin (Figs. 59–4 and 59–5). Slight "tunneling" peripherally is completely acceptable to keep the skin incision central on the breast; circumareolar incisions should be avoided except for central masses or for patients with large areolas so that significant exposure can be achieved. Minimizing skin sacrifice during mastectomy is more important as women increasingly select reconstruction, especially immediate reconstruction.[19] Skin-sparing mastectomy is more suitable with earlier small cancers and may involve only sacrifice of the nipple and areola with a "racket" type incision, the "handle" of which extends laterally.[4]

After exposing the localization wire within the breast and pulling it into the excision site, the presumed area of the mammographic lesion surrounding the tip of the hooked wire should be widely circumscribed by the incision into the breast substance. Breast biopsies should be performed sharply with a knife to completely encompass the suspected area and produce a single, coherent, unfragmented specimen (Fig. 59–6). Electrocautery should be avoided because the resulting tissue destruction may distort or destroy pathological findings in extremely small lesions, and it makes margin analysis particularly difficult or impossible. Paradoxically, the biopsy specimen for nonpalpable lesions may need to be larger than the local excision of a palpable lesion; it is unclear to the surgeon exactly where the lesion may be in relationship to the wire or within the excised tissue during the actual resection, because it cannot be felt or completely localized.

The careful handling of the excised tissue specimen after wire localization and biopsy of a mammographically detected lesion is critical; it is as important as the sympathetic management of the patient herself during these biopsies. After removal of the coherent, intact surgical specimen with the accompanying localization wire, the tissue should be carefully marked

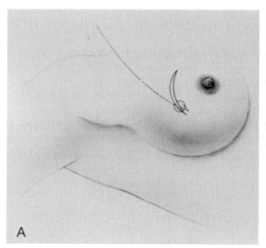
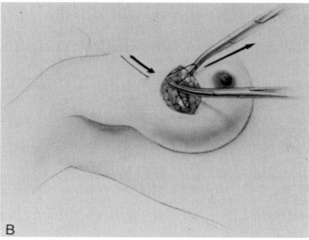

Figure 59–6   **A,** *Central circular incisions are also used for lesions removed after mammographic wire localization.*   **B,** *The wire is grasped beneath the skin by a Kelly clamp, and then the exterior portion is flipped into the wound. The wire, now completely within the biopsy incision, can be used for more accurate localization by gentle traction to demonstrate the area of the engaged hooked end near the lesion to be removed.*

with India ink by the surgeon[6] to define the excision margins for the pathologist. Multicolored India inks make margin analysis highly accurate if the surgeon places the inks carefully and promptly on removal to ensure proper specimen orientation. Evaluation of the adequacy of the removal of the primary cancer is only possible if the tissue is removed as a single piece and not excised in fragments or with a markedly irregular or a "chewed-up" margin. In almost all situations (but always if calcifications are the reason for the biopsy), the specimen should be examined radiologically after inking and compared with the preoperative mammogram to ensure removal of the entire radiological lesion. A frozen section should usually not be performed, because it is difficult to freeze fatty tissue, margin analysis is not accurate, and very small or noninvasive cancers may be destroyed or distorted by the tissue sectioning required for rapid analysis. If the area of calcification or lesion is extremely small in size (less than 5 mm), a frozen section should be strictly avoided so that the entire tissue can be carefully analyzed by permanent sections. The histological definition of cellular details is critical for very small lesions, and the destruction of even a portion of the tissue sample by frozen section analysis required for hormonal assay or margin assessment can complicate precise histopathology. Patients with invasive cancers of very small size have such outstandingly good prognoses that estrogen and progesterone receptor determinations are of minimal value in planning adjuvant therapy, and histochemical staining for estrogen receptor activity is now highly accurate, should be the standard analysis, and can be performed later.[16] Patients do not benefit from frozen section because no other therapeutic maneuvers are planned at the time of initial biopsy/lumpectomy. When reliable, nondestructive analysis of margins can be accomplished, frozen section is acceptable, but equally careful final pathology analysis of the fixed specimen with re-excision is more accurate.

There are additional reasons why all breast cancer diagnosis and treatments should be performed as a two-step surgical process, with the local anesthesia biopsy/lumpectomy procedure separated completely from any general anesthesia for axillary dissection or mastectomy. If the mass is of significant size or is palpable within the tissue removed at local excision and confirmed by postlumpectomy mammogram of the specimen, then the tissue block may be incised after inking for visual gross lesion inspection for size and margin, but because frozen section will not change what is done at that time, it should be avoided. Every biopsy of an early breast cancer should attempt to fulfill the requirements of a lumpectomy to minimize the need for later re-excision, but because accurate margin analysis is difficult and unreliable at frozen section, little is to be gained by operating room rapid analysis at the present time. A single small metallic clip placed at the base of the lumpectomy space provides useful information for the radiologist later.

To re-emphasize, a single-step process combining initial biopsy and definitive mastectomy or axillary dissection under general anesthesia is to be condemned. Only after careful histological analysis of the removed specimen by permanent section with specialized stains (if necessary) can final decisions be made about the presence of invasion, size, nuclear grade, lymphatic vessel involvement, and other histological features, the adequacy of local excision, the histological status of the margins, the extent of EIC, the suitability for conservative therapy, the need for axillary dissection, the need for radiation therapy, and any further specific prognostic aspects of the cancer. In addition, patients usually require prolonged discussion and presentation of data before they can make informed and adequate decisions and evaluate the cosmetic appearance after lumpectomy.

For simplicity and psychological comfort, patients should go into the operating room initially only for biopsy under local anesthesia (beginning the multiple-step process). Most patients are fearful of general anesthesia, not knowing whether they will wake up with a mastectomy or a preserved breast (one-step approach). A comprehensive discussion of therapeutic options should be postponed until proof has been obtained that cancer exists, the full details of the histology have been carefully documented and explained, and the patient has participated in the decisions. Such a detailed discussion can only occur after a preliminary biopsy/lumpectomy and detailed pathologic analysis (DCIS versus invasive cancer, size, EIC, etc.). In some situations, the eventual cosmetic result can only be evaluated at the postoperative visit after lumpectomy, particularly when a major tissue excision has been required because of a larger cancer or a re-excision has been required. Because the majority of patients in premenopausal age groups do not have cancer as the cause of the mammographic changes, enormous savings in time and effort by the surgeon and patient can be achieved by performing only the biopsy/lumpectomy at the first step and avoiding complicated discussions until later actual proof of cancer is obtained and definition of risks outlined. Even with cancers diagnosed by stereotactic biopsy, full details of the pathology are not known, and patient discussion cannot be complete. In postmenopausal patients with lesions detected by screening, the extra time that occurs by separating the initial surgery from the final decisions is extremely helpful in achieving emotional and practical accommodation to the diagnosis by the patient, especially when recognizing that the majority of suspicious lesions will be cancer and that options of therapy exist. Although many believe that older women may prefer the simplicity of mastectomy, with the increasing proportion of very small cancers detected at screening, most of these women could have simplified therapy.

After the results of the biopsy report and careful review of the histology with the pathologist, the patient can be apprised of the size of the primary cancer, the extent of the surrounding intraductal carcinoma, the adequacy of the margins, the likelihood of positive nodes, the chance of a cure based on size and grade, and the suitability of various therapeutic options. Because most of these mammographically detected breast cancers will be of small size with an excellent prognosis, it is possible and desirable from the first patient contact to provide a very positive outlook and a supportive environment for the patient when discussing outcome and therapeutic management.

A recent detailed analysis of the effect of specimen margin on local recurrence after breast preservation and radiation therapy provides important information (see Table 59–9).[83] If the invasive cancer is without an EIC –, even if margins are focally positive, local recurrence is uncommon. In EIC + cases, local recurrence is less than 10 percent if margins are negative, even though close. The most favorable patients for breast preservation, those *without* an extensive intraductal component (EIC –) and a negative margin (47 percent of cases), have only a 1.5 percent local recurrence rate. Fifty-six percent of patients, regardless of EIC status, have only a 2.5 percent local recurrence rate, and 83 percent of patients have less than a 5 percent local recurrence rate. The remaining 17 percent of patients have more than a focally positive margin and a 28 percent local recurrence rate. These patients should have a re-excision to negative margins if they wish to attempt breast preservation, or else they should consider mastectomy. We must keep in mind, however, that although as surgeons we might consider a 28 percent local recurrence high, many patients might understand that this means a 72 percent chance of keeping the breast without reduced survival. Extrapolating from this data should encourage surgeons to achieve a histologically negative margin if patients are EIC +, but if there is only a focally positive margin in patients without an extensive intermediate component, local recurrence rates are less than 5 percent and re-excision is not mandatory.

Re-excisions are required in at least 20 to 30 percent of patients with cancer, whether DCIS or invasive, reflecting the inability of frozen sections to detect accurately the presence and extent of EIC, the obscure involvement of margins by either invasive or intraductal carcinoma, the inaccuracy of frozen section estimation of margins, and the balance between initial extensive resection and cosmetic appearance. Margin evaluations are much less satisfactorily obtained at frozen section and are indeed unnecessary in the multiple-step process of diagnosis and treatment we advocate. Re-excisions should be kept to a reasonable minimum, because the cosmetic result may be adversely affected by re-excisions or large-volume initial biopsy specimens. However, in the balance between adequate excision and cosmetic appearance, re-excision rates are perfectly acceptable in up to 20 or 30 percent of the patients who actually have cancer, keeping the initial excision within reasonable volume limits for cosmetic purposes.

If the mammographically detected carcinoma is less than 5 mm in diameter (T1a) or 6 to 10 mm in diameter (T1b), and the initial excision or re-excision margins were adequate (≥1 cm minimum), EIC –, and with no adverse prognostic factors present, it may well be that no further therapy is required, particularly if the patient is postmenopausal.[101] Discussion about therapy selection in such patients should center on the risk:gain analysis of adding adjuvant radiation therapy to further reduce already low local recurrence rates in such a tiny primary breast cancer,[101] the projected low incidence of axillary lymph node metastases,[12] the risk:benefit ratio of axillary dissection,[11] and the marginal gain from adjuvant systemic therapy. Because of the excellent prognosis (more than 90 or even 95 percent long-term disease free survival),[58] therapy can frequently be markedly simplified.[11, 12] The use of radiation therapy to reduce local recurrence in such extremely small primary cancers has not been extensively studied, but in unpublished information from NSABP protocol B-06,[26] in palpable lesions of 1 cm or less in size, the addition of radiation therapy (5000 rad to entire breast without a local boost) contributes only a small reduction in local breast recurrence, from 24 percent in the nonirradiated breast to about 15 percent in the irradiated breast at 8 years.

In the study by Greening and associates,[36] patients after quadrant resection without radiotherapy had a 10 percent local recurrence rate if selected by age and tumor size. Veronesi and colleagues[101] reported only a 7 percent breast recurrence after quadratectomy for invasive cancers 1.5 cm or less in diameter without radiotherapy. Other series also demonstrate only small differences in local recurrence for selected patients comparing postexcision radiotherapy to observation.[53, 75] Use of radiation therapy in all patients with very small breast cancers may not be worth the financial costs and morbidity, but this should be a judgment made after discussions among the patient, the surgeon, and the radiotherapist. Although standard therapy,[35] when only a 10 or 15 percent reduction in local breast recurrence is achieved, radiotherapy can be avoided with significant gains in simplicity of management and marked reduction in cost.[11, 12] With 6000 cGy breast radiotherapy, charges range from $12,000 in the Northeast to $18,000 to $24,000 in Florida and California. Actual costs, although not well defined, are clearly less. Clear cosmetic advantages accrue to patients not receiving radiation therapy; they have essentially no breast edema, fibrosis, or long-term tenderness. For the 15 to 20 percent of patients that recur, subsequent local re-excision and radiotherapy at that time is usually possible. By such selective use of radiotherapy, significant gains occur in terms of reduced morbidity and cost without any reduction in survival. Furthermore, by avoiding axillary dissection in such patients, the risks of general anesthesia and arm and breast edema (10 to 15 percent incidence) can be avoided, shoulder function can be maintained, and entirely outpatient management can be utilized.[12, 101] This also saves considerable expense, because an axillary dissection under general anesthesia costs approximately $10,000. Thus, if 100 women undergoing local excision only of a T1a or T1b invasive breast cancer detected by mammography do not have adjuvant radiotherapy or axillary dissection, as much as $2 million can be saved with no reduction in survival. There is no reduction in eventual breast preservation either, because patients initially radiated usually require mastectomy for recurrence, whereas patients who are not initially radiated can usually have breast-conserving surgery again, followed by radiotherapy (Table 59–10).

Radiation therapy of the primary intact breast after breast preservation techniques should not be extended to include regional lymphatic drainage basins such as axillary apex, supraclavicular space, or interval mammary lymph nodes. Tangent fields are used for the breast to a total dose of 4500 cGy or less, followed by a local boost of 1600 cGy to bring the local dose to at least 6000 cGy in the style advocated by the Harvard Joint Center for Radiation Therapy.[74] Achieving at least 6000 cGy to the local area has been demonstrated to minimize local recurrence.[74] This policy of limited radiation, avoiding deliberate regional nodal radiation, again reflects the fact that lymph node metastases are "indicators but not governors."[7] Because internal mammary, axillary apex, or supraclavicular nodes are seldom involved with small breast cancer nodal spread, require separate radiation portals, and do not govern survival, nodal radiotherapeutic treatment should be avoided. Nodal recurrence is both very uncommon and well treated by later systemic or local therapy. Added morbidity in terms of arm and breast edema results from extensive adjuvant radiation therapy to the lymphatics of the supraclavicular space and axillary apex, and survival is not enhanced; thus, complications can be avoided by limiting radiotherapy, when utilized, to the breast itself.

TABLE 59–10.   RADIATION AFTER BREAST CONSERVATION: COST-BENEFIT*

	% Recurrence	% Mastectomy	% Retained Breast	Total
No RT Initially				
No further therapy			70	
Recurrence (15%) or new primary (15%)	30			
Mastectomy @ $10,000		10		$100,000
Excision and RT @ $15,000			20	$300,000
Total charges				$400,000
RT Initially @ $12,000				$1,200,000
No further therapy			85	
Recurrence (5%) or new primary (10%)	15			
Mastectomy @ $10,000		10		$100,000
Excision @ $3,000			5	$15,000
Total charges				$1,315,000

*100 patients ≤1 cm cancer with adequate negative margin.

In a number of recent studies,[17, 61, 76] the incidence of axillary lymph node metastases in patients with cancers 1 cm or less in diameter was 10 percent or less. Many of these patients have only micrometastasis,[33, 80] and the majority have minimal axillary involvement if nodes are positive.[12, 41] Of patients with palpable cancers,[28] two thirds had only one to three positive lymph nodes in the 27 percent of patients with axillary metastases. In our recent report, only 10 percent of patients in the years 1989 to 1993 with T1a and T1b cancers had axillary metastases, and 70 percent of these had only one or two positive nodes, almost half of which were micrometastases.[12] Thus, whether axillary dissection is justified in very small cancers (T1a and T1b) detected by screening is an open question.[60, 88] For T1c lesions, the incidence of lymph node metastases may be only 13 percent when discovered by mammography only, but it is more than 25 percent when palpable, and the risk of local recurrence in the breast may be substantial after local excision only. In the NSABP B-06 study,[29] breast recurrence was more than 25 percent if axillary nodes were negative and more than 35 percent if nodes were positive in T1c cancers if radiotherapy was not used. Local breast recurrences in such patients were reduced substantially by radiation therapy. If axillary nodes were positive, these patients also received adjuvant systemic therapy, and the reduction in local breast recurrence in those patients was quite dramatic, from about 35 percent to about 5 percent with the combination of radiation and chemotherapy. Thus, for patients with T1c primary invasive cancers detected by palpation, standard therapy should probably include radiation therapy to the breast, even if EIC-, unless an extensive resection or quadratectomy is performed.[101] However, if the cancer is of low grade or of tubular, colloid, or papillary type, the patient can avoid radiation with only a minimal risk of a local recurrence in the breast if no radiotherapy is used, provided that adequate negative operative margins are obtained. A slightly wider local resection, such as a quadratectomy, is as successful in reducing local recurrence risk as adding radiation therapy, but a 1-cm margin will probably be adequate. If a very wide excision can be performed with a satisfactory cosmetic result, that may well be an easier and less costly local treatment, with a better cosmetic outcome, than the addition of adjuvant breast radiation. The axillary nodes are almost always negative in such low-grade breast cancers. Axillary dissection or preferably sentinel node biopsy should be considered in T1c patients with palpable cancers, because of the much higher likelihood of positive axillary nodes and the increased absolute benefit of adjuvant therapy if nodes are positive. However, if adjuvant therapy is to be used because of primary cancer features, axillary dissection can be avoided in the clinically negative axilla regardless of axillary lymph node status, because the discovery of metastatic nodes will not alter the selection of therapy. In addition, recent data support the effectiveness of sentinel node biopsy as a method of harvesting a single physiologically defined lymph node under local anesthesia that acts as the surrogate for the entire node basin (see Chapter 56). Therefore, any case in which axillary dissection is to be considered or is necessary can be initially evaluated by sentinel node biopsy. Definition of a sentinel node can be achieved in 95 percent of cases, with a nearly 100 percent accuracy of predicting the regional node status on the basis of the physiologically defined sentinel node.

The entire thrust of sophisticated breast cancer management during the past decades has emphasized accurate staging. This has been stimulated by the need for separation by stage to prognosticate, and thus select appropriate therapy, particularly systemic adjuvant therapy. If such adjuvant therapy is to be administered regardless of exact anatomical stage, then accurate axillary staging operations are not required and are not necessarily a service to the patient. Thus, if prognostic features of the primary cancer itself (such as large size, ER negativity, extremely poor histology, lymphatic permeation, flow cytometry, thymidine labeling index, oncogene expression, or other features) indicate that adjuvant systemic therapy will be selected, then avoidance of an axillary dissection merely to conform to traditional anatomical staging criteria is justified.[94] Breast cancer management can be simplified enormously, because adequate axillary staging operations to obtain the 10 nodes required can only be performed under general anesthesia and involve hospitalization, wound drainage, considerable (though temporary) shoulder stiffness, numbness and disability from sacrifice of the brachiocutaneous nerve. Sentinel node biopsy under local anesthesia will be the best compromise between obtaining important prognostic information and reducing costs and morbidity. As a matter of fact, improved nodal sampling for prognostication can be achieved by enabling identification of internal mammary lymph nodes or anatomical "skip" axillary nodes that are not in the low axilla, and subjecting a single lymph node to more intense or sophisticated analysis.[33]

Sophisticated analysis of bone marrow with monoclonal antibodies[60] may provide more accurate staging of systemic disease, encourage the use of breast-conservation procedures in patients with defined metastases, and eliminate the need for axillary lymph node dissections.

The traditional anatomical staging of breast cancer (which includes axillary lymph node dissection) will have to be altered in the near future to reduce the morbidity of the staging, expedite decision making, and reduce unnecessary costs. Although modification by recognition of a single sentinel node biopsy defies the traditional criteria, it reflects the inevitable result of current prognostic indicator development and the need to rationalize the more widespread use of adjuvant therapy in breast cancer management of node-negative patients in a period of rapidly improving clinical presentation.

Clinically Detected Invasive Breast Cancer

For palpable T1 breast cancers and for those lesions more than 2 cm in diameter but with clinically negative axillary nodes (T2N0), decision algorithms similar to those for mammographically detected cancers are appropriate. For palpable breast cancers, histological confirmation can usually be obtained by needle aspiration or core cutting biopsy of the mass in the physician's office on the first patient visit. However, although the rapid diagnosis of breast cancer in such situations can usually be obtained in the office, the details of the local pathology (EIC; grade; type) cannot be determined without adequate total removal of the breast cancer itself. Thus, lumpectomy should be carried out promptly under local anesthesia to assess the features of the primary cancer (multiple-step process). Although there is usually a correlation between the palpable size of the cancer and the pathological measurement of the invasive component of the cancer, in some situations a small sclerosing invasive breast cancer can present with a mass apparently considerably larger by palpation, and even by mammography, than the actual invasive cancer itself. In addition, a small invasive cancer may be surrounded by DCIS that presents as a larger mass. Thus, even the exact size of the primary invasive cancer cannot be determined until after a gross total removal and careful histological examination. Clearly, the excision procedure should satisfy all the described requirements of a lumpectomy with at least a 1-cm gross margin surrounding the palpable cancer, attention to placement of a cosmetically appropriate incision (see Figures 59–3, 59–4, and 59–5), sharp knife excision of a coherent intact tissue specimen, inking of the specimen for margin analysis, careful control of bleeding in the residual biopsy cavity, avoidance of drains, and closure of the skin over the residual breast tissue defect, usually without breast tissue re-approximation performed in the usual fashion with buried absorbable sutures. Exceptions to the multiple-step procedure may be acceptable in elderly patients in whom office needle biopsy provides cytologic proof of breast cancer and preliminary discussion regarding therapy indicates that mastectomy is desired or more feasible. In these situations, mastectomy can be performed forthwith, because details of the local breast cancer excision margin, histology, and prognostic indicators will not alter the selection of treatment. However, for any patient who wishes to explore the option of breast preservation, the lumpectomy/biopsy should be performed as a separate procedure so that features of the primary cancer can be completely documented before discussion with the patient about options for therapy. In perhaps one quarter to one third of such patients, local excision with or without radiation therapy may not be suitable because of EIC surrounding the primary cancer, inability to obtain tumor-free margins, poor cosmetic outcome in a small breast by the removal of a relatively large carcinoma, or occurrence of multiple primary cancers. In such situations more suitable for mastectomy, immediate reconstruction of the breast can be offered, but the preliminary consultation and coordination of operative schedules with the plastic surgeon may require some extra time. A considerable body of literature currently indicates the complete suitability and the lack of adverse consequences of immediate reconstruction at the time of mastectomy.[47] Many reconstructions at the present time use a subpectoral implant that thrusts the entire operative field forward just under the skin so that local recurrences are not hidden from examination but can be readily detected. However, the safety, ease, and better cosmetic appearance of a pedical or free rectus abdominal or latissimus flap make these suitable options, despite the burying of the deep operative field and the risk of obscuring local recurrence.

Axillary dissection or initial sentinel node biopsy should be considered standard therapy in patients with larger primary breast cancers; nevertheless, because these patients will almost certainly receive adjuvant systemic therapy (polychemotherapy if premenopausal or tamoxifen if postmenopausal), the value and usefulness of axillary dissection is eliminated except to fulfill the rigid requirements of the anatomical staging system. Axillary lymph node metastases are "indicators but not governors of survival,"[8] and therefore axillary dissection is only a staging and not a therapeutic procedure for clinically negative axillas. Thus, in the absence of palpable axillary lymphadenopathy, a patient undergoing lumpectomy, radiation therapy, and adjuvant systemic therapy regardless of node status may, indeed should, avoid axillary dissection after thorough explanation of options, risks, and benefits. If the patient would not receive adjuvant therapy if axillary nodes were negative, but would be treated if nodes were positive, axillary dissection, or preferably sentinel node biopsy, is clearly indicated. For clinical research trials in which detailed anatomical staging is critical for evaluation of results, axillary dissections may still be recommended. If unusual therapeutic measures would be offered if more than four or ten node metastases were present, axillary dissection can be limited to these patients with a positive sentinel node.

Extensive data indicate proportionally reduced recurrence and mortality rates after use of adjuvant systemic therapy in node-negative patients (both premenopausal and postmenopausal) and particularly reduced mortality in node-positive patients of approximately 15 percent (with tamoxifen in postmenopausal patients) to 33 percent (with polychemotherapy in premenopausal patients).[42] When overall survival expectations at 10 years are less than 75 percent, benefits clearly outweigh the risks of using adjuvant therapy.[34] Therefore, patients with larger primary invasive breast cancer (T2 or T3), lymph node metastases, or poor prognostic indicators in the primary cancer generally should be advised to receive adjuvant therapy. It should be kept in mind, however,

that an absolute reduction in recurrence of 5 percent means that 95 percent of such patients receive *no* benefit. A proportional 33 percent reduction in a patient with an expected 15 percent recurrence or mortality yields only a 5 percent absolute gain. Therefore, the proportionality of benefit must be kept constantly in mind, because absolute gains may be very small in cancers with relatively good prognoses.

In this time of rapidly evolving management changes in primary breast cancer resulting from mammographic screening, it is critical that patients be fully informed of the various therapeutic options, risks, and benefits so they can make suitable personal judgments regarding what they think is appropriate therapy. Although some patients will choose standard therapy from a desire to conform and achieve maximal benefit from conventional wisdom, many patients are willing to explore variations in management and therapy for perceived gains in simplicity and reduced morbidity risk when they receive sympathetic and supportive guidance, empathy, and information by the surgeon. The current headlong rush into bone marrow or stem cell transplantation, despite incomplete or absent data, merely displays this willingness on the part of many women to explore therapeutic alternatives or assume risks. It is important to involve patients in therapeutic decisions, particularly in early breast cancer, because a wide variety of more conservative or less aggressive or morbid options are currently available and more may be developed in the next decade. Patients usually assume that a "recurrence" of the breast cancer equals death, so that ipsilateral in-breast recurrence causes undo fright, when in reality such recurrence causes no increased risk of death. The real risk of death from disease after local recurrence is only a small fraction of the recurrence risk and is not caused by the recurrence. In-breast recurrence is a risk indicator and not apparently a generating focus for further metastases.[27] Because the word "cancer" terrifies most patients, careful detailed explanation of realistic prognostic figures and outcomes is particularly important in patients with very early disease; their outlook may be extremely favorable, but their assumptions about outcome may be very gloomy because of the word "cancer." Patients frequently are frightened of a diagnosis of minuscule DCIS discovered mammographically with no risk of death, yet they may be heavy cigarette smokers, incurring large risks to their life apparently without regret or recognition. Although it is vitally important to point out to patients risks and benefits of their management decisions, it is also important to have them recognize and act on the basis of their personal philosophy regarding their physical body as well as their approach to life. (Are they risk takers? Are they body conscious? Are their breasts of major social, sexual, or psychological importance?) Discussions about their breast cancer and the selection of variations in therapy should be conducted at length and, if at all possible, with other people present for support and reiteration of data and details. Despite careful explanation, emotion-laden material may not be comprehended or remembered by anxious patients or even their families, and repeated discussion may be needed. Unsophisticated, angry, hostile, or ignorant patients may require great sensitivity and considerable time to resolve therapy selection.

Patients frequently urge the surgeon to do what is "best." These pleas should resolutely be deflected, because the "best" therapy is completely relative. What is "best" for one patient is hardly "best" for someone else, and whenever true options exist in terms of equivalent survival the patient must make the ultimate therapeutic selection with guidance. The patient's decision is required not only for achieving ultimate satisfaction and feelings of being in control, but also for the surgeon's protection to avoid even the suggestion that the physician is autocratically dictating therapy to an uninformed patient. Such autocratic dictation of therapy by surgeons is inappropriate in the realm of contemporary breast cancer management, where even the unsophisticated public recognizes from publicity in the press that there are options available. Before 1970, there was only one realistic therapeutic alternative available for patients with breast cancer, but currently there are innumerable variations in treatment, with at least 50 combinations and permutations. For each individual patient, the therapeutic options may be numerous, and arbitrary imposition of a therapeutic pathway by physicians or surgeons should be avoided. Individualization should be the key element of decisions. Such an approach, however, not only places a larger burden on patients and families, but also implies a burden of time, empathy, and flexibility on surgeons. Patients are frequently initially uncomfortable making decisions about their treatment, particularly when confronting a cancer diagnosis, but usually become more settled and relaxed as they are helped along by supportive surgeons.

Follow-Up

For patients with mastectomy, routine subsequent physical examination can be performed at 6-month intervals initially and, after a few years, at yearly intervals. Examination should focus on the mastectomy area and regional nodes. Ample evidence exists that detailed laboratory based follow-up is costly and of no help in improving prognosis.[92, 97] Symptom-based follow-up management is perfectly satisfactory, conserves patient and system resources, and results in identical survival. Thus, routine blood studies, chest radiographs, and bone scans are not performed, and indeed are specifically avoided. Instead, management using specific symptomatic or physical examination indicators (backache, cough, fatigue, mass, etc.) is practiced. Radiological tests may be used effectively to rule out metastatic disease when patients have symptoms. If metastatic or recurrent disease is discovered, a complete work-up is undertaken before therapy selection to completely delineate the disease state.

For patients with breast-preserving local therapy, however, follow-up of the breast must be more detailed, frequent, and careful, because local recurrence is not infrequent, and treatment by mastectomy or by repeated local excision if radiation therapy was not previously used is possible with excellent survival expectations. Breast physical examination should be performed every 3 months, perhaps alternating between surgeon and radiotherapist. Mammography should be performed every 6 months for the first 2 or 3 years, with the understanding that a prominent postlumpectomy scar or radiation fibrosis can exactly mimic recurrent cancer. A high index of suspicion must be maintained, and any worrisome mass or thickening of breast tissue should undergo needle aspiration, stereotactic, or core-cutting biopsy after evaluation by mammography. Open biopsy is used cautiously, because late surgical incisions in the radiated breast exacerbate scar formation and mass development that continue the diagnostic problem. Mammographic changes that suggest recurrent or new cancer (i.e., clustered calcification or later mass) may require localization and biopsy. The time sequence for locally recurrent disease is prolonged, although after 10 years, most cancers that arise are new primary cancers, not true recurrences, and appear in other areas of the same breast or the opposite breast. Keep in mind that initial breast-conservation surgery keeps in place large volumes of high-risk breast tissue, and significant numbers of patients in the future will have two, three, or even four separate primary cancers. This provides yet further reason to avoid radiotherapy initially, because it may be required later, and radiation scarring and fibrosis makes breast examination less accurate.

A summary of expected disease-free survival at 10 years from the various entities discussed in this chapter is given in Table 59–11.

TABLE 59–11. ESTIMATE OF DISEASE-FREE SURVIVAL AT 10 YEARS

T Category	Lesion Size (cm)	N Category	Disease-Free Survival at 10 Years (%)
Tis		N0	100
T1a	0–0.5	N0	99
		pN1ai + micrometastasis	95
		pN1bi + macrometastasis	80
T1b	0.6–1.0	N0	95
		pN1ai + micrometastasis	90
		pN1bi + macrometastasis	75
T1c	1.1–2	N0	90
		pN1bii + 1–3 macrometastases	70
		pN1biii + >3 macrometastases	<50
T2	2.1–3	N0	80
		N1	<50

Compiled from Rosen PP, et al: J Clin Oncol 7:355–366, 1989; Seidman H, et al: CA 5(37):258–290, 1987; Wilkinson LH, et al: Arch Surg 117:579–582, 1982.

References

1. Abrams JS, Phillips PH, Friedman MA: *Commentary* Meeting Highlights: A Reappraisal of Research Results for the Local Treatment of Early Stage Breast Cancer. J Natl Cancer Inst 87:1837–1845, 1995.
2. Alex JC, Krag DN: The gamma-probe-guided resection of radio labeled primary lymph nodes. Surg Oncol Clin North Am 5:33–41, 1996.
3. American Joint Committee on Cancer. Handbook for Staging of Cancer: From the Manual for Staging of Cancer, 4th Edition. Philadelphia, JB Lippincott, 1993.
4. Beasley ME: Immediate breast reconstruction with a pedicled TRAM flap. *In* Hartrampf CR (ed): Hartrampf's Breast Reconstruction with Living Tissue. New York, Raven Press, 1991, pp 161–174.
5. Bostwick DG: Anatomy and pathology of prostate cancer prostatic intra epithelial neoplasia. *In* Vogelzang NJ, Scardino PT, Shipley WU, Coffey DS (eds): Comprehensive Textbook of Genitourinary Oncology. Baltimore, Williams & Wilkins, 1996, pp 639–644.
6. Cady B: Duct carcinoma in situ. Surg Oncol Clin North Am 2(1):75–91, 1993.
7. Cady B: Lymph node metastases: Indicators but not governors of survival. Arch Surg 119:1067–1072, 1984.
8. Cady B: New diagnostic, staging, and therapeutic aspects of early breast cancer. Cancer 65:634–647, 1990.
9. Cady B: The need to reexamine axillary lymph node dissection in invasive breast cancer. Cancer 73:505–508, 1994.
10. Cady B, Rossi R: An expanded view of risk group definition in differentiated thyroid carcinoma. Surgery 104:947–953, 1988.
11. Cady B, Stone MD, Wayne J: New therapeutic possibilities in primary invasive breast cancer. Ann Surg 218:338–349, 1993.
12. Cady B, Stone MD, Schuler JG, Thakur R, Wanner MA, Lavin PT: The new era in breast cancer invasion, size, and nodal involvement dramatically decreasing as a result of mammographic screening. Arch Surg 131:301–308, 1996.
13. Calle R, Vilcoq JR, Pilleron JP: Conservative treatment of operable breast cancer by irradiation with or without limited surgery: Ten year results. In Harris JR, Hellman S, Silen W (eds): Conservative Management of Breast Cancer. Philadelphia, JB Lippincott 1985, pp 3–9.
14. De Koning HJ, Fracheboud J, Boer R, et al: Nation-wide breast cancer screening in the Netherlands; support for breast-cancer mortality reduction. National Evaluation Team for Breast Cancer Screening (NETB). Int J Cancer 60:777–780, 1995.
15. Delouche G, Bachelot F, Premont M, Kurtz JM: Conservation treatment of early breast cancer: Long term results and complications. Int J Radiat Oncol Biol Phys 13:29–34, 1987.
16. DeRosa CM, Ozzello L, Habif DV, Konrath JG, Greene GL: Immunohistochemical assessment of estrogen and progesterone receptors in stored imprints and cryostat sections of breast carcinomas. Ann Surg 210:224–228, 1989.
17. Dowlatshahi K, Snider HC, Kim R: Axillary node status in nonpalpable breast cancer. Ann Surg Oncol 2:424–428, 1995.
18. Dupont WD, Page DL: Risk factors for breast cancer in women with proliferative breast disease. N Engl J Med 312:146–151, 1985.
19. Eberlein TJ, Crespo LP, Smith BL, et al: Prospective evaluation of immediate reconstruction after mastectomy. Ann Surg 218:23–36, 1993.
20. Fallowfield LJ: Has psychosocial oncology helped in the management of women with breast cancer? Breast 2:107–113, 1996.
21. Fallowfield LJ, Hall A, Maguire GP, Baum M: Psychological outcomes of different treatment policies in women with early breast cancer outside a clinical trial. Br Med J 301:575–580, 1990.
22. Fallowfield LJ, Phil D, Baum M: Psychosocial problems associated with the diagnosis and treatment of breast cancer. *In* Bland KI, Copeland EM (eds): The Breast: Comprehensive Management of Benign and Malignant Diseases. Philadelphia, WB Saunders 1991, pp 1081–1092.
23. Farrow JH: Current concepts in the detection and treatment of the earliest of the breast cancers. Cancer 25:468–477, 1970.
24. Feuer EJ, Wun LM: How much of the recent rise in breast cancer incidence can be explained by increases in mammography utilization? Am J Epidemiol 136:1423–1426, 1992.
25. Findlay P, Lippman M, Danforth D, et al: A randomized trial comparing mastectomy to radiotherapy in the treatment of stage I-II breast cancer: A preliminary report. Proc Am Soc Clin Oncol 5:246–263, 1986.
26. Fisher B: Unpublished presentation in Milan, Italy, 1989.
27. Fisher B, Anderson S, Fisher ER, Redmond C, Wickerham DL, et al: Significance of ipsilateral breast tumour recurrence after lumpectomy. Lancet 338:327–331, 1991.
28. Fisher B, Costantio J, Fisher B, Palekar AS, Redmond C, et al: Pathologic findings from the National Surgical Adjuvant Breast Project (NSABP) Protocol B-17: Intraductal carcinoma (ductal carcinoma in situ). Cancer 75:1310–1319, 1995.
29. Fisher ER, Sass R, Fisher B, Wickerham C, Paik SM: Pathologic findings from the National Surgical Adjuvant Breast Project (protocol 6). I. Intraductal carcinoma (DCIS) Cancer 57:197–208, 1986.
30. Fowble BL, Solin LJ, Goodman RL: Results of conservative surgery and radiation for intraductal non-invasive breast cancer. Am J Clin Oncol 10:110–111, 1987. Abstract.
31. Frykberg E, Santiago F, Betsill WL, O'Brien PH: Lobular carcinoma *in situ* of the breast. Surg Gynecol Obstet 164:285–301, 1987.
32. Gallagher WJ, Koener FC, Wood WC: Treatment of intraductal carcinoma with limited surgery: Long-term follow-up. J Clin Oncol 7:373–380, 1989.
33. Giuliano AE, Dale PS, Turner RR, Morton DL, Evans SW: Improved axillary staging of breast cancer with sentinel lymphadenectomy. Ann Surg 222:394–401, 1995.
34. Goldhirsch A, Gelber RD, Simes RJ, Glasziou P, Coates AS: Costs and benefits of adjuvant therapy in breast cancer: A quality-adjusted survival analysis. J Clin Oncol 7:36–44, 1989.
35. Goldhirsch A, Wood WC, Senn HJ, Glick JH, Gelber RD: Commentary Meeting Highlights: International Consensus Panel on the Treatment of Primary Breast Cancer. J Natl Cancer Inst 87:1441–1445.
36. Greening WP, Montgomery CV, Gordon AB, Gowing NEF: Quadrantic excision and axillary node dissection without radiation therapy: The long-term results of a selective policy in the treatment of Stage I breast cancer. Eur J Surg Oncol 14:221–225, 1988.
37. Gump F, Jica DL, Ozzella L: Ductal carcinoma *in situ* (DCIS): a revised concept. Surgery 102:190–195, 1987.
38. Haagensen CD, Bodian C, Haagensen D (eds): Breast Carcinoma Risk and Detection. Philadelphia, WB Saunders, 1981, p 267.
39. Haagensen CD, Lane N, Lattes R, Bodian C: Lobular neoplasia (so called lobular carcinoma *in situ*) of the breast. Cancer 42:737–769, 1978.
40. Hatschek T, Fagerberg G, Stal O, Sullivan S, Carstensen J, et al: Cytometric characterization and clinical course of breast cancer diagnosed in a population-based screening program. Cancer 64:1074–1081, 1989.
41. Hellman S: Karnofsky Memorial Lecture. Natural History of Small Breast Cancers. J Clin Oncol 12:2229–2234, 1994.
42. Henderson IC, Mouridsen H: Effects of adjuvant Tamoxifen and of cytotoxic therapy on mortality in early breast cancer: An overview of 61 randomized trials among 28,896 women. N Engl J Med 319:1681–1692, 1988.
43. Hermann RE, Esselstyne Jr CB, Grundfest-Broniatowski S, et al: Partial mastectomy without radiation is adequate treatment for patients with Stage 0 and I carcinoma of the breast. Surg Gynecol Obstet 177:247–253, 1993.
44. Hetelekidis S, Schnitt SJ, Morrow M, Harris JR: Management of ductal carcinoma in situ. CA Cancer J Clin 45:244–253, 1995.
45. Hetelekidis S, Silver B, Nixon A, Love S, Eberlein T, et al: Is wide excision alone adequate treatment for selected patients with DCIS? Int J Radiat Oncol Biol Phys 32(suppl 1):263, 1995. Abstract.

46. Joensuu H, Taikkanen S: Cured of breast cancer? J Clin Oncol 13:62–69, 1995.

47. Johnson CH, van Heerden JA, Donohue JH, Martin JK, Jackson IT, et al: Oncological aspects of immediate breast reconstruction following mastectomy for malignancy. Arch Surg 124:819–824, 1989.

48. Kotwall CA, Maxwell JG, Covington DL, Churchill P, Smith SE, et al: Clinico-pathologic factors and patient perceptions associated with surgical breast-conserving treatment. Ann Surg Oncol 3:169–175, 1996.

49. Kurtz JM, Amalric R, Brandone H, Ayme Y, Jacquemier J, et al: Local recurrence after breast conserving surgery and radiotherapy: Frequency, time course, and prognosis. Cancer 63:1912–1917, 1989.

50. Kurtz JM, Jacquemier J, Torhorst J, Spitalier JM, Amalric R, et al: Conservation therapy for breast cancers other than infiltrating ductal carcinoma. Cancer 63:1630–1635, 1989.

51. Lagios MD: Ductal carcinoma in situ: Controversies in diagnosis, biology, and treatment. Breast J 1:68–78, 1995.

52. Lagios MD, Margolin R, Westdahl PR, Rose MR: Mammographically detected duct carcinoma *in situ*. Cancer 63:618–624, 1989.

53. Lagios MD, Richard UE, Rose MR, Yee E: Segmental mastectomy without radiotherapy: Short-term follow-up. Cancer 52:2173–2179, 1983.

54. Lagios MD, Silverstein MJ: Duct carcinoma in situ: The success of breast conservation therapy. A shared experience of two single institutional non-randomized prospective studies. Surg Oncol Clin North Am 1997. In Press.

55. Lagios MD, Westdahl PR, Margolin FR, Rose MR: Duct carcinoma *in situ*: Relationship of extent of non-invasive disease to the frequency of occult invasion, multicentricity, lymph node metastases, and short-term treatment failures. Cancer 50:1309–1314, 1982.

56. Leitner SP, Swern AS, Weinberger D, Duncan LJ, Hutter RVP: Predictors of recurrence for patients with small (one centimeter or less) localized breast cancer (T1a,bN0M0). Cancer 76:2266–2274, 1995.

57. Lennington WJ, Jensen RA, Dalton LW, Page DL: Ductal carcinoma in situ of the breast: Heterogeneity of individual lesions. Cancer 73:118–124, 1994.

58. Letton AH, Mason EM, Ramshaw BJ: Twenty-year review of a breast cancer screening project ninety-five percent survival of patients with nonpalpable cancers. Cancer 77:104–106, 1996.

59. Love SM, Gelman RS, Silen W: Fibrocystic "disease" of the breast--a nondisease? N Engl J Med 307:1010–1014, 1982.

60. Mansi JL, Berger U, McDonnell T, Pople A, Rayter Z, et al: The fate of bone marrow micro metastases in patients with primary breast cancer. J Clin Oncol 7:445–449, 1989.

61. Meterissian S, Fornage BD, Singletary SE: Clinically occult breast carcinoma: Diagnostic approaches and role of axillary node dissection. Ann Surg Oncol 2(4):314–318, 1995.

62. Miller BA, Feuer EJ, Hankey BF: The increasing incidence of breast cancer since 1982; relevance of early detection. Cancer Causes Control 2:67–74, 1991.

63. Moffat FL, Ketcham AS: Breast conserving surgery and selective adjuvant radiation therapy for stage I and II breast cancers. Semin Surg Oncol 8:172–176, 1992.

64. Morrow M, Schmidt C, Cregger B, Hassett C, Cox S: Preoperative evaluation of abnormal mammographic findings to avoid unnecessary breast biopsy. Arch Surg 129:1091–1096, 1994.

65. Neilsen M, Jensen J, Anderson J: Precancerous and cancerous breast lesions during lifetime and at autopsy. Cancer 54:612–615, 1984.

66. Newcomb PA, Lantz PM: Recent trends in breast cancer incidence, mortality, and mammography. Breast Cancer Res Treat 28:97–106, 1993.

67. Ohtake T, Abe R, Kimijima I, Fukushima T, Tsuchiya A, et al: Intraductal extension of primary invasive breast carcinoma treated by breast-conservative surgery: Computer graphic three-dimensional reconstruction of the mammary duct-lobular systems. Cancer 76:32–45, 1995.

68. Osteen RT, Cady B, Chmiel JS, et al: 1991 national survey of carcinoma of the breast by the commission on cancer. J Am Coll Surg 178:213–219, 1994.

69. Page DL, Dupont WD, Rogers LW, Jensen RA, Schuyler PA: Continued local recurrence of carcinoma 15-25 years after a diagnosis of low grade ductal carcinoma in situ of the breast treated only by biopsy. Cancer 76:1197–1200, 1995.

70. Page DL, Dupont WD, Rogers LW, Rados MS: Atypical hyperplastic lesions of the female breast: A long-term follow-up study. Cancer 55:2698–2708, 1985.

71. Pierce SM, Schnitt S, Gelman R, Love S, Eberlein T, Harris JR: Wide excision without radiation therapy in selected patients with early stage breast cancer. Proc Am Soc Clin Oncol 12:70, 1993. Abstract.

72. Recht A, Connolly JC, Schnitt SJ, et al: The effect of young age on tumor recurrence in the treated breast after conservative surgery and radiotherapy. Int J Radiat Oncol Biol Phys 14:3–10, 1988.

73. Recht A, Danoff BF, Solin LJ, et al: Intraductal carcinoma of the breast: Results of treatment with excisional biopsy and irradiation. J Clin Oncol 3:1339–1343, 1985.

74. Recht A, Houlihan MJ: Conservative surgery without radiotherapy in the treatment of patients with early-stage invasive breast cancer: A review. Ann Surg 222(1):9–18, 1995.

75. Reed MW, Morrison JM: Wide local excision as the sole primary treatment in elderly patients with carcinoma of the breast. Br J Surg 76:898–900, 1989.

76. Reger V, Beito G, Jolly PC: Factors affecting the incidence of lymph node metastases in small cancers of the breast. Am J Surg 157:501–502, 1989.

77. Rosen PP, Braun DW, Kinne DE: The clinical significance of pre-invasive breast carcinoma. Cancer 46:919–925, 1980.

78. Rosen PP, Groshen S, Saigo PE, Kinne DW, Hellman S: A long-term follow-up study of survival in stage 1 (T1N0M0) and stage II (T1N1M0) breast carcinoma. J Clin Oncol 7:355–366, 1989.

79. Rosen PP, Lieberman PH, Braun DW, et al: Lobular carcinoma *in situ* of the breast: Detailed analysis of 99 patients with average follow-up of 24 years. Am J Surg Pathol 2:225–251, 1978.

80. Rosen PP, Saigo PE, Braun DW, Weathers E, Fracchia AA, Kinne DW: Axillary micro- and macro metastases in breast cancer: Prognostic significance of tumor size. Ann Surg 194:585–591, 1981.

81. Rosner D, Dedwant RN, Vana J, et al: Non-invasive breast carcinoma: Results of a national survey by the American College of Surgeons. Ann Surg 192:139–147, 1980.

82. Saccani Jott G, Petit JY, Contesso G: Minimal breast cancer: A clinically meaningful term? Semin Oncol 4:384–392, 1986.

83. Schnitt SJ, Abner A, Gelman R, Connolly JL, Recht A, Duda RB, Eberline TJ, Mayzel K, Silver B, Harris JR: The relationship between microscopic margins of resection and the risk of local recurrence in patients with breast cancer treated with breast-conserving surgery and radiation therapy. Cancer 74:1746–1751, 1994.

84. Schnitt SJ, Silen W, Sadowsky NL, Connolly JL, Harris JR: Ductal carcinoma *in situ* (intraductal carcinoma) of the breast. N Engl J Med 318:898–903, 1988.

85. Schwartz GF: Sub-clinical ductal carcinoma in situ of the breast: Selection for treatment by local excision and surveillance alone. Breast J 2(1):41–44, 1996.

86. Seidman H, Gelb SK, Silverberg E, Laverda N, Lubera JA: Survival experience in the breast cancer detection demonstration project end results. CA Cancer J Clin 5:258–290, 1987.

87. Shapiro S: Determining the efficacy of breast cancer screening. Cancer 63:1873–1880, 1989.

88. Silverstein MJ, Gierson ED, Waisman JR, Senofsky GM, Colburn WJ, et al: Axillary lymph node dissection for T1a breast carcinoma: Is it indicated? Cancer 73:664–667, 1994.

89. Silverstein MJ, Lagios MD, Craig PH, Waisman JR, Lewinsky BS, et al: A prognostic index for ductal carcinoma in situ of the breast. Cancer 77:2267–2274, 1996.

90. Slovak ML, Wolman SR: Breast cancer cytogenetics: Clues to genetic complexity of the disease. Breast J 2:124–140, 1996.

91. Solin LJ, Yeh IT, Kurtz J: Ductal carcinoma in situ (intraductal carcinoma) of the breast treated with breast-conserving surgery and definitive irradiation: Correlation of pathologic

parameters with outcome of treatment. Cancer 71(8):2532–2542, 1993.

92. Stierer M, Rosen HR: Influence of early diagnosis on prognosis of recurrent breast cancer. Cancer 64:1128–1131, 1989.
93. Sunshine JA, Moseley HS, Fletcher WS, Krippaehe WW: Breast carcinoma in situ: A retrospective review of 112 cases with a minimum 10 year follow-up. Am J Surg 150:44–51, 1985.
94. Swain SM: Ductal carcinoma *in situ*: Incidence, presentation, guidelines to treatment. Oncology 3(3):25–31, 1989.
95. Tabar L, Fagerberg G, Chen HH, Duffy SW, Smart CR: Efficacy of breast cancer screening by age. New results from the Swedish Two-County Trial. Cancer 75:2507–2517, 1995.
96. Tinnemans JGM, Wobbes T, Holland R, Hendriks JHCL, et al: Treatment and survival of female patients with nonpalpable breast carcinoma. Ann Surg 209:249–253, 1989.
97. Tomlin R, Donegan WL. Screening for recurrent breast cancer—its effectiveness and prognostic value. J Clin Oncol 5:62–67, 1987.
98. Uppsala-Onebro Breast Cancer Study Group Sector: Resection with or without postoperative radiotherapy for Stage I breast cancer: A randomized trial. J Natl Cancer Inst 82:277–282, 1990.
99. van de Vijver MJ, Peterse JL, Mooi WJ, Wisman P, Lomans J, Dalesio O, Nusse R: Neu-protein over expression in breast cancer: Association with comedo-type ductal carcinoma *in situ* and limited prognostic value in stage II breast cancer. N Engl J Med 319:1239–1282, 1988.
100. Veronesi U: Rationale and indications for limited surgery in breast cancer: Current data. World J Surg 11:493–498, 1987.
101. Veronesi U, Luini A, DelVecchio M, Greco M, Galimberti V, et al: Radiotherapy after breast-preserving surgery in women with localized cancer of the breast. N Engl J Med 328:1587–1590, 1993.
102. Winchester DP, Menck HR, Osteen RT, Kraybill W: Treatment trends for ductal carcinoma in situ of the breast. Ann Surg Oncol 2:207–213, 1995.
103. Wun LM, Feuer EJ, Miller BA: Are increases in mammographic screening still a valid explanation for trends in breast cancer incidence in the United States? Cancer Causes Control 6:135–144, 1995.
104. Zafrani B, Fourquet A, Vilcoq RJ, Legal M, Calle R: Conservative management of intraductal breast carcinoma with tumorectomy and radiation therapy. Cancer 57:1299–1301, 1986.

CHAPTER 60
ADJUVANT RADIATION THERAPY FOR PRIMARY MANAGEMENT OF APPARENTLY REGIONALLY CONFINED BREAST CANCER

Seymour H. Levitt, M.D. / Gilbert H. Fletcher, M.D.*

EVOLUTION OF CLINICAL DATA

Two sets of clinical data had a profound impact on the management of apparently confined breast cancer: prognostic factors based on the clinical features of the disease both in the breast and the axilla, and the demonstration that the internal mammary chain nodes are a primary route of spread. These data forced clinicians to consider radiotherapy as an effective complement or option to surgery, which had once been the universal treatment of choice for breast cancer.

Criteria of Clinical Operability

The Halsted operation extended the mastectomy by removing the whole of the sternal head of the pectoralis major muscle with division of the clavicular head and the pectoralis minor muscle, thus giving better access to the lymph nodes in the infraclavicular fossa. In his first 50 cases, Halsted also dissected the supraclavicular nodes, a procedure he later abandoned as a routine but continued to practice in many cases. All of Halsted's first 50 patients were found to have invasion of the axillary lymph nodes.

Until World War II, the radical mastectomy was regarded as the routine treatment in most cases of cancer confined to the breast and the axillary nodes on the same side. The first critical appraisal of the radical mastectomy was done by Haagensen and Stout. Their paper, published in 1943, is a milestone in the evaluation of the effectiveness of the surgical procedure.[22] It demonstrated that, in patients with criteria of clinical inoperability, the radical mastectomy was not only futile but also possibly harmful, because almost all patients died within 5 years and the incidence of local/regional failures was 47 percent. Haagensen and Stout[22] noted the following (Table 60–1):

From these correlations we have drawn up rules for judging operability in breast carcinoma as follows: women of all age-groups, who are in good enough general condition to run the risk of major surgery, should be treated by radical mastectomy, except as follows:

1. When the carcinoma is one which developed during pregnancy or lactation.
2. When extensive edema of the skin over the breast is present.
3. When satellite nodules are present in the skin over the breast.
4. When intercostal or parasternal tumor nodules are present.
5. When there is edema of the arm.
6. When proved supraclavicular metastases are present.
7. When the carcinoma is the inflammatory type.
8. When distant metastases are demonstrated.
9. When any two, or more, of the following signs of locally advanced carcinoma are present:
   a. Ulceration of the skin.
   b. Edema of the skin of limited extent (less than one-third of the skin over the breast involved).
   c. Fixation of the tumor to the chest wall.
   d. Axillary lymph nodes measuring 2.5 cm or more in transverse diameter, and proved to contain metastases by biopsy.
   e. Fixation of axillary lymph nodes to the skin or the deep structures of the axilla, and proved to contain metastases by biopsy.

If these criteria had actually been followed in judging operability in the series of 640 radical mastectomies which we have reported, the fate of 109 of the patients would not have been affected.

In his book *Diseases of the Breast,* Haagensen elaborated on the clinical features of the primary tumor and the axillary status as prognostic factors, particularly in local/regional failures.[21] A high incidence of local/regional recurrences was also reported in another series.[49] These two analyses prompted us to combine the surgical procedure with preoperative or postoperative irradiation or to use irradiation alone to cut down on this high recurrence rate (Table 60–2).[18]

---

*Deceased.

TABLE 60–1.   HAAGENSEN-STOUT CRITERIA OF OPERABILITY APPLIED TO PRESBYTERIAN HOSPITAL SERIES OF RADICAL MASTECTOMIES, 1915–1934

Group	No. of Cases	5-Year Local Recurrence		5-Year Clinical Cures		Permanent Cures
		No.	*Percent*	*No.*	*Percent*	
Cases in which radical mastectomy was actually performed (1914–1934)	640	161	25.2	231	36.1	Many still well
Cases that would now be classified as inoperable	109	52	47.7	3	2.8	None
Cases that would now be classified as operable	531	109	20.5	228	42.9	Many still well

From Haagensen CD, Stout AP: Carcinoma of the breast: II. Criteria of operability. Ann Surg 118:859–870; 1032–1051, 1943. Reprinted by permission.

Internal Mammary Chain Nodes

The invasion of the internal mammary chain nodes was recorded for the first time in an autopsy report from Middlesex Hospital Cancer Ward on October 22, 1806. Halsted was probably the first to attempt to excise the internal mammary nodes as part of the surgical attack on breast cancer. In 1922, Sampson Handley, a surgeon at Middlesex Hospital, explored the mediastinum in six patients and found involvement of the chain in two. In 1927, Handley again documented his belief in the importance of the internal mammary chain route of metastases:

> It is the fact that in more than half of my recurrent cases, before I began the prophylactic use of radium, the return of the disease manifested itself either by an enlargement of the gland of the lower and inner angle of the posterior triangle, or by the appearance of nodules, later merging in sternal recurrence, upon the deep fascia at the inner end of the first, second, or third intercostal spaces. The position of these recurrences accurately along the line of the internal mammary artery shows, I think, beyond doubt that they are due to invasion of the lymphatic glands which lie along its course.[26]

Richard Handley, son of Sampson Handley, began in 1946 to excise the nodes at the first three intercostal spaces at the completion of the radical mastectomy. In 1949, he reported his findings in 50 patients, correlating the involvement of the chain with the histological status of the axilla and the location of the tumor in the breast.[24, 25]

Treatment of the internal mammary chain nodes by dissecting them became very popular in con-

junction with conventional radical mastectomy (extended radical mastectomy). The survival benefits of the treatment were controversial, and so an intercontinental randomized trial of radical mastectomy versus radical mastectomy plus dissection of the chain nodes was structured. Initially, it seemed to show survival benefits in patients with histologically positive axillary nodes and the tumor located in the inner quadrants. With longer follow-up, the statistical difference disappeared in most patients, but was maintained in the patients treated at the Institut Gustave Roussy.[31, 32] The results of irradiation of the internal mammary nodes have also not been consistent. Possible reasons for this inconsistency include the difficulty of diagnosing internal mammary nodal involvement and inadequate radiation technique.[33]

HISTORY OF BREAST IRRADIATION

Pioneer Era (1896–1930)

After the discovery of x-rays by Roentgen in 1895, Emil Grubbe, a Chicago medical student, developed a severe dermatitis of the skin of his hand while testing Crookes' tubes with that hand. A physician who had seen Grubbe's lesion referred a patient with breast cancer to him for irradiation, because of the apparent biological damaging effect of the recently discovered x-rays.

From 1900 until the 1920s, the practice was to give one treatment that produced a brisk skin erythema. The dose was called Haut (skin) Erythema Dosis or HED. Later, the HED was measured to be approximately 1000 roentgen. It was believed that the dose killing the epithelium of the skin would kill cancer. In the 1920s, after the Coolidge tube was invented, somewhat more systematic treatments of breast cancer were done with external irradiation. Technical advances were made in external irradiation treatment planning, such as the introduction of tangential fields for irradiating the breast. Inoperable lesions were irradiated and some regression resulted, a phenomenon that was noticed with interest. Also at this time, irradiation began to be used preoperatively or postoperatively. The rationale for preoperative irradiation was the same as it is today, that by diminishing

TABLE 60–2.   EFFECTIVENESS OF LOCAL/REGIONAL IRRADIATION IN BREAST CANCER

Site of Recurrence	Incidence of Recurrence (%)	
	No Irradiation	*Irradiation*
Supraclavicular	20–26	1.5
Parasternal	9	0
Chest wall	35–45	10

Data from Fletcher GH: Textbook of Radiotherapy. 3rd ed. Philadelphia, Lea & Febiger, 1980.

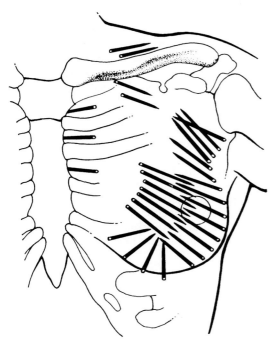

Figure 60–1   *Diagram showing usual distribution of needles. (From Keynes G: The radium treatment of breast cancer. Br J Surg 19:415–480, 1932. Reprinted by permission.)*

the tumor cell population, the spread of cancer would be less likely during the surgical procedure.

In the early 1920s, radium needles were made available in the Surgical Department of St. Bartholomew's Hospital in England. Geoffrey Keynes, a surgeon, began in 1922 to treat patients who had recurrent disease and found that the tumor in nearly every instance disappeared. The method was extended to treatment of primary disease in 1924, initially for very advanced or inoperable tumors and later for operable lesions (Fig. 60–1).[29] In 1937, Keynes reported that long-term, disease-free survival rates were comparable to those obtained with radical mastectomy and considered this method an alternative to radical mastectomy. He also carefully mentioned the disadvantages, specifically the development of fibrosis and neuropathies.[30]

Preoperative Irradiation Followed by Radical Mastectomy

In the 1930s, Baclesse gave, at best estimate, a radiation dose to 21 patients of at least 5000 roentgen over an 8- to 13-week period. The surgery was performed 4 to 8 weeks after irradiation. In one third of the surgical specimens, no tumor at all could be detected, and only two specimens had cancer cells with no marked morphological changes.[7] As a result, preoperative irradiation had some popularity in the 1930s and 1940s, but since 1950, the interest in preoperative irradiation has been limited, and few series of patients have been available for analysis. At the University of Texas M. D. Anderson Cancer

Center, patients with lesions of borderline clinical operability or with large ecchymoses after an outside biopsy were treated with preoperative irradiation, first with 250 kV and later with cobalt 60. An analysis of the long-term results showed a lower percentage than expected of patients with histologically positive axillary nodes and a low incidence of local/regional failures. Survival rates were similar to those in patients given postoperative irradiation.[44] Similarly, a study conducted by the Stockholm Breast Cancer Study Group from 1971 to 1976 to compare preoperative and postoperative radiation after modified radical mastectomy found no significant differences between the two treatments.[45]

Irradiation After Radical Mastectomy

In 1949 in Manchester, England, a randomized trial comparing the results of radical mastectomy with and without postoperative irradiation was started using two different techniques. The quadrate technique essentially irradiated the chest wall, and the other technique irradiated the peripheral lymphatics but did not irradiate the chest wall. No survival benefits were seen with either technique, although there was a diminution of local/regional failure rates with both techniques. Paterson and Russell concluded that one could wait for failures to appear before treating them.[42]

Since 1948 at M. D. Anderson Cancer Center, postoperative irradiation has been given to the lymphatics of the apex of the axilla, supraclavicular area, and internal mammary chain with an en face L-shaped portal.[17] Because of the variable location of the nodes, they may be only marginally covered unless an en face portal or sophisticated techniques are used to identify their location. Kilovoltage was first used, then cesium 137, cobalt 60, and finally, since 1963, electron beam. An analysis of the incidence of failures in the supraclavicular area in patients with initially clinically negative supraclavicular nodes showed that approximately 5000 rad in 4 weeks reduced the incidence of failures at this site to almost zero (Table 60–3),[16] compared with 25 percent rates

TABLE 60–3.   INCIDENCE OF DISEASE DEVELOPING IN THE SUPRACLAVICULAR AREA AFTER RADICAL MASTECTOMY* AT M. D. ANDERSON CANCER CENTER, JANUARY 1955–DECEMBER 1967

Treatment	No.	Percent
Postoperative irradiation		
250 kV: 4000 rad skin dose in 4 weeks (<3500 rad node dose)	6/89	7
Cesium 137, cobalt 60, electron beam: 5000 to 5500 rad given in 4 weeks	4/273	1.5
Preoperative irradiation		
Cobalt 60: 4000 rad given in 4 weeks	4/121	3

*When axillary nodes are positive in the surgical specimen.
Modified from Fletcher GH: Local results of irradiation in the primary management of localized breast cancer. Cancer 29:545–551, 1972.

at Manchester and Memorial Hospital, New York, where no postoperative irradiation was given. Since 1963, the chest wall has been irradiated with an electron beam if there was a heavy involvement of the axilla in the surgical specimen, aggressive features of the disease in the breast, or both. An analysis of the disease-free survival rates and the local/regional failures was done in 1991.[19]

At M. D. Anderson, the chest wall is treated with low energy beams of 6 or 7 MeV and the internal mammary nodes are treated with energies of 12 to 13 MeV. Energy beams of 9 or 10 MeV are used to treat the supraclavicular field and axillary apex.[35] Current radiation technique emphasizes the importance of appropriately treating the chest wall to avoid the increased risk of cardiac morbidity and mortality reported in patients treated with inappropriate mediastinal irradiation.[45] (See *Levitt and Tapley's Technological Basis of Radiation Therapy* for more specific information on modern radiation technique.[35]) Recent long-term studies report increased local control, disease-specific survival, and overall survival in patients treated with modern radiation techniques after radical mastectomy.[4, 12, 45]

Simple Mastectomy and Postoperative Irradiation

In 1941 in Edinburgh, McWhirter initiated the use of simple mastectomy followed by postoperative irradiation for operable breast cancer instead of a radical mastectomy. In 1948, he reported 5-year survival rates comparable to the ones obtained with radical mastectomy.[36] The so-called McWhirter technique was the first challenge to the radical mastectomy, which had been considered the only curative procedure. The historical importance of the Edinburgh experiment cannot be overemphasized, because it justified the use of surgical procedures less extensive than the classical radical procedures.

At the M. D. Anderson Cancer Center, simple mastectomy followed by irradiation has been used since 1948 in patients with stage III and stage IV disease. Later, dissection of the lateral axilla was added. The results showed approximately ten percent local/regional failures and disease-free survival rates of 35 percent in patients without clinically positive supraclavicular nodes.[37]

Irradiation Alone

Baclesse was the first to explore the use of external irradiation alone for the curative treatment of breast cancer. Between 1936 and 1945, 145 patients, some with operable and some with inoperable lesions, were treated with irradiation alone. Only 10 of the patients had had the tumor removed by an excisional biopsy. Baclesse reported on this series in 1948, including detailed sketches of the treatment portals.[5] It can be estimated that doses of 7000 to 9000 roentgen were given to a large mass in the breast in 16 weeks. The supraclavicular area received a 5000-

roentgen skin dose in 12 weeks if there were no palpable nodes; in-between doses were given to the intermediately sized axillary nodes. A correlation was made between the size of the tumor mass and the amount of irradiation necessary to control it. For instance, doses as low as 4100 rad produced control in relatively small tumors, whereas in large tumors higher doses and a minimum of 3 months of treatment time were necessary. It is of interest that 9 of the 10 patients whose tumor had been removed by excisional biopsy were alive, disease free, 5 years or more after removal. Baclesse concluded in 1959 that in properly selected patients, the percentage of cures was not significantly different from that obtained by more conventional methods, and although it was not a method to replace all others, radiotherapy was an alternative to consider for those patients who refused mutilating surgery.[6]

At M. D. Anderson Cancer Center, patients with unresectable lesions or who met Haagensen's criteria of clinical inoperability were treated with irradiation alone by the Baclesse technique, initially with 250 kV and later with cobalt 60. The total dose in some patients was as high as 10,000 rad. In 1965, an analysis confirmed that gross masses can be controlled with very large doses, with significant survival rates.[20] A later analysis showed that fibrosis and sometimes ulceration developed in all patients.[48]

Conservation Surgery Followed by Irradiation

In 1945, Mustakiallio initiated careful dissection of early tumors, leaving only sound tissue, followed with 2100 rad (6 × 350) to the breast through tangential portals.[38] The axilla was treated through front and back portals and the supraclavicular area through a direct portal. In 1969, an analysis of long-term results showed survival rates comparable to those obtained with radical mastectomy, but with a 20 percent recurrence rate in the breast.[43]

In 1955, at Guy's Hospital in London, a randomized clinical trial of radical mastectomy versus wide excision (extended tylectomy) followed by postoperative irradiation was initiated.[3] The doses were inadequate by present standards. Fifteen local/regional failures occurred in 112 patients with clinical stage I disease (clinically negative axilla) and 30 failures occurred in 70 patients with clinical stage II disease (clinically positive axilla). The incidence of failures in the axilla in patients with clinically positive nodes corresponds with the expected percentage of patients who would have had histologically positive axillary nodes had a radical mastectomy been performed.

These early trials were precursors to several randomized clinical trials initiated in the 1970s and 1980s that compared conservative surgery with radiation to radical mastectomy (Table 60–4).[27] All these studies reported comparable survival results between the two treatments, which resulted in a 1991 report from the National Cancer Institute that stated "[b]reast conserving treatment (excision of the pri-

TABLE 60–4.   MODERN RANDOMIZED TRIALS OF CONSERVATIVE SURGERY AND IRRADIATION COMPARED WITH MASTECTOMY

Investigations	Dates of Trial	No. of Patients	Survival Equivalent
Gustave-Roussy[47]	1972–1979	179	Yes
MCI, Milan[52]	1973–1980	701	Yes
NSABP Protocol B-06[15]	1976–1984	1843	Yes
NCI, Bethesda[50]	1980–1986	112	Yes
EORTC[51]	1980–1986	903	Yes
Guy's Hospital[23]	1981–1986	399	Yes
Danish Breast Cancer Group[8]	1983–1987	619	Yes

MCI = Milan Cancer Institute; NSABP = National Surgical Adjuvant Breast and Bowel Project; NCI = National Cancer Institute; EORTC = European Organization for Research and Treatment of Cancer.

From Harris JR, Morrow M, Bonadonna G: Cancer of the Breast. *In* DeVita VT, et al (eds): Principles and Practice of Oncology. 4th ed. Philadelphia, JB Lippincott, 1993, pp 1264–1332.

mary tumor and adjacent breast tissue followed by radiation therapy) is an appropriate method of primary therapy for the majority of women with stage I and II breast cancer and is preferable because it provides survival equivalent to total mastectomy and axillary dissection while preserving the breast."[39] Four major randomized clinical trials have been published that compare the results between conservative surgery with or without radiation.[14, 34, 53, 54] Based on current information, radiation as an adjuvant to conservative surgery is considered standard treatment for early breast cancer.[1, 14]

Evolution of the Concept of Radiosensitivity of Breast Cancer

Until relatively recently, the concept of radiosensitivity had been based on histology; within the same histology, there were subsets of tumors that, for no obvious reasons, were radiosensitive or radioresistant. This was best expressed by Paterson on the radiosensitivity of breast cancer.[41]

A few fall into the highly radiosensitive group already discussed; the majority seem to respond in a surprising way to doses at the 4/5000 r level. But on the other hand, there are cases which definitely do not respond to even 7000 r. The breast group of tumors, as a whole, lacks the interesting consistency of the true squamous epitheliomata, and promises to present an interesting research problem for the pathologist and therapist jointly.

Baclesse must be credited with demonstrating that breast cancer can be eradicated by irradiation only. His work on breast cancer has great significance, because it established the correlation among dose, control, and size of the tumor. The fact that he gave much smaller doses to clinically negative lymphatic areas is important, but the effectiveness of these doses on subclinical disease cannot be assessed, because he did not report the incidence of failures in electively irradiated areas; at that time, the 5-year survival rate was the only analyzed end point.

Elective irradiation of the supraclavicular areas has shown that 4500 to 5000 rad given in 5 weeks eradicates more than 90 percent of occult deposits (see Table 60–3). These data are the basis of the regimen in which 5000 rad is given to the breast after a segmental resection of the tumor. A boost is given if the margins are poor.[16]

Current advances in radiation physics and molecular biology will allow for greater precision in applying the knowledge gained from the radiosensitivity of cells. One major area of research is the use of agents that enhance the ability of radiation to kill tumor cells and to protect normal cells.[28]

Curability of Breast Cancer

At the middle of this century, after investigating breast cancer mortality since 1900, some epidemiologists concluded that survival rates of patients with breast cancer were not at all affected by any treatment.[40] In their study, the 5-year survival rate was used as an index. Other authors have constructed

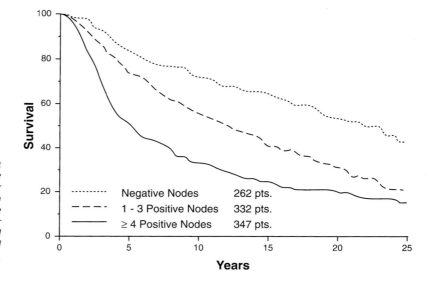

Figure 60–2 *Comparative overall survival rates among breast cancer patients with negative nodes, one to three positive nodes, and four or more positive nodes treated by radical mastectomy and postoperative radiotherapy with no adjuvant chemotherapy from 1963 to 1977 at the M. D. Anderson Hospital (analysis 1991). (From Fletcher GH: Is breast cancer curable? In Fletcher GH, Levitt SH [eds]: Non-Disseminated Breast Cancer: Controversial Issues in Management. Berlin, Springer-Verlag, 1993, pp 1–3.)*

·········· Negative Nodes	262 pts.	
- - - - 1 - 3 Positive Nodes	332 pts.	
—— ≥ 4 Positive Nodes	347 pts.	

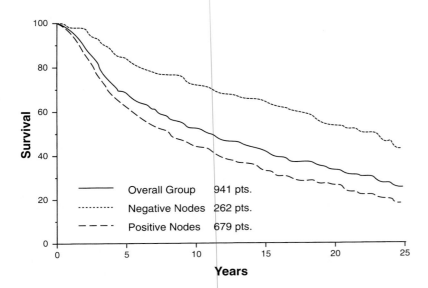

Figure 60–3   *Comparative survival rates among node-negative, node-positive, and overall group of breast cancer patients treated by radical mastectomy and postoperative radiotherapy with no adjuvant chemotherapy from 1963 to 1966 at the M. D. Anderson Hospital (analysis 1991). (From Fletcher GH: Is breast cancer curable? In Fletcher GH, Levitt SH [eds]: Non-Disseminated Breast Cancer: Controversial Issues in Management. Berlin, Springer-Verlag, 1993, pp 1–3.)*

mathematical models of the behavior of breast cancer and have concluded that at any one time the same proportion of patients experiences failure, so that eventually all patients die from breast cancer.[11, 13] Other studies have indicated that less than 15 percent of breast cancer patients with positive axillary lymph nodes will be free of disseminated disease.[10] However, some models of breast cancer survival suggest that a fraction of patients are cured by therapy.[46] There are data in the literature showing that patients with histologically positive axillary nodes can survive a long time. For instance, of 1958 breast cancer patients treated at Memorial Hospital in New York City in the years 1940 to 1943, 184 were known to be alive for an average of 30.6 years; 60 of them had had positive axillary nodes.[2] At M. D. Anderson Cancer Center, an analysis done in 1991 of the results in patients who had received postoperative irradiation between 1963 and 1977 showed that the survival curves flatten out after 15 years, which indicates that not all patients with histologically positive

nodes die from disease. This suggests that 40 percent of patients with histologically positive axillary nodes are alive and free of disease after 20 years (Figs. 60–2 and 60–3).[19]

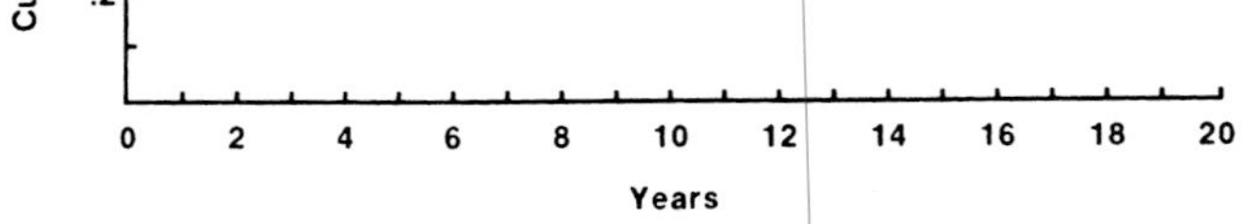

A graph in the second edition of *Diseases of the Breast* compares the mortality of breast cancer patients 20 years after treatment with the mortality of the general population (Fig. 60–4).[21] After 15 years, the curves are parallel, indicating that a certain proportion of patients is cured. In another series comparing the mortality of breast cancer patients with the mortality of the general population, some patients were also shown to be cured.[9]

Acknowledgments

The original version of this chapter was supported in part by grants CA06294 and CA16672 awarded by the National Cancer Institute, U.S. Department of Health and Human Services.

THE NATURAL HISTORY OF BREAST CARCINOMA

Figure 60–4   *Cumulative probabilities of survival for 662 women treated by radical mastectomy for carcinoma of the breast are compared with age-adjusted survival rates for women in the general population of New York State. (From Haagensen CD: Diseases of the Breast. 2nd ed. Philadelphia, WB Saunders, 1971. Reprinted by permission.)*

References

1. Abrams JS, Phillips PA, Friedman MA: Meeting highlights: A reappraisal of research results for the local treatment of early stage breast cancer. J Natl Cancer Inst 87:1837–1845, 1995.
2. Adair F, Berg J, Joubert L, Robbins GF: Long-term follow-up of breast cancer patients: The 30-year report. Cancer 33:1145–1150, 1974.
3. Atkins H, Hayward JL, Klugman DJ, Wayte AB: Treatment of early breast cancer: A report after ten years of clinical trials. Br Med J 20:423–429, 1972.
4. Auquier A, Rutqvist LE, Host H, Rotstein S, Arriagada R: Postmastectomy megavoltage radiotherapy: The Oslo and Stockholm trials. Eur J Cancer 28:433–437, 1992.
5. Baclesse F: La roentgentherapie scule dans le traitement des cancers due scin operables et inoperables: Troisieme rapport. Presented at the Association Francaise de Chirurgie, 51st Congress Francais de Chirurgie, Paris, 1948.
6. Baclesse F: Roentgen therapy alone in cancer of the breast. Acta Un Int Contra Cancrum 15:1023, 1959.
7. Baclesse F, Gricouroff G, Tailhefer A: Essai de roentgentherapie du cancer cu scin suivie d'operation large: Resultat histologiques. Bull Cancer 28:729–743, 1939.
8. Blichert-Toft M, Rose C, Andersen JA, et al: Danish random-

ized trial comparing breast conservation therapy with mastectomy: Six years of life table analysis. J Natl Cancer Inst Monogr 11:19–26, 1992.

9. Brinkley D, Haybittle JL: The curability of breast cancer. Lancet 2:95–97, 1975.

10. Bross IDJ, Blumenson LE: Predictive design of experiments using deep mathematical models. Cancer 28:1637–1646, 1971.

11. Cutler SJ, Axtell SJ: Partitioning of a patient population with respect to different mortality risk. Am Stat Assoc J 6:701–712, 1963.

12. Cuzick J, Stewart H, Rutqvist L, Houghton J, Edwards R, Redmond C, et al: Cause-specific mortality in long-term survivors of breast cancer who participated in trials of radiotherapy. J Clin Oncol 12:447–453, 1994.

13. Ederer F, Cutler SJ, Goldberg IS, Eisenberg H: Causes of death among long-term survivors from breast cancer in Connecticut. J Natl Cancer Inst 30:933–947, 1963.

14. Fisher B, Anderson S, Redmond CK, et al: Reanalysis and results after 12 years of follow-up in a randomized clinical trial comparing total mastectomy with lumpectomy with or without irradiation in the treatment of breast cancer. N Engl J Med 333:1456–1461, 1995.

15. Fisher B, Redmond C, Poisson R, et al: Eight year results of a randomized clinical trial comparing mastectomy and lumpectomy with or without irradiation in the treatment of breast cancer. N Engl J Med 320:822–828, 1989.

16. Fletcher GH: Local results of irradiation in the primary management of localized breast cancer. Cancer 29:545–551, 1972.

17. Fletcher GH: Textbook of Radiotherapy. 2nd ed. Philadelphia, Lea & Febiger, 1973.

18. Fletcher GH: Textbook of Radiotherapy. 3rd ed. Philadelphia, Lea & Febiger, 1980.

19. Fletcher GH: Is breast cancer curable? In Fletcher GH, Levitt SH (eds): Non-Disseminated Breast Cancer: Controversial Issues in Management. Berlin, Springer-Verlag, 1993, pp 1–3.

20. Fletcher GH, Montague ED: Radical irradiation of advanced breast cancer. AJR 93:573–584, 1965.

21. Haagensen CD: Diseases of the Breast. 2nd ed. Philadelphia, WB Saunders, 1971.

22. Haagensen CD, Stout AP: Carcinoma of the breast: II. Criteria of operability. Ann Surg 118:859–870; 1032–1051, 1943.

23. Habibollahi F, Fentiman I, Chandry M: Conservation treatment of operable breast cancer. Proc Am Soc Clin Oncol 6:59, 1987. Abstract.

24. Handley RS: A surgeon's view of the spread of breast cancer. Cancer 24:1231–1234, 1969.

25. Handley RS, Thackray AC: The internal mammary lymph chains in carcinoma of the breast. Lancet 2:276–278, 1949.

26. Handley WS: Parasternal invasion of the thorax in breast cancer and its suppression by the use of radium tubes as an operative precaution. Surg Gynecol Obstet 45:721–728, 1927.

27. Harris JR, Morrow M, Bonadonna G: Cancer of the breast. In DeVita VT, Hellman S, Rosenberg SA (eds): Principles and Practices of Oncology. 4th ed. Philadelphia, JB Lippincott, 1993, pp 1264–1332.

28. Hellman S, Weichselbaum R: Radiation oncology and the new biology. Cancer J Sci Am 1(3):174–179, 1995.

29. Keynes G: The radium treatment of carcinoma of the breast. Br J Surg 19:415–480, 1932.

30. Keynes G: Conservative treatment of cancer of the breast. Br Med J 2:643–647, 1937.

31. Lacour J, Le MG, Hill C, Kramer A, Contesso G, Sarrazin D: Is it useful to remove internal mammary nodes in operable breast cancer? Eur J Surg Oncol 13:309–314, 1987.

32. Le MG, Arriagada R, de Vathaire F, Dewar J, Fontaine F, Lacour J, et al: Can internal mammary chain treatment decrease the risk of death for patients with medial breast cancers and positive axillary lymph nodes? Cancer 66:2313–2218, 1990.

33. Levitt SH: The importance of locoregional control in the treatment of breast cancer and its impact on survival. Cancer 74:1840–1846, 1994.

34. Liljegren G, Holmberg L, Adami HO, Westman G, Graffman S, Bergh J, for the Uppsala-Orebro Breast Cancer Study Group: Sector resection with or without postoperative radiotherapy for stage I breast cancer: Five-year results of a randomized trial. J Natl Cancer Inst 86:717–722, 1994.

35. McNeese MD, Fletcher GH, Levitt SH, Khan FM: Breast cancer. In Levitt SH, Khan FM, Potish RA (eds): Levitt and Tapley's Technological Basis of Radiation Therapy: Practical Clinical Applications. 2nd ed. Philadelphia, Lea & Febiger, 1992, pp 232–247.

36. McWhirter R: The value of simple mastectomy and radiotherapy in the treatment of cancer of the breast. Br J Radiol 21:599–610, 1948.

37. Montague ED, Spanos WJ Jr, Fletcher GH: Die Entwicklung der Behandlungsmethoden bei der Primartherapie des nicht-metastasierten Mammakarzinoma. In Frischbier HJ (ed): Die Erkrandungen den weiblichen Brustdruse. Stuttgart, Georg Thieme Verlag, 1982, pp 201–208.

38. Mustakiallio S: Uber die Moeglichkeiten der roentgentherapie bei der Behandlung des Bruskrebes. Acta Radiol (Stockh) 26:503–511, 1945.

39. National Institute of Health Consensus Conference: Treatment of early stage breast cancer. JAMA 265:391–395, 1991.

40. Park WW, Lees JC: The absolute curability of cancer of the breast. Surg Gynecol Obstet 93:129–152, 1951.

41. Paterson R: The radical x-ray treatment of carcinomata. Br J Radiol 9:671–679, 1936.

42. Paterson R, Russell M: Clinical trials in malignant disease: Part III. Breast cancer: Evaluation of postoperative radiotherapy. J Fac Radiol 10:175–180, 1959.

43. Rissanen PM: A comparison of conservative and radical surgery combined with radiotherapy in the treatment of stage I carcinoma of the breast. Br J Radiol 42:423–426, 1969.

44. Rodger A, Montague ED, Fletcher GH: Preoperative or postoperative irradiation as adjuvant treatment with radical mastectomy in breast cancer. Cancer 51:1388–1392, 1983.

45. Rutqvist LE: What have we learned from the Stockholm trials on adjuvant radiation therapy in early-stage breast cancer? In Fletcher GH, Levitt SH (eds): Non-Disseminated Breast Cancer: Controversial Issues in Management. Berlin, Springer-Verlag, 1993, pp 83–92.

46. Rutqvist LE, Wallgren A, Nilsson B: Is breast cancer a curable disease? A study of 14,731 women with breast cancer from the cancer registry of Norway. Cancer 53:1793–1800, 1984.

47. Sarrazin D, Le M, Arriagada R, et al: Ten-year results of a randomized trial comparing a conservative treatment of mastectomy in early breast cancer. Radiother Oncol 14:177–184, 1989.

48. Spanos WJ, Montague ED, Fletcher GH: Late complications of radiation only for advanced breast cancer. Int J Radiat Oncol Biol Phys 6:1473–1476, 1980.

49. Spratt JS: Locally recurrent cancer after radical mastectomy. Cancer 20:1051–1053, 1967.

50. Straus K, Lichter A, Lippman M, et al: Results of the National Cancer Institute early breast cancer trial. J Natl Cancer Inst Monogr 11:27–32, 1992.

51. van Dongen JA, Bartelink H, Fentiman IS, et al: Randomized clinical trial to assess the value of breast-conserving therapy in stage I and II breast cancer, EORTC 10801 trial. J Natl Cancer Inst Monographs 11:15–18, 1992.

52. Veronesi U, Banfi A, Salvadori B: Breast conservation is the treatment of choice in small breast cancer: Long-term results of a randomized trial. Eur J Cancer 26:668–670, 1990.

53. Veronesi U, Luini A, Galimberti V, Zurrida S: Conservation approaches for the management of stage I/II carcinoma of the breast: Milan Cancer Institute trials. World J Surg 18:70–75, 1994.

54. Whelan T, Clark R, Roberts R, Levine M, Foster G, for the Investigators of the Ontario Clinical Oncology Group: Ipsilateral breast tumor recurrence postlumpectomy is predictive of subsequent mortality: Results from a randomized trial. Int J Radiat Oncol Biol Phys 30:11–16, 1994.

CHAPTER 61
ADJUVANT RADIOTHERAPY AFTER MODIFIED RADICAL MASTECTOMY

Michael P. Hagan, M.D., Ph.D. / Nancy Price Mendenhall, M.D.

INDICATIONS FOR TREATMENT

Historical

Based on the incidence and pattern of local/regional recurrences after radical or modified radical mastectomy for operable breast cancer in historical series, Fletcher identified subsets of patients with a significant risk of local/regional recurrence and established the following indications for elective irradiation after radical or modified radical mastectomy[11, 24, 31]:

1. Patients with outer quadrant lesions smaller than 5 cm and no involvement of axillary nodes do not receive postoperative irradiation.

2. Patients with histologically negative axillary nodes and central or medial breast cancers smaller than 2 cm receive irradiation to the internal mammary nodes only.

3. Patients with positive axillary nodes (but fewer than 20 percent of nodes involved) or patients with central or medial tumors larger than 2 cm receive peripheral lymphatic irradiation (i.e., the internal mammary and the supraclavicular and axillary apex nodes).

4. Patients with more than 20 percent of nodes involved receive not only peripheral lymphatic irradiation but also chest wall irradiation, regardless of the size of the primary lesion or its location in the breast. The whole axilla is not irradiated unless the dissection is incomplete, axillary nodes larger than 2.5 cm are present, or extranodal disease is histologically verified or clinically suspected because of mat-

ted adenopathy before surgery. The chest wall is also irradiated if the primary tumor is larger than 5 cm, grave signs are present (skin edema, erythema, or ulceration or fixation to skin, pectoral fascia, or chest wall), the surgical margins are close or involved, or the primary tumor has extensive vascular or lymphatic space invasion.

Current

Because of the prognostic significance of the number of involved nodes and more variability in the type of axillary procedures performed, most clinicians today base management decisions on the *number* of involved nodes rather than the *percentage*. Since Fletcher's guidelines were published, additional information has led to modification of the indications used at the University of Florida for postmastectomy irradiation (Table 61–1). Two areas, in particular, warrant discussion: the role of internal mammary chain (IMC) irradiation and the role of peripheral lymphatic irradiation alone.

In recent years there has been controversy over the role of internal mammary node irradiation. The incidence of internal mammary node involvement is related to tumor size and status of the axilla. In patients undergoing extended radical mastectomy with internal mammary node dissection in a prospective randomized trial of radical versus extended radical mastectomy (Table 61–2),[35] fewer than 10 percent of patients with a "negative" axilla and a T1 or T2 tumor had internal mammary node involvement, re-

TABLE 61–1. RADIATION TREATMENT VOLUMES RECOMMENDED AT THE UNIVERSITY OF FLORIDA

Primary Tumor	Negative	Micrometastases	Status of Axilla		
			1 to 3 Positive Nodes	≥4 Positive Nodes	Extensive Axillary Disease*
T1	—	—	PL; consider CW	CW + PL	CW + PL + Ax
T2	—	Consider CW + PL	PL; consider CW	CW + PL	CW + PL + Ax
T1/T2 with poor histological features†	Consider CW + PL	Consider CW + PL	CW + PL	CW + PL	CW + PL + Ax
Close/positive margins	CW	CW + PL	CW + PL	CW + PL	CW + PL + Ax
T3	CW + PL	CW + PL	CW + PL	CW + PL	CW + PL + Ax
T4	CW + PL	CW + PL	CW + PL	CW + PL	CW + PL + Ax
Primary grave signs‡	CW + PL + Ax	CW + PL + Ax	CW + PL + Ax	CW + PL + Ax	CW + PL + Ax

*Extranodal axillary disease; clinically matted or fixed nodes; nodes ≥2.5 cm.
†Poorly differentiated lesions; extensive vascular, lymphatic, or perineural invasion; multifocal disease.
‡Skin edema, erythema, ulceration, or fixation; pectoral fascia or chest wall fixation.
Key: CW, chest wall; PL, peripheral lymphatics (supraclavicular and axillary apex and internal mammary nodes); Ax, whole axillary irradiation with posterior axillary boost.

TABLE 61–2.   PREVALENCE OF INTERNAL MAMMARY NODE INVOLVEMENT DOCUMENTED AT EXTENDED MASTECTOMY AS A FUNCTION OF TUMOR SIZE AND LOCATION AND AXILLARY STATUS

	Status of Axillary Nodes					
	Negative		Positive		Total	
	(%)	*(n)*	*(%)*	*(n)*	*(%)*	*(n)*
T1–2, lateral	8	89	22	93	15	182
T1–2, medial	9	57	35	63	23	120
T3, lateral	25	4	64	11	53	15
T3, medial	18	11	43	14	32	25
Total	9	161	30	181	21	342

Adapted from Veronesi U, Valagussa P: Inefficiency of internal mammary nodes dissection in breast cancer surgery. Cancer 47:170–175, 1981.

gardless of whether the tumor was located in the medial or lateral part of the breast. For this reason, internal mammary node irradiation currently is not usually given to such patients unless there is extensive vascular or lymphatic space invasion or an aggressive histological pattern evidenced by high nuclear or histological grade or mitotic rate. For patients with T3 tumors or positive axillary nodes, however, the prevalence of internal mammary node involvement ranged from 20 percent to 60 percent, depending on the site of the tumor. Based on the overall incidence of internal mammary node involvement in the extended radical mastectomy arm of the trial, a 20 percent rate of internal mammary node recurrence was expected in the radical mastectomy study arm, but clinically overt internal mammary node recurrence was detected in only 4 percent of patients. Indeed, internal mammary node recurrence has rarely been reported in other series that assessed local/regional recurrence.[13] This discrepancy between the known incidence of internal mammary node involvement as documented pathologically and the incidence of clinically detected recurrence in the internal mammary nodes has led some investigators to conclude that subclinical disease in the internal mammary nodes is clinically insignificant; thus, the controversy over whether or not internal mammary node irradiation is indicated. Another interpretation of the discrepancies between observed and expected local-regional recurrence rates is that our ability to detect local/regional disease clinically, particularly in the internal mammary nodes, is limited (Figs. 61–1 and 61–2), especially when observations are limited to the first site of failure. This underreporting of local/regional disease recurrence may confound our interpretation of trials designed to determine the relationship between uncontrolled local/regional disease and distant metastases. Clinicians who believe that the role of irradiation is to eradicate subclinical disease remaining after mastectomy recommend treating internal mammary nodes of patients who have T3 tumors or involved axillary nodes with high-risk T1 and T2 tumors. Those who believe that the

role of irradiation is to eliminate clinically overt recurrences may not recommend internal mammary node irradiation.

Few data are available on the role of IMC or peripheral lymphatic irradiation alone without treating the chest wall. The two experiences with this approach from M. D. Anderson and Oslo II are discussed below and detailed in Table 61–3 and Table 61–4.[12] The M. D. Anderson experience with peripheral lymphatic irradiation was clearly successful in patients with fewer than 4 involved lymph nodes; whether the addition of chest wall treatment would have improved results for these lower risk patients is not known. In Oslo II, not only was local/regional disease control improved but also freedom from distant metastases[2]; whether further benefits would have been observed with the addition of chest wall treatment is also not known. If there is a role for peripheral lymphatic irradiation without chest wall treatment, it appears to be in the patients who have fewer involved nodes.

The chest wall is treated in all patients with T3 or T4 tumors, close or positive surgical margins, grave primary signs (skin erythema, edema, or ulceration or tumor fixation to skin, pectoral fascia, or chest wall), or more than four positive axillary lymph nodes (see Table 61–1). The peripheral lymphatics (internal mammary, supraclavicular, and axillary apical nodes) are treated in all patients with T3 or T4 tumors or any positive axillary lymph nodes, other than micrometastatic disease. Consideration is given to peripheral lymphatic or chest wall irradiation for patients with micrometastases or small tumors with unfavorable histological features such as high grade; invasion of lymphatic, vascular, or perineural spaces; or multicentric disease. The whole axilla is treated in patients with extensive axillary disease, as indicated by clinically fixed or matted lymph nodes, extensive extracapsular disease, or lymph nodes larger than 2.5 cm in diameter.

TREATMENT

Different techniques are acceptable for adjuvant postmastectomy irradiation. All successful techniques include a device for patient immobilization, a method for reproducible daily patient positioning, and treatment fields tailored to the individual patient's anatomy, using physical landmarks and radiographic tools (e.g., computed tomography [CT], ultrasound) for delivery to the areas at risk for disease. Examples of three techniques are provided (Figs. 61–3, 61–4, and 61–5).

Internal Mammary Chain Field

The IMC nodes lie in a parasternal position within the first six intercostal spaces. Approximately 85 percent of these nodes (on average, four per patient) lie in the first three interspaces within a space 1 to 4 cm lateral to the sternum and 3 to 4 cm deep to the

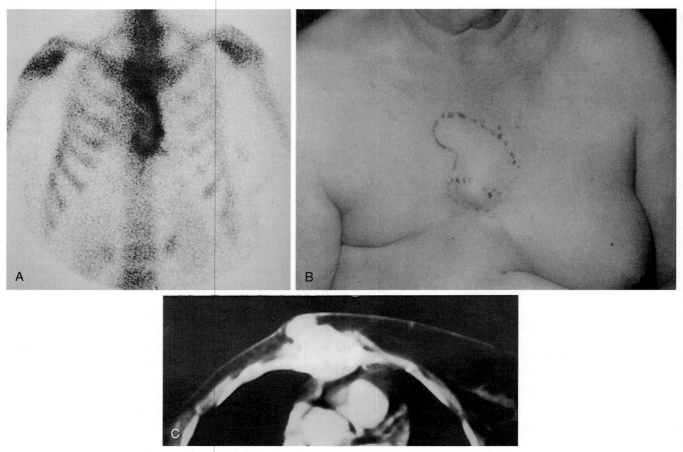

Figure 61–1   *This 71-year-old woman presented with chest wall pain 6 years after modified radical mastectomy for a >5-cm T3N0 breast cancer. Plain film demonstrated a destructive lesion of the sternum.*   **A,** *Bone scan demonstrated abnormal uptake only in the sternum. She was referred to the radiation oncology department for palliation of a presumed isolated bone metastasis.*   **B,** *On physical examination there was a parasternal mass.*   **C,** *A CT scan demonstrated soft tissue involvement centered around the parasternal area that was thought to be most consistent with an internal mammary node recurrence that had infiltrated the sternum. Localized radiation provided complete pain relief and resolution of the soft tissue mass; the patient survived another 6 years.*

skin surface.[26] Chest wall thickness may be determined from a cross-table lateral roentgenogram obtained at simulation (see Fig. 61–3C), CT, (see Fig. 61–4), or ultrasonography of the chest wall.[3, 5, 21]

Knowledge of the thickness of the chest wall provides a maximum potential depth for the IMC nodes, so that appropriate electron beam energy may be chosen.

The IMC nodes are usually treated with an en face

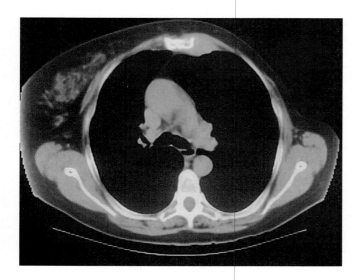

Figure 61–2   *This 68-year-old woman presented with dyspnea and a nonproductive cough 5 years after a modified radical mastectomy and 10 cycles of CMF chemotherapy for stage II breast cancer with three positive nodes. A CT was performed that showed several small pulmonary nodules and a clinically unsuspected parasternal mass that was thought to be consistent with an internal mammary node recurrence.*

TABLE 61–3.   LOCAL/REGIONAL RECURRENCE SITES IN PATIENTS TREATED AT THE M. D. ANDERSON HOSPITAL WITH RADICAL MASTECTOMY, POSTOPERATIVE RADIATION THERAPY, BUT NO ADJUVANT CHEMOTHERAPY (1963–1977)

Area Irradiated	Positive Axillary Nodes (n)	Total Patients (n)	Patients with Recurrence at Site (n)				Recurrence at Site (%)	
			CW	SC	AX	CW + LN	LN (%)	CW (%)
Peripheral lymphatics	0	210*	9	0	0	2	1	5
	1–3	230	20	1	0	4	2	10
	≥4	89	16	1	1	1	3	19
Peripheral lymphatics and chest wall	0	52	0	0	1	1	4	2
	1–3	102	9	0	1	0	1	9
	≥4	258	25	5	2	4	4	11

*Includes 27 patients treated with IMC irradiation only.
Key: CW, chest wall; SC, supraclavicular region; AX, axilla; LN, any regional lymph node areas (SC, AX, IMC).
Adapted from Fletcher GH, McNeese MD, Oswald MJ: Long-range results for breast cancer patients treated by radical mastectomy and postoperative radiation without adjuvant chemotherapy: An update. Int J Radiat Oncol Biol Phys 17:11–14, 1989.

electron field (see Fig. 61–3A). The lateral border is placed 6 cm from midline, and the medial border slopes from midline at the inferior border of the field to 1 cm contralateral to midline at the superior border of the field (see Fig. 61–3A and B). If the mastectomy incision extends across the midline, it may be necessary to modify the field shape to include the mastectomy incision in the field (see Fig. 61–3A). The inferior border is placed below the third interspace. The superior border is placed above the first interspace or matches the inferior border of the supraclavicular field. With inferior medial quadrant primaries, the fourth through sixth interspaces may be included (see dotted line in Fig. 61–3B). The internal mammary chain can be treated together with the chest wall within opposed tangential fields; however, it is necessary to extend the tangential fields across the midline to secure coverage of the internal mammary nodes (see Fig. 61–4). Without CT planning or lymphoscintigraphy it is not possible to be certain that these nodes are adequately covered by the tangential field. If the internal mammary chain nodes

are included in the tangents, the volume of exposed lung (as well as the heart with left-sided lesions) increases, and management of subsequent contralateral breast carcinomas is complicated. The technique of tangential chest wall fields, combined with an en face electron internal mammary field, provides excellent coverage of all areas at risk without excessive exposure of heart, lung, or contralateral breast (see Fig. 61–5).

An en face IMC field is treated with electrons or with a combination of electrons and photons when the patient is very large or partial skin sparing is desired. An electron beam energy (usually 10 to 14 MeV) or a combination of energies is selected so that the lymph nodes are contained within the 90 percent isodose volume. A given dose of 50 Gy may be delivered, or a dose of 45 Gy may be specified to the 90 percent isodose line. It is important to limit the dose to the heart from the IMC field by covering only the first three interspaces whenever possible (see Fig. 61–3B), particularly for patients who were or will be exposed to doxorubicin HCl.

TABLE 61–4.   RANDOMIZED TRIALS OF RADICAL MASTECTOMY WITH OR WITHOUT ADJUVANT RADIATION THERAPY (RT)

Trial	Subjects (n)	Accrual Period	Radiotherapy	Dose (Gy)	LRR* at 10 yr		Overall Survival at 10 yr	
					RT	No RT	RT	No RT
Manchester[23]	1461	1949–55	Chest wall and axilla or regional lymph nodes (orthovoltage)	32.5–45	19	32	39	42
NSABP-02[10]	428	1961–68	Regional lymph nodes (orthovoltage)	35–45	3†	15†	56†	62†
Oslo I[15]	546	1964–67	Chest wall and regional lymph nodes (orthovoltage)	25–41	7	16	75 / 49	76 (stage I) / 43 (stage II)
Oslo II[15]	541	1968–72	Regional lymph nodes (⁶⁰Co)	50	5	13	75 / 58	80 (stage I) / 53 (stage II)
Stockholm‡[30]	644	1971–76	Chest wall and regional lymph nodes (⁶⁰Co and electrons)	45	9§	33§	66	62

*LRR (local/regional recurrence) is reported as first site of failure unless otherwise indicated.
†Only 5-year follow-up data (regional recurrences) have been reported.
‡Patients treated with modified radical mastectomy.
§Overall incidence of local/regional recurrence after 16 years' follow-up (mean duration).

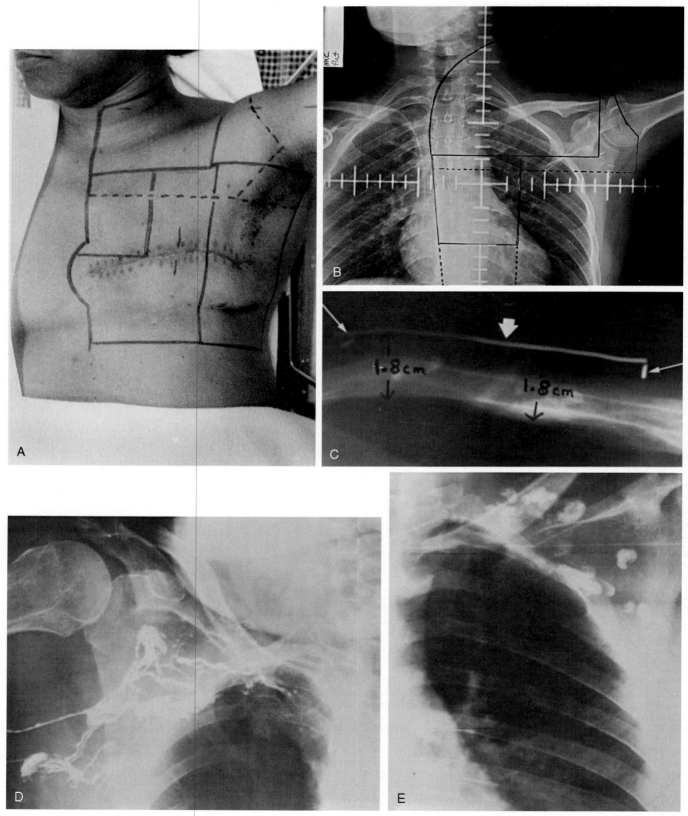

Figure 61–3   *See legend on opposite page*

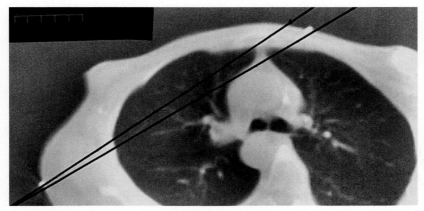

Figure 61–4 *The chest wall and IMN fields may be treated with tangential fields. To ensure adequate coverage of the IMN and an adequate deep margin on the medial and lateral aspects of the chest wall, CT planning is necessary. The shape of the chest wall is variable among patients, and adequate coverage of the IMN cannot reliably be predicted by setting the medial tangent 3 cm beyond midline. In the case mentioned earlier, the shallow medial tangent is 3 cm across midline, providing a margin of coverage of the IMN of less than 1 cm. The deeper tangent provides adequate coverage of the IMN, but extends more than 3 cm across midline as shown. CT planning is also helpful in documenting the volume of heart and lung exposed to radiation. As IMN coverage below the third interspace is not necessary in most patients, a significant amount of heart and lung sparing can be achieved through careful CT planning with customized blocking.*

Axillary Apex and Supraclavicular Node Field

The supraclavicular–axillary apex portal covers the lymph nodes in the axillary apex, which lie beneath the pectoral muscle in the infraclavicular fossa, and the lymph nodes in the supraclavicular fossa, which are superficial laterally but deep to the insertion of the sternocleidomastoid muscle medially.

The medial border of the supraclavicular field is 1 cm across the midline at the level of the sternal notch, extending superiorly to the thyrocricoid groove, extending laterally to include the supraclavicular fossa and axillary apex to the superior limits of surgical dissection in the axilla, and extending inferiorly to the first costal cartilage (see Fig. 61–3A

and *B*). If a full axillary dissection has been performed with removal of level I, II, and III nodes or if there are no indications for full axial irradiation after level I and II dissection, the lateral border of the field can be placed just lateral to the coracoid process, where the pectoralis minor muscle inserts. Clips placed in the axilla at the superior level of axillary dissection are useful in setting the lateral border. When photons are used, the axillary apical-supraclavicular portal can be angled 15 degrees laterally to avoid or decrease irradiation of the esophagus and spinal cord. When electrons are used, the field is not angled.

High-energy photons are used for the supraclavicular–axillary apex field because of the varying target depth for nodes at risk (4-MeV and 6-MeV photons).

Figure 61–3 *En face electron and photon technique.* **A,** *Field lines are drawn on the patient based on anatomical landmarks, then confirmed with fluoroscopy or CT. The lateral border of the internal mammary node (IMN) field is drawn 6 cm lateral to midline; the inferior border is placed on the fourth rib to encompass the third intercostal space; the medial border is placed at midline inferiorly and 1 cm across midline superiorly, so that the IMN field width is 7 cm superiorly and 6 cm inferiorly. The superior border of the IMN field abuts the inferior border of the supraclavicular field. If the whole axilla is irradiated, the inferior border of the supraclavicular-axillary field is at the second rib, and the lateral border includes the lateral edge of the pectoral muscle and splits the humerus [see dotted line in* **B**]. *The medial border is 1 cm contralateral to midline, and the superior border is at the thyrocricoid junction. The supraclavicular field may be angled to decrease esophageal and spine irradiation and to increase axillary coverage. If whole axillary irradiation is not indicated, the lateral border of the supraclavicular–axillary apex field just encompasses the coracoid process (or surgical clips left at the superior extent of the axillary dissection); the inferior border is at the first rib. Chest wall fields are then drawn that abut the supradural field superiorly and the internal mammary field medially, and include the entire chest wall flaps with at least a 5-cm margin inferiorly and a 2-cm margin on the incision medially and laterally.* **B,** *The standard IMN field includes only the nodes in the first three interspaces and avoids significant cardiac irradiation. If the risk of disease in the lower internal mammary nodes is judged to be high because of a large inferior medial tumor, the field may be extended caudally to include the fourth through the sixth interspaces (see dotted lines). The extension of the supraclavicular field to include the entire axilla is also indicated by dotted lines.* **C,** *After field lines are drawn on the patient, a cross-table x-ray film is taken with solder placed on the skin at midline (arrowhead) and at the superior and inferior field borders of the IMN. The distance between the skin surface and posterior surface of the sternum is calculated and used to select an appropriate electron energy or mix of electrons and photons for the IMN field. Alternatively, this depth may be obtained through ultrasound or CT planning.* **D,** *This photograph shows opacification of the axillary lymph nodes by hand lymphangiogram and demonstrates that the axillary lymph nodes are located very close to the chest wall in the low axilla, then wrap around the chest wall medially in the axillary apex.* **E,** *When the entire axilla is irradiated, the midplane position of the low axillary lymph nodes and the thickness of the patient are such that a posterior axillary field is required to supplement the dose from the anterior supraclavicular-axillary field. The low axillary lymph nodes (see* **D**) *lie at the midaxillary line close to the chest wall, so adequate coverage with irradiation requires a margin of lung. The superior border splits the clavicle and humerus, the inferior matches the inferior border of the supraclavicular-axillary field, and the lateral includes axillary soft tissues but does not flash the skin or lateral border of the latissimus dorsi muscle. (**E,** From Miller RR: The lymphomatous diseases. In Fletcher GH: Textbook of Radiotherapy. 3rd ed. Philadelphia, Lea & Febiger, 1980, pp 584–636. Reprinted by permission.)*

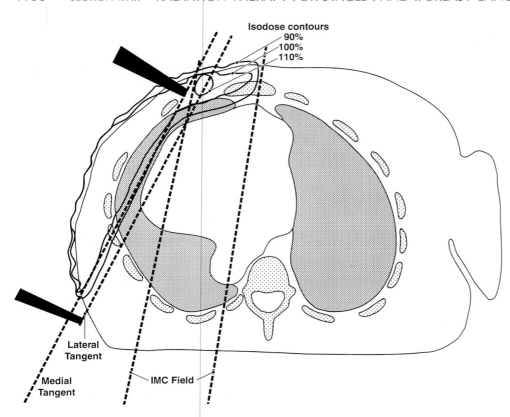

Isodose contours
90%
100%
110%

Lateral Tangent

Medial Tangent

IMC Field

Figure 61–5 *In some cases, the amount of heart or lung exposure precludes using tangential fields for the chest wall and IMN. In these cases, a combination of tangential photon fields for the chest wall and an en face IMN field treated with electrons or a mixture of electrons and photons may be used. To achieve an adequate dose throughout the target volume, it may be necessary to set the deep border of the lateral tangential field 1 cm deeper than the medial field deep border; the lateral field will actually exit into the IMN field dose distribution.*

Some 20 percent to 40 percent of the dose may be delivered with electrons, which effectively decreases the dose to the lung and the incidence of acute symptomatic pneumonitis.[20] In elective irradiation of subclinical disease, the supraclavicular–axillary apex portal receives 1.8 to 2 Gy per day. A posterior axillary boost field may be used to supplement the dose at the midaxilla in patients with indications for treatment of the whole axilla (see Fig. 61–3E).

Whole Axilla and Supraclavicular Node Field

The commonly involved axillary lymph nodes lie in the anterior half of the axilla. The most inferior axillary nodes lie at the midaxillary line, close to the chest wall (see Fig. 61–3D).[19] The apical axillary nodes, which are related to the medial aspect of the axillary vein, are anterior to the midcoronal plane. Thus, the target depth from the anterior skin surface ranges from 5 to 8 cm in the low to central axilla to 0.5 to 1 cm in the supraclavicular area and 1 to 4 cm beneath the sternocleidomastoid muscle insertion. Both the apical and the interpectoral nodes lie deep to the pectoralis muscle, which varies considerably in thickness among patients.

When indications call for treatment of the whole axilla, the standard axillary apex and supraclavicular field (see earlier) may be extended laterally and inferiorly to incorporate the entire axilla. The medial and superior field borders are the same, but the lateral border crosses the acromioclavicular joint and

splits the humeral head to cover the soft tissues of the axilla, and the inferior border of the field is extended to the second costal cartilage. If the whole axilla-supraclavicular field is angled, coverage in the lateral soft tissues of the axilla is increased and the beam may exit through the axillary skin (see Fig. 61–3A and B) without tangentially irradiating the skin of the axilla. The entire dose to the whole axilla-supraclavicular field is delivered with photons. To achieve an adequate skin dose in the superior chest wall flap, bolus material is applied to the skin below the clavicle. A posterior field is added to increase the dose to the middle and lower axilla, which can be underdosed from the anterior supraclavicular field because of its relative depth in comparison to the more superficial axillary apex and supraclavicular fossa.

The posterior axillary field and the supraclavicular field may be treated isocentrically with the patient lying supine, with a half-beam block to eliminate beam divergence into the chest wall fields. The posterior axillary field may also be treated through a direct posterior field with the patient prone and immobilized with a customized upper torso body mold. The medial border of the posterior axillary field includes a 1-cm rim of lung and is limited by the intersection of the clavicle and the first rib; the superior border splits the clavicle and the humeral head; the lateral border includes the soft tissues of the axilla; and the inferior border coincides with the superior edge of the anterior chest wall field (see Fig. 61–3D and E). The posterior axillary field is treated with high-energy photons. The total dose at midplane is 45 Gy for subclinical disease and 50 Gy for extensive extranodal disease. If gross residual disease is left in the axilla, the dose may be boosted through a reduced anterior or appositional field to 60 Gy. When the posterior axillary field is used, care is taken to ensure that the added dose contributions from the posterior and anterior portals throughout the treatment volume do not exceed a daily dose of 2 Gy. This may require treatment of the posterior axillary field on all or most treatment days.

Chest Wall Field

The main site of clinically overt recurrence after mastectomy is the subcutis and skin of the chest wall flap. The interpectoral nodes may be at risk after simple mastectomy or modified radical mastectomy if not dissected, particularly with large, superior, central primary tumors or extensive axillary disease.

In general, the superior and inferior chest wall flaps are included with at least a 5-cm margin beyond the mastectomy scar, except at the extreme lateral and medial borders, where 2- to 3-cm margins are acceptable (see Fig. 61–3A). Chest wall irradiation may be delivered through en face or rotational electron-beam fields or opposed tangential photon fields (see Figs. 61–3, 61–4, and 61–5).

In patients whose risk is limited to skin and subcutis, the electron-beam technique is usually chosen because of technical simplicity, less lung exposure, and better coverage of internal mammary nodes with a separate portal with higher-energy electrons. One to three adjoining fields are planned using electron energies chosen to match the tissue depth over each region. Tissue-equivalent bolus material is applied to the skin during treatment to increase the skin dose to at least 90 percent of the specified dose; this approach produces brisk erythema in most patients after delivery of 50 Gy. For patients whose interpectoral nodes are at risk, higher-energy electrons or a tangential photon technique may be used. If higher-energy electrons are used with en face or rotational techniques, CT planning and tissue compensation may be required to avoid excessive pulmonary exposure. There is often significant dose inhomogeneity between abutting electron fields or in the junction between the IMC field and tangential photon fields. An excellent technique for minimizing dose inhomogeneity is the "Rotterdam technique" (see Fig. 61–5).[36] For this technique, en face IMC treatment is combined with tangential chest wall fields. The fields abut at the skin surface, creating a region of low dose deep to the matchline. This dose inhomogeneity is eliminated through oblique angulation of the electron beam and a 1-cm deep extension of the lateral tangential field that results in overlap between the lateral edge of the IMC field and the deep edge of the lateral tangential field. When opposed tangential photon fields are used, bolus material should be applied as needed to achieve a brisk erythema by the end of treatment. With either technique, the match-

lines for abutting fields can be changed during treatment, to "feather" the dose inhomogeneity at the junction line.

For patients judged to be at particularly high risk for chest wall recurrence because of extensive axillary node involvement or close surgical margins, the dose to a 2-cm strip of skin along the mastectomy scar is boosted for an additional 10 Gy in four to five fractions.

RESULTS OF TREATMENT

The goal of adjuvant irradiation after mastectomy is eradication of local and regional disease. The primary end point by which the efficacy of this treatment must be measured then is freedom from local/regional failure. It is expected that uncontrolled local/regional disease will eventually metastasize and that complete eradication of local/regional disease may improve chances of survival. Therefore, adjuvant irradiation should also be evaluated for its impact on freedom from distant disease, cause-specific survival, and overall survival.

Efficacy of Postoperative Radiation Therapy Without Systemic Therapy

Nonrandomized Studies

Retrospective studies of mastectomy followed by adjuvant irradiation show decreased rates of local/regional recurrences (LRR) as compared with surgery alone. Fletcher and colleagues reported on 941 patients treated at M. D. Anderson Hospital, with a 10-year minimum follow-up period.[12] Seventy percent of patients had axillary metastases, averaging 6.7 involved nodes per patient. The LRR rates for node-negative and node-positive patients were 5 percent and 11 percent, respectively. During the period of the study the indications used for chest wall irradiation changed, so some patients were treated with chest wall irradiation while others were not. The analysis of results in patients with a 10-year minimum follow-up is shown in Table 61–3.[12] The chest wall recurrence rate for patients with four or more positive axillary nodes was 11 percent after chest wall irradiation and 19 percent without chest wall irradiation. In patients with fewer than four involved nodes, the chest wall recurrence rate was similar, with or without chest wall irradiation. At the University of Florida, the crude 10-year incidence of recurrence was 6 percent in the chest wall and 3 percent in the regional nodes in node-positive patients treated with adjuvant postmastectomy irradiation. For similar cases reported from the Joint Center for Radiation Therapy, LRR in the irradiated chest wall after 10 years was 3 percent.[34]

Prospective Randomized Trials

Five prospective randomized trials (Manchester Quadrate and Peripheral [Q&P] Trial, National Surgical Adjuvant Breast and Bowel Project [NSABP], Oslo I, Oslo II, Stockholm I) of adjuvant irradiation with radical mastectomy without systemic therapy were conducted between 1950 and 1975 (Table 61–4).[10, 15, 23, 30] These early trials moved clinical research in breast cancer to a more scientific level, but the results are difficult to interpret because of problems with radiation techniques, patient selection, and trial design. In the earliest trials orthovoltage machines were used and doses were smaller than the 45 Gy to 50 Gy now regarded as necessary for control of subclinical disease.[10, 15, 23] In most of the early trials, only some of the areas at risk for subclinical disease (chest wall and regional nodes) were treated and, even in the treated areas, techniques were unlikely to deliver adequate doses.[10, 15, 23] Some trials included large proportions of node-negative patients who were at low risk for residual subclinical disease and thus were unlikely to benefit from adjuvant irradiation.[15, 30] In these trials the overall sample sizes were too small to have the power to detect small but significant differences in outcomes.[15, 30] Although LRR was clearly reduced to approximately one third by irradiation (e.g., from 30 percent to 45 percent without irradiation to 10 percent to 15 percent with irradiation), the impact of adjuvant irradiation on the other end points (e.g., disease-free survival, freedom from distant metastases, and overall survival) is less clear.

Stockholm I from the Radiumhemmet Karolinska Hospital is the only one of these early trials that treated all volumes at risk for subclinical disease with doses likely to be sufficient for subclinical disease and with treatment techniques likely to include most of the target volume. Nine hundred-sixty patients were randomized to one of three treatment arms, in conjunction with modified radical mastectomy: preoperative irradiation, postoperative irradiation, or observation. In the irradiation arms, a dose of 45 Gy was delivered to the chest wall and peripheral lymphatics, including the ipsilateral IMC, with supervoltage equipment. In some patients the chest wall was treated with en face electrons and in others

with tangential photon fields planned without the benefit of CT. During the initial period of the study, bilateral IMCs were treated. Only 37 percent of the postoperative and control groups had positive axillary lymph nodes and thus were at significant risk for LRR. After a median follow-up of 16 years, 20 percent of patients treated with surgery alone developed LRR as the site of first treatment failure, as compared with 4 percent of the those who received adjuvant irradiation. Results for the postoperative and control groups, according to their axillary lymph node status, are shown in Table 61–5.[30] Local/regional recurrence was reduced in both node-positive and node-negative irradiated patients. In addition, both the incidence of distant metastases and the rate of death due to breast cancer were significantly improved for node-positive patients who received irradiation. Auquier and associates performed joint analysis of data from the Oslo II trial (which delivered 50 Gy to the regional nodes only and not to the chest wall) and Stockholm I trial after 13 to 16 years of follow-up, which showed significant improvement in both local/regional disease control ($p < .0001$) and overall disease-free survival ($p < .001$) for irradiated patients.[2] In irradiated node-positive patients, a significant reduction in distant metastases was seen ($p < .01$) as was a trend toward improvement in overall survival ($p < .06$).

Cuzick and coworkers published two metaanalyses of trials testing the role of adjuvant irradiation during the era before use of systemic chemotherapy became routine.[6, 7] In the first report there appeared to be an excess of mortality in irradiated patients.[6] In the second report,[7] which included more follow-up information, there was no overall excess of mortality in irradiated patients; however, some subsets of irradiated patients clearly had excessive mortality rates and other subsets clearly had reduced mortality rates. In particular, excessive cardiac-related mortality was observed in trials using treatment techniques that exposed a significant amount of heart to full-dose irradiation.[15, 29] Two such techniques include the

TABLE 61–5.   STOCKHOLM TRIAL RESULTS ANALYZED BY PATHOLOGICAL LYMPH NODE STATUS[30]

Type of Event	Radiotherapy (n %)		Surgery Alone (n %)		Relative Hazard (mean/range)	p
pN0						
Cases (n)	204		197			
Local/regional recurrence	10	5	45	23	0.25 (0.15–0.42)	<.001
Distant metastasis	52	26	49	25	1.02 (0.69–1.50)	.94
Death	66	33	74	38	0.87 (0.63–1.21)	.40
Death due to breast cancer	47	23	43	22	1.05 (0.70–1.59)	.80
pN+						
Cases (n)	118		120			
Local/regional recurrence	18	15	58	48	0.29 (0.18–0.45)	<.001
Distant metastasis	61	52	83	69	0.66 (0.48–0.92)	.02
Death	72	61	84	70	0.82 (0.60–1.12)	.21
Death due to breast cancer	59	50	81	68	0.70 (0.50–0.98)	.04

*Log rank test.
Adapted from Rutqvist LE, Pettersson D, Johansson H: Adjuvant radiotherapy versus surgery alone in operable breast cancer: Long-term follow-up of a randomized clinical trial. Radiother Oncol 26:104–110, 1993.

treatment of en face unilateral or bilateral internal mammary node fields with photons, and in patients with left-sided breast cancers the treatment of the chest wall and internal mammary nodes through deep tangential fields with photons.[15, 29] Patients with left-sided breast cancers who were treated with en face electron techniques did not have an excess of cardiac-related mortality, nor did patients with right-sided lesions treated with deep tangents.[29] The overview clearly demonstrated an improved breast cancer–specific mortality rate in more recent trials, particularly for premenopausal stage II disease patients.

Effect of Adjuvant Systemic Therapy on Local/Regional Control

Three studies have documented a substantial risk of LRR after mastectomy and adjuvant chemotherapy. Stefanik and associates, in a retrospective review of 117 patients who received adjuvant cyclophosphamide, methotrexate, and fluorouracil (CMF) for node-positive disease after mastectomy, documented an incidence of LRR at 5 years of 19 percent in the overall patient population and 38 percent in patients with four or more positive nodes. Sykes' group retrospectively reviewed 400 stage II or III patients treated with cyclophosphamide and doxorubicin and reported a 15 percent isolated LRR rate at an average follow-up time of 5 years.[32, 33] Finally, in 627 node-positive patients treated on Eastern Cooperative Oncology Group trials involving adjuvant systemic therapy, Fowble and coworkers reported an overall relapse rate of 35 percent at 3 years; 31 percent of these were isolated LRRs.[13]

Prospective randomized trials from University Hospital of South Manchester (West Didsbury, UK), Guy's Hospital (London), and Osaka University Medical School (Osaka, Japan), with 2 to 3 years of follow-up information, suggest an early (though possibly transient) reduction in LRR from adjuvant chemotherapy.[16, 17, 28] In the NSABP-05 trial, adjuvant treatment with melphalan resulted in 14 percent LRR at 10 years, as compared with 24 percent after placebo treatment.[9] In a trial from Milan, patients were randomized to treatment with CMF. Early results indicated improvement in both relapse-free survival and LRR, but at 10 years the difference in LRR had disappeared (15 percent for controls, 12 percent for CMF-treated patients).[4] It appears from current data that the impact of adjuvant chemotherapy alone on LRR is minimal, and possibly transient.

Efficacy of Combined Chemotherapy and Radiation

Several prospective, randomized studies have examined the effectiveness of radiotherapy in patients who also received adjuvant chemotherapy. At the Mayo Clinic, 293 patients with positive axillary nodes or unfavorable local signs were randomized to receive one of three regimens[1]: melphalan; cyclophosphamide,

fluorouracil, and prednisone (CFP); or CFP plus irradiation. Irradiation was given in a split-course fashion with a 1-month break after 25 Gy. Although there was no difference in disease-free survival between the group who received CFP alone and the irradiated group, the incidence of LRR was significantly decreased by the addition of radiation therapy (54 percent versus 12 percent, $p < .01$). In a study from the Harvard Joint Center for Radiation Therapy, patients with one to three positive nodes or a tumor larger than 5 cm were considered to be at moderate risk of recurrence and were treated with either CMF or MF chemotherapy.[14] Patients who had four or more positive nodes or one or more positive nodes in the axillary apex were considered at high risk and received either 15 or 30 weeks of cyclophosphamide and doxorubicin. The moderate- and high-risk groups were secondarily randomized to receive either adjuvant irradiation or no further treatment. The irradiated treatment volume did not routinely include the internal mammary nodes. After median follow-up periods of 45 to 53 months, 17 percent of patients receiving chemotherapy alone experienced a local/regional failure, as compared with only 5 percent of irradiated patients ($p = .03$). In a three-arm trial from Glasgow, Scotland, after mastectomy patients received adjuvant orthovoltage irradiation, CMF therapy, or both. At 5 years, the LRR rate was reduced by more than half in the treatment arms that included irradiation.[18] Subset analysis further revealed a significant improvement in disease-specific survival for irradiated patients with four or more involved lymph nodes.

Two recent trials are of special interest because the radiation techniques, doses, and prescribed treatment volumes are likely to have adequately treated all areas at risk for subclinical disease (Table 61–6). In the British Columbia Randomized Trial, radiation was delivered with a five-field technique including an en face internal mammary field, opposed tangential chest wall photon fields, anterior supraclavicular axillary field, and a posterior axillary field.[25] In this study, 10-year disease-free survival was improved with the addition of radiotherapy to adjuvant CMF treatment (56 percent versus 41 percent, $p = .007$). Systemic disease-free survival in patients with four or more positive nodes was 41 percent with irradiation versus 21 percent without irradiation ($p = .04$); in patients with one to three positive nodes, systemic disease-free survival was 68 percent with irradiation and 53 percent without ($p = .06$). In another report of the British Columbia study, patients with extensive extracapsular spread of disease had not only better disease-free survival ($p = .003$) with the addition of radiotherapy, but also a better overall rate of survival ($p = .03$). In all patients there was a strong trend ($p = .07$) at 10 years to improved overall survival (64 percent versus 54 percent) with the addition of radiation.[25, 25a] In another study (Table 61–6), the Danish Breast Cancer Cooperative Group randomized 2028 high-risk premenopausal patients to receive CMF with or without irradiation or tamoxifen.[22]

TABLE 61–6.   TRIALS OF RADIATION THERAPY (RT) IN PATIENTS RECEIVING ADJUVANT SYSTEMIC THERAPY

Trial	Group	Follow-up (yr)	Patients (n)	Treatment	LRR (%)	(p)	RFS/DFS (%)	(p)	Systemic DFS (%)	(p)	OS (%)	(p)
DBCG[8, 22a, 27]	Postmenopausal	7 or 10	2030	TAM + RT	—		43		—		53	
				TAM	—		33	.0004	—		53	.59
				TAM + CMF	—		36		—		53	
	Premenopausal	7 or 10	2028	CMF* + RT	9 (10 yr)		46 (10 yr)		—		54	
												.001
				CMF*	32 (10 yr)		34 (10 yr)	.001	—	.001	45	
				CMF + TAM‡	43 (7 yr)		38 (7 yr)		—		51 (7 yr)	
BCRT[25, 25a]	All patients	10	318	CMF† + RT	13		56		58		64	
						.003		.007		.006		.09
				CMF	25		41		43		54	
	1–3 involved nodes	10	183	CMF + RT	10		—		68		—	
						.55				.06		
				CMF	16		—		53		—	
	≥4 involved nodes	10	112	CMF + RT	21		—		44		—	
						.04				.05		
				CMF	41		—		24		—	
	Extracapsular + nodal disease	10	70	CMF + RT	—		55		—		52	
								.003				.03
				CMF	—		13		—		33	

*One cycle of CMF given before RT; total of nine cycles, 10-year results.
†Four cycles of CMF given before RT; total of six cycles.
‡Seven-year results.
Key: LRR, local/regional recurrence; RFS, relapse-free survival; DFS, disease-free survival; OS, overall survival; DBCG, Danish Breast Cancer Cooperative Group Trial 82; TAM, tamoxifen; CMF, cyclophosphamide, methotrexate, and fluorouracil; BCRT, British Columbia Randomized Trial Report.

In this study, the chest wall and peripheral lymphatics were treated; the internal mammary nodes were treated within tangential photon chest wall fields, but CT planning was used to ensure adequate coverage of all areas at risk for subclinical disease. After follow-up of 10 years, overall survival was significantly improved for patients who received CMF and irradiation (54 percent versus 45 percent, $p = .001$) as well as LRR and disease-free survival.[8, 22a] In a second trial, the Danish Breast Cancer Cooperative Group randomized 2030 postmenopausal patients to receive tamoxifen, with or without irradiation; disease-specific survival was significantly improved for patients receiving combined treatment, but overall survival rates were not affected.[27]

SUMMARY

In patients at moderate to high risk for LRR after radical or modified radical mastectomy because of tumor size greater than 5 cm, positive axillary lymph nodes, close or positive surgical margins, or one or more grave signs, LRR is reduced by the addition of adjuvant radiotherapy. With improved radiation treatment planning and techniques used in modern trials, reduced rates of LRR have translated into modest but significant gains in (1) freedom from distant metastases, (2) disease-free survival, and (3) overall survival, without causing excessive injury to normal tissues.

References

1. Ahmann DL, O'Fallon JR, Scanlon PW, Payne WS, Bisel HF, Edmonson JH, Frytak S, Hahn RG, Ingle JN, Rubin J, Creagan ET: A preliminary assessment of factors associated with recurrent disease in a surgical adjuvant clinical trial for patients with breast cancer with special emphasis on the aggressiveness of therapy. Am J Clin Oncol 5:371–381, 1982.
2. Auquier A, Rutqvist LE, Host H, Rotstein S, Arriagada R: Post-mastectomy megavoltage radiotherapy: The Oslo and Stockholm trials. Eur J Cancer 28:433–437, 1992.
3. Bernardino ME, Spanos W Jr: A simple technique for determining internal mammary chain depth by sonography. Int J Radiat Oncol Biol Phys 7:671–673, 1981.
4. Bonadonna G, Valagussa P, Rossi A, Tancini G, Brambilla C, Zambetti M, Veronesi U: Ten-year experience with CMF-based adjuvant chemotherapy in resectable breast cancer. Breast Cancer Res Treat 5:95–115, 1985.
5. Cheung AYC, Chang KS: Effects of a sonographic technique for determining chest wall thickness in treatment planning for breast carcinoma. Int J Radiat Oncol Biol Phys 15:223–225, 1988.
6. Cuzick J, Stewart H, Peto R, Baum M, Fisher B, Host H, Lythgoe JP, Ribeiro GG, Scheurlen H, Wallgren A: Overview of randomized trials of postoperative adjuvant radiotherapy in breast cancer. Cancer Treat Rep 71:15–29, 1987.
7. Cuzick J, Stewart H, Rutqvist L, Houghton J, Edwards R, Redmond C, Peto R, Baum M, Fisher B, Host H, Lythgoe J, Ribeiro G, et al: Cause-specific mortality in long-term survivors of breast cancer who participated in trials of radiotherapy. J Clin Oncol 12:447–453, 1994.
8. Dombernowsky P, Hansen PS, Mouridsen HT, Overgaard M, Rose C, Zedeler K: Randomized trial of adjuvant CMF + radiotherapy (RT) vs CMF alone vs + tamoxifen (TAM) in pre- and menopausal stage II breast cancer. Ann Oncol 5(Suppl 8): 2, 1994. Abstract.
9. Fisher B, Redmond C, Fisher ER, Bauer M, Wolmark N, Wickerham DL, Deutsch M, Montague E, Margolese R, Foster R: Ten-year results of a randomized clinical trial comparing

radical mastectomy and total mastectomy with or without radiation. N Engl J Med 312:674–681, 1985.

10. Fisher B, Slack NH, Cavanaugh PJ, Gardner B, Ravdin RG: Postoperative radiotherapy in the treatment of breast cancer: Results of the NSABP clinical trial. Ann Surg 172:711–732, 1970.

11. Fletcher GH: Textbook of Radiotherapy. 3rd ed. Philadelphia, Lea & Febiger, 1980.

12. Fletcher GH, McNeese MD, Oswald MJ: Long-range results for breast cancer patients treated by radical mastectomy and postoperative radiation without adjuvant chemotherapy: An update. Int J Radiat Oncol Biol Phys 17:11–14, 1989.

13. Fowble B, Gray R, Gilchrist K, Goodman RL, Taylor S, Tormey DC: Identification of a subgroup of patients with breast cancer and histologically positive axillary nodes receiving adjuvant chemotherapy who may benefit from postoperative radiotherapy. J Clin Oncol 6:1107–1117, 1988.

14. Griem KL, Henderson IC, Gelman R, Ascoli D, Silver B, Recht A, Goodman RL, Hellman S, Harris JR: The 5-year results of a randomized trial of adjuvant radiation therapy after chemotherapy in breast cancer patients treated with mastectomy. J Clin Oncol 5:1546–1555, 1987.

15. Host H, Brennhovd IO, Loeb M: Postoperative radiotherapy in breast cancer: Long-term results from the Oslo study. Int J Radiat Oncol Biol Phys 12:727–732, 1986.

16. Howell A, Bush H, George WD, Howat JMT, Crowther D, Sellwood RA, Rubens RD, Hayward JL, Bulbrook RD, Fentiman IS, Chaudary M: Controlled trial of adjuvant chemotherapy with cyclophosphamide, methotrexate, and fluorouracil for breast cancer. Lancet 2:307–311, 1984.

17. Koyama H, Wada T, Takahashi Y, Nishizawa Y, Iwanaga T, Aoki Y, Terasawa T, Kosaki G, Kajita A, Wada A: Surgical adjuvant chemotherapy with mitomycin-C and cyclophosphamide in Japanese patients with breast cancer. Cancer 46: 2373–2379, 1980.

18. McArdle CS, Crawford D, Dykes EH, Calman KC, Hole D, Russell AR, Smith DC: Adjuvant radiotherapy and chemotherapy in breast cancer. Br J Surg 73:264–266, 1986.

19. Million RR: The lymphomatous diseases: Hodgkin's disease. *In* Fletcher GH (ed): Textbook of Radiotherapy. 3rd ed. Philadelphia, Lea & Febiger, 1980, pp 584–621.

20. Montague ED, Schell SR, Romsdahl MM, Ames FC: Conservation surgery and irradiation in the treatment of breast cancer. Front Radiat Ther Oncol 17:76–83, 1983.

21. Munzenrider JE, Tchakarova I, Castro M, Carter B: Computerized body tomography in breast cancer. I. Internal mammary nodes and radiation treatment planning. Cancer 43: 137–150, 1979.

22. Overgaard M, Christensen JJ, Johansen H, Nybo-Rasmussen A, Rose C, van der Kooy P, Panduro J, Laursen F, Kjaer M, Sorensen NE: Evaluation of radiotherapy in high-risk breast cancer patients: Report from the Danish Breast Cancer Cooperative Group (DBCG 82) Trial. Int J Radiat Oncol Biol Phys 19:1121–1124, 1990.

22a. Overgaard M, Hansen PS, Overgaard J, Rose C, Andersson M, Bach F, Kjaer M, Gadeberg CC, Mouridsen HT, Jensen MB, Zedeler K: Danish Breast Cancer Cooperative Group 82b Trial: Postoperative radiotherapy in high-risk premenopausal women with breast cancer who receive adjuvant chemotherapy. N Engl J Med 337(14):949–955, 1997.

23. Palmer MK, Ribeiro GG: Thirty-four year follow up of patients with breast cancer in clinical trial of postoperative radiotherapy. Br Med J Clin Res Ed 291:1088–1091, 1985.

24. Patterson R: Clinical trials in malignant disease: Principles of random selection. J Facul Radiol 9:80–83, 1958.

25. Ragaz J, Jackson SM, Plenderleith IH, Wilson K, Basco V, Knowling M, Worth A, Spinelli J, Ng V: Can adjuvant radiotherapy (XRT) improve the overall survival (OS) of breast cancer (BR CA) patients in the presence of adjuvant chemotherapy (CT)? 10-yr analysis of the British Columbia randomized trial. (Abstract.) Proc Annu Meet Am Soc Clin Oncol 12:A40, 1993.

25a. Ragaz J, Jackson SM, Plenderleith IH, Wilson K, Basco V, Knowling M, Worth A, Spinelli J, Ng V: Can adjuvant radiotherapy (XRT) improve the overall survival (OS) of breast cancer (BR CA) patients in the presence of adjuvant chemotherapy (CT)? 10-yr analysis of the British Columbia randomized trial. (Abstract.) Proc Annu Meet Am Soc Clin Oncol 12:A40, 1993.

26. Recht A, Siddon RL, Kaplan WD, Andersen JW, Harris JR: Three-dimensional internal mammary lymphoscintigraphy: Implications for radiation therapy treatment planning for breast carcinoma. Int J Radiat Oncol Biol Phys 14:477–481, 1988.

27. Rose C, Dombernowsky P, Hansen P: A randomized trial of adjuvant (ADJ) tamoxifen (TAM) + radiotherapy (RT) vs TAM alone vs TAM + CMF in postmenopausal stage II breast cancer. Eur J Cancer 30A(Suppl 2):S28, 1994. Abstract.

28. Rubens RD, Hayward JL, Knight RK, Bulbrook RD, Fentiman IS, Chaudary M, Howell A, Bush H, Crowther D, Sellwood RA, George WD, Howat JMT: Controlled trial of adjuvant chemotherapy with melphalan for breast cancer. Lancet 1: 839–843, 1983.

29. Rutqvist LE, Lax I, Fornander T, Johansson H: Cardiovascular mortality in a randomized trial of adjuvant radiation therapy versus surgery alone in primary breast cancer. Int J Radiat Oncol Biol Phys 22:887–896, 1992.

30. Rutqvist LE, Pettersson D, Johansson H: Adjuvant radiation therapy versus surgery alone in operable breast cancer: Long-term follow-up of a randomized clinical trial. Radiother Oncol 26:104–110, 1993.

31. Spratt JS: Locally recurrent cancer after radical mastectomy. Cancer 20:1051–1053, 1967.

32. Stefanik D, Goldberg R, Byrne P, Smith F, Ueno W, Smith L, Bachenheimer L, Beiser C, Dritschilo A: Local-regional failure in patients treated with adjuvant chemotherapy for breast cancer. J Clin Oncol 3:660–665, 1985.

33. Sykes HF, Sim DA, Wong CJ, Cassady JR, Salmon SE: Local-regional recurrence in breast cancer after mastectomy and Adriamycin-based adjuvant chemotherapy: Evaluation of the role of postoperative radiotherapy. Int J Radiat Oncol Biol Phys 16:641–647, 1989.

34. Uematsu M, Bornstein BA, Recht A, Abner A, Come SE, Shulman LN, Silver B, Harris JR: Long-term results of postoperative radiation therapy following mastectomy with or without chemotherapy in stage I-III breast cancer. Int J Radiat Oncol Biol Phys 25:765–770, 1993.

35. Veronesi U, Valagussa P: Inefficacy of internal mammary nodes dissection in breast cancer surgery. Cancer 47:170–175, 1981.

36. Woudstra E, van der Werf H: Obliquely incident electron beams for irradiation of the internal mammary lymph nodes. Radiother Oncol 10:209–215, 1987.

CHAPTER 62
CONSERVATIVE SURGERY AND RADIATION FOR STAGES I AND II BREAST CANCER

Barbara Fowble, M.D. / Cynthia Rosser / Alexandra Hanlon, M.S.

Many prospective randomized trials have established the equivalence of conservative surgery and radiation with mastectomy for the treatment of early-stage invasive breast cancer. However, support for the development and initiation of these trials was provided by the clinical efforts of single institutions. Retrospective series continue to contribute to our knowledge of the natural history of breast cancer and its treatment and outcome. In this chapter, we review the experience of the University of Pennsylvania and Fox Chase Cancer Center with conservative surgery and radiation for stages I and II breast cancer. Prior publications reflect the experience of the two institutions combined.* Some publications have reported outcome only from patients treated at the University of Pennsylvania.† More recent studies by one of the authors (B.F.) include only patients from the University of Pennsylvania treated or followed by her as well as all patients treated at Fox Chase Cancer Center.[4–7, 15]

Our data base for patients treated with conservative surgery and radiation was established in 1982. Data management and statistical support have been independent, thereby limiting the possibility for physician bias. The data base has proved to be a unique resource for clinical research and has provided us with the opportunity to examine the natural history of breast cancer and the outcome of our treatment approach. Colleagues in diagnostic radiology, pathology, surgery, radiation oncology, and medical oncology have collaborated with us in this endeavor.

TEN-YEAR RESULTS

The 10-year results of conservative surgery and radiation for stages I and II breast cancer from the University of Pennsylvania and Fox Chase Cancer Center were published in 1991.[10] In this study, 697 women were treated between the years 1977 and 1985. The series was relatively contemporary in that 47 percent of patients underwent a re-excision, margins of resection were assessed in 50 percent, all patients had an axillary dissection, and 77 percent of axillary node–positive patients received adjuvant chemotherapy, primarily CMF (cyclophosphamide, methotrexate, and 5-fluorouracil). The median follow-up was 4.8 years. The 10-year actuarial overall

survival was 83 percent for all patients, 87 percent for clinical stage I patients, and 77 percent for clinical stage II patients. The 10-year actuarial overall survival was 86 percent for axillary node–negative patients, compared with 74 percent for axillary node–positive patients. The cumulative probability for a recurrence in the treated breast (without simultaneous distant metastases) was 6 percent at 5 years and 16 percent at 10 years. Treatment-related complications included a 5 percent incidence of moderate to severe arm edema and a 1 percent incidence of rib fracture. There were no instances of pericarditis, and fewer than 1 percent of patients experienced symptomatic pneumonitis or brachial plexopathy. Good to excellent cosmesis was noted in 93 percent of patients.

We have recently performed a separate analysis of our 10-year results in patients treated or followed by one of the authors (B.F.) at University of Pennsylvania and in all patients treated at Fox Chase Cancer Center. Between 1970 and 1992, 1569 women with clinical stages I to II breast cancer underwent an excisional biopsy, axillary node dissection, and radiation. The median age of the patient population was 55 years (range, 22 to 89 years). Sixty-six percent of patients had primary tumors 2 cm or less and 72 percent had negative axillary nodes. Three hundred and thirty-seven patients had one to three positive nodes, 75 had four to nine positive nodes, and 32 had ten or more positive nodes. Eight hundred and sixty-nine patients (55 percent) had a re-excision. The final resection margin status was unknown in 19 percent, negative in 62 percent, close (<2 mm) in 9 percent, and positive in 10 percent. Radiation consisting of tangential fields to the breast was applied to 76 percent of patients, with doses ranging from 4600 to 5000 cGy delivered in 180 to 200 cGy fractions. One hundred and seventy-three patients received treatment to the breast and supraclavicular nodes, and 200 received treatment to the breast, supraclavicular, and axillary nodes. A boost (electrons, external beam, or iridium 192 implant) dose of 400 to 2250 cGy (median, 1600 cGy) was given to 99 percent of the patients. Thirteen percent of axillary node–negative patients and 68 percent of axillary node–positive patients received adjuvant chemotherapy (with or without tamoxifen), which in 84 percent consisted of CMF. Two hundred and eighty patients received tamoxifen alone.

The 5- and 10-year actuarial rates of breast recurrence without simultaneous distant metastases were 5 percent and 12 percent. The 10-year overall and

---

*See references 9–14, 18, 20–22, 26, and 27.
†See references 1, 2, 8, 16, 19, 23, and 28.

cause-specific survival were 79 percent and 83 percent for all patients, 82 percent and 86 percent for axillary node–negative patients, and 70 percent and 75 percent for axillary node–positive patients. Treatment-related complications included symptomatic pneumonitis (<1 percent), rib fracture (<1 percent), pericarditis (<1 percent), and brachial plexopathy (<1 percent). Arm edema of any degree was noted in 15 percent of the patients, which was mild in the majority. Good to excellent cosmesis (physician assessment) was observed in 92 percent.

The discussion that follows focuses on the knowledge we have gained through our analysis in the areas of patient selection, surgical and radiotherapeutic technique, integration with adjuvant therapy, and the significance of a local/regional recurrence.

PATIENT SELECTION

Tumor Size, Extent, and Location

We have not observed an increased risk of breast recurrence with increasing tumor size for tumors up to 4 to 5 cm in patients in whom an excisional biopsy has been performed.[10] The 10-year actuarial rate of breast recurrence in our most recent analysis was 13 percent for clinical T1 tumors and 10 percent for clinical T2 tumors (p = .90). Therefore, patients with tumors less than 4 to 5 cm in size have been considered candidates for conservative surgery and radiation, provided that an adequate excision can be performed.

Several series have reported an increased risk of breast recurrence in patients with clinical evidence of more than one malignancy in a single breast (gross multicentric or multifocal disease). This presentation is considered a contraindication to conservative surgery and radiation. We reviewed the pathological findings and clinical outcome of 57 of these patients treated with modified radical mastectomy at Fox Chase Cancer Center and University of Pennsylvania.[14] We identified that 40 percent of these patients had pathological evidence of involvement of more than one quadrant of the breast. Forty-six percent had positive axillary nodes, with 21 percent having four or more positive nodes. These findings suggested that the increased risk of breast recurrence in patients with clinical gross multicentric disease treated with conservative surgery and radiation was related to a significant residual tumor burden that was not controlled with moderate doses of radiation. Our study demonstrated no increased risk of local/regional recurrence in patients with clinical gross multifocal or multicentric disease treated with mastectomy. Indications for postmastectomy radiation in these patients included four or more positive nodes or a positive or close mastectomy margin.

Subareolar cancers (tumors within 2 cm of the nipple-areolar complex) may involve the nipple-areolar complex in up to 50 percent of cases and have been associated with a higher incidence of pathological multicentricity. We reported a 5-year actuarial breast recurrence rate of 8 percent and a 5-year overall survival of 91 percent in 70 patients with subareolar tumors undergoing conservative surgery and radiation.[12] Three percent had resection of the nipple-areolar complex. The outcomes of these patients were compared with those of 495 patients with outer quadrant tumors, 202 patients with inner quadrant tumors, and 119 patients with central tumors. There were no significant differences among the groups in terms of the 5-year actuarial breast recurrence rate, overall relapse-free rate, or disease survival rate. We concluded that patients with subareolar tumors are candidates for conservative surgery and radiation, provided that an adequate excision is achieved. Sacrifice of the nipple-areolar complex is often not required.

Race

Black women with early-stage breast cancer have a decreased survival when compared with white women.[4, 22] There is little information regarding the outcome of black women treated with breast conservation therapy. We initially reported the outcome in 75 black and 615 white women treated with conservative surgery and radiation.[22] We reported no increased risk of breast recurrence at 5 years in black women but did note a significant increase in the incidence of regional node failure (supraclavicular) and distant metastases. The 5-year actuarial overall survival was 82 percent for black women compared with 91 percent for white women (p = .01). There was no significant difference in the cosmetic results at 5 years for the two groups of patients. We have subsequently reported our experience with 124 black women and 1330 white women.[4] We again observed no increased risk of breast recurrence at 10 years in black women but did note an increased risk of failure in the supraclavicular nodes for both axillary node–negative and –positive patients. The 10-year actuarial cause-specific survival was 89 percent for white women compared with 65 percent for black women (p = .0001). The addition of chemotherapy or tamoxifen in axillary node–positive women diminished the cause-specific survival differences between the two races. The 5-year cause-specific survival was 90 percent for white women and 86 percent for black women who received chemotherapy, and 90 percent and 100 percent for tamoxifen alone. Therefore, being a woman of color is not a contraindication to conservative surgery and radiation. Race by itself, however, may be an indication for adjuvant systemic therapy.

Patient Age

Young age (<35 to 40 years) has been associated with an increased risk of breast recurrence in a number of series. In 1994, we reported the outcome of 980 women with stages I and II breast cancer treated with conservative surgery and radiation at the University of Pennsylvania.[8] Women 35 years or younger had a statistically significant increased risk of breast and regional node failure at 5 and 8 years when compared with women 36 to 50 years and women older than 50 years. The 8-year actuarial breast recurrence rate was 24 percent for the women 35 years or younger compared with 14 percent for women 36 to 50 years and 12 percent for women older than 50 years (p = .001). However, for women 35 years or younger who received adjuvant chemotherapy, there was no increased risk of breast recurrence. Re-excision did not decrease the risk of a breast recurrence in axillary node–negative women younger than 35 years who did not receive chemotherapy. Young age was associated with a statistically significant increase in regional node failure and distant metastases and a statistically significant decrease in cause-specific survival. We have also observed an increased risk of distant metastases in women 35 years or younger with axillary node–negative minimally invasive (≤1 cm) breast cancer.[23] Young age by itself may be an indication for adjuvant chemotherapy, and the addition of chemotherapy may decrease the risk of a breast recurrence in women 35 years or younger treated with conservative surgery and radiation.

Current studies are evaluating the role of minimal local-regional treatment (surgery or radiation) in women 65 years or older with early-stage breast cancer. In 1995, we reported our results of conservative surgery and radiation in 173 women 65 years or older with stages I and II breast cancer and compared their outcome to that of 385 women 50 to 64 years of age.[28] Thirty-four percent of women 65 years or older had T2 tumors, 13 percent were estrogen receptor–negative, and 24 percent had positive axillary nodes. The 10-year actuarial breast recurrence rate was 13 percent for women 65 years or older and 10 percent for women 50 to 64 years of age. The 10-year rate of death from breast cancer was 13 percent for both groups of patients. For women 65 years or older, the 10-year rate of death from intercurrent disease was 11 percent, compared with 2 percent for women 50 to 64 years. The 10-year actuarial overall survival was 77 percent for women 65 years or older and 85 percent for those 50 to 64 years (p = .14). This study suggests that women 65 years or older do not have more indolent breast cancers and that patterns of survival, local control, and distant metastases are similar to women 50 to 64 years of age. Given the current life expectancy of women, breast conservation therapy should include radiation until the results of the ongoing studies are available. With appropriate treatment, the probability of death from breast cancer in a woman older than 65 years is almost equal to that from intercurrent disease.

Family History

It has been suggested that women with hereditary breast cancer should undergo mastectomy rather than breast-conservation therapy. Unfortunately,

there is a paucity of information regarding the results of conservative surgery and radiation in women with a positive family history of breast cancer. We reported outcome in 264 women with a positive family history and in 517 women with a negative family history.[21] A positive family history was associated with a statistically significant decreased incidence of positive axillary nodes. At 5 and 10 years, there were no statistically significant differences in breast recurrence rate, overall, or relapse-free survival for the two groups. In particular, women 35 years or younger with a positive family history of breast cancer did not have an increased risk of breast recurrence at 5 years (9 percent); however, women 35 years or younger without a positive family history did have an increased risk of breast recurrence (17 percent). As the number of affected relatives increased, the breast recurrence rate decreased, and overall survival increased. It is estimated that 50 to 60 percent of families with three or more affected members will have *BRCA1* linked breast cancer. In our series, there were no breast recurrences at 5 years in the 14 women with three or more affected members, and the 5-year overall survival was 100 percent, with a relapse-free survival of 88 percent. At the present time, a positive family history should not be a contraindication to conservative surgery and radiation. However, more information is needed in patients with hereditary breast cancer.

Histology

Most of the information on outcome of patients with stages I and II breast cancer treated with conservative surgery and radiation relates to patients with the most common histology, that is, invasive ductal carcinoma. A distinct pathological entity of extensive intraductal component (EIC) was first described by investigators at Harvard. This entity consists of patients whose primary tumor contains an *in situ* ductal component of 25 percent or more and in whom ductal carcinoma *in situ* (DCIS) is present in the normal surrounding breast tissue. In an initial report[9, 30] with pathology review by a single pathologist of 275 patients at the University of Pennsylvania, the 5- and 10-year actuarial breast recurrence rates were 22 percent and 22 percent for EIC-positive tumors, and 4 percent and 11 percent for EIC-negative tumors (p = .03). An additional definition of EIC-positive tumors also includes tumors that are primarily DCIS but with areas of focal invasion. We identified 39 women with microinvasive (≤2 mm or <10 percent of the primary tumor) ductal cancers treated with conservative surgery and radiation.[27] The 5-year actuarial breast recurrence rate was 19 percent in these patients and was significantly higher than the 5-year actuarial rate of 6 percent for invasive ductal cancers (p = .006). Negative margins of resection decreased the incidence of breast recurrence (5 percent negative margins, 35 percent unknown, 67 percent close or positive). We have also examined a number of pathological factors for their potential association with an increased risk of breast recurrence in patients with invasive ductal cancers.[30] In univariate analysis, higher histological grade, marked inflammatory response, necrosis in DCIS, retrograde cancerization of the lobules, the presence of background fibrocystic changes, atypical ductal hyperplasia, and an EIC predicted for an increased risk of breast recurrence at 10 years. In multivariate analysis, only moderate to marked necrosis in the associated DCIS and the presence of fibrocystic changes were significant. In a subsequent analysis of patients treated at University of Pennsylvania and Fox Chase Cancer Center,[29] we found no increased risk of breast recurrence at 5 years for invasive lobular cancers; invasive ductal and lobular cancers; medullary, colloid, or tubular cancers.

Positive Axillary Nodes

We have reported no increased risk of breast recurrence in patients with positive axillary nodes.[10] However, most of these patients have also received adjuvant chemotherapy, tamoxifen, or both. In our most recent analysis, the 10-year actuarial rate of breast recurrence was 13 percent for axillary node–negative patients and 9 percent for axillary node–positive patients ($p = .22$).

SURGICAL CONSIDERATIONS

Surgery for the primary tumor consists of an excisional biopsy with the goal of achieving microscopic negative margins of resection (≥ 2 mm). The correlation between the pathological margin status and the subsequent risk of an ipsilateral breast recurrence remains controversial. Factors that confound the issue include variations in the definition of a positive or close margin, the extent of the surgical resection (limited excision versus wide excision versus quadrantectomy), histology, patient age, and the addition of adjuvant chemotherapy or tamoxifen. Even for small mammographically detected cancers, negative margins of resection are difficult to obtain at the time of initial excision. We recently reported that only 24 percent of 353 mammographically detected T1 tumors had negative margins of resection after needle localization biopsy.[15] Close or positive margins were noted in 48 percent, and unknown margins were noted in 29 percent. Breast size correlated with negative margins (35 percent large breasts negative versus 18 percent small).

In an earlier analysis,[26] patients with positive or close margins did not have an increased risk of breast recurrence at 5 years when compared with patients with negative margins. However, patients with positive margins were carefully selected with focal involvement only. Patients with positive or close margins received a somewhat higher dose of radiation to the primary site (6000 versus 6500 versus 6400 cGy).

In our recent analysis, we observed similar findings at 5 years. The 5-year actuarial rate of breast recurrence was 4 percent for patients with negative margins, 9 percent for close margins, and 4 percent for positive margins. However, the 10-year actuarial rates of breast recurrence were 8 percent for negative margins, 18 percent for close margins, and 17 percent for positive margins. These findings emphasize the importance of long-term follow-up and the fact that early results may underestimate differences in outcome.

We have routinely recommended re-excision for patients with positive or unknown margins and in cases where close margins exist in more than one limited area. Re-excision is also indicated for patients whose mammographic presentation is one of malignant-appearing calcifications, and in whom a postbiopsy mammogram reveals residual calcifications. We recently reported that 47 percent of 420 patients who underwent re-excision had residual tumor.[16] A positive re-excision was significantly correlated with increasing tumor size, detection as a palpable mass, invasive lobular histology, and positive axillary nodes. The re-excision margin was positive in 9 percent and correlated significantly with positive axillary nodes and detection as a palpable mass.

Radiotherapy Technique

Radiation in general has consisted of 4600 to 5000 cGy to the breast with tangential fields, followed by a boost to the primary site of an additional 1000 to 2000 cGy. The boost volume was determined with computed tomography or stereo-shift radiographs in patients whose biopsy site was delineated with surgical clips.[24, 25] In a recent analysis, we compared outcome in terms of the 10-year actuarial risk of a true or marginal breast recurrence for 556 patients with clips and 808 patients without clips, all of whom received boost treatment.[5] The 10-year actuarial true or marginal breast recurrence rate was 5 percent for patients without clips compared with 11 percent for patients with clips. This difference appeared to be related to surgical techniques. Patients treated with more limited excisions and unknown margins accounted for a significant percent of the failures in the patients with clips. Delineation of the surgical bed with clips is important to accurately direct the boost treatment as well as to minimize the area treated. However, more precise definition of this region will not compensate for an inadequate surgical excision.

Indications for treatment of the axillary nodes with radiation in patients with early-stage invasive breast cancer have included an undissected clinically negative axilla, inadequate axillary dissection (≤ 3 nodes removed), or extensive axillary node involvement. Indications for supraclavicular node irradiation include four or more positive axillary nodes and one to three positive nodes in women 35 years or younger or black women. These indicators show an increased risk of supraclavicular node failure.[4, 8, 13, 22] Controversy continues to exist regarding the role of supraclavicular irradiation in all patients with one to three positive axillary nodes. Routine irradiation of the internal mammary nodes is not indicated in axillary node–negative or –positive patients with stages I and II breast cancer. The incidence of clinical internal mammary node failure is extremely low, and this pattern of failure is not significantly diminished by the addition of such treatment.[13] Regional node irradiation is not indicated in patients with negative axillary nodes.

Integration with Adjuvant Therapy

A concurrent regimen of chemotherapy and radiation was developed at University of Pennsylvania and Fox Chase Cancer Center. It was assumed that prompt initiation of both local/regional treatment and systemic therapy was important for long-term outcome. Ten-year results of this approach were reported in 1992.[20] During radiation, patients received two 28-day cycles of cyclophosphamide and 5-fluorouracil with or without tamoxifen; after radiation, either methotrexate or doxorubicin was added for an additional six cycles. Two hundred and nine patients received concurrent chemotherapy and radiation (11 percent node-negative, 65 percent one to three positive nodes, and 24 percent ≥4 positive nodes). The 10-year actuarial overall survival, cause-specific, and distant disease-free survival were 79 percent, 82 percent, and 66 percent. Good to excellent cosmesis was achieved in 84 percent. Two percent developed symptomatic pneumonitis and rib fractures. There were no radiation-related cardiac events. We had previously reported that the median volume of heart included in left-sided tangents was 9 percent compared with 53 percent for tangents and photon treatment of the internal mammary nodes.[1] The medial aspect of the left breast was treated with electrons when indicated to minimize the volume of heart within the tangential fields. No attempt was made to routinely treat the internal mammary nodes. In our earlier 10-year report, we noted that adjuvant chemotherapy significantly decreased the risk of an isolated (without distant metastases) breast recurrence at 5 and 10 years.[10] In our most recent analysis, the 10-year actuarial rate of a breast recurrence was 9 percent in the 443 patients who received chemotherapy, compared with 13 percent for 1126 patients who did not (p = .06).

The role of tamoxifen in decreasing the risk of an ipsilateral breast recurrence has been reported by several series. We recently evaluated the impact of adjuvant tamoxifen on breast recurrence, cosmesis, and complications in 154 women with estrogen receptor–positive tumors who received tamoxifen. We compared their outcome to 337 women with estrogen receptor–positive tumors who did not receive tamoxifen.[7] The 5-year actuarial rate of breast recurrence was 4 percent for the tamoxifen patients and 7 percent for the patients who did not receive tamoxifen

(p = .21). Tamoxifen resulted in a greater decrease in the 5-year actuarial rate of breast recurrence (4 percent versus 21 percent; p = .08) in axillary node–positive patients when compared with axillary node–negative patients (6 percent versus 7 percent; p = .29). Cosmesis was good to excellent in 85 percent of the tamoxifen patients and 88 percent of the patients who did not receive tamoxifen. Breast edema and hyperemia were more commonly observed in the tamoxifen patients.

Patterns and Significance of Local/Regional Failure

Ten years after conservative surgery and radiation for stages I and II breast cancer, 10 to 15 percent of patients will experience a recurrence in the treated breast.[10] We[3, 11] have reported that the majority of these recurrences occur in the vicinity of the primary tumor; however, after 5 years almost 50 percent occur in a separate quadrant. In our series, only 10 percent of the recurrences were noninvasive, and 12 percent presented with simultaneous distant metastases. Approximately one third of recurrences were detected solely by mammography. This percentage may seem low for a group of patients who have been followed carefully. However, we recently reported that in 1994 only one third to one half of all early-stage breast cancers treated with conservative surgery and radiation were diagnosed solely by mammography, depending on the patient's age.[17] Therefore, there is little evidence to suggest that the pattern of detection of an initial cancer is any different from that of a recurrence. We have also reported that the method of detection of the breast recurrence does not correlate with subsequent outcome.[18] We developed an algorithm for follow-up mammography after conservative surgery and radiation for early-stage invasive breast cancer.[19] We recommend that the first mammogram be performed 9 to 12 months after radiation to allow for resolution of the radiation changes. Breast recurrences within the first year of treatment are infrequent. If there are no suspicious findings, a 12-month follow-up mammogram program is initiated. Six-month follow-up mammograms are recommended only for patients with a nodular scar or ambiguous calcifications.

In our series, salvage mastectomy resulted in a 5-year survival and disease-free survival of 84 percent and 59 percent. The only significant prognostic factor for survival or disease-free survival was the initial tumor size. This factor, however, correlated with the extent of the recurrence. Five-year overall and disease-free survival of less than 80 percent were reported for a recurrence interval of 3 years or less, age 35 years or less, initial T2 tumor, initial positive axillary nodes, and skin or vascular-lymphatic invasion. We could not identify any pathological features that would predict for a recurrence of which surgical treatment could be less than a mastectomy.

The most common site of a regional node failure

in patients treated with conservative surgery and radiation is the axilla,[13] followed by the supraclavicular nodes. We reported a 3 percent 5-year actuarial rate of isolated regional node failure. Salvage therapy was relatively effective for an isolated axillary failure. A second axillary dissection resulted in regional control in 100 percent of patients, compared with only 50 percent for those who underwent excision of gross disease. Fifty percent of the patients with an isolated axillary failure were alive without evidence of disease. None of the patients with a supraclavicular failure was alive without disease.

SUMMARY

Our experience with conservative surgery and radiation in the treatment of stages I and II breast cancer has evolved during the last 15 years. We have learned the importance of long-term follow-up, surgical and radiotherapeutic techniques in minimizing recurrence rates and complications, and documentation of outcome to better define patient selection and modify treatment. Most important, we have had the opportunity to observe and record the natural history of breast cancer in patients treated with breast-conservation therapy. Our future efforts will continue to address those questions that remain unanswered.

References

 1. Danoff BF, Galvin JM, Cheng E, Brookland RK, Powlis WD, Goodman RL: The clinical application of CT scanning in the treatment of primary breast cancer. In Ames FC, Blumenschein GR, Montague ED (eds): Current Controversies in Breast Cancer. Austin, University of Texas Press, 1984, pp 391–397.
 2. Danoff BF, Goodman RL, Glick JH: The effect of adjuvant chemotherapy on cosmesis and complications in patients with breast cancer treated by definitive irradiation. Int J Radiat Oncol Biol Phys 9:1625, 1983.
 3. DiPaola RS, Orel SG, Fowble BL: Ipsilateral breast tumor recurrence following conservative surgery and definitive radiation therapy. Oncology 8:59–75, 1994.
 4. Fein D, Fowble B, Hanlon A, Goldstein L, Hoffman J, Sigurdson E, Eisenberg B: Race influences patterns of failure and cause-specific survival in women with Stage I–II breast cancer. Proc Am Soc Clin Oncol 15:98, 1996. Abstract.
 5. Fein DA, Fowble BL, Hanlon AL, Hoffman JP, Sigurdson ER, Eisenberg BL: Does the placement of surgical clips within the excision cavity influence local control for patients treated with breast conservation surgery and irradiation? Int J Radiat Oncol Biol Phys 34:1009–1017, 1996.
 6. Fein DA, Fowble BL, Hanlon AL, Hooks MA, Hoffman JP, Sigurdson ER, Jardines LA, Eisenberg BL: Identification of a group of women with T1 T2 breast cancer at low risk for positive axillary nodes. Proc Soc Surg Oncol March 21–24, 1996, p 13. Abstract.
 7. Fowble B, Fein DA, Hanlon AL, Eisenberg BL, Hoffman JP, Sigurdson ER, Daly MB, Goldstein LJ: The impact of tamoxifen on breast recurrence, cosmesis, complications, and survival in estrogen receptor positive early stage breast cancer. Int J Radiat Oncol Biol Phys 35:669–677, 1996.
 8. Fowble B, Schultz DJ, Overmoyer B, Solin LJ, Fox K, Jardines L, Orel S, Glick JH: The influence of young age on outcome in early stage breast cancer. Int J Radiat Oncol Biol Phys 30:23–33, 1994.
 9. Fowble B, Solin LJ, Schultz DJ. Conservative surgery and radiation for early breast cancer. In Fowble B, Goodman RL, Glick JH, Rosato EF (eds): Breast Cancer Treatment: A Comprehensive Guide to Management. St. Louis, Mosby, 1991, pp 105–150.
10. Fowble B, Solin LJ, Schultz DJ, Goodman RL: Ten year results of conservative surgery and irradiation for stage I and II breast cancer. Int J Radiat Oncol Biol Phys 21:269–277, 1991.
11. Fowble B, Solin LJ, Schultz DJ, Rubenstein J, Goodman RL: Breast recurrence following conservative surgery and radiation: Patterns of failure, prognosis and pathologic findings from mastectomy specimens with implications for treatment. Int J Radiat Oncol Biol Phys 19:833–842, 1990.
12. Fowble B, Solin LJ, Schultz DJ, Weiss MC: Breast recurrence and survival related to primary tumor location in patients undergoing conservative surgery and radiation for early-stage breast cancer. Int J Radiat Oncol Biol Phys 23:933–939, 1992.
13. Fowble B, Solin LJ, Schultz DJ, Goodman RL: Frequency, sites of relapse and outcome of regional node failures following conservative surgery and radiation for early breast cancer. Int J Radiat Oncol Biol Phys 17:703–710, 1989.
14. Fowble B, Yeh I-T, Schultz DJ, Solin LJ, Rosato EF, Jardines L, Hoffman J, Eisenberg B, Weiss MC, Hanks G: The role of mastectomy in patients with stage I–II breast cancer presenting with gross multifocal or multicentric disease or diffuse microcalcifications. Int J Radiat Oncol Biol Phys 27:567–573, 1993.
15. Hooks M, Eisenberg B, Sigurdson E, Hoffman J, Hanlon A, Fein D, Fowble B: Mammographically detected breast cancer: Resection margin status at needle localization biopsy and implications for re-excision. Proc Soc Surg Oncol March 21–24, 1996, p 41. Abstract.
16. Jardines L, Fowble B, Schultz D, Mackie J, Buzby G, Torosian M, Daly J, Weiss M, Orel S, Rosato E: Factors associated with a positive re-excision following excisional biopsy for invasive breast cancer. Surgery 118:803–809, 1995.
17. Orel SG, Fowble BL, Patterson EA, Kessler H: Trends in method of detection of early stage breast cancer in young women vs. older women. Radiology 197P:343, 1995. Abstract.
18. Orel SG, Fowble BL, Solin LJ, Delray JS, Conant EF, Troupin RH: Breast cancer recurrence after lumpectomy and radiation therapy for early-stage disease: Prognostic significance of detection method. Radiology 188:189–194, 1993.
19. Orel SG, Troupin RH, Patterson EA, Fowble BL: Breast cancer recurrence after lumpectomy and irradiation: Role of mammography in detection. Radiology 183:201–206, 1992.
20. Overmoyer B, Fowble B, Solin L, Goldstein L, Glick J: The long term results of conservative surgery and radiation with concurrent chemotherapy for early stage breast cancer. Proc Am Soc Clin Oncol 11:90, 1992. Abstract.
21. Peterson M, Fowble B, Solin LJ, Schultz DJ: Family history status as a prognostic factor for women with early stage breast cancer treated with conservative surgery and radiation. Breast J 1:202–209, 1995.
22. Pierce L, Fowble B, Solin LJ, Schultz DJ, Rosser C, Goodman RL: Conservative surgery and radiation therapy in black women with early stage breast cancer. Cancer 69:2831–2841, 1992.
23. Russo SA, Fowble B, Fox K, Solin LJ, Schultz DJ: The identification of a subset of patients with axillary node negative invasive breast cancer ≤1 cm who may benefit from adjuvant systemic therapy. Breast J 1:163–172, 1995.
24. Solin LJ, Chu JCH, Larsen R, Fowble B, Galvin JM, Goodman RL: Determination of depth for electron breast boosts. Int J Radiat Oncol Biol Phys 13:1915, 1987.
25. Solin LJ, Danoff BF, Schwartz GF, Galvin JM, Goodman RL: A practical technique for the localization of the tumor volume in definitive irradiation of the breast. Int J Radiat Oncol Biol Phys 11:1215, 1985.
26. Solin LJ, Fowble B, Schultz DJ, Goodman RL: The significance of pathology margins of the tumor excision on the outcome of patients treated with definitive irradiation for early-stage breast cancer. Int J Radiat Oncol Biol Phys 21:279–287, 1991.
27. Solin LJ, Fowble BL, Yeh I-T, Kowalyshyn MJ, Schultz DJ,

Weiss MC, Goodman RL: Microinvasive ductal carcinoma of the breast treated with breast conserving surgery and definitive irradiation. Int J Radiat Oncol Biol Phys 23:961–966, 1992.

28. Solin LJ, Schultz DJ, Fowble BL: Ten-year results of the treatment of early-stage breast carcinoma in elderly women using breast-conserving surgery and definitive breast irradiation. Int J Radiat Oncol Biol Phys 33:45–51, 1995.

29. Weiss MC, Fowble BL, Solin LJ, Yeh I-T, Schultz DJ: Outcome of conservative therapy for invasive breast cancer by histologic subtype. Int J Radiat Oncol Biol Phys 23:941–947, 1992.

30. Yeh IT, Fowble B, Viglione MJ, LiVolsi VA, Schultz DJ: Pathologic assessment and pathologic prognostic factors in operable breast cancer. *In* Fowble B, Goodman RL, Glick JH, Rosato EF (eds): Breast Cancer Treatment: A Comprehensive Guide to Management. St. Louis, Mosby, 1991, pp 167–208.

CHAPTER 63

CONSERVATION SURGERY AND RADIATION: THE M. D. ANDERSON CANCER CENTER EXPERIENCE

Kelly K. Hunt, M.D. / S. Eva Singletary, M.D. / Terry L. Smith, M.S. / Merrick I. Ross, M.D. / Eric A. Strom, M.D. / Marsha D. McNeese, M.D. / Frederick C. Ames, M.D.

Conservation surgery plus radiation therapy is generally accepted as an alternative to mastectomy for many patients with operable breast cancer, on the basis of data from several prospective randomized trials (reviewed in other chapters).[4, 5, 17, 18] Before the mid 1970s, however, patients were seldom considered for conservation surgery plus radiation unless they refused mastectomy or were considered medically unable to undergo operation under general anesthesia. Previously published reports from our institution summarize our early experience with breast conservation in the treatment of operable breast cancer.[10–13] This chapter reviews the techniques, results, and complications of treatment after 1976 of patients who were prospectively treated for invasive or noninvasive breast cancer with breast-conserving surgery and radiation therapy at the University of Texas M. D. Anderson Cancer Center.

PATIENTS AND METHODS

From 1955 through December 1992, 1075 patients with 1100 operable breast cancers were treated with conservative surgery plus radiotherapy at the M. D. Anderson Cancer Center. Before 1976, however, few patients were offered tumor excision (segmental mastectomy) plus radiation as an alternative to mastectomy. Before that time, some patients were treated with protracted high-dose radiation without excision or were treated with breast conservation plus radiation because they refused mastectomy. In many instances, the biopsy carried out before referral served as the only tumor excision. Through 1975, therefore, only a few patients with operable invasive breast cancer had been treated with excision plus radiation comparable to current practice. After a review of that earlier period, we modified our treatment approach and increasingly considered patients for elective breast conservation plus radiation as an alternative to mastectomy.[10–13] The results of treatment and complications in 928 patients with stage 0, I, or II breast cancer prospectively treated with conservation surgery plus radiation between 1976 and 1992 are reviewed in this chapter. Patients who underwent breast-conserving surgery after tumor downstaging with induction chemotherapy were not included in this review.

SURGICAL TECHNIQUE

Most patients underwent excision of all gross tumor in a procedure that attempted to achieve histologically proved negative surgical margins. More than one third of these patients, however, were referred after biopsy and removal of most or all of the tumor. In these patients, a re-excision was often performed when feasible if surgical margins were involved or if they could not be assessed. Our previous review revealed an increased rate of local recurrence in such patients if the surgical margins were unknown.[10] This was most often the case when the surgeon performed the biopsy as a diagnostic procedure with no intent to consider treatment by excision plus radiation. Some patients refused re-excision, and in some others, it was not technically feasible for cosmetic reasons. Among patients who underwent re-excision under these circumstances, more than 50 percent had residual cancer at the biopsy site.[12] In addition, axillary lymph node dissection for staging was recommended to all patients with invasive breast cancer, and most underwent a Level I–II axillary dissection through a separate incision.

In the latter part of our series, radiopaque hemoclips were placed at the margins of resection to assist the radiotherapist in treatment planning. The importance of hemoclips in determining the appropriate treatment fields can be demonstrated in the treatment planning film shown in Figure 63–1. In the case illustrated in Figure 63–1, if the surgical incision alone (marked with a radiopaque wire) was used to determine the fields for a boost dose to the tumor bed (marked with radiopaque hemoclips), a significant portion of the tumor bed would have been missed by the boost.

RADIATION THERAPY

The breast was treated through medial and lateral tangential fields of cobalt 60 or 6 mV photons to 45 to 50 Gy in 25 fractions over 5 weeks. The dose was calculated at a point approximately two thirds of the distance from the areola to the base of the breast, based on breast contours and computed tomographic (CT) treatment planning.[12] If there was tumor in a re-excision specimen, a boost of 10 Gy in 5 days was delivered through reduced fields with electrons of

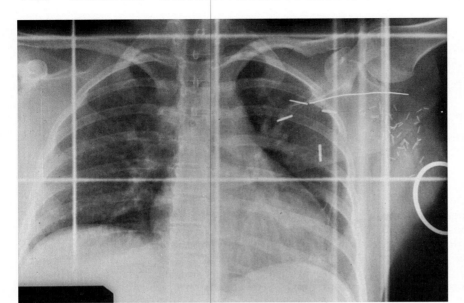

Figure 63–1 *Radiation therapy treatment planning films in a patient following segmental mastectomy and axillary lymph node dissection for a left upper outer quadrant breast cancer. The margins of excision of the primary tumor were marked by the surgeon with four large radiopaque hemoclips. The surgical incision is marked with a radiopaque wire. If the surgical incision alone was used for planning the boost dose, a significant portion of the primary tumor bed would have been missed by the boost.*

appropriate energy. Other indications for a boost dose included vascular or lymphatic invasion, nuclear anaplasia (Black's nuclear grade I), or four or more involved lymph nodes. Additionally, if the margins contained tumor, if the tumor was close (less than 2 mm) to the margin, or if the status of the margins were unknown and re-excision was not performed, an interstitial implant or electron beam boost was used to deliver 15 to 20 Gy.

Patients with lateral T1N0 tumors received radiation to the breast only. In some patients with central, medial, and node-positive tumors, the internal mammary and supraclavicular nodes were treated to 45 to 50 Gy. Generally, electrons were used to treat the nodal areas to avoid heart and lung damage. Rarely, the axilla was treated in patients with large nodes (>3 cm) or extranodal extension. As treatment evolved, less emphasis was placed on nodal irradiation in patients with fewer than four positive axillary lymph nodes.[9, 16]

We have seen breast necrosis after radiation in one patient with scleroderma and one with systemic lupus erythematosus and are currently reluctant to irradiate patients who have systemic collagen vascular diseases, with the exception of patients with rheumatoid arthritis.[7]

SYSTEMIC ADJUVANT THERAPY

After 1976, many patients with histologically positive axillary lymph nodes were considered for systemic adjuvant therapy using doxorubicin-based, combination chemotherapy regimens. For patients with four or more disease-positive nodes, radiation was usually delayed until at least three cycles of the planned course of chemotherapy had been administered. Most patients who received systemic therapy before the early 1980s did so after the completion of the planned radiation therapy, following a 2- to 3-week rest. Cur-

rently, patients receive systemic chemotherapy after surgery and radiation therapy is performed at the completion of their systemic treatment. Details of chemotherapy regimens used at the M. D. Anderson Cancer Center have been previously reported.[1]

RESULTS

As of January 1996, the estimated 5-year and 10-year disease-specific survival rates were 99 percent and 97 percent, respectively, for stage 0 patients, 94 percent and 87 percent for stage I patients, and 90 percent and 83 percent for stage II patients. Estimated 5-year and 10-year survival rates for stage II patients by nodal status are listed in Table 63–1. Survival rates were slightly decreased in node-positive patients but were higher in the small group of patients whose nodal status was unknown or clinically negative at the time of their treatment.

With a median follow-up of 88 months, local/regional recurrence rates were 9.5 percent for stage 0 patients, 9.2 percent for stage I patients, and 10.6 percent for stage II patients. Estimated local/regional

TABLE 63–1. SURVIVAL IN STAGE II PATIENTS BY NODAL STATUS AFTER BREAST CONSERVATION THERAPY

Stage	Nodal Status	No. of Patients	No. of Deaths*	Disease-Specific Survival Rates (Percent)	
				5 Year	10 Year
II	Negative	145	22	90	82
II	Positive	204	32	88	81
II	Unknown	38	4	97	94
II	All	387	58	90	83

*Number of deaths as of last follow-up, December 1995.

TABLE 63–2. LOCAL/REGIONAL RECURRENCE-FREE SURVIVAL IN STAGE 0, I, AND II BREAST CANCER PATIENTS AFTER BREAST CONSERVATION THERAPY

Stage	Nodal Status	Total No. of Patients	No. of Local/ Regional Recurrences (Percent)	Local/Regional Recurrence- Free Survival (Percent)	
				5 Year	10 Year
0	Negative	84	8 (9.5)	98	90
I	Negative	457	42 (9.2)	93	88
II					
	Negative	145	14 (9.7)	91	86
	Positive	204	19 (9.3)	92	85
	Unknown	38	8 (21.1)	86	74
II	All	387	41 (10.6)	91	84

recurrence-free survival rates by stage are listed in Table 63–2. In our series, a total of 142 patients received systemic chemotherapy and 123 patients received adjuvant hormonal therapy.

COMPLICATIONS

A representative sample of the complications of conservation surgery plus radiation therapy in this series was derived from patients who received radiation therapy in the calendar year 1990 (Table 63–3). We chose the year 1990 because treatment delivered during that time was similar to current practice. In addition, patients treated in 1990 have been followed at least 5 years, allowing us to obtain accurate data on long-term complications. A concerted effort was made to register all probable treatment complications, even if they were minor or produced no symptoms.

TABLE 63–3. COMPLICATIONS AFTER CONSERVATION SURGERY PLUS RADIATION THERAPY FOR STAGE 0, I, AND II BREAST CANCER PATIENTS TREATED IN 1990

Complication	No. of Patients Any Severity (Percent)*	No. of Patients Moderate to Severe (Percent)
Pneumonitis (fibrosis)	5 (6)	0
Breast skin fibrosis	19 (23)	1 (1)
Axillary fibrosis	1 (1)	0
Rib fracture	0	0
Loss of motion	7 (9)	0
Fat necrosis	1 (1)	0
Neuropathy	0	0
Arm edema	10 (12)	4 (5)
Breast edema†	13 (16)	0
Other‡	9 (11)	1 (1)

* A total of 90 patients received radiation therapy in 1990, but 8 were excluded because their follow-up was performed at other institutions.

† Breast edema and hyperpigmentation changes were generally of a mild nature, and in most cases were resolved within 2 to 3 years.

‡ Includes pigmentation changes of the breast skin and areola, telangiectasias of the breast skin, and skin dimpling.

Ninety patients received radiation therapy during 1990, but 8 of them received the majority of their follow-up care outside our institution and could not be accurately assessed for long-term complications. Although 42 of the 82 evaluable patients (51 percent) had some type of complication, most were asymptomatic or had only minor symptoms. For example, 5 patients (6 percent) had evidence of apical fibrosis on chest roentgenogram, but none were symptomatic. Fibrosis in the breast, skin, or axilla or at field junctions was observed in 21 patients (26 percent) but was of a mild degree and had not resulted in significant morbidity in 20 of the 21 patients. More recently, these complications have been minimized by using improved techniques that minimize overlap at field junctions. Overall, although 42 patients (51 percent) had measurable changes resulting from treatment, only 7 percent had symptoms that were judged to be significant and were persistent. Of these patients, 4 had arm edema, 1 had severe breast fibrosis, and 1 had fibrosis at the treatment site with breast pain and tenderness. The risk of these complications can probably be minimized by altering the radiation techniques described earlier in this report and elsewhere.[2, 8, 10–14] At present, patients with clinical stage I or II disease undergo Level I–II axillary dissection and do not receive irradiation to the axilla unless extensive nodal or extranodal disease is found. This has minimized arm edema. Cosmesis was judged to be good or excellent in more than 80 percent of all patients.

SUMMARY

Long-term results of prospective, randomized trials have proved that breast conservation is an effective therapy for early stage breast cancer.[3, 5, 18] Physicians at the M. D. Anderson Cancer Center have treated breast cancer patients with breast-conserving methods since 1955, but most patients treated with breast conservation before 1976 either refused mastectomy or were not believed to be good surgical candidates. The current treatment approach includes segmental mastectomy to achieve pathologically negative margins and Level I–II axillary lymph node dissection for patients with invasive disease. Patients who are candidates for systemic adjuvant chemotherapy are evaluated for accrual to currently active treatment protocols that are designed to evaluate different chemotherapy regimens in addition to the appropriate sequencing of radiation and chemotherapy. Patients who are not eligible for protocols generally receive their chemotherapy after surgery, with radiation therapy given at the completion of chemotherapy.

Local effects from treatment with conservation surgery plus radiation therapy for breast cancer are generally mild and frequently asymptomatic. We found that 5 percent of patients had moderate lymphedema of the upper extremity and 1 patient had significant breast fibrosis. We did not find any severe or disabling complications. As one would expect, overall survival decreased with increasing stage of disease, and local/regional recurrence rates were only slightly different among stages. Overall survival rates were 90 percent or better at 5 years for all groups except node-positive patients, who had an 88 percent 5-year survival rate. Our local/regional recurrence-free survival rates are similar to those reported in other series and support the use of conservation treatment for patients with early-stage breast cancer.[6, 15]

Acknowledgments

The authors would like to acknowledge Bobbie Lester for her assistance in data collection and data base management. This manuscript was reviewed by the Department of Scientific Publications at the University of Texas M. D. Anderson Cancer Center.

References

1. Buzdar AU, Hortobagyi GN, Kau S-W, et al: Breast cancer adjuvant therapy at the M. D. Anderson Cancer Center: Results of four prospective studies. *In* Salmon SE (ed): Adjuvant Therapy of Cancer VII. Philadelphia, JB Lippincott, 1993, p 220.
2. Chu JCH, Solin LJ, Hwang CC, et al: A nondivergent three field matching technique for breast irradiation. Int J Radiat Oncol Biol Phys 19:1037, 1990.
3. Early Breast Cancer Trialists' Collaborative Group: Effects of radiotherapy and surgery in early breast cancer. N Engl J Med 333:1444, 1995.
4. Fisher B, Bauer M, Margolese R, et al: Five-year results of a randomized clinical trial comparing total mastectomy and segmental mastectomy with or without radiation in the treatment of breast cancer. N Engl J Med 312:665, 1985.
5. Fisher B, Anderson S, Redmond CK, et al: Reanalysis and results after 12 years of follow-up in a randomized clinical trial comparing total mastectomy with lumpectomy with or without irradiation in the treatment of breast cancer. N Engl J Med 333:1456, 1995.
6. Fisher B, Anderson S, Fisher ER, et al: Significance of ipsilat-
eral breast tumour recurrence after lumpectomy. Lancet 338:327, 1991.
7. Fleck R, McNeese MD, Ellerbroek NA, et al: Consequences of breast irradiation in patients with pre-existing collagen vascular diseases. Int J Radiat Oncol Biol Phys 17:829, 1989.
8. McCune K, Parsons L, Schoenfeld L, et al: A technique for evaluating cast foam positioning and immobilization devices used in breast cancer radiotherapy. Int J Radiat Oncol Biol Phys 16:119, 1991.
9. McNeese MD, Fletcher GH, Levitt SH, et al: Technique related to tumor extent in cancer of the breast. *In* Levitt S (ed): Technological Basis of Radiation Therapy: Practical Clinical Applications. New York, Lea & Febiger, 1992, p 232.
10. Montague ED, Gutierrez AE, Barker JL, et al: Conservation surgery and irradiation for the treatment of favorable breast cancer. Cancer 43:1058, 1979.
11. Montague ED, Schell SR, Romsdahl MM, et al: Conservation surgery and irradiation in clinically favorable breast cancer: The M. D. Anderson experience. *In* Harris JR, Hellman S, Silen W (eds): Conservative Management of Breast Cancer: New Surgical and Radiotherapeutic Techniques. Philadelphia, JB Lippincott, 1983, p 53.
12. Montague ED: Conservation surgery and radiation therapy in the treatment of operable breast cancer. Cancer 53:700, 1984.
13. Montague ED, Ames FC, Schell SR, et al: Conservation surgery and irradiation as an alternative to mastectomy in the treatment of clinically favorable breast cancer. Cancer 54:2668, 1984.
14. Siddon RL, Buck BA, Harris JR, et al: Three-field technique for breast irradiation using tangential field corner blocks. Int J Radiat Oncol Biol Phys 9:583, 1983.
15. Stotter AT, McNeese MD, Ames FC, et al: Predicting the rate and extent of locoregional failure after breast conservation therapy for early breast cancer. Cancer 64:2217, 1989.
16. Strom EA, McNeese MD, Fletcher GH: Treatment of the peripheral lymphatics: Rationale, indications, and techniques. *In* Fletcher GH, Levitt SH (eds): Medical Radiology: Non-Disseminated Breast Cancer—Controversial Issues in Management. Berlin Heidelberg, Springer-Verlag, 1993, p 57.
17. Veronesi U, Saccozzi R, Del Vecchio M, et al: Comparing radical mastectomy with quadrantectomy, axillary dissection, and radiotherapy in patients with small cancers of the breast. N Engl J Med 305:6, 1981.
18. Veronesi U, Salvadori B, Luini A, et al: Breast conservation is a safe method in patients with small cancer of the breast: Long-term results of three randomised trials on 1,973 patients. Eur J Cancer 31A:1574, 1995.

CHAPTER 64

PATTERNS OF FAILURE IN SMALL BREAST CANCERS TREATED BY CONSERVATIVE SURGERY AND RADIOTHERAPY AT THE INSTITUT GUSTAVE-ROUSSY

Rodrigo Arriagada, M.D. / Karen Goset, M.D. / Serge Koscielny, Ph.D.

Breast-conserving surgery combined with radiotherapy has been widely used in the treatment of early breast cancer. The rationale is to treat the entire breast to decrease the rate of local recurrence. The results are equivalent to those achieved with radical surgery, as has been clearly established by randomized trials* and more recently by a comprehensive meta-analysis based on individual patient data.[12] This chapter describes the pattern of failure in patients at the Institut Gustave-Roussy homogeneously treated for early breast cancer with a conservative approach and to analyze which factors could predict the main causes of treatment failure.

PATIENTS AND METHODS

This series comprised 959 patients with unilateral invasive breast cancer, staged as T0–T2, N0–N1, M0 tumors,[29] integrally treated at the Institut Gustave-Roussy (IGR) between June 1970 and December 1984. They were treated conservatively if the tumor, measured by the pathologist at the time of surgery, was 20 mm or less (1970–1979) or 25 mm or less (1980–1984). The exceptions were 42 patients who were included because they were medically unfit for more extensive surgery or had declined mastectomy. In addition, 44 patients with multiple invasive adenocarcinoma (38 with two tumors, 5 with three tumors, and 1 with four tumors) were treated conservatively for similar reasons.

Surgery

All patients underwent tumorectomy at the IGR. The adequacy of margins was confirmed by the pathologist at the time of surgery. Surgical margins were considered clear if, on definitive paraffin section, invasive tumor or *in situ* components were absent within 2 mm of the margins at any point. If widespread ductal carcinoma *in situ* was subsequently found in the specimen, it was recommended that the patient should proceed to a mastectomy. These patients were not included in this series.

The policy for the axilla was to perform a lower axillary dissection and remove at least seven nodes.

These were examined by the pathologist at the time of surgery, and if any of them were involved by tumor (node positive), a complete axillary dissection was performed.

Radiotherapy

All patients received radiotherapy. A dose of 45 Gy in 18 sessions in 30 days was delivered at the breast and regional nodes if indicated. This was followed by a booster dose on the tumor bed of 15 Gy in 6 sessions in 10 days. Target volumes included the breast and chest wall for patients with histologically negative axillary nodes. If the patient had positive histological axillary nodes, the supraclavicular, axillary, and internal mammary nodes were included. Furthermore, it was found that the combination of axillary clearance and radiotherapy was associated with excessive morbidity,[10] so after 1981, node-positive patients treated by axillary clearance received no axillary irradiation.

The treatment was delivered with cobalt 60 radiation beams, and for the booster dose of some medial tumors, 8 or 10 MeV electron beams of a linear accelerator were used. Details about the radiation technique have been published elsewhere.[27] Briefly, the fields were planned according to the following principles for patients receiving a complete local/regional radiotherapy:

1. One anterior supraclavicular and axillary field. This large field was used three times per week (three fractions of 2.5 Gy).
2. One anterior supraclavicular field and one posterior axillary field. Both delivered one fraction of 2.5 Gy once a week when the previous large field was not treated.
3. Two sets of two tangential mammary fields with wedge filters. The first set allowed the internal mammary chain and the whole mammary gland to be irradiated to a total dose of 45 Gy. The second set, performed in a second step, involved smaller fields and was devoted to the booster irradiation of the tumor bed at a total dose of 60 Gy. For both sets of mammary fields, the irradiation was delivered four times per week.
4. Since 1980, treatment of the internal mammary chain for most patients was given with a mixed direct

---

*See references 2, 4, 15, 19, 20, 26, 31, and 32.

beam (50 to 50 percent) of cobalt 60 photons and electrons of appropriate energy. This anterior field matched with the internal tangential field.

The patients were treated lying on their backs. Patients were adjusted on a declined plane to bring the anterior part of the chest wall as horizontal as possible.

Systemic Treatment

Varied adjuvant systemic treatment was given in 132 node-positive patients and 4 node-negative patients. This therapy comprised, alone or in combination, ovarian irradiation in 25 patients, tamoxifen in 48 patients, immunotherapy with polyadenylic-polyuridylic acid[23] in 84 patients, and chemotherapy in 21 patients.

Follow-up

After treatment, all patients were followed regularly: every 4 months for the first 2 years, every 6 months for the next 3 years, and annually after 5 years. A careful clinical examination at each visit was supplemented by annual mammography and chest radiography.

Statistical Analysis

Patterns and risk of failure were analyzed using three procedures: log-rank test of censored curves of tumor events, a model assuming competing risks,[1, 3, 5, 21, 22] and a Cox's proportional hazards model[8] adjusted on prognostic factors. The model assuming competing risks includes all events synonymous with relapse by using cumulative incidence functions. These incidence estimates are subdivided into separate components that when summed, represent the overall event rates. In this context, events are considered as competing events and no assumption of independence is necessary. Event-specific cumulative incidence curves were estimated from the decomposition of the event-free survival curves, and a computer program (COMPETE), developed at the IGR[21, 22] was used for the calculations. Events analyzed were breast recurrence, distant metastasis, contralateral breast cancer and other new primary malignancies, and death. The rates of the first events or first cause of failure obtained with this method are compared with the usual censoring method and with the total relapse rates in which other events, except death, are ignored.

Prognostic factors were analyzed, selecting as criteria overall survival, breast recurrence, and distant metastasis rates. Covariates shown to be significant ($p \leq 0.10$) in univariate analyses were included in Cox's proportional hazards models[8] to estimate the independent prognostic value of each covariate. Other than clinical covariates, we used the quality of the surgical excision, three levels of a modified histological Scarff-Bloom-Richardson-based grading

system,[7] the number of positive axillary lymph nodes (0, 1 to 3, 4 or more), and the level of hormone receptors (≤ 10 fm/mg protein was defined as negative).

RESULTS

Clinical and Histological Findings

The distribution of main clinical and histological characteristics are shown in Table 64–1. The mean age of patients was 52 years (SD, 11; range, 22–82). Fifty-two percent of patients were postmenopausal. Mean length of follow-up was 152 months (SD, 46 months). At the end date for follow-up (January 1, 1995) only 14 percent of patients alive had been followed less than 10 years. Clinically, the tumors were small: the mean clinical size was 18.5 mm (SD, 7; range, 0–45). The macroscopic tumor diameter was less than 20 mm in 62 percent, and the mean macroscopic tumor diameter was 17 mm (SD, 6; range 0–45). The distribution of Bloom grade was 28 percent, 53 percent, and 19 percent for grades 1, 2, and 3, respectively. The grade was not established in 54 patients. The surgical tumor resection was considered complete in 84 percent of patients. The mean number of examined axillary lymph nodes was 13 (SD, 5; range, 1–31). Sixty-three percent of patients had histological negative axillary nodes.

Treatment Compliance

The mean total radiation dose to the breast was 45.1 Gy (SD, 0.8; range, 40–50), and the mean total dose to the tumor bed was 59.6 Gy (SD, 1.6; range, 45–66).

Local/Regional Control

There were 129 local recurrences in the breast (including 3 associated with ipsilateral axillary or supraclavicular nodal relapses), and there were 24 regional recurrences entirely outside the breast. In 20 cases, local/regional recurrences were associated with synchronous metastatic relapse (defined as appearing within the 3 months before or after the diagnosis of local recurrence). The 10-year actuarial rate of breast relapse was 12.4 percent, using the usual censoring method, and 9.8 percent by using the competing risk approach. Table 64–2 summarizes the pattern of failure in the whole population, including type of events and according to the methodology of including competing events or censoring or ignoring other events.

Figure 64–1 shows the overall survival, the event-free survival, the distant metastases, local recurrence, contralateral breast cancer, and new primary malignancy rates with a follow-up of 10 years, according to the competing risk approach. Considering the 129 relapses within the breast, including 19 cutaneous relapses, the actuarial (censoring) rate of relapse within the breast increased by approximately

TABLE 64–1. PATIENT CHARACTERISTICS AND UNIVARIATE ANALYSIS OF COVARIATES*

Factor	Level	No. of Patients	No. of Events	10-Year Rates (Percent)	p Value
Age (years)	<40	135	26	22	$<10^{-4}$
	40 < 50	291	45	14	
	50 < 60	299	20	8	
	60 +	234	11	5	
Menopausal status	Pre	451	71	15	$<10^{-4}$
	Post	483	27	7	
	Unknown	25	6		
Side	Right	443	51	12	0.32
	Left	516	51	10	
Clinical T size (mm)	<20	400	37	8	0.07
	20 +	510	60	13	
	Unknown	49	5		
Histological T size (mm)	<20	596	61	10	0.08
	20 +	363	41	12	
Multiple tumors	No	915	94	11	0.11
	Yes	44	8	20	
Histological grade	I	254	23	7	0.003
	II	475	47	11	
	III	176	26	17	
	Unknown	54	6		
No. of involved nodes	0	607	62	10	0.31
	1–3	276	34	12	
	4 +	76	6	15	
Estrogen receptors (fm/mg protein)	≤10	56	5	12	0.87
	>10	521	52	11	
	Unknown	382	45		
Progesterone receptors (fm/mg protein)	≤10	82	5	7	0.24
	>10	493	52	11	
	Unknown	384	45		
Clear surgical margins	Yes	801	78	10	0.03
	No	154	24	18	
	Unknown	4	0		

*End point is breast recurrence as first site of failure. Patients with other events (distant metastases, contralateral breast cancer, or other primary malignancy) are censored at the date of the event.

1 percent per annum, being 5 percent at 5 years and 9.9 percent at 10 years (see Table 64–2).

After breast relapse, 34 patients were deemed inoperable because of an inflammatory relapse (3) or the presence of distant metastases (31). The treatment of the relapse could not be determined for 13 patients (7 returned abroad and 6 were lost to follow-up within 3 months after diagnosis of the relapse). The remaining 82 patients underwent surgery (7 partial surgery, 75 mastectomy). All 82 patients remained in local control, although 23 died of distant metastases.

Twenty-four patients relapsed in sites outside the breast: 5 axillary and 19 supraclavicular relapses. The mean time for axillary relapse was 54 months (SD, 61 months), although 1 was observed after 5 years (146 months). The probability of axillary relapse at 5 years was only 0.45 percent (95 percent confidence interval, 0 to 0.9 percent). Only 1 of the node-positive patients who underwent complete axillary dissection (without axillary radiotherapy) relapsed in the axilla but with synchronous distant metastases.

TABLE 64–2. TEN-YEAR CUMULATIVE INCIDENCE RATES ACCORDING TO THREE METHODS OF ESTIMATING EVENT OCCURRENCE IN 959 PATIENTS

Event at 10 Years (Percent)	Assuming Competing Events	Censoring Other Events	Ignoring Other Events
Breast recurrence	7.9	9.9	12.4
Distant metastasis	18.9	20.7	23.4
Contralateral breast cancer	5.8	7.1	7.6
New primary malignancy	3.2	3.8	3.8
Intercurrent death	3.4	4.5	
Any first event*	39.2		
Overall death*	—	—	21.6

*These are the complementary values of event-free and overall survival, respectively.

Survival

Overall survival was 91 percent at 5 years and 79 percent at 10 years. The equivalent figures for disease-free survival were 76 percent and 61 percent, respectively. Both curves are shown in Figure 64–1.

Distant Metastatic Relapses and Contralateral Breast Cancers

The distant metastasis relapse rate was 19 percent at 10 years, according to the competing risk approach

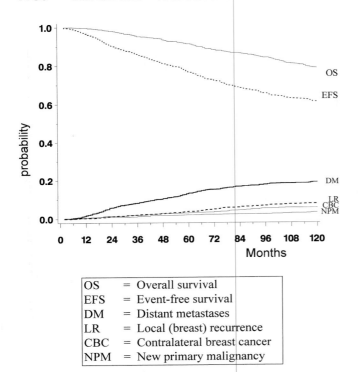

OS	= Overall survival
EFS	= Event-free survival
DM	= Distant metastases
LR	= Local (breast) recurrence
CBC	= Contralateral breast cancer
NPM	= New primary malignancy

Figure 64–1 *Pattern of failure of 959 patients with conservatively treated breast cancer according to a competing risk approach. Other than overall survival and event-free survival, events included are distant metastasis, local recurrence, contralateral breast cancer, and new primary malignancy.*

(see Fig. 64–1). Two hundred and forty-three patients developed distant metastases, and of these, 191 died of breast cancer. A total of 84 patients developed contralateral breast cancer, an incidence (0.8 percent per year) that was not significantly different from that of patients developing relapse within the treated breast.

New Primary Malignancies

Forty-five patients developed new primary malignancies other than contralateral breast cancer: 16 skin (14 basal cell carcinomas and 2 melanomas); gastrointestinal tract (9); uterus (7); hematological disease (3); ovary (2); thyroid (2); pancreas, lung, brain, tongue (1 each); and 2 not specified.

Prognostic Factors

Univariate analysis for breast recurrence is shown in Table 64–1. Significant factors were age, menopausal status, histological grade, and clear surgical margins. The presence of multiple tumors and clinical or histological tumor size were of borderline significance. All these factors, excluding menopausal status (because of the high correlation with age), were included in a multivariate analysis shown in Table 64–3. The strongest prognostic factors were age, histological grade, and histological tumor size. A patient younger than 40 years had a relative risk of local recurrence of 4.22 as compared with patients 60 years or older. The effect of age decreased continuously after 40 years. A patient with histological grade III tumor had a twofold risk of breast recurrence as compared with a patient with a grade I tumor. The surgical margin and multiple tumors factors did not reach statistical significance.

Univariate analyses for distant metastases and death rates are shown in Table 64–4. Highly significant factors were histological tumor size, clinical tumor size, histological grade, and number of involved nodes. Because clinical size is highly correlated to histological size, only the latter factor was included in the multivariate analysis. Age and menopausal status were of borderline significance. Because these factors are highly correlated, only age in four groups

TABLE 64–3. MULTIVARIATE ANALYSIS FOR THE 902 PATIENTS WITH KNOWN HISTOLOGICAL GRADE AND SURGICAL MARGIN STATUS

Factor	Level	No. of Patients	No. of Events	Relative Risk (95 Percent CI)	p Value
Age (yr)	<40	124	25	4.22 (2.06–8.66)	0.0001
	40 < 50	264	40	2.94 (1.51–5.74)	0.002
	50 < 60	288	20	1.31 (0.63–2.74)	0.47
	60 +	226	11	1†	
Histological grade	I	252	23	1†	
	II	474	47	1.24 (0.74–2.06)	0.29
	III	176	26	1.89 (1.05–3.38)	0.03
Histological T size (mm)	<20	555	56	1	
	20 +	347	40	1.55 (1.01–2.37)	0.04
Factors Not Included in the Final Model					
Clear surgical margins	Yes	759	74	1†	
	No	143	22	1.37 (0.84–2.23)	0.20
Multiple tumors	No	856	87	1	
	Yes	41	8	1.51 (0.72–3.15)	0.28
Total‡		902	96		

*End point is breast recurrence as first site of failure. Patients with other events (distant metastases, contralateral breast cancer, or other primary malignancy) are censored at the date of the event. Menopausal status was not included in the model as it is highly correlated with age.
†Reference category.
‡Except for model including multiple tumors, where totals were 897 and 95, respectively.

TABLE 64–4. UNIVARIATE ANALYSES OF COVARIATES*

Factor	Level	No. of Patients	Distant Metastases			Overall Death		
			No. of Events	10-Year Rates (Percent)	p Value	No. of Events	10-Year Rates (Percent)	p Value
Age (yr)	<40	135	30	25	0.99	43	27	0.15
	40 < 50	291	44	15		60	16	
	50 < 60	299	57	20		64	20	
	60 +	234	45	22		77	27	
Menopausal status	Pre	451	76	18	0.25	101	19	0.01
	Post	483	96	21		138	24	
	Unknown	25	4			5		
Side	Right	443	84	19	0.53	118	24	0.34
	Left	516	92	19		126	20	
Clinical T size (mm)	<20	400	56	15	0.003	83	17	0.001
	20 +	510	110	23		147	25	
	Unknown	49	10			14		
Histological T size (mm)	<20	596	76	14	$<10^{-4}$	122	16	$<10^{-4}$
	20 +	363	100	29		122	31	
Multiple tumors	No	915	168	19	0.99			
	Yes	44	8	21				
Histological grade	I	254	23	8	$<10^{-4}$	30	6	$<10^{-4}$
	II	475	100	24		134	25	
	III	176	44	27		68	34	
	Unknown	54	9			12		
No. of involved nodes	0	607	69	12	$<10^{-4}$	115	16	$<10^{-4}$
	1–3	276	70	26		91	27	
	4 +	76	37	52		38	43	
Estrogen receptors (fm/mg protein)	≤10	56	12	24	0.83	18	29	0.29
	>10	521	113	25		143	24	
	Unknown	382	51			83		
Progesterone receptors (fm/mg protein)	≤10	82	17	24	0.81	25	28	0.60
	>10	493	110	23		137	24	
	Unknown	384	49			82		
Clear surgical margins	Yes	801	145	19	0.54	198	21	0.52
	No	154	29	21		45	25	
	Unknown	4	2			1		

*End points are distant metastasis as first site of failure, and death. Patients with other events (breast recurrence, contralateral breast cancer, or other primary malignancy) are censored at the date of the event.

was included in the multivariate analyses. Number of involved nodes, histological grade, and tumor size were significant prognostic factors of distant metastasis and death rates. Age was also significant for death (Table 64–5) with a decreased death rate for the groups between 40 and 60 years. Surgical margins and multiple tumors did not reach significance in these models.

Cosmetic Results and Complications

The final cosmetic result[11] was considered good in 55 percent, moderate in 27 percent, and poor in 18 percent of patients. Complications were observed as follows: important arm edema in 5 percent of patients, clinical radiation pneumonitis in 1.3 percent, painful rib fractures in 1.3 percent, and tenderness of the chest wall in 6 percent. Five patients (1 percent) developed motor deficit in the ipsilateral upper extremities compatible with a brachial plexopathy.

DISCUSSION

Patients with small breast tumors (≤ 25 mm) can be managed by tumorectomy, axillary dissection, and radiotherapy with an acceptable local control rate, i.e., 90 percent at 10 years. These results were obtained in patients with relatively small tumors (mean macroscopic size, 17 mm) by using a meticulous surgical technique, adhering rigidly to a consistent radiotherapy protocol, and following the patients assiduously. Deviations from this treatment plan might well be associated with less favorable results. In this series, tumors with a histological size greater than 20 mm had a slightly higher risk of local recurrence than did smaller tumors (see Table 64–3). These results do not exclude the possibility that patients with larger tumors (>30 mm) may be at increased risk of local relapse. Further studies are necessary to define the upper limit of tumor size suitable for conservation therapy and to determine whether the tumorectomy must be macroscopically complete. The National Surgical Adjuvant Breast and Bowel Project and the European Organization for Research and Treatment of Cancer trials[15, 31] included patients with tumor of a clinical size up to 4 and 5 cm, respectively. No deleterious effect of tumor size has been described, but a longer follow-up would be necessary to ascertain this point.

Patients with extensive ductal carcinoma *in situ*

TABLE 64–5.   MULTIVARIATE ANALYSIS FOR 902 PATIENTS WITH KNOWN HISTOLOGICAL GRADE AND SURGICAL MARGINS*

Factor	Level	No. of Patients	Distant Metastasis			Overall Death		
			No. of Events	Relative Risk (95 Percent CI)	p Value	No. of Events	Relative Risk (95 Percent CI)	p Value
Histological T size	<20	555	73	1†		114	1†	
	20+	347	96	1.72 (1.25–2.36)	0.001	117	1.54 (1.17–2.03)	0.002
Histological grade	I	252	22	1†		29	1†	
	II	474	103	2.15 (1.36–3.41)	0.001	134	2.42 (1.60–3.64)	0.0001
	III	176	44	2.44 (1.46–4.09)	0.001	68	3.38 (2.16–5.29)	0.0001
No. of involved nodes	0	565	68	1†		110	1†	
	1–3	264	66	1.89 (1.34–2.67)	0.0003	85	1.51 (1.13–2.02)	0.005
	4+	73	35	4.11 (2.70–6.23)	0.0001	36	2.50 (1.69–3.68)	0.0001
Age (yr)	<40	124				41	0.89 (0.60–1.32)	0.56
	40 < 50	264				54	0.57 (0.40–0.81)	0.002
	50 < 60	288				62	0.58 (0.42–0.82)	0.002
	60+	226				74	1†	
Total		902	169			231		
Factors Not Included in the Final Model								
Age (yr)	<40	124	28	1.24 (0.77–2.00)	0.37			
	40 < 50	264	40	0.78 (0.51–1.19)	0.25			
	50 < 60	288	56	0.94 (0.64–1.40)	0.78			
	60+	226	45	1†				
Clear surgical margins	Yes	759	144	1†	0.48	190	1†	
	No	143	25	0.86 (0.56–1.31)		41	0.94 (0.67–1.33)	0.75
Multiple tumors	No	856	163	1		223	1†	
	Yes	41	5	0.48 (0.19–1.16)	0.10	7	0.54 (0.25–1.14)	0.11

*End points are distant metastasis as first cause of failure, and death. Clinical T size was not included in the model because it is highly correlated with histological T size.

†Reference category.

were not included in this series because they were treated by mastectomy; thus, we are not able to evaluate this factor in the analysis of breast recurrence.[24] In contrast to an earlier series,[9] clear surgical margin was not a significant predictive factor of local recurrence, and histological grading became significant. These differences may be partially explained by the fact that the present study included only patients primarily undergoing surgery at the IGR; we excluded those receiving a previous tumorectomy in other hospitals. These findings are similar to those published by van Dongen and coworkers[31] in a European trial that showed a trend for involved margins to be associated with a lower local control rate, but did not reach statistical significance. The negative effect of involved margins could be offset by higher local radiation doses.[28] However, changes in the prognostic value of analyzed factors depending on the time of follow-up and the methodology of analyses show the need for large numbers of patients with a long follow-up in each patient category to decrease statistical variability.

In the present series, low age was confirmed as a significant factor for local recurrence, and this negative effect is decreasing continuously up to 60 years of age. The pattern of failure described by the use of a competing risk approach (see Fig. 64–1) is consistent with that found in the randomized trial conducted in our institute using the same methodology.[2]

Patients with breast recurrence treated with total mastectomy had good local control as in other series.[17] There was good local control within the axilla.

After complete axillary dissection in node-positive patients, only one axillary relapse occurred. This confirms the adequacy of complete axillary dissection as a therapeutic modality. Irradiation after axillary clearance is thus unnecessary and, in addition, is associated with excessive morbidity.[10]

The need for postoperative radiotherapy to obtain a high rate of local control has been confirmed by randomized trials.[6, 30, 33] Furthermore, a good local/regional control may have an impact on overall survival, as suggested by recent studies.[2, 14, 34]

The rate of development of tumors in the contralateral breast was similar to that of relapse within the treated breast. This confirms the importance of careful long-term follow-up of these patients to detect local relapse or a new breast tumor. The reported rate could be decreased with the more systematic use of tamoxifen, which has been done in more recent years.[13, 16, 25]

Overall survival depends on the rate of distant metastatic relapse. The method of therapy (mastectomy or conservation treatment) has little effect on local control and hence survival.[12] Independent prognostic factors of death were number of involved axillary nodes, histological grade, histological tumor size, and age (see Table 64–5).

Breast conservation offers an acceptable rate of local control for patients with small primary tumors. The upper size limit for a safe treatment should be analyzed in randomized series with a large number of patients in each tumor size category and a long follow-up.[15, 31] The increasing use of adjuvant systemic therapies, such as tamoxifen and cytotoxics, could help to decrease the breast recurrence rate.[13, 18] Higher local radiation doses for high-risk patients, such as those with young age, large primary tumor, and high histologic grade, should be still tested prospectively.

References

1. Arriagada R, Kramar A, Le Chevalier T, De Cremoux H, for the French Cancer Centers' Lung Group: Competing events determining relapse-free survival in limited small-cell lung carcinoma. J Clin Oncol 10:447–451, 1992.
2. Arriagada R, Le MG, Rochard F, Contesso G, for the IGR Breast Cancer Group: Conservative treatment versus mastectomy in early breast cancer: Patterns of failure with fifteen-years of follow-up. J Clin Oncol 14:1558–1564, 1996.
3. Arriagada R, Rutqvist LE, Kramar A, Johansson H: Competing risks determining event-free survival in early breast cancer. Br J Cancer 66:951–957, 1992.
4. Blichert-Toft M: Danish randomized trial comparing breast conservation therapy with mastectomy: Six years of life-table analysis. J Natl Cancer Inst Monogr 11:19–25, 1992.
5. Castiglione M, Gelber RD, Goldhirsh A, for the International Breast Cancer Study Group: Adjuvant systemic therapy for breast cancer in the elderly: Competing causes of mortality. J Clin Oncol 8:519–526, 1990.
6. Clark RM, McCulloch PB, Levine MN, Lipa M, Wilkinson RH, Mahoney LJ, Basrur VR, Nair BD, McDermot RS, Wong CS, Corbett PJ: Randomized clinical trial to assess the effectiveness of breast irradiation following lumpectomy and axillary dissection for node-negative breast cancer. J Natl Cancer Inst 84:683–689, 1992.
7. Contesso G, Mouriesse H, Friedman S, Genin J, Sarrazin D, Rouesse J: The importance of histologic grade in long-term prognosis of breast cancer: A study of 1,010 patients, uniformly treated at the Institut Gustave-Roussy. J Clin Oncol 5:1378–1386, 1987.
8. Cox DR: Regression models and life tables (with discussion). J R Stat Soc 34:187–220, 1972.
9. Dewar JA, Arriagada R, Benhamou S, Benhamou E, Bretel JJ, Pellae-Cosset B, Marin JL, Petit JY, Contesso G, Sarrazin D: Local relapse and contralateral tumour rates in patients with breast cancer treated with conservative surgery and radiotherapy (Institut Gustave-Roussy 1970–1972). Cancer 76:2260–2265, 1995.
10. Dewar JA, Sarrazin D, Benhamou S, Petit JY, Benhamou E, Arriagada R, Fontaine F, Castaigne D, Contesso G: Management of the axilla in conservatively-treated breast cancer: 592 patients treated at the Institut Gustave-Roussy. Int J Radiat Oncol Biol Phys 13:475–781, 1987.
11. Dewar JA, Benhamou S, Benhamou E, Arriagada R, Petit JY, Fontaine F, Sarrazin D: Cosmetic results following lumpectomy, axillary dissection and radiotherapy for small breast cancers. Radiother Oncol 12:273–280, 1988.
12. Early Breast Cancer Trialists' Collaborative Group: Effects of radiotherapy and surgery in early breast cancer: An overview of the randomized trials. N Engl J Med 333:1444–1455, 1995.
13. Early Breast Cancer Trialists' Collaborative Group: Systemic treatment of early breast cancer by hormonal, cytotoxic, or immune therapy: 133 randomised trials involving 31,000 recurrences and 24,000 deaths among 75,000 women. Lancet 339:1571–1585, 1992.
14. Fisher B, Anderson S, Fisher ER, Redmond C, Wickerman DL, Wolmark N, Mamounas EP, Deutsch M, Margolese R: Significance of ipsilateral breast tumor recurrence after lumpectomy. Lancet 338:327–331, 1991.
15. Fisher B, Anderson S, Redmond CK, Wolmark N, Wickerham DL, Cronin WM: Reanalysis and results after 12 years of follow-up in a randomized clinical trial comparing total mastectomy with lumpectomy with or without irradiation in the treatment of breast cancer. N Engl J Med 333:1456–1461, 1995.
16. Fisher B, Redmond C: New perspective on cancer of the contralateral breast: A marker for assessing tamoxifen as a preventive agent. J Natl Cancer Inst 83:1278–1281, 1991.
17. Fowble B, Solin LJ, Schultz DJ, Rubenstein J, Goodman RL: Breast recurrence following conservative surgery and radiation: Patterns of failure, prognosis, and pathologic findings from mastectomy specimens with implications for treatment. Int J Radiat Oncol Biol Phys 19:833–842, 1990.
18. Goldhirsch A, Gelber RD, Price KN, Castiglione M, Coates AS, Rudenstam CM, Collins J, Lindtner J, Hacking A, Marini G, Byrne M, Cortes-Funes H, Schnurch G, Brunner KW, Tattersall MHN, Forbes J, Senn HJ: Effect of systemic adjuvant treatment on first sites of breast cancer relapse. Lancet 343:377–381, 1994.
19. Hayward JL: The Guy's Hospital trials on breast conservation. In, Harris JR, Hellman S, Silen W (eds): Conservative Management of Breast Cancer. Philadelphia, JB Lippincott, 1983, pp 78–90.
20. Jacobson JA, Danforth DN, Cowan KH, D'Angelo T, Steinberg SM, Pierce L, Lippman ME, Lichter AS, Glatstein E, Okunieff P: Ten-year results of a comparison of conservation with mastectomy in the treatment of stage I and II breast cancer. N Engl J Med 332:907–911, 1995.
21. Kramar A, Arriagada R: Analysing local and distant recurrence. J Clin Oncol 8:2086–2087, 1990. Letter.
22. Kramar A, Pejovic MH, Chassagne DA: A method of analysis taking into account competing events: Application to the study of digestive complications following irradiation for cervical cancer. Stat Med 6:785–794, 1987.
23. Lacour J, Lacour F, Spira A, Michelson M, Petit JY, Delage G, Sarrazin D, Contesso G, Viguier J: Adjuvant treatment with polyadenylic-polyuridylic acid in operable breast cancer: Updated results of a randomised trial. Br Med J 288:589–592, 1984.
24. Recht A, Silver B, Schmitt S, Connolly J, Hellman S, Harris JR: Breast relapse following primary radiation therapy for early breast cancer: I. Classification, frequency and salvage. Int J Radiat Oncol Biol Phys 11:1211–1216, 1985.
25. Rutqvist LE, Cedermark B, Glas U, Mattsson A, Skoog L, Somell A, Theve T, Wilking N, Askergren J, Hjalmar ML, Rotstein S, Perbeck L, Ringbord U: Contralateral primaries among breast cancer patients included in a randomized trial of adjuvant tamoxifen. J Natl Cancer Inst 83:1299–1306, 1991.
26. Sarrazin D, Le MG, Arriagada R, Contesso G, Fontaine F, Spielmann M, Rochard F, Le Chevalier T, Lacour J: Ten-year results of a randomized trial comparing a conservative treatment to mastectomy in early breast cancer. Radiother Oncol 14:177–184, 1989.
27. Sarrazin D, Le MG, Fontaine MF, Arriagada R: Conservative treatment versus mastectomy in T1 or small T2 breast cancer: A randomized clinical trial. In Harris JR, Hellman S, Silen W (eds): Conservative Management of Breast Cancer. Philadelphia, JB Lippincott, 1983, pp 101–111.
28. Schmidt-Ullrich R, Wazer DE, Tercilla O, Safaii H, Marchant DJ, Smith TJ, Homer MA, Robert NJ: Tumor margin assessment as a guide to optimal conservation surgery and irradiation in early stage breast carcinoma. Int J Radiat Oncol Biol Phys 17:733–738, 1989.
29. UICC: TNM: Classification of Malignant Tumours. 3rd ed. Geneva, 1979.
30. Uppsala-Orebro Breast Cancer Study Group: Sector resection with or without postoperative radiotherapy for stage I breast cancer: A randomized trial. J Natl Cancer Inst 82:277–281, 1990.
31. Van Dongen JA, Bartelink H, Fentiman IS, Lerut T, Mignolet F, Olthuis G, Van Der Schueren E, Sylvester R, Tong D, Winter J, Van Zijl K: Factors influencing local relapse and survival and results of salvage treatment after breast-conserving therapy in operable breast cancer: EORTC trial 10801, breast conservation compared with mastectomy in TNM stage I and II breast cancer. Eur J Cancer 28A:801–805, 1992.

32. Veronesi U, Banfi A, Salvadori B, Luini A, Saccozzi R, Zucali R, Marubini E, Del Veccio M, Boracchi P, Marchini S, Merson M, Sacchini V, Riboldi G, Santoro G: Breast conservation is the treatment of choice in small breast cancer: Long-term results of a randomized trial. Eur J Cancer 26:668–670, 1990.

33. Veronesi U, Luini A, Del Vecchio M, Greco M, Galimberti V, Merson M, Rilke F, Sacchini V, Saccozzi R, Savio T, Zucali R, Zurrida S, Salvatori B: Radiotherapy after breast-preserving surgery in women with localized cancer of the breast. N Engl J Med 328:1587–1591, 1993.

34. Whelan T, Clark R, Roberts R, Levine M, Foster G, McCulloch PB, Basrur VR, Lipa M, Wilkinson RH, Mahoney LJ, Nair BD, McDermot, Wong CS, Corbett PJ: Ipsilateral breast tumor recurrence postlumpectomy is predictive of subsequent mortality: Results from a randomized trial. Int J Radiat Oncol Biol Phys 30:11–16, 1994.

CHAPTER 65

CONSERVATION SURGERY AND IRRADIATION IN STAGES I AND II DISEASE: THE EUROPEAN EXPERIENCE

Umberto Veronesi, M.D.

The major development in Europe of conservative breast cancer treatments occurred in the 1970s. The first and main reason for the new course was a change in the conception of the natural history of breast cancer. Instead of being regarded as a mainly local/regional disease, breast cancer was now seen as a disease that may spread early in the body, so that the extent of the removal of the primary carcinoma has little influence on its prognosis. A second reason was the change in the patient population, resulting from the introduction of large-scale information campaigns, screening programs, and new diagnostic tools such as mammography. Before 1970, only a minority of patients had tumors less than 2 cm in diameter; since the early 1970s, the number of early cases has increased to 30 to 50 percent of all cases, at least in Western countries. A third reason was the observation of the failure of the aggressive surgical and radiotherapeutic procedures used in the 1960s, with many trials showing that super-radical operations and intense postoperative radiotherapy did not improve the prognosis of breast cancer patients. A final factor was the changed attitude of women in the decision-making process. Breast cancer patients today ask their surgeon for a complete description of the range of options available and the related benefits and risks to treat their disease.

The main randomized trials (with more than 300 patients accrued) conducted in Europe on breast-conservative treatments are here reviewed.

THE GUY'S HOSPITAL TRIAL

The first randomized trial of conservative treatment was conducted at Guy's Hospital in London between 1961 and 1970, and involved 370 patients.[1] The patients were randomized in two groups, the first group being treated with radical mastectomy plus radiotherapy to the axilla, supraclavicular triangle, and internal mammary chain (25–27 Gy), the second treated with breast resection plus radiotherapy on the breast (35–38 Gy) and on the regional nodes as in the mastectomy groups. The early results published in 1972 showed a significant increase of local/regional recurrences and a reduced survival in stage II patients,[1] but a more recent report by Hayward from Guy's Hospital in 1988[3] of stage I patients confirmed that mastectomy was superior to conservative treatment.

THE MILAN TRIALS

In 1968, at the meeting of the World Health Organization (WHO) Committee of Investigators on Breast Cancer Diagnosis and Treatment, a paper presented by Veronesi and associates proposed a randomized international study that would compare radical mastectomy with a conservative procedure consisting of a large breast resection (quadrantectomy) with a complete axillary dissection followed by radiotherapy (QUART) on the same breast. Although the project was endorsed by the Committee by the end of 1969, attempts to organize a coordinated international trial failed. Eventually, in 1973 the trial was implemented at the Milan Institute; the preliminary results were published in 1981,[8] and the extended analysis of these results were made available in 1990[10] and 1995.[9]

Only patients with clinical or mammographic evidence of a breast cancer smaller than 2 cm in diameter were selected for the trial. In addition, eligibility was contingent on the absence of clinically metastatic nodes. If the excisional biopsy and frozen section examination showed a carcinoma measuring up to 2 cm in diameter, the patient was randomized to one of two treatment groups and received either the Halsted mastectomy or a conservative treatment (QUART). Patients with noninfiltrating carcinoma were excluded, as were patients who were older than 70 years or who had had previous malignant disease of any type. From 1973 to 1975, patients with histologically proved nodal metastases were further randomized to receive radiotherapy to the supraclavicular and internal mammary nodes or no further treatment. From 1976 to 1980, 211 patients with histologically proven axillary metastases were given adjuvant combination chemotherapy consisting of cyclophosphamide, methotrexate, and 5-fluorouracil (CMF) for 1 year.

Patients randomized to conservative treatment were treated with the quadrantectomy technique. The term *quadrantectomy* refers to an extensive breast resection that removes a good portion of the quadrant of the breast containing the primary carcinoma, including the overlying skin and the fascia of the major pectoral muscle. This type of operation, although conservative, is considered a "locally radical" operation and not just a "debulking" operation, as are many conservative procedures.

When the primary cancer was located in the upper outer quadrant, the operation was performed en bloc, whereas when the primary site was in one of the other quadrants, the axillary dissection was performed through a separate incision. In all cases, to obtain a complete axillary dissection, the minor pectoralis muscle was resected, and all the axillary lymph nodes up to the apex of the axilla were removed. In more recent years, this technique has been substituted with one that preserves the minor pectoralis muscle.

Irradiation of the breast was an important part of the treatment. A dose of 50 Gy was delivered through two opposing tangential fields with high-energy photons (a cobalt unit or a 6-MeV linear accelerator), and another dose of 10 Gy was given with orthovoltage radiotherapy as a booster to the skin surrounding the scar.

Chemotherapy in node-positive patients was started 15 to 30 days after surgery; in the quadrantectomy group in most cases, it was begun simultaneously with radiotherapy. The average dosage of drugs administered was similar in the mastectomy and conservation therapy groups.

From 1973 to early 1980, 701 evaluable patients were entered into the trial; 349 were treated with the Halsted mastectomy and 352 with QUART. There were no significant differences between the two groups in any of the characteristics considered (i.e., age, menopausal status, tumor site by quadrant, dimensions of the primary cancer, incidence of axillary metastases and previous biopsy) thus making the two series perfectly comparable.

Fifteen patients in the QUART group and 8 in the Halsted group had local recurrences. Eleven of the 15 patients with local recurrence in the QUART group underwent mastectomy, and 4 were treated with a breast re-excision. Ten of the fifteen are alive and well as of mid-1996, and 5 died of distant metastases. Of the 8 patients with local recurrences in the Halsted group, 6 died of the disease. Ten patients treated with the conservative technique had a second cancer in the ipsilateral breast 4 to 10 years after the operation. The diagnosis of a second primary tumor in the ipsilateral breast was recorded after careful clinicopathological evaluation by surgeons, radiologists, and pathologists. Contralateral primary breast cancers were observed in 26 of the QUART patients and in 30 of the Halsted patients. By July 1995, there had been 127 deaths in the quadrantectomy group and 125 in the Halsted group.

The curves for overall survival and local recurrence rates are shown in Figures 65–1 and 65–2. No differences between the two groups were recorded after 18 years of follow-up. Evaluation of disease-free survival by subgroups according to the presence or absence of

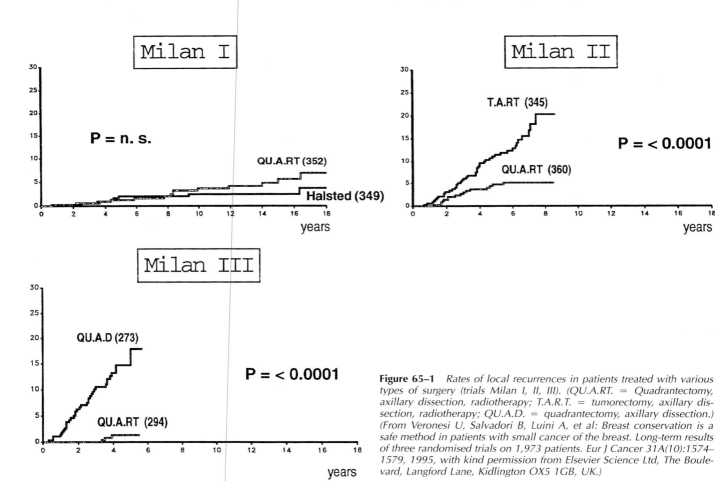

Figure 65–1   *Rates of local recurrences in patients treated with various types of surgery (trials Milan I, II, III). (QU.A.RT. = Quadrantectomy, axillary dissection, radiotherapy; T.A.R.T. = tumorectomy, axillary dissection, radiotherapy; QU.A.D. = quadrantectomy, axillary dissection.) (From Veronesi U, Salvadori B, Luini A, et al: Breast conservation is a safe method in patients with small cancer of the breast. Long-term results of three randomised trials on 1,973 patients. Eur J Cancer 31A(10):1574–1579, 1995, with kind permission from Elsevier Science Ltd, The Boulevard, Langford Lane, Kidlington OX5 1GB, UK.)*

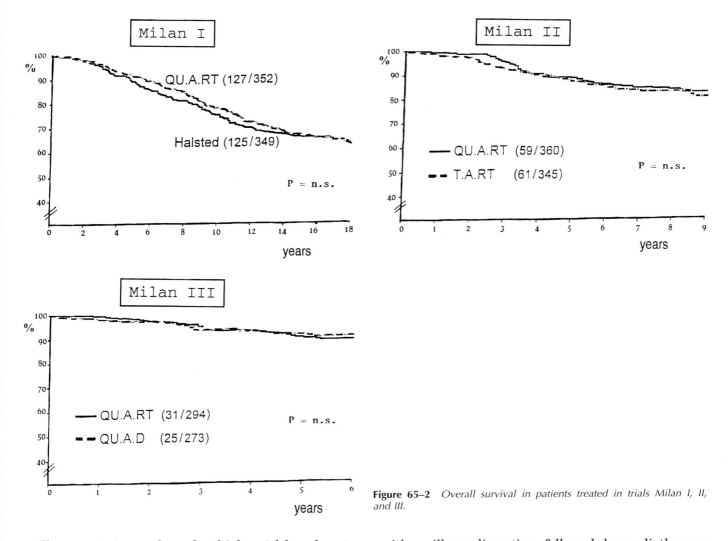

Figure 65–2 *Overall survival in patients treated in trials Milan I, II, and III.*

axillary metastases showed a higher (although not significant) survival in the patients treated with the conservative procedure in the subgroup of patients with positive axillary nodes.

In conclusion, the results of the first Milan trial showed that a less-mutilating procedure can replace mastectomy without modifying the long-term survival rate.

The Milan trial was the first controlled study demonstrating the same efficacy for a conservative treatment as for the Halsted mastectomy. After the Milan results were published, quadrantectomy and other nonmutilating operations were extensively introduced into surgical practice in most European countries. However, the main question of the efficacy for a combination of a "radical" local surgical procedure (quadrantectomy) with a "radical" local radiotherapy still remained. Therefore, a new trial was designed in Milan to compare the classic QUART procedure with a procedure consisting of intensive radiotherapy preceded by a lumpectomy—a very limited resection serving as a debulking rather than a radical procedure.

Thus, the new procedure to be compared with QUART consisted of a lumpectomy (or tumorectomy)

with axillary dissection followed by radiotherapy (TART) administered by external irradiation with high energy (45 Gy) and by implantation of wires of iridium 192. The radioactive implantation was performed after the completion of the external irradiation, and therefore generally occurred about 2 months after the operation.

The study enrolled 705 evaluable patients from 1985 to 1987. The two series of randomized patients (360 treated with QUART and 345 treated with TART) were comparable as to site and size of the primary tumor, age, menopausal status, and rate of axillary metastases. The margins of resection were examined by pathologists and found to be positive in 13 percent of the lumpectomy and 2 percent of the quadrantectomy specimens. According to the study protocol, however, these findings did not modify the therapeutic plan.[7]

After an average follow-up of 7 years, there were 20 local recurrences in the QUART patients and 49 in the TART patients. Moreover, in 5 QUART patients and in 9 TART patients a second primary carcinoma appeared in other quadrants of the breast. Fourteen of the 20 patients with local recurrences in the QUART group were treated with total mastectomy and 6 were treated with re-excision. The 49 patients who suffered local recurrences among the TART patients were treated with total mastectomy in 23 cases and with quadrantectomy in 26 cases.

Therefore, the total number of patients who lost a breast did not differ greatly between the QUART and TART groups: 14 in the quadrantectomy group and 23 in the tumorectomy group. In other words, in the case of local failure, tumorectomy, which exposes patients to an increased risk of local recurrences, has the advantage of less frequently requiring a mastectomy compared to quadrantectomy.

Overall survival was identical in both groups.

A third trial was initiated in 1987 to determine whether radiotherapy is needed after quadrantectomy or can be administered only at the appearance of a local recurrence. The new trial compared QUART to quadrantectomy and axillary dissection without radiotherapy (QUAD). The advantages of QUAD are not only that the treatment is easier, simpler, and less expensive, but that it is also better tolerated by the patient. In addition, the follow-up of the operated breast is much easier, because the breast is deprived of the postirradiation fibrotic component that often complicates the discovery of a recurrence. Moreover, the late toxic effects of radiotherapy on the chest wall and cardiac muscle are avoided.

Radiotherapy, according to the trial design, was administered only in the case of a local recurrence. The trial, therefore, tested if delaying the radiotherapeutic treatment from the immediate postoperative period (when the hypothetical residual cancer cells are occult) to a later time (when overt recurrences appear) reduces the efficacy of radiotherapy in controlling the disease locally. The early results were published in 1993[7] and 1995.[9] Of 273 patients treated with quadrantectomy followed by radiotherapy, 8 suffered a local recurrence; among the patients treated only with quadrantectomy there were 34 local recurrences. In addition, there were 2 second primary ipsilateral carcinomas in the QUART group and 9 among the patients treated with quadrantectomy without radiation.

Of the 8 QUART patients with local recurrence, 2 were treated with mastectomy and 6 with re-excision. Among the 34 patients with recurrence treated only with quadrantectomy, 10 underwent mastectomy and 24 had a re-excision followed by radiotherapy. Total local control of the disease was achieved in all patients but 1, who had a second appearance of the disease and required a mastectomy.

Most of the local recurrences among the 567 evaluable patients in the trial occurred in women younger than 55 years (45 of 353 [12.7 percent]). In older women, the incidence was much lower (9 of 214 [4.2 percent]).

Overall survival was the same in both groups.

THE EORTC TRIAL

In 1980, the European Organization for Research and Treatment of Cancer (EORTC) started a random-
ized trial to evaluate the value of breast-conserving therapy in breast cancer patients with the specific aim of evaluating the results in stage II patients.[6] The trial accrued 878 patients, 745 of whom were classified as stage II, mainly because of tumor sizes greater than 2 cm. The conservative surgical treatment consisted of a wide excision with a margin of 1 cm of healthy tissue and complete axillary dissection. Surgery was followed by radiotherapy on the breast (50 Gy in 5 weeks), with an additional booster dose of 25 Gy on the resection site, and with iridium implant. The study was multicentric, with eight institutes participating, two of which contributed about 60 percent of the total number of patients. End points consisted of survival, local control, time to distant metastases, cosmetics, and quality of life. Patients were randomized, with 452 in the conservative treatment group and 426 undergoing modified radical mastectomy. The number of axillary nodes investigated by the pathologists was equal in both groups. At 8 years follow-up, there were 33 local regional recurrences in the mastectomy group and 45 in the breast-conservative group. In the breast-conservative group, local recurrences were more frequently observed in patients with large tumors (≥ 2 cm) than in patients with small tumors (≤ 2 cm). Node-positive patients suffered an increased incidence of local relapses compared with node-negative patients, despite the administered adjuvant chemotherapy.

The overall survival curves were superimposable (Fig. 65–3). The distant disease-free survival also did not differ between groups. The quality-of-life evaluation, measured as body image and treatment satisfaction, was clearly in favor of patients treated conservatively.

THE DANISH TRIAL

In 1983, the Danish Breast Cancer Cooperative Group initiated a randomized clinical trial comparing breast-conservative therapy with mastectomy in patients with invasive breast carcinoma. The trial was multicentric, involving 20 surgical units throughout Denmark. Randomization was conducted mainly with the use of one-wing information according to the principle of Zelen.[11] In a procedure accepted by the National Ethics Committee, randomization took place before the surgeon explained the type of treatment to the patient, and consent was requested only for the type of surgery to which the patient had been randomized. From January 1983 to March 1989, 905 patients were assigned to either breast-conservation therapy (450) or mastectomy (455). The breast-preserving surgical technique consisted of a segmental mastectomy, including skin and deep fascia when the tumor was peripheral and in lumpectomy in the case of central location. Radiotherapy was administered on the breast with a dose of 50 Gy in 25 fractions over 5 weeks plus a boost of 10 Gy on the tumor bed. If the resection margins were positive, the booster dose was increased to 25 Gy. Patients in both arms

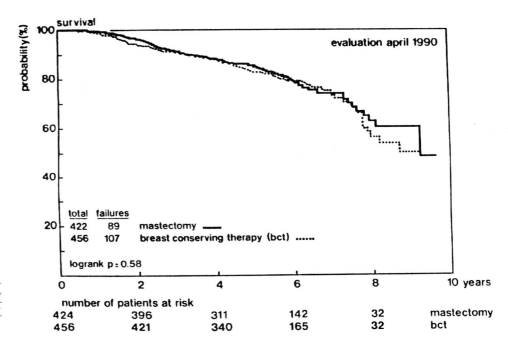

Figure 65–3 *Survival after breast-conserving therapy and radical mastectomy in I and II breast cancer in the EORTC Trial. (From van Dongen JA, et al: Monogr Natl Cancer Inst 11:15–28, 1992.)*

of the study who showed positive axillary nodes were treated with additional radiotherapy on the supraclavicular and axillary nodes with a target dose of 55 Gy. At 6 years of observation, the probability of recurrence free-survival was 70 percent in the conservative arm and 66 percent in the mastectomy arm. The number of local/regional recurrences in the breast-conservation group was very limited (18 [4.5 percent]), and lower than that observed in the mastectomy group (23 [5.5 percent]). Overall survival was identical in the two groups (Fig. 65–4).

The cosmetic outcome, based on the evaluation of

Survival % (N=859) March 1990

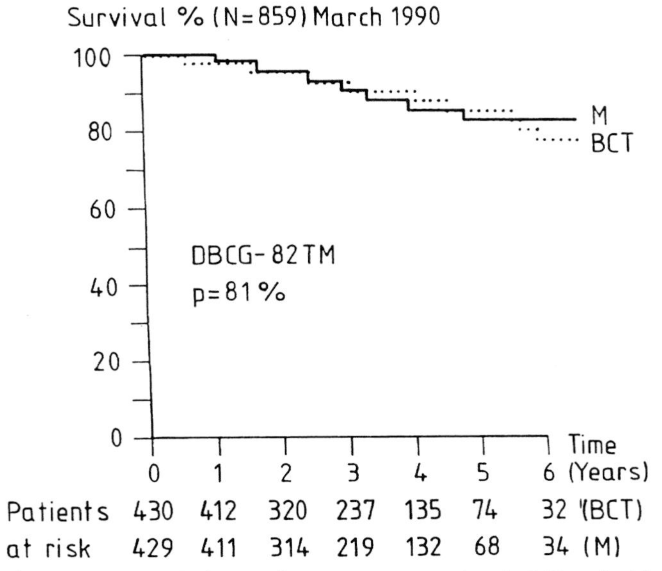

Figure 65–4 *Survival according to treatment options in 859 evaluable randomly assigned patients. (BCT = breast conservation; M = mastectomy [Danish trial].) (From Blichert-Toft M, et al: J Natl Cancer Inst Monographs 11:19–25, 1992.)*

one surgeon and one oncologist, was graded excellent and satisfactory in 72 percent of patients, fair in 27 percent, and poor in only 1 percent.[2]

THE UPPSALA-OREBRO TRIAL

In October 1981, the Uppsala-Orebro Breast Cancer Study Group started a prospective randomized trial to evaluate the necessity of postoperative radiotherapy after breast-conservation treatment.[5] Patients were operated on with sector resection (a wide excision similar to quadrantectomy) and axillary dissection and were randomly assigned to receive postoperative radiotherapy (to a total mean dose of 54 Gy to the breast) or no further treatment. The aim was to determine whether a strictly standardized surgical technique could produce an acceptably low level of local recurrence rates without routine adjuvant radiotherapy. Patients randomly assigned to postoperative radiotherapy were treated with a total mean dose of 54 Gy in 27 fractions, 5 days a week, with a cobalt unit or with a linear accelerator. No booster dose was given to the scar region.

Accrual stopped in September 1988 after 381 patients were enrolled, 187 to postoperative radiotherapy and 194 to simple follow-up. During the 5-year observation period, 43 patients had local recurrences. Six had been treated with postoperative radiotherapy, and 37 had not received radiotherapy. The estimated recurrence-free survival after 5 years was 90.0 percent in the groups receiving radiotherapy and 87.1 percent in the groups without radiotherapy. During the period of study and follow-up, 25 women died of breast cancer, 12 treated with surgery alone and 13 with surgery and radiotherapy. Overall survival was equal in both groups of patients.

The authors concluded that despite a carefully conducted "sector" resection without radiotherapy, the rate of local recurrences is approximately 20 percent, whereas with radiotherapy, recurrences are rare. In cases of local recurrence, a second resection may be performed, followed by radiotherapy.[4]

FUTURE DEVELOPMENTS

The experience in conservative treatments accumulated in Europe since the 1970s and the results of controlled therapeutic trials have made it possible to reach two important conclusions. First, certain breast-preserving treatments, such as sector resection and quadrantectomy, are definitely safe. Second, patients treated with inadequate local/regional surgery or inadequate radiotherapy may be exposed to an excess of local/regional recurrences, which in turn might produce lower overall survival.[3] Therefore, in the next few years, an effort should be made to identify the point at which additional reduction of treatment may become dangerous.

Although the future trend definitely favors increasingly reduced surgery, the adequacy of new techniques must be carefully tested and evaluated. Future trials will address the extent of the surgical act (limited excision versus extensive resection, axillary dissection versus axillary sampling); the type of radiotherapy (immediate versus delayed, whole breast versus limited direct field, boost versus no boost, and regional node irradiation versus no nodal irradiation); the comparison with other forms of surgery providing good cosmetic results (conservative treatments versus total mastectomy plus immediate reconstruction); the size of the primary tumor to be submitted to conservative procedures; and the pathological patterns requiring differentiated conservative techniques (intraductal noninfiltrating carcinoma, Paget's disease, and minimal carcinomas).

The introduction of conservative procedures in early breast cancer has created an atmosphere of confidence on the part of women toward surgeons and radiotherapists involved in the treatment of breast cancer. With this comes high expectations regarding further progress that clinical scientists must try to fulfill.

References

1. Atkins H, Hayward JL, Kligman DJ, Wayte AB: Treatment of early breast cancer: A report after ten years of a clinical trial. Br Med J 2:423–529, 1972.
2. Blichert-Toft M, Rose C, Andersen JA, et al: Danish randomized trial comparing breast conservation therapy with mastectomy: Six years of life-table analysis. J Natl Cancer Inst Monogr 11:19–25, 1992.
3. Hayward JL: The Guy's trial of treatment of early breast cancer. World J Surg 1:314–316, 1988.
4. Liljegren G, Holmberg L, Adami HO, et al: Sector resection with or without postoperative radiotherapy for stage I breast cancer: Five-year results of a randomized trial. Uppsala-Orebro Breast Cancer Study Group. J Natl Cancer Inst 86:717–722, 1994.
5. Uppsala-Orebro Breast Cancer Study Group: Sector resection with or without postoperative radiotherapy for stage I breast cancer: A randomized trial. J Natl Cancer Inst 82:277–282, 1990.
6. van Dongen JA, Bartelink H, Fentiman IS, et al: Randomized clinical trial to assess the value of breast-conserving therapy in stage I and II breast cancer, EORTC 10801 trial. Monogr Natl Cancer Inst 11:15–18, 1992.
7. Veronesi U, Luini A, Del Vecchio M, et al: Radiotherapy after breast-preserving surgery in women with localized cancer of the breast. N Engl J Med 328:1587–1591, 1993.
8. Veronesi U, Saccozzi R, Del Vecchio M, et al: Comparing radical mastectomy with quadrantectomy, axillary dissection, and radiotherapy in patients with small cancers of the breast. N Engl J Med 305:6–11, 1981.
9. Veronesi U, Salvadori B, Luini A, et al: Breast conservation is a safe method in patients with small cancer of the breast: Long-term results of three randomised trials on 1,973 patients. Eur J Cancer 31:1574–1579, 1995.
10. Veronesi U, Volterrani F, Luini A, et al: Quadrantectomy versus lumpectomy for small size breast cancer. Eur J Cancer 26:671–673, 1990.
11. Zelen M: A new design for randomized clinical trials. N Engl J Med 300:1242–1245, 1979.

ADJUVANT SYSTEMIC MODALITIES FOR THERAPY OF STAGES I AND II BREAST CANCER

CHAPTER 66

ADJUVANT SYSTEMIC THERAPY OF BREAST CANCER

Karen A. Johnson, M.D., Ph.D., M.P.H. / Barnett S. Kramer, M.D., M.P.H. / Michael J. Anderson, M.D.

HISTORICAL ASPECTS AND THEORY

Since the late 1950s, the evaluation of systemic adjuvant therapy for breast cancer through randomized clinical trials has been a major priority in cancer research. Even though clinical application of the adjuvant concept has been evolving for more than a century, a great deal of recently collected information has helped to refine the use of adjuvant therapy in clinical practice.

As described in 1889, the first approach to adjuvant therapy in treatment of breast cancer was oophorectomy used as an endocrine therapy to involute the breast before or at the time of mastectomy.[249] In 1934, others applied these same concepts using radiation-induced castration.[263] In addition to these clinical approaches, preclinical animal models showed a curative effect of adjuvant chemotherapy[94, 246] and reinforced the theoretical basis for the introduction of adjuvant cytotoxic chemotherapy in the late 1950s. Interest in this approach was spurred by the developing awareness of the relative plateau in cure rates of breast cancer.[10, 72] Clinicians realized that the Halsted radical mastectomy,[145] based on anatomical principles of tumor confinement and sequential contiguous spread, was inadequate for cure in many patients, even when all clinically apparent disease could be surgically extirpated. The realization that "curative cancer surgery" resulted in a recurrence rate at 5 years of 20 percent in patients with negative nodes and approximately 70 percent in patients with positive nodes underscored the shortcoming of even the most aggressive local therapy.[104] This led to the important realization that the outcome of therapy for breast cancer patients could be improved only by control of subclinical distant disease for a substantial proportion of "early stage" patients.

Early Theoretical Constructs and Resulting Trials

The scientific background for the use of systemic therapy as an adjuvant to the primary surgical treatment of breast cancer began with the observation by Ashworth in 1869, of blood-borne tumor cells post mortem.[6] Although there were scattered similar observations by others, the medical community showed no significant interest in this phenomenon until the observation in 1955 of tumor cells in the mesenteric venous blood in patients with colorectal carcinoma.[124] This piqued the interest of a number of investigators,[89, 95] and in the ensuing few years, cancer cells in the peripheral blood were demonstrated in a number of clinical circumstances. When tumor cells were observed in the peripheral blood after procedures such as pelvic[235] and rectal[171] examination, surgical scrubbing of a tumor prior to surgery,[171] and cancer surgery,[80] the notion developed that blood-borne metastases were spawned by manipulation of the tumor at the time of surgery. Because Halsted's theory of anatomical tumor confinement still prevailed, it was believed that in spite of impeccable surgical technique, neoplastic cells dislodged during the mastectomy procedure and caused metastatic disease. Consequently, researchers set out to test whether the administration of chemotherapy during the perioperative period destroyed these circulating cells and prolonged survival in experimental animals. There were reports of successful destruction of peripherally disseminated cells with the administration of chemotherapeutic agents in experimental animals.[69, 184, 185] The prolonged survival of animals transplanted with mammary adenocarcinoma and then treated with a combination of surgery and 6-mercaptopurine versus surgery or chemotherapy alone provided supportive experimental evidence.[95, 112, 253]

The first randomized adjuvant chemotherapy trial in breast cancer was begun in 1958.[121] It was performed at the National Institutes of Health Cancer Chemotherapy National Service Center and was conducted by the forerunner of the National Surgical Adjuvant Breast and Bowel Project (NSABP). It was designed to determine the efficacy of chemotherapy added to the Halsted radical mastectomy for improvement in survival and freedom from relapse for patients with breast cancer. This trial (NSABP B-01)

TABLE 66–1. SURIVIVAL RATES AT 5 AND 10 YEARS AFTER RADICAL MASTECTOMY

Premenopausal Patients	Effect of TSPA			
	% at 5 Yr		% at 10 Yr	
	Placebo	*TSPA*	*Placebo*	*TSPA*
All	60	73*	49	58
Negative nodes	83	82	76	73
Positive nodes	41	61	28	41
1–3	67	67	50	48
≥4	24	57†	14	35

* $p < 0.01$.
† $p < 0.05$.
Abbreviation: TSPA = thiotepa.
From Fisher B, Redmond C, Fisher ER, Wolmark N: Systemic adjuvant therapy in treatment of primary operable breast cancer: National Surgical Adjuvant Breast and Bowel Project Experience. NCI Monogr 1:35–43, 1986. Reprinted with permission.

evaluated the hypothesis that chemotherapy administered in the perioperative period could destroy tumor cells disseminated at the time of surgery and thus extend the disease-free survival and overall survival of certain patients with breast cancer. After definitive surgery, patients were randomly assigned to receive perioperative adjuvant thiotepa or placebo.[104] The first patient was entered into NSABP B-01 in April 1958, and patient entry was terminated after accrual of 826 acceptable patients in October 1961.[104] Eligible for inclusion were stage I and II patients between 30 and 70 years of age who had undergone a Halsted radical mastectomy en bloc. Stage IIIA patients were also eligible if the axillary lymph nodes were movable in relation to the chest wall. Three doses of thiotepa were given intravenously, one at the time of surgery and the other two on postoperative days 1 and 2.

Analysis of the data did not reveal an overall difference in recurrence rate at 5 years in patients receiving thiotepa vs. placebo, however, variation in recurrence rates suggested a beneficial effect of thiotepa in premenopausal women with four or more positive nodes. There was also a difference in survival favoring the treatment group in the same patient subset at 5 and 10 years after surgery (Table 66–1). The importance of this study was minimized at the time of evaluation because of the disappointment that all patients were not cured with the administration of chemotherapy. In retrospect, however, this was the first demonstration that the natural history of breast cancer could be altered by systemic chemotherapy at the time of surgery. Moreover, the study was the first to show the importance of patient subsets in the evaluation of breast cancer therapy.[95]

A similar randomized trial of a short course of adjuvant chemotherapy performed by the Scandinavian Adjuvant Chemotherapy Study Group[207] began in 1965 and ended in 1975. As in NSABP B-01, the goal of adjuvant therapy was the eradication of tumor cells disseminated at surgery, which were

thought to result in metastatic disease years later. The treated group, consisting of 507 patients who received cyclophosphamide 5 mg/kg/day IV for 6 days beginning on the day of surgery, was compared with 519 patients in a control group. Results after a median follow-up time of 17 years showed a significant disease-free survival advantage of 13.5 percent for the treated group.[167] A beneficial effect on crude survival was first apparent at 6 years, but decreased as the age of the patients advanced.[167]

Current Theory

Parallel to these first adjuvant chemotherapy trials, a number of principles were being developed that related directly to the administration of systemic adjuvant chemotherapy. Among these principles were a better understanding of micrometastases, population cell kinetics, drug kill of tumor cells, and prognostic features of breast cancer. Initially, the origin of metastatic disease was attributed to the release of tumor cells into the systemic circulation by manipulation of the primary tumor during surgery. This point of view was challenged by a group of investigators who produced evidence that pre-existing micrometastases at the time of surgery had a greater bearing on disease outcome than did tumor cells disseminated as a result of surgery (Fig. 66–1).[80, 95, 119, 245, 257] The presence and number of positive axillary nodes was an indicator of subclinical body burden of disease and of the presence of micrometastases at the time of diagnosis. This new paradigm cast doubt on the view of regional nodes as protective "barriers" to tumor spread.

Clinical evidence now supports the concept that pre-existing micrometastases are predominantly responsible for the eventual appearance of detectable metastatic disease. The Ludwig Breast Cancer Study Group reported on the timing and duration of adjuvant chemotherapy for patients with node-positive breast cancer.[174] The study randomized 1229 pre- and postmenopausal patients with positive axillary lymph nodes into three treatment groups. The basic chemotherapy regimen was cyclophosphamide, meth-

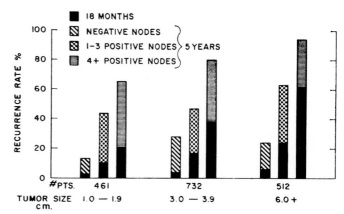

Figure 66–1 *Tumor size, nodal involvement, and recurrence rate. (From Fisher B, et al: Cancer 24:1071, 1969. Reprinted by permission.)*

otrexate, and fluorouracil (CMF). One group received a single cycle of CMF beginning 36 hours after surgery, a second group received six cycles of conventionally timed CMF beginning 25 to 32 days after surgery, and a third group received both chemotherapy regimens. At 42 months of follow-up, disease-free survival and overall survival significantly favored the longer treatments. The authors concluded that the single perioperative treatment was not as effective as longer courses and that starting the treatment perioperatively was no more effective than beginning 4 weeks after mastectomy. Pre-existent micrometastases, rather than tumor cells released during surgery, appeared to be the overriding clinical problem.

There is also the notion that chemosensitivity of tumor cells is related to their proliferative status. This concept, based on growth fraction of tumor cell populations, holds that tumors are composed of three cellular compartments.[190, 257] According to this model, a compartment of proliferating cells (A) with clonogenic potential is responsible for tumor growth when cellular proliferation exceeds cell loss. There is a second compartment (B) that is nonproliferative but retains the potential for proliferation. This compartment is in equilibrium with compartment A and is recruited to replace a depleted clonogenic proliferative compartment. A third compartment (C) is composed of permanently nonproliferative, nonclonogenic cells that contribute only to tumor volume. A tumor's growth fraction is defined as the ratio A:B + C. The greater the value of the growth fraction, the more rapidly the tumor increases in size. Furthermore, tumor growth approximates the Gompertz equation,[246, 257] that is, an exponentially increasing doubling time with increase in tumor mass. This relationship also reflects a decreasing growth fraction or a decrease in clonogenic proliferating cell number with tumor size. Because chemotherapeutic agents interfere primarily with mitotically active cells, there is more potential for cell kill in smaller tumor masses with their associated larger growth fractions. This result was shown in laboratory experiments[143] with the B16 transplantable mouse melanoma that revealed a direct relationship between cell numbers in the range of 10^3 to 10^9 and a cure rate achievable with chemotherapy. Theoretically, when cell kill follows first-order kinetics,[246, 283] a constant percentage of cells die regardless of population size, as long as the tumor cell population is metabolically homogeneous relative to the chemotherapeutic agent applied. This concept further defines a small mitotically active cell population as most vulnerable to total cell kill.

These theoretical ideas, along with preclinical and clinical evidence, gave credence to the potential for surgical adjuvant chemotherapy to eliminate small metastatic foci of tumors with a high growth fraction. Experiments in mouse tumor models in administering chemotherapy after surgical excision of the primary tumor yielded evidence in favor of adjuvant chemotherapy in several different tumor types.[247, 258]

The appropriateness of administering chemotherapy when the tumor cell burden is at a minimum, is further supported by a mathematical model developed by Goldie and Coldman to predict tumor response to cytotoxic therapy based on spontaneous mutation rates.[139, 140] In this model, a given tumor maintains a constant mutation rate during its growth history. The theory states that, like microbial populations, drug-resistant phenotypes occur spontaneously, at a definite frequency. With the passage of time, the total population of resistant cells increases in mass, making chemotherapeutic cure less likely. This theory also predicts, however, that there is a period early in the growth of the tumor during which cure is possible with chemotherapeutic agents that would be ineffective in the later stages of the tumor's development. Within each tumor, there are various other forms of tumor cell heterogeneity, including factors such as growth rate, karyotype, cell surface properties, antigenicity, and metastatic potential.[92] The cellular heterogeneity is a consequence of the emergence of new clonal subpopulations, the outcome of which is to render the cells less responsive to the host's (and the clinician's) attempts at control. Some known mechanisms of drug resistance, such as gene amplification and pleiotropic drug resistance, also increase in likelihood with tumor growth.[141] This body of theoretical and laboratory evidence argues for adjuvant chemotherapy directed at a small population of subclinical metastatic cells present at the time of diagnosis in an attempt to destroy a relatively uniform cell population early in its exponential phase of growth.

In a retrospective look at NSABP B-01, it is perhaps more surprising that any benefit was found in survival in any subgroup from the short course of thiotepa therapy than that there was a lack of universal cure, which was the desired result. By current standards, thiotepa is not considered a particularly useful agent for breast cancer. The choice of thiotepa was a result of its modest effectiveness in the palliation of breast cancer[104]; at the time there was not a long list of drugs from which to choose. In addition, knowledge of the prognostic factors for breast cancer was limited.

As the primary importance of nodal status as a prognostic indicator was becoming recognized,[15] the utility of grouping patients by the number of positive nodes (1 to 3, more than 3, or more than 10) was also being demonstrated.[27, 100, 104, 273] Although recent work has emphasized that node-positive patients form a prognostic continuum,[233] grouping patients remains the practical way to use this prognostic factor. In classifying lymph node status, the lymph node–negative category is the fourth category that is traditionally recognized.[60] Nodal involvement by metastatic breast cancer is the single most significant prognostic factor, even though a number of other factors are recognized to further refine prognostication. In the absence of axillary lymph node metastases at the time of breast cancer diagnosis, the most important prognostic factors for predicting breast cancer recurrence are tumor size, nuclear and histological grade, estrogen receptor status, and proliferation indicators.[186, 255] Although theoretically all these indicators should be considered in studies of adjuvant chemotherapy for breast cancer, nodal status was the important indicator that dominated studies of adjuvant therapy throughout the 1970s.

ADJUVANT CHEMOTHERAPY TRIALS

Many subsequent trials of systemic adjuvant therapy have been initiated since the first such trial in 1958. The largest studies with the longest follow-up data are those by the NSABP and the National Cancer Institute in Milan, Italy.[282]

NSABP

Between 1958 and 1986, 12 randomized studies were initiated by the NSABP to evaluate the efficacy of various adjuvant therapy regimens. More than 9000 women with stage I or II breast cancer were entered into these trials,[112] which were designed to compare treatments and define the basic biology of breast cancer. Performed in sequence, each subsequent study was influenced by the results of its predecessor. The population of patients was similar among all the studies.[112] Patients were included who had had a radical mastectomy (Halsted or modified) and an axillary dissection to establish nodal status. Aside from nodal involvement, no other evidence of metastatic disease was permitted. Detailed descriptions of each study that include the specific criteria of patient selection, randomization, drug administration and modification, host and tumor characteristics and statistical procedures have been reported and are summarized in Table 66–2.*

The investigators of NSABP adjuvant chemotherapy trials have periodically reviewed the results from

---

*References 96, 97–99, 101–104, 106–109, 111, 113, 115, 116, 120.

these early trials.[93, 112, 122] The data for 10 years of follow-up are available for B-01 and B-05. The first protocol (B-01) compared women treated with Halsted radical mastectomy and perioperative thiotepa with those treated with the same surgical procedure and placebo. Statistically significant increases in disease-free survival and overall survival were noted only for premenopausal patients at 10 years as well as 5 years, with the greatest effect in women with 4 or more nodes.[120] Recognizing that perioperative chemotherapy was inadequate, 2 years of single-agent therapy with melphalan was used in the next protocol, B-05, for breast cancer patients with axillary nodes positive for tumor.

Melphalan given at a dosage of 0.15 mg/kg orally daily for 5 days every 6 weeks for 17 courses (2 years of therapy) was compared with placebo.[112] At 10 years of follow-up there was a statistically significant improvement for women aged 49 years or younger in disease-free survival and overall survival in the melphalan-treated group. In this age group, benefit accrued to women with poorly differentiated tumors as delineated by nuclear grade. Although no advantage was seen for women older than 50 years as a group, the subgroup of older women with poorly differentiated tumors also experienced a survival advantage. The only trials that compared chemotherapy with an untreated control group were B-01 and B-05. In all subsequent chemotherapy trials, an alternative combination therapy was compared to a previously tested regimen, used in the control group. The NSABP also made comparisons across protocols, using a justification that is controversial, but depends on the assumption that patients in a group demonstrating no benefit or detriment from therapy are appropriate as surrogates for untreated patients.[103]

After a combination of melphalan and 5-fluorouracil (5-FU) was found to be superior to melphalan alone, a sequence of four protocols compared L-PAM/5-FU with and without each of the following agents: methotrexate, tamoxifen, *C. parvum* (renamed *Propionibacterium acnes*), and doxorubicin. The last of this series of studies was opened in 1981.

TABLE 66–2.   NSABP RANDOMIZED BREAST CANCER TRIALS OF SYSTEMIC ADJUVANT THERAPY, 1958–1986[112]

Trial	Start Date	Therapy	Patients	Nodal Status	Ref
B-01	4/58	Thiotepa vs. Placebo	826	Either	104,120
B-05	9/72	L-PAM vs. Placebo	370	Positive	96,99
B-07	2/75	L-PAM ± F	741	Positive	103
B-08	4/76	L-PAM/F ± M	737	Positive	111,116
B-09	1/77	L-PAM/F ± T	1891	Positive	106,107
B-10	5/77	L-PAM/F ± *P. acnes*	264	Positive	102
B-11	6/81	L-PAM/F ± A	707	Positive	115
B-12	6/81	L-PAM/F/T ± A	1106	Positive	115
B-13	8/81	MF vs. Placebo	425	Negative	109
B-14	1/82	T vs. Placebo	1379	Negative	97
B-15	10/84	CMF vs. AC vs. AC + CMF	472	Positive	101
B-16	10/84	PAFT vs. ACT vs. TAM	338	Positive	113

Abbreviations: A = doxorubicin; C = cyclophosphamide; F = 5-fluorouracil; L-PAM = melphalan; M = methotrexate; P = prednisone; T = tamoxifen.

From the early NSABP studies, the following conclusions were made[25, 112]:

1. The natural history of breast cancer can be altered by adjuvant chemotherapy prolonging disease-free survival and overall survival in premenopausal women.

2. Regardless of age, or nodal involvement, there was a significant overall survival advantage for women with poorly differentiated tumors treated with adjuvant chemotherapy.

3. An advantage in disease-free survival and overall survival for postmenopausal women treated with melphalan and 5-FU did not achieve statistical significance.

4. A variety of factors, including age, tumor size, nodal status, differentiation, and estrogen receptor and progesterone receptor content influenced survival outcomes in breast cancer patients treated with systemic adjuvant therapy.

Milan Trial

In 1973, the Milan Cancer Institute began to study a combination chemotherapy regimen in treatment of women with breast cancer and positive axillary lymph nodes.[19] The primary tumor of patients included in the study could be clinically classified as T1, T2, or the subset of T3 lesions that were not fixed to the chest wall. Surgery consisted of a conventional Halsted radical mastectomy or an extended radical mastectomy. The CMF drug combination was chosen because of its activity in patients with advanced breast cancer.[22] Cyclophosphamide (100 mg/m^2 PO qd, days 1 through 14), methotrexate (40 mg/m^2 IV days 1 and 8), and 5-FU (600 mg/m^2 IV days 1 and 8) were administered on a 28-day schedule for 12 cycles. Patients older than 65 years received lower doses of methotrexate and 5-FU.

This prospective randomized study included 207 patients who were treated with CMF and 179 controls who received no further treatment. The 10-year follow-up reports[20, 21, 31] showed a persistent disease-free survival advantage in the CMF-treated group ($p < 0.001$) and a favorable overall survival trend ($p = 0.10$). The advantage in disease-free survival and overall survival, although suggestive in postmenopausal women, was statistically significant only in the premenopausal subset.

At a median follow-up of 19.4 years, there was a 29% reduction ($p = 0.004$) in risk of relapse for the CMF-treated women as a group.[29] No benefit in disease-free or overall survival was observed for postmenopausal women. In contrast, the survival advantage for premenopausal and perimenopausal women was substantial, with 47 percent of the CMF-treated group alive at 20 years compared with 22 percent of the control group. As observed at 10 years of follow-up, the number of histologically positive axillary lymph nodes remained prognostically important at the 20-year analysis, with the greatest benefit in disease-free and overall survival seen in the treated group with 1 to 3 positive nodes. The investigators concluded that although the CMF regimen demonstrated a prolonged therapeutic advantage in a percentage of premenopausal women with micrometastic disease, the lack of response to CMF by postmenopausal women in the first Milan trial was related to the way it was given, because subsequent studies have shown that postmenopausal women may expect to obtain results similar to those for premenopausal women, as demonstrated in multiple later studies.[33, 43, 194, 285] Subsequent Milan Cancer Institute studies of adjuvant breast cancer chemotherapy evaluated 12 versus 6 cycles of CMF, sequential non–cross-resistant chemotherapy combinations, and adjuvant therapy for patients with negative axillary nodes.

Additional Controlled Trials

In addition to the early NSABP and Milan controlled trials, there have been a number of other studies that have evaluated the effectiveness of systemic adjuvant therapy. Tables 66–3 and 66–4 summarize the larger adjuvant chemotherapy studies in node-positive women that included a local/regional treatment control group. With certain exceptions, results from these studies are similar. Although both the NSABP and Milan trials reported a disease-free and overall survival advantage in premenopausal women, advantages for postmenopausal women were not clearly demonstrated. Early results inconsistent with the prevailing assumption that premenopausal but not postmenopausal women benefited from systemic adjuvant therapy, came from the Clinical Oncology Study Group of Eastern Switzerland (OSAKO) trial,[251] which showed a significant disease-free survival advantage in postmenopausal women but not in premenopausal patients. In addition, the Guy's/Manchester melphalan study failed to show a significant advantage in either disease-free survival or overall survival in premenopausal women given chemotherapy.[241] The largest of the trials, which evaluated only premenopausal women, was that performed by the Danish Breast Cancer Cooperative Group.[36] Total mastectomy with partial axillary dissection followed by local radiation therapy was performed before randomization to one of the following: no further treatment, 12 monthly courses of cyclophosphamide (130 mg/m^2 PO days 1 to 14), or CMF (cyclophosphamide 80 mg/m^2 PO days 1 to 14, methotrexate 30 mg/m^2 IV days 1 and 8, and 5-FU 500 mg/m^2 IV days 1 and 8). Increases in total survival and disease-free survival at 7 years for the cyclophosphamide- and CMF-treated groups compared with controls were statistically significant.

Tables 66–3 and 66–4 summarize the data related to menopausal status from trials that included a local/regional treatment control group. In each study in which disease-free survival was evaluated in premenopausal women, results favored the chemotherapy-treated group and were often statistically significant. Overall survival was affected significantly

TABLE 66–3.   EARLY ADJUVANT CHEMOTHERAPY STUDIES WITH A LOCAL/REGIONAL TREATMENT CONTROL GROUP IN PREMENOPAUSAL NODE-POSITIVE PATIENTS

Author	Study Population	No. of Patients	Chemotherapy	Treatment Duration	Follow-up	Disease-Free Survival (%)		Overall Survival (%)	
						Control	Chemotherapy	Control	Chemotherapy
Fisher et al.[112] (NSABP B-05)	Age ≤49 yr	120	L-PAM	2 yr	10 yr	30*	46*	38*	61*
Bonadonna et al.[21, 31] (Milan)	Age ≤49 yr	189	CMF	1 yr	10 yr	31‡	48‡	45	59
Senn et al.[251] (OSAKO)	Premenopausal and perimenopausal	118	ChMFPBCG	6 mo	8 yr	Not significant		Not significant	
Rubens et al.[241] (Guy's/Manchester)	Premenopausal	156	L-PAM	96 wk	5–7.5 yr	52	62	Not significant	
						Not significant			
Padmanabhan et al.[211] (Guy's/Manchester)	Premenopausal	211	CMF	1 yr	5 yr	52†	70†	68	74
								Not significant	
Morrison et al.[195] (West Midlands)	Premenopausal	228	AVCMFL	24 wk	54 mo	53	65*	Not significant	
Brinckner et al.[36] (Danish Cancer Group)	Premenopausal	1032§	C	1 yr	68 mo	42‡	62‡	55	70
								Not significant	
			CMF	1 yr	68 mo	42‡	62‡	55*	70*
Smith et al.[260] (Glasgow)	Premenopausal	322‖	CMF	13 mo	42 mo	Significant		Not significant	

Abbreviations: A = doxorubicin; BCG = bacille Calmette-Guérin; C = cyclophosphamide; Ch = chlorambucil; F = 5-fluorouracil; L = leucovorin; L-PAM = melphalan; M = methotrexate; V = vincristine.
  * $p < 0.05$ for chemotherapy vs. control.
  † $p < 0.005$ for chemotherapy vs. control.
  ‡ $p < 0.0005$ for chemotherapy vs. control.
  § Randomization to observation, C, or CMF.
  ‖ Both premenopausal and postmenopausal patients.

only in premenopausal women in the NSABP, Milan, and Danish trials. In postmenopausal women, although there was a trend in improvement in disease-free survival in some studies, this was less pronounced than that in the premenopausal group. The findings of these studies supported the belief that there is a definite and statistically significant disease-free survival advantage for premenopausal women with positive axillary nodes given chemotherapy, and that a statistically significant overall survival advantage was shown for premenopausal

women given chemotherapy in the NSABP, Milan, and Danish trials. An understanding of the effect of chemotherapy in node-positive postmenopausal women has been extended by subsequent studies.

Heterogeneous Results of Clinical Trials

Even if the biological effects of adjuvant chemotherapy on tumor cells were uniform irrespective of patient age, the efficacy of adjuvant chemotherapy on overall survival is not likely to be uniform over the

TABLE 66–4.   EARLY ADJUVANT CHEMOTHERAPY STUDIES WITH A LOCAL/REGIONAL TREATMENT CONTROL GROUP IN POSTMENOPAUSAL NODE-POSITIVE PATIENTS

Author	Study Population	No. of Patients	Chemotherapy	Treatment Duration	Follow-up	Disease-Free Survival (%)		Overall Survival (%)	
						Control	Chemotherapy	Control	Chemotherapy
Fisher et al.[112] (NSABP B-05)	Age ≥50 yr	229	L-PAM	2 yr	10 yr	29*	32*	44*	41*
Bonadonna et al.[21, 31, 77] (Milan)	Age ≥50 yr	202	CMF	1 yr	10 yr	32*	38*	50*	52*
Senn et al.[251] (OSAKO)	Postmenopausal	114	ChMFPBCG	6 mo	8 yr	42†	56†	53*	65*
Rubens et al.[241] (Guy's/Manchester)	Postmenopausal	214	L-PAM	96 wk	5–7.5 yr	45*	51*	Not significant	
Padmanabhan et al.[211] (Guy's/Manchester)	Postmenopausal	228	CMF	1 yr	5 yr	55*	59*	65*	70*
Morrison et al.[195] (West Midlands)	Postmenopausal	234	AVCMFL	24 wk	54 mo	Not significant		Not significant	
Smith et al.[260] (Glasgow)	Postmenopausal	322‡	CMF	13 mo	42 mo	No data		Not significant	
Wallgren et al.[230] (Stockholm-Gotland)	Postmenopausal	163	Ch or CMF	1 yr	49 mo	55†	48†	Not significant	
Tormey et al.[99, 266, 270] (ECOG)	Postmenopausal	155	CMFP	1 yr	5 yr	57*	60*	Not significant	

Abbreviations: A = doxorubicin; BCG = bacille Calmette-Guérin; C = cyclophosphamide; Ch = chlorambucil; F = 5-fluorouracil; L = leucovorin; L-PAM = melphalan; M = methotrexate; P = prednisone; V = vincristine.
  * Not significant.
  † $p < 0.5$ for chemotherapy vs. control.
  ‡ Both premenopausal and postmenopausal patients.

entire age spectrum because of competing causes of death. With advancing age, larger numbers of women will die as a result of causes other than breast cancer. Using the examples of Zelen and Gelman,[286] white women aged 50 to 54 years experience a 10-year death rate of 5.3 percent from all causes other than breast cancer. Node-positive breast cancer has a 10-year death rate of about 70 percent. Therefore, there will be approximately 13.2 breast cancer deaths relative to each death from other causes (70/5.3) in the 10-year period. This ratio will fall with increasing patient age at diagnosis of breast cancer and will alter the statistical efficiency of the study for any given number of patients included.

The issue of competing causes of death becomes more problematic in studies in which a larger proportion of older postmenopausal women are included. The result of including such a population of women in a study is to decrease the statistical efficiency of the trials with postmenopausal patients. A larger sample of postmenopausal women compared with premenopausal women is needed for equivalent statistical efficiency. A Southwestern Oncology Group (SWOG) study is illustrative of the phenomenon.[209] Premenopausal and postmenopausal women with primary breast cancer and positive axillary nodes were randomized after stratification according to menopausal status and nodal involvement (1 to 3 nodes and 4 or more nodes) to receive CMF plus vincristine and prednisone (CMFVP) for 1 year or melphalan for 2 years. After 8 years median follow-up, overall disease-free survival was superior in all subsets but was not statistically significant in postmenopausal women. When deaths from other causes before recurrence are taken into account, a significant benefit for CMFVP is found in postmenopausal women as well.

As efforts were being applied to improve the effectiveness of systemic adjuvant chemotherapy in postmenopausal women, several factors were scrutinized for their role in eroding the benefit of adjuvant therapy observed in postmenopausal compared with premenopausal women. Among the most important of these factors are the potential for differences in tumor biology, hormonal milieu, and dose intensity.

Heterogeneity between premenopausal and postmenopausal groups of women with respect to the nuclear and/or histological grade of their tumors may confound the interpretation of results from adjuvant trials. Multiple reports have identified nuclear and/or histological grade as a prognostic factor for breast cancers that are likely to be treated with systemic adjuvant therapy.[110, 256] Other studies, such as NSABP B-05, have indicated that the effect of adjuvant chemotherapy varies with age. The NSABP B-05 study revealed a significant disease-free survival and overall survival advantage for women 49 years or younger and those 50 years or older with high nuclear grade tumor histologies treated with melphalan.[99] At 10 years' follow-up, no advantage from melphalan was seen in all patients 50 years or older, but a significant overall survival advantage was observed

in the same age group of patients with poorly differentiated tumors. There was no survival benefit in either age group with good nuclear grade. If postmenopausal women as a group have tumors that are less aggressive for reasons related to histological and nuclear grade or other factors, such a biological gradient will reduce the observed effectiveness of adjuvant therapy in postmenopausal women by diluting the chance to see an effect.

Multiple studies support the concept that aggressive disease affords an opportunity to see a large absolute benefit for adjuvant therapy. If an assumption is made that adjuvant therapy leads to a proportional reduction in disease recurrence on the order of 25 percent, then in groups at high risk of recurrence the opportunity to see an effect is enhanced by higher risk, resulting in a larger number of events.[74] Studies consistent with this hypothesis include the Danish Breast Cancer Group Study,[198] in which premenopausal women with aggressive disease (4 or more nodes, tumor larger than 5 cm, and anaplasia grade 3 of 3) showed a statistically significant improvement in disease-free survival when treated with CMF versus control. The Vienna Study[159] reported an overall survival difference in favor of women with undifferentiated and estrogen receptor (ER)-negative tumors given chemotherapy (79 percent versus 41 percent, p <0.001; and 84 percent versus 37 percent, p <0.05, respectively). No effect was seen in survival in patients with well or moderately differentiated tumors or in patients with ER-positive tumors. Data were not presented according to menopausal status. It is reported, however, that the ER-positive rate and median ER concentration increase with postmenopausal status and age.[55, 114, 146] Furthermore, ER-negative tumors are frequently poorly differentiated.[114] These data support the thesis that premenopausal women respond favorably as a group to adjuvant chemotherapy compared with controls because of an increased incidence of ER-negative, poorly differentiated tumors.

Certain studies support the premise that prophylactic surgical castration may increase disease-free survival and overall survival in breast cancer patients who are premenopausal or younger than age 50.[86,189] This evidence suggests that adjuvant chemotherapy, to some degree, may act in premenopausal women by causing a temporary, if not permanent, amenorrhea.[217] Several studies have determined that amenorrhea occurring in premenopausal women during the administration of cytotoxic chemotherapy is caused by primary ovarian failure and not by alteration of pituitary or adrenal function.[84] There are no significant pituitary, ovarian, or adrenal hormonal profile alterations caused by chemotherapy in postmenopausal women.[84] Amenorrhea is permanent in the majority of the approximately 80 percent of premenopausal women who have disruption of menses during chemotherapy.[84, 211] There is however, an inverse relationship between age and duration of treatment required to induce cessation of menses, with some younger women showing no evidence of ovarian suppression.

Studies supporting the concept that chemotherapy given to premenopausal women with breast cancer is effective, at least in part, because of induction of amenorrhea, include the Guy's/Manchester study, which randomized premenopausal and postmenopausal women to local control versus CMF adjuvant chemotherapy.[211] In this study, only premenopausal women benefited from treatment, with a statistically significant disease-free survival. Menstrual history was recorded in the premenopausal patients in 87 of 102 treated with CMF and in 89 of 109 controls. Of these women, 53 of 87 patients (61 percent) treated with CMF became permanently amenorrheic, as did 10 of 89 controls (11 percent). Among premenopausal women with CMF-induced amenorrhea, there was a significant increase in disease-free survival and overall survival compared with controls ($p = 0.0001$ and 0.01, respectively) and with CMF-treated women without amenorrhea ($p = 0.02$ and 0.01, respectively). There was no significant difference in either parameter between CMF treated women without amenorrhea and controls. The early results from this trial were updated in 1990, to the point where the median survival was 8 years.[229] Although the earlier results were confirmed, it was noted that among the premenopausal women younger than 40 years old, chemotherapy-induced amenorrhea did not affect outcome.

An Eastern Cooperative Oncology Group (ECOG) trial[271] that randomized premenopausal and postmenopausal women to 12 monthly cycles of intermittent CMF, CMF plus prednisone (CMFP), or CMFP plus continuous tamoxifen also determined a statistically significant disease-free survival and overall survival for patients who developed amenorrhea during therapy. A study of premenopausal and postmenopausal patients with one to three tumor-bearing axillary lymph nodes randomized 491 patients to receive CMF or CMFP for 12 4-week cycles in Ludwig I.[176, 177] Of the 399 women who had menses during the 6 months before trial entry, 85 percent experienced amenorrhea for at least 3 months during treatment. Disease-free survival at 6 years for the amenorrhea-induced group was 75 percent, compared with 62 percent for the group that continued menses ($p = 0.006$). Re-establishment of menstrual function occurred in 20 percent of the patients who had experienced amenorrhea during treatment. Disease-free survival for these patients was 75 percent, compared with 78 percent for patients who did not resume menses.

Patients in Ludwig V (now International Trial V) were also evaluated for the impact of amenorrhea induced by adjuvant chemotherapy.[136] In this trial, 575 patients with node-positive disease received either a single cycle of perioperative CMF or prolonged therapy with six 28-day cycles of CMF.[174] In women who received prolonged chemotherapy with six 28-day cycles of CMF, the estimated disease-free survival at 4 years was 68 percent for women who developed amenorrhea and 61 percent for those who did not. This difference was interpreted as reflecting, in part, the endocrinological impact of adjuvant therapy. However, looking at women who did not develop amenorrhea, those who received extended treatment had a 4-year disease-free survival of 61 percent compared to 39 percent for those who received a single perioperative cycle of CMF. This latter comparison was thought to reflect the relatively greater magnitude of the chemotherapy effect.

Additional information concerning treatment-induced amenorrhea as a factor that mediates the effect of adjuvant chemotherapy in premenopausal women has been provided by a retrospective analysis of a trial conducted by the Danish Breast Cancer Cooperative Group comparing observation versus adjuvant chemotherapy with cyclophosphamide or CMF in 1032 premenopausal and perimenopausal women.[36] It was determined that CMF and cyclophosphamide were equally effective in improving disease-free survival when compared with the local-treatment-only control groups. A statistically significant survival advantage was evident in the treated groups and was slightly more pronounced in the patients who received CMF. Amenorrhea occurred in 70 percent of patients who received cyclophosphamide, 63 percent of patients who received CMF, and 13 percent of the control group. When comparing the amenorrheic women with the women who continued menses within each group of patients, only in the cyclophosphamide-treated women was there a statistical advantage to disease-free survival for the women who ceased to menstruate. In both the control and CMF groups, there was no statistical difference between the women who continued or ceased menstruation. The authors believe that these data support the hypothesis that the results of adjuvant chemotherapy occur in part because of chemical castration (the cyclophosphamide group) and in part through a purely cytotoxic effect that is additive to the effect of chemical castration (the CMF group). This view is supported by the results from NSABP B-05,[118] which divided the premenopausal group into those age 39 years or younger and those 40 to 49 years of age. The treated women in the younger group demonstrated a greater improvement in disease-free survival at 4 years relative to controls (69 percent versus 32 percent; $p = 0.01$) than did those in the older age group (61 percent versus 48 percent; $p = 0.09$). Amenorrhea, however, occurred in 73 percent of patients in the 40- to 49-year age group and in only 22 percent of women age 39 years or younger ($p < 0.001$). The dichotomy of results from ovarian suppression on disease-free survival benefit is used as evidence by NSABP to support the conclusion that although chemical castration may account for some of the effectiveness of adjuvant chemotherapy in premenopausal women, other factors are primarily responsible.

Not every review supports the hypothesis that chemotherapy-induced amenorrhea improves survival in premenopausal women. Data from the initial CMF trial in Milan did not confirm an enhanced effect on disease-free survival in premenopausal women with amenorrhea.[20, 21] With stratification according to more than versus less than or equal to 3 nodes, the 9-year disease-free survival of the 19 patients who did not experience drug-induced amenorrhea was no different from that for the 13 who experienced amenorrhea.[24] The analysis was limited to women younger than 40 years, since only 2 patients older than 40 years comprised the subgroup that maintained menstrual function.

To summarize the evidence concerning an effect of chemotherapy-induced amenorrhea on survival, there are several observations that suggest that amenorrhea is unlikely to be entirely responsible for the survival benefit from adjuvant chemotherapy in premenopausal women. For example, cytotoxic therapy is effective in women who (1) do not develop amenorrhea, (2) have ER-negative tumors, and (3) at age 40 or younger enjoy a greater benefit from cytotoxic chemotherapy in spite of the fact that they are less susceptible to chemotherapy-related amenorrhea.

In addition to differences in tumor biology and susceptibility to induction of ovarian failure, a third reason that has been cited for diminished efficacy of chemotherapy in a postmenopausal treatment population has been a dose-response effect, as suggested by the Milan group. In a retrospective analysis of 901 women[26] all of whom had received CMF in previous prospective Milan studies, the authors determined a dose-response effect, indicating that CMF was effective only when given in a full or nearly full dose. Women receiving 85 percent or more of the planned dose had a 5-year disease-free survival of 77 percent compared with a 5-year disease-free survival of 45 percent in those receiving 65 percent or less of the planned dose (45 percent disease-free survival in the control population). The Milan update of this information at 9 years confirmed these initial findings.[24] Furthermore, this relationship was true in both of the subgroups of premenopausal and postmenopausal women. The analysis of the Milan data indicated that a higher proportion of women in the premenopausal group received 85 percent or more of the planned dose than did those in the postmenopausal group. When similar groups of women were compared (i.e., similar dose and similar number of involved axillary lymph nodes), the disease-free survival was the same in a statistically significant comparison regardless of menopausal status. The Milan investigators used this information to suggest that "menopausal status should probably no longer be regarded as an important prognostic factor."[26] It must be borne in mind, however, that any retrospective dose-response analysis might be misleading, because it cannot establish a cause-and-effect relationship between dose and outcome. Factors that decrease the ability to give chemotherapy at full dose may also be associated with more aggressive disease and poorer outcome.[28]

Nevertheless, other groups examined their data in an attempt to confirm the Milan experience by showing a poor response to a CMF regimen among postmenopausal node-positive breast cancer patients whose delivered dose was substantially less than the planned dose.[175, 241, 277, 280] In the Ludwig III study, CMFP plus tamoxifen (*CMFP + T*) was compared with prednisone and tamoxifen and no further treatment.[175] For the CMF-treated subpopulation in this study, response was analyzed according to whether more than 84 percent of planned dose was received versus 65 to 84 percent or less than 64 percent. Differences in disease-free survival among these levels were not statistically significant. It has been pointed out that because prednisone and tamoxifen were part of the regimen these results may not be strictly comparable to those with CMF alone.[24]

In the Stockholm-Gotland study, although patients receiving greater than 86 percent of the ideal dose had a rate of recurrence approximately 70 percent of that for patients receiving lower doses, this difference was not statistically significant.[280] Finally, in a study analyzed similarly to that of the Milan group, the Southeastern Cancer Study Group randomized premenopausal and postmenopausal women to CMF for 6 to 12 months or to local/regional radiation therapy followed by 6 months of CMF. No significant differences in relapse rates, regardless of number of nodes involved or menopausal status, were detected.[277]

In keeping with the results of the Southeastern Cancer Study Group, several other prospective studies of adjuvant chemotherapy in postmenopausal women have modified the notion that postmenopausal women cannot obtain a survival benefit comparable to that obtained by premenopausal women. In 1981, the Milan group launched a trial for women with resectable breast cancer and 1 to 3 positive nodes.[194] One group of women received intravenous CMF every 3 weeks for 12 cycles. This approach was used specifically to improve compliance and document delivery of cyclophosphamide. Dose reductions were avoided by delaying 1 to 2 weeks for myelosuppression rather than keeping on schedule by adjusting with smaller doses. Among the 243 women who were treated with this approach, relapse-free survival at 5 years for the 70 postmenopausal women did not differ from the 173 premenopausal women in the group. In a contemporaneous study for women with resectable breast cancer and more than 3 positive nodes, the approach was to use intravenous CMF either sequentially or alternating with doxorubicin. Although the outcome was superior for doxorubicin followed by sequential CMF, it was noted that the difference between median relapse-free survival at 10 years in postmenopausal patients (72 months) was not statistically different from the median survival for premenopausal patients (99 months). A third trial using cyclophosphamide, doxorubicin, and 5-FU with three variations in dose and schedule also demonstrated that postmenopausal women in the two arms with higher doses experienced a survival effect as great as that observed for premenopausal women.[285]

Optimal Adjuvant Chemotherapy Regimen

In 1958 the NSABP initiated sequential randomized clinical trials to assess the efficacy of various adjuvant chemotherapy regimens.[112] The NSABP B-07 compared women treated with melphalan to those treated with melphalan and 5-FU. The addition of 5-FU to melphalan resulted in a statistically insignificant improvement in disease-free survival in both premenopausal and postmenopausal women and prompted a comparison of melphalan and 5-FU with melphalan, 5-FU, and methotrexate. The addition of methotrexate failed to show any advantage. This NSABP experience and the Milan CMF report[19] established the precedent for clinical trials comparing single-agent and multi-agent adjuvant chemotherapy.

There have been few studies by other groups similar to the NSABP clinical trials that have compared a single agent with a combination of drugs including the single agent.[147] Two of these studies showed no statistical difference in disease-free survival or overall survival in women treated with monotherapy versus combination therapy.[51, 142] A third study, the Danish Breast Cancer Cooperative Group Study comparing cyclophosphamide with CMF therapy in premenopausal and perimenopausal women, also found no statistically significant difference in outcome between treatment groups.[36] Noteworthy facts about this Danish study are that the intended ideal CMF dose was 20 percent to 25 percent less than the Milan CMF dose and that the hematological toxicity of cy-

clophosphamide was slightly greater than that of CMF. This indicates that the two regimens were not equitoxic, making a comparison difficult.

Several studies have compared melphalan with CMF or a regimen similar to CMF (Table 66–5). The studies were heterogeneous, and none included a no-treatment control arm. Four of five comparisons defined a subgroup that benefited by receiving the combination chemotherapy.[3, 75, 209, 231] Although one of the five studies showed no difference in outcome between melphalan and combination chemotherapy,[44, 58] the entire body of evidence indicates that the CMF combination is a superior regimen to melphalan alone.

Clinical investigators have compared the CMF combination to CMF plus additional agents in several studies. In Ludwig I, CMF was compared with CMFP in premenopausal women with one to three positive nodes.[135] At 4 years, the disease-free survival and overall survival were virtually identical in the two arms of therapy. Although there was less hematological toxicity with CMFP, more severe infections (eight of ten patients), greater weight gain (8 percent versus 4 percent), and cushingoid appearance (17 percent) occurred in the CMFP regimen.

The Eastern Cooperative Oncology Group initiated a study comparing 12 monthly cycles of CMF with CMFP in premenopausal women.[271] There was no significant overall or disease-free survival difference between the two regimens. Moreover, as in the Ludwig I study, toxicity was significantly increased by the addition of prednisone to the adjuvant regimen. Finally, the Cancer and Leukemia Group B (CALGB) performed a study comparing CMF to CMF + methanol extraction residue (MER) of Calmette-Guérin bacillus, or to CMFVP in premenopausal and perimenopausal women.[269] The CMF + MER arm was

TABLE 66–5. EARLY RANDOMIZED TRIALS COMPARING MELPHALAN AND REGIMENS SIMILAR TO CMF IN NODE-POSITIVE PATIENTS

Author	Study Population	No. of Patients	Chemotherapy	Treatment Duration	Follow-up (yr)	Disease-Free Survival (%)		Overall Survival (%)	
						Melphalan	*CMF*	*Melphalan*	*CMF*
Davis et al.[75]	Premenopausal and postmenopausal	254	L-PAM vs. CMFV	1 yr	4.5	54†	66†	No significant difference	
Osborne et al.[209, 231] (SWOG)	Premenopausal and postmenopausal	366	L-PAM vs. CMFVP	2 yr vs. 1 yr	10	35†	43†	48†	56†
Ahmann[3]	Premenopausal and postmenopausal	293	L-PAM vs. CFP	60 wk	2	31*‡	44*	40*‡	70*
Cohen et al.[44, 58]	Premenopausal and postmenopausal	194	L-PAM vs. CFP vs. CFP + BCG	1 yr	2	No significant difference		No data	
Carpenter et al.[46]	Premenopausal and postmenopausal	171	L-PAM vs. CMF	56 wk vs. 48 wk	3	No significant difference		90*	74*

Abbreviations: BCG = bacille Calmette-Guérin; C = cyclophosphamide; F = 5-fluorouracil; L = leucovorin; L-PAM = melphalan; M = methotrexate; P = prednisone; T = tamoxifen; V = vincristine.
*$p < 0.05$
†$p < 0.005$
‡Results pertain to premenopausal patients only. Results for postmenopausal patients were not statistically significant.

discontinued before the end of the trial because of side effects from MER. The comparison of CMFVP with CMF revealed no significant difference in disease-free survival or overall survival. Separate analysis suggested the possibility that CMFVP was superior to CMF in those patients with 4 or more involved nodes (median disease-free survival, 55.3 percent versus 35.3 percent; $p = 0.010$). Among patients with 4 or more involved nodes, the benefit was limited to both premenopausal and postmenopausal groups with 10 or more positive nodes. The disease-free survival advantage was not translated into a survival benefit. Both regimens were well tolerated.[272] The suggestion of these three studies is that there is no definite advantage in disease-free or overall survival by the addition of prednisone or vincristine and prednisone to the CMF regimen. Toxicity may be greater with the CMFP and CMFVP regimens.

Several studies have been conducted evaluating the use of doxorubicin in adjuvant chemotherapy regimens (Table 66–6). One of these trials was conducted by the West Midlands Oncology Association and evaluated node-positive patients randomized after surgery to no further therapy or to therapy using vincristine, doxorubicin, cyclophosphamide, methotrexate, and 5-FU with leucovorin every 21 days for eight cycles.[195] After a median follow-up of 7 years for 569 patients,[196] the recurrence rate continued to be significantly reduced in treated patients versus controls. Although recurrence-free survival was prolonged in both the premenopausal and postmenopausal subpopulations, the trend achieved statistical significance only in premenopausal patients. Treatment conferred no benefit in overall survival to any subgroup.

Additional studies have compared a doxorubicin-containing regimen to another adjuvant chemotherapy regimen. The French Adjuvant Trial for Breast Cancer compared CMF therapy with therapy using a combination of doxorubicin, vincristine, cyclophosphamide, and 5-FU in a randomized group of 249 node-positive premenopausal and postmenopausal women.[181] Both the CMF and the doxorubicin-containing regimens were administered for 12 months. At 10 years, the difference in both disease-free survival and overall survival was statistically superior in premenopausal patients treated with the doxorubicin-containing regimen.[193] No difference in relapse-free or overall survival was demonstrated for postmenopausal patients. The Southeastern Cancer Study Group conducted a trial comparing 6 months of CMF to a doxorubicin-containing regimen in node-positive patients.[46] Cyclophosphamide, doxorubicin, and 5-FU (CAF) were given at doses of 500/50/500 mg/m². Both regimens were adjusted by 15 percent up or down as needed to achieve a granulocyte nadir between 800 and 1200/µl. At 5 years of median follow-up, there was no significant difference in overall survival.[47] This analysis had a 77 percent power to detect a 10 percent difference, so the authors concluded that any potential advantage with CAF is likely to be small.

The NSABP has evaluated the addition of doxorubicin to two regimens[115] and followed up on these studies by comparing four cycles of doxorubicin and cyclophosphamide (AC) given every 3 weeks with 6 cycles of conventional CMF.[101] In NSABP B-09, premenopausal and postmenopausal node-positive patients were randomized after surgery to melphalan plus 5-FU (PF) versus melphalan, 5-FU, and tamoxifen (PFT). In two later trials, NSABP randomized the subset of patients responsive to PFT between PFT and PFT plus doxorubicin (PAFT); those patients who showed no difference in their responses to PF and PFT in B-09 were termed *tamoxifen-nonresponsive* and randomized between PF and PF plus doxorubicin (PAF). Preliminary results indicated that the addition of doxorubicin to PF and PFT increases the disease-free survival resulting from either regimen alone[112]; however, the difference for PAFT versus PFT was not sustained. When the results for both studies were more mature with follow-up through 6 years, the *tamoxifen-nonresponsive* patients of NSABP B-11 who were randomized to PAF continued to have a statistically significant improvement in relapse-free and overall survival compared with patients randomized to PF.[115] But, there was no longer a significant difference between patients randomized to PFT versus PAFT on NSABP B-12. Both of the patient populations included in these two studies were addressed by subsequent trials examining the value of therapy with doxorubicin. In NSABP B-15, node-positive breast cancer patients were randomized to two months of therapy with AC (four cycles every 3 weeks) versus six cycles of conventional CMF if they were either 49 years or younger, regardless of receptor status, or 50 to 59 years old with a progesterone receptor (PR) level less than 10 fmol/mg.[101] There was no significant difference in relapse-free survival or overall survival, but patients preferred the shorter regimen.

A third arm of this study demonstrated that no benefit was obtained by following the 2 months of AC therapy with an additional 6 months of CMF. Node-positive patients aged 50 to 59 with a PR level above 10 fmol/mg and patients 60 years or more in age regardless of receptor status were entered on NSABP B-16.[113] Initially, this trial compared tamoxifen versus doxorubicin, cyclophosphamide, and tamoxifen (ACT) to PFT, but only 75 patients entered the PFT arm before it was modified to include doxorubicin. Four cycles of AC administered over 2 months simultaneously with tamoxifen, which continued for 5 years, was superior to tamoxifen alone for a statistically significant increase in relapse-free and overall survival at 3 years of follow-up. In the group of patients treated with PFT or PAFT there was also a statistically significant advantage in relapse-free survival at 3 years compared with tamoxifen, but a difference in overall survival was not apparent.

The Milan group also developed several trials based on the use of doxorubicin in node-positive patients. For one to three positive nodes, 12 cycles of intravenous CMF were compared with 8 cycles of

TABLE 66–6. RANDOMIZED TRIALS OF DOXORUBICIN-CONTAINING ADJUVANT REGIMENS IN NODE-POSITIVE PATIENTS

Trial	Study Population	No. of Patients	Chemotherapy	Treatment Duration	Follow-up (yr)	Disease-Free Survival (%)		Overall Survival (%)	
						Doxorubicin	Other	Doxorubicin	Other
Misset et al.[193] (Oncofrance Group)	Premenopausal and postmenopausal	249	CMF vs. AVCF	2 yr	10	54*	43*	67*	51*
Carpenter[43] (Southeastern Cancer Study Group)	Premenopausal and postmenopausal	528	CMF vs. CAF					74†	68†
Morrison et al.[196] (West Midlands Oncology Association)	Premenopausal and postmenopausal	569	AVCMFL vs. no adjuvant	6 mo	7	34*(Crude)	24*(Crude)	51†(Crude)	49†(Crude)
Fisher et al.[115] (NSABP B-11)	Premenopausal and postmenopausal	707	PF vs. PAF	2 yr	5	51*	44*	65†	59†
Fisher et al.[115] (NSABP B-12)	Premenopausal and postmenopausal	1106	PFT vs. PAFT	2 yr	5	64†	63†	77†	78†
Fisher et al.[101] (NSABP B-15)	Premenopausal and postmenopausal	2194	CMF vs. AC	2 vs. 6 mon	3	62†	63†	83†	82†

Abbreviations: A = doxorubicin; C = cyclophosphamide; F = 5-fluorouracil; L = leucovorin; M = methotrexate; P = prednisone; T = tamoxifen; V = vincristine; Vbl = vinblastine.
* $p < 0.05$
† not significant.

CMF followed by single-agent doxorubicin; no difference in outcome was observed.[194] For patients with more than three positive nodes, four courses of doxorubicin were followed with 8 cycles of CMF. This regimen was compared with 2 cycles of CMF followed by a cycle of doxorubicin and repeated for a total of 12 cycles.[43] Relapse-free survival and overall survival were superior when doxorubicin was given first, and all subgroups of patients received benefit. Although some of the data from studies evaluating the addition of doxorubicin to adjuvant regimens are encouraging, this strategy must be further studied to determine the conditions for which inclusion of doxorubicin or a doxorubicin-containing regimen in treatment of stage II breast cancer is a desirable practice. Whether an anthracycline other than doxorubicin has potential in adjuvant regimens is also the subject of ongoing study. Coombes and associates have reported the results for a comparison of 5-FU, epirubicin, and cyclophosphamide (FEC) with CMF, both given intravenously on days 1 and 8 every 28 days for six cycles.[64] In a group of 399 node-positive, operable breast cancer patients, those randomized to FEC had a statistically significant improvement in relapse-free and overall survival compared with patients treated with CMF.

Optimal Duration of Adjuvant Chemotherapy

A practical and clinically relevant problem in adjuvant chemotherapy administration is the optimal duration of therapy. Shorter courses diminish short-term toxicity of treatment and possibly decrease the chance of long-term toxicities. Patient compliance may also be enhanced. Five vanguard studies evaluated the question of outcome related to duration of therapy.

Two studies evaluated short versus long courses of CMF.[262, 277] The Milan group entered a total of 466 patients in a prospective randomized study from 1975 to 1978.[262] Within 4 weeks of surgery, patients younger than 70 years of age with T1 to T3a breast cancer and histologically positive nodes were randomized to receive either 6 or 12 cycles of CMF. Patients were stratified according to the number of nodes involved (1 to 3 or more than 3), and both premenopausal and postmenopausal women were entered into the study. No disease-free or overall survival advantage was seen between the two treatment groups. The authors concluded that the results of the study were sufficiently mature to say that 6 cycles of CMF are equivalent to 12 cycles with regard to overall and disease-free survival. Subsequent observation up to 14 years confirmed that relapse-free survival and overall survival were similar between these two groups of patients.[18]

A second study of duration of adjuvant CMF administration was performed by the Southeastern Cancer Study Group.[277] Patients were entered on study as in the Milan protocol with similar stratification according to the number of involved nodes (one to three and more than three). CMF was administered as originally described by Bonadonna and colleagues.[19] There were 620 patients entered on study. The one group with an improved disease-free survival was the premenopausal group with one to three positive nodes who received 12 months of CMF.[278] The authors of this study concluded that there was an improvement in disease-free survival with the longer course of CMF administered to this subset of patients.

A different perspective on duration of adjuvant chemotherapy has been provided by a prolonged low-dose CMF trial conducted jointly by the European Organization for Research and Treatment of Cancer (EORTC) and the Dutch Breast Cancer Working Party.[53] The goal in this trial was to evaluate a regimen delivering an amount of chemotherapy equivalent to 12 cycles of conventional CMF, but given over 2 years, with the intent of reducing toxicity without losing efficacy. There were 452 node-positive breast cancer patients aged 70 or less, who were randomized between low-dose CMF or no further therapy. Although there was no direct comparison with conventional CMF, the authors reported after a median follow-up time of 10 years that low-dose CMF for 2 years significantly prolonged overall survival and was probably as effective as shorter-term CMF. Nevertheless, the toxicity, including nausea, vomiting, alopecia, stomatitis, infection, and neutropenia, led the authors to conclude that shorter-term CMF at conventional doses is preferable.

Several studies have evaluated treatment duration for drug regimens other than CMF. The Dana-Farber Cancer Institute initiated a study in 1974 that closed to entry in 1985 and evaluated 286 patients given cyclophosphamide 500 mg/m^2 IV and doxorubicin 45 mg/m^2 IV on day 1 of a 3-week cycle for 5 versus 10 courses.[148] No significant differences were observed in either overall survival or disease-free survival among the patients randomized to the two arms of the study, either at initial report[148] or at a median follow-up of 9.1 years.[252] The Southwest Oncology Group randomized 411 patients with positive axillary nodes and ER-negative tumors to 1 versus 2 years of CMFVP.[232] There was no benefit to patients given the longer course of chemotherapy at a median follow-up of more than 8 years. Finally, the Swiss Group SAKK (Schweizerische Arbeitsgruppe für Klinische Krebsforschung) reported data for 351 evaluable patients who received 6 monthly 14-day cycles of oral chlorambucil, methotrexate, and 5-FU (LMF) or 12 monthly courses of LMF followed by 1 course every other month for a total of 18 courses during a period of 24 months.[163] After a mean observation time of 6 years, there was no difference in overall survival or disease-free survival between the two groups. It is noteworthy that the overall recurrence rate of 62.1 percent raises the issue of whether the LMF regimen had any activity at all. Because the study lacked an untreated control group, this question cannot be answered. There is no evidence from any of these studies that the longer course of chemotherapy benefited overall survival. Only one study showed an advantage in disease-free survival in a subgroup of patients receiving the longer course of chemotherapy (premenopausal with one to three positive nodes),[277] but the authors have questioned the validity of the result on the basis of a small number of events in a retrospective subset analysis. Therefore, the early studies evaluating longer versus shorter duration of a single adjuvant regimen seem consistent in their findings of no added benefit from courses of chemotherapy longer than five or six cycles.

The evidence that addresses a duration of treatment shorter than 5 or 6 cycles is limited. Two trials mentioned earlier tested the adequacy of a single postoperative cycle with CMF. In Ludwig V, there was a clear advantage for 6 cycles of CMF compared with 1 cycle,[174] and in the Scandinavian SACS 2 trial, 12 cycles of CMF were superior to a single cycle.[207] An Eastern Cooperative Oncology Group study with 803 postmenopausal node-positive women compared 4 versus 12 cycles of CMFPT with or without long-term tamoxifen.[91] Although the group continuing tamoxifen for 5 years had a longer time to relapse, there was no difference between 4 versus 12 cycles of CMFPT with respect to relapse-free and overall survival. Similarly, in a trial conducted by the German Breast Cancer Study Group,[248] no differences in survival have emerged from a comparison of 3 versus 6 cycles of CMF. In this trial, 473 patients after modified radical mastectomy were randomized according to a factorial design to no further treatment versus tamoxifen (20 mg/day × 2 yr) and CMF for 3 versus 6 cycles. Although no differences in relapse-free survival or overall survival are apparent, a difference might become apparent with additional follow-up. At a median follow-up of 56 months, the German trial had 80 percent power to detect a 30 percent reduction in risk of recurrence. A Canadian trial has provided an unfavorable profile for a 12-week regimen that was compared with 36 weeks of CMFVP.[169] In this comparison, 437 patients with stage II breast cancer were randomized, but accrual was stopped prematurely because of a high recurrence rate for patients treated with the 12-week regimen. Although this trial did not strictly compare duration of therapy, because the shorter course of therapy included two additional drugs (doxorubicin and tamoxifen), the decrease in relapse-free survival for the 12-week regimen was statistically significant.

Combinations of Non–Cross-Resistant Regimens

There is a continuing interest in improving the result of adjuvant therapy for breast cancer by adding non–cross-resistant chemotherapy to an established regimen such as CMF. A theoretical foundation for this approach has been provided by the Goldie-Coldman hypothesis, which relates drug sensitivity of tumors to spontaneous mutation rates. According to this model, the mutation rate for a given tumor is maintained throughout its growth history,[139, 140] and truly

non–cross-resistant combinations should afford a broader spectrum of cytolytic activity. The Norton-Simon hypothesis, which defends more intense schedules and higher doses in the use of adjuvant chemotherapy, also supports the use of non–cross-resistant regimens.[208] Under conditions where the tumor burden is high, the Norton-Simon hypothesis also predicts that the most efficient treatment would use moderately intense therapy, followed by intensifying therapy later in the course of treatment. However, predictions from these mathematical models depend on a variety of assumptions that cannot be directly tested. Randomized prospective studies are necessary to test the predictions of such models.

A study from Milan evaluated the concept of non–cross-resistant combinations in widely metastatic breast cancer.[34] This prospective study of 110 patients randomized initial therapy between CMF and doxorubicin plus vincristine (AV) and found no significant difference between the treatment groups in the response rate, median duration of response, or median survival. Effective secondary treatment after crossover for progressive or relapsed disease occurred in 35 percent of those in the AV group and in 20 percent of those in the CMF group. The authors concluded that there is no cross-resistance between CMF and AV.

Similar regimens were used in a Milan study of adjuvant chemotherapy in postmenopausal women.[35] Six-year results were reported for patients treated with CMFP for 6 cycles followed by AV for 4 cycles. In an attempt to clinically evaluate the Norton-Simon hypothesis, patients were randomized to receive a standard dose regimen or progressive dose intensification of all drugs except prednisolone and vincristine. Although no difference in outcome was seen between the two randomized groups, there was a better-than-expected disease-free survival and overall survival when the results were retrospectively compared with adjuvant CMF therapy in previous Milan studies of postmenopausal patients.

Given the difficulties of reaching a meaningful conclusion on the basis of historical controls, a direct comparison was subsequently made between 8 cycles of CMF followed by 4 cycles of single-agent doxorubicin without vincristine versus 12 cycles of CMF.[43] In the absence of benefit for an AV combination in metastatic disease, vincristine was dropped to avoid neurotoxicity. In the direct comparison, there were no significant differences between the two treatment groups at a median follow-up of 5 years.

The Milan group has tested an additional variation in sequencing 8 cycles of CMF with 4 cycles of doxorubicin. When the 4 cycles of doxorubicin are followed with 8 cycles of CMF, this sequence gives a statistically significant improvement in relapse-free survival and overall survival compared with four blocks of alternating therapy with 2 cycles of CMF followed by 1 cycle of doxorubicin.[33] Interpretation of this result is complicated by the asymmetry of the therapy.[76] It is not apparent how 4 cycles of doxorubicin followed by 8 cycles of CMF would compare with 4 cycles of doxorubicin only or 12 cycles of CMF.

The Cancer and Leukemia Group B evaluated 897 node-positive stage II patients randomized to receive initial treatment with CMFVP followed by further randomization to additional CMFVP versus vinblastine, doxorubicin, thiotepa, and halotestin (VATH).[214] At a median follow-up of 2 years, disease-free survival was significantly superior in patients who received VATH. Furthermore, the disease-free survival advantage for patients who received VATH was present in patients at highest risk for relapse, including postmenopausal patients with 4 or more positive nodes, patients with 10 or more positive nodes, and ER-negative patients. At a median follow-up of 11.5 years, there was a statistically significant increase in overall survival as well as an ongoing increase in relapse-free survival in favor of patients who received VATH. Again, the advantage was present for patients with either four or more involved lymph nodes, ER-negative tumors, or in postmenopausal women.[215] These results are consistent with a beneficial effect predicted by the Norton-Simon hypothesis when a period of moderate therapy is followed by intensification. This concept is being pursued with a regimen that is a successor to CMFVP-VATH. In this regimen, the course of CMFVP has been reduced from 8 to 4 months and the 6 months of VATH is replaced by 4 months of intensive, escalating 3-day cycles of doxorubicin.[17] For the present, there are no convincing data to dictate use of non–cross-resistant regimens in preference to 6 cycles of adjuvant CMF or 4 cycles of adjuvant AC as demonstrated by NSABP B-15.

Dose Intensity

Although dose intensity was raised as an issue that could explain some of the survival differences between premenopausal and postmenopausal women treated with multi-agent adjuvant chemotherapy in early studies of adjuvant therapy for node-positive patients, the concept of dose intensity may have implications for all patients. Dose intensity is defined as the amount of drug given per unit of time, typically mg/m²/wk. Some theoretical foundations for a consideration of dose intensity or rate were established by Hryniuk and associates, who analysed data from more than 6000 stage II breast cancer patients treated with adjuvant chemotherapy in randomized trials.[154] Patients receiving cyclophosphamide, methotrexate, 5-FU, or melphalan were categorized according to nodal and menopausal status. The analysis was retrospective and combined data from more than a dozen trials, according to the following assumptions:

1. Each of the drugs in a regimen was of equivalent activity.
2. Differences in drug scheduling could be ignored.
3. A dose intensity of zero could be assigned to missing drugs in partial CMF combinations.

4. Vincristine and prednisone did not contribute to the outcome of therapy in breast cancer.
5. For purposes of calculation of equivalent activity of dose cyclophosphamide equaled 40 times the milligrams of melphalan.

It was concluded that dose intensity correlated with disease-free survival rate for all four of the prognostic groups that were evaluated (i.e., women younger than 50 years with one to three and more than three positive nodes, and those 50 years or older with one to three and more than three positive nodes). The authors distinguished between intended and actual dose intensity and acknowledged methodological difficulties in dose calculation and retrospective analysis of clinical trials.

These methodological difficulties are in part illustrated by the NSABP report that in the studies comparing melphalan to control and melphalan plus 5-FU to control, women receiving 85 percent or more of the dose of placebo had a significantly better disease-free survival than women receiving less than 65 percent of placebo.[223] Another example is the report of the Coronary Drug Project Research Group, which sought to evaluate the efficacy of several lipid-influencing drugs on the long-term treatment of coronary artery disease.[66] Patients who took at least 80 percent of placebo had a highly statistically significant (p less than 10^{-12}) lower 5-year mortality than those who took less than 80 percent of placebo. These results highlight the potential for confounding that might occur as a result of an inability to control for factors related to dose delivery. Consequently, the limited amount of prospective data addressing the issue of dose intensity is relatively important and deserves special consideration.

Issues of dose intensity are highlighted by a study from CALGB.[285] Randomization began in January 1985 for stage II, node-positive breast cancer patients. Accrual of 1572 women finished in 1991, and results were published after a median of 3.4 years of follow-up. In this study of dose as well as dose intensity, one group of women received cyclophosphamide (600 mg/m²), doxorubicin (60 mg/m²), and 5-FU (600 mg/m² for 2 doses) every 28 days for four cycles. In a second protocol arm, described as being of moderate dose intensity, the same overall amount of medication was delivered in 6 cycles by reducing the individual doses by one-third. Patients treated on the third arm of the study received doses that provided half the medication in the first two arms (300 mg, 30 mg, 300 mg × 2) over four cycles. For both premenopausal and postmenopausal women treated with the high- and moderate-dose therapy, disease-free and overall survival were significantly lengthened over survival in the third group. Although the observed survival differences between the high- and moderate-dose therapy suggested a trend in favor of higher doses, statistical significance was not reached; however, the possibility of meaningful divergence after longer follow-up cannot be ruled out. The authors concluded that the results could be consistent with either a dose-response effect or a threshold effect related to dose or dose intensity. When the doses of CAF were reduced to the level used in the low-dose, low-intensity arm of this trial, there was a detrimental effect on survival for both premenopausal and postmenopausal patients.

In a companion study to the CALGB dose and dose intensity protocol, *ERBB2* levels, DNA index, S-phase fraction, and *P53* accumulation were determined for 442 randomly selected patients and correlated with response to the CAF adjuvant chemotherapy.[199] Of the markers evaluated, there was a significant dose-response effect in favor of increased relapse-free survival and overall survival for tumors that overexpressed *ERBB2*. This effect was not seen with the other markers. When *ERBB2* expression was minimal or absent, there was no difference in survival related to treatment level. These results have been viewed with caution because of small numbers and short follow-up. Nevertheless the results are useful in suggesting the potential for markers to assist in guiding therapeutic strategies for adjuvant therapy.

Results of the CALGB dose-intensity study also lend themselves to a discussion of the complexities of evaluating dose delivery. One assessment of the CALGB trial concluded that it did not isolate the main variables of interest, namely dose size, dose intensity, or total dose.[65] Because a difference in outcome could not be demonstrated for the two groups that received the higher total dose, but both of these groups obtained superior results compared with the low-dose group, it was suggested that total dose might be the basis for the results. This conclusion would favor the delivery of a target dose consistent with the moderate dose-intensity regimen rather than using the higher dose intensity arm regimen with its higher potential toxicity.

In addition to the CALGB study, another investigation of dose delivery has been performed in the adjuvant setting by the NSABP.[83] In NSABP B-22, 2238 patients with positive axillary nodes were randomized to one of three arms for an assessment of dose intensity and increased total dose. The standard NSABP AC regimen for four cycles was used in one arm of the study and modified for the other two arms by doubling the standard dose of cyclophosphamide. In the second arm, cyclophosphamide was stopped after 2 cycles, so that total cyclophosphamide dose was the same as that for the first arm. In the third arm, the higher dose of cyclophosphamide was continued for all 4 cycles, an amount that was twice the standard. All the patients received four doses of doxorubicin (60 mg/m^2 every 3 weeks). After 3 years of follow-up, the preliminary results showed that there was no difference in relapse-free or overall survival, suggesting that intensification or increasing the total dose of cyclophosphamide did not provide additional benefit. With more follow-up, this conclusion could change. For the next generation of studies, it can be expected that hematopoietic growth factors will be used to achieve even higher increments in

dose and dose intensity. Such an approach is being used in NSABP B-25, in which the regimen from NSABP B-22 with the highest cyclophosphamide dose is modified by once again doubling the cyclophosphamide dose and using granulocyte colony-stimulating factor (G-CSF) for hematopoietic support.

The question remains as to whether any of the dose-intense regimens will offer an advantage over a standard AC or CAF regimen. Several candidate regimens have been developed in pilot works with a view to such a comparison. The Johns Hopkins Oncology Center has demonstrated the feasibility of using a five drug regimen over 16 weeks, using weekly treatment, sequential antimetabolites, and periods of continuous infusion 5-FU.[2] This regimen is now being compared with a standard version of CAF[40] in an Intergroup (CALGB, ECOG, SWOG) Trial for node-positive, hormone receptor–negative patients.

It is widely agreed that breast cancer patients with 10 or more axillary lymph nodes involved with tumor are at high risk of relapse.[73] Even after doxorubicin-containing adjuvant therapy, this particular group of women has a recurrence rate of about 60 percent at 5 years.[41] With only modest benefit accruing to these women from conventional adjuvant chemotherapy, dose-intensive adjuvant therapy has become a focus of the effort to improve outcomes.

Within the range of conventional chemotherapy, the dose-response effect may be smaller than what can be achieved at the higher doses with bone marrow support. For high-risk women (defined by ten nodes or more), a definitive approach to dose intensity may involve late intensification followed by high-dose therapy that requires autologous bone marrow transplantation (ABMT) and/or peripheral blood stem cell (PBSC) support. This concept is being tested by two Intergroup protocols.[234] One of these compares "standard" CAF with CAF followed by high-dose therapy with cyclophosphamide and thiotepa. After this high-dose therapy, there is a comparison of bone marrow reconstitution with autologous bone marrow, peripheral blood stem cells, or both. The other Intergroup trial for stage II or III breast cancer patients with ten or more axillary nodes starts with CAF and randomizes between high-dose cyclophosphamide, cisplatin, and carmustine with ABMT versus lower doses of the same drugs with G-CSF. Pilot experience for the transplant regimen in 85 women has been previously described.[216] At a median follow-up of 2.5 years, event-free survival was 72 percent. This result is promising compared with historical controls and similar women in other trials. The possible increase in event-free survival must be balanced against adverse outcomes, which included 12 percent mortality and 31 percent pulmonary toxicity in the pilot. A preliminary report of pilot work by the Milan group describes a high-dose regimen with three courses; the first with high-dose cyclophosphamide; the second with high-dose methotrexate with leucovorin rescue, vincristine, and cisplatin; and the third with high-dose melphalan plus peripheral blood progenitor cell infusion.[23, 133] After a median follow-up of 50 months, for the 67 patients 55 years or older with ten or more axillary nodes involved with tumor, the relapse-free survival was 56 percent with an overall survival of 78 percent. A randomized trial is now ongoing and compares a modification of the Milan pilot regimen with doxorubicin followed sequentially by CMF. Results from these high-dose trials should help to clarify certain aspects of the controversy surrounding dose-delivery options in adjuvant chemotherapy. It has been suggested that some of the improvement observed in phase II trials of ABMT is derived from patient selection factors such as the exclusion of women with occult metastatic disease. In one series of 44 women with ten or more positive axillary lymph nodes who were referred for possible participation in a transplantation trial, further evaluation identified occult metastases in 7.[68]

NODE-NEGATIVE PATIENTS

With evidence that the biology of the natural history of stage II breast cancer can be altered with chemotherapy and hormonal therapy, investigators have extended their efforts to improve outcomes of patients with stage I disease. Although these patients have a relatively good prognosis, the relapse rate is still considerable. Moreover, women with stage I disease account for 40 percent to 50 percent of the total of newly diagnosed breast cancer patients. In a surgical study of 512 patients treated for breast cancer from 1965 to 1979 with negative lymph nodes (both axillary and internal mammary), the 10-year disease-free survival was 73 percent, and the overall survival was 80 percent.[279] Some patients had primary tumors larger than 2 cm, but none had been treated with adjuvant CMF. Similar results have been reported for node-negative breast cancer patients first seen and treated between 1964 and 1970 before adjuvant chemotherapy was established in the United States. For 474 women with T1N0 (primary tumor less than 2 cm, negative nodes) breast cancer, relapse-free survival was 79 percent at a median follow-up of 18 years.[239] In the subcategory of tumors 1 cm or less, the relapse-free survival was 88 percent. For 293 T2N0 (primary tumor larger than 2 cm but 5 cm or less) patients, recurrence-free survival was 69 percent after a median follow-up of 20 years.[238] These figures suggest that in the most favorable categories, the percentage of women destined to relapse may be less than 10 percent, and the chance for women in the least-favorable categories to relapse may be more than 40 percent.

Recognizing that it would be optimal to restrict the use of adjuvant therapy in node-negative patients to those who would otherwise relapse, there has been an attempt to evaluate patients for the prognostic features that indicate a high probability of breast cancer recurrence. In breast cancer without nodal involvement by tumor, the most important prognostic factors[186] are tumor size,[48] ER status,[9, 187] nuclear and histological grade,[123, 150] proliferation status,[54, 132, 255] and DNA content.[54, 90] Although a case has been made for the value of each of these markers, in practical terms, comprehensive multivariate models are rare, and the bulk of the variation in survival can be accounted for by a limited number of factors. Tumor size is usually available and relatively reproducible with prognosis codified through the TNM system. In contrast, ER status and tumor grade may not be as formally stratified for good versus poor prognoses; nevertheless, this constellation of factors, along with age[78] provides the basis for one set of current treatment recommendations.[138] A variety of other factors have been investigated for their role in determining outcome in stage I patients and are potentially valuable for research that examines their contribution to the natural history of node-negative disease or response to therapy.

Additional markers that have been cited for prognostic significance in predicting early relapse in stage I breast cancer include labeling index, mitotic index, diffuse hyperplasia of regional lymph nodes or a pattern of germinal center predominance in lymph nodes, extensive tumor necrosis, and family history of breast cancer.[1, 9, 123, 156]

The thymidine labeling index has been found to have predictive value independent of stage and estrogen receptor content and to select a subgroup of stage I patients with a relapse expectancy of approximately 50 percent at 4 years.[191, 192] Similarly, DNA flow cytometry measurements of both S-phase analysis and ploidy status have been shown to be predictors of relapse in node-negative patients.[54]

Recent interest in prognostic factors has focused on HER2/neu[259] and tumor angiogenesis.[127] The literature contains conflicting reports on the role of HER2/neu in node-negative disease, with some series indicating an effect on survival only in node-positive disease,[144, 268] and others finding increased mortality with overexpression regardless of nodal status.[212] Angiogenesis has been evaluated by quantitatively determining intratumoral microvessel density using antibody methodology. With this technique, it has been demonstrated that increased levels of tumor angiogenesis are associated with decreased relapse-free survival and overall survival in stage I breast cancer.[16] These results are based on median follow-up of 78 months in 211 node-negative breast cancer patients. Ultimately, the risk of breast cancer recurrence may be a function of the presence of distant micrometastases at the time of diagnosis. An overview of a dozen studies examining the detection of micrometastases in the bone marrow indicates that the prevalence ranges from 4 to 48 percent in early-stage breast cancer patients.[210] According to most of the studies reviewed, patients with bone marrow micrometastases appear to be more likely to relapse. Perhaps, as knowledge of the prognostic factors mentioned here is extended by further research, more specific decisions will be possible as to which node-negative patients should be recommended for adjuvant therapy and which therapies are most appropriate.

The NIH Consensus Conference of 1985 on Adjuvant Chemotherapy and Endocrine Therapy for breast cancer commented on patients with negative nodes. For both premenopausal and postmenopausal women with stage I disease, there was no therapy routinely recommended, but treatment could be considered for certain high-risk patients in each menopausal category.[201] Studies on which to base firm recommendations were unavailable at the time. Ten years later, more data are available and recommendations have followed. A consensus panel at the Fifth International Conference on Adjuvant Therapy of Primary Breast Cancer specified three levels of risk for premenopausal and postmenopausal women who were further categorized by ER status.[138] Low-risk individuals were defined as women more than age 35 who have tumors smaller than 1 cm, with grade 1 histology and a positive ER status. Moderate-risk women have tumors from 1 to 2 cm, of histological grade 1 to 2 with positive ER status. High-risk women have tumors with one of three features: negative ER status or ER positive with size larger than 2 cm, histological grade 2 to 3. Treatment recommendations were developed for the resulting eight categories of node-negative breast cancer patients as well as for an elderly population. Adjuvant chemotherapy was recommended for all categories of women at high risk of recurrence, except for postmenopausal women with positive ER status. For this latter category, tamoxifen was the first choice with or without chemotherapy. The 1995 St. Gallen's recommendations are summarized in Table 66–7.

Of the nine studies listed in Table 66–8, six have described a disease-free survival benefit for node-negative women given adjuvant therapy. In the majority of these, the benefit is statistically significant in all or a subset of patients treated. All the studies included both premenopausal and postmenopausal women in the study group. In three of the studies, an overall survival benefit was observed in the treated population. Jakesz and colleagues[160] and Bonadonna and associates[32] administered CMF in differing schedules to premenopausal and postmenopausal patients. Both studies realized an overall survival benefit in the treated group in a small number of patients. The control group in the Bonadonna study exhibited high-risk characteristics, with a disease-free survival of less than 50 percent at 5 years and an overall survival of approximately 65 percent at almost 5 years. These results are significantly worse than those for the majority of studies of stage I breast cancer patients. The disparity in survival between the treated patients and the control group and the statistical significance, however, are impressive.

Three of the studies listed in Table 66–7 had a profound impact on patterns of care for node-negative breast cancer patients with respect to chemotherapy. NSABP B-13 is a study of premenopausal and postmenopausal node-negative, ER-negative women in which 339 women were randomized to receive sequential methotrexate and 5-FU for 12 courses and 340 to receive surgical therapy alone.[109] At 4 years of follow-up, 80 percent of the treated women were disease-free, whereas 71 percent of the control population were disease-free ($p = 0.003$); there was no difference in survival outcome between premenopausal and postmenopausal women. The Ludwig Breast Cancer Study group reported the Ludwig V study in which 848 premenopausal and postmenopausal women who received one course of CMF with leucovorin on days 1 and 8 begun within 36 hours after surgery were compared with 427 control patients who received no adjuvant therapy after surgery, which consisted of either total mastectomy with axillary clearance or modified radical mastectomy.[178] At 4 years median follow-up, disease-free survival was statistically superior at 77 percent (± 2 percent) for the treated group compared with 73 percent (± 2 percent) for the control group. A trend in overall survival favored the treated group. The largest benefit in disease-free survival was realized by the ER-negative group compared to the control group, both premenopausal and postmenopausal women benefited in disease-free survival by receiving chemotherapy.

Finally, the Intergroup Study (INT 0011), which included ECOG, CALGB, and SWOG, randomized ER-negative and ER-positive patients with tumors 3 cm or larger to CMFP for six cycles or to no adjuvant therapy.[180] A disease-free survival benefit independent of ER and menopausal status was realized, with 84 percent of 196 treated patients and 69 percent of 210 control patients disease-free at a median follow-up of 3 years ($p = 0.0001$).

For NSABP B-13, Ludwig V, and INT 0011, more than 2000 node-negative breast cancer patients were treated with adjuvant chemotherapy. At the time of their most recently reported analyses, the increase in relapse-free survival was statistically significant in all three trials, and overall survival was significantly increased in two of three. In the third study, NSABP B-13, an increase in overall survival was statistically significant for the subset of patients who were 50 years of age or older.[105] Early results from these studies became available in the late 1980s, and results from NSABP B-13 and INT 0011 were cited in a 1988 Clinical Alert from the National Cancer Institute of the United States.[56] For more than a year after release of the Clinical Alert, the proportion of node-negative patients receiving adjuvant therapy was increased more than the level projected from trends previous to the Alert.[161]

Further improvement in the application of adjuvant chemotherapy in node-negative disease can be expected to occur with better understanding of prognostic variables in node-negative breast cancer patients. This development would facilitate rational treatment selection according to risk for recurrence.

TOXICITY OF ADJUVANT CHEMOTHERAPY

The disease-free and overall survival benefits of adjuvant therapy must be balanced against acute,

TABLE 66–7. RANDOMIZED TRIALS COMPARING LOCAL THERAPY WITH AND WITHOUT ADJUVANT CHEMOTHERAPY IN NODE-NEGATIVE PATIENTS

Author or Study	Study Population	No. of Patients	Chemotherapy	Treatment Duration	Median Follow-up (yr)	Disease-Free Survival (%)		Overall Survival (%)	
						Chemotherapy	Control	Chemotherapy	Control
Nissen Meyer[206]	Premenopausal and postmenopausal	609	C	6 day	20	64*	55*	Not analyzed	
Jungi et al.[164]	Premenopausal and postmenopausal	254	ChMFBCG	6 mo	14	No significant difference		75†	50†
Morrison et al.[197]	Premenopausal and postmenopausal	574	ChMF	3 yr	7	No significant difference		No significant difference	
Jakesze et al.[160]	Premenopausal and postmenopausal	128	CMFVbl	1 yr	6	No significant difference		74†	90†
Bonadonna et al.[24] (Milan)	Premenopausal and postmenopausal	90	CMF	18 wk	8	80‡	39‡	84‡	58‡
Williams et al.[284]	Premenopausal and postmenopausal; ER-negative tumors	52	CAV	1 yr	6	95§	68§	No significant difference	
NSABP-13[109]	Premenopausal and postmenopausal; ER-negative tumors	737	MF	6 mo	5	76‡	67‡	No significant difference	
Intergroup Study[179]	Premenopausal and postmenopausal; ER-negative tumors; ER-positive tumors ≥3 cm	406	CMFP	6 mo	4.5	83‡	61‡	86*	80*
Ludwig[178]	Premenopausal and postmenopausal	1275	CMFL	Day 1 (starting within 36 hr after surgery) and then day 8 after surgery	4	77 ± 2†	73 ± 2†	90 ± 1*	86 ± 2*

Abbreviations: A = doxorubicin; BCG = bacille Calmette-Guérin; C = cyclophosphamide; Ch = chlorambucil; F = 5-fluorouracil; L = leucovorin; M = methotrexate; P = prednisone; V = vincristine; Vbl = vinblastine.
*No significant difference.
†$p < 0.05$ for chemotherapy vs. control.
‡$p < 0.005$ for chemotherapy vs. control.
§Seven patients who were randomized to treatment arm refused chemotherapy and were included in the control group. Results were statistically significant when analyzed for treatment delivered.

TABLE 66–8. ROUTINE ADJUVANT TREATMENT FOR BREAST CANCER PATIENTS WITH NEGATIVE LYMPH NODES AS DISCUSSED AT THE 5TH INTERNATIONAL CONFERENCE ON THE ADJUVANT TREATMENT OF PRIMARY BREAST CANCER

	Low Risk, ER-Positive*	Good Risk, ER-Positive†	High Risk‡
Premenopausal	None vs. tamoxifen§	Tamoxifen	ER-positive: Chemotherapy plus tamoxifen§ ER-negative: Chemotherapy
Postmenopausal	None vs. tamoxifen§	Tamoxifen	ER-positive: Tamoxifen plus chemotherapy§ ER-negative: Chemotherapy plus tamoxifen§

*Low risk: >35 years old, tumor < 1 cm, ER-positive, and grade 1 histology.
†Good risk: Tumor 1–2 cm, ER-positive, and grade 1–2 histology.
‡High risk: Either tumor > 2 cm, ER-negative, grade 2–3 histology.
§Therapy is under investigation.

delayed, and psychological toxicities caused by treatment. Acute toxicity secondary to CMF-based regimens has been reported for 2500 women representing the Milan experience[25] and for 533 premenopausal women who received CMF, CMFP, or CMFPT and 223 postmenopausal women who received CMFP or CMFPT while participating in ECOG trials.[270] Acute toxicities included weight gain (3 to 4 kg in almost 50 percent of women treated, severe alopecia in less than 10 percent, nausea and vomiting in more than 90 percent, leukopenia less than 2500/mm^3 in ten percent, thrombocytopenia less than 75,000/mm^3 in less than 10 percent, and hemorrhagic cystitis in less than 15 percent. Systemic infection was reported by ECOG as occurring in one percent of patients receiving CMF. The Milan report emphasized that none of the women treated with CMF required intensive supportive therapy for life-threatening toxicity. The addition of prednisone added toxicities of edema, cushingoid appearance, and increased weight gain. An increased incidence of thromboembolic disease during the months patients received CMFVP has also been reported in premenopausal and postmenopausal women.[168] Persistent amenorrhea has been reported in 40 percent of women younger than 40 years and in 95 percent of women older than 40 years who receive CMF.[25]

The primary concern with delayed toxicity is secondary malignancy. The risk of leukemia following adjuvant therapy with melphalan has been reported by the NSABP.[117] In this report of 8483 women entered on NSABP trials since 1971, the cumulative risk of leukemia for surgical controls was 0.06 percent after 10 years in patients free of metastases (3 of 2068 patients). For 5299 women treated with a 2-year course of melphalan, however, the cumulative risk for leukemia for patients free of metastases or a second primary was 1.11 ± 0.30 percent at 10 years; when combined with the incidence of myeloproliferative syndrome, the risk was 1.54 ± 0.36 percent. There were 26 cases of acute myelogenous leukemia and 7 cases of myeloproliferative syndrome in the treated women. The results indicated an increased risk of hematological malignancy following treatment in this setting with 2 years of melphalan.

The Milan group reported the incidence of all sec-

ond malignancies after adjuvant therapy with CMF.[274] From 1973 to 1978, 845 premenopausal and postmenopausal women were entered on two studies evaluating CMF as adjuvant therapy. Of 666 women who received either 6 months or 12 months of CMF, there were no cases of leukemia. Furthermore, the incidence of second malignancies in general, including breast cancer, was equivalent to that in the 179 patients who did not receive therapy. Median follow-up for the group was more than 10 years. However, Henderson cautioned that the population sample of the Milan study is too small to conclude that there is absolutely no danger in developing second malignancies after CMF.[149]

In reviewing the various factors that might contribute to acute nonlymphocytic leukemia (ANLL) after therapy with CMF, investigators from Milan raised the issue of duration of therapy and intercurrent radiation therapy.[274] These issues have been addressed with a case-control study of 90 patients with leukemia from a cohort of 82,700 women who were diagnosed with breast cancer between 1973 and 1985 in five areas of the United States.[71] From this analysis, it was concluded that risk of ANLL was significantly increased by radiation therapy (relative risk, 2.4; 95 percent confidence interval [CI] = 1.0 to 5.8), by therapy with alkylating agents (relative risk, 10.0; 95 percent CI = 3.9 to 25.2), and by the combination of these two therapies (relative risk, 17.4; 95 percent CI = 6.4 to 47.0). Cumulative dose of alkylating agent and duration of therapy were also significantly associated with ANLL. In addition to cyclophosphamide, other alkylating agents that have been linked with leukemia include thiotepa, chlorambucil, nitrogen mustard, and melphalan.[240]

Recent results from NSABP B-25 have confirmed the potential for developing ANLL in the setting of dose-intense adjuvant chemotherapy.[79] In this study, 2548 node-positive breast cancer patients were randomized to therapy with doxorubicin, cyclophosphamide, and tamoxifen with G-CSF support. In this trial, doses of cyclophosphamide were increased two to four times above the standard level. Six cases of acute myeloid leukemia occurred in patients aged 50 or older within 18 months of starting chemotherapy. Because of concern about the potential for leukemogenesis in the setting of chemotherapy, a monitoring plan for second malignancies is in place in the United States for federally sponsored chemotherapy protocols for cancer treatment.

To the extent that the anthracycline doxorubicin is used as part of adjuvant chemotherapy regimens, it will be accompanied by a second serious consequence of chemotherapeutic treatment, namely doxorubicin-associated cardiotoxicity.[173] Anthracycline cardiotoxicity is dose-dependent, and the possibility that concurrent chest irradiation increases the risk has been investigated. Valagussa and coworkers reported on outcomes for more than 800 breast cancer patients who were randomized in three Milan trials of doxorubicin-containing adjuvant chemotherapy.[275] In their studies, less than 0.8 percent of patients developed doxorubicin-related congestive heart failure and 3 of these patients had received radiation treatment to the left chest wall. For a doxorubicin target dose of 300 mg/m^2, the expected level of treatment-associated cardiomyopathy is 1 percent or less. This result has been confirmed by the experience of other groups, including the NSABP[115] and the M. D. Anderson Cancer Center.[42] Shapiro and Henderson have pointed out that the length of follow-up for this problem in adjuvant study populations does not allow a full assessment of delayed cardiac toxicity.[254] Consequently, any movement to routinely incorporate doxorubicin in adjuvant therapy would need to weigh the potential cardiac toxicity against an as-yet undefined but possibly small advantage in reducing breast cancer recurrence and mortality over non–anthracycline containing regimens.

Ongoing attention is being given to the quality of life for patients who receive adjuvant chemotherapy. Analysis of the Ludwig Breast Cancer Study III evaluated time without symptoms and toxicity (TWiST).[129] The Ludwig III Study randomized 463 postmenopausal women 65 years old or younger to no therapy, therapy with 12 months of prednisone plus tamoxifen (P + T), or CMFP + T. Periods during which the patient experienced side effects from therapy were subtracted from overall survival and compared with the control group. It was determined that the CMFP + T group had a significantly longer TWiST than did controls, with values at 72 months of follow-up of 37.9 months for controls, 42.4 months for P + T, and 44.3 months for CMFP + T. The TWiST after relapse was not calculated. This was a symptom-related evaluation that did not include psychological or stress-related phenomena.

TWiST methodology has been upgraded so that comparisons of adjuvant trials based on time without symptoms and toxicity can be adjusted for quality of life (QOL). The integration of these two outcomes with respect to adjuvant therapy has depended on the development of appropriate QOL instruments. One of these, the Breast Cancer Chemotherapy Questionnaire (BCQ),[170] can be used to produce Q-TWiST (quality-adjusted survival relative to TWiST). The BCQ correlates well with global assessments of physical and emotional function. A variety of other instruments and approaches have been used to integrate QOL data into assessments of adjuvant chemotherapy.[131] Q-TWiST has been applied to the INT 0011,[131] Ludwig III,[137] and Ludwig V[130] trials of adjuvant chemotherapy. For Ludwig V, in a comparison of a single perioperative cycle of chemotherapy with six or seven postoperative cycles, Q-TWiST projected that for patients surviving 3.5 years, the burden of a longer period of adjuvant therapy was offset by better control of disease. Time past 3.5 years was consistent with improvement in both quantity and quality of life. In the future, methods such as Q-TWiST should permit a more refined approach in assessing the usefulness of adjuvant chemotherapy.

META-ANALYSIS OF ADJUVANT CHEMOTHERAPY FOR BREAST CANCER

Meta-analysis (or overview analysis) is a statistical methodology that has been used to evaluate issues in medicine that remain unresolved in spite of extensive evaluation. Previously used in the field of psychology and in the analysis of cardiovascular studies,[88] it is now being applied to analyze adjuvant therapies of breast cancer. This approach to research analysis is a structured review of medical data. A number of review articles on the subject have appeared.[88, 128, 224] The analysis must be of adequate sample size relative to the degree of expected treatment benefit, and systematic bias must be minimized. Before selection of individual clinical trials, study criteria must be strictly established and the question to be answered by the meta-analysis must be specific. Variability of trials must be minimal to diminish the possibility of effective therapies being cancelled by ineffective therapies in the results of the overview analysis. Although debated, it has been stated that all eligible trials, not just published trials, should be included, and that the quality of individual trials should meet minimal criteria. Objective end points of analysis should be selected. For example, overall survival is a more unbiased outcome parameter than disease-specific survival or disease-free survival. An objective of the overall analysis is to minimize the effects of minor, random variations by increasing the sample size. Statistical issues and techniques are discussed in review articles of the subject.[88, 128, 224]

Richard Peto and colleagues from the Clinical Trials Unit, Oxford University, reported findings of a meta-analysis of adjuvant chemotherapy at the National Institutes of Health Consensus Development Conference on Adjuvant Chemotherapy and Endocrine Therapy for Breast Cancer in 1985. This report was not published with the Proceedings for the NIH Consensus Conference, but it was nevertheless influential in developing the recommendations for therapy adopted at the conference.[220] Afterward, qualitative discussions of the information ensued.[60, 225] Summary portions of this overview were incorporated in Henderson's monograph.[147] Peto's 1985 overview analysis evaluated published and unpublished randomized clinical trials in which chemotherapy was included in only one arm of the study.[147] Nearly 15,000 women were included in the trials, 25 percent of whom died within the first 5 years of follow-up. In the analysis of all trials evaluating patients receiving chemotherapy, odds of death decreased 14 ± 3 percent in the group receiving chemotherapy. All age groups benefited, but women younger than 50 years benefited by an odds-of-death reduction of 24 ± 5 percent versus 8 ± 4 percent for women older than 50 years. When the analysis was restricted to CMF, women younger than 50 years realized an odds-of-death reduction of 34 ± 6 percent versus 17 ± 6 percent for women older than 50 years. The absolute effect of all chemotherapy was to increase the overall survival by 9 percent at 5 years for women younger than 50 years and by 3 percent for women older than 50 years.

A follow-up to the 1985 overview was published in 1988 by the Early Breast Cancer Trialists Collaborative Group, which analyzed 61 randomized trials of 28,896 women.[85] This study evaluated outcome by mortality in trials that began randomization of patients before January 1, 1985, to tamoxifen or cytotoxic chemotherapy for early breast cancer. Data were collected on age, nodal status, date of entry, and date of death. Four comparison groups of patients were evaluated: tamoxifen versus controls, all chemotherapy versus controls, multiple agent chemotherapy versus single agent chemotherapy, and short-term chemotherapy versus longer administration of the same chemotherapy.

Out of 61 randomized trials, there were 31 trials of chemotherapy versus no chemotherapy, with 9069 patients participating. At the time of analysis, 2872 were dead. The treated group exhibited an overall 14 ± 4 percent reduction in odds of death with an even greater effect in younger women. Women younger than 50 years at entry demonstrated a 22 ± 6 percent reduction in annual odds of death, whereas there was no definite advantage for women older than 50 years at entry. Ten trials examined the issue of multi-agent versus single-agent chemotherapy in 3005 women entered. Multi-agent chemotherapy conferred a 21 ± 9 percent reduction in annual odds of death compared with single-agent chemotherapy. When evaluating regimens of multi-agent chemotherapy, there was a suggestion that CMF was better than other regimens, but this was not statistically significant. Adding tamoxifen to chemotherapy did not improve survival. There was no improvement in survival with the more prolonged (6 to 24 mo) versus shorter (3 to 6 mo) regimens. For women with no nodal involvement (1589 women in the chemotherapy trials), although the proportional reduction in mortality was similar to that for women with positive nodes, the amount of information was limited and not statistically significant.

An update of the overview of adjuvant chemotherapy from the Early Breast Cancer Trialists' Collaborative Group was published in 1992. At this point,

the number of trials contributing data for a comparison of cytotoxic chemotherapy versus no chemotherapy had increased to 44.[87] Data were analyzed for 18,403 patients, of whom 6582 were dead. The results of this analysis show that the women treated with polychemotherapy enjoy a highly statistically significant advantage, with a 21 percent reduction in the average annual odds of recurrence and an 11 percent reduction in the average annual odds of death compared with control groups. The relative reduction in recurrence rate in the treated group is confined to the first 5 years, after which the difference is maintained but not enlarged. The impact of treatment on mortality continues beyond the first 5 years, with the result that the difference in survival is twice as great at 10 years compared with 5 years. One of the conclusions from this overview is that women with the greater risk of recurrence (node-positive) obtain a greater absolute benefit from adjuvant chemotherapy. The latest in a series of updates to the overview is expected soon. Given the methodology used to generate the overview results, it is useful to remember that the incorporation of data from diverse sources is likely to produce a result reflecting heterogeneous conditions that are less than ideal. Overview results of adjuvant chemotherapy are likely to underestimate its potential benefit giving a conditional assessment of effectiveness rather than an optimized estimate of efficacy.

ADJUVANT HORMONAL THERAPIES

Rationale

For a variety of reasons, there is continued interest in adjuvant hormonal manipulations for early-stage breast carcinoma. With the initial hope in the early 1970s that a large percentage of women with early-stage breast cancer would be cured with adjuvant chemotherapy, enthusiasm for hormonal therapies waned. In part, this was a result of the paradigm that hormonal therapy was "cytostatic" and would not be as effective as "cytolytic" chemotherapy. However, it is by no means clear, given the results presented earlier in this chapter, that adjuvant chemotherapy is effective because it totally eliminates occult micrometastases. In most trials, the breast cancer-specific survival curves do not become completely flat at any point. One of several possible explanations for this observation is that chemotherapy may extend survival in uncured patients rather than achieve cure. Furthermore, the stigma of the term *cytostatic*, which has been attached to hormonal agents based on in vitro studies, is not consistent with the observation of complete tumor regressions and dramatic partial remissions that occur in many trials of hormonal agents in metastatic breast cancer.

It is accepted that some of the benefits of adjuvant chemotherapy in premenopausal women with breast cancer are mediated through "chemically induced castration." A previously described study from the Danish Breast Cancer Cooperative Group supports this hypothesis.[36] More than 1000 women with breast cancer and axillary node involvement who had undergone total mastectomy with axillary sampling were randomly assigned to receive either radiation alone (RT), RT plus single-agent oral cyclophosphamide, or RT plus CMF. Adjuvant chemotherapy was given in the latter two groups for 12 months. Both of these groups had a significant improvement in disease-free and overall survival compared with controls but were not significantly different when compared with each other. In a retrospective analysis of the RT + cyclophosphamide arm of the study, it was found that disease-free survival was not improved in the subset of women who did not undergo chemotherapy-induced amenorrhea. By contrast, disease-free survival was virtually identical for women who did versus those who did not undergo treatment-induced amenorrhea in the adjuvant CMF arm.

Similar results were reported by Howell and colleagues[153] in a randomized study of low-dose (20 percent less than standard) CMF versus no adjuvant therapy in 327 women who had undergone total mastectomy and axillary dissection. In this study, disease-free survival was better in patients who had chemotherapy-induced amenorrhea than in control patients; disease-free survival was intermediate in treated patients who had no amenorrhea. There were no significant differences in overall survival in the study. In an Eastern Cooperative Oncology Group study in premenopausal women comparing CMF versus CMF plus prednisone versus CMF plus prednisone and tamoxifen, patients who developed amenorrhea had improved disease-free survival as well as overall survival when compared with those who did not have cessation of menses.[269]

Other trials failed to support the hypothesis that the effects of adjuvant chemotherapy are mediated through a chemical castration. Neither the Milan trial of adjuvant CMF versus no adjuvant therapy in node-positive women[30] nor the NSABP trial of adjuvant melphalan versus placebo[118] in node-positive women revealed significant differences in the benefits to treated women when analyzed for cessation of menses in premenopausal women. It therefore seems clear that not all of the effects of adjuvant chemotherapy are mediated through a chemical castration. It is possible, nevertheless, that hormonal effects of chemotherapy play some role in the benefits in premenopausal women.

The ability to routinely assay tumor tissue from primary resections for estrogen and progesterone receptor content may heighten the ability to identify those women most likely to benefit from adjuvant hormonal therapy. Because the receptor content could not be measured at the time of many of the early trials, it was not known whether there were subsets of patients who benefited more than others. The conclusion that a receptor assay can be used to predict response to adjuvant hormonal manipulations depends on a correlation between the receptor content of the primary tumor and the subclinical metastases that are present at the time of diagnosis,

as well as concordance in receptor status among the multiple subclinical metastases. Allegra and colleagues found an 85 percent concordance rate in ER status in 23 cases in which multiple metastases were assayed simultaneously.[4] In another study, receptor status was compared between primary breast tumors and metastatic tumors that subsequently came to clinical attention.[151] The concordance rate was only 46 percent. In this instance, the comparison is complicated by an interval of time to recurrence during which ER status may have changed. Another complicating factor is the possibility of false-negative receptor assays. Such results may in part account for recent observations in some adjuvant trials (discussed in following sections) that adjuvant tamoxifen carries some benefit even in ER-negative women. On the other hand, tamoxifen may exert its effect through several alternative mechanisms that may not involve the ER.[202]

Trials of Adjuvant Ovarian Ablation

Oophorectomy was first proposed as an adjuvant therapy for primary breast cancer in 1889.[249] Remission of advanced breast cancer after bilateral oophorectomy was first reported in 1896,[13] and the first therapeutic radiation-induced castration was reported in 1905.[77] The first clinical trial of prophylactic radiation castration was reported in 1939.[264] However, early clinical trials of the concept in the 1940s and 1950s gave no definitive information, because they were not internally controlled.[7, 82] In the 1992 overview, data were available for 10 trials of ovarian ablation started before 1985, with 3072 women randomized. The six studies of adjuvant ovarian ablation in the absence of chemotherapy are summarized in Table 66–9. In one of the trials, allocation to treatment versus control was by month of birth.[59] In three of these studies, the method of ovarian ablation was external beam radiation,[59, 189, 205] and in the other three, surgical oophorectomy was performed.[37, 204, 222] The two modalities of castration are not necessarily equivalent, because in one of the trials of adjuvant ovarian radiation in premenopausal women, 12.7 percent of the irradiated patients subsequently had return of menses.[59] However, in a randomized trial of 112 premenopausal women with breast cancer, prophylactic surgical castration was compared with ovarian radiation. Disease-free survival was very similar with 7 years of follow-up, and crude survival was virtually identical.[205]

Of the three randomized trials of adjuvant oophorectomy in operable breast carcinoma, one showed a statistically significant improvement in disease-free survival and overall survival.[37] In that trial, reported by Bryant and Wier, premenopausal women with clinicopathological stages I and II invasive breast cancer were randomly assigned after mastectomy to no therapy versus prophylactic bilateral oophorectomy. Analysis was performed on 359 patients. Disease-free survival at 5 and 10 years of follow-up was 73 percent and 69 percent, respectively, in the

TABLE 66–9.   CONTROLLED TRIALS OF ADJUVANT CASTRATION FOR EARLY-STAGE BREAST CANCER

Authors	Study Population	No. of Patients	Follow-up (yr)	Relapse-Free Survival (%)		Overall Survival (%)	
				Castration	*Controls*	*Castration*	*Controls*
Surgical Oophorectomy Studies							
Nevinny et al.[204]	Premenopausal or postmenopausal, node negative or positive	143	63 pts followed >5 years	68	54	78	74
Ravdin et al.[222] (NSABP)	Premenopausal, node negative or positive	236	Up to 5	44	45 (Placebo grp)	71	79 (Placebo grp)
Bryant and Weir[37]	Premenopausal, stage I or II	359	10	69*	53	71*	60
Ovarian Radiation Studies							
Nissen-Meyer[205]	Premenopausal (stage I); postmenopausal (stage I, II)	346	More than 15	Significantly improved crude survival and DFS			
Cole[59]	Premenopausal and perimenopausal, node negative or positive (pts allocated by birth month)	598	Up to 15	Not significantly different overall		45	40
Meakin[188, 189]	Age <45 yr (ovarian RT vs. none)	137	Up to 15	No significant differences found			
	Premenopausal, age ≥45 yr (none vs. ovarian RT ± prednisone)	208		Significantly better survival and DFS for RT + prednisone vs. no adjuvant*			
	Postmenopausal (none vs. ovarian RT ± prednisone)	360		No significant differences found			

*Statistically significant difference between treated group and controls.
Abbreviations: RT = radiotherapy; pts = patients; grp = group; DFS = disease-free survival.

oophorectomy group, compared with 65 percent and 53 percent, respectively, in the controls. Crude survival at 5 and 10 years was 81 percent and 71 percent in the adjuvant therapy group versus 77 percent and 60 percent in the controls. These differences were statistically significant. Survival differences at 10 years favoring the oophorectomy group occurred in both stage I and II patients, although not in women with four or more involved axillary nodes. It should be noted that there was a design flaw in this study. Patients were randomized prior to giving consent for oophorectomy. If a patient assigned to the operation refused (or if her physician refused on her behalf), her randomization card was replaced in the randomization deck, and she was not analyzed with the other patients who underwent castration. This could have led to unintentional bias.[49] The authors do not state how many women fell into this category, but characterized the number as few.

The remaining two randomized trials of prophylactic surgical castration show no differences in either disease-free or overall survival.[204, 222] However, follow-up in both of these trials was only 5 years. In the positive trial discussed previously, survival differences did not become apparent for 5 years.[37]

There have been two randomized trials[188, 205] of prophylactic radiation-induced castration and one trial in which patients were allocated by month of birth[59] (see Table 66–9). One of them, conducted at the Princess Margaret Hospital, has been reported after up to 15 years of follow-up and suggests improved disease-free survival as well as overall survival in certain subgroups.[188] A total of 779 premenopausal and postmenopausal women with clinical stage I, II, or III operable breast cancer were entered in the study. After surgery and local radiation, women younger than 45 years were randomized to receive no further treatment versus ovarian radiation (2000 rad in five fractions). Women aged 45 years or older were randomized to no further treatment versus ovarian radiation plus or minus prednisone 7.5 mg per day for up to 5 years. No differences were observed in either disease-free survival or overall survival in postmenopausal women. In premenopausal women younger than 45 years, disease-free and overall survival were superior in the castrated women, but differences were not statistically significant. In premenopausal women 45 years or older, disease-free survival and overall survival were significantly better ($p = 0.04$ and 0.02, respectively) for the castrated women who received prednisone compared with the controls. Differences did not become significant until after 3 to 5 years. Women who received ovarian radiation alone had an intermediate outcome. Recognizing a potential source of bias, the authors reported that the prolongation of survival for the group receiving radiation and prednisone remained significant despite inclusion of 23 ineligible patients and 51 eligible patients who did not receive the treatment to which they were assigned.[129]

A second randomized trial showed similar results favoring ovarian radiation.[205] Nissen-Meyer, reporting from the Norwegian Radium Hospital, conducted a study comparing prophylactic to therapeutic (at recurrence) ovarian radiation. A total of 177 postmenopausal women (stage I and II) and 169 premenopausal women ("good risk" only patients) were entered. With more than 15 years' follow-up, disease-free survival and crude survival were significantly improved in both pre- and postmenopausal patients. Finally, a third large study of ovarian radiation in 598 premenopausal and perimenopausal women with stages I and II cancer showed no significant advantages for the radiation arm after 15 years of follow-up.[59]

Perhaps the best summary of the effect of adjuvant ovarian ablation on relapse-free survival and overall survival is provided by the 1992 overview.[86] For the sake of consistency, the analysis used age as a surrogate for menopausal status. At 15 years of follow-up, women under age 50 who received ovarian ablation had a proportional improvement of 26 percent (SD 6) in recurrence-free survival and 25 percent (SD 7) in overall survival. When adjuvant cytotoxic chemotherapy was used in addition to ovarian ablation, the reduction in recurrence and mortality was still significant, but the benefit was smaller. There was no advantage from ovarian ablation in women over age 50.

Adjuvant Tamoxifen Trials

The rationale for the use of tamoxifen as adjuvant therapy in premenopausal women is supported by two randomized trials of tamoxifen versus oophorectomy, which suggest that the two interventions have similar efficacy in premenopausal women with metastatic breast cancer. A crossover-designed trial in 54 premenopausal women with advanced carcinoma (ER-positive or ER-unknown) showed response rates that were not statistically different between the two treatments—37 percent for oophorectomy versus 27 percent for tamoxifen.[158] Time to progression and survival were virtually identical, although interpretation of survival results is complicated by the crossover design. The statistical power of the study was low, but a large advantage for the oophorectomy group was thought to be unlikely.

Similar results were reported by Buchanan and colleagues in a randomized trial of 107 patients.[39] The response rate to oophorectomy was 21 percent compared with 24 percent for tamoxifen. The median duration of response for tamoxifen was 20 months compared with 7 months for oophorectomy; this difference approached but did not achieve statistical significance ($p = 0.056$).[39] Another comparison of tamoxifen versus ovarian ablation has been provided by the Christie Hospital's adjuvant tamoxifen trial.[227, 228] In this study, premenopausal women with clinical stage T1–T3a, N1–N2b, M0 tumors were ran-

domized to 1 year of tamoxifen (20 mg/day) or to radiation-induced menopause. After 10 years of follow-up, there was a non–statistically significant trend in overall survival favoring the women treated with tamoxifen of 93 percent versus 82 percent for the group with induced menopause ($p = 0.09$).

In elderly women with metastatic disease, tamoxifen appears to have activity that is roughly equivalent to combination chemotherapy. Taylor and associates[265] reported a trial in 181 women aged 65 or older with advanced breast cancer who were randomly assigned to treatment with tamoxifen or to a regimen of CMF. Response rates to tamoxifen were 45 percent versus 38 percent for CMF. Although survival favored the tamoxifen treatment group, the difference was not statistically significant. Moreover, tamoxifen appeared to show efficacy similar to that of CMF in ER-negative and ER-positive patients.

In North America, adjuvant trials have tended to concentrate on the use of chemotherapy in premenopausal women, using tamoxifen as a single agent for postmenopausal women. This dichotomy may be related to the belief that premenopausal women may have enough circulating endogenous estrogens to overcome the effects of tamoxifen. As will be discussed, however, the 1992 overview analysis has suggested that premenopausal breast cancer patients may benefit from the use of adjuvant tamoxifen. For premenopausal women younger than 50, the relative reduction in the odds of death was 6 percent (SD, 5), and for premenopausal women between the ages of 50 and 59, the reduction was 23 percent (SD, 9). Of the trials incorporated in the overview, two European studies are noteworthy for results consistent with the conclusion that the survival advantage and mortality reduction from adjuvant tamoxifen may occur irrespective of menopausal status.[8, 12] In certain subsets of premenopausal women in which tamoxifen may be particularly effective, e.g., those with ER-positive tumors, the therapeutic index for tamoxifen may be superior to that of chemotherapy by virtue of its lower acute toxicity.

As summarized in 1992, there were 40 randomized trials comparing adjuvant treatment with tamoxifen versus the same without tamoxifen.[86] Of these, 12 trials comparing adjuvant tamoxifen to either no adjuvant therapy or to placebo have been summarized in Table 66–10. All but one has demonstrated a statistically significant advantage in relapse-free survival for women randomized to tamoxifen. Several of the trials showing improvement in relapse-free survival were placebo-controlled, which increases the reliability of their findings.[70, 97, 213] Because the ultimate goal of adjuvant therapy is to extend survival, the trials showing significant survival advantages will be discussed in more detail.

In the Nolvadex Adjuvant Trial Organization (NATO) study, reported in 1985[11] and updated in 1988,[12] 1285 premenopausal women with positive axillary nodes and postmenopausal women with positive or negative axillary nodes were randomized either to tamoxifen 10 mg orally twice daily or to

TABLE 66–10. RANDOMIZED TRIALS COMPARING LOCAL THERAPY WITH AND WITHOUT ADJUVANT TAMOXIFEN

Author or Study	Study Population	No. of Patients	Duration of Tamoxifen (yrs)	Follow-Up (yrs)	Relapse-Free Survival (%)		Overall Survival (%)	
					Tamoxifen	Control	Tamoxifen	Control
Node Negative								
Fisher et al.[97]	ER-positive, age ≤ 70 yr, stage T1–T3	2644	At least 5§	Up to 4	83†	77†	93	92
Rutqvist et al.[242]	Postmenopausal, tumor ≤ 3 cm, age < 71 yr	891	At least 2	Median 4.4	0.68(0.49–0.94) Observed: Expected Ratio Favoring T		.88(0.58–1.33) Observed: Expected Ratio	
Wallgren et al.[280]	Postmenopausal, tumor ≤ 3 cm	158	2	Mean 4.1	0.75(0.43–1.30) Observed: Expected Ratio		Not available	
Node Negative and Positive								
Rose et al.[236, 237]	Postmenopausal, tumor > 5 cm or skin/fascia invasion	1650	1	Up to 6	44*	40*	51	51
Bartlett et al.[8]	Postmenopausal and premenopausal, node negative	1312	At least 5§	2.5–8	≈60†	≈40†	≈62†	≈45†
Baum et al.[11, 12]	Postmenopausal and premenopausal, node negative	1285	2	Up to 8	0.64(0.53–0.77) Observed: Expected Ratio Favoring T		0.71(0.58–0.88) Observed: Expected Ratio Favoring T	
Rebeiro and Swindell[226]	Postmenopausal, stages I–III	588	1	Up to 10	71* (Does not include local relapses)	65*	≈62	≈54
Palshoff et al.[213]	Premenopausal, postmenopausal	213 155	2	Median 3.7	Pre 68* Post 83*	61* 68*	0.86 (0.53–1.40) 0.74 (0.37–1.49)	
Node-Positive Studies								
Ludwig[175]	Postmenopausal	629	1	Up to 5	58†	44†	75	80
Pritchard et al.[219]	Postmenopausal	391	2	Median 5.8	≈43†	≈27†	Not available	
Senanayake[250]	Local therapy for curative intent possible	197	2	Up to 5 Median 2	81* (crude)	68* (crude)	89‡ (crude)	82‡ (crude)
Cummings et al.[70]	Age > 65 yr	170	2	41 mo (median)	76†	52†	80	70

*p < 0.05 for tamoxifen vs. control.
†p < 0.005 for tamoxifen vs. control.
‡p = 0.06 for tamoxifen vs. control.
§Patients receiving tamoxifen were randomized after 5 years to continue or to receive placebo.
Abbreviations: Pre = premenopausal women; post = postmenopausal women; T = tamoxifen.

no adjuvant therapy after mastectomy and axillary dissection. Overall survival was superior in the treated group ($p = 0.0001$), representing a 0.71 observed:expected mortality ratio in the tamoxifen group. Only 524 of the primary tumors (46 percent) were assayed for ER content. Interestingly, the hazard ratios for disease-free survival and overall survival were similar for patients with ER-positive and ER-negative tumors, when the separation was based on levels less than 30 fmol versus higher levels.[256] The result was unchanged by using lower cutoff points, but the comparison was statistically weakened. Regression analysis also showed no interaction between treatment effect and either menopausal or nodal status. Results were virtually identical at the 6- and 8-year updates of the trial, though significant differences in survival did not emerge until the third and fourth years.

In the Scottish trial begun in 1978, node-negative premenopausal and node-negative or node-positive postmenopausal women who had undergone definitive local therapy were randomized to receive prophylactic tamoxifen 20 mg daily for 5 years versus thera-

peutic tamoxifen at first relapse.[8] A total of 1312 eligible patients younger than 80 years were randomized, and a full report was made, with follow-up ranging from 2.5 to 8 years. Estrogen receptor status was available in 57 percent of patients. As in the NATO trial, there was a statistically significant reduction in mortality for the adjuvant tamoxifen arm ($p = 0.002$; hazard ratio = 0.71). Again as in the NATO trial, there was a consistent benefit regardless of ER, nodal, or menopausal status.

Initial results have been reported from a trial performed by the International Adjuvant Trial Organization (IATO) in node-positive patients with early breast cancer.[250] After "definitive" local therapy, 399 node-positive patients were randomized to one of four arms: no adjuvant therapy, tamoxifen 40 mg orally per day for 2 years, CMF, and CMF plus tamoxifen. After a median follow-up of 2 years (range, 3 months to about 5 years), the tamoxifen arm showed an improved survival ($p = 0.06$) and disease-free survival ($p = 0.02$) compared with the control arm. The remaining two study arms gave very similar results to the tamoxifen alone arm but were associated with more toxicity. No information was given on the effects of treatments in subgroups.

Duration of Treatment with Adjuvant Tamoxifen

When adjuvant tamoxifen is used, a question remains concerning the optimal duration of treatment. The answer is not yet known, but an upper limit has been suggested by information from NSABP B-14 and the Scottish adjuvant tamoxifen trial. Both of these trials examined the use of adjuvant tamoxifen beyond 5 years. In the NSABP trial of adjuvant tamoxifen, women with node-negative, ER-positive primary tumors were randomized to receive tamoxifen versus placebo for 5 years. A registration group was also treated with tamoxifen for 5 years, yielding a pool of 1166 women who were subsequently randomized to receive an additional 5 years of tamoxifen versus placebo.[57] After an average follow-up of 43 months beyond the initial 5-year period of tamoxifen treatment, the relapse-free survival in the two groups was compared. After 5 years of disease-free survival while taking tamoxifen therapy, 92 percent of the women who were subsequently treated with placebo remained disease free, compared with 86 percent who continued to take tamoxifen. This difference was based on an interim analysis and did not reach statistical significance; however, it was concluded that continued use of tamoxifen was unlikely to produce additional benefit compared with that obtained from the initial 5 years of tamoxifen therapy. As a result, the NSABP stopped protocol therapy in the B-14 study.

In the Scottish trial of adjuvant tamoxifen, there was a group of patients who were also randomized to additional tamoxifen beyond an initial 5 years of treatment. Unlike NSABP B-14, the Scottish trial included node-positive women, and ER levels were not required. From the initial pool of 1312 women, 342 patients participated in the second randomization for tamoxifen beyond 5 years, with 173 assigned to indefinite use of 20 mg of tamoxifen daily. With a median follow-up of 6.2 years, relapse-free survival since rerandomization was 62 percent for those who continued tamoxifen compared with 70 percent for those who discontinued tamoxifen. This evidence falls short of statistical significance, but is consistent with a trend that favors stopping tamoxifen at 5 years. The results from the Scottish trial and NSABP B-14 suggest that 5 years of adjuvant tamoxifen in a routine clinical setting is a reasonable standard of practice. Future results from ongoing tamoxifen studies may provide clarification about optimizing the duration of adjuvant tamoxifen according to patient characteristics.

Tamoxifen Toxicity

Tamoxifen in the adjuvant setting is a very well-tolerated medication. One of the most instructive sources of information about tamoxifen toxicity is the NSABP B-14 trial for node-negative women.[52] Because this trial was randomized and placebo-controlled, it allows a direct comparison of toxicities between tamoxifen and placebo. In this setting, tamoxifen-associated symptoms and their frequency have been reported as hot flushes (62 percent), fluid retention (31 percent), vaginal discharge (28 percent), nausea (23 percent), and skin rash (18 percent). Without the placebo comparison, these results would give a misleading picture of tamoxifen symptoms.[52] For example the frequency of fluid retention and nausea was no different in placebo-treated patients than in patients treated with tamoxifen. Forty-six percent of women on placebo reported having hot flushes, 14 percent had vaginal discharge, and 14 percent had skin rashes. The high prevalence of hot flushes, vaginal discharge, and skin rashes without tamoxifen therapy needs to be considered when symptoms from this therapy are discussed. Less frequent toxicities associated with tamoxifen include leukopenia, thrombocytopenia, and visual abnormalities. Retinopathy has been reported with long-term (more than 1 year) use of tamoxifen,[165] but usually at doses in the range of 60 to 100 mg/m^2, far above those used in the adjuvant setting.[14] The phenomenon of tamoxifen "flare" (increase in bone pain or hypercalcemia shortly after starting therapy) is associated with widespread bony metastases and has not been reported in the adjuvant setting.

Two life-threatening toxicities associated with tamoxifen therapy, thrombophlebitis and endometrial cancer, present the greatest concern to physicians and their patients who take tamoxifen. In the NSABP B-14 trial, the NSABP observed thromboembolic events in 1.5 percent of the patients taking tamoxifen, compared with 0.2 percent in the placebo arm. Most of these events were limited to reports of venous thrombosis, but 0.4 percent involved pulmonary emboli and 0.1 percent deaths.[221] Similarly, Scottish investigators reported that nonusers of tamoxifen in their adjuvant trial had significantly fewer thromboembolic events, with a hazard ratio of 0.4 (95 percent CI = 0.18–0.9).[183]

It has been reported by the NSABP that in women taking tamoxifen as part of the B-14 study, the risk of developing endometrial cancer was two per thousand per year.[98] This level was about three times the rate that would be expected on the basis of Surveillance, Epidemiology, and End Results (SEER*) registry figures. Indeed, an additional source has reported the relative risk for endometrial cancer in tamoxifen users to be between two and three per thousand.[276] Excess endometrial cancer was also reported in the Stockholm adjuvant tamoxifen trial.[126] The details of this association have yet to be worked out; for example, an assessment of the role of prior hormonal therapy has not yet been made. Not all sources of data indicate that endometrial cancer is increased in the

---

*The SEER registry is a data base collecting cancer data from population-based cancer registries covering approximately 15 percent of the population of the United States.[230]

setting of tamoxifen therapy. In a case-control study, Cook and associates found that for a duration of tamoxifen use less than 2 years, the relative risk of several second primary cancers, including endometrial cancers, was less than 1, with the 95 percent confidence interval overlapping 1.[61] This result is consistent with no association between tamoxifen and endometrial cancer, under the conditions of the analysis. This kind of information must be balanced with other observations such as those from a series of 111 patients who were randomized to tamoxifen or placebo in a British tamoxifen trial.[166] In this group, 16 percent of the women taking tamoxifen were reported to have atypical hyperplasia on uterine sampling. Having reviewed the issue of endometrial cancer in breast cancer patients being treated with tamoxifen, the American College of Obstetrics and Gynecology has recently prepared an advisory statement, recommending an annual gynecologic evaluation of patients using tamoxifen, with the decision about screening, e.g., endometrial sampling, to be left to the discretion of the physician.[261]

Among the many toxicity concerns that have surfaced as a result of the extensive experience from using tamoxifen for breast cancer patients, liver toxicity is rare. There have been occasional reports of liver necrosis[50] and hepatocellular carcinoma in patients using tamoxifen.[126] At this time, four cases of hepatocellular carcinoma have been reported in the tamoxifen arms of two breast cancer trials evaluating adjuvant tamoxifen therapy.[5, 244] In these trials there were also three cases of liver cancer in the control arms, leaving doubt as to whether there is any difference in the frequency of liver cancer in the two groups.

Although tamoxifen toxicity has been a focus of much attention associated with tamoxifen therapy, there are beneficial outcomes beyond the reported increases in relapse-free and overall survival. In the Scottish trial of adjuvant tamoxifen, the women treated with tamoxifen experienced fewer cardiac events.[182, 183] A similar experience was reported by Swedish investigators.[243] Another benefit that is anticipated from tamoxifen therapy in postmenopausal women is the maintenance of bone density.[172] One subset of women, however, who may not experience this benefit are premenopausal women. Powles and associates reported that a group of 125 premenopausal women taking 20 mg of tamoxifen daily experienced on average a significant loss in bone mineral density from lumbar spine and hip of about 1 percent a year during an observation period of 3 years.[218] In the same study, tamoxifen had the opposite effect in postmenopausal women. When survival benefits related to adjuvant tamoxifen therapy are considered in the context of its other potential benefits and the various toxicities noted above, tamoxifen has an overwhelmingly favorable therapeutic index for breast cancer patients.

Other Adjuvant Hormonal Therapies

There have been few trials of other forms of adjuvant hormonal therapy for breast cancer, and even fewer

have been randomized. A 2-year course of aminoglutethimide plus hydrocortisone has been tested by the Collaborative Breast Cancer Project in a randomized placebo-controlled study of 354 node-positive postmenopausal women.[63, 162] The aminoglutethimide successfully suppressed circulating levels of dehydroepiandrosterone over the 2-year period that patients were treated.[62, 63] However, there was no advantage in relapse-free or overall survival after a median of 8 years of follow-up. Interim analyses showed an advantage from aminoglutethimide therapy compared with placebo for relapse-free survival up to the 4-year point, and a marginal benefit in relapse-free survival in that subset of patients who were ER-positive. Given the reported toxicities, which included 2 percent agranulocytosis and 17 percent ataxia (versus 0 and 4 percent, respectively, with placebo) and the lack of survival benefit, aminoglutethimide is not an attractive candidate for adjuvant hormonal therapy. Newer, more specific aromatase inhibitors have not been evaluated in the adjuvant setting. Limited data are available for a randomized comparison of adjuvant high-dose medroxyprogesterone acetate (MPA) compared with no adjuvant treatment in 216 node-negative early breast cancer patients.[125] Treatment with MPA was given intramuscularly in doses of 500 mg per day, such that either 25 or 28 doses were delivered in a period of 4 to 5 weeks. Afterward, MPA was given twice weekly for an additional 5 months. An interim report for median follow-up time of at least 32 months showed a statistically significant advantage in relapse-free survival of 94 percent for MPA versus 73 percent without MPA. Overall survival for the MPA-treated group was 99 percent compared with 89 percent without MPA.

A Copenhagen Breast Cancer Trial compared a study of diethylstilbestrol versus tamoxifen versus controls in postmenopausal women with operable breast cancer.[213] There were no significant differences in disease-free survival or overall survival, and more than 40 percent of the women receiving diethylstilbestrol discontinued therapy because of toxicity. It is not likely that these alternate forms of hormonal therapy will be developed extensively in the adjuvant setting, unless their risk-benefit profile compares favorably with that of tamoxifen.

Trials Evaluating the Addition of Hormonal Therapy to Chemotherapy

A somewhat separate issue is whether hormonal manipulations can improve the therapeutic efficacy of adjuvant chemotherapy. There are theoretical arguments both for and against this hypothesis. Hormonal therapy may act on a different subpopulation of malignant cells than those affected by "cytolytic" agents. On the other hand, endocrine treatments may theoretically interfere with the impact of cytotoxic chemotherapy by reducing the growth fraction or altering the transport of cytotoxic drugs into malignant cells. Although there are in vitro data to support these possibilities, none of this information resolves the issue. A number of randomized trials have been performed comparing chemotherapy with chemohormonal therapy.* Some have shown a trend toward enhanced survival with chemohormonal treatment,[250, 281] whereas others have shown a trend toward worsened survival.[155] The NSABP trial of melphalan and 5-FU with and without tamoxifen showed opposite trends in survival for patients age 49 or younger versus those older than 49.[106] Thus, the issue of the impact of hormonal therapy on concomitant chemotherapy remains unresolved.

Because of the scarcity of information about using hormonal therapy either concurrently or sequentially with chemotherapy, results from an overview analysis could become especially useful. In the 1992 overview, there were insufficient numbers of women under the age of 50 for a comparison to be made.[87] For women older than age 50, when chemotherapy was used with tamoxifen, the reduction in odds of recurrence and death were 26 and 14 percent, respectively. These values compare with an odds reduction of 22 percent in recurrence and 10 percent in death in women who only received chemotherapy. It is expected that an update of the overview will provide additional detail about any improvement in outcome that can be obtained by using both therapies. Ongoing studies are also expected to provide new data addressing this issue; for example, the Adjuvant Breast Cancer (ABC) trial was launched in 1993, by four collaborating groups of breast cancer trialists in the United Kingdom.[38] The underlying premise of this trial is that all participants receive adjuvant tamoxifen therapy for 5 years. For premenopausal participants, there is a randomization for ovarian suppression versus none, chemotherapy versus none, or randomization for both modalities. Postmenopausal patients are randomized for the addition of chemotherapy.

SUMMARY

In 1985, the recommendation made at the National Institutes of Health Consensus Development Conference on Adjuvant Chemotherapy and Endocrine Therapy for Breast Cancer[201] was that adjuvant tamoxifen should be considered standard therapy for postmenopausal women with hormone receptor–positive tumors and axillary node involvement. Given the availability of additional results since 1985, the rationale for using hormonal therapy in ER-positive patients has been strengthened. For a number of years, an international consensus panel has met to develop guidelines and recommendations related to adjuvant systemic therapy for breast cancer. The 4th International Conference on Adjuvant Therapy of Primary Breast Cancer took place in 1992 and provided conclusions incorporating the results from the most recent overview analysis performed

by the Early Breast Cancer Trialists' Collaborative Group.[134] The question of adjuvant therapy was revisited at the 5th International Conference, which took place in March 1995 at St. Gallen, Switzerland.[138]

Node-Positive Postmenopausal Women

Consistent with previous recommendations that adjuvant tamoxifen was the treatment of choice for node-positive, ER-positive postmenopausal breast cancer patients, the international experts continued to view tamoxifen as the mainstay of treatment, but noted that the question of an advantage from tamoxifen and chemotherapy versus tamoxifen alone remains the subject of ongoing research. However, the use of chemotherapy in physiologically elderly, node-positive women was not a consideration. On the basis of the recent Clinical Announcement, 5 years of tamoxifen as adjuvant therapy is generally appropriate, unless evidence becomes available to recommend a different duration of therapy.[57]

In node-positive postmenopausal women who are ER-negative, the mainstay of treatment is chemotherapy. Whether the use chemotherapy and tamoxifen is more beneficial than chemotherapy alone has not been decided.

Node-Positive Premenopausal Women

For node-positive, ER-positive premenopausal women, the options from St. Gallen for treating these patients were numerous; however, chemotherapy was one of two therapies recognized for routine use. Whether the results from chemotherapy may be enhanced by adding tamoxifen or ovarian ablation remains a research question. Ovarian ablation was noted as a second standard therapy for ER-positive women in this category. Benefit from adding tamoxifen to ovarian ablation is the subject of ongoing research.

For premenopausal women with positive nodes and ER-negative tumors, chemotherapy was the sole adjuvant option advised by the international consensus panel. In general, either 6 cycles of CMF or 4 cycles of an anthracycline-based regimen are appropriate as adjuvant chemotherapy.[138]

Node-Negative Women With Low Risk

Node-negative women at low risk of recurrence were defined as individuals older than 35 years with well-differentiated tumors that are ER-positive and smaller than 1 cm. No therapy was recognized as being routinely appropriate for this category of patients. On the basis of ER positivity, the international experts advised that tamoxifen be considered optional.

Node-Negative Women With Moderate Risk

Node-negative women at moderate risk of recurrence were defined as patients with tumors between 1 and

---

*See references 106, 155, 157, 177, 250, 267, 269 and 281.

2 cm in size, ER-positive, and of histological grade 1 or 2. The international panel noted that tamoxifen was the standard therapy for women in this category. On the basis of ongoing research, oophorectomy chemotherapy, or a gonadotropin-releasing hormone were cited as interventions that may prove to be useful for this category of ER-positive, premenopausal women in the future.

Node-Negative Women With High Risk

Node-negative women at high risk of recurrence were described as patients with tumors characterized by any one of several factors, including size greater than 2 cm, a histological grade of 2 or 3, and ER negativity. Chemotherapy was noted as the routine treatment for premenopausal women at high risk of recurrence. In conjunction with chemotherapy, for high-risk premenopausal women who were ER-positive, tamoxifen, oophorectomy, and a gonadotropin-releasing hormone analogue are the subjects of ongoing research that might find future application in this setting. For postmenopausal women, the standard therapy was noted as tamoxifen for ER-positive tumors, or chemotherapy for ER-negative tumors. Chemoendocrine therapy may be a future consideration when the results of ongoing studies become available.

With the information currently available, physicians are able better than ever to provide an estimate of the risk of breast cancer recurrence and the impact of adjuvant therapy on preventing recurrence. Just as there is heterogeneity in tumor biology, there is also variability among patients in risk of recurrence and the acceptability of any particular adjuvant therapy in terms of its projected benefits and toxicities. Because the number of women who could obtain a survival benefit from adjuvant therapy is large, adjuvant systemic therapy has been seen as an important advance in breast cancer control, however, the number of women who can be expected to have recurrence after adjuvant therapy is also large. For the immediate future, it appears that efforts to improve adjuvant therapy will focus on high-dose and dose-intense treatments.

In addition, several new agents active against advanced breast cancer, such as taxanes like paclitaxel and taxotere may find application in the adjuvant setting. At the M.D. Anderson Cancer Center, a randomized phase II trial is in progress comparing 4 cycles of paclitaxel followed by four cycles of FAC with 8 cycles of FAC as adjuvant therapy for stage II and III breast cancer patients.[152] A feasibility study of a dose-intense regimen for adjuvant therapy in the cooperative group setting using cyclophosphamide and doxorubicin followed by paclitaxel as a non–cross-resistant agent has been described.[81] Ultimately, an understanding of disease progression at the molecular level may permit specific and individualized therapies.

References

1. Aaltomaa S, Lipponen P, Eskelinen M, et al: Prognostic factors in axillary lymph node-negative (pN-) breast carcinomas. Eur J Cancer 27:1255–1259, 1991.

2. Abeloff MD, Beveridge RA, Donehower RC, et al: Sixteen-week dose-intense chemotherapy in the adjuvant treatment of breast cancer. J Natl Cancer Inst 82:570–574, 1990.

3. Ahmann DL, O'Fallon JR, Scanlon PW, et al: A preliminary assessment of factors associated with recurrent disease in a surgical adjuvant clinical trial for patients with breast cancer with special emphasis on the aggressiveness of therapy. Am J Clin Oncol 5:371–381, 1982.

4. Allegra JA, Barlock A, Huff KK, et al: Changes in multiple or sequential estrogen receptor determinations in breast cancer. Cancer 45:792–794, 1980.

5. Andersson M, Storm HH, Mouridsen HT: Incidence of new primary cancers after adjuvant tamoxifen therapy and radiotherapy for early breast cancer. J Natl Cancer Inst 83:1013–1017, 1991.

6. Ashworth TR: A case of cancer in which cells similar to those in the tumors were seen in the blood after death. Aust Med J 14:146, 1869.

7. Bailar JC III, Louis TA, Lavori PW, et al: Studies without internal controls. N Engl J Med 311:156–162, 1984.

8. Bartlett K, Eremin O, Hutcheon A, et al: Adjuvant tamoxifen in the management of operable breast cancer: The Scottish trial. Lancet 2:171–175, 1987.

9. Bauer T, O'Ceallaigh D, Ellgeston J, et al: Prognostic factors in patients with Stage I, estrogen receptor-negative carcinoma of the breast. Cancer 52:1423–1431, 1983.

10. Baum M: The curability of breast cancer. Br Med J 1:439, 1976.

11. Baum M, Brinkley CM, Dossett JA, et al: Controlled trial of tamoxifen as single adjuvant agent in management of early breast cancer: Analysis at six years by Nolvadex Adjuvant Trial Organization. Lancet 1:836–840, 1985.

12. Baum M, Brinkley CM, Dossett JA, et al: Controlled trial of tamoxifen as a single agent in the management of early breast cancer: Analysis at eight years by Nolvadex Adjuvant Trial Organization. Br J Cancer 57:608–611, 1988.

13. Beatson GT: On the treatment of inoperable cases of carcinoma of the mamma: Suggestions for a new method of treatment with illustrative cases. Lancet 2:104–107, 1896.

14. Beck M, Mills PV: Ocular assessment of patients treated with tamoxifen. Cancer Treat Rep 63:1833–1834, 1979.

15. Berg JW, Robbins GF: Factors influencing short and long term survival of breast cancer patients. Surg Gynecol Obstet 1311–1316, 1966.

16. Bevilacqua P, Barbareschi M, Verderio P, et al: Prognostic value of intratumoral microvessel density, a measure of tumor angiogenesis, in node-negative breast carcinoma: Results of a multiparametric study. Breast Cancer Res Treat 36:205–217, 1995.

17. Bhardwaj S, Holland JF, Norton L: An intensive sequenced adjuvant chemotherapy regimen for breast cancer. Cancer Invest 11:6–9, 1993.

18. Bonadonna G: Evolving concepts in the systemic adjuvant treatment of breast cancer. Cancer Res 52:2127–2137, 1992.

19. Bonadonna G, Brusamolino E, Valagussa P, et al: Combination chemotherapy as an adjuvant treatment in operable breast cancer. N Engl J Med 294:405–410, 1976.

20. Bonadonna G, Rossi A, Valagussa P: Adjuvant CMT chemotherapy in operable breast cancer: Ten years later. Lancet 1:976–977, 1985.

21. Bonadonna G, Rossi A, Valagussa P: Adjuvant CMT chemotherapy in operable breast cancer: Ten years later. World J Surg 9:707–713, 1985.

22. Bonadonna G, Rossi A, Valagussa P: The CMF program for operable breast cancer with positive axillary nodes. Cancer 39:2904–2915, 1977.

23. Bonadonna G, Valagussa P: Dose-intense adjuvant treatment of high-risk breast cancer. J Natl Cancer Inst 82:542–543, 1990.

24. Bonadonna G, Valagussa P: Adjuvant systemic therapy for resectable breast cancer. J Clin Oncol 3:259–275, 1985.

25. Bonadonna G, Valagussa P: Current status of adjuvant chemotherapy for breast cancer. Semin Oncol 14:8–22, 1987.

26. Bonadonna G, Valagussa P: Dose-response effect of adjuvant chemotherapy in breast cancer. N Engl J Med 304:10–15, 1981.

27. Bonadonna G, Valagussa P: Contribution of prognostic factors to adjuvant chemotherapy in breast cancer. Recent Results Cancer Res 96:34–45, 1984.
28. Bonadonna G, Valagussa P: Comment on "The methodologic dilemma in retrospectively correlating the amount of chemotherapy received in adjuvant therapy protocols with disease-free survival." Cancer Treat Rep 67:527–529, 1983.
29. Bonadonna G, Valagussa P, Moliterni A, et al: Adjuvant cyclophosphamide, methotrexate, and fluorouracil in node-positive breast cancer: The results of 20 years of follow-up. N Engl J Med 332:901–906, 1995.
30. Bonadonna G, Valagussa P, Rossi A, et al: Ten-year experience with CMF-based adjuvant chemotherapy in resectable breast cancer. Breast Cancer Res Treat 5:95–115, 1985.
31. Bonadonna G, Valagussa P, Tancini G, et al: Current status of Milan adjuvant chemotherapy trials for node-positive and node-negative breast cancer. NCI Monogr 1:45–49, 1986.
32. Bonadonna G, Valagussa P, Zambetti M, et al: Milan adjuvant trials for stage I-II breast cancer. In Salmon S (ed): Adjuvant Therapy of Cancer. Orlando, Grune & Stratton, 1987, pp 211–222.
33. Bonadonna G, Zambetti M, Valagussa P: Sequential or alternating doxorubicin and CMF regimens in breast cancer with more than three positive nodes: Ten-year results. JAMA 273:542–547, 1995.
34. Brambilla C, Delena M, Rossi A, et al: Response and survival in advanced breast cancer after two noncross-resistant combinations. Br Med J 1:801–804, 1976.
35. Brambilla C, Rossi A, Valagussa P, et al: Adjuvant chemotherapy in postmenopausal women: Results of sequential noncross-resistant regimens. World J Surg 9:728–737, 1985.
36. Brincker H, Rose C, Rank F, et al, Danish Breast Cancer Cooperative Group: Evidence of a castration-mediated effect of adjuvant cytotoxic chemotherapy in premenopausal breast cancer. J Clin Oncol 5:1771–1778, 1987.
37. Bryant AJS, Weir JA: Prophylactic oophorectomy in operable instances of carcinoma of the breast. Surg Gynecol Obstet 153:660–664, 1981.
38. Brunt AM, ABC Trial Steering Committee: The UKCCCR adjuvant breast cancer (ABC) trial. Clin Oncol 6:209–210, 1994.
39. Buchanan RB, Blamey KR, Durrant A, et al: A randomized comparison of tamoxifen with surgical oophorectomy in premenopausal patients with advanced breast cancer. J Clin Oncol 4:1326–1330, 1986.
40. Bull J, Tormey DC, Li SH, et al: A randomized comparative trial of adriamycin versus methotrexate in combination drug therapy. Cancer 41:1649–1657, 1978.
41. Buzdar AU, Kau S-W, Hortobagyi GN, et al: Clinical course of patients with breast cancer with ten or more positive nodes who were treated with doxorubicin-containing adjuvant therapy. Cancer 69:448–452, 1992.
42. Buzdar A, Kau S, Smith T, et al: Ten year results of FAC adjuvant chemotherapy trial in breast cancer. Am J Clin Oncol 12:123–128, 1989.
43. Buzzoni R, Bonadonna G, Valagussa P, Zambetti M: Adjuvant chemotherapy with doxorubicin plus cyclophosphamide, methotrexate, and fluorouracil in the treatment of resectable breast cancer with more than three positive axillary nodes. J Clin Oncol 9:2134–2140.
44. Caprini JA, Oviedo MA, Cunningham MP, et al.: Adjuvant chemotherapy in stage II and III carcinoma of the breast. JAMA 244:243–246, 1981.
45. Carpenter JT, Maddox WA, Laws HL, et al: Favorable factors in the adjuvant therapy of breast cancer. Cancer 50:18–23, 1982.
46. Carpenter JT, Velez-Garcia E, Aron BS, et al: Prospective randomized comparison of cyclophosphamide, doxorubicin (adriamycin) and fluorouracil (CAF) vs. cyclophosphamide, methotrexate and fluorouracil (CMF) for breast cancer with positive axillary nodes: A Southeastern Cancer Study Group Study. Proc Am Soc Clin Oncol 10:45, 1991.
47. Carpenter JT, Velez-Garcia E, Aron BS, et al: Five-year results of a randomized comparison of cyclophosphamide, doxorubicin (adriamycin) (CAF) vs. cyclophos-
phamide, methotrexate and fluorouracil (CMF) for node postive breast cancer: A Southeastern Cancer Study Group Study. Proc Am Soc Clin Oncol 13:66, 1994.
48. Carter CL, Allen C, Henson DE: Relation of tumor size, lymph node status, and survival in 24,740 breast cancer cases. Cancer 63:181–187, 1989.
49. Chalmers TC, Celano P, Sacks HS, et al: Bias in treatment assignment in controlled clinical trials. N Engl J Med 309:1358–1361, 1983.
50. Ching CK, Smith PG, Long RG: Tamoxifen-associated hepatocellular damage and agranulocytosis. Lancet 339:940, 1992.
51. Chlebowski RT, Weiner JM, Reynolds R, et al: Long term survival following relapse after 5-FU but not CMF adjuvant breast cancer therapy. Breast Cancer Res Treat 7:23–29, 1986.
52. Chlebowski RT, Butler J, Nelson A, et al: Breast cancer chemoprevention—Tamoxifen: Current issues and future prospective. Cancer 72:1032–1037, 1993.
53. Clahsen PC, van de Velde CJH, Welvaart K, et al: Ten-year results of a randomized trial evaluating prolonged low-dose adjuvant chemotherapy in node-positive breast cancer: A joint European Organization for Research and Treatment of Cancer—Dutch Breast Cancer Working Party study. J Clin Oncol 13:33–41, 1995.
54. Clark GM, Dressler LG, Owens MA, et al: Prediction of relapse or survival in patients with node-negative breast cancer by DNA flow cytometry. N Engl J Med 320:627–633, 1989.
55. Clark GM, Osborne CK, McGuire WL: Correlations between estrogen receptor, progesterone receptor, and patient characteristics in human breast cancer. J Clin Oncol 2:1102–1109, 1984.
56. Clinical Alert. National Cancer Institute, May 18, 1988.
57. Clinical Announcement. Adjuvant therapy of breast cancer—tamoxifen update. National Cancer Institute, November 30, 1995.
58. Cohen E, Scanlon EF, Caprini JA, et al: Follow-up adjuvant chemotherapy and chemoimmunotherapy for stage II and III carcinoma of the breast. Cancer 49:1754–1761, 1982.
59. Cole MP: A clinical trial of an artificial menopause in carcinoma of the breast. In Namer M, Lalanne CM (eds): Hormones and Breast Cancer. 55. Paris, INSERM, 1975, pp 143–150.
60. Consensus Conference: Adjuvant chemotherapy for breast cancer. JAMA 254:3461–3463, 1985.
61. Cook LS, Weiss NS, Schwartz SM, et al: Population-based study of tamoxifen therapy and subsequent ovarian, endometrial, and breast cancers. J Natl Cancer Inst 87:1359–1364, 1995.
62. Coombes RC, Chilvers C, Powles TJ: Adjuvant aminoglutethimide therapy for postmenopausal patients with primary breast cancer. In Jones SE, Salmon SE (eds): Adjuvant Therapy of Cancer. Vol 4. Orlando, Grune & Stratton, 1984, pp 349–357.
63. Coombes RC, Chilvers C, Dowsett M, et al: Adjuvant aminoglutethimide therapy for postmenopausal patients with primary breast cancer: Progress report. Cancer Res 42 (Suppl):3415s–3419s, 1982.
64. Coombes RC, Bliss JM, Wils J, et al: Adjuvant cyclophosphamide, methotrexate, and fluorouracil versus fluorouracil, epirubicin, and cyclophosphamide chemotherapy in premenopausal women with axillary node-positive operable breast cancer: Results of a randomized trial. J Clin Oncol 14:35–45, 1996.
65. Coppin CML, Goldie JH: Adjuvant therapy for breast cancer. N Engl J Med 331:742, 1994. Letter.
66. Coronary Drug Project Research Group: Influence of adherence to treatment and response of cholesterol on mortality in the Coronary Drug Project. N Engl J Med 303:1038–1041, 1980.
67. Creech RH, Dayal H, Alberts R, et al: A comparison of L-PAM and low dose CMF as adjuvant therapy for breast cancer patients with nodal metastases. Proc American Association for Cancer Research 24:148, 1983.

68. Crump M, Goss PE, Prince M, et al: Outcome of extensive evaluation before adjuvant therapy in women with breast cancer and 10 or more positive axillary lymph nodes. J Clin Oncol 14:66–69, 1996.

69. Cruz EP, McDonald GO, Cole WH: Prophylactic treatment of cancer: The use of chemotherapeutic agents to prevent tumor metastasis. Surgery 40:291–296, 1986.

70. Cummings FJ, Gray R, Davis TE, et al: Adjuvant tamoxifen treatment of elderly women with stage II breast cancer: A double-blind comparison with placebo. Ann Intern Med 103:324–329, 1985.

71. Curtis RE, Boice JD, Stovall M, et al: Risk of leukemia after chemotherapy and radiation treatment for breast cancer. N Engl J Med 326:1745–1751, 1992.

72. Cutler SJ, Myers H, Green SB: Trend in survival rates in patients with cancer. N Engl J Med 293:122, 1975.

73. Davidson NE, Abeloff MD: Adjuvant systemic therapy in women with early-stage breast cancer at high risk for relapse. J Natl Cancer Inst 84:301–305, 1992.

74. Davidson NE, Abeloff MD: Adjuvant therapy of breast cancer. World J Surg 18:112–116, 1994.

75. Davis HL, Metter GE, Romirez G, et al: An adjuvant trial of L-phenylalanine (L-PAM) vs cyclophosphamide (C), methotrexate (M), 5-fluorouracil (F), and vincristine (V) (CMF-V) following mastectomy for operable breast cancer. Proc Am Soc Clin Oncol 22:426, 1981.

76. Day RS: Treatment sequencing, asymmetry, and uncertainty: Protocol strategies for combination chemotherapy. Cancer Res 46:3876–3885, 1986.

77. DeCoumelles F: Action atrophique glandulaire des rayons. CR Acad Sci (D) (Paris) 140:606, 1905.

78. De La Rochefordiere A, Asselain B, Campana F, et al: Age as prognostic factor in premenopausal breast carcinoma. Lancet 341:1039–1043, 1993.

79. DeCillis A, Anderson S, Wickerham DL, et al: Acute myeloid leukemia (AML) in NSABP B-25. Proc Am Soc Clin Oncol 14:98, 1995.

80. Delarue NC: The free cancer cell. Can Med Assoc J 82:1175–1182, 1960.

81. Demetri GD, Berry D, Younger J, et al: Dose-intensified cyclophosphamide/doxorubicin (CD) followed by taxol (T) as adjuvant systemic chemotherapy for node-positive breast cancer (CALGB 9141): Randomized comparison of two dose levels of G-CSF. Proc Am Soc Clin Oncol 13:65, 1994.

82. Diehl LF, Perry DJ: A comparison of randomized concurrent control groups with matched historical control groups: Are historical controls valid? J Clin Oncol 4:1114–1120, 1986.

83. Dimitrov N, Anderson S, Fisher B, et al: Dose intensification and increased total dose of adjuvant chemotherapy for breast cancer (BC): Findings from NSABP B-22. Proc Am Soc Clin Oncol 13:64, 1994.

84. Dnistrian AM, Schwartz MK, Fracchia AA, et al: Endocrine consequences of CMF adjuvant therapy in premenopausal and postmenopausal breast cancer patients. Cancer 51:803–807, 1983.

85. Early Breast Cancer Trialists' Collaborative Group: Effects of adjuvant tamoxifen and of cytotoxic therapy on mortality in early breast cancer: An overview of 61 randomized trials among 28,896 women. N Engl J Med 319:1681–1692, 1988.

86. Early Breast Cancer Trialists' Collaborative Group: Systemic treatment of early breast cancer by hormonal, cytotoxic, or immune therapy: 133 randomised trials involving 31,000 recurrences and 24,000 deaths among 75,000 women. Lancet 339:1–15, 1992.

87. Early Breast Cancer Trialists' Collaborative Group: Systemic treatment of early breast cancer by hormonal, cytotoxic, or immune therapy: 133 randomised trials involving 31,000 recurrences and 24,000 deaths among 75,000 women. Lancet 339:71–85, 1992.

88. Ellenberg SS: Meta-analysis: The quantitative approach to research review. Semin Oncol 15:472–481, 1988.

89. Engell HC: Cancer cells in the blood: A five to nine year follow-up study. Ann Surg 147:457–461, 1959.

90. Ewers S-B, Baldetorp B, Killander D, et al: Flow cytometry DNA ploidy and number of cell populations in the primary breast and their correlation to the prognosis. Acta Oncol 28:913–918, 1989.

91. Falkson HC, Gray R, Wolberg WH, et al: Adjuvant trial of 12 cycles of CMFPT followed by observation or continuous tamoxifen versus four cycles of CMFPT in postmenopausal women with breast cancer: An Eastern Cooperative Oncology Group phase III study. J Clin Oncol 8:599–607, 1990.

92. Fidler IJ, Poste G: The cellular heterogeneity of malignant neoplasma: Implications for adjuvant chemotherapy. Semin Oncol 12:207–221, 1985.

93. Fisher B: A biological perspective of breast cancer: Contributions of the National Surgical Adjuvant Breast and Bowel Project clinical trials. CA Cancer J Clin 41:97–111, 1991.

94. Fisher B: Biological and clinical considerations regarding the use of surgery and chemotherapy in the treatment of primary breast cancer. Cancer 40:574, 1977.

95. Fisher B: The clinical scientific basis of adjuvant chemotherapy in breast cancer. Recent Results Cancer Res 96:8–17, 1984.

96. Fisher B, Carbone P, Economou SG, et al: L-phenylalanine mustard (L-PAM) in the management of primary breast cancer: A report of early findings. N Engl J Med 292:117–122, 1975.

97. Fisher B, Costantino J, Redmond C: A randomized clinical trial evaluating tamoxifen in the treatment of patients with node-negative breast cancer who have estrogen-receptor-positive tumors. N Engl J Med 320:479–484, 1989.

98. Fisher B, Costantino JP, Redmond CK, et al: Endometrial cancer in tamoxifen-treated breast cancer patients: Findings from the National Surgical Adjuvant Breast and Bowel Project (NSABP) B-14. J Natl Cancer Inst 86:527–537, 1994.

99. Fisher B, Fisher ER, Redmond C: Ten year results from the NSABP clinical trial evaluating the use of L-phenylalanine mustard (L-PAM) in the management of primary breast cancer. J Clin Oncol 4:929–941, 1986.

100. Fisher B, Bauer M, Wickerham L, Redmond CK, Fisher E, Cruz A, Foster R, Gardner B, Lerner H, Margolese R, Poisson R, Shibata H, Vold H: Relation of number of positive axillary nodes to the prognosis of patients with primary breast cancer: An NSABP update. Cancer 52:1551–1557, 1983.

101. Fisher B, Brown AM, Dimitrov NV, et al: Two months of doxorubicin-cyclophosphamide with and without interval reinduction therapy compared with 6 months of cyclophosphamide, methotrexate, and fluorouracil in positive-node breast cancer patients with tamoxifen-nonresponsive tumors: Results from the National Adjuvant Breast and Bowel Project B-15. J Clin Oncol 8:1483–1496, 1990.

102. Fisher B, Brown A, Wolmark N, et al: Evaluation of the worth of Corynebacterium parvum in conjunction with chemotherapy as adjuvant treatment for primary breast cancer: Eight-year results from the National Surgical Adjuvant Breast and Bowel Project B-10. Cancer 66:220–227, 1990.

103. Fisher B, Glass A, Redmond C, et al: L-phenylalanine mustard (L-PAM) in the management of primary breast cancer: An update of earlier findings and a comparison with those utilizing L-PAM plus 5-fluorouracil (5-FU). Cancer 39:2883–2903, 1977.

104. Fisher B, Ravdin RG, Ausman RK, Slack NH, More GE, Rudolf JN: Surgical adjuvant chemotherapy in cancer of the breast: Results of a decade of cooperative investigation. Ann Surg 168:337–356, 1968.

105. Fisher B, Redmond C, and Others for the National Surgical Adjuvant Breast and Bowel Project: Systemic therapy in node-negative patients: Updated findings from NSABP clinical trials. J Natl Cancer Inst Monogr 11:105–116, 1992.

106. Fisher B, Redmond C, Brown A, et al: Adjuvant chemotherapy with and without tamoxifen in the treatment of primary breast cancer: 5-year results from the National Surgical Adjuvant Breast and Bowel Project Trial. J Clin Oncol 4:459–471, 1986.

107. Fisher B, Redmond C, Brown A, et al: Treatment of primary breast cancer with chemotherapy and tamoxifen. N Engl J Med 305:1–6, 1981.

108. Fisher B, Redmond C, Brown A, et al: Influence of tumor estrogen and progesterone receptor levels on the response to

tamoxifen and chemotherapy in primary breast cancer. J Clin Oncol 1:227–241, 1983.

109. Fisher B, Redmond C, Dimitrov N, et al: A randomized clinical trial evaluating sequential methotrexate and 5-fluorouracil for the treatment of node negative breast cancer patients with estrogen receptor negative tumors. N Engl J Med 320:473–478, 1989.

110. Fisher B, Redmond C, Fisher ER, Caplan R, and National Surgical Adjuvant Breast and Bowel Project Investigators: Relative worth of estrogen or progesterone receptor and pathologic characteristics of differentiation as indicators of prognosis in node negative breast cancer patients: Findings from National Surgical Adjuvant Breast and Bowel Project Protocol B-06. J Clin Oncol 6:1076–1087, 1988.

111. Fisher B, Redmond C, Fisher ER, and NSABP Investigators: The contribution of recent NSABP clinical trials of primary breast cancer therapy to an understanding of tumor biology: An overview of findings. Cancer 46:1009–1025, 1980.

112. Fisher B, Redmond C, Fisher ER, Wolmark N: Systemic adjuvant therapy in treatment of primary operable breast cancer: National Surgical Adjuvant Breast and Bowel Project Experience. NCI Monogr 1:35–43, 1986.

113. Fisher B, Redmond C, Legault-Poisson S, et al: Postoperative chemotherapy and tamoxifen compared with tamoxifen alone in the treatment of positive-node breast cancer patients aged 50 years and older with tumors responsive to tamoxifen: Results from the National Surgical Adjuvant Breast and Bowel Project B-16. J Clin Oncol 8:1005–1018, 1990.

114. Fisher ER, Redmond CK, Liu H, et al: Correlation of estrogen receptor and pathologic characteristics of invasive breast cancer. Cancer 45:349–353, 1980.

115. Fisher B, Redmond C, Wickerham L: Doxorubicin-containing regimens for the treatment of stage II breast cancer: The National Surgical Adjuvant Breast and Bowel Project experience. J Clin Oncol 7:572–582, 1989.

116. Fisher B, Redmond C, Wolmark N, et al: Disease-free survival at intervals during and following completion of adjuvant chemotherapy: The NSABP experience from three breast cancer protocols. Cancer 48:1273–1280, 1981.

117. Fisher B, Rockette H, Fisher ER, et al: Leukemia in breast cancer patients following adjuvant chemotherapy or postoperative radiation: The NSABP experience. J Clin Oncol 3:1640–1658, 1985.

118. Fisher B, Sherman B, Rockette H, Redmond C, Margolese R, Fisher ER: L-phenylalanine mustard (L-PAM) in the management of premenopausal patients with primary breast cancer. Cancer 44:847–857, 1979.

119. Fisher B, Slack N, Bross IDJ, and Cooperating Investigators: Cancer of the breast: Size of neoplasm and prognosis. Cancer 24:1071–1080, 1969.

120. Fisher B, Slack N, Katrych D, et al: Ten year follow-up results of patients with carcinoma of the breast in a cooperative clinical trial evaluating surgical adjuvant chemotherapy. Surg Gynecol Obstet 140:528–534, 1975.

121. Fisher B, Wickerham DL, Beazley R, Bornstein R, et al: The use of adjuvant therapy for primary breast cancer: An overview. In Margolese R (ed): Contemporary Issues in Clinical Oncology. New York, Churchill Livingstone, 1983, pp 93–121.

122. Fisher B, Wickerham DL, Redmond C: Recent developments in the use of systemic adjuvant therapy for the treatment of breast cancer. Semin Oncol 19:263–277, 1992.

123. Fisher E: Prognostic and therapeutic significance of pathologic features of breast cancer. NCI Monogr 1:29–34, 1986.

124. Fisher ER, Turnbull RB Jr: Cytologic demonstration and significance of tumor cells in the mesenteric venous blood in patients with colorectal carcinoma. Surg Gynecol Obstet 100:102–108, 1955.

125. Focan C, Baudoux A, Beauduin M, et al: Adjuvant treatment with high dose medroxyprogesterone acetate in node-negative early breast cancer. Acta Oncol 28:237–240, 1989.

126. Fornander T, Rutqvist LE, Cedermark B, et al: Adjuvant tamoxifen in early breast cancer: Occurrence of new primary cancers. Lancet 1:117–120, 1989.

127. Gasparini G, Harris AL: Clinical importance of the determi-

nation of tumor angiogenesis in breast carcinoma: Much more than a new prognostic tool. J Clin Oncol 13:765–782, 1995.

128. Gelber RD, Goldhirsch A: The concept of an overview of cancer clinical trials with special emphasis on early breast cancer. J Clin Oncol 4:1696–1703, 1986.

129. Gelber RD, Goldhirsch A, for the Ludwig Breast Cancer Study Group: A new endpoint for the assessment of adjuvant therapy in postmenopausal women with operable breast cancer. J Clin Oncol 4:1772–1779, 1986.

130. Gelber RD, Goldhirsch A, Cavalli F, et al: Quality-of-life–adjusted evaluation of adjuvant therapies for operable breast cancer. Ann Intern Med 114:621–628, 1991.

131. Gelber RD, Goldhirsch A, Hurny C, et al: Quality of life in clinical trials of adjuvant therapies. J Natl Cancer Inst Monogr 11:127–135, 1992.

132. Gentili C, Sanfilippo O, Silvestrini R: Cell proliferation and its relationship to clinical features and relapse in breast cancers. Cancer 48:974–979, 1981.

133. Gianni AM, Siena S, Bregni M, et al: 5-Year results of high-dose sequential (HDS) adjuvant chemotherapy in breast cancer with ≥10 positive nodes. Proc Am Soc Clin Oncol 14:90, 1995.

134. Glick JH, Gelber RD, Goldhirsch A, et al: Meeting highlights: Adjuvant therapy for primary breast cancer. J Natl Cancer Inst 84:1476–1485, 1992.

135. Goldhirsch A, Gelber R: Adjuvant treatment for early breast cancer: The Ludwig breast cancer studies. NCI Monogr 1:55–70, 1986.

136. Goldhirsch A, Gelber RD, Castiglione M: The magnitude of endocrine effects of adjuvant chemotherapy for premenopausal breast cancer patients. Ann Oncol 1:183–188, 1990.

137. Goldhirsch A, Gelber RD, Simes J, et al: Costs and benefits of adjuvant therapy in breast cancer: A quality-adjusted survival analysis. J Clin Oncol 7:36–44, 1989.

138. Goldhirsch A, Wood WC, Senn H-J, et al: Meeting highlights: International consensus panel on the treatment of primary breast cancer. J Natl Cancer Inst 87:1441–1445, 1995.

139. Goldie JH, Coldman AJ: A mathematic model for relating the drug sensitivity of tumors to their a/spontaneous mutation rate. Cancer Treat Rep 63:1727–1731, 1979.

140. Goldie JH, Coldman AJ: Quantitative model for multiple levels of drug resistance in clinical tumors. Cancer Treat Rep 67:923–931, 1983.

141. Goldie JH, Coldman AJ: Genetic instability in the development of drug resistance. Semin Oncol 12:222–230, 1985.

142. Gough MH, Durrant KR, Girard-Saunders AM, et al: A randomized controlled trial of prophylactic cytotoxic chemotherapy in potentially curable breast cancer. Br J Surg 72:182–185, 1985.

143. Griswold DP Jr: The potential for murine tumor models in surgical adjuvant chemotherapy. Cancer Chemother Rep 5 (Part 2):187–204, 1975.

144. Gusterson BA, Gelber RD, Goldhirsch A, et al: Prognostic importance of c-erbB-2 expression in breast cancer. J Clin Oncol 10:1049–1056, 1992.

145. Halsted WS: Results of operations for the cure of cancer of the breast performed at Johns Hopkins Hospital from June, 1889–January, 1894. Ann Surg 20:497, 1894.

146. Harlan LC, Coates RJ, Block G, et al: Estrogen receptor status and dietary intakes in breast cancer patients. Epidemiology 4:25–31, 1993.

147. Henderson IC: Adjuvant chemotherapy and endocrine therapy in patients with operable cancer. In DeVita VT Jr, Hellman S, Rosenberg SA (eds): Cancer: Principles and Practice of Oncology. 2nd Ed. Philadelphia, JB Lippincott, 1985: Update, March 1987.

148. Henderson IC, Gelman RS, Harris FR, et al: Duration of therapy in adjuvant chemotherapy trials. NCI Monogr 1:95–98, 1986.

149. Henderson IC: Second malignancies from adjuvant chemotherapy? Too soon to tell. J Clin Oncol 5:1135–1137, 1987.

150. Henson DE, Ries L, Freedman LS, et al: Relationship among outcome, stage of disease, and histologic grade for 22,616 cases of breast cancer: The basis for a prognostic index. Cancer 68:2142–2149, 1991.

151. Holdaway IM, Bowditch JV: Variation in receptor status between primary and metastatic breast cancer. Cancer 52:479–485, 1983.

152. Holmes FA: Update: The M.D. Anderson Cancer Center experience with paclitaxel in the management of breast carcinoma. Semin Oncol 22(Suppl 8):9–15, 1995.

153. Howell A, George WD, Crowther D, et al: Controlled trial of adjuvant chemotherapy with cyclophosphamide, methotrexate, and fluorouracil for breast cancer. Lancet 2:307–311, 1984.

154. Hryniuk WM, Levine MN, Levin N: Analysis of dose intensity for chemotherapy in early (stage II) and advanced breast cancer. NCI Monogr 1:87–94, 1986.

155. Hubay CA, Gordon NH, Pearson OH, et al: Eight-year follow-up of adjuvant therapy for stage II breast cancer. World J Surg 9:738–749, 1985.

156. Huseby R, Ownby H, Frederick J, et al: Node-negative breast cancer treated by modified radical mastectomy without adjuvant therapies: Variables associated with disease recurrence and survivorship. J Clin Oncol 6:83–88, 1988.

157. Ingle JN, Everson LK, Wieand HS, et al: Randomized trial of observation versus adjuvant therapy with cyclophosphamide, 5-fluorouracil, prednisone with or without tamoxifen following mastectomy in post menopausal women with node positive breast cancer. J Clin Oncol 6:1388–1396, 1988.

158. Ingle JN, Krook JE, Green SJ, et al: Randomized trial of bilateral oophorectomy versus tamoxifen in premenopausal women with metastatic breast cancer. J Clin Oncol 4:178–185, 1986.

159. Jakesz R, Kolb R, Reiner G, et al: Effect of adjuvant chemotherapy in stage I and II breast cancer is dependent on tumor differentiation and estrogen status. Proc Am Soc Clin Oncol 4:69, 1985.

160. Jakesz R, Kolb R, Reiner G, et al: Adjuvant chemotherapy in node-negative breast cancer patients. In Salmon S (ed): Adjuvant Therapy of Cancer. Vol 5. Orlando, Grune & Stratton, 1987, pp 223–233.

161. Johnson TP, Ford L, Warnecke RB, et al: Effect of a National Cancer Institute clinical alert on breast cancer practice patterns. J Clin Oncol 12:1783–1788, 1994.

162. Jones AL, Powles TJ, Law M, et al: Adjuvant aminoglutethimide for postmenopausal patients with primary breast cancer: Analysis at 8 years. J Clin Oncol 10:1547–1552, 1992.

163. Jungi WF, Alberto P, Brunner KW, et al: Short- or long-term chemotherapy for node-positive breast cancer: LMF 6 versus 18 cycles. ASKK study 27/76. Recent Results Cancer Res 96:175–177, 1984.

164. Jungi WF, Senn HJ: Swiss adjuvant trials in women with node-negative breast cancer. J Natl Cancer Inst Monogr 11:71–76, 1992.

165. Kaiser-Kupfer MI, Lippman ME: Tamoxifen retinopathy. Cancer Treat Rep 62:315–320, 1978.

166. Kedar RP, Bourne TH, Powles TJ, et al: Effects of tamoxifen on uterus and ovaries of postmenopausal women in a randomised breast cancer prevention trial. Lancet 343:1318–1321, 1994.

167. Kjellgren K, Nissen-Meyer R, Norin T: Perioperative adjuvant chemotherapy in breast cancer. Acta Oncol 28:899–901, 1989.

168. Levine MN, Gent M, Hirsh J, et al: The thrombogenic effect of anti-cancer drug therapy in women with stage II breast cancer. N Engl J Med 318:404–407, 1988.

169. Levine MN, Gent M, Hryniuk WM, et al: A randomized trial comparing 12 weeks versus 36 weeks of adjuvant chemotherapy in stage II breast cancer. J Clin Oncol 8:1217–1225, 1990.

170. Levine MN, Guyatt GH, Gent M, et al: Quality of life in stage II breast cancer: An instrument for clinical trials. J Clin Oncol 6:1798–1810, 1988.

171. Long L, Jonasson O, Roberts S, McGrath R, McGrew E, Cole W: Cancer cells in the blood: Results of simplified isolation technique. Arch Surg 80:910–919, 1960.

172. Love RR, Mazess RB, Barden HS, et al: Effects of tamoxifen on bone mineral density in postmenopausal women with breast cancer. N Engl J Med 326:852–856, 1992.

173. Lowenthal EA, Carpenter JT Jr: The use of anthracyclines in the adjuvant treatment of breast cancer. Cancer Treat Rev 21:199–214, 1995.

174. Ludwig Breast Cancer Study Group: Combination adjuvant chemotherapy for node-positive breast cancer: Inadequacy of a single perioperative cycle. N Engl J Med 319:677–684, 1988.

175. Ludwig Breast Cancer Study Group: Randomized trial of chemoendocrine therapy, endocrine therapy, and mastectomy alone in postmenopausal patients with operable breast cancer and axillary node metastasis. Lancet 1:1256–1260, 1984.

176. Ludwig Breast Cancer Study Group: Adjuvant combination chemotherapy with or without prednisone in premenopausal breast cancer patients with metastases in 1 to 3 axillary lymph nodes: A randomized trial. Cancer Res 45:4454–4459, 1985.

177. Ludwig Breast Cancer Study Group: Adjuvant chemotherapy (CMF) with or without low-dose prednisone (P) in premenopausal patients with metastases in 1 to 3 axillary lymph nodes: Ludwig Trial I (LBCS I). Proc Am Soc Clin Oncol 4:53, 1985.

178. Ludwig Breast Cancer Study Group: Prolonged disease-free survival after one course of perioperative adjuvant chemotherapy for node-negative breast cancer patients. N Engl J Med 320:491–496, 1989.

179. Mansour EG, Eudey L, Tormey DC, et al: Chemotherapy versus observation in high-risk node-negative breast cancer patients. J Natl Cancer Inst Monogr 11:97–104, 1992.

180. Mansour EG, Gray R, Shatila AH, et al: Efficiency of adjuvant chemotherapy in high risk node negative breast cancer: An intergroup study (INT-0011) N Engl J Med 320:485–490, 1989.

181. Mathe G, Misset JL, Plagne R, et al: Adriamycin, vincristine, cyclophosphamide and 5-fluorouracil (AVCF) compared with cyclophosphamide, methotrexate and 5-fluorouracil (CMF) in premenopausal breast carcinoma: Personal results. Drugs Exp Clin Res 12:143–145, 1986.

182. McDonald CC, Stewart HJ, for the Scottish Breast Cancer Committee: Fatal myocardial infarction in the Scottish adjuvant tamoxifen trial. Br Med J 303:435–437, 1991.

183. McDonald CC, Alexander FE, Whyte BW, et al: Cardiac and vascular morbidity in women receiving adjuvant tamoxifen for breast cancer in a randomised trial. Br Med J 311:977–980, 1995.

184. McDonald GO, Long EP, Cruz WH: The effect of cancer inhibitor drugs on the "take" of Walker carcinosarcoma 256 in rats. Surg Forum 7:486–489, 1956.

185. McDonald GO, Livingston C, Boyles CT, Cole W: The prophylactic treatment of malignant disease with nitrogen mustard and triethylenethiophosphoramide (Thio-TEPA). Ann Surg 145:624–629, 1957.

186. McGuire WL, Clark GM: Prognostic factors and treatment decisions in axillary-node-negative breast cancer. N Engl J Med 326:1756–1761, 1992.

187. McGuire W, Clark G, Dressler L, et al: Role of steroid hormone receptors as prognostic factors in primary breast cancer. NCI Monogr 1:19–223, 1986.

188. Meakin JW, Allt WC, Beale FA, et al: Ovarian irradiation and prednisone following surgery and radiotherapy for carcinoma of the breast. Breast Cancer Res Treat 3 (Suppl):45–48, 1983.

189. Meakin JW: Review of Canadian trials of adjuvant endocrine therapy for breast cancer. NCI Monogr 1:111–113, 1986.

190. Mendelsohn ML: The growth fraction: A new concept applied to tumors. Science 132:1486, 1960.

191. Meyer J: Cell kinetics in selection and stratification of patients for adjuvant therapy of breast carcinoma. NCI Monogr 1:25–28, 1986.

192. Meyer J, Friedman E, McCrate M, et al: Prediction of early course of breast carcinoma by thymidine labeling. Cancer 51:1879–1886, 1983.

193. Misset JL, Gil-Delgado M, Chollet PH, et al: Ten year results of the French trial comparing adriamycin, vincristine, 5-fluorouracil and cyclophosphamide to standard CMF as adjuvant therapy for node positive breast cancer. Proc Am Soc Clin Oncol 11:54, 1992.

194. Moliterni A, Bonadonna G, Valagussa P, et al: Cyclophospha- mide, methotrexate, and fluorouracil with and without doxo- rubicin in the adjuvant treatment of resectable breast cancer with one to three positive axillary nodes. J Clin Oncol 9:1124–1130, 1991.
195. Morrison JM, Howell A, Grieve RJ, et al: The West Midlands Oncology Association trials of adjuvant chemotherapy for operable breast cancer. *In* Jones SE, Salmon SE (eds): Adjuvant Therapy of Cancer. Vol. 4. New York, Grune & Stratton, 1984, pp 253–261.
196. Morrison JM, Howell A, Kelly KA, et al: West Midlands Oncology Association trials of adjuvant chemotherapy in op- erable breast cancer: Results after a median follow-up of 7 years: I. Patients with involved axillary lymph nodes. Br J Cancer 60:911–918, 1989.
197. Morrison JM, Howell A, Kelly KA, et al: West Midlands Oncology Association trials of adjuvant chemotherapy in op- erable breast cancer: Results after a median follow-up of 7 years: II. Patients without involved axillary lymph nodes. Br J Cancer 60:919–923, 1989.
198. Mouridsen HT, Rose C, Brincker H, et al: Adjuvant systemic therapy in high-risk breast cancer: The Danish Breast Can- cer Cooperative Group's trials of cyclophosphamide or CMF in premenopausal and tamoxifen in post-menopausal pa- tients. *In* Senn H (ed): Recent Results in Cancer Research: Adjuvant Chemotherapy in Breast Cancer. New York, Springer-Verlag, 1984, pp 117–127.
199. Muss HB, Thor AD, Berry CA, et al: c-*erb*B-2 expression and response to adjuvant therapy in women with node-positive early breast cancer. N Engl J Med 330:1260–1266, 1994.
200. National Cancer Institute: Clinical alert. National Cancer Institute. Bethesda, National Cancer Institute, May 18, 1988.
201. National Institutes of Health Consensus Development Panel on Adjuvant Chemotherapy and Endocrine Therapy for Breast Cancer: Introduction and conclusions. NCI Monogr 1:1–4, 1986.
202. Nayfield SG, Karp JE, Ford LG, et al: Potential role of tamoxifen in prevention of breast cancer. J Natl Cancer Inst 83:1450–1459, 1991.
203. Nayfield SG, Gorin MB: Tamoxifen-associated eye disease: A review. J Clin Oncol 14:1018–1026, 1996.
204. Nevinny HB, Nevinny D, Rosoff CB, et al: Prophylactic oophorectomy in breast cancer therapy: A preliminary report. Am J Surg 117:531–536, 1969.
205. Nissen-Meyer R: Primary breast cancer: The effect of pri- mary ovarian irradiation. Am Oncol 2:343–346, 1991.
206. Nissen-Meyer R, Host H, Kjellgren K, et al: Treatment of node-negative breast cancer patients with short course of chemotherapy immediately after surgery. NCI Monogr 1:125–128, 1986.
207. Nissen-Meyer R, Host H, Kjellgren K, Mansson B, Norin T: Neoadjuvant chemotherapy in breast cancer: As single perioperative treatment and with supplementary long-term chemotherapy. *In* Salmon S (ed): Adjuvant Therapy of Can- cer. Vol 5. Orlando, Grune & Stratton 1987, pp 253–261.
208. Norton L, Simon R: Tumor size, sensitivity to therapy, and design of treatment schedules. Cancer Treat Rep 61:1307–1317, 1977.
209. Osborne CK, Rivkin SE, McDivitt RW, et al: Adjuvant ther- apy of breast cancer: Southwest Oncology Group studies. NCI Monogr 1:71–74, 1986.
210. Osborne MP, Rosen PP: Detection and management of bone marrow micrometastases in breast cancer. Oncology 8:25–31, 1994.
211. Padmanabhan N, Howell A, Rubens RD: Mechanism of action of adjuvant chemotherapy in early breast cancer. Lancet 2:411–414, 1986.
212. Paik S, Hazan R, Fisher ER, et al: Pathologic findings from the National Surgical Adjuvant Breast and Bowel Project: Prognostic significance of *erb*B-2 protein overexpression in primary breast cancer. J Clin Oncol 8:103–112, 1990.
213. Palshoff T, Mouridsen HT, Daehnfeldt JL: Adjuvant endo- crine therapy of primary operable breast cancer: Report on the Copenhagen breast cancer trials. Eur J Cancer 2 (Suppl):183–187, 1980.
214. Perloff M, Norton L, Korzun A, et al: Advantage of an adria- mycin combination plus halotestin after initial cyclophospha- mide, methotrexate, 5-fluorouracil, vincristine and predni- sone (CMFVP) for adjuvant therapy of node-positive stage II breast cancer. Proc Am Soc Clin Oncol 5:70, 1986.
215. Perloff M, Norton L, Korzun A, et al: Postsurgical adjuvant chemotherapy of stage II breast carcinoma with or without crossover to a noncross-resistant regimen: A CALGB study. J Clin Oncol 14:1589–1598, 1996.
216. Peters WP, Ross M, Vredenburgh JJ, et al: High-dose chemo- therapy and autologous bone marrow support as consolida- tion after standard-dose adjuvant therapy for high-risk pri- mary breast cancer. J Clin Oncol 11:1132–1143, 1993.
217. Pourquier H: The results of adjuvant chemotherapy are pre- dominantly caused by the hormonal changes such therapy induces: In favor. *In* VanScoy-Mosher MB (ed): Medical On- cology: Controversies in Cancer Treatment. Boston, GK Hall, 1981, pp 83–99.
218. Powles TJ, Hickish T, Kanis JA, et al: Effect of tamoxifen on bone mineral density measured by dual-energy x-ray absorp- tiometry in healthy premenopausal and postmenopausal women. J Clin Oncol 14:78–84, 1996.
219. Pritchard KE, Meakin JW, Boyd NF, et al: Adjuvant tamoxi- fen in postmenopausal women with axillary node positive breast cancer: An update. *In* Salmon SE (ed): Adjuvant Ther- apy of Cancer. Vol 5. Orlando, Grune & Stratton, 1987, pp 391–400.
220. Proceedings of the NIH Consensus Development Conference on Adjuvant Chemotherapy and Endocrine Therapy for Breast Cancer. NCI Monogr 1:1, 1986.
221. Protocol P-1: A clinical trial to determine the worth of tamox- ifen for preventing breast cancer. National Surgical Adjuvant Breast and Bowel Project, Pittsburgh, September 23, 1994.
222. Ravdin RG, Lewison EF, Slack NH, et al: Results of a clinical trial concerning the worth of prophylactic oophorectomy for breast cancer. Surg Gynecol Obstet 131:1055–1064, 1970.
223. Redmond C, Fisher B, Wieand HS: The methodologic di- lemma in retrospectively correlating the amount of chemo- therapy received in adjuvant therapy protocols with disease- free survival. Cancer Treat Rep 67:519–526, 1983.
224. Redmond CK, Rockett HE: Meta-analysis: Considerations of its worth and its limitations. *In* Salmon SE (ed): Adjuvant Therapy of Cancer. Vol 5. Orlando, Grune & Stratton, 1987, pp 467–475.
225. Review of mortality results in randomized trials in early breast cancer. Lancet 2:1205, 1984.
226. Ribeiro G, Swindell R: The Christie Hospital tamoxifen (Nol- vadex) adjuvant trial for operable breast cancer: 7 year re- sults. Eur J Cancer Clin Oncol 21:897–900, 1985.
227. Ribeiro G, Swindell R: The Christie Hospital adjuvant ta- moxifen trial: Status at 10 years. Br J Cancer 57:601–603, 1988.
228. Ribeiro G, Swindell R: The Christie Hospital Adjuvant Ta- moxifen Trial. J Natl Cancer Inst Monogr 11:121–125, 1992.
229. Richards MA, O'Reilly SM, Howell A, et al: Adjuvant cyclo- phosphamide, methotrexate, and fluorouracil in patients with axillary node-positive breast cancer: An update of the Guy's/Manchester Trial. J Clin Oncol 8:2032–2039, 1990.
230. Ries LAG, Miller BA, Hankey B, Kosary CL, Harras A, Edwards BK (eds): SEER Cancer Statistics Review, 1973–1991: Bethesda, National Cancer Institute, NIH Publ. no. 94–2789, 1994, p 129.
231. Rivkin SE, Green S, Metch B, et al: Adjuvant CMFVP versus melphalan for operable breast cancer with positive axillary nodes: 10-year results of a Southwest Oncology Group Study. J Clin Oncol 7:1229–1238, 1989.
232. Rivkin SE, Green S, Metch B, et al: One versus 2 years of CMDVP adjuvant chemotherapy in axillary node-positive and estrogen receptor-negative patients: A Southwest Oncol- ogy Group study. J Clin Oncol 11:1710–1716, 1993.
233. Robert NJ, Gray R, Gelber RD, Goldhirsch A, Abeloff M, Tormey DC, for the Eastern Cooperative Oncology Group and the International Breast Cancer Study Group: Node positive (N+) breast cancer: Which patients (PTS) are at high risk? Proc Am Soc Clin Oncol 10:59, 1991.

234. Robert NNJ: Adjuvant therapy in breast cancer. Obstet Gynecol Clin N Am 21:693–707, 1994.
235. Roberts S, Watne A, McGrath R, McGrew E, Cole WH: Technique and results of isolation of cancer cells from the circulating blood. Arch Surg 76:334–336, 1958.
236. Rose C, Mouridsen HT, Thorpe SM, et al: Anti-oestrogen treatment of postmenopausal breast cancer patients with high risk of recurrence: 72 months of life-table analysis and steroid hormone receptor status. World J Surg 9:765–774, 1985.
237. Rose C, Thorpe SM, Andersen KW, et al: Beneficial effect of adjuvant tamoxifen therapy in primary breast cancer patients with high oestrogen receptor values. Lancet 1:16–19, 1985.
238. Rosen PP, Groshen S, Kinne DW: Prognosis in $T_2N_0M_0$ Stage I breast carcinoma: A 20-year follow-up study. J Clin Oncol 9:1650–1661, 1991.
239. Rosen PP, Groshen S, Saigo PE, et al: Pathological prognostic factors in stage I ($T_1N_0M_0$) and stage II ($T_1N_1M_0$) breast carcinoma: A study of 644 patients with median follow-up of 18 years. J Clin Oncol 7:1239–1251, 1989.
240. Rosner F, Carey RW, Zarrabi MH: Breast cancer and acute leukemia: Report of 24 cases and review of the literature. Am J Hematol 4:151–172, 1978.
241. Rubens RD, Knight RK, Fentiman IS, et al: Controlled trial of adjuvant chemotherapy with melphalan for breast cancer. Lancet 1:839–843, 1983.
242. Rutqvist LE, Cedemark B, Glas U, et al: The Stockholm trial on adjuvant tamoxifen in early breast cancer: Correlation between estrogen receptor level and treatment effect. Breast Cancer Res Treat 10:255–266, 1987.
243. Rutqvist LE, Mattsson A: Cardiac and thromboembolic morbidity among postmenopausal women with early-stage breast cancer in a randomized trial of adjuvant tamoxifen. J Natl Cancer Inst 85:1398–1406, 1993.
244. Rutqvist LE, Johansson H, Signomklao T, et al: Adjuvant tamoxifen therapy for early stage breast cancer and second primary malignancies. J Natl Cancer Inst 87:645–651, 1995.
245. Salsbury HJ: The significance of the circulating cancer cell. Cancer Treat Rev 2:55–72, 1975.
246. Schabel FM: Concepts for systemic treatment of micrometastases. Cancer 35:15, 1975.
247. Schabel FM: Surgical adjuvant chemotherapy of metastatic murine tumors. Cancer 40:558–568, 1977.
248. Schumacher M, Bastert G, Bihar G, et al: Randomized 2 × 2 trial evaluating hormonal treatment and the duration of chemotherapy in node-positive breast cancer patients. J Clin Oncol 12:2086–2093, 1994.
249. Schinzinger A: Ueber carcinoma mammae. Verh Dtsch Ges Chir 18:28–29, 1889.
250. Senanayake F: Adjuvant hormonal chemotherapy in early breast cancer: Early results from a controlled trial. Lancet 2:1148–1149, 1984.
251. Senn JH, Jungi WF: Swiss adjuvant trials with LMF (+BCG) in N− and N+ breast cancer patients. In Jones SE, Salmon SE (eds): Adjuvant Therapy of Cancer. Vol 4. Orlando, Grune & Stratton, 1984, pp 261–270.
252. Shapiro CL, Henderson IC, Gelman RS, et al: A randomized trial of 15 vs. 30 weeks (wks) of adjuvant chemotherapy in high risk breast cancer patients: Results after a median follow-up of 9.1 years. Proc Am Soc Clin Oncol 10:44, 1991.
253. Shapiro DM, Fugmann RA: A role for chemotherapy as an adjunct to surgery. Cancer Res 17:1098–1101, 1957.
254. Shapiro CL, Henderson IC: Late cardiac effects of adjuvant therapy: Too soon to tell? Ann Oncol 5:196–198, 1994.
255. Sigurdsson H, Baldetorp B, Borg A, Dalber M, Ferno M, Killander D, Olsson H: Indicators of prognosis in node-negative breast cancer. N Engl J Med 322:1045–1053, 1990.
256. Singh L, Wilson AJ, Baum M, et al: The relationship between histological grade, oestrogen receptor status, events and survival at 8 years in the NATO ("Nolvadex") trial. Br J Cancer 57:612–614, 1988.
257. Skipper HE: Kinetics of mammary tumor cell growth and implication for therapy. Cancer 28:1479–1499, 1971.
258. Skipper HE: Adjuvant chemotherapy. Cancer 41:936–940, 1971.
259. Slamon D, Clark G, Wong S, et al: Human breast cancer: Correlation of relapse and survival with amplification of the HER-2/neu oncogene. Science 235:177–182, 1987.
260. Smith DC, Crawford C, Dykes EH, et al: Adjuvant radiotherapy and chemotherapy in breast cancer. In Jones SE, Salmon SE (eds): Adjuvant Therapy of Cancer. Vol IV. Orlando, Grune & Stratton, 1984, pp 283–289.
261. Tamoxifen and Endometrial Cancer: ACOG Committee Opinion. Washington, DC, American College of Obstetricians and Gynecologists, Feb 1996.
262. Tancini G, Bonadonna G, Valagussa P, et al: Adjuvant CMF in breast cancer: Comparative 5-year results of 12 versus 6 cycles. J Clin Oncol 1:2–10, 1983.
263. Taylor GW: Artificial menopause in carcinoma of the breast. N Engl J Med 211:1138–1140, 1934.
264. Taylor GW: Evaluation of ovarian sterilization for breast cancer. Surg Gynecol Obstet 68:452–456, 1939.
265. Taylor SG IV, Gelman RS, Falkson G, et al: Combination chemotherapy compared to tamoxifen as initial therapy for stage IV breast cancer in elderly women. Ann Intern Med 104:455–461, 1986.
266. Taylor SG IV, Olsen JE, Cummings FJ, et al: Observation compared to adjuvant chemohormonal therapy in postmenopausal breast cancer: The ECOG trial. Proc Am Soc Clin Oncol 4:61, 1985.
267. Taylor SG, Kalish LA, Olson JE, et al: Adjuvant CMFP versus CMFP plus tamoxifen versus observation alone in postmenopausal, node-positive breast cancer patients: Three-year results of an Eastern Cooperative Oncology Group study. J Clin Oncol 3:144–154, 1985.
268. Toikkanen S, Helin H, Isola J, et al: Prognostic significance of HER-2 oncoprotein expression in breast cancer: A 30-year follow-up. J Clin Oncol 10:1044–1048, 1992.
269. Tormey DC: Clinical results III: Experience of randomized trials without surgical controls. In Senn JH (ed): Recent Results in Cancer Research: Adjuvant Chemotherapy of Breast Cancer. New York, Springer-Verlag, 1984, pp 155–165.
270. Tormey DC, Gray R, Taylor SG IV, et al: Postoperative chemotherapy and chemohormonal therapy in women with node-positive breast cancer. NCI Monogr 1:75–80, 1986.
271. Tormey DC, Taylor SG IV, Kalish LA, et al: Adjuvant systemic therapy in premenopausal (CMF, CMFP, CMFPT) and postmenopausal (observation, CMFP, CMFPT) women with node positive breast cancer. In Jones SE, Salmon SE (eds): Adjuvant Therapy of Cancer. Vol 4. Orlando, Grune & Stratton, 1984, pp 359–368.
272. Tormey DC, Weinberg VE, Holland JF, et al: A randomized trial of five and three drug chemotherapy and chemoimmunotherapy in women with operable node positive breast cancer. J Clin Oncol 1:138–145, 1983.
273. Valagussa P, Bonadonna G, Veronesi U: Patterns of relapse, and survival following radical mastectomy. Cancer 41:1170–1178, 1978.
274. Valagussa P, Tancini G, Bonadonna G: Second malignancies after CMF for resectable breast cancer. J Clin Oncol 5:1138–1142, 1987.
275. Valagussa P, Zambetti M, Biasi S, et al: Cardiac effects following adjuvant chemotherapy and breast irradiation in operable breast cancer. Ann Oncol 5:209–216, 1994.
276. van Leeuwen FE, Benraadt J, Coebergh JWW, et al: Risk of endometrial cancer after tamoxifen treatment of breast cancer. Lancet 343:448–452, 1994.
277. Velez-Garcia E, Moore M, Vogel CL, et al: Post surgical adjuvant chemotherapy with or without radiation therapy in women with breast cancer and positive axillary nodes: The Southeastern Cancer Study Group (SECSG) experience. In Jones SE, Salmon SE (eds): Adjuvant Therapy of Cancer. Vol 4. Orlando, Grune & Stratton, 1984, pp 273–283.
278. Velez-Garcia E, Carpenter JT Jr, Moore M, et al: Postsurgical adjuvant chemotherapy with or without radiotherapy in women with breast cancer and positive axillary nodes: Progress report of a Southeastern Cancer Study Group (SEG)

trial. *In* Salmon SE (ed): Adjuvant Therapy of Cancer. Vol 5. Orlando, Grune & Stratton, 1987, pp 347–355.

279. Veronesi U, Cascinelli N, Greco M, et al: Prognosis of breast cancer patients after mastectomy and dissection of internal mammary nodes. Ann Surg 202:702–707, 1985.

280. Wallgren A, Baral E, Beling U, et al: Tamoxifen and combination chemotherapy as adjuvant treatment in postmenopausal women with breast cancer. *In* Senn HJ (ed): Recent Results in Cancer Research: Adjuvant Chemotherapy of Breast Cancer. New York, Springer-Verlag, 1984, pp 197–203.

281. Wallgren A, Baral E, Carstensen J, et al: Should adjuvant tamoxifen be given for several years in breast cancer? *In* Jones SE, Salmon SE (eds): Adjuvant Therapy for Cancer. Vol 2. Orlando, Grune & Stratton, 1984, pp 331–337.

282. Weiss RB, DeVita VT: Multimodal primary cancer treatment (adjuvant chemotherapy): Current results and future prospects. Ann Intern Med 91:251–260, 1979.

283. Wilcox WS: The last surviving cancer cell: The chance of killing it. Cancer Chemother Rep 50:541–542, 1966.

284. Williams C, Buchanan R, Hall V, Taylor I, et al: Adjuvant chemotherapy for T1-2, NO, MO estrogen receptor negative breast cancer: Preliminary results of a randomized trial. *In* Salmon S (ed): Adjuvant Therapy of Cancer. Vol 5. Orlando, Grune & Stratton, 1987, pp 233–242.

285. Wood WC, Budman DR, Korzun AH, et al: Dose and dose intensity of adjuvant chemotherapy for stage II, node-positive breast carcinoma. N Engl J Med 330:1253–1259, 1994.

286. Zelen M, Gelman R: Assessment of adjuvant trials in breast cancer. NCI Monogr 1:11–17, 1986.

SECTION XX

MANAGEMENT OF ADVANCED LOCAL AND REGIONAL DISEASE

CHAPTER 67

SURGICAL PROCEDURES FOR ADVANCED LOCAL AND REGIONAL MALIGNANCIES OF THE BREAST

Kelly K. Hunt, M.D. / Stephen S. Kroll, M.D. / Raphael E. Pollock, M.D., Ph.D.

Surgery has an important role in the palliative treatment of local and advanced malignancy of the breast. It is the quickest and most effective way to establish a durable, complete response for local disease control. There are, however, some significant limitations of surgery. Surgical treatment of stage III breast cancer fails to treat distant micrometastases that are present in virtually all such patients and even fails locally in 10–20 percent of patients who live 2 years or longer. Nevertheless, the integration of surgery, chemotherapy, and radiotherapy in the treatment of these advanced problems has resulted in improvements in palliation and even cure. In order to understand the remarkable successes of current multimodality therapy for advanced breast disease, it is critical to examine the rationale and evolution of this therapeutic approach.

Locally advanced breast cancer encompasses four distinct clinical entities occurring in patients without clinically evident distant metastases: (1) locally recurrent (persistent) breast carcinoma, (2) inflammatory breast carcinoma, (3) stage IIIA breast cancer, and (4) stage IIIB breast carcinoma. Inflammatory and locally recurrent carcinoma are discussed elsewhere in this book. Stage IIIA disease includes (1) any tumor with metastases to homolateral axillary lymph nodes that are fixed to each other or to other structures and (2) any tumor equal to or greater than 5 cm with metastasis to nonfixed ipsilateral axillary nodes.[18] Stage IIIB disease includes (1) any tumor with direct extension to the chest wall or skin with any form of axillary or internal mammary node involvement and (2) any tumor with internal mammary node involvement (Fig. 67–1).[18] The most recent, at the time of this writing, staging schema proposed by the American Joint Committee for Cancer (AJCC) has designated ipsilateral infra- or supraclavicular node involvement as M1, instead of N3, and designates this clinical presentation as stage IV disease.[1] Likewise, a primary tumor equal to or greater than 5 cm without lymph node involvement is now considered stage IIB rather than stage IIIA disease.[1]

These staging changes have important ramifications as most clinical research studies to date have been based on earlier staging schemes. Any clinical series prior to 1987 will therefore possibly include some patients who would currently, at the time of this writing, be considered either stage IIB or IV, rather than stage III. Because it is not feasible to retrospectively restage these studies, our discussion will be based on these earlier staging categories, except where otherwise indicated. Historically, stage IIIA tumors have been considered operable whereas stage IIIB tumors have not.

HISTORICAL CONSIDERATIONS

Unimodality Approaches

The awareness of differences in natural biology (and therefore therapy) for locally advanced breast cancer stems from Haagensen and Stout's[11] pioneering insights derived from nearly 30 years of cumulative experience in breast cancer management. Based on a review of 1135 breast cancer patients treated with radical mastectomy at Presbyterian Hospital in New York (1915–1942), it was recognized that patients with certain features of locally advanced breast cancer were beyond cure, even by radical surgery.[11] Haagensen's "grave signs" included edema of the skin of the breast, skin ulceration, chest wall fixation, an axillary lymph node greater than 2.5 cm in diameter, and fixed axillary nodes. Patients with two or more signs had a 42 percent local recurrence rate and a 2 percent 5-year disease-free survival; hence Haagenson and Stout[11] recommended that these patients be treated with palliative radiotherapy alone.

In 1949 Baclesse[2] used radiotherapy alone to achieve local tumor control in selected patients with advanced breast cancer. In 1965 Fletcher and Montague[9] from the M. D. Anderson Cancer Center reported a 70 percent local control rate of advanced breast cancer using radiotherapy alone. Distant metastasis occurred an average of 18 months later, and patients' 5-year overall survival rate was 25 percent. Another retrospective review of the 1960s and 1970s included Harris and coworkers'[12] report on the Joint Center for Radiation Therapy experience in which a

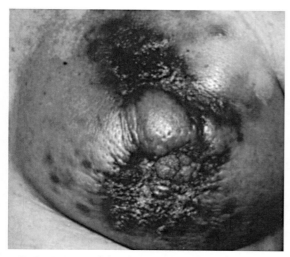

Figure 67–1 *Patient with locally advanced breast cancer. Note prominent skin retraction and nipple distortion caused by large underlying primary tumor.*

54 percent rate of 5-year local tumor control and a 30 percent rate of 5-year overall survival were achieved using radical radiation therapy alone. The National Cancer Institute in Milan, Italy, published their experience with radiation therapy in the treatment of locally advanced breast cancer in 1973.[29] This study, also retrospective, reported an encouraging 50 percent control rate. However, 45 percent of these "controlled" patients experienced relapse within 18 months of beginning radiotherapy. Of these relapses, 82 percent were at a distant site. An overall 21 percent rate of 5-year survival was achieved. It should be kept in mind that supervoltage radiotherapy, as was administered at that time, was not benign. Fibrosis and skin ulceration, pathological fractures, and severe lymphedema of the ipsilateral arm were common and debilitating occurrences.

More recently, the Alabama Breast Project examined the efficacy of modified radical mastectomy versus radical mastectomy as unimodality therapy for stage III breast carcinoma in patients with a minimum of 10 years follow-up.[21] In this study, stage III patients treated by modified radical mastectomy represented only 6 percent of the total study population but 20 percent of the total local recurrences. In contrast, the stage III radical mastectomy patients represented 5 percent of the total study population but 6 percent of the total local recurrences. Radical mastectomy significantly decreased the rate of local recurrence and improved survival as compared with modified mastectomy, albeit with greater morbidity. Observations such as those in the Alabama experience led to the realization that multimodality therapy might yield comparable survival rates but without the associated severe morbidities of unimodal radical interventions.

Multimodality Approaches

The unimodality experiences all demonstrated that good local control rates by surgery or radiotherapy alone did not correlate with good prognosis and ultimate survival. Clearly, hematogenous metastases were not being controlled with either radical surgery or radical radiotherapy alone.[6] Consequently, in the early 1970s a change in treatment strategies occurred that incorporated systemic chemotherapy as an integral part of the primary management of locally advanced breast cancer.[7] Several major prospective multimodality trials were initiated, including the National Cancer Institute (Milan, Italy) trial begun in 1973 and the M. D. Anderson Cancer Center trial begun in 1974.

In the Milan trial, patients with IIIA or IIIB breast cancer were given four cycles of doxorubicin and vincristine, followed by 60 Gy to the breast and a 10 Gy boost to the area of residual tumor. Patients who demonstrated a complete response were randomized to (1) no further treatment or (2) six more courses of chemotherapy. An 89 percent objective response rate occurred with this neoadjuvant chemotherapy regimen: 15.5 percent complete response, 54.5 percent major response (greater than 50 percent tumor size reduction), and 19 percent minor response (less than 50 percent tumor size reduction). Of the patients responding to induction chemotherapy, 83 percent had a complete response after the addition of radiotherapy. This combined chemotherapy-radiotherapy approach resulted in an overall 53 percent rate of 3-year survival in these patients.[7]

In 1975 the National Cancer Institute group in Milan, Italy began a second trial that ultimately enrolled 277 consecutive stage IIIA and IIIB patients.[28] In this trial, patients received three courses of doxorubicin and vincristine preoperatively. They were randomized to radiotherapy or surgery (radical or modified radical mastectomy). After these treatments, the patients then received six additional courses of chemotherapy. The best local control was achieved when surgery was interposed between chemotherapy courses; an 82.3 percent complete local control rate was achieved in these cases. In contrast, when chemotherapy and radiotherapy were employed without surgery, the rate of complete local control was significantly smaller at 63.9 percent. Freedom from disease progression was continuous for 5 years or longer in 25 percent of the patients who received chemotherapy followed by surgery followed by more chemotherapy, which was significantly better than the 4.9 percent rate achieved with a regimen of chemotherapy followed by radiotherapy. Likewise, the overall 5-year survival rate was higher for the chemotherapy-surgery-chemotherapy group than for the chemotherapy-radiotherapy group: 49.4 percent versus 19.7 percent.

In 1974 a multimodality treatment protocol for locally advanced breast cancer was initiated at the M. D. Anderson Cancer Center.[16] It was postulated that the combined use of all three modalities (chemotherapy, surgery, and radiotherapy) would result in control of micrometastases and reduce local tumor bulk, thereby avoiding the need for either radical radiotherapy or radical mastectomy.

Between 1974 and 1985, 174 patients with stage III noninflammatory (operable and inoperable) breast cancer were treated with combination chemotherapy consisting of fluorouracil, doxorubicin (Adriamycin), and cyclophosphamide (FAC) as the initial form of therapy. After three cycles of induction chemotherapy, patients were assessed for clinical response and classified as showing (1) complete response; (2) major response; (3) minor response; (4) nonresponse, resectable; or (5) nonresponse, unresectable. Complete responders and unresectable nonresponders were treated with radiotherapy, followed by an additional 6 to 12 courses of chemotherapy. Major responders, minor responders, and resectable nonresponders were treated with mastectomy (total or partial) and Level 1–2 axillary node dissection, followed next by chemotherapy, and lastly by radiotherapy.

The specific chemotherapy and radiotherapy protocols used are discussed in the text that follows. The median follow-up when this study was reported was 95 months. A complete remission was achieved in 16.7 percent of the patients, and 70.7 percent of the patients had a major partial response after the initial three cycles of FAC. All but six of the 174 patients treated were eventually rendered disease-free after induction chemotherapy and local treatment.

The stage IIIA patients had a 19 percent complete response rate and a 73 percent partial response rate after induction chemotherapy. The complete response rate was 100 percent after induction chemotherapy followed by local therapies. At 5 years, an 84 percent survival rate and a 78 percent disease-free survival rate had been achieved.

In the 122 stage IIIB patients, induction chemotherapy yielded a 7 percent complete response, an 80 percent partial response, and a 96 percent complete response rate after induction chemotherapy plus local therapy.

Only three (1.7 percent) of 174 stage III patients had progression of their disease while receiving FAC induction chemotherapy. These initial responses translated into a 5-year 33 percent disease-free survival rate and a 56 percent overall survival rate. Figure 67–2 summarizes the 5-year survival rates resulting from radical surgery alone or radiotherapy alone compared with those resulting from multimodality approaches.

PATIENT MANAGEMENT

The latest revision of the AJCC staging system for breast cancer undoubtedly influences the manner in which certain subsets of patients are managed. Because ipsilateral supraclavicular or infraclavicular adenopathy is now categorized as stage IV disease, the tendency is to treat these individuals by chemotherapy alone.[18] Because the multimodality experience suggests that some of these patients are potentially curable, it is hoped that the astute clinician will use multimodality programs for patients if the

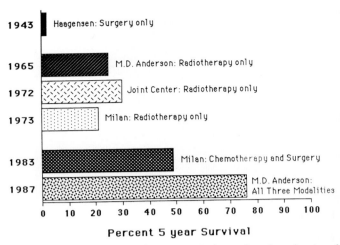

Figure 67–2 *Comparison of 5-year survival rates for selected series of patients with locally advanced breast cancer.*

presence of ipsilateral periclavicular nodes is the only reason the patient is classified as stage IV.

A complete staging work-up includes a thorough history and physical examination, a complete blood count (CBC) with differential and platelet counts, a biochemical survey (SMA-12), chest roentgenogram, bilateral mammogram, bone scan, and liver imaging (liver ultrasonography or computerized tomography). Patients with bone pain, abnormal results on bone scan, or elevated alkaline phosphatase levels should have pertinent bone radiographs taken to rule out distant disease. Needle core biopsy should be performed for both histopathological examination and hormone receptor studies.

There is a biological rationale for the sequence of modalities as used in the treatment of locally advanced breast cancer at the University of Texas M. D. Anderson Cancer Center (Fig. 67–3). Three to

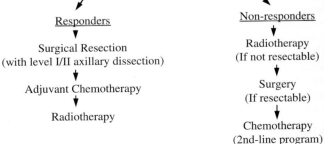

Figure 67–3 *M. D. Anderson algorithm for the treatment of stage III breast carcinoma.*

TABLE 67–1.   M. D. ANDERSON CHEMOTHERAPY PROTOCOL FOR STAGE III BREAST CANCER

1. 5-Fluorouracil 500 mg/m² IV on days 1 and 4.
2. Doxorubicin (Adriamycin) 50 mg/m² on days 1–3 as a 72-hour continuous infusion.
3. Cyclophosphamide 500 mg/m² IV on day 1.
4. Chemotherapy repeated at 21-day intervals.
5. Dose modification based on hematological toxicity as defined by weekly CBC with differential and platelet counts. If the lowest platelet count is <50,000/mm³, the doses of all drugs are reduced 20 percent.
6. Adjuvant chemotherapy is initiated after surgical treatment has been completed.
7. Adjuvant chemotherapy is continued as above until a total dose of 450–500 mg/m² doxorubicin has been administered.

Note: Patients are accrued to currently active prospective, randomized treatment protocols whenever possible. When patients are not eligible to be treated on protocol, they are treated with the FAC regimen as described above.

TABLE 67–2.   CRITERIA FOR BREAST CONSERVATION SURGERY AFTER INDUCTION CHEMOTHERAPY FOR LOCALLY ADVANCED BREAST CANCER

1. Resolution of skin edema (dermal lymphatic involvement).
2. Residual tumor size of less than 5 cm.
3. Absence of extensive intramammary lymphatic invasion.
4. Absence of extensive suspicious-looking microcalcifications.
5. No known evidence of multicentricity.
6. Patient's desire for breast preservation.

From Singletary SE, Dhingra K, Yu D-H: New strategies in locally advanced breast cancer. *In* Pollock RE (ed): Advances in Surgical Oncology. Norwell, MA, Kluwer Academic Publishers, 1997.

four courses of induction chemotherapy are used first in an attempt to achieve early control of distant micrometastases (Table 67–1). Even though distant disease may be undetectable by current clinical diagnostic procedures, its presence is suggested by the high percentage of distant failures that occurred even when complete local control was achieved with radiotherapy and surgery in the prechemotherapy era, as discussed previously. In addition, the use of induction chemotherapy may decrease primary tumor bulk sufficiently to convert some inoperable patients into candidates for mastectomy or breast conserving therapy. The third reason for using induction chemotherapy is that tumor responsiveness has been shown to correlate with overall survival, as will be discussed later. Consequently, tumor responsiveness to induction chemotherapy may serve as an in vivo chemosensitivity assay to indicate the potential effectiveness of postoperative adjuvant chemotherapy.

If the tumor has increased in size after three courses of induction chemotherapy, surgical resection is considered if feasible. Otherwise, radiotherapy is used, followed by surgical resection. If the tumor has responded to induction chemotherapy, surgery is then used as the second modality. The issue of response versus progression of the primary tumor is assessed by physical examination, repeat mammograms, and ultrasonography (Fig. 67–4). Criteria used for grading tumor regression are those of the Union Internationale Contre le Cancer (UICC).[14]

The surgical procedure is either a total mastectomy or lumpectomy with Level 1–2 axillary dissection, defined as dissection of the nodal tissues between the latissimus dorsi muscle and lateral pectoralis minor muscle (Level 1) as well as the nodal tissues posterior to the pectoralis minor muscle (Level 2). Patients are considered for breast conservation surgery if they meet specific criteria after downstaging with induction chemotherapy (Table 67–2). Surgical resection is generally performed 3 weeks after the last chemotherapy treatment in order to avoid granulocyte and platelet nadir effects commonly observed about 2 weeks after myelosuppressive chemotherapy. In the event of prolonged myelosuppression, the CBC with

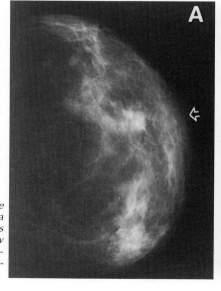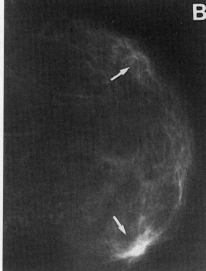

Figure 67–4   *Mammography before and after three courses of FAC induction chemotherapy showing a marked response of the primary tumor.*   **A** *shows the pretreatment mammogram with the open arrow denoting skin thickening.*   **B** *shows the mammogram after induction chemotherapy. The arrows denote small areas of residual tumor in the breast.*

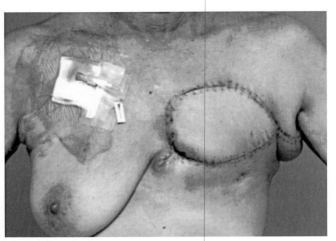

Figure 67–5   *The same patient as in Figure 67–1 after preoperative induction chemotherapy. Full-thickness chest wall resection and mastectomy site have been reconstructed using a pedicle flap. Note the presence of a percutaneous subclavian chemotherapy catheter to be used for postoperative adjuvant chemotherapy.*

differential is followed until the granulocyte count is ≥1000/mm³, at which time surgical resection is performed. The technique of mastectomy is discussed elsewhere in this book. Occasionally, an en bloc chest wall resection is required for some stage IIIB lesions. The surgical goal is to achieve the best possible local control on the chest wall and the axilla so as to avoid the complex and difficult problems of chest wall recurrence (Fig. 67–5).

The mastectomy performed includes a Level 1 and 2 axillary dissection for pathological node assessment. Because of the documented low incidence of "skip metastasis" (metastatic deposits in Level 3 nodes without Level 1–2 disease)[3] and because the patient will be receiving axillary radiotherapy, the possibility of uncontrolled axillary disease is minimal. In addition, the Level 1–2 dissection avoids the functional and cosmetic difficulties that can result from axillary radiotherapy in an already completely dissected axilla.[26] Surgery is used before radiotherapy because, having the tumor debulked surgically allows for better radiotherapeutic local control in the adjuvant setting.[22] There have been no significant increases in infection or wound-healing problems in postoperative patients treated by this multimodality approach.[5]

The last reason for using surgery after induction chemotherapy but before radiotherapy is that it provides the opportunity for pathological assessment of primary tumor response at a point in the clinical course where operability has been achieved. The importance of this pathological assessment was suggested by Feldman and coworkers,[8] who examined 90 patients with locally advanced breast cancer treated from 1974 to 1981 at the M. D. Anderson Cancer Center. All patients had at least 5 years of posttreatment follow-up. Group A consisted of patients whose mastectomy specimen showed no macroscopic cancer on gross pathological examination (15 of 90 patients);

Group B patients had residual pathological macroscopic disease (75 of 90 patients).

The rate of relapse after 5-year follow-up was significantly higher for Group B patients, as was death from recurrent breast cancer at 6-year follow-up (Group A had a 93 percent 5-year survival rate versus a 30 percent 5-year survival rate for Group B; $p <0.01$). The median disease-free survival was more than 5 years for Group A and only 22 months for Group B. At the M. D. Anderson Cancer Center, pathological assessment of response to induction chemotherapy is used as an indicator of whether to continue "first-line" FAC chemotherapy as a postoperative adjuvant or consider "second-line" agents.

After surgical therapy, adjuvant chemotherapy is given. Initially 12 courses were used, but no significant improvement in survival was noted when compared with six courses.[16] Therefore, six courses of adjuvant chemotherapy are now standard (see Table 67–1). Patients are accrued to currently active prospective, randomized treatment protocols whenever possible. Treatment strategies that are under investigation at the time of this writing at the M. D. Anderson Cancer Center include (1) dose-intensive chemotherapy with growth factor support or hematopoietic stem cell support, (2) non–cross-resistant chemotherapeutic regimens, and (3) comparison of new selected regimens (paclitaxel) versus standard FAC induction chemotherapy.[25]

At the completion of chemotherapy, radiotherapy is then performed (Table 67–3). The rationale for this sequence is based on the awareness that radiotherapy and doxorubicin are poorly tolerated if given simultaneously.[16] In addition, local control is equally good with early or late radiotherapy; however, more distant failures have been observed with postoperative radiotherapy given before adjuvant chemotherapy.

The use of hormonal therapy has not yet been evaluated in the context of prospective multimodality trials of locally advanced breast disease except in combination with chemotherapy. The addition of hormonal therapy to standard chemotherapy regimens and the use of estrogenic recruitment have not, as

TABLE 67–3.   M. D. ANDERSON RADIOTHERAPY POSTMASTECTOMY IRRADIATION PROTOCOL FOR STAGE III BREAST CARCINOMA

1. The chest wall and peripheral lymphatics are treated to 50 Gy in 25 fractions.
2. The mastectomy scar receives a boost of 10–16 Gy.
3. The chest wall is treated with either tangential photon-beam or electron-beam fields, depending on patient anatomy.
4. The peripheral lymphatics are usually treated with electrons.
5. The dissected axilla is treated only in patients with N2 or supraclavicular disease or pathological evidence of extranodal extension.
6. Patients with inflammatory carcinoma are treated on an accelerated, hyperfractionated (twice-daily) schedule.

From Eric A. Strom, M.D., personal communication.

yet, shown improved survival or freedom from local/regional relapse over other neoadjuvant regimens.[17] An accurate understanding of the natural biology of locally advanced breast carcinoma, coupled with the ability to integrate extirpative and reconstructive surgery with the other available modalities, has radically improved our capacities to treat and even cure these formerly lethal problems.

RECONSTRUCTION OF DEFECTS FOLLOWING MASTECTOMY

The success of chemotherapy in controlling distant disease places an important new emphasis on local control of stage III breast cancer. Although in many patients local control can be achieved with a standard mastectomy, at times skin invasion or chest wall fixation may mandate more radical ablative procedures. Such procedures are possible only if closure of the wound can be achieved. Fortunately, if wound closure by primary approximation of the wound edges is impossible, reconstructive techniques can be used to bring additional tissues into the wound and allow healing to occur. The surgeon performing the ablative procedure is then free to excise whatever is required to achieve local control of the tumor.

The choice of reconstructive method depends on the size and type of the defect that will be presented to the reconstructive surgical team. Such defects are best considered by dividing them into two groups: those in which the chest wall is intact and those in which it is not.

Intact Chest Wall

If the defect involves only skin and subcutaneous tissue, in some cases it can be repaired with a skin graft. This rather simple maneuver will provide coverage that is reasonably functional and will stand up to postoperative radiotherapy once it has fully healed (Fig. 67–6). Unfortunately, it is also rather unattrac-

tive and less durable than a myocutaneous flap. In addition, skin grafts require an extended period of time for recipient site healing and healing of the donor site. For these reasons, and because of advances in the ability to cover wounds with flaps, skin grafts are rarely used at the M. D. Anderson Cancer Center.

Most larger defects are best reconstructed with myocutaneous flaps.[4] Flaps provide durable skin coverage of normal quality and thickness and heal in a manner similar to a wound closed primarily. Although the use of a flap requires sacrifice of muscle function, that loss is generally well tolerated and may even go unnoticed by the patient. Because of these advantages, flaps have grown in popularity and have become the cornerstone of chest wall and breast reconstruction at the M. D. Anderson Cancer Center. Many flaps are available for the reconstruction of mastectomy defects, but the latissimus dorsi and the rectus abdominis myocutaneous flaps are the ones most commonly used because of their suitability and reliability.

Latissimus Dorsi Myocutaneous Flap

The latissimus dorsi myocutaneous flap was first described in 1897 by the Italian surgeon Tansini.[27] This flap, which consists of a skin paddle based on the underlying latissimus dorsi muscle, is supplied with blood by both the thoracodorsal artery and by branches of the posterior intercostal arteries close to the spine (Fig. 67–7). The flap can survive on either of these two blood supplies; for chest wall and breast reconstruction the larger and dominant thoracodorsal pedicle is used. The flap is isolated on its thoracodorsal vascular leash and rotated around its attachment point in the axilla. From there it will easily reach to the sternum and will generally fill a defect 8 cm in width and up to 20 cm in length (Fig. 67–8).

The two chief advantages of the latissimus dorsi flap are its lack of donor site morbidity and its reliable blood supply. Perhaps because of similar actions by the teres major and minor, patients notice little morbidity from use of the latissimus dorsi muscle in a flap. This flap is rarely lost perioperatively unless the thoracodorsal vessels have been damaged during the mastectomy. Even in that event, the flap will often survive on collateral flow between the thoracodorsal vessel and its serratus branch.

The chief disadvantage of the latissimus flap is its limited size. Although the muscular portion of the flap can be quite wide, the skin of the donor site in the back does not stretch well. If more than 8 to 10 cm of skin is mobilized in flap development, primary closure of the donor site can no longer be achieved. Although larger donor defects can be skin grafted, the use of skin grafts will compromise the ultimate cosmetic result.

Rectus Abdominis Flaps

The rectus abdominis myocutaneous flaps are large flaps of great usefulness. There are four versions of

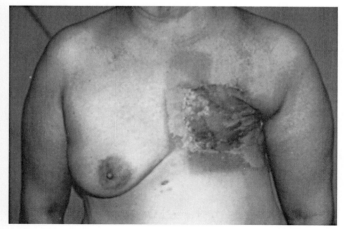

Figure 67–6 *Patient with skin graft on left chest wall. Note the thin cover and poor cosmetic appearance.*

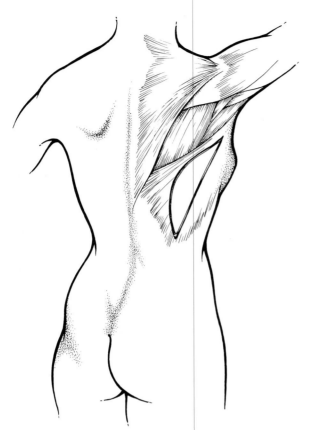

Figure 67–7 *Drawing of the plan for a latissimus dorsi myocutaneous flap. (Note underlying latissimus muscle.) The shape of the skin paddle can be altered to fit the defect.*

the flap that can be used for chest wall reconstruction: the vertical rectus abdominis flap, the single-pedicle transverse rectus abdominis myocutaneous (TRAM) flap, the double-pedicle TRAM flap, and the free TRAM flap.

The vertical rectus abdominis flap was the earliest

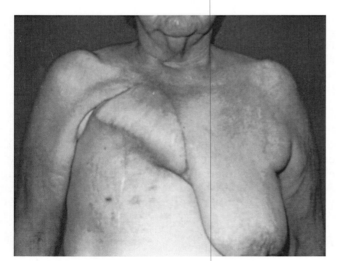

Figure 67–8 *Patient with healed latissimus dorsi myocutaneous flap reconstruction of full-thickness chest wall defect.*

of the rectus flaps to be described and is the easiest technically.[23] The skin paddle is positioned vertically over the contralateral rectus abdominis muscle, where it is abundantly supplied with blood from the underlying muscle by way of perforating vessels (Fig. 67–9). Fortuitously, in most females the abdominal skin is lax or redundant. Consequently, large amounts of skin can be mobilized and the donor site can still be closed primarily. The width of the skin paddle can frequently be greater than 15 cm.

The single-pedicle TRAM flap has become justifiably popular for postmastectomy breast reconstruction (Fig. 67–10).[13] Adaptation of this technique, which uses a transversely oriented skin paddle, has been hindered by the less robust nature of its blood supply. Because a large part of the skin paddle does not lie directly over the muscle, the flap is dependent on the integrity of a small number of perforating vessels that exist where the skin and the muscle overlap. In most healthy patients this blood supply is adequate, and a large flap may be obtained. In smoking patients, diabetic patients, and patients with multiple abdominal scars, circulation may be inadequate and may limit the size and viability of the flap.

Despite its decreased reliability, the single-pedicle TRAM flap is useful for nonsmoking patients with an intact chest wall. Situated low on the rectus muscle, this flap has a long leash and a long axis of

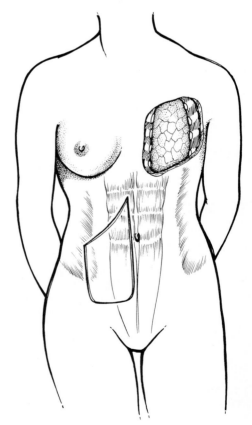

Figure 67–9 *Drawing of plan for a vertical rectus abdominis myocutaneous flap for chest wall reconstruction.*

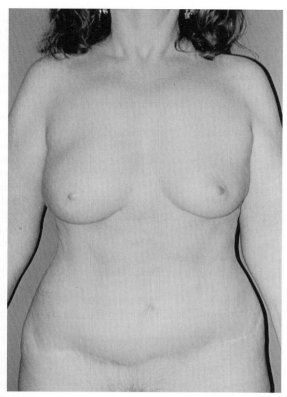

Figure 67–10   *Right breast reconstruction with a single-pedicle TRAM flap. This patient did not have a chest wall defect.*

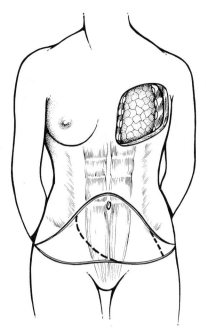

Figure 67–11   *Drawing of plan for a double-pedicle TRAM flap to be used for chest wall reconstruction.*

rotation, allowing it to rotate quite far laterally or high into the axilla. If the chest wall is intact, the viability of the flap is less critical, and a slightly higher risk of flap loss can therefore be tolerated.

The double-pedicle TRAM flap is a variation on the single-pedicle TRAM in which the blood supply is doubled by basing the flap on both rectus abdominis muscles (Fig. 67–11).[19] The double-pedicle TRAM flap avoids the blood supply problems of the single-pedicle TRAM flap and combines the reliability of the vertical rectus with the mobility and improved postoperative appearance of the TRAM concept. The decreased abdominal strength from the loss of two rectus muscles is usually well tolerated. Because the blood supply is better, the flap can often be made quite large. In some cases, not only reconstruction of the chest wall cover but also an approximation of the missing breast can be accomplished (Figs. 67–12 and 67–13).

The free TRAM flap is based on the deep inferior epigastric vessels, and uses microvascular anastomoses to re-establish blood supply to the flap.[10, 15, 24] The advantages of this method include more robust flap perfusion (provided the anastomoses remain patent) and reduced muscle sacrifice in the donor site. Because less muscle is harvested, patients have less postoperative pain and tend to recover from their surgery more quickly. At the M. D. Anderson Cancer Center, where, at the time of this writing, almost 600 free TRAM flaps have been used for breast reconstruction, the flap loss rate is less than 1 percent. The authors of this chapter would therefore not hesi-

tate to use a free TRAM flap for chest wall reconstruction, provided that the defect was not full-thickness, and provided that the requisite equipment and personnel were available.

Chest Wall Not Intact

When the underlying chest wall is not intact, the reconstruction problems are no different from those

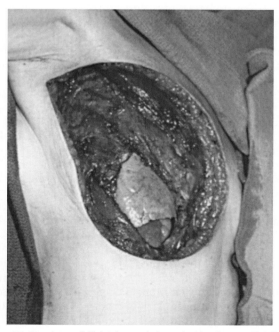

Figure 67–12   *Large full-thickness defect of right chest wall following mastectomy and chest wall resection.*

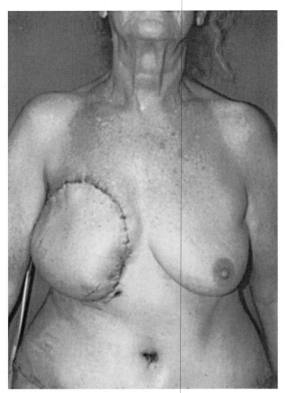

Figure 67–13   *Right chest wall and breast mound reconstruction of patient shown in Figure 67–12.*

when the chest wall is intact, except that flap reliability becomes more critical. Because an open pleural cavity is poorly tolerated, flap reliability over a full-thickness defect of the chest wall is of utmost importance. For this reason, free flaps are rarely used at the M. D. Anderson Cancer Center for repair of such defects if a pedicled myocutaneous flap is available. In this situation, the safest and most reliable technique is desired, and even a 1 percent flap loss rate should be avoided if possible. For these patients, a double-pedicled TRAM flap may be a good alternative, providing very reliable coverage at the cost of a somewhat increased sacrifice of muscle in the donor site.

As in the case of partial-thickness chest wall defects, the latissimus dorsi myocutaneous flap is often the best choice for small defects that are within its arc of rotation. The flap is very reliable, and the thickness of the flap is similar to that of the normal chest wall, so the flap blends in well cosmetically. The underlying muscle can be sutured to muscle around the edges of the rib cage defect to provide a two-layer closure so that even if some skin loss occurs, the underlying muscle can survive and protect the underlying mesh or chest cavity. For defects lower on the chest wall that would be difficult to reach with the latissimus, or for very large defects that the latissimus flap would not cover, the vertical rectus abdominis flap and the double-pedicle TRAM flap are good options. Both of these flaps are quite reliable; although there is only one layer of closure,

the flaps are fairly thick. This bulkiness helps to stabilize the chest wall and compensate for the loss of ribs. Also, in selected cases the bulk can be used to simulate a missing breast.

Reconstruction of the rib cage is not usually necessary after resection of one or two ribs. If good flap coverage and respirator support are provided, sufficient scar tissue will form to stabilize the chest wall without additional support. If a larger area of structural support will be lost, it is usually advisable to stabilize the chest wall with Marlex or Prolene prosthetic mesh. Provided that the mesh is completely covered by viable tissue, it is usually well tolerated and will allow the patient to be weaned from the respirator and discharged from the hospital earlier than otherwise would be the case.[20] Although infection can occur in such cases, it has been uncommon, provided that the overlying flap is well vascularized and that pre-existing infection was not present.

Other methods and techniques that can be used in chest wall reconstruction include random and axial skin flaps, omental flaps, other myocutaneous flaps, and microvascular free flaps other than the TRAM. However, the methods previously discussed in this chapter have been so successful and versatile that these other approaches are rarely needed. Because variation is inherent in both human anatomy and the biological behavior of tumors, there will always be exceptional situations requiring alternative strategies. Nevertheless, appropriate use of the latissimus dorsi flap and the various rectus abdominis flaps will allow successful reconstruction of almost all defects encountered in the treatment of locally advanced breast cancer.

References

1. American Joint Committee on Cancer. Manual for Staging of Cancer, 4th ed. Philadelphia, JB Lippincott, 1992, p 149.
2. Baclesse F: Roentgen therapy as the sole method of treatment of cancer of the breast. AJR 62:311, 1949.
3. Boova RS, Bonanni R, Rosato FE: Patterns of axillary nodal involvement in breast cancer. Predictability of level one dissection. Ann Surg 196:642, 1982.
4. Bostwick J, Vasconez LO, Jurkiewicz MJ: Breast reconstruction after a radical mastectomy. Plast Reconstr Surg 61:682, 1978.
5. Broadwater JR, Edwards MJ, Kuglen C: Mastectomy following preoperative chemotherapy. Ann Surg 213:126, 1991.
6. Davila E, Vogel CL: Management of locally advanced breast cancer (stage III): A review. Int Adv Surg Oncol 7:297, 1984.
7. DeLena M, Zucali R, Viganotti G: Combined chemotherapy-radiotherapy approach in locally advanced (T_{3b}–T_4) breast cancer. Cancer Chemother Pharmacol 1:53, 1978.
8. Feldman LD, Hortobagyi GN, Buzdar AU: Pathological assessment of response to induction chemotherapy in breast cancer. Cancer Res 46:2578, 1986.
9. Fletcher GH, Montague ED: Radical irradiation of advanced breast cancer. AJR 93:573, 1965.
10. Grotting JC, Urist MM, Maddox WA, Vasconez LO: Conventional TRAM flap versus free microsurgical TRAM flap for immediate breast reconstruction. Plast Reconstr Surg 83:842, 1989.
11. Haagensen CD, Stout AP: Carcinoma of the breast: II. Criteria of operability. Ann Surg 118:859; 1032, 1943.
12. Harris JR, Sawicka J, Gelman R: Management of locally ad-

vanced carcinoma of the breast by primary radiation therapy. Int J Radiat Oncol Biol Phys 9:345, 1983.

13. Hartrampf CR, Scheflan M, Black PW: Breast reconstruction with a transverse abdominal island flap. Plast Reconstr Surg 69:216, 1982.

14. Hayward JL, Carbone PP, Heuson J-C: Assessment of response to therapy in advanced breast cancer: A project of the programme on clinical oncology of the International Union Against Cancer, Geneva, Switzerland. Cancer 39:1289, 1977.

15. Holmstron H: The free abdominoplasty flap and its use in breast reconstruction. Scand J Plast Reconstr Surg 13:423, 1979.

16. Hortobagyi GN, Ames FC, Buzdar AU: Management of stage III primary breast cancer with primary chemotherapy, surgery and radiation therapy. Cancer 62:2507, 1988.

17. Hunt KK, Ames FC, Singletary SE: Locally advanced noninflammatory breast cancer. Surg Clin North Am 76:393, 1996.

18. Hutter RVP: At last—worldwide agreement on the staging of cancer. Arch Surg 122:1235, 1987.

19. Ishii CH, Bostwick J, Raine TJ: Double-pedicle transverse rectus abdominis myocutaneous flap for unilateral breast and chest-wall reconstruction. Plast Reconstr Surg 76:901, 1985.

20. Kroll SS, Walsch G, Ryan B, King R: Risks and benefits of using Marlex mesh in chest wall reconstruction. Ann Plast Surg 31:303, 1993.

21. Maddox WA, Carpenter JT, Laws HT: Does radical mastectomy still have a place in the treatment of primary operable breast cancer? Arch Surg 122:1317, 1987.

22. Montague ED, Fletcher GH: Local regional effectiveness of surgery and radiation therapy in the treatment of breast cancer. Cancer 55:2266, 1985.

23. Robbins TH: Rectus abdominis myocutaneous flap for breast reconstruction. Aust N Z J Surg 49:527, 1979.

24. Schusterman MA, Kroll SS, Miller MJ: The free TRAM flap for breast reconstruction: A single center's experience with 211 consecutive cases. Ann Plast Surg 32:234, 1994.

25. Singletary SE, Dhingra K, Yu D-H: New strategies in locally advanced breast cancer. In Pollock RE (ed): Advances in Surgical Oncology, Norwell, Kluwer Academic Publishers, 1996.

26. Spanos WJ, Montague ED, Fletcher GH: Late complications of radiation only for advanced breast cancer. Int J Radiat Oncol Biol Phys 6:1473, 1980.

27. Tansini I: Sopra il mio nuovo processo di amputazione della mammella. Gazetta Medica Italiana 57:141, 1906.

28. Valagussa P, Zambetti M, Bignami P: T_{3b}–T_4 breast cancer: Factors affecting results in combined modality treatments. Clin Exp Metastasis 1:191, 1983.

29. Zucali R, Uslenghi C, Kenda R: Natural history and survival of inoperable breast cancer treated with radiotherapy and radiotherapy followed by radical mastectomy. Cancer 37:1422, 1976.

CHAPTER 68

MANAGEMENT OF LOCAL/REGIONAL RECURRENCE: ROLE OF RADIATION ONCOLOGY

Michael P. Hagan, M.D., Ph.D. / Nancy Price Mendenhall, M.D.

Local/regional recurrence (LRR) refers to a second clinical manifestation of breast cancer in either the primary site (breast, chest wall, incision, or skin flaps) or regional lymphatics, including first-echelon (axillary, internal mammary, Rotter's) or second-echelon (supraclavicular) lymph nodes.

PRESENTATION

LRR can be easily overlooked both because of the subtlety of presentation and because of denial on the part of the patient.[53] As a result, diagnosis is frequently made after the disease has become extensive, or secondarily after the presentation of distant disease. The extent of disease at discovery is often greater than is apparent on physical examination.[12, 43, 54] Some of the more common clinical presentations, shown in Figures 68–1 through 68–11, are described in the sections that follow.

Chest Wall Recurrence

Chest wall recurrence most commonly appears as single or multiple, millimeter-size, painless nodules. Although the nodules are occasionally in the skin, they are usually found under the skin, frequently in close proximity to the scar (Figs. 68–1 and 68–2).[10, 41] Early diagnosis requires meticulous palpation of the skin flaps. Eventually, however, the lesion will progress to distort, infiltrate, or ulcerate the overlying skin. Less commonly, erythema or violaceous discoloration of the skin, without palpable nodularity or skin thickening (Fig. 68–3), may be the only sign of recurrence. Advanced signs of recurrence include skin induration, widespread nodularity, pruritic or nonpruritic erythematous macules and papules (Fig. 68–4), obvious inflammatory skin changes, ridging, and carcinoma *en cuirasse* (Fig. 68–5). As the disease progresses, tumor may extend beyond the chest wall (Figs. 68–5 and 68–6).[41] Rarely, an ipsilateral pleural effusion may signal chest wall recurrence in the intercostal musculature.[69]

Regional Lymphatic Recurrence

Regional recurrence most commonly is detected as a painless, mobile mass during examination of the supraclavicular fossa (Fig. 68–7). Occasionally, however, LRR may not be discovered until new or worsened arm edema or brachial plexopathy develops (Figs. 68–8 and 68–9). Signs of LRR in the axillary apex include a mobile mass or vague fullness palpa-

ble in the infraclavicular area deep to the pectoralis major muscle (Figs. 68–9 and 68–10). Axillary recurrence after complete axillary dissection is distinctly uncommon. Signs and symptoms of axillary disease, in addition to the presence of a mass, include pain, decreased range of motion, and new onset of arm edema.

Internal mammary node recurrence most often is presented as a painless subcutaneous parasternal mass, with or without skin involvement (Fig. 68–10).[55] Less commonly, an abnormality on chest roentgenogram or CT scan is the first sign of an internal mammary node recurrence (Figs. 68–10 and 68–11). Patients with advanced disease may present with symptoms secondary to destruction of the sternum or rib (Fig. 68–11), pleural effusion, or anterior mediastinal involvement with superior vena cava syndrome.[55]

A recurrence in Rotter's (interpectoral) nodes, though rare, is most frequently discovered in a patient who has had a modified radical mastectomy for a large tumor located in the superior mid-breast. The recurrence is presented as a submuscular mass

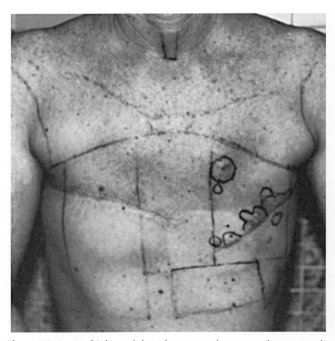

Figure 68–1 *Multiple nodules of recurrent breast carcinoma ranging from 0.25 cm to 1 cm in diameter were palpable in the chest wall flap along the mastectomy incision in this 44-year-old woman 6 months after diagnosis of inflammatory carcinoma (T4 N2) treated with three courses of preoperative chemotherapy, simple extended mastectomy, and an additional 4 months of postoperative chemotherapy.*

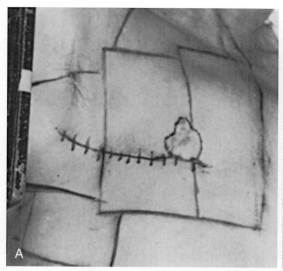
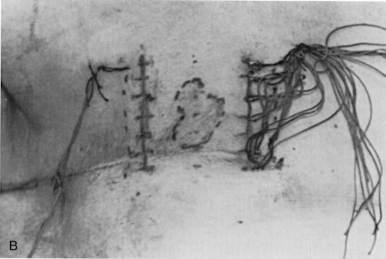

Figure 68–2   *This 64-year-old woman underwent a right modified radical mastectomy in March 1984 and 6 months of postoperative chemotherapy for an estrogen and progesterone receptor–negative, 3-cm breast carcinoma with metastatic involvement of 15 of 18 nodes retrieved. In June 1985, a small nodule was noted in the superior chest wall flap, just above the mastectomy incision. Bone scan demonstrated multiple asymptomatic bone metastases. The nodule was excised, and the patient was placed on tamoxifen. In July 1986, the tumor progressed to a 2.5-cm area of tender multiple confluent nodules.   **A,** External-beam treatment portals are shown with the tumor nodules encircled. Because distant metastases were present, a short course of therapy was indicated. A dose of 30 Gy in 10 fractions over 15 days was delivered to the chest wall with 8 MeV electrons with bolus, to the supraclavicular fossa with 8 MV x-rays, and to the internal mammary chain nodes with 14 MeV electrons.   **B,** The chest wall recurrence was given an additional 20 Gy over 50 hours with an interstitial radium needle implant. Complete regression of the chest wall tumor was obtained. The chest wall and regional lymphatics remained free of tumor until the patient's death from progression of distant metastases in March 1987.*

palpable deep to the pectoralis major.[10, 57] Distinguishing this lesion as a nodal rather than chest wall recurrence is frequently impossible.

NATURAL HISTORY

Incidence

After the introduction of the radical mastectomy, Halsted's students reported a 32 percent incidence of LRR.[42] Much attention was subsequently focused on the details of the surgical procedure with the hope of improving control of local disease and therefore survival rates. Neither careful dissection of the overlying skin nor grafting eliminated LRR.[13, 31, 70] Results are mixed as to the significance of the mastectomy technique.[44, 66] Since 1960 most series reporting on results of mastectomy for operable disease indicate an incidence of LRR of 10–30 percent.[9, 14, 19, 67] The use of adjuvant irradiation after mastectomy reduces

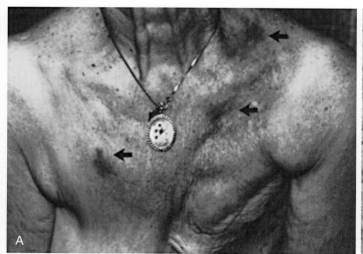
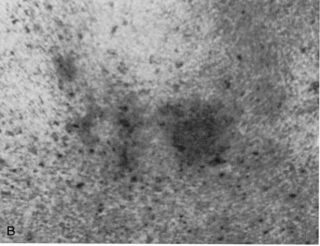

Figure 68–3   *This 72-year-old woman initially had left axillary adenopathy of unknown origin. Mammogram and physical examination did not confirm any obvious primary tumor in the breast. She was treated with preoperative irradiation to the left breast and regional lymphatics followed by modified radical mastectomy.   **A,** One and a half years after the initial treatment, multiple nonpalpable areas (arrows) of purplish skin discoloration were observed and were proved by biopsy to be recurrent breast carcinoma.   **B,** Detail of recurrent disease involving the skin.*

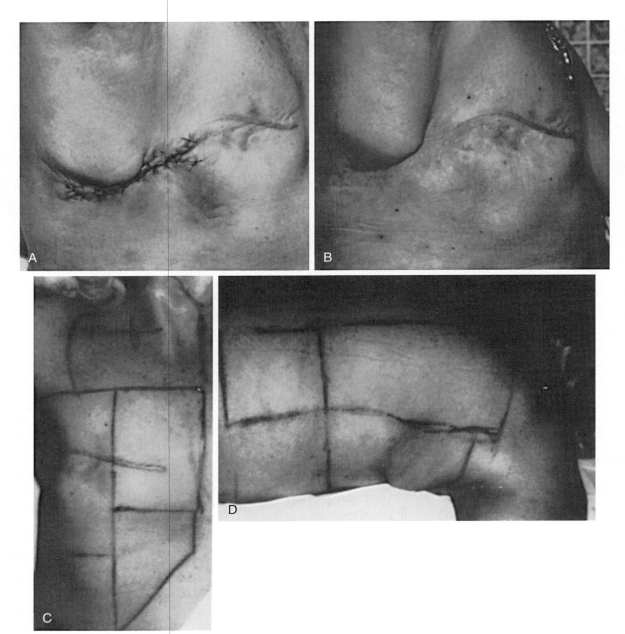

Figure 68–4   *Three years after modified radical mastectomy for a node-negative (T stage unknown) breast cancer, this 77-year-old woman had an extensive chest wall recurrence. For 6 months before biopsy of the chest wall, the patient had repeatedly reported skin erythema, thickening, and tenderness to her physician, who noted these findings but attributed them to irritation from her brassiere.   **A,** Photograph obtained after biopsy shows marked leathery induration and erythema of skin along the lateral portion of the mastectomy incision and multiple satellite nodules in the inferior chest wall flap and along the medial portion of the mastectomy incision.*

*The estrogen receptor level in the recurrent tumor was 301 fmol per mg of protein and the progesterone receptor level was <1 fmol per mg. Because of the extent of the recurrence, radiotherapy was not thought to be feasible, so the patient was placed on tamoxifen.   **B,** Regression of erythema and nodularity was judged to be 75 percent at 3 months after administration of tamoxifen. Tattoos indicate sites of previous satellite nodules.*

*   **C,** After the response to tamoxifen, the chest wall was treated with radiation using ⁶⁰Co and 14 MeV electrons for the supraclavicular fossa, 8 MeV electrons with bolus for the chest wall fields, and 14 MeV electrons for the internal mammary chain field with the patient supine. Because of the posterior extent of the recurrence, posterior lateral chest wall fields were also treated, with the patient in a prone position **D.** The initial treatment plan was 50 Gy to the peripheral lymphatic areas and 60 Gy to the entire chest wall, followed by an interstitial implant to the mastectomy scar and tattooed satellite nodules.*

Moist desquamation of the chest wall precluded delivery of more than 56 Gy. The peripheral lymphatic areas received 50 Gy. The patient died with metastatic disease 5.5 years after completing radiotherapy, without evidence of further local or regional disease.

LRR by approximately a factor of 3 (see Chapter 61, Adjuvant Radiotherapy after Modified Radical Mastectomy).[33, 49, 56, 64] The impact of systemic therapy is less clear.

Pattern of Recurrence

LRR is a component of one third of all first recurrences after mastectomy. Approximately one half of LRRs are isolated. Additionally, LRRs are identified in 10–20 percent of patients who already have distant metastases.[4, 6, 15, 64] Because of the subtlety of presentation (see Fig. 68–4), the low sensitivity of the typical follow-up evaluation, and the long natural history of breast cancer, reported incidences are likely to be underestimates of the true rate of uncontrolled LRR.[4, 40]

The distribution of sites of recurrence reported in several series is shown in Table 68–1.* Recurrence in the chest wall predominates. Over one half of all isolated recurrences are found in the skin, subcutis, or, rarely, the deeper chest wall structures.[2, 13, 14, 70, 72] Similar distributions are seen after either radical or modified radical mastectomy.[52]

---

*See references 4, 10, 18, 30, 36, 46, 59, 65.

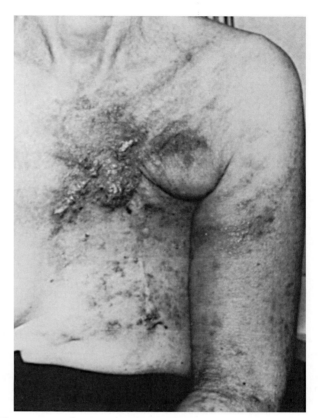

Figure 68–6   *This patient underwent left modified radical mastectomy, three courses of adjuvant chemotherapy, and postoperative irradiation for T2 N1 carcinoma with histologic involvement of all 23 nodes. Progressive arm edema developed 8 months after treatment, requiring aggressive treatment with a Jobst stocking and pump. At 16 months, a pruritic rash involving the left chest wall flaps developed. The multiple flat and raised erythematous papules, confluent over the mastectomy incision, were confirmed on biopsy to be recurrent breast carcinoma. The tumor did not respond to CAF chemotherapy or mitomycin but progressed to involve the skin of the entire anterior chest wall and left upper extremity (as shown) as well as patchy areas of the skin of the back before her death as a result of pericardial and pleural effusions.*

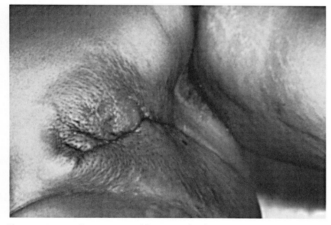

Figure 68–5   *This 48-year-old woman had a 10-cm left breast mass in December 1987. Needle aspiration showed infiltrating ductal carcinoma. The patient was staged as IIIA and treated with three courses of CAF chemotherapy. A residual 7-cm mass was present in the breast at the time of simple mastectomy with dissection of the lower (Level 1) axillary contents in March 1988. Pathology revealed residual infiltrating ductal carcinoma that did not extend beyond the capsule of the lymph nodes. Postoperative chemotherapy was recommended but not given. Two weeks after a normal physical examination in June 1988, the patient went to the emergency room with the sudden onset of massive arm edema and a tender reddened area on the chest wall. She had pain in the upper aspect of the left arm. Physical examination revealed extensive carcinoma en cuirasse involving the left anterior chest wall with scattered nodules of tumor on the inferior chest wall flap and posterior to the mastectomy incision on the lateral portion of the back. There was massive edema of the arm with palpable tumor filling the infraclavicular axillary apical area.*

CT scan of the chest confirmed tumor involving the axillary apex and surrounding the brachial plexus. Bone scan demonstrated diffuse metastatic disease. Chemotherapy was recommended for palliation.

Time to Recurrence

The time to local recurrence or the initial disease-free interval varies inversely with initial stage of disease; in a study by Gilliland and coworkers,[26] the median time to local recurrence was 6.2 years, 4.3 years, and 2.1 years for patients with stage I, II, and III disease, respectively. Both Donegan and colleagues[19] and Crowe and colleagues[15] have analyzed the time course for LRR in large populations of patients with recurrent breast cancer. Their results (Fig. 68–12A) show that approximately 70 percent of LRRs occurred in the first 3 years. A logarithmic plot of the same data (Fig. 68–12B) reveals a single exponential for each set of data, consistent with a simple Poisson distribution with a half-time for recurrence of 26 months extending over the initial 6 years. Although 80–90 percent of LRRs occur within 6 years of the initial treatment, LRRs have been reported after much longer intervals.[17, 40, 45]

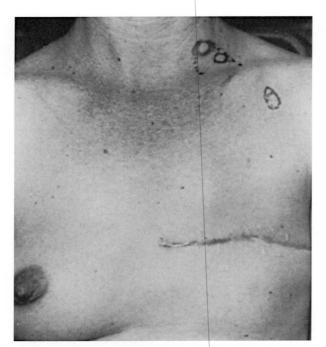

Figure 68–7   *This 35-year-old woman had a left modified radical mastectomy in May 1985 for a stage I (T1 N0) estrogen and progesterone receptor–negative adenocarcinoma of the breast with close surgical margins and lymphatic space invasion within the specimen. In August 1986, she had biopsy-proven recurrent disease in the left supraclavicular and infraclavicular nodes, as shown. The lymph nodes ranged from 0.5 cm to 1.5 cm in diameter and were located in the medial supraclavicular fossa, deep to the insertion of the sternocleidomastoid muscle and just beneath the clavicle in the midclavicular line. She received three courses of chemotherapy (CMF) with little response, radiation to the chest wall and lymphatic areas with complete regression of the tumor, and then another course of chemotherapy, during which contralateral axillary nodal disease and distant metastases developed. She died of progressive disease in May 1987.*

Prognostic Indicators

Many tumor and patient characteristics have been examined for prognostic significance. These include lymph node status, tumor size and site, receptor status, histological grade, percent of cells in the S-phase, *HER2/neu* overexpression, and skin changes at original presentation* as well as nodule size and site, number of nodules, and the disease-free interval at the time of recurrence.† From these analyses a consistent picture has emerged in which the risk of LRR and survival are related to both the original tumor burden indicated by the size of the primary tumor and the amount of axillary disease, and the tumor burden at recurrence indicated by the size and number of nodules.‡ Potential prognostic factors are usually identified from univariate analysis, but those factors related to tumor burden are robust indicators under multivariate analyses as well.‡

Prognosis for survival is best in patients with small recurrences involving a single site and presenting more than 2 years after initial management.[1, 5, 30, 59] Several reports show that both 5- and 10-year survival rates are higher in patients with only a single site of recurrence rather than multiple sites.[1, 11, 23, 50] Halverson and coworkers[30] reported a 5-year survival rate of 19 percent for patients with multifocal disease compared with 36–59 percent for patients with unifocal recurrences. Likewise, Schwaibold and coworkers[59] reported a 5-year survival rate of 77 percent for patients with a single focus of disease, compared with 44 percent for patients with multifocal recurrence. The data are less clear concerning the specific site of recurrence. Although Schwaibold and coworkers[59] found that site of recurrence had no prognostic significance, in some series patients with chest wall recurrences have done better than patients with recurrences at other sites.[1, 30, 65]

Disease-free interval (DFI), the most consistently reported single prognostic indicator, probably reflects tumor burden and tumor biology.[30] The value of the DFI as a predictor of second recurrence and survival was reported by Shimkin and associates[62] as early as 1954. Aberizk and coworkers[1] confirmed the importance of the DFI by showing that 5- and 10-year survival rates were significantly higher for patients with recurrence after a 2-year interval. Other investigators have confirmed the prognostic significance of

---

*See references 7, 8, 14, 26, 28, 47, 53, 71.
†See references 3, 4, 7, 11, 18, 30, 46, 59.
‡See references 3, 4, 11, 13, 30, 35, 46, 59.

TABLE 68–1.   **SITES OF LOCAL/REGIONAL RECURRENCE**

| | | Percent with Isolated Recurrence (Percent with Any Recurrence at Site) | | | |
Researchers	No. of Patients	*Chest Wall*	*Supraclavicular Fossa*	*Axilla*	*Internal Mammary or Parasternal*
Bedwinek et al[7]	129	47 (60)	19	8	8
Chen et al[10]	194	55 (65)	12	8	10
Deutsch et al[18]	107	44 (57)	17 (29)	8 (17)	10 (14)
Halverson et al[29]	224	60 (70)	13	8	6
Kamby et al[36]	312	— (61)	—	— (27)	—
Mendenhall et al[46]	47	53	11	6	11
Schwaibold et al[59]	128	67 (83)	9 (16)	4 (11)	3
Toonkel et al[65]	124	63 (77)	0 (9)	12 (21)	4 (10)

Adapted from Bedwinek JM: Natural history and management of isolated local-regional recurrence following mastectomy. Semin Radiat Oncol 1994; 4:260–269, p 261.

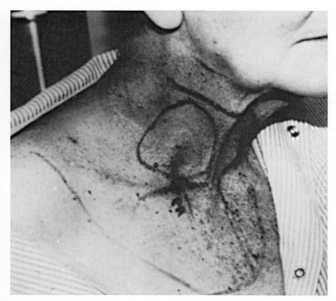

Figure 68–8 *This patient had a modified radical mastectomy in 1974 for a T3 N1 M0 carcinoma of the left breast (3 of the 9 nodes retrieved were involved) followed by 2.5 years of adjuvant melphalan. In March 1980, she noted numbness and tingling in the right hand that did not respond to physical therapy. In October 1980, a biopsy-proven recurrence was found in the right supraclavicular fossa with an estrogen receptor level of 62 fmol per mg of protein. Her symptoms resolved with tamoxifen but recurred, together with weakness and pain in the right arm, in May 1983. In July 1983, Horner's syndrome developed. She was treated for 1 year with chemotherapy (CMF). A 4 × 5 cm mass was noted in the medial right supraclavicular fossa and low neck, as shown; progression was suspected and she was referred for radiotherapy. On radiographic studies, the lesion extended from C3 to T2 with involvement of the bodies and transverse processes of C5 and C6 and grossly invaded the spinal canal. She had resolution of her paresthesias, improvement in the arm weakness, and regression of the tumor mass with 60 Gy of radiation delivered in 1.2-Gy fractions twice a day. Pleural effusions developed 1 year after irradiation, however, and she died in February 1986.*

the DFI in multivariate analyses.[5, 30, 59] In these studies, overall survival at 5 years is 30–35 percent for patients with recurrence within the first 2 years compared with 50–67 percent for patients with later recurrences.[30, 59]

TREATMENT

Patient Selection

Uncontrolled LRR can be painful and can present problems involving hygiene and infection that alienate the patient from family and friends. As an obvious sign of treatment failure, LRR can be psychologically devastating to the patient. Therefore, patients with any LRR should be treated with the goal of achieving local control in order to improve the quality of remaining life.

LRR is isolated (i.e., not associated with clinically apparent distant metastases at the time of diagnosis) in approximately one half of patients.[12, 72] Nevertheless, LRR has been regarded as a harbinger of distant

metastases. In the series reported by Gilliland and coworkers,[26] distant metastases eventually developed in every patient, and all died of breast cancer. Most series with a long-term follow-up report a 10-year disease-free survival (DFS) of 7–17 percent after initial recurrence.[1, 10, 30, 46, 65] Careful selection, however, can identify subsets of patients with a better prognosis. In general, patients with a long initial DFI and limited recurrence should be treated aggressively. For patients whose disease is controlled locally after an initial DFI of at least 2 years and complete excision, the 5-year overall survival rate and DFS rate can be greater than 50 percent. Overall survival rate and DFS rate at 10 years will likely exceed 30 percent and 20 percent, respectively.

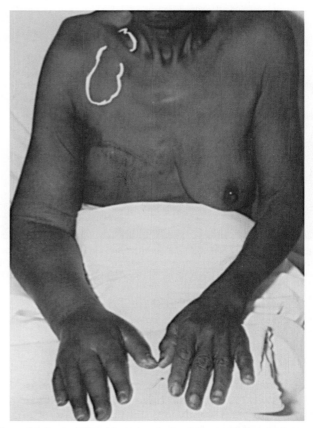

Figure 68–9 *In 1967, this patient had a right modified radical mastectomy followed by 1 year of adjuvant chemotherapy for a breast carcinoma of unknown stage. Progressive arm edema developed in 1982, which was treated with pain medications. In 1984, she had surgery for presumed right carpal tunnel syndrome with progressive neurological loss in the right hand. In March 1987, she went to the emergency room with a nonfunctioning right upper extremity with severe arm edema (despite a stocking), severe arm pain, and ulnar and radial nerve neuropathies. Recurrent carcinoma was confirmed with biopsy after a CT scan demonstrated a mass high in the right axilla, involving the pectoralis major muscle, with extension along the brachial plexus. Obvious disease was palpable in the right supraclavicular fossa. The tumor did not respond to tamoxifen, megestrol acetate, or combination chemotherapy, and the patient was referred for irradiation in March 1988. She then had supraclavicular disease fixed to underlying tissues and infraclavicular disease fixed to the anterior chest wall (shown outlined in white). Bone scan was negative, and on CT scan of the chest, the disease was localized to the supraclavicular and infraclavicular fossae with no evidence of other adenopathy or lung metastases.*

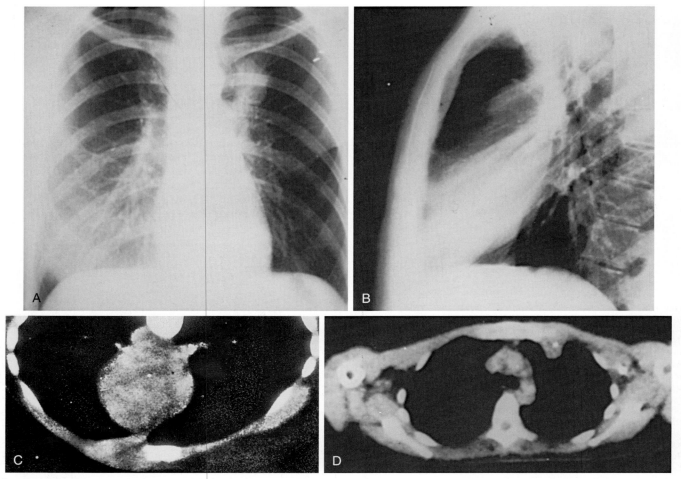

Figure 68–10   *This patient had a left modified radical mastectomy in May 1977 for a T1 N0 upper outer quadrant breast carcinoma. Posteroanterior and lateral chest roentgenograms obtained on routine follow-up in 1978 were normal. She noted a rapidly growing parasternal nodule in July 1979. She also reported a several-month history of mild upper extremity pain and paresthesias relieved by arm elevation. Physical examination showed a 7.5 × 8.5 cm left parasternal nodule in the second interspace, a 1 × 2 cm subcutaneous nodule in the first interspace, and a tethered 5 × 5 cm node high in the left axilla. Biopsy confirmed recurrent breast carcinoma.   **A** and **B,** posteroanterior and lateral chest roentgenograms in August 1979 demonstrated an anterior mediastinal mass at the level of the first and second intercostal spaces.   **C** and **D,** CT scan sections from August 1979 showed destruction of the sternum by a mass consistent with internal mammary adenopathy and also demonstrated the subpectoral (infraclavicular) mass that was palpable high in the axilla.*

Illustration continued on opposite page

Only palliative treatment may be appropriate for patients who are elderly, have extensive LRR, or are in poor medical condition. Palliation can often be obtained with hormonal manipulation, chemotherapy, or a brief course of irradiation; therapy in this setting should be relatively short and of low morbidity (see Fig. 68–2). Patients with synchronous distant metastases and asymptomatic LRR may be considered for observation. When local/regional treatment is delayed for delivery of systemic therapy, or when observation is selected, the patient should have frequent follow-up examinations, and irradiation should be instituted promptly if disease progression is noted.

Work-Up

At time of presentation of LRR, initial studies should include chest roentgenogram, bone scan, liver function tests, and CT of the chest. The chest CT has

identified additional sites of disease in one quarter to two thirds of patients.[34, 43, 54, 58] Lymphoscintigraphy may help identify patients with low-volume internal mammary node or axillary node disease,[21, 22, 52] but this procedure is not available in many institutions. When results of initial studies are equivocal, other tests, such as plain roentgenograms for suspected bone lesions, magnetic resonance imaging of the neck and shoulder girdle, or CT scans of the abdomen, may be useful. A CT scan of the head should be performed if neurological signs or symptoms are present.

Biopsy

When planning the biopsy, it is important to take into consideration the overall management plan. To facilitate decisions regarding systemic therapy, tissue should be submitted for assay of estrogen and proges-

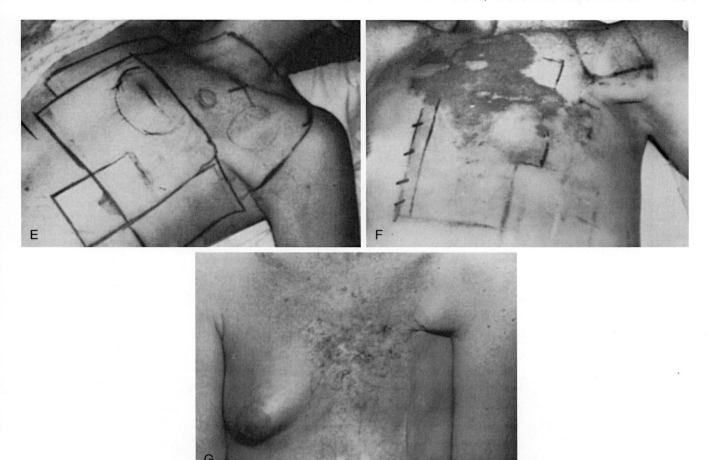

Figure 68–10   Continued.   **E,** *Radiation treatment fields are shown; the three palpable recurrent nodules are circled. The patient received comprehensive chest wall and regional lymphatic irradiation and concomitant chemotherapy (CMF), which was continued for 1 year. Following 50 Gy to the entire chest wall and supraclavicular fossa, the dose to the parasternal area was boosted through a shrinking-field technique with 14 MeV, 12 MeV, and 10 MeV electrons to 75 Gy, and the dose to the left infraclavicular mass was boosted with 17 MV x-rays with a shrinking-field technique to 65 Gy.*   **F,** *A moist desquamation occurred at the end of treatment, most pronounced in areas of previous sun exposure. Her treatment was complicated by radiation pneumonitis, requiring prolonged steroid therapy, and symptomatic pericarditis, which was managed with aspirin.*   **G,** *She was alive and well and remained without evidence of disease until 1994 (15 years) when a 1-cm nodule of recurrent or new breast cancer arose just below the radiation field. The node was excised and the adjacent skin was treated with electrons. She continues (August 1996) with no evidence of disease, 17 years after treatment for LRR, with only moderate telangiectasia and hyperpigmentation in the treatment field.*

terone receptor levels (which may differ from those in the original tumor). When total excision of a gross tumor nodule can easily be accomplished, it should be done, as this surgery may improve disease control and allow the radiation oncologist to use a lower dose or lesser penetration of radiation. An unnecessarily large or aggressive surgical procedure may require prolonged healing before definitive treatment with radiation can be started. An ill-planned incision that potentially contaminates additional tissue can necessitate extension of radiation portals and place the patient at increased risk for complications. Therefore, close coordination between the surgeon and the radiation therapist is necessary. In selected cases, chest wall resection may be appropriate (see Fig. 68–11).[61]

Radiation Therapy

No Prior Irradiation

Irradiation combined with local excision is the mainstay of management if the initial treatment did not include irradiation. Examples are shown in Figures 68–2, 68–4, 68–10, and 68–11.

Local Resection. Although local excision alone is associated with a high rate (67–76 percent) of second recurrence,[6, 16, 25] a complete excision may improve the rate of local control achieved by aggressive irradiation.[1, 10, 11, 30, 59] Data from Halverson and coworkers[29] from Mallinckrodt Institute, shown in Table 68–2, demonstrate improved local control when complete excision is followed by higher dose irradiation, a phenomenon confirmed in several other studies.[1, 41, 59, 63] When excision is possible, irradiation can be delayed for 2–3 weeks to permit wound healing.

Treatment Volume. Small local-field irradiation is associated with a high rate of in-field and marginal failures.[1, 3, 9] Therefore, the treatment volume for patients selected for aggressive treatment should include the chest wall, undissected first- and second-

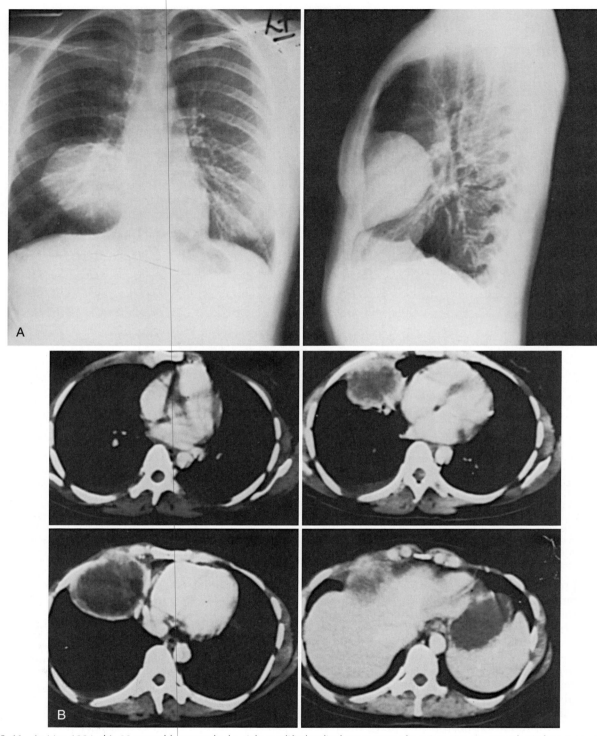

Figure 68–11   In May 1984, this 29-year-old woman had a right modified radical mastectomy for a 3 × 2.5-cm metaplastic breast carcinoma with squamous differentiation. Eight lymph nodes retrieved contained no tumor, and estrogen and progesterone receptor levels were negative. Chest roentgenogram was normal.   **A,** In November 1984, she had right anterior chest wall pain, and chest roentgenogram demonstrated a 10-cm mass in the right lower chest.   **B,** CT scan showed involvement of the anterior right fifth rib, as did bone scan. The mass was located in a parasternal position adherent to the right pericardium. Biopsy confirmed recurrent tumor. Metastatic evaluation was negative.

Illustration continued on opposite page

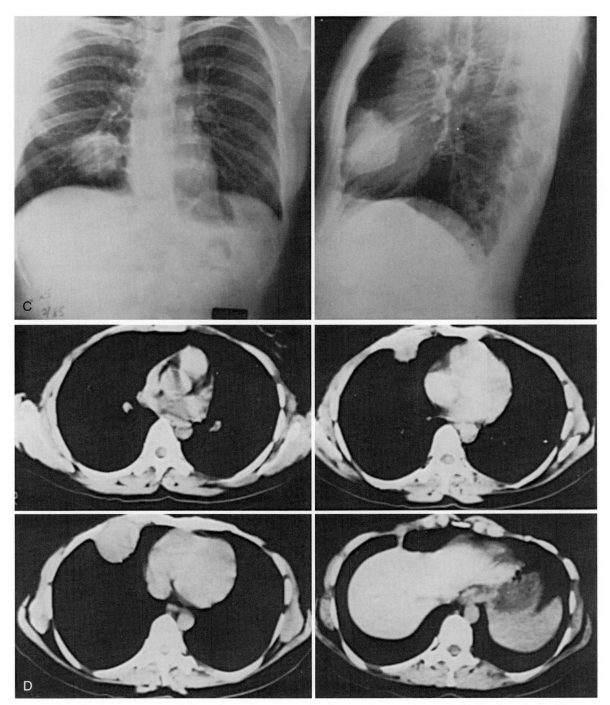

Figure 68–11   Continued. *After six courses of chemotherapy (CAF) completed in March 1985, she was judged to have had a 50 percent reduction in the tumor as apparent on chest roentgenogram (**C**) and CT scan (**D**), with stabilization of response after the third course of chemotherapy. In April 1985, she underwent resection of the residual mass, which grossly appeared to be a large, necrotic internal mammary lymph node that had grown into the anterior fifth rib and into the thoracic cavity, invading lung and adherent to pericardium. With the chest wall resection, a margin of lung was removed, which on histological examination was positive; tumor was also noted in the marrow of one of the resected ribs. Other margins were negative. A myocutaneous flap from the right latissimus dorsi was used to close the defect.*

Illustration continued on following page

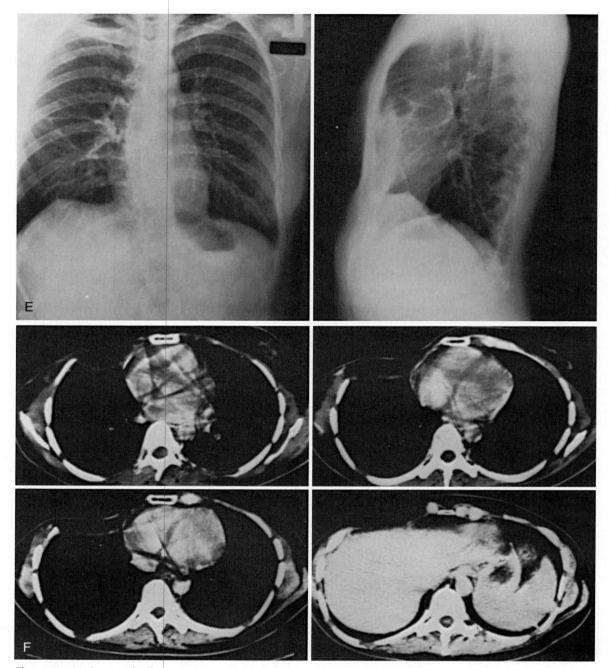

Figure 68–11   Continued. *Chest roentgenogram* (**E**) *and CT scan* (**F**) *after surgery are shown.*

Illustration continued on opposite page

echelon nodes, and occasionally the previously dissected axilla. The axilla may require treatment because of LRR or an initial presentation that included one of the following conditions: incomplete axillary dissection, nodes 2.5 cm or more in diameter, clinically matted nodes, or extensive extranodal disease.[24] Treatment of the internal mammary node chain is controversial. If the internal mammary node chain is treated, a technique should be selected that minimizes the radiation dose to the heart and lung. Generally, an *en face* field with electron beam of appropriate energy is the best technique for assuring coverage of these nodes and limiting radiation exposure of other structures.

Time-Dose Factors. All areas at risk for subclinical involvement are given 50 Gy in 5 weeks at 2 Gy per fraction. The dose to areas around surgical incisions, including sites of biopsy, is boosted with an additional 10 Gy delivered at 2.0–2.5 Gy per fraction. For areas of gross involvement, the boost dose is increased to 15–25 Gy at 2.0–2.5 Gy per fraction. The boost may be delivered by interstitial implant when technically suitable.

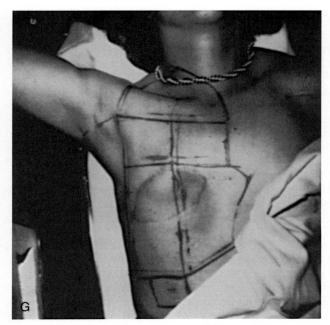

Figure 68–11 Continued.   **G,** External-beam treatment portals. From May through July 1985, the patient received 50 Gy in 25 fractions over 5 weeks to the supraclavicular fossa (with 40 Gy from ^{60}Co and 10 Gy from 10 MeV electrons), the internal mammary nodes (with 12 MeV electrons), and the medial and lateral chest walls (6 MeV electrons). An additional 10 Gy was delivered to the internal mammary nodes, myocutaneous flap, and incision (with 6 MeV and 12 MeV electrons) for a total dose of 60 Gy. To spare the underlying heart, beeswax bolus was shaped to fit the chest wall defect during treatment of the portion of the medial chest wall that was included in the internal mammary chain portal. She received two courses of CMF chemotherapy concurrently and two more courses after irradiation, finishing treatment in August 1985. In November 1985, restaging studies (chest roentgenogram, bone scan, and CT scan of the chest) were negative. In December 1985, however, a brain metastasis developed, which was treated aggressively with craniotomy and radiation. Thereafter metastatic disease developed in the thyroid (March 1986), left supraclavicular area (May 1986), and lung (July 1986). She remained free of local/regional disease until her death in August 1986.

Prior Irradiation

Retreatment with irradiation is not likely to be successful, may result in severe complications, and is generally not advised.

Hyperthermia

The role of hyperthermia in the treatment of LRR is unclear. In previously unirradiated patients, combined irradiation and hyperthermia has resulted in a high rate of local control with good durability at 2 years.[60] It is unclear, however, whether results with combined irradiation and hyperthermia are better than with radiotherapy alone. The RTOG reported 85 percent local control for LRRs less than 4 cm in depth treated with hyperthermia and 60 Gy, but the follow-up period was short, and 24 percent of patients experienced ulceration and subcutaneous necrosis.[60] In a randomized study, the local control rate with combined hyperthermia and low-dose irradiation (32 Gy) was 62 percent for lesions smaller than 3 cm and

40 percent with irradiation alone.[51] Irradiation alone, when used at definitive doses in other studies, has resulted in local control rates of 50–80 percent for lesions of a similar size.[10, 29, 59]

Hyperthermia with or without low-dose irradiation (24–32 Gy) may be useful for recurrences in previously irradiated tissues.[20, 38, 68] However, disease control is usually short-lived,[20, 27, 37, 68] and complications requiring surgical management are frequent.[20, 27]

Systemic Therapy

It is unlikely that chemotherapy alone will eradicate LRR (see Fig. 68–8).[32, 35] Chemotherapy or hormonal therapy should be used alone only in patients who are not suitable for irradiation. Furthermore, the authors of this chapter (Hagan and Mendenhall) do not recommend a lengthy delay in the start of irradiation to permit a prolonged course of chemotherapy. On occasion, however, a patient who is not initially a candidate for radical irradiation will respond to systemic therapy and thus become a candidate for definitive radiotherapy (see Fig. 68–4). Since knowledge of the original extent of the LRR is critical for planning radiation treatment, it is imperative that the radiation oncologist examine the patient before systemic treatment or surgical excision.

In patients who have not previously received systemic therapy, it is rational to use adjuvant hormonal manipulation for postmenopausal patients or patients with positive estrogen receptors and to use chemotherapy for premenopausal patients or those with negative estrogen receptors. It is not possible, however, to use a doxorubicin-containing regimen concurrently with irradiation. Occasionally, it has been difficult to complete the full course of irradiation, including the boost, with concomitant cyclophosphamide, methotrexate, and fluorouracil (CMF). For patients with surgical resection of all gross tumor who require only modest doses of irradiation, radiation usually can be delivered concomitantly with CMF. For patients with gross residual disease after biopsy, chemotherapy may be delayed until completion of irradiation. Alternatively, two or three courses

TABLE 68–2. DEPENDENCE OF SECOND RECURRENCE ON EXTENT OF SURGERY AND RADIATION DOSE

	No. of Second Recurrences/ No. of Initial Recurrences			
		*Gross Residual**		
Dose (Gy)	*Locally Excised*	<3 cm	3–5 cm	>5 cm
<50	1/9	2/7	2/4	5/6
50–59.9	2/47 (4%)	3/14	1/7	8/19
≥60	4/24 (17%)	0/15	6/12	11/23

*Size of initial recurrence.
Data from Halverson KJ, Perez CA, Kuske RR, et al: Isolated local/regional recurrence of breast cancer following mastectomy: Radiotherapeutic management. Int J Radiat Oncol Biol Phys 19:851–855, 1990.

of chemotherapy may be given prior to irradiation so that information on the tumor's responsiveness to chemotherapy can be obtained (see Fig. 68–8). The response achieved with 2 to 3 months of chemotherapy or hormonal therapy may significantly reduce gross tumor and facilitate subsequent irradiation (see Figs. 68–4 and 68–12).

The role of standard chemotherapy is unclear when LRR develops after standard adjuvant chemotherapy [CMF or cyclophosphamide, doxorubicin HCl, and fluorouracil (CAF)]. The role of high-dose chemotherapy with stem cell rescue for LRR is being investigated at the time of this writing.

For patients whose tumors contain estrogen or progesterone receptors, hormonal therapy may be started once the diagnosis is secure, and this hormonal therapy may be given concurrently with irradiation. The first choice is usually tamoxifen. If the patient has already received tamoxifen, Megace (megestrol acetate) can be considered. Other treatment choices are oophorectomy or radioablation of the ovaries.

RESULTS OF TREATMENT

Radiation Therapy

Although most patients treated with aggressive irradiation obtain an initial complete response, another LRR eventually develops in a large proportion of them. The data from several series are summarized in Table 68–3.[1, 10, 18, 30, 46, 59, 65] Most patients who experience a second LRR do so in the first 5 years. Series reporting long-term follow-up, however, show that 79–90 percent of patients with disease controlled at 5 years continue to have control of local/regional disease at 10 years.[1, 48, 65]

Control of LRR

In patients with LRR on the chest wall, the adjacent chest wall and regional lymphatics are at high risk for subclinical disease.[4, 10, 29, 39] If the original radiation treatment volume includes only the LRR without elective treatment of the entire chest wall and regional lymph nodes, the predominant pattern of failure will be in the adjacent chest wall and regional lymphatics.[10, 30, 59] Clinically evident recurrence in an initially uninvolved axilla or IMC is unlikely.[29, 59] When sites at risk for subclinical disease are treated, the original site of LRR becomes the most likely site of failure.[4]

Data from the Mallinckrodt Institute (shown in Table 68–2)[29] and other series[1, 59] suggest that the addition of complete surgical resection of the LRR before radiotherapy increases the probability of disease control. Furthermore, local control is independent of the size of the lesion after a complete excision followed by adequate irradiation.[59] In several series, however, complete excision has been possible in only 33–60 percent of patients treated with definitive irradiation.[1, 6, 59] When gross disease remains *in situ*, a radiation boost dose to a total of 65–75 Gy will achieve local control in approximately 50 percent of patients.[29]

Local control of LRR with radiotherapy appears to depend on the site or sites of the recurrence. Halverson and coworkers,[29] Toonkel and coworkers,[65] and others have reported better disease control rates for patients with nodal recurrences or isolated chest wall recurrences than for those with multiple sites of involvement.[1, 10, 18, 59] Even in the most favorable-prognosis patients whose isolated recurrences are completely resected and whose radiotherapy treatment volumes are comprehensive, the reported 5-year second-recurrence rates vary from 25 percent to 52 percent.[30, 59]

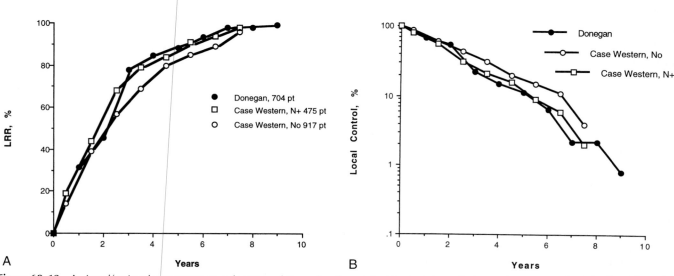

Figure 68–12   A, *Local/regional recurrence as a function of time after the original treatment.*   **B,** *Same data presented as the logarithm of the percentage remaining locally controlled. Data are from the series reported by Crowe and associates[15] (node-negative patients, N_0, and node-positive, N^+) and Donegan and colleagues.[19]*

Approximately 25 percent of patients with LRR survive 10 years after their treatment,[1, 10, 29, 46, 48, 65] and one half of them remain disease-free.[29, 46, 48, 65] Schwaibold and coworkers[59] reported better DFS rates in patients whose LRR was controlled for 5 years (64 percent versus 24 percent). Mendenhall and coworkers[46] reported a lower incidence of distant metastases (20 percent versus 60 percent; $p = 0.26$) at 5 years in patients whose LRR was controlled. The relationship between local disease control and survival is less clear.[6, 18, 29, 59, 65] Local/regional control should be pursued aggressively, regardless of its impact on survival, because it offers a considerable improvement in the quality of life for the breast cancer patient.

Systemic Therapy

Control of LRR

Little information exists on the efficacy of chemotherapy or hormonal treatment as sole or adjuvant treatment for LRR. The only prospective randomized trial of chemotherapy is a study involving 32 patients treated with irradiation with or without single-agent dactinomycin.[48] Follow-up was short, a median of 15–18 months, and details of the irradiation were not reported. Although the use of dactinomycin increased the rate of local control from 59 percent to 80 percent, the difference was not statistically significant. Two retrospective studies reported complete response rates of 28 percent and 46 percent after chemotherapy alone for LRR.[32, 35] In a case control study by Halverson and coworkers,[30] a trend was seen toward improved local/regional control with chemotherapy and radiotherapy over radiotherapy alone, but this result has not been confirmed in other studies.[18, 35, 59]

A Swiss multicenter study is the only reported multiarm prospective randomized trial of hormone therapy for LRR.[9] Originally a four-arm study was designed, but only "good-risk" patients accrued in numbers sufficient for analysis. These 113 good-risk patients had either positive estrogen receptor recurrences or recurrences limited to three or fewer nodules, each less than 3 cm in its largest dimension,

and disease-free intervals greater than 12 months. In all patients, the recurrence was grossly resected and the chest wall irradiated with up to 50 Gy. Patients were then randomized. Local/regional control after 3 years was 77 percent for excision plus irradiation versus 91 percent with the addition of tamoxifen.

Beck and colleagues[3] from the Mountain States Tumor Institute, reported a complete-response rate of 64 percent for patients receiving hormone therapy or chemotherapy alone; the results in patients receiving hormone therapy were not reported separately, and the durability of control was poor.

Survival Rates

As discussed previously, distant disease will develop in most patients experiencing LRR. Therefore, it would seem appropriate to deliver systemic therapy to all such patients. Although several cooperative groups initiated randomized trials of chemotherapy to address this issue, all had to close because of poor accrual.[4] The Swiss multicenter trial detailed earlier reported a DFS of 59 percent with combined local therapy and tamoxifen versus 36 percent without tamoxifen, but there was no overall survival difference between the arms of the study. In a matched cohort study reported by Halverson and coworkers,[30] hormone manipulation combined with irradiation resulted in both increased DFS and overall survival rates.

The only existing data relevant to cytotoxic chemotherapy in the setting of LRR are retrospective. Janjan and colleagues[35] compared outcome in patients receiving combination chemotherapy, irradiation, or both at the M. D. Anderson Cancer Center. DFS did not differ among the three groups. The interpretation of these data was confounded by substantial clinical differences among the treatment groups. For example, 32 percent of the radiation-only group had four or more positive nodes at presentation compared with 16 percent in the chemotherapy group and 19 percent in the combined-modality group. In another retrospective study, Beck and coworkers[3] showed that overall and DFS rates were 35 percent and 23 percent, respectively, for patients treated with systemic therapy for LRR. Although these values

TABLE 68–3. LOCAL CONTROL AND SURVIVAL FROM TIME OF RECURRENCE

Researchers	No. of Patients	Local/Regional Control (%)		Overall Survival (%)		Disease-Free Survival (%)	
		5-Year	10-Year	5-Year	10-Year	5-Year	10-Year
Aberizk et al[1]	90	42	35	50	26	30	7
Chen et al[10]	194	60	—	51	26	—	—
Deutsch et al[18]	107	45	—	35	—	12*	—
Halverson et al[29]	224	57	—	43	26	26	14
Mendenhall et al[46]	47	68	61	50	34	41	17
Schwaibold et al[59]	128	43	—	49	—	24	—
Toonkel et al[65]	121	58	46	38	26	26	15
Weighted average		53		48	27	25	13

*Crude survival.

were substantially better than those reported for radiation treatment alone, undoubtedly selection factors were involved, as the results for radiation treatment are not comparable to those of other series (see Table 68–3). Thus, with the exception of tamoxifen treatment for patients with positive estrogen and progesterone receptor recurrences presenting after a 12-month disease-free interval, there is no clear evidence that systemic treatment is efficacious in treatment of LRR.

References

1. Aberizk WJ, Silver B, Henderson IC, et al: The use of radiotherapy for treatment of isolated locoregional recurrence of breast carcinoma after mastectomy. Cancer 58:1214–1218, 1986.
2. Auchincloss H: The nature of local recurrence following radical mastectomy. Cancer 11:611–619, 1958.
3. Beck TM, Hart NE, Woodard DA, et al: Local or regionally recurrent carcinoma of the breast: Results of therapy in 121 patients. J Clin Oncol 1:400–405, 1983.
4. Bedwinek JM: Natural history and management of isolated local-regional recurrence following mastectomy. Semin Radiat Oncol 4:260–269, 1994.
5. Bedwinek JM: Radiation therapy of isolated local-regional recurrence of breast cancer: Decisions regarding dose, field size, and elective irradiation of uninvolved sites. Int J Radiat Oncol Biol Phys 19:1093–1095, 1990. Editorial.
6. Bedwinek JM, Fineberg B, Lee J, et al: Analysis of failures following local treatment of isolated local-regional recurrence of breast cancer. Int J Radiat Oncol Biol Phys 7:581–585, 1981.
7. Bedwinek JM, Lee J, Fineberg B, et al: Prognostic indicators in patients with isolated local-regional recurrence of breast cancer. Cancer 47:2232–2235, 1981.
8. Bonadonna G, Valagussa BS, Rossi A, et al: Ten-year experience with CMF-based adjuvant chemotherapy in resectable breast cancer. Breast Cancer Res Treat 5:95–115, 1985.
9. Borner M, Bacchi M, Goldhirsch A, et al: First isolated locoregional recurrence following mastectomy for breast cancer: Results of a phase III multicenter study comparing systemic treatment with observation after excision and radiation. Swiss Group for Clinical Cancer Research. J Clin Oncol 12:2071–2077, 1994.
10. Chen KK-Y, Montague ED, Oswald MJ, et al: Results of irradiation in the treatment of locoregional breast cancer recurrence. Cancer 56:1269–1273, 1985.
11. Chu FCH, Lin F-J, Kim JH, et al: Locally recurrent carcinoma of the breast: Results of radiation therapy. Cancer 37:2677–2681, 1976.
12. Ciatto S, Rosselli del Turco M, Pacini P, et al: Early detection of local recurrences in the follow-up of primary breast cancer. Tumori 70:179–183, 1984.
13. Conway H, Neumann CG: Evaluation of skin grafting in the technique of radical mastectomy in relation to local recurrence of carcinoma. Surg Gynecol Obstet 88:45–49, 1949.
14. Crile G Jr: The incidence of local recurrence of carcinoma of the breast. Surg Gynecol Obstet 156:497–498, 1983. Editorial.
15. Crowe JP Jr, Gordon NH, Antunez AR, et al: Local-regional breast cancer recurrence following mastectomy. Arch Surg 126:429–432, 1991.
16. Dahlstrom KK, Andersson AP, Andersen M, et al: Wide local excision of recurrent breast cancer in the thoracic wall. Cancer. 72:774–777, 1993.
17. Danckers UF, Hamann A, Savage JL: Postoperative recurrence of breast cancer after thirty-two years: A case report and review of the literature. Surgery 47:656–662, 1960.
18. Deutsch M, Parsons JA, Mittal BB: Radiation therapy for local-regional recurrent breast cancer. Int J Radiat Oncol Biol Phys 12:2061–2065, 1986.
19. Donegan WL, Perez-Mesa CM, Watson FR: A biostatistical study of locally recurrent breast carcinoma. Surg Gynecol Obstet 122:529–540, 1966.
20. Dragovic J, Seydel HG, Sandhu T, et al: Local superficial hyperthermia in combination with low-dose radiation therapy for palliation of locally recurrent breast cancer. J Clin Oncol 7:30–35, 1989.
21. Ege GN: Internal mammary lymphoscintigraphy: The rationale, technique, interpretation and clinical application: A review based on 848 cases. Radiology 118:101–107, 1976.
22. Ege GN, Elhakim T: The relevance of internal mammary lymphoscintigraphy in the management of breast carcinoma. J Clin Oncol 2:774–781, 1984.
23. Fentiman IS, Matthews PN, Davison OW, et al: Survival following local skin recurrence after mastectomy. Br J Surg 72:14–16, 1985.
24. Fletcher GH: Textbook of Radiotherapy, 3rd ed. Philadelphia, Lea and Febiger, 1980.
25. Flook D, Webster DJT, Hughes LE, et al: Salvage surgery for advanced local recurrence of breast cancer. Br J Surg 76:512–514, 1989.
26. Gilliland MD, Barton RM, Copeland EM III: The implications of local recurrence of breast cancer as the first site of therapeutic failure. Ann Surg 197:284–287, 1983.
27. Gonzalez-Gonzalez D, van Dijk JDP, Blank LECM: Chestwall recurrences of breast cancer: Results of combined treatment with radiation and hyperthermia. Radiother Oncol 12:95–103, 1988.
28. Haagensen CD: Disease of the Breast, 2nd ed, revised reprint. Philadelphia, WB Saunders, 1971.
29. Halverson KJ, Perez CA, Kuske RR, et al: Isolated local-regional recurrence of breast cancer following mastectomy: Radiotherapeutic management. Int J Radiat Oncol Biol Phys 19:851–858, 1990.
30. Halverson KJ, Perez CA, Kuske RR, et al: Survival following locoregional recurrence of breast cancer: Univariate and multivariate analysis. Int J Radiat Oncol Biol Phys 23:285–291, 1992.
31. Handley RS, Thackray AC: Conservative radical mastectomy (Patey's operation). Ann Surg 170:880–882, 1969.
32. Hoogstraten B, Gad-el-Mawla N, Maloney TR, et al: Combined-modality therapy for first recurrence breast cancer: A Southwest Oncology Group study. Cancer 54:2248–2256, 1984.
33. Host H, Brennhovd IO, Loeb M: Postoperative radiotherapy in breast cancer—long-term results from the Oslo study. Int J Radiat Oncol Biol Phys 12:727–732, 1986.
34. Jacobs CG, Zinreich ES, Fishman EK, et al: Computed tomography in radiotherapy planning of the axillary region. J Comput Tomogr 10:221–225, 1986.
35. Janjan NA, McNeese MD, Buzdar AU, et al: Management of locoregional recurrent breast cancer. Cancer 58:1552–1556, 1986.
36. Kamby C, Andersen J, Ejlertsen B, et al: Pattern of spread and progression in relation to the characteristics of the primary tumour in human breast cancer. Acta Oncol 30:301–308, 1991.
37. Kapp DS, Barnett TA, Cox RS, et al: Hyperthermia and radiation therapy of local-regional recurrent breast cancer: Prognostic factors for response and local control of diffuse or nodular tumors. Int J Radiat Oncol Biol Phys 20:1147–1164, 1991.
38. Kapp DS, Cox RS, Barnett TA, et al: Thermoradiotherapy for residual microscopic cancer: Elective or post-excisional hyperthermia and radiation therapy in the management of local-regional recurrent breast cancer. Int J Radiat Oncol Biol Phys 24:261–277, 1992.
39. Kenda R, Lozza L, Zucali R: Results of irradiation in the treatment of chest wall recurrent breast cancer. Radiother Oncol 24:S41, 1992. Abstract 155.
40. LaRaja RD, Meo MA, Alcindor F: Local chest wall recurrence of breast cancer forty years after mastectomy: A case report. Breast 7:203, 1994.
41. Leggett CAC: Local recurrence of carcinoma of the breast. Aust N Z J Surg 50:298–300, 1980.
42. Lewis D, Reinhoff WF Jr: A study of the results of operations for the cure of cancer of the breast: Performed at the Johns Hopkins Hospital from 1889 to 1931. Ann Surg 95:336–400, 1932.
43. Lindfors KK, Meyer JE, Busse PM, et al: CT evaluation of

local and regional breast cancer recurrence. AJR Am J Roentgenol 145:833–837, 1985.

44. Maddox WA, Carpenter JT Jr, Laws HT, et al: Does radical mastectomy still have a place in the treatment of primary operable breast cancer? Arch Surg 122:1317–1320, 1987.

45. Mamby CC, Love RR, Heaney E, et al: Metastatic breast cancer 39 years after primary treatment. Wis Med J 92:567–569, 1993.

46. Mendenhall NP, Devine JW, Mendenhall WM, et al: Isolated local-regional recurrence following mastectomy for adenocarcinoma of the breast treated with radiation therapy alone or combined with surgery and/or chemotherapy. Radiother Oncol 12:177–185, 1988.

47. Moot SK, Peters GN, Cheek JH: Tumor hormone receptor status and recurrences in premenopausal node negative breast carcinoma. Cancer 60:382–385, 1987.

48. Olson CE, Ansfield FJ, Richards MJS, et al: Review of local soft tissue recurrence of breast cancer irradiated with and without actinomycin-D. Cancer 39:1981–1983, 1977.

49. Overgaard M, Christensen JJ, Johansen H, et al: Evaluation of radiotherapy in high-risk breast cancer patients: Report from the Danish Breast Cancer Cooperative Group (DBCG 82) trial. Int J Radiat Oncol Biol Phys 19:1121–1124, 1990.

50. Patanaphan V, Salazar OM, Poussin-Rosillo H: Prognosticators in recurrent breast cancer: A 15-year experience with irradiation. Cancer 54:228–234, 1984.

51. Perez CA, Pajak T, Emami B: Randomized phase III study comparing irradiation and hyperthermia with irradiation alone in superficial measurable tumors: Final report by the Radiation Therapy Oncology Group. Am J Clin Oncol 14:133–141, 1991.

52. Recht A, Siddon RL, Kaplan WD, et al: Three-dimensional internal mammary lymphoscintigraphy: Implications for radiation therapy treatment planning for breast carcinoma. Int J Radiat Oncol Biol Phys 14:477–481, 1988.

53. Rosenman J, Bernard S, Kober C, et al: Local recurrences in patients with breast cancer at the North Carolina Memorial Hospital (1970–1982). Cancer 57:1421–1425, 1986.

54. Rosenman J, Churchill CA, Mauro MA, et al: The role of computed tomography in the evaluation of post-mastectomy locally recurrent breast cancer. Int J Radiat Oncol Biol Phys 14:57–62, 1988.

55. Rubin P, Bunyagidj S, Poulter C: Internal mammary lymph node metastases in breast cancer: Detection and management. Am J Roentgenol Radium Ther Nucl Med 111:588–598, 1971.

56. Rutqvist LE, Cedermark B, Glas U, et al: Radiotherapy, chemotherapy, and tamoxifen as adjuncts to surgery in early breast cancer: A summary of three randomized trials. Int J Radiat Oncol Biol Phys 16:629–639, 1989.

57. Scanlon EF: Local recurrence in the pectoralis muscles following modified radical mastectomy for carcinoma. J Surg Oncol 30:149–151, 1985.

58. Scatarige JC, Fishman EK, Zinreich ES, et al: Internal mammary lymphadenopathy in breast carcinoma: CT appraisal of anatomic distribution. Radiology 167:89–91, 1988.

59. Schwaibold F, Fowble BL, Solin LJ, et al: The results of radiation therapy for isolated local-regional recurrence after mastectomy. Int J Radiat Oncol Biol Phys 21:299–310, 1991.

60. Scott R, Gillespie B, Perez CA, et al: Hyperthermia in combination with definitive radiation therapy: Results of a phase I/II RTOG study. Int J Radiat Oncol Biol Phys 15:711–716, 1988.

61. Shah JP, Urban JA: Full-thickness chest wall resection for recurrent breast carcinoma involving the bony chest wall. Cancer 35:567–573, 1975.

62. Shimkin MB, Lucia EL, Low-Beer BVA, et al: Recurrent cancer of the breast: Analysis of frequency, distribution, and mortality at the University of California Hospital, 1918 to 1947, inclusive. Cancer 7:29–46, 1954.

63. Stadler B, Kogelnik HD: Local control and outcome of patients irradiated for isolated chest wall recurrences of breast cancer. Radiother Oncol 8:105–111, 1987.

64. Tennvall-Nittby L, Tenegrup I, Landberg T: The total incidence of loco-regional recurrence in a randomized trial of breast cancer TNM stage II: The South Sweden Breast Cancer Trial. Acta Oncol 32:641–646, 1993.

65. Toonkel LM, Fix I, Jacobson LH, et al: The significance of local recurrence of carcinoma of the breast. Int J Radiat Oncol Biol Phys 9:33–39, 1983.

66. Turner L, Swindell R, Bell WGT, et al: Radical versus modified radical mastectomy for breast cancer. Ann R Coll Surg Engl 63:239–243, 1981.

67. Valagussa P, Bonadonna G, Veronesi U: Patterns of relapse and survival following radical mastectomy: Analysis of 716 consecutive patients. Cancer 41:1170–1178, 1978.

68. Van der Zee J, Treurniet-Donker AD, The SK, et al: Low-dose reirradiation in combination with hyperthermia: A palliative treatment for patients with breast cancer recurring in previously irradiated areas. Int J Radiat Oncol Biol Phys 15:1407–1413, 1988.

69. Weichselbaum R, Marck A, Hellman S: Pathogenesis of pleural effusion in carcinoma of the breast. Int J Radiat Oncol Biol Phys 2:963–965, 1977.

70. White WC: The problem of local recurrence after radical mastectomy for carcinoma. Surgery 19:149–153, 1949.

71. Wong WW, Vijayakumar S, Weichselbaum RR: Prognostic indicators in node-negative early-stage breast cancer. Am J Med 92:539–548, 1992.

72. Zimmerman KW, Montague ED, Fletcher GH: Frequency, anatomical distribution and management of local recurrences after definitive therapy for breast cancer. Cancer 19:67–74, 1966.

CHAPTER 69

LOCALLY ADVANCED BREAST CANCER: ROLE OF MEDICAL ONCOLOGY

Sreeni R. Chittoor, M.D. / Sandra M. Swain, M.D.

Locally advanced breast cancer includes a heterogenous group of patients with varying biology and range of prognoses. This group includes large operable tumors and those considered inoperable but without distant metastases. One could consider locally advanced breast cancer synonymous with stage III disease as defined by the current American Joint Committee on Cancer (AJCC)/Union Internationale Contre le Cancer (UICC) TNM staging of breast cancer (1992)[21] (Table 69–1). However, it should be noted that interpretation of published data on locally advanced breast cancer over the past 25 years remains difficult because the AJCC breast cancer staging system has changed several times since its inception in 1962.

STAGING

The 1992 clinical staging systems for breast cancer used by the UICC and AJCC are now identical, being based on the TNM (T = tumor; N = nodes; M = metastases) system. They differ from their 1983 staging systems (Table 69–2)[20] in that T3, N0 is now considered stage IIB and supraclavicular lymph node metastases are considered stage IV. These changes correlate with the survival data for these two subsets. Patients with large tumors and pathologically negative nodes have a survival rate of 77 percent, whereas those with pathologically positive nodes have a survival rate of 48–58 percent.[177]

INCIDENCE

The percentage of patients with stage III disease in 1985–1986 was 10.9 percent compared with 8.1 percent in 1991.[140] This small decrease may reflect a change in the staging of breast cancer. Current stage IIB breast cancer patients were considered stage III in the past. Twelve percent of women aged 0–21 years presented with stage III disease compared with 7 percent of women aged 60–69 and 70–79. The Surveillance, Epidemiology and End Results (SEER) program reported a 5.4 percent incidence of stage III breast cancer at the time of diagnosis in white females in 1992 versus 8.9 percent in black females.[169] Ten percent of low-income patients presented with stage III disease compared with 7 percent of high-income patients. Stage III disease is diagnosed in approximately 13,000 women annually, making it still a major health problem.

HISTORICAL PERSPECTIVE

A significant percentage of breast cancers during the mid 1800s were locally advanced. William Stewart Halsted's[92] study published in 1894 popularized radical mastectomy, which significantly reduced local recurrence rates. This study involved his first 50 patients. The local recurrence rate was 6 percent, and the 3-year survival rate was 45 percent. Half a century later, Haagensen and Stout,[88] in their landmark publication in 1943, analyzed the experience at Columbia-Presbyterian Hospital in New York. They reviewed 1135 cases of breast cancer treated with radical mastectomy during the period of 1915 to 1942. Based on their analysis, they developed the Columbia Clinical Classification System, which was one of the earliest attempts to correlate treatment and prognosis.

Haagensen and Stout[88] were able to identify clinical features of breast cancer that were associated with a greater than 50 percent chance of local recurrence and zero percent chance of 5-year cure. These clinical features are shown in Table 69–3. Patients with these clinical features were included in stage D of the Columbia Clinical Classification and were considered "categorically inoperable." Five features of locally advanced breast cancer that were called "grave signs" are shown in Table 69–4. Any one of these signs placed the patient in stage C of the Columbia Clinical Classification but any one of these signs alone did not make the patient inoperable. If two or more of these signs were present, patients were placed in stage D and were considered "categorically inoperable." This categorization was based on the fact that only one patient in their series with two "grave signs" was disease-free at 5 years. Haagensen and Stout[88] noted a 5-year clinical cure in 5–38 percent of stage C patients treated by radical mastectomy, and local recurrences ranged from 13 percent to 40 percent.

It became apparent that radical mastectomy for locally advanced breast cancer was inadequate treatment and was associated with a poor survival rate. This observation led to the use of primary radiation therapy. In 1965, Baclesse[15] published his 5-year results on the treatment of 431 breast carcinoma patients treated with 200 kV roentgen rays as the sole modality of therapy. He treated 95 patients who were classified as Columbia Clinical Classification stage C, and the survival rate was 41 percent. This survival rate was comparable to that of Haagensen and

TABLE 69–1.   AJJC/UICC TNM 1992 CLINICAL STAGING SYSTEM

Stage	Tumor	Nodes	Metastases
IIIA	T0, T1, T2	N2	M0
	T3	N1, N2	M0
IIIB	T4	Any N	M0
	Any T	N3	M0

T1 = tumors ≤2 cm.
T2 = tumors >2 cm and ≤5 cm.
T3 = tumors >5 cm.
T4 = tumors of any size with direct extension to chest wall or skin.
T4a = extension to the chest wall.
T4b = edema (including peau d'orange) or ulceration of the skin of the breast or satellite skin nodules confined to the same breast.
T4c = Both T4a and T4b.
T4d = inflammatory carcinoma.
N0 = no regional lymph node metastasis.
N1 = metastasis to movable ipsilateral axillary nodes.
N2 = metastasis to ipsilateral axillary nodes fixed to one another or to other structures.
N3 = metastasis to ipsilateral internal mammary lymph nodes.
M0 = no distant metastases.

Stout's[88] study in regard to radical mastectomy for the same patient subgroup (42.9 percent). Baclesse[15] also treated 200 stage D patients with radiation treatment, and the 5-year survival rate for them was 13 percent. However, six of the 27 patients who survived 5 years were not disease-free.

These observations along with the experiences of others suggest that locally advanced breast cancer is a systemic disease with micrometastases present at the time of diagnosis. Hence local therapy alone is insufficient to cure most patients with this disease.

PROGNOSTIC FACTORS

Size of the Primary Tumor

There is a direct relationship of primary tumor size to the extent of axillary nodal metastases and consequently tumor recurrence rate. From a study of 2578 patients, Fisher and coworkers[71] concluded that patients with tumors greater than 6 cm had a 63 per-

TABLE 69–2.   AJCC/UICC TNM 1983 CLINICAL STAGING SYSTEM

Stage	Tumor	Nodes	Metastases
IIIA	T0, T1, T2, T3	N2	M0
	T3	N0, N1, N2	M0
IIIB	Any T	N3	M0
	Any T4	Any N	M0

T1 = tumors ≤2 cm.
T2 = tumors >2 cm and ≤5 cm.
T3 = tumors >5 cm.
T4 = tumors of any size with direct extension to chest wall or skin.
T4a = fixation to the chest wall.
T4b = edema (including peau d'orange), ulceration of the skin of the breast, or satellite skin nodules confined to the same breast.
T4c = both of the T4a and T4b.
T4d = inflammatory carcinoma.
N0 = axillary nodes not considered to contain growth.
N1 = axillary nodes considered to contain growth.
N2 = axillary nodes fixed.
N3 = metastases to ipsilateral supraclavicular or infraclavicular nodes or arm edema.
M0 = no distant metastases.

TABLE 69–3.   LOCALLY ADVANCED BREAST CANCER: HAAGENSEN AND STOUT'S "CATEGORICALLY INOPERABLE" PATIENTS

- Extensive edema of the skin, covering more than one third of the surface of the breast.
- Satellite tumor nodules in the skin over the breast.
- Inflammatory carcinoma—defined by involvement of greater than one third of the breast with edema or erythema.
- Parasternal tumor with internal mammary nodal metastases.
- Supraclavicular nodal metastases.
- Edema of the arm.
- Distant metastases.

cent incidence of axillary nodal involvement compared with a 38 percent incidence in patients with 1.0–1.9 cm tumors. Of the 63 percent of patients with axillary nodal metastases, 35 percent had one to three nodes involved, and 65 percent had four or more nodes involved. Patients with one to three nodes involved had a recurrence rate of 63 percent, and those with four or more nodes involved had a recurrence rate of 94 percent.

Haagensen[90] reported a 52 percent incidence of nodal involvement in patients with primary tumors greater than 5 cm compared with 28 percent in patients with primary tumors less than 1 cm. The 5-year relapse rate reported by Valagussa and colleagues[196] was 37 percent for patients with positive nodes and tumors less than 2 cm and 79 percent for patients with positive nodes and tumors greater than 5 cm. Nemoto and associates[135] reported a 65 percent incidence of axillary nodal involvement in patients with tumors greater than 5 cm compared with 24 percent in those with tumors less than 1 cm. Koscielny and colleagues[107] noted a direct relationship between the size of the primary tumor and prognosis in 2648 breast cancer patients treated at the Institut Gustave-Roussy between 1954 and 1972. The likelihood of distant metastases increased with the size of the primary tumor.

Negative Axillary Lymph Nodes

Of 488 patients with stage III disease treated by mastectomy, Fracchia and coworkers[80] reported that 58 (11.8 percent) had no nodal metastases. These patients had a 10-year survival rate of 75.3 percent.[80] Toonkel and coworkers[191] analyzed 58 patients with T3 tumors and negative axillary nodes at mastectomy and found that the 5-year survival rate was 72 percent and the 10-year survival rate was 57 percent.[191] Fisher and associates[71] patients with tu-

TABLE 69–4.   LOCALLY ADVANCED BREAST CANCER: HAAGENSEN AND STOUT'S "GRAVE SIGNS"

- Edema of less than one third of the skin of the breast.
- Ulceration of the skin.
- Fixation of the tumor to the chest wall.
- Involved axillary lymph nodes greater than 2.5 cm in diameter.
- Fixed axillary lymph nodes.

mors greater than 6 cm and negative axillary nodes had a recurrence rate of 24 percent and a 5-year survival rate of 75 percent compared with a 5-year survival rate of 15 percent for patients with the same tumor size but with four or more involved lymph nodes.

Thus, a small group of patients with locally advanced breast cancer and pathologically negative lymph nodes do have a favorable prognosis, and attempts should be made to identify these patients. Although the recurrence rate for patients with large tumors is lower if they have negative nodes, it is higher than for patients with small tumors. In 27–32 percent of patients with clinically nonpalpable axillary nodes, histological involvement is seen at nodal dissection.[37, 40, 90, 165]

Estrogen Receptor Status

Estrogen receptor status probably has little impact on prognosis for patients with locally advanced breast cancer. Stewart and colleagues[182] reported a significant increase in the median disease-free and overall survival rates for 124 operable patients who had T3a, N0–N1 lesions and pathologically negative nodes with positive estrogen receptors as compared with patients who had negative receptors ($p < 0.05$).[182] However, in patients with inoperable breast carcinoma (T3b–T4, N0–N1, M0 or TX, N2–N3, M0) estrogen receptor status had no effect on prognosis. Robertson and coworkers[153] studied the prognostic factors in 60 patients with operable locally advanced breast carcinoma. Survival rates in these patients from time of initial therapy correlated significantly with estrogen receptor status ($p = 0.01$) and progesterone receptor status ($p = 0.04$).[153]

Thymidine Labeling Index

Silvestrini and coworkers[172] evaluated pretreatment labeling index in 52 patients with locally advanced breast cancer and found that a high labeling index was associated with a higher recurrence rate, a shorter time to disease progression, and a shorter 4-year survival rate (37 percent) when compared with the 4-year survival rates of patients with tumors demonstrating low labeling index (68 percent). However, the relapse-free survival rates were comparable, with 24 percent for a low labeling index and 19 percent for a high labeling index. This study suggests that evaluating tumor cell kinetics could allow aggressive therapy to be offered to a subset of patients who are at high risk for relapse.

Gardin and associates[81] noted a significantly better objective response following primary chemotherapy in patients with a high thymidine labeling index compared with those with a low pretreatment thymidine labeling index ($p = 0.06$). They also noted that patients with tumors that continued to have a high thymidine labeling index following primary chemotherapy benefited from subsequent adjuvant systemic therapy.

DIAGNOSIS

One important rationale for the use of primary chemotherapy, as will be discussed in more detail later in this chapter, relates to the prevention of kinetic changes occurring in residual malignant cells following removal of the primary tumor. It may be important to use a diagnostic modality that will least perturb the primary tumor. The usual methods of evaluating the primary tumor in studies related to primary chemotherapy are discussed next.

Fine Needle Aspiration

Fine needle aspiration (FNA) is used in the evaluation of palpable lesions. It is easy to perform, fast, cost effective, and associated with minimal kinetic alteration in the primary tumor specimen. In one study, the sensitivity of cytologic interpretation for diagnosing malignancy on adequate material was 94 percent and the specificity was 98 percent.[93]

FNA has been used for more than 20 years at the Karolinska Institute in Sweden. The rate of a false-negative cytology report is less than 10 percent, and false-positive diagnosis never occurs.[200] The success of this technique depends on an experienced physician performing the aspiration and an experienced pathologist preparing the smear and interpreting the specimen. Some disadvantages with FNA may relate to the inability to adequately assess morphology and status of estrogen and progesterone receptors. FNA cannot differentiate invasive from noninvasive tumors. Therefore, it may be necessary to aspirate both the primary tumor and palpable lymph nodes for confirmation of invasive tumor. Core needle biopsy may be required if no enlarged lymph nodes are detected. Techniques are now available to perform flow cytometric studies and other prognostic indicators on FNA specimens.

Incisional Biopsy

Incisional biopsy establishes the tissue diagnosis but theoretically may increase the labeling index of the residual primary tumor.[72] Also, the resulting changes, such as hemorrhage and edema, following an incisional biopsy might make response to chemotherapy difficult to assess.

PRETREATMENT EVALUATION

Pretreatment evaluation should include a complete patient history and physical examination with clear measurements of any palpable masses. All patients should also have a complete blood count, liver function studies, and chest roentgenograms (posteroanterior and lateral views). A bone scan is recommended for patients with locally advanced breast cancer because an abnormal finding can be found in 20–25 percent of asymptomatic women with locally advanced breast cancer.[60] A bilateral mammogram is essential, and attention should be paid to the contra-lateral breast to exclude an occult synchronous primary tumor or contralateral metastases.

ASSESSMENT OF DISEASE RESPONSE

Mammography

Mammography provides a valuable adjunct to clinical examination in assessing response to treatment for breast cancer. Moskovic and coworkers[128] reviewed sequential mammograms of 48 patients with large operable breast cancers undergoing primary chemotherapy. Clinical and mammographic findings were in concurrence in 79 percent of the patients.[128] In the study published by Semiglazov and coworkers[170] discussed later in this chapter, the response rate in patients undergoing a combination of clinical examination and mammography was 35 percent versus 12.4 percent in those undergoing clinical examination only.

Digital mammography has the capability of achieving spatial resolution of images as small as 1/20th of a millimeter.[67] This technique has the potential to detect areas of breast tissue that harbor occult cancer. Technetium-labeled sestamibi imaging has been shown to have a negative predictive value of 97 percent and a positive predictive value of 78.9 percent. In contrast, mammography has a positive predictive value of 25 percent.[102] Multicenter clinical trials are under way, and depending on their results, this technique could be useful in the future.

Ultrasonography

Powles and coworkers[149] noted that there was a better correlation of tumor shrinkage to clinical response on ultrasonography than on mammography. This better correlation could be due to unchanging microcalcifications and persistence of architectural distortion seen at mammography after response. Although ultrasonographic technique has been considered less accurate than mammographic technique, Fornage and colleagues[77] reported that sonographic measurement of established breast carcinoma correlated with pathological examination more closely than mammographic measurement. Furthermore, some reports suggest that duplex Doppler ultrasonography has a very high sensitivity and specificity for the detection of breast carcinoma.[32, 163] Newer ultrasonographic techniques are also being developed to adequately visualize dense breast tissue and detect small breast tumors using higher frequencies. These newer techniques would also decrease the scanning time and have the potential to reduce the cost of ultrasonographic breast examination.

Magnetic Resonance Imaging

Gadolinium-enhanced magnetic resonance imaging (MRI) has been used successfully in the diagnosis of recurrent malignancy in previously irradiated or surgically treated breast tissue. A recently developed MRI technique for evaluating breast cancer has shown better pathological correlation than conventional imaging techniques. This new MRI technique utilizes a new pulse sequence called RODEO (Rotating Delivery of Excitation Off-resonance) that produces high-resolution images emphasizing the gadolinium contrast-enhancement qualities of cancers over the background tissues, including fat and normal breast parenchyma.

In a study of 39 patients with locally advanced breast cancer receiving primary chemotherapy, RODEO MRI was able to accurately predict the extent of residual disease in 30 of 31 cases reviewed (97 percent).[1] By incorporating this technique, one may be able to better select women for breast conservation following primary chemotherapy without compromising local control.

However, MRI does have a high false-positive rate of about 37 percent. Also, misinterpretation of data may occur because of a flare response caused by hyperemia surrounding the tumor that may not resolve for several months following chemotherapy.

Molecular Markers

Assessing the percentage of tumor cells in the S phase by flow cytometry may help predict their responsiveness to chemotherapy. Tumors with a low S phase prior to treatment may not respond well to primary chemotherapy, and alternative treatment modalities may need to be considered.[31]

Tumors that overexpress *ERBB2* may be resistant to alkylator-based chemotherapy regimens.[6, 24, 87] In vitro studies suggest that *ERBB2* and topoisomerase II co-amplification correlate with sensitivity to chemotherapeutic agents.[176] Breast cancers with overexpression of *ERBB2* are relatively more sensitive to doxorubicin, which may be due to induction of topoisomerase II.[94] One large adjuvant study in node-positive patients suggested that patients with tumors overexpressing *ERBB2* derived greater benefit, as indicated by longer disease-free and overall survival rates, when given higher doses of chemotherapy containing doxorubicin.[133] It may be possible to select a subgroup of patients who will benefit from more intensive chemotherapeutic intervention or specific drugs such as doxorubicin.

McDermott and coworkers[125] quantified levels of *ERBB2* extracellular domain in the serum before and after chemotherapy. Persistent levels of this oncogene following adjuvant chemotherapy corresponded to earlier recurrence.[125]

Bcl-2 expression and mutant *p53* have been correlated with resistance to chemotherapy. When these proteins are expressed, the tumor cells are able to avoid apoptosis (programmed cell death). These proteins may allow the cancer cells to become resistant to chemotherapy, as one of the main mechanisms of cell killing by cytotoxic agents is by inducing apoptosis.[121, 136]

TABLE 69–5. RATIONALE FOR THE USE OF PRIMARY CHEMOTHERAPY

- Potential ability to convert inoperable tumors to operable ones.
- Assessment of tumor response to chemotherapy in vivo.
- Chemotherapeutic ablation of primary tumor may favorably alter the growth characteristics of residual micrometastases.

The area of molecular pathology is an exciting and rapidly expanding field. The study of locally advanced breast cancers will add to the understanding of the biology and characteristics of breast cancer.

Primary Chemotherapy

In this chapter the term *primary chemotherapy* is defined as chemotherapy given before local treatment of breast cancer. Other terms used for this modality of intervention include *preoperative chemotherapy, neoadjuvant chemotherapy,* and *induction chemotherapy.* The rationale for primary chemotherapy incorporates several important concepts and is summarized in Table 69–5. An increase has been reported in the labeling index of metastases following either removal of the primary tumor or radiation of the primary tumor sufficient to retard growth.[72, 73] This stimulation of cell growth in metastatic lesions is hypothesized to be due to a serum growth factor.[75] Based on the Goldie-Coldman hypothesis, as the tumor cell population increases, so does the number of drug-resistant phenotypic variants giving rise to spontaneous somatic mutations.[83] It is hypothesized that primary chemotherapy may prevent kinetic alterations in micrometastatic lesions and concomitant increase in the resistant cells.

Primary chemotherapy can change an inoperable tumor to an operable one. Also, reduction in the tumor size by primary chemotherapy may allow the use of conservative surgery with breast conservation.[97, 167, 184] Primary chemotherapy allows assessment of treatment efficacy in vivo. Therefore, if patients do not respond to the initial course of primary chemotherapy, a treatment change to a non–cross-resistant regimen can be implemented.

MANAGEMENT OF LOCALLY ADVANCED NONINFLAMMATORY BREAST CANCER

Local Therapy

Surgery

As discussed earlier, Haagensen and Stout[88] reported a zero percent 5-year cure rate in patients who were classified as "categorically inoperable." Donegan[60] reported a 50 percent local recurrence rate in patients with "inoperable disease" treated by surgery alone and a 22 percent 5-year survival rate. Arnold and Lesnick,[10] in their retrospective analysis, reported a

5-year survival rate of 77 percent for patients with clinical T3, N0 disease and a 65 percent survival rate for those with T4, N0 disease. The local recurrence rate for the 50 patients treated by mastectomy was 27 percent.[10] Fracchia and coworkers[80] reported a 10-year survival rate of 75 percent in women with large node-negative tumors (T3, N0), but the survival rate was 21 percent when patients had T3 tumors with positive axillary lymph nodes. Therefore, it is clear that surgery alone is inadequate treatment, although it is an integral part of combined-modality treatment.

Radiotherapy

Following Baclesse's[15] publication in 1965, several studies on the use of primary radiation therapy alone have been published. Comparison of the various studies remains difficult because of different patient entry criteria, radiation doses, and radiation treatment techniques.

The Joint Center for Radiation Therapy experience was reported by Bruckman and associates[34] in 1979 and by Sheldon and associates[171] in 1987. The former study included 116 patients with stage III disease. A subset of 54 of these patients was treated with external beam therapy (5000–6500 cGy megavoltage to the breast and lymph nodes) and interstitial iridium implant (1500–3500 cGy). The local recurrence rate was 24 percent. In this series, the local control was 76.5 percent if the patients had either excisional biopsy or an interstitial implant and 47 percent if the patients had neither. Doses greater than 6000 cGy were associated with a 78 percent local control rate versus 39 percent for doses less than 6000 cGy.

Sheldon and associates[171] in 1987 updated this series, noting a 5-year survival rate of 41 percent and a 10-year survival rate of 23 percent. The relapse-free survival rate was 30 percent at 5 years and 19 percent at 10 years. Dose was an important factor for local control, with a 5-year local control rate of 83 percent for 6000 cGy or more and 70 percent for less than 6000 cGy.

Treurniet-Donker and coworkers[192] reported a 70 percent local control rate at 3 years in patients treated with megavoltage radiation compared to a 40 percent local control rate in those treated with orthovoltage radiation. In contrast, Bedwinek and coworkers[22] found no difference in the local control rate when doses were increased from 4000 cGy to 7000 cGy.

Zucali and colleagues[204] retrospectively evaluated and reported histological findings after radiation therapy and radical mastectomy in an attempt to determine the efficacy of radiation therapy. Of the 454 consecutive patients with stage III disease evaluated, 133 patients with T3 or T4 disease were given either roentgenographic therapy (4000–4500 cGy to the breast and 3000 cGy to the nodes) or cobalt therapy (6000–7000 cGy to the breast and nodes) and then underwent radical mastectomy. Most patients who had surgery had a complete clinical response to radiation and therefore were a highly select group of patients with a better prognosis than the others. Only 25 percent of the mastectomy specimens were free of tumor, 32 percent had histologically negative axillary lymph nodes, and 10 percent had neither residual tumor in the breast nor axillary nodal involvement. Other small series examining irradiated breasts have found residual tumor in 62 percent[195] to 100 percent[114] of the cases.

It can be concluded from these studies that patients with a large tumor burden are not treated adequately by radiation alone. A combination of radiation and some type of surgery seems more likely to achieve optimal local control.

Surgery and Radiotherapy

Radiotherapy given preoperatively or postoperatively with some form of surgery was undertaken at many institutions in an attempt to achieve adequate local control without affecting cosmesis. Preoperative radiation treatment followed by surgery resulted in local control rates of 11–45 percent and the development of subsequent distant metastases in 65–89 percent of the patients.[179] Surgery followed by radiation resulted in local control rates of 70–86 percent and 5-year survival rates of 30–45 percent.[179]

Combined-Modality Therapy

Local Therapy Alone versus Combined-Modality Therapy

Table 69–6 summarizes randomized trials, comparing local treatment versus combined-modality treatment. Local treatment consisted of radiation alone,

surgery alone, or a combination of radiation and surgery.

Grohn and coworkers[85] in 1984 and Klefström and coworkers[103] in an update in 1987 reported the results of a randomized study of 119 patients with operable T3, N0–N2 lesions. All patients underwent modified radical mastectomy. Patients were then randomized to receive postoperative radiotherapy (40 patients), chemotherapy (40 patients), or a combination of radiotherapy and chemotherapy (39 patients). Chemotherapy consisted of six cycles of vincristine, doxorubicin, and cyclophosphamide given every 4 weeks. The doses of chemotherapy were as follows: vincristine 1.2 mg/m^2 intravenously (IV) on day 1, doxorubicin 45 mg/m^2 IV on day 1, and cyclophosphamide 200 mg/m^2 orally for 5 days. The first 60 patients entered in this trial received levamisole 150 mg orally for 2 consecutive days weekly for 1 year. The next 59 patients did not receive levamisole.

The crude 5-year disease-free survival was 22 percent for those given radiotherapy, 30 percent for those given chemotherapy, and 67 percent for those given both radiotherapy and chemotherapy. Patients who received the combination treatment had a significant disease-free survival ($p < 0.001$) and overall survival benefit ($p < 0.001$). The 5-year analysis also revealed a disease-free survival benefit in patients receiving levamisole ($p < 0.035$), but there was no benefit in overall survival.

In the initial report by Grohn and coworkers,[85] 25 of 34 premenopausal patients had chemotherapy-induced amenorrhea. Six of the 25 patients (25 percent) developed metastatic disease compared with four of nine (44 percent) premenopausal women without menstrual disturbances. This result raises the

TABLE 69–6.   RANDOMIZED TRIALS: LOCAL THERAPY ALONE VERSUS COMBINED-MODALITY THERAPY

Author (Year)	Stage	Treatment Design	Number of Patients	Relapse-Free Survival	Overall Survival
Klefström[103] (1983)	T3, N0–N2	S → RT ± LVM	40	22% 5-year RFS	NA
Update		S → CT ± LVM	40	30% 5-year RFS	NA
Grohn[85] (1983)		S → RT → CT ± LVM	39	67% 5-year RFS	NA
Schaake-Koning[161] (1985)	T3B–T4, Any N, M0 or T1–T3 with a positive axillary apex biopsy	RT	45	14 months median	37% 5-year actuarial survival for all groups
		RT → CT	34	26 months median	
		CT → RT → CT	39	20 months median	
Rubens[156] (1989)	T3B–T4, Any N, M0 or T1–T3 with a positive axillary apex biopsy	RT	91	$p = 0.12$ months median (ns)	
		RT → HT	92		
		RT → CT	88		
		RT → CT → HT	92		
Derman[59] (1989)	T3, T4, N0–N3 excluding IBC	RT	87	27.0 months median	49.0 months median
		RT → CT (1)	91	53.0 months median	61.0 months median
		RT → CT (2)	42	56.0 months median	63.0 months median
Caceres[42] (1980)	T3, T4, N0–N3	RT	34	11.0 months median	19.9 months median
		RT + S	27	8.9 months median	17.8 months median
		RT + CT	26	14.6 months median	24.6 months median

CT = chemotherapy.
HT = hormonal therapy.
IBC = inflammatory breast cancer.
LVM = levamisole.
ns = not significant.
RFS = relapse-free survival.
RT = radiation therapy.
S = surgery.

issue of improved therapeutic response from chemotherapy following ovarian ablation. Even though the numbers are small, this is the only randomized trial to show a statistically significant overall survival benefit with a combination of radiotherapy and chemotherapy versus either modality alone following mastectomy for operable stage III patients (T3, N0–N2).

Schaake-Koning and colleagues[161] reported results on 118 inoperable patients younger than 65 years with T3b–T4, any N, M0, or T1–T3 disease with positive results on axillary apex biopsy. Biopsy of the apex node (the highest axillary lymph node) was frequently performed as a part of staging in this study because involvement of this lymph node has been associated with a poor prognosis after mastectomy. Patients with supraclavicular or infraclavicular nodal involvement or inflammatory disease that could not be confined to standard radiation fields were excluded.

The randomization was as follows: radiotherapy alone (arm I, 45 patients); radiotherapy followed by 12 cycles of cyclophosphamide, methotrexate, and fluorouracil (CMF) and tamoxifen (arm II, 34 patients); and primary chemotherapy with doxorubicin and vincristine (AV) for two cycles alternating with two cycles of CMF followed by radiotherapy and then four cycles of AV alternating with four cycles of CMF and tamoxifen given for the entire treatment period (arm III, 39 patients).

The median follow-up was 66 months. The relapse-free survival was 14 months for arm I, 26 months for arm II, and 20 months for arm III ($p = 0.11$). The actuarial 5-year survival was 37 percent for all treatment arms.

This study concluded that chemohormonal treatment therapy did not improve survival compared with radiotherapy alone. However, caution must be exercised in this interpretation for the following reasons:

1. The number of randomized patients was small.
2. The relapse-free survival rates in the CMF arm of patients and in the arm of patients receiving the alternating drug regimens with an anthracycline were similar.
3. Radiotherapy alone was given to six of the eight patients with T1 tumors, and this therapy may therefore have improved the results in that arm of patients.
4. Patients receiving primary chemotherapy followed by radiotherapy did not receive a boost dose of radiation, making results not directly comparable with those of radiation given to patients in arms I and II.
5. The relapse-free survival rate, however, was shortest (though not significantly so) in the radiotherapy-alone arm of patients (arm I), which suggests that chemotherapy could have delayed recurrence.

The European Organization for Research and Treatment of Cancer (EORTC) performed a randomized study of 363 evaluable patients with inoperable disease (comparable to the patients studied by Schaake-Koning and associates[161]).[156] Patients were randomized as follows: radiotherapy alone (91 patients); radiotherapy and endocrine therapy (92 patients); radiotherapy and chemotherapy (88 patients); and radiotherapy, endocrine therapy, and chemotherapy (92 patients). Endocrine therapies were given irrespective of estrogen receptor status and were given together with the chemotherapy in the combined-treatment arm of patients.

Premenopausal patients underwent ovarian ablation followed by treatment with prednisolone 2.5 mg three times a day for 5 years. Postmenopausal women received tamoxifen 10 mg twice daily for 5 years. Chemotherapy consisted of 12 cycles of CMF. Only 54 percent of patients received 12 cycles of chemotherapy, and 91 percent received dose reductions. There was a prolongation of disease-free survival in all systemic-treatment arms of the study compared with radiation therapy alone, and this prolongation of disease-free survival was largely attributable to a decrease in local regional recurrence. The effect of endocrine treatment on the time to local regional failure was significant in patients with positive estrogen receptors ($p = 0.002$), whereas the effect of chemotherapy was significant in patients with negative estrogen receptors ($p = 0.042$).

A trend toward increased overall survival was seen in the patients receiving endocrine treatment and chemotherapy, but there was no statistically significant difference among the four treatment arms of the study ($p = 0.12$). This study concluded that systemic treatment had a significant effect on local control but not on overall survival of poor-prognosis patients with locally advanced disease. The lack of significant effect on overall survival could be due to inadequate doses of chemotherapy given in this trial.

Derman and coworkers[59] in 1989 reported results on 198 evaluable patients with locally advanced breast cancer (T3, T4, N0–N3) excluding inflammatory breast cancer. A total of 220 patients were randomized. Local treatment consisted of (1) primary radiotherapy if the tumor was inoperable or (2) surgery followed by radiotherapy if the tumor was operable. Patients were randomized to an arm of local treatment alone (87 patients) versus an arm of local treatment plus systemic treatment with two dosages of CMF-combination chemotherapy (133 patients). Of the patients in the local-treatment-alone arm, 53 percent also underwent surgery, whereas 50 percent of the patients in the systemic-treatment arm underwent surgery, suggesting that a large proportion of women in the local-treatment arm had better-prognosis tumors. The median disease-free survival rate for premenopausal women given radiotherapy alone was 27 months; for those given the two chemotherapy regimens, it was 53 months. The median survival rates for these three groups were 49 months, 61 months, and 63 months, respectively. Thus, premenopausal patients receiving systemic treatment had a significant increase in the disease-free survival rate without an increase in the overall survival rate. The median disease-free survival rate for postmenopausal women was 30 months, and the overall survival rate was 56 months. This difference between rates was not statistically significant.

Caceres and colleagues[42] in 1980 published the results of their study of patients with T3, T4, N0–N3 disease in abstract form. Patients were randomized as follows: radiotherapy (34 patients), radiotherapy plus total mastectomy (27 patients), and radiotherapy plus CMF chemotherapy (26 patients). The details of radiotherapy and chemotherapy were not given. The median survival rate was prolonged with combined radiotherapy and chemotherapy (24.6 months) versus radiotherapy alone (19.9 months) or radiotherapy plus total mastectomy (17.8 months). Local control was best in patients receiving both radiotherapy and total mastectomy.

These studies suggest that compared with local therapy alone, combined-modality therapy in patients with locally advanced breast cancer improved disease-free survival rates. This improvement may be due to a decrease in local regional recurrence.

Maintenance versus No-Maintenance Chemotherapy

In 1978, DeLena and colleagues[57] reported the results of a randomized study of patients with locally advanced breast carcinoma who received combined-modality treatment. The 110 patients with T3b–T4, NX, M0 disease, including inflammatory cancer, were treated with four cycles of doxorubicin and vincristine. The dose of doxorubicin was 75 mg/m^2 IV on day 1 and vincristine 1.4 mg/m^2 IV on days 1 and 8 every 3 weeks. Responders to chemotherapy received radiotherapy. Complete responders following radiotherapy were randomized to maintenance chemotherapy with six more cycles of chemotherapy or observation.

The objective response rate to primary chemotherapy was 70 percent, with 15.5 percent showing complete response and 54.5 percent partial response. The median disease-free survival rate was 19 months for all patients who received maintenance chemotherapy and 11 months for all who were randomized to the observation arm ($p = 0.02$). The 3-year survival rate was 52 percent for all patients, a significant improvement when compared historically with local treatment alone. This study concluded that maintenance chemotherapy increased disease-free survival and overall survival rates.

Radiotherapy versus Surgery Following Primary Chemotherapy

DeLena and colleagues[58] in 1981 reported the results of a study that attempted to determine whether surgery combined with chemotherapy could improve local control and survival compared with radiotherapy and chemotherapy. Table 69–7 summarizes these trials. A total of 132 women, excluding those with inflammatory disease or supraclavicular nodal involvement, were treated with three cycles of primary chemotherapy. Patients were randomized prior to primary chemotherapy to receive either radiotherapy (group A, 57 patients) or mastectomy (group B, 51 patients) following primary chemotherapy.

Chemotherapy consisted of doxorubicin 60 mg/m^2 IV on day 1 and vincristine 1.2 mg/m^2 IV on days 1 and 8 repeated every 3 weeks. Doxorubicin was decreased to 50 mg/m^2 after local therapy, for a total of seven more cycles. Patients who had no objective response or who experienced progression of disease during primary chemotherapy received CMF. In 50 percent of patients in group A, there was an objective

TABLE 69–7. RANDOMIZED TRIALS: RADIOTHERAPY VERSUS SURGERY AS LOCAL TREATMENT

Author (Year)	Stage	Treatment Design	Number of Patients	Median Relapse-Free Survival (Months)	Median Overall Survival (Months)
DeLena[58] (1981)	Stage III (T3, T4, N0–N2) excluding IBC or supraclavicular lymph node involvement	RT ⟋ ⟍ CT ⟍ CT ⟍ ⟋ S	67 (57 received RT) 65 (51 received S)	22.0 ⎱ ⎬ 48 15.0 ⎰	49.1
Perloff[145] (1988)	T3, N1–N2 T4, N0–N2	CT → S ⟍ CT ⟋ CT → RT	43 44	29.2 24.4	39.3 39.0
Papaioannou[141] (1983)	T3, N0–N2 excluding T4	CT → S → CT CT → S → RT → CT	57 48	NA NA (Crude recurrence rate)	NA NA

CT = chemotherapy.
HT = hormonal therapy.
IBC = inflammatory breast cancer.
NA = not available.
RT = radiation therapy.
S = surgery.

response to primary chemotherapy; 1 percent a complete response and 49 percent a partial response. In contrast, 54 percent of those in group B had an objective response; 6 percent a complete response and 48 percent a partial response. The median duration of remission was 22 months for group A and 15 months for group B ($p = 0.50$). The median survival rate was 48 months for both groups. The local regional recurrence rate was 31 percent in group A and 30 percent in group B, a difference that was not significant.

Perloff and coworkers[145] in 1988 reported the results of a randomized study in 113 evaluable patients with locally advanced breast cancer. Patients with clinical T3, N0 disease were excluded. The objective of this study was to determine the modality of therapy for optimal local control. All patients were treated with three monthly cycles of CAFVP regimen—cyclophosphamide (100 mg/m² orally on days 1–14), doxorubicin (25 mg/m² IV on days 1 and 8), fluorouracil (500 mg/m² IV on days 1 and 8), vincristine (1.4 mg/m² IV on days 1 and 8), and prednisone (40 mg/m² orally on days 1–14). Patients with operable tumors were randomized to either mastectomy or radiation therapy, followed in either case with 2 years of CAFVP (with methotrexate substituted for doxorubicin after a total dose of 550 mg/m²).

There was a 69 percent objective response rate in these 113 patients following primary chemotherapy. Four of the 91 patients eligible for randomization refused it. Of the rest, 43 patients were randomized to surgery and 44 patients to radiotherapy. The median relapse-free survival period was 29.2 months for patients who underwent surgery and 24.4 months for patients who underwent radiotherapy ($p = 0.50$). The median survival was 39 months for both groups, and the local recurrence rate was 27 percent after radiotherapy and 19 percent after surgery.

DeLena and associates[58] excluded patients with inflammatory breast cancer and included T3, N0 patients. In contrast, Perloff and coworkers[145] excluded patients with clinical T3, N0 disease. However, in both studies, the modality of local therapy did not affect survival.

Papaioannou and coworkers,[141] in an attempt to determine optimal local treatment for patients with locally advanced breast cancer after primary chemotherapy, randomized patients to either receive postoperative radiotherapy or not. Patients with T4 tumors were excluded. The planned treatment was two cycles of primary chemotherapy with cyclophosphamide, doxorubicin, vincristine, methotrexate, and fluorouracil (CAVMF) plus hormonal manipulation and mastectomy, then randomization to radiotherapy or observation alone. After local therapy, all patients received 10 additional cycles of chemotherapy and tamoxifen.

There were 205 patients entered, with 78 patients (38 percent) excluded entirely from analysis and 22 others receiving less than 6 months follow-up. Of the patients assigned to the mastectomy and radiotherapy arm, 42 were excluded, 14 of them having re-

fused radiotherapy. Of the patients assigned to the observation-only arm, 36 were excluded. More patients in the radiotherapy arm had negative nodes than those in the observation-only arm, and fewer patients in the radiotherapy arm had four or more positive nodes. The local recurrence rate was similar for both arms: 8.3 percent for the radiotherapy arm and 10.5 percent for the observation arm. The crude recurrence rate was 27 percent for the radiotherapy arm and 21 percent for the observation arm, not a significant difference. It should be noted that because of the large number of exclusions in this study, no firm conclusions should be drawn.

Randomized Studies—Operable Locally Advanced Breast Cancer

The objectives of randomized studies on patients with operable locally advanced breast cancer were to determine the respective values of postoperative chemotherapy, hormonal therapy, radiotherapy, and a combination of therapies. Table 69–8 summarizes these randomized trials.

Olson and colleagues[139] published the results of their randomized trial in an abstract form in 1989. This study was performed to establish the role of radiotherapy following surgery and chemotherapy in patients with stage III breast carcinoma. Between 1982 and 1987, 426 patients were entered in this trial. Those who were disease-free following modified or standard radical mastectomy were treated for 6 months with six cycles of cyclophosphamide 100 mg/m² orally on days 1–14, doxorubicin 30 mg/m² IV on days 1 and 8, fluorouracil 500 mg/m² IV on days 1 and 8, tamoxifen 20 mg orally every day, and halotestin 20 mg orally every day. Patients were then restaged, and those who were disease-free were randomized to undergo local regional radiotherapy or observation. The observation group received radiotherapy only when there was local regional recurrence.

Following completion of chemotherapy, 381 of the 426 patients were evaluable. Of these, 332 patients were randomized to radiotherapy (RT) versus observation (OBS). There were 301 evaluable patients analyzed at a median follow-up of 3.1 years. Radiotherapy after surgery and chemotherapy for resectable stage III breast cancer had no significant effect on survival (80 percent for RT versus 78 percent for OBS, with $p = 0.76$), disease-free survival (69 percent for RT versus 61 percent for OBS, with $p = 0.26$), or distant relapse (18 percent for both RT and OBS). Radiotherapy did, however, result in fewer local-regional failures (7 percent for RT versus 16 percent for OBS).

Spangenberg and coworkers[180] randomized 131 patients following surgery to either radiotherapy followed by monochemotherapy with cyclophosphamide for 2 years (B1) or polychemotherapy with CMF vinblastine for 2 years (B2). This study included patients with T3-T4, N0-N1 lesions. Patients with N2 or N3 nodes and peau d'orange or chest wall fixation

TABLE 69–8. RANDOMIZED TRIALS: OPERABLE LOCALLY ADVANCED BREAST CANCER

Author (Year)	Stage (TNM)	Treatment Design	Number of Patients	Relapse-Free Survival	Overall Survival
Spangenberg[180] (1986)	Operable stage III (N2, N3, chest wall fixation and peau d'orange excluded)	RT → MONO CT / S \ POLY CT	131	40.4% 5-year RFS 26.8% 5-year RFS	5-Year OS 62.5% 5-year OS 56.3%
Alagaratnam and Wong[4] (1986)	T3, T4, N0–N3 (stage III)	HT / S → RT \ CT	40 31	35 months median[a] 28 months median[a]	NA NA
Casper[45] (1987)	T2, N2; T3, N1–N3; T4N1–N3 (T3, N0, IBC, residual tumor after surgery excluded)	CT(1) / S \ CT(2)	21 20	23 months median \ $p = 0.05$ 15 months median	33 months median \ $p = 0.26$ 18 months median

CT = chemotherapy.
HT = hormonal therapy.
IBC = inflammatory breast cancer.
OS = overall survival.
RFS = relapse-free survival.
RT = radiation therapy.
S = surgery.
[a]Median determined approximately, based on survival curves in published studies.

were excluded. All patients also received hormonal therapy or ovarian ablation. The 5-year disease-free survival rate was 40.4 percent for the B1 arm and 26.8 percent for the B2 arm, not a significant difference. The 5-year local recurrence rate was 11.7 percent for B1 and 22.5 percent for B2. The 5-year median survival rate was 62.5 percent for B1 and 56.3 percent for B2—again, not a significant difference. The conclusion from this study was that polychemotherapy after local therapy did not increase survival in operable patients. These findings are perhaps due to the low intensity of chemotherapy in both arms of the study. Also, most of the chemotherapy was oral, with the issue of compliance not addressed.

In 1986, Alagaratnam and Wong[4] published the results of their randomized trial in patients with operable locally advanced breast cancer. All patients had mastectomy followed by radiotherapy. At 3 weeks following radiotherapy, 40 patients were randomized to receive tamoxifen 40 mg per day until relapse and 31 patients were randomized to a doxorubicin-containing regimen for 9 or 10 cycles. The median disease-free survival was about 35 months for the tamoxifen arm of the study and 28 months for the chemotherapy arm. This study was small and had a selection bias in that randomization did not occur prior to any treatment nor was the number of patients who refused randomization given.

Casper and coworkers[50] randomized 41 women with T2, N2, T3, N1–N3 and T4, N1–N3 breast cancer following modified radical or radical mastectomy to receive two different adjuvant chemotherapy regimens, one of which contained doxorubicin. The median disease-free survival for patients on regimen A was 23 months compared with 15 months for those

on regimen B ($p = 0.05$). The median overall survival was 33 months for patients on regimen A and 18 months for those on regimen B. This study reported improved disease-free survival rates, but no change in overall survival rates, with a doxorubicin-containing chemotherapy regimen.

These randomized trials revealed a modest increase in survival when chemotherapy was used in conjunction with local therapy. Local treatment alone did not affect overall survival but might have affected local control.

Primary Chemotherapy versus Adjuvant Chemotherapy

Scholl and coworkers[164] published the preliminary results of a randomized trial (S6) in 1994. The purpose of their trial was to assess whether there was a survival advantage with primary chemotherapy versus adjuvant chemotherapy. A total of 414 premenopausal women with locally advanced breast cancer (T2–T3, N0–N1, M0) were randomized to receive either four cycles of primary chemotherapy followed by local-regional treatment (group I) or four cycles of adjuvant chemotherapy after local regional treatment (group II).

Chemotherapy consisted of doxorubicin 25 mg/m² IV on days 1 and 8, cyclophosphamide 500 mg/m² IV on days 1 and 8, and fluorouracil 500 mg/m² IV on days 1, 3, 5, and 8. Chemotherapy cycles were repeated every 28 days. Local-regional treatment consisted of radiotherapy and surgery. Radiotherapy was given both to eradicate the tumor and preserve the breast. Techniques were used to reduce the radiation dose directed to the cardiac area. Patients who presented with a persisting mass after radiation treatment had either a wide surgical excision of the residual tumor, when technically or cosmetically feasible, or a mastectomy. Breast conservation was identical for both groups at the end of primary local-regional treatment.

The median follow-up was 54 months for the 390 patients who were evaluable. Total breast preservation was 82 percent in the primary-chemotherapy arm and 77 percent in the adjuvant-chemotherapy arm. This difference was not statistically significant. The 5-year actuarial local control rates were 73 percent in the primary-chemotherapy arm and 81 percent in the adjuvant-chemotherapy arm ($p = 0.21$). The 5-year breast preservation rates were 61 percent in the primary-chemotherapy arm and 63 percent in the adjuvant-chemotherapy arm ($p = 0.95$). The 5-year probability of survival was 86 percent for the primary-chemotherapy arm and 78 percent for the adjuvant-chemotherapy arm; this difference was statistically significant ($p = 0.039$). There were no differences in the disease-free survival rates or local recurrence rates for the two groups. This study revealed a survival advantage with primary chemotherapy but also showed that breast conservation was possible to avoid mastectomy.

Mauriac and colleagues[124] randomized 272 women with breast cancers larger than 3 cm to either (1) mastectomy and axillary node dissection followed by adjuvant chemotherapy for node-positive, estrogen receptor/progesterone receptor (ER/PR)–negative patients (group A, 138 patients) or (2) primary chemotherapy followed by local regional treatment based on patient response to chemotherapy (group B, 134 patients). Chemotherapy consisted of a total of six cycles: three cycles with epirubicin 50 mg/m^2 IV, vincristine 1 mg/m^2 IV, and methotrexate 20 mg/m^2 IV, followed by three cycles with mitomycin C 10 mg/m^2 IV, thiotepa 20 mg/m^2 IV, and vindesine 4 mg/m^2 IV.

In group A, 104 patients received chemotherapy. In group B, all 134 patients received chemotherapy. In group B, 84 patients had breast preservation. After a median follow-up of 34 months, relapse-free survival was no different for the two groups, but overall survival was better for the primary-chemotherapy group ($p = 0.04$). There were no deaths related to chemotherapy-related toxicity. Dose reductions because of treatment-related toxicities were equivalent in both group A and group B patients. In the adjuvant-chemotherapy group, 5 percent (seven patients) had local-regional recurrences and 16 percent (22 patients) had metastatic disease. In the primary-chemotherapy group, 8 percent (11 patients) had local-regional recurrences and 11 percent (15 patients) had metastatic relapses. Six of these 11 patients who had recurrences in the breast in the primary-chemotherapy group underwent either mastectomy or lumpectomy. This study concluded that patients receiving primary chemotherapy can receive conservative local treatment even for large primary breast tumors and enjoy a possible increase in survival.

Semiglazov and coworkers[170] randomized 271 patients with stage IIA–IIIB breast cancer (T3, N1, M0; T3 N0, M0; T2, N1, M0; and T1–2, N2, M0) to receive primary chemotherapy and radiotherapy (group I, 137 patients) versus primary radiotherapy (group II, 134 patients). After initial preoperative treatment with either primary chemotherapy and radiotherapy or primary radiotherapy alone, all patients underwent mastectomy with axillary node dissection and then received four to six cycles of chemotherapy.

Chemotherapy consisted of thiotepa 20 mg intramuscularly (IM) on days 1, 3, 5, 7, 9, and 11 (120 mg total dose/cycle); methotrexate 40 mg/m^2 IV on days 1 and 8; and fluorouracil 500 mg/m^2 IV on days 1 and 8 (TMF) given every 4–6 weeks. The estimated 5-year disease-free survival rate was 81 percent for group I and 71.6 percent for group II ($p < 0.05$).

Of interest, a complete histological response at mastectomy was seen in 29.1 percent of patients in group I and in 19.4 percent of patients in group II. This study showed significantly improved results from combined-modality treatment (radiotherapy and chemotherapy) prior to mastectomy versus radiotherapy alone as local treatment. Table 69–9 summarizes the findings from the Mauriac, Scholl, and Semiglazov studies.

Powles and colleagues[149] conducted a prospective randomized study of 200 patients with operable breast cancer (T0, T1, T2, T3, N0, N1a, and N2b) to determine if breast conservation could be accomplished following primary chemoendocrine therapy. Patients were randomized to either (1) surgery followed by chemoendocrine therapy (control arm) or (2) four cycles of chemoendocrine therapy before and four cycles after surgery. Chemoendocrine therapy initially consisted of mitoxantrone, mitomycin, methotrexate, and tamoxifen but was changed to mitoxantrone and methotrexate with tamoxifen because of toxicity. The median follow-up was 28 months.

There was a dramatic decrease in the size of the primary tumor following primary chemotherapy, increasing the number of patients with tumors less than 2 cm to 81 percent from 9 percent preoperatively. There were no significant differences between the survival rates of the two arms of the study. Only 13 percent of the patients receiving primary chemoendocrine therapy required mastectomy versus 28 percent in the control arm ($p < 0.005$). This study suggests that primary chemotherapy does allow for an increase in conservative surgery. Future studies will compare this treatment with adjuvant treatment in a large number of patients to assess the effect on disease-free survival and overall survival rates.

At the time of this writing, the NSABP B-18 study is evaluating the role of primary chemotherapy in women with operable breast cancer.[74] As of April 1993, 1313 patients had been entered into this study, and patients were randomized to (1) surgery followed by chemotherapy or (2) primary chemotherapy followed by surgery. Preliminary results published in abstract form suggested that primary chemotherapy in patients with operable breast cancer resulted in

TABLE 69–9. RANDOMIZED TRIALS: PRIMARY CHEMOTHERAPY VERSUS ADJUVANT CHEMOTHERAPY

Author (Year)	TNM Stage	Treatment Design	Number of Patients	Disease-Free Survival	Overall Survival
Mauriac[124] (1991)	T2–T3, N0–N1	S → CT / CT → S	138 / 134	84% / p = ns / 88%	85% / 34 months median p = 0.04 / 95%
Scholl[164] (1994)	T2–T3, N0–N1	RT → S → CT / CT → RT → S	190 / 200	55% / 5-year DFS p = 0.4 / 59%	78% / 5-year OS p = 0.04 / 86%
Semiglazov[170] (1994)	T2, N1; T1–T2, N2; T3, N0; T3, N1	CT + RT → S → CT / RT → S → CT	137 / 134	81% / 5-year DFS p <0.05 / 71.6%	86.1% / 5-year OS p >0.05 / 78.3%

CT = chemotherapy.
DFS = disease-free survival.
ns = not significant.
OS = overall survival.
RT = radiation therapy.
S = surgery.

objective response rates of 80 percent, with 37 percent complete responses. These patients would be candidates for breast conservation. This is the largest study of its kind, and a preliminary review of data suggests that there is no significant difference in the disease-free and overall survival of these two treatment arms (Dr. Bernard Fisher, personal communication, April 1997).

These studies show that primary chemotherapy may not only decrease the size of breast tumors, rendering inoperable tumors operable, but may also allow breast conservation. These studies further suggest that primary chemotherapy may improve survival rates, although that issue is yet to be definitively settled.

Nonrandomized Studies

Several nonrandomized studies have treated various subsets of locally advanced breast cancer with a multimodality approach. The 5-year disease-free survival rates ranged from 28 percent to 78 percent, and the 5-year overall survival rates ranged from 38 percent to 80 percent depending on the stage subset.

Buzdar and coworkers[41] updated the M.D. Anderson Cancer Center experience and published the results of three studies that took place from April 1974 to August 1994. Patients had T1–T3 or T4 tumors or T1–T2 disease with either N2 or N3 (or M1 supraclavicular or infraclavicular nodes) disease. The initial study ran from April 1974 to April 1985. Of the 191 patients, 174 were evaluable; 48 had stage IIIA disease and 126 had stage IIIB disease. Inflammatory cancer was excluded.

Several changes occurred in the treatment regimen over the 11-year period. All patients received primary chemotherapy with fluorouracil 500 mg/m² IV on days 1 and 8, doxorubicin 50 mg/m² IV on day 1, and cyclophosphamide 500 mg/m² IV on day 1 (FAC), cycled every 3 weeks for a total of three to six cycles. The first 52 patients also received bacillus Calmette-Guérin (BCG) immunotherapy.

Patients with objective response and nonresponders who were inoperable received radiotherapy. The remaining patients received a combination of radiotherapy and chemotherapy. Chemotherapy was given for a total duration of 2 years between 1974 and 1981, after which time it was given for only 1 year. Methotrexate was substituted after a total dose of 450 mg/m² of doxorubicin. The median follow-up was 131 months. The objective response rate was 88 percent, with 17 percent having complete response (29 patients) and 71 percent partial response (123 patients). At 15 years, 54 percent of patients with stage IIIA disease and 24 percent of patients with stage IIIB disease were estimated to be disease-free.

The second study ran from April 1985 to May 1989. The role of alternate non–cross-resistant drugs was evaluated. Patients received three cycles of primary chemotherapy with vincristine, doxorubicin, cyclophosphamide, and prednisone (VACP) followed by surgery. Those who had a complete histological response or residual disease of less than 1 cm³ received the same chemotherapy postoperatively for a total of nine cycles. Patients who had an objective response with greater than 1 cm³ of residual tumor were randomized to either continue five cycles of the same chemotherapy or receive five cycles of alternate chemotherapy with vinblastine, methotrexate, fluorouracil, and folinic acid (VbMF).

All patients responding to primary chemotherapy received radiotherapy following completion of chemotherapy. Patients who initially had minimal response or no response to primary chemotherapy received radiotherapy followed by surgery and five cycles of alternate chemotherapy. Of 200 patients, 193 were evaluable. The median follow-up was 80 months. The objective response rate to primary chemotherapy was 84 percent, with 18 percent having complete response (34 patients) and 66 percent partial response (127 patients). Then 106 patients were randomized to alternate therapy or VbMF. Even though there was a slight improvement in the disease-free and overall survival rates for patients who were treated with alternate therapy compared with the agents used for primary chemotherapy, this improvement was not significant ($p = 0.5$ and $p = 0.3$, respectively).

In the first and second studies, the local regional failure was 7 percent for stage IIIA patients and 26 percent for stage IIIB patients. Also in these studies, 58 patients had either supraclavicular or infraclavicular disease (M1), and approximately 24 percent of these patients were disease-free after 15 years. Following primary chemotherapy, patients with histologically negative axillae had disease-free and overall survival rates similar to those of patients with node-negative breast cancer.

In the third study, which ran from June 1989 to December 1991, 207 patients received chemotherapy (FAC) similar to that of the first study except that the doxorubicin was given as a 72-hour infusion. Furthermore, the feasibility of breast conservation was evaluated in this study. Local excision and axillary node dissection were performed in 25 percent of the patients with T3 tumors (15 of 60 patients) and in 6 percent of the patients with T4 tumors (5 of 82 patients). With a median follow-up of 43 months, three patients with T3 tumors and one with a T4 tumor had recurrences in the breast. Five patients had distant metastases. The researchers concluded that aggressive combined-modality therapy had increased disease-free and overall survival rates in both stage IIIA and stage IIIB patients compared with historical controls at the same institution treated with local therapy only. They also concluded that (1) initial response to primary chemotherapy was an important prognostic factor for long-term disease-free and overall survival rates and (2) patients with supraclavicular and infraclavicular lymph node involvement should not be considered incurable but should be offered combined-modality therapy.

The National Cancer Institute (NCI) analyzed the data on 107 patients with locally advanced breast cancer treated there from April 1980 to February 1988 with primary chemotherapy including an attempted hormonal synchronization.[148, 178, 184] The rationale for this approach was based on the prior laboratory studies demonstrating that antiestrogen-based inhibition of breast cancer cell growth can be reversed by estrogen rescue.[61, 118, 134] Weichselbaum and colleagues[202] found that antiestrogen treatment followed by estrogen rescue could increase the sensitivity of breast cancer cells to cytotoxic drug therapy. It has also been demonstrated by flow cytometry that tamoxifen has caused G1 arrest in *MCF7* human breast cancer cells and that subsequent estrogen treatment can induce a synchronous wave of DNA synthesis in human breast cancer cells.[3, 84] Based on this hypothesis, the cell cycle–specific agents methotrexate and fluorouracil were administered in this study after tumor cells were synchronized by tamoxifen and recruited by estrogen, thus making them more susceptible to cytotoxic agents. Previously published studies have demonstrated a significantly high complete-response rate in patients treated with hormonal synchronization.[5, 119]

The NCI study included 48 patients (45 percent) with clinical stage IIIA disease, 46 (43 percent) with clinical stage IIIB inflammatory breast cancer (IBC), and 13 (12 percent) with clinical stage IIIB noninflammatory disease (non-IBC). (This is according to the AJCC 1983 staging system.) Patients received primary chemotherapy to the best response (median of five cycles) prior to local therapy.

The chemotherapy regimen consisted of cyclophosphamide 500 mg/m^2 IV on day 1, doxorubicin 30 mg/m^2 IV on day 1, tamoxifen 40 mg orally on days 2–6, conjugated estrogen (Premarin) 0.625 mg orally every 12 hours in three doses on days 7–8, and methotrexate 300 mg/m^2 IV on day 8 followed in 1 hour by fluorouracil 500 mg/m^2 on day 8 and leucovorin 10 mg/m^2 orally every 6 hours in six doses starting day 9. A 25 percent dose escalation of either methotrexate or fluorouracil in alternate cycles was used to achieve maximum doses of these drugs.

An incisional biopsy was performed at the site of the original lesion at the time of best response, and if negative results on the biopsy were obtained, patients received radiotherapy along with chemotherapy. If tumor cells remained, patients then had mastectomy and radiation as local therapy. Following local therapy, all patients received six additional cycles of chemotherapy.

Following primary chemotherapy, objective response rate was 92 percent in patients with stage IIIA disease, 98 percent in patients with stage IIIB-IBC disease, and 85 percent in patients with IIIB–non-IBC disease. Complete clinical response was seen in 50 percent of stage IIIA patients, 57 percent of stage IIIB-IBC patients, and 31 percent of stage IIIB–non-IBC patients. Of those with a complete clinical response, 58 percent of patients with IIIA or IIIB-IBC disease and 50 percent of those with IIIB–non-IBC disease had a complete histological response. This represented 29 percent (31 of 107) of the entire study group.

After a median follow-up of 64 months, the 5-year actuarial local regional failure rate was 3 percent for stage IIIA, 21 percent for stage IIIB-IBC ($p = 0.02$), and 33 percent for stage IIIB–non-IBC patients ($p = 0.03$). The 5-year actuarial local-regional failure rate as the first site of failure was 5 percent for positive-biopsy patients (treated with mastectomy and radiation) and 23 percent for negative-biopsy patients (treated with radiation alone) ($p = 0.07$).

Five-year relapse-free survival and overall survival were not significantly different for positive-biopsy patients who subsequently underwent mastectomy and radiotherapy than for negative-biopsy patients who underwent radiotherapy only. The 5-year actuarial relapse-free survival was 55 percent for stage IIIA patients compared with 33 percent for stage IIIB-IBC ($p = 0.01$) patients and 31 percent for stage IIIB–non-IBC patients ($p = 0.03$). The 5-year actuarial survival was 61 percent for stage IIIA patients, 36 percent for stage IIIB-IBC patients, and 31 percent for stage IIIB–non-IBC patients.

Baillet and colleagues[16] evaluated the role of exclusive radiotherapy and interstitial brachytherapy boost as local regional treatment of locally advanced breast cancer in 135 patients following primary chemotherapy. In this study, 108 patients had T3 tumors, 27 had T4 tumors of less than 5 cm, and 81 had palpable nodes. Complete clinical regression occurred in 20 percent of the patients following primary chemotherapy, in 72 percent following radiotherapy, and in 100 percent following brachytherapy boost.

The mean follow-up was 8 years. Local regional failure occurred in 29 patients (21 percent). Of these, 14 patients did not have distant metastases. Nine patients had subsequent local control as a result of either mastectomy or lumpectomy. Breast preservation was possible in 90 percent of the patients. The actuarial survival rate at 5 years was 64 percent and at 10 years was 50 percent. Patients with T3 lesions had a survival rate of 66 percent at 5 years and 52 percent at 10 years. Patients with T4 lesions had a survival rate of 56 percent at 5 years and 47 percent at 10 years. The 34 patients with inflammatory breast carcinoma had a survival rate of 53 percent at 5 years and 43 percent at 10 years. Baillet and colleagues[16] concluded that patients with large breast tumors could receive conservative surgery followed by radiotherapy and primary chemotherapy without requiring a mastectomy.

Anderson and colleagues[7] studied the response to systemic therapy prior to surgery that included endocrine therapy, chemotherapy, or both. In this study of 88 patients with operable breast cancers (T2, T3, N0, N1, M0), 38 were premenopausal women and 50 were postmenopausal. Following biopsy for diagnosis, estrogen receptor concentration was determined. A total of 41 patients received endocrine therapy only that consisted of (1) ovarian ablation followed by luteinizing hormone–releasing hormone if patients were premenopausal and (2) either tamoxifen or an aromatase inhibitor, aminoglutethimide, if they were postmenopausal. A total of 27 patients received chemotherapy only that consisted of cyclophosphamide, doxorubicin, vincristine, and prednisone. The 20 patients remaining who did not respond to initial endocrine therapy received chemotherapy and endocrine therapy.

Following primary systemic therapy, 82 patients underwent mastectomy, and the remaining six patients were able to have breast preservation. The median follow-up was 24 months. Of the 61 patients who received endocrine therapy, 24 (39 percent) had a response. All 24 patients had estrogen receptor concentration of more than 20 fmol/mg of cytosol protein. Response to chemotherapy was seen in 34 patients (72 percent), and these patients had estrogen receptor concentration of less than 20 fmol/mg of cytosol protein.

The overall survival rate at 3 years was 86 percent, and 81 percent remained free from local relapse. The researchers concluded that treatment for operable locally advanced breast cancer may need to be individualized and systemic endocrine therapy considered for patients with strongly positive estrogen receptors. However, the response rate to endocrine therapy was much lower than that seen with chemotherapy. This issue will be discussed in a later section.

The main objective of a study by Fabian and coworkers[65] was to determine whether there would be a significant increase in the proliferation of the tumor cell population following a high physiological dose of estradiol. A total of 50 women with locally advanced breast cancer or metastatic breast cancer, or both, were entered into this study. Premenopausal women were required to be estrogen receptor positive and to have undergone oophorectomy 2 or more weeks prior to the study entry. Postmenopausal women were eligible regardless of their estrogen receptor status. Of these 50 women, 28 had locally advanced breast cancer (T4, N2–N3). Nine of the 28 women were premenopausal, and 19 were postmenopausal; 22 were estrogen receptor positive, and six were estrogen receptor negative.

Estradiol vaginal suppositories were given for 96 hours (days 1–4). Chemotherapy was begun 72 to 96 hours after estradiol administration and consisted of a combination of cyclophosphamide, doxorubicin, and fluorouracil, with or without vinblastine according to the choice of the investigator. Patients received three cycles of primary chemotherapy prior to mastectomy and then received three to four cycles of additional chemotherapy followed by radiotherapy. Two cycles of concurrent chemotherapy were administered while patients received radiotherapy.

Mastectomy was performed in 25 of the 28 patients with locally advanced breast carcinoma. Biopsy data were available for 19 of 28 patients with locally advanced breast cancer; the median baseline S-phase fraction and proliferative index were 14.3 percent and 16.5 percent, respectively. Of these 28 patients with locally advanced breast cancer, 26 (93 percent), including all six estrogen receptor negative patients, had a complete response. The 5-year disease-free survival estimate was 30 percent, and the 5-year overall survival estimate was 49 percent. These results are not markedly different from those of studies that used chemotherapy and radiotherapy with or without surgery but did not attempt hormonal recruitment.

Fabian and coworkers[65] concluded that this disappointing disease-free survival rate may be related to the time of administration of chemotherapy, which was 72–96 hours after estrogen administration rather than 48 hours, at which time the majority of the patients had an increased proliferative index.

They further noted a greater relative increase in the proliferative index following administration of estradiol in those patients with an initial proliferative index of less than 10 percent versus one greater than 10 percent. Another possibility entertained was that the expression of multidrug resistance in patients with locally advanced breast carcinoma may have been increased by estrogen.

Conte and coworkers[52] also used estrogen recruitment in a primary chemotherapy regimen for the treatment of locally advanced breast cancer. They treated 39 patients with T3b–T4, N1–N3 lesions with three cycles of diethylstilbestrol (DES) 1 mg orally on days 1–3 followed by fluorouracil 600 mg/m^2 IV on day 4, doxorubicin 50 mg/m^2 IV on day 4, and cyclophosphamide 600 mg/m^2 IV on day 4 (FAC). Patients then underwent mastectomy followed by three cycles of DES-FAC alternating with DES-CMF for three cycles. The objective response rate was 71.8 percent, with a 15.4 percent complete response and a 56.4 percent partial response. The 3-year relapse-free survival rate was 53.5 percent, and the overall survival rate was 60 percent.

Biopsies obtained serially for evaluation of tumor cell kinetics showed a significant increase in the thymidine labeling index in 39 percent of the patients and in the primer-dependent alpha DNA polymerase in 70 percent of the patients after DES administration; this increase did not depend on the presence of estrogen receptor. Conte and coworkers[52] found that tumor cells in vivo were stimulated by estrogen regardless of the estrogen receptor status. Estrogen, then, may be important in recruiting cells into cell cycle, thus facilitating cytotoxic action by chemotherapeutic agents.

Hobar and associates[96] treated 40 patients who had stage IIIA and IIIB breast cancer with primary chemotherapy. Primary chemotherapy was followed by mastectomy in 28 patients, and in some cases by postoperative radiotherapy. There was a 75 percent objective response rate to primary chemotherapy in the 28 patients who underwent surgery. At mastectomy, 18 percent had no residual tumor in the breast, and 11 percent had no tumor either in the breast or the axilla. Local control rates were 92 percent in stage IIIA patients and 88 percent in stage IIIB patients. The 5-year actuarial survival rate for the 34 patients who complied with primary chemotherapy was 46 percent.

Piccart and colleagues[146] treated 59 patients with locally advanced breast cancer (T3b or T4) with concurrent radiotherapy and chemohormonal therapy. Chemohormonal therapy consisted of doxorubicin 75 mg/m^2 IV on day 1, vincristine 1.4 mg/m^2 IV on days 1 and 8, cyclophosphamide 100 mg/m^2 orally on days 29–42, methotrexate 60 mg/m^2 IV on days 29 and 36, and fluorouracil 600 mg/m^2 IV on days 29 and 36. Tamoxifen 40 mg/day was given continuously throughout the entire study. Doses of 50 percent of doxorubicin and vincristine (AV) alternating with cyclophosphamide, methotrexate, and fluorouracil (CMF) were administered while the patients were receiving concurrent radiation. Mastectomy was planned for day 56. Postoperative chemotherapy consisted of five cycles each of AV alternating with CMF, planned to be given at 100 percent doses. Each cycle lasted for 56 days. All tumors were operable.

The objective response rate was 68 percent, and 10 percent of the patients had no residual disease at mastectomy. Relapse occurred in 68 percent of the patients, and the local/regional recurrence rate was 20 percent. The median survival was 4 years. Because of hematological toxicity, only 60 percent of the patients received 80 percent or more of the prescribed drug doses of doxorubicin and CMF following local-regional treatment. Piccart and colleagues[146] concluded that concurrent chemotherapy and radiotherapy was feasible but is associated with increased toxicity. If dose intensity is important, chemotherapy should precede radiation treatment.

Smith and coworkers[175] evaluated the role of infusional chemotherapy in 50 patients with large operable breast cancers having a mean tumor diameter of 6 cm. Median patient age was 44 years. In 21 of these patients (42 percent), axillary nodes were clinically involved. All patients received fluorouracil 200 mg/m^2 per day, given as a continuous infusion for 6 months. Epirubicin 50 mg/m^2 IV and cisplatin 60 mg/m^2 IV were given every 3 weeks for a total of six courses.

The overall response rate was 98 percent (49 patients), with a complete response of 66 percent (33 patients). Four patients (6 percent) had a mastectomy, and 31 patients (62 percent) were able to have conservative surgery. In 27 percent (11 patients), there was a complete histological response.

During a median follow-up of 15 months, five patients (10 percent) experienced a relapse, two of them (4 percent) in the breast. This study showed that primary infusional chemotherapy can achieve a higher complete response rate and allow mastectomy to be avoided. However, the median follow-up in this study was short; infusional chemotherapy should be compared with conventional chemotherapy in a randomized trial to see if there is a true clinical benefit.

Histological Response

Buzdar and colleagues[41] updated the results of seven prospective studies (752 patients) conducted at their institution since 1974. They reported that the initial response to primary chemotherapy was an important prognostic factor in determining the disease-free and overall survival rates, with complete and partial responders having better prognoses. Feldman and coworkers[69] reported that histological response to primary chemotherapy was the single most important prognostic factor for both disease-free and overall survival rates in patients with locally advanced breast cancer. Table 69–10 summarizes the various studies with complete clinical and histological responses. Although complete response rates ranged from 5 percent to 66 percent, histologically negative disease occurred in only 1.5 percent to 29 percent.

TABLE 69–10.   COMPLETE CLINICAL AND HISTOLOGICAL RESPONSE IN LOCALLY ADVANCED BREAST CANCER FOLLOWING PRIMARY CHEMOTHERAPY

Author (Year)	Treatment Design	Number of Patients	Complete Clinical Response (%)	Complete Histological Response
Conte[52] (1987)	CT + S + RT	39	15%	8%
Hortobagyi[97] (1988)	CT ± S + RT + CT	174	17%	8%
Hobar[96] (1988)	CT + S ± RT + CT	36	8%	11%
Piccart[146] (1988)	RT/CT + S + CT	59	5%	10%
Cocconi[51] (1990)	CT + S + CT + RT	49	8%	14%
Singletary[173] (1992)	CT + S + CT + RT	143	16%	10%
Pierce[148] (1992)	CT ± S + RT + CT	107	49%	29%
Rasbridge[151] (1994)	CT ± S ± RT	47	NR	9%
Schwartz[167] (1994)	CT + S + RT + CT	189	85% objective response	10%
Bonnadonna[28] (1995)	CT + S ± RT ± CT	227	21%	4%
	Two studies	210	12%	1.5%
Semiglazov[170] (1994)	CT + RT + S + CT	137	35%	29.1%
	RT + S + CT	134	27.6%	19.4%
Sataloff[160] (1995)	CT + S + CT + RT	36	33%	39% (complete or near complete)
Smith[175] (1995)	ICT ± S ± RT	50	66%	27%
Powles[149] (1995)	CT/HT + S + RT + CT/HT	101	19%	10%
Chollet[48] (1995)	CT + S	40	49%	23%

CT = chemotherapy.
HT = hormonal therapy.
ICT = infusional chemotherapy.
NR = no response.
RT = radiation therapy.
S = surgery.

These statistics suggest that there is a large component of resistant tumor remaining in such patients that has not responded to different therapeutic modalities. Future work should be aimed at discovering interventions that will overcome this resistance.

Hormonal Therapy

The role of tamoxifen in treating locally advanced breast cancer was evaluated in two studies. Veronesi and coworkers[198] treated 46 postmenopausal women with "inoperable" T3–T4 breast cancers with tamoxifen 10–20 mg daily for at least 6 weeks. Eight patients (17 percent) had an objective response after the first course of treatment, and 14 (30 percent) had an objective response after subsequent evaluations. No patients with inflammatory disease responded. The median survival was 10 months.

Campbell and coworkers[44] treated 51 postmenopausal women who had locally advanced breast cancer with tamoxifen 10–20 mg daily. Estrogen receptor values were assessed in 40 patients. The objective response rate was 45 percent, with 14 percent showing a complete clinical response. Responses were seen in 63 percent of the estrogen receptor positive patients versus 33 percent of the estrogen receptor negative patients and 36 percent of those in whom the estrogen receptor status was unknown. The median overall survival determined from the graphs for the tamoxifen responders was 48 months; for the nonresponders it was 18 months.

Gazet and associates[82] conducted a randomized pilot study comparing endocrine therapy and chemotherapy as primary treatment for locally advanced breast carcinoma. A total of 60 patients aged 34 to 69 with T3, T4, N0–N2, M0 lesions were entered into this study from December 1986 to January 1989. Following histological diagnosis, patients in the endocrine-therapy arm (30 patients) received luteinizing hormone–releasing hormone analogue, goserelin, 3.6 mg subcutaneously every 4 weeks if patients were premenopausal and 4-hydroxyandrostenedione 250 mg every 2 weeks IM if patients were postmenopausal. In the chemotherapy arm of the study, 30 patients received mitoxantrone and methotrexate given IV every 3 weeks for four cycles and mitomycin IV every 6 weeks for two cycles.

Following 12 weeks of therapy, wide local excision or mastectomy was performed if the patient had operable disease. If not, radiation therapy was begun. Radiation therapy was also offered as an alternative to surgery for complete responders. Following local therapy, chemotherapy was continued for 12 weeks and endocrine therapy for 65 weeks. At 12 weeks following primary therapy, 53 percent of patients (16 patients) in the chemotherapy arm had an objective response, of whom eight had a complete response. Of the 30 patients in the endocrine-therapy arm, 10 percent (three patients) had an objective response, and there were no complete responders.

Seven patients in the chemotherapy arm underwent surgery as local therapy, whereas 16 patients in the endocrine arm underwent surgery. Examination on completion of the trial at 65 weeks showed no significant difference in the disease-free survival, local recurrence, or death rates for patients receiving chemotherapy versus endocrine therapy. This study is interesting in that it is the only randomized trial comparing endocrine therapy and chemotherapy in these types of patients. However, the study has significant limitations, including the fact that it involved a small number of patients.

These studies show a low overall response rate (10–45 percent) with hormonal therapy alone. As discussed previously, even in a group of patients who were estrogen receptor positive, response to endocrine therapy was only 39 percent.[7] This 39 percent is in comparison to up to 90–95 percent objective responses seen with combination chemotherapy. Also, the overall survival rate in patients receiving tamoxifen alone is poor in these studies. Thus, tamoxifen may increase survival only after combination chemotherapy. Combined-modality therapy incorporating chemotherapy with local/regional therapy should be the standard of care for locally advanced breast cancer.

Breast Conservation in Locally Advanced Breast Cancer

There has been growing interest in breast conservation for patients with locally advanced breast cancer. Numerous researchers report excellent local-regional control. The ability to offer patients conservative surgery correlates with initial tumor size in most studies.

Jacquillat and coworkers[100] reported the results of a nonrandomized trial in 250 patients between 1980 and 1986 in which 36 patients had stage IIIA disease and 58 had stage IIIB disease. Diagnoses were confirmed by needle biopsies. This study enrolled patients in all T stages. Patients received combined-modality treatment and surgery was avoided whenever possible. Primary chemotherapy varied according to the risk group, but at least three cycles were given prior to local treatment. Chemotherapy consisted of a combination of vinblastine, thiotepa, methotrexate, and fluorouracil by infusion, and prednisone was given orally on days 1–5 of each cycle. Doxorubicin was given IV for high-risk patients. Radiotherapy was subsequently administered to the breast and regional lymph nodes.

Clinical complete responses were seen in 30 percent of patients following primary chemotherapy, and subsequent radiotherapy produced a complete response in all patients, with none requiring mastectomy. The 5-year actuarial local-regional recurrence rates were 13 percent for patients with T2 disease, 18 percent for those with T3 disease, and 19 percent for those with T4 disease. The 5-year disease-free survival rates and overall survival rates were 46 percent and 60 percent, respectively, for stage IIIA patients and 52 percent and 58 percent, respectively, for stage IIIB patients. Good to excellent cosmetic results were seen, with the rate of breast preservation at 5 years being 94 percent. In this study, intensive primary chemotherapy without surgery resulted in substantial local control and good overall outcomes.

Calais and colleagues[43] treated 158 patients with T2 tumors larger than 3 cm or T3, N0–N1 carcinoma of the breast. Primary chemotherapy consisted of three cycles of mitoxantrone, vindesine, cyclophosphamide, and fluorouracil given to 106 patients. The remaining 52 patients received the same combination except that mitoxantrone was replaced by epirubicin. Patients were evaluated after three cycles of chemotherapy, and nonresponders were treated by mastectomy and radiotherapy in addition to six cycles of chemotherapy (teniposide, mitomycin, and methotrexate). Responders with tumors smaller than 3 cm underwent lumpectomy with a 1 cm margin. In patients with N1 tumors, limited axillary lymph node dissection was performed. When tumors were larger than 3 cm, modified radical mastectomy was performed. Radiotherapy was then directed at the breast and the supraclavicular and axillary nodes. Breast-conserving treatment was performed in 49 percent of the patients. Local failure rates were 8 percent for patients treated with conservative therapy and 6 percent for patients treated with mastectomy. The 5-year survival rate was 73 percent (90 percent in responders and 57 percent in nonresponders: $p < 0.03$)

Singletary and coworkers[173] analyzed the clinical, mammographic, and histological response in 143 patients with AJCC (1988) stage IIB disease (17 percent), IIIA disease (36 percent), IIIB disease (41 percent), and stage IV disease with positive supraclavicular lymph nodes (6 percent). The treatment consisted of three cycles of vincristine, doxorubicin, cyclophosphamide, and prednisone (VACP) given every 3 weeks and followed by total mastectomy and axillary lymph node dissection. Patients with histologically confirmed complete remission and those with less than 1 cm³ of residual tumor received five additional cycles of VACP. Those with no response to primary chemotherapy received five cycles of methotrexate, fluorouracil, and vinblastine (MFVb).

The 120 patients with partial responses were randomly assigned to receive five additional cycles of VACP or MFVb. All patients received radiotherapy to the chest wall. Of 33 patients, 14 (42 percent) had a complete histological response and 15 (45 percent) had negative nodes. During a median follow-up of 34 months, 30 patients had no evidence of local recurrence. Also, none of the 33 patients who underwent breast conservation had evidence of local recurrence. This study showed that primary chemotherapy can significantly decrease tumor size in patients with locally advanced breast cancer, thus allowing breast conservation surgery.

Schwartz and coworkers[167] analyzed results in 189 women with T2, T3, and T4 breast cancer who received three cycles of primary chemotherapy with cyclophosphamide, methotrexate, and fluorouracil. Doxorubicin was substituted for methotrexate after three cycles in the nonresponders. An average of seven cycles of chemotherapy were delivered. A total of 103 patients (64 percent) underwent mastectomy, and 55 patients (34 percent) had breast conservation surgery. Breast radiotherapy was administered to women who had breast conservation, and chemotherapy was continued for a total of 12 cycles or for an additional 6 months, whichever was longer. Of the 189 women, 85 percent responded to chemotherapy. The mean follow-up was 53 months for the mastectomy group and 29 months for the breast conservation group.

The 5-year disease-free survival rate was 61 percent for all responders, 56 percent for the mastectomy group, and 77 percent for the breast conservation group. The 5-year overall survival was 69 percent for all responders, 67 percent for the mastectomy group, and 80 percent for the breast conservation group. Four patients had an isolated local recurrence after mastectomy and one after breast conservation. Excellent local control was achieved in patients with large primary tumors after wide excision and radiation. Schwartz and coworkers[167] concluded that breast conservation should be considered as an alternative to mastectomy in patients with locally advanced breast cancer.

Bonadonna and colleagues[27] administered primary chemotherapy to 165 women with breast cancer tumors 3 cm or greater in diameter. Chemotherapy consisted of three or four cycles of cyclophosphamide, fluorouracil, and either methotrexate, doxorubicin, or epirubicin. Of the 161 evaluable patients, 157 had a decrease in tumor size. Of the 157 women who underwent surgery, 127 (81 percent) had tumor shrinkage to less than 3 cm, allowing breast conservation surgery. The degree of response was inversely related to the size of the primary tumor, and the frequency of response was greater when estrogen receptor was negative. Tumor response was unrelated to age, menopausal status, ploidy, thymidine labeling index, drug combinations used, or number of treatment cycles in excess of three cycles. This study again demonstrates that primary chemotherapy allows breast conservation in most women with large breast tumors, depending on initial tumor size.

Sataloff and associates[160] conducted a retrospective single-institution study of 36 patients with locally advanced breast cancer in stages IIB, IIIA, and IIIB according to the 1992 AJCC staging system. Of these 36 patients, 23 received three cycles of cyclophosphamide, doxorubicin, and fluorouracil and 13 patients received cyclophosphamide, methotrexate, and fluorouracil as primary chemotherapy. Following primary chemotherapy, all patients underwent modified radical mastectomy.

Patients received postoperative chemotherapy 2 weeks following surgery for a total of 6 months or 12 months depending on whether they had noninflammatory or inflammatory locally advanced breast carcinoma. Patients received radiotherapy following completion of chemotherapy. There was a 53 percent partial clinical response (19 patients) and a 33 percent complete clinical response (12 patients). Of 36 patients, 14 (39 percent) had a complete or near complete histological response. Patients who had minimal or no residual tumor cells on histological evaluation had a 65 percent 5-year disease-free sur-

vival rate and a 79 percent overall survival rate compared with a 44 percent 5-year disease-free survival rate and a 66 percent overall survival rate for the group overall.

Therefore, it can be concluded that there is a subset of patients with locally advanced breast cancer who will be candidates for breast conservation following primary chemotherapy. Tumor size predicts which patients will be able to undergo breast conservation surgery. Also, it appears that a generous wide local excision is necessary to optimize local control.

Treatment Recommendations for Locally Advanced Noninflammatory Breast Cancer

The optimal management of locally advanced breast cancer involves a multidisciplinary approach in which the medical, surgical, and radiation oncologists work closely with the pathologist and diagnostic radiologist. Combined-modality therapy should be the standard of care for these patients. Treatment goals should include not only optimal disease-free and overall survival rates but also adequate local control and satisfactory cosmetic outcome.

Following confirmation of diagnosis with fine needle aspiration or incisional biopsy and clinical staging, four cycles of primary chemotherapy with a doxorubicin-containing regimen are recommended until best response is obtained. Then a modified radical mastectomy or breast conservation surgery may be performed, depending on the extent of clinical response from primary chemotherapy. Surgery should be followed by approximately six cycles of either the same chemotherapy regimen or, depending on the nodal status and extent of residual disease, a change to non–cross-resistant therapy. Postoperative radiotherapy should be given either following completion of the adjuvant phase of chemotherapy or concurrently.[25] Prolonged chemotherapy after surgery before adjuvant radiation therapy may increase the risk of local recurrence.[38, 152]

If no clinical response or progression is noted during or following primary chemotherapy, patients can have a mastectomy if the tumor is operable, followed by radiotherapy. If the tumor is inoperable, preoperative radiotherapy may decrease tumor size, facilitating surgical resection. Following local therapy, such patients can be treated with non–cross-resistant chemotherapy regimens or can be enrolled in other investigational studies.

INFLAMMATORY BREAST CANCER

Definition

Inflammatory breast cancer is the most aggressive form of locally advanced breast carcinoma and is frequently mistaken for other diseases. It is a clinicopathological entity characterized by diffuse brawny induration and the presence of erythema and edema (peau d'orange) of the skin of the breast with a raised edge reminiscent of erysipelas. This feature may or may not be associated with an underlying palpable mass.[21] Dermal lymphatic invasion may be present but is not necessary for the diagnosis of true inflammatory breast cancer.

Incidence

Inflammatory breast cancer is uncommon, accounting for 1–4 percent of all breast cancers.[89, 115, 189] The SEER program presented an analysis of data from 1975 to 1981 in which overall incidence was 5.1 percent.[115] Among the 60,479 cases of breast cancer reported, 153 had both the clinical and pathological features of inflammatory breast cancer and 2937 had the clinical features alone. There were also 81 cases with only the pathological finding of dermal lymphatic invasion; these were considered to be cases of "occult" inflammatory breast cancer and were not included in the incidence figures. The incidence of inflammatory breast carcinoma that included occult inflammatory breast carcinoma in the African American population was 10.1 percent according to the SEER data.[115] This incidence was substantially higher than that seen in white women (6.2 percent) and in other non-white women (5.1 percent). In Tunisia, however, inflammatory breast cancer constitutes up to 55 percent of all breast cancer cases.[129]

The average age at which inflammatory breast carcinoma is diagnosed is similar to the age at which the more common invasive breast carcinomas are diagnosed—it ranges from 45 years to 54 years.[89, 112, 183, 189] This disease has been reported in a 12-year-old child[46] and in males[193] but is extremely rare in both children and males. Even though early reports suggested that inflammatory breast carcinoma was associated in most cases with pregnancy and lactation,[104, 166, 199] several later series showed that although inflammatory breast cancer can occur during pregnancy, it is not more common in these patient groups.[89]

Staging

Inflammatory breast cancer is classified as a T4 tumor and is considered stage IIIB breast carcinoma according to the UICC/TNM staging classification.[21] Haagensen's Columbia Clinical Classification designates inflammatory breast carcinoma as stage D.[89] The investigators at the Institut Gustave-Roussy (Villejuif, France) developed a classification for breast carcinoma called *pousée evolutive* (PEV),[110] shown in Table 69–11, which differs from TNM staging, is descriptive, and takes recent tumor growth and inflammatory signs into consideration. Inflammatory breast carcinoma is included in the PEV2 and PEV3 categories.

Historical Perspective

In the 1814 report by Bell,[23] the extremely unfavorable prognosis of inflammatory breast cancer was

TABLE 69–11.   POUSÉE EVOLUTIVE (PEV) STAGING FOR BREAST CANCER

PEV Category	Clinical Findings
PEV-0	A tumor without recent increase in volume and without inflammatory signs.
PEV-1	A tumor showing marked increase in volume during the previous two months but without inflammatory signs.
PEV-2	A tumor in which breast tissue, particularly the skin, is affected by subacute inflammation and edema involving less than half of the breast surface.
PEV-3	A tumor with acute and subacute inflammation and edema involving more than half of the breast surface.

emphasized. In subsequent publications, Klotz[104] in 1869, Von Volkmann and Brust[199] in 1875, Leicht[113] in 1909, Schumann[166] in 1911, and Learmonth[111] in 1916 emphasized the clinical features by using terms such as *acute mammary carcinoma, mastitis carcinomatosa,* and *carcinoma mastoiditis.* The term *inflammatory breast carcinoma* was first used by Lee and Tannenbaum[112] in 1924. They described this condition in detail so that it would be better recognized by all physicians:

> [T]he breast of the affected side usually increases in size. . . . This enlargement is more often diffuse . . . as the disease progresses the skin becomes deep red or reddish purple and to the touch is brawny and infiltrated. The inflamed areas present a distinct raised periphery after the fashion of erysipelas.[112]

Lee and Tannenbaum[112] described 28 cases of inflammatory breast carcinoma with these characteristics. They concluded that inflammatory breast carcinoma was a distinct entity often mistaken for other diseases of the breast. Even though the clinical signs were characteristic, the pathology of the tumor varied and was not of any specific histology.

Prognosis

Metastatic Disease

The single most important prognostic variable in cases of breast cancer is the presence and extent of axillary nodal involvement, which is indicative of systemic microscopic metastatic disease. The majority of patients with inflammatory breast cancer have clinically evident involvement of the lymph nodes. Haagensen[89] noted axillary nodal involvement in 100 percent of his 30 patients treated by radical mastectomy. In his larger series, 81 of 89 patients had positive nodes, 50 percent of these being greater than 2.5 cm.

Taylor and Meltzer's[189] 25 patients with primary inflammatory cancer included 10 with supraclavicular nodal involvement. Only five of these patients had disease localized to the breast and axilla, and four of these five patients had clinically evident nodal involvement.

Lee and Tannenbaum,[112] in describing their 18 patients, stated that axillary nodes were involved early. In 17 of their patients (98 percent), gross axillary nodal involvement was present, and several patients had clinically positive supraclavicular nodal disease. Knight and coworkers[105] treated 18 patients with primary chemotherapy, and 14 (78 percent) had axillary nodal metastases at mastectomy. Meyer and coworkers[126] reported that 86 percent of 61 patients with inflammatory breast carcinoma treated with radical mastectomy had carcinoma involving the axillary nodes. Rogers and Fitts[154] reported a 95 percent incidence of clinical axillary nodal involvement and a 43 percent incidence of supraclavicular nodal involvement in their 46 patients. Droulias and associates[62] reported that 89 percent of their 67 patients had clinically positive nodes. Barber and colleagues[17] reported a 100 percent incidence of clinically positive nodes, many accompanied by supraclavicular nodal involvement.

Patients with inflammatory breast carcinoma more frequently present with distant metastatic disease at time of diagnosis than patients with other breast carcinomas. Taylor and Meltzer[189] found visceral or bone metastases in nine of 25 (36 percent) of their patients with inflammatory breast carcinoma. Haagensen[89] reported that 15 of 89 patients with inflammatory breast carcinoma (17 percent) had distant metastases at presentation (nine lung, five bone, and one brain).

In the 59 patients DeLarue and coworkers[56] reviewed, 21 (36 percent) had metastases at time of diagnosis. In the 114 patients Bozzetti and coworkers[30] reviewed at the National Cancer Institute of Milan, 20 (17 percent) had distant metastases. The SEER data revealed metastatic disease in 24 percent of the 3171 white patients in whom inflammatory breast carcinoma was diagnosed from 1975 to 1981.[115] From 17 percent to 36 percent of patients with inflammatory breast carcinoma have distant metasta-

ses at the time of presentation in contrast to about 5 percent of patients with noninflammatory breast cancer.[115]

Hormone Receptors and Labeling Index

Table 69–12 shows the results of hormone assays in patients with inflammatory breast carcinoma. Paradiso and colleagues[142] published a retrospective study evaluating the prognostic role of hormone receptors and proliferative activity (thymidine labeling index) in patients with inflammatory breast carcinoma. Patients with locally advanced breast carcinoma from their institution served as a control. Evaluated were 28 patients with inflammatory breast carcinoma and 50 patients with locally advanced breast carcinoma; 50 percent of the patients with inflammatory breast carcinoma and 38 percent of the patients with locally advanced breast carcinoma were premenopausal.

Treatment regimens for both series consisted of primary chemotherapy or hormone therapy followed by local therapy with radiation or surgery followed by additional systemic therapy. Median follow-up was 18 months for patients with inflammatory breast carcinoma and 16 months for patients with locally advanced breast carcinoma.

Estrogen receptors were positive in 44 percent of the women with inflammatory breast carcinoma versus 64 percent of those with locally advanced carcinoma. Progesterone receptors were positive in 30 percent of women with inflammatory breast carcinoma versus 51 percent of those with locally advanced breast carcinoma. Patients with inflammatory breast carcinoma had a high percentage of cells in S-phase (high labeling index) compared with patients with locally advanced breast carcinoma (3.5 percent versus 1.6 percent, $p = 0.006$). The time to progression was not affected by hormone receptor status or labeling index after 36 months of follow-up. The overall survival rate was longer for patients with inflammatory breast cancer and positive progesterone receptors than for those with negative progesterone receptors (31 months versus 18 months, $p =$

TABLE 69–12.   HORMONE RECEPTORS IN PATIENTS WITH INFLAMMMATORY BREAST CANCER

Author (Year)	Number of Patients	ER Positive (%)	PR Positive (%)
DeLarue[56] (1981)	59	39 (66)	20 (34)
Harvey[95] (1982)	16	5 (31)	— (—)
Kokal[106] (1985)	22 (ER status determined on 7)	0 (0)	0 (0)
Keiling[101] (1985)	78	18 (23)	12 (15)
Schäfer[162] (1987)	21	10 (48)	5 (24)
Paradiso[142] (1989)	27	12 (44)	8 (30)
Fields[70] (1989)	107	20 (19)	16 (15)
Maloisel[123] (1990)	43	12 (28)	12 (28)
Attia-Sobol[12] (1993)	109	22 (20)	12 (11)
Bonnier[29] (1995)	144	59 (41)	45 (32)
Buzdar[41] (1995)	178	40 (22)	— (—)

ER = estrogen receptor.
PR = progesterone receptor.

0.04). This survival advantage was also seen in patients with a low labeling index as compared with a high labeling index ($p = 0.06$). Paradiso and colleagues[142] concluded that hormone receptor status and cell kinetics could be used as an important prognostic tool for appropriate treatment planning in patients with inflammatory breast carcinoma.

ERBB2 and Epidermal Growth Factor Receptor

The *ERBB2* oncogene overexpression has been found by several investigators to be associated with shorter survival rates, particularly in patients with positive lymph nodes.[158, 174] Guerin and colleagues[86] studied specimens from 80 patients with inflammatory breast carcinoma and 151 patients with noninflammatory breast carcinoma. They found that 41 percent of the specimens from inflammatory breast carcinomas had a threefold to 30-fold amplification of *ERBB2* compared with 19 percent of specimens from noninflammatory breast carcinomas. In 91 percent of both groups there was *ERBB2* overexpression, epidermal growth factor receptor expression, or both when the patient had 10 or more positive nodes. Yet only 50 percent of noninflammatory breast cancer specimens from patients with no positive nodes had these features. This finding implies that overexpression of *ERBB2* or expression of epidermal growth factor receptor is more common in tumors from patients with a worse prognosis, such as inflammatory breast cancer or noninflammatory breast cancer with many positive nodes.

THE TUNISIAN EXPERIENCE

Investigators from Tunis, Tunisia, noted a remarkably high incidence of inflammatory breast carcinoma there as compared with the United States.[187] Of the breast cancer cases diagnosed between 1969 and 1974 in Tunisia, 49 percent belonged to the PEV3 group, which percentage is similar to that reported in studies in the United States. The Tunisian investigators described rural residence, blood type A, and recent pregnancy as risk factors in premenopausal women for development of inflammatory breast carcinoma.[129] Older age, rural residence, blood type A, late menarche, and delay in diagnosis were risk factors for postmenopausal women. These investigators also suggested that clinical inflammatory signs were sufficient to make a diagnosis of inflammatory breast carcinoma and that the presence of dermal lymphatic invasion was not necessary.[53]

PATHOLOGY

There is no consistent histological type of breast carcinoma associated with inflammatory breast disease. The histology ranges from infiltrating ductal to medullary. Haagensen's[91] series of 40 patients included 19 (47 percent) with the large cell undifferentiated type.

In 1887, Bryant[36] made the initial observation that dermal lymphatic invasion by tumor was present in inflammatory carcinoma. This observation was reported by other investigators, making it an integral part of the diagnosis.[112, 113, 189] Some have found involvement of subepidermal capillaries or venules, but most researchers agree that the disease is primarily of the lymphatic vessels.[50, 89] Lymphatic blockage with subsequent capillary congestion is thought to be responsible for the edema and erythema seen clinically.[189]

A controversy exists in the literature as to whether inflammatory carcinoma is a clinical or pathological diagnosis. Several investigators have attempted to define the disease more specifically. Ellis and Teitelbaum[63] in 1974 proposed the name "dermal lymphatic carcinomatosis of the breast" and suggested making the presence of dermal lymphatic invasion mandatory for the diagnosis. They reviewed the literature regarding all patients diagnosed with inflammatory cancer who were disease-free at 5 years. They found eight such patients, seven of whom had pathological material available for review at the Mayo Clinic. Four of these seven patients had lymphatic invasion from the breast tumor, and six had axillary nodal involvement. The skin of the breast of four patients was found not to contain carcinoma in the dermal lymphatics. Slides of the skin were not available from three patients, two of whom were still disease-free. Therefore, six patients were disease-free, and four of these patients had negative skin biopsy results. Two other patients were described: no pathological material was available for one; the other had no evidence of dermal lymphatic invasion. Ellis and Teitelbaum[63] concluded that an improved disease-free survival was likely if no dermal lymphatic invasion was present.

Saltzstein[159] in 1974 described four patients who had no clinical evidence of inflammatory carcinoma but had dermal lymphatic invasion histologically. These patients all died rapidly. He suggested the term *clinically occult inflammatory carcinoma* and concluded that inflammatory carcinoma was a histological rather than clinical diagnosis.

Lucas and Perez-Mesa[122] attempted to clarify this controversy in a retrospective review of inflammatory carcinoma. Of 79 patients, they excluded 21 because of inadequate material, leaving 58 patients with clinical inflammatory disease and an additional 15 with occult disease in the study. They also included patients with secondary inflammatory carcinoma if there had been an acute onset of inflammation of the breast with a long-standing tumor. For 39 patients with clinical and pathological evidence of inflammatory carcinoma, median survival was about 16 months. For 19 patients with clinical signs alone, median survival was about 14 months. For 15 patients with pathological evidence alone, median survival was about 40 months. These patients were not treated homogeneously but were treated with different modalities of therapy, both local and systemic. Lucas and Perez-Mesa[122] concluded that patients with clinical evidence of inflammation, regardless of pathological findings, had an equally poor prognosis and therefore were justifiably included in the diagnosis of inflammatory carcinoma.

Levine and coworkers[115] presented the SEER data in an attempt to make the criteria for the diagnosis more uniform. There were 153 patients with both clinical and pathological diagnoses who had a 3-year relative survival rate of 34 percent; 2937 patients with clinical features alone had a 3-year survival rate of 60 percent, and 81 patients with pathological features alone had a 3-year survival rate of 52 percent. These survival rates suggest that prognosis is better for patients with a clinical diagnosis alone. The shortcomings of this analysis include the fact that it was a retrospective review, the data were from many different investigators, many clinical characteristics may not have been noted, skin biopsies were not routinely done, and patients were treated with many different modalities of therapy.

Bonnier and colleagues[29] studied the clinical findings, biological data, and treatment outcomes in 144 patients between 1976 and 1993 and identified three different entities of inflammatory breast carcinoma (IBC): true IBC, occult IBC, and pseudo IBC (Table 69–13). Classifications were based on the different biological characteristics and treatment outcomes of these entities. The patients in this study by Bonnier and colleagues[29] had either clinical features as defined by Haagensen[89] or dermal lymphatic tumor emboli or both. The mean patient age was 53 years. Evaluation included a mammary skin biopsy, a full axillary dissection or lymph node biopsy, and a tumor biopsy.

Patients were divided into three groups. Group A,

true IBC, included patients with typical features of IBC as described previously. Ipsilateral axillary lymph nodes were often palpable early, and lymph node involvement was consistent. Tumor emboli were often found in the subdermal lymphatics. Patients with true IBC were classified as having *primary* IBC if there was concurrent appearance of the tumor and inflammatory signs and *secondary* IBC if inflammatory signs and symptoms appeared later than the tumor.[189]

Group B (occult IBC) included patients with dermal lymphatic tumor emboli but no inflammatory signs.[159] Group C (pseudo IBC) included patients with symptoms and signs that resembled those of the patients in group A. However, there were subtle differences: tumors were better circumscribed and more readily palpable. Subdermal lymphatics were never involved in this group of patients, and there was little or no axillary lymph node involvement.

Group A had 109 patients (75.7 percent), group B had 19 patients (13.2 percent), and group C had 16 patients (11.1 percent). Patients received combined-modality treatment regimens. Modified radical mastectomy was performed either as initial treatment or after local treatment failure in 30 patients in group A, in six patients in group B, and in 10 patients in group C. Disease recurred in 85 patients in group A, in 11 patients in group B, and in one patient in group C. There was no difference between the disease-free and overall survival rates for group A versus group B. Patients in group C (pseudo IBC) had a very favorable outcome compared with patients in group A and group B, with better disease-free survival and overall survival rates ($p = 0.007$ and $p = 0.002$, respectively).

Bonnier and coworkers[29] concluded that the presence of dermal lymphatic emboli is sufficient but not necessary for the diagnosis of true IBC. They noted that there was no difference with regard to biological features or outcomes in patients with true IBC versus occult IBC. They suggested that true IBC should be suspected based on clinical findings and that diagnosis should be confirmed by pathological demonstration of dermal lymphatic emboli or extensive lymph node involvement. Patients presenting with rapidly growing tumors without inflammatory signs should have a skin biopsy to demonstrate dermal lymphatic emboli, which will confirm a diagnosis of occult IBC.

The issue of whether the presence of dermal lymphatic invasion influences the disease-free survival rate has been addressed in two other small studies. Burton and colleagues[39] treated patients with CAFV (cyclophosphamide, doxorubicin, fluorouracil, and vincristine) chemotherapy and found that the median disease-free survival for the 12 patients with carcinoma in the dermal lymphatics was 17 months compared with 15 months for the five patients without dermal lymphatic invasion. In Schäfer and coworkers'[162] series of 21 patients treated with chlorambucil, methotrexate, fluorouracil, and doxorubicin, the median distant disease-free survival rate was 22.5 months for patients with dermal lymphatic inva-

TABLE 69–13.   INFLAMMATORY BREAST CANCER (IBC)

True IBC	Pseudo IBC
• Dermal lymphatic emboli are present with or without inflammatory changes. In some cases, dermal lymphatic emboli cannot be found. • Tumor is not sharply delineated. • Erythema and edema involve more than one third of the skin over the breast. • Extensive lymph node involvement is usually present. • Distant metastases are more common at initial presentation. • Intensive chemotherapy is required, and mastectomy is contraindicated. • Outcome is usually not favorable.	• Inflammatory changes are present without dermal lymphatic invasion. • Tumor is better delineated. • Erythema is confined to the lesion, and edema is less extensive. • Lymph nodes are involved in about 50 percent of the cases. • Distant metastases are less common at initial presentation. • Patient can be treated with conventional chemotherapy, and mastectomy is often indicated. • Outcome is usually favorable despite large tumor size.

sion and 12 months for patients without invasion, not a significant difference.

In conclusion, in patients with clinical inflammatory signs, the presence of dermal lymphatic invasion is not necessary to confirm the diagnosis of IBC. Survival rates are poor in patients who present with the "classical" clinical signs as described by Haagensen regardless of the presence or absence of dermal lymphatic invasion.

Clinical Features

The most common symptoms of IBC include heaviness in the breast, a slight burning sensation, aching, and an increase in the size, tenderness, firmness, and redness of the breast. There is usually no fever, but these patients are often treated with a course of antibiotics for a presumed infection, thereby delaying the diagnosis.

Clinical signs include erythema and edema of the breast, especially in the dependent lower part. The skin color varies from a reddish purple to faint pink, and these changes may occur beyond the normal extent of the breast. The breast is enlarged and warm and tender to the touch. It frequently lacks an associated mass. Nipple retraction may be present later in the course of the disease.

Haagensen[89] described the clinical features of IBC in a series of 89 patients. The diagnosis was not made unless redness was present over at least one third of the breast. A tumor mass was present in 57 percent of the patients, erythema in 57 percent, breast enlargement in 48 percent, edema of the skin in 13 percent, warmness of the skin in 8 percent, nipple retraction in 13 percent, and pain in 29 percent. Many investigators rely on these criteria for the diagnosis of IBC.

Taylor and Meltzer[189] described the primary type of IBC as having features matching Haagensen's description. The secondary type of IBC, also reported by Taylor and Meltzer,[189] occurred in a breast with a localized tumor present for some time, with the eventual occurrence of inflammatory signs late in the course of the disease.

Piera and colleagues[147] in 1986 described 50 patients who had locally advanced breast carcinoma with an inflammatory component. They reported these patients to have rates of survival and disease progression similar to those of patients with IBC. They suggested that such patients should be considered as having IBC and treated accordingly.

Differential Diagnosis

The following diseases are often confused with IBC, leading to a delay in diagnosis.

1. *Bacterial infections of the breast:* Mastitis and abscess are usually seen only in lactating breasts. Infections are usually associated with fever, localized tenderness, and leucocytosis, and these features rarely occur in patients with IBC.

2. *Radiation dermatitis and fibrosis:* Erythema and inflammation in the intact breast usually occur 2–4 weeks after the treatment has begun, and these areas correspond to the fields of treatment. Radiation fibrosis, however, which occurs much later, can more closely mimic IBC and may be difficult to distinguish from an aggressive tumor recurrence. Physical examination in either case can reveal areas of thickening and masslike lesions with skin edema.

3. *Lymphoma, leukemia, or sarcoma:* These conditions involving the breast may be clinically indistinguishable from IBC and may require cytologic or histological examination for an accurate diagnosis.

4. *Carcinoma en cuirasse:* This is a slow-growing tumor that produces red discoloration of the skin. It is not, however, associated with signs of acute inflammation.

5. *Tuberculosis and syphilis involving the breast:* These conditions are now rarely encountered in the United States.

MANAGEMENT OF INFLAMMATORY BREAST CANCER

Local Treatment

Surgery

Surgery has produced disappointing results in patients with inflammatory breast carcinoma. In 1916, Learmonth[111] reviewed 45 cases reported in the literature and found that only one patient was disease-free after 5 years. Most of these cases were initially treated as mastitis, and the cancer was very advanced by the time diagnosis was made. Learmonth[111] recommended that the most radical operation possible should be performed, with thorough removal of the axillary nodes and the supraclavicular nodes if deemed necessary.

Taylor and Meltzer[189] in 1938 treated six patients with inflammatory breast carcinoma with radical mastectomy. These patients all developed either local, regional, or contralateral breast recurrences fairly rapidly. The average survival was 21 months, with a range of 11 to 34 months.

Haagensen and Stout[89] were convinced that radical mastectomy should not be done in patients with classical IBC. They reported that 20 breast cancer patients with inflammatory signs treated by radical mastectomy had a local recurrence rate of 50 percent and a mean survival of 15.5 months. Haagensen[89] then presented his data on 30 patients treated by radical mastectomy before the criteria for operability had been established. The mean survival was 19 months, and the only 5-year survivor experienced recurrence and died 68 months after surgery.

Table 69–14 summarizes the results described by several physicians treating inflammatory breast carcinoma by surgery. Treves,[194] in his review of 114 patients in whom radical mastectomy was performed, noted that only four patients (3.5 percent) were alive

TABLE 69–14.   SURGICAL TREATMENT OF INFLAMMATORY BREAST CANCER

Author (Year)	Treatment Design	Number of Patients	Overall Survival
Taylor and Meltzer[189] (1938)	RM	6	19 months mean
Meyer[126] (1948)	RM or SM	61	6% 5-year survival
Haagensen[89] (1956)	RM	30	19 months mean
Treves[194] (1959)	RM	114	NA (only 3.5% alive at 5 years)
Stocks and Patterson[183] (1976)	RM ± hormones	10	32 months mean
Bozzetti[30] (1981)	RM	8	12 months mean

NA = not available.
RM = radical mastectomy.
SM = simple mastectomy.

at 5 years. In 1959, he wrote an editorial stating that radical mastectomy was contraindicated in this disease based on six reports in the literature showing, he believed, that the disease was disseminated at the time of diagnosis in most patients.

Radiotherapy

In the late 1800s and early 1900s, IBC was often not diagnosed until it had reached a point that precluded surgical treatment alone. Many patients who were considered inoperable were then treated with radiation therapy alone. Table 69–15 summarizes the reports on patients treated with radiation as the primary modality of therapy. In many of these series, patients underwent hormonal manipulation, which was a popular modality at that time. It is difficult to compare early results of radiation therapy to more recent outcomes because of the differences in the techniques and stages of disease treated.

Wang and Griscom[201] treated a series of 33 patients with IBC from 1944 to 1959 with radiation therapy alone. Six of these patients had metastatic disease. Orthovoltage radiation was used in 23 patients and supervoltage radiation in 10. The average dose was 2600 cGy in 30 days for the orthovoltage-treated patients and 5200 cGy for the supervoltage group. Sixteen of these patients were also treated with hormonal manipulation. The orthovoltage-treated tumors were controlled locally for a mean of 9.8 months compared with 27.4 months for the supervoltage-treated tumors. There was a local recurrence rate of 67 percent for all patients. Mean survival was 14.3 months for the orthovoltage-treated patients and 30 months for the supervoltage-treated patients. Overall survival from the date of diagnosis averaged 20.5

TABLE 69–15.   RADIATION THERAPY FOR INFLAMMATORY BREAST CANCER

Author (Year)	Treatment Design	Number of Patients	Survival
Lee & Tannenbaum[112] (1924)	RT	13	11 months mean
Taylor and Meltzer[189] (1938)	RT	19	9.2 months mean
Chris[50] (1950)	RT	5	9 months mean
Rogers and Fitts[154] (1956)	RT	24	4% 5-year OS
Dao and McCarthy[55] (1957)	RT	3	4 months mean
Wang and Griscom[201] (1964)	RT	17 ⎫	20.5 months mean
	RT ± HT	16 ⎭	
Haagensen[89] (1971)	RT ± HT	38	16.3 months mean
Zucali[204] (1976)	RT—x ray	21 ⎫	14 months mean
	RT—cobalt	37 ⎭	
	Other	12	
Droulias[62] (1976)	RT	31	23 months mean
Nussbaum[138] (1977)	RT	15	15 months mean
Bruckman[34] (1979)	RT ± hormones and chemotherapy	18	13% 5-year RFS (actuarial)
Chu[49] (1980)	RT	28	28.5 months mean
Barker[19] (1980)	RT	80	19% 2-year OS
Bozzetti[30] (1981)	RT—x ray	20	16.5 months mean
	RT—cobalt	12	12 months mean
Roüessé[155] (1986)	RT + oophorectomy	60	33 months median
Perez and Fields[144] (1987)	RT	28	18 months median

HT = hormonal therapy.
OS = overall survival.
RFS = relapse-free survival.
RT = radiation therapy.

months. Wang and Griscom[201] concluded that supervoltage treatment was preferred because of better dose delivery to the tumor, which resulted in better local control.

Chu and coworkers[49] treated 62 IBC patients with radical radiotherapy. Of these 62 patients, 14 received hormonal manipulation and 20 received adjuvant chemotherapy (four patients received single-agent therapy, and 16 received CMFVP or CMF). Megavoltage therapy was used in 26 patients, orthovoltage in 29, and both megavoltage and orthovoltage in seven. Patients received different tumor doses. Mean survival for the 28 patients who were treated by radiation therapy alone was 28 months; for the whole group, mean survival was 24 months (median 18 months). Chu and colleagues[49] noted that doses of 6000 cGy were needed for optimal local control in patients with tumors larger than 10 cm. An increase in the dose did not decrease the local recurrence rate but did prolong time to local recurrence. This study also included six patients treated with twice-daily fractionation, and their local recurrence rate of 33 percent suggests that better local control may be achieved by using this schedule.

Barker and coworkers[19] described their experience at M.D. Anderson Cancer Center from July 1948 through July 1972 in treating 80 patients with IBC. Conventional once-daily radiation was used in 69 patients and twice-daily fractionation in 11 patients. The local recurrence rate was 46 percent in the once-daily group compared with 27 percent in the twice-daily group. The 2-year disease-free survival was 17 percent in patients treated with conventional once-daily radiation and 27 percent in those treated with twice-daily fractionation. Barker and coworkers[19] concluded that twice-daily fractionation may improve local control.

Perez and Fields[144] analyzed 95 patients with IBC treated at Washington University in St. Louis. Radiotherapy alone was used in 28 of these patients. The median disease-free survival was 8 months, and the overall survival was 18 months. The local recurrence rate was 68 percent (19 patients), with 18 of these patients also having distant metastases.

It can be concluded from the preceding studies that a tumor dose of 6000 cGy is necessary for optimal local control and twice-daily fractionation may improve local control. However, radiation therapy alone has little impact on survival.

Surgery and Radiotherapy

The combination of surgery and radiotherapy has been used in an effort to improve local control. The results of some of these studies are summarized in Table 69–16.

Perez and Fields[144] treated 12 patients with radiotherapy and mastectomy. The median disease-free survival rate was 24 months, and the median overall survival rate was 42 months. The disease-free sur-

TABLE 69–16. RADIATION AND SURGERY AS TREATMENT OF INFLAMMATORY BREAST CANCER

Author (Year)	Treatment Design	Number of Patients	Mean Survival in Months
Lee and Tannenbaum[112] (1924)	M + RT	4	24
Meyer[126] (1948)	M + RT	47	28
Chris[50] (1950)	M + RT (3 preop/postop RT, 1 postop RT)	4	10.8
Rogers and Fitts[154] (1956)	SM (10) RM (10) Postop RT (18) Preop RT (6)	20	21
Dao and McCarthy[55] (1957)	RM + Postop RT (3) Preop RT + RM (2) Preop RT + HT (1)	6	12
Barber[17] (1961)	RM + Postop RT	42	25
Zucali[204] (1976)	X ray + RM	3	14
	Cobalt + RM	9	(For the entire group)
		(70 total)	
Barker[18] (1976)	SM + Postop RT	17	<12
Droulias[62] (1976)	M + RT	5	29
Nussbaum[138] (1977)	SM + RT	7	15
		(54 total)	(For the entire sample)
Bozzetti[30] (1981)	RM + Postop RT	24	18
Rao[150] (1982)	M + RT	7	7
		(36 total)	(For the entire group)
Haagensen[90] (1986)	RM + Postop RT	2	16
Perez and Fields[144] (1987)	M + RT	12	42 (median)

HT = hormone therapy.
M = mastectomy.
Preop = preoperative.
Postop = postoperative.
RM = radical mastectomy.
RT = radiation therapy.
SM = simple mastectomy.

vival rate was significantly better than that seen in a previous series of 28 patients from the same institute who were treated with radiotherapy alone ($p = 0.01$).

Barker and colleagues[18] treated 17 patients with simple mastectomy followed by radiotherapy. The local recurrence rate was 63 percent, and none of these patients were alive at 5 years.

The mean survival rates for several other series ranged from 7 months to 29 months. Thus, overall survival rates are still poor, even with the combination of radiation therapy and mastectomy, and these survival rates are not significantly different from those for patients treated with either surgery or radiation therapy alone.

Combined-Modality Treatment

The previous discussion supports the hypothesis that IBC is a systemic disease by the time it can be diagnosed and that local therapy alone is inadequate. Several investigators have treated this disease with a combined-modality treatment approach. These studies are summarized in Table 69–17.

In a study by DeLena and associates,[57] discussed previously, 36 patients with IBC were treated with primary chemotherapy before local therapy. The objective response rate was 67 percent (20 percent complete response and 47 percent partial response), and the median survival was 25 months. The 3-year survival was 25 percent. These percentages include patients who did and who did not receive maintenance chemotherapy. Results were not significantly different from this group's previous experience with radiotherapy alone, when the response rate was 28 percent. Although this study did not show a benefit for IBC patients receiving chemotherapy as compared with historical controls receiving radiotherapy alone, it did suggest that maintenance chemotherapy increased disease-free survival rates overall for patients with locally advanced breast cancer. In the 16 IBC patients who were postmenopausal, substantial dose reductions were made. Also, not all IBC patients received maintenance therapy. Therefore, these data are not conclusive as regards to IBC patients but have stimulated other investigators to take a more aggressive approach in treating these patients.

Buzdar and coworkers[41] reported the results of 178 patients treated at the M.D. Anderson Cancer Center since April 1974. Patients were divided into four groups: group A (January 1974–September 1978), with 40 patients; group B (September 1978–December 1981), with 23 patients; group C (August 1982–February 1987), with 43 patients; and group D (March 1987–September 1993), with 72 patients.

All patients received primary chemotherapy with fluorouracil, doxorubicin, and cyclophosphamide. Following this, patients in group A received radiotherapy as a local treatment modality, and chemotherapy was subsequently given for 24 months. Group B patients underwent mastectomy as a local treatment modality, followed by chemotherapy and consolida-tion radiotherapy. Mastectomy was employed in an attempt to reduce the dose of radiation needed for optimal control. Group C patients were treated similarly to group B patients except that vincristine and prednisone were added to the chemotherapy regimen, and doxorubicin was given as a continuous infusion over 48 hours to prevent cardiac toxicity. In group D patients, the role of alternate therapy with non–cross-resistant drugs was evaluated.

The median follow-up was 198 months for group A, 176 months for group B, 110 months for group C, and 34 months for group D. The objective response rate to primary chemotherapy was 80 percent in group A, 57 percent in group B, 65 percent in group C, and 75 percent in group D. The objective response rate overall was 72 percent, with a complete response rate of 12 percent. The local regional failure rate was 18 percent (seven patients) in group A, 26 percent (six patients) in group B, 14 percent (six patients) in group C, and 19 percent (14 patients) in group D.

The median disease-free survival rate for all patients in the four groups was 21 months, and the median overall survival rate was 40 months. There was no significant difference in the disease-free versus the overall survival rate among the various groups. Patients who had a complete or a partial response following primary chemotherapy had superior disease-free and overall survival rates compared with those who had less than a partial response. There was no difference in response rates to the various chemotherapy regimens. Furthermore, the addition of mastectomy to radiotherapy in groups B and C did not decrease the local recurrence rate. However, mastectomy following primary chemotherapy resulted in the use of lower radiation doses, as the gross residual disease was resected, thus eliminating the late complications of high doses of radiation therapy.

Perez and Fields[144] in 1987 reported another large nonrandomized series of patients treated for IBC. They compared the treatment outcomes of different combined-modality treatment approaches in 95 patients at a single institution. The details of the chemotherapy were not given, but it was stated that patients received two or three cycles of FAC (fluorouracil, doxorubicin, and cyclophosphamide) prior to mastectomy. The median disease-free survival for patients receiving radiotherapy alone (28 patients) was 8 months compared with 41 months for patients receiving chemotherapy (c), surgery (s), radiotherapy (r), and more chemotherapy (c) (CSRC) (32 patients, $p < 0.0001$). The median overall survival for radiotherapy alone was 18 months versus 47 months for the CSRC group ($p = 0.0002$).

There was a significant increase in the survival rate for patients who received CSRC versus those who received chemotherapy and radiotherapy alone (23 patients, $p = 0.02$). There was also a decrease in the local recurrence rate for patients who received a combination of the three modalities of therapy. The local recurrence rate was 16 percent for the CSRC group, 57 percent for the radiotherapy and chemo-

TABLE 69–17.   COMBINED-MODALITY TREATMENT OF INFLAMMATORY BREAST CANCER

Author (Year)	Treatment	Number of Patients	Relapse-Free Survival	Overall Survival
DeLena[57] (1978)	CT + RT ± CT	36	NA	25 months median
Krutchik[109] (1979)	CT + RT + CT	32	NA	24 months median
Chu[49] (1980)	RT + HT	14	NA	15 months median
	RT + CT	16	NA	>26 months median
Zylberberg[205] (1982)	CT + S + CT ± RT	15	66% crude	>56 months median; 70% 5-year
Pawlicki[143] (1983)	CT ± S + RT	72	10% 3-year	28% 3-year
Loprinzi[120] (1984)	S + CT + RT + CT	9	29.5 months	>25 months median; 55% 5-year
Fastenberg[66] (1985)	CT ± RT ± S	63	24 months	43 months median
Keiling[101] (1985)	CT + S + CT	41	58 months; 54%	63% 5-year
Knight[105] (1986)	CT	18	NA	23 months median
Fowble[78] (1986)	CT1 or CT2	16 (19 total)	65% 3-year	84% 3-year OS
Israel[98] (1986)	HD-CT + S + CT	25	33 months median	62% 5-year
Jacquillat[99] (1987)	CT + RT + CT ± HT	66	Observed 73% 4-year	62% 4-year OS
Schäfer[162] (1987)	CT	21	NA	43 months median
Burton[39] (1987)	CT	22	16.4 months	23.6 months median
Schwartz[168] (1987)	CT ± TAM ± CT	17	NA	>85% 5-year OS
Conte[52] (1987)	HT + CT	14	15 months	NA
Perez[144] (1987)	CT + RT	23	18 months	25 months median
	CT + S + RT	32	41 months	46 months median
Perloff[145] (1988)	CT	14	17.5 months	26.9 months median
Swain[185] (1989)	CT + RT + S + CT + HT	45	23 months	36 months median; 61% stage IIIA (actuarial); 36% IIIB (actuarial)
Noguchi[137] (1988)	IA-CT + S + CT	28	53% 10-year	47% 10-year OS
Brun[35] (1988)	CT + RT + S + CT	26	12 months	31 months median
Roüessé[155] (1989)	CT1 + RT + CT + HT	91	28% 4-year	38 months median for CT1; 44% 4-year OS
	CT2 + RT + CT + HT	79	46% 4-year	66% 4-year OS
Fields[70] (1989)	CT + S + RT + CT	37	NA	49 months median; 44% 5-year OS
	RT + C	23	NA	10% 5-year
Maloisel[123] (1990)	CT + S + CT + RT + HT	43	NA	46 months median; 75% 5-year OS
Arriagada[11] (1990)	CT + RT + CT	99	NA	55% 5-year OS
Armstrong[9] (1993)	CT + S ± RT ± CT	24	58% (actuarial)	75% (actuarial)
Attia-Sobol[12] (1993)	CT ± S + RT + CT	109	45 months median; 44% 5-year	70 months median; 55% (actuarial)
Mourali[130] (1993)	RT → CT / CT \ S → CT	34 / 34 (83 entered into study)	27 months median for both groups	18% 5-year; 14% 10-year survival for both groups
Chevallier[47] (1993)	CT + RT ± CT ± S	178	22% 5-year; 13% 10-year	37 months median; 32% 5-year OS; 23% 10-year OS
Fein[68] (1994)	CT + S + RT / RT ± S ± CT	33 / 17	50% 5-year OS \ ↘ p = 0.0002 ↗ / 7% 5-year	39% 5-year for both groups
Thomas[190] (1995)	CT + RT + CT ± HT	125	38% 5-year	50% 5-year OS
Buzdar[41] (1995)	CT ± RT ± S + CT ± RT	178	21 months	40 months median; 30% 5-year OS

CT = chemotherapy.
HD-CT = high-dose chemotherapy.
HT = hormonal therapy.
IA-CT = intra-arterial chemotherapy.
NA = not available.
OS = overall survival.
RT = radiation therapy.
S = surgery.

therapy group, 33 percent for the radiotherapy and mastectomy group, and 68 percent for the radiotherapy-alone group. Firm conclusions cannot be drawn from this study as patients were selected for treatment and not randomized.

The largest series of patients with IBC was reported by Rouësse and colleagues[155] in 1986 from the Institut Gustave-Roussy in Villejuif, France. The difficulty in comparing the findings on these 230 patients with the findings in North American literature lies in the different classification systems. Although the PEV classification was used, it was stated that all patients would have been classified as T4b in the UICC/TNM classification.

Three different protocols were used in the study by Rouësse and coworkers.[155] Group C, treated from 1973 to 1975, received radiotherapy only. Group A, treated from 1976 to 1980, received three cycles of doxorubicin (40 mg/m^2 IV on day 1), vincristine (1 mg/m^2 IV on day 2), and methotrexate (3 mg/m^2 subcutaneously for six doses every 12 hours beginning on day 3) (AVM), all repeated every 3 to 4 weeks prior to radiotherapy for three courses, then for one cycle during radiotherapy and five cycles after radiotherapy. Group B, treated from 1980 to 1982, received three cycles of doxorubicin (50 mg/m^2 IV on day 1), vincristine (0.6 mg/m^2 IV on day 2), cyclophosphamide (200 mg/m^2 IM on days 3–5), and fluorouracil (300 mg/m^2 IM on days 3–5) every 4 weeks for three courses, followed by radiotherapy with one cycle of AVM and then five more cycles of AVM.

Groups A and B both received maintenance with vincristine (1 mg/m^2 IV on day 1), cyclophosphamide (200 mg/m^2 IM on days 2–4), and fluorouracil (300 mg/m^2 IM on days 2–4) every 4 weeks for four to 12 cycles. The median number of maintenance cycles was nine for group A patients and 10 for group B patients. Radiation treatment was the same for all three groups, including 4500 cGy to the breast and draining lymph nodes with a 2000–3000 cGy boost to the tumor.

All patients had hormonal manipulation consisting of radiocastration for premenopausal or perimenopausal women and tamoxifen 20 mg daily for 1 year (after 1973) for postmenopausal women. Patient characteristics were similar in all three groups. There were 60 patients in group C, 91 in group A, and 79 in group B. Patients classified as PEV2 and PEV3 were equally distributed, with 68 percent and 32 percent, respectively, in the control group; 69 percent and 31 percent, respectively, in group A; and 73 percent and 27 percent, respectively, in group B.

The objective response rate to primary chemotherapy was 14 percent in group A and 27 percent in group B (p = 0.04). The 4-year disease-free survival and overall survival rates were, respectively, 16 percent and 28 percent for group C, 28 percent and 44 percent for group A, and 46 percent and 66 percent for group B (p <0.005 in group C versus A, p <0.00001 in group C versus B, and p <0.01 in group A versus B).

There was a survival difference between group C

and A (p = 0.03), group A and B (p <0.001), and group C and B (p = 0.0001).

Rouësse and coworkers[155] also analyzed the disease-free survival and overall survival rates in 91 patients who did not relapse either during maintenance chemotherapy or within 3 months of the termination of treatment. They looked at the length of administration of maintenance therapy as patients received different numbers of cycles. They stated that there was no difference in the disease-free survival or overall survival rates in relation to the duration of chemotherapy. At 4 years, the disease-free survival rates for patients with PEV2 and PEV3 disease were as follows: 8 percent and 0 percent (p = 0.00001) for group C, 35 percent and 11 percent (p = 0.005) for group A, and 52 percent and 30 percent (p = 0.11) for group B. There was an improvement in the disease-free survival rate for the PEV3 group, which received more intensive chemotherapy (group B versus A, p = 0.03). However, when patients with N2, N3 disease were analyzed, there was no significant difference in the disease-free survival rate for the group receiving more intensive chemotherapy (6 percent for group C, 18 percent for group A, and 15 percent for group B; p = not significant). There was, however, a benefit seen for patients with N0–N1 disease. The 4-year disease-free survival rate was 6 percent for group C, 30 percent for group A, and 53 percent for group B (p = 0.00001 for all groups). The majority of patients actually fell into the N0–N1 category: 70 percent of group C, 76 percent of group A, and 82 percent of group B had N0–N1 disease.

The conclusions from this study were that more aggressive chemotherapy prolonged the disease-free survival rate for patients with PEV3 disease, which is similar to IBC according to UICC/TNM classification. Patients with N0–N1 disease benefited from more dose-intensive chemotherapy. However, patients with a larger tumor burden (N2–N3 disease) did not benefit from the more aggressive regimen used in this study. A high-dose intensive primary chemotherapy regimen or a different approach may be needed for these patients.

Morvan and coworkers[127] presented their data on a 15-year follow-up of 71 patients with T4d IBC between 1979 and 1984. Diagnosis was based on clinical findings with histological confirmation. Tumor emboli in lymphatics were found in 60 percent of the patients. All patients received four cycles of primary chemotherapy followed by radical mastectomy and axillary lymph node dissection. Patients subsequently received 14 cycles of chemotherapy and radiotherapy. Doxorubicin was given every three cycles at a dose of 60 mg/m^2. Premenopausal patients underwent oophorectomy, and all patients received tamoxifen for 18 months at the end of chemotherapy. The median follow-up was 170 months. There was an objective response rate of 64 percent, with 51 percent complete response and 13 percent partial response. The overall survival rate was 41 percent at 5 years, 27 percent at 10 years, and 25 percent at 15 years. The only significant prognostic factor that had a major impact on survival was the response of inflammatory signs to primary chemotherapy ($p = <0.001$).

Mourali and colleagues[130] reported the results of a randomized trial using primary chemotherapy in patients with IBC. The TNM and PEV (*pousée evolutive*) staging system was used, and all patients belonged to PEV2 and PEV3 categories. Of the 83 patients entered into this study, 38 patients (45.8 percent) were in the PEV2 category and 45 patients (54.2 percent) were in the PEV3 category. Almost half, 49 patients, were premenopausal, 30 were postmenopausal, and four had unknown menopausal status.

Treatment consisted of three cycles of primary chemotherapy followed by randomization to radiotherapy or surgery for local control. Radiotherapy or surgery was followed by 15 additional cycles of chemotherapy. Chemotherapy consisted of cyclophosphamide 100 mg/m² given orally every day from day 1 to day 14, methotrexate 40 mg/m² IV on days 1 and 8, and fluorouracil 600 mg/m² IV on days 1 and 8. This cycle was repeated every 28 days.

Among the 83 patients, 68 patients were randomized to radiotherapy or surgery—34 patients to surgery and 34 patients to radiotherapy (11 of these patients, four of those assigned to radiotherapy and seven of those assigned to surgery, were considered protocol violations).

A total of 57 patients completed the entire protocol with a minimum follow-up of 10 years. The disease-free interval for this series was compared historically with that of a previous series from the same institution. The median disease-free interval was based on local/regional treatment alone and was 36 months for PEV-2 patients and 21 months for PEV-3 patients. In contrast, the median disease-free interval was 26 months for PEV-2 patients and 16 months for PEV-3 patients in the previous series from the same institution.

The two most important prognostic factors predicting disease-free survival were initial tumor size and initial response to chemotherapy. This study also suggested that surgery and radiotherapy achieved equivalent long-term survival rates after primary chemotherapy. Mourali and colleagues[130] concluded that postmenopausal patients can benefit from chemotherapy just as much as premenopausal patients. This study is interesting in that it is the only randomized study on IBC but is limited in its application by the small number of patients and by the protocol violations.

Fields and colleagues[70] reviewed the outcome of 107 patients who had either clinical or histopathological evidence of IBC. Treatment modalities included radiotherapy alone, radiotherapy and chemotherapy, radiotherapy and surgery, and combined radiotherapy, surgery, and chemotherapy. They evaluated 15 different factors of prognostic significance by univariate and multivariate analyses. In this study, 45 percent of patients (47 of 105) experienced local-regional recurrence; 19 percent of these patients had been

treated with mastectomy and 70 percent had not ($p = <0.0001$). Factors suggesting prognostic value for relapse-free survival included mastectomy, discrete tumor mass, and white race. The latter was of marginal significance. Multivariate analysis showed that mastectomy and chemotherapy had prognostic value for survival.

Fields and coworkers[70] also noted that the prognostic significance of clinical or histopathological criteria was similar. The diagnosis of IBC could be based on either set of criteria. It was concluded that mastectomy is an important component of local treatment and contributed significantly to local control in this retrospective analysis.

Attia-Sobol and coworkers[12] retrospectively reviewed 109 patients with IBC between 1978 and 1987. In this study, 62 patients had clinical evidence of IBC and had T4d lesions, whereas 47 patients were considered to have "neglected" locally advanced breast carcinoma, and these patients presented with secondary evidence of clinical inflammatory signs. All patients received six cycles of primary chemotherapy with cyclophosphamide, doxorubicin, vincristine, and fluorouracil. Patients who had a complete response received radiotherapy followed by chemotherapy. Patients who had a partial response underwent a total mastectomy followed by radiotherapy and chemotherapy. Patients with no change or with progressive disease had preoperative radiotherapy and surgery.

The median follow-up was 120 months. The median overall survival was 70 months, and actuarial 5-year survival was 55 percent. The median disease-free survival was 45 months, and actuarial 5-year disease-free survival was 44 percent.

No difference was noted between the patients with neglected locally advanced breast cancer and the patients with IBC in terms of disease-free survival or overall survival rates.

In 23 patients, primary chemotherapy was followed by radiotherapy only, whereas 74 patients had a modified radical mastectomy followed by radiotherapy. Six patients with progressive or persistent disease received preoperative irradiation. Relapse occurred in 62 percent of patients (68 patients), of whom 24 percent (26 patients) had local-regional recurrence. There was local/regional recurrence in 15 percent of the patients treated with radiotherapy alone and in 27 percent of the patients treated with radiotherapy and surgery. The investigators concluded that primary chemotherapy was effective in improving survival rates both for patients with IBC and for patients with locally advanced breast carcinoma as compared with historical controls.

Chevallier and associates[47] reported on three studies that included 178 patients with IBC. The median follow-up for the three studies was 67 months. In the first study, 64 patients received primary chemotherapy with either (1) cyclophosphamide, methotrexate, and fluorouracil or (2) cyclophosphamide, doxorubicin, vincristine, and fluorouracil. Patients then received radiotherapy. Surgery was used only as a salvage treatment in patients who had local-regional relapse after surgery. The objective response rate was 56.2 percent, with no significant difference between the results of the two regimens. The median disease-free survival was 16.7 months, and the median overall survival was 25 months.

In the second study, three different doxorubicin-containing regimens were used for primary chemotherapy. In 23 patients who had stable disease, supraclavicular lymph node involvement, or progressive disease, radiotherapy alone was given for local/regional control. Of the 60 patients in the study, 38 had surgery and 22 had radiotherapy alone. The objective response rate in this study was 73.5 percent. The median disease-free survival was 19 months, and the median overall survival was 45.7 months. Again, objective responses for the various chemotherapy regimens were not significantly different ($p = 0.96$).

In the third study, estrogen recruitment along with a chemotherapy combination was used in 31 patients. Following response to primary chemotherapy, all patients underwent surgery and radiotherapy. The objective response rate was 93.5 percent. The median disease-free survival was 22 months, and the median overall survival was 32.6 months.

For the first study, the disease-free survival rates at 5 years and 10 years were 18 percent and 11 percent, respectively. The overall survival rates at 5 years and 10 years were 29 percent and 20 percent, respectively. For the second study, the disease-free survival rate at 5 years was 28 percent, and the 5-year overall survival rate was 39 percent. For the third study, 5-year and 10-year results are not available. For patients in all three studies, the 5-year and 10-year disease-free survival rates were 22 percent and 13 percent, respectively, and the 5-year and 10-year overall survival rates were 32 percent and 23 percent, respectively. Thus, in spite of a better response rate in the second and third studies, there were no significant differences in the disease-free and overall survival rates of patients who received intensive chemotherapy.

Arriagada and coworkers[11] evaluated the response rates in 99 patients with IBC who received alternating radiotherapy and chemotherapy schedules. All patients received three courses of a primary chemotherapy regimen (CT1). CT1 was followed by local-regional radiotherapy given in three courses (RT1, RT2, and RT3) alternated with a second chemotherapy regimen (CT2). The first two courses of radiotherapy (RT1 and RT2) involved treatment of the supraclavicular lymph nodes, internal mammary chain, whole breast, and tumor. The third course of radiotherapy (RT3) was an irradiation boost given to the residual tumor and axillary lymph nodes. Patients received three additional courses of the second regimen of chemotherapy (CT2).

The median follow-up was 46 months. The objective response after CT1 was 70 percent, with a 10 percent complete response and a 60 percent partial response. The objective response after CT1-RT3 was 93 percent, with a 75 percent complete response

and an 18 percent partial response. The 4-year overall survival rate was 55 percent, the local control rate was 72 percent, and the rate of distant metastases was 53 percent. Isolated local recurrence was seen in only 4 percent of the patients. Arriagada and coworkers[11] concluded that combined-modality therapy with chemotherapy and radiotherapy is highly effective in producing local control.

Noguchi and colleagues[137] took a different approach in treating their IBC patients with intra-arterial infusional chemotherapy. These 28 patients received intra-arterial infusional chemotherapy, surgical ablation, extended radical mastectomy, and adjuvant chemotherapy. At mastectomy, 13 patients (46 percent) had complete histological necrosis of the tumor. The median follow-up was 111 months. The local recurrence rate was 32 percent, which is not much different from that seen after radiotherapy and surgery. Leukopenia, with a white blood cell count of less than $3000/mm^3$ occurred in 75 percent of the patients treated with intra-arterial therapy alone. The median 10-year disease-free survival rate was 53 percent, and the median overall survival rate was 47 percent.

Thomas and colleagues[190] treated 125 patients with an alternating schedule of radiotherapy and chemotherapy. The pattern of failure with this alternating chemoradiotherapy schedule was evaluated. The mean age of patients was 52 years, and 48 percent of patients were premenopausal. All patients had T4d tumors; 67 percent had N1 disease, and 11 percent had N2 disease. Primary chemotherapy (CT1) consisted of doxorubicin or epirubicin 50 mg/m² IV on day 1, vincristine 0.6 mg/m² IV on day 2, cyclophosphamide 200 mg/m² IV on days 3–5, methotrexate 10 mg/m² IV on days 3–5, and fluorouracil 300 mg/m² IV on days 3–5 (AVCMF) every 4 weeks for three courses. After a 1-week rest period, three courses of local/regional radiotherapy (RT1, RT2, and RT3) were alternated with a second chemotherapy regimen (CT2). The first two courses of local/regional radiotherapy (RT1 and RT2) involved treating the supraclavicular, axillary, and internal mammary lymph nodes as well as the whole breast. The RT program (RT3) included a boost to the residual breast tumor and the axillary lymph nodes in the case of N1 or N2 disease. The second chemotherapy regimen (CT2) consisted of doxorubicin or epirubicin 50 mg/m² IV on day 1, cyclophosphamide 500 mg/m² IV on day 1, and fluorouracil 500 mg/m² IV on day 1 (FAC or FEC). Hormonal manipulation included ovarian irradiation for premenopausal women and tamoxifen for postmenopausal women.

The median follow-up was 72 months. The disease-free and overall survival rates were 38 percent and 50 percent, respectively, at 5 years. Local failure as the first sign of recurrence occurred in 18 percent of the patients, and distant metastases developed within a year. The tumor size and histological grade affected relapse-free survival. Grade 1 histology was rarely seen in IBC in this series. Local control with this alternating chemoradiotherapy schedule was similar to that obtained historically with surgery alone. The advantage with this regimen was that full doses of radiation and chemotherapy could be delivered because of different toxicity profiles associated with these modalities.

Armstrong and coworkers[9] performed a pilot study in 24 patients with inoperable locally advanced breast cancer of whom 83 percent had IBC. There were two important aspects to this treatment regimen. First was the use of the principles of dose intensity using a multidrug non–cross-resistant chemotherapy regimen, and second was the assessment of histological response to primary chemotherapy. The median follow-up was 45 months. The median age of the patients was 41.5 years. The chemotherapy regimen consisted of eight cycles, each of 2 weeks duration given over a 16-week period. The treatment consisted of cyclophosphamide 100 mg/m^2 per day orally on days 1–7, doxorubicin 40 mg/m^2 IV on day 1, vincristine 1 mg IV on day 1, methotrexate 100 mg/m^2 IV on day 1, leucovorin 10 mg/m^2 orally every 6 hours for six doses on day 2, fluorouracil 600 mg/m^2 IV on day 2, and fluorouracil 300 mg/m^2 per day given as a continuous infusion on days 8 and 9. Maximal response was noted at a median of 3 months. A median number of eight cycles was completed.

Following primary chemotherapy, a partial clinical response was noted in 15 patients (63 percent), and a complete response was noted in nine patients (37 percent), for an objective response rate of 100 percent. All patients had surgery performed, 20 patients (83 percent) undergoing a modified radical mastectomy and four patients (17 percent) undergoing a simple mastectomy. On pathological evaluation, 46 percent of the patients had no gross evidence of disease and 29 percent had no microscopic evidence of disease in the breast.

Therapy after mastectomy was not standardized; 79 percent of patients had radiotherapy, and 75 percent had adjuvant chemotherapy. The actuarial 5-year relapse-free and overall survival rates were 58 percent and 75 percent, respectively. The only significant variable affecting relapse was histological response to primary chemotherapy. All deaths that occurred in the study were in patients who had macroscopic residual disease after primary chemotherapy.

Fein and associates[68] did a retrospective analysis of 50 patients who had clinical or histological evidence of IBC and were treated with a curative intent between October 1964 and March 1989. Average patient age was 55 years, and 31 patients were post-menopausal, three were perimenopausal, and 15 were premenopausal. In 59 percent of the patients, a mass greater than 5 cm was presented. Patients received local/regional treatment modalities alone or combined-modality treatment with radiotherapy, surgery, and systemic chemotherapy. Those who received combined-modality treatment ($n = 33$) had a 5-year relapse-free survival of 50 percent compared with 7 percent for those ($n = 17$) who received fewer than

three modalities ($p = 0.0002$). A tumor size of greater than 5 cm was the only clinical factor that had an negative impact on the relapse-free survival.

Neither primary chemotherapy nor doxorubicin-containing chemotherapy contributed to an improvement in the disease-free survival rate. As this was a retrospective analysis, selection factors may have negatively influenced the outcomes from primary chemotherapy and doxorubicin-containing chemotherapy. There was, however, an increase in the local recurrence rate when local-regional treatment was delayed.

Hormonal Therapy

Hormonal therapy with testosterone, estrogen, tamoxifen, or hormonal ablation (oophorectomy, adrenalectomy, or hypophysectomy) have all been used alone or in combination with local therapies in the treatment of patients with IBC.

Two large series have been reported of patients with advanced breast cancer treated with adrenalectomy. Yonemoto and coworkers[203] treated 14 patients with IBC (11 considered primary) from 1956 to 1966. Haagensen's[88] criteria were used for diagnosis. A majority of patients had other treatments in addition to adrenalectomy: 10 patients had bilateral oophorectomy, and the other four previously had ovarian ablation. Four of the primary cases received radiotherapy, hormonal therapy, or chemotherapy before adrenalectomy. There was an objective response rate of 50 percent lasting 6 months. The median survival for the entire series was 12 months. Only one of the patients with inflammatory disease was alive after 5 years.

Fracchia and colleagues[79] treated 500 patients with adrenalectomy. There were 27 patients with primary inoperable inflammatory carcinoma. Of these, 21 were treated with combined adrenalectomy and oophorectomy and six with adrenalectomy alone. There were 12 responses (57 percent) in the combined group and two responses (33 percent) in the adrenalectomy-only group. These responses were not clearly defined. Disease-free and overall survival rates were not discussed.

Two other studies using tamoxifen have been discussed previously. In the study reported by Veronesi and coworkers,[198] none of the patients with IBC responded to tamoxifen. Campbell and coworkers[44] reported a 45 percent objective response rate in patients with locally advanced breast carcinoma.

These studies suggest that patients with IBC can have an objective response to hormonal therapy, but the survival duration is short. Administering hormonal therapy alone is not recommended for treating this disease.

Breast Preservation in Patients with Inflammatory Breast Carcinoma

Patients with IBC pose a therapeutic challenge, as there is a greater than 50 percent local recurrence rate following surgery and a 50–75 percent local-regional recurrence rate following primary radiotherapy. Primary chemotherapy in these patients has produced not only high objective responses but also a marked improvement in 5-year survival rates, ranging from 25 percent to 40 percent. Roüessé and colleagues[155] reported the results of treatment of 230 patients with IBC, all of whom had breast conservation. Mourali and associates[130] randomized patients to surgery or radiotherapy following primary chemotherapy and reported that surgery and radiotherapy were equivalent in their effects on long-term survival after primary chemotherapy. One important prognostic factor predicting disease-free survival rates was initial response to primary chemotherapy. The M.D. Anderson Cancer Center experience reported by Buzdar and colleagues[41] showed that the addition of mastectomy to combined-modality therapy did not decrease the risk of local recurrence. Buzdar and colleagues[41] noted, however, delayed effects of irradiation in patients who had breast conservation, as these patients required higher doses of radiation. Arriagada and coworkers[11] treated patients with alternating chemotherapy and radiotherapy schedules and found that this regimen was highly effective in producing local control.

IBC is characterized by diffuse edema and erythema of the skin of the breast with or without an easily defined underlying mass. Some of these changes persist following primary chemotherapy and radiotherapy, making local surgical excision difficult. Furthermore, in up to 80 percent of the patients, residual tumor is found in the mastectomy specimens after primary chemotherapy and radiotherapy. For these reasons, radiotherapy with a tumor dose of 6000 cGy is necessary. Twice-daily fractionation may improve local control and is being evaluated. Whether twice-daily fractionation will translate into improved survival rates when given in a multimodality-treatment setting remains unclear.

In conclusion, mastectomy may not be necessary for patients with IBC if aggressive radiotherapy is given for local control. Also, no residual macroscopic disease should be present in patients chosen for this therapeutic option.

Treatment Recommendations for Inflammatory Breast Cancer

The treatment principles for IBC are similar to those for locally advanced breast carcinoma. Combined-modality therapy should be the standard of care, and treatment goals should include an increase in disease-free and overall survival rates as well as satisfactory cosmetic outcome.

Diagnosis should be confirmed by fine needle aspiration or incisional biopsy. Following clinical staging, primary chemotherapy with a doxorubicin-containing regimen is recommended until best response is noted. Three to four cycles of primary chemotherapy may be required. Depending on the extent of clinical response to primary chemotherapy, a modified radical

mastectomy or breast conservation surgery would be the next step. Surgery should be followed by six cycles of either the same chemotherapy regimen or, depending on the nodal status and extent of residual disease, a change to non–cross-resistant therapy such as a taxane. Postoperative radiotherapy should be given following completion of the adjuvant phase of chemotherapy. If patients do not demonstrate a response to primary chemotherapy containing doxorubicin, a regimen containing a taxane should be implemented. If there is still no response, then radiotherapy should be directed at the involved fields. High-dose chemotherapy with hematopoietic rescue should be considered if the patient is eligible to be entered into a clinical trial and has been shown to be sensitive to conventional-dose chemotherapy.

HIGH-DOSE CHEMOTHERAPY WITH HEMATOPOIETIC RESCUE

High-dose chemotherapy with hematopoietic rescue has been shown to produce a higher rate of overall response and of complete response in patients with metastatic breast carcinoma.[8] Given the disappointing results with conventional-dose chemotherapy in patients with IBC and in some patients with locally advanced breast carcinoma, high-dose chemotherapy is now being studied as a first-line or consolidation therapy for patients with these diseases. Patient accrual has been an issue because of the relative rarity of IBC. There have been several small studies addressing this disease, but many of the high-dose therapy protocols include a mixture of locally advanced and metastatic breast carcinoma cases.

Extra and coworkers[64] randomized 67 patients with IBC using primary chemotherapy consisting of four to six cycles of cyclophosphamide 1200 mg/m^2 IV and epirubicin 75 mg/m^2 IV given every 2 weeks followed by mastectomy (66 patients), radiotherapy (4500 cGy), and six cycles of chemotherapy (54 patients) or intensification with autologous bone marrow transplant (13 patients). Complete response on histological evaluation of the mastectomy specimens was seen in seven patients (10 percent). The actuarial 4-year disease-free survival rate was 54 percent. The outcome was influenced more by histological response than by the use of an autologous bone marrow transplant. The overall survival rate was 66 percent.

Israel and colleagues[98] treated 25 IBC patients with high-dose cyclophosphamide and fluorouracil. Treatment consisted of three cycles of fluorouracil given at a daily dose of 600 mg/m^2 in a 1-hour infusion for 5 consecutive days and cyclophosphamide administered at a dose of 1.2–1 gm/m^2 IV on day 1 of each cycle. These cycles were repeated every 3 weeks. Total mastectomy was performed 3 weeks after the beginning of the third cycle of chemotherapy. Chemotherapy was resumed 3 weeks after mastectomy and continued for 2 years. The median disease-free survival was 46 months, and the projected actuarial survival for the whole group was greater than 70 percent at 6 years.

Ayash and associates[13] reported the results of their pilot study on women with either locally unresectable breast carcinoma or IBC. These 16 women received four 2-week cycles of dose-intensive doxorubicin (90 mg/m[2] IV) and granulocyte colony-stimulating factor (5 μg/kg/day) followed by cyclophosphamide 6000 mg/m[2] IV, thiotepa 500 mg/m[2] IV, and carboplatin 800 mg/m[2] IV with hematopoietic rescue. Local therapy consisted of mastectomy and radiotherapy. Patients then received tamoxifen if estrogen receptors were positive or borderline positive for 5 years. During a median follow-up of 9 months following surgery, no relapses were noted.

Muldar and coworkers[132] treated 29 patients with untreated stage III breast carcinoma with methotrexate, doxorubicin, fluorouracil, vincristine, and prednisone. Complete responders received high-dose chemotherapy with cyclophosphamide and etoposide followed by autologous bone marrow transplantation. Of these 29 patients, 18 were evaluable. The median follow-up was 25 months. The disease-free survival rate was 70 percent, and the overall survival rate was 75 percent.

The Japanese autologous bone marrow transplantation experience with stage II and III breast cancer patients was reported by Tajima and coworkers.[188] Beginning in 1980, 173 patients were treated in an adjuvant setting using high-dose cyclophosphamide, doxorubicin, and either cisplatin or nimustine followed by autologous bone marrow rescue. The 5-year overall survival rate in these patients was 79 percent. An update reported that 36 patients, 24 of them with stage III disease, 11 with stage II disease, and one with stage I disease, had a 5-year disease-free survival rate of 55 percent and an overall survival rate of 66 percent.

Bezwoda and colleagues,[26] in a randomized trial, compared high-dose with conventional-dose chemotherapy as a first-line treatment for metastatic breast carcinoma. A survival benefit was noted for patients receiving high-dose chemotherapy versus those receiving conventional-dose chemotherapy ($p = .01$). This study was small, with 90 patients randomized and with a median follow-up of 72 weeks. However, it is the only randomized study of high-dose versus conventional-dose therapy reported.

The groups of patients who are rendered disease-free or are highly responsive after conventional-dose therapy and local therapy are ideal for testing the hypothesis of a clinical benefit with high-dose chemotherapy. Randomization with uniform staging before randomized trials comparing high-dose and conventional-dose chemotherapy is essential before this modality should be offered routinely to patients with locally advanced breast carcinoma. Also, patients should all receive local radiation therapy as part of the treatment after high-dose chemotherapy is given.

TREATMENT-RELATED TOXICITIES

The treatment modalities in the management of locally advanced breast cancer can either separately or in combination lead to various toxicities. These toxicities should be taken into consideration when multimodality therapy is planned.

Neutropenia secondary to conventional-dose chemotherapy resulting in infection-related admissions is rare. Granulocyte colony-stimulating factors should be considered in planning further treatment if neutropenia occurs. The availability of 5-HT$_3$ receptor-selective antagonists (ondansetron and granisetron) for the prevention and treatment of chemotherapy-induced nausea and vomiting has significantly improved the quality of life in patients receiving chemotherapy for breast cancer.

There are side effects unique to certain chemotherapeutic drugs used in the treatment of breast cancer. Cyclophosphamide given in high doses or prolonged use of oral cyclophosphamide can be associated with hemorrhagic cystitis due to acrolein, which is an active metabolite of cyclophosphamide. Hemorrhagic cystitis can be prevented by the use of mesna (sodium 2-mercapto ethane sulfonate), which inactivates the alkylating metabolites.[33] Doses of cyclophosphamide exceeding 1.55 gm/m[2] are associated with cardiac toxicity. Two factors that may further increase the risk of cardiac toxicity are prior therapy with doxorubicin or a patient age greater than 50 years.[181]

Prolonged myelosuppression and mucositis resulting from methotrexate can be prevented by the administration of leucovorin. Methotrexate administration to patients with renal dysfunction can result in fatal myelosuppression. Methotrexate administration to patients with pleural effusion or ascites can result in prolonged toxicity resulting from the "slow-release" effect of the drug from the fluid that has accumulated in the third space. High-dose methotrexate administration without adequate hydration and urinary alkalinization is associated with acute renal failure.

Administering the doxorubicin as a 48–96-hour infusion.[41] Dexrazoxane, a cardioprotective agent, can minimize the risk of cardiac toxicity if the cumulative dose of doxorubicin exceeds 300 mg/m[2].[186]

Administration of fluorouracil as a continuous infusion may be associated with mucositis, diarrhea, and hand-foot syndrome (swelling of the palms and soles with erythema and paresthesia). Paresthesia, peripheral neuropathy, and disabling neurotoxicity may be seen in older patients receiving weekly vincristine. Mitomycin is associated with microangiopathic hemolytic anemia and renal failure (hemolytic-uremic syndrome). The incidence of renal failure increases with the total dose of drug administered.[197] Also, there is a higher incidence of interstitial pneumonitis in patients receiving mitomycin C and vinca alkaloids.[108] Furthermore, mitomycin C can exacerbate the cardiac toxicity associated with doxorubicin.[14]

Radiotherapy may be associated with skin changes such as edema, erythema, and sometimes moist desquamation. These skin changes can be more severe in patients receiving concurrent chemotherapy and radiotherapy. Radiotherapy also has a profound lympholytic effect and may result in a significant decrease in lymphocyte count.[117] Therefore, dose modifications made in patients receiving radiotherapy and chemotherapy should be based on absolute granulocyte count rather than total leukocyte count.[117]

Concurrent radiotherapy and chemotherapy are associated with a higher incidence of radiation pneumonitis (8.8 percent) than is the case for sequential radiation and chemotherapy (1.3 percent).[116] Randomized trials from the 1950s and 1960s reported an increased incidence of radiation-induced ischemic heart disease exacerbated by doxorubicin.[157] The risk of complications can be minimized by modifying radiotherapy techniques and ensuring careful sequencing of radiotherapy and chemotherapy.

In an attempt to address the complications following primary chemotherapy, Danforth and coworkers[54] reviewed the perioperative course of 54 patients with locally advanced breast carcinoma who underwent mastectomy following primary chemotherapy. These patients received primary chemotherapy as discussed previously[148, 178, 184] and underwent surgery at a median of 20 days after completing the last chemotherapy regimen. Total mastectomy with or without axillary node dissection was performed in 53 patients and Halsted's radical mastectomy in one. All received a median of seven cycles (6 months) of primary chemotherapy.

Statistics on postoperative complications, median hospital stay, intraoperative blood loss, and wound catheter drainage were all comparable to those reported for patients undergoing modified radical mastectomy without primary chemotherapy. Patients were able to resume systemic chemotherapy at a median of 16 days and radiotherapy at a median of 33 days after mastectomy. Danforth and colleagues[54] concluded that intense primary chemotherapy did not increase postoperative complications or lengthen the hospital stay for patients undergoing mastectomy following primary chemotherapy for locally advanced breast cancer. They recommended that patients receiving doxorubicin-containing chemotherapy should undergo mastectomy approximately 4 weeks after the last dose of doxorubicin to minimize the morbidity of mastectomy resulting from chemotherapy-induced myelosuppression.

Pierce and colleagues[148] retrospectively reviewed the cosmetic outcome in 25 women who received multimodality therapy for locally advanced breast carcinoma. These patients received primary chemotherapy as was discussed previously[178, 184] and were treated locally with radiation alone. Cosmetic outcome was determined based on the breast size, breast edema, retraction, fibrosis, and skin changes, including telangiectasia and pigmentation. Cosmetic scores were assigned using the following criteria: excellent—treated breast almost identical to the untreated breast; good—minimal difference between the treated and untreated breast; fair—obvious difference between the treated and untreated breast but without major distortion; and poor—major functional

and aesthetic sequelae in the treated breast. The median follow-up was 49 months. Cosmetic outcome was good in 44 percent of the patients, fair in 44 percent, and poor in 12 percent. The patients with a fair to poor cosmetic outcome suffered marked fibrosis and retraction of the treated breast. Breast examination of three patients with a poor outcome was difficult. One patient required mastectomy for severe breast pain. Four of 25 patients (16 percent) developed rib fractures. All patients with poor cosmesis had presented with IBC.

In summary, combined-modality therapy is well tolerated in patients with locally advanced breast cancer. Supportive measures have improved, with dramatic results. Long-term complications have not been adequately studied because in the past so many of these patients succumbed to their disease. More attention to long-term complications will be important as treatment improves survival rates.

FUTURE DIRECTIONS

In spite of the advances made in the treatment of locally advanced breast cancer, more than 50 percent of these patients die of metastatic disease. Different treatment modalities are needed to improve their prognosis. Newer drugs, including taxanes and vinorelbine, are being administered preoperatively in an attempt to increase responses and to improve overall outcomes. A novel therapeutic approach being tested is the use of techniques to block certain oncogenes or certain growth factors such as *ERBB2* or epidermal growth factor receptor.

In vitro studies suggest that *ERBB2* is at least associated with, if not responsible for, decreased sensitivity to the various chemotherapeutic agents. This relative resistance to chemotherapy can be overcome by interfering with the *ERBB2* signal transduction pathway. This therapeutic approach could be developed by combining conventional drugs with agents that block *ERBB2*—for example, antisense oligodeoxynucleotides or monoclonal antibodies.

Inhibition of tumor-associated tissue angiogenesis might be an effective therapy in the treatment of patients with breast cancer. Several factors have been identified that stimulate angiogenesis. Agents are being developed that specifically block the effect of these angiogenic factors. These compounds could be used after conventional therapy in an attempt to prevent recurrence.

Locally advanced breast carcinoma is a fertile area for research into the biology of breast cancer and the assessment of molecular markers. Fortunately, the therapeutic efficacy in vivo of the various new treatment modalities, including agents inhibiting angiogenesis, tumor vaccines, monoclonal antibodies, and gene therapy, can be tested with immediately apparent results.

References

1. Abraham DC, Jones RC, Jones SE, et al: Evaluation of neoadjuvant chemotherapeutic response in locally advanced

breast cancer by magnetic resonance imaging. Presented at the 48th Annual Cancer Symposium of the Society of Surgical Oncology, Boston, Massachusetts, March 23–26, 1995.

2. Ahern V, Barraclough B, Bosch C, Langlands A, Boyages J: Locally advanced breast cancer: Defining an optimum treatment regimen. Int J Radiat Oncol Biol Phys 28:867–875, 1994.

3. Aitken SC, Lippman ME: Hormonal regulation of net DNA synthesis in MCF-7 human breast cancer cells in tissue culture. Cancer Res 42:1727–1735, 1982.

4. Alagaratnam TT, Wong J: Tamoxifen versus chemotherapy as adjuvant treatment in stage III breast cancer. Aust N Z J Surg 56:39–41, 1986.

5. Allegra JC, Woodcock TM, Richman SP, et al: A phase II trial of tamoxifen, Premarin, methotrexate and 5-fluorouracil in metastatic breast cancer. Breast Cancer Res Treat 2:93–100, 1982.

6. Allred DC, Clark GM, Tandon AK, et al: HER-2/neu in node-negative breast cancer: Prognostic significance of overexpression influenced by the presence of in-situ carcinoma. J Clin Oncol 10:599–605, 1992.

7. Anderson EDC, Forrest APM, Hawkins RA, Anderson TJ, Leonard RCF, Chetty U: Primary systemic therapy for operable breast cancer. Br J Cancer 63:561–566, 1991.

8. Antman K, Gale RP: Advanced breast cancer: High-dose chemotherapy and bone marrow autotransplant. Ann Intern Med 108:570–574, 1988.

9. Armstrong DK, Fetting JH, Davidson NE, Gordon GB, Huelskamp AM, Abeloff MD: Sixteen-week dose-intense chemotherapy for inoperable, locally advanced breast cancer. Breast Cancer Res Treat 28:277–284, 1993.

10. Arnold DJ, Lesnick GJ: Survival following mastectomy for stage III breast cancer. Am J Surg 137:362–366, 1979.

11. Arriagada R, Mouriesse H, Spielmann M, et al: Alternating radiotherapy and chemotherapy in non-metastatic inflammatory breast cancer. Int J Radiat Oncol Biol Phys 19:1207–1210, 1990.

12. Attia-Sobol J, Ferriere JP, Cure H, et al: Treatment results, survival and prognostic factors in 109 inflammatory breast cancers: Univariate and multivariate analysis. Eur J Cancer 29A:1081–1088, 1993.

13. Ayash L, Lynch J, Cruz J, et al: High-dose multimodality therapy for locally unresectable or inflammatory (stage IIIb) breast cancer. Proc Am Soc Clin Oncol 12:A158, 1993.

14. Bachur NR, Gordon SL, Gee RV: A general mechanism for microsomal activation of quinone anticancer agents to free radicals. Cancer Res 38:1745–1750, 1978.

15. Baclesse F: Five-year results in 431 breast cancers treated solely by roentgen rays. Ann Surg 161:103–104, 1965.

16. Baillet F, Rozec C, Ucla L, Chauveinc L, Housset M, Weil M: Treatment of locally advanced breast cancer without mastectomy: 5- and 10-year results of 135 tumors larger than 5 centimeters treated by external beam therapy, brachytherapy, and neoadjuvant chemotherapy. Ann N Y Acad Sci 30:264–270, 1993.

17. Barber KW, Dockerty MG, Clagett OT: Inflammatory carcinoma of the breast. Surg Gynecol Obstet 112:406–410, 1961.

18. Barker JL, Nelson AJ, Montague ED: Inflammatory carcinoma of the breast. Radiology 121:173–176, 1976.

19. Barker JL, Montague ED, Peters LJ: Clinical experience with irradiation of inflammatory carcinoma of the breast with and without elective chemotherapy. Cancer 45:625–629, 1980.

20. Beahrs OH, Myers NH (eds): Manual for Staging of Cancer, 2nd ed. Philadelphia, JB Lippincott, 1983, pp 127–133.

21. Beahrs OH, Henson DE, Hutter RVP, Kennedy BJ (eds): American Joint Committee on Cancer Manual for Staging of Cancer. Philadelphia, JB Lippincott, 1992, pp 149–154.

22. Bedwinek J, Rao DV, Perez C, et al: Stage III and localized stage IV breast cancer: Irradiation alone versus irradiation plus surgery. Int J Radiat Oncol Biol Phys 8:31–36, 1982.

23. Bell CA: A system of operative surgery. Surgery 11:136, 1814.

24. Benz CC, Scott GK, Sarup JC, et al: Estrogen-dependent, tamoxifen-resistant tumorigenic growth of MCF-7 cells transfected with HER2/neu. Breast Cancer Res Treat 24:85–89, 1992.

25. Berg CD, Swain SM: Results of concomitantly administered chemoradiation for locally advanced noninflammatory breast cancer. Semin Radiat Oncol 4:226–235, 1994.

26. Bezwoda WR, Seymour L, Dansey RD: High-dose chemotherapy with hematopoietic rescue as primary treatment for metastatic breast cancer: A randomized trial. J Clin Oncol 13:2483–2489, 1995.

27. Bonadonna G, Veronesi U, Brambilla C, et al: Primary chemotherapy to avoid mastectomy in tumors with diameters of three centimeters or more. J Natl Cancer Inst 82:1539–1545, 1990.

28. Bonadonna G, Valagussa P, Zucali R, et al: Primary chemotherapy in surgically resectable breast cancer. CA Cancer J Clin 45:227–243, 1995.

29. Bonnier P, Charpin C, Lejeune C, et al: Inflammatory carcinomas of the breast: A clinical, pathological, or a clinical and pathological definition? Int J Cancer 62:382–385, 1995.

30. Bozzetti F, Saccozzi R, DeLena M, Salvadori B: Inflammatory cancer of the breast: Analysis of 114 cases. J Surg Oncol 18:355–361, 1981.

31. Briffod M, Spyratos F, Hacene K: Evaluation of breast carcinoma chemosensitivity by flow cytometric DNA analysis and computer-assisted image analysis. Cytometry 13(3):250–258, 1992.

32. Britton PD, Coulden RA: The use of duplex Doppler ultrasound in diagnosis of breast cancer. Clin Radiol 42:399–401, 1990.

33. Brock N, Pohl J, Stekar J: Detoxification of urotoxic oxazaphosphorines by sulfhydryl compounds. J Cancer Res Clin Oncol 100:311, 1981.

34. Bruckman JE, Harris JR, Levene MB, Chaffey JT, Hellman S: Results of treating stage III carcinoma of the breast by primary radiation therapy. Cancer 43:985–993, 1979.

35. Brun B, Otmezguine Y, Feuilhade F, et al: Treatment of inflammatory breast cancer with combination chemotherapy and mastectomy versus breast conservation. Cancer 61:1096–1103, 1988.

36. Bryant T: Diseases of the Breast. London, Cassell and Co Ltd, 1887, pp 171–194.

37. Bucalossi P, Veronesi V, Zingo L, et al: Enlarged mastectomy for breast cancer: Review of 1213 cases. Am J Roentgenol Radium Ther Mucl Med 111:119–122, 1971.

38. Buchholz TA, Austin-Seymour MM, Moe RE, et al: Effect of delay in radiation in the combined modality treatment of breast cancer. Int J Radiat Oncol Biol Phys 26:23–35, 1993.

39. Burton GV, Cox EB, Leight GS, et al: Inflammatory breast carcinoma: Effective multimodal approach. Arch Surg 122:1329–1332, 1987.

40. Butcher H: Radical mastectomy for mammary carcinoma. Ann Surg 170:833–884, 1969.

41. Buzdar AU, Singletary SE, Booser DJ, et al: Combined-modality treatment of stage III and inflammatory breast cancer. Surg Oncol Clin North Am 4(4):715–734, 1995.

42. Caceres B, Zaharia M, Lingan M, et al: Combined therapy of stage III adenocarcinoma of the breast. Proc Am Acad Cancer Res 798:199, 1980.

43. Calais G, Descamps P, Chapet S, et al: Primary chemotherapy and radiosurgical breast-conserving treatment for patients with locally advanced operable breast cancer. Int J Radiat Oncol Biol Phys 26:37–42, 1993.

44. Campbell FC, Morgan DAL, Bishop HM, et al: The management of locally advanced carcinoma of the breast by Nolvadex (tamoxifen): A pilot study. J Clin Oncol 10:111–115, 1984.

45. Casper ES, Guidera CA, Bosl GJ, et al: Combined-modality treatment of locally advanced breast cancer: Adjuvant combination chemotherapy with and without doxorubicin. Breast Cancer Res Treat 9:39–44, 1987.

46. Chamadol W, Pesie M, Puapairoj A: Inflammatory carcinoma of the breast in a 12-year-old Thai girl. J Med Assoc Thai 70:543–548, 1987.

47. Chevallier B, Bastit P, Graic Y, et al: The Centre H. Becquerel studies in inflammatory non-metastatic breast cancer: Combined-modality approach in 178 patients. Br J Cancer 67:594–601, 1993.

48. Chollet PH, Charrier S, Brain E, et al: Neoadjuvant chemo-

therapy in breast cancer: High pathological response rate induced by intensive anthracycline-based regimen. Proc Am Soc Clin Oncol 14:A218, 1995.

49. Chu AM, Wood WC, Doucette JA: Inflammatory breast carcinoma treated by radical radiotherapy. Cancer 45:2730–2737, 1980.

50. Chris SM: Inflammatory carcinoma of the breast: A report of 20 cases and a review of the literature. Br J Surg 38:163–174, 1950.

51. Cocconi G, diBlasio, Bisagni G, et al: Neoadjuvant chemotherapy or chemotherapy and endocrine therapy in locally advanced breast carcinoma. Am J Clin Oncol 13:226, 1990.

52. Conte PF, Alama A, Bertelli G: Chemotherapy with estrogenic recruitment and surgery in locally advanced breast cancer: Clinical and cytokinetic results. Int J Cancer 40:490–494, 1987.

53. Costa J, Webber BL, Levine PL, et al: Histopathological features of rapidly progressing breast carcinoma in Tunisia: A study of 94 cases. Int J Cancer 30:35–37, 1982.

54. Danforth D, Lippman M, McDonald H, et al: Effect of preoperative chemotherapy on mastectomy for locally advanced breast cancer. Am Surg 56:6–11, 1990.

55. Dao TL, McCarthy JD: Treatment of inflammatory carcinoma of the breast. Surg Gynecol Obstet 105:289–294, 1957.

56. DeLarue JC, Levin F, Mouriesse H, et al: Oestrogen and progesterone cytosolic receptors in clinically inflammatory tumors of the human breast. Br J Cancer 44:911–916, 1981.

57. DeLena M, Zucali R, Viganotti G, Valagussa P, Bonadonna G: Combined chemotherapy-radiotherapy approach in locally advanced (T_{3b}-T_4) breast cancer. Cancer Chemother Pharmacol 1:53–59, 1978.

58. DeLena M, Virion M, Zucali R, et al: Multimodality treatment for locally advanced breast cancer: Results of chemotherapy-radiotherapy versus chemotherapy-surgery. Cancer Clin Trials 4:229–236, 1981.

59. Derman DP, Browde S, Kessel IL, et al: Adjuvant chemotherapy for stage III breast cancer: A randomized trial. Int J Radiat Oncol Biol Phys 17:257–261, 1989.

60. Donegan WL: Cancer of the Breast, 3rd ed. Philadelphia, WB Saunders, 1979, p 263.

61. Donehower R, Allegra JC, Lippman ME, Chabner B: Combined effects of methotrexate and 5-fluoropyrimidine on human breast cancer cells in serum-free culture. Eur J Cancer 16:655–661, 1980.

62. Droulias CA, Sewell CW, McSweeney MB, Powell R: Inflammatory carcinoma of the breast: A correlation of clinical, radiologic and pathologic findings. Ann Surg 184:217–222, 1976.

63. Ellis DL, Teitelbaum SL: Inflammatory carcinoma of the breast: A pathologic definition. Cancer 33:1045–1047, 1974.

64. Extra JM, Bourstyn E, Espie M: Intensive induction chemotherapy followed by mastectomy in inflammatory breast carcinoma. Proc Am Soc Clin Oncol 12:A233, 1993.

65. Fabian CJ, Kimler BF, McKittrick R, et al: Recruitment with high physiological doses of estradiol preceding chemotherapy: Flow cytometric and therapeutic results in women with locally advanced breast cancer—a Southwest Oncology Group study. Cancer Res 54:5357–5362, 1994.

66. Fastenberg NA, Buzdar AU, Montague ED, et al: Management of inflammatory carcinoma of the breast. A combined-modality approach. Am J Clin Oncol 8:134–141, 1985.

67. Feig SA, Yaffe MJ: Digital mammography, computer-aided diagnosis, telemammography. Radiol Clin North Am 33(6):1205–1230, 1995.

68. Fein DA, Mendenhall NP, Marsh RDW, Bland KI, Copeland EM, Million RR: Results of multimodality therapy for inflammatory breast cancer: An analysis of clinical and treatment factors affecting outcome. Am Surg 60(3):220–225, 1994.

69. Feldman LD, Hortobagyi GN, Buzdar AU, et al: Pathological assessment of response to induction chemotherapy in breast cancer. Cancer Res 46:2578–2581, 1986.

70. Fields JN, Kuske RR, Perez CA, Fineberg BB, Bartlett N: Prognostic factors in inflammatory breast cancer. Cancer 63:1225–1232, 1989.

71. Fisher B, Slack NH, Bross IDJ: Cancer of the breast: Size of the neoplasm and prognosis. Cancer 24:1071–1081, 1969.

72. Fisher B, Gunduz N, Saffer E: Influence of the interval between primary tumor removal and chemotherapy on kinetics and growth of metastases. Cancer Res 43:1488–1492, 1983.

73. Fisher B, Saffer EA, Deutsch M: Influence of irradiation of a primary tumor on the labeling index and estrogen receptor index in a distant tumor focus. Int J Radiat Oncol Biol Phys 12:879–885, 1986.

74. Fisher B, Rockette II, Robidoux A, et al: Effect of preoperative therapy for breast cancer on local-regional disease: First report of NSABP B-18. Proc Am Soc Clin Oncol 13:64, 1994.

75. Fisher B, Gunduz N, Coyle J, Rudock C, Saffer E: Presence of a growth-stimulating factor in serum following primary tumor removal in mice. Cancer Res 49:1996–2001, 1989.

76. Fonseca GA, Valero V, Buzdar A, et al: Decreased cardiac toxicity by TLC D-99 (liposomal doxorubicin) in the treatment of metastatic breast carcinoma. Proc Am Soc Clin Oncol 14:A96, 1995.

77. Fornage BD, Toubas O, Morel M: Clinical mammographic and sonographic determination of preoperative breast cancer size. Cancer 60(4):765–771, 1987.

78. Fowble B, Glover D, Rosato EF, et al: Combined-modality treatment of inflammatory breast cancer. Int J Radiat Oncol Biol Phys 12:11–12, 1986.

79. Fracchia AA, Randall HT, Farrow JH: The results of adrenalectomy in advanced breast cancer in 500 consecutive patients. Surg Gynecol Obstet 125:747–756, 1967.

80. Fracchia AA, Evans JF, Eisenberg BL: Stage III carcinoma of the breast: A detailed analysis. Ann Surg 19:705–710, 1980.

81. Gardin G, Alama A, Rosso R, et al: Relationship of variations in tumor cell kinetics induced by primary chemotherapy to tumor regression and prognosis in locally advanced breast cancer. Breast Cancer Res Treat 32(3):311–318, 1994.

82. Gazet JC, Ford HT, Coombes RC: Randomized trial of chemotherapy versus endocrine therapy in patients presenting with locally advanced breast cancer (a pilot study). Br J Cancer 63:279–282, 1991.

83. Goldie JH, Coldman AJ: A mathematical model for relating the drug sensitivity of tumors to their spontaneous mutation rate. Cancer Treat Res 63:1727–1733, 1979.

84. Green MD, Whybourne AM, Taylor IW, Sutherland RL: Effects of antiestrogens on the growth and cell cycle kinetics of cultured human mammary carcinoma cells. In Sutherland RL, Jordan VC (eds): Nonsteroidal Antiestrogens. New York, Academic Press, 1981, pp 397–413.

85. Gröhn P, Heinonen E, Klefström P, et al: Adjuvant postoperative radiotherapy, chemotherapy, and immunotherapy in stage III breast cancer. Cancer 54:670–674, 1984.

86. Guerin M, Gabillot M, Mathieu M-C, et al: Structure and expression of c-erbB-2 and EGF receptor genes in inflammatory and non-inflammatory breast cancer: Prognostic significance. Int J Cancer 43:201–208, 1989.

87. Gusterson BA, Gelber RD, Goldhirsh A, et al: Prognostic importance of c-erbB2 expression in breast cancer. J Clin Oncol 10:1049–1056, 1992.

88. Haagensen CD, Stout AP: Carcinoma of the breast. II: Criteria of operability. Ann Surg 118:859–870, 1032–1051, 1943.

89. Haagensen CD: Diseases of the Breast, 2nd ed. Philadelphia, WB Saunders, 1971, pp 576–584.

90. Haagensen CD: Diseases of the Breast, 3rd ed. Philadelphia, WB Saunders, 1986, p 656.

91. Haagensen CD: Diseases of the Breast, 3rd ed. Philadelphia, WB Saunders, 1986, pp 808–814.

92. Halsted WS: The results of operations for the cure of cancer of the breast performed at Johns Hopkins Hospital from June 1889 to January 1894. Johns Hopkins Hospital Bulletin 4:497–555, 1894.

93. Hammond S, Keyhani-Rofagha S, O'Toole RV: Statistical analysis of fine needle aspiration cytology of the breast: A review of 678 cases plus 4,265 cases from the literature. Acta Cytol 31(3):276–280, 1987.

94. Harris LN, Tang C, Perez C, et al: Induction to sensitivity to doxorubicin and etoposide by transfection of MCF-7 breast

cancer cells with gp-30 (heregulin), an activator of the *erb*-b2/*erb*-b4 signalling pathway. At Fifth Meeting on the Molecular Basis of Cancer, June 1994.

95. Harvey H, Lipton A, Lawrence B, et al: Estrogen receptors in inflammatory breast carcinoma. J Surg Oncol 21:42–44, 1982.

96. Hobar PC, Jones RC, Schouten J, Lietch AM, Hendler F: Multimodality treatment of locally advanced breast carcinoma. Arch Surg 123:951–955, 1988.

97. Hortobagyi GN, Ames FC, Buzdar AU, et al: Management of stage III primary breast cancer with primary chemotherapy, surgery, and radiation therapy. Cancer 62:2507–2516, 1988.

98. Israel L, Breau J, Morere JF: Two years of high-dose cyclophosphamide and 5-fluorouracil followed by surgery after 3 months for acute inflammatory breast carcinoma: A phase II study of 25 cases with a median follow-up of 35 months. Cancer 57:24–28, 1986.

99. Jacquillat C, Weil M, Auclerc G, et al: Neoadjuvant chemotherapy in the conservative management of breast cancer: A study of 205 patients. *In* Adjuvant Therapy of Cancer, Vol. 5. New York, Grune & Stratton, 1987, pp 403–409.

100. Jacquillat C, Weil M, Baillet F, et al: Results of neoadjuvant chemotherapy and radiation therapy in the breast-conserving treatment of 250 patients with all stages of infiltrative breast cancer. Cancer 66:119–129, 1990.

101. Keiling R, Guiochet N, Calderoli H, et al: Preoperative chemotherapy in the treatment of inflammatory breast cancer. *In* Primary Chemotherapy in Cancer Medicine. New York, Alan R Liss, 1985, pp 95–104.

102. Khalkhali I, Cutrone JA, Mena IG, et al: Scintimammography: The complementary role of technetium-99 sestamibi prone breast imaging for the diagnosis of breast cancer. Radiology 196:421–426, 1995.

103. Klefström P, Gröhn P, Heinonen E, et al: Adjuvant postoperative radiotherapy, chemotherapy, and immunotherapy in stage III breast cancer. Cancer 60:936–942, 1987.

104. Klotz HH: Ueber mastitis carcinomatosa gravidarum et lactantium. Germany, Halle, 1869.

105. Knight CD, Martin JK, Welch JS: Surgical considerations after chemotherapy and radiation therapy for inflammatory breast cancer. Surgery 99:385–391, 1986.

106. Kokal W, Hill C, Porudomisky D, et al: Inflammatory breast carcinoma: A distinct entity? J Surg Oncol 30:152–155, 1985.

107. Koscielny S, Tubiana M, Le MG, et al: Breast cancer: Relationship between the size of the primary tumour and the probability of metastatic dissemination. Br J Cancer 49:709–715, 1984.

108. Kuedke D, McLaughlin TT, Daughaday C, et al: Mitomycin C and vindesine associated pulmonary toxicity with variable clinical expression. Cancer 55:542–547, 1985.

109. Krutchik A, Buzdar A, Blumenschein G, et al: Combined chemoimmunotherapy and radiation therapy of inflammatory breast cancer. J Surg Oncol 11:325–332, 1979.

110. Lacour J, Hourtoule FG: La place de la chirurgie dans le traitement des formes evolutives du cancer du sein. Mem Acad Chir 93:635–643, 1967.

111. Learmonth GE: Acute mammary carcinoma (Volkmann's mastitis carcinomatosa). Can Med Assoc J 6:499–511, 1916.

112. Lee BJ, Tannenbaum NE: Inflammatory carcinoma of the breast: A report of twenty-eight cases from the Breast Clinic of the Memorial Hospital. Surg Gynecol Obstet 39:580–595, 1924.

113. Leicht A: Peau d'orange in acute mammary carcinoma: Its causes and diagnosis value. Lancet 1:861–863, 1909.

114. Lenz M: Tumor dosage and results in roentgen therapy of cancer of the breast. Am J Roentgenol Radiat Ther 56:67–74, 1946.

115. Levine PH, Steinhorn SC, Ries LG, Aron JL: Inflammatory breast cancer: The experience of the surveillance, epidemiology, and end results (SEER) program. J Natl Cancer Inst 74:291–297, 1985.

116. Lingos TK, Recht A, Vicini F, et al: Radiation pneumonitis in breast cancer patients treated with conservative surgery and radiation therapy. Int J Radiat Oncol Biol Phys 21:355–360, 1991.

117. Lippman ME, Lichter AS, Edwards BK, et al: The impact of primary irradiation treatment of localized breast cancer on the ability to administer systemic adjuvant chemotherapy. J Clin Oncol 2:21, 1984.

118. Lippman M, Bolan G, Huff K: The effects of estrogens and antiestrogens on hormone-responsive human breast cancer in long-term tissue culture. Cancer Res 36:4595–4601, 1976.

119. Lippman ME, Cassidy J, Wesley M, Young RC: A randomized attempt to increase the efficacy of cytotoxic chemotherapy in metastatic breast cancer by hormonal synchronization. J Clin Oncol 2:28–36, 1984.

120. Loprinzi C, Carbone P, Tormey D, et al: Aggressive combined-modality therapy for advanced local-regional breast carcinoma. J Clin Oncol 2:157–163, 1984.

121. Lowe SW, Ruley HE, Jacks T, et al: p53-dependent apoptosis modulates the cytotoxicity of anticancer agents. Cell 74:957–967, 1993.

122. Lucas FV, Perez-Mesa C: Inflammatory carcinoma of the breast. Cancer 41:1595–1605, 1978.

123. Maloisel F, Dufour P, Bergerat J, et al: Results of initial doxorubicin, 5-fluorouracil, and cyclophosphamide combination chemotherapy for inflammatory carcinoma of the breast. Cancer 65:851–855, 1990.

124. Mauriac L, Durand M, Avril A, Dilhuydy JM: Effects of primary chemotherapy in conservative treatment of breast cancer patients with operable tumors larger than 3 cm. Ann Oncol 2:347–354, 1991.

125. McDermott J, Mehta RR, Das Gupta TK: Plasma c-*erb*-b2 levels and response to chemotherapy in breast cancer patients. Proc Am Assoc Cancer Res 36:212, 1995. Abstract 1265.

126. Meyer AC, Dockerty MB, Harrington SW: Inflammatory carcinoma of the breast. Surg Gynecol Obstet 87:417–424, 1948.

127. Morvan F, Espie M, Mignot L, et al: Fifteen years' follow-up for T4d (inflammatory) breast cancer patients. Proc Am Soc Clin Oncol 14:A265, 1995.

128. Moskovic EC, Mansi JL, King DM, et al: Mammography in the assessment of response to medical treatment of large primary breast cancer. Clin Radiol 47:339–344, 1993.

129. Mourali N, Muenz LR, Tabbane F, et al: Epidemiologic features of rapidly progressing breast cancers in Tunisia. Cancer 46:2741–2746, 1980.

130. Mourali N, Tabbane F, Muenz LR, et al: Ten-year results utilizing chemotherapy as primary treatment in nonmetastatic, rapidly progressing breast cancer. Cancer Invest 11:363–370, 1993.

131. Muldar NH, Devries EGE, Sleijfer DT, et al: Intensive induction chemotherapy and intensification with autologous bone marrow infusion in patients with stage IIIb and IV breast cancer: An update. Proc Am Soc Clin Oncol 9:25, 1990.

132. Muldar NH, Mulder POM, Sleijfer DT, et al: Induction chemotherapy and intensification with autologous bone marrow reinfusion in patients with locally advanced and disseminated breast cancer. Eur J Cancer 29A(5):668–671, 1993.

133. Muss HB, Thor AD, Berry DA, et al: c-*erb*-b2 expression and response to adjuvant treatment in women with node-positive early breast cancer. N Engl J Med 330:1260–1266, 1994.

134. Nawata H, Chong M, Bronzert D, Lippman M: Estradiol in dependent growth of subline of MCF-7 human breast cancer cell line in culture. J Biol Chem 256:6895–6902, 1981.

135. Nemoto T, Vana J, Bedwani RN, et al: Management and survival of female breast cancer: Results of a national survey by the American College of Surgeons. Cancer 45:2917–2924, 1980.

136. Neville AM, Bettelheim R, Gelber RD, et al: Factors predicting treatment responsiveness and prognosis in node-negative breast cancer. J Clin Oncol 10(5):696–705, 1992.

137. Noguchi S, Miyauchi K, Nishizawa Y, et al: Management of inflammatory carcinoma of the breast with combined-modality therapy including intra-arterial infusion chemotherapy as induction therapy. Cancer 61:1483–1491, 1988.

138. Nussbaum H, Kagan A, Gilbert H, et al: Management of inflammatory breast carcinoma. Breast 3:25–29, 1977.

139. Olson JE, Neuberg D, Pandya K, Richter M, Falkson G: The management of resectable stage II breast cancer: The East-

ern Cooperative Oncology Group trial. Proceedings of ASCO 8:23, 1989. Abstract 85.

140. Osteen RT: Breast cancer. *In* Steele GD, Osteen RT, Winchester DP (eds): National Cancer Data Base: Annual Review of Patient Care 1994. Atlanta, GA, The American Cancer Society, 1994, pp 56–71.

141. Papaioannou A, Lissaios B, Vasilaros S, et al: Pre- and postoperative chemoendocrine treatment with or without postoperative radiotherapy for locally advanced breast cancer. Cancer 51:1284–1290, 1983.

142. Paradiso A, Tommasi S, Brandi M, et al: Cell kinetics and hormone receptor status in inflammatory breast carcinoma: Comparison with locally advanced disease. Cancer 64:1922–1927, 1989.

143. Pawlicki M, Skolyszewski J, Brandys A: Results of combined treatment of patients with locally advanced breast cancer. Tumori 69:249–253, 1983.

144. Perez CA, Fields JN: Role of radiation therapy for locally advanced and inflammatory carcinoma of the breast. Oncology 1:81–93, 1987.

145. Perloff M, Lesnick GJ, Korzun A, et al: Combination chemotherapy with mastectomy or radiotherapy for stage III breast carcinoma: A Cancer and Leukemia Group B Study. J Clin Oncol 6:261–269, 1988.

146. Piccart MJ, De Valeriola D, Paridaens R, et al: Six-year results of a multimodality treatment strategy for locally advanced breast cancer. Cancer 62:2501–2506, 1988.

147. Piera JM, Alonso MC, Ojeda MB, et al: Locally advanced breast cancer with inflammatory component: A clinical entity with a poor prognosis. Radiother Oncol 7:199–208, 1986.

148. Pierce LJ, Lippman M, Ben-Baruch N, et al: The effect of systemic therapy upon local-regional control in locally advanced breast cancer. Int J Radiat Oncol Biol Phys 23:949–960, 1992.

149. Powles TJ, Hickish TF, Makris A, et al: Randomized trial of chemoendocrine therapy started before or after surgery for treatment of primary breast cancer. J Clin Oncol 13(3):547–552, 1995.

150. Rao D, Bedwineck J, Perez C, et al: Prognostic indicators in stage III and localized stage IV breast cancer. Cancer 50:2037–2043, 1982.

151. Rasbridge SA, Gillett CE, Seymour AM, et al: The effects of chemotherapy on morphology, cellular proliferation, apoptosis, and oncoprotein expression in primary breast carcinoma. Br J Cancer 70:335–341, 1994.

152. Recht A, Come SE, Gelman RS, et al: Integration of conservative surgery, radiotherapy, and chemotherapy for the treatment of early-stage, node-positive breast cancer: Sequencing, timing, and outcome. J Clin Oncol 9:1662–1667, 1991.

153. Robertson JF, Ellis IO, Pearson D, et al: Biological factors of prognostic significance in locally advanced breast cancer. Breast Cancer Res Treat 29(3):259–264, 1994.

154. Rogers CS, Fitts WT: Inflammatory carcinoma of the breast: A critique of therapy. Surgery 39:367–370, 1956.

155. Rouëssé S, Sarrazin D, Mouriesse H, et al: Primary chemotherapy in the treatment of inflammatory breast carcinoma: A study of 230 cases from the Institut Gustave-Roussy. J Clin Oncol 4:1765–1771, 1986.

156. Rubens RD, Bartelink H, Engelsman E, et al: Locally advanced breast cancer: The contribution of cytotoxic and endocrine treatment to radiotherapy. An EORTC Breast Cancer Co-operative Group Trial (10792). Eur J Cancer Clin Oncol 25(4):667–678, 1989.

157. Rutqvist LE, Lax I, Fornander T, et al: Cardiovascular mortality in a randomized trial of adjuvant radiation therapy versus surgery alone in primary breast cancer. Int J Radiat Oncol Biol Phys 22:887–896, 1992.

158. Sainsbury JRC, Fardon JR, Needham GK: Epidermal-growth-factor receptor status as predictor of early recurrence of and death from breast cancer. Lancet 1:1398–1402, 1987.

159. Saltzstein SL: Clinically occult inflammatory carcinoma of the breast. Cancer 34:382–388, 1974.

160. Sataloff DM, Mason BA, Prestipino AJ, Seinige UL, Lieber CP, Baloch Z: Pathologic response to induction chemotherapy in locally advanced carcinoma of the breast: A determinant of outcome. J Am Coll Surg 180:297–306, 1995.

161. Schaake-Koning C, Van Der Linden EH, Hart G, et al: Adjuvant chemo- and hormonal therapy in locally advanced breast cancer: A randomized clinical study. Int J Radiat Oncol Biol Phys 11:1759–1763, 1985.

162. Schäfer P, Alberto P, Forni M, et al: Surgery as part of a combined-modality approach for inflammatory breast carcinoma. Cancer 59:1063–1067, 1987.

163. Schoenberger SG, Sutherland CM, Robinson AE: Breast neoplasms: Duplex sonographic imaging as an adjunct in diagnosis. Radiology 168:665–668, 1988.

164. Scholl SM, Fourquet A, Asselain B, et al: Neoadjuvant versus adjuvant chemotherapy in premenopausal patients with tumors considered too large for breast conserving surgery: Preliminary results of a randomized trial: S6. Eur J Cancer 30A(5):645–652, 1994.

165. Schottenfeld D, Nash AG, Robbins GF, et al: Ten-year results of the treatment of primary operable breast carcinoma. Cancer 38:1001–1007, 1976.

166. Schumann EA: A study of carcinoma mastoiditis. Ann Surg 54:69–77, 1911.

167. Schwartz GF, Birchansky CA, Komarnicky LT, et al: Induction chemotherapy followed by breast conservation for locally advanced carcinoma of the breast. Cancer 73(2):362–369, 1994.

168. Schwartz GF, Cantor RI, Biermann WA: Neoadjuvant chemotherapy before definitive treatment for stage III carcinoma of the breast. Arch Surg 122:1430–1434, 1987.

169. Surveillance, Epidemiology, and End Results (SEER) Program. J Natl Cancer Inst No. 19, October 4, 1995.

170. Semiglazov VF, Topuzov EE, Bavli JL, et al: Primary (neoadjuvant) chemotherapy and radiotherapy compared with primary radiotherapy alone in stage IIb–IIIa breast cancer. Ann Oncol 591–595, 1994.

171. Sheldon T, Hayes DF, Cady B, et al: Primary radiation therapy for locally advanced breast cancer. Cancer 60:1219–1225, 1987.

172. Silvestrini R, Daidone MG, Valagussa P, et al: Cell kinetics as a prognostic marker in locally advanced breast cancer. Cancer Treat Res 71:375–379, 1987.

173. Singletary SE, McNeese MD, Hortobagyi GN: Feasibility of breast-conservation surgery after induction chemotherapy for locally advanced breast carcinoma. Cancer 69:2849–2852, 1992.

174. Slamon DJ, Clark GM, Wong SG, et al: Human breast cancer correlation of relapse and survival with amplification of the HER-2/*neu* oncogene. Science 235:177–182, 1987.

175. Smith IE, Walsh G, Jones A, et al: High complete rates with primary neoadjuvant infusional chemotherapy for large early breast cancer. J Clin Oncol 13:424–429, 1995.

176. Smith K, Houlbrook S, Greenall J, et al: Topoisomerase II∝ co-amplification with *erb*-B2 in human primary breast cancer and breast cancer cell lines: Relationship to *m*-AMSA and mitoxantrone sensitivity. Oncogene 8:933–938, 1993.

177. Sondik EJ, Young JL, Horn JW, et al: CDCPC 1985 annual cancer statistics review. NIH publication No. 86-2789, Bethesda, US Department of Health and Human Services, 1986.

178. Sorace RA, Bagley CS, Lichter AS, et al: The management of nonmetastatic locally advanced breast cancer using primary induction chemotherapy with hormonal synchronization followed by radiation therapy with or without debulking surgery. World J Surg 9:775–785, 1985.

179. Sorace RA, Lippman ME: Locally advanced breast cancer. *In* Lippman ME, Lichter AS, Danforth DN Jr (eds): Diagnosis and Management of Breast Cancer. Philadelphia, WB Saunders, 1988, pp 272–295.

180. Spangenberg JP, Nel CJC, Anderson JD, Doman MJ: A prospective study of the treatment of stage III breast cancer. S Afr J Surg 24:57–60, 1986.

181. Steinherz LJ, Steinherz PG: Cyclophosphamide cardiotoxicity. Cancer Bull 37:231–234, 1985.

182. Stewart JF, King RJB, Winter PJ, et al: Oestrogen receptors: Clinical features and prognosis in stage III breast cancer. Eur J Cancer Clin Oncol 18:1315–1320, 1982.

183. Stocks LH, Patterson FMS: Inflammatory carcinoma of the breast. Surg Gynecol Obstet 143:885–889, 1976.

184. Swain SM, Sorace R, Bagley C, et al: Neoadjuvant chemotherapy in the combined-modality approach of locally advanced nonmetastatic breast cancer. Cancer Res 47:3889–3894, 1987.
185. Swain SM, Lippman ME: The treatment of patients with inflammatory breast cancer. In Rosenberg SA, Hellman S, Devita VT (eds): Important Advances in Oncology 1989. Philadelphia, JB Lippincott, 1989, pp 129–150.
186. Swain S, Whaley F, Gerber M, et al: Delayed administration of dexrazoxane provides cardioprotection for patients with advanced breast cancer treated with doxorubicin-containing therapy. J Clin Oncol 15:1333–1340, 1997.
187. Tabbane F, Muenz L, Jaziri M, et al: Clinical and prognostic features of a rapidly progressing breast cancer in Tunisia. Cancer 40:376–382, 1977.
188. Tajima T, Tokuda Y, Kubota M, et al: Adjuvant chemotherapy supported by autologous bone marrow transplantation in breast cancer. Proc Am Soc Clin Oncol 9:31, 1990.
189. Taylor GW, Meltzer A: Inflammatory carcinoma of the breast. Ann Surg 33:33–49, 1938.
190. Thomas F, Arriagada R, Spielmann M, et al: Pattern of failure in patients with inflammatory breast cancer treated by alternating radiotherapy and chemotherapy. Cancer 76:2286–2296, 1995.
191. Toonkel LM, Fix I, Jacobson LH, et al: Locally advanced breast carcinoma: Results with combined regional therapy. Int J Radiat Oncol Biol Phys 12:1583–1587, 1986.
192. Treurniet-Donker AD, Hop WCJ, Hoed-Sijtsema S: Radiation treatment of stage III mammary carcinoma: A review of 129 patients. Int J Radiat Oncol Biol Phys 6:1477–1482, 1981.
193. Treves N: Inflammatory carcinoma of the breast in the male patient. Surgery 34:810–820, 1953.
194. Treves N: The inoperability of inflammatory carcinoma of the breast. Surg Gynecol Obstet 109:240–242, 1959.
195. Vaeth JM, Clark JC, Green JP, et al: Radiotherapeutic management of locally advanced carcinoma of the breast. Cancer 30:107–112, 1972.
196. Valagussa P, Bonadonna G, Veronesi V, et al: Patterns of relapse and survival following radical mastectomy. Cancer 41:1170–1178, 1978.
197. Valavaara R, Nordman E: Renal complications of mitomycin C therapy with special reference to the total dose. Cancer 55:47–50, 1985.
198. Veronesi A, Frustaci S, Tirelli U, et al: Tamoxifen therapy in postmenopausal advanced breast cancer: Efficacy at the primary tumor site in 46 evaluable patients. Tumori 67:235–238, 1981.
199. VonVolkmann R, Brust K: Beitrage zur chirurgie. Breitkopf und Hartel, Leipzig, 1875, pp 319–334.
200. Wallgren A, Arner O, Bergstrom J, et al: Preoperative radiotherapy in operable breast cancer: Results in the Stockholm breast cancer trial. Cancer 42:1120–1125, 1978.
201. Wang CC, Griscom NT: Inflammatory carcinoma of the breast: Results following orthovoltage and supervoltage radiation therapy. Clin Radiol 15:168–174, 1964.
202. Weichselbaum RR, Hellman S, Piro AJ, et al: Proliferation kinetics of a human breast cancer cell line in vitro following treatment with 17β-estradiol and 1-β-D-arabinofuranosylcytosine. Cancer Res 38:2339–2345, 1978.
203. Yonemoto RH, Keating JL, Byron RL, et al: Inflammatory carcinoma of the breast treated by bilateral adrenalectomy. Surgery 68:461–467, 1970.
204. Zucali R, Uslenghi C, Kenda R, Bonadonna G: Natural history of survival of inoperable breast cancer treated with radiotherapy and radiotherapy followed by radical mastectomy. Cancer 37:1422–1431, 1976.
205. Zylberberg B, Salat-Baroux J, Ravina J, et al: Initial chemoimmunotherapy in inflammatory carcinoma of the breast. Cancer 49:1537–1543, 1982.

SECTION XXI
MANAGEMENT OF SYSTEMIC DISEASE

CHAPTER 70
DETECTION OF OCCULT MICROMETASTATIC DISEASE

Bonnie S. Reichman, M.D. / Michael P. Osborne, M.D., M.S.

In 1996, it was estimated that there were 184,300 new cases of breast cancer and 44,300 deaths.[1] The National Cancer Institute's Surveillance, Epidemiology and End Results (SEER) program reported a nearly 5 percent decline in the breast cancer death rate between 1989 and 1992.[2] This benefit has been attributed to early detection and administration of adjuvant treatments. Unfortunately, despite gains in detection and treatment, breast cancer remains the leading cause of cancer in women and is second to lung cancer as the cause of cancer death. Clinically occult microscopic metastases present at initial diagnosis and treatment, which subsequently grow, and cause death from breast cancer.

Most metastases from breast cancer are initiated when the primary tumor is less than 0.125 cm[3].[3] Tumor cells metastasize and disseminate shortly after primary tumor vascularization.[4] The skeletal system is the most common site of hematogeneous dissemination, with clinically evident metastasis present in approximately 50 percent of patients at relapse and 50 to 70 percent at autopsy. The microenvironment of the reticuloendothelial system and other marrow components present in the osseous medulli provides the fertile soil for the "seed and soil" hypothesis for tumor cell growth and replication.[5] The precise mechanisms for micrometastatic tumor cell embolization, adhesion, and growth in the bone marrow microenvironment and the tropism for breast cancer metastases to bone are under evaluation.[6]

In operable breast cancer, the probability of distant metastases currently is best predicted by the presence or absence of lymph node metastasis and maximum tumor diameter in lymph node–negative patients.[7, 8] Many other prognostic factors have been described but as yet have not been confirmed to be highly predictive or generally applicable.[9]

Pretreatment or perioperative screening tests for the detection of metastatic disease at initial diagnosis have not been particularly useful. Bone metastases, detected by bone scan, are seen in less than 5 percent of patients with stage I or II disease.[10–12] Routine light microscopic evaluation of bone marrow aspirates and biopsies at the time of perioperative staging in asymptomatic patients rarely identifies metastatic disease.[13–15]

The detection of bone marrow micrometastases at initial presentation could be considered an adverse prognostic factor. This would identify a subgroup of patients who are at increased risk for relapse and could be targeted for more intensive adjuvant treatment. The use of high-dose chemotherapy with autologous hematopoietic support also underscores the need for highly sensitive methods that may detect microscopic tumor cells in the hematopoietic transplant.

IMMUNOLOGIC TECHNIQUES

A polyclonal antisera against human milk fat globule membrane, epithelial membrane antigen (EMA), has been found in a wide variety of normal and neoplastic tissue, including the breast.[16] Primary and metastatic breast cancers almost always express EMA, and it is not expressed by normal and neoplastic—hematopoietic, osseous, and other connective tissue cells.[17, 18] Cells positive for EMA have the morphological and cytologic characteristics of breast cancer cells. Subsequently, it was noted that EMA stained solitary malignant cells in bone marrow. Staining was initially described in 9 of 24 (38 percent) of patients with known bone metastases, 4 of 20 (20 percent) with nonosseous systemic metastases, and 2 of 20 (10 percent) with primary operable breast cancer.[19] Researchers at the Ludwig Institute subsequently demonstrated that the detection of EMA-positive cells in the bone marrow of stage I, II or III breast cancer correlated with the development of metastases and shortened survival.[20–26] The presence of EMA staining cells in the marrow correlated with established prognostic factors: tumor diameter, axillary lymph node involvement, vascular invasion, and estrogen reception status.[22–25] In addition, the presence of EMA positivity predicted for relapse in bone and other distant sites.[24–30] The rate of relapse also correlated with the number of EMA-positive cells detected.[31]

In an effort to improve sensitivity and specificity, either single monoclonal antibodies or "cocktails" of multiple monoclonal antibodies have been used that recognize membrane and cytoskeletal antigens. Cytoskeletal antigens are expressed by epithelial tumors and are not expressed by normal bone marrow cells. Epithelial cells are not found in the bone marrow of normal volunteers or patients with nonepithelial cancers. Epithelial membrane antigen is expressed by nonepithelial cells, including lymphoid cells.[32-34] Thus, cytokeratins are a more sensitive marker of differentiation than EMA. Increasing the number of bone marrow sites sampled does not necessarily increase the yield of positivity. These studies are summarized in Table 70–1.[35]

Using these techniques, it has been possible to detect one to two cancer cells per 1×10^6 normal bone marrow cells.[36] The use of pooled aspirates separated by Ficoll-Hypaque density gradient allows for concentration of extrinsic cells in the interface. Cytospin preparations of these nucleated cells are subsequently immunostained. The use of cytospins or smears allows for the examination of large numbers of cells. It has been suggested that at least 1 million cells should be examined. This technique is more sensitive and less time consuming than routine paraffin processing of bone marrow biopsies, and slides may be stored for several years. Osborne and Rosen review the methodology.[35] Further research to develop more specific monoclonal antibodies is required.

CLINICAL IMPLICATIONS

In general, bone marrow positivity has correlated with standard prognostic factors such as T stage and lymph node status. However, results have been conflicting regarding correlation with other prognostic variables such as hormone receptor status and *ERBB2*. Cote and Osborne and their associates have correlated the tumor cell burden in the bone marrow,

as evidenced by the number of bone marrow positive cells, with prognosis.[31, 37] No clear relationship exists between the number of sites sampled and positivity.[38-40] Menard and colleagues also collected peripheral blood before and after surgery and determined that contamination by circulating tumor cells is not the cause of bone marrow positivity.[41] Similarly, Porro, Diel, and Singhal and their associates[38, 42, 43] found no difference in the rate of positivity in specimens obtained preoperatively versus postoperatively. A National Cancer Institute workshop on micrometastases in 1992 recommended that at least 1×10^6 cells be examined.[44]

Data on the use of bone marrow metastases to predict recurrence are presented in Table 70–2. Time to recurrence and overall survival are consistently shorter among bone marrow–positive patients as compared with bone marrow–negative patients. The presence of bone marrow micrometastases appears to predict for skeletal metastases. This appears to be significant despite differences in patient population, adjuvant treatments, and lack of appropriate controls. Cote and coworkers[31] indicated that the tumor burden identified as the number of positive bone marrow micrometastases cells was predictive for recurrence; the presence of at least ten positive cells significantly predicted early occurrence. This was the only factor in a multivariate analysis comparing bone marrow metastasis, axillary lymph node status, and tumor size that independently predicted early recurrence. Subsequent, more detailed statistical analysis demonstrated that the number of micrometastatic cells (<14 or >14) was important in multivariate analysis, and the predictive power of early relapse was significantly enhanced when combined with a maximum tumor diameter of more than 2.0 cm or axillary lymph node metastases.[37]

TABLE 70–1.   RESULTS OF ANTIBODY DETECTION OF OCCULT BONE MARROW MICROMETASTASES

Author	Antibody Used	No. of Patients	% BMM Positive	No. BMM Positive
Untch et al.[45]	CK, EMA, TAG12	170	33	56
Ellis et al.[46]	34BH11, 34BE12	6	33	2
Giai et al.[47]	AB/3	39	3	1
Coombes et al.[23]	EMA	269	22	60
Mansi et al.[26]	EMA	350	25	89
Osborne et al.[37]*	T16, C26, AE-1	348	32	111
Diel et al.[42]	2E11	260	44	115
Menard et al.[41]	MBr1, MBr8, MOr8, MOv12, MluC1, CK2	197	31	62
Harbeck et al.[49]†	EMA, CK, TAG12	100	38	38
Kirk et al.[39]	LICR. LON. M8.4	25	48	12
Manegold et al.[40]	PKK1	50	8	4
Porro et al.[38]	MBr1	159	16	25
Schlimok et al.[48]	CK2	187	28	53
Redding et al.[22]	EMA	110	28	31
Dearnaley et al.[27]	EMA	37	27	10
Cote et al.[30]	C26, T16, AE-1	51	35	18
Cote et al.[31]	C26, T16, AE-1	49	37	18

BMM = bone marrow micrometastasis.
* Extension of study reported by Cote and associates.[31]
† Extension of study reported by Untch and associates.[25]

TABLE 70–2. RELATIONSHIP BETWEEN BONE MARROW MICROMETASTASIS AND RELAPSE

Author	Median Follow-up	Relapse BMM Positive (%)	Relapse BMM Negative (%)	p Value
Coombes et al.[23]	22 mo	19/60 (32)	34/195 (17)	$p<.05$
Mansi et al.[26]	76 mo (34–108)	43/89 (48)	64/261 (25)	$p<0.005$
Dearnaley et al.[27]	9.5 yr	10/11 (91)	8/26 (31)	$p<0.05$
Cote et al.[31]	30 mo (12–38)	7/18 (39)	5/31 (16)	$p=0.094$†
Diel et al.[42]	24 mo (12–73)	22/81 (27)	4/130 (3)	$p<.0005$
Kirk et al.[39]	15 mo	4/12 (33)	5/13 (38)	NS
Untch et al.[25]	13.1 mo (3–27)	8/15 (53)	3/30 (10)	$p=0.003$†
Harbeck et al.[49]*	34 mo	15/38 (39)	9/62 (15)	$p=0.016$

NS = not significant; BMM = bone marrow micrometastasis.
* Extension of study reported by Untch and associates.[25]
† This p value was derived using Fisher's exact test based on the proportions provided by the authors.

DIRECTIONS FOR FUTURE RESEARCH

More research in the format of carefully designed clinical trials is needed to delineate the prognostic value of bone marrow micrometastases. Many centers have been trying to identify the clinical relevance of bone marrow immunostaining as a prognostic variable. Reported rates of bone marrow metastases range from 2.6 to 48 percent (see Table 70–1). Differences in rates of bone marrow positivity may be attributed to case selection, number and site of aspiration, number of cells examined, type and number of antibodies used, and variations in the technical methods used. Standardization of technical methods would aid in defining the utility of the potentially significant prognostic variable. The majority of studies suggest that the presence and number of breast cancer micrometastases in the bone marrow at the time of diagnosis or initial treatment are predictive of early distant relapse. The meta-analysis of randomized clinical trials of adjuvant systemic therapy reported by Peto and associates clearly demonstrated the beneficial effect of adjuvant chemotherapy.[50] This benefit may be further enhanced by using this technology to identify patients at substantial risk of systemic disease. This approach, combined with standard prognostic factors of tumor diameter and axillary lymph node status, may permit the planning and administration of systemic therapeutic strategies superior to those that have been used to date. This technology may help us to delineate which operable breast cancer patients should be treated with lesser or greater intensity.

The criteria for determining bone marrow positivity have not been fully defined. Available data have been limited regarding the prognostic significance of small numbers of micrometastatic cells. At present, no studies reported have addressed the utility of this method in "good prognosis" patients who have small tumors and negative axillary lymph nodes. It is unclear whether all patients with micrometastases will ultimately develop clinical recurrence.

It was recommended at the St. Gallen Conference on adjuvant systemic treatment that the majority of patients with invasive breast cancer are eligible for systemic therapy if the invasive tumor exceeds 1.0 cm or, in the case of special tumor types such as medullary, colloid, and tubular, 2 to 3 cm.[51] It would be exceedingly difficult to demonstrate a beneficial effect of systemic therapy in those patients who are not currently recommended to receive adjuvant treatment. Because the overall relapse rate in these patients is less than 10 percent at 10 years, the sample size required to demonstrate a significant relapse or mortality reduction caused by adjuvant systemic therapy would be extremely large.

The longitudinal evaluation of bone marrow to determine the efficacy of systemic therapy is unlikely to be useful, because micrometastatic cells may spontaneously disappear without treatment on repeated examination.[52] It has not been clearly determined whether malignant cells in the bone marrow are truly clonogenic foci or represent cells in transit.

The detection of bone marrow micrometastases may be useful in predicting prognosis in other tumors such as colorectal cancer,[28, 53, 54] gastric cancer,[55] lung cancer,[56–60] neuroblastoma,[61–67] and melanoma.[68] Investigation of this technique in urological cancers is in progress.[69, 70] New technology such as reverse transcriptase–polymerase chain reaction has been applied to the detection of bone marrow micrometastases and regional lymph node metastasis.[71–73]

The characteristics of the primary tumor that correlate with bone marrow micrometastases require further investigation. Expressions of the laminin receptor,[74] and of a parathyroid hormone-related protein[75, 76] are associated with bone marrow micrometastases and the likelihood of overt bone metastases, respectively. Additional studies are required to determine the proliferative,[77–79] endocrine,[80] molecular biological,[79] and immunological[81] characteristics of micrometastases that correlate with recurrence. This technology may lead to the development of immunotherapeutic strategies using an immunocytotoxic approach[28] as well as techniques for purging bone marrow or peripheral blood progenitor cells of patients undergoing autologous hematopoietic recovery after high-dose chemotherapy.[82–85] In this setting, the significance of the presence of tumor cell contamination of the bone marrow or peripheral blood progenitor cells remains controversial. Contamination might have greater significance in the setting of adjuvant treatment than for stage IV disease. The utility of detecting micrometastases as an indicator for intensive adjuvant therapy will ultimately be determined by results of randomized clinical trials.

References

1. Parker SL, Tong T, Bolden S, et al: Cancer statistics - 1996. CA Cancer J Clin 65:5–27, 1996.
2. Smigel K: Breast cancer death rates decline for white women. J Natl Cancer Inst 87:173, 1995.
3. Liotta LA, Stetler-Stevenson WG: Principles of molecular cell biology of cancer: Cancer metastases. In DeVita VT, et al (eds): Cancer: Principles and Practice of Oncology. Philadelphia, JB Lippincott, 1993, pp 134–147.
4. Werdner N, Semple NJ, Welch WR, Folkman J: Tumor angiogenous and metastasis: Correlation in invasive breast carcinoma. N Engl J Med 324:1–8, 1991.
5. Paget S: The distribution of secondary growth in cancer of the breast. Lancet 1:571–573, 1889.
6. Orr F, Kostenuik P, Sanchez-Sweatman O, et al: Mechanisms involved in the metastasis of cancer to bone. Br Cancer Res Treat 25:151–163, 1993.
7. Fisher B, Bauer M, Wickerham L, et al: Relation of number of positive axillary nodes to the prognosis of patients with primary breast cancer. Cancer 52:1551–1557, 1983.
8. Rosen P, Groshen S, Saigo PE, et al: A long-term follow-up study of survival in Stage I (T1N0M0) breast carcinoma. J Clin Oncol 7:355–366, 1989.
9. McGuire WL, Tandon AK, Allred DC, et al: Projecting breast cancer probabilities. J Natl Cancer Inst 82:1006–1015, 1990.
10. Khansur T, Haick A, Patel B: Evaluation of bone scan as a screening work-up in primary and local-regional recurrence of breast cancer. Am J Clin Oncol 10:167–170, 1987.
11. Gerber F, Goddreau J, Kirchner P: Efficacy of preoperative and postoperative bone scanning in the management of breast carcinoma. N Engl J Med 297:300–303, 1977.
12. Lee Y: Bone scanning in patients with early breast carcinoma: Should it be a routine staging procedure? Cancer 47:486–495, 1981.
13. Ingle J, Torney D, Tan H: The bone marrow examination in breast cancer: Diagnostic considerations and clinical usefulness. Cancer 41:670–674, 1978.
14. Landys K: Prognostic value of bone marrow biopsy in breast cancer. Cancer 49:513–518, 1982.
15. Ceci G, Franciosi V, Nizzoli R, et al: The value of bone marrow biopsy in breast cancer at time of diagnosis: A prospective study. Cancer 61:96–98, 1988.
16. Heyderman E, Steele K, Ormerod M: A new antigen on the epithelial membrane: Its immunoperoxidase localization in normal and neoplastic tissue. J Clin Pathol 32:35–39, 1979.
17. Sloane J, Ormerod M: Distribution of epithelial membrane antigen in normal and neoplastic tissues and its value in diagnostic tumor pathology. Cancer 47:1786–1795, 1981.
18. Sloane J, Ormerod MC, Neville AM: Potential pathological application of immunocytochemical methods to the detection of micrometastases. Cancer Res 40:3079–3082, 1980.
19. Dearnaley D, Sloane J, Ormerod M, et al: Increased detection of mammary carcinoma cells in marrow smears using antisera to epithelial membrane antigen. Br J Cancer 44:85–90, 1981.
20. Coombes R, Dearnaley D, Buckman R, et al: Detection of bone metastases in patients with breast cancer. Invasion Metastasis 2:177–184, 1982.
21. Dearnaley D, Ormerod M, Sloane J, et al: Detection of isolated mammary carcinoma cells in marrow of patients with primary breast cancer. J R Soc Med 76:359–364, 1983.
22. Redding W, Coombes R, Monoghan P, et al: Detection of micrometastases in patients with primary breast cancer. Lancet 2:1271–1274, 1983.
23. Coombes R, Berger U, Mansi J, et al: Prognostic significance of micrometastases in bone marrow in patients with primary breast cancer. Natl Cancer Inst Monogr 1:51–53, 1986.
24. Mansi J, Berger U, Easton D, et al: Micrometastases in bone marrow in patients with primary breast cancer: Evaluation as an early predictor of bone metastases. Br Med J 295:1093–1096, 1987.
25. Untch M, Harbeck N, Eirmann W: Micrometastases in bone marrow in patients with breast cancer. Br Med J 296:290, 1988.
26. Mansi J, Easton D, Berger U, et al: Bone marrow micrometastases in primary breast cancer: Prognostic significance after 6 years' follow-up. Eur J Cancer 27:1552–1555, 1991.
27. Dearnaley D, Ormerod M, Sloane J: Micrometastases in breast cancer: Long-term follow-up of the first patient cohort. Eur J Cancer 27:236–239, 1991.
28. Schlimok G, Funke I, Holzmann B, et al: Micrometastatic cancer cells in bone marrow: In vitro detection with anti-cytokeratin and in vivo labeling with anti-17-1A monoclonal antibodies. Proc Natl Acad Sci USA 84:8672–8676, 1987.
29. Cote R, Rosen P, Osborne M, et al: Monoclonal antibodies detect occult bone marrow metastases in operable breast cancer. Lab Invest 56:16, 1987.
30. Cote R, Rosen P, Hakes T, et al: Monoclonal antibodies detect occult breast carcinoma metastases in the bone marrow of patients with early stage disease. Am J Surg Pathol 12:333–340, 1988.
31. Cote R, Rosen P, Lesser M, et al: Prediction of early relapse in patients with operable breast cancer by detection of occult bone marrow micrometastases. J Clin Oncol 9:1749–1756, 1991.
32. Delson G, Gatter K, Stein H, et al: Human lymphoid cells express epithelial membrane antigen: Implications for diagnosis of human neoplasms. Lancet 2:1124–1128, 1985.
33. Pinkus G, Kurtin P: Epithelial membrane antigen—a diagnostic discriminant in surgical pathology: Immunohistochemical profile in epithelial, mesenchymal and hematopoietic neoplasms using paraffin sections and monoclonal antibodies. Hum Pathol 6:929–940, 1985.
34. Rabkin MS, Kjeldsberg CR: Epithelial membrane antigen staining patterns of histiocytic lesions. Arch Pathol Lab Med 111:337–338, 1987.
35. Osborne MP, Rosen PP: Detection and management of bone marrow micrometastases in breast cancer. Oncology 8:25–29, 1994.
36. Osborne MP, Wong GY, Asina S, et al: Sensitivity of immunocytochemical detection of breast cancer cells in human bone marrow. Cancer Res 51:2706–2709, 1991.
37. Osborne MP, Wong GY, Gonzalez A, et al: Bone marrow micrometastases (BMM) in breast cancer: The effect of systemic tumor cell (TC) burden on early relapse. Proc Am Soc Clin Oncol 12:75, 1993.
38. Porro G, Menard S, Tagliabue E, et al: Monoclonal antibody detection of carcinoma cells in bone marrow biopsy specimens from breast cancer patients. Cancer 61:2407–2411, 1988.
39. Kirk S, Cooper G, Hoper M, et al: The prognostic significance of marrow micrometastases in women with early breast cancer. Eur J Surg Oncol 16:481–485, 1990.
40. Manegold C, Krempien B, Kaufmann M, et al: The value of bone marrow examination for tumor staging in breast cancer. J Cancer Res Clin Oncol 114:425–428, 1988.
41. Menard S, Squicciarini P, Luini A, et al: Immunodetection of bone marrow micrometastases in breast carcinoma patients and its correlation with primary tumour prognostic features. Br J Cancer 69:1126–1129, 1994.
42. Diel I, Kaufmann M, Goerner R, et al: Detection of tumor cells in bone marrow of patients with primary breast cancer: A prognostic factor for distant metastasis. J Clin Oncol 10:1534–1539, 1992.
43. Singhal H, Cote RJ, Potter C, et al: Bone marrow micrometastases (BMM) in breast cancer: Relationship to local-regional disease status. Proc Am Soc Clin Oncol 13:103, 1994.
44. National Cancer Institute Conference on Cancer Micrometastasis: Biology, Methodology and Clinical Significance. Bethesda, June 25, 1992.
45. Untch M, Nestle-Kramling C, Konecy G, et al: Prognostic significance of tumor cells in bone marrow in early breast cancer. Breast Cancer Res Treat 27:157, 1993.

46. Ellis G, Ferguson M, Yamanaka E, et al: Monoclonal antibodies for detection of occult carcinoma cells in bone marrow of breast cancer patients. Cancer 63:2509–2514, 1989.
47. Giai M, Natoli C, Sismondi P, et al: Bone marrow micrometastases detected by a monoclonal antibody in patients with breast cancer. Anticancer Res 10:119–121, 1990.
48. Schlimok G, Lindermann F, Holzman K, et al: Prognostic significance of disseminated tumor cells in bone marrow of patients with breast and colorectal cancer: A multivariate analysis. National Cancer Institute Conference on Cancer Micrometastasis: Biology, Methodology and Clinical Significance. Bethesda, June 25, 1992.
49. Harbeck N, Untch M, Pache L, Wiermann W: Tumor cell detection in the bone marrow of breast cancer patients at primary therapy: Results of a 3 year median follow-up. Br J Cancer 69:566–571, 1994.
50. Early Breast Cancer Trialists' Collaborative Group: Systemic treatment of early breast cancer by hormonal, cytoxic, or immune therapy: 133 randomized trials involving 31,000 recurrences and 24,000 deaths among 75,000 women. Part II. Lancet 339:71–85, 1992.
51. Goldhirsh A, Wood WC, Senn HJ, et al: Fifth international conference on adjuvant therapy of breast cancer: St. Gallen, March 1995. International consensus panel on the treatment of primary breast cancer. Eur J Cancer 31A:17554–17559, 1995.
52. Mansi JL, Berger V, McDonall T, et al: The fate of bone marrow micrometastases in patients with primary breast cancer. J Clin Oncol 7:445–449, 1989.
53. Schlimok G, Funke I, Bock B, et al: Epithelial tumor cells in bone marrow of patients with colorectal cancer: Immunocytochemical detection, phenotypic characterization, and prognostic significance. J Clin Oncol 8:831–837, 1990.
54. Lindermann F, Schlimok G, Dirschedl P, et al: Prognostic significance of micrometastatic tumor cells in bone marrow of colorectal cancer patients. Lancet 340:685–689, 1992.
55. Schlimok G, Funke I, Pantel K, et al: Micrometastatic tumour cells in bone marrow of patients with gastric cancer: Methodological aspects of detection and prognostic significance. Eur J Cancer 27:1461–1464, 1991.
56. Stahel R, Mabry M, Skarin A, et al: Detection of bone marrow metastasis in small-cell lung cancer by monoclonal antibody. J Clin Oncol 3:455–461, 1985.
57. Bezwoda W, Lewis D, Livini N, et al: Bone marrow involvement in anaplastic small cell lung cancer: Prognosis, hematologic features and prognostic implications. Cancer 58:1762–1765, 1986.
58. Leonard R, Duncan L, Hay F: Immunocytochemical detection of residual marrow disease at clinical remission predicts metastatic relapse in small cell lung cancer. Cancer Res 50:6545–6548, 1990.
59. Skov B, Hirsch F, Bobrow L: Monoclonal antibodies in the detection of bone marrow metastases in small cell lung cancer. Br J Cancer 65:593–596, 1992.
60. Pantel K, Izbicki J, Angstrwurm M: Immunocytochemical detection of bone marrow micrometastases in operable non–small cell lung cancer. Cancer Res 53:1027–1031, 1993.
61. Jonak ZL, Kennett RH, Bechtol KB: Detection of neuroblastoma cells in human bone marrow using a combination of monoclonal antibodies. Hybridoma 1:349–368, 1982.
62. Cheung NK, Van Hoff DD, Strandjord SE, et al: Detection of neuroblastoma cells in bone marrow using G_{D2} specific monoclonal antibodies. J Clin Oncol 4:363–369, 1986.
63. Favrot MC, Frappaz D, Maritaz O, et al: Histological, cytological and immunological analyses are complementary for the detection of neuroblastoma cells in bone marrow. Br J Cancer 54:637–641, 1986.
64. Beck D, Maritaz O, Gross N, et al: Immunocytochemical detection of neuroblastoma cells infiltrating clinical bone marrow samples. Eur J Pediatr 147:609–612, 1988.
65. Combaret V, Favrot MC, Kremens B, et al: Immunological detection of neuroblastoma cells in bone marrow harvested for autologous transplantation. Br J Cancer 59:844–847, 1989.
66. Oppedal BR, Storm-Methisen I, Kemshead JT, et al: Bone marrow examination in neuroblastoma patients: A morphological, immunocytochemical, and immunohistochemical study. Hum Pathol 20:800–805, 1989.
67. Rogers DW, Treleaven JG, Kemshead JT, et al: Monoclonal antibodies for detecting bone marrow invasion by neuroblastoma. J Clin Pathol 42:422–426, 1989.
68. Dantas ME, Brown JP, Thomas MR, et al: Detection of melanoma cells in bone marrow using monoclonal antibodies. Cancer 52:949–953, 1983.
69. Mansi J, Berger U, Wilson P, et al: Detection of tumor cells in bone marrow of patients with prostatic carcinoma by immunocytochemical techniques. J Urol 139:545–548, 1988.
70. Oberneder R, Kriegman M, Riesenberg R, et al: Diagnostic and prognostic significance of micrometastatic cells in cancer of prostate, kidney and bladder. National Cancer Institute Conference on Cancer Micrometastasis: Biology, Methodology and Clinical Significance. Bethesda, June 25, 1992.
71. Datta YH, Adams PT, Drobyski WR, et al: Sensitive detection of occult breast cancer by the reverse-transcriptase polymerase chain reaction. J Clin Oncol 12:475–482, 1994.
72. Fields KK, Perkins JB, Ballester OF, et al: Time of relapse following high dose chemotherapy for the treatment of poor prognosis breast cancer: Durable remissions beyond 24 months. Breast Cancer Res Treat 32:63, 1994.
73. Noguchi S, Aihara T, Nakamori S, et al: The detection of breast carcinoma micrometastases in axillary lymph nodes by means of reverse transcriptase-polymerase chain reaction. Cancer 74:1595–1600, 1994.
74. Menard S: Bone marrow micrometastases in breast cancer: Correlation with tumor biology. National Cancer Institute Conference on Cancer Micrometastasis: Biology, Methodology and Clinical Significance. Bethesda, June 25, 1992.
75. Bundred NJ, Walker RA, Ratcliffe WA, et al: Parathyroid hormone related protein and skeletal morbidity in breast cancer. Eur J Cancer 28:690–692, 1992.
76. Bouizar Z, Spyratos F, Deytieux S, et al: Polymerase chain reaction analysis of parathyroid hormone-related protein gene expression in breast cancer patients and occurrence of bone metastases. Cancer Res 53:5076–5078, 1993.
77. Ginsbourg M, Musset M, Misset J, et al: Simultaneous detection in the bone marrow of mammary cancer metastatic cells and of their labeling index as respective markers of the residual minimum submacroscopic disease and its proliferative condition (preliminary results). Biomed Pharmacother 40:386–388, 1986.
78. Ginsbourg M, Musset M, Misset J, et al: Identification of mammary metastatic cells: I. The bone marrow as a marker of minimal residual disease and of their proliferative index as a factor of prognosis—an immunocytologic study with monoclonal antibodies. J Med Oncol Tumor Pharmacother 1:51–54, 1988.
79. Pantel K, Schlimok G, Braun S, et al: Differential expression of proliferation-associated molecules in individual micrometastatic carcinoma cells. J Natl Cancer Inst 85:1419–1424, 1993.
80. Berger U, Mansi JL, Wilson P, et al: Detection of estrogen receptor in bone marrow from patients with metastatic breast cancer. J Clin Oncol 5:1779–1782, 1987.
81. Pantel K, Schlimok G, Kutter D, et al: Frequent down-regulation of major histocompatibility cell I antigen expression on individual micrometastatic carcinoma cells. Cancer Res 51:4712–4715, 1991.
82. Coombes RC, Buckman R, Forrester JA, et al: In vitro and in vivo effects of a monoclonal antibody-toxin conjugate for use in autologous bone marrow transplantation for patients with breast cancer. Cancer Res 40:4217–4220, 1986.
83. Anderson IC, Shpall EJ, Leslie DS, et al: Elimination of malignant clonogenic breast cancer cells from human bone marrow. Cancer Res 49:4659–4664, 1989.
84. Vredenburgh J, Simpson W, Memoli V, et al: Reactivity of anti-CD15 monoclonal antibody PM-81 with breast cancer and elimination of breast cancer cells from human bone marrow by PM-81 and immunomagnetic beads. Cancer Res 51:2451–2455, 1991.
85. Wong JR, Ho C, Mauch P, et al: A novel method of purging carcinoma contaminated bone marrow using lipophilic cation rhodamine 123. Int J Radiat Oncol Biol Phys 24:207, 1992.

CHAPTER 71

PALLIATIVE RADIOTHERAPY FOR DISSEMINATED BREAST CANCER

Robert A. Zlotecki, M.D., Ph.D. / Nancy Price Mendenhall, M.D.

Radiotherapy is extremely effective in the treatment of localized metastasis from primary breast cancer. Once distant metastasis has occurred, however, the potential for cure, and thus for survival, is limited. The primary goal of treatment once metastasis has occurred, therefore, is palliative, and only those patients who are either symptomatic or likely to develop irreversible symptoms require treatment.

In planning palliative treatment, an assessment of the patient's overall prognosis and functional performance status must be made, based on the extent and site(s) of metastases, the disease-free interval (between time of initial diagnosis and treatment and the occurrence of metastasis), the estrogen and progesterone status of the tumor, the age and general medical condition of the patient, the prior therapy, the potential responsiveness of the tumor to treatment, and the probability of treatment-related side effects and complications during the expected life span of the patient.

Patients with metastatic breast cancer can be expected to encounter multiple problems during the course of their disease that may require treatment with radiotherapy. As treatment is planned for each local metastatic site, it must be anticipated that at a later date additional treatments may be required at adjacent sites. If this unfortunate but all too frequent occurrence is not anticipated, the junctions between adjacent treatment fields may be overdosed or underdosed. More than one radiotherapy technique may be indicated (for example, localized external-beam plus systemic radioisotope treatment). Thus, the potential additive side effects of combined treatments must be anticipated.

Treatments of the more common presentations of disseminated breast cancer are discussed in this chapter; treatment of local-regional recurrence, with or without disseminated disease, is discussed in Chapter 68.

BONE METASTASES

Bone metastasis is the most common problem for which radiotherapy is required in the treatment of disseminated breast cancer. Breast cancer represents the primary tumor site in 40–60 percent of all bone metastases in most reported series.*

The median survival for patients with metastatic breast cancer ranges from 4 months to 15 months in most series,* with 2-year survival rates of only 15–20 percent. In general, patients with bone metastases from breast cancer survive somewhat longer than patients with bone metastases from other cancers.[162] Gilbert and coworkers[51] reported a median survival of 15 months from time of treatment of first bone metastasis from breast cancer but also found that 15 percent of patients with metastatic breast cancer died within less than 3 months of treatment.

Toma and coworkers[160] reported on a series of 110 patients who were treated nonsurgically for metastasis to either the vertebrae or other bone sites; three quarters of these patients had primary cancers of the breast. Interestingly, the clinical and radiographic objective responses were better in the patients with vertebral metastases than in the patients with metastases to other sites. The average survival time after diagnosis of bone metastasis was 40.4 months in this series; thus the investigators recommended early and aggressive treatment to provide durable, effective palliation and to maintain acceptable quality of life in the patients. In the Radiation Therapy Oncology Group (RTOG) study of single-dose hemibody radiotherapy for multiple bone metastases, in which more than 80 percent of the patients had severe and constant pain and many patients were considered terminal, two patients remained alive more than 5 years after treatment.

Mechanism of Pain Relief

The mechanisms by which radiotherapy relieves pain are not fully known. Pain secondary to bone metastasis is believed to be due either to invasion or stretching of the periosteum, through which nerve fibers conducting pain sensation pass. The rapidity of response to low doses of radiotherapy given to large fields and the effectiveness of many different dose regimens have led some researchers to hypothesize that palliation from radiotherapy may also depend on humoral factors, such as prostaglandins, through which pain may also be mediated, rather than only on tumor shrinkage and relief of periosteal tension.[25, 166, 178] The humoral theory for pain relief may correlate with the effectiveness of biphosphonate agents in relieving bone pain and preventing hypercalcemia through inhibition of osteoclast activity and tumor-induced osteolysis.[111, 167]

---

*See references 17, 63, 75, 93, 122, 139, 160, and 164.

*See references 7, 42, 49, 51, 75, 136, 162, and 168.

External-Beam Radiotherapy

Response Rates

Various treatment regimens with external-beam radiotherapy are favored at different institutions, and all produce excellent palliation, with complete response (CR) rates in the range of 50–60 percent and overall response rates, defined as CR plus partial-response (PR) rates, in the range of 70–90 percent (Table 71–1).*

Dose

Trodella and coworkers[164] noted no significant differences in overall response rates with various total or daily doses, but concluded that 3 Gy daily fractions produced the best ratio of complete responses to par-

---

*See references 2, 16, 49, 51, 75, 113, 123, 139, 159, 164, and 168.

tial responses (Fig. 71–1). The results of four prospective studies (from Odense University Hospital in Denmark, the Royal Marsden Hospital in London, the RTOG, and Rush-Presbyterian Medical Center in Chicago) of various dose-fractionation schemes for palliation of bone metastases are summarized in Table 71–2.[67, 92, 122, 162] Doses tested included extremely hypofractionated regimens with large doses delivered in one or two fractions (8 Gy × 1, 10 Gy × 2), moderately hypofractionated regimens delivering a daily dose of 3, 4, or 5 Gy for 1 week, an intermediate regimen of 30 Gy in ten fractions over 2 weeks, and one relatively high-dose regimen of 40.5 Gy delivered in 15 fractions of 2.7 Gy over 3 weeks. The conclusion from these reports was that there was no demonstrable benefit for protracted courses of treatment in the overall population of patients with bone metastases. Reanalysis of the RTOG data, however, by Blitzer[10] (Table 71–3) with different statistical techniques and an emphasis on the parameters of complete pain relief before retreatment and complete relief from

TABLE 71–1. NONCONTROLLED TRIALS OF VARIOUS RADIOTHERAPY REGIMENS FOR PALLIATION OF BONE METASTASES

Researchers	No. Patients (No. Areas Treated)	Dose/No. Fractions/ Duration	CR (%)[a]	CR + PR (%)[a]	Percent Requiring Retreatment	Overall Survival	Percent with Breast Cancer
Vargha et al,[168] Mt. Sinai Hospital, New York, 1969	119 (132)	4–18 Gy/1f/1day	59	96 (98)	2	4 months median	39
Thomas,[159] University Hospital, Leiden, 1976	65	ND	ND	71	ND	ND	100
Jensen and Roesdahl,[75] Radiumcenter, Copenhagen, 1976	64 (104)	3–7 Gy/1f/1day	62	85	6	4 months median	84
Qasim,[123] Weston Park Radiotherapy Hospital, Sheffield, 1977	315	8–10 Gy/1f/1day 20 Gy/5f/5days	55 56	83 84	10 15	ND ND	38
Penn,[113] London Hospital, Exeter, 1976	144 (223)	8–15 Gy/1f/1day 30 Gy/10f/2weeks	53 50	89 94	5 4	16% 2-year 20% 2-year	100
Allen et al,[2] Swedish Hospital, Seattle, 1976	110 (152)	10 Gy/2f/2days 20 Gy/8f/12days 20 Gy/5f/7days	ND	77 (85)	15	ND	60
		40 Gy/20f/45days 20 Gy/4f/4days 40 Gy/16f/25days	ND	78 (82)	18	ND	
		32 Gy/8f/10days 30 Gy/5f/7days 40 Gy/10f/12days	ND	80 (86)	14	ND	
Gilbert et al,[51] Kaiser Permanente, Los Angeles, 1977	158	30–40 Gy/3–4weeks 20 Gy/5f 13 Gy/2f	ND	73	ND	12 months median	43
Garmatis and Chu,[49] Memorial Sloan-Kettering, New York, 1978	75 (158)	20–25Gy/8–10f/2 weeks	20	75	ND	15 months median	100
Schocker and Brady,[139] Hahnemann Medical College, Philadelphia, 1982	(384)	20–50 Gy/1–4.5weeks	72	86	17	ND	53
Trodella et al,[164] Universita Cattolica del Sacra Cuore, Rome, 1984	79	20–40 Gy/ at 2–4 Gy/f	52 (67)	89 (95)	ND	ND	54

[a]Figures in parentheses represent results for only the patients with breast cancer.
CR = complete response.
PR = partial response.
f = fraction.
ND = no data.

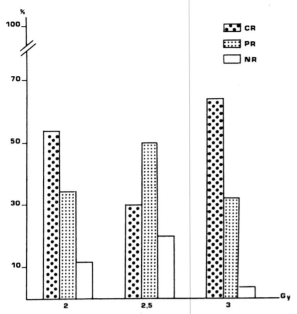

Figure 71–1 *Relationship of therapeutic response and daily dose in Gy for bone metastases (3 Gy = 300 cGy). The graph shows the percentage of complete, partial, and no responses obtained with various fraction (daily dose) sizes in a retrospective study of the effectiveness of various treatment regimens for palliation of bone metastases conducted at the Universita Cattolica del Sacro Cuore. CR = complete response, PR = partial response, NR = no response. (From Trodella L, Ausili-Cefaro G, Turriziani A, Marmiroli L, Cellini N, Nardone L: Pain in osseous metastases: Results of radiotherapy. Pain 18(4):392, 1984.)*

pain without narcotics has shown a benefit for the two more protracted, higher-dose treatment regimens (30 Gy in ten fractions and 40.5 Gy in 15 fractions) over the lower-dose, hypofractionated regimens (15, 20, or 25 Gy in five fractions). The complete

pain-relief parameter in this RTOG study was based on subjective reports by the patient, and the combined pain-relief parameter was based not only on the patient's subjective response but also on narcotic intake.

Time to Response

The time to response is usually rapid. Trodella and coworkers[164] reported that 60 percent of all patients respond within 5–7 days after beginning treatment. Tong and coworkers[162] reported that 96 percent of all patients achieving at least a minimal response to radiotherapy did so within 4 weeks of treatment, as did 50 percent of all patients achieving a complete response.

Duration of Response

Duration of response is difficult to assess, but one study found that more than 70 percent of patients who responded did not relapse in the treated site before death.[162] In an attempt to assess the durability of response, several studies have documented the percentage of patients responding to treatment who require retreatment of the same lesion. Retreatment rates range from 2 percent to 18 percent.[2, 75, 113, 123, 168] Retreatment rates underestimate the relapse rate, which ranges from 8.6 percent to 25 percent when documented.[2, 113] Two prospective randomized trials comparing different dose schedules have addressed the issue of duration of response.[92, 162] Madsen,[92] reporting on a trial conducted at the Royal Marsden Hospital of 8 Gy in one fraction compared with 30 Gy in ten fractions over 2 weeks, found no difference in durability of response between the two regimens. Tong and colleagues,[162] reporting on an RTOG trial

TABLE 71–2. PROSPECTIVE RANDOMIZED TRIALS OF VARIOUS RADIOTHERAPY REGIMENS FOR PALLIATION OF BONE METASTASES

Researchers	No. Patients	Type of Lesion	Dose/ No. Fractions/ Duration	CR (%)	CR + PR (%)	CR + PR in Breast Cancer Patients
Price et al,[122] Royal Marsden Hospital, London, 1986	288	ND	8 Gy/1f/1day	45	72	88%
			30 Gy/10f/2weeks	28	64	
Tong et al,[162] RTOG, 1982	1016	Solitary	40.5 Gy/15f/3weeks	61	92	*
			20 Gy/5f/1week	53	90	
		Multiple	30 Gy/10f/2weeks	57	92	
			15 Gy/5f/1week	49	89	
			20 Gy/5f/1week	56	89	
			25 Gy/5f/1week	40	87	
Madsen,[92] Odense University Hospital, Denmark, 1983	157	ND	24 Gy/6f/3weeks	ND	47	4/10
			20 Gy/2f/1week	ND	48	6/10
Hendrickson et al,[67] Rush-Presbyterian-St. Luke's, Chicago, 1976	86	ND	9 Gy/1f/1day	ND		
			12 Gy/2f	ND	86	82%
			15 Gy/5f	ND		
			20 Gy/10f	ND		
			20 Gy/5f	ND	70	
			30 Gy/10f	ND		

Note: For all dose-fractionation schedules, breast and lung cancer metastases responded significantly better than did other histological types.
CR = complete response.
PR = partial response.
f = fraction.
ND = no data.

TABLE 71–3. RESULTS OF RADIOTHERAPY OF BONE METASTASES

	Complete Pain Relief (Pain Score Only)	Preretreatment Complete Pain Relief (Pain Score Only)	Retreated	Complete Combined (Pain + Narcotic)
Solitary group				
2.7 Gy × 15 fractions	61% (45/74)	61% (45/74)	11% (8/74)	55% (38/69)
4.0 Gy × 5 fractions	53% (38/72)	49% (35/72)	24% (17/72)	37% (25/68)
Multiple group				
3.0 Gy × 10 fractions	57% (96/167)	55% (92/167)	12% (20/167)	46% (72/158)
3.0 Gy × 5 fractions	49% (70/143)	47% (67/143)	23% (33/143)	36% (48/135)
4.0 Gy × 5 fractions	56% (87/155)	52% (81/155)	15% (24/155)	40% (59/147)
5.0 Gy × 5 fractions	49% (72/148)	46% (68/148)	16% (23/148)	28% (39/137)
B_1 = *coefficient for number of fractions*				
Estimate	.0409	.0511	.0790	.0834
p value	.07	.02	.02	.0003

From Blitzer PH. Reanalysis of the RTOG study of the palliation of symptomatic osseous metastasis. Cancer 55:1468–1472, 1985, p 1469.

of various dose regimens stratified by whether the patient had solitary or multiple metastases, found no difference in duration of response between short, hypofractionated regimens and more protracted regimens delivering higher doses.

Schocker and Brady,[139] analyzing the same RTOG data, noted that retreatment rates appeared to be higher in the shorter, more hypofractionated regimens. In a reanalysis of the RTOG data with multivariate techniques, Blitzer[10] concluded that there was a significantly increased rate of retreatment following the shorter, hypofractionated regimens as well as a significant improvement in the rate of complete pain relief with the higher-dose, more protracted regimens (see Table 71–3). The rate of retreatment after the more protracted regimens was 11 percent and 12 percent for 40.5 Gy and 30 Gy, respectively, compared with 23 percent, 24 percent, 15 percent, and 16 percent for various treatment schedules that delivered 15 Gy, 20 Gy, and 25 Gy, respectively. For isolated bone metastases or a limited number of symptomatic sites, external-beam radiotherapy provides excellent palliation that lasts for the duration of the patient's life.

Pathological Fractures and Bone Healing After Radiotherapy

In the RTOG study of dose-fractionation regimens for the treatment of bone metastases, the rate of pathological fracture after radiotherapy was 8 percent when all sites were studied, 13 percent when only long bones were considered, and 6 percent when only spinal sites were considered.[162] In this study, the rate of pathological fracture in patients with a solitary metastasis was significantly higher after 40.5 Gy than after 20 Gy (18 percent versus 4 percent, p = .02). Other studies have not found a correlation between the risk of pathological fracture and the dose of radiotherapy.[113, 123]

Pathological fracture is a complication of malignancy that can frequently be avoided by attention to risk factors and prophylactic surgical intervention. Roentgenographic and clinical features that indicate a high risk of fracture include a lytic lesion greater than 2 cm in diameter on either anteroposterior or lateral view of the proximal femur, an avulsion fracture of the lesser trochanter, or destruction of more than 50 percent of the cortex at any level.

Persistent stress pain after radiotherapy may indicate fracture. The initial response of bone to radiotherapy is focal hyperemia, leading to localized osteoporosis and structural weakening. In a patient receiving radiotherapy for a bone metastasis, the period at highest risk for fracture is 10–18 days after beginning radiotherapy. Once a fracture has occurred, radiotherapy may interfere with the normal healing mechanism, resulting in nonunion.[12, 63] Bonarigo and Rubin[12] demonstrated that radiotherapy interferes with the chondrogenetic phase of osteoblastic proliferation required for fracture healing. In patients at risk for a pathological fracture, therefore, surgical intervention is best performed prophylactically before radiotherapy.

If fracture does not occur, frequently bone healing takes place after radiotherapy through a mechanism different from that required for fracture healing, not requiring a chondrogenetic phase.[63] Several researchers have reported roentgenographic evidence of healing of bone metastases from breast cancer and other malignancies after radiotherapy in 25–85 percent of cases.[16, 26, 49, 63] Bouchard[16] noted that there is no roentgenographic evidence of bone repair for at least 2 months after beginning radiotherapy and that optimum healing usually requires 6 months to 12 months.

The University of Kansas reported a series of 60 consecutive patients with bone metastasis who underwent 64 orthopedic stabilization procedures. Adjuvant postoperative radiotherapy was given to 35 of these patients. Multivariate analysis of prognostic and technical factors suggested that these patients receiving adjuvant radiotherapy were significantly more likely to regain normal use of their extremities and to undergo fewer reoperations on the same site.[163]

Side Effects and Complications

Side effects and complications of treatment are related to the site, treatment volume, and dose-fractionation regimen. Transient acute reactions of incidentally irradiated mucosa occur, causing sore throat with treatment of the cervical spine, dysphagia with treatment of the thoracic spine, and nausea, vomiting, and occasionally diarrhea with treatment of the lumbar spine. Transient erythematous skin reactions are most pronounced with orthovoltage treatment, are moderate with cobalt treatment, and are insignificant with higher-energy photon radiotherapy from accelerators.

Several researchers have reported more severe, though transient, nausea and vomiting lasting from a few hours up to 2 days with large single doses of radiotherapy to either the lumbar spine or pelvis[92, 113, 123, 168] than generally is observed with moderately fractionated treatment regimens. Additionally, Penn[113] reported a transient myelitis and Madsen[92] reported a permanent myelitis after a large single dose (10 Gy or 12 Gy) of radiotherapy to the lumbar spine.

Systemic Radioisotope Therapy

The use of systemic radioisotope administration either in addition to or as a replacement for external-beam radiotherapy has been revisited with the introduction of strontium chloride Sr^{89} (^{89}Sr) therapy. This therapy has proved effective in the treatment of bone metastasis from hormonally resistant prostate cancers in several randomized prospective trials and in the treatment of breast cancers and other blastic lesions.[115, 116, 124, 131] The rate of response for radioisotope treatment alone has been similar to that for external-beam radiotherapy, with an effective duration of approximately 3 months. In the treatment of patients with blastic bone metastasis from breast and prostate cancers,[89]Sr has been reported to provide pain relief in up to 80 percent of patients, with one fifth of patients becoming pain-free.[131] In a study of ^{89}Sr compared with hemibody radiotherapy or local radiotherapy as reported by Quilty and coworkers,[124] 65–70 percent of patients experienced some relief of pain with ^{89}Sr therapy, and 30–40 percent were able to significantly decrease their need for narcotic analgesics. When used in combination with local-field radiotherapy, systemic radioisotope therapy has demonstrated a potential benefit in delaying the symptomatic progression of disease at metastatic sites not initially symptomatic.[115, 124, 130, 131]

Patients treated with systemic radioisotope therapy (^{89}Sr) have a somewhat slower response for relief of pain, with a median time to response of 9 days (range, 3–25 days).[146] The duration of pain relief from radioisotope therapy has been reported in the range of 1.5–4 months.[115, 124, 146]

The main toxicity of systemic radioisotope therapy is bone marrow suppression, primarily transient thrombocytopenia and neutropenia with up to a 20–30 percent decrease in blood counts. The nadir occurs at 5–6 weeks, and partial to full recovery occurs by 12 weeks. Although this has not been a significant problem with the standard 4.0 mCi doses currently used, patients should be monitored closely. Robinson and coworkers[132] have recommended that baseline complete white blood cell and platelet counts be greater than 2.4 K and 60 K, respectively, with follow-up checks made every 2 weeks until stabilization.

Single-Dose Hemibody Radiotherapy

Several reports have documented the effect of single-dose hemibody radiotherapy on patients with widespread metastases.[7, 42, 118, 136, 140] Treatment is delivered to either the upper hemibody or the lower hemibody through equally weighted anterior and posterior fields. Doses of 4–8 Gy have been given to the upper hemibody and 8–10 Gy to the lower hemibody. The responses achieved with this approach are summarized in Table 71–4. Complete response rates have ranged from 20 percent to 65 percent and total response rates from 60 percent to 100 percent.

The time to response has been very short. Salazar and coworkers[136] reported that 50 percent of responses occurred within 48 hours and 80 percent within 1 week. Bartelink and coworkers[7] also noted that most responses occurred within 48 hours. In the study by Schorcht and coworkers,[140] the duration of response varied in different subsets of patients from 0 to 7.8 months; patients with long disease-free intervals before diagnosis of disseminated disease and a limited number of involved organ systems did best. In the study by Bartelink and coworkers,[7] the median duration for both complete and partial responses was approximately 3 months.

Salazar and coworkers,[136] analyzing data from the RTOG trial of hemibody radiotherapy, defined the parameter of *net pain relief* as the proportion of remaining life with relief of pain. The mean survival time for patients obtaining some pain relief was 30 weeks and the mean duration of pain relief was 15 weeks. Thus, the net pain relief was 50 percent. In the same RTOG study, 50 percent of patients did not require retreatment.[136]

The duration of response reported by Fitzpatrick and Garrett[42] was substantially longer, as was patient survival, possibly because all patients had had little or no prior therapy and all were premenopausal or perimenopausal and may have also benefited from ovarian ablation. In fact, 41 percent of premenopausal patients in their study showed indirect effects of the lower hemibody radiotherapy (i.e., tumor response in areas not treated). RTOG study 8206[118] has evaluated the use of hemibody radiotherapy as an adjuvant to local radiotherapy alone and documented an increase in time to disease progression and time to new disease occurrence within the irradiated hemibody field.

There were no occurrences of radiation pneumonitis or treatment-related fatalities associated with hemibody radiotherapy in the RTOG study with hemibody irradiation doses of 8 Gy. (Upper hemibody irradiation fields incorporated partial lung shielding to limit the dose to the lung to 7 Gy.) Significant,

TABLE 71–4. SINGLE-FRACTION HEMIBODY RADIOTHERAPY FOR MULTIPLE BONE METASTASES

Researchers	No. Patients and Dose	CR (%)	CR + PR (%)	Time to Response (hours)	Median Duration of Response (months)	Median Survival
Bartelink et al,[7] Antoni van Leeuwenhoek Hospital, Amsterdam, 1980	21 patients 8 Gy lower 6 Gy upper	57	100	<48	3	ND
Fitzpatrick and Garrett,[42] Princess Margaret Hospital, Toronto, 1981	34 patients 8–10 Gy lower	65	82	ND	17 (CR) 2 (PR)	58 weeks
Schorcht et al,[140] Medical Academy Carl Gustav Carus, Dresden, 1984	23 patients 8 Gy lower 4–8 Gy upper	ND	60	ND	5–7[a] 0–1[b] 7–8[c] 2–5[d]	7.7 months
Salazar et al,[136] ROTG 78-10, 1986	168 patients 8–10 Gy lower 6–7 upper	20	73	48	4	7.5 months
Poulter et al,[118] RTOG 82-06, 1992	229 patients 8 Gy lower and upper (7 Gy maximum to lung)	ND	ND	ND	12.6 months median time to new disease	33% at 12 months

[a]In patients with involvement of one or two systems.
[b]In patients with involvement of three or four systems.
[c]In patients with disease-free interval >2 years.
[d]In patients with disease-free interval ≤2 years.
CR = complete response.
PR = partial response.
ND = no data.

but transient hematopoietic toxicity did occur.[118] The morbidity of hemibody radiotherapy includes transient nausea, vomiting, diarrhea, bone marrow suppression, and occasional pneumonitis (Tables 71–5 and 71–6). When irradiation doses significantly greater than 6–7 Gy are delivered to the upper hemibody and lungs, pneumonitis has been reported and can be fatal.[46, 121, 137]

Treatment Recommendations

Because response rates are good with a variety of dose-fractionation regimens, high-dose, protracted treatment regimens that may occupy a significant proportion of most patients' lives are not indicated in the majority of cases. Because of the risk of severe late complications with high-dose, hypofractionated

TABLE 71–5. OVERALL TOXICITY OF MIDBODY RADIOTHERAPY AND LOWER HEMIBODY RADIOTHERAPY

	Acute (%)		Subacute (%)
Scale	Nausea and Vomiting	Diarrhea	Hematological
0 None	51	80	62
1 Mild	18	7	7
2 Moderate	22	10	21
3 Severe	7	1	3
4 Life-threatening	2	2	7
5 Fatal	0	0	0

From Salazar OM, Rubin P, Hendrickson FR, Komaki R, Poulter C, Newall J, Asbell SO, Mohiuddin M, van Ess J: Single-dose half-body irradiation for palliation of multiple bone metastases from solid tumors. Final Radiation Therapy Oncology Group report. Cancer 58:29–36, 1986, p 33.

regimens[62, 151] and the possibility of more durable responses with higher-dose, protracted regimens,[10] the majority of patients at the University of Florida are treated with an intermediate regimen of 30 Gy in ten fractions over 2 weeks.

Treatment is more aggressive in patients with a favorable presentation whose survival may be prolonged. For example, a patient with a solitary bone metastasis, high performance status, otherwise good health, and a high estrogen-receptor level or a long disease-free interval, may survive 5 to 10 years. In selected good-prognosis patients, a dose of 45–50 Gy over 5–5½ weeks is delivered. The objective of this regimen is to provide prolonged effective palliation to the treated site for the remainder of the patient's life in a single course of treatment, based on the conclusions of the RTOG reanalysis by Blitzer.[10]

For patients with a very poor prognosis and multiple metastases, hemibody or sequential hemibody radiotherapy is the recommended regimen of radiotherapeutic treatment. This approach saves the very ill patient many difficult trips to the radiotherapy clinic to receive treatment but still provides effective, rapid, and durable pain relief. The dose delivered to the upper hemibody is 6 Gy and to the lower hemibody is 8 Gy. Most patients are observed overnight in the hospital and are treated aggressively for the transient, but often significant, nausea and vomiting that may occur. When sequential treatment is given, a period of 4–6 weeks is usually required for marrow recovery before radiotherapy of the remaining body half should be given. For patients with very poor prognosis or performance status and localized symptoms of bone metastasis, a single localized treatment fraction of 8 Gy or 10 Gy may be administered.

TABLE 71–6. OVERALL TOXICITY OF UPPER HEMIBODY RADIOTHERAPY

	Acute (%)			Subacute (%)	
Scale	Nausea and Vomiting	Fever	Diarrhea	Hematological	Pneumonitis
0 None	45	87	94	37	97
1 Mild	13	5	3	5	3[a]
2 Moderate	26	8	3	26	0
3 Severe	16	3	0	21	0
4 Life-threatening	0	0	0	11	0
5 Fatal	0	0	0	0	0

[a]One patient; pneumonitis not fatal, lasted 1 week, treated symptomatically.
From Salazar OM, Rubin P, Hendrickson FR, Komaki R, Poulter C, Newall J, Asbell SO, Mohiuddin M, van Ess J: Single-dose half-body irradiation for palliation of multiple bone metastases from solid tumors. Final Radiation Therapy Oncology Group report. Cancer 58:29–36, 1986, p 34.

The use of ^{89}Sr systemic radiation treatment can also be considered for patients with multiple painful metastatic foci that demonstrate adequate tracer uptake by bone scan evaluation. If lesions are present in the spine or weight-bearing bones, the addition of localized external-beam radiotherapy may be warranted to further diminish the risk of pathological fracture resulting from early disease progression.

BRAIN METASTASES

One of the more common indications for palliative radiotherapy is brain metastasis. In most series reporting results of palliative irradiation for brain metastases, breast cancer is the primary malignancy in 20–40 percent of cases (Table 71–7).*

---

*See references 13, 27, 37, 52, 60, 70, 80, 104, 108, 149, and 171.

Response Rates

Response rates on the order of 60 percent are reported by most researchers (see Table 71–7). The median duration of survival after radiotherapy for brain metastases is approximately 5 months and is highly dependent on the presence or absence of systemic disease.[13, 105] The response rates for symptomatic palliation obtained in two RTOG studies are shown in Table 71–8.[15] The duration of response is difficult to assess. In one study, control of symptoms was documented at last follow-up in only 55 of the 242 patients for whom information was available.[171] In the RTOG trials, it was estimated that patients' symptoms remained palliated for 75 percent of their remaining life span.[15] As can be anticipated based on clinical experience, those patients with minimal intracranial disease burden but with progressive systemic disease can be predicted to have the highest

TABLE 71–7. NONCONTROLLED STUDIES OF PALLIATION OF BRAIN METASTASES WITH RADIOTHERAPY

Researchers	No. Patients	Percent with Breast Cancer	Response Rate (%)	Median Duration of Survival
Chu and Hilaris,[27] Memorial Hospital, New York, 1961	218	39	86[a]	6.7 months[b] 2.2 months[c]
Order et al,[108] Yale, New Haven, 1968	108	14	60	6.3 months
Hindo et al,[70] Presbyterian-St. Luke's, Chicago, 1970	54	21	65	5.6 months
Nisce et al,[104] Memorial Hospital, New York, 1971	560	39	80[a]	6 months[a]
Gilbert et al,[52] Southern California Permanente, Los Angeles, 1978	90	23	48 (10/21)	3–7 months
West and Maor,[171] M. D. Anderson Cancer Center, Houston, 1980	350	42	75	5.7 months
Snee et al,[149] Western General Hospital, Edinburgh, 1985	90	100	81	4 months
Eqawa et al,[37] National Cancer Center Hospital, Tokyo, 1986	254	11	44[d]	4.6 months
Komarnicky et al,[80] Thomas Jefferson University Hospital, Philadelphia, 1991 (RTOG 79-16)	859	12	ND	3.9 weeks[e]
Boogerd et al,[13] The Netherlands Cancer Institute, Amsterdam, 1993	137	100	ND	16 weeks[f]
Haie-Meder et al,[60] Institut Gustave-Roussy, Villejuif, France, 1993	216	25–33	ND 2–3 months median	4.2 months ± 5.3 months[g]

[a]Of breast cancer patients who completed prescribed treatment.
[b]In responders.
[c]In nonresponders.
[d]Breast cancer only.
[e]Patients treated by 3 Gy × 10; 5 Gy × 6; 5 Gy × 6 + misonidazole; 3 Gy × 10 + misonidazole.
[f]Patients treated with courses of radiotherapy/resection.
[g]Radiotherapy by 6 Gy in 3 fractions (two courses); 6 Gy in three fractions + 25 Gy in ten fractions.
ND, no data.

TABLE 71–8. SPECIFIC NEUROLOGICAL SYMPTOM RELIEF WITH BRAIN RADIOTHERAPY

Symptom	First Study			Second Study		
	No. Pts.	CR (%)	CR + PR (%)	No. Pts.	CR (%)	CR + PR (%)
Headache	500	52	82	482	69	82
Motor loss	454	32	74	456	37	61
Impaired mentation	355	34	71	425	52	69
Cerebellar dysfunction	218	39	75	259	50	64
Cranial nerve	215	40	71	244	44	59
Increased intracranial pressure	165	57	83	ND	ND	ND
Convulsions, general	108	66	86			
Convulsions, focal	85	58	76	134	87	90
Sensory loss	175	41	77	ND	ND	ND
Lethargy	237	39	69	ND	ND	ND

CR = complete response.
PR = partial response.
ND = no data.
From Borgelt BB, Gelber R, Kramer S, Brady LW, Chang CH, Davis LW, Perez CA, Hendrickson FR: The palliation of brain metastases: Final results of the first two studies by the Radiation Therapy Oncology Group. Int J Radiat Oncol Biol Phys 6:1–9, 1980, p 6. Copyright 1980 by Elsevier Science Inc.

probability of functional central nervous system capacity until the time of death.

Dose

The Princess Margaret Hospital conducted a prospective randomized trial of various dose-fractionation schemes in patients irradiated for brain metastases.[43] The two regimens tested were 10 Gy delivered in a single fraction and 30 Gy delivered in ten fractions over 2 weeks. There was no statistically significant difference in response rates, with responses obtained in 57 percent of the patients receiving 10 Gy and 64 percent of the patients receiving 30 Gy.

The RTOG conducted two prospective randomized trials evaluating the efficacy of various dose-fractionation schemes.[15] In the first study, patients were randomized to receive 30 Gy in either 2 or 3 weeks or 40 Gy in either 3 or 4 weeks. In the second trial, patients were randomized to receive 20 Gy in 1 week, 30 Gy in 2 weeks, or 40 Gy in 3 weeks. No benefit was demonstrated for any regimen. A subset analysis performed on favorable subgroups of patients, including ambulatory breast cancer patients with no soft-tissue metastases, also showed no advantage with any of the dose-fractionation regimens tested.[50]

A third trial compared conventional fractionation with an accelerated hyperfractionation scheme employing multiple daily treatments. Patients received either 30 Gy delivered in ten fractions over 2 weeks or 30 Gy delivered in 15 fractions, three a day, over 1 week.[32] No difference was found between conventional treatment and multiple daily fractions in terms of response rate, neurological improvement, survival, or morbidity.

A prospective trial conducted at the Institut Gustave-Roussy, France, randomized 216 patients to receive either 18 Gy given in three fractions over 3 days or the same fractionation followed by a second course of treatment after a 1-month time interval. The second treatment course either was identical to the first or consisted of 25 Gy in ten fractions over 14

days. No differences were noted for overall survival, neurological response, or the incidence of complications. Again, the factors most prognostic for overall survival were the presence of multiple versus solitary brain metastasis and the presence of extracranial metastases.[60]

The use of misonidazole as a radiosensitizer was evaluated by the RTOG (protocol 7916) in the treatment of patients with brain metastases. Although the majority of patients in this study had primary lung cancers, 12 percent had breast cancers as their primary malignancy. No differences were found in any treatment arm, either by the use of misonidazole or the radiation dosage fractionation scheme used (ten fractions of 3 Gy each versus six fractions of 5 Gy each). It was the conclusion of this randomized study that the treatment of choice for the majority of patients still remains a conventional palliative course of 30 Gy in ten daily fractions.[80]

Corticosteroids

Borgelt and coworkers[15] have suggested that patients treated with steroids and radiation may obtain a more rapid response than patients treated with radiation only. In a comprehensive review of the role of glucocorticoid treatment for brain metastases and epidural spinal cord compression, Weissman[170] found that steroids decrease or prevent peritumoral edema. The primary role of steroids is to rapidly improve or stabilize neurological deficits until definitive treatment is underway. Steroids are also useful in managing steroid-reversible neurological deficits in patients after completion of definitive therapy and at the time of tumor progression. It is not clear that steroids are beneficial for neurologically intact patients, but their routine use has been adopted at many centers as a prophylaxis against transient swelling and edema of the tumor or tumors when radiation treatment is initiated.

Weissman[170] recommends a starting dose of 16 mg per day of dexamethasone with tapering of the dose once definitive treatment is underway. It is recommended that the overall steroid course should last no longer than 14–21 days for most patients. The dose may be escalated to 100 mg per day in patients with progressive neurological deficits; after a 7-day trial, the dose should be tapered to the lowest dose that will maintain stable neurological function.

The only indication for long-term steroid treatment is the presence of a steroid-reversible deficit, not a fixed neurological deficit. The potential toxicity from prolonged steroid therapy includes not only weight gain, change in facial appearance, striae, acne, and emotional and sleep disturbances, but also life-threatening problems such as diabetes, susceptibility to infections, peripheral edema, gastrointestinal perforation, and psychosis.

Side Effects and Complications

In most series, overall side effects are minimal and limited to transient alopecia. Treatment regimens using high-dose single-fraction or hypofractionated therapy tend to produce more of both acute and late complications than conventional-fractionation regimens. In the prospective randomized trial from Princess Margaret Hospital comparing two dose-fractionation schemes, acute complications consisting of headache, nausea, vomiting, increased neurological deficit, and decrease in the level of consciousness occurred in 47 percent of patients receiving 10 Gy and in 27 percent of patients receiving 30 Gy.[43] In a study of patients treated with 10 Gy in a single fraction, Hindo and coworkers[70] reported deaths within 48 hours of treatment in three of 54 patients, all of whom had severe neurological deficits. Sundaresan and coworkers[154] reported three cases of radiation necrosis resulting in severe debility or death after treatment regimens employing high doses per fraction and high overall doses (39 Gy in 11 fractions to the whole brain).

Solitary Brain Metastasis

Historically, long-term survivors were reported after aggressive treatment of solitary metastasis from breast cancer as well as renal carcinoma,[36] and several reports suggested a benefit to surgical resection with and without postoperative whole-brain radiotherapy.[36, 48, 169] Postoperative mortality, in early reports from the 1960s, was on the order of 15 percent.[128, 169] Smalley and coworkers[147] demonstrated that whole-brain radiotherapy after surgical resection results in a decrease in the subsequent incidence of brain relapse and may prolong survival. In the group of 1895 patients treated in the two RTOG trials of various dose-fractionation schemes discussed earlier, 218 patients had undergone prior surgery (either biopsy or surgical resection of a solitary metastasis).[66] When these patients were stratified according to neurological function at presentation, no improvement in neurological function was seen with the addition of surgery. Palliation of headache and

motor-loss symptoms, however, was greater in patients whose metastasis was surgically resected before radiotherapy. The greatest advantage was observed in patients with no extracerebral disease.

Two prospective trials have evaluated the relative roles and potential benefits of neurosurgical resection and postoperative whole-brain radiotherapy for solitary brain metastasis (Table 71–9).[105, 110] Patchell and coworkers[110] from the University of Kentucky randomized patients to either surgical resection followed by whole-brain radiotherapy (36 Gy in 12 fractions) or treatment by radiotherapy alone. The majority of patients in this study had non–small-cell carcinoma of the lung as the primary malignancy. Combined surgery plus radiotherapy showed a significant advantage over radiotherapy for three outcome measures. First, local recurrence was less frequent in the surgically treated patients (20 percent compared with 52 percent in the radiotherapy-alone group). Second, overall survival was longer in the surgical group (40 weeks median versus only 15 weeks in the radiotherapy-alone group). Finally, surgically treated patients were also functionally independent for a longer time (38 weeks versus 8 weeks in the radiotherapy-alone patients). The researchers concluded that surgical resection of solitary metastases produced both a significant functional and survival benefit in this patient population.

Noordijk and colleagues[105] of the University Hospital Leiden (Leiden, Netherlands) also conducted a randomized trial of neurosurgery plus radiotherapy compared with radiotherapy alone. Radiotherapy was delivered at 2 Gy twice daily, amounting to a total dosage of 40 Gy in 2 weeks. The most significant finding regarding the treatment groups was for the patients with no active extracranial disease. Median survival was 12 months for patients treated by surgical resection plus radiotherapy compared with 7 months for those treated by radiotherapy alone. The investigators concluded that for patients with solitary brain metastasis and either no extracranial disease or stable extracranial disease, surgical resection may provide a significant survival advantage.

Radiosurgery and Brachytherapy

A limited experience has been reported from several centers on the use of single-fraction high-dose (20–30 Gy) radiotherapy of brain metastases using stereotactic radiosurgery delivered by either linear accelerator or gamma knife technology.* There is also a limited experience with interstitial implantation of brain metastases by stereotactic placement of afterloading catheters.[69, 119] Both approaches offer the potential for selective high-dose radiotherapy of the tumor volume with minimal exposure of normal brain tissue, and both can be applied to either the primary treatment of metastatic lesions or the retreatment of recurrent lesions.

Currently, stereotactic radiosurgery is the predom-

---

*See references 20, 44, 47, 77, 88, 99, 100, and 152.

TABLE 71–9. CONTROLLED STUDIES OF PALLIATION OF BRAIN METASTASES WITH SURGERY OR RADIOTHERAPY

Researchers	No. Patients	Percent with Breast Cancer	Median Duration of Survival	
			Surgery and Radiotherapy	Radiotherapy Alone
Patchell et al,[110] University of Kentucky Medical Center, Lexington, 1990	48	3/48 (6)	40 weeks	15 weeks
Noordijk et al,[105] University Hospital Leiden, 1994	66	12/66 (18)	10 months	6 months

inant treatment used for the majority of patients, based on satisfactory response and control rates without the need for surgical penetration of the cranium. Control of the metastatic lesions has been reported to be in the range of 80–88 percent, with median patient survival durations of 4–6.5 months, depending on patient selection criteria in each series. The necessity of additional whole-brain radiotherapy to achieve effective prophylaxis of the entire brain parenchyma and ensure regional control within the cranium has been emphasized in both the Stanford University and University of Florida series.[20, 47] Further experience and follow-up will be required to define the patient population, indications, and treatment parameters to best optimize the use of stereotactic radiosurgery as a radiotherapy technique.

Retreatment

Several studies have reported responses in one third to one half of patients given a second course of radiotherapy for recurrent brain metastases.[43, 81, 104, 108] Responses lasting an average of 1.5–2.6 months were obtained in 50–69 percent of patients undergoing second and third courses of radiotherapy at Rush-Presbyterian Medical Center.[142] In a study from the University of Colorado, however, Hazuka and Kinzie[65] found neurological improvement in only 27 percent of the 44 patients undergoing retreatment. The median survival after a second course of radiotherapy was only 8 weeks. Brain necrosis occurred in three patients, causing death in two. The investigators concluded that retreatment was seldom worthwhile.

The Institut Gustave-Roussy tested a regimen in which half the patients were randomized to receive a repeat course of radiotherapy after a 1-month treatment break. No differences in neurological response or complications were seen between single-course and repeat-course treatment protocols, and the most significant prognostic factor was the extent of disease.[60] Radiosurgical techniques have been applied to the treatment of recurrent lesions, with principles of treatment similar to those discussed earlier for the treatment of solitary brain metastasis.[90] Further follow-up is necessary to determine the ultimate value of this approach.

Treatment Recommendations

Steroid therapy is initiated for all symptomatic patients to achieve as rapid a clinical response as possible. The steroid dosage is tapered off after radiotherapy is started and symptomatic improvement is evident. The standard course of radiotherapy for the majority of patients is to irradiate the whole brain with up to 30 Gy in ten fractions of 3 Gy daily, administered over 2 weeks. In patients who have solitary lesions, as determined by contrast-enhanced magnetic resonance imaging (MRI), and who are judged to have a favorable prognosis because of a long disease-free interval, control of the primary disease, and no evidence of extracerebral metastases, surgical resection is performed if feasible before whole-brain radiotherapy. For patients treated after neurosurgical resection, the whole brain is irradiated with up to 45 Gy in 25 fractions at 1.8 Gy once daily; the dose to the tumor bed is boosted with an additional 5–10 Gy (Fig. 71–2). If surgical resection is incomplete or not feasible, consideration may be given to using radiosurgical techniques to deliver the boost dosage after completing whole-brain radiotherapy.

SPINAL CORD COMPRESSION

Evaluation

Spinal cord compression complicates the course of disseminated cancer in 5 percent of cases and represents a true oncologic emergency.[129] Breast cancer accounts for the primary malignancy in 15–25 percent of cases of spinal cord compression secondary to metastatic cancer.* The first symptom of epidural cord compression is pain in 80–95 percent of cases (Table 71–10).[6, 21, 53, 98] The pain may be axial, radicular, or referred and is characteristically aggravated by movement but not alleviated by recumbency. At the time of diagnosis, sensory and motor symptoms are common; sphincter dysfunction is less common and indicates an advanced lesion and a poor prognosis.[174] A high index of suspicion is imperative, as the outcome of treatment is dependent on early diagnosis

---

*See references 8, 21, 31, 53, 76, 86, 98, 173, and 177.

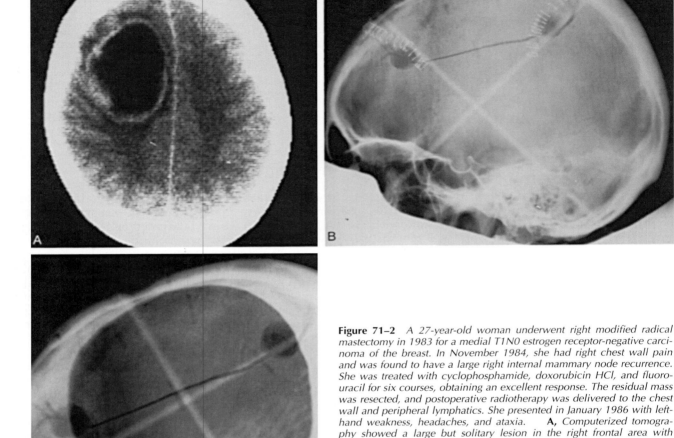

Figure 71–2   *A 27-year-old woman underwent right modified radical mastectomy in 1983 for a medial T1N0 estrogen receptor-negative carcinoma of the breast. In November 1984, she had right chest wall pain and was found to have a large right internal mammary node recurrence. She was treated with cyclophosphamide, doxorubicin HCl, and fluorouracil for six courses, obtaining an excellent response. The residual mass was resected, and postoperative radiotherapy was delivered to the chest wall and peripheral lymphatics. She presented in January 1986 with left-hand weakness, headaches, and ataxia.   **A,** Computerized tomography showed a large but solitary lesion in the right frontal area with moderate mass effect. Craniotomy was performed with gross resection of the fluid-filled cystic mass, which was consistent histologically with her primary breast cancer. After surgery, all neurological signs and symptoms resolved.   **B,** Postoperatively, she received 45 Gy to the whole brain in 25 fractions over 5 weeks, followed by   **(C)** a 5-Gy boost dose to the tumor bed delivered in three fractions through reduced lateral and anterior portals with wedge filters. Although other sites of distant disease developed, there was no further evidence of disease in the brain at the time of her death in August 1986.*

and initiation of treatment while neurological symptoms are minimal.[19, 53, 59, 97]

Cord compression from metastatic disease may result from direct tumor extension through intervertebral foramina from mediastinal or retroperitoneal lymph nodes, soft-tissue extension from metastatic disease in vertebral bodies, vertebral collapse from tumor destruction, or intramedullary metastases. Most cord compressions in patients with metastatic breast cancer are complications of vertebral metastases (85 percent of cases) or metastases in the paravertebral spaces (10–15 percent of cases). Metastasis to the epidural space and intramedullary metastases are rare.[22, 53, 176]

Results of Treatment

Spinal cord compression traditionally has been treated by radiotherapy alone[53, 103, 112] or by laminec-tomy with or without postoperative radiotherapy.[173] Studies retrospectively comparing results in patients treated with these three approaches have failed to conclusively demonstrate a better result with the addition of laminectomy.[29, 53, 174] Two studies specifically addressing the role of radiotherapy after laminectomy have shown better motor recovery with laminectomy plus postoperative radiotherapy than with laminectomy alone.[174, 177]

White and coworkers[173] noted that a substantial number of patients who recovered the ability to ambulate after surgery subsequently lost it because of local recurrence. In a prospective study of surgical resection for spinal metastasis in which 44 percent of patients were nonambulatory before decompression, all achieved ambulation postoperatively.[153] The surgical complication rate for this group of patients was 15 percent.[153] The only prospective randomized trial comparing laminectomy and postoperative ra-

TABLE 71–10. SIGNS AND SYMPTOMS OF EPIDURAL SPINAL CORD COMPRESSION IN 130 PATIENTS

Sign/Symptom	First Symptoms No. Patients	Symptoms at Diagnosis No. Patients
Pain	125 (96%)	125 (96%)
Weakness	2 (2%)	99 (76%)
Autonomic dysfunction	0	74 (57%)
Sensory loss	0	66 (51%)
Ataxia	2 (2%)	4 (3%)
Herpes zoster	0	3 (2%)
Flexor spasms	0	2 (2%)

From Gilbert RW, Kin JH, Posner JB: Epidural spinal cord compression from metastatic tumor: Diagnosis and treatment. Ann Neurol 3:40–51, 1978, p 42.

diotherapy with radiotherapy alone demonstrated no advantage with either regimen for pain relief, improved ambulation, or sphincter function.[179]

The results of several studies relating prognosis for ambulation to initial functional status are shown in Table 71–11.[86, 97, 173, 174, 177] Recovery of ambulation is rare in patients who are paraplegic at presentation.* It is likely that the only paraplegic patients with a reasonable chance of recovery are those in whom the paralysis is of very short duration,[94] usually less than 24 hours. Therefore, as soon as the diagnosis of cord compression is made, emergent treatment is indicated.

A second important prognostic factor is the degree of blockage of cerebrospinal flow demonstrated at myelography (Table 71–12). In a trial of radiotherapy with or without preceding laminectomy,[179] six of seven patients who had neither paraplegia nor complete blockage at myelography were ambulatory after treatment. In contrast, only eight of 19 patients with

*See references 6, 61, 150, 161, 173, 174, and 177.

complete myelographic block but no clinical paraplegia were ambulatory after treatment. Four months after treatment, four of seven patients without complete block remained ambulatory, compared with only six of 19 patients with complete block. Other factors indicating a poor prognosis are rapid progression of symptoms, vertebral collapse, elevated protein in the cerebrospinal fluid, and complete sensory loss.[102]

Side Effects and Complications

The risks and potential complications of surgical resection are significant, and patient selection should be careful.[64] Early series reported laminectomy mortality rates of 8 percent,[177] but subsequent series showed few nontumor-related deaths with surgery or radiotherapy.[179] Side effects and complications of radiotherapy are similar to those observed after palliative radiotherapy for bone metastases.

Treatment Recommendations

Patients suspected of having cord compression require immediate imaging of the spinal canal to either confirm or rule out the diagnosis of epidural disease with compression. At one time, myelography was the standard for evaluation of spinal cord compression, but now magnetic resonance imaging (MRI) is considered the diagnostic test of choice at most centers. MRI has been shown to be equal to myelography in the detection of epidural disease and, in some cases, superior for the evaluation of vertebral and paravertebral lesions.[22, 24, 87, 148, 155] MRI has the advantage of being a fast, safe, and noninvasive technique, but when it is not available or when patients cannot tolerate the procedure (because of claustrophobia or excessive motion), then myelography should be obtained promptly.

TABLE 71–11. RESULTS OF TREATMENT OF SPINAL CORD COMPRESSION

Pretherapy Function	Posttherapy Function (Percent of Patients Treated)		
	Ambulatory	Nonambulatory	Paraplegic
Ambulatory			
Memorial Hospital, New York[173]	64	22	14
Massachusetts General Hospital, Boston[177]	53	37	10
Long Beach VA Hospital, California[174]	1/3 patients	—	2/3 patients
Rambam Medical Center, Haifa, Israel[86]	66	—	—
Policlinico-Monteluce, Perugia, Italy[97]	97	3	—
Nonambulatory			
Memorial Hospital, New York[173]	34	47	19
Massachusetts General Hospital, Boston[177]	37	30	33
Long Beach VA Hospital, California[174]	71	14	14
Rambam Medical Center, Haifa, Israel[86]	30	—	—
Policlinico-Monteluce, Perugia, Italy[97]	74	22	4
Paraplegic			
Memorial Hospital, New York[173]	10	14	76
Massachusetts General Hospital, Boston[177]	0	11	89
Long Beach VA Hospital, California[174]	31	26	43
Rambam Medical Center, Haifa, Israel[86]	16	—	—
Policlinico-Monteluce, Perugia, Italy[97]	33	—	67

TABLE 71–12.   EFFECT OF MYELOGRAPHIC BLOCK ON 29 PATIENTS WITH SPINAL EPIDURAL MESTASTASES: MOTOR PERFORMANCE

	No Block		Block	
Results	*No. Patients*	*No. Ambulatory*	*No. Patients*	*No. Ambulatory*
Immediate results				
Ambulatory	4	4 (100%)	7	4 (57%)
Not ambulatory	3	2 (67%)	12	4 (33%)
Paraplegic	0	0	3	0
At 4 months				
Ambulatory	4	3 (75%)	7	2 (29%)
Not ambulatory	3	1 (33%)	12	4 (33%)
Paraplegic	0	0	3	0

From Young RF, Post EM, King GA: Treatment of spinal epidural metastases. Randomized prospective comparison of laminectomy and radiotherapy. J Neurosurg 53:741–748, 1980, p 744.

Neurosurgical evaluation for decompressive laminectomy should be considered in cases of previously irradiated areas of disease, compression secondary to vertebral collapse, diagnosis when the primary tumor is not known, compression secondary to relatively less radioresponsive tumors (e.g., melanoma and sarcoma), and symptomatic progression during the course of radiotherapy.[141, 144, 156, 179] The majority of patients with breast cancer do not require laminectomy and should be started on a course of treatment with corticosteroids and radiotherapy after a diagnosis of malignancy is confirmed and the full extent of the disease is determined.[41, 117, 145, 179] A dose of 30 Gy delivered in ten fractions of 3 Gy over 2 weeks is generally given. In patients who are paraplegic or have severe weakness, 4–5 Gy may be given once or twice, followed by smaller fractions (2.5–2.75 Gy) for the remainder of the treatment course, as experimental and clinical data suggest that higher initial daily doses are safe and may result in better responses.[134]

In planning the radiotherapy treatment portal(s), it is important to carefully review the imaging studies to determine disease extent, as the clinical examination may frequently indicate a sensory level deficit two to three vertebral levels below the actual lesion. The precise localization of the compressive lesion is critical, as it has been shown that a high proportion of the recurrences after radiotherapy are in lesions outside the treatment field that were present at the time of diagnosis but were missed by the treatment portal.[89] Another study demonstrated that 75 percent of portals planned on the basis of clinical findings and plain roentgenograms were inadequate to cover the disease apparent on myelography.[23]

If radiotherapy must be administered without the availability of MRI or myelographic imaging, then bone-detail radiographs of the entire spine and nuclear bone scan should be performed to ensure that the site of probable cord compression is limited to a single location.[114, 126] The policy at the University of Florida Dept. of Radiation Oncology is that the treatment portals should include two vertebral bodies above and below the lesion defined at MRI or myelography and any immediately adjacent asymptomatic lesions. Once treatment has been initiated, the patients must be monitored closely; if the neurological defect progresses during the course of radiotherapy, decompressive laminectomy should be considered, as some patients may still regain function and potentially the ability to ambulate.[29]

As in the treatment of brain metastases, corticosteroids also play an important role in the treatment of symptomatic spinal cord compression. When spinal cord compression is either suggested clinically or detected by radiological imaging, the patient should be started promptly on a course of corticosteroid therapy with the goal of improving neurological function by decreasing localized edema and inflammation. Dexamethasone is the most common agent used, but the best dosage remains controversial. Laboratory data have shown a dose-related benefit to steroid use, which has led some researchers to recommend intravenous loading doses as high as 100 mg.[33, 117] Doses of 10–100 mg as an immediate intravenous loading dose followed by 4–24 mg four times a day have been suggested by Byrne,[21] and the authors of this chapter (Zlotecki and Mendenhall) agree with this recommendation. Again, it is most important to initiate tapering of the steroid dosage as soon as possible to minimize the risks of acute and late side effects of glucocorticoid therapy.

CHOROID METASTASES

Evaluation

Metastatic cancers are the most common intraocular tumors, and the most common intraocular site affected by metastases is the choroid.[11, 40] Within the choroid, the posterior pole on the temporal side of the macula is the site most frequently affected by metastatic spread.[28, 127, 138] Breast cancer is the primary malignancy, accounting for 60–70 percent of all metastatic choroid lesions.* Choroid metastases usually occur in conjunction with widespread metastases in other sites, but they are the first sign of distant metastases in 20–30 percent of cases.[28, 96, 158]

---

*See references 11, 34, 40, 45, 54, 71, 73, 109, 125, and 175.

Bilateral involvement occurs in 25–40 percent of cases.* The incidence of intracranial metastasis in patients with choroidal metastasis is no greater than in patients with breast cancer metastatic to other sites.[35] In a series of 152 patients presenting with ocular complaints and a history of breast cancer at the M.D. Anderson Cancer Center, 38 percent were found to have choroid metastases.[101] In 98 asymptomatic patients with a history of breast cancer, 9 percent were discovered to have incidental choroid metastases on screening examination. All patients found to have incidental choroid metastases had known stage IV disease, for a 14 percent rate of choroid involvement in asymptomatic stage IV disease.

Choroid metastasis represents a significant clinical problem because of its potential to produce debilitating complications of blindness or glaucoma. Blindness results from mechanical elevation and detachment of the retina by the metastatic tumor, and glaucoma may result from increased intraocular pressure resulting from either rapid tumor growth, venous congestion from pressure on choroid vessels, or blockage of the iris angle by tumor or anterior motion of the lens.[107] Initially, the most common symptoms are blurred vision, scotomata, pain, and photophobia.[28] Choroid metastases may exhibit rapid growth, leading to blindness within days or weeks of initial presentation; thus, prompt diagnosis and treatment are necessary to prevent an irreversible and symptomatic disability.

Results of Treatment

One third to one half of patients will have a marked response or a complete resolution of symptoms after radiotherapy.[28, 34, 106, 109, 125, 158] Another third will obtain a partial response or a stabilization of disease, and in only a few patients will the disease progress after radiotherapy.[28, 34, 35, 109, 125] Chu and coworkers[28] noted that 100 percent of patients responded to radiotherapy when lesions occupied less than half a quadrant of the eye ground. Also, 77 percent of patients with lesions involving more than half of a quadrant with minimal or no retinal detachment responded. In contrast, only 37 percent of patients with moderate to massive retinal detachment showed improvement. Most responses to radiotherapy occur within 3–4 weeks, but when retinal detachment has occurred, responses may be delayed because of slow resorption of subretinal fluids.[158]

Treatment Recommendations

Although there are reports of response to hormonal therapy[30, 38, 78] and chemotherapy,[57, 78] radiotherapy has proved both effective and safe. In patients with choroidal metastasis, radiotherapy is the preferred treatment; chemotherapy or surgery should be re-

served for the lesions not responsive to radiotherapy or recurring after radiotherapy.

The standard treatment technique for choroid metastasis is conventional external-beam photon radiotherapy. Doses of 30 Gy in ten fractions over 2 weeks or 40 Gy in 20 fractions over 4 weeks have been demonstrated to be effective. Lesions confined to the posterior pole are adequately treated with a single lateral 4 × 4 cm field. The anterior field edge is positioned posterior to the lens, which is the most radiosensitive structure in the eye.

The field is angled 5 degrees posteriorly to avoid divergent irradiation of the contralateral lens. For patients with bilateral involvement, opposed lateral fields are used with either a 5-degree posterior tilt on both fields or anterior half-beam blocks placed to eliminate divergence.

Side effects and complications of standard photon beam therapy are rare.[28, 91, 101, 109] In a series from the Karolinska Hospital, only three of 21 eyes treated developed signs of radioretinopathy, and in only one case was vision compromised.[106] Electron-beam[28] and proton-beam[58] radiotherapy have been used in attempts to limit irradiation of normal tissue structures. Electron-beam therapy suffers from the disadvantage of producing a very significant skin reaction, which does not occur with standard high-energy photon radiotherapy. Proton-beam radiotherapy is generally inaccessible to most patients, very expensive, and not necessary for effective palliation.

Responses to both chemotherapy[18, 85] and hormonal therapy[30, 38, 78] have been reported, so patients diagnosed incidentally with asymptomatic choroid metastases who are already undergoing systemic therapy may be observed closely before focal ocular radiotherapy is begun. Radiotherapy should be instituted at the first sign of progression, however, as results may depend on the extent of tumor.[28]

LIVER METASTASES

The prognosis for patients with hepatic metastases is quite poor. The median survival in 390 patients with untreated liver metastases was 75 days, with only 7 percent of patients surviving more than a year.[74] The signs and symptoms most often associated with liver metastases are abdominal pain, nausea and vomiting, fevers and night sweats, ascites, anorexia, abdominal distention, jaundice, weakness, and fatigue.

Conventional Radiotherapy

In an excellent discussion of the role of radiotherapy in the treatment of liver metastases, Kinsella[79] emphasized that the primary limitation in the use of radiotherapy in the treatment of hepatic metastases is the limited tolerance of normal liver parenchyma to radiotherapy. The clinical syndrome indicating acute radiation damage is radiation hepatitis, which usually occurs within 2–6 weeks of treatment and

---

*See references 28, 34, 73, 96, 101, 125, 133, and 158.

can be fatal.[72] This syndrome and its relation to radiation parameters of treatment volume, dose, and fraction size (daily dose) have been studied by Ingold and coworkers[72] from Stanford University. The syndrome is uncommon after doses to the whole liver of less than 30–35 Gy delivered in fractions of 2 Gy or less per day. Other data suggest that the threshold for radiation hepatitis may be as low as 25 Gy when the daily dose is greater than 2 Gy.[172] When smaller volumes of liver are treated, doses as high as 55 Gy can be administered without severe toxicity.[72] Treatment regimens employing dose-fractionation schemes and three-dimensional conformal radiotherapy techniques that might limit the potential for radiation hepatitis are being investigated by Lawrence and coworkers.[82]

Several series have documented excellent palliative results with radiotherapy.[120, 143, 165] Total response rates ranged from 70 percent to 90 percent with up to 44 percent obtaining complete pain relief.[120, 143] Improvement in jaundice and ascites was occasionally noted as well.[120] Sherman and coworkers[143] noted that pain relief usually persisted for most of the remainder of the patient's life. The RTOG conducted a prospective nonrandomized study of optimal doses for patients with either solitary or multiple liver metastases.[14] For patients with solitary liver metastases, participating investigators were allowed a choice of 20.4 Gy in 19 fractions or 30 Gy in 15 fractions to the entire liver, each with an optional 20 Gy boost dose to the metastasis. For patients with multiple liver metastases, the options were 30 Gy in 15 fractions, 25.6 Gy in 16 fractions, 20 Gy in ten fractions, or 21 Gy in seven fractions. The median survival for this patient population was 11 weeks; 22 percent of patients died less than 4 weeks after treatment, and 20 percent lived more than 6 months after treatment. No differences in outcome were noted among the various regimens. A higher proportion of patients with multiple metastases completed the treatment regimen of 21 Gy in seven fractions, in contrast to a more protracted regimen. Response rates for various signs and symptoms of hepatic metastases are shown in Table 71–13. Patients with mild symptoms before treatment spent 80 percent of their remaining life with mild or no pain; patients with moderate or severe pain spent 63 percent of their remaining life with only mild or no pain.

Continued efforts have been made by the RTOG to improve the effectiveness of hepatic radiotherapy. An analysis of two RTOG studies of liver metastases (RTOG 7605 and 8003) was performed to identify the patient characteristics associated with a favorable prognosis for survival. The probability of surviving at least 6 months was influenced by performance score, primary tumor site, and the presence or absence of extrahepatic metastases.[83] The feasibility of radiotherapy dose escalation to the whole liver was then tested in this "good prognosis" population of patients with hepatic metastasis from primary gastrointestinal tract cancers. An accelerated hyperfractionated dosage scheme was used. The whole liver

TABLE 71–13.   THERAPEUTIC BENEFIT OF HEPATIC RADIOTHERAPY (FOURTH-WEEK ASSESSMENT)

Sign/Symptom	No. Patients Responding[a]/No. Patients Evaluable[b]	Percent with Improvement
Abdominal pain	43/78 (55%)	24%
Nausea/vomiting	17/35 (49%)	34%
Fever/night sweats	10/22 (45%)	27%
Ascites	7/21 (33%)	29%
Anorexia	18/65 (28%)	9%
Abdominal distension	13/49 (27%)	10%
Jaundice	8/30 (27%)	17%
Weakness/fatigue	15/81 (19%)	7%

[a]Patients dying within 4 weeks were considered to be nonresponders.
[b]Includes all patients with symptoms initially present.
From Borgelt BB, Gelber R, Brady LW, Griffin T, Hendrickson FR: The palliation of hepatic metastases: Results of the Radiation Therapy Oncology Group pilot study. Int J Radiat Oncol Biol Phys 7:587–591, 1981, p 589. Copyright 1981 by Elsevier Science Inc.

was treated with twice-daily doses of 1.5 Gy separated by 4-hour interfraction intervals. The use of three progressively larger dosages of radiation to the entire liver (27, 30, and 33 Gy) did not prolong median survival or decrease the frequency with which liver metastases were the cause of death. None of 122 patients who received 27 or 30 Gy to the entire liver developed radiation hepatitis, but five of 51 patients who received 33 Gy developed clinical or biochemical evidence of late liver injury with an actuarial risk of severe (grade III) radiation hepatitis of 10 percent (± 7.3 percent SE) at 6 months.[135]

Investigational Radiotherapy Methods

In an effort to increase the effectiveness of radiotherapy in the treatment of hepatic metastases, several approaches have been investigated.

Radiotherapy in Combination with Misonidazole

The RTOG has tested the benefit of misonidazole, a hypoxic cell sensitizer, in conjunction with conventional radiation.[84] Patients were allocated in a prospective random fashion to receive 21 Gy in seven fractions to the entire liver for metastatic disease, with or without misonidazole. The dose of misonidazole was 1.5 gm/m² given 4 hours before each dose of radiation. The patient population was stratified by primary site, extent of metastatic disease, and Karnofsky's performance rating. The end points of the study were relief of hepatic pain, improvement in Karnofsky status, decrease in alkaline phosphatase level, decrease in liver and tumor size, and increase in duration of survival. The addition of misonidazole did not significantly improve the therapeutic response to radiotherapy in any of the parameters studied. Abdominal pain was relieved in 80 percent of symptomatic patients; 54 percent of patients had complete pain relief. Palliation of pain occurred at a median time of 1.7 weeks after beginning treatment.

The median duration of response was 13 weeks in symptomatic patients. The use of radiotherapy in combination with the administration of radiosensitizing agents remains investigational at the time of this writing. The treatment of primary and metastatic liver tumors originating from the gastrointestinal tract with hepatic arterial infusional chemotherapy (floxuridine or other radiosensitizers) in combination with focal radiotherapy treatment may eventually be applied to primary breast cancers metastatic to the liver.[79]

Infusion of Radioactive Microspheres

Microscopic liver metastases derive their blood supply from the portal system, whereas large, established hepatic metastases derive their blood supply preferentially from the hepatic arterial system.[1, 9] It is reasonable, therefore, to assume that large, solitary hepatic metastases could be selectively treated by infusing a cytotoxic agent into the appropriate branch of the hepatic artery, and this has been the principle for hepatic arterial infusional chemotherapy for treatment of metastatic colorectal cancers. Extensive work has been done with intra-arterial infusion of fluorouracil, both with portal vein infusion as adjuvant therapy in patients with colorectal carcinoma[157] and with hepatic arterial infusion for known hepatic metastases.[5, 57] In a similar fashion, the radioactive isotope ^{32}P has been injected into both the superior mesenteric and the celiac arteries in an attempt to eradicate subclinical liver metastases in patients with colorectal carcinoma.[55, 95] Under investigation at the time of this writing is the use of radioactive ^{90}Y-labeled glass microspheres, which are selectively injected under angiographic guidance into the hepatic arteries of patients with known liver metastases.[3, 4, 55, 68, 95] Yttrium 90, a beta-particle-emitting radioisotope with a half-life of only 64 hours, is incorporated into inert glass microspheres that are 15 microns in diameter. When selectively infused via the hepatic arterial system using angiographic techniques, the microspheres are trapped within the tumor capillaries to essentially embolize the tumor microcirculation with radioactive particles. This process allows selective delivery of high doses (50 Gy) of radiotherapy to the tumor with little irradiation of the surrounding liver parenchyma.

Andrews and coworkers[4] treated a series of 24 patients by this technique with no hematological, hepatic, or pulmonary toxicity encountered at nominal absorbed radiation doses to the whole liver of up to 150 Gy. Response data showed progressive disease in eight patients, stable disease in seven, minimal response in four, and partial response in five at 16 weeks. Three long-term survivors were reported at 2 or more years.[4]

Grady and coworkers[56] also treated patients with metastatic liver disease with ^{90}Y-labeled microspheres and hyperthermia. Most of the patients treated in this manner had colorectal carcinoma. Response rates of 65 percent were reported, but treatment-related morbidity was high, with some treatment-related deaths.

Radioactive Isotope–Labeled Immunoglobulin

Treatment of primary liver cancer with radiolabeled antibody is being investigated at the time of this writing.[39] If tumor-associated antigens can be identified for metastases from breast cancer and highly specific antibodies developed, this approach may be useful in the future for treating patients with metastatic breast cancer.

Treatment Recommendations

For patients expected to have a very short survival because of poor performance status or widespread metastasis, single fractions of 6–8 Gy can be delivered to the liver with good results. Effective palliation can often be achieved without treating the entire liver. If radiotherapy produces a good response, retreatment can be performed in 1–2 weeks. For most patients with a long expected survival, a more conventional treatment regimen of 21–30 Gy in fractions of 3 Gy is prescribed. The whole liver is treated with equally weighted anterior and posterior portals; the left kidney, if in the treatment volume, is blocked from the posterior portal after 18 Gy.

References

1. Ackerman NB, Lien WM, Kondi ES, Silverman NA: The blood supply of experimental liver metastases. I. The distribution of hepatic artery and portal vein blood to "small" and "large" tumors. Surgery 66:1067–1072, 1969.
2. Allen KL, Johnson TW, Hibbs GG: Effective bone palliation as related to various treatment regimens. Cancer 37:984–987, 1976.
3. Anderson JH, Goldberg JA, Bessent RG, Kerr DJ, McKillop JH, Stewart I, Cooke TG, McArdle CS: Glass yttrium-90 microspheres for patients with colorectal liver metastases. Radiother Oncol 25:137–139, 1992.
4. Andrews JC, Walker SC, Ackermann RJ, Cotton LA, Ensminger WD, Shapiro B: Hepatic radioembolization with yttrium-90 containing glass microspheres: Preliminary results and clinical follow-up. J Nucl Med 35:1637–1644, 1994.
5. Ansfield FJ, Ramirez G, Davis HL Jr, Wirtanen GW, Johnson RO, Bryan GT, Manalo FB, Borden EC, Davis TE, Esmaili M: Further clinical studies with intrahepatic arterial infusion with 5-fluorouracil. Cancer 36:2413–2417, 1975.
6. Barron KD, Hirano A, Araki S, Terry RD: Experiences with metastatic neoplasms involving the spinal cord. Neurology 9:91–106, 1959.
7. Bartelink H, Battermann J, Hart G: Half-body irradiation. Int J Radiat Oncol Biol Phys 6:87–90, 1980.
8. Bates T: A review of local radiotherapy in the treatment of bone metastases and cord compression. Int J Radiat Oncol Biol Phys 23:217–221, 1992.
9. Blanchard RJW, Grotenhuis I, LaFave JW, Perry JF Jr: Blood supply to hepatic V2 carcinoma implants as measured by radioactive microspheres. Proc Soc Exp Biol Med 118:465–468, 1965.
10. Blitzer PH: Reanalysis of the RTOG study of the palliation of symptomatic osseous metastasis. Cancer 55:1468–1472, 1985.
11. Bloch RS, Gartner S: The incidence of ocular metastatic carcinoma. Arch Ophthalmol 85:673–675, 1971.

12. Bonarigo BC, Rubin P: Nonunion of pathologic fracture after radiation therapy. Radiology 88:889–898, 1967.

13. Boogerd W, Vos VW, Hart AA, Baris G: Brain metastases in breast cancer; natural history, prognostic factors and outcome. J Neurooncol 15:165–174, 1993.

14. Borgelt BB, Gelber R, Brady LW, Griffin T, Hendrickson FR: The palliation of hepatic metastases: Results of the Radiation Therapy Oncology Group pilot study. Int J Radiat Oncol Biol Phys 7:587–591, 1981.

15. Borgelt B, Gelber R, Kramer S, Brady LW, Chang CH, Davis LW, Perez CA, Hendrickson FR: The palliation of brain metastases: Final results of the first two studies by the Radiation Therapy Oncology Group. Int J Radiat Oncol Biol Phys 6:1–9, 1980.

16. Bouchard J: Skeletal metastases in cancer of the breast. Study of the character, incidence, and response to roentgen therapy. Am J Roentgenol Radium Ther 54:156–171, 1945.

17. Brage ME, Simon MA: Evaluation, prognosis, and medical treatment considerations of metastatic bone tumors. Orthopedics 15:589–596, 1992.

18. Brinkley JR Jr: Response of a choroidal metastasis to multiple-drug chemotherapy. Cancer 45:1538–1539, 1980.

19. Bruckman JE, Bloomer WD: Management of spinal cord compression. Semin Oncol 5:135–140, 1978.

20. Buatti JM, Friedman WA, Bova FJ, Mendenhall WM: Treatment selection factors for stereotactic radiosurgery of intracranial metastases. Int J Radiat Oncol Biol Phys 32:1161–1166, 1995.

21. Byrne TN: Spinal cord compression from epidural metastases. N Engl J Med 327:614–619, 1992.

22. Byrne TN, Waxman SG: Spinal Cord Compression: Diagnosis and Principles of Management. Philadelphia, F. A. Davis, 1990.

23. Calkins AR, Olson MA, Ellis JH. Impact of myelography on the radiotherapeutic management of malignant spinal cord compression. Neurosurgery 19:614–616, 1986.

24. Carmody RF, Yang PJ, Seeley GW, Seeger JF, Unger EC, Johnson JE: Spinal cord compression due to metastatic disease: Diagnosis with MR imaging versus myelography. Radiology 173:225–229, 1989.

25. Carr DB, Carr JM: Role of brain opiates in pain relief. In Stoll BA, Parbhoo S (eds): Bone Metastasis: Monitoring and Treatment. New York, Raven Press, 1983, pp 375–393.

26. Cheng DS, Seitz CB, Eyre HJ: Nonoperative management of femoral, humeral, and acetabular metastases in patients with breast carcinoma. Cancer 45:1533–1537, 1980.

27. Chu FCH, Hilaris BB: Value of radiation therapy in the management of intracranial metastases. Cancer 14:577–581, 1961.

28. Chu FCH, Huh SH, Nisce LZ, Simpson LD: Radiation therapy of choroid metastasis from breast cancer. Int J Radiat Oncol Biol Phys 2:273–279, 1977.

29. Cobb CA III, Leavens ME, Eckles N: Indications for nonoperative treatment of spinal cord compression due to breast cancer. J Neurosurg 47:653–658, 1977.

30. Cogan DG, Kuwabara T: Metastatic carcinoma to eye from breast. Effect of endocrine therapy. Arch Ophthalmol 52:240–249, 1954.

31. Constans JP, de Divitiis E, Donzelli R, Spaziante R, Meder JF, Haye C: Spinal metastases with neurological manifestations. Review of 600 cases. J Neurosurg 59:111–118, 1983.

32. D'Elia F, Bonucci I, Biti GP, Pirtoli L: Different fractionation schedules in radiation treatment of cerebral metastases. Acta Radiol Oncol 25:181–184, 1986.

33. Delattre JY, Arbit E, Thaler HT, Rosenblum MK, Posner JB: A dose-response study of dexamethosone in a model of spinal cord compression caused by epidural tumor. J Neurosurg 70(6):920–925, 1989.

34. Dobrowsky W: Treatment of choroid metastases. Br J Radiol 61(722):140–142, 1988.

35. Doig RG, Olver IN, Jeal PN, Bishop JF: Symptomatic choroidal metastases in breast cancer. Aust N Z J Med 22(4):349–352, 1992.

36. Dosoretz DE, Blitzer PH, Russell AH, Wang CC: Management of solitary metastasis to the brain: The role of elective brain irradiation following complete surgical resection. Int J Radiat Oncol Biol Phys 6(12):1727–1730, 1980.

37. Egawa S, Tukiyama I, Akine Y, Kajiura Y, Yanagawa S, Watai K, Nomura K: Radiotherapy of brain metastases. Int J Radiat Oncol Biol Phys 12(9):1621–1625, 1986.

38. Ellis RA, Scheie HG: Regression of metastatic lesions of breast carcinoma following sterilization. Arch Ophthalmol 48:455–459, 1952.

39. Ettinger DS, Order SE, Wharam MD, Parker MK, Klein JL, Leichner PK: Phase I-II study of isotopic immunoglobulin therapy for primary liver cancer. Cancer Treat Res 66(2):289–297, 1982.

40. Ferry AP, Font RL: Carcinoma metastatic to the eye and orbit. I. A clinicopathologic study of 227 cases. Arch Ophthalmol 92(4):276–286, 1974.

41. Findlay GFG: Adverse effects of the management of malignant spinal cord compression. J Neurol Neurosurg Psychiatry 47:761–768, 1984.

42. Fitzpatrick PJ, Garrett PG: Metastatic breast cancer: Ovarian ablation with lower half-body irradiation. Int J Radiat Oncol Biol Phys 7:1523–1526, 1981.

43. Fitzpatrick PJ, Keen CW: The Princess Margaret and Ontario Cancer Foundation experience. In Weiss L, Gilbert HA, Posner JB (eds): Brain Metastasis. Proceedings of the Workshop on Brain Metastasis. New York, GK Hall, 1978, pp 286–302.

44. Flickinger JC, Kondziolka D, Lunsford LD, Coffey RJ, Goodman ML, Shaw EG, Hudgins WR, Weiner R, Harsh GR IV, Sneed PK, Larson DA: A multi-institutional experience with stereotactic radiosurgery for solitary brain metastasis. Int J Radiat Oncol Biol Phys 28:797–802, 1994.

45. Freedman MI, Folk JC: Metastatic tumors to the eye and orbit. Patient survival and clinical characteristics. Arch Ophthalmol 105(9):1215–1219, 1987.

46. Fryer CJH, Fitzpatrick PJ, Rider WD, Poon P: Radiation pneumonitis: Experience following a large single dose of radiation. Int J Radiat Oncol Biol Phys 4(11–12):931–936, 1978.

47. Fuller BG, Kaplan ID, Alder J, Cox RS, Bagshaw MA: Stereotaxic radiosurgery for brain metastases: The importance of adjuvant whole-brain irradiation. Int J Radiat Oncol Biol Phys 23(2):413–418, 1992.

48. Galicich JH, Sundaresan N, Thaler HT: Surgical treatment of single brain metastasis. Evaluation of results by computerized tomography scanning. J Neurosurg 53(1):63–67, 1980.

49. Garmatis CJ, Chu FCH: The effectiveness of radiation therapy in the treatment of bone metastases from breast cancer. Radiology 126:235–237, 1978.

50. Gelber RD, Larson M, Borgelt BB, Kramer S: Equivalence of radiation schedules for the palliative treatment of brain metastases in patients with favorable prognosis. Cancer 48:1749–1753, 1981.

51. Gilbert HA, Kagan AR, Nussbaum H, Rao AR, Satzman J, Chan P, Allen B, Forsythe A: Evaluation of radiation therapy for bone metastases: Pain relief and quality of life. AJR 129(6):1095–1096, 1977.

52. Gilbert H, Kagan AR, Wagner J, Fuchs K, Nussbaum H, Rao AR: The Southern California Permanente Medical Group experience: Functional results. In Weiss L, Gilbert HA, Posner JB (eds): Brain Metastasis. Proceedings of the Workshop on Brain Metastasis. New York, GK Hall, 1978, pp 303–313.

53. Gilbert RW, Kim JH, Posner JB: Epidural spinal cord compression from metastatic tumor: Diagnosis and treatment. Ann Neurol 3(1):40–51, 1978.

54. Giri DV: Metastatic carcinoma of the choroid secondary to mammary carcinoma in a man. Schweiz Med Wochenschr 69:1069–1072, 1939.

55. Grady ED: Internal radiation therapy of hepatic cancer. Dis Colon Rectum 22(6):371–375, 1979.

56. Grady ED, McLaren J, Auda SP, McGinley PH: Combination of internal radiation therapy and hyperthermia to treat liver cancer. South Med J 76(9):1101–1105, 1983.

57. Grage TB, Vassilopoulos PP, Shingleton WW, Jubert AV, Elias EG, Aust JB, Moss SE: Results of a prospective randomized study of hepatic artery infusion with 5-fluorouracil versus

intravenous 5-fluorouracil in patients with hepatic metastases from colorectal cancer: A Central Oncology Group study. Surgery 86(4):550–555, 1979.

58. Gragoudas ES: Current treatment of metastatic choroidal tumors. Oncology (Huntingt) 3(6):103–110, 1989.

59. Greenberg HS, Kim JH, Posner JB: Epidural spinal cord compression from metastatic tumor: Results with a new treatment protocol. Ann Neurol 8(4):361–366, 1980.

60. Haie-Meder C, Pellae-Cosset B, Laplanche A, Lagrange JL, Tuchais C, Nogues C, Arriagada R: Results of a randomized clinical trial comparing two radiation schedules in the palliative treatment of brain metastases. Radiother Oncol 26(2):111–116, 1993.

61. Hall AJ, Mackay NN: The results of laminectomy for compression of the cord or cauda equina by extradural malignant tumour. J Bone Joint Surg Br 55(3):497–505, 1973.

62. Halle JS, Rosenman JG, Varia MA, Fowler WC, Walton LA, Currie JL: 1000 cGy single-dose palliation for advanced carcinoma of the cervix or endometrium. Int J Radiat Oncol Biol Phys 12(11):1947–1950, 1986.

63. Harrington KD: Impending pathologic fractures from metastatic malignancy: Evaluation and management. Instr Course Lect 35:357–381, 1986.

64. Harrington KD: Anterior decompression and stabilization of the spine as a treatment for vertebral collapse and spinal cord compression from metastatic malignancy. Clin Orthop 233:177–197, 1988.

65. Hazuka MB, Kinzie JJ: Brain metastases: Results and effects of re-irradiation. Int J Radiat Oncol Biol Phys 15:433–437, 1988.

66. Hendrickson FR, Lee MS, Larson M, Gelber RD: The influence of surgery and radiation therapy on patients with brain metastases. Int J Radiat Oncol Biol Phys 9:623–627, 1983.

67. Hendrickson FR, Shehata WM, Kirchner AB: Radiation therapy for osseous metastasis. Int J Radiat Oncol Biol Phys 1(3–4):275–278, 1976.

68. Herba MJ, Illescas FF, Thirlwell MP, Boos GJ, Rosenthall L, Atri M, Bret PM: Hepatic malignancies: Improved treatment with intraarterial Y-90. Radiology 169(2):311–314, 1988.

69. Heros DO, Kasdon DL, Chun M: Brachytherapy in the treatment of recurrent solitary brain metastases. Neurosurgery 23(6):733–737, 1988.

70. Hindo WA, DeTrana FA III, Lee MS, Hendrickson FR: Large-dose increment irradiation in treatment of cerebral metastases. Cancer 26(1):138–141, 1970.

71. Hoogenhout J, Brink HM, Verbeek AM, Van Gasteren JJ, Beex LV: Radiotherapy of choroidal metastases. Strahlenther Onkol 165(5):375–379, 1989.

72. Ingold JA, Reed GB, Kaplan HS, Bagshaw MA: Radiation hepatitis. Am J Roentgenol Radium Ther Nucl Med 93:200–208, 1965.

73. Jaeger EA, Frayer WC, Southard ME, Kramer S: Effect of radiation therapy on metastatic choroidal tumors. Trans Am Acad Ophthalmol Otolaryngol 75(1):94–101, 1971.

74. Jaffe BM, Donegan WL, Watson F, Spratt JS Jr: Factors influencing survival in patients with untreated hepatic metastases. Surg Gynecol Obstet 127(1):1–11, 1968.

75. Jensen NH, Roesdahl K: Single-dose irradiation of bone metastases. Acta Radiol Ther Phys Biol 15(4):337–339, 1976.

76. Khan FR, Glicksman AS, Chu FCH, Nickson JJ: Treatment by radiotherapy of spinal cord compression due to extradural metastases. Radiology 89(3):495–500, 1967.

77. Kihlstrom L, Karlsson B, Lindquist C: Gamma knife surgery for cerebral metastases: implications for survival based on 16 years experience. Stereotact Funct Neurosurg 61(Suppl 1):45–50, 1993.

78. King EF: Two cases of secondary carcinoma of choroid. Trans Ophthalmol Soc UK 74:229–234, 1954.

79. Kinsella TJ: The role of radiation therapy alone and combined with infusion chemotherapy for treating liver metastases. Semin Oncol 10(2):215–222, 1983.

80. Komarnicky LT, Phillips TL, Martz K, Asbell S, Isaacson S, Urtasun R: A randomized phase III protocol for the evaluation of misonidazole combined with radiation in the treatment of patients with brain metastases (RTOG-7916). Int J Radiat Oncol Biol Phys 20(1):53–58, 1991.

81. Kurup P, Reddy S, Hendrickson FR: Results of re-irradiation for cerebral metastases. Cancer 46(12):2587–2589, 1980.

82. Lawrence TS, Ten Haken RK, Kessler ML, Robertson JM, Lyman JT, Lavigne ML, Brown MB, DuRoss DJ, Andrews JC, Ensminger WD, Lichter AS: The use of 3-D dose volume analysis to predict radiation hepatitis. Int J Radiat Oncol Biol Phys 23(4):781–788, 1992.

83. Leibel SA, Guse C, Order SE, Hendrickson FR, Komaki RU, Chang CH, Brady LW, Wasserman TH, Russell KJ, Asbell SO, Phillips TL, Russell AH, Pajak TF: Accelerated fractionation radiation therapy for liver metastases: Selection of an optimal patient population for the evaluation of late hepatic injury in RTOG studies. Int J Radiat Oncol Biol Phys 18(3):523–528, 1990.

84. Leibel SA, Pajak TF, Massullo V, Order SE, Komaki RU, Chang CH, Wasserman TH, Phillips TL, Lipshutz J, Durbin LM: A comparison of misonidazole sensitized radiation therapy to radiation therapy alone for the palliation of hepatic metastases: Results of a Radiation Therapy Oncology Group randomized prospective trial. Int J Radiat Oncol Biol Phys 13(7):1057–1064, 1987.

85. Letson AD, Davidorf FH, Bruce RA Jr: Chemotherapy for treatment of choroidal metastases from breast carcinoma. Am J Ophthalmol 93(1):102–106, 1982.

86. Leviov M, Dale J, Stein M, Ben-Shahar M, Ben-Arush M, Milstein D, Goldsher D, Kuten A: The management of metastatic spinal cord compression: A radiotherapeutic success ceiling. Int J Radiat Oncol Biol Phys 27(2):231–234, 1993.

87. Li KC, Poon PY: Sensitivity and specificity of MRI in detecting malignant spinal cord compression and in distinguishing malignant from benign compression fractures of vertebrae. Magn Reson Imaging 6(5):547–556, 1988.

88. Loeffler JS, Alexander E: Radiosurgery for the treatment on intracranial metastases. In Alexander E, Loeffler JS, Lunsford D (eds): Stereotactic Radiosurgery. New York, McGraw-Hill, 1993, pp 197–206.

89. Loeffler JS, Glicksman AS, Tefft M, Gelch M: Treatment of spinal cord compression: A retrospective analysis. Med Pediatr Oncol 11(5):347–351, 1983.

90. Loeffler JS, Kooy HM, Wen PY, Fine HA, Cheng CW, Mannarino EG, Tsai JS, Alexander E III: The treatment of recurrent brain metastases with stereotactic radiosurgery. J Clin Oncol 8(4):576–582, 1990.

91. Macmichael IM: Management of choroidal metastases from breast carcinoma. Br J Ophthalmol 53(11):782–785, 1969.

92. Madsen EL: Painful bone metastasis: Efficacy of radiotherapy assessed by the patients: a randomized trial comparing 4 Gy × 6 versus 10 Gy × 2. Int J Radiat Oncol Biol Phys 9(12):1775–1779, 1983.

93. Maher EJ: The use of palliative radiotherapy in the management of breast cancer. Eur J Cancer 28(2–3):706–710, 1992.

94. Makin WP: Treatment of spinal cord compression due to malignant disease. Br J Radiol 61(728):715, 1988. Abstract.

95. Mantravadi RVP, Spigos DG, Grady ED, Tan WS, Karesh SG, Capek V: Treatment of hepatic malignancies by intravascular administration of radioisotopes. In Winkler C (ed): Nuclear Medicine in Clinical Oncology: Current Status and Future Aspects. Berlin, Springer-Verlag, 1986, pp 365–371.

96. Maor M, Chan RC, Young SE: Radiotherapy of choroidal metastases: Breast cancer as primary site. Cancer 40(5):2081–2086, 1977.

97. Maranzano E, Latini P, Checcaglini F, Perrucci E, Aristei C, Panizza BM, Ricci S: Radiation therapy of spinal cord compression caused by breast cancer: Report of a prospective trial. Int J Radiat Oncol Biol Phys 24(2):301–306, 1992.

98. Maranzano E, Latini P, Checcaglini F, Ricci S, Panizza BM, Aristei C, Perrucci E, Beneventi S, Corgna E, Tonato M: Radiation therapy in metastatic spinal cord compression. A prospective analysis of 105 consecutive patients. Cancer 67(5):1311–1317, 1991.

99. Mehta MP: Radiosurgery for brain metastases. In DeSalles AF, Goetsch SJ (eds): Stereotactic Surgery and Radiosurgery. Madison, WI, Medical Physics Publishing Corporation, 1993, pp. 353–368.

100. Mehta MP, Rozental JM, Levin AB, Mackie TR, Kubsad SS,

Gehring MA, Kinsella TJ: Defining the role of radiosurgery in the management of brain metastases. Int J Radiat Oncol Biol Phys 24(4):619–625, 1992.

101. Mewis L, Young SE: Breast carcinoma metastatic to the choroid. Analysis of 67 patients. Ophthalmology 89:147–151, 1982.

102. Millburn L, Hibbs GG, Hendrickson FR: Treatment of spinal cord compression from metastatic carcinoma. Review of the literature and presentation of a new method of treatment. Cancer 21(3):447–452, 1968.

103. Mones RJ, Dozier D, Berrett A: Analysis of medical treatment of malignant extradural spinal cord tumors. Cancer 19(12):1842–1853, 1966.

104. Nisce LZ, Hilaris BS, Chu FCH: A review of experience with irradiation of brain metastasis. Am J Roentgenol Radium Ther Nucl Med 111(2):329–333, 1971.

105. Noordijk EM, Vecht CJ, Haaxma-Reiche H, Padberg GW, Voormolen JHC, Hoekstra FH, Tans JTJ, Lambooij N, Metsaars JAL, Wattendorff AR, Brand R, Hermans J: The choice of treatment of single brain metastasis should be based on extracranial tumor activity and age. Int J Radiat Oncol Biol Phys 29(4):711–717, 1994.

106. Nylén U, Kock E, Lax I, Lundell G, af Trampe E, Wilking N: Standardized precision radiotherapy in choroidal metastases. Acta Oncol 33(1):65–68, 1994.

107. De Ocampo G, Espiritu R: Bronchogenic metastatic carcinoma of the choroid. Am J Ophthalmol 52:107–110, 1961.

108. Order SE, Hellman S, von Essen CF, Kligerman MM: Improvement in quality of survival following whole-brain irradiation for brain metastasis. Radiology 91(1):149–153, 1968.

109. Orenstein MM, Anderson DP, Stein JJ: Choroid metastasis. Cancer 29(4):1101–1107, 1972.

110. Patchell RA, Tibbs PA, Walsh JW, Dempsey RJ, Maruyama Y, Kryscio RJ, Markesbery WR, Macdonald JS, Young B: A randomized trial of surgery in the treatment of single metastases to the brain. N Engl J Med 322(8):494–500, 1990.

111. Paterson AHG, Powles TJ, Kanis JA, McCloskey E, Hanson J, Ashley S: Double-blind controlled trial of oral clodronate in patients with bone metastases from breast cancer. J Clin Oncol 11(1):59–65, 1993.

112. Patterson RH Jr: Metastatic disease of the spines: Surgical risk versus radiation therapy. Clin Neurosurg 27:641–644, 1980.

113. Penn CRH: Single-dose and fractionated palliative irradiation for osseous metastases. Clin Radiol 27:405–408, 1976.

114. Portenoy RK, Galer BS, Salamon O, Freilich M, Finkel JE, Milstein D, Thaler HT, Berger M, Lipton RB: Identification of epidural neoplasm: Radiography and bone scintigraphy in the symptomatic and asymptomatic spine. Cancer 64(11):2207–2213, 1989.

115. Porter AT, McEwan AJB: Strontium-89 as an adjuvant to external-beam radiation improves pain relief and delays disease progression in advanced prostate cancer: Results of a randomized controlled trial. Semin Oncol 20(3 Suppl 2):38–43, 1993.

116. Porter AT, McEwan AJB, Powe JE, Reid R, McGowan DG, Lukka H, Sathyanarayana JR, Yakemchuk VN, Thomas GM, Erlich LE, Crook J, Gulenchyn KY, Hong KE, Wesolowski C, Yardley J: Results of a randomized phase-III trial to evaluate the efficacy of strontium-89 adjuvant to local-field external-beam irradiation in the management of endocrine-resistant metastatic prostate cancer. Int J Radiat Oncol Biol Phys 25(5):805–813, 1993.

117. Posner JB: Back pain and epidural spinal cord compression. Med Clin North Am 71:185–205, 1987.

118. Poulter CA, Cosmatos D, Rubin P, Urtasun R, Cooper JS, Kuske RR, Hornback N, Coughlin C, Weigensberg I, Rotman M: A report of RTOG 8206: A phase III study of whether the addition of single-dose hemibody irradiation to standard fractionated local-field irradiation is more effective than local-field irradiation alone in the treatment of symptomatic osseous metastases. Int J Radiat Oncol Biol Phys 23(1):207–214, 1992.

119. Prados M, Leibel S, Barnett CM, Gutin P: Interstitial brachytherapy for metastatic brain tumors. Cancer 63(4):657–660, 1989.

120. Prasad B, Lee MS, Hendrickson FR: Irradiation of hepatic metastases. Int J Radiat Oncol Biol Phys 2(1–2):129–132, 1977.

121. Prato FS, Kurdyak R, Saibil EA, Carruthers JS, Rider WD, Aspin N: The incidence of radiation pneumonitis as a result of single-fraction upper half-body irradiation. Cancer 39(1):71–78, 1976.

122. Price P, Hoskin PJ, Easton D, Austin D, Palmer SG, Yarnold JR: Prospective randomized trial of single and multifraction radiotherapy schedules in the treatment of painful bony metastases. Radiother Oncol 6(4):247–255, 1986.

123. Qasim MM: Single-dose palliative irradiation for bony metastasis. Strahlentherapie 153(8):531–532, 1977.

124. Quilty PM, Kirk D, Bolger JJ, Dearnaley DP, Lewington VJ, Mason MD, Reed NSE, Russell JM, Yardley J: A comparison of the palliative effects of strontium-89 and external-beam radiotherapy in metastatic prostate cancer. Radiother Oncol 31(1):33–40, 1994.

125. Reddy S, Saxena VS, Hendrickson F, Deutsch W: Malignant metastatic disease of the eye: Management of an uncommon complication. Cancer 47(4):810–812, 1981.

126. Redmond J III, Friedl KE, Cornett P, Stone M, O'Rourke T, George CB: Clinical usefulness of an algorithm for the early diagnosis of spinal metastatic disease. J Clin Oncol 6(1):154–157, 1988.

127. Reese AB: Metastatic tumors of the eye and adnexa. In Reese AB (ed): Tumors of the Eye. 3rd ed. Hagerstown, MD, Harper & Row, 1976, pp 423–431.

128. Richards P, McKissock W: Intracranial metastases. Br Med J 1:15–18, 1963.

129. Richter MP, Coia LR: Palliative radiation therapy. Semin Oncol 12(4):375–383, 1985.

130. Robinson RG: Strontium-89—precursor-targeted therapy for pain relief of blastic metastatic disease. Cancer 72:3433–3435, 1993.

131. Robinson RG, Preston DF, Baxter KG, Dusing RW, Spicer JA: Clinical experience with strontium-89 in prostatic and breast cancer patients. Semin Oncol 20(3 Suppl 2):44–48, 1993.

132. Robinson RG, Preston DF, Spicer JA, Baxter KG: Radionuclide therapy of intractable bone pain: Emphasis on strontium-89. Semin Nucl Med 22(1):28–32, 1992.

133. Rose MA, Feldman EL: Choroidal metastases from breast cancer. In Harris JR, Hellman S, Henderson IC, Kinne DW (eds): Breast Diseases. Philadelphia, JB Lippincott, 1987, pp 506–508.

134. Rubin P, Miller G: Extradural spinal cord compression by tumor. Part I: Experimental production and treatment trials. Radiology 93(6):1243–1260, 1969.

135. Russell AH, Clyde C, Wasserman TH, Turner SS, Rotman M: Accelerated hyperfractionated hepatic irradiation in the management of patients with liver metastases: Results of the RTOG dose escalating protocol. Int J Radiat Oncol Biol Phys 27(1):117–123, 1993.

136. Salazar OM, Rubin P, Hendrickson FR, Komaki R, Poulter C, Newall J, Asbell SO, Mohiuddin M, van Ess J: Single-dose half-body irradiation for palliation of multiple bone metastases from solid tumors. Final Radiation Therapy Oncology Group report. Cancer 58(1):29–36, 1986.

137. Salazar OM, Rubin P, Keller B, Scarantino C: Systemic (half-body) radiation therapy: response and toxicity. Int J Radiat Oncol Biol Phys 4(11–12):937–950, 1978.

138. Sanders TE: Metastatic carcinoma of the iris. Am J Ophthalmol 21:646–651, 1938.

139. Schocker JD, Brady LW: Radiation therapy for bone metastasis. Clin Orthop 169:38–43, 1982.

140. Schorcht J, Herrmann T, Friedrich S, Jochem I, Winkler C: Single exposure of high-dose half-body irradiation in cases of carcinoma of the breast. Radiobiol Radiother (Berl), 25:531–535, 1984.

141. Shaw B, Mansfield FL, Borges L: One-stage posterolateral decompression and stabilization for primary and metastatic vertebral tumors in the thoracic and lumbar spine. J Neurosurg 70(3):405–410, 1989.

142. Shehata WM, Hendrickson FR, Hindo WA: Rapid-fraction-

ation technique and re-treatment of cerebral metastases by irradiation. Cancer 34(2):257–261, 1974.

143. Sherman DM, Weichselbaum R, Order SE, Cloud L, Trey C, Piro AJ: Palliation of hepatic metastasis. Cancer 41(5):2013–2017, 1978.

144. Shimizu K, Shikata J, Iida H, Iwasaki R, Yoshikawa J, Yamamuro T: Posterior decompression and stabilization for multiple metastatic tumors of the spine. Spine 17:1400–1404, 1992.

145. Siegal T, Siegal T: Current considerations in the management of neoplastic spinal cord compression. Spine 14:223–228, 1989.

146. Silberstein EB, Williams C: Strontium-89 therapy for the pain of osseous metastases. J Nucl Med 26:345–348, 1985.

147. Smalley SR, Schray MF, Laws ER Jr, O'Fallon JR: Adjuvant radiation therapy after surgical resection of solitary brain metastasis: Association with pattern of failure and survival. Int J Radiat Oncol Biol Phys 13(11):1611–1616, 1987.

148. Smoker WRK, Godersky JC, Knutzon RK, Keyes WD, Norman D, Bergman W: The role of MR imaging in evaluating metastatic spinal disease. AJR Am J Roentgenol 149(6):1241–1248, 1987.

149. Snee MP, Rodger A, Kerr GR: Brain metastases from carcinoma of breast: A review of 90 cases. Clin Radiol 36(4):365–367, 1985.

150. Solisio EO, Akbiyik N, Alexander LL: Spinal cord compression from metastatic breast carcinoma: Treatment by radiation therapy alone. J Natl Med Assoc 71(3):229–230, 1979.

151. Spanos WJ Jr, Wasserman T, Meoz R, Sala J, Kong J, Stetz J: Palliation of advanced pelvic malignant disease with large-fraction pelvic radiation and misonidazole: Final report of RTOG Phase I/II study. Int J Radiat Oncol Biol Phys 13(10):1479–1482, 1987.

152. Sturm V, Kober B, Höver KH, Schlegel W, Boesecke R, Pastyr O, Hartmann GH, Schabbert S, zum Winkel K, Kunze S, Lorenz WJ: Stereotactic percutaneous single-dose irradiation of brain metastases with a linear accelerator. Int J Radiat Oncol Biol Phys 13(2):279–282, 1987.

153. Sundaresan N, Digiacinto GV, Hughes JE, Cafferty M, Vallejo A: Treatment of neoplastic spinal cord compression: Results of a prospective study. Neurosurgery 29(5):645–650, 1991.

154. Sundaresan N, Galicich JH, Deck MDF, Tomita T: Radiation necrosis after treatment of solitary intracranial metastases. Neurosurgery 8(3):329–333, 1981.

155. Sze G, Abramson A, Krol G, Liu D, Amster J, Zimmerman RD, Deck MD: Gadolinium-DTPA in the evaluation of intradural extramedullary spinal disease. AJR Am J Roentgenol 150(4):911–921, 1988.

156. Tabbara IA, Sibley DS, Quesenberry PJ: Spinal cord compression due to metastatic neoplasm. South Med J 83(5):519–523, 1990.

157. Taylor I, Brooman P, Rowling JT: Adjuvant liver perfusion in colorectal cancer: Initial results of a clinical trial. Br Med J 2(6098):1320–1322, 1977.

158. Thatcher N, Thomas PR: Choroidal metastases from breast carcinoma: A survey of 42 patients and the use of radiation therapy. Clin Radiol 26(4):549–553, 1975.

159. Thomas P: Radiotherapy of metastases of mammary carcinoma. Radiol Clin Basel 45(2–4):306–313, 1976.

160. Toma S, Venturino A, Sogno G, Formica C, Bignotti B, Bonassi S, Palumbo R: Metastatic bone tumors. Nonsurgical treatment. Outcome and survival. Clin Orthop 295:246–251, 1993.

161. Tomita T, Galicich JH, Sundaresan N: Radiation therapy for spinal epidural metastases with complete block. Acta Radiol Oncol 22(2):135–143, 1983.

162. Tong D, Gillick L, Hendrickson FR: The palliation of symptomatic osseous metastases: Final results of the study by the Radiation Therapy Oncology Group. Cancer 50:893–899, 1982.

163. Townsend PW, Rosenthal HG, Smalley SR, Cozad SC, Hassanein RES: Impact of postoperative radiation therapy and other perioperative factors on outcome after orthopedic stabilization of impending or pathologic fractures due to metastatic disease. J Clin Oncol 12(11):2345–2350, 1994.

164. Trodella L, Ausili-Cefaro G, Turriziani A, Marmiroli L, Cellini N, Nardone L: Pain in osseous metastases: Results of radiotherapy. Pain 18(4):387–396, 1984.

165. Turek-Maischeider M, Kazem I: Palliative irradiation for liver metastasis. JAMA 232(6):625–628, 1975.

166. Twycross RG: Analgesics and relief of bone pain. In Stoll BA, Parbhoo S (eds): Bone Metastasis. Monitoring and Treatment. New York, Raven Press, 1983, pp 289–310.

167. Van Holten-Verzantvoort ATM, Kroon HM, Bijvoet OLM, Cleton FJ, Beex LVAM, Blijham G, Hermans J, Neijt JP, Papapoulos SE, Sleeboom HP, Vermey P, Zwinderman AH: Palliative pamidronate treatment in patients with bone metastasis from breast cancer. J Clin Oncol 11(3):491–498, 1993.

168. Vargha ZO, Glicksman AS, Boland J: Single-dose radiation therapy in the palliation of metastatic disease. Radiology 93(5):1181–1184, 1969.

169. Vieth RG, Odom GL: Intracranial metastases and their neurosurgical treatment. J Neurosurg 23:375–383, 1965.

170. Weissman DE: Glucocorticoid treatment for brain metastases and epidural spinal cord compression: A review. J Clin Oncol 6(3):543–551, 1988.

171. West J, Maor M: Intracranial metastases: Behavioral patterns related to primary site and results of treatment by whole-brain irradiation. Int J Radiat Oncol Biol Phys 6(1):11–15, 1980.

172. Wharton JT, Delclos L, Gallager S, Smith JP: Radiation hepatitis induced by abdominal irradiation with the cobalt 60 moving-strip technique. Am J Roentgenol Radium Ther Nucl Med 117(1):73–80, 1973.

173. White WA, Patterson RH Jr, Bergland RM: Role of surgery in the treatment of spinal cord compression by metastatic neoplasm. Cancer 27(3):558–561, 1971.

174. Wild WO, Porter RW: Metastatic epidural tumor of the spine. A study of 45 cases. Arch Surg 87:825–830, 1963.

175. Willis RA: Secondary tumors in sundry unusual situations. In Willis RA (ed): The Spread of Tumours in the Human Body. St. Louis, CV Mosby, 1952, pp 296–298.

176. Winkelman MD, Adelstein DJ, Karlins NL: Intramedullary spinal cord metastasis. Diagnostic and therapeutic considerations. Arch Neurol 44(5):526–531, 1987.

177. Wright RL: Malignant tumors in the spinal extradural space: Results of surgical treatment. Ann Surg 157:227–231, 1963.

178. Yarnold JR: Role of radiotherapy in the management of bone metastases from breast cancer. J R Soc Med 78(Suppl 9):23–25, 1985.

179. Young RF, Post EM, King GA: Treatment of spinal epidural metastases. Randomized prospective comparison of laminectomy and radiotherapy. J Neurosurg 53(6):741–748, 1980.

CHAPTER 72
CHEMOTHERAPY FOR METASTATIC BREAST CANCER

George W. Sledge, Jr., M.D.

NATURAL HISTORY

In the year this chapter was composed, it is estimated that 44,300 American women will die of breast cancer; the age-adjusted death rate for breast cancer is 22.0 per 100,000 population.[1] The great majority of the patients who succumb to this disease do so not because of the primary cancer but because of metastatic disease. In addition to the mortality caused by metastatic breast cancer, the disease results in significant morbidity and expense. Metastatic breast cancer robs the patient of her comfort, her dignity, and ultimately her life.

Metastatic breast cancer represents part of a continuum of disease, beginning with noninvasive (*in situ*) cancer and ending with life-ending disseminated breast cancer. It is important to realize that, although metastatic breast cancer is almost uniformly fatal, it is not monoform. Important differences exist in terms of site of recurrence, response to therapy, and survival of patients with metastatic disease.

Site of Recurrence

Breast cancer metastases, like the metastases of many malignancies, are site specific. While autopsy series reveal that virtually every organ may fall prey to metastasis from breast cancer, the clinician regularly deals with a more limited spectrum of recurrence in which soft tissue (lymph node and chest wall), bone, liver, and lung metastases predominate. Metastases to the brain, pleura, and pericardium, though less common, may have devastating consequences and require specific treatments. These are discussed elsewhere in this text.

Site of recurrence is not random. Studies from several centers reveal that steroid receptor status is an important predictor of site of recurrence.[2–5] In general, patients with estrogen receptor (ER)–positive tumors are more likely to suffer recurrence in bones, whereas those with ER–negative tumors are more likely to develop metastases in liver or brain. The ER–negative tumor therefore represents a prognostic "double whammy": the patient has a hormone-insensitive tumor in a site where progression may rapidly prove fatal. In addition to steroid receptor status, tumor histopathology is also a determinant of site of recurrence. Lobular carcinomas more frequently recur in gastrointestinal, peritoneal and pericardial, endocrine organ, and female reproductive system sites; breast sarcomas (cystosarcoma phylloides)

most often have a lung-predominant pattern of recurrence.[6–8] The biology underlying such site specificity is still poorly understood.

Predictors of Survival After Recurrence

On average, a patient with metastatic breast cancer lives about 16 to 24 months after the recurrence is discovered. It is important to recognize, however, that for some the disease takes a rapid and aggressive course that is essentially unaffected by therapy. Others may live quite long with excellent quality of life. Just as there are predictors of site of recurrence of breast cancer, several factors predict survival after recurrence.

Predictors of Initial Relapse

It should come as no surprise that several of the predictors of relapse are also predictors of survival after relapse. While physicians and patients often think of micro- and overt metastatic disease as being somehow different, they are simply points on a continuum. Initial lymph node positivity (or initial stage), high histological grade, and steroid receptor negativity have all been correlated with impaired survival after relapse.[3, 9–16] To what extent the effect of steroid receptor status is confounded by response to hormone therapy after metastasis is unclear, though it is reasonable to expect some such effect.

Factors Associated with Metastasis

In addition to the importance of factors that initially predict relapse, the fact of metastasis is itself a potent determinant of survival. The duration of metastasis-free survival (the period between initial diagnosis and relapse—the disease-free interval) is strongly associated with survival after relapse.[9, 11, 12, 15] Since metastasis-free survival reflects tumor burden and aggressiveness, this correlation makes sense. The number and site(s) of initial metastasis also correlate with survival after relapse.[3, 10, 15, 17–21] Visceral (particularly liver and brain) metastases portend short survival, whereas soft tissue and bone metastasis are associated with longer median survival. This effect is confounded with steroid receptor status: The ER-positive patient is more likely to suffer recurrence in bone, and the ER-negative patient a liver or brain metastasis.[3] Patient performance status at the time of initiation of chemotherapy is also correlated with survival duration.[17, 18, 21]

Chemotherapy

At first glance it might seem obvious that chemotherapy should prolong survival of patients with metastatic breast cancer. Many chemotherapy regimens induce objective responses in more than half of patients, and 10 percent to 20 percent, on average, experience complete clinical remissions. Responding patients routinely live longer than nonresponders, and treatment-related deaths are rare.

Despite these facts, doubts about the survival benefit of chemotherapy persist. Median duration of response is generally short (6 to 12 months for modern chemotherapy regimens), and the superior survival of responding patients might have more to do with underlying prognostic factors (e.g., disease volume, steroid receptor status, performance status) than with the response itself. Comparisons of survival results at single institutions in the prechemotherapy and the modern eras have not always suggested that survival has improved, and even the positive analyses have suggested that chemotherapy confers modest rather than dramatic survival benefits that are generally measurable in months rather than years.[22–27]

Such comparisons over time have their own problems: the passage of time introduces many confounding variables beside those related to changes in therapy. Ideally, this question might be resolved through a prospective, randomized trial that compares treated and untreated patients with metastatic breast cancer. Such a trial would be impossible to perform, for ethical reasons: leaving aside the issue of survival, chemotherapy clearly has major palliative benefits. A surrogate for such a trial has been suggested: if chemotherapy improves survival, then one would expect the more active arm of any randomized trial comparing two chemotherapy regimens to demonstrate superior overall survival rates. An overview of randomized chemotherapy trials has suggested that this is, indeed, the case, as the relationship between relative response rates and survival is statistically significant.[28]

Previous Therapy

In several series previous adjuvant therapy reduced survival for patients receiving chemotherapy. The reasons for this are unclear. One reasonable explanation—indeed the first that springs to mind—is that previous adjuvant chemotherapy renders a tumor resistant because the cells that survive are "naturally selected" for their failure to respond to the treatment. Thus cells of recurrent lesions will also be less responsive to therapy and patients will therefore die sooner. Exposure of cell populations to chemotherapeutic agents in the laboratory certainly accomplishes such selection, and the rate of spontaneous drug resistance has been calculated for many specific drugs. In the clinic, however, patients who previously received adjuvant chemotherapy and then suffered a relapse exhibit sensitivity to the adjuvant

TABLE 72–1. EFFECT OF PRIOR ADJUVANT CHEMOTHERAPY ON RESPONSE TO CHEMOTHERAPY FOR METASTATIC DISEASE

Adjuvant Therapy	Reference	Patients (n)	Responses (n/%)	MDR/TTP (mo)
CMF	31	83	32/39	17
None		55	21/38	16
CMF	29	26	6/23	2
None		51	24/47	4
CMF	30	137	44/32	6
None		340	163/48	9

Key: MDR, median duration of response; TTP, time to progression.

combination chemotherapy that is similar or only modestly inferior to that of a chemotherapy-naive population (Table 72–1).[29–31] One possible explanation is that the association between previous adjuvant therapy and curtailed survival is a spurious one based on confounding variables. Patients who previously received adjuvant therapy generally did so because their primary tumors were more aggressive, and those are the tumors most likely to kill rapidly after recurrence. Another explanation, difficult to document, is that cumulative toxicity of chemotherapeutic agents limits both dose and duration of therapy after recurrence, thus impairing the delivery of life-prolonging therapy.

Miscellaneous Factors

A number of other factors have been associated with survival after metastasis. Advanced age has been associated with improved survival; African-American ancestry is associated with impaired survival.[32, 33] The presence of invasive lobular carcinoma (as opposed to invasive ductal carcinoma) has been reported by some authors to confer improved survival chances after metastasis.[34]

INITIAL EVALUATION OF THE PATIENT WITH METASTATIC BREAST CANCER

When metastatic breast cancer is suspected, several steps should routinely be taken. A careful examination of these steps allows the physician to avoid numerous subsequent pitfalls and the patient to avoid considerable morbidity. These steps are summarized in Table 72–2.

Confirming the Existence of Metastasis

Because it represents a death sentence for most patients, the diagnosis of metastatic breast cancer should not be made casually. Misdiagnosis can have devastating consequences. Two common pitfalls are worth mentioning in this regard. First, although diagnostic tests are useful and important, they are never perfect. The computed tomography (CT) scan may be misread; the "positive" bone scan finding

TABLE 72–2 INITIAL APPROACH TO THE PATIENT WITH METASTATIC DISEASE

Confirm the existence of metastasis
↓
Determine disease sites
↓
Review initial disease characteristics
↓
Review previous therapy
↓
Determine disease morbidity and tempo
↓
Evaluate the general medical and social condition

may be an old traumatic fracture or an osteoporotic compression fracture; the elevated Carcino Embryonic Antigen (CEA) level may reflect the patient's smoking habit rather than metastasis. Even the pathologist can err. Second, breast cancer does not render a person immune to other problems. Both malignant and nonmalignant lesions can be incorrectly labeled metastatic breast cancer, to the patient's detriment. An old proverb says that to a hammer everything appears to be a nail; the oncologist, confronted with the breast cancer patient, should not assume that the patient's every problem is breast cancer.

In the terms of the courts, metastasis should be confirmed beyond a reasonable doubt: not beyond *all* doubt, as not every recurrence demands a biopsy, but certainly beyond a reasonable doubt. Whenever there is any serious question about the diagnosis of metastatic breast cancer, biopsy is warranted to confirm the diagnosis. Biopsy is also warranted when the initial pathology study was inadequate, as, for instance, when steroid receptor analysis was not obtained or when an initial diagnosis of a noninvasive cancer is followed by the apparent development of metastatic disease.

Demonstrating Sites of Metastasis

The sites of metastasis should be identified and documented. Determining the sites of metastasis is important for several reasons: it can have prognostic significance (patients who have disease at multiple sites or liver metastasis, have relatively poorer prognosis than those who have isolated, extravisceral disease); it can help determine therapy (some specific disease sites require specific therapeutic approaches); it can give the physician some sense of the aggressiveness or tempo of the disease; and it can be useful in determining response to therapy. It also spares the physician unnecessary dilemmas. For instance, if at the time of recurrence the presence of bone metastasis is not documented, a flare reaction to hormonal manipulation might be misinterpreted as disease progression and could rob the patient of the benefits derived from a well-tolerated hormonal manipulation.

Breast cancer metastasis is often site specific (i.e., it commonly spreads to a limited number of specific organs). These potential sites should be evaluated when metastasis is suspected: soft tissues, bone, liver, and lungs. Soft tissue involvement (e.g., supraclavicular lymphadenopathy or chest wall recurrence) is often readily detectable on physical examination. Bony metastasis may be evaluated with radionuclide bone scan and plain film x-rays, and occasionally by magnetic resonance imaging (MRI). The possibility of liver metastasis may be evaluated with CT; ultrasonography is clearly inferior as a means of imaging the liver. Lung metastasis may be evaluated with either plain chest films or chest CT. Less common sites of metastasis (e.g., the brain) may be evaluated if the patient's symptoms so indicate.

Reviewing Characteristics of the Primary Lesion

For patients with breast cancer, the past is often prologue. In particular, the steroid receptor status of the primary tumor is crucial for determining which form of systemic therapy will prove most useful as initial therapy. As there is general concordance between the steroid receptor status of a primary tumor and that of its metastases, an adequate steroid receptor determination performed on the primary tumor obviates the need for steroid receptor analysis of metastases.[35] Occasionally, the pathology of the primary tumor is such that it can affect the therapy of metastases. While the overwhelming majority of primary breast tumors are adenocarcinomas, occasionally a sarcoma or a lymphoma is detected. These cancers are treated quite differently from adenocarcinomas of the breast, and they have different prognostic implications. Finally, the lymph node status of the primary tumor is a powerful determinant, not only of recurrence, but of survival after recurrence.

Reviewing Previous Therapy

Therapy given after the primary diagnosis can limit subsequent treatment options and should always be considered carefully. Did the patient previously receive radiotherapy, and, if so, in what dose, and to what fields? Did the patient receive adjuvant hormone therapy?—adjuvant chemotherapy? If so, what drugs were given and to what cumulative doses? How long ago did treatment end? Such questions can be crucial in determining appropriate therapy for metastatic or recurrent disease. For instance, a patient with a chest wall recurrence may be treated differently if she previously received chest radiotherapy. A patient who has received adjuvant hormone therapy with tamoxifen until a month before recurrence should not receive tamoxifen as first-line hormone therapy for metastatic disease, regardless of steroid receptor status. A patient who received prior adjuvant chemotherapy with regimens containing doxorubicin may still be responsive to doxorubicin yet may rapidly surpass the anthracycline "speed limit" above which further therapy may cause cardiac toxicity. A patient who suffers relapse within months of adjuvant chemotherapy is far less likely to benefit from further chemotherapy than one who "relapses" several years later.

Determining Disease Morbidity and Tempo

The physician should consider the patient's condition. Is the patient symptomatic? Symptomatic patients, particularly those with impaired performance status, are likely to have more advanced, more aggressive, and less responsive disease than those whose metastases are discovered coincidentally. Rapidly progressive, increasingly symptomatic disease has different therapeutic implications than indolent, asymptomatic metastasis.

Evaluating the Patient's Medical and Social Condition

Journal articles describing phase II or III trial results necessarily treat patients as anonymous and largely interchangeable; indeed, clinical trials are regularly structured to exclude troublesome cases, leaving a relatively homogenous clinical population. In the clinic, the physician is confronted with individuals and their unique problems. The ability afforded clinical researchers of excluding problem patients is not a luxury enjoyed by practicing physicians. Does the patient have any underlying condition that might affect the choice of therapy (e.g., heart disease, impaired renal function)? For instance, the presence of hypertensive cardiomyopathy necessarily limits the use of an anthracycline or anthracenedione. A pregnant patient who wishes to carry the fetus to term cannot be treated with methotrexate. What are the patient's goals and concerns about her disease and its therapy? The experienced physician is aware that more goes into treatment decisions than is encompassed by simple treatment algorithms. It is wise to recognize and face patient concerns and desires at the outset of therapy. A patient's fears about hair loss or her desire to attend her child's high school graduation on a given day, are quite real and important to her, even if they do not fit the formulaic prescriptions of medical textbooks.

THE TREATMENT DECISION PROCESS

Once the factors discussed above have been evaluated, the treatment of the patient's metastatic disease can proceed. The initial decision the physician faces is whether to treat the patient with local or systemic therapy. The initial presentation of metastatic breast cancer may mandate a localized rather than a systemic form of therapy. Examples of this abound—brain metastasis, epidural cord compression, pericardial effusion, among others. Prompt resolution of these problems is necessary to prevent death (in the case of brain metastasis and pericardial

effusion) or severely impaired quality of life (epidural cord compression). Management of these problems is discussed elsewhere in this text.

Once local issues of importance have been resolved, the physician should consider systemic therapy. The approach to systemic therapy (either chemotherapy or hormone therapy) should, in general, be grounded in the realization that, for the vast majority of patients systemic therapy will not effect cure. Given this, appropriate therapeutic goals for most patients include maximizing quantity and quality of life and minimizing treatment-related toxicity. In general, this approach implies choosing less toxic regimens as long as such regimens offer the hope of a clinical response and palliation of symptoms.

Because hormone manipulations are generally less toxic than chemotherapy, and because responses to hormone therapy may be of relatively long duration, it is reasonable to employ hormonal manipulation as initial therapy whenever it stands a reasonable chance of working. One decides whether hormone therapy is likely to prove beneficial by examining steroid receptor status. Breast cancers that are ER- or PR-positive are relatively likely to respond to hormone therapy. Conversely, patients with ER- and PR-negative tumors are relatively unlikely to benefit from a hormonal manipulation and should be considered candidates for chemotherapy.

There are, of course, exceptions. The steroid receptor–negative tumor that is small in volume, located in soft tissue, and indolent in nature can be considered for hormone therapy, on the off chance that it might respond. Similarly, an elderly patient whose tumor relapses after a long disease-free interval might be considered for hormone therapy, despite a reported steroid receptor–negative tumor. In contrast, for a patient with rapidly progressive, multiorgan metastatic breast cancer, the 2 to 3 months' wait to evaluate a hormone response might seem dangerously long should hormonal therapy fail, so chemotherapy should be considered despite a steroid receptor–positive tumor. The type of the steroid receptors (the ERs and PRs in particular) and the use of hormone therapy for treatment of metastatic breast cancer are discussed in Chapter 25.

CHEMOTHERAPY

General Principles

The principles underlying the use of chemotherapy for metastatic breast cancer were largely established by Skipper and Schabel in the 1960s and have since remained essentially unchanged. Skipper and Schabel proposed that the doubling time of cancer cells is constant over time. Virtually all chemotherapy agents share the common effect of affecting division of cancer cells. Chemotherapeutic agents work by first-order kinetics, killing a constant *fraction* rather than a constant *number* of tumor cells (the "log kill hypothesis"). The ability of a drug or combination of drugs to defeat a malignancy thus depends on tumor mass (how many "logs" of tumor there are), antitumor efficacy (how many "logs" of tumor are killed with each each cycle of therapy), and the rapidity of tumor cell regrowth after each cycle of therapy.[36-40]

Rationale for Drug Combinations

The discovery of single agents with significant activity against metastatic breast cancer in the 1950s and early 1960s led naturally to combining them. The first such combination was reported by Greenspan in 1963.[41] This and subsequent combinations were accompanied regularly by significantly improved overall response rates, and the use of combination chemotherapy became standard for metastatic disease.

Combination chemotherapy is so universally applied that it may be difficult either to remember or defend the principles employed to support its use. In general, these can be stated as follows: The existence of somatic cell (inherited) drug resistance is the major barrier to cure of (or tumor response in) metastatic breast cancer. Drug resistance can be partial (i.e., may be overcome by increasing the dose) rather than complete, but this is of little help because dose-dependent toxicity to normal tissues prevents full exploitation of the dose-response curve. Because resistance may be drug specific and because different subpopulations in a given tumor may exhibit different degrees and types of resistance, the use of combinations of drugs capable of eliminating different subpopulations of a tumor should result in increased (additive or synergistic) tumor cell kill. The increased cell kill should increase the likelihood of remission (expressed either as the response rate for a population or the completeness of response for an individual), which in turn should translate to improved survival. Finally, the use of agents whose toxicities do not overlap should allow this to be accomplished with relatively less toxicity than when single agents are "pushed" to the maximum tolerated dose.

In practice, the benefits of combination chemotherapy, while real, are balanced by equally real problems. The reasons are multifold and involve the assumptions underlying the use of drug combinations. It is now widely recognized that drug resistance often involves multiple drugs of different classes, so that the assumed benefits of combining drugs of several different classes may be nullified by a common mechanism of resistance. The discovery of P glycoprotein (coded for by the multidrug resistance gene, *MDR1*), and subsequently of other genes that code for multidrug resistance, has demonstrated at a molecular level why combinations often fail to produce additive or synergistic tumor cell kill. More practically, combinations regularly involve some degree of overlapping toxicity, or even novel and unexpected toxicities. These necessarily result in therapeutic compromises, as toxicity is avoided by decreasing the concentrations of the component drugs. This, in turn, lowers tumor cell kill, and, presumably, response rates fail.

In addition, the gompertzian nature of tumor growth, as discussed above, may suggest that a tumor near its plateau growth phase may, with either partial or complete remission be returned to the rapid-growth portion of its growth curve. As a result, the impressive increases in response rates seen with combination therapy are not associated with significantly increased times to treatment failure or overall survival times.

Randomized trials comparing sequential single-agent chemotherapy with combination chemotherapy are rare. Cheblowski and colleagues compared sequential single-agent therapy with combination chemotherapy. Combination chemotherapy provided clearly higher response rates, but overall survival was not superior, though the number of patients enrolled in the trial was insufficient to rule out a modest survival benefit.[42] Smalley and coworkers, on the other hand, showed doubling of median survival time (48 versus 24 weeks; $p < .05$) for combination as opposed to sequential single-agent chemotherapy.[43]

Changes in technology represent a new challenge to the concept of combination chemotherapy. Jones and associates demonstrated that large-dose, single-agent chemotherapy with doxorubicin can produce response rates equivalent to the best achieved with standard combination chemotherapy.[44] Similarly, the response rates of the taxanes (paclitaxel and docetaxel) reported in phase II trials of previously untreated patients appear roughly similar to those of prior combination regimens; whether combination regimens containing taxane will prove superior to single-agent taxane regimens remains to be determined. While in the past the toxicity of high-dose, single-agent therapy was limiting, in terms of both dose intensity and treatment duration, the advent of hematopoietic colony–stimulating factors and of the cardioprotectant dexrazoxane (discussed below) may render such concerns less pressing in the future.

The Importance of Drug Resistance

Clinical manifestations of drug resistance abound in patients with metastatic breast cancer. Drug resistance can be primary: some 10 percent to 15 percent of patients suffer progressive disease during initial treatment for metastatic disease. In addition, tumors that initially respond to a regimen eventually progress, despite continued therapy with that regimen. This is a common finding even following complete clinical remission. Second- or third-line chemotherapy regimens are virtually always associated with lower response rates, despite the use of new agents.

The existence of clinical drug resistance, and particularly of cross-resistance to agents of different classes, has led to a large body of theoretical and laboratory work, in attempts to elucidate the nature of drug resistance. Many of these studies have concentrated on the presence of somatic cell (inherited, genetic) forms of resistance.

Goldie, Coldman, and colleagues suggested in the late 1970s and early 1980s that the development in a tumor of drug-resistant clones was the primary cause of death from cancer.[45–47] Arguing by analogy from the Luria-Delbruck hypothesis, they made three suggestions: (1) The development of drug-resistant clones is a lethal event. (2) Cancer cells undergo spontaneous somatic cell mutations at a given rate per generation (e.g., 1 cell/10^5 cells per generation). (3) Mutations represent stochastic events that can occur at any time but are more likely to occur as tumors grow larger, and similarly in fast-growing tumors or tumors with a high spontaneous mutation rate are more likely to occur early. The relation between the probability of a lethal mutation to drug resistance can be expressed as:

$$P = e^{-a(N-)}$$

where P is the probability of cure, e is the base of natural logarithms, a is the mutation rate per cell generation, and N represents the total number of cells present in the tumor.

Goldie and Coldman argued from their analysis that the use of alternating, non–cross-resistant chemotherapy regimens would provide superior results.[45–47] These predictions, unfortunately, have not been confirmed in prospective, randomized trials in either the adjuvant or metastatic setting.[48, 49]

Drug resistance has been explored extensively at the cellular and molecular levels. While drug resistance for specific agents (e.g., methotrexate resistance mediated by dihydrofolate reductase [DHFR] pathway) has been amply demonstrated, more recent interest has focused on mediators of multiple-drug resistance. The best-described of these is P glycoprotein (P-gp), a transmembrane, energy-dependent efflux pump encoded by the *MDRL* gene, described in the early 1980s.[50] This protein confers resistance to several natural products, including the vinca alkaloids, doxorubicin, the taxanes, and the epipodophyllotoxins. P-gp has been identified in some studies as a prognostic factor in breast cancer.[51, 52] Recently, another protein that confers multidrug resistance, the "multidrug resistance–associated protein" (MRP), has been described. Like P-gp, it is a member of the ATP-binding cassette supergene family.[53, 54] Its role in breast cancer is currently unknown.

In addition, somatic cell resistance is clearly not the only barrier to cure of breast cancer. Norton and Simon, beginning in the mid-1970s, described the growth of breast cancer in terms of gompertzian kinetics.[55–60] In this model, the rate of tumor growth decreases (owing to either decreasing tumor growth fractions or increasing cell loss) as tumor cell population increases, eventually reaching an asymptotic plateau. This change in tumor growth rate is described by the mathematical formulation:

$$N(t) = N(0) \exp \{In[N(\infty)/N(0)] [1 - \exp (-bt)]\},$$

where $N(0)$ is the tumor size at time $t = 0$ and $N(\infty)$ is the plateau size that is approached as t approaches infinity; b is a variable for growth rate. As examined by Norton and Simon, and subsequently by Norton in numerous publications, application of gompertzian kinetics predicts tumors to be most resistant at an early point in their growth and again at a late point, and most sensitive during the middle portion of their natural history, where the tumor growth fraction is greatest and cell loss relatively minimal.[55–60] Furthermore, gompertzian models predict that, for tumors treated at or near their asymptotic plateau, (in the absence of total cell elimination significant cell kill is associated with rapid tumor regrowth, as cells re-enter the exponential portion of the growth curve.[59, 60] This phenomenon, frequently seen in human tumors, but poorly documented has recently been confirmed in a multicellular tumor spheroid system using radiation-treated tumors.[61]

More recently, Retsky and colleagues have proposed as a modification to gompertzian kinetics a stochastic growth model, characterized by an irregular pattern of tumor growth in which plateaus or dormant periods are separated by gompertzian growth spurts. In this approach, drug resistance is a consequence of spontaneous changes in the growth rate or rate of decay of growth, such that the tumor is kinetically resistant to chemotherapy during growth plateaus.[62–64]

Chemotherapeutic Agents

Standard Agents

While a huge number of agents have been utilized to treat metastatic breast cancer, the actual therapeutic repertoire of the practicing oncologist is limited to a handful of active drugs. A listing of the agents most commonly used is shown in Table 72–3, with representative response rates. These agents are discussed below.

Antitumor Antibiotics

Doxorubicin (Adriamycin) is one of the most useful of the standard agents for metastatic breast cancer.

TABLE 72–3. STANDARD CHEMOTHERAPEUTIC AGENTS FOR METASTATIC BREAST CANCER

Agent	Response Rate (%)
Doxorubicin	
Prior therapy	28
No prior therapy	52
Mitoxantrone	
Prior therapy	13
No prior therapy	31
Methotrexate	34
5-Fluorouracil	28
Vinblastine	20
Paclitaxel	
Prior therapy	34
No prior therapy	59
Cyclophosphamide	32
Mitomycin C	41

Data from references 181 and 182.

In the pre-taxane era it was generally considered the most active single agent for the treatment of metastatic breast cancer. Like its sister drug, epirubicin, it functions as a DNA intercalator. Primary toxicities include hair loss, emesis, mucositis, and neutropenia. Cardiac toxicity may be either acute (arrhythmias, generally asymptomatic and transient) or chronic (congestive cardiomyopathy). Doxorubicin-induced cardiomyopathy is related to cumulative dose, individual dose, and underlying risk factors, including history of congestive heart failure, chest wall irradiation, and advanced age. Because peak serum dose is thought to be associated with increased risk of congestive heart failure, infusion time has been prolonged in an attempt to ameliorate this toxicity.[65]

Doxorubicin has been a mainstay of combination regimens, and has commonly been used for salvage therapy when the initial methotrexate-based regimens (e.g., cyclophosphate, methotrexate, and 5-fluorouracil [CMF]) failed. Phase II trials have demonstrated that high-dose doxorubicin (in the range of 75 to 90 mg/m^2) results in increased response rates, albeit at the price of increased dose-related toxicity.[66]

Epirubicin (4'-epiadriamycin, epidoxorubicin) is a semisynthetic L-arabino derivative of doxorubicin in which the aminosugar daunosamine is replaced with acosamine.[67] Epirubicin is characterized by a modestly better therapeutic index than doxorubicin, with less myelosuppression, less nausea and vomiting, less hair loss, and a significantly lower risk of congestive heart failure. At either equimolar or equitoxic doses, its activity is similar against metastatic breast cancer.[67] The drug has been administered intravenously in a wide range of doses, generally every 3 weeks. Dose-escalation trials with this agent (both alone and in combination with other agents) have demonstrated increased response rates with increasing dose but no improvement in overall survival.[68–73] Epirubicin, inexplicably, is not approved for use in the United States.

Mitomycin C works principally by alkylation of DNA, producing cross-linking and adduct formation.[74] As a single agent, it is given intravenously in doses of 10 to 20 m/m^2 every 4 to 8 weeks. Mitomycin has been used primarily for salvage, owing in large part to its peculiar and often dangerous side effects. These include myelosuppression, which unlike is delayed in onset, peaking at 4 to 5 weeks; the (fortunately) relatively rare hemolytic-uremic syndrome; and phlebitis and extravasation necrosis of the skin. Mitomycin has most often been combined with vinblastine. Used for salvaging, this combination produces response rates as high as 40 percent.[74, 75] The taxanes have largely supplanted mitomycin's role for salvaging; a randomized trial comparing paclitaxel, 175 mg/m^2 every 3 weeks, with mitomycin C, 12 mg/m^2 every 6 weeks, revealed a significantly higher response rate and significantly longer median time to progression for paclitaxel.[76]

Anthracenediones

The anthracenedione mitoxantrone, a member of the anthraquinone chemical class, is a synthetic DNA intercalator that bears comparison to doxorubicin and epirubicin. Interest in this compound came about in large part because it lacks the amino sugar thought responsible for doxorubicin's cardiotoxicity. Randomized trials comparing mitoxantrone with doxorubicin for metastatic breast cancer have demonstrated similar but somewhat inferior overall response rates, though with considerably less cardiotoxicity, alopecia, emesis, and mucositis.[77, 78] The modestly inferior response rates have not been associated with inferior overall survival rates for either single-agent or combination chemotherapy comparisons, making this agent an acceptable alternative to doxorubicin for metastases.[77–81] In recent years, mitoxantrone has been combined effectively with fluorouracil and leucovorin with relatively high reported response rates and acceptable toxicity.[82, 83]

The greatest benefit of this agent, its relatively milder cardiotoxicity, is lost when the dose is increased significantly: an intensive single-agent trial reported cardiotoxicity (as determined by MUGA scan–documented decrease in left ventricular ejection fraction) in 37 percent of patients treated with mean total doses of 83.0 mg/m^2.[84] This increased toxicity was not accompanied by an impressive improvement in response rates. Mitoxantrone has seen limited use as a component of large-dose chemotherapy combinations.

Antimetabolites

5-Fluorouracil. The fluorinated pyrimidine 5-fluorouracil (5-FU) has long been a mainstay of combination chemotherapy for breast cancer. Typically, it is administered as a brief IV infusion, though other routes of administration have been utilized. Oral administration results in poor absorption (25 percent to 30 percent) that is often erratic. Given a single agent, response rates of 28% may be obtained in previously untreated patients. In recent years, when continuous infusion 5-FU was utilized as salvage therapy, response rates ranged from 4 percent to 53 percent in reported trials.[85] This large range reflects the effect on response of previous therapy and other patient selection factors.

Methotrexate. The antifol methotrexate, like 5-FU, has frequently been used for metastases, particularly in the pre-doxorubicin era. When small doses are administered orally absorption is acceptable (75 percent to 95 percent), but typically it is administered intravenously. As described elsewhere in this chapter, randomized trials comparing combinations in which doxorubicin is substituted for methotrexate consistently demonstrate lower response rates (and lower overall toxicity) for the regimens containing methotrexate, though the effect on overall survival is only modest.

Microtubule Inhibitors

Vinca Alkaloids. The vinca alkaloids are a family of drugs derived from the periwinkle plant. They function through their effects as inhibitors of microtubule synthesis. The two standard vincas, vinblastine and vincristine, both have significant single-agent activity against metastatic breast cancer but significantly different toxicity profiles. While toxicities overlap, vinblastine is characterized by relatively more myelotoxicity and relatively less neurotoxicity than vincristine. Thus, vinblastine has been the vinca of choice for metastatic breast cancer. While the vincas were a mainstay of early combination regimens (for instance, the Cooper regimen, CMFVP, and vinblastine, Adriamycin [doxorubicin], thiotepa, and halotestin [VATH]), interest and use waned after the discovery in randomized trials that the addition of vinblastine to other active agents added nothing except toxicity for patients with metastatic breast cancer.[86-90]

The most recent addition to the vinca alkaloid family is vinorelbine (5′ nor-anhdrovinblastine, Navelbine), a semisynthetic vinca alkaloid that differs from vinblastine by a modification of the cantharine moiety of the molecule. Several recent phase II trials suggest that this agent is effective for metastatic breast cancer and tolerated well, having significant first- and second-line activity.[91-94] Vinorelbine response rates of 41 percent as first-line chemotherapy (Table 72–4) for metastatic breast cancer have been reported, results generally superior to those obtained with other vinca alkaloids. As salvage chemotherapy, it produced response rates between 15 percent and 36 percent. It is not clear whether this superiority is real or is some artifact of patient selection. A prospective, randomized trial whose subjects were heavily pretreated compared intraveneous vinorelbine (30 mg/m² weekly) with intravenous melphalan (25 mg/m² every 4 weeks). The superiority of vinorelbine, in terms of time to treatment failure and overall survival was demonstrated.[95] Vinorelbine is generally given in intravenous doses of 30 mg/m² weekly.

Taxanes

The taxanes are among the newest standard agents for metastatic breast cancer. Paclitaxel, the parent taxane, was approved by the U.S. Food and Drug Administration for use in metastatic breast cancer in 1994. Despite this, the taxanes rapidly found a place in the treatment of advanced breast cancer, because of their activity and their novel mechanism of action. The taxanes work through their effects on microtubules. In contrast to the vinca alkaloids (which inhibit microtubule formation), the taxanes promote microtubule formation, resulting in microtubules that are excessively stable, and therefore dysfunctional.[96-98] In vitro data suggest that cytotoxicity is related to both concentration and duration of exposure. Both taxanes appear to work through similar mechanism.

The two agents have similar mechanisms of action, but they differ considerably in toxicity. Both agents are characterized by toxicities that include myelosuppression, alopecia, gastrointestinal toxicity, anaphylactoid reactions, and cardiac arrhythmias. Docetaxel, in addition, is associated with progressive, and sometimes dose-limiting, development of peripheral edema, and occasionally with pericardial effusions and an excess of skin reactions.

Both agents are among the most active ones available for metastatic breast cancer. Paclitaxel has been given in a broader spectrum of doses and schedules than docetaxel. Initial trials of paclitaxel suggested an objective response rate of 56 percent to 62 percent when administered over 24 hours in doses of 200 to 250 mg/m².[99, 100] Subsequent trials using shorter infusion durations generally resulted in lower objective response rates overall (Table 72–5). A recent prospective, randomized trial showed no difference in overall response rates comparing shorter (3 hours) and longer (24 hours) durations of infusion but did demonstrate a survival advantage with longer infusion times. Ongoing trials are comparing 3- with 96-hour infusion times, and 24- with 96-hour infusions. In contrast, docetaxel has been administered mostly in a single dosage (100 mg/m² over 1 hour every 3 weeks). Response rates have been consistently in the 55 percent to 70 percent range (see Table 72–4) when it was given as first-line therapy for metastatic breast cancer. The fact that both agents show significant second-line activity in patients who previously received anthracycline-based chemotherapy, suggests a relative absence of cross-resistance.

Only recently have the taxanes been combined with other active agents to treat metastatic breast

TABLE 72–4. VINORELBINE IN METASTATIC BREAST CANCER

Dosage	Patients (n)	RR (%)	MDR/TTP	Prior Therapy	Reference
30 mg/m²/wk	100	16	5 mo/3 mo	Yes	195
30 mg/m²/wk	115	15	NS/12w	Yes	95
30 mg/m²/wk	45	41	9 mo/6 mo	No	91
20–25 mg/m²/wk	70	36	29 wk/18 wk	Yes	92
5.5–10 mg/m²/d × 5 q 21–28 d	64	36	6 mo/NS	Yes	93
30 mg/m²/wk	107	34	34 wk/18 wk	Yes	94
30 mg/m²/wk	157	41	NS/6 mo	No	196
130 mg/wk PO	17	0	——/——	Yes	197

Key: NS, not stated; MDR, median duration of response; RR, response rate; TTP, time to progression.

TABLE 72–5. TAXANES IN PATIENTS PREVIOUSLY UNTREATED FOR METASTATIC BREAST CANCER

Drug/Dosage	n	Response Rate (%)	MDR	PFS/TTP	Reference
Paclitaxel					
250 mg/m²/24 hr	25	56	5 + mo	7 mo	99
250 mg/m²/24 hr	28	62	NS	NS	100
250 mg/m²/3 hr	25	32	7 mo	NS	183
Docetaxel					
100 mg/m²/1 hr	35	67	44 + wk	NS	184
100 mg/m²/1 hr	34	53	9 mo	NS	185
100 mg/m²/1 hr	32	63	4.6 mo	NS	
100 mg/m²/1 hr	37	54	26 wk	NS	186
75 mg/m²/1 hr	15	40			187

Key: MDR, median duration of response; PFS, progression-free survival; TTP, time to progression.

cancer. A recent trial by Gianni and associates reported a 94 percent overall response rate in previously untreated patients who received paclitaxel and doxorubicin in combination, though use of this combination has been hampered by reported increased risk of congestive cardiomyopathy.[101] Similarly, the combination of cisplatin and paclitaxel has been reported to result in an 85 percent overall response rate.[102] Whether paclitaxel or docetaxel in combination with other active agents will have a significant impact remains to be seen; a current Eastern Cooperative Oncology Group trial is comparing single-agent paclitaxel, single-agent doxorubicin, and the combination of paclitaxel and doxorubicin.

Alkylating Agents

The alkylating agents have a long history in the treatment of metastatic breast cancer, where they play a significant role in virtually every disease stage, including regular use in standard adjuvant and metastatic regimens and in large-dose chemotherapy regimens. As a group, they are characterized by their ability to damage negatively charged, electron-rich, nucleophilic sites on biological molecules, adding alkyl groups and forming DNA adducts that alter DNA form and function.[103] Their activity is cell cycle dependent but not cell cycle specific. Resistance to alkylators is almost always relative rather than absolute and generally can be overcome (at least in vitro) by increasing the dose.[104–106]

Cyclophosphamide is the alkylating agent most often used to treat breast cancer, generally in combination with the anthracycline doxorubicin and/or antimetabolites such as methotrexate and 5-FU. It can be administered orally (absorption from the gut is essentially complete) or intravenously. An EORTC trial comparing oral and intravenous cyclophosphamide (in the context of the CMF regimen) has suggested that oral administration results in a higher overall remission rate.[107] In recent years, cyclophosphamide has seen extensive use in the setting of large-dose chemotherapy, as its predominant dose-limiting myelotoxicity may be countered through stem cell rescue.

Platinum Compounds

The platinum compounds cisplatin and carboplatin in essence function as alkylating agents. Cisplatin has been tested extensively against metastatic breast cancer, as both first-line and salvage therapy. It is only minimally active for salvage, but several phase II front-line trials have demonstrated significant activity (composite 50 percent response rate).[108, 109] Despite this relatively high level of activity, the agent has been little used as a standard chemotherapeutic agent, owing to inconvenience of administration, cumulative toxicity, and diminished quality of life. Carboplatin demonstrated a lower level of activity as front-line therapy for metastatic breast cancer, with response rates of 35 percent in previously untreated patients.[110] It is worth noting, however, that the trials in which carboplatin was originally examined based dosing on body surface area, whereas more recently the more precise approach of area under the curve (AUC) dosing has been adopted.

Although the platinum compounds have been little used as standard outpatient chemotherapy, owing to their relatively greater toxicity and inconvenience, they have found regular application in the setting of high-dose chemotherapy and autologous stem cell transplantation. This role is based in part on retrospective analyses of platinum-based therapy that suggest a relatively steep dose-response curve and, more importantly, on laboratory data that suggest that resistance to platinum compounds is dose dependent and rarely complete.[104, 106, 108]

Investigational Agents and Approaches

An enormous number of chemotherapeutic agents have been investigated for activity against breast cancer in a phase II setting. Every oncology textbook published in the past 20 years will list large numbers of "promising new agents" for the treatment of metastatic breast cancer, few of which ever came to be used in routine clinical practice. One is reminded of François Villon's famous lament: *Ou sont les neiges d'antan?* ("Where are the snows of yesteryear?")

The reasons for this depressing litany of failed

agents are many. Certainly the most common reason is drug inactivity. Chemotherapeutic agents have generally been tested in previously treated patients when the twin rocks of multiple-drug resistance and toxicity have dashed the hopes of many new agents. Only in recent years has phase II testing switched to less heavily pretreated patients. A more significant problem has been that the nature of the drug-testing process has generally involved a brute force, highly empirical screen of large numbers of chemical agents, rather than a biology-driven, mechanistic, first-principle approach. One of the more appealing aspects of recent approaches has been the increasing investigation of rationally designed agents directed against specific tumor processes or problems. The coming years should tell whether this approach will bear significant fruit.

Novel Chemotherapeutic Agents

Gemcitabine

Gemcitabine is a new nucleoside analog (2′, 2′-difluorodeoxycytidine) with multiple biochemical effects, including inhibition of ribonucleotide reductase, and competition with deoxycytidine for incorporation into DNA as a fraudulent base. In a recent phase II trial, an overall response rate of 25 percent was reported in a mixture of previously treated and untreated patients.[111] While this response rate is not striking, the drug is tolerated well and may prove useful in combination therapy.

Campothecins

The campothecins interfere with topoisomerase I activity. At present, topotecan is the only one of the campothecins for which results with metastatic breast cancer have been reported. Chang and colleagues reported responses in 5 of 14 (36 percent) of patients, most of whom had previously received one chemotherapy regimen for metastatic disease.[112] Preliminary evidence suggests that clinical activity can be predicted by western blot or immunohistochemical staining of topoisomerase I in tumor tissue.

Liposomal Doxorubicin

As discussed above, doxorubicin has been known for many years to be one of the most active agents for the treatment of breast cancer. Yet the nonhematopoietic toxicities of doxorubicin have limited its dose and duration of therapy. The use of liposome-encapsulated doxorubicin was formulated in an attempt to overcome these old obstacles, but its pharmacokinetics are basically altered: prolonged circulation time, reduced clearance, and small volume of distribution.[113] Phase I trials of liposomal doxorubicin have shown that hand-foot syndrome and stomatitis are dose limiting; curiously enough, no alopecia is observed.[114]

Growth Inhibitors

Unregulated growth is a first constant of lethal cancers. Put quite simply, cancers that do not grow cannot kill. The evidence for this statement is based on a plethora of laboratory and clinical data. Inhibition of cancer cell growth therefore represents an important goal and a useful therapeutic target. The seeming paradox of ER negativity portending poorer prognosis, increased biological aggressiveness, and growth autonomy was explained with the discovery of the polypeptide growth factors and their unique cell surface receptors. These included the insulin-like growth factors (IGFs), the epidermal growth factors (EGFs), and the fibroblast growth factors (FGFs). The realization that polypeptide growth factor–receptor amplification was associated with poorer prognosis (e.g., EGF receptor, Her-2/neu), and that oncogenes (e.g., *ERBB1* for the EGF receptor) coded for portions of common growth factor receptors, implied the biological significance of these systems.[115]

The existence of novel and heretofore unnoticed growth factor receptors also implied the existence of new therapeutic targets. Recent attention has focused on the EGF-receptor family, which include the parent EGF receptor as well as *ERBB2* (*HER2*/neu), *ERBB3,* and *ERBB4.* Members of this receptor family are characterized by an external (extracellular) ligand receptor domain, a transmembrane portion, and an internal domain containing a tyrosine kinase that is responsible for initiation of intracellular actions of the receptor.

The external (extracellular) domain is an obvious therapeutic target, particularly given the frequent overexpression by breast cancers of cell membrane receptor sites (for EGF and heregulin). The external domain can be attacked in several ways. First, agents that block or prevent ligand binding (e.g., false ligands, monoclonal antibodies) can be used in a way that is analogous to the use of tamoxifen for the ER. Second, using either ligand or antibody directed against the external domain, linked toxins can be brought into contact with and internalized by the cancer cells.[116, 117] Such toxins include classic chemotherapeutic agents, cell poisons such as ricin or diphtheria toxins, and radionuclides. Third, the external domain can be used to attract immune effector systems, as was recently examined in phase I trials through the use of bispecific antibodies that recognize both breast cancer cell and monocyte or macrophage cells.[118]

The internal (tyrosine kinase) domain of members of the EGF receptor family is another potential target for therapy. Agents with the ability to affect the tyrosine kinase domain of members of the EGF family that were recently identified have in vitro activity against breast cancer cells.[119] Trials to examine such agents are in development.

A third, quite fascinating, approach was recently identified. Investigators have combined antibodies directed against growth factor receptors with chemotherapeutic agents such as cisplatin and etoposide, with resultant increased cell kill.[120] This is, perhaps, not particularly surprising at first glance, but the mechanism by which this effect occurs is novel. The antibody used against the cell surface receptor has a stimulating effect. Studies using antisense to EGF mRNA demonstrate that a functioning growth factor receptor pathway is necessary for chemotherapy-induced apoptosis (programmed cell death).[121]

Several recent clinical trials have explored these points of attack. Baselga and colleagues used naked monoclonal antibody directed against HER2/NEU (*ERBB2*), and responses were reported in 11.6 percent of patients with advanced breast cancer.[122] Pegram and coworkers used monoclonal anti-HER2/NEU antibody in combination with cisplatin in patients with advanced breast cancer. Objective responses were observed in 25 percent of patients.[123] Valone and associates recently presented the results of a phase I study employing a bispecific monoclonal antibody (for HER2/NEU and monocyte/macrophage cells) in breast cancer patients.[118] As these trials have observed responses from cancers that were refractory to multiple chemotherapy regimens, it will be interesting to examine this approach in less heavily pretreated patients.

Modulation of Drug Resistance

The discovery of the mechanisms underlying multiple drug resistance, described above, has led to novel attempts to overcome such resistance. The P-glycoprotein efflux pump may be inhibited by several agents, including cyclosporine A, PSC-833, quinine, quinidine, tamoxifen, dexverapamil, beproidil, and progesterone. In vitro, inhibition with any of these agents increases the efficacy of natural products. In patients with metastatic breast cancer, conflicting results have been seen. Wishart and associates were unable to demonstrate any clinical benefit in a prospective, randomized trial that compared epirubicin to epirubicin plus quinidine.[124] In contrast, Belpomme and colleagues demonstrated clinical benefit when verapamil was added to vindesine and 5-FU in a randomized trial.[125] Further trials using drugs specifically designed to inhibit the P-gp efflux pump are under way.

Antisense-Oligonucleotide Therapy

The growth, invasion, and metastasis of breast cancer cells result from complex but specific regulatory processes within cancer cells. These include activation of cellular oncogenes and their protein products. A new way of blocking these products is to prevent translation of messenger RNA (mRNA) into protein. This can be accomplished with antisense oligonucleotides.[126] Antisense oligonucleotides to several protooncogene sense RNAs that have been made were shown to inhibit breast cancer growth in vitro, including FOS, ERBB2, and WNT-1.[127–130] In addition, antisense oligonucleotides may be utilized to modulate multidrug resistance and to affect crucial intra-

cellular enzymatic processes.[131, 132] These agents are currently entering clinical trials. While many practical concerns remain about their use (e.g., destruction by DNase in vivo, the large doses required, the need for parenteral administration, and the relatively short half-life in vivo), antisense technology offers the prospect of treating the cause, rather than the consequences, of the malignant process.[126]

Combination Chemotherapy

Standard Outpatient Regimens

A large number of combination chemotherapy regimens have been utilized for the management of metastatic breast cancer. A representative, but by no means inclusive, sampling of these regimens is shown in Table 72–6. Despite frequent assertions to the contrary, choice of regimen for the individual patient is often an arbitrary decision based on the bias (or place and time of training) of the physician, the physician's gut feeling about the likelihood of success of a regimen, and the physician's understanding of its tolerability for the patient.

Standard combination chemotherapy regimens can be expected to induce remissions in 45 percent to 75 percent of previously untreated patients. Patients remain in remission for 6 to 12 months on average. About 10 percent to 20 percent of responses are complete (i.e., disease cannot be appreciated in sites of previously documented disease). With all but a very

TABLE 72–6. COMBINATION CHEMOTHERAPY REGIMENS FOR METASTATIC BREAST CANCER

Drugs	Dosage	Reference
Cyclophosphamide	600 mg/m² IV d1	260
Methotrexate	40 mg/m² IV d1	
5-Fluorouracil	600 mg/m² IV d1	
	Repeat q 21 d	
Cyclophosphamide	100 mg/m² PO d1–14	261
Doxorubicin	40 mg/m² IV d1&8	
5-Fluorouracil	600 mg/m² IV d1&8	
	Repeat q 21 d	
5-Fluorouracil	500 mg/m² IV d1&8	262
Doxorubicin	50 mg/m² IV d1	
Cyclophosphamide	500 mg/m² IV d1	
	Repeat q 21 d	
Cyclophosphamide	100 mg/m² PO d1–14	138
Doxorubicin	30 mg/m² d1&8	
5-Fluorouracil	500 mg/m² IV d1&8	
	Repeat q 28 d	
Mitomycin	20 mg/m² IV d1	75
Vinblastine	0.15 mg/kg IV d1&22	
	Repeat q 6–8wk	
Mitoxantrone	12 mg/m² IV d1	82
5-Fluorouracil	350 mg/m² IV d1–3	
Leucovorin	300 mg/m² IV d1–3 over 1 hr before 5-FU	
	Repeat q 21 d	
Vinblastine	4.5 mg/m² IV d1	263
Doxorubicin	45 mg/m² IV d1	
Thiotepa	12 mg/m² IV d1	
Fluoxymesterone	30 mg/d PO d1–21	
	Repeat q 21 d	

small percentage of complete remissions, disease eventually recurs, generally in sites of previously documented disease.

Choice of regimens is rarely based on the manifest superiority of one over another with respect to either quality of life or survival benefit. Quality of life comparisons derived from randomized comparisons are vanishingly rare in the literature of metastatic breast cancer. As for survival comparisons, a retrospective analysis of clinical trials published in the *Proceedings of the American Society of Clinical Oncology* from 1984 to 1993, only three of 141 randomized controlled trials (with 26,281 patients) of advanced breast cancer reported a significant ($p<.05$) survival benefit.[133] As this represented a smaller number of positive trials than would have been predicted by chance alone, one may question whether a decade of clinical research succeeded in defining optimal therapy for metastatic breast cancer, let alone advancing the level of care.

Comparison of Regimens Containing Doxorubicin and Methotrexate

Numerous chemotherapy trials in the pre-taxane era compared doxorubicin- and methotrexate-based regimens.[18, 134–138] The hypothesis tested in these trials was that doxorubicin, by virtue of its superior activity as single-agent for front-line and salvage chemotherapy, would favorably affect survival, time to progression, and quality of life for patients with metastatic breast cancer.

These trials, taken as a whole, demonstrated that regimens containing doxorubicin produce superior response rates as compared with methotrexate-based regimens. In several of these studies, superior response rates were associated with modest improvements in survival and time to progression. In 1993 A'Hern and coworkers performed meta-analysis of regimens in which patients were randomized to receive either doxorubicin or methotrexate as part of the regimen.[139] This analysis demonstrated a significant benefit in terms of response (odds of response 0.56, $p<.001$), time to treatment failure (hazard ratio = 0.69, $p<.001$), and survival (hazard ratio 0.78, $p<.001$). These hazard ratios correlated with increase in survival (from approximately 14 months to 18 months), and increased median time to treatment failure (from 5 months to 7 months). Quality of life or palliative effect of the doxorubicin regimens was not evaluated in any published trial, an important consideration given the generally greater toxicity of those regimens. It is reasonable to consider a doxorubicin regimen as first-line chemotherapy, particularly for patients with aggressive, symptomatic disease, whom the superior response of the doxorubicin regimen would be most likely to benefit. It is equally reasonable to use CMF-like regimens for patients with poorer performance status, advanced age, or a history of heart disease.

Duration of Therapy. For patients who respond to induction chemotherapy, it is reasonable to ask what is an appropriate duration of therapy. For the vast majority of patients, metastatic breast cancer is incurable. In this context, questions about length of life, disease-free survival, quality of life, and therapeutic toxicity all take on different valences than in an adjuvant setting. Does prolonging therapy beyond a set number of cycles prolong disease-free or overall survival for the patient with metastatic breast cancer? If so, at what cost, in terms of quality of life and financial resources? Such questions are clearly important but, as yet, good answers elude us.

Several prospective, randomized trials have attempted to answer questions about duration.[140–143] A summary of these trials is shown in Table 72–7. In general, these trials have suggested that prolongation of therapy extends the time to disease progression. The survival effect for prolonged treatment duration, however, is small, when, indeed, there is any.[140–143] Surprisingly, only one of the four published randomized trials directly examined the effect of treatment duration on quality of life.[142] This trial demonstrated significantly better quality of life for patients who received continuous, as opposed to intermittent (i.e., short initial duration) treatment. The results of this trial are limited by the fact that the duration of therapy in the intermittent chemotherapy arm (three cycles of either AC or CMFP) was quite short; some responders may not have expressed the maximal possible response (and therefore benefit) before therapy was discontinued. They are also, of course, limited to the specific regimens employed; a more toxic or less efficacious regimen would necessarily alter cost (toxicity)–benefit (symptomatic improvement) ratio of chemotherapy.

Dose Effects. It has long been known that dose is an important factor in the outcome of chemotherapy, but only since the mid-1980s has this issue been addressed critically.[144] Beginning in the early 1980s, Hryniuk and Bush proposed the dose intensity hypothesis.[145] This can be summarized as follows:

1. Dose intensity, both of individual drugs and of combinations can be calculated in terms of dose per unit of time (commonly milligrams per square meter of body surface per week).
2. The dose intensity of a given regimen correlates with the response rate for that regimen.
3. Relatively modest changes in dose intensity can produce significant changes in response.
4. Increased response rates are associated with improved survival.

While the Hryniuk and Bush approach has been applied to many tumor types, it was first used with methotrexate-based regimens for metastatic breast cancer.[145] Comparing calculated dose intensities for published regimens, Hryniuk and Bush demonstrated a statistically significant correlation between dose intensity and response and a similar correlation between response and survival. This retrospective analysis of dose-response effects has been criticized on several grounds.[146] These include its retrospective

TABLE 72–7.   RANDOMIZED TRIALS OF TREATMENT DURATION IN METASTATIC BREAST CANCER

Regimen	Randomization	TTP	OS	P Value	Reference
D 50 mg/m²	Continue to progression				142
C 750 mg/m² q 21 d	vs.	6 mo	10.7 mo		
or	3 cycles; re-treat upon			6.19	
C 100 mg/m²/d for 14 days	progression				
M 40 mg/m²/d1&8					
F 600 mg/m² d1&8		4 mo	9.4 mo		
Pr 40 mg/m²/d for 14 days q 28 d					
C 600 mg/m²	18 mo	52 wk	67 wk		140
E 60 mg/m² q 3wk	vs.			.068	
F 600 mg/m²	6 mo	39 wk	58 wk		
+					
T 30 mg/d PO each day					
Mx 14 mg/m² q 3 wk for 4 courses	Re-treat upon	26 wk	52 wk		143
	progression				
	vs.			NS	
	Continue to progression				
		22 wk	49 wk		
C 500 mg/m²					
A 50 mg/m²					
F 500 mg/m² q 3 wk for 6 courses					
(induction)					
Followed by:					
C 100 mg/m² × 14 d PO	Continue to progression	9.4 mo	19.6 mo		141
M 40 mg/m² d1&8	vs.			0.68	
F 500 mg/m² d1&8 q 4 wk	Re-treat upon	3.2 mo	21.1 mo		
	progression				

Key: D, doxorubicin; C, cyclophosphamide; M, methotrexate; F, 5-fluorouracil; Pr, prednisone; T, tamoxifen; Mx, mitoxantrone; TTP, time to progression; OS, overall survival.

nature and the comparison of trials using different inclusion and exclusion criteria, different schedules of administration, and even different drugs—in short, a classic "apples and oranges" comparison eschewed in basic statistics courses.

The provocative nature of the dose intensity hypothesis, and the promise it held for improving treatment outcome in breast cancer, naturally led to the development of prospective, randomized trials that would test the hypothesis in a statistically clean fashion. A summary of these trials is shown in Table 72–8. These studies clearly suggest that increases in dose intensity are associated with increased response rates. They have, however, failed to demonstrate improved overall survival for the more dose-intense arm. At least for conventional chemotherapy regimens, increases in dose intensity fail to deliver the promised improvements in survival. It should be added that virtually no study of the dose intensity hypothesis has examined the effect of increasing dose intensity on quality of life. As with questions about duration of therapy, increasing dose intensity might either improve quality of life (by decreasing tumor volume) or impair it (by increasing dose-related toxicity).

These results, it should be emphasized, do not represent a final rejection of the dose intensity hypothesis. The relative increases in dose intensity achieved in such trials—about twofold on average—may simply be too small to overcome drug resistance to commonly used chemotherapeutic agents. In addition, achieved dose intensity—the serum or plasma levels of a drug following administration of a given dose—are known from pharmacological studies to vary tremendously. High-dose chemotherapy plus autologous stem cell rescue, discussed below, is another promising approach to the question of dose effects.

High-Dose Chemotherapy with Autologous Bone Marrow Transplantation

High-dose chemotherapy with autologous transplantation is based on principles similar to those advanced for the dose intensity argument. These principles are a logical extension of several of the first principles underlying the use of chemotherapy. In essence, these can be stated as follows:

1. *Drug resistance is the major barrier to cure.* A large body of theoretical, laboratory and clinical data suggest that the development of somatic cell resistance is the prime determinant of mortality from cancer.[45, 47]

2. *Increased doses overcome drug resistance.* While some tumors develop extreme drug resistance to some agents (defined as resistance to drug levels several orders of magnitude greater than those that are clinically achievable), and while resistance to some drugs or classes of drugs may be essentially absolute (e.g., methotrexate) laboratory data suggest

TABLE 72–8. RANDOMIZED DOSE INTENSITY TRIALS IN METASTATIC BREAST CANCER

Regimen	RDI	N	ORR	P Value	OS	P Value	Reference
D 70 mg/m² q 3 wk	2	24	58		20 mo		188
vs.		24	25	<.02	8 mo	<.01	
D 35 mg/m² q 3 wk							
E 40 mg/wk	2	26	34		42 wk		68
vs.		27	37	NS	84 wk	NS	
E 20 mg/wk							
"good-risk" patients							
D 75 mg/m² q 3 wk	1.87	44	25				189
vs.		27	37	NS	NR	NR	
D 60 mg/m² q 3 wk	1.33						
vs.		32	32				
D 40 mg/m² q 3 wk							
"poor-risk" patients							
D 50 mg/m² q 3 wk	2	34	24				
vs.				NR	NR	NR	
D 25 mg/m² q 3 wk		34	6				
C 600 mg/m² q 3 wk	1.5	58	40				190
E 60 mg/m² q 3 wk				NS	NR	NS	
vs.							
C 600 mg/m² q 3 wk		67	40				
E 40 mg/m² q 3 wk							
E 100 mg/m² q 3 wk	2	102	41		44 wk		71
Pr 50 mg 5×/d q 3 wk							
vs.				.006		NS	
E 50 mg/m² q 3 wk		100	23		46 wk		
Pr 50 mg 5×/d q 3 wk							
P 120 mg/m² q 3 wk	2	19	21				191
vs.				NS	NR	NR	
P 60 mg/m² q 3 wk		18	0				
C 600 mg/m²							192
M 40 mg/m² q 3 wk	2	67	30		15.6 mo		
F 600 mg/m²				.03		.026	
vs.							
C 300 mg/m²		66	11				
M 20 mg/m² q 3 wk					12.8 mo		
F 300 mg/m²							
F 500 mg/m² d1–5	2.5						193
D 70 mg/m² d1	1.4	32	78		20 mo		
C 1200 mg/m² d1	2.4			NS		NS	
vs.							
F 500 mg/m² d1&8		27	78		20 mo		
D 50 mg/m² d1							
C 500 mg/m² d1							
E 50 mg/m² d1&8	2.0						73
C 500 mg/m² q 3 wk	1.0		67.2				
F 500 mg/m²	1.0						
vs.		160		<.02	NR	NS	
E 50 mg/m² d1							
C 500 mg/m² q 3 wk			43.1				
F 500 mg/m²							
V 0.625 mg/m²/wk	2						194
M 15 mg/m²/wk	3						
F 300 mg/m²/wk	1.33						
C 60 mg/m²/PO	2.8	106	59		14 mo		
Pr 30 mg/m²/d for 14 days							
20 mg/m²/d for 14 days							
10 mg/m²/d							
vs.				<.05		NS	
C 120 mg/m² IV 5×							
M 4 mg/m² IV 5×							
F 180 mg/m² IV 5×							
V 0.625 IV d1&5		98	40		14 mo		
Pr 40 mg/m² 5×							
Repeat every 28 d							

Key: C, cyclophosphamide; D, doxorubicin; F, fluorouracil; M, methotrexate; E, epirubicin; P, cisplatin; Pr, prednisone; NS, not significant; NR, not reported; RDI, relative dose intensity of more dose intense: less dose intense regimen for individual drugs in regimen; ORR, objective response rate; OS, overall survival (weeks or months).

that alkylating agents in particular are rarely associated with extreme drug resistance.

3. *Myelosuppression represents the major practical barrier to increased dose.* The use of high-dose chemotherapy, particularly in the era before the use of hematopoietic growth factors, was associated with excessive morbidity and not a little mortality.

4. *Myelosuppression can be overcome through the use of supportive care measures (stem cell rescue).* The use of stem cell rescue techniques (either autologous bone marrow transplantation or peripheral stem cell rescue) allows reconstitution of marrow damaged by large-dose combination alkylator therapy.

High-dose chemotherapy trials with stem cell rescue initially used single agents, usually in heavily pretreated patients. The results of such trials were almost uniformly poor (Table 72–9). The heavily pretreated patients in early combination high-dose trials suffered a similar fate, though higher complete remission rates were observed (Table 72–10). Subsequent combination trials performed in patients pretreated less heavily (Table 72–11) achieved relatively consistent results. As a group, they have demonstrated overall and complete remission rates higher than those usually obtained with standard-dose chemotherapy regimens: on average, slightly more than half of patients who receive transplantation enter a clinical complete remission. While most such patients suffer relapse and die, some 10 percent to 25 percent

of transplant patients remain alive and disease-free 5 years after institution of therapy. As with the results for response rates, these results appear to be more impressive than those obtained with standard chemotherapy trials.

There are problems, however, with too easy acceptance of the single-institution trials. Candidates for high-dose chemotherapy differ in significant ways from the average patient with metastatic breast cancer. The process of selection for high-dose chemotherapy, which in most institutions involves exclusions for age, poor performance status, impaired organ function, and (for practical purposes) financial impoverishment, is selection biased and may distort outcome. A retrospective analysis of patients treated with standard-dose anthracycline-based chemotherapy at M.D. Anderson Hospital has demonstrated that application of standard inclusion and exclusion criteria used for stem cell transplantation *select* a group of patients who are likely to have higher overall response rates, superior times to progression, and better overall survival.[147] The wise words of Fyodor Dostoyevsky in his novel *The Possessed* bear remembering: "Its impossible to avoid being biased as long as there is any possibility of choice. The very selection of items constitutes advice on how they should be interpreted."

The ideal solution to this problem would be the completion of prospective, randomized trials. At present, two such trials have been reported.[148, 149] The first compared a standard-dose regimen of cyclophos-

TABLE 72–9. HIGH-DOSE TRIALS OF SINGLE AGENTS FOR FAILED TREATMENT OR REFRACTORY BREAST CANCER

| | | | | Median Duration of Response (mo) | | | | | |
| | | | | CR | | RR | | | |
Investigator	Institution	Drug	n	#	%	#	%	V	mg/m²
Nonalkylating agents									
Fraschini[198]	MDAH	Etoposide	15	0	0	1	7	NA	900–1350
Mulder[199]	Groningen	Etoposide	3	0	0	1	33	1.5	1000–1500
Wolff[200]	Vanderbuilt	Etoposide	3	0	0	0	0	——	1500–2700
Total		Etoposide	21	0	0	2	10		
Ariel[201]	NY Med Col	Hydrea	8	0	0	3	38	NA	40000
Tannir[202]*	MDAH	AMSA	16	0	0	2	13	7, 11	600–750
Total			45	0	0	7	16		
Alkylating agents									
Shea[203]	DFCI	Carboplatin	2	0	0	1	50	NA	500–2400
Peters[202]*	Duke	Dibromodulcitol	7	0	0	1	14	1	1500–4800
Tannir[202]*	MDAH	Mitomycin C	15	0	0	1	7	<3	30–50
Schilcher[204, 205]*	Wayne State	Mitomycin C	2	0	0	0	0	——	60
LeMaistre[206]	NATG	Thiotepa	18	1	6	8	44	4 (2–7)	180–1575
Lazarus[207]	Case Western	Thiotepa	2	0	0	1	50	4	270–810
Slease[208]	Oklahoma	Cyclophosphamide	6	0	0	3	50	3,4,8	7800
Collins[202]*	Seattle	Cyclophosphamide	2	0	0	1	50	NA	5000
Corringham[202]*	R Free Hospital, London	Melphalan	4	3	75	3	75	9–23 +	120–140
Maraninchi[209, 210]	Marseilles	Melphalan	4	1	25	1	25	24	140
Knight[211]	San Antonio	Melphalan	6	1	17	3	50	(1–4)	180
Lazarus[212, 213]	NATG	Melphalan	6	0	0	4	67	(2–14)	120–225
Total			74	6	8	27	36		

*Findings reported in reference 202.

n, number of patients treated; #, number with response; CR, complete response; RR, overall response rate; V, vincristine.

TABLE 72–10.   HIGH-DOSE TRIALS OF COMBINATIONS IN FAILED TREATMENT OR REFRACTORY BREAST CANCER

Author	Institution	Regimen	n	CR #	CR %	RR #	RR %	Median Duration Response (mo)
Combination chemotherapy								
Eder[220]	DFCI	CT	7	0	0	5	71	2 (1–3)
Mukaiyama[221]	Tokyo (JFCR)	CT	4	1	25	2	50	3
Fay[83]	NATG	CT	9	1	11	9	100	4 (3–11)
Peters[222]	Duke	CTcP	6	1	17	3	50	2
Kaizer[219]	Rush	CTcP	9	1	11	6	67	(1–9)
Eder[223]	DFCI	CTCb	4	0	0	4	100	1–3 +
Vaughan†	Nebraska	CT ± H	7	0	0	4	57	(1–6)
Eder[220]	DFCI	CTL	1	0	0	1	100	3
Kaminer[224, 225]	Chicago	CT/LorB	19	2	11	14	74	3 (1–12)
Lazarus[212]	ECOG	LE	4	2	50	4	100	1–4 +
Peters[222]	Duke	CLcP	8	3	38	7	88	(2–6)
Maraninchi†	Marseilles	CL	5	3	60	3	60	(3–8)
Maraninchi[226]	Marseilles	CL/Mitox.	2	1	50	2	100	(3–25 +)
Langleben[90]	McGill	CLP/Mitox.	4	2	50	3	75	6–11 +
Dunphy†	MDAH	TE/Mitox.	28	7	25	22	79	(3–10 +)
Spitzer†	MDAH	T/Mitox.	24	3	13	16	67	6 +
Mulder[227]	Groningen	Mitox/Cor L	2	2	100	2	100	11 + − 25 +
Spitzer[228]	MDAH	T/Mitox.	24	3	13	16	67	6 +
Tajima[218]	Tokai	ACU/EcP	16	1	6	7	44	4 (2–42)
Tobias†	DFCI	CA	3	0	0	1	33	NA
Lazarus[212]	Case W Res	BP	3	0	0	0	0	—
Eder[215]	DFCI	CBcP	14	3	21	10	71	5
Slease[208]	Oklahoma	CB	10	2	20	8	80	(2–7)
Robinson[229]	Denver	FMV/HN/Ad	1	0	0	1	100	NA
Slease[208]	Oklahoma	CcPEB	3	0	0	1	33	2
Jacobs †	Pittsburg	CcPE	4	0	0	2	50	NA
Kessinger†	Nebraska	CcPE	3	0	0	3	100	4
Bearman†	Seattle	BU/C	4	1	25	1	25	10
Total			228	39	17	157	69	
TBI Regimens								
Stewart[230]	Seattle	C	5	2	40	2	40	(5–6)
Kessinger†	Nebraska	CcP	5	0	0	3	60	(3–9)
Niederwieser[202]	Innsbruck	C*	4	4	100	4	100	(3–34)
Bearman†	Seattle	C	2	0	0	2	100	3
Douer[231]	UCLA	CA/Vbl	2	1	50	1	50	5
Vaughan†	Nebraska	CT	1	0	0	0	0	—
Total			19	7	37	12	63	

*3 in CR prior to BMT (2 liver Tx & 1 lobectomy)
†Findings reported in reference 202.
Key: CR, complete response; RR, overall response rate; n, number of patients; #, number of patients with response; MDR, median duration response.

TABLE 72–11   HIGH-DOSE TRIALS OF COMBINATION THERAPY IN PATIENTS WITH NO PRIOR CHEMOTHERAPY FOR STAGE 4 BREAST CANCER

Investigator No.	Institution	Agents	n	CR #	CR %	RR n	RR %
Peters[214]	Duke	CBcP	21	11	52	14	67
Eder[215]	DFCI*	CBcP	4	3	75	4	100
Tajima[215–218]	Tokai	CAU	23	7	30	17	74
Kaizer[219]	Rush	CTcP	5	4	80	5	100
Total			53	25	47	40	75

*One patient reported in both Duke and DFCI data is shown here with DFCI.
Key: CR, complete response; RR, overall response rate; n, number of patients; #, number of patients with response.
Modified from Sledge GWJ, Antman KH: Progress in chemotherapy for metastatic breast cancer. Semin Oncol 19:317–332, 1992.

phamide, mitoxantrone, and vinblastine with a large-dose regimen of cyclophosphamide, mitoxantrone, and etoposide followed by stem cell rescue. The high-dose–stem cell rescue arm of the trial showed significantly higher complete remission, disease-free survival, and overall survival rates, findings that would support the hypothesis that high-dose chemotherapy has advantages for patients with metastatic breast cancer. However, The relatively small number of patients entered into the trial (90 in all), the poor complete remission rate in the definitely atypical "standard" arm (only 4 percent, and the relatively unimpressive median duration of survival (22 months) observed in the high-dose arm, all suggest that a final answer to this question awaits the results of a larger prospective, randomized trial.

The second trial presents different challenges. It did not directly address whether high-dose chemotherapy is superior to standard therapy. Instead, Peters and coworkers randomized patients entering a complete remission after adriamycin-based chemotherapy to receive high-dose chemotherapy either immediately after standard chemotherapy, or at the time of disease progression. While (as expected) disease-free survival was superior for patients who immediately received high-dose therapy, overall survival was significantly better for those who received high-dose chemotherapy. This apparently counterintuitive result remains to be explained, but it argues against immediate resort to high-dose chemotherapy for metastatic disease.

It is clear that only a minority of patients who undergo high-dose chemotherapy with autologous stem cell transplantation benefit from it with prolonged disease-free survival. In general, analysis of prognostic factors for long-term survival after high-dose chemotherapy suggests a striking parallel to prognosis for all patients with metastatic breast cancer. Patients with disease at a single site fare better than those with multiple sites of disease; patients with hepatic metastases fare poorly; patients who fail to achieve complete remission after induction therapy fare worse; and patients with a short disease-free interval between initial diagnosis and eventual relapse do poorly.[150, 151]

Schedule Effects. Closely related to dose effects, and frequently difficult to disentangle from them, are effects of dosing schedule. Dose effect trials have asked, How much drug is best? Schedule effect trials ask, How are the regimens best given? How a regimen is given can, of course, affect how much is given, and vice versa, making a clean separation of the two difficult. Analyses of schedule, therefore, need to control adequately for differences in dose intensity.

While a large and ever growing body of literature attests to the seemingly infinite number of schedules in which individual drugs may be administered (reviewed above), amazingly few trials compare different schedules for combination regimens. Schedules of anthracycline-based regimens are the most thoroughly investigated, which is perhaps surprising

given that experimental data do not suggest schedule-based differences in response. Hortobagyi and colleagues investigated three different fluorouracil-adriamycin cyclophosphamide (FAC) schedules: constant doxorubicin doses but with administration times that included bolus and 48- and 96-hour infusions.[65] No differences in response were seen, though the long infusions were associated with somewhat lower rates of congestive cardiomyopathy. In a Finnish trial, weekly CEF, administered with the same dose intensity (mg/m^2/week) as monthly CEF, was inferior in terms of response, duration of response, and overall survival.[152]

For nonanthracycline regimens, a randomized EORTC trial that compared bolus cyclophosphamide with oral cyclophosphamide (in the setting of CMF chemotherapy) clearly demonstrated the superiority of oral cyclophosphamide for response rate and overall survival.[107] The regimens used, however, varied considerably, not only in schedule but in dose intensity, and this makes it difficult to judge the effect of schedule per se.

Chemohormonal Therapy

The patient with breast cancer has, of course, more options for systemic therapy of metastatic breast cancer than chemotherapy. For many patients (indeed, a majority), the presence of a positive ER means that the patient is potentially hormone sensitive. Given that chemotherapy and hormone therapy do not necessarily attack the same cells in a cancer, it is reasonable to ask whether addition of hormone therapy to chemotherapy might improve cell kill, prolong time to treatment failure, and improve overall survival time.

This hypothesis has been tested in a fairly large number of prospective, randomized trials (Table 72–12).[153–159]

The results of these trials have varied considerably with regard to response rate and time to progression. In general, however, such trials have shown no clear survival benefit for the addition of hormone therapy to chemotherapy. There are important practical objections to combining chemotherapy with hormone therapy. When two such disparate treatment approaches are combined and a clinical response is seen, investigators are left with the problem of deciding whether the patient is responding to chemotherapy or hormone therapy. While hormone therapy may be continued indefinitely, chemotherapy duration is frequently limited by the patient's tolerance and drug toxicity. Prolonging an ineffective therapy, whose ineffectiveness is masked by the success of the active therapy, exposes the patient to unnecessary expense and cumulative toxicity.

Chemoprotective Agents

The dose and duration of chemotherapeutic agents are often limited by both acute and cumulative toxicities. As these toxicities are potential barriers to the

TABLE 72–12.   RANDOMIZED TRIALS COMPARING CHEMOTHERAPY AND CHEMOHORMONAL THERAPY FOR METASTATIC BREAST CANCER

Regimen	Reference No.	Patients (n)	RR (%)	TTF/TTP	OS
DA vs	258	135	36†	110 d†	270 d
DAT			55	170 d	340
AC	153	339	45.1	11 mo	NS
T			22.1	3 mo	
ACT			51.3	9 mo	
CAF	155	474	55	9.5 mo	19.9 mo
CAFT			64	11.4 mo	20.6 mo
CMF	154	220	49†	7 mo†	19 mo
CMFT			75	14 mo	24
CFP	156	131	68	287 d	544 d
CFPT			61	158 d	394
CMF	157	117	45.5†	13.3 mo	22.5
CMFT			70.6	16.3 mo	24.7
CMFMp			67.7	12.7 mo	21.7
CMF	158	145	51†	24 wk	111 wk
CMFT			74	48 wk	78 wk
AV/CMF	159	69	61		15 mo
AV/CMF +N			53		8
CMFVP	259	42	56	7.8 mo	13.2 mo
CMFVP/ Ov			74	9.5 mo	19.9
CMFVP	259	96	54	10.6 mo	19.2 mo
CMFVP +DES			63	8.4 mo	26.7
CMFVP	259	75	63	10.0 mo	22.8
CMFVP +MPA			53	8.9 mo	18.1

Key: RR, response rate; TTF/TTP, time to treatment failure or to progression; OS, overall survival; C, cyclophosphamide; M, methotrexate; F, 5-fluorouracil; T, tamoxifen; A, adriamycin (doxorubicin); Mp, methylprednisolone; V, vincristine; P, prednisone; Ov, ovariectomy; DES, diethylstilbestrol; MPA, medroxyprogesterone acetate; NS, not significant.
*Except where indicated by a dagger († = $P \leq .05$), all differences in RR, TTF/TTP, and OS have a P value $>.05$.

success of chemotherapy for metastatic disease, efforts have focused on means of decreasing such toxicities, thus improving the therapeutic ratio.

Dexrazoxane

Dexrazoxane (Zinecard, ADR-529, ICRF-187) is a potent intracellular chelating agent derived from EDTA. Originally evaluated as a chemotherapeutic agent for the treatment of solid tumors, including breast cancer, it was found to be inactive. It has proven successful in reducing anthracycline-induced cardiac toxicity, particularly dose-related congestive heart failure. Whereas the mechanism of this action is unclear, it is thought to be related to its ability to interfere with iron-mediated free radical generation in myocardial cells, the presumed mechanism of anthracycline-induced cardiomyopathy.[160, 161]

Three prospective, randomized trials performed in the setting of metastatic breast cancer have demonstrated that dexrazoxane significantly reduces the incidence of congestive cardiomyopathy, allowing larger cumulative doxorubicin doses than may be achieved in the absence of the cardioprotectant.[162, 163] In one of these studies, the response rates of patients with metastatic breast cancer who received dexrazoxane were lower than those of patients who did not receive the cardioprotectant. While similar results have not been seen in the other breast cancer trials, the Food and Drug Administration has restricted the use of this agent to patients who receive more than 300 mg/m² of doxorubicin in all. In this setting it is administered in proportions of 10:1 with doxorubicin. The ability of this agent to reduce the cardiotoxicity of doxorubicin is unquestioned, but its use begs the question of whether prolonged therapy with doxorubicin has any significant benefit for survival or quality of life. Prospective trials are currently under way to address this question.

Hematopoietic Colony-Stimulating Factors (CSFs)

Recent years have seen the development and extensive use of hematopoietic colony-stimulating factors (e.g., granulocyte CSF and granulocyte-macrophage CSF) as chemoprotectants. Prospective, randomized trials have demonstrated the ability of these agents to stimulate granulopoiesis and to decrease febrile neutropenia. While the efficacy of CSFs in this regard is unchallenged, their exact role in the day-to-day management of patients receiving chemotherapy is less clear. Standard chemotherapy regimens (such as those shown in Table 72–6) frequently induce neutropenia but result in febrile neutropenias in only a minority of patients. Such patients are probably best served by simple dose reductions or delay of subsequent cycles.

In a sense, extended use of CSFs is hostage to the dose intensity issue. Regimens with greater dose intensities of myelosuppressants clearly produce neutropenias that can, in turn, be prevented or ameliorated by CSFs. But as discussed elsewhere in this chapter, the modest increases in dose intensity achieved in outpatient chemotherapy regimens have not clearly been accompanied by prolonged survival or improved quality of life. In the absence of demonstrable clinical benefit, the use of such regimens, and thus of CSFs, should be held in abeyance. The American Society of Clinical Oncology recently presented general guidelines for the use of CSFs.[164] These recommendations are summarized in Table 72–13.

Bisphosphonates for Bone Metastasis

Many patients with metastatic breast cancer suffer bone metastases, often when no other sites of overt metastatic disease are apparent. Such metastases may compromise quality of life long before they threaten its duration. Systemic chemotherapy and local radiotherapy, while they frequently ameliorate bone symptoms, can themselves directly impair bone marrow function and, in any event, are often limited in dose, and eventually in effectiveness.

Bisphosphonates are a novel alternative to chemotherapy and radiotherapy for bone metastasis.[165] These agents, originally used for the treatment of malignant hypercalcemia, inhibit osteoclasts and retard or prevent osteoclast-mediated bone resorption. In vivo laboratory studies suggest that bisphosphonates may selectively reduce tumor burden in bone.[166] Phase II trials of bisphosphonates in metastatic breast cancer have demonstrated that their

administration can reduce pain, increase mobility, and decrease analgesic requirements.[167–169] In some cases, bisphosphonate administration may result in recalcification of lytic bone metastases.[169] Prospective, randomized trials that compared bisphosphonate administration with control or placebo demonstrated statistically significant reductions in pain, analgesic requirements, radiation therapy requirements, and incidence of fractures in patients with metastatic breast cancer and other malignancies.[170–174]

While dose, schedule, and type of bisphosphonates have varied considerably in published trials, dose-finding studies of intravenous pamidronate suggest a dose-response effect, and dose intensities of at least 20 mg/week are most effective at ameliorating symptoms.[175] Duration of infusion has also varied considerably, though pharmacokinetic evidence suggests that bone retention of pamidronate is independent of infusion rate.[176] A reasonable dose of pamidronate would be 90 mg infused over 2 hours every 4 weeks.[174] Complications of therapy are generally mild and may include transient infusion site reactions, fever, nausea and vomiting, electrolyte abnormalities (hypocalcemia, hypokalemia, and hypophosphatemia), and (rarely) cardiac arrhythmias.[177]

THE CURABILITY OF METASTATIC DISEASE

While metastatic breast cancer is eventually fatal for most of its victims, a small fraction of patients enter clinically complete remission and remain in remission, off all therapy, quite long. Such occurrences are, for the average physician, anecdotal, but these are powerful anecdotes, nevertheless. They are a source of encouragement for patients, who have no wish to be robbed of hope, and to clinical scientists, whose hope is to turn the anecdotal into the commonplace. The extent to which routine clinical practice should be guided by such anecdotes, rather than by the grim realization of the common fate of patients with metastatic breast cancer, depends, of course, on the interaction of doctor and patient.

The frequency of long-term disease-free survival (to use a more precise, if less euphonious, term than "cure") varies by study. The best evidence for its existence comes from the M.D. Anderson Cancer Center, where 3.1 percent of patients treated with doxorubicin-based (generally FAC-type) chemotherapy remained in complete remission at 5 years, and more than half of those longer than 10 years.[178] Other series have reported lower rates of long-term disease-free survival, generally in fewer than 1 percent of patients.[179, 180]

It seems likely that one major barrier to cure is the low induction rate of complete remission associated with most currently used regimens. Achievement of a clinical complete remission represents no more than a 2- or 3-log reduction in mass of a tumor with as many as 10^{12} cancer cells, but this is a necessary precondition for cure. More recent years have

---

TABLE 72–13. GUIDELINES FOR USE OF COLONY-STIMULATING FACTORS

Primary CSF administration
  1. Primary administration of hematopoietic CSF should be reserved for patients whose therapy is expected to produce febrile neutropenia ≥40%.
  2. Special circumstances in which CSFs may be used include
     • Pre-existing neutropenia due to disease, extensive previous chemotherapy, previous irradiation therapy to the pelvis, or other significant marrow-containing areas.
     • A history of recurrent febrile neutropenias during earlier chemotherapy regimens of similar or lesser dose intensity.
     • Conditions that enhance the risk of serious infection (e.g., decreased immune function, open wounds, active tissue infections).
Secondary CSF administration
  1. After a documented febrile neutropenia in an earlier cycle.
  2. Where prolonged neutropenia necessitates excessive dose reduction or delay in chemotherapy.
Progenitor-cell transplantation (autologous bone marrow transplantation): All patients.*

*High-dose chemotherapy is an indication for CSF.

seen the introduction of many high-dose chemotherapy regimens for metastatic breast cancer, and these regimens regularly induce complete remission in some 50 percent to 60 percent of treated patients. The majority of patients who enter complete remission after high-dose chemotherapy eventually suffer relapse, a fraction (generally some 10 percent to 25 percent) remain alive and disease-free 5 years after therapy. Whether these patients will be long-term disease-free survivors remains to be seen with further follow-up.

References

1. Parker SL, Tong T, Bolden S, Wingo PA: Cancer statistics, 1996. CA 46(1):5–27, 1996.
2. Singhakowinta A, Potter HG, Burcker TR, et al: Estrogen receptor and natural course of breast cancer. Ann Surg 183:84–88, 1976.
3. Clark GM, Sledge GW Jr, Osborne CK, McGuire WL: Survival from first recurrence: Relative importance of prognostic factors in 1,015 breast cancer patients. J Clin Oncol 5:55–61, 1987.
4. Cambell FC, Blamey RW, Elston CW, Nicholson RI, Griffiths K, Haybittle JL: Oestrogen-receptor status and sites of metastasis in breast cancer. Br J Cancer 44:456–459, 1981.
5. Stewart JF, King RJB, Sexton SA, Mills RR, Rubens RD, Hayward JL: Oestrogen receptors, sites of metastatic disease and survival in recurrent breast cancer. Eur J Cancer 17:449–453, 1981.
6. Lamovec J, Bracko M: Metastatic pattern of infiltrating lobular carcinoma of the breast: An autopsy study. J Surg Oncol 48:28–33, 1991.
7. Bumpers H, Hassett JJ, Penetrante R, Hoover E: Endocrine organ metastases in subjects with lobular carcinoma of the breast. Arch Surg 128:1344–1347, 1993.
8. Borst M, Ingold J: Metastatic patterns of invasive lobular versus invasive ductal carcinoma of the breast. Surgery 114:637–641, 1993.
9. Hietanen P, Miettinen M, Makinen J: Survival after first recurrence in breast cancer. Eur J Clin Oncol 22:913–919, 1986.
10. Falkson G, Gelman RS, Leone L, Galkson CI: Survival of premenopausal women with metastatic breast cancer. Long-term follow-up of Eastern Cooperative Group and Cancer and Leukemia Group Studies. Cancer 66:1621–1629, 1990.
11. Goldhirsch A, Gelber RD, Castiglione M: Relapse of breast cancer after adjuvant treatment in premenopausal and perimenopausal women: Patterns and prognoses. J Clin Oncol 6:89–97, 1988.
12. Rouesse BJ, Friedman S, Sarrazin D, et al: Primary chemotherapy in the treatment of inflammatory breast carcinoma: A study of 230 cases from the Institut Gustave-Roussy. J Clin Oncol 4:1765–1771, 1986.
13. Howat JMT, Harris M, Swindell R, Barnes DM: The effect of oestrogen and progesterone receptors on recurrence and survival in patients with carcinoma of the breast. Br J Cancer 51:263–270, 1985.
14. Paterson AHG, Zuck VP, Szafran O, Lees AW, Hanson J: Influence and significance of certain prognostic factors on survival in breast cancer. Eur J Cancer Clin Oncol 18:937–943, 1982.
15. Vincent MD, Powles TJ, Skeet R, et al: An analysis of possible prognostic features of long term and short term survivors of metastatic breast cancer. Eur J Cancer 22:1059–1065, 1986.
16. Kamby C, Rose C, Ejlertsen B, et al: Stage and pattern of metastases in patients with breast cancer. Eur J Cancer Clin Oncol 23:1925–1934, 1987.
17. Falkson G, Gelman RS, Tormey DC, Cummings FJ, Carbone PP, Falkson HC: The Eastern Cooperative Oncology Group experience with cyclophosphamide, adriamycin, and 5-fluorouracil (CAF) in patients with metastatic breast cancer. Cancer 56:219–224, 1985.
18. Cummings FJ, Gelman R, Horton J: Comparison of CAF versus CMFP in metastatic breast cancer: Analysis of prognostic factors. J Clin Oncol 3:932–940, 1985.
19. Falkson G, Gelman R, Falkson CI, Glick J, Haris J: Factors predicting for response, time to treatment failure, and survival in women with metastatic breast cancer treated with DAVTH: A prospective Eastern Cooperative Oncoloy Group Study. J Clin Oncol 9:2153–2161, 1991.
20. Falkson G, Gelman RS, Tormey DC, Falkson C, Walter JM, Cummings FJ: Treatment of metastatic breast cancer in premenopausal women using CAF, with or without oophorectomy: An Eastern Cooperative Oncology Group Study. J Clin Oncol 5:881–889, 1987.
21. Marschke RFJ, Ingle JN, Schaid DJ, et al: Randomized clinical trial of CFP versus CMFP in women with metastatic breast cancer. Cancer 63:1931–1937, 1989.
22. Devitt J, Advent D: Effect of current palliative treatment on the survival of patients with breast cancer. Can J Surg 20:46–50, 1977.
23. Paterson AHG, Szafran O, Cornish F, Lees AW, Hanson J: Effect of chemotherapy on survival in metastatic breast cancer. Breast Cancer Res Treat 1:357–363, 1982.
24. Fey MF, Brunner KW, Sonntag RW: Prognostic factors in metastatic breast cancer. Cancer Clin Trials 4:237–247, 1981.
25. Todd M, Shoag M, Cadman E: Survival of women with metastatic breast cancer at Yale from 1920 to 1980. J Clin Oncol 1:406–408, 1983.
26. Powles T, Coombes R, Smith I, Jones J, Ford H, Gazet J: Failure of chemotherapy to prolong survival in a group of patients with metastatic breast cancer. Lancet 1:580–582, 1980.
27. Ross M, Buzdar A, Smith T, et al: Improved survival of patients with metastatic breast cancer receiving combination chemotherapy. Cancer 55:341–346, 1985.
28. A'Hern RP, Ebbs SR, Baum MB: Does chemotherapy improve survival in advanced breast cancer? A statistical overview. Br J Cancer 57:615–618, 1988.
29. Houston SJ, Richards MA, Bentley AE, Smith P, Rubens RD: The influence of adjuvant chemotherapy on outcome after relapse for patients with breast cancer. Eur J Cancer 29A:1513–1518, 1993.
30. Bonneterre J, Mercer M: Response to chemotherapy after relapse in patients with or without previous adjuvant chemotherapy for breast cancer. Cancer Treat Rev 19:21–30, 1993.
31. Valagussa PT, Bonadonna G: Salvage treatment of patients suffering relapse after adjuvant CMF chemotherapy. Cancer 58:1411–1417, 1986.
32. Alberts A, Falkson G, van der Merwe R: Metastatic breast cancer—age has a significant effect on survival. S African Med J 79:239–241, 1991.
33. Kimmick G, Muss H, Case L, Stanley V: A comparison of treatment outcomes for black patients and white patients with metastatic breast cancer. The Piedmont Oncology Association experience. Cancer 67:2850–2854, 1991.
34. du Toit R, Locker A, Ellis I, et al: An evaluation of differences in prognosis, recurrence patterns and receptor status between invasive lobular and other invasive carcinomas of the breast. Eur J Surg Oncol 17:251–257, 1991.
35. Hahnel R, Twaddle E: The relationship between estrogen receptors in primary and secondary breast carcinomas and in sequential primary breast carcinomas. Breast Cancer Res Treat 5:155–163, 1985.
36. Skipper HE: Criteria associated with destruction of leukemia and solid tumor cells in animals. Cancer Res 27:2636–2645, 1967.
37. Skipper HE: Kinetics of mammary tumor cell growth and implications for therapy. Cancer 28:1479–1499, 1971.
38. Skipper HE: Stepwise progress in the treatment of disseminated cancers. Cancer 51:1773–1776, 1983.
39. Skipper HE: Tumor differences, drug differences, treatment design differences, and effects on therapeutic outcome (degree and duration of therapeutic response). *In* Ragaz J, Simpson-Herren L, Lippman ME, Fisher B (eds): Effects of Ther-

apy on Biology and Kinetics, Part A: Pre-Clinical Aspects. New York, Wiley-Liss, 1990, pp 81–98.

40. Skipper HE: Combination therapy: Some concepts and results. Cancer Chemother Rep 4:137–145, 1974.

41. Greenspan E, Fieber M, Lesnick G, Edelman S: Response of advanced breast carcinoma to the combination of the antimetabolite methotrexate and the alkylating agent thio-TEPA. J Mt Sinai Hosp 30:246–267, 1963.

42. Chlebowski R, Irwin L, Pugh R, et al: Survival of patients with metastatic breast cancer treated with either combination or sequential chemotherapy. Cancer Res 39:4503–4506, 1979.

43. Smalley R, Murphy S, Huguley CJ, Bartolucci A: Combination versus sequential five-drug chemotherapy in metastatic carcinoma of the breast. Cancer Res 36:3911–3916, 1976.

44. Jones RB, Holland JF, Bhardwaj S, Norton L, Wilfinger C, Strashun A: A Phase I-II study of intensive-dose adriamycin for advanced breast cancer. J Clin Oncol 5:172–177, 1987.

45. Goldie JH, Coldman AJ: A mathematic model for relating drug sensitivity of tumors to spontaneous mutation rate. Cancer Treat Rep 63:1727–1733, 1979.

46. Goldie JH, Coldman AJ, Gudauskas GA: Rationale for the use of alternating non–cross-resistant chemotherapy. Cancer Treat Rep 66:439–449, 1982.

47. Goldie JH, Coldman AJ: The genetic origin of drug resistance in neoplasms: Implications for systemic therapy. Cancer Res 44:3643–3653, 1984.

48. Bonadonna G, Zambetti M, Valagussa P: Sequential or alternating doxorubicin and CMF regimens in breast cancer with more than three positive nodes. Ten-year results. JAMA 273:542–547, 1995.

49. Henderson IC, Hayes DF, Come S, Harris JR, Canellos G: New agents and new medical treatments for advanced breast cancer. Semin Oncol 14:34–64, 1987.

50. Kartner N, Riordan J, Ling V: Cell surface P-glycoprotein associated with multidrug resistance in mammalian cell lines. Science 221:1285–1288, 1983.

51. Verrelle P, Meissonnier F, Fonck Y: Clinical relevance of immunohistochemical detection of multidrug resistance P-glycoprotein in breast cancer. J Natl Cancer Inst 83:111, 1991.

52. Linn S, Giaccone G, van Diest P: Prognostic relevance of P-glycoprotein expression in breast cancer. Ann Oncol 6:679–685, 1995.

53. Cole S, Bhardaj G, Gerlach J: Overexpression of a transporter gene in a multidrug resistant human lung cancer cell line. Science 258:1650, 1992.

54. Grant C, Valdimarsson G, Hipfner D: Overexpression of multidrug resistance–associated protein (MRP) increases resistance to natural product drugs. Cancer Res 54:357, 1994.

55. Norton L, Simon R: Tumor size, sensitivity to therapy, and design of treatment schedules. Cancer Treat Rep 61:1307–1317, 1977.

56. Norton L, Simon R: Growth curve of an experimental solid tumor following radiotherapy. J Natl Cancer Inst 58:1735–1741, 1977.

57. Norton L: Implications of kinetic heterogeneity in clinical oncology. Semin Oncol 12:231–249, 1985.

58. Norton L, Simon R: The Norton-Simon hypothesis revisited. Cancer Treat Rep 70:163–169, 1986.

59. Norton L: A Gompertzian model of human breast cancer growth. Cancer Res 48:7067–7071, 1988.

60. Norton L: Biology of residual breast cancer after therapy: A kinetic interpretation. In Ragaz J, Simpson-Herren L, Lippman ME, Fisher B (eds): Effects of Therapy on Biology and Kinetics of the Residual Tumor, Part A: Pre-Clinical Aspects. New York, Wiley-Liss, 1990, pp 109–132.

61. Durand RE: Repopulation: A significant factor in tumor response to multifraction therapy. Proc Am Assoc Cancer Res 33:428, 1992. (Abstract 2553)

62. Speer JF, Petrovsky VE, Retsky MW, Wardell RH: A stochastic numerical model of breast cancer growth that simulates clinical data. Cancer Res 44:4124–4130, 1984.

63. Retsky MW, Schwartzendruber DE, Wardwell RH, Bame PD: Is Gompertzian or exponential kinetics a valid description of

individual human cancer growth? Med Hypotheses 33:95–106, 1990.

64. Retsky MW, Wardell RH, Swartzendruber DE, Headley DL: Prospective computerized simulation of breast cancer: Comparison of computer predictions with nine sets of biological and clinical data. Cancer Res 47:4982–4987, 1987.

65. Hortobagyi G, Fryee E, Buzdar A: Decreased cardiac toxicity of doxorubicin administered by continuous intravenous infusion in combination chemotherapy for metastatic breast carcinoma. Cancer 63:37–45, 1989.

66. Jones RB, Holland JF, Bhardwaj S, et al: A phase I-II study of intensive-dose adriamycin for advanced breast cancer. J Clin Oncol 5:172–177, 1987.

67. Bonadonna G, Gianni L, Santoro A, et al: Drugs ten years later: Epirubicin. Ann Oncol 4:359–369, 1993.

68. Ebbs SR, Saunders JA, Graham H, A'Hern RPA, Bates T, Baum M: Advanced breast cancer. A randomised trial of epidexorubicin at two different dosages and two administration systems. Acta Oncol 28:887–892, 1989.

69. Colajori E, Tosello C, Pannuti F, et al: Randomized multinational trial comparing epirubicin 50 mg/m^2 vs 100 mg/m^2 in combination with 5-fluorouracil and cyclophosphamide as front-line treatment of metastatic breast cancer. Ann Oncol 5(suppl. 8):26, 1994. (Abstract 0127)

70. Marschner N, Kreienberg R, Souchon R, et al: Evaluation of the relevance of epirubicin dose intensity in combination with a fixed dose of cyclophosphamide in metastatic breast cancer. Ann Oncol 5(Suppl. 8):26, 1994. (Abstract 0126)

71. Habeshaw T, Jones R, Stallard S, et al: Epirubicin (Epi) at 2 dose levels with prednisolone (P) as treatment for advanced breast cancer (ABC): Results of a randomised trial. Proc Am Soc Clin Oncol 9:43, 1990.

72. Focan C, Closon MT, Andrien JM, et al: Dose response relationship with epirubicin (E) as first line chemotherapy for advanced breast cancer (BC). A randomized trial. Ann Oncol 1(Suppl.):S18, 1990.

73. Focan C, Andrien JM, Closon MT, et al: Dose-response relationship of epirubicin-based first-line chemotherapy for advanced breast cancer: A prospective randomized trial. J Clin Oncol 11:1253–1263, 1993.

74. Doll C, Weiss R, Issell B: Mitomycin: Ten years after approval for marketing. J Clin Oncol 3:276–286, 1985.

75. Konits P, Aisner J, van Echo D, et al: Mitomycin C and vinblastine chemotherapy for advanced breast cancer. Cancer 48:1295–1298, 1981.

76. Dieras V, Marty M, Morvan F: A phase II randomized study of taxol versus mitomycin C in patients with advanced breast cancer. Proc Am Soc Clin Oncol 13:111, 1994.

77. Neidhart JA, Gochnour D, Roach R, Hoth D, Young D: A comparison of mitoxantrone and doxorubicin in breast cancer. J Clin Oncol 4:672–677, 1986.

78. Henderson IC, Allegra JC, Woodcock T, et al: Randomized clinical trial comparing mitoxantrone with doxorubicin in previously treated patients with metastatic breast cancer. J Clin Oncol 7:560–571, 1989.

79. Bennett JM, Muss HB, Doroshow JH, et al: A randomized multicenter trial comparing mitoxantrone, cyclophosphamide, and fluoruracil with doxorubicin, cyclophosphamide, and fluorouracil in the therapy of metastatic breast cancer. J Clin Oncol 6:1611–1620, 1988.

80. Leonard RCF, Cornbleet MA, Kaye SB, et al: Mitoxantrone versus doxorubicin in combination chemotherapy for advanced carcinoma of the breast. J Clin Oncol 5:1056–1063, 1987.

81. Pavesi L, Preti P, Da Prada G, Pedrazzoli P, Poggi G, Robustelli della Cuna G: Epirubicin versus mitoxantrone in combination chemotherapy for metastatic breast cancer. Anticancer Res 15:495–501, 1995.

82. Hainsworth J, Andrews M, Johnson D, et al: Mitoxantrone, fluorouracil, and high-dose leucovorin: An effective, well-tolerated regimen for metastatic breast cancer. J Clin Oncol 9:1731–1736, 1991.

83. Jones SE, Mennel RG, Brooks B, et al: Phase II study of mitoxantrone, leucovorin, and infusional fluorouacil for treatment of metastatic breast cancer. J Clin Oncol 9:1736–1739, 1991.

84. Shpall EJ, Jones RB, Holland JF, et al: Intensive single-agent mitoxantrone for metastatic breast cancer. J Natl Cancer Inst 80:204–208, 1988.
85. Ng JSY, Cameron DA, Leonard RCF: Infusional 5-fluorouracil in breast cancer. Cancer Treat Rev 20:357–364, 1994.
86. Ahmann D, Bisel H, Hahn R, et al: An analysis of a multiple drug program in the treatment of patients with advanced breast cancer utilizing 5-fluorouracil, cyclophosphamide and prednisone with or without vincristine. Cancer 36:1925–1935, 1985.
87. Tucker WG: Treatment of adenocarcinoma with combinations of cyclophosphamide (NSC26271) and 5-fluorouracil (NSC19893). Cancer Chemother Rep 59:425–427, 1975.
88. Steiner R, Stewart JF, Cantwell BJM, Minton MJ, Knight RK, Rubens RD: Adriamycin alone or combined with vincristine in the treatment of advanced breast cancer. Eur J Cancer Clin Oncol 19:1553, 1983.
89. Chlebowski R, Pugh R, Weiner J, et al: Doxorubicin and CCNU with or without vincristine in patients with advanced breast cancer. Cancer 52:606–609, 1983.
90. Segaloff A, Carter AC, Escher GC, et al: An evaluation of the effect of vincristine added to cyclophosphamide, 5-fluorouracil, methotrexate, and prednisone in advanced breast cancer. Breast Cancer Res Treat 5:311–319, 1985.
91. Romero A, Rabinovich MG, Vallejo CT, et al: Vinorelbine as first-line chemotherapy for metastatic breast carcinoma. J Clin Oncol 12:336–341, 1994.
92. Gasparini G, Caffo O, Barni S, et al: Vinorelbine is an active antiproliferative agent in pretreated advanced breast cancer patients: A phase II study. J Clin Oncol 12:2094–2101, 1994.
93. Toussaint C, Izzo J, Spielmann M, et al: Phase I/II trial of continuous infusion vinorelbine for advanced breast cancer. J Clin Oncol 12:2102–2112, 1994.
94. Weber BL, Vogel C, Jones S, et al: Intravenous vinorelbine as first-line and second-line therapy in advanced breast cancer. J Clin Oncol 13:2722–2730, 1995.
95. Jones S, Winer E, Vogel C, et al: Randomized comparison of vinorelbine and melphalan in anthracycline-refractory advanced breast cancer. J Clin Oncol 13:2567–2574, 1995.
96. Rowinsky EK, Donehower RC: Paclitaxel (Taxol). N Engl J Med 332:1004–1014, 1995.
97. Rowinsky EK, McGuire WP, Donehower RC: The current status of taxol. Principles and Practice of Gynecologic Oncology Updates 1:1–16, 1993.
98. Rowinsky EK, McGuire WP: Taxol: Present status and future prospects. Contemp Oncol March:29–36, 1992.
99. Holmes FA, Walters RS, Theriault RL, et al: Phase II trial of taxol, an active drug in the treatment of metastatic breast cancer. J Natl Cancer Inst 83:1797–1805, 1991.
100. Reichman BS, Seidman AD, Crown JPA, et al: Paclitaxel and recombinant human granulocyte colony–stimulating factor as initial chemotherapy for metastatic breast cancer. J Clin Oncol 11:1943–1951, 1993.
101. Gianni L, Munzone E, Capri G, et al: Paclitaxel by 3-hour infusion in combination with bolus doxorubicin in women with untreated metastatic breast cancer: High antitumor efficacy and cardiac effects in a dose-finding and sequence-finding study. J Clin Oncol 13:2688–2699, 1995.
102. Gelmon KA, O'Reilly S, Plenderleith IH, et al: Bi-weekly paclitaxel and cisplatin in the treatment of metastatic breast cancer. Proc Am Soc Clin Oncol 13:71, 1994. (Abstract #88)
103. Berger NA: Alkylating agents. In DeVita VT, Hellman S, Rosenberg SA, (eds): Cancer: Principles & Practice of Oncology, ed 4. Philadelphia, JB Lippincott, 1993.
104. Teicher B, Cucchi C, Lee J, et al: Alkylating agents. In vitro studies of cross-resistance patterns in human tumor cell lines. Cancer Res 46:4379–4383, 1986.
105. Frei E III, Teicher BA, Holden SA, Cathcart KNS, Wang Y: Preclinical studies and clinical correlation of the effect of alkylating dose. Cancer Res 48:6417–6423, 1988.
106. Frei E III, Cucchi C, Rosowsky A, et al: Alkylating agent resistance: In vitro studies of human cell lines. Proc Natl Acad Sci USA 82:2158–2162, 1985.
107. Engelsman E, Klijn J, Rubens R, et al: "Classical" CMF versus a 3-weekly intravenous CMF schedule in postmeno-

108. pausal patients with advanced breast cancer. Eur J Cancer 27:966–970, 1991.
108. Sledge GW, Roth BJ: Cisplatin in the management of breast cancer. Semin Oncol 16:110–115, 1989.
109. Sledge GW, Loehrer PJ, Roth BJ, Einhorn LH: Cisplatin as first line therapy for metastatic breast cancer. J Clin Oncol 6:1811–1814, 1988.
110. Martin M, Diaz-Rubio E, Casado A, et al: Carboplatin: An active drug in metastatic breast cancer. J Clin Oncol 10:433–437, 1992.
111. Carmichael J, Possinger K, Phillip P, et al: Advanced breast cancer: A phase II trial with gemcitabine. J Clin Oncol 13:2731–2736, 1995.
112. Chang A, Garrow G, Boros L, Asbury R, Pandya K, Keng P: Clinical and laboratory studies of topotecan in breast cancer. Proc Am Soc Clin Oncol 14:105, 1995.
113. Gabizon A, Barenholz Y, Bialer M: Prolongation of the circulation time of doxorubicin encapsulated in liposomes containing a polyethylene glycol–derivatized phospholipid: Pharmacokinetic studies in rodents and dogs. Pharm Res 10:703–708, 1993.
114. Uziely B, Jeffers S, Isacson R, et al: Liposomal doxorubicin: antitumor activity and unique toxicities during two complementary phase I studies. J Clin Oncol 13:1777–1785, 1995.
115. Rajkumar T, Gullick WJ: The type I growth factor receptors in human breast cancer. Breast Cancer Res Treat 29:3–9, 1994.
116. Kihara A, Pastan I: Cytotoxic activity of chimeric toxins containing the epidermal growth factor–like domain of heregulins fused to PE38KDEL, a truncated recombinant form of *Pseudomonas* exotoxin. Cancer Res 55:71–77, 1995.
117. Arteaga CL, Hurd SD, Dugger TC, Winnier AR, Robertson JB: Epidermal growth factor receptors in human breast carcinoma cells: A potential selective target for transforming growth factor alpha-*Pseudomonas* exotoxin 40 fusion protein. Cancer Res 54:4703–4709, 1994.
118. Valone FH, Kaufman PA, Guyre PM, et al: Phase Ia/Ib trial of bisepecific antibody MDX-210 in patients with advanced breast or ovarian cancer that overexpress the proto-oncogene HER-2/neu. J Clin Oncol 13:2281–2292, 1995.
119. Zhang L, Chang C, Bacus SS, Hung M-C: Suppressed transformation and induced differentiation of HER-2/neu–overexpressing breast cancer cells by emodin. Cancer Res 55:3890–3896, 1995.
120. Arteaga CL, Dugger TC, Winnier AR: Anti-epidermal growth factor receptor (EGFR) monoclonal antibodies sensitize human carcinoma cells to etoposide and restore etoposide sensitivity to drug resistant carcinoma cells in culture. Proc Am Soc Clin Oncol 13:125, 1994.
121. Dixit M, Andrews PA, Arteaga CL: EGF receptor antisense RNA abrogates cisplatin-induced programmed cell death in human breast carcinoma cells. Proc Am Soc Clin Oncol 14:155, 1995.
122. Baselga J, Tripathy D, Mendelsohn J, et al: Phase II study of recombinant human anti-HER2 monoclonal antibody (rhuMab HER2) in stage IV breast cancer: HER2-shedding dependent pharmacokinetics and antitumor activity. Proc Am Soc Clin Oncol 14:103, 1995. (Abstract 113)
123. Pegram M, Lipton A, Pietras R, et al: Phase II study of intravenous recombinant humanized anti-p185 HER-2 monoclonal antibody (rhuMab HER-2) plus cisplatin in patients with HER-2/neu overexpressing metastatic breast cancer. Proc Am Soc Clin Oncol 14:106, 1995.
124. Wishart G, Bisset D, Jodrell P: Quinidine as a resistance modulator of epirubicin in advanced breast cancer: Mature results of a placebo-controlled randomized trial. J Clin Oncol 12:1771, 1994.
125. Belpomme D, Pujade-Lorraine E, Gauthier S: Continuous low dose racemic verapamil significantly increases response rate and survival in patients treated with VDS and 5-FU (VF) for anthracycline resistant metastatic breast carcinoma. Proc Am Soc Clin Oncol 36:219, 1995.
126. Askari F, McDonnell W: Antisense-oligonucleotide therapy. N Engl J Med 334:316–318, 1996.
127. Arteaga C, Holt J: Tissue-targeted antisense c-fos retroviral

vector inhibits established breast cancer xenografts in nude mice. Cancer Res 56:1098–1103, 1996.

128. Liu XJ, Pogo BG-T: Inhibition of the erbB-2 protein expression by antisense oligonucleotide. Proc Am Assoc Cancer Res 36:623, 1995.

129. Vaughn JP, Marks JR, Iglehart J: A study of antisense down-regulation of the erbB-2 receptor. Proc Am Assoc Cancer Res 36:515, 1995.

130. DuMontelle J, Myers W: Inhibition of expression of the endogenous mammary oncogene Wnt-1 by antisense oligonucleotides. Proc Am Assoc Cancer Res 36:515, 1995.

131. Ramachandran C, Wellham L, Krishan A: Reversal of multi-drug resistance by MDR-1 antisense phosphorothioate oligodeoxy nucleotides in SW620 Ad300 human colon carcinoma cells in vitro and in xenografts. Proc Am Assoc Cancer Res 36:412, 1995.

132. Szemraj J, Walaszek Z, Hanausek M, Adams A: Growth inhibition of breast cancer cell lines by a β-glucuronidase antisense oligonucleotide. Proc Am Assoc Cancer Res 36:515, 1995.

133. Chlebowski RT, Lillington LM: A decade of breast cancer clinical investigation: Results as reported in the Program/Proceedings of the American Society of Clinical Oncology. J Clin Oncol 12:1789–1795, 1994.

134. Aisner J, Weinberg V, Perloff M, et al: Chemotherapy versus chemoimmunotherapy (CAF v VAFVP v CMF +/− MER) for metastatic carcinoma of the breast: A CALGB study. J Clin Oncol 5:1523–1533, 1987.

135. Muss H, White D, Richards F, et al: Adriamycin versus methotrexate in five-drug combination chemotherapy for advanced breast cancer. Cancer 42:2141–2148, 1978.

136. Tormey D, Wenberg V, Leone L, et al: A comparison of intermittent vs. continuous and Adriamycin vs methotrexate 5-drug chemotherapy for advanced breast cancer. Am J Clin Oncol 7:231–239, 1984.

137. Smalley R, Lefante J, Bartolucci A, et al: A comparison of cyclophosphamide, Adriamycin, and 5-fluorouracil (CAF) and cyclophosphamide, methotrexate, 5-fluorouracil, vincristine, and prednisone (CMFVP) in patients with advanced breast cancer. Breast Cancer Res Treat 3:209–220, 1983.

138. Bull JM, Tormey DC, Li S-H, et al: A randomized comparative trial of adriamycin versus methotrexate in combination drug therapy. Cancer 41:1649–1657, 1978.

139. A'Hern R, Smith I, Ebbs S: Chemotherapy and survival in advanced breast cancer: The inclusion of doxorubicin in Cooper type regimens. Br J Cancer 67:801–805, 1993.

140. Ejlertsen B, Pfeiffer P, Pedersen D, et al: Decreased efficacy of cyclophosphamide, epirubicin and 5-fluorouracil in metastatic breast cancer when reducing treatment from 18 to 6 months. Eur J Cancer 29A:527–531, 1993.

141. Muss HB, Case LD, Richards F, et al: Interrupted versus continuous chemotherapy in patients with metastatic breast cancer. N Engl J Med 325:1342–1348, 1991.

142. Coates A, Gebski V, Bishop JF, et al: Improving the quality of life during chemotherapy for advanced breast cancer. A comparison of intermittent and continuous treatment strategies. N Engl J Med 317:1490–1495, 1987.

143. Harris AL, Cantwell BMJ, Carmichael J, et al: Comparison of short-term and continuous chemotherapy (mitoxantrone) for advanced breast cancer. Lancet 1:186–190, 1990.

144. Frei E, Canellos GP: Dose: A critical factor in cancer chemotherapy. Am J Med 69:585–594, 1980.

145. Hryniuk WM, Bush H: The importance of dose intensity in chemotherapy of metastatic breast cancer. J Clin Oncol 2:1281–1287, 1984.

146. Henderson IC, Hayes DF, Gelman R: Dose-response in the treatment of breast cancer: A critical review. J Clin Oncol 6:1501–1515, 1988.

147. Rahman Z, Frye D, Buzdar A, Hortobagyi G: A retrospective analysis to evaluate the impact of selection process for high-dose chemotherapy on the outcome of patients with metastatic breast cancer. Proc Am Soc Clin Oncol 14:95, 1995.

148. Bezwoda WR, Seymour L, Dansey RD: High-dose chemotherapy with hematopoietic rescue as primary treatment for metastatic breast cancer: A randomized trial. J Clin Oncol 13:2483–2489, 1995.

149. Peters W, Jones R, Vredenburgh J, et al: A large, prospective, randomized trial of high-dose combination alkylating agents (CPB) with autologous cellular support (ABMS) as consolidation for patients with metastatic breast cancer achieving complete remission after intensive doxorubicin-based induction therapy (AFM). Proc Am Soc Clin Oncol 15:121, 1996. (Abstract 149)

150. Dunphy F, Spitzer G, Fornoff J, et al: Factors predicting long-term survival for metastatic breast cancer patients treated with high-dose chemotherapy and bone marrow support. Cancer 73:2157–2167, 1994.

151. Ayash L: Cancer. High dose chemotherapy with autologous stem cell support for the treatment of metastatic breast cancer. Cancer 74(1 Suppl):532–535, 1994.

152. Blomqvist C, Elomaa I, Rissanen P, Hietanen P, Nevasaari K, Helle L: FEC (5-fluorouracil-epirubicin-cyclophosphamide) monthly versus FEC weekly in metastatic breast cancer. First results of a randomized trial. Acta Oncol 31:231–236, 1992.

153. Australia–New Zealand Breast Cancer Trials Group: A randomized trial in postmenopausal patients with advanced breast cancer comparing endocrine and cytotoxic therapy given sequentially or in combination. J Clin Oncol 4:186–193, 1986.

154. Mouridsen HT, Rose C, Engelsman E, Sylvester R, Rotmensz N: Combined cytotoxic and endocrine therapy in postmenopausal patients with advanced breast cancer. A randomized study of CMF vs CMF plus tamoxifen. Eur J Cancer Clin Oncol 21:291–299, 1985.

155. Perry MC, Kardinal CG, Korzun AH, et al: Chemohormonal therapy in advanced carcinoma of the breast: Cancer and Leukemia Group B Protocol 8081. J Clin Oncol 5:1534–1545, 1987.

156. Krook JE, Ingle JN, Green SJ, et al: Randomized clinical trial of cyclophosphamide, 5-FU, and prednisone with or without tamoxifen in postmenopausal women with advanced breast cancer. Cancer Treat Rep 69:355–361, 1985.

157. Viladiu P, Alonso MC, Avella A, et al: Chemotherapy versus chemotherapy plus hormonotherapy in postmenopausal advanced breast cancer patients. A randomized trial. Cancer 56:2745–2750, 1985.

158. Cocconi G, De Lisi V, Boni C, et al: Chemotherapy versus combination of chemotherapy and endocrine therapy in advanced breast cancer. A prospective randomized study. Cancer 51:581–588, 1983.

159. Rubens RD, Begent RHJ, Knight RK, Sexton SA, Hatward JL: Combined cytotoxic and progestogen therapy for advanced breast cancer. Cancer 42:1680–1686, 1978.

160. Myers CE, Gianni L, Zweier J, Muindi J, Sinha BK, Eliot HM: Role of iron in Adriamycin biochemistry. Fed Proc 45:2792–2797, 1986.

161. Olson RD, Musklin PS: Doxorubicin cardiotoxicity: Analysis of prevailing hypothesis. FASEB J 4:3076–3076, 1990.

162. Speyer JL, Green MD, Zeleniuch-Jacquotte A, et al: ICRF-187 permits longer treatment with doxorubicin in women with breast cancer. J Clin Oncol 10:117–127, 1992.

163. Speyer JL, Green MD, Kramer E, et al: Protective effect of the bispiperazinedione ICRF-187 against doxorubicin-induced cardiac toxicity in women with advanced breast cancer. N Engl J Med 319:745–752, 1988.

164. ASCO: American Society for Clinical Oncology recommendations for the use of hematopoietic colony-stimulating factors: Evidence-based, clinical practice guidelines. J Clin Oncol 12:2471–2508, 1994.

165. Shapiro C: Bisphosphonates in breast cancer patients with skeletal metastases. Hematol Oncol Clin North Am 8:153–163, 1994.

166. Sasaki A, Boyce B, Story B, et al: Bisphosphonate risedronate reduces metastatic human breast cancer burden in bone in nude mice. Cancer Res 55:3551–3557, 1995.

167. Tyrrell CT, Bruning PF, May-Levin F, et al: Pamidronate infusions as single-agent therapy for bone metastases: A phase II trial in patients with breast cancer. Eur J Cancer 31A:1976–1980, 1995.

168. Coleman RE, Woll PJ, Miles M, Scrivener W, Rubens RD:

Treatment of bone metastases from breast cancer with (3-amino-1,1-hydroxypropylidene)-1,1-bisphosphonate (APD). Br J Cancer 58:621–625, 1988.

169. Morton AR, Cantrill JA, Pilai GV, McMahon A, Anderson DC, Howell A: Sclerosis of lytic bone metastases after amino-hydroxypropylidene bisphosphonate (APD). Br Med J 297:772–773, 1988.

170. Conte P, Giannessi P, Latreille J, et al: Delayed progression of bone metastases with pamidronate therapy in breast cancer patients: A randomized, multicenter phase III trial. Ann Oncol 5 (Suppl 7):S41–44, 1994.

171. van Holten-Verzantvoort A, Kroon H, Bijvoet O, et al: Palliative pamidronate treatment in patients with bone metastases from breast cancer. J Clin Oncol 11:491–498, 1993.

172. Paterson A, Powles T, Kanis J, McCloskey E, Hanson J, Ashley S: Double-blind controlled trial of oral clodronate in patients with bone metastases from breast cancer. J Clin Oncol 11:59–65, 1993.

173. Robertson AG, Reed NS, Ralston SH: Effect of oral clodronate on metastatic bone pain: A double-blind, placebo-controlled study. J Clin Oncol 13:2427–2430, 1995.

174. Hortobagyi G, Theriault R, Porter L, et al: Efficacy of pamidronate in reducing skeletal complications in patients with breast cancer and lytic bone metastases. N Engl J Med 335:1785–1791, 1996.

175. Thurlimann B, Morant R, Jungi W, Radziwill A: Pamidronate for pain control in patients with malignant osteolytic bone disease: A prospective dose-effect study. Support Care Cancer 2:61–65, 1994.

176. Leyvraz S, Hess U, Flesch G, et al: Pharmacokinetics of pamidronate in patients with bone metastases. J Natl Cancer Inst USA 84:788–792, 1992.

177. Fischer DS, Knobf MT, Durivage HJ: The Cancer Chemotherapy Handbook, ed 4. St. Louis, Mosby–Year Book, 1993.

178. Greenberg PAC, Hortobagyi GN, Smith TL, Ziegler LD, Frye DK, Buzdar AU: Long-term follow-up of patients with complete remission following combination chemotherapy for metastatic breast cancer. J Clin Oncol 14:2197–2205, 1996.

179. Decker DA, Ahmann DL, Bisel HF: Complete responders to chemotherapy in metastatic breast cancer. JAMA 242:2075–2079, 1979.

180. Nemoto T: Metastatic breast cancer: Prolonged complete remission or possible cure with chemotherapy. Proc Am Soc Clin Oncol 2:110, 1983.

181. Livingston R, Carter S: Single Agents in Cancer Chemotherapy. New York, IFI Plenum, 1970.

182. Kardinal CG: Chemotherapy of breast cancer. In Perry M (ed): The Chemotherapy Sourcebook. Baltimore, Williams & Wilkins, 1992.

183. Seidman AD, Tiersten A, Hudis C, et al: Phase II trial of paclitaxel by 3-hour infusion as initial and salvage chemotherapy for metastatic breast cancer. J Clin Oncol 13:2575–2581, 1995.

184. Chevalier B, Fumoleau P, Kerbrat P, et al: Docetaxel is a major cytotoxic drug for the treatment of advanced breast cancer: A phase II trial of the clinical screening cooperative group of the European Organization for Research and Treatment of Cancer. J Clin Oncol 13:314–322, 1995.

185. Valero V, Holmes FA, Waaltrs RS, et al: Phase II trial of docetaxel: A new, highly effective antineoplasic agent in the management of patients with anthracyclne-resistant metastatic breast cancer. J Clin Oncol 13:2886–2894, 1995.

186. Hudis CA, Seidman AD, Crown JPA, et al: Phase II and pharmacologic study of docetaxel as initial chemotherapy for metastatic breast cancer. J Clin Oncol 14:58–65, 1996.

187. Trudeau M, Eisenhauer E, Higgins B, et al: Docetaxel in patients with metastatic breast cancer: A phase II study of the National Cancer Institute of Canada-Clinical Trials Group. J Clin Oncol 14:422–428, 1996.

188. Carmo-Pereira J, Costa FO, Henriquies E, et al: A comparison of two doses of adriamycin in the primary chemotherapy of disseminated breast carcinoma. Br J Cancer 56:471–473, 1987.

189. O'Bryan RM, Baker LH, Gottlieb JE, et al: Dose response evaluation of adriamycin in human neoplasia. Cancer 39:1940–1948, 1977.

190. Becher R, Wandl U, Kloke O, et al: Randomized study of different doses of epirubicin and identical doses of cyclophosphamide in advanced breast cancer. Proc Am Soc Clin Oncol 9:47, 1990.

191. Forastiere A, Hakes TB, Wittes JT, Wittes RE: Cisplatin in the treatment of metastatic breast carcinoma. A prospective randomized trial of two dosage schedules. Am J Clin Oncol 5:243–247, 1982.

192. Tannock IF, Boyd NF, DeBoer G, et al: A randomized trial of two dose levels of cyclophosphamide, methotrexate, and fluorouracil chemotherapy for patients with metastatic breast cancer. J Clin Oncol 6:1377–1387, 1988.

193. Hortobagyi GN, Bodey GP, Buzdar AU, et al: Evaluation of high-dose versus standard FAC chemotherapy for advanced breast cancer in protected environment units: A prospective randomized study. J Clin Oncol 5:354–364, 1987.

194. Hoogstraten B, George SL, Samal B, et al: Combination chemotherapy and adriamycin in patients with advanced breast cancer. Cancer 38:13–20, 1976.

195. Degardin M, Bonneterre J, Hecquet B, et al: Vinorelbine (Navelbine) as a salvage treatment for advanced breast cancer. Ann Oncol 5:423–426, 1994.

196. Fumoleau P, Delgado FM, Delozier T, et al: Phase II trial of weekly intravenous vinorelbine in first-line advanced breast cancer chemotherapy. J Clin Oncol 11:1145–1252, 1993.

197. Queisser W, Doss A, Wander H, et al: Phase II study of vinorelbine by oral route (in a hard gelatine capsule) for metastatic breast cancer patients. A trial of the phase I/II study group of the Association for Medical Oncology of the German Cancer Society. Onkologie 14:35–39, 1991.

198. Fraschini G, Esparza L, Holmes F, Tashima C, Theriault R, Hortobagyi G: High-dose etoposide in metastatic breast cancer. Breast Cancer Res Treat 14:142, 1989. (Abstract 39)

199. Mulder NH, Meinesz AP, Sleijfer DT, et al: High-dose etoposide with or without cyclophosphamide and autologous bone marrow transplantation in solid tumors. In McVie JG, Dalesio O, Smith IE (eds): Autologous Bone Marrow Transplantation and Solid Tumors. New York, Raven Press, 1984, pp 125–130.

200. Wolff S, Fer M, McKay C: High-dose VP-16-213 and autologous bone marrow transplantation for refractory malignancies: A phase I study. J Clin Oncol 1:701–705, 1983.

201. Ariel I: Treatment of disseminated cancer by intravenous hydroxyurea and autogenous bone-marrow transplants: Experiences with 35 patients. J Surg Oncol 7:331–335, 1975.

202. Sledge GWJ, Antman KH: Progress in chemotherapy for metastatic breast cancer. Semin Oncol 19:317–332, 1992.

203. Shea TC, Flaherty M, Elias A, et al: A phase I clinical and pharmacological study of high-dose carboplatin and autologous bone marrow support. J Clin Oncol 7:651–661, 1989.

204. Schilcher RB, Young JD, Ratanathorathorn V, Baker LH: High dose mitomycin C and autologous bone marrow transplantation: Clinical results and pharmacokinetics. Blut 45:183, 1982.

205. Schilcher RB, Young JD, Ratanatharathorn V, Karanes C, Baker LH: Clinical pharmacokinetics of high dose mitomycin C. Cancer Chemother Pharmacol 13:186–190, 1984.

206. Le Maistre CF, Herzig GP, Herzig RH, et al: High dose thiotepa and autologous bone marrow rescue for the treatment of refractory breast cancer. Breast Cancer Res Treat 10:89, 1987. (Abstract)

207. Lazarus HM, Reed MD, Spitzer TR, Rabaa MS, Blumer JL: High-dose IV thiotepa and cryopreserved autologous bone marrow transplantation for therapy of refractory cancer. Cancer Treat Rep 71:689–695, 1987.

208. Slease RB, Benear JB, Selby GB, et al: High-dose combination alkylating agent therapy with autologous bone marrow rescue for refractory solid tumors. J Clin Oncol 6:1314–1320, 1988.

209. Maraninchi D, Abecasis M, Gastaut J, et al: High-dose melphalan with autologous bone marrow rescue for the treatment of advanced adult solid tumors. Cancer Treat Rep 68:471–474, 1984.

210. Maraninchi D, Gastaut JA, Herve P, et al: High-dose melphalan and autologous marrow transplantation in adult solid

tumors: Clinical responses and preliminary evaluation of different strategies. *In* McVie JG, Dalesio O, Smith IE (ed): Autologous Bone Marrow Transplantation and Solid Tumors. New York, Raven 1984, pp 145–150.

211. Knight WA, Page CP, Kuhn JG, et al: High dose L-PAM with autologous bone marrow infusion for advanced, steroid hormone receptor negative breast cancer. Breast Cancer Res Treat 4:336, 1984. (Abstract)

212. Lazarus J, Herzig R, Graham-Pole J, et al: Intensive melphalan chemotherapy and cryopreserved autologous bone marrow transplantation for the treatment of refractory cancer. J Clin Oncol 2:359–367, 1983.

213. Herzig R, Phillips G, Lazarus H, et al: Intensive chemotherapy and autologous bone marrow transplantation for the treatment of refractory malignancies. *In* Dicke K, Spitzer G, Zander A (eds): Autologous Bone Marrow Transplantation; Proceedings of the First International Symposium. Houston: University of Texas, MD Anderson Cancer Center Press, 1985, pp 197–202.

214. Peters WP, Shpall EJ, Jones RB, et al: High-dose combination alkylating agents with bone marrow support as initial treatment for metastatic breast cancer. J Clin Oncol 6:1368–1376, 1988.

215. Eder JP, Antman K, Peters W, et al: High dose combination alkylating agent chemotherapy with autologous bone marrow support for metastatic breast cancer. J Clin Oncol 4:1592–1597, 1986.

216. Tajima T, Sonoda K, Tokuda Y, et al: High-dose chemotherapy supported by autologous bone marrow transplantation in solid tumors. Tokai J Exp Clin Med 8:41–51, 1988.

217. Tajima T, Tokuda Y, Ohta M, et al: Role of autologous bone marrow transplantation in cancer chemotherapy. Low Temp Med 15:44–50, 1989.

218. Tajima T, Sonoda H, Kubnota M, et al: High-dose combination chemotherapy with autologous bone marrow transplantation in breast carcinoma. Jpn J Cancer Chemother 10:840–847, 1983.

219. Kaizer H, Ghalle R, Adler SS, Korenblit AD, Richman CM: High dose chemotherapy and bone marrow transplantation in the treatment of metastatic breast cancer. J Cell Biochem 14A:321, 1990.

220. Eder JP, Antman K, Elias A, et al: Cyclophosphamide and thiotepa with autologous bone marrow transplantation with solid tumors. J Natl Cancer Inst 80:1221–1226, 1988.

221. Mukaiyama T, Ogawa M, Horikoshi N, et al: A study to overcome drug resistance using high-dose chemotherapy with autologous bone marrow transplantation. Jpn J Cancer Chemother 16:2013–2018, 1989.

222. Peters W, Jones R, Shpall E, Shogan J: Dose intensification using high-dose combination alkylating agents and autologous bone marrow support for the treatment of breast cancer. *In* Dicke K, Spitzer G, Jagannath S, Evinger-Hodges M (eds): Autologous Bone Marrow Transplantation; Proceedings of the Fourth International Symposium. Houston, University of Texas, MD Anderson Cancer Center Press, 1989, pp 389–399.

223. Eder JP, Elias A, Shea TC, et al: A Phase I/II study of cyclophosphamide, thiotepa and carboplatin with autologous bone marrow transplantation in solid tumor patients. J Clin Oncol 8:1239–1245, 1990.

224. Kaminer L, Williams S, Beschorner J, Golick J, O'Brian S, Bitran J: High dose chemotherapy with autologous hematopoietic stem cell support in the treatment of refractory Stage IV breast carcinoma. Breast Cancer Res Treat 12:122, 1988. (Abstract 62)

225. Kaminer L, Williams S, Beschorner J, O'Brien S, Golick J, Bitran J: High dose chemotherapy with autologous hematopoietic stem cell support in the treatment of Stage IV breast carcinoma. Proc Am Soc Clin Oncol 8:45, 1989. (Abstract 174)

226. Maraninchi D, Piana L, Blaise D, et al: Phase I and II studies of high dose alkylating agents in poor risk patients with breast cancer with bone marrow transplantation. *In* Dicke K, Spitzer TR, Jaggannath S (eds): Autologous Bone Marrow Transplantation: Proceedings of the 3rd International Symposium. Houston, University of Texas M.D. Anderson Hospital Press, 1987, pp 475–480.

227. Mulder POM, Sleijfer DT, Willemse PHB, de Vries EGE, Uges DRA, Mulder NH: High-dose cyclophosphamide or melphalan with escalating doses of mitoxantrone and autologous bone marrow transplantation for refractory solid tumors. Cancer Res 49:4654–4658, 1989.

228. Spitzer G, F Dunphy I, Ellis J, et al: High-dose intensification for stage IV hormonally-refractory breast cancer. *In* Dicke K, Spitzer G, Jagannath S, Evinger-Hodges M (eds): Autologous Bone Marrow Transplantation: Proceedings of the Fourth International Symposium. Houston, University of Texas, M.D. Anderson Cancer Center Press. 1989, pp 399–405.

229. Robinson W, Hartmann D, Mangalik A, et al: Autologous nonfrozen bone marrow transplantation after intensive chemotherapy: A pilot study. Acta Haematol 66:145–153, 1981.

230. Stewart P: Autologous bone marrow transplantation in metastatic breast cancer. Breast Cancer Res Treat 2:85–92, 1982.

231. Douer YD, Champlin R, Ho W, et al: High-dose combined-modality therapy and autologous bone marrow rescue for refractory solid tumors. Am J Med 71:973–976, 1981.

232. Gisselbrecht C, Lepage E, Espie M, et al: Cyclophosphamide, total body irradiation with autologous bone marrow support for metastatic breast cancer. Proc Am Soc Clin Oncol 6:65, 1987. (Abstract 255)

233. Gisselbrecht C, LePage E, Extra J, et al: Inflammatory and metastatic breast cancer: Cyclophosphamide and total body irradiation (TBI) with autologous bone marrow transplantation (ABMT). *In* Dicke K, Spitzer G, Jagannath S, Evinger-Hodges M (eds): Autologous Bone Marrow Transplantation; Proceedings of the Fourth International Symposium. Houston, University of Texas, MD Anderson Cancer Center Press, 1989, pp 363–367.

234. Livingston R, Schulman S, Griffin B, et al: Combination chemotherapy & systemic irradiation consolidation for poor prognosis breast cancer. Cancer 9:1249–1254, 1987.

235. Vincent MD, Trevor J, Powles R, Coombes R, McElwain T: Late intensification with high-dose melphalan and autologous bone marrow support in breast cancer patients responding to conventional chemotherapy. Cancer Chemother Pharmacol 21:255–260, 1988.

236. Spitzer G, Buzdar A, Hortobagyi G, et al: High-dose chemotherapy intensification and autologous bone marrow transplantation with emphasis on breast carcinoma. *In* Spitzer G, Dicke K (eds): Autologous Bone Marrow Transplantation: Proceedings of the 3rd International Symposium. Houston, University of Texas, M D Anderson Hospital Press, 1987, pp 455–463.

237. Spitzer G, Buzdar A, Auber M, et al: High dose cyclophosphamide/VP-16/platinum intensification for metastatic breast cancer. Breast Cancer Res Treat 10:89, 1987.

238. Spitzer G, Farha P, Valdiviesco M, et al: High dose intensification therapy with autologous bone marrow support for limited small cell bronchogenic carcinoma. J Clin Oncol 4:4–13, 1986.

239. Spitzer G, Dicke KA, Latam J, et al: High-dose combination chemotherapy with autologous bone marrow transplantation in adult solid tumors. Cancer 45:3075–3085, 1980.

240. Jones RB, Shpall EJ, Ross M, Bast R, Affronti M, Peters WP: AFM induction chemotherapy, followed by intensive alkylating agent consolidation with autologous bone marrow support (ABMS) of advanced breast cancer. Proc Am Soc Clin Oncol 9:9, 1990.

241. Jones RB, Shpall EJ, Shogan J, et al: The Duke AFM program: Intensive induction chemotherapy for metastatic breast cancer. Cancer 66:431–436, 1990.

242. Jones RB, Shpall EJ, Ross M, Bass R, Affronti M, Peters WP: AFM induction chemotherapy, followed by intensive alkylating agent consolidation with autologous bone marrow support (ABMS) for advanced breast cancer, current results. Proc Am Soc Clin Oncol 9:9, 1990. (Abstract 30)

243. Jones RB, Shpall EJ, Shogan J, Gockerman J, Peters WP: AFM induction chemotherapy followed by intensive consolidation with autologous bone marrow support for advanced breast cancer. Proc Am Soc Clin Oncol 7:8, 1988. (Abstract 29)

244. Williams S, Mick R, Dresser R, Golick J, Beschorner J, Bitran J: High dose consolidation therapy with autologous stem cell rescue in stage IV breast cancer. J Clin Oncol 7:1824–1830, 1989.

245. Bitran JD, Williams SF: A phase II study of induction chemotherapy followed by intensification with high dose chemotherapy with autologous bone marrow rescue (ABMR) in stage IV breast cancer. Breast Cancer Res Treat 10:88, 1987. (Abstract)

246. Kennedy MJ, Beveridge RA, Rowley SD, Gordon GB, Abeloff MD, Davidson NE: High-dose chemotherapy with reinfusion of purged autologous bone marrow following dose-intense induction as initial therapy for metastatic breast cancer. J Natl Cancer Inst 83:920–926, 1991.

247. Kennedy MJ, Beveridge R, Rowley S, et al: High dose consolidation chemotherapy and rescue with purged autologous bone marrow following dose-intense induction for metastatic breast cancer. Proc Am Soc Clin Oncol 8:19, 1989. (Abstract 69)

248. Kennedy M, Beveridge R, Rowley S, Abeloff M, Davidson N: Dose-intense cytoreduction followed by high dose consolidation chemotherapy and rescue with purged autologous bone marrow for metastatic breast cancer. Breast Cancer Res Treat 14:133, 1989. (Abstract 3)

249. Beveridge RA, Abeloff MD, Donehower RC, Damron DJ, Fetting JH, Waterfield W: Sixteen week dose intense chemotherapy for breast cancer. Proc Am Soc Clin Oncol 7:13, 1988.

250. Rosti G, Tumolo S, Figoli F, et al: High dose chemotherapy and autologous bone marrow transplantation in advanced breast cancer. Breast Cancer Res Treat 10:110, 1987. (Abstract)

251. Rosti G, Galligioni E, Argnani M, et al: Autologous bone marrow transplantation as intensification therapy in breast cancer: An Italian cooperative experience. *In* Dicke K, Spitzer G, Jagannath S, Evinger-Hodges M (eds): Proceedings of the Fourth International Symposium. Houston, University of Texas, MD Anderson Cancer Center Press, 1989, pp 357–363.

252. Leoni M, Rosti G, Flamini E, et al: High-dose chemotherapy and ABMT in advanced breast cancer: A pilot study. Bone Marrow Transplant 3:299, 1988. (Abstract)

253. Willemse PHB, de Vries EGE, Sleijfer DT, Mulder POM, Sibinga CTS, Mulder NH: Intensive induction chemotherapy and intensification with autologous bone marrow reinfusion in patients with stage IIIB and IV breast cancer. Breast Cancer Res Treat 12:147, 1988. (Abstract 163)

254. Mulder NH, Sleijfer DT, de Vries EG, Willemse PH: Intensive induction chemotherapy and intensification with autologous bone marrow reinfusion in patients with stage IIIB and IV breast cancer. Proc Am Soc Clin Oncol 7:8, 1988. (Abstract 26)

255. Mulder N, Dolsma W, Mulder P, et al: Long-term results of induction- and intensification chemotherapy supported with autologous bone marrow reinfusion in patients with disseminated or T4 breast cancer. Anticancer Res 15:1565–1568, 1995.

256. Mulder NH, Mulder POM, Sleijfer DT, et al: Induction chemotherapy and intensification with autologous bone marrow reinfusion in patients with locally advanced and disseminated breast cancer. Eur J Cancer 29A:668–671, 1993.

257. Slease R, Selby G, Saez R, Keller A, Benear J, Epstein R: Autologous bone marrow transplantation for metastatic breast carcinoma in complete or partial remission. Breast Cancer Res Treat 14:147, 1989. (Abstract 58)

258. Tormey DC, Falkson G, Crowley J, Falkson HC, Voelkel J, Davis TE: Dibromodulcitol and adriamycin ± tamoxifen in advanced breast cancer. Am J Clin Oncol 5:33–39, 1982.

259. Brunner KW, Sonntag RW, Alberto P, et al: Combined chemo- and hormonal therapy in advanced breast cancer. Cancer 39:2923–2933, 1977.

260. Weiss R, Valagussa P, Moliterni A, et al: Adjuvant chemotherapy after conservative surgery plus irradiation versus modified radical mastectomy. Am J Med 83:455–463, 1987.

261. Bonadonna G, Brusamolino E, Valagussa P, et al: Combination chemotherapy as an adjuvant treatment in operable breast cancer. N Engl J Med 294:405–410, 1976.

262. Hortobagyi G, Gutterman J, Blumenschein G, et al: Combination chemoimmunotherapy of metastatic breast cancer with 5-fluorouracil, Adriamycin, cyclophosphamide and BCG. Cancer 43:1225–1233, 1979.

263. Hart R, Perloff M, Holland J: One-day VATH (vinblastine, Adriamycin, thiotepa and Halotestin) therapy for advanced breast cancer refractory to prior chemotherapy. Cancer 48:1522–1527, 1981.

CHAPTER 73
ENDOCRINE THERAPY OF BREAST CANCER

William J. Gradishar, M.D. / V. Craig Jordan, Ph.D., D.Sc.

In 1997 in excess of 185,000 new cases of breast cancer will be diagnosed in the United States, and approximately 44,000 deaths from breast cancer will occur.[1] Breast cancer is a disease that affects women of all ages and at all stages of their reproductive life. Because of greater patient awareness and the widespread use of screening mammography, the majority of new breast cancer cases are detected at a very early stage; however, 5 to 10 percent of all newly diagnosed cases present with metastatic disease. A variety of therapeutic strategies have been investigated to improve the outcome of patients with advanced disease, but, unfortunately, few patients have been cured. The realistic goals of treatment for metastatic breast cancer are prolongation of survival and palliation of symptoms. Endocrine therapy remains one of primary treatment options for the majority of patients with metastatic breast cancer. This chapter will review the evolution of hormonal therapy (Table 73–1) from surgical ablative approaches to modern pharmacological strategies based on an understanding of how hormones, specifically estrogens, influence the growth of certain breast cancers.

HISTORICAL BACKGROUND OF BREAST CANCER TREATMENT

In 1836 Sir Astley Cooper of St. Bartholomew's Hospital in London observed that advanced breast cancer appeared to wax and wane during the course of a woman's menstrual cycle.[2] In 1889 Albert Schinzinger[3] in Freiburg suggested that breast cancer in younger women followed a more aggressive course than in older women. In an effort to alter the course of breast cancer in younger women, he proposed making young women older by removing the ovaries. He believed that the breasts would atrophy and the tumor contained in the breast would also shrink.

George Thomas Beatson[4, 5] studied the phenomenon of lactation in preparation for writing his doctoral thesis. He determined that there was a connection between the ovary and breast that was not based on a special nerve supply. In animals, lactation was maintained by rendering the ovaries nonfunctional (i.e., oophorectomy or immediate pregnancy after calving). Thus, Beatson believed that one organ was controlling the function of another without a direct connection. This hypothesis was all the more remarkable because it was formulated at a time before Starling coined the term *hormone* and before there was any detailed knowledge of the endocrine system.

The first reported bilateral oophorectomy as treatment for advanced breast cancer was performed by Beatson on June 15, 1895, at the Glasgow Cancer Hospital. The patient was a 33-year-old premenopausal woman with recurrent breast carcinoma involving the chest wall that had developed 6 months after she had undergone a mastectomy. The chest wall disease completely resolved 8 months following the bilateral oophorectomy. The disease was controlled for 49 months following the operation before a recurrence was detected. The patient died 2 years later.[4, 5]

Boyd,[6] at the Charing Cross Hospital in London, subsequently reported on a series of 54 patients with advanced breast cancer who were treated with bilateral oophorectomy. Approximately one third of the patients had tumor regression and these women gained approximately 1 year of additional life. Lett and Thompson[7–9] reported similar response rates and survival advantages for responding patients who were treated with bilateral oophorectomy. After the first two decades of the twentieth century, interest in surgical oophorectomy waned, as other techniques became available.

In 1922 DeCourmelles[10] administered radiation therapy to the ovaries in an effort to induce menopause as a treatment for locally advanced and metastatic breast cancer. Several other reports suggested that radiation was safe and as effective as bilateral oophorectomy in treating advanced breast cancer. The only difference between the two procedures appeared to be that tumor regression often was not observed for several months following radiation therapy. Block and coworkers[11] later showed that this latent effect of radiation correlated with estrogen production in that the ovaries reached basal levels several months following treatment.

The modern era of endocrine therapy began with the award of the Nobel Prize for medicine to Charles Huggins[12] from the University of Chicago for introducing the concept of hormone-dependency of certain human tumors. He reported the beneficial effects of castration in men with prostate cancer and subsequently showed that the effect of castration was mediated by reducing testosterone levels.[13] Huggins and coworkers also resurrected the concept of surgical oophorectomy as a means to remove endogenous estrogen in premenopausal women with advanced breast cancer. Once synthetic corticosteroids became available in the early 1950s, bilateral surgical adrenalectomy also became feasible as a means of removing other sources of steroid hormones. In an early report by Huggins and Bergenstal,[12] three of six patients with advanced breast cancer appeared to benefit from bilateral adrenalectomy. Other investigators

TABLE 73–1. **LANDMARKS IN THE DEVELOPMENT OF HORMONAL THERAPIES FOR ADVANCED BREAST CANCER**

Year	Concept	Reference
1895	Bilateral oophorectomy in premonopausal patients	4, 5
1938	Synthesis of diethylstilbestrol (DES)	17
1944	Treatment of postmenopausal patients with DES	255
1950–1953	Surgical hypophysectomy and bilateral adrenalectomy introduced as treatment for premenopausal patients	12–16
1958–1967	Synthesis of nonsteroidal antiestrogens	25, 46
1960–1966	Discovery of the estrogen receptor	19, 20
1972–1975	Development of the estrogen receptor assay for breast cancer	21, 22
1971–1978	Testing and registration of tamoxifen for treatment of advanced breast cancer	26–29

subsequently reported that bilateral adrenalectomy produced objective responses in 30 to 40 percent of cases, but, most importantly, these were usually in premenopausal women who had previously responded to oophorectomy.[14, 15]

Hypophysectomy was introduced in 1953 by Luft and Olivecrona[16] in Stockholm as alternative treatment to surgical adrenalectomy for patients with advanced breast cancer. Multiple studies have reported response rates of approximately 40 percent, which is comparable to those attained with surgical adrenalectomy. Regrettably, the morbidity and mortality of these surgical procedures was not insignificant. Santen and coworkers[14] reported on randomized clinical trial that showed equivalent response rates in patients treated with surgical adrenalectomy and medical adrenalectomy in the form of aminoglutethimide with hydrocortisone replacement. The patients undergoing adrenalectomy through medical therapy experienced less morbidity; as a result, surgical adrenalectomy has been abandoned as treatment for breast cancer. However, the major therapeutic breakthrough has resulted from our knowledge of estrogen action and the successful development of antiestrogens. Drug development originated with the pioneering studies of Sir Charles Dodds[17] in the 1930s and his discovery of the nonsteroidal estrogen diethylstilbestrol (DES).

In 1944 Sir Alexander Haddow[18] reported that four of 13 patients with advanced disease responded to high-dose estrogen therapy and that older patients were more likely to respond. Nevertheless, extensive studies to discover why some patients responded to hormonal manipulation whereas others did not were unsuccessful. The first clues came with the laboratory studies of Elwood Jensen[19] at the University of Chicago, who discovered why estrogen target tissues (e.g., uterus, vagina) respond to estrogen. Jensen and Jacobson[19] synthesized tritiated estradiol and injected small quantities into immature female rats. Radioactivity was taken up and retained by estrogen-target tissues such as the uterus, vagina, and pituitary gland, whereas the radioactivity taken up by nontarget tissues such as muscle was not retained. They suggested that an estrogen receptor must be present to regulate estrogen action in estrogen target tissues.[19]

The estrogen receptor protein was subsequently identified by Toft and coworkers[20] as an extractable protein from estrogen target tissues. These findings led to the development of estrogen receptor assays by Jensen and coworkers[21] that could be used to predict which patients would or would not respond to endocrine therapy. In unselected cases, 30 to 35 percent of patients will respond to endocrine therapy; however, if endocrine therapy is administered only to patients with positive estrogen receptors 55 to 60 percent of patients will respond.[21, 22] Although this test was most important for selecting women for endocrine ablation, the discovery of antiestrogens revolutionized the approach to breast cancer treatment.

In 1958 Lerner and coworkers[23] reported the biological properties of the first nonsteroidal antiestrogen, MER-25. The compound was found to be an antiestrogen in all species tested. The discovery was initially thought to be important because MER-25 was found to be a contraceptive in laboratory animals, but its evaluation as a "morning-after pill" was disappointing because the drug had low potency and the high doses necessary for it to work were associated with unacceptable side effects on the central nervous system. A successor compound, MRL-41, or clomiphene, was a more potent antiestrogen and an effective antifertility drug in animals, but paradoxically it induced ovulation in subfertile women.[24] Clomiphene demonstrated modest activity in the treatment of advanced breast cancer, but further development stopped after the introduction of tamoxifen into clinical trials.

Harper and Walpole[25] found that in the laboratory, tamoxifen, like clomiphene, was an antiestrogen with antifertility properties. The compound was then evaluated in a number of clinical situations, but clinical development progressed successfully only for the treatment of breast cancer.[26, 27] In 1971 Cole and coworkers[28] reported the preliminary results of a clinical trial using tamoxifen as a treatment for advanced breast cancer in which ten of 46 patients (22 percent) showed objective responses, with few side effects in any of the treated patients. These results compared favorably to those of treatment with DES, but tamoxifen had fewer side effects.[28, 29] Tamoxifen is now the most widely prescribed cancer therapy in the world and is the endocrine therapy of choice for the treatment of breast cancer.

GENERAL TREATMENT STRATEGIES FOR BREAST CANCER

The combined data from numerous clinical trials of different forms of endocrine therapy in patients with metastatic breast cancer reveal similar overall response rates. The decision to choose one endocrine therapy over another must take into consideration the comparative efficacy, ease of administration, and toxicity of therapy as well as the menopausal status of the patient.

Most breast cancers express hormone receptors, either estrogen receptors or progesterone receptors or both. The estrogen receptor can be isolated from the primary tumor or a metastatic lesion[30] and is measured by a ligand-binding method[31] or by monoclonal antibodies used to measure estrogen receptors by flow cytometry.[32] Alternatively, tissue sections can be used to determine cellular heterogeneity using immunohistochemistry,[33] or the estrogen receptors can be quantitated using an estrogen receptor immunoassay.[34] The progesterone receptor is an estrogen-regulated protein that can be synthesized only if the estrogen receptor system is functional. In 1975 Horwitz and coworkers[35, 36] hypothesized that the presence of the progesterone receptor in breast tumors would be a sensitive predictor of response to hormone therapy, and it is now accepted that a patient has an 80 percent probability of a response to endocrine therapy if the tumor is positive for both estrogen and progesterone receptors.

The cutoff point to determine whether a tumor is estrogen receptor (ER) or progesterone receptor (PR) positive (+) or negative (−) has been the subject of considerable debate, especially because the immunohistochemical assays are subjective, and the results are usually described as a percentage of tumor cells staining positive. In general, assay methods that do quantitate the receptor are considered to be positive if the result is greater than 10 fmol/mg cytosol protein.

Hormone receptor status has important implications for treatment and for the likelihood that a patient will respond to hormonal therapy (Table 73–2).[37, 38] Witliff[37] reported that of patients with tumors that are ER + /PR +, 75 to 80 percent will respond to hormonal therapy. Objective tumor responses will be observed in 25 to 30 percent and 40-45 percent of patients with ER + /PR − and ER−/PR+ tumors, respectively. In addition, 10 percent of patients with ER−/PR− tumors will respond to hormonal therapy.[37, 38]

TABLE 73–2. ANTITUMOR RESPONSE TO HORMONAL THERAPY ACCORDING TO RECEPTOR STATUS IN PATIENTS WITH ADVANCED DISEASE

Receptor Status	Response Rate (%)
ER+/PR+	75–80
ER+/PR−	25–30
ER−/PR+	40–45
ER−/PR−	<10

From McGuire WL, Clark GM: Prognostic factor for recurrence and survival in axillary node-negative breast cancer. J Steroid Biochem 34:145–148, 1989; Witliff J: Steroid hormone receptors. In Pesce AJ, Kaplan LA (eds): Methods in Clinical Chemistry. St. Louis, Mosby, 1987, p 767.

According to several studies, the values of receptor assays increase with age. Allegra[39] reported that 44 percent of breast cancer patients in the age group of 40 to 49 years express the ER, while 69 percent of those who are 70 years old express the ER. In Witliff's[37] study of 1314 women, 72 percent of premenopausal and 83 percent of postmenopausal breast cancer patients had a positive ER, positive PR, or both. More patients in both age groups have a ER+/PR+ status (45 percent premenopausal and 63 percent postmenopausal) than have a ER−/PR− status (28 percent premenopausal and 17 percent postmenopausal). These data suggest that the majority of breast cancer patients are potential candidates for hormonal therapy. The fact that 10 percent of patients with ER−/PR− tumors do respond to hormonal therapies is important to consider, particularly in treating patients who have asymptomatic metastatic disease or those who have progressive disease after receiving first- and second-line cytotoxic chemotherapy.

In the absence of hormone receptor results, a number of other predictors of response to endocrine therapy have been used. Patients with prolonged disease-free intervals after primary treatment and those with metastatic disease in soft-tissue, bone, and lung sites but not in visceral or central nervous system sites are more likely to respond to hormonal therapies.[40] Response to hormonal therapies is also more likely in older patients, which fact correlates with the observation that median receptor levels increase with age.

Tamoxifen is considered the first-line hormonal therapy for metastatic breast cancer. Upon disease progression during tamoxifen treatment, patients may gain additional benefit from second-line hormonal therapy. Most patients who respond to one hormone therapy can be expected to respond to subsequent maneuvers, although the duration of response to subsequent maneuvers is generally shorter. Wilson[41] has reviewed second-line endocrine therapy after first-line oophorectomy or tamoxifen. He described response rates ranging from 19 to 38 percent for a variety of therapies, including adrenalectomy, hypophysectomy, aminoglutethimide, DES, androgens, and progestins. Similarly, Rose and Mouridsen[42] have reported that 35 to 53 percent of tamoxifen responders attain a response to second-line aminoglutethimide or a progestin. In a retrospective analysis by Iveson and coworkers,[43] 42 percent of 55 patients receiving a third-line endocrine therapy benefited as determined by objective response, disease stabilization, or symptom improvement.

CURRENT THERAPIES AND DRUGS IN DEVELOPMENT FOR BREAST CANCER

Antiestrogens

Tamoxifen

As discussed previously, tamoxifen was identified as an effective postcoital contraceptive in rats and was believed to have clinical potential as a "morning-after pill."[25] Unfortunately, when tamoxifen was initially evaluated in patients, it was found to induce ovulation rather than reduce fertility. Tamoxifen continues to be marketed in some countries for the induction of ovulation in subfertile women.

The first preliminary clinical evaluation of tamoxifen to treat advanced breast cancer was conducted by Cole and colleagues[28] at the Christie Hospital in Manchester. The efficacy of tamoxifen proved to be equivalent to that of androgens or high-dose estrogens in postmenopausal women, but the side effects of tamoxifen were mild in comparison. Similarly Ward[29] conducted a small-dose response study of tamoxifen and found side effects to be insignificant. Tamoxifen was subsequently shown to cause the regression of carcinogen-induced rat mammary tumors,[44, 45] and this model was used to develop the treatment strategies (e.g., long-term adjuvant therapy, prevention) that are being used today.

Tamoxifen is now the most successful and widely used endocrine therapy for the treatment for breast cancer (Fig. 73–1).[46] It has been approved by the Food and Drug Administration for the treatment of metastatic breast cancer in postmenopausal women, ER-positive, metastatic breast cancer in premenopausal women, and metastatic breast cancer in men.

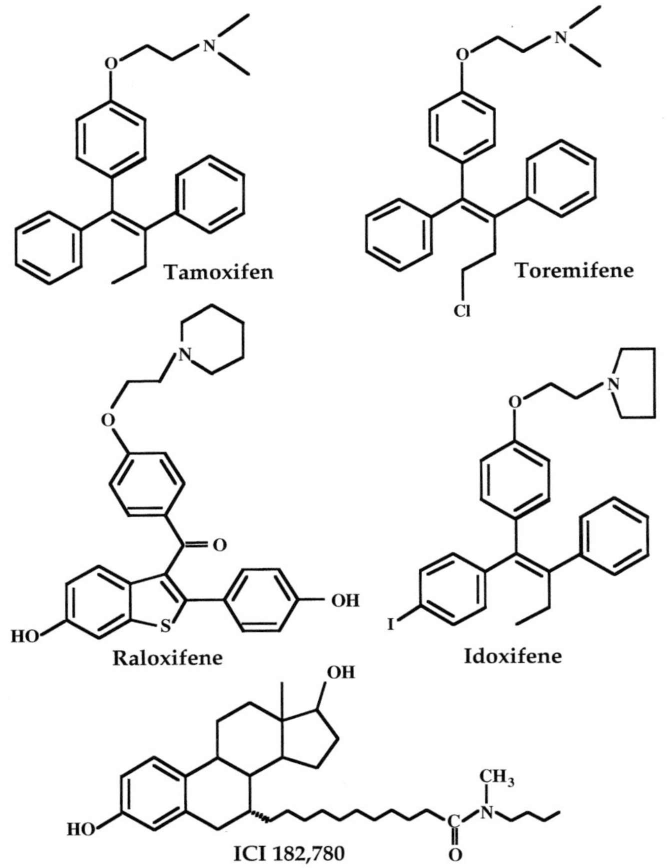

Figure 73–1 *Structure of the triphenylethylene antiestrogen tamoxifen and the new antiestrogens undergoing clinical evaluation.*

Tamoxifen has also been approved as an adjuvant therapy, either alone or following chemotherapy, for early stage, hormone receptor-positive breast cancer in pre- and postmenopausal women.

Tamoxifen's antitumor effect is believed to be mediated primarily through the ER, although other potential mechanisms of action may contribute.[47–50] The recognition of the ER as a nuclear transcription factor that binds estrogens or antiestrogens and programs breast cancer cells to replicate or not has focused enormous interest on the basic mechanism of antiestrogen action.[50] A generally accepted model for estrogen and antiestrogen effects in breast cancer is illustrated in Figures 73–2 and 73–3. Estradiol or any estrogen binds to the nuclear ER, which then produces a change in shape to fully expose the DNA binding domain on the protein complex. The activated receptor complex then dimerizes and binds to an estrogen response element (ERE) located in the promoter region of estrogen-responsive genes. Once bound to the ERE, the ER acts as an anchor for other transcription factors or associated proteins that, when assembled and associated with RNA polymerase, produce a transcription complex. The estrogen-responsive gene is then transcribed and subsequently translated to proteins that are involved either in growth responses or differentiation responses (such as progesterone receptor synthesis).

Type I antiestrogens, like tamoxifen, appear to form a receptor complex that is incompletely converted to the fully activated form (see Fig. 73–3).[51–56] As a result of the imperfect changes in the tertiary structure of the protein, the complex is only partially active in initiating the programmed series of events necessary to initiate gene activation.[51, 57] Tamoxifen also potentially inhibits tumor growth through mechanisms not mediated by the ER.[58] Tamoxifen increases antibody synthesis,[59] enhances natural killer cell activity, inhibits suppressor T-cell activity,[60] inhibits protein kinase C,[61, 62] and calmodulin-dependent cAMP phosphodiesterase,[63, 64] inhibits angiogenesis,[65] and decreases the synthesis of breast cancer mitogens, including insulin growth factor I (IGF-I), transforming growth factor α (TGFα), epidermal growth factor (EGF), and platelet-derived growth factor (PDGF).[58, 66–68]

In most of the early clinical trials of tamoxifen in patients with advanced disease, a daily oral dose of 20 to 40 mg was administered. No significant increase in tumor response was observed with higher daily doses.[69–73] With the daily oral administration of one 20 mg tablet or two 10 mg tablets of tamoxifen, steady-state plasma concentrations are reached after approximately 4 weeks.[74] Tamoxifen and its major metabolite, *N*-desmethyltamoxifen, remain in a patient serum for 6 weeks after discontinuing therapy.[75] With the oral administration of tamoxifen at 20 mg/day, a significant degree of variability in serum drug concentration has been documented among patients and in the same patient at different time points, but a correlation between drug concentration and tumor response has never been confirmed.[70, 72, 76]

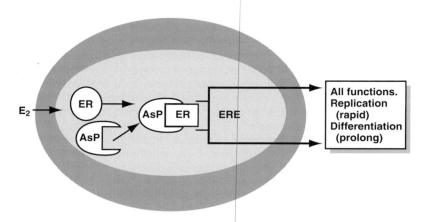

Figure 73–2 *A molecular model of estrogen actions in the breast cancer cell. Estradiol (E₂) binds to the nuclear estrogen receptor (ER), which changes shape to bind to estrogen response elements (EREs) that control the transcription of estrogen-responsive genes involved in growth or differentiation responses. Associated proteins (ASP) that are necessary to produce a transcriptional unit for the transcription of genes may modify the cellular responses to estrogen.*

Tamoxifen and the metabolites that have been identified in patients are all antiestrogens that inhibit estradiol binding to the ER.[77, 78] Tamoxifen undergoes hepatic metabolism through hydroxylation and conjugation. N-desmethyltamoxifen is the principal metabolite of tamoxifen. It has a binding affinity for the ER similar to that of tamoxifen and a biological half-life twice that of tamoxifen (14 days versus 7 days).[77] The long half-life is due to binding to plasma proteins and enterohepatic recirculation. 4-Hydroxytamoxifen is present in low plasma concentrations but has a binding affinity for the ER that is 25-fold to 50-fold greater than that of tamoxifen. Tamoxifen is believed to undergo extensive first-pass metabolism and is excreted primarily by the biliary system.[75]

Data from the first clinical trial of tamoxifen revealed a response rate of 22 percent in hormonally pretreated women.[28] Initially tamoxifen use was restricted largely to postmenopausal women with metastatic breast cancer. Clinical trials of tamoxifen conducted in this patient population have shown response rates of 15 to 53 percent, with a median duration of response of 20 months.[28, 29, 70, 79–91]

The patient characteristics that predict a response to tamoxifen are similar to those for other endocrine therapies. Tumors expressing ER have a 50 percent probability of responding to tamoxifen compared with less than 10 percent for ER-negative tumors.[37] Response to tamoxifen is more likely in patients who have responded to prior hormonal therapy, have had a long disease-free interval from primary treatment to relapse, are older, and have sites of disease primarily in the soft tissues, bone, and lung.

Tamoxifen has been shown to be just as effective in inducing tumor responses as other forms of hormonal therapy, including endocrine ablative therapies (e.g., adrenalectomy, hypophysectomy),[92, 93] estrogens,[94–97] progestins,[98–100] androgens,[101] and aminoglutethimide.[102] Yet, tamoxifen is associated with less toxicity than these other forms of endocrine therapy.

Tamoxifen is an extremely well tolerated drug and only rarely will it have to be discontinued because of

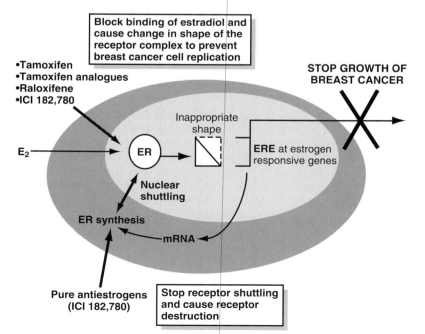

Figure 73–3 *A molecular model of antiestrogen action in the breast cancer cell. All antiestrogens can bind to the ER but cause an inappropriate change in shape so that binding to the EREs is imperfect. The pure antiestrogens have an additional mechanism of action by promoting the cytoplasmic destruction of the newly synthesized ER.*

toxicity. Its most common side effect is hot flashes, which are tolerated well by most patients.[103–105] Other side effects include nausea, vomiting, weight gain, and vaginal bleeding or discharge. Occasionally patients complain of nonspecific neurological symptoms (i.e., depression, headache, insomnia, fatigue, irritability, and dizziness), thromboembolic disease, and visual disturbances caused by optic neuritis, retinopathy, or macular edema.[103–105] Rarely patients with metastatic bone disease will report increased bone pain (tumor flare), with or without hypercalcemia, within 1 to 2 weeks of initiating tamoxifen therapy.[106–107] This phenomenon is believed to be due to tamoxifen's mild estrogenic effect, and it should be treated with supportive measures, including analgesics and possibly low-dose prednisone Tamoxifen should not be discontinued because of this side effect as the symptoms usually dissipate within a few weeks.

Tamoxifen retains some estrogenic effect on certain target tissues that may be beneficial or potentially deleterious. In rats, tamoxifen produces sufficient estrogen-like effects in bone to prevent osteoporosis following oophorectomy.[108, 109] In postmenopausal patients receiving long-term tamoxifen therapy, primarily in the adjuvant setting, a detrimental effect on bone density has not been observed.[110, 111] Tamoxifen also causes a significant decrease in circulating cholesterol, primarily LDL cholesterol.[112, 113] During the past 5 years, a number of case reports and clinical trial results have associated tamoxifen therapy with an increased incidence of endometrial carcinoma.[114, 115] Several analyses of the data have concluded that there is only a modest increase in endometrial carcinoma incidence during tamoxifen therapy (i.e., 2/1000 tamoxifen-treated women per year versus 1/1000 women per year for the normal female population at risk).[116–118] The potential risks and benefits associated with tamoxifen therapy may be more relevant to patients receiving adjuvant treatment, as survival is expected to be longer in these patients, and cure, rather than palliation, is the goal of adjuvant therapy. Nevertheless, patients should be monitored for pre-existing endometrial carcinoma.

Tamoxifen is approved by the Federal Drug Administration for the treatment of ER-positive, advanced breast cancer in premenopausal women. The few published phase II clinical trials in this patient population report response rates between 20 and 45 percent (mean 30 percent), with a median duration of response of 2.5 to 36 months.[79, 85, 91, 119–124] Tumor regression is more likely to occur in patients with soft-tissue and bony disease. For patients with ER- and PR-positive tumors, response rates range between 45 and 75 percent. Small randomized trials comparing results of tamoxifen with those of oophorectomy in premenopausal patients with metastatic disease show no difference in overall response rates, duration of response, or survival rates.[125, 126]

Premenopausal women often continue to menstruate regularly while receiving tamoxifen therapy; however, between 16 and 39 percent of patients ex-perience complete amenorrhea, and the frequency increases with longer use.[84, 122, 123] Long-term or short-term tamoxifen therapy causes an increase in ovarian estrogen (estrone and estradiol) and progesterone synthesis.[127–129] Serum levels of steroids often double over those observed during normal menstrual cycles. There is no evidence that these menstrual or hormonal alterations correlate with tumor response.[84, 122, 123]

Laboratory evidence suggests that tamoxifen can exert an agonist effect on human mammary tumors. This effect may be mediated by selection of a clone of tumor cells that respond to tamoxifen as an estrogen or by the metabolic conversion of tamoxifen to an estrogenic metabolite that acts as mitogen. Gottardis and coworkers[130, 131] demonstrated a tamoxifen withdrawal effect in an animal model of human disease. Nude mice were inoculated with ER-positive, MCF-7 cells, which rapidly proliferate if the animals are treated with estrogen while tumor growth is inhibited if the animals are also treated with tamoxifen. After several months, even in the presence of tamoxifen the tumors begin to grow again. When tamoxifen therapy was withdrawn, tumor regression was observed. This laboratory observation has been corroborated clinically; tamoxifen withdrawal responses have been observed in 10 to 30 percent of advanced breast cancer patients with documented disease progression on tamoxifen therapy.[132] These findings suggest that clones of tumor cells that respond to tamoxifen as an agonist may become the dominant population in a tumor over time.

New Antiestrogens

Numerous compounds classified as antiestrogens are being evaluated in clinical trials. These antiestrogens can be broadly classified three ways: triphenylethylenes or tamoxifen analogues, pure antiestrogens, and targeted antiestrogens.

Tamoxifen Analogues

Toremifene

Toremifene (Farnesdon) or chlorotamoxifen (see Fig. 73–1) is approved by the Federal Drug Administration for the treatment of metastatic breast cancer in postmenopausal women. In animal models, toremifene is effective in controlling the growth of carcinogen-induced mammary carcinomas,[133–136] but it appears to be approximately one third less potent than tamoxifen.[137] This finding is consistent with the larger dose of toremifene (60 mg/day orally) that is used clinically compared with the dose of tamoxifen (20 mg/day orally). Toremifene exhibits weak estrogen-like properties in postmenopausal patients. Luteinizing hormone (LH) and follicle-stimulating hormone (FSH) are slightly depressed during therapy, and sex hormone binding globulin (SHBG) is increased.[138–140]

Although toremifene exhibits antiestrogenic effects

on the vaginal mucosa of estrogen-primed women,[141, 142] it has no effect in blocking short-term estrogen action in the uterus.[142] Toremifene and tamoxifen produce the same estrogen-like effects on the histology of the postmenopausal endometrium[143]; however, no data are available on the incidence of endometrial cancer during toremifene treatment. Unlike tamoxifen, toremifene does not produce liver tumors in rats, but the clinical relevance of this laboratory finding has been questioned.[117]

Clinical trials with toremifene were initiated in the early 1980s. In postmenopausal patients with advanced disease refractory to tamoxifen, toremifene infrequently induced objective responses (response rate 0 to 33 percent),[144–149] suggesting that it has cross-resistance to tamoxifen. In postmenopausal patients with advanced disease who had not received prior hormonal or cytotoxic chemotherapy, treatment with toremifene (20 to 240 mg/day orally) resulted in response rates of 21 to 68 percent, including up to 26 percent complete clinical responses.[150–158]

Toremifene has been directly likened to tamoxifen as a first-line therapy for patients with advanced disease. In the largest trial, 648 previously untreated metastatic breast cancer patients with positive hormone receptors or receptors of unknown status were randomized to receive tamoxifen (20 mg/day orally) or two different doses of toremifene (60 or 200 mg/day orally).[159] Tamoxifen produced a response rate of 19 percent and a median survival of 32 months. Toremifene produced a response rate of 21 percent with the 60 mg dose and 23 percent with the 200 mg dose. Median survival of toremifene-treated patients was 38 months for the 60 mg dose) and 30 months for the 200 mg dose. The median time to disease progression was not statistically different between treatment arms. Response rates, time to disease progression, and overall survival rates for patients on each treatment arm were better for ER-positive patients than for ER-negative patients. Toxicity associated with toremifene in this trial, as well as in others, was mild, similar to that of tamoxifen. The data from this large randomized trial support the use of toremifene as an alternative first-line therapy to tamoxifen in postmenopausal patients with advanced disease and positive hormone receptors.[159]

Droloxifene

Droloxifene, or 3-hydroxytamoxifen (see Fig. 73–1), has been tested for the treatment of metastatic breast cancer, but this drug is currently being developed for the treatment of osteoporosis in postmenopausal women. In the laboratory droloxifene appeared promising because it has a tenfold higher binding affinity for ER-positive breast cancer cells than tamoxifen.[160] The principal pharmacological advantage of droloxifene appears to be reduced estrogenic activity compared with tamoxifen in animal uterine weight tests,[161] an absence of DNA adduct formation in laboratory assays of carcinogenesis,[162] and an inability to produce rat liver tumors.[162]

Several clinical trials have been published in which patients previously treated with chemotherapy or hormone therapy, or both, received daily oral doses of droloxifene ranging from 20 to 300 mg.[163–169] Response rates ranged from 0 to 70 percent, with most occurring in peri- or postmenopausal patients. Trials evaluating different doses of droloxifene have not convincingly demonstrated a dose-response effect.[166, 168, 169] In all trials reported, droloxifene has been extremely well tolerated, with hot flashes, fatigue, and nausea being the most commonly cited side effects. Two episodes of pulmonary emboli were documented. Hypercoagulability, increased levels of sex hormone binding globulin and decreased gonadotropin levels are evidence of the estrogenic properties of droloxifene.

Droloxifene is rapidly absorbed and excreted and does not appear to accumulate the way tamoxifen and toremifene do. Droloxifene has a short biological half-life of approximately 27 to 28 hours.[170, 171] As a result, droloxifene can be cleared from a patient's body within a few days, whereas up to 6 weeks may be required to achieve total clearance of tamoxifen.

Idoxifene

Idoxifene (see Fig. 73–1) has a binding capacity for the ER that is about twice that of tamoxifen, and this binding capacity translates to a modest increase, compared with tamoxifen, in the ability to inhibit the growth of ER-positive breast cancer cells in culture.[172] Idoxifene was designed to be "metabolically resistant" with an iodine atom at the 4 position of tamoxifen to prevent toxicity through 4-hydroxylation and a pyrrolidine side chain to avoid theoretical toxicities associated with demethylation.[173, 174] Ideally the drug will avoid the toxicology problems with liver carcinogenicity produced by tamoxifen in animals,[175] although additional studies are required. Only one clinical trial using idoxifene in humans has been published. Coombes and coworkers[176] reported the results of a phase I clinical trial in which 20 patients with advanced breast cancer (ER-positive or ER of unknown status) were treated with one of four dose levels of idoxifene. In this heavily pretreated population of patients, partial responses were observed in 14 percent, and toxicity was mild.

Pure Antiestrogens

The antiestrogens ICI 164,384 and ICI 182,780 (see Fig. 73–1) are derivatives of 17-beta-estradiol with an optimal binding affinity for the ER, but these structural analogues are unique because they do not have any estrogenic properties and they have a novel subcellular mechanism of action. ICI 182,780 differs slightly from ICI 164,384 by possessing fluorine atoms in the side chain to decrease phase I metabolism.[177, 178]

Initially it was believed that pure antiestrogens prevent the dimerization of receptor complexes, thereby preventing binding to estrogen response elements (ERE).[179] As a result, it was thought that if receptor complexes do not bind to any EREs, then genes cannot be activated, and this fact would explain why the compound was a "pure" antiestrogen. Now, a different mechanism has been proposed (see Fig. 73–3). The pure antiestrogen-ER complex can bind to EREs, but the transcriptional unit is inactive.[53, 160, 180, 181] In addition, pure antiestrogens appear to provoke the complete destruction of the ER in breast cancer cells in culture,[182] mouse uterus,[183] and in breast tumors *in situ*.[184] Under normal circumstances, the ER is synthesized in the cytoplasm and transported to the nucleus, where it functions as a transcription factor. A pure antiestrogen binds to the newly synthesized receptor in the cytoplasm and prevents transport to the nucleus.[185] The paralyzed receptor complex is then rapidly destroyed.[185] The complete destruction of available ER will prevent any estrogen events from occurring. Normal cells will become quiescent, whereas hormone-dependent tumors will rapidly regress because senescent tumor cells cannot be replaced by replication.

The pure antiestrogen ICI 164,384 has been used extensively in laboratory studies, but the more potent ICI 182,780 is being evaluated as a second-line therapy for the treatment of breast cancer after the failure of long-term adjuvant tamoxifen. ICI 182,780 is a potent inhibitor of the growth of ER-positive breast cancer cells in culture[186] and causes a more complete inhibition of growth than does tamoxifen.[187] The growth of ER-negative breast cancer cell lines is unaffected by ICI 182,780. Pure antiestrogens will inhibit the growth of tamoxifen-stimulated breast and endometrial tumors in the laboratory, but growth of tamoxifen-stimulated tumors will resume after prolonged therapy with pure antiestrogens.[131, 188]

Laboratory evidence also suggests that more complete estrogen blockade and tumor growth inhibition can be achieved with a combination of the luteinizing hormone-releasing hormone analogue, goserelin, and ICI 164,384 than can be achieved with goserelin alone.[189] This observation may have clinical applications as a strategy to treat premenopausal patients with advanced disease.

There have been no reports of genotoxicity or carcinogenesis with ICI 182,780. Patients with breast tumors treated with ICI 182,780 for a few days have a significant decrease in Ki67, PR, and ER, whereas no effect on LH, FSH, or SHBG has been observed.[184] Only two clinical reports on ICI 182,780 have been published. DeFriend and coworkers[184] found no significant toxicity associated with preoperative, intramuscular (IM) injection of ICI 182,780. Howell and coworkers[190] treated a group of 19 tamoxifen-resistant, advanced breast cancer patients with ICI 182,780 (250 mg/month, IM). A 37 percent partial response rate was reported, involving soft-tissue, bone, and visceral sites of disease. In addition, 32 percent of patients maintained stable disease status. The lack of cross resistance in 69 percent of patients suggests that ICI 182,780 may be useful as a first-line therapy for advanced disease or as a second-line

therapy for advanced disease when tamoxifen has been previously administered. At present ICI 182,780 is available only as a depot injection. Further development of pure antiestrogens will necessitate the availability of a sustained-release preparation or the development of an orally active drug.

Targeted Antiestrogens

Raloxifene

Raloxifene (see Fig. 73–1), originally named keoxifene, is being developed as a treatment for osteoporosis and undergoing testing for treatment of ER-positive, advanced breast cancer. The drug is referred to as a selective estrogen receptor modulator (SERM), which builds on the original concept that targeted antiestrogens can have estrogenic effects on the cardiovascular system and bone but an antiestrogenic effect on the breast and uterus.[191, 192] Raloxifene is an antiestrogen in the immature rat uterine weight test but has little agonist action on the uterus when administered alone. Raloxifene maintains bone density in the ovariectomized rat,[108, 193, 194] but the drug also reduces circulating cholesterol.[195] There is no evidence that raloxifene causes the formation of DNA adducts or induces hepatocarcinogenesis.

A single phase II clinical trial of raloxifene in female patients with metastatic breast cancer refractory to tamoxifen therapy has been reported.[196] In 14 patients treated with raloxifene (200 mg/day orally) for up to 8 months, the drug was well tolerated, with no significant clinical or laboratory abnormalities detected, but no objective responses were observed. Raloxifene will not be available for the treatment of breast cancer, although there is every reason to believe from the pharmacological profile of the drug that it would be an effective agent.

Aromatase Inhibitors

The aromatase enzyme is the rate-limiting step in estrogen biosynthesis that converts androstenedione to estrone.[197] In premenopausal women the most important site of aromatase is the ovary. Other sites of the aromatase enzyme include adipose tissue, liver, muscle, and hair follicles. In the ovary of premenopausal women, FSH stimulates the granulosa cell compartment to synthesize more aromatase, and LH stimulates the theca cell compartment to synthesize androstenedione, the substrate for aromatase.[198–200] Inhibition of ovarian aromatase in premenopausal women results in decreased estradiol production, which signals the pituitary to increase FSH and LH secretion. The reflex rise in gonadotropins overcomes the inhibition of the aromatase system. As a result, strategies to inhibit the aromatase system are more rational for treating postmenopausal women, in whom the primary source of estrogen production is the extraovarian conversion of adrenal androstenedione to estrone.[199, 200]

In postmenopausal women the precursor of estrogen biosynthesis, androstenedione, is secreted by the adrenals. Androstenedione is converted to estrone by the peripheral cytochrome P450 mono-oxygenase system. Estrone is then converted to estradiol by the enzyme 17β-hydroxysteroid dehydrogenase. Several investigators have also demonstrated aromatase activity in human breast tumors, although the activity is generally considered too low to be of biological significance.[201–203] A small amount of androstenedione is also secreted by the ovaries so that a precise measurement of estradiol will reveal slightly higher levels in surgically oophorectomized women compared with women who undergo natural menopause.[204] The treatment strategies to be considered are either block adrenal steroidogenesis and peripheral aromatase enzymes or specifically peripheral aromatase.

Aminoglutethimide

Aminoglutethimide was originally developed as an anticonvulsant agent in the 1950s, but it was withdrawn from the market in 1966 after adrenal insufficiency developed in two children being treated with the drug.[205, 206] This serendipitous finding was the primary reason that aminoglutethimide was re-evaluated as a potential breast cancer treatment. The first clinical use of aminoglutethimide as a breast cancer treatment was an effort to produce a "medical adrenalectomy" by blocking cholesterol side-chain cleavage, leading to a decrease in adrenal steroid synthesis. Subsequent in vitro and in vivo experiments confirmed that aminoglutethimide prevents estrogen biosynthesis primarily by two mechanisms: the inhibition of cholesterol side-chain cleavage in the adrenal glands (e.g., inhibition of the enzyme desmolase), leading to decreased production of adrenal glucocorticoids and inhibition of the peripheral aromatase system and thus resulting in decreased conversion of androstenedione to estrogens (Fig. 73–4).[207–209] In addition, aminoglutethimide blocks a number of other enzymes, including 11-, 18-, and 21-hydroxylase. Thyroid hormone (T_4) synthesis is also lowered, resulting in a reflex rise in thyroid-stimulating hormone (TSH) in a small fraction of patients.[210]

Adrenal synthesis of cortisol is inhibited by the action of aminoglutethimide, which can lead to the clinical features of Addison's disease. The decrease in cortisol synthesis is associated with a reflex rise in adrenocorticotropic hormone (ACTH) levels that may not fully compensate for the decreased cortisol levels; however, increased adrenal steroidogenesis may reverse the therapeutic goal intended with the use of aminoglutethimide. As a result, glucocorticoid replacement (i.e., hydrocortisone) is often administered along with aminoglutethimide. The conversion of androstenedione to estrone is decreased by 98 percent in postmenopausal women treated with the aminoglutethimide/glucocorticoid regimen, and both urinary and plasma estrogen levels are decreased to a similar degree.[209]

The results from numerous clinical trials involving the combination of aminoglutethimide and replacement glucocorticoids in patients with metastatic breast cancer have been published.[197, 211, 212] The dose of aminoglutethimide has varied from 250 mg/day to 1000 mg/day. Response rates in previously untreated patients have varied from 20 to 56 percent, with a mean duration of response of approximately 11 to 12 months, results similar to those of tamoxifen treatment. Although described as previously untreated, many of the patients in these trials previously received additive hormonal treatment in the form of androgens and estrogens or oophorectomy.[197, 211, 212]

Several studies have demonstrated that aminoglutethimide plus glucocorticoids as first-line therapy in metastatic breast cancer achieves response rates and response duration similar to those achieved with tamoxifen, but tamoxifen has fewer associated side effects. Some studies have reported that patients with ER-positive tumors have higher response rates (54 percent) than patients with ER-negative tumors (12 percent).[31] Sites of disease most likely to respond to aminoglutethimide therapy include the soft tissues, lymph nodes, bones, and lungs.

A prospective randomized trial conducted by the Eastern Cooperative Oncology Group (ECOG) demonstrated response rates of 45 percent for treatment with aminoglutethimide and 27 percent for treatment with tamoxifen.[102] The survival rate was the same for both groups of patients, but toxicities were more common in the patients treated with aminoglutethimide.

A wide variety of side effects are associated with aminoglutethimide treatment, and in up to 10 per-

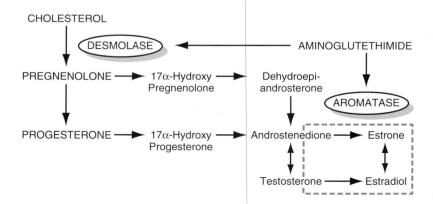

Figure 73–4 *Mechanism of action of aminoglutethimide in the adrenal cortex at the desmolase enzyme and in peripheral tissue at the aromatase enzyme.*

cent of patients therapy must be discontinued because of toxicity.[197, 211, 212] Skin rashes are very common, occurring in up to one third of patients. The skin rash, usually morbilliform and maculopapular, generally develops during the first week of treatment and spontaneously resolves after 1 week. Lethargy, drowsiness, and fatigue are reported in up to two thirds of patients, but the incidence of these side effects increases with increasing doses of aminoglutethimide and decreases with the co-administration of glucocorticoids. Reversible ataxia has been reported in one third of patients receiving a daily dose of 1000 mg of aminoglutethimide. Rarely, cytopenias, Stevens-Johnson syndrome, depression, and hypotension have been reported. Some side effects (e.g., lethargy, skin rash, ataxia, and dizziness) are more prominent at the initiation of therapy and subside with long-term administration.

In an effort to reduce the side effects associated with aminoglutethimide therapy, lower daily doses (125 or 250 mg/day) of the drug have been administered along with glucocorticoids.[197, 211, 212] Response rates were similar to those resulting from higher doses; however, lethargy was observed less frequently with lower daily doses of aminoglutethimide. Clinical trials have also attempted to determine if glucocorticoid replacement can be eliminated from the treatment regimen without adding toxicity. Low-dose aminoglutethimide (125 or 250 mg/day) administered without glucocorticoids causes a decrease in serum/urine estradiol levels (inhibition of aromatase) to a degree similar to that resulting from higher doses of aminoglutethimide. In addition, there appears to be no clear dose-response relationship with aminoglutethimide at doses varying between 250 and 1000 mg/day. A randomized trial comparing aminoglutethimide alone (500 mg/day) with aminoglutethimide (500 mg/day) plus glucocorticoids demonstrated similar response rates, response duration, and survival rates for the two groups.[213] These results suggest that glucocorticoids do not add to the antitumor effect of aminoglutethimide, but the co-administration of glucocorticoids may attenuate the side effects associated with aminoglutethimide treatment. In general, daily doses of aminoglutethimide in excess of 250 to 500 mg/day with or without concurrent glucocorticoid treatment are unlikely to provide additional clinical benefit.

Anastrozole

Aminoglutethimide is an effective treatment for some breast cancers, but because of its lack of specificity, its low potency, and its associated side effects, other compounds have been under development.[214] The ideal drug would inhibit aromatase without inhibiting adrenal steroid synthesis and would have few side effects. The second-generation aromatase inhibitors were developed with the rationale that steroid substrate analogues would possess more specificity for the aromatase enzyme than aminoglutethimide.[215, 216]

Anastrozole (Arimidex) is a potent, selective aromatase inhibitor approved by the Federal Drug Administration as a treatment for metastatic breast cancer in postmenopausal women who have not been helped by tamoxifen (see Fig. 73–5). In animal studies, anastrozole was selective for the aromatase enzyme while not inhibiting enzymes in the adrenal gland that controls steroid hormone synthesis.[217] In five phase I clinical trials of anastrozole evaluating both single- and multiple-dose schedules, the drug was well tolerated and toxicity was mild. For all doses, anastrozole did not effect cortisol or aldosterone secretion at baseline or in response to ACTH. As a result, it can be concluded that glucocorticoid or mineralocorticoid replacement therapy is not necessary with anastrozole treatment.

Anastrozole has been evaluated in two randomized clinical trials comparing anastrozole (1 mg or 10 mg/day orally) to megestrol acetate (160 mg/day orally) as a treatment for postmenopausal women with advanced breast cancer who had disease progression following tamoxifen therapy for either advanced or early stage breast cancer.[217, 218] Some of the patients in these trials had previously received cytotoxic chemotherapy. Most patients were ER-positive; ER-negative patients were enrolled only if response to prior tamoxifen therapy was documented.

Approximately one third of the patients in each treatment group on both trials had either an objective response or stabilization of disease for greater than 24 weeks. There was no evidence that the higher dose of anastrozole was superior to the 1 mg dose. Anastrozole was well tolerated at both doses and was not associated with the weight gain seen in patients receiving megestrol acetate. The recommended dose of anastrozole is one 1 mg tablet daily.

Other Aromatase Inhibitors in Clinical Trial

4-Hydroxyandrostenedione, or formestane, irreversibly binds to aromatase with a high degree of specificity.[215] This type of inhibitor is commonly referred to as a "suicide inhibitor" because it can produce prolonged inhibition of the enzyme, the duration of which is dependent on new enzyme synthesis or persistent levels of the inhibitor. In vitro studies have demonstrated that formestane produces a 30-fold greater inhibition of aromatase than aminoglutethimide.[215] Since formestane inhibits only aromatase en-

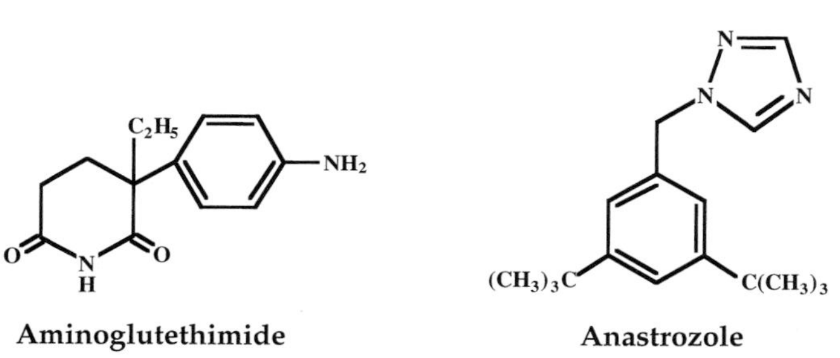

Figure 73–5 *The formula of aminoglutethimide and the specific aromatase inhibitor anastrozole.*

zymes without affecting the cytochrome P450-related enzymes, concurrent glucocorticoid replacement therapy is not necessary. Because of the rapid clearance of formestane when it is administered orally, the drug is administered intramuscularly. The administration of formestane, 250 mg IM every other week, achieves 85 percent inhibition of peripheral aromatase and 65 percent suppression of estradiol. Higher IM doses of formestane achieve similar results. Formestane does not appear to significantly alter LH, FSH, SHBG, dehydroepiandrosterone sulfate, testosterone, 5α-reductase, or androstenedione when administered IM.[215, 216, 219]

Most investigators report few side effects with formestane treatment, though one trial did report local reactions (e.g., pain, sterile abscesses, inflammation) in 13 percent of patients related to the IM injection.[216] Other rare side effects include fatigue, nausea or vomiting, and neutropenia. Formestane administered IM every 4 days or every 14 days, in doses of 250 to 500 mg, produces response rates ranging from 14 to 46 percent in patients with advanced breast cancer. One randomized clinical trial reported higher response rates in patients receiving 500 mg of formestane (IM every 2 weeks) compared to patients receiving 250 mg of the drug, but the time to disease progression and overall survival rates were identical for both groups.[219] Generally response rates are higher in patients who have previously responded to tamoxifen; rarely tumor regression has been observed in patients unresponsive to tamoxifen.[219] Other members of the steroid class of inhibitors of aromatase include testolactone, atamestane, and 6-methyleneandrostenedione. In general, response rates observed with these compounds are similar to those for aminoglutethimide, but toxicity appears less.[211, 214]

Fadrozole,[220] letrozole,[220, 221] and vorozole[222, 223] are orally active, nonsteroidal aromatase inhibitors currently under evaluation in clinical trials. All three compounds effectively suppress blood and urine levels of estradiol and estrone. Letrozole and vorozole do not appear to have a significant effect at any dose on aldosterone, testosterone, androstenedione, 17α-hydroxyprogesterone, or TSH levels. Cortisol and aldosterone output are diminished at higher doses of fadrozole.[220] The drugs are well tolerated, and tumor responses have been observed in postmenopausal women who previously responded to tamoxifen.

Luteinizing Hormone-Releasing Hormone Agonists

The primary effectiveness of luteinizing hormone-releasing hormone (LHRH) agonists for the treatment of breast cancer is to produce a reversible chemical castration.[224–228] Naturally occurring LHRH is a decapeptide with a short biological half-life that is secreted in a pulsatile fashion from the hypothalamus into the portal circulation. LHRH causes the secretion of LH and FSH from the pituitary, which in turn stimulate the ovaries to synthesize and secrete estrogen.[229]

Synthetic analogues of LHRH have been developed with substitutions at the 6,9, and/or 10 positions in the peptide sequence, which results in a protein more biologically active by prolonging the duration of action compared to the native protein.[230, 231] Immediately following the initiation of therapy with one of the LHRH analogues in a premenopausal woman, plasma levels of estradiol and gonadotropins rise, but long-term use paradoxically suppresses ovarian function, and plasma estradiol levels fall to castrate levels.[224, 232] This finding is in contrast to the striking rise in plasma estradiol levels and cyclic secretion of LH and FSH observed in premenopausal women treated with tamoxifen.[128] Withdrawal or exhaustion of the LHRH analogue depot returns the plasma estradiol levels to pretreatment levels, and menstrual periods generally return within 1 to 2 months.[233] Serum levels of gonadotropin, testosterone, androstenedione, and estradiol fell to 10 percent of pretreatment levels following treatment of premenopausal women with one analogue, goserelin.[234, 235] In contrast, levels of the adrenal hormones, estrone and dehydroepiandrosterone, did not change.

Laboratory and clinical observations have been reported that suggest a direct effect by the LHRH agonists on cancer cells. Eidne and coworkers[236] have demonstrated the presence of gonadotropin-releasing hormone binding sites on several breast cancer cell lines. Miller and coworkers[237] have reported growth inhibition of breast cancer cell lines by an LHRH agonist. Supporting a nonhormonal antitumor effect by LHRH agonists are the clinical reports that occasionally identify postmenopausal or ER-negative patients who attain objective responses after treatment with LHRH agonists.[238–240]

Of the many LHRH agonists that have been synthesized, buserelin, leuprolide (Lupron), and goserelin (Zoladex®) have been most extensively studied in clinical trials. All of these agents can be administered in a subcutaneous preparation, but buserelin can also be administered intranasally, and goserelin and leuprolide are available in a depot preparation requiring a single monthly intramuscular injection.[230, 231] Goserelin was recently approved by the Federal Drug Administration for the treatment of breast cancer in premenopausal women.

Some of the initial clinical trials with LHRH agonists were conducted in postmenopausal women. One study using leuprolide for the treatment of 31 heavily pretreated postmenopausal patients with advanced disease reported a 39 percent objective response rate.[239] Other clinical trials that followed evaluating goserelin, leuprolide, and buserelin in the postmenopausal patient population, reported objective response rates of only 8 to 20 percent.[241–244] A relatively low response rate in postmenopausal women would be expected, as the ovaries produce only a small quantity of estrogen in this patient population.

Results in premenopausal patients are more promising.[233, 245–249] An early phase II study of a depot preparation of goserelin in 134 pre- and perimenopausal women with advanced disease reported an objective response rate of 44 percent, including 10 percent complete responders.[233] Serum concentrations of estradiol fell into the range of castrated or postmenopausal women within 2 to 3 weeks of starting therapy. In responders, the median time to response was 4 months, and the median duration of response was 8 months. Although objective responses were more likely to occur in patients with ER-positive tumors (49 percent), objective responses were also observed in 33 percent of patients with ER-negative tumors.[233] A significant fraction of responses were detected in both visceral and bony sites of disease. The most common side effect was hot flashes, occurring in 63 percent of patients.

Blamey and coworkers[246] reported results on 333 pre- and perimenopausal women with advanced breast cancer treated with a monthly subcutaneous depot injection (3.6 mg) of goserelin.[246] Mean serum LH and estradiol concentrations were suppressed by day 22 after the first injection. Objective responses were detected in 36 percent of patients, and median duration of response was 44 weeks. Hot flashes and loss of libido occurred in 75 percent and 47 percent of patients, respectively.[246] Objective clinical responses were observed in patients initially presenting with advanced disease and in patients who had developed recurrent disease following a disease-free interval after initial diagnosis, including patients previously treated with adjuvant hormone or chemotherapy. Tumor regression was observed in visceral sites of disease, including lung (28 percent) and liver (24 percent).[246] Other studies have reported objective response rates in up to 50 percent of premenopausal women treated with LHRH agonists.[233, 245–251] Whether treatment with LHRH agonists effectively results in an oophorectomy is debatable, because objective tumor responses to surgical oophorectomy have been reported following disease progression while patients were receiving goserelin.[233]

Other treatment strategies have attempted to provide maximal estrogen blockade by combining the use of tamoxifen and LHRH agonists.[252–254] Jonat and coworkers[254] reported the results of a randomized trial comparing the results of goserelin with and without tamoxifen in 318 pre- or perimenopausal patients with advanced breast cancer. There was a modest benefit in favor of combination therapy in time to progression but not in survival rate. In 115 patients with skeletal metastases only, significant differences in favor of combination therapy were seen in response rate, time to progression, and survival rate. Other studies have demonstrated the feasibility of the "total estrogen blockade" approach, but enhanced efficacy has not been demonstrated, and toxicity may be increased.[252, 253]

Additive Hormonal Therapies

With the exception of progestins, other additive hormone therapies are rarely used in practice today primarily because other forms of endocrine therapy are more effective and are associated with fewer side effects.

Androgens

Androgenic agents such as testosterone, fluoxymesterone, testolactone, and calusterone have been used to treat postmenopausal women with hormone-responsive breast cancer.[255–257] Patients with ER-positive breast tumors respond better than those with ER-negative tumors. Objective response rates of up to 21 percent in unselected patients and 46 percent in patients with ER-positive tumors have been reported. The mechanism of action of androgens is unknown but probably involves blocking the stimulating effect of estrogen. The high incidence of androgenic side effects (e.g., hirsutism, male-pattern baldness, acne, fluid retention, and so forth) make these compounds second-line agents in the treatment of breast cancer.[256, 257] In addition, tumor flare and hypercalcemia occur more commonly with these androgens than with other hormonal therapies.[258] Danazol is a weak androgen that is associated with milder side effects compared with other androgens. Clinical trials of danazol in women with advanced disease have reported objective response rates as high as 25 percent.[259–263]

Estrogens

Treatment with high-dose estrogens such as DES and ethinyl estradiol is effective as a therapy for advanced breast cancer.[255] The mechanism of action for estrogen's antitumor effect is unknown. The high dose of DES used (15 mg/day) produces beneficial effects in ER-positive breast cancer patients, possibly by downregulating the ER and thereby decreasing the effect of estrogen.[22, 264] Objective response rates of up to 26 percent in unselected patients and 65 percent in patients with ER-positive tumors have been reported.[265, 266] High-dose estrogen therapy is associated with toxicities, including vaginal bleeding, breast tenderness, cholestatic jaundice, nausea, vomiting, and depression. Treatment with estrogens is accompanied by flare in about 10 percent of patients and withdrawal response after subsequent relapse in about 5 percent of patients.[267]

Progestins

Megestrol acetate (Megace) and medroxyprogesterone acetate are the progestins most widely used to treat advanced breast cancer.[197, 255, 268] They are associated with response rates similar to those of other hormonal treatments. Progestins have several mechanisms of action that might explain the observed antitumor effect in breast cancer patients. Treatment with progestins downregulate the expression of the ER (and the PR), potentially making the cell less sensitive to the effects of estrogen.[269] Progestins can also bind to androgen and glucocorticoid receptors that are expressed by some breast cancer cells, and this receptor binding may cause downstream events that inhibit growth.[270] Progestin interaction with the progesterone receptor may have an antiestrogenic effect by increasing the oxidative activity of 17β-hydroxysteroid dehydrogenase, thereby facilitating the conversion of estradiol to the weaker estrogen, estrone.[271] Higher doses of progestins are capable of suppressing the hypothalamic-pituitary-adrenal axis, resulting in inhibition of steroidogenesis, with a resulting fall in circulating estrogens.[272]

Megestrol acetate is an orally active progesterone derivative with better gastrointestinal absorption and bioavailability than medroxyprogesterone acetate. Standard-dose megestrol acetate (160 mg/day) administered orally results in blood levels five to ten times higher than those detected in patients treated with 1000 mg of oral medroxyprogesterone acetate.[272, 273] Because of the poor bioavailability of oral medroxyprogesterone acetate, the agent is most commonly administered intramuscularly.

In multiple clinical trials of standard-dose megestrol acetate in previously treated, primarily postmenopausal patients with advanced disease, the objective response rate was approximately 27 percent, including complete remissions in 5 percent of patients.[272, 274–285] The main side effect was weight gain, which occurred in 20 percent of patients.[272, 274–282] Less common side effects included hypertension, congestive heart failure, thrombophlebitis, and pulmonary embolism. Medroxyprogesterone acetate has been evaluated in a similar group of patients in which response rates were as high as 40 percent, but in addition to the side effects described for megestrol acetate, intramuscular injections were associated with local skin reactions and gluteal abscesses.[286] In addition, up to 15 percent of patients developed cushingoid features.

Megestrol acetate (160 mg/day) has been compared to medroxyprogesterone acetate (1000 mg/day) in two clinical trials. Wander and coworkers[283] reported equivalent response rates for megestrol acetate and medroxyprogesterone acetate (25 percent and 29 percent, respectively). Willemse and colleagues,[282] reported a higher response rate (45 percent) for medroxyprogesterone acetate, predominantly in bony sites, than for megestrol acetate (12 percent). Progression-free survival and overall survival rates were not significantly different for the two treatment groups.

Several trials have investigated whether dose escalation of megestrol acetate is associated with improved clinical outcome.[284, 285, 287] Muss and coworkers[284] studied 172 women treated with megestrol acetate (160 mg/day or 800 mg/day). The majority of women were postmenopausal and had received prior tamoxifen therapy for advanced disease or in the adjuvant setting. Treatment with high-dose megestrol acetate was associated with improved response rates (27 percent versus 10 percent), time to treatment failure (22 months versus 16 months) and overall survival (22 months versus 16 months) compared

with standard-dose megestrol acetate. Weight gain of more than 20 pounds occurred in 13 percent and 43 percent of the standard-dose and high-dose groups, respectively.

Two other clinical trials evaluating dose escalation of megestrol acetate failed to demonstrate an improvement in response rates or overall survival rates for patients receiving doses of 160 mg/day versus 1600 mg/day.[285, 287] In addition, quality-of-life instruments were incorporated into one trial and clearly indicated that increased daily doses of megestrol acetate were associated with decreased levels of function and increased levels of distress.[289] The results of these trials support the standard-dose regimen (160 mg/day) of megestrol acetate for the treatment of advanced breast cancer.

Randomized clinical trials have also directly compared the efficacy of tamoxifen with that of megestrol acetate.[276, 278, 280, 281, 284, 290] Overall response rates attained by the two agents are comparable, ranging from 7 to 32 percent for megestrol acetate and 7 to 42 percent for tamoxifen. Only one report suggested a difference in median survival and time to disease progression, and this difference favored tamoxifen. Several of these trials incorporated a crossover design so that upon documentation of disease progression while receiving one drug, patients would "cross over" to the other treatment.[274–278, 280, 284] Results of these trials showed a 14 percent response rate for tamoxifen in megestrol acetate nonresponders and a 20 percent response rate for megestrol acetate in tamoxifen nonresponders. A summary of the treatment effects of commonly used hormonal therapies is outlined in Table 73–3.

Antiprogestins

Progestin antagonists are at a relatively early stage of development for the treatment of breast cancer. In

TABLE 73–3.   EFFECTS OF STANDARD HORMONAL TREATMENTS IN PATIENTS WITH ADVANCED BREAST CANCER

Menopausal Status	Response Rates (%)	Comments
Postmenopausal		
Androgens	21	RR higher in ER+ tumors (46%)
Estrogens	26	RR higher in ER+ tumors (65%)
Aromatase inhibitors	20–56	RR highest in ER+ tumors
Premenopausal		
Oophorectomy	30	
LHRH agonists	30–50	RR highest in ER+ tumors
Pre- or postmenopausal		
Antiestrogens	15–53	RR correlates with ER content of tumor
Progestins	20–54	

RR = response rates.

addition, the controversy that surrounds their use as an abortifacient has limited their availability for clinical trials. Mifepristone (RU 486) is a steroidal compound that antagonizes the effect of glucocorticoids and progestins by binding with high affinity to their receptors.[291, 292] Mifepristone exhibits both a growth-inhibitory and growth-stimulatory effect depending on the cell line and culture conditions. Mifepristone also inhibits estrogen-stimulated growth in cultured cell lines and the development of tumor formation induced by DMBA in rats.[291, 292]

Only two small clinical trials using mifepristone have been reported.[293, 294] The first was a series from France in which 22 oophorectomized or postmenopausal women who had been previously treated with chemotherapy, hormone therapy, or both, received 200 mg/day of mifepristone.[293] Partial regression or stabilization of disease was demonstrated in 53 percent of patients after 4 to 6 weeks of treatment. In the second trial, 11 postmenopausal women with advanced disease received 200 to 400 mg/day of mifepristone for 3 to 34 weeks following disease progression while receiving tamoxifen.[294] Six of 11 patients had short-term stabilization of disease, and one attained an objective response. As in the other trial, responses appeared to be associated with the presence of progestin in the tumors. Interestingly, high doses of mifepristone have estrogen-like effects in laboratory models of breast cancer. It is possible the high-dose mifepristone acts as an estrogen such as DES. Because of the antiglucocorticoid effects of mifepristone, treated patients developed high-serum ACTH, cortisol, and androstenedione levels that in turn caused an increase in the serum estradiol level as a result of peripheral aromatization.[291, 292]

Tumor Cell Synchronization by Hormonal Therapy

Drugs such as tamoxifen decrease the tumor growth fraction by preventing cells from progressing beyond the G_0, G_1 phases of the cell cycle. As a result, pretreatment with tamoxifen prior to cytotoxic chemotherapy may attenuate the effects of the chemotherapy that would act on the most rapidly growing subset of cells in the tumor. In contrast, growth-stimulating hormones such as estrogen may increase the tumor growth fraction by recruiting cells out of the G_0 phase of the cell cycle and making them more susceptible to the cytotoxic effects of chemotherapy. The strategy of "priming" the tumor in an effort to synchronize the cells into a proliferating phase of the cell cycle prior to receiving chemotherapy has proved effective in in vitro and in vivo models.[295–298]

This strategy has been employed in several clinical trials.[299–305] An NCI trial randomized patients to receive (1) cyclophosphamide and doxorubicin on day 1 and methotrexate and fluorouracil on day 8; or (2) the identical chemotherapy schedule but with the addition of tamoxifen on days 2 through 6 and Premarin for 3 consecutive days starting on day 7.[299] The time to disease progression was longer on the

hormonally synchronized arm (17.5 months versus 11.1 months), but response rates and survival rates were identical. Lippman and coworkers[299] utilized hormonal depletion followed by estrogen recruitment prior to administering chemotherapy. Postmenopausal patients were treated with aminoglutethimide and hydrocortisone continuously and then randomized to receive placebo or estradiol prior to CAF (cyclophosphamide, Adriamycin [doxorubicin], and fluorouracil) chemotherapy. Response rates, response duration, and survival rates were similar in the "primed" and control groups.[299]

In the randomized trial reported by Conte and coworkers,[301] patients were randomized to receive (1) cyclophosphamide, epidoxorubicin, and fluorouracil (FEC) on day 1; or (2) cyclophosphamide on day 1; DES on days 5 to 7, and epidoxorubicin and fluorouracil on day 8. Since the treatment regimens differ by more than simply the addition of DES, the contribution of DES to recruitment or synchronization of tumor cells is impossible to identify.[300]

Paridaens and coworkers[302] reported the results of a randomized trial in which women with advanced breast cancer and positive hormone receptors were treated with aminoglutethimide and hydrocortisone (and surgical castration if they were premenopausal) to suppress estrogen synthesis. Patients were then randomized to receive placebo or ethinylestradiol exactly 24 hours before receiving CAF chemotherapy. Response rates, time to progression, and median survival duration were identical for both treatment groups. The results from these trials and others have not validated the concept of hormonal recruitment, and it should be viewed only as an investigational treatment approach.

Combination Chemohormonal Therapy

Although breast tumors are often classified as hormone receptor-positive or -negative based on the criteria established for a particular assay, a breast tumor is rarely ever composed of a homogenous population of cells. Nenci[306] reported that the cytosolic assay for ER can be interpreted as positive when only 20 percent of the cell population expresses ER. This interpretation implies that within any breast tumor a mixture of ER-positive and ER-negative cells exists. As previously discussed, breast tumors that are hormone receptor-positive are more likely to respond to hormone therapy than those that are hormone receptor-negative.[31] In an effort to improve the outcome for patients with advanced disease, clinical trials have been conducted combining chemotherapy with hormonal therapy.[307–312] This strategy is based on the assumption that chemotherapy kills tumor cells indiscriminately, irrespective of hormone receptor status. But this notion has been debated, because results from some clinical trials suggest that ER-positive tumors respond better to chemotherapy than ER-negative tumors, whereas other trials have shown the opposite results.[313, 314]

In a prospective randomized trial, Cancer and Leukemia Group B (CALGB) evaluated CAF chemotherapy versus CAF-plus-tamoxifen therapy in patients with advanced disease.[310] A secondary objective of this study was to determine the response to CAF in ER-positive and ER-negative patients. Response rates were identical in both subsets of patients (56 percent). This lack of differential response implies that chemotherapy and hormonal therapy may compete for the same population of ER-positive cells. In addition, the results suggest that chemotherapy kills breast cancer cells indiscriminately, regardless of ER status.

A large clinical trial involving 339 postmenopausal women with advanced breast cancer randomized patients to receive (1) doxorubicin and cyclophosphamide (AC), followed after failure by tamoxifen; or (2) tamoxifen, followed after failure by AC or by concurrent AC and tamoxifen.[312] The ER status was unknown for the majority of patients enrolled in the study. There was no difference in response rates or survival rates for the two treatment arms. No subset of patients in this study benefited from initial chemotherapy. In the CALGB study cited earlier, 474 patients were randomized to receive CAF and tamoxifen or CAF alone until relapse.[310] In each treatment arm, approximately one third of patients were classified as ER-positive and one third as ER-negative. In addition, 70 percent of patients were postmenopausal. Regardless of the ER status or menopausal status, the addition of tamoxifen conferred no significant advantage in response rate, response duration, time to treatment failure, or overall survival rate over CAF alone.

Cocconi and colleagues[309] reported similar findings from a trial involving 145 postmenopausal patients with advanced disease who were randomized to received (1) concurrent cyclophosphamide, methotrexate, and fluorouracil (CMF); or (2) tamoxifen or CMF followed by CMF and tamoxifen after of relapse. Although the response rate in the patients receiving initial combined-modality therapy was higher (74 percent versus 51 percent) than in patients receiving delayed combined therapy, there was no difference in the survival rate. Trials with similar designs have shown no advantage for combined chemohormonal therapy.[307, 308]

In contrast to the previously mentioned studies, Kiang and coworkers[311] reported the results of a clinical trial in which 81 postmenopausal women with advanced disease were randomized to receive DES alone or cyclophosphamide and fluorouracil (CF) and DES. Patients had ER-positive tumors or tumors with an unknown ER status. An additional 31 patients with ER-negative tumors were randomized to receive CF or CF and DES. In patients with ER-positive tumors, survival was significantly longer for those receiving combined therapy than for those receiving DES alone (median survival was 72 and 29 months, respectively). Among the 41 patients with tumors of unknown receptor status, a survival advantage from combined therapy over chemotherapy was seen in the first 2 years but subsequently disap-

peared. The survival rate for 31 patients with ER-negative tumors was uniformly short regardless of therapy.

The findings from this trial suggest that combined chemohormonal therapy may offer a survival advantage to postmenopausal patients with ER-positive tumors; however, most clinical trials have not confirmed the advantage to combined chemohormonal therapy, and laboratory data has suggested that antagonism rather than synergism occurs between certain chemotherapy drugs and tamoxifen.[313] Furthermore, the toxicity of combined chemohormonal therapy is greater than of either modality alone.

Conclusions

Endocrine therapy has been used for the treatment of breast cancer for over a century, but only in recent decades has a mechanistic model of hormonal influence on the development and progression of breast cancer been defined. Multiple forms of hormonal therapy have been evaluated, from surgical ablative techniques to modern pharmacological approaches that employ rational drug design in an effort to block the influence of estrogen on tumor growth. The response rates and response duration to these different endocrine therapies are similar, but as they are administered with palliative intent, selection of one therapy over another should be based on ease of administration and lack of toxicity. Currently available endocrine therapies and those under development provide treatment options for the majority of patients with advanced breast cancer.

References

1. Parker SL, Tong T, Bolden S, Wingo PA: Cancer statistics, 1996. CA Cancer J Clin 65:5–27, 1996.
2. Brock RC: The life and works of Astley Cooper. London, E& S Livingston, Ltd, 1952.
3. Schinzinger A: Quoted by Trendelenburg F: Die ersten 25 Jahre der Deutschen Gesellschaft fur Chirurgie. Berlin, J Springer, 1923, p 254.
4. Beatson GT: On the treatment of inoperable cases of carcinoma of the mammary: Suggestions for a new method of treatment, with illustrative cases. Lancet ii:104–107; 162–165, 1896.
5. Beatson GT: The treatment of cancer of the breast by oophorectomy and thyroid extract. Br Med J ii:1145–1148, 1901.
6. Boyd S: An oophorectomy in cancer of the breast. BMJ 2:1161–1167, 1900.
7. Yarbro JW: Cancer research and the development of cancer centers. *In* Gross SC and Garb S (eds): Cancer Treatment and Research in Humanistic Perspective. New York, Springer, 1985, pp 3–15.
8. MacMahon CE, Cahil JL: The evolution of the concept of the use of surgical castration in the palliation of breast cancer in premenopausal females. Ann Surg 184:713–716, 1976.
9. Ravdin RG, Lewison EF, Slack NH, Dao TL, Gardner B, State D, Fisher B: Results of a clinical trial concerning the worth of prophylactic oophorectomy for breast carcinoma. Surg Gynecol Obstet 31:1055–1064, 1970.
10. DeCourmellers FV: La radiotherapie indirecte, ou dirigée par les correlations organiques. Arch Elect Med 32:264, 1922.
11. Block GE, Vial AB, Pullen FW: Estrogen excretion following operative and irradiation castration in cases of mammary cancer. Surgery 43:415–422, 1958.

12. Huggins C, Bergenstal DM: Inhibition of human mammary and prostatic cancer by adrenalectomy. Cancer Res 12:134–141, 1952.
13. Huggins C, Hodges CV: Studies on prostatic cancer. Effect of castration, of estrogen and of androgen injection on serum phosphatases in metastatic carcinoma of the prostate. Cancer Res 1:293–297, 1941.
14. Santen RJ, Worgul TJ, Samoljik E, Interrante A, Boucher AE, Lipton AM, Harvey HA, White DS, Smart E, Cox C, Well S: A randomized trial comparing surgical adrenalectomy with aminoglutethimide plus hydrocortisone in women with advanced breast cancer. N Engl J Med 305:545–551, 1981.
15. Huggins C, Dao TLY: Adrenalectomy and oophorectomy in the treatment of advanced carcinoma of the breast. JAMA 151:1388–1394, 1953.
16. Luft R, Olivecrona H: Hypophysectomy in man. J Neurosurg 10:301–316, 1953.
17. Dodds EC, Lawson W, Noble RL: Biological effects of the synthetic oestrogen substance 4:4-dihydroxy a beta-diethylstilbene. Lancet i:1389–1391, 1938.
18. Haddow A: Stilbestrol for advanced breast cancer. Br Med J 2:393–8, 1944.
19. Jensen EV, Jacobson HI: Basic guides to the mechanism of estrogen action. Recent Prog Horm Res 18:387–414, 1962.
20. Toft D, Shyamala G, Gorski J: A receptor molecule for estrogens: Studies using cell-free system. Proc Natl Acad Sci 57:1740–1743, 1967.
21. Jensen EV, Block GE, Smith S, Kyser K, DeSombre ER: Estrogen receptors and breast cancer response to adrenalectomy. NCI Monograph 34:55–70, 1971.
22. McGuire WL, Carbone PP, Vollmer EP (eds): Estrogen receptors in human breast cancer. New York, Raven Press, 1975.
23. Lerner LJ, Holthaus JF, Thompson CR: A nonsteroidal estrogen antagonist 1-(p-2-diethylamino-ethoxyphenyl)-1-phenyl-2-p-methoxyethanol. Endocrinology 63:295–318, 1958.
24. William S, Merrell Company: Clomiphene citrate (clomid). Clin Pharmacol Ther 8:891–897, 1967.
25. Harper MJK, Walpole AL: A derivative of triphenylethylene: Effect on implantation and mode of action in rats. J Reprod Fertil 13:101–119, 1967.
26. Jordan VC: Antiestrogenic and antitumor properties of tamoxifen in laboratory animals. Cancer Treat Rep 60:1409–1419, 1976.
27. Jordan VC: The development of tamoxifen for breast cancer therapy. In Jordan VC (ed): Long-Term Tamoxifen Treatment for Breast Cancer. Madison, WI, University of Wisconsin Press, 1994, pp 3–26.
28. Cole MP, Jones CTA, Todd IDH: A new antiestrogenic agent in late breast cancer. An early appraisal of ICI 46–474. Br J Cancer 25:270–275, 1971.
29. Ward HWC: Antiestrogen therapy for breast cancer: A trial of tamoxifen at two dose levels. BMJ 1:13–14, 1973.
30. McGuire WL, Clark GM: Prognostic factor for recurrence and survival in axillary node-negative breast cancer. J Steroid Biochem Mol Biol 34:145–148, 1989.
31. Witliff J: Steroid hormone receptors. In Pesce AJ, Kaplan LA (eds): Methods in Clinical Chemistry. St. Louis, Mosby, 1987, p 767.
32. Oxenhandler RW, McCune R, Subtelney A, Truelove C, Tyrer HW: Flow cytometry determination of estrogen receptor in intact cells. Cancer Res 44:2516–2523, 1984.
33. Taylor CR, Cooper CL, Kurman RJ, Goebelsmann U, Markland FS: Detection of estrogen receptor in breast and endometrial carcinoma by the immunoperoxidase technique. Cancer 47:2634–26340, 1981.
34. Jordan VC, Jacobson HI, Keenan EJ: Determination of estrogen receptors in breast cancer using monoclonal antibody technology in the United States. Cancer Res 46:4237S–4240S, 1986.
35. Horwitz KB, McGuire KB: Specific progesterone receptors in human breast cancer. Steroids 25:497–505, 1975.
36. Horwitz KB, McGuire WL: Predicting response to endocrine therapy in human breast cancer: A hypothesis. Science 189:726–727, 1975.
37. Wittliff JL: Steroid-hormone receptors in breast cancer. Cancer 53:630–643, 1984.
38. McGuire WL, Chamness GC, Fuqua SAW: Mini-review—Estrogen receptor variants in clinical breast cancer. Mol Endocrinol 5:1571–1577, 1991.
39. Allegra JC: Role of hormone receptors in determining treatment of breast cancer. In The Management of Breast Cancer through Endocrine Therapies. Amsterdam, Excerpta Medica, 1984, pp 1–13.
40. Rozencwieg M, Heuson JC: Breast cancer: Prognostic factors and clinical evaluation. In Staquet MS (ed): Cancer Therapy: Prognostic Factors and Criteria of Response. New York, Raven Press, 1975, pp 139–147.
41. Wilson AJ: Response in breast cancer to a second hormonal therapy. Rev Endocrine-Related Cancer 14:5–11, 1983.
42. Rose C, Mouridsen HT: Preferred sequence of endocrine therapies in advanced breast cancer. In Santen RJ, Juhos E (eds): Endocrine-dependent Breast Cancer: Critical Assessment of Recent Advances. Bern, Switzerland, Hans Huber Publishers, 1988, p 81.
43. Iveson TJ, Ahern J, Smith IE: Response to third-line endocrine treatment for advanced breast cancer. Eur J Cancer 29A:572–574, 1993.
44. Jordan VC: Antitumor activity of the antiestrogen ICI 46,474 (tamoxifen) in the dimethylbenzanthracene (DMBA)-induced rat mammary carcinoma model. J Steroid Biochem 5:354, 1974.
45. Nicholson RI, Golder MP: The effect of synthetic antioestrogens on the growth and biochemistry of rat mammary tumours. Eur J Cancer 11:571–579, 1975.
46. Jordan VC: The development of tamoxifen for breast cancer therapy: A tribute to the late Arthur L. Walpole. Breast Cancer Res Treat 11:197–209, 1988.
47. Jordan VC, Koerner S: Tamoxifen (ICI 46 474) and the human carcinoma 8S estrogen receptor. Eur J Cancer 11:205–206, 1975.
48. Jordan VC, Dowse LJ: Tamoxifen as an antitumour agent: Effect on oestrogen binding. J Endocrinol 68:297–303, 1976.
49. Wolf DM, Fuqua SAW: Mechanisms of action of antiestrogens. Cancer Treat Rev 21:247–71, 1995.
50. Green S, Chambon P: The oestrogen receptor: From perception to mechanism. In Parker MG (ed): Nuclear Hormone Receptors. New York, Academic Press, 1991, pp 15–38.
51. Tate AC, Greene GL, DeSombre ER, Jordan VC: Differences between estrogen and antiestrogen—Estrogen receptor complexes identified with an antibody raised against the estrogen receptor. Cancer Res 44:1012–1018, 1984.
52. Martin PM, Berthois Y, Jensen EV: Binding of antiestrogen exposes an occult antigenic determinant in the human estrogen receptor. Proc Natl Acad Sci U S A 85:2533–2537, 1988.
53. Pham TA, Elliston JF, Nawaz Z, McDonnell DP, Tsai MJ, O'Malley BW: Antiestrogens can establish nonproductive receptor complexes and alter chomatin structure at target enhancers. Proc Natl Acad Sci U S A 88:3125–3129, 1991.
54. Tzukerman MT, Esty A, Santiso-Mere D, Danielian P, Parker MG, Stein RB, Pike JW, McDonnell DP: Human estrogen receptor transactivational capacity is determined by both cellular and promoter context and mediated by two functionally distinct intramolecular regions. Mol Endocrinol 8:21–30, 1994.
55. McDonnell DP, Clemm DL, Hermann T, Goldman ME, Pike JW: Analysis of estrogen receptor function reveals three distinct classes of antiestrogens. Mol Endocrinol 9:659–669, 1995.
56. Allan GF, Leng X, Tsai ST, O'Malley BW: Hormone and antihormone induce distinct conformational changes which are central to steroid receptor activation. J Biol Chem 267:19513–19520, 1992.
57. Metzger D, White J, Chambon P: The human estrogen receptor functions in yeast. Nature 334:31–36, 1988.
58. Colletta AA, Benson JR, Baum M: Alternative mechanisms of action of anti-oestrogens. Breast Cancer Res Treat 31:5–9, 1994.
59. Nagy E, Berczi I: Immunomodulation by tamoxifen and pergolide. Immunopharmacology 12:145–153, 1986.
60. Paavonen T, Andersson LC: The oestrogen antagonists, tamoxifen and Fc-1157a, display oestrogen-like effects on hu-

man lymphocyte functions in vitro. Clin Exp Immunol 61:467–74, 1985.

61. O'Brian CA, Liskamp RM, Solomon DH, Weinstein IB: Inhibition of protein kinase C by tamoxifen. Cancer Res 45:2462–2465, 1985.

62. Su HD, Mazzei GJ, Vogler WR, Kuo JF: Effect of tamoxifen, a nonsteroidal antiestrogen, on phospholipid/calcium-dependent protein kinase and phosphorylation of its endogenous substrate proteins from the rat brain and ovary. Biochem Pharmacol 34:3649–3653, 1985.

63. Gulino A, Barrera G, Vacca A, Farina A, Ferretti C, Serepanti I, Dianzani MO, Frati L: Calmodulin antagonism and growth-inhibiting activity of triphenylethylene antiestrogens in MCF-7 human breast cancer cells. Cancer Res 46:6274–6278, 1986.

64. Greenberg DA, Carpenter CL, Messing RO: Calcium channel antagonist properties of the antineoplastic antiestrogen tamoxifen in the PC12 neurosecretory cell line. Cancer Res 47:70–74, 1987.

65. Gagliardi A, Collins DC: Inhibition of angiogenesis by antiestrogens. Cancer Res 53:533–535, 1993.

66. Jordan VC: Growth factor regulation by tamoxifen is demonstrated in patients with breast cancer. Cancer 72:1–2, 1993.

67. Murphy LC: Antiestrogen action and growth factor regulation. Breast Cancer Res Treat 31:61–71, 1994.

68. Winston R, Kao PC, Kiang DT: Regulation of insulin-like growth factors by antiestrogen. Breast Cancer Res Treat 31:107–115, 1994.

69. Rose C, Theilade K, Boesen E, Salimtschik M, Dombernowsky P, Brunner N: Treatment of advanced breast cancer with tamoxifen: Evaluation of the dose-response relationship at two dose levels. Breast Cancer Res Treat 2:395, 1982.

70. Bratherton DG, Brown CH, Buchanan R, Hall V, Kingsley Pillers EM, Wheeler TK, William CJ: A comparison of two doses of tamoxifen (Nolvadex) in postmenopausal women with advanced breast cancer: 10 mg bd versus 20 mg bd. Br J Cancer 50:199–205, 1984.

71. Manni A, Arafah BM: Tamoxifen-induced remission in breast cancer by escalating the dose to 40 mg daily after progression on 20 mg daily: A case report and review of the literature. Cancer 48:873–875, 1981.

72. Watkins SM: The value of high-dose tamoxifen in postmenopausal breast cancer patients progressing on standard doses: A pilot study. Br J Cancer 57:320–321, 1988.

73. Stewart JF, Minton MJ, Rubens RD: Trial of tamoxifen at a dose of 40 mg after disease progression during tamoxifen therapy at a dose of 20 mg daily. Cancer Treat Rep 66:1445–1446, 1982.

74. Adams HK, Patterson JS, Kemp JV: Studies on the metabolism and pharmacokinetics of tamoxifen in normal volunteers. Cancer Treat Rep 64:761–764, 1980.

75. Langan-Fehey SM, Jordan VC, Fritz NF, Robinson SP, Waters D, Tormey DC: Clinical pharmacology and endocrinology of long-term tamoxifen therapy. In Jordan VC: Long-term Tamoxifen Treatment for Breast Cancer. Madison, WI, University of Wisconsin Press, 1994, pp 27–56.

76. Fabian C, Sternson L, El-Serafi M, Cain L, Hearne E: Clinical pharmacology of tamoxifen in patients with breast cancer: Correlation with clinical data. Cancer 48:876–882, 1981.

77. Fromson JMS, Pearson S, Bramah S: The metabolism of tamoxifen (ICI 46,474). Part 2. In female patients. Xenobiotica 3:711–714, 1973.

78. Kemp JV, Adams HK, Wakeling AE, Slater R: Identification and biological activity of tamoxifen and its metabolites. Cancer Treat Rep 64:741–744, 1980.

79. Hoogstraten B, Fletcher WS, Gad-el-Mawla N, Maloney T, Altman SJ, Vaughn CB, Foulkes MA: Tamoxifen and oophorectomy in the treatment of recurrent breast cancer. A Southwest Oncology Group study. Cancer Res 42:4788–4791, 1982.

80. Kiang DT, Kennedy BJ: Tamoxifen therapy in advanced breast cancer. Ann Intern Med 87:687–690, 1977.

81. Lerner HJ, Band PR, Israel L, Leung BS: Phase II study of tamoxifen. Report of 74 patients with stage IV breast cancer. Cancer Treat Rep 60:1431–1435, 1976.

82. Tormey DC, Lippman ME, Edwards BK, Cassidy JG: Evaluation of tamoxifen doses with and without fluoxymestrone in advanced breast cancer. Ann Intern Med 98:139–144, 1983.

83. Morgan LR, Schein PS, Wooley V, Hoth D, MacDonald J, Lippman M, Posey LE, Beazley RW: Therapeutic use of tamoxifen in advanced breast cancer: Correlation with biochemical parameters. Cancer Treat Rep 60:1437–1443, 1976.

84. Manni A, Pearson OH: Antiestrogen-induced remissions in premenopausal women with stage IV breast cancer: Effects on ovarian function. Cancer Treat Rep 64:779–785, 1980.

85. Litherland S, Jackson IM: Anti-estrogens in the management of hormone dependent cancer. Cancer Treat Rev 15:183–194, 1988.

86. Rose C, Mouridsen HT: Treatment of advanced breast cancer with tamoxifen. Recent Results Cancer Res 91:230–42, 1984.

87. Petru E, Schmahl D: On the role of additive hormone monotherapy with tamoxifen, medroxyprogesterone acetate and aminoglutethimide in advanced breast cancer. Klin Wochenschr 65:959–966, 1987.

88. Ingle JN, Malliard JA, Schaid DJ, Krook JE: A double-blind trial of tamoxifen plus placebo in postmenopausal women with metastatic breast cancer. A collaborative trial of the North Central Cancer Treatment Group and Mayo Clinic. Cancer 68:34–39, 1991.

89. Wiggans RG, Woolley PV, Smythe T, Hoth D, Macdonald JS, Green L, Schein PS: Phase-II trial of tamoxifen in advanced breast cancer. Cancer Chemother Pharmacol 3:45–48, 1979.

90. Manni A, Trujillo JE, Marshal JS, Brodkey J, Pearson OH: Antihormone treatment of stage IV breast cancer. Cancer 43:444–450, 1979.

91. Heuson JC: Current overview of EORTC clinical trials with tamoxifen. Cancer Treat Rep 60:1463–1466, 1976.

92. Kiang DT, Frenning DIT, Vosika GJ, Kennedy BT: Comparison of tamoxifen and hypophysectomy in breast cancer treatment. Cancer 45:1322–1325, 1980.

93. Nemoto T, Patel J, Rosner D, Dao TL: Tamoxifen (Nolvadex) versus adrenalectomy in metastatic breast cancer. Cancer 53:1333–1335, 1984.

94. Ribeiro GG: A clinical trial to compare the use of tamoxifen vs stilbestrol in the treatment of postmenopausal women with advanced breast cancer. In Reviews on Endocrine-related Cancer (Suppl 9), Wilmington, DE, Stuart Pharmaceuticals, 1980, pp 409–413.

95. Ingle JN, Ahmann DL, Green SJ, Edmonson JH, Bisel HF, Kvols LK, Nichols WC, Creagan ET, Hahn RG, Rubin J, Frytak S: Randomized clinical trial of diethylstibesterol versus tamoxifen in postmenopausal women with advanced breast cancer. N Engl J Med 304:16–21, 1981.

96. Beex L, Pieters G, Smals A, Koenders A, Benraad T, Kloppenberg P: Tamoxifen versus ethinyl estradiol in the treatment of postmenopausal women with advanced breast cancer. Cancer Treat Rep 65:179–185, 1981.

97. Matelski H, Greene R, Huberman M, Zipoli T: Randomized trial of estrogen vs tamoxifen therapy for advanced breast cancer. Am J Clin Oncol 8:128–133, 1985.

98. Muss HB, Paschold EH, Black WR, Cooper MR, Capizzi RL, Christian R, Cruz JM, Jackson DV, Stuart JJ, Richards F, White DR, Zekan PJ, Spurr CL, Pope E, Case D, Morgan T, Wells HB: Megestrol acetate v. tamoxifen in advanced breast cancer: A phase III trial of Piedmont Oncology Association (POA). Semin Oncol 12(Suppl 1):55–61, 1985.

99. Van Veelen H, Willemse PHB, Tjabbes T, Schweitzer MJ, Sleijfer DT: Oral high-dose medroxyprogesterone acetate versus tamoxifen: A randomized crossover trial in postmenopausal patients with advanced breast cancer. Cancer 58:7–13, 1986.

100. Castiglione-Gertsch M, Pampallona S, Varini M, Cavalli F, Brunner K, Senn HJ, Goldhirsch A, Metzger U: Primary endocrine therapy for advanced breast cancer: To start with tamoxifen or with medroxyprogesterone acetate. Ann Oncol 4:735–740, 1993.

101. Westerberg H: Tamoxifen and fluoxymesterone in advanced breast cancer: A controlled clinical trial. Breast Cancer Treat Rep 64:117–121, 1980.

102. Gale KE, Andersen JW, Tormey DC, Mansour EG, Davis TE, Horton J, Wolter JM, Smith TJ, Cummings FJ: Hormonal

treatment for metastatic breast cancer. An Eastern Cooperative Group Phase III trial comparing aminoglutethimide to tamoxifen. Cancer 73:354–361, 1994.

103. Cummings FJ, Gray R, Davis TE, Harris JE, Falkson G, Arseneau J: Adjuvant tamoxifen treatment of elderly women with stage II breast cancer: A double-blind comparison with placebo. Ann Intern Med 103:324–329, 1985.

104. Fisher B, Constantino J, Redmond C, Poisson R, Bowman D, Couture J, Dimitrov NV, Wolmark N, Wickerham DL, Fisher ER: A randomized clinical trial evaluating tamoxifen in the treatment of patients with node-negative breast cancer who have estrogen receptor positive tumors. N Engl J Med 320:479–484, 1989.

105. Fitsch M, Wolf D: Symptomatic side effects of tamoxifen therapy. In Jordan VC (ed): Long-Term Tamoxifen Treatment for Breast Cancer. Madison, WI, University of Wisconsin Press, 1994, pp 235–256.

106. Plotkin D, Lechner JJ, Jung WE, Rosen PJ: Tamoxifen flare in advanced breast cancer. JAMA 240:2644–2646, 1978.

107. Legault-Poisson S, Jolivet J, Poisson R: Tamoxifen-induced tumour stimulation and withdrawal response. Cancer Treat Rep 63:1839–1841, 1979.

108. Jordan VC, Phelps E, Lindgren JU: Effects of antiestrogens on bone in castrated and intact female rate. Breast Cancer Res Treat 10:31–35, 1987.

109. Turner RT, Wakley GK, Hannon KS, Bell NH: Tamoxifen prevents the skeletal effects of ovarian hormone deficiency in rats. J Bone Miner Res 2:449–456, 1987.

110. Love RR, Mazess RB, Barden HS, Epstein S, Newcomb PA, Jordan VC, Carbone PP, DeMets DL: Effects of tamoxifen on bone mineral density in postmenopausal women with breast cancer. N Engl J Med 326:852–856, 1992.

111. Turken S, Siris E, Selding E, Flaster E, Hyman G, Lindsay R: Effect of tamoxifen on spinal bone density in women with breast cancer. J Natl Cancer Inst 81:1086–1088, 1989.

112. Thangaraju M, Kumar M, Gandhirajan R, Sachdanandem P: Effect of tamoxifen on plasma lipids and lipoproteins in postmenopausal women with breast cancer. Cancer 73:659–663, 1994.

113. Fornander T, Rutquist LE, Wilking N, Carlström K, von Schoultz B: Oestrogenic effects of adjuvant tamoxifen in postmenopausal breast cancer. Eur J Cancer 29A:497–500, 1993.

114. Fisher B, Constantino JP, Richmond CK, Fisher ER, Wickerham DL, Cronin WM: Endometrial cancer in tamoxifen-treated breast cancer patients: Finding from the National Surgical Adjuvant Breast and Bowel Project (NSABP) B-14. J Natl Cancer Inst 86:527–537, 1994.

115. Magriples U, Naftolin F, Schwartz PE, Carcangiu ML: High-grade endometrial carcinoma in tamoxifen-treated breast cancer patients. J Clin Oncol 11:485–490, 1993.

116. Jordan VC, Assikis VJ: Endometrial carcinoma and tamoxifen: Clearing up a controversy. Clin Cancer Res 1:467–472, 1995.

117. Jordan VC, Morrow M: Should clinicians be concerned about the carcinogenic potential of tamoxifen? Eur J Cancer 30A:1714–1721, 1994.

118. Catherino WH, Jordan VC: A risk-benefit assessment of tamoxifen therapy. Drug Safety 8:381–97, 1993.

119. Sawka CA, Pritchard KI, Paterson AHG, Sutherland DJ, Thomson DB, Shelley WE, Meyers RE, Mobbs BG, Malkin A, Meakin JW: Role and mechanism of action of tamoxifen in premenopausal women with metastatic breast carcinoma. Cancer Res 46:3152–3156, 1986.

120. Wada T, Koyama H, Terasawa T: Effect of tamoxifen in premenopausal Japanese women with advanced breast cancer. Cancer Treat Rep 65:728–729, 1981.

121. Yoshida M, Murai H, Miura S: Tamoxifen therapy for premenopausal and postmenopausal Japanese females with advanced breast carcinoma. Jpn J Clin Oncol 12:57–64, 1982.

122. Margreiter R, Wiegle J: Tamoxifen (Nolvadex) for premenopausal patients with advanced breast cancer. Breast Cancer Res Treat 4:45–84, 1984.

123. Planting AST, Alexieva-Figusch J, Blonk-vdWijst J, van Putten WL: Tamoxifen therapy in premenopausal women with metastatic breast cancer. Cancer Treat Rep 69:363–368, 1985.

124. Hoogstraten B, Gad-el-Mawla N, Maloney TR, Fletcher WS, Vaugh CB, Tranum BL, Athens JW, Constanzi JJ, Foulkes M: Combined-modality therapy for first recurrence of breast cancer. A Southwest Oncology Group study. Cancer 54:2248–2256, 1984.

125. Buchanan RB, Blamey RW, Durrant KR, Howell A, Paterson AG, Preece PE, Smith DC, Williams CJ, Wilson RG: A randomized comparison of tamoxifen with surgical oophorectomy in premenopausal patients with advanced breast cancer. J Clin Oncol 4:1326–1330, 1986.

126. Ingle JN, Krook JE, Green SJ, Kubista TP, Everson LK, Ahmann DL, Chang MN, Bisel HF, Windschitl HE, Twito DI, Pfeifle DM: Randomized trial of bilateral oophorectomy versus tamoxifen in premenopausal women with advanced breast cancer. J Clin Oncol 4:178–185, 1986.

127. Groom GV, Griffiths K: Effects of the anti-oestrogen tamoxifen on plasma levels of luteinizing hormone, follicle-stimulating hormone, prolactin, oestradiol and progesterone in normal pre-menopausal women. J Endocrinol 70:421–428, 1976.

128. Jordan VC, Fritz NF, Langan-Fahey S, Thompson M, Tormey DC: Alteration of endocrine parameters in premenopausal women with breast cancer during long-term adjuvant therapy with tamoxifen as the single agent. J Natl Cancer Inst 83:1488–1491, 1991.

129. Delrio G, De Placido S, Pagliarulo C, d'Istria M, Fasano S, Marinelli A, Citarella F, DeSio L, Contegiacomo A, Iaffaioli RV: Hypothalamic-pituitary-ovarian axis in women with operable breast cancer treated with adjuvant CMF and tamoxifen. Tumori 72:53–61, 1986.

130. Gottardis MM, Jordan VC: Development of tamoxifen-stimulated growth of MCF-7 tumors in athymic mice after long-term antiestrogen administration. Cancer Res 48:5183–5187, 1988.

131. Gottardis MM, Jiang SY, Jeng MH, Jordan VC: Inhibition of tamoxifen-stimulated growth of an MCF-7 tumor variant in athymic mice by novel steroidal antiestrogens. Cancer Res 49:4090–4093, 1989.

132. Canney PA, Griffiths T, Latief TN, Priestman TJ: Clinical significance of tamoxifen withdrawal response. Lancet i:36, 1987. Letter.

133. DiSalle E, Zaccheo T, Ornati G: Antioestrogenic and antitumour properties of the new triphenylethylene derivative toremifene in the rat. J Steroid Biochem 36:203–206, 1990.

134. Huovinen R, Warri A, Collan Y: Mitotic activity, apoptosis and TRPM-2 messenger RNA expression in DMBA-induced rat mammary carcinoma treated with antiestrogen toremifene. Int J Cancer 55:685–691, 1993.

135. Huovinen R, Kellokumpu-Lehtinen P-LI, Collan Y: Evaluating the response to antiestrogen toremifene treatment in DMBA-induced rat mammary carcinoma. Int J Exp Pathol 75:257–263, 1994.

136. Huovinen RL, Alanen KA, Collan Y: Cell proliferation in dimethylbenzanthracene-induced rat mammary carcinoma treated with antiestrogen toremifene. Acta Oncol 34:479–485, 1995.

137. Robinson SP, Mauel DA, Jordan VC: Antitumor actions of toremifene in the 7,12-dimethylbenzanthracene (DMBA)-induced rat mammary tumor model. Eur J Cancer 24:1817–1821, 1988.

138. Hamm JT, Tormey DC, Kohler PC, Haller D, Green M, Shemano I: Phase I study of toremifene in patients with advanced cancer. J Clin Oncol 9:2036–2041, 1991.

139. Kivinen S, Maenpaa J: Effect of toremifene on clinical hematological and hormonal parameters at different dose levels in healthy postmenopausal volunteers: Phase I study. J. Steroid Biochem 36:217–220, 1990.

140. Szamel I, Hindy I, Vincze B, Eckhardt S, Kangas L, Hajba A: Influence of toremifene on the endocrine regulation in breast cancer patients. Eur J Cancer 30A:154–158, 1994.

141. Homesley HD, Shemano I, Gamms RA, Harry DS, Hickox PG, Rebar RW, Bump RC, Mullin TJ, Wentz AC, O'Toole RV: Antiestrogenic potency of toremifene and tamoxifen in postmenopausal women. Am J Clin Oncol 16:117–122, 1993.

142. Maenpaa J, Sonderatram KO, Granroos M, Taina E, Hajba A, Kangas L: Effect of toremifene on estrogen-primed vaginal

mucosa in postmenopausal women. J Steroid Biochem 36:221–223, 1990.

143. Tomas E, Kauppila A, Blanco G, Apaja-Sarkkinen M, Laatikainen T: Comparison between the effects of tamoxifen and toremifene on the uterus in postmenopausal breast cancer patients. Gynecol Oncol 59:261–266, 1995.

144. Ebbs SR, Roberts J, Baum M: Response to toremifene (Fc-1157a) therapy in tamoxifen-failed patients with breast cancer. Preliminary communication. J Steroid Biochem 36:239, 1990.

145. Hindy I, Juhos E, Szanto J, Szamel I: Effect of toremifene in breast cancer patients. Preliminary communication. J Steroid Biochem 36:225–226, 1990.

146. Jonsson P-E, Malmberg M, Bergejung L, Ingvar C, Ericsson M, Ryden S, Nilsson I, Terje IJ: Phase II study of high-dose toremifene in advanced breast cancer progressing during tamoxifen treatment. Anticancer Res 11:873–876, 1991.

147. Asaishi K, Tominaga T, Abe O: Efficacy and safety of high-dose NK 622 (toremifene citrate) in tamoxifen-failed patients with breast cancer [in Japanese]. Gan To Kagaku Ryoho 20:91–99, 1993.

148. Vogel CL, Shemano I, Schoenfelder J, Gams RA, Green MR: Multicenter phase II efficacy trial of toremifene in tamoxifen-refractory patients with advanced breast cancer. J Clin Oncol 11:345–350, 1993.

149. Pyrhonen S, Valavaara R, Vuorinen J, Hajba A: High-dose toremifene in advanced breast cancer resistant to or relapsed during tamoxifen treatment. Breast Cancer Res Treat 29:223–228, 1994.

150. Valavaara R, Pyrhonen S, Heikkinen M, Rissanen P, Blanco G, Tholix E, Nordman E, Taskinen P, Holsti L, Hajba A: Toremifene, a new antiestrogenic treatment of advanced breast cancer. Phase II study. Eur J Cancer 24:785–790, 1988.

151. Valavaara R, Pyrhonen S: Low-dose toremifene in the treatment of estrogen-receptor-positive advanced breast cancer in postmenopausal women. Curr Ther Res 46:966–973, 1989.

152. Gunderson S: Toremifene, a new antiestrogenic compound in the treatment of advanced breast cancer. Phase II study. Eur J Cancer 24:785–790, 1990.

153. Modig H, Borgstrom M, Nilsson I, Westman G: Phase II clinical study of toremifene in patients with metastatic breast cancer. J Steroid Biochem 36:235–236, 1990.

154. Hietanen T, Baltina D, Johansson R, Numminen S, Hakala T, Helle L, Valavaara R: High-dose toremifene (240 mg daily) is effective as first-line hormonal treatment in advanced breast cancer—an ongoing phase-II multicenter Finnish-Latvian cooperative study. Breast Cancer Res Treat 16(Suppl):37–40, 1990.

155. Valavaara R: Phase II experience with toremifene in the treatment of ER-positive breast cancer of postmenopausal women. Cancer Invest 8:275–276, 1990.

156. Nomura Y, Tominaga T, Abe O: Clinical evaluation of NK 22 (toremifene citrate) in advanced or recurrent breast cancer—A comparative study by a double-blind method with tamoxifen [in Japanese]. Gan To Kagaku Ryoho 20:247–258, 1993.

157. Konstantinova MM, Gershanovich ML: Results of comparative clinical evaluation of antiestrogens toremifene and tamoxifen in locally advanced and disseminated breast cancer [in Russian]. Vopr Onkol 36:1182–1186, 1990.

158. Stenbygaard LE, Herrstedt J, Thomsen JF, Svendsen KR, Engelholm SA, Dombernowsky P: Toremifene and tamoxifen in advanced breast cancer—A double-blind cross-over trial. Breast Cancer Res Treat 25:57–63, 1993.

159. Hayes DF, Van Zyl JA, Hacking A, Goedhals L, Bezwoda WR, Maillard JA, Jones SE, Vogel CL, Berris RF, Shemano I, Schoenfelder J: Randomized comparison of tamoxifen and two separate doses of toremifene in postmenopausal patients with metastic breast cancer. J Clin Oncol 113:2556–2566, 1995.

160. Sabbah M, Grouilleux F, Sola B, Redeuilh G, Baulieu EE: Structural differences between the hormone and antihormone estrogen receptor complexes bound to the hormone response elements. Proc Natl Acad Sci U S A 88:390–394, 1991.

161. Loser R, Seibel K Roos W, Eppenberger U: In vivo and in vitro antiestrogenic action of 3-hydroxy-tamoxifen, tamoxifen and 4-hydroxy-tamoxifen. Eur J Cancer Clin Oncol 21:885–900, 1985.

162. Kawamura I, Mizota T, Lacey E, Tanaka Y, Manda T, Shimomura K, Kohsaka M: The estrogenic and antiestrogenic activities of droloxifene in human breast cancers. Jpn J Pharmacol 63:27–34, 1993.

163. Ahlemann LM, Staab HJ, Loser R: Inhibition of growth of human cancer by intermittent exposure to the antiestrogen droloxifene. Tumor Diag Ther 9:41–46, 1988.

164. Abe O: Japanese early phase II study of droloxifene in the treatment of advanced breast cancer. Am J Clin Oncol 14:540–451, 1991.

165. Abe O, Enomote K, Fujiwara K, Izuo M, Iino Y, Tominaga T, Hayashi K, Takatani O, Kugai N, Yoshida M: Phase I study of FK 435. Jpn J Cancer Clin 36:903–913, 1990.

166. Bellmunt J, Sole L: European early phase II dose finding study of droloxifene in advanced breast cancer. Am J Clin Oncol 14:536–539, 1991.

167. Haarstad H, Gundersen S, Wist E, Raabe N, Mella O, Kvinnsland S: Droloxifene—a new antiestrogen phase II study in advanced breast cancer. Acta Oncol 31:425–428, 1992.

168. Rausching W, Pritchard KI: Droloxifene, a new antiestrogen: Its role in metastatic breast cancer. Breast Cancer Res Treat 31:83–94, 1994.

169. Buzdar AU, Kau S, Hortobagyi GN, Theriault RL, Booser D, Holmes FA, Walters R, Krakoff IH: Phase I trial of droloxifene in patients with metastatic breast cancer. Cancer Chemother Pharmacol 33:313–316, 1994.

170. Winterfeld G, Hauff P, Grolich M, Arnold W, Fichtner I, Staab HJ: Investigations of droloxifene and other hormonal manipulations on N-nitrosomethylurea–induced rat mammary tumours. J Cancer Res Clin Oncol 119:91–96, 1992.

171. Metzler M, Schiffmann D: Structural requirements for the in vitro transformation of Syrian hamster embryo cells by stilbene estrogens and triphenylethylene-type antiestrogens. Am J Clin Oncol (Suppl 2) 14:S30–S35, 1991.

172. Chander SK, McCague R, Lugmani Y, Newton C, Dowsett M, Jarman M, Coombes RC: Pyrrolidino-4-iodotamoxifen and 4-iodotamoxifen, new analogues of the antiestrogen tamoxifen for the treatment of breast cancer. Cancer Res 51:5851–5858, 1991.

173. McCague R, LeClercq G, Legros N, Goodman J, Blackburn GM, Jarman M, Foster AM: Derivatives of tamoxifen. Dependency of estrogenicity on the 4 substituent. J Med Chem 32:2527–2533, 1989.

174. McCague R, Parr IB, Haynes BP: Metabolism of the 4 iodo derivative of tamoxifen by isolated rat hepatocytes. Demonstration that the iodine atom reduces metabolic conversion and identification of four metabolites. Biochem Pharmacol 40:2277–2283, 1990.

175. Furr BJA, Jordan VC: The pharmacology and clinical uses of tamoxifen. Pharmacol Ther 25:127–205, 1984.

176. Coombes RC, Haynes BP, Dowsett M, Quigley M, English J, Judson IR, Griggs LJ, Potter GA, McCague R, Jarman M: Idoxifene: Report of a phase I study in patients with metastatic breast cancer. Cancer Res 55:1070–1074, 1995.

177. Parker MG: Action of "pure" antiestrogens in inhibiting estrogen receptor action. Breast Cancer Res Treat 26:131–137, 1993.

178. Wakeling AE, Bowler J: Biology and mode of action of pure antiestrogens. J Steroid Biochem 30:141–148, 1988.

179. Fawell SE, White R, Hoare S, Sydenham M, Page M, Parker MG: Inhibition of estrogen receptor DNA binding by the pure antiestrogen ICI 164 384 appears to be mediated by impaired receptor dimerization. Proc Natl Acad Sci U S A 87:6883–6887, 1990.

180. Pink JJ, Jordan VC: Models of estrogen receptor regulation by estrogens and antiestrogens in breast cancer cell lines. Cancer Res 56:2321–2330, 1996.

181. Wolf PM, Fuqua SAW: Mechanisms of action of antiestrogens. Cancer Treat Rev 21:247–271, 1995.

182. Dauvois S, Danielian PS, White R, Parker MG: Antiestrogen

ICI 164,384 reduces cellular estrogen receptor by increasing its turnover. Proc Natl Acad Sci U S A 89:4037–4041, 1992.

183. Gibson MK, Nemmas LA, Beckman WC, Davis VL, Curtis SW, Korach KS: The mechanism of ICI 164,384 antiestrogenicity involves rapid loss of estrogen receptor in uterine tissue. Endocrinology 129:2000–2010, 1991.

184. DeFriend DJ, Howell A, Nicholson RI, Anderson E, Dowsett M, Mansel RE, Blamey RW, Bundred NJ, Robertson JF, Saunders C: Investigation of a pure new antiestrogen (ICI 182,780) in women with primary breast cancer. Cancer Res 54:408–414, 1994.

185. Davois S, White R, Parker MG: The antiestrogen ICI 182 780 disrupts estrogen receptor nucleocytoplasmic shuttling. J Cell Sci 106:1377–1388, 1993.

186. Wakeling AE, Dukes M, Bowler J: A potent specific pure antiestrogen with clinical potential. Cancer Res 51:3867–3873, 1991.

187. Thompson EW, Katz D, Shima TB, Wakeling AE, Lippman ME, Dickson RB: ICI 164,384, a pure antagonist of estrogen stimulated MCF-7 cell proliferation and invasiveness. Cancer Res 49:6929–6934, 1989.

188. Gottardis MM, Ricchio MD, Satyaswaroop PG, Jordan VC: Effect of steroidal and nonsteroidal antiestrogens on the growth of a tamoxifen-stimulated human endometrial carcinoma (EnCa101) in athymic mice. Cancer Res 50:3189–3192, 1990.

189. Nicholson RI, Walker KJ, Bouzukar N, Wills RJ, Gee JM, Rushmere NK, Davies P: Estrogen deprivation in breast cancer. Clinical, experimental and biological aspects. Ann N Y Acad Sci 595:316–327, 1990.

190. Howell A, DeFriend D, Robertson J, Blamey R, Walton P: Response to a specific antioestrogen (ICI 182,780) in tamoxifen-resistant breast cancer. Lancet 345:29–30, 1995.

191. Lerner LJ, Jordan VC: Development of antiestrogens and their use in breast cancer. Eighth Cain Memorial Lecture. Cancer Res 50:4177–4189, 1990.

192. Tonetti D, Jordan VC: The development of targeted antiestrogens to prevent diseases in women. Mol Med Today 2:218–223, 1996.

193. Evans G, Bryant HU, Magee D, Sato M, Turner RT: The effects of raloxifene on tibia histomorphometry in ovariectomized rats. Endocrinology 134:2283–2288, 1994.

194. Sato M, Kim J, Short LL, Slemenda CW, Bryant HU: Longitudinal and cross-sectional analysis of raloxifene effects on tibiae from ovariectomized rats. J Pharmacol Exp Ther 272:1251–1259, 1995.

195. Black LJ, Sato M, Rowley ER, Magee DE, Bekele A, Williams DC, Cullinan GJ, Bendele R, Kauffman RF, Bensch WR: Raloxifene (LY139481 HCl) prevents bone loss and reduces serum cholesterol without causing uterine hypotrophy in ovariectomized rats. J Clin Invest 93:63–69, 1994.

196. Buzdar AU, Marcus C, Holmes F, Hug V, Hortobagyi G: Phase II evaluation of LY156758 in metastatic breast cancer. Oncology 45:344–345, 1988.

197. Santen RJ, Manni A, Harvey H, Redmond C: Endocrine treatment of breast cancer in women. Endocrine Rev 11:221–265, 1990.

198. Richards JS, Hickey GJ, Chen S, Shively JE, Hall PF, Gaddy-Kurten D, Kurten R: Hormonal regulation of estradiol biosynthesis, aromatase activity, and aromatase mRNA in rat ovarian follicles and corpora lutea. Steroids 50:393–409, 1987.

199. Judd HL, Judd GE, Lucas WE, Yen SCC: Endocrine function of the postmenopausal ovary: Concentration of androgens and estrogens in ovarian and peripheral vein blood. J Clin Endocrinol Metab 39:1020–1024, 1974.

200. Santen RJ, Boucher AE, Santner SJ, Henderson IC, Harvey HA, Lipton A: Inhibition of aromatase as a treatment of breast carcinoma in postmenopausal women. J Lab Clin Med 109:278–289, 1987.

201. Reed MJ: The role of aromatase in breast tumors. Breast Cancer Res Treat 30:7–17, 1994.

202. O'Neil JS, Miller WR: Aromatase activity in breast adipose tissue from women with benign and malignant breast diseases. Br J Cancer 56:601–604, 1987.

203. Abul-Hajj YJ, Iverson R, Kiang DT: Aromatization of androgens by human breast cancer. Steroids 33:205–222, 1979.

204. Samojlik E, Veldhuis JD, Wells SA, Santen RJ: Preservation of androgen secretion during estrogen suppression with aminoglutethimide in the treatment of metastatic breast cancer. J Clin Invest 65:602–612, 1980.

205. Council on Drugs: New drugs and developments in therapeutics. JAMA 179:55–58, 1963.

206. Camacho AM, Brough AJ, Cash R, Wilroy RS: Adrenal toxicity associated with the administration of an anticonvulsant drug. J Pediatr 68:852–853, 1966.

207. Lonning PE, Kuinnsland S: Mechanism of action of aminoglutethimide as endocrine therapy for breast cancer. Drugs 35:685–710, 1988.

208. Dexter RN, Fishman LM, Ney RC, Lidde GW: Inhibition of adrenal corticosteroid synthesis by aminoglutethimide. Studies on mechanism of action. J Clin Endocrinol 27:473–480, 1967.

209. Santen RJ, Santner SJ, Davis B, Veldluis J, Samojlik E, Ruby E: Aminoglutethimide inhibits extraglandular estrogen production in postmenopausal women with breast carcinoma. J Clin Endocrinol Metab 47:1257–1265, 1978.

210. Santen RJ, Wells SA, Cohn N, Demers LM, Misbin RI, Foltz EL: Compensatory increase in TSH secretion without effect on prolactin secretion in patients treated with aminoglutethimide. J Clin Endocrinol Metab 45:739–746, 1977.

211. Höffken K: Experience with aromatase inhibitors in the treatment of advanced breast cancer. Cancer Treat Rev 19:37–44, 1993.

212. Cocconi G: First-generation aromatase inhibitors—Aminoglutethimide and testololactone. Breast Cancer Res Treat 30:57–80, 1994.

213. Cocconi G, Bisagni G, Ceci G, Bacchi M, Boni C, Brugia M, Carpi A, DiConstanzo F, Franciosi V, Gori S, Indelli M, Passalacqua R: Low-dose aminoglutethimide with and without hydrocortisone replacement as a first-line endocrine treatment in advanced breast cancer: A prospective randomized trial of the Italian Oncology Group for Clinical Research. J Clin Oncol 10:984–989, 1992.

214. Goss PE, Gwyn KM: Current perspectives on aromatase inhibitors in breast cancer. J Clin Oncol 12:2460–2470, 1994.

215. Dowsett M, Coombes RC: Second-generation aromatase inhibitor—4-hydroxy-androstenedione. Breast Cancer Res Treat 30:81–87, 1994.

216. Coombes RC, Hughes SWM, Dowsett M: 4-Hydroxy-androstenedione: A new treatment for postmenopausal patients with breast cancer. Eur J Cancer 28A:1941–1945, 1992.

217. Plourde PU, Dyroft M, Dukes M: Arimidex: A potent and selective fourth-generation aromatase inhibitor. Breast Cancer Res Treat 30:103–111, 1994.

218. Jonat W, Howell A, Blomquist C, Eirmann W, Winblad G, Tyrell C, Mauriac L, Roche H, Lundgren S, Hellmund R, Azab M: A randomized trial comparing two doses of the new selective aromatase inhibitor anastrozole (Arimidex) with megestrol acetate in postmenopausal patients with advanced breast cancer. Eur J Cancer 32A:404–412, 1996.

219. Bajetta E, Zilembo N, Buzzoni R, Noberasco C, DiLeo A, Bartoli C, Merson M, Sacchini V, Moglic D, Celio L, Nelli P: Endocrinological and clinical evaluation of two doses of formestane in advanced breast cancer. Br J Cancer 70:145–150, 1994.

220. Demers LM: Effects of fadrozole (CGS 16949A) and letrozole (CGS 20267) on the inhibition of aromatase activity in breast cancer patients. Breast Cancer Res Treat 30:95–102, 1994.

221. Lipton A, Demers LM, Harvey HA, Kambic KB, Grossberg H, Brady C, Adlercruetz H, Trunet PF, Santen RJ: Letrozole (CGS 20267): A phase I study of a new potent oral aromatase inhibitor of breast cancer. Cancer 75:2132–82138, 1995.

222. Wouters W, Snoeck E, De Coster R: Vorozole, a specific nonsteroidal aromatase inhibitor. Breast Cancer Res Treat 30:89–94, 1994.

223. Johnston SRD, Smith IE, Doody D, Jacobs S, Robertshaw H, Dowsett M: Clinical and endocrine effects of the oral aromatase inhibitor vorozole in postmenopausal patients with advanced breast cancer. Cancer Res 54:5875–5881, 1994.

224. Robin D, McNeil LW: Pituitary and gonadal desensitization after continuous luteinizing hormone-releasing hormone infusion in normal females. J Clin Endocrinol Metab 51:873–876, 1980.
225. Harvey HA, Lipton A, Max DT, Pearlman HG, Diaz-Perches R, de la Garza J: Medical castration produced by the GnRH analogue leuprolide to treat metastatic breast cancer. J Clin Oncol 3:1068–1072, 1985.
226. Santen RJ, Bourguignon JP: Gonadotropin-releasing hormone: Physiologic and therapeutic aspects, agonists, and antagonists. Horm Res 28:88–103, 1987.
227. Davidson NE: Ovarian ablation as a treatment for young women with breast cancer. Monogr Natl Cancer Instit 16:95–99, 1994.
228. Klijn JGM, de Jong FH, Lambert SWJ, Blankenstein MA: LHRH-agonist treatment in clinical and experimental human breast cancer. J Steroid Biochem 23:867–873, 1985.
229. Schally AV: Aspects of hypothalamic regulation of the pituitary gland. Its implications for the control of reproductive processes. Science 202:18–28, 1978.
230. Furr BJA, Woodburn JR: Luteinizing hormone-releasing hormone and its analogues: A review of biological properties and clinical uses. J Endocrinol Invest 11:535–557, 1988.
231. Conn PM, Crowley WF: Gonadotropin-releasing hormone and its analogues. N Engl J Med 324:93–103, 1991.
232. Belchetz PE, Plant TM, Nakai Y, Keogh EJ, Knobil E: Hypophysial responses to continuous and intermittent delivery of hypothalamic gonadotropin-releasing hormone. Science 202:631–633, 1978.
233. Kaufman M, Jonat W, Kleeberg U, Eiermann W, Jänicke F, Hilfrich J, Kreienberg R, Albrecht M, Weitzel HK, Schmid H: Goserelin, a depot gonadotrophin-releasing hormone agonist in the treatment of premenopausal patients with metastatic breast cancer. German Zoladex Trial Group. J Clin Oncol 7:1113–1119, 1989.
234. Bajetta E, Zilembo N, Buzzoni R, Celio L, Zampino MG, Colleoni M, Oriana S, Attili A, Sacchini V, Martinetti A: Goserelin in premenopausal advanced breast cancer: Clinical and endocrine evaluation of responsive patients. Oncology 51:262–269, 1994.
235. Walker KJ, Turkes A, Williams MR, Blamey RW, Nicholson RI: Preliminary endocrinological evaluation of a sustained-release formulation of the LH-releasing hormone agonist D-Ser (But)-Azgly-LHRH in premenopausal women with advanced breast cancer. J Endocrinol 111:349–353, 1986.
236. Eidne KA, Flanagan CA, Harris NS, Millar RP: Gonadotropin-releasing hormone (GnRH)–binding sites in human breast cancer cell lines and inhibitory effects of GnRH antagonists. J Clin Endocrinol Metab 64:425–432, 1987.
237. Miller WR, Scott WN, Morris R, Fraser HM, Sharpe RM: Growth of human breast cancer cells inhibited by a luteinizing hormone-releasing hormone agonist. Nature 313:231–233, 1985.
238. Waxman H, Harland SJ, Coombes RC, Wrigley PF, Malpas JS, Powlest T, Lister TA: The treatment of postmenopausal women with advanced breast cancer with buserelin. Cancer Chemother Pharmacol 15:171–173, 1985.
239. Harvey HA, Lipton A, Max DT, Pearlman HG, Diaz-Perches R, de la Gerza J: Medical castration produced by the GnRH analogue leuprolide to treat metastatic breast cancer. J Clin Oncol 3:1068–1072, 1985.
240. Dowsett M, Jacobs S, Aherne J, Smith IE: Clinical and endocrine effects of leuprorelin acetate in pre- and postmenopausal patients with advanced breast cancer. Clin Ther 14A:97–103, 1992.
241. Plowman PN, Nicholson RI, Walker KJ: Remission of postmenopausal breast cancer during treatment with the luteinising hormone-releasing agonist ICI 118630. Br J Cancer 54:903–904, 1986.
242. Lissoni P, Barni S, Crispino S, Paolorossi F, Esposti D, Esposti G, Fraschini F, Tancini G: Endocrine and clinical effects of an LHRH analogue in pretreated advanced breast cancer. Cancer Treat Rev 15:183–194, 1988.
243. Harris AL, Carmichael J, Cantwell BMJ, Dowsett M: Zoladex: Endocrine and therapeutic effects in postmenopausal breast cancer. Br J Cancer 59:97–99, 1989.
244. Saphner T, Troxel AB, Tormey DC, Neuberg D, Robert NJ, Pandya KJ, Edmonson JH, Rosenbluth RJ, Abeloff MD: Phase II study of goserelin for patients with postmenopausal metastatic breast cancer. J Clin Oncol 11:1529–1535, 1993.
245. Williams MR, Walker KJ, Turkes A, Blamey RW, Nicholson RI: The use of an LH-RH agonist (ICI 118630, Zoladex) in advanced premenopausal breast cancer. Br J Cancer 53:622–636, 1986.
246. Blamey RW, Jonat W, Kaufmann B, Bianco AR, Namer M. Goserelin depot in the treatment of premenopausal advanced breast cancer. Eur J Cancer 28A:810–814, 1992.
247. Blamey RW, Jonat W, Kaufmann M, Bianco AR, Namer M. Survival data relating to the use of goserelin depot in the treatment of premenopausal advanced breast cancer. Eur J Cancer 29A:1498, 1993. Letter.
248. Kaufman M, Jonat W, Schachner-Wunschmann E, Bastert G: The depot GnRH analogue goserelin in the treatment of pre-menopausal patients with metastatic breast cancer—A 5-year experience and further endocrine therapies. Onkologie 14:22–30, 1991.
249. Dixon AR, Robertson JF, Jackson L, Nicholson RI, Walker KJ, Blamey RW: Goserelin (Zoladex) in premenopausal advanced breast cancer: Duration of response and survival. Br J Cancer 62:868–870, 1990.
250. Brambilla C, Escobedo A, Artioli R, Lechuga MJ, Motta M: Treatment of pre-menopausal advanced breast cancer with goserelin—A long-acting luteinizing hormone-releasing hormone agonist. Anticancer Drugs 3:3–8, 1992.
251. Santen RJ, Manni A, Harvey H: Gonadotropin-releasing hormone (GnRH) analogs for the treatment of breast and prostate carcinoma. Breast Cancer Res Treat 7:129–145, 1986.
252. Buzzoni R, Biganzol L, Bajetta E, Celio L, Fornasiero A, Mariani L, Zilembo N, DiBartolomeo M, DiLeo A, Archangel G: Combination goserelin and tamoxifen therapy in premenopausal advanced breast cancer: A multicentric study by the ITMO group. Italian Trials in Medical Oncology. Br J Cancer 71:1111–1114, 1995.
253. Boccardo F, Rubagotti A, Perrotta A, Amoroso D, Balestreno M, DeMatteis A, Zola P, Sismondi P, Francini G, Petrioli R: Ovarian ablation versus goserelin with or without tamoxifen in pre-peri menopausal patients with advanced breast cancer: Results of a multicentric Italian study. Ann Oncol 5:337–342, 1994.
254. Jonat W, Kaufmann M, Blamey RW, Howell A, Collins JP, Coates A, Eiermann W, Janicke F, Njordenskold B, Forbes JF, Kolvenberg GJ: A randomised study to compare the effect of the luteinising hormone-releasing hormone (LHRH) analogue goserelin with or without tamoxifen in pre- and perimenopausal patients with advanced breast cancer. Eur J Cancer 31A:137–142, 1995.
255. Henderson IC, Canellos GP: Cancer of the breast: The past decade. N Engl J Med 302:17–30, 78–90, 1980.
256. Goldenberg IS, Waters N, Ravdin RS, Ansfield FJ, Segaloff A: Androgenic therapy for advanced breast cancer in women. A report of the Cooperative Breast Cancer Group. JAMA 223:1267–1268, 1973.
257. Manni A, Arafah BM, Pearson OH: Androgen-induced remissions after antiestrogen and hypophysectomy in stage IV breast cancer. Cancer 48:2507–2509, 1981.
258. Clarysse A: Hormone-induced tumor flare. Eur J Cancer 21:545–547, 1985. Editorial.
259. Peters TG, Lewis JD, Wilkinson EJ, Fuhrman TM: Danazol therapy in hormone-sensitive mammary carcinoma. Cancer 40:2797–2800, 1977.
260. Coombes RC, Dearnaley D, Humphreys J, Gazet JC, Ford HT, Nash AG, Mashiter K, Powles TJ: Danazol treatment of advanced breast cancer. Cancer Treat Rep 64:1073–1076, 1980.
261. Coombes RC, Perez D, Gazet JC, Ford HT, Powles TJ: Danazol treatment for advanced breast cancer. Cancer Chemother Pharmacol 10:194–195, 1987.
262. Brodovsky HS, Holroyde CP, Laucius JF, Dugery C, Serbin J: Danazol in the treatment of women with metastatic breast cancer. Cancer Treat Rep 71:875–876, 1987.
263. Pronzato P, Amoroso D, Ardizzoni A, Bertelli G, Conte PF,

Michelotti A, Rosso R: A phase II study of danazol in metastatic breast cancer. Am J Clin Oncol 10:407–409, 1987.

264. Kiang DT, Kennedy BJ: "Intranuclear" castration effect of high-dose estrogen. Proc Am Assoc Cancer Res 17:194, 1976.

265. Report of the Council on Drugs: Androgens and estrogens in the treatment of disseminated mammary carcinoma: Retrospective study of nine hundred forty-four patients. JAMA 172:135–147, 1960.

266. Carter AC, Sedransk N, Kelly RM, Ansfield FJ, Ravdin RG, Talley RW, Potter NR: Diethylstibestrol: Recommended dosages for different categories of breast cancer patients. Report of the Cooperative Breast Cancer Group. JAMA 237:2079–2085, 1977.

267. Powles TJ: Current controversies in the endocrine therapy of advanced breast cancer. Oncology 49(Suppl 2):18–21, 1992.

268. Miller WR: Endocrine treatment for breast cancer: Biological rationale and current progress. J Steroid Biochem Mol Biol 37:467–480, 1990.

269. Clark JH, Peck EJ: Female sex steroids: Receptors and function. Monogr Endocrinol 14:1–245, 1979.

270. Teulings FA, Van Glise HA, Henkelman MS, Portengen H, Alexieva-Figusch J: Estrogen, androgen, glucocorticoid and progesterone receptors in progestin-induced regression of human breast cancer. Cancer Res 40:2557–2561, 1980.

271. Liu HC, Tseng L: Estradiol metabolism in isolated human endometrial epithelial glands and stroma cells. Endocrinology 104:1674–1681, 1979.

272. Alexieva-Figush J, Blankenstein MA, Jop WCJ, Klijn JG, Lamberts SW, de Jong FH, Docter R, Adlercreutz H, van Gilse HA: Treatment of metastatic breast cancer patients with different dosages of megesterol acetate: Dose relations, metabolic and endocrine effects. Eur J Cancer 20:33–40, 1984.

273. Canetta R, Florentine S, Hunter H: Megestrol acetate. Cancer Treat Rev 10:141–157, 1983.

274. Alexevia-Figush J, Van Gilse HA, Hop WCJ, Phoa CH, Blonk J, Treurniet RE: Progestin therapy in advanced breast cancer: Megestrol acetate. An evaluation of 160 treated cases. Cancer 46:2369–2372, 1980.

275. Alexevia-Figush J, Van Putten WLJ, Van Gilse HA, Blonk J, Wijst VD, Klijn JGM: Sequential treatment of metastatic breast cancer with tamoxifen after megestrol acetate therapy and vice versa. Med Oncol Tumor Pharmacother 2:69–75, 1985.

276. Allegra JC, Bertino J, Bonomi P, Carpenter J, Catalano R, Creech R, Dana B, Durivage H, Einhorn L, Ettinger D, Greco FA, Greenwald E, Henderson I: Metastatic breast cancer: Preliminary results with oral hormonal therapy. Semin Oncol 12:61–64, 1985.

277. Benghiat A, Cassidy SA, Davidson HE, Mancero FS, Pickard JG, Tyrrell CJ: Megestrol acetate in the treatment of advanced post-menopausal breast cancer. Eur J Surg Oncol 12:43–45, 1986.

278. Bonomi P, Johnson P, Anderson K, Wolter J, Bunting N, Strauss A, Roseman D, Shorey W, Economou S: Primary hormonal therapy of advanced breast cancer with megestrol acetate: Predictive value of estrogen receptor levels. Semin Oncol 12:48–54, 1985.

279. Ettinger DS, Allegra J, Bonomi P, Brodwer H, Byrne P, Carpenter J, Catalano R, Creech R, Dana B: Megestrol acetate vs tamoxifen in advanced breast cancer: Correlation of hormone receptors and response. Semin Oncol 13:9–14, 1986.

280. Ingle JN, Ahmann DL, Reen SJ, Edmonson JH, Creagan ET, Hahn RG, Rubin J: Randomized clinical trial of megestrol acetate versus tamoxifen in paramenopausal or castrated women with advanced breast cancer. Am J Clin Oncol 5:155–160, 1982.

281. Paterson AHG, Hanson J, Pritchard KI, Sanregret E, Dahrouge S, McDermot RS, Fine S, White DF, Trudeau M, Stewart DJ, Unger W: Comparison of antiestrogen and progestogen therapy for initial treatment and consequences of their combination for second-line treatment of recurrent breast cancer. Semin Oncol 17(Suppl 9):52–62, 1990.

282. Willemse P, Van des Ploeg E, Sleijfer D, Tjabbes T, Van Veelen H: A randomized comparison of megestrol acetate (MA) and medroxyprogesterone acetate (MPA) in patients with advanced breast cancer. Eur J Cancer 26:337–343, 1990.

283. Wander HE, Kleeber VR, Gärtner E: Megestrol-azetat versus medroxyprogesteronazetat in der behandlung metastasierender mammakarzinome. Onkologie 10:104–106, 1987.

284. Muss HB, Case LD, Capizzi RL, Cooper MR, Cruz J, Jackson D, Richards F, Powell BL, Spurr CL, White D: High- versus standard-dose megestrol acetate in women with advanced breast cancer: A phase III trial of the Piedmont Oncology Association. J Clin Oncol 8:1797–1805, 1990.

285. Abram JS, Cirrincione C, Aisner J, Berry D, Henderson IC, Panasci L, Ellerton J, Muss H, Kirschner J, Nowak W, Wood W: A phase III dose-response trial of megestrol acetate (MA) in metastatic breast cancer. Proc Am Soc Clin Oncol 11:56, 1992. Abstract 50.

286. Mattsson W: Current status of high-dose progestin treatment in advanced breast cancer. Breast Cancer Res Treat 3:231–235, 1983.

287. Abrams JS, Gutheil J, Aisner J: Potential applications of high-dose megestrol acetate in breast cancer. Oncology 49(Suppl 2):12–17, 1992.

288. Parnes HL, Abrams JS, Tchekmedyian NS, Tait N, Aisner J: A phase I/II study of high-dose megestrol acetate in the treatment of metastatic breast cancer. Breast Cancer Res Treat 18:171–177, 1991.

289. Kornblith AB, Hollis DR, Zuckerman E, Lyss AP, Canellos GP, Cooper MR, Herndon JE, Phillips CA, Abrams J, Aisner J, Norton L, Henderson C, Holland JC: Effect of megestrol acetate on quality of life in a dose-response trial in women with advanced breast cancer. J Clin Oncol 11:2081–2089, 1993.

290. Morgan LR: Megestrol acetate vs tamoxifen in advanced breast cancer in postmenopausal patients. Semin Oncol 12:43–47, 1985.

291. Horwitz KB: The molecular biology of RU486. Is there a role for antiprogestins in the treatment of breast cancer? Endocrine Rev 13:146–163, 1992.

292. Gaillard RC, Riondel A, Muller AF, Herrmann W, Baulieu E-E: RU486: A steroid with antiglucocorticosteroid activity that only disinhibits the human pituitary-adrenal system at a specific time of day. Proc Natl Acad Sci U S A 81:3879–3882, 1984.

293. Maudelonde T, Romieu G, Ulmann A, Pujol H, Grenier J, Khalaf S, Cavalie G, Rochefort H: First clinical trial on the use of the antiprogestin RU486 in advanced breast cancer. In Klijn JGM, Paridaens R, Foekens JA (eds): Hormonal Manipulation of Cancer: Peptides, Growth Factors and New (Anti-)Steroidal Agents. New York, Raven Press, 1987, p 55.

294. Klijn JGM, de Jong FH, Bakker GH, Lamberts SW, Rodenburg CJ, Alexieva-Figusch J: Antiprogestins, a new form of endocrine therapy for human breast cancer. Cancer Res 49:2851–2856, 1989.

295. Hug V, Johnston D, Finders M, Hortobagyi G: Use of growth-stimulatory hormones to improve the in vitro therapeutic index of doxorubicin for human breast tissues. Cancer Res 46:147–152, 1986.

296. Markaverich BM, Medina D, Clark JH: Effects of combination estrogen: Cyclophosphamide treatment on the growth of MXT transplantable mammary tumor in the mouse. Cancer Res 43:3208–3211, 1983.

297. Lippman M, Bolan G, Huff KK: The effects of estrogens and antiestrogens in hormone-responsive human breast cancer in long-term tissue culture. Cancer Res 36:4595–4601, 1976.

298. Conte PF, Gardin G, Pronzato P, Miglietta L, Rosso R, Amadori D, Gentilini P, Monzeglio C, Galotti P, Dimicheli R: In vivo manipulation of human breast cancer growth by estrogens and growth hormone. J Steroid Biochem Mol Biol 37:1103–1108, 1990.

299. Lippman ME, Cassidy J, Wesley M, Young RC: A randomized attempt to increase the efficacy of cytotoxic chemotherapy in metastatic breast cancer by hormonal synchronization. J Clin Oncol 2:28–36, 1984.

300. Lippman ME: Hormone stimulation and chemotherapy for breast cancer. J Clin Oncol 5:331–332, 1987.

301. Conte PF, Pronzato P, Rubagotti A, Alama A, Amadori D,

Demicheli R, Gardin G, Gentilini P, Jacomuzzi A, Lionetto R: Conventional versus cytokinetic polychemotherapy with estrogenic recruitment in metastatic breast cancer: Results of a randomized cooperative trial. J Clin Oncol 5:339–347, 1987.

302. Paridaens R, Heuson JC, Julien JP, Veyret C, Van Zyl J, Klijn JGM, Sylvester R, Mignolet F: Assessment of estrogenic recruitment before chemotherapy in advanced breast cancer: A double-blind randomized study. J Clin Oncol 11:1723–1728, 1993.

303. Benz C, Gandara D, Miller B, Drakes T, Monroe S, Wilbur B, DeGregorio M: Chemoendocrine therapy with prolonged estrogen priming in advanced breast cancer: Endocrine pharmacokinetics and toxicity. Cancer Treat Rep 71:283–289, 1987.

304. Lipton A, Santen RJ, Harvey HA, Manni A, Simmonds MA, White-Hershey D, Bartholomew MJ, Walker BK, Dixon RH, Valdevia DH: A randomized trial of aminoglutethimide +/− estrogen before chemotherapy in advanced breast cancer. Am J Clin Oncol 10:65–70, 1987.

305. Allegra JC, Woodcock TM, Richman SP, Bland KI, Witliff JL: A phase II trial of tamoxifen, Premarin, methotrexate, and 5-fluorouracil in metastatic breast cancer. Breast Cancer Res Treat 2:93–100, 1982.

306. Nenci I: Charting steroid-cell interactions in normal and neoplastic tissues. *In* Gurpride E, Calandra R, Levy C (eds): Hormones and Cancer. New York, Alan R. Liss, 1984, pp 23–26.

307. Mouridsen HT, Rose C, Engelsmann E, Sylvester R, Rotmensz N: Combined cytotoxic and endocrine therapy in postmenopausal patients with advanced breast cancer: A randomized study of CMF vs. CMF plus tamoxifen. Eur J Cancer Clin Oncol 21:291–299, 1985.

308. Tormey DC, Kline JC, Palta M, Davis TE, Love RR, Carbone PP: Short-term high-density systemic therapy for metastatic breast cancer. Breast Cancer Res Treat 5:177–188, 1985.

309. Cocconi G, De Lisi V, Boni C, Mori P, Malacarne P, Amadori D, Giovanelli E: Chemotherapy versus combination of chemotherapy and endocrine therapy in advanced breast cancer. A prospective randomized study. Cancer 51:581–858, 1983.

310. Perry MC, Kardinal CG, Korzun AH, Ginsberg SJ, Raich PC, Holland JF, Ellison RR, Kopel S, Shilling A, Aisner J: Chemohormonal therapy in advanced carcinoma of the breast: Cancer and Leukemia Group B Protocol 8081. J Clin Oncol 5:1534–1545, 1987.

311. Kiang DT, Gay J, Goldman A, Kennedy BJ: A randomized trial of chemotherapy and hormonal therapy in advanced breast cancer. N Engl J Med 313:1241–1246, 1985.

312. Australian and New Zealand Breast Cancer Trials Group, Clinical Oncological Society of Australia: A randomized trial in postmenopausal patients with advanced breast cancer comparing endocrine and cytotoxic therapy given sequentially or in combination. J Clin Oncol 4:186–193, 1986.

313. Hug V, Hortobagyi GN, Drewinko B, Finder M: Tamoxifencitrate counteracts the antitumor effects of cytotoxic drugs in vitro. J Clin Oncol 3:1672–1677, 1985.

314. Hug V, Thames H, Clark J: Chemotherapy and hormonal therapy in combination. J Clin Oncol 6:173–177, 1988.

CHAPTER 74

MANAGEMENT OF OSSEOUS METASTASES AND IMPENDING PATHOLOGICAL FRACTURES

Dempsey S. Springfield, M.D.

Carcinoma of the breast has an affinity for the skeleton. Of the patients who succumb to this disease, the incidence of skeletal involvement has been reported to be as great as 73 percent.[1] Clinically, breast metastases are not uncommon, but less than half of patients with metastatic breast carcinoma will have clinically symptomatic skeletal lesions. These lesions should be treated when recognized and can usually be successfully managed with irradiation alone.[44] Delay in the recognition of bone metastasis may necessitate surgical stabilization in addition to irradiation to adequately treat impending or completed pathological fractures. It is therefore important for the physician managing a patient with breast carcinoma to be aware of the significant percentage of patients who develop bone metastasis and the advantages of early diagnosis and therapy. The clinician should be cognizant of the possibility for the development of metastatic disease and should not be complacent in its recognition. It is discouraging to see a patient with bone metastasis that has been ignored until the fracture is clinically evident or the pathological progression of the osseous lesion is extensive and symptomatic (impending fracture). It is equally important for the patient to be aware of the significance of pain in an extremity, and all patients should be encouraged to report such symptoms to their physician, who should then obtain high-quality roentgenograms.

A plain film radiograph does not always identify a metastatic lesion, but the majority of significant metastatic deposits are seen. The risk of fracture is predicted from the plain radiograph. The technetium 99m bone scan is very sensitive and often reveals occult metastatic foci in bone. However, it is not absolutely essential to obtain bone scans, because repeat roentgenographs can be taken at monthly intervals if clinically indicated. Should a metastatic lesion be present, it will in time become obvious on the plain radiograph and can usually be managed with irradiation. The physician must be cognizant of musculoskeletal pain in the patient with breast carcinoma, because the pain often is secondary to metastatic spread of disease.

Any bone can be involved with metastatic breast carcinoma; however, the spine, pelvis, skull, ribs, and femur, in decreasing order, are the most common sites affected.[44] The lumbar spine is the single most commonly involved osseous metastatic site, because approximately 20 percent of the osseous metastases involve this area. Metastatic frequencies for the ribs, pelvis, thoracic spine, skull, and femur are 15 percent, 14 percent, 13 percent, 12 percent and 11 percent, respectively. The humerus is not a common site for metastatic deposits (5.5 percent).[44] However, when a pathological fracture occurs in this bone, the patient loses significant function and experiences pain, and the fracture usually does not heal spontaneously. Therefore, the humerus should be included in the bones that must be evaluated closely for the possibility of metastatic deposits.

Skull and rib lesions can be irradiated whenever metastases are discovered, and early diagnosis has less importance than in long bone lesions. The early discovery of lumbar or thoracic spine lesions permits the metastatic foci to be best managed with irradiation as a solitary modality with little or negligible risk of neurological compromise. If treatment is delayed, lower extremity paralysis may develop, and recovery is less frequently obtained even with surgical decompression. Lesions of the pelvis, femur, or humerus are important to identify and treat as early as possible to eliminate the pathological fracture that may occur should the metastatic foci be left untreated.

Patients with metastatic breast carcinoma to osseous sites often survive for considerable periods with established disease. For this reason, the physician should not withhold therapy for palliative purposes. This is of particular significance for patients with metastatic disease confined to the skeleton because they frequently have a more indolent course than patients with metastases to both bone and other organ systems. Sherry and coinvestigators[37] observed a median survival of 48 months for 86 patients with metastatic breast carcinoma confined to the skeleton; however, median survival was only 17 months for patients with disease metastatic to other sites. With a response rate of 87 percent, the group with only bone metastases responded better to hormonal and chemotherapy than those with metastases to other sites.

Metastatic tumor in the skeleton results in bone destruction with secondary bone formation. Usually bone destruction exceeds bone formation, and the net effect of the metastatic lesion is bone loss. On occasion bone formation predominates, and the lesion is seen on the radiograph as an osteoblastic abnormality. Metastases from breast carcinoma only rarely produce sufficient stroma for membranous bone formation, as is common with metastatic prostatic carcinoma, and the osteoblastic activity occasionally seen with metastatic breast carcinoma is reactive bone from adjacent periosteal and endosteal osteoblasts.

There are two mechanisms that initiate bone destruction in metastatic carcinoma.[11] First, in the presence of the metastatic foci, there is stimulation of local osteoclasts as the result of the secretion of a variety of osteoclast stimulating factors. Thereafter the stimulated osteoclast resorbs the contiguous local bone, initiating net loss of bone matrix. The second mechanism of destruction is resorption of local bone by the carcinoma. This event occurs in the later phrases of metastatic destruction. Both mechanisms of bone loss are probably mediated through prostaglandin E_2 production, and the administration of prostaglandin inhibitors can diminish the degree of bone resorption and the subsequent net total loss of bone integrity.

Galasko[11] has completed a series of in vitro experiments with tissue cultures of breast carcinoma incubated with mouse calvarium to determine the osteolytic effect of the breast carcinoma cells. These experiments revealed that two thirds of breast tumors are osteolytic, while one third do not produce osteolysis in the cultured osseous cells. In the predominant cell lines that were osteolytic, the addition to cell media of prostaglandin inhibitors of diphosphonates reduced the amount of lysis of the calvarium. The addition of these two inhibitors of bony lysis was more than additive. This work suggests that patients with osteolytic breast carcinoma may best be treated with nonsteroidal anti-inflammatory agents that have prostaglandin inhibitor activity; however, this therapeutic treatment has only been infrequently initiated, and clinical experience is limited.

During the past few years, more work has been done in investigating the use of drugs to inhibit the osteolytic effects of breast carcinoma cells on the skeleton. Bisphosphonates have been used in the more recent experimental studies[33] and clinical studies.[27, 28, 39] In animal experiments, risedronate, the third-generation bisphosphonate, reduced the number of bone metastasis and prolonged the life expectancy of nude mice with injected breast cancer cells.[33] In humans, the bisphosphonate clodronate has been used and shown to decrease the incidence of hypercalcemia, bone pain, and vertebral fractures.[27, 28, 29] The frequency of long bone fractures was not reduced but this factor may be a reflection of the relative small size of the patient populations examined and more work is needed. The date, it is not clear what role the bisphosphonates should play in the management of a patient with metastatic breast cancer, but there seems to be an important place for them.

The strength of the bone matrix can be rapidly diminished by the osteolytic process of the metastatic lesion and subsequent destruction. Biomechanical studies provide data that the orthopedic surgeon uses to determine bone stability when a destructive lesion is confirmed.[10, 31] The strength and integrity of the bone matrix is best predicted by the extent of the defect in the bone cortex (e.g., partial versus full-thickness) and, if present, the size of the defect in relation to the diameter of the affected bone. Osteolytic defects that do not penetrate the cortex rarely lead to a pathologic fracture, although the strength of the bone is reduced. When the cortex is completely eroded, the bone strength is dramatically reduced. Fortunately the "extra" strength in the unaffected, normal bone is significant; thus small defects (less than 50 percent of the diameter of the bone) usually will not cause sufficient reduction in strength for the lesion to be considered an impending fracture. Defects larger than this or any defect in osteoporatic bone will weaken the bone to the degree that the bone can break with normal activity. This pathological or spontaneous fracture occurs with minimal stress, such as occurs with torque of the skeleton (twisting) in bed with the foot in a stationary position.[11] With spontaneous fractures, the bone fails in tension, and because torsion initiates significant tension, pathological fractures are most commonly seen with torsional stresses of the axial skeleton and long bones.

Metastatic lesions that, on measurement, are smaller than the diameter of the bone are called *stress-risers*. These neoplastic lesions reduce the strength of the bone to 40 percent or less of its inherent strength.[31] Whether this defect is a small drill-type hole or a pathological defect just less than the diameter of the bone, the percentage weakening of the bone is essentially identical. Holes from osteolytic metastases with diameters that are measurably greater than the diameter of the affected bone are called *open-section defects* and reduce the inherent strength of the bone as much as 90 percent.

Often a bone can tolerate a stress-riser without becoming excessively weak, and should the underlying process be arrested, the involved segment will regain its original strength within 4 to 6 weeks. If the metastatic foci can be controlled with irradiation, the involved bony area can compensate for the osteolytic defect without filling the defect with bone. Thus a small defect can be treated successfully with irradiation alone; even if the bone does not remodel on the radiograph, it is uncommon for the bone to fracture. Patients should be protected during the treatment. Crutch walking is recommended if the lesion is in a lower extremity. We recommend prophylactic internal fixation for defects with a measured diameter that is less than 50 percent of the diameter of the bone only for patients who continue to have local pain 1 month after completion of their irradiation. Those lesions that are osteolytic, painful, and are equal to or greater than 50 percent of bone diameter have such a high risk for fracture that they are considered to be impending fractures, and immediate operative stabilization is recommended. Those bones with metastatic lesions producing a diffuse, permeative destruction are at significant risk for pathological fracture and should be internally stabilized prophylactically. Irradiation is given postoperatively.

The orthopedist should be more aggressive surgically with any lesion in the periacetabulum, proximal femur, and distal femur than with a lesion in the wing of the ilium, pubis, and scapula[3, 19] because of the added risk of fracture in the weight-bearing bones and the difficulty of treatment after such fractures occur compared with treatment before fracture. As a rule, if the patient undergoes surgery before the fracture, the technical procedure is considerably simplified for the surgeon, and morbidity and mortality for the patient are minimized. Furthermore, the patient does not suffer the intense pain associated with the fracture or experience the complications inherent with the restrictions of immobilization with bed rest. On occasion the orthopedist may be more aggressive than is absolutely essential, but the advantages of prophylactic fixation cannot be over-emphasized. Some radiotherapists suggest that the majority of patients with metastatic foci, even those with large destructive lesions, are best managed with irradiation alone.[8] The results of the study performed by Cheng and colleagues[8, 40] suggest that only patients with diffusely mottled destruction of the femoral neck require internal stabilization before irradiation; these management principles are disputed by the orthopedic community.

Although orthopedists and radiotherapists disagree as to the necessity for operative intervention in patients with impending fractures, they do agree with respect to the role of surgery in patients with a pathological fracture secondary to metastatic disease. Pathological fractures should have open reduction and internal fixation as soon as medically feasible, provided the operative procedure will result in sufficient stabilization to allow the patient pain-free movement. Early operative stabilization of the pathological fracture will permit the patient to be out of bed quickly and decrease the risk of superimposed illness that occurs with the immobilization of bed rest and pain medications. Irradiation is given postoperatively.

Before surgery in the patient with a metastatic breast lesion, a thorough physical examination is essential. It is incumbent on the surgeon to be certain of the necessity of the procedure as determined by a risk-benefit determination with operative planning. Patients with metastatic breast carcinoma not uncommonly have elevated serum calcium levels; prolongation of clotting parameters, myeloplastic anemia, and pulmonary compromise as a consequence of this systemic illness. These parameters must be evaluated in addition to the routine preoperative parameters before anesthetic induction. Additional metastatic bone lesions that require surgery can often be confirmed by palpating the entire skeleton, including the spine. Radiographs of the potentially involved bones (humerus, pelvis, and femur) are recommended, and if possible, a preoperative technetium 99m bone scan should be done. The technetium scan is an excellent method to evaluate the entire skeleton for metastatic deposits, as it is uncommon for a metastatic deposit from breast carcinoma not to be associated with increased activity on a technetium scan.

There is no consensus as to how long a patient's life expectancy should be before operative treatment of a bone metastasis is indicated. My experience is that unless the patient is moribund, he or she will usually benefit from treatment and when the patient's expected survival is longer than the interval expected for recovery from the operation, I believe surgery is indicated.

Without operation treatment of a pathological fracture, the patient remains in pain, often bedridden, and in need of narcotics. After the surgical stabilization of the fractured bone, most patients can be mobilized in 3 to 4 days and their narcotic requirements reduced. For patients with impending fractures, recovery is expeditious, and unless there are specific contraindications to surgery, operative stabilization is recommended, especially for osseous lesions of the lower extremity.

Operative stabilization of pathological fractures has become an accepted axiom in orthopedic management during the past decade, and results have dramatically improved, principally as a consequence of the availability and use of polymethylmethacrylate (PMMA).* PMMA is used primarily to enhance the fixation of metal devices placed in fractures that otherwise would not be of adequate strength to secure fixation screws; it is also used to replace a segment of the bone, improving the stability of the reconstruction.[2, 17, 19, 41] Before the availability of PMMA, it was not often possible to sufficiently stabilize a pathological fracture to allow the patient unrestricted activity, and the failure rate of internal fixation in these patients was unacceptably high.

Fractures of long bones are best treated with internal fixation devices either without or, more commonly, with PMMA.[6] Intramedullary rods or plates and fixation screws can be operatively placed depending on the bone that is fractured. Preferably, the fracture is reduced using closed techniques; thereafter an intramedullary rod is positioned for fixation without exposing the fracture site. When the fracture site must be exposed, either for reduction or to augment fixation with PMMA, the site of the gross (metastatic) tumor should be excised and rigid fixation applied. The first goal of the operation is to relieve pain and permit ambulation of the patient in the immediate postoperative period. The second goal of the operation is to provide sufficient stability and bone apposition so that a union will be achieved. If osseous union is not achieved, the internal fixation device will fail if the patient lives 18 months or more. The surgeon should assume the patient will live long enough to break the fixation device. Therefore the surgeon should aim for internal fixation that is immediately adequate for ambulation and sufficient to allow bone repair. Patients with insufficient bone matrix for primary healing should have bone grafting at the time of internal fixation. Also, metastatic breast carcinoma can be dangerously vascular. Although metastatic breast lesions are not extensively vascularized, it is important to consider preoperative angiography with therapeutic embolization to reduce

---

*See references 9, 12, 18, 21, 29, 35, and 42.

the blood loss expected at the time of the stabilization of the fracture.[7]

All patients with metastatic carcinoma to bone that initiates an impending or pathological fracture should have irradiation following operative stabilization.[5, 34] The usual recommended dose of irradiation varies between 2000 cGy in 5 fractions given over 5 days and 3500 cGy in 10 fractions given over 14 days. This therapeutic dose usually controls progression of the metastatis but does not inhibit osseous repair and fracture union. Because bone pain is the usual indication for irradiation of metastatic lesions and patients are asymptomatic after successful stabilization, radiotherapists occasionally think irradiation is not necessary. It is. If the lesion is not irradiated, further destruction of the bone matrix may occur, and the fixation will be lost.

SPECIFIC ANATOMICAL SITES FOR METASTASES

Spine

Metastatic involvement of the vertebrae by breast carcinoma is common, usually asymptomatic, and therefore not recognized except at autopsy. When symptomatic, however, as a consequence of a pathological fracture, it is difficult to determine whether the vertebral body is simply osteoporotic or a metastasis is present. If the patient has other metastases, it should be assumed that the spinal lesion represents an additional metastatic deposit, and the patient should be treated with irradiation. When metastatic disease has not been confirmed radiologically or histologically, a biopsy is required. A prebiopsy magnetic resonance imaging (MRI) scan is of value to localize the extent of disease within the vertebral body and to determine the extent and location of any extraosseous disease. The biopsy can be successfully completed with a needle using computed tomography (CT) guidance; however, when an open biopsy is the preferred approach, we recommend posterior exposure of the metastatic site with the biopsy done through the pedicle of the area with maximal involvement.

On occasion, the patient with metastatic breast carcinoma develops progressive neurological compromise following anterior compression of the cord by the tumor. These neurological events may result after irradiation either from latent growth of the neoplasm or, more commonly, following collapse of the vertebral body with resultant sharp kyphosis. With these neurological symptoms, an anterior decompression and fusion is recommended.[15, 16] The anterior decompression should be radical, with removal of as much tumor as is technically possible. This will reduce the late risk of progressive neurological compromise. Cortical allografts or prostactic vertebral bodies are advised to replace the resected vertebral body.

Periacetabulum

The periacetabular metastasis is a difficult orthopedic problem to treat successfully, especially if the

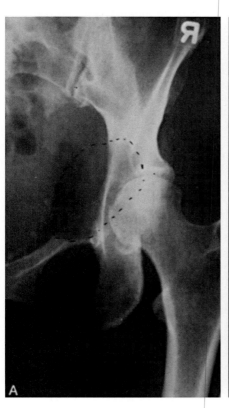 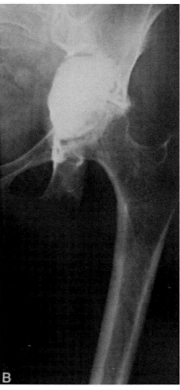

Figure 74–1   A, *Radiograph of the hip with outline of the acetabular metastatic lesion. The patient had mild groin pain. The radiograph changes are subtle, and the clinician reviewing these films must carefully scrutinize for details of bony destruction. A technetium bone scan often indicates because areas of greatest concern, almost all metastatic breast lesions have increased uptake.*   **B,** *Plain x-ray film of the patient following curettage and polymethylmethacrylate (PMMA) packing of the cavity. The patient became asymptomatic after curettage and packing and was treated with 3000 rads postoperatively.*

patient's femoral head begins to advance and protrude into the pelvis. When sufficient acetabular bone exists, irradiation is the treatment of choice after a limited curettage and packing with PMMA (Fig. 74–1).[8] More extensive disease requires reconstruction of the hip joint with replacement of the acetabulum and femoral head (Fig. 74–2).[14, 20]

Femur

The proximal femur is the most common metastatic location that requires surgical intervention.* The combination of frequent involvement, large stress and torque forces placed on the bone, the consequences of a fracture, and the numerous devices available to stabilize the bone explain the frequency of surgical intervention. When the femoral head is damaged, it is best to replace it with a prosthesis.[22] The operation is a routine orthopedic procedure and can be done with minimal blood loss and without excess morbidity to the patient. It is important for the surgeon to have available a comprehensive set of hip prostheses in the event there is greater destruction of bone than was indicated on the preoperative radiographs. Both calcar femorale replacement and long-stem prosthetic devices should be available as well. If involvement of the calcar femorale is established, it should be resected, and when metastases in the femoral shaft are evident radiographically or

---

*See references 13, 22, 23, 24, 26, 30, 32, and 38.

at surgery, the stem of the prosthesis should extend beyond them.

Habermann and colleagues[13] reported that 19 of 23 patients with metastatic breast carcinoma and fractures of the femoral neck had acetabular involvement; however, even if this disease is not apparent on the plain roentgenogram, the effectiveness of the hemiarthroplasty will not be altered. If acetabular disease is apparent on the roentgenogram and the patient has a fractured femoral head or neck, a total hip replacement is recommended. Often the acetabular component may require augmentation with a protrusio ring.

Metastatic deposits of the femoral neck can be managed with either a proximal femoral replacement or internal fixation with or without PMMA. When the femoral head is uninvolved and the hip joint is normal, the neck fracture should be treated with reduction and internal fixation. If reduction cannot be obtained, hemiarthroplasty should be performed.

Involvement of the proximal femur, either the intratrochanteric or subtrochanteric area, is especially dangerous. The normal forces of torque and stress experienced by the bone with walking are as great as three times body weight.[10] When the metastatic lesion is discovered before fracture, an internal fixation device can be placed with little difficulty; this practice is recommended in the majority of patients. The Zickel nail is the only device designed specifically for subtrochanteric fractures and is recommended when the patient has a subtrochanteric frac-

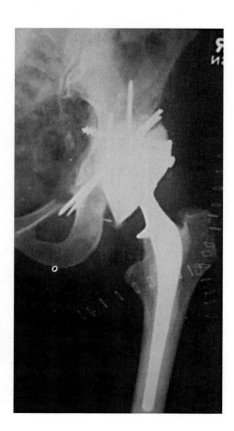

Figure 74–2 *This woman had extensive acetabular destruction secondary to metastatic breast carcinoma and required an acetabular reconstruction. The lesion and involved bone were curetted. Following removal of gross tumor, the defect was replaced by PMMA reinforced with metal pins, and a prosthetic hip was used for the reconstruction. She also received postoperative irradiation. Thereafter, the patient could ambulate asymptomatically with the aid of a cane. The metal acetabular component is a protrusio ring and is applied to enhance stability of the acetabular components.*

ture of the femur (Fig. 74–3).[24, 32, 36, 43] This device is best used without PMMA. Avulsion fractures of the lesser trochanter have been reported as indicative of a metastasis, and with the presentation of this unusual injury, metastatic carcinoma should be suspected.

Femoral shaft metastases are best treated with an intramedullary rod. PMMA is indicated when the rod is not able to provide sufficient stabilization to permit early ambulation. When numerous metastatic lesions are present within the femur or when the femur is diffusely involved with disease, PMMA augmentation of the intramedullary rod is indicated. A technique has been developed for the introduction of an intramedullary rod and PMMA into the femur from either the greater trochanteric approach or the knee (Fig. 74–4).[25] This method allows the stabilization of the entire femur with a limited surgical exposure. The use of intramedullary rods with proximal and distal screw fixation has become popular and is an excellent method of obtaining stability.

Carcinoma metastatic to the distal femur is less common than to more proximal areas and, when seen, the more proximal sites should be examined carefully; as a rule, metastatic disease involves the bone from proximal to distal. Internal fixation of the fractured distal femur is best accomplished with a supracondylar blade plate (Fig. 74–5). PMMA is used

to replace completely destroyed bone or to improve the fixation of screws.

Humerus

Disease metastatic to the humerus is better tolerated than carcinomatous foci in the lower extremity, unless the patient needs crutches for ambulation. When the patient has bone pain in the absence of a fracture, irradiation is recommended. If the patient has a humeral fracture, it is best treated with internal fixation and postoperative irradiation. With internal fixation, the bone is exposed, the gross disease curetted, and plate fixation completed (Fig. 74–6). Intramedullary fixation is an alternative, but it usually does not provide sufficiently rigid stabilization.

POSTOPERATIVE CARE

Postoperatively, the patient should be encouraged to use the extremity as soon as possible. An active rehabilitation program is important to maximize the patient's recovery. Patients with skeletal metastases are at greater risk of developing the complications of osteoporosis, kidney stones, and pulmonary emboli (the most dangerous) with bed rest. The generalized weakness and loss of will associated with pain and

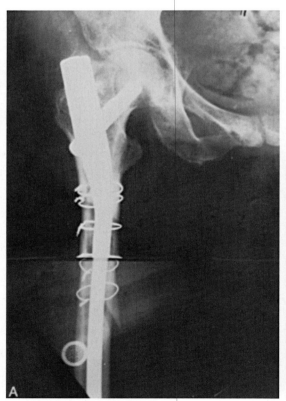
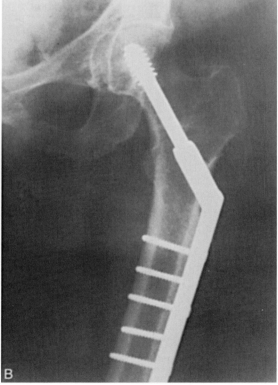

Figure 74–3 *This patient with metastatic breast carcinoma had acute pain in her proximal thigh and sustained a fall.* **A,** *On her initial radiograph, a subtrochanteric femur fracture was diagnosed and she had internal fixation with a Zickel nail and five circulage wires. The Zickel nail was designed specifically for subtrochanteric femoral fractures and has been frequently placed for internal fixation of pathological subtrochanteric fractures.* **B,** *Radiograph of the same patient, who was evaluated and diagnosed with an "impending fracture" of the opposite femur. Thereafter, the patient had prophylactic internal fixation with a sliding hip screw and side plate. Both proximal femurs were irradiated postoperatively.*

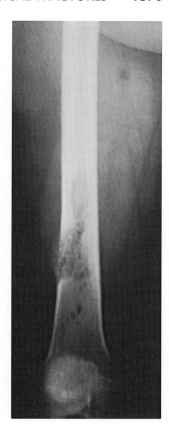

Figure 74–4   *This woman had extensive destruction of the distal femur in the absence of a demonstrable fracture. She was considered to have an "impending fracture" and underwent prophylactic internal fixation. The method of bone fixation necessitated the introduction of an intramedullary rod through the intracondylar notch exposed with an arthrotomy of the knee. PMMA was injected into the medullary canal to enhance the strength of fixation. Thereafter, the patient was asymptomatic and received postoperative irradiation.*

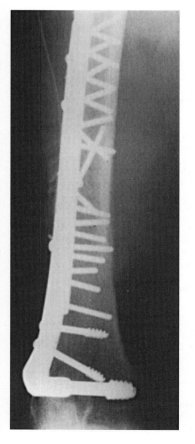

Figure 74–5   *The method of internal fixation of a distal femoral lesion using a supracondylar plate and screws. This fixation technique requires extensive exposure of the bone for placement of the device and is indicated when the metastatic lesion requires curettage or biopsy.*

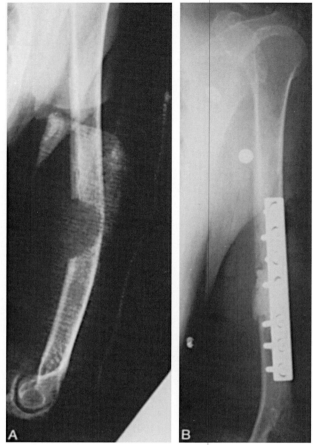

Figure 74–6 *This woman's arm was painful for 2 months prior to x-ray study.* **A,** *The breast metastasis has destroyed the majority of the bone in the mid-diaphysis of the humerus.* **B,** *The lesion was exposed and curetted and the bone replaced with PMMA. The entire construct was secured with a large bone plate and screws. A bone graft was placed to assist in osseous repair and union.*

prolonged bed rest can be devastating to a patient with metastatic breast carcinoma. An aggressive program that allows early stabilization of fractures with a return to activity will improve the quality of life. Finally, the patient who has had a bone metastasis is at significantly increased risk for a second focus to develop; close follow-up reduces the possibility of yet another pathological fracture if the lesion is identified early.

References

1. Abrams HL, Spiro R, Goldstein N: Metastasis in carcinoma. Cancer 3:74–85, 1950.
2. Anderson JJ, Erickson JM, Thompson RC, Chao LY: Pathologic femoral shaft fractures comparing fixation techniques using cement. Clin Orthop 131:273–278, 1978.
3. Beals RK, Lawton GD, Snell WE: Prophylactic internal fixation of the femur in metastatic breast cancer. Cancer 28:1350–1354, 1971.
4. Bertin KC, Horstman J, Coleman SS: Isolated fracture of the lesser trochanter in adults. An initial manifestation of metastatic disease. J Bone Joint Surg 66A:770–773, 1984.
5. Blake DD: Radiation treatment of metastatic bone disease. Clin Orthop 73:89–100, 1970.
6. Broos P, Reynders P, van den Bogert W, Vanderschot P: Surgical treatment of metastatic fracture of the femur improvement of quality of life. Acta Orthop Belg 59 (Suppl 1): 52–56, 1993.
7. Carpenter PR, Ewing JW, Cook AJ, Kuster A: Angiographic assessment and control of potential operative hemorrhage with pathologic fractures secondary to metastasis. Clin Orthop 123:6–8, 1977.
8. Cheng DS, Seitz CB, Eyre HJ: Nonoperative management of femoral, humeral and acetabular metastases in patients with breast carcinoma. Cancer 45:1533–1537, 1980.
9. Coran AG, Banks HH, Aliapoulios MA, Wilson RE: The management of pathologic fractures in patients with metastatic carcinoma of the breast. Surg Gynecol Obstet 127:1225–1230, 1968.
10. Fielding JW, Cochran GVB, Zickel RE: Biomechanical characteristics and surgical management of subtrochanteric fracture Orthop Clin North Am 5:629–650, 1974.
11. Galasko CSB: Mechanism of lytic and blastic metastatic disease of bone. Clin Orthop 169:20–27, 1982.
12. Gristina AG, Adair DM, Spurr CL: Intraosseous metastatic breast cancer treatment with internal fixation and study of survivors. Ann Surg 197:128–134, 1983.
13. Habermann ET, Sachs R, Stern RE, Hirsh DM, Anderson WJ: The pathology and treatment of metastatic disease of the femur. Clin Orthop 169:70–82, 1982.
14. Harrington KD: The management of acetabular insufficiency secondary to metastatic malignant disease. J Bone Joint Surg 63A:653–664, 1981.
15. Harrington KD: Metastatic disease of the spine. J Bone Joint Surg 68A:1110–1115, 1986.
16. Harrington KD: The use of methylmethacrylate for vertebral body replacement and anterior stabilization of pathological fracture-dislocations of the spine due to metastatic malignant disease. J Bone Joint Surg 63A:36–46, 1981.
17. Harrington KD, Sim FH, Eric JE, Johnston JO, Dick HW, Gristina AG: Methylmethacrylate as an adjuvant in internal fixation of pathological fractures. Experience with three hundred and seventy-five cases. J Bone Joint Surg 58A:1047–1055, 1976.
18. Heisterberg L, Johansen TS: Treatment of pathological fractures. Acta Orthop Scand 50:787–790, 1979.
19. Jensen TM, Dillon WL, Reckling FW: Changing concepts in the management of pathological and impending pathological fractures. J Trauma 16:496–502, 1976.
20. Johnson JTH: Reconstruction of the pelvic ring following tumor resection. J Bone Joint Surg 60A:747–751, 1978.
21. Krebs H: Management of pathologic fractures of long bones in malignant disease. Arch Orthop Trauma Surg 92:133–137, 1978.
22. Lane JM, Sculco TP, Zolan S: Treatment of pathologic fractures of the hip by endoprosthetic replacement. J Bone Joint Surg 62A:954–959, 1980.
23. Levy RN, Sherry HS, Siffert RS: Surgical management of metastatic disease of bone at the hip. Clin Orthop 169:62–69, 1982.
24. Mickelson MR, Bonfiglio M: Pathologic fractures in the proximal part of the femur treated by Zickel nail fixation. J Bone Joint Surg 58A:1067–1070, 1976.
25. Miller GJ, Vander Griend RA, Blake P, Springfield DS. Performance evaluation of a cement augmented intramedullary fixation system for pathologic lesions of the femoral shaft. Clin Orthop 221:246–254, 1987.
26. Murray JA, Parrish FF: Surgical management of secondary neoplastic fractures about the hip. Orthop Clin North Am 5:887–901, 1974.
27. Paterson AH, Ernst DS, Powles TJ, Ashley S, McCloskey EV, Kanis JA: Treatment of skeletal disease in breast cancer with clodronate. Bone 12(Suppl 1) s25–s30, 1991.
28. Paterson AH, Powles TJ, Kanis JA, McCloskey E, Hanson J, Ashley S: Double-blind controlled trial of oral clodronate in patients with bone metastases from breast cancer. J Clin Oncol 11:59–65, 1993.
29. Perez CA, Bradfield JS, Morgan HC: Management of pathologic fractures. Cancer 29:684–693, 1972.
30. Poigenfurst J, Marcove RC, Miller TR: Surgical treatment of

fractures through metastasis in the proximal femur. J Bone Joint Surg 50B:743–756, 1968.
31. Pugh J, Sherry HS, Futterman B, Frankel VH: Biomechanics of pathologic fractures. Clin Orthop 169:109–114, 1982.
32. Sangeorzan BJ, Ryan JR, Saleiccioli GG: Prophylactic femoral stabilization with the Zickel nail by closed technique. J Bone Joint Surg 68A:991–999, 1986.
33. Sasaki A, Boyce BF, Story B, Wright KR, Chapman M, Boyce R, Mundy GR, Yoneda T: Bisphosphonate risedronate reduces metastatic human breast cancer burden in bone in nude mice. Cancer Res 55:3551–3557, 1995.
34. Schocker JD, Brady LW: Radiation therapy for bone metastasis. Clin Orthop 169:38–43, 1982.
35. Schurman DJ, Amstutz HC: Orthopaedic management of patients with metastatic carcinoma of the breast. Surg Gynecol Obstet 137:831–836, 1973.
36. Schurman DJ, Amstutz HC: Treatment of neoplastic subtrochanteric fractures. Clin Orthop 97:108–113, 1973.
37. Sherry MM, Greco FA, Johnson DH, Hainsworth SD: Metastatic breast cancer confined to the skeletal system. An indolent disease. Am J Med 81:381–386, 1986.
38. Snell WM, Beals RK: Femoral metastases and fractures from breast cancer. Surg Gynecol Obstet 119:22–25, 1964.
39. Theriault RL, Hortobagye GN: Bone metastasis in breast cancer. Anticancer Drugs 3:455–462, 1992.
40. Tong D, Gillick L, Hendrickson FR: The palliation of symptomatic osseous metastasis. Cancer 50:893–899, 1982.
41. Wang GJ, Reger SI, Maffeo C, McLaughlin RE, Stemp WG: The strength of metal reinforced methylmethacrylate fixation of pathologic fractures. Clin Orthop 135:287–290, 1978.
42. Welch CE. Pathologic fracture due to malignant disease. Surg Gynecol Obstet 62:735–744, 1936.
43. Zickel RE, Mouradian WH: Intramedullary fixation of pathologic fractures and lesions of the subtrochanteric region of the femur. J Bone Joint Surg 58A:1061–1066, 1976.
44. Zimskind PD, Surver JM: Metastasis to bone from carcinoma of the breast. Clin Orthop 11:202–215, 1958.

CHAPTER 75

MANAGEMENT OF PLEURAL METASTASES IN BREAST CANCER

Karen A. Johnson, M.D., Ph.D., M.P.H. / Barnett S. Kramer, M.D., M.P.H. /
Jeffrey M. Crane, M.D.

Pleural effusions and metastatic pleural disease are a common problem in patients with disseminated breast cancer. Historically, about 50 percent of patients with metastatic breast cancer were observed to develop malignant pleural effusion.[27] In 1950 Abrams and coworkers[1] reported that there were pleural metastases in 65 percent of 167 patients with breast cancer in a series of 1000 consecutive autopsied cancer patients. Four subsequent U.S. autopsy studies between 1955 and 1982 yielded similar results, with pleural findings in about 50 percent of the breast cancer patients.[46] Given the incidence of breast cancer and the relative frequency of the pleura as a metastatic site, carcinoma of the breast is the most common cause of malignant pleural effusions in U.S. women, occurring in 37 percent of the women in one series of 472 patients with malignant effusions at Duke Medical Center.[38]

Although the interval from initial diagnosis to time of recognized pleural metastases ranges from zero to more than 20 years,[23, 62] when pleural metastases occur, they are usually an indication of widespread systemic disease. In one well-studied series of breast cancer patients, at first recurrence, when pleural disease was present, at least one additional metastatic site was identified in 80 percent of patients, and two thirds of these had two or three additional metastatic sites.[39] When the pleurae were not involved, first recurrence was much more likely to involve a single site (70 percent).

Consistent with the concept that pleural metastases presage extensive disease, the mean or median survival after diagnosis of malignant pleural effusion has generally been reported to be short, ranging from 6 to 15.7 months in a number of series;[18, 23, 52, 62] however, in some subsets of patients, survival may be substantially longer.[65] Factors associated with a relatively better prognosis are (1) absence of other metastatic sites[10] and (2) estrogen receptor positivity of the tumor.[20] A disease-free interval of less than 12 months from time of original diagnosis is indicative of a poor prognosis.[10]

Debate exists about the routes followed by breast cancer cells metastasizing to the pleura. Although breast metastases to the pleura have been observed as the result of direct tumor extension,[54] the usual mechanisms of dissemination are postulated to be hematogenous and lymphatic spread. In addressing this issue, laterality of the effusion compared with the side of original breast cancer diagnosis can pro-

vide insight. Using eight reports with 493 breast cancer patients,* compilation shows that effusions were ipsilateral in 62 percent of cases, contralateral in 25 percent, and bilateral in 13 percent.

Because of the great potential for variation in observations of this nature, it is useful to remember that in clinical practice, pleural effusion from breast cancer is more frequently observed to be ipsilateral than contralateral, and that bilateral effusions are relatively infrequent. Several observers have interpreted the predominance of ipsilateral effusions as supporting a mechanism of regional, nonhematogenous dissemination.[83, 89] One such explanation invokes spread of tumor to the pleura through the lymphatics of the chest wall. Hematogenous dissemination is thought to involve increased capillary permeability secondary to blood-borne metastases, which would be associated with bilateral pleural disease. The opportunity to verify these ideas is limited, but practical experience suggests that both mechanisms are operating. In the clinic, pleural disease is highly associated with mediastinal disease as well as parenchymal metastases.[39] Parenchymal metastases follow lymphangitic as well as hematogenous patterns of spread.[28] At autopsy, pleural disease occurs with extensive involvement of both blood vessels and lymphatics in the chest.[83]

Multiple investigations have been carried out with the hope that an understanding of the way pleural effusions develop might lead to more rational treatment,[24] but the algorithm for treatment remains at a plateau. In general, a new pleural effusion in a breast cancer patient may respond to systemic therapy for metastatic disease (see Chapters 72 and 73), especially in women with no prior systemic therapy for metastatic disease; nevertheless, tumor resistance to systemic treatment eventually occurs, either naturally or in conjunction with treatment, and pleural effusions in this setting are managed palliatively.

PATHOPHYSIOLOGY

The pathophysiology of pleural effusions has been recently reviewed.[7] The pleural cavity is a potential space, normally containing 10 ml or less of low-protein fluid (approximately 2 gm/dl). The formation of this fluid is the result of a net hydrostatic-oncotic

---

*See references 18, 23, 24, 44, 60, 62, 78, and 89.

pressure of the capillaries of the parietal pleura moving fluid into the pleural space. In the normal state, fluid is thought to enter the space at a rate of about 20 ml/day and to leave through lymphatic stomata in the parietal pleura.[47]

Accumulation of pleural fluid may result when any one of several pathophysiological events occur. These fall into the following categories:

1. Increased capillary permeability, usually related to inflammatory processes.
2. Increased hydrostatic pressure, as in congestive heart failure.
3. Increased negative intrapleural pressure, as in atelectasis.
4. Decreased oncotic pressure, as in any hypoalbuminemic state.
5. Increased oncotic pressure of pleural fluid, usually related to an inflammatory process or malignancy.
6. Impaired visceral lymphatic drainage, such as found in tumor infiltration of hilar or mediastinal lymph nodes or lymphatic interstitial spread.

Obviously, some of the causes of disturbed physiology of the pleurae are not malignant. Hence it is important to document the cause of an effusion in any patient with breast cancer before attributing it to metastatic disease.

A malignant pleural effusion is defined by the presence of malignant cells on cytologic examination of pleural fluid or on histological examination of a pleural biopsy in the setting of a pleural effusion.[69] When this direct evidence of malignancy is absent, but pleural pathology is indirectly related to malignancy, the resulting effusions have been called "para-malignant effusions" (Table 75–1). Causes include mediastinal lymphatic obstruction, postobstructive pneumonia or atelectasis, pulmonary embolism, superior vena cava syndrome, low oncotic pressure, and chylothorax from disruption of the lymphatics or following radiation therapy to the mediastinum.[69] The precise incidence of these "para-malignant" conditions is unknown in patients presenting with pleural effusions, as most are described in case reports. However, the medical history, physical examination, and supporting laboratory data should aid in differentiating

TABLE 75–1   CAUSES OF PARAMALIGNANT EFFUSIONS

Mediastinal lymph node obstruction
Bronchial obstruction with pneumonia
Bronchial obstruction with atelectasis
Pulmonary embolism
Superior vena cava syndrome
Chylothorax
Mediastinal radiation
Drug reactions
   Methotrexate
   Procarbazine
   Cyclophosphamide

Adapted from Sahn SA: Malignant pleural effusions. Clin Chest Med 6:113–125, 1985.

these conditions from metastatic involvement of the pleura.

Attempts to define the causes of a pleural effusion begin with a characterization of the nature of the fluid as either a transudate or an exudate. There are only three circumstances in which tests of pleural fluid are diagnostic: (1) the presence of malignant cells, (2) bacteria on stain or culture, and (3) the presence of lupus erythematosus cells.[19, 36] Most of the remaining tests of pleural fluid lack sufficient sensitivity, specificity, or predictive accuracy to be considered definitive. Therefore, the history, physical examination, and ancillary laboratory investigations will guide the clinician in selecting the most appropriate algorithm for diagnosis and management.

SIGNS AND SYMPTOMS

Metastatic breast cancer involving the pleura rarely presents as adenocarcinoma of occult primary site, because at presentation most patients are known to have breast cancer.* Although as many as 25 percent of patients are asymptomatic, cough is the most common symptom. Dyspnea on exertion may be noted by 50 percent of patients.[69, 75] The accumulated fluid may be as much as 1 l in up to 60 percent of patients.[18] Approximately 10 percent of patients will have a massive effusion, opacifying the entire hemithorax. In such cases, shift of the mediastinum into the contralateral hemithorax helps distinguish massive effusion from bronchial obstruction with lung collapse, which does not cause this kind of shift.

DIAGNOSTIC TESTS

For patients presenting with pleural effusions, the initial diagnostic maneuver is thoracentesis. The gross appearance of the pleural fluid may be suggestive of the cause. Typically, malignant processes produce bloody fluid. However, although serous fluid may suggest a nonmalignant etiology, this is not always the case. Malignant effusions are serous in approximately 10 to 20 percent of cases.[18, 19] Turbid, nonbloody fluid suggests a parapneumonic etiology, possibly secondary to bronchial obstruction with a postobstructive pneumonia present.[75, 79] Typically, a malignant effusion has fewer than 4000 leukocytes per μl, and lymphocytes predominate (>50 percent).[69]

It is helpful to determine whether the pleural fluid is a transudate or an exudate,[48] as malignant effusions are usually exudative.[18, 19, 69, 79] A transudate is typically caused by diseases that alter hydrostatic or osmotic forces, with normal pleural surfaces.[19] As such, further evaluation of a transudative effusion by pleural biopsy is usually not helpful.[19] There are exceptions, however, as 10 to 20 percent of malignant effusions are transudative.[48, 69, 79] Hence if a nonmalignant cause for the effusion cannot be determined, a pleural biopsy or thoracoscopy is sometimes indicated.[76, 90]

Exudates are caused by diseases that influence the permeability of the pleural tissues to protein, decrease the lymphatic flow from the pleural surface, or decrease pressure in the pleural space. In these instances, further characterization of the pleural exudate usually will provide additional discriminating information about the etiology of the exudate. A simple, two-stage evaluation of pleural fluid is a sensitive, specific, and relatively cost-effective laboratory approach.[48, 59] First, pleural fluid:serum protein and pleural fluid:serum lactate dehydrogenase (LDH) ratios are determined. Light and coworkers[48] have demonstrated that a pleural fluid:serum protein ratio greater than 0.5 predicts an exudate with 97 percent accuracy. If the ratio is less than or equal to 0.5, a transudate is predicted with 83 percent accuracy. Similarly, a pleural fluid:serum LDH ratio greater than 0.6 indicates an exudate with an accuracy of 98 percent; if the ratio is less than or equal to 0.6, a transudate is predicted with an accuracy of 77 percent.[48] If the first stage of this evaluation is consistent with an exudate, then a second stage of further evaluation is justified. Little additional information is gained from further evaluation of a transudate. Pleural fluid pH has been found to be decreased in approximately one third of nonmesothelioma malignant effusions.[21, 29]

The implications of a low pleural fluid pH are shorter survival and less success with pleurodesis;[69] however, there is evidence that talc may be more effective than other agents used for pleurodesis in the low pH environment.[3, 74] Pleural fluid pH of less than 7.3 is usually accompanied by low glucose with a fluid:serum ratio of less than 0.5. These abnormalities relate to inhibition of glucose transport from blood to pleural fluid and an efflux-block to the end products of glucose metabolism, leading to a buildup of acidic products in the pleural space secondary to overwhelming malignant disease.[70] With these abnormalities, when survival is judged to be a matter of weeks, repeated thoracentesis has been recommended as the preferred treatment of the effusion.[29, 72]

In the patient with known metastatic breast cancer, a pleural fluid cytology specimen often will be positive. Cytology findings in different malignant effusions are of variable diagnostic accuracy, ranging from 42 to 92 percent in published series.* False-positive results in pleural fluid cytology specimens for metastatic carcinoma of various types are infrequent; Grunze[30] reported a false-positive rate of only 2 percent. The number and volume of samples available for cytologic review influence the diagnostic accuracy of the procedure. It is recommended that the sample volume be at least 250 ml (though not more than 1500 ml taken at one procedure). In the series reported by Salyer and colleagues[73] and Winklemann

and Pfitzer,[90] a single sample of fluid had a diagnostic yield of approximately 53 percent; the second sample, 64 percent; and a third sample increased the cumulative accuracy to 69 percent.[73, 90] Diagnostic yield is also increased when an effusion has low pH and low glucose.[70]

Automated flow cytometry analysis for aneuploidy may also enhance the accuracy of cytologic examination of pleural fluid.[85] Pleural fluid carcinoembryonic antigen, though a poor screening test, may be helpful in the diagnostically difficult effusion.[53, 63] If cytology specimens from three thoracenteses are negative but malignancy is still suspected, then biopsy of the pleura, with diagnostic thoracoscopy, if available, has been proposed.[16, 33, 69, 73, 76, 90]

THERAPY

Therapy for breast cancer metastatic to the pleura or leading to pleural effusions may be broadly divided into three categories: local, systemic, and a combination of the two. The decision to treat the patient is contingent on the physician's knowledge of the growth rate of the patient's cancer, the patient's performance status, and on the patient's prior exposure to chemotherapeutic agents.

A variety of cytotoxic and hormonal therapies are currently available for advanced metastatic breast cancer. The appearance of a malignant pleural effusion is indicative of extensive systemic disease in nearly all patients. Although no presently available therapy for systemic disease is curative, there is effective palliative systemic treatment that may improve the pleural disease. Breast cancer is a chemo-, hormone-, and relatively radioresponsive neoplasm. The treatment given to the patient with a malignant effusion is directed at symptomatic control of the local process as well as, in many cases, the systemic spread of tumor. Systemic therapy in advanced breast cancer is addressed elsewhere in this text (Chapters 72 and 73) and will not be further covered in this section.

Local therapy for the malignant pleural effusion may be useful to control the effusion until systemic therapy has a chance to work, or when systemic therapy is ineffective. However, not all malignant effusions in breast cancer require local therapy. Local treatment is aimed solely at palliation and should be reserved for relief of the symptoms that are being caused by the effusion. Choice of treatment will often depend on the life expectancy and performance status of the patient.[29, 73]

Therapeutic and diagnostic thoracentesis is best used initially, not only for diagnosis but also to relieve the patient's distressing pulmonary symptoms. After initial thoracentesis with removal of the pleural fluid, the rate of reaccumulation may be determined (typically 2 to 3 weeks in malignant effusions). However, repeated attempts at thoracentesis are rarely effective in the long-term control of malignant pleural effusions, and several investigators have

---

*See references 21, 30, 36, 38, 77, 79, and 90.

found a 97 to 100 percent frequency of fluid reaccumulation within 1 month.[6, 45, 75] Furthermore, repeated thoracentesis can lead to a number of complications, including reexpansion pulmonary edema, severe bradycardia or hypotension, and traumatic pneumothorax or hemothorax, as well as hypoproteinemia and loculation of the fluid remaining in the affected hemithorax, making later attempts at pleurodesis difficult. Sclerosis of the pleural space should be considered if there is rapid symptomatic fluid accumulation and the patient's life expectancy is at least several months.

Most studies of pleurodesis in malignant pleural effusions use tube thoracostomy as a means of delivering the therapy and draining reaccumulated fluid. Most of these studies focus on a variety of tumor types. Nevertheless, a large percentage of patients in most series have breast cancer. The data presented here will attempt to highlight information related specifically to breast cancer. Tube thoracostomy alone has been advanced as an effective means of controlling recurrent malignant pleural effusions. However, the support for this is derived from a study with incomplete data on response rates. If a specific definition of success (i.e., no fluid reaccumulation for at least 1 month) is applied, then only a minority of patients (11 to 43 percent) respond to tube thoracostomy alone.[6, 27, 35, 91]

Sclerosing agents are usually necessary in conjunction with tube thoracostomy and drainage. This procedure allows the apposition of pleural surfaces and facilitates the action of the instilled sclerosing agent. Several studies have compared thoracentesis with instillation of a sclerosing agent (mechlorethamine, a nitrogen mustard) to tube drainage and sclerosing agent instillation.[6, 27] These studies support the importance of pleural surface apposition. Treatment with mechlorethamine using tube thoracostomy for drainage successfully sclerosed the pleural space for more than 1 month in 66 percent of patients, whereas instillation via thoracentesis needle was successful in only 27 percent of patients. In these studies, it was felt that prior to the instillation of the sclerosing agent, pleural fluid drainage should be less than 50 to 100 ml per day. The less pleural fluid present before therapy, the better is the apposition of the surfaces and the more even the distribution of the sclerosing agent instilled.

Those patients in whom collapsed lobes fail to reexpand following 24 hours of tube thoracostomy drainage and prior to sclerosing therapy should undergo bronchoscopy or thoracoscopy. Many of these patients will have collapse secondary to bronchial obstruction or to a trapped, tumor-encased lung. The use of a sclerosing agent in these cases is to be discouraged, as the results are uniformly poor.

Sclerosing agents affect the pleural surface by direct reaction, causing an inflammatory response in the pleural tissues that leads to fibrotic sclerosis.[29] There is little apparent antitumor effect of the various agents used, and many are not antineoplastic agents. Several reviews of the subject summarize the trials published using the various agents and address the relative merits and disadvantages of each agent.[33]

For years, tetracycline (15 to 20 mg/kg or 1 gm) administered via tube thoracostomy was considered by many to be the initial agent of choice for pleurodesis of malignant pleural effusions.[9, 82] Its use yielded a 70 percent or better response rate in several studies in which patient follow-up was available for more than 1 month.[11, 69, 87, 91]

Since 1991 the injectable tetracycline hydrochloride used for pleurodesis in the United States has been commercially unavailable.[12, 34] Although the use of tetracycline was previously widespread, experts have pointed out that multiple instillations, which extend hospitalization, are usually required and that there are problems with translating the results from uncontrolled retrospective case series into current clinical practice.[66, 68] In a rare prospective multi-institutional trial that randomized patients to bleomycin or tetracycline, the median time to recurrence or progression was 32 days for tetracycline and 46 days for bleomycin, with similar toxicities.[67] Although this particular study does not end the controversy about the best agent to use for intrapleural therapy, follow-up studies will address unresolved questions. A National Cancer Institute intergroup pleurodesis trial will compare bleomycin (60 units), intrapleural talc (5 gm by slurry), and doxycycline (500 mg)—the latter as an alternative to tetracycline.[66] Until further results become available, any of these three options is likely to be used in practice. Of the three, bleomycin, which is a relatively expensive agent, and talc have received recommendations for approval by Food and Drug Administration Advisory Committees. When repeated instillations are required, as is likely with doxycycline, cost is increased by the need for additional days of hospitalization.

As a sclerosing agent, doxycycline gives results similar to tetracycline. In several studies, the complete response rate at a month or more of follow-up was 75 percent (58/77).[41, 51, 55, 64] Side effects of pain or fever are seen in approximately 50 percent of patients. When the tube thoracostomy has low output (less than 100 ml/day) and the lung is fully expanded, a solution of 500 mg of doxycycline (or 10 mg/kg) in 30 ml of normal saline is instilled via the chest tube.[70] The tube is then clamped for 2 to 4 hours, with the patient encouraged to change position, although intensive maneuvers do not appear to be necessary.[22, 50] After several hours, the chest tube is unclamped and reconnected to suction (-20 cm H_2O). After 24 hours, the chest tube can be removed if drainage is less than 100 ml per day. If drainage continues at a high level, a repeat dose of 500 mg of doxycycline should be instilled.

Depending on the study, the use of bleomycin as a sclerosing agent in treating malignant pleural effusions is effective in 65 to 85 percent of patients.[13, 58] Bleomycin is instilled in the same fashion as doxycycline, and the usual dose of 1.00 U/kg in 50 ml of normal saline is used in younger patients.[80] Because of two episodes of possible drug-related deaths in elderly patients receiving more than 40 U/m² of bleomycin solution into the pleural space, this should be considered the maximum dose in the elderly.[84] The toxicity of bleomycin may be less than tetracycline; several investigators used no pretreatment and reported pain in only 4 percent of patients and fever in 16 percent.[33]

Hausheer and Yarbro[33] have extensively reviewed the use of other sclerosing agents, including mechlorethamine,[6, 9, 27] quinacrine,[14, 15, 75, 87] thiotepa,[5] and fluorouracil.[81] Expense, toxicity, or unacceptable therapeutic yields render these agents less desirable alternatives to doxycycline or bleomycin as initial therapy. Patients who fail despite treatment with doxycycline and bleomycin, however, may be candidates for talc pleurodesis.

Talc (2.5 to 6 gm by insufflation) may be the most effective sclerosing agent available, achieving complete response rates above 90 percent.[4, 25, 31, 32, 61] However, delivery of talc into the pleural space is often accomplished at thoracoscopy during general anesthesia or with heavy intravenous sedation and supplemental oxygen. Patients with malignant effusions may not be good candidates for such a procedure, so chest tube instillation of sclerosing agents is usually favored. Unlike doxycycline and bleomycin, talc is not cleared from the pleural space, an attribute that may contribute to the effectiveness of this agent.[49] Although experience with tube instillation of talc is limited,[2, 17, 88] good response rates with low rates of pain (7 percent) and fever (16 percent)[86] justify the controlled comparison of talc with doxycycline and bleomycin.

PROGNOSIS

Pleurectomy is rarely indicated and should be used only in those patients who fail to respond to other methods of controlling pleural effusions, who can tolerate major surgery, and whose life expectancy is reasonably long.[52] Pleurectomy, in competent hands, is nearly 100 percent effective in controlling malignant effusions, but perioperative mortality is approximately 10 percent, and the rate of complications postoperatively is approximately 20 percent and includes air leaks, bleeding, respiratory insufficiency, and pulmonary embolism.[37]

External-beam radiotherapy is not effective as a sole-treatment modality because of the large surface area being exposed, the radiosensitivity of the underlying lung relative to the metastatic breast cancer cells, and the complex dosimetry associated with treating these curved surfaces.[80]

In the literature reviewed here, a variety of treatment modalities have been used to treat malignant pleural effusions from breast cancer. From the time of diagnosis of the pleural effusion, median survival was about 10 months. Ongoing studies may identify an agent of choice, but until that time, the use of doxycycline, bleomycin, or talc by the methods de-

scribed herein should control 70 to 90 percent of malignant effusions for 1 month or more. New experimental approaches to the local management of malignant pleural effusion involve intrapleural immunotherapy with interleukin-2[8] and pleurodesis with OK-432, a biological response modifier that increases intercellular adhesion molecule-1.[42, 56] Nevertheless, pleural disease identifies a systemic problem that must ultimately be resolved on a systemic level.

References

1. Abrams HC, Spiro R, Goldstein N: Metastases in carcinoma: Analysis of 1000 autopsied cases. Cancer 3:74–85, 1950.
2. Adler RH, Sayek I: Treatment of malignant pleural effusion: A method using tube thoracostomy and talc. Ann Thorac Surg 22:8–15, 1976.
3. Aelony Y: Pleurodesis, pH, and thoracoscopic talc poudrage. Chest 104:1317–1319, 1993.
4. Aelony Y, King R, Boutin C: Thoracoscopic talc poudrage pleurodesis for chronic recurrent pleural effusions. Ann Int Med 15:778–782, 1991.
5. Andersen AP, Brinker H: Intracavitary thiotepa in malignant pleural and peritoneal effusions. Acta Radiol 7:369–378, 1969.
6. Anderson CB, Philpott GW, Ferguson TB: The treatment of malignant pleural and peritoneal effusions. Cancer 33:916–922, 1974.
7. Andrews CO, Gora ML: Pleural effusions: Pathophysiology and management. Ann Pharmacother 28:894–903, 1994.
8. Astoul P, Bertault-Peres P, Durand A, et al: Pharmacokinetics of intrapleural recombinant interleukin-2 in immunotherapy for malignant pleural effusion. Cancer 73:308–313, 1994.
9. Austin EH, Flye MW: The treatment of recurrent malignant pleural effusions. Ann Thorac Surg 28:190–203, 1979.
10. Banerjee AK, Willetts I, Robertson FR, et al: Pleural effusion in breast cancer: A review of the Nottingham experience. Eur J Surg Oncol 20:33–36, 1994.
11. Bayly TC, Kisner DL, Sybert A, et al: Tetracycline and quinacrine in the control of malignant pleural effusions: A randomized trial. Cancer 41:1188–1192, 1978.
12. Berger R: Pleurodesis for spontaneous pneumothorax: Will the procedure of choice please stand up? Chest 106:992–994, 1994.
13. Bitran JD, Brown C, Desser RK, et al: Intracavitary bleomycin for the control of malignant effusions. J Surg Oncol 16:273–277, 1981.
14. Borda I, Krant M: Convulsions following intrapleural administration of quinacrine hydrochloride. JAMA 201:1049–1050, 1967.
15. Borja ER, Pugh RP: Single-dose quinacrine and thoracostomy in the control of pleural effusion in patients with neoplastic diseases. Cancer 31:899–902, 1973.
16. Canto A, Rivas J, Saumench J, et al: Points to consider when choosing a biopsy method in cases of pleurisy of unknown origin. Chest 84:176–179, 1983.
17. Chambers JS: Palliative treatment of neoplastic pleural effusion with intercostal intubation and talc instillation. West J Surg Obstet Gynecol 66:26, 1958.
18. Chernow B, Sahn SA: Carcinomatous involvement of the pleura: An analysis of 96 patients. Am J Med 63:695–702, 1977.
19. Chetty KG: Transudative pleural effusions. Clin Chest Med 6:49–54, 1985.
20. Clark GM, Sledge GW, Osborne CK, et al: Survival from first recurrence: Relative importance of prognostic factors in 1,015 breast cancer patients. J Clin Oncol 5:55–61, 1987.
21. Clarkson B: Relationship between cell type, glucose concentration, and response to treatment in neoplastic effusions. Cancer 17:914–928, 1964.
22. Dryzer SR, Allen ML, Strange C, et al: A comparison of rotation and no rotation in tetracycline pleurodesis. Chest 104:1763–1766, 1993.
23. Fentiman IS, Millis R, Sexton S, et al: Pleural effusion in

breast cancer: A review of 105 cases. Cancer 47:2087–2092, 1981.
24. Fentiman IS, Rubens RD, Hayward JL: The pattern of metastatic disease in patients with pleural effusions secondary to breast cancer. Br J Surg 69:193–194, 1982.
25. Fentiman IS, Rubens RD, Hayward JL: A comparison of intracavitary talc and tetracycline for the control of pleural effusions secondary to breast cancer. Eur J Cancer Clin Oncol 1986:1079–1081, 1986.
26. Fenton KN, Richardson JD: Diagnosis and management of malignant pleural effusions. Am J Surg 170:69–74, 1995.
27. Fracchia AA, Knapper WH, Carey JT, et al: Intrapleural chemotherapy for effusion from metastatic breast carcinoma. Cancer 26:626–629, 1970.
28. Goldsmith HS, Bailey HD, Callahan EL, et al: Pulmonary lymphangitic metastases from breast carcinoma. Arch Surg 94:483–488, 1967.
29. Good JT Fr, Taryle DA, Sahn SA: Pleural fluid pH in malignant effusions: Pathophysiology and prognostic implication. Chest 74:338, 1978.
30. Grunze H: The comparative diagnostic accuracy, efficiency, and specificity of cytologic techniques used in the diagnosis of malignant neoplasms in serous effusions of the pleural and pericardial cavities. In Symposium on Diagnostic Accuracy of Cytologic Technics, vol 8. 1984, pp 150–163.
31. Harley HRS: Malignant pleural effusions and their treatment by intercostal talc pleurodesis. Br J Dis Chest 73:173–177, 1979.
32. Hartman DL, Gaither JM, Kesler KA, et al: Comparison of insufflated talc under thoracoscopic guidance with standard tetracycline and bleomycin pleurodesis for control of malignant pleural effusions. Cardiovasc Surg 105:743–748, 1993.
33. Hausheer FH, Yarbro JW: Diagnosis and treatment of malignant pleural effusion. Semin Oncol 12:54–75, 1985.
34. Heffner JE, Unruh LC: Tetracycline pleurodesis: Adios, farewell, adieu. Chest 101:5–7, 1992.
35. Izbicki R, Weyhing BT III, Baker L, et al: Pleural effusions in cancer patients; a prospective randomized study of pleural drainage with the addition of radiophosphorus to pleural space vs. drainage alone. Cancer 36:1511–1518, 1975.
36. Jay SJ: Diagnostic procedures for pleural disease. Clin Chest Med 6:33, 1985.
37. Jensik R, Cagle JE, Milloy F, et al: Pleurectomy in the treatment of pleural effusion due to metastatic malignancy. J Thorac Cardiovasc Surg 46:322–330, 1963.
38. Johnston WW: The malignant pleural effusion: A review of cytopathologic diagnoses of 584 specimens from 472 consecutive patients. Cancer 56:905–909, 1985.
39. Kamby C, Vejborg I, Kristensen B, et al: Metastatic pattern in recurrent breast cancer: Special reference to intrathoracic recurrences. Cancer 62:2226–2233, 1988.
40. Keller SM: Current and future therapy for malignant pleural effusion. Chest 103:63S–67S, 1993.
41. Kitamura S, Sugiyama Y, Izumi T, et al: Intrapleural doxycycline for control of malignant pleural effusion. Curr Ther Res 30:515–521, 1981.
42. Kitsuki H, Uchiyama A, Yoshida T, et al: OK-432–induced enhancement of ICAM-1 expression on tumor cells positively correlates to therapeutic effects for malignant effusion. Clin Immunol Immunopathol 71:89–95, 1994.
43. Koldsland S, Svennevig JL, Lehne G, et al: Chemical pleurodesis in malignant pleural effusions: A randomised prospective study of mepacrine versus bleomycin. Thorax 48:790–793, 1993.
44. Kreisman H, Wolkove N, Finkelstein HS, et al: Breast cancer and thoracic metastases: Review of 119 patients. Thorax 38:175–179, 1983.
45. Lambert CJ, Shah HH, Urschel HC Jr, et al: The treatment of malignant pleural effusion by closed trocar tube drainage. Ann Thorac Surg 3:1–5, 1967.
46. Lee Y-T: Breast carcinoma: Pattern of metastasis at autopsy. J Surg Oncol 23:175–180, 1983.
47. Light RW: Pleural diseases. Dis Mon 38:266–331, 1992.
48. Light RW, MacGregor MI, Luchsinger PC, et al: Pleural effusions: The diagnostic separation of transudates and exudates. Ann Int Med 77:507–513, 1972.
49. Loddenkemper R, Boutin C: Thoracoscopy: Present diagnostic and therapeutic indications. Eur Respir J 6:1544–1555, 1993.
50. Lorch DG, Gordon L, Wooten S, et al: Effect of patient positioning on distribution of tetracycline in the pleural space during pleurodesis. Chest 93:527–529, 1988.
51. Mansson T: Treatment of malignant pleural effusion with doxycycline. Scand J Infect Dis. 53:29–34, 1988.
52. Martini N, Bains MS, Beattie EJ: Indications for pleurectomy in malignant effusion. Cancer 35:734–738, 1975.
53. McKenna JM, Chandrasekhar AJ, Henkins RE: Diagnostic value of carcino-embryonic antigen in exudative pleural effusions. Chest 78:587–590, 1980.
54. Meyer PC: Metastatic carcinoma of the pleura. Thorax 21:437–443, 1966.
55. Muir JF, Defouilloy C, Ndarurinze S, et al: The use of intrapleural doxycycline by lavage-drainage in recurrent effusions of neoplastic origin. Rev Mal Respir 4:29–33, 1987.
56. Nakano, Dato M, Watanabe T, et al: OK-432 chemical pleurodesis for the treatment of persistent chylothorax. Hepatogastroenterology 41:568–570, 1994.
57. Ostrowski MJ: An assessment of the long-term results of controlling the reaccumulation of malignant effusions using intracavity bleomycin. Cancer 57:721–727, 1986.
58. Paladine W, Cunningham TJ, Sponzo R, et al: Intracavitary bleomycin in the management of malignant effusions. Cancer 38:1903–1908, 1976.
59. Peterman TA, Speichler CE: Evaluating pleural effusions: A two-stage laboratory approach. JAMA 25:1051–1053, 1984.
60. Porter EH: Pleural effusion and breast cancer. Br Med J 1:251–252, 1965.
61. Prorok J, Nealon TF: Pleural symphysis by talc poudrage in the treatment of malignant pleural effusion. Bull Soc Chir 27:630, 1968.
62. Raju RN, Kardinal CG: Pleural effusion in breast carcinoma: Analysis of 122 cases. Cancer 48:2524–2527, 1981.
63. Rittgers RA, Lowenstein MS, Feinerman AE, et al: Carcinoembryonic antigen levels in benign and malignant pleural effusions. Ann Int Med 88:631, 1978.
64. Robinson LA, Fleming WH, Galbraith TA: Intrapleural doxycycline control of malignant pleural effusions. Ann Thorac Surg 55:1115–1122, 1993.
65. Rosato RE, Wallach MW, Rosato FR: The management of malignant effusions from breast cancer. J Surg Oncol 6:441–449, 1974.
66. Ruckdeschel JC: Controversy over sclerotherapy for malignant pleural effusions: To the editor. Ann Intern Med 121:150, 1994.
67. Ruckdeschel JC, Moores D, Lee JY, et al: Intrapleural therapy for malignant pleural effusions: A randomized comparison of bleomycin and tetracycline. Chest 100:1528–1535, 1991.
68. Rusch VM: The optimal treatment of malignant pleural effusions. Chest 100:1483–1484, 1991.
69. Sahn SA: Malignant pleural effusions. Clin Chest Med 6:113–125, 1985.
70. Sahn SA: Pleural effusion in lung cancer. Clin Chest Med 14:189–200, 1993.
71. Sahn SA, Good JT Jr: Pleural fluid pH in malignant effusions: Diagnostic, prognostic, and therapeutic implications. Ann Int Med 108:345–349, 1988.
72. Sahn SA, Good JT, Potts DE: The pH of sclerosing agents: A determinant of pleural symphysis. Chest 76:198–200, 1979.
73. Salyer WR, Effleston JC, Erozan YS: Efficacy of pleural needle biopsy and pleural fluid cytopathology in the diagnosis of malignant neoplasm involving the pleura. Chest 67:536–539, 1975.
74. Sanchez-Armengol A, Rodriguez-Panadero F: Survival and talc pleurodesis in metastatic pleural carcinoma, revisited: Report of 125 cases. Chest 104:1482–1485, 1993.
75. Sarma PR, Moore MR: Approach to the management of pleural effusion in malignancy. South Med J 71:133–136, 1978.
76. Scerbo J, Keltz H, Stone DJ: A prospective study of closed pleural biopsies. JAMA 218:377–380, 1971.
77. Stiksa G, Korsgaard R, Simonsson BG: Treatment of recurrent pleural effusion by pleurodesis with quinacrine. Scand J Resp Dis 60:197, 1979.
78. Stoll BA, Ellis F: Treatment by oestrogens of pulmonary metastases from breast cancer. Br Med J 2:796–800, 1953.

79. Storey DD, Dines DE, Coles DT: Pleural effusion: A diagnostic dilemma. JAMA 236:2183–2186, 1976.

80. Strober SJ, Klotz E, Kuperman A, et al: Malignant pleural disease—A radiotherapeutic approach to the problem. JAMA 226:2183–2186, 1973.

81. Suhrland LG, Weisberger AS: Intracavitary 5-fluorouracil in malignant effusions. Arch Int Med 116:431, 1965.

82. The treatment of malignant pleural and pericardial effusions. Med Lett Drugs Ther 23:59, 1981.

83. Thomas JM, Redding WH, Sloane JP: The spread of breast cancer: Importance of the intrathoracic lymphatic route and its relevance to treatment. Br J Cancer 40:540–547, 1979.

84. Trotter JM, Stuart JFB, McBeth JG, et al: The management of malignant effusions with bleomycin. Br J Cancer 40:310, 1979.

85. Unger KM, Raber M, Bedrosian CWM, et al: Analysis of pleural effusions using automated flow cytometry. Cancer 52:873–877, 1983.

86. Walker-Renard PB, Vaughn LM, Sahn SA: Chemical pleurodesis for malignant pleural effusions. Ann Intern Med 120:56–64, 1994.

87. Wallach HW: Intrapleural tetracycline for malignant pleural effusions. Chest 68:510–512, 1975.

88. Webb WR, Ozman V, Moulder PV, et al: Iodized talc pleurodesis for the treatment of pleural effusions. J Thorac Cardiovasc Surg 103:881–886, 1992.

89. Weichselbaum R, Marck A, Hellman S: Pathogenesis of pleural effusion in carcinoma of the breast. Int J Radiat Oncol Biol Phys 2:963–965, 1977.

90. Winkelmann M, Pfitzer P: Blind pleural biopsy in combination with cytology of pleural effusions. Acta Cytol 25:373–376, 1981.

91. Zaloznik AJ, Oswald SJ, Langin M: Intrapleural tetracycline in pleural effusions: A randomized study. Cancer 51:752–755, 1983.

CHAPTER 76

MANAGEMENT OF CENTRAL NERVOUS SYSTEM METASTASES IN BREAST CANCER

Karen A. Johnson, M.D., Ph.D., M.P.H. / Barnett S. Kramer, M.D., M.P.H. / Jeffrey M. Crane, M.D.

As a cause of central nervous system (CNS) metastases, carcinoma of the breast has been first in women and second only to lung cancer overall.[75] In autopsy series, CNS metastases (primarily to brain, dura, and meninges) occur in about 30 percent of breast cancer patients.[1, 112] In one series, two thirds of the CNS metastases found at autopsy were not recognized before death.[108] CNS metastases nearly always occur in the setting of widespread disease.[31, 48, 108] In Tsukada's autopsy series, only three percent of CNS metastases were the sole site of metastatic spread, and 70 percent of patients with recognized CNS disease died of causes other than CNS failure.[108] In another series of 101 breast cancer patients with brain metastases, 70 percent had progressive extracranial disease at the time of death.[31]

Metastatic disease of the CNS may be conveniently divided into three sites. The major site of metastases is the intracranial portion of the CNS. This site includes the extradural and subdural sites of metastases as well as the cerebrum, cerebellum, midbrain, and choroid plexus. The second most common anatomical site is the leptomeninges, an area of involvement that many investigators believe increases in frequency as more patients with cancer survive longer.[7, 79, 117] The third site of CNS metastases is the spinal cord. Extradural spinal metastases account for 97 percent of cases in this site.[79]

The time to development of CNS metastases of breast cancer is variable. CNS disease is occasionally symptomatic at the time of initial diagnosis, and metastases have been found as late as 19 years after the primary diagnosis.[36, 71] The disease-free interval which also reflects the underlying rate of growth of the primary disease is an important prognostic factor. Metastases to one site in the CNS predict increased likelihood of metastatic involvement at other CNS sites.[79, 108] Although a combination of therapeutic modalities may secure symptomatic relief of CNS metastases, survival is usually short after the appearance of symptomatic CNS metastases.[108] Equally important, however, is the fact that once signs or symptoms of CNS metastases are detected, prompt and appropriate therapeutic palliation can frequently alleviate the disturbing symptoms and prevent unfortunate sequelae. It is the rare patient who survives longer than 5 years.[56]

ANATOMICAL SITES OF SPREAD

Intracranial Disease

Of breast cancer patients with metastatic CNS disease, the majority have intracranial tumors (62 percent of 309 patients in Tsukada and coworkers investigation).[108] Presenting symptoms may be nonlocalizing (e.g., increased intracranial pressure) or focal (e.g., a single metastasis). In Tsukada's series, the cranial dura was involved in approximately 54 percent of patients, the leptomeninges in 19 percent, and the spinal cord in 10 percent. The incidence of cranial dural involvement was increased threefold when vertebral body metastases were present.[108] On average, each patient had 2.4 sites of CNS involvement. The prevalence of metastases to the cranial dura was roughly 50 percent, regardless of whether the diagnosis was made ante mortem or post mortem; however, the incidence of solitary intracranial metastases varied according to the time of diagnosis. Among the patients with intracranial CNS disease at autopsy, 42 percent had solitary parenchymal metastases. When there was an ante mortem diagnosis of intracranial CNS metastases, only 16 percent of patients had a solitary lesion. There was evidence of a time trend in favor of ante mortem diagnosis of brain metastases in the two decades covered by the Tsukada's series. From 1959 to 1969, 26 percent of patients with CNS metastases were diagnosed before death, in contrast with 38 percent in the period from 1970 to 1979.

Diagnosis

Although CNS metastases may be asymptomatic, Posner has stressed that careful examination of patients with systemic cancer often discloses signs of CNS disease not noticed by the patients themselves.[79] As an example, he notes that, although only 40 percent of patients with documented intracranial metastases complain of focal weakness, two thirds of them may be found to have focal weakness on physical examination. Similarly, impaired cognitive function was found by careful mental status examination in three fourths of patients, but barely a third complained of behavioral or mental changes. The clinician must be vigilant for changes that indicate the onset of symptomatic CNS disease, since devastating sequelae can rapidly ensue once symptoms become obvious. One group of investigators attempted to use computed tomography (CT) for early diagnosis of occult disease in asymptomatic patients and found the approach unhelpful.[60] Although each patient had a series of at least four studies, with and without contrast, the yield of positive scans in the absence of symptoms was low, for a variety of reasons; for example, one subject with a normal scan developed proven cerebral metastases only 4 months later. The investigators concluded that CT should be reserved for symptomatic patients. The majority of breast cancer patients with symptomatic brain metastases have concurrent extra-CNS disease and eventually die of it. In one series of 101 such patients, 70 percent were receiving systemic chemotherapy at the time their CNS metastases were diagnosed.[31] Very few breast cancer patients have CNS disease that is sufficiently anatomically limited that they may be considered candidates for curative surgical or radiotherapeutic measures. Even though most therapeutic interventions are considered *palliative,* it must be emphasized that the intervention frequently improves the quality, and occasionally the quantity, of life. Appropriate and prompt treatment may prevent the potentially crippling sequelae of progressive CNS metastases.

Headache is a presenting complaint in approximately 50 percent of patients with intracranial (including dural) metastases.[19, 79] Many of these patients describe the headache in terms that strongly indicate elevated intracranial pressure. Classically, the headache is worse on awakening in the morning and abates within 30 minutes of arising, returning again the next morning. Papilledema is reported by Posner to be present in only 25 percent of patients with symptomatic metastatic intracranial disease.[79] Its absence, therefore, is not helpful. In addition to headache, the most common findings associated with intracranial malignancy include mental status changes, focal weakness or hemiparesis, ataxia, cranial nerve involvement, and seizures.[34] Focal or generalized seizures are a presenting complaint in about 15 percent of patients and are relatively more frequent in patients with leptomeningeal metastases.[79, 108]

Diagnostic evaluation with CT or magnetic resonance imaging (MRI) is indicated when a breast cancer patient has unexplained signs or symptoms of intracranial disease.[22] In many institutions, CT with contrast is the initial test of choice. CT is capable of defining mass lesions as well as peritumor edema as small as 5 mm. There is no current "gold standard" by which to determine negative predictive accuracy or sensitivity of CT, except at necropsy. Necropsy studies of patients who succumbed to small cell lung cancer, however, indicate that, in symptomatic patients, CT of the brain has positive and negative predictive accuracies of 98 percent and 99 percent, respectively.[25] Furthermore, in symptomatic patients with suspected spinal cord compression by metasta-

ses, the frequency of concomitant intracranial metastases encourages prompt CT of the brain.[108] Radionuclide brain scanning has generally been replaced by brain CT, as have cerebral arteriography and pneumonencephalography.[3] Plain skull roentgenograms have little or no role in the diagnosis of intracranial CNS metastases.[48, 108]

In a patient with breast cancer who has signs and symptoms of CNS metastases, the CT finding of a solitary intracranial mass usually indicates metastasis; however, other causes of a solitary lesion should be considered, such as brain abscess, cerebral infarcts from either thrombotic or embolic arterial occlusion, chronic subdural hematomas or effusions, or primary brain tumors (such as gliomas or meningiomas).[7] A potential association between breast cancer and meningioma based on hormonal factors has been discussed in the literature.[96] These can often be excluded on the basis of CT appearance. Multiple intracranial lesions seen on CT in a patient with breast cancer are nearly always secondary to metastatic disease. If no intracranial mass lesion is seen in a symptomatic patient with breast cancer, diagnoses that should be considered include leptomeningeal metastases, endocrine-related paraneoplastic encephalopathy, carcinomatous neuromyopathy (such as subacute cerebellar degeneration), and, rarely, sensorimotor neuropathy syndrome or progressive multifocal leukoencephalopathy.[7]

Several patterns consistent with parenchymal brain lesions have been described.[29] The most common are circumscribed lesions that undergo homogeneous enhancement after administration of contrast material or, less often, heterogenous enhancement in conjunction with edema and a mass effect. Protocols have been developed for delayed scanning of late-enhancing lesions, a procedure that is associated with a reduced rate of false-negative studies.[91] Delayed CT with a double dose of contrast is also more sensitive than studies that use less contrast medium.[26, 86] Although CT with contrast does not detect every lesion, results nevertheless compare favorably with unenhanced MRI in demonstrating intracranial metastases[106]; however, recent reports suggest that gadolinium-enhanced MRI is superior to contrast-enhanced CT for evaluating intraparenchymal brain lesions.[26, 105] In most situations, CT is adequate for meeting the diagnostic needs for the anticipated interventions. Nevertheless, it has been suggested that equivocal findings or solitary lesions on contrast-enhanced CT should be followed up with contrast-enhanced MRI, since management decisions could be altered by more sensitive MRI findings.[26]

Management

Because cure of intracranial metastases is rarely possible, the goal of treatment is almost always palliation. When intracranial metastases from breast cancer are left untreated, median survival is approximately 4 to 6 weeks.[31, 66, 79] With treatment, overall median survival is typically reported to be 16 weeks; about 20 percent of patients survive a year.[12, 34] In the selected subset of patients who have a solitary brain metastasis, aggressive, combined modality therapy is associated with increased survival. Kocher and associates reported that, for patients with a single brain metastasis median survival was 1 year for persons who underwent surgery followed by whole-brain irradiation, as compared with 3.2 months for patients who received radiation only.[56] In this series, three of eight breast cancer patients treated with combined therapy for a single metastasis survived longer than 5 years. Critical appraisal of various treatment modalities suffers from the lack of controlled studies; however, it appears that certain patient variables predict a better chance of survival after therapy: a relapse-free interval longer than 5 years, a solitary brain metastasis, few sites of extracranial metastases, chemotherapy after diagnosis of the brain metastases, and Karnofsky performance status of 70 or more (i.e., ambulatory and self-sufficient).[12, 31, 53, 56] Obviously, patient selection factors can play a role in the better outcomes for these patients, apart from the effects of therapy.

Several comprehensive reviews have outlined the therapeutic options, once intracranial metastases are diagnosed.[21, 34, 79] Coia and associates have reported the results of an international consensus workshop on the treatment of brain metastases. The resulting treatment algorithm, summarized in Table 76–1, lists six diagnostic issues and the indicated interventions. Confirmation of cranial metastases with diagnostic imaging is the starting point for intervention. Once metastases are imaged, intervention with steroids is indicated.

Corticosteroids are the treatment used most often for intracranial metastases. Corticosteroids, by themselves, improve symptoms of brain metastases in 60 percent to 75 percent of patients, often within 24 hours.[79] Used alone, however, their effect is only temporary, and related to the reduction of tumor-associated edema. Although corticosteroids decrease the permeability of tumor capillaries, there has been no demonstration of oncolytic effect on breast cancer metastases. Glucocorticoids are favored, but no particular type has been proven more efficacious than another. Nevertheless, there is evidence that the CNS pharmacokinetics of systemically administered dexamethasone are more favorable than those of prednisone.[4] At the time of diagnosis, dexamethasone is usually begun with a loading dose of 10 mg given intravenously, followed by 16 mg per day in three or four daily oral or parenteral doses.[21] This dose may be increased to as much as 100 mg daily if symptomatic improvement is not apparent within 24 hours. Steroid therapy is usually continued through the institution of a more definitive therapy, after which the dose may be tapered to the minimum effective dose. There is no evidence that steroids are of any benefit in patients without CNS symptoms.[48] Used alone, the glucocorticoids exert their effect for an average of 1 to 2 months. If no other treatment is given, extension in survival may be approximately 1 month over that of untreated patients, but this result has not been verified in randomized controlled trials.[7] The side effects of steroids are numerous; the most bothersome are steroid-associated myopathy and insomnia. There is a possibility of an enhanced tendency to develop peptic ulcer disease with perforation. Glucose intolerance may also occur and may improve with lower doses of steroid.[7, 79] One report suggested that breast cancer patients treated with corticosteroid therapy for CNS metastases may be at increased risk of developing *Pneumocystis carinii* pneumonia.[90] However, the most common type of opportunistic infections in neuro-oncology patients taking glucocorticoids are *Candida* pharyngitis and mucositis.[57]

When corticosteroid therapy is being started, an assessment is also made of the need to treat impending herniation. This decision is the second major issue in the treatment pathway (Table 76–1). Occasionally, a patient with brain metastases exhibits rapid neurological decompensation, suggesting tentorial or cerebellar herniation, and prompt use of osmotically active agents may stabilize (and often improve) the patient's symptoms.[7] Mannitol, 20 percent in distilled water, 1–2 gm/kg body weight, or urea, 30 percent, 1.5 gm/kg body weight, given intravenously may stabilize the patient's condition enough to permit initiation of radiation or surgery, as indicated. In the presence of diminishing alertness and rapid development of stupor or coma and impaired breathing, emergency treatment with intubation, mannitol, and dexamethasone may be applied presumptively before a confirmatory CT scan is obtained.

A third major decision point in treatment requires determining whether seizures have occurred. Unless seizures have occurred, the routine use of diphenylhydantoin or another anticonvulsant to prevent seizures in all patients with brain metastases is not recommended. At presentation, approximately 15 percent of patients will have experienced seizures. Another 10 percent may be expected to develop seizures after the initial diagnosis of intracranial me-

TABLE 76–1.   TREATMENT OF BRAIN METASTASES

Diagnostic Finding	Response
Brain metastases on CT or MRI	Institute corticosteroids
Impending herniation	Start osmotherapy (mannitol)
Seizures	Start anticonvulsant (diphenylhydantoin)
Unconfirmed malignant diagnosis	Establish diagnosis by biopsy
Solitary metastasis	Decide whether surgical resection is practical and indicated
Multiple or recurrent metastases, patient not a candidate for surgery or radiotherapy	Decide whether whole-brain irradiation is indicated

Adapted with permission of the publisher from Coia LR: Int J Radiat Oncol Biol Phys 23:229–238, 1992. Copyright 1992 by Elsevier Science Inc.

tastases.[20] The seizures are associated with cerebral metastases and dysfunction. In a series of 195 patients with intracranial metastases, none who had posterior fossa lesions developed seizures.[20] In this retrospective series, patients were just as likely to develop seizures, whether they were treated with diphenylhydantoin or not. In two thirds of the patients who developed seizures while being treated with diphenylhydantoin, the medication levels were subtherapeutic. Although diphenylhydantoin is preferred over other anticonvulsants because of relatively less sedation, once-a-day dosing, and low cost, the potential toxicities of this medication (e.g., nystagmus, ataxia) argue against "automatic" use in patients with brain metastases.[21, 79, 100] Patients who take diphenylhydantoin while receiving whole-brain irradiation are at risk for erythema multiforme and Stevens-Johnson syndrome.[30] Regardless of whether or not an anticonvulsant is used, it is our opinion that patients with documented brain metastases should not drive or operate heavy machinery.

A fourth question involves the likelihood of a malignant cause for radiographically documented intracranial lesions. Most breast cancer patients who have an intracranial lesion already have a tissue diagnosis for their primary breast cancer; however, in the absence of recurrent breast cancer outside the CNS, a solitary brain lesion raises the possibility of an alternative diagnosis and supports the need for biopsy if it can safely be accomplished. In one surgical series examining solitary brain lesions suggestive of metastatic disease, 11 percent were something other than metastases on tissue diagnosis.[74]

At the critical point where a diagnosis of solitary intracranial metastasis is being entertained, it may be appropriate to perform MRI if the initial assessment relied on CT evidence. More than one metastatic deposit does not entirely rule out a role for surgical resection, but the circumstances in which this approach would be used are limited.[80] The role of surgery for brain metastases is usually confined to the fewer than 5 percent of breast cancer patients whose metastases are solitary and surgically approachable and preferably, who have no apparent metastases outside the CNS and no evidence of leptomeningeal involvement.[7, 80] If there is other metastatic disease outside the CNS, surgery may be considered if the disease is inactive or responds to systemic therapy. Other considerations are performance status and age. Patients with a Karnofsky performance status of 70 or better, and patients aged 60 or younger are more likely to have favorable outcomes after a surgical approach. In several series of patients undergoing resection of brain metastases from a variety of tumor types, those with breast cancer did better in general than the group as a whole.[13, 14, 19] A randomized trial of therapy for patients with brain metastases is rare, but such an approach was used for 48 patients who were randomized for either removal of the lesion followed by radiation therapy or stereotaxic needle biopsy followed by radiation for solitary brain metastases from a

variety of solid tumors (three from breast cancer).[74] Overall survival in the surgically treated patients averaged 40 weeks, versus 15 weeks for patients who received radiation only. In addition to increased survival, surgical treatment achieved better local control of the metastases and patients' quality of life was better. The operative mortality rate—defined as death within 30 days of surgery—was 4 percent in the resection group. This result was the same as the 30-day mortality rate for in the radiation-only group.

Results are also available from a second randomized trial that compared surgery followed by radiation therapy with radiation therapy alone for solitary brain metastasis.[70] Median survival was 10 months versus 6 months, in favor of the patients who had resection of the metastasis. Of the 63 evaluable patients with solid tumors contributing to this report, 12 had a diagnosis of breast cancer. This study confirmed that patients with active extracranial disease are poor candidates for surgery, and survival was no different when the treatment was radiation therapy alone. In this trial, age was a strong prognostic factor. For patients older than 60 years, the hazard ratio of dying was 2.74 ($P = .0030$). For these patients, stereotaxically directed, high-intensity external-beam radiation ("radiosurgery") may be a preferable alternative to surgery.

Because occult CNS metastases are likely to accompany documented solitary metastases, whole-brain irradiation is usually given after surgical removal of the solitary lesion.[7, 19, 48] Another source of residual disease is tumor left at the margins of resection.[7, 19] Postcraniotomy autopsy series have shown the continued presence of tumor at the margins of resection in 25 percent to 42 percent of cases when death occurred within 30 days of supposed complete surgical resection. In one case series, 25 breast cancer patients with solitary metastases who underwent surgical removal followed by radiation therapy had a mean survival time of 28 months.[87] Nine similar patients who had only surgical excision of their metastases without subsequent radiation therapy had mean survival of only 15 months, and their disease courses were characterized by a higher rate of intracranial relapse. Another series found a 21 percent brain relapse rate with irradiation, as compared with a relapse rate of 85 percent when surgery alone was used.[95] The same pattern was observed in another series of 98 patients who had a single brain metastasis: patients who received radiation had a median survival of 21 months, 6 months longer than their counterparts who did not receive radiation.[28] In view of the extended survival, the authors suggested a potential benefit from hyperfractionation of the whole-brain radiation, which might minimize delayed neurotoxicity. The results from these two series indicate longer survival, as compared with earlier studies in which the reported median survival for surgery and radiation was 9 to 12 months.[19, 81, 103] Of course, any apparent improvement observed in unrandomized series could well be the result of patient selection and other sources of bias.

Although as many as 90 percent of patients may report symptomatic improvement after combined surgery and postoperative whole-brain irradiation, many authors have noted a high risk of recurrence in the brain.[22] Sundaresan and Galicich noted that, of eight breast cancer patients who underwent surgery, six had a solitary metastasis, and five of these six suffered relapse in the CNS within 2 years of craniotomy and radiation therapy.[103] In a series of 21 patients with stable systemic disease who underwent repeat craniotomy for recurrence of metastatic disease, median survival after the second procedure was 9 months.[104] Recurrence of a solitary lesion involved the original site in 14 of 21 patients.

In addition to resection of individual lesions and biopsy to confirm diagnosis, CNS metastases provide several other indications for surgery. These include rapid relief of symptoms from mass effect in emergency circumstances. Occasionally surgical placement of a ventricular shunt is necessary when obstructive hydrocephalus is present in a candidate for surgical reversal of the obstruction.[103] Also, if meningeal carcinomatosis is evident, the placement of an Ommaya reservoir may be indicated for delivery of chemotherapy.[82]

Increases in survival associated with surgical excision of a solitary metastasis have provoked debate about what constitutes appropriate therapy for a single brain metastasis. A less invasive approach to treating solitary metastases involves the use of stereotaxic radiosurgery. Usually performed on an outpatient basis, radiosurgery often reaches lesions that are surgically inaccessible. In a retrospective analysis of 248 consecutive patients treated with radiosurgery, the median overall survival from the time of treatment was a little over 9 months.[2] It was concluded that radiosurgery was not as effective as surgery (both followed by whole brain irradiation) for controlling brain metastases. The benefits of radiosurgery are also limited by systemic disease and age. In an overlapping report covering 300 patients treated with radiosurgery, survival was decreased in the presence of active systemic disease (relative risk of mortality 4.43, $p = .0001$) and age over 60 (relative risk 1.618, $p = .002$).[63]

Once the management questions are settled with regard to corticosteroids, mannitol, diphenylhydantoin, surgery, and radiosurgery (as described above), the last remaining issue is radiation therapy, including the appropriate dose and schedule. In the United States, the standard treatment schedule for patients with brain metastases is 30 Gy in 10 fractions over 2 weeks, *or* less commonly, 20 Gy in five fractions over 1 week.[22] Most patients with multiple brain metastases receive whole-brain irradiation. Patients with a solitary brain metastasis who are treated with whole-brain irradiation have been treated with a boost of an additional 5 to 10 Gy to the lesion[7, 38, 48]; however, the benefit of this practice is debatable. From a series of 164 consecutive patients who received cranial irradiation amounting to 35 Gy in 15 daily fractions, there were 50 patients with solitary

metastases who received a boost of 15 Gray in eight daily fractions.[51] No difference in overall survival was observed between the patients who received the boost and those who did not.

In the mid 1970s, a National Cooperative Study sponsored by the Radiation Therapy Oncology Group (RTOG) evaluated more than 1000 patients with a variety of metastatic intracerebral metastases for the effects of different schedules and doses of radiation therapy steroids and chemotherapy, and of primary tumor site and status.[48] Hendrickson's review of the results concluded that a total of 3000 rad delivered to the whole brain given in 10 or 15 fractions was equal to 4000 rad in 15 or 20 fractions. There were no differences in median survival or in the proportion of patients with symptomatic improvement. Headaches or convulsions resolved completely in 55 percent and 67 percent, respectively, whereas no more than 15 percent were unchanged or had worsening of these symptoms. Impaired mentation and motor loss were completely resolved in approximately a third of the patients, and partially resolved in 40 percent. For patients with multiple intracranial metastases, whole-brain irradiation is associated with extension of survival for an average of 3 to 6 months.[79] Efforts to enhance the effectiveness of radiation therapy with radiosensitizers have generally been unsuccessful.[34] Cranial irradiation is associated with a number of early side effects, including desquamation of skin, hair loss, and somnolence.[22] For long-term survivors, severe radiation dementia may be observed (prevalence up to 5 percent).[27]

Intercurrent systemic chemotherapy is advocated for patients with brain metastases and evidence of active extra-CNS systemic disease. Failure to control extra-CNS disease may often be the rate-limiting factor for survival. Other chapters in this text outline the use of chemotherapy that can yield a 40 percent to 70 percent response rate in previously untreated metastatic breast cancer. However, since chemotherapy does not cross the blood-brain barrier in therapeutic amounts, it is not likely to prevent CNS relapse.

Once intracranial metastases have developed, the lesions are characterized by various degrees of disruption to the blood-brain barrier, a circumstance that may facilitate a response to chemotherapy. Although a number of reports describe the responsiveness to chemotherapy of breast cancer metastatic to brain, many of the reports are difficult to interpret because of intercurrent use of radiation therapy. Rosner and colleagues reported the results for a series of 100 patients, most of whom were treated with a combination of cyclophosphamide, 5-fluorouracil, plus prednisone *or* methotrexate.[85] In this series, 23 patients received—and failed to respond to—radiation therapy. Among the 100 patients, 50 responded to chemotherapy, 10 completely. These results suggests that chemotherapy might have a role in treating brain metastases, which do not respond to radiation therapy.

There are many case reports on the responsiveness

to endocrine therapy for brain metastases from breast cancer. Responses to tamoxifen, megestrol acetate, and bromocriptine have been described.* Being lipophilic drugs, tamoxifen and its metabolites do not depend on the disruption of the blood-brain barrier for entry into brain tissue. For brain tumors derived from hormone-responsive primary breast lesions, agents like tamoxifen may be a secondary tool that can be used to advantage in selected patients. The fact that patients with brain metastases are more likely to have ER-negative primary tumors limits this approach.[102]

Recurrence of symptomatic metastases after radiation of the brain is not uncommon (prevalence 5 percent in the RTOG national study and as high as 83 percent in other studies).[31, 48] Retreatment may still be possible. However, CNS metastases were the primary cause of death in 60 percent of the patients who had recurrence.[31, 99] Median survival following re-treatment may be 8 to 14 weeks.[47, 59] At some centers, patients have been re-treated as many as two or three times.[93] With retreatment, the risk of brain necrosis is elevated.[59]

Prognosis

Although survival after the diagnosis of brain metastases is relatively limited, relief of neurological symptoms to improve quality of remaining life is a realistic goal. Rapid improvement in symptoms may be seen in as many as 90 percent of patients after administration of corticosteroids. Sustained improvement with extension of survival by several months is associated with cranial irradiation. Longer-term survival is possible for patients with solitary lesions in the setting of quiescent systemic disease.

Leptomeninges

As with both childhood and some adult leukemias, leptomeningeal involvement appears to be increasing in frequency in association with breast cancer.[7, 62, 79] Metastatic involvement of the leptomeninges has been found in approximately 6 percent of breast cancer patients at autopsy.[108, 112] Solitary leptomeningeal metastases are rare; Tsukada's group found only three cases in 309 patients with CNS metastases (1044 breast cancer patients in all).[108] Of 59 patients found at autopsy to have leptomeningeal involvement, 32 had had symptoms, whereas none of the three patients with solitary meningeal spread did. About one third of breast cancer patients with symptomatic intracranial metastases also have intercurrent leptomeningeal metastases.[37, 108] In this situation, both areas require medical attention.

Diagnosis

Leptomeningeal carcinomatosis is the widespread dissemination of cancer in the subarachnoid space, which can occur as a diffuse process, or with multifo-

cal seeding.[39, 62, 71] Since this spread may occur microscopically, asymptomatic disease may be found at necropsy.[108] The lag time from initial diagnosis of breast cancer to diagnosis of leptomeningeal metastases ranges in the literature from 3 months to 17 years.[71, 117]

Leptomeningeal spread of breast cancer usually presents with signs and symptoms similar to those of intracranial metastases, but with additional symptoms and signs of cranial neuropathies or of spinal root compression.[62, 71, 117] Although headache is the most common presenting complaint, only about a third of patients report it at diagnosis and only about 50 percent at any time during the course of the illness. Global symptoms of hydrocephalus can occur as a result of tumor obstruction of CSF circulation.[79] Meningeal carcinomatosis can also extend to involve the parenchyma of the brain, nerve roots within the spinal canal, or the parenchyma of the spinal cord.[52] In this way neurological symptoms that originate in the neuroaxis may be produced by a variety of mechanisms. Cranial neuropathies or lower motor neuron signs (i.e., facial paralysis or urinary incontinence) may be caused by invasion of the nerves in the subarachnoid space. Focal neurological problems such as seizures or hemiplegia can arise from direct invasion of the brain parenchyma or disruption of circulation normally provided by pial blood vessels. Central hypoventilation has also been described as a consequence of meningeal spread of breast cancer.[65]

Posner, in a review of patients with various types of primary cancer, states "the diagnosis of meningeal carcinomatosis is suggested by the fact that patients have neurological symptoms or signs of either widespread or multifocal invasion of the neuroaxis rather than a single focal lesion."[79] The physician should be especially aware of the potential for metastases to the leptomeninges in breast cancer patients who have other CNS metastases or vertebral body metastases and multifocal symptoms. Nuchal rigidity, pain in the back or neck, lower extremity weakness, decreased deep tendon reflexes, or other spinal root signs are often present, and as many as 55 percent of patients demonstrate extensor plantar response, poor attention span, diplopia, or papilledema. The cranial nerves are involved in 78 percent of these patients at presentation and in 94 percent during the course of the illness. Most frequently involved is the constellation of III, IV, VI (46 percent at presentation, 70 percent during the course of illness), followed by VII (42 percent and 44 percent) and VIII (30 percent and 38 percent), although involvement of each of the cranial nerves has been reported.[71] Dysarthria and gait abnormalities are occasionally seen in these patients.[62, 71, 113]

The diagnosis of leptomeningeal carcinomatosis is confirmed by the finding of malignant cells in CSF but is not excluded by their absence.[37] Multiple lumbar punctures may be necessary to detect malignant cells. In one series, the diagnosis was established in 82 of 90 patients by the third lumbar puncture.[113] However, in most instances there is at least one of

---

*See references 17, 23, 41, 77, 88, 101, and 110.

the following abnormalities: elevated CSF pressure (over 150 mm H_2O in 64 of 90 patients); an increased number of white blood cells (65 of 90 patients, more than 5 cells/mm³ predominantly lymphocytes); elevated CSF protein level (above 50 mg/dl in 80 of 90 patients) or decreased CSF glucose (less than 40 mg/100 mL in 37 of 90 patients).[113] In two separate series, only one of 137 different CSF samples was completely normal (including chemistry analysis, cell count, and cytologic analysis), in patients ultimately proven to have leptomeningeal carcinomatosis.[71, 113] Measurement of CSF concentration of carcinoembryonic antigen (CEA) is possible, but its role in diagnosis and management of meningeal carcinomatosis of metastatic breast cancer is unclear.[72, 113, 115]

In Tsukada's group's autopsy series of 1044 breast cancer patients, 17 of 59 cases of leptomeningeal metastases were not clinically suspected ante mortem.[108] Intracerebral metastases frequently are found on brain CT in patients with leptomeningeal metastases. CT findings of hydrocephalus or of contrast enhancement of the basal cisterns or cerebral sulci suggest leptomeningeal spread; however, CT is not capable of demonstrating microscopic spread of metastases into the leptomeninges. Unlike contrast-enhanced CT scanning, gadolinium-enhanced MRI is able to demonstrate the diffuse abnormalities associated with meningeal carcinomatosis. In a group of 30 patients with leptomeningeal disease, MRI with gadolinium showed enhancement of the inner table of the skull in two thirds.[107]

Myelography occasionally indicates concomitant extradural spinal cord spread. In one series of various types of carcinomatous meningitis, 7 of 18 patients had multiple nodular defects noted on nerve roots later confirmed at laminectomy to be metastases.[71] Although electroencephalography is not diagnostically useful, it has been performed in a series of patients with leptomeningeal carcinomatosis from various primary cancers. Seventy-five percent of these studies were abnormal: the predominant finding was nonspecific diffuse slow waves.[108, 113]

Management

The treatment of leptomeningeal carcinomatosis is directed at preventing further neurological deterioration and possibly reversing evolving signs and symptoms. Once metastatic disease has caused a deficit, complete reversal with therapy is rare.[79] Indeed, even in the occasional patient with carcinomatous meningitis who survives more than 2.5 years after intensive therapy, post mortem examination frequently discloses persistent metastatic leptomeningeal involvement. Untreated patients usually succumb within 6 weeks of diagnosis.[62, 71, 113] However, length of survival may not be substantively related to treatment. Some data suggest that the perceived benefit of treatment is confounded by the factors used to select patients for intervention.[10, 98]

When intracranial metastases are suspected but the symptoms also indicate leptomeningeal carcinomatosis, the intracranial lesions are addressed first. Until diagnostic imaging is completed, lumbar puncture is avoided when brain metastases are suspected because of the potential for cerebral herniation. When it has been determined radiographically that a patient has brain metastases, elevated intracranial pressure must be controlled before lumbar puncture can be performed. Also, when papilledema is present 72 hours of dexamethasone therapy is given before lumbar puncture. If leptomeningeal carcinomatosis is then confirmed, some groups treat intracranial metastases using radiation intercurrently with intraventricular chemotherapy for carcinomatous meningitis.[94]

If there is no evidence of brain parenchymal metastases on CT or MRI and papilledema is absent, then the diagnostic work-up for leptomeningeal disease may proceed in the usual way.

A variety of treatments for leptomeningeal carcinomatosis have been reported[67]; none have been compared in controlled trials. The entire neuroaxis must be treated to effect long-term control of symptomatic disease.[113] Because myelosuppression results from irradiation of the entire craniospinal axis, it is recommended that only the site of primary neurological symptoms receive radiation in patients who are receiving chemotherapy (e.g., whole-brain ports for cranial neuropathies). The usual dose of radiation is 3000 to 4000 rad.[117] The remainder of the neuroaxis is then treated with intrathecal or intraventricular (via Ommaya reservoir) administration of methotrexate, 12 mg twice weekly via lumbar intrathecal route or 6.25 mg/m² (12 mg maximum) if given via Ommaya in preservative-free 0.9 percent saline.[79] At some institutions, oral leucovorin is given routinely after each intraventricular methotrexate treatment.[94] Another approach is to give leucovorin only if bone marrow suppression occurs after methotrexate therapy.[10]

The decision to place an Ommaya reservoir is usually contingent on an acceptable prognosis and functional status of the individual patient.[82, 117] Central instillation through the Ommaya reservoir permits more thorough exposure of the meningeal surfaces to methotrexate and allows intermittent therapeutic drug monitoring to ensure adequate therapeutic levels of methotrexate and avoidance of toxic CNS levels as well as weekly cytologic assessment of CSF.[8, 9, 82, 92] When malignant cells are cleared from the CSF and symptoms have abated, the interval between doses lengthens until maintenance methotrexate is given about once a month.[79, 117] Should evidence of progressive leptomeningeal disease occur during the therapeutic course, despite confirmation of adequate methotrexate levels at the site of meningeal disease, cytosine arabinoside, 50 mg/m² twice weekly, or thiotepa, 10 mg total, may be substituted for methotrexate.[8, 9, 44]

Administration of methotrexate via repetitive lumbar punctures fails to deliver drug to the subarachnoid space in 5 percent to 10 percent of treatments, reaching instead the subepidural or epidural space.[92]

Furthermore, it has been noted that neoplastic meningitis results in disordered CSF circulation,[43, 69] even in the absence of extradural blockage, with the consequence that the physician may be delivering a subtherapeutic (below 10^{-6} mg/L) dose of methotrexate to the field of neoplastic meningeal involvement. Consequently in patients with leptomeningeal carcinomatosis whose prognosis is potentially good, methotrexate should be given via Ommaya reservoir.

To improve the management of patients with carcinomatous meningitis, efforts to optimize the use of intraventricular chemotherapy remain a focus of research. In a randomized comparison of methotrexate and thiotepa for a series of 52 patients (25 with a breast cancer diagnosis) not previously treated for carcinomatous meningitis, these drugs, as single agents, were found to be comparable in efficacy and toxicity.[42] In another randomized trial that examined the use of methotrexate alone versus the combination of methotrexate and cytosine arabinoside, results favored the single agent but the difference in response to therapy was not statistically significant.[50] However, several series have demonstrated that dose-limiting myelosuppression is more likely to be a problem when combination intraventricular chemotherapy is employed.[35, 109]

The response to treatment depends on the status of the patient's extra-CNS disease and the level of neurological function or degree of deficits prior to therapy.[116] Durable results are most often observed in patients who are diagnosed early in the course of their meningeal disease and who can tolerate combined therapy. It is uncommon for the leptomeninges to be the only site of progressive metastatic disease, and effective systemic treatment of breast cancer is necessary but not sufficient for extended survival. In two series of breast cancer patients, treated for leptomeningeal disease as outlined previously, the overall response rate was approximately 65 percent and median survival for responders was 4.5 to 7.2 (range 1 to 29) months. Nonresponders succumb (median survival of 1 month), generally, to CNS disease, whereas approximately half of responders die as a result of extra-CNS disease.[71, 113] The overall survival at 1 year in treated patients is only about 10 to 15 percent.[71, 113, 116]

Several toxicities can be associated with treatment. The use of combined whole-brain irradiation and intraventricular methotrexate may rarely result in brain necrosis or multifocal leukoencephalopathy. Also, occasional marrow suppression is reported with methotrexate but is reversible with folinic acid. More commonly, intrathecal (via lumbar puncture) or intraventricular (via Ommaya reservoir) methotrexate therapy results in aseptic meningitis or arachnoiditis. Except in accomplished and experienced hospitals, the rate of complications with insertion and maintenance of the Ommaya device is approximately 20 percent. Though usually mild, complications can include infections or catheter migration, either of which can produce new neurological signs.[113]

Prognosis

When leptomeningeal metastases from breast cancer cause severe neurological signs, there is less chance of extended survival. Since the benefit of treatment is unclear, investigational studies could help to improve the care of breast cancer patients with leptomeningeal carcinomatosis.

Spinal Cord

In a number of series, lung cancer and breast cancer are the two most common causes of symptomatic spinal cord compression.[6, 16, 24, 36] The true incidence of spinal cord metastases in breast cancer is not known, as no studies have studied post mortem spinal cords systematically in a large cohort of breast cancer patients. Thus, information is not available on the frequency of asymptomatic breast cancer with metastases to the spinal cord. In Tsukada's series, the cord was examined only when clinical symptoms were referrable to that site; 32 cases of spinal cord metastases were found among 96 cords examined; eight were found to be the sole site of CNS involvement.[108] Seventy-five percent of spinal cord metastases were associated with metastases in other CNS sites. In Barron and colleagues' analysis of 127 necropsied cases of symptomatic involvement of the spinal cord and cauda equina by a variety of metastatic neoplasms, there were 20 cases of metastatic breast cancer.[6] Their review of all cases of breast cancer at autopsy at Montefiore Hospital indicated an incidence of 6.5 percent metastatic involvement of the spinal cord and its dura. Compiling several series has shown up to a 12 percent incidence of cord metastases from breast cancer.[1, 6, 108]

Posner reports that more than 97 percent of metastatic disease affecting the spinal cord is extradural.[79] Edelson and colleagues series further substantiates the rarity of metastatic intramedullary disease.[33] Batson described the important role of the plexus of veins around the vertebral bodies, with their anastomoses to the dural sinuses in metastasis to the CNS, in association with vertebral body disease. In Barron's group's 20 cases of breast cancer metastatic to the spinal cord, he noted the following four characteristics[6]:

1. Carcinoma of the breast was always an established diagnosis at the time of spinal cord disease.
2. The median duration of pain was often longer than with other carcinomas metastatic to the cord; however, once neurological signs were present, progression to hemiparesis or hemiplegia was rapid.
3. The onset of spinal cord metastases in breast cancer typically came late in the course of disease.
4. In patients with back pain, myelographic abnormalities, and breast cancer, the plain films of the spine were usually (94 percent) abnormal.

Diagnosis

Early diagnosis of extradural metastatic tumor tests the skills of every physician who treats these patients. Although breast cancer patients may have pain secondary to a benign musculoskeletal problem, back pain can also be the first indication of metastasis to a vertebral body or spinal epidural space.[6, 16, 24, 79] Extremely variable in onset, spinal cord compression has been reported to occur up to 19 years after the original diagnosis.[36] Despite advances in other aspects of oncology, the prognosis of patients with neurological impairment from extradural spinal cord compression has remained static over the past several decades.[24, 78] Irreversible paraplegia occurs in approximately one third of cancer patients with spinal cord compression.[36] Patients who could not walk before treatment rarely walk again.[6, 16, 24, 36] Knowing this, the physician must diagnose compressive metastatic tumor in the early stage of back pain and when there is minimal or no neurological deficit. Once suspected, the diagnosis of spinal cord compression must be pursued until it is either confirmed or excluded. An algorithmic approach follows.[78]

Metastatic breast cancer reaches the epidural space, leading to compression of the spinal cord by invading the vertebral body or growing directly into the spinal canal or growing from the paravertebral gutter through the intravertebral foramina.[24, 79] Also, tumor deposits in the subarachnoid space may occur via hematogenous spread or seeding of the CSF via leptomeningeal metastases. All mechanisms are important, and in the latter two instances it should be noted that plain roentgenograms and radionuclide scans will likely be normal. No more than 3 percent of cord compression syndromes in cancer patients result from intramedullary metastases.[24, 33] Intervertebral discs are rarely involved unless extension from adjacent osseous metastases is present.[40]

Localized back pain, by far the most common early symptom, lasts weeks to months and is present in 90 percent to 95 percent of patients who are ultimately found to have epidural spinal cord compression (ESCC).[6, 24, 36, 78, 79] The pain may have a radicular component and is commonly exacerbated by recumbency, movement, coughing, or Valsalva's maneuver. Once neurological signs other than local pain begin, development of other deficits often follows quickly (often within days).[79]

The cord level of disease affects the presentation. In Barron's group's series of 127 patients with various types of cancer metastatic to the cord (of which breast cancer was the second most prevalent type), 14 of 14 patients with cervical spine ESCC presented with pain.[6] Thoracic cord involvement, when painful, is usually central, not radiating or bandlike.[6, 36] However, 37 percent of patients with thoracic spine ESCC presented without back pain.[6] This latter group often presented with paraplegia or paraparesis. Patients with cauda equina metastases commonly present with severe pain sometimes of months' duration and radiating into one or both legs, with late development of sphincter disturbances. In contrast, sphincter disturbance in the absence of radiculopathy is characteristic of conus medullaris lesions.[6, 78] A benign condition such as herpes zoster or herniated nucleus pulposus can mimic malignant cord compression. When myelography discloses ESCC at the level of an intervertebral disc without neighboring vertebral body disease, more confirmatory evidence of metastatic ESCC may be needed. Metastases to the intervertebral disc space are rare, and patients so affected are also at risk for benign processes such as extradural abscess or herniation of the nucleus pulposus.[40] Radiation therapy is clearly not the best treatment for these processes.

Plain films of the painful area should always be performed in a patient with breast cancer and focal or radicular back pain. A routine roentgenogram of the spine correctly predicts the presence or absence of epidural solid tumor in more than 80 percent of cases and is more specific than bone scintigraphy.[46, 78, 83] Moreover, a negative plain film in a patient with a normal neurological examination virtually eliminates (0 of 20 patients in Rodichok and colleagues' series) spinal epidural metastases as the cause of back pain in a patient with a solid tumor.[78, 83, 99]

Traditionally, the diagnosis of cord compression has been made with myelography.[6, 16, 36, 78, 79, 83] Myelography is useful not only for diagnosis but also for defining the extent of cord compression.[36, 79, 83, 84, 99] The degree of myelographic block (i.e., more than or less than 75 percent) also reflects the prognosis, the higher degree of block corresponding to a 93 percent chance of myelopathy. One impediment to myelography is a complete block that prevents cephalad passage of the contrast material from the lumbar injection site. In this instance, imaging of the upper boundary of the lesion is accomplished with cisternal puncture. After myelography, contrast is left in the thecal sac to enable assessment of the response to therapy.

As an adjunct to myelography, CT with contrast provides accurate detail about the presence of epidural masses and their relationship to surrounding structures. CT can be useful in case of plexopathy as an initial study to evaluate soft tissue metastases and the paravertebral gutter. When CT demonstrates a vertebral lesion or paraspinal mass, follow-up with MRI is indicated.

In many institutions the diagnosis of cord compression is established with MRI rather than myelography. MRI is very accurate, and the quality of imaging has improved since the earliest studies applied this technique to diagnosis and assessment of epidural metastases.[15, 45, 58] In recent years, MRI has been accepted as close to ideal for investigating metastatic spinal lesions.[76] It affords direct, noninvasive, full-length imaging of the cord with remarkable detail.[114] With a single study, MRI provides information comparable to what previous efforts to upgrade the findings from conventional myelography achieved by adding contrast CT to produce CT myelography.[73] In a direct comparison of MRI and myelography for assessing spinal cord compression, the sensitivity and specificity of MRI were found to be 0.92 and 0.90, respectively, as compared with 0.95 and 0.88 for the sensitivity and specificity of myelography.[18]

For epidural lesions that did not cause cord compression, MRI had sensitivity and specificity of 0.73 and 0.90, as compared with 0.49 and 0.88 for myelography. On the basis of this comparison, the authors concluded that MRI is an acceptable alternative to myelography.

Management

The appropriate treatment for any spinal cord compression depends on the type of primary tumor, the level of the block, the rapidity of onset, and the degree of block. Patients present with symptoms ranging from localized back pain to full-blown myelopathy, and a method of determining urgency is helpful. A useful system has been outlined by Portenoy and associates.[78] Three different degrees of myelopathy are associated with different levels of urgency. The initial evaluation and the three algorithms are illustrated in Figures 76–1 through 76–4.

Patients with new or progressing signs of ESCC, such as ascending numbness, paraparesis, or sphincter disturbance are in category I (see Fig. 76–2). This evaluation proceeds as a response to a medical emergency. The recommended approach is intravenous injection of 100 mg of dexamethasone before emergency myelography. In the presence of bone lesions without evidence of cord involvement, the lesion could be treated with local radiotherapy or with systemic therapy and analgesics.

Category II (Fig. 76–3) includes patients with evidence of stable or mild ESCC or radiculopathy or plexopathy without evidence of ESCC, which requires prompt evaluation (24 to 48 hours). When signs or symptoms of ESCC are absent, plexopathy may obscure the diagnosis of intercurrent radiculopathy or paraspinal mass. Patients with plexopathy may be evaluated with either CT or MRI. If a bony lesion of epidural mass is detected on CT, definitive imaging with MRI is indicated.

Patients who present with back pain and no evi-

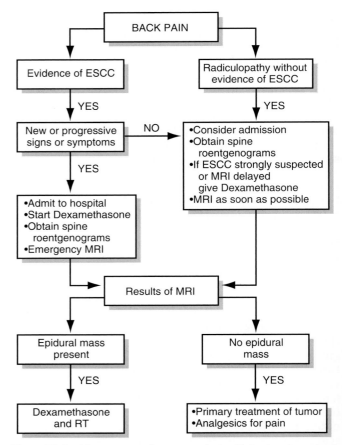

Figure 76–2 *Management of cancer patient with back pain and evidence of ESCC or radiculopathy. (Adapted from Portenoy RK, et al: Neurology 37:135, 1987. Reprinted with permission.)*

dence of neurological deficit (category III) may undergo nonemergent evaluation as outpatients. The approach to these patients, however, must be prompt and directed at ruling out ESCC. Plain roentgenograms of the painful vertebral areas, including oblique areas, should be obtained initially (Fig. 76–4). In breast cancer, bone abnormalities on plain films corresponding to the symptomatic site very likely represent epidural disease. If, based on historical characteristics of the patient's pain, suspicion remains high, despite a normal plain film, CT of the vertebrae in the symptomatic area may be indicated.

As summarizzed above, the patient who presents with a history of new or progressing signs or symptoms of ESCC has the criteria for category I (Fig. 76–2). As outlined, treatment would begin immediately using dexamethasone. In a randomized comparison of 100 mg and of 10 mg of dexamethasone as an initial intravenous bolus for patients with ESCC, no differences could be determined with respect to pain, ambulation, or bladder function.[111] The initial bolus is followed by doses of 16 mg per day given in four doses until the necessary diagnostic procedures have been accomplished. If an epidural lesion is identified, dexamethasone is then given orally and tapered over the course of the radiation therapy. Radiation ther-

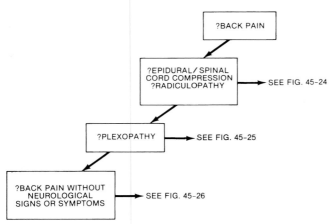

Figure 76–1 *Initial evaluation of back pain in the cancer patient. (From Portenoy RK, et al: Neurology 37:135, 1987. Reprinted with permission.)*

apy and dexamethasone are the standard therapeutic measures for most breast cancer patients with metastatic ESCC.[36, 79, 99] Breast cancer is a moderately radiosensitive tumor. A commonly recommended regimen is 400 rad per day for 3 days followed by 200 rad daily to a total dose of 3000 to 4000 rad.[54, 79] However, with the antiedema effects of corticosteroids, others report that it is not necessary to give the first few doses at higher fractionation.[16, 54, 55] Using radiotherapy and dexamethasone alone in breast cancer ESCC, approximately 50 percent of patients respond (as defined by preservation or restoration of neurological function for at least 4 weeks).[5, 36, 54, 99] Prognosis is determined primarily by severity and rapidity of onset of motor dysfunction, again emphasizing the need for prompt diagnosis and therapy.[5, 16, 54, 99] In one series, the response to high-dose dexamethasone was seen to have prognostic value, in that 67 percent of patients with various primary tumors who had an objective response to steroids, improved with radiotherapy.[5]

Current indications for surgical decompression include a lesion in a posterior site in the canal, progression of signs during or after radiation therapy, recurrence in an area previously irradiated heavily, and severe vertebral body instability.[5, 16, 24, 32, 36, 99] It has been suggested that, for the subgroup of patients who are not ambulatory at presentation, restoration

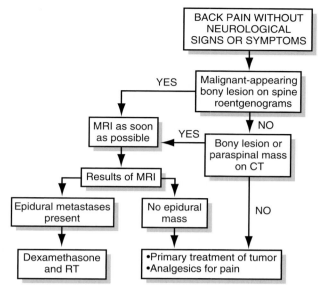

Figure 76–4 *Management of cancer patient with back pain and no neurological signs or symptoms. (Adapted from Portenoy RK, et al: Neurology 37:137, 1987. Reprinted with permission.)*

to ambulatory status is more likely if they are treated with both laminectomy and radiotherapy.[97] This result, however, may reflect a selection bias. After surgical decompression, radiation should be given to any patient who has not previously received radiation to the area, as complete resection of tumor is virtually never possible. Added radiation is intended to decrease the risk of local recurrence.[24, 32, 36, 68, 99]

Although the median survival time for breast cancer patients with ESCC may be on the order of 4 months, the length of survival may be related to the status of extra-CNS disease.[49] Consequently, the option of systemic therapy should be considered when that is appropriate. There have been case reports of resolution of spinal epidural metastases in breast cancer patients treated with chemotherapy and/or hormone therapy.[11] For patients who have not been heavily pretreated with chemotherapy or whose epidural disease is not responsive to radiation therapy, systemic therapy should be considered.

Prognosis

There are few situations in oncology in which rapid diagnosis and treatment enhance therapeutic benefits as much as in spinal cord compression. Undiagnosed and untreated, the consequences are devastating. Although there are no randomized prospective trials comparing surgical decompression and radiation therapy with radiation therapy alone, retrospective analysis indicates that both short- and long-term outcomes for the two approaches are very similar.[5, 6, 24, 32, 36, 99] As outlined previously, however, there are specific indications for surgical decompression followed by radiation.

In two trials of radiation therapy in patients with a variety of primary cancers, patients with tumors

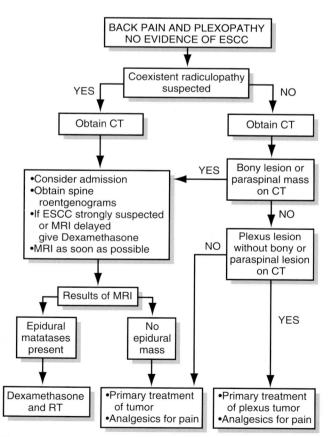

Figure 76–3 *Management of cancer patient with suspected plexopathy. (Adapted from Portenoy RK, et al: Neurology 37:136, 1987. Reprinted with permission.)*

considered radiosensitive (including breast cancer, in 181 of 730 cases) had a favorable response (ability to ambulate) in 47 percent to 67 percent of cases.[24, 36] Pretreatment neurological status grade (ambulatory, paraparetic, paraplegic) also has a profound influence on outcome. Patients who were ambulatory before treatment remained ambulatory in 79 percent of cases; those who were paraparetic remained or regained complete ambulatory ability in 34 percent of cases; and paraplegic patients had no full recovery of ambulation.[5, 6, 16, 32, 54, 99] These results are qualitatively similar to those from smaller trials of breast cancer patients only. In two series involving a total of 126 breast cancer patients with ESCC, patients who were walking before therapy maintained ambulation after therapy in 96 percent to 97 percent of cases.[49, 64] For patients who were unable to walk before receiving therapy, 45 percent to 69 percent regained ambulation. Hill and colleagues noted that the most important predictor of survival in their series was the patients' ability to walk after treatment.[49] In the Italian series, those who could walk after treatment had a 66 percent chance of surviving 1 year, as compared with 10 percent for "nonwalking" patients.[64]

As with other metastatic tumors, overall survival is not significantly affected by local therapy. However, relieving the signs and symptoms of this complication and preventing paraplegia or reversing paraparesis are important goals for the physician.

References

1. Abrams HL, Spiro R, Goldstein N: Metastases in carcinoma: Analysis of 1000 autopsied cases. Cancer 3:74–85, 1950.
2. Alexander E, Moriarty TM, Davis RB, et al: Stereotactic radiosurgery for the definitive, noninvasive treatment of brain metastases. J Natl Cancer Inst 87:34–40, 1995.
3. Baker HL, Houser OW, Campbell JK: National Cancer Institute study: Evaluation of computed tomography in the diagnosis of intracranial neoplasms. Radiology 136:91–96, 1980.
4. Balis FM, Lester CM, Chrousos GP, et al: Differences in cerebrospinal fluid penetration of corticosteroids: Possible relationship to the prevention of meningeal leukemia. J Clin Oncol 5:202–207, 1987.
5. Barcena A, Lobato RD, Rivas JJ, et al: Spinal metastatic disease: Analysis of factors determining functional prognosis and the choice of treatment. Neurosurgery 15:820–827, 1984.
6. Barron KD, Hirona A, Araki S, et al: Experiences with metastatic neoplasms involving the spinal cord. Neurology 9:91–106, 1959.
7. Black P: Brain metastasis: Current status and recommended guidelines for management. Neurosurgery 5:5:617–631, 1979.
8. Blasberg RG: Methotrexate cytosine arabinoside, and BCNU concentration in brain after ventriculocisternal perfusion. Cancer Treat Rep 61:625–631, 1977.
9. Blasberg RG, Patlak CS, Shapiro WR: Distribution of methotrexate in the cerebrospinal fluid and brain after intraventricular administration. Cancer Treat Rep 61:633–641, 1977.
10. Boogerd W, Hart AAM, van der Sande JJ, et al: Meningeal carcinomatosis in breast cancer: Prognostic factors and influence of treatment. Cancer 67:1685–1695, 1991.
11. Boogerd W, van der Sande JJ, Kroger R, et al: Effective systemic therapy for spinal epidural metastases from breast carcinoma. Eur J Cancer Clin Oncol 25:149–153, 1989.
12. Boogerd W, Vos VW, Hart AAM, et al: Brain metastases in breast cancer; natural history, prognostic factors and outcome. J Neuro-Oncol 15:165–174, 1993.
13. Borgelt B, Gelber R, Kramer S, et al: Final results of the first two studies by the Radiation Therapy Oncology Group. Int J Radiat Oncol Biol Phys 6:1–19, 1980.
14. Borgelt B, Gelber R, Larson D, et al: Ultra-rapid high dose irradiation schedules for the palliation of brain metastases: Final results of the first two studies by the Radiation Therapy Oncology Group. Int J Radiat Oncol Biol Phys 7:1633–1638, 1981.
15. Bosley TM, Cohen DA, Schatz NJ, et al: Comparison of metrizamide computed tomography and magnetic resonance imaging in the evaluation of lesions at the cervicomedullary junction. Neurology 35:485–492, 1985.
16. Bruckman JE, Bloomer WD: Management of spinal cord compression. Semin Oncol 5:135–140, 1978.
17. Carey RW, Davis JM, Servas NT: Tamoxifen-induced regression of cerebral metastases in breast carcinoma. Cancer Treat Rep 65:793–795, 1981.
18. Carmody RF, Yang PJ, Seeley GW, et al: Spinal cord compression due to metastatic disease: Diagnosis with MR imaging versus myelography. Radiology 173:225–229, 1989.
19. Chan RC, Steinbok P: Solitary cerebral metastasis: The effect of craniotomy on the quality and duration of survival. Neurosurgery 11:254–257, 1982.
20. Cohen N, Strauss G, Lew R, et al: Should prophylactic anticonvulsants be administered to patients with newly diagnosed cerebral metastases? A retrospective analysis. J Clin Oncol 6:1621–1624.
21. Coia LR, Aaronson N, Linggood R, et al: A report of the consensus workshop panel on the treatment of brain metastases. Int J Radiat Oncol Biol Phys 23:223–227, 1992.
22. Coia LR: The role of radiation therapy in the treatment of brain metastases. Int J Radiat Oncol Biol Phys 23:229–238, 1992.
23. Colomer R, Casas D, Del Campo JM, et al: Brain metastases from breast cancer may respond to endocrine therapy. Breast Cancer Treat Res 12:83–86, 1988.
24. Constans JP, DeDiviths E, Donzelli R, et al: Spinal metastases with neurological manifestations. J Neurosurg 59:111–118, 1983.
25. Crane JM, Nelson MJ, Ihde DC, et al: A comparison of computed tomography and radionuclide scanning for detection of brain metastases in small cell lung cancer. J Clin Oncol 2:1017–1024, 1984.
26. Davis PC, Hudgins PA, Peterman SB, et al: Diagnosis of cerebral metastases: Double-dose delayed CT vs contrast-enhanced MR imaging. Am J Neuroradiol 12:301–307, 1991.
27. DeAngelis L, Delattre J-Y, Posner JB: Radiation-induced dementia in patients cured of brain metastases. Neurology 39:789–796, 1989.
28. DeAngelis LM, Mandell LR, Thaler HT, et al: The role of postoperative radiotherapy after resection of single brain metastases. Neurosurgery 24:798–805, 1989.
29. Delattre J, Krol G, Thaler H, et al: Distribution of brain metastases. Arch Neurol 45:741–744, 1988.
30. Delattre J, Safai B, Posner J: Erythema multiforme and Stevens-Johnson syndrome in patients receiving cranial irradiation and phenytoin. Neurology 38:194–198, 1988.
31. Distefano A, Yong Yap Y, Hortobagyi GN, et al: The natural history of breast cancer patients with brain metastases. Cancer 44:1913–1918, 1979.
32. Dunn RC, Kelly WA, Wohns RNW, et al: Spinal epidural neoplasia: A 15 year review of the results of surgical therapy. J Neurosurg 52:47–51, 1980.
33. Edelson RN, Deck MDF, Posner JB: Intramedullary spinal cord metastases: Clinical and radiographic findings in 9 cases. Neurology 22:1222–1231, 1972.
34. Flowers A, Levin VA: Management of brain metastases from breast carcinoma. Oncology 7:21–26, 1993.
35. Giannone L, Greco FA, Hainsworth JD: Combination intraventricular chemotherapy for meningeal neoplasia. J Clin Oncol 4:68–73, 1986.
36. Gilbert RW, Jae-Ho K, Posner JB: Epidural spinal cord compression from metastatic tumor: Diagnosis and treatment. Ann Neurol 3:40–51, 1978.
37. Glass JP, Melamed M, Chernik NL, et al: Malignant cells in

cerebrospinal fluid (CSF): The meaning of a positive CSF cytology. Neurology 29:1369–1375, 1979.

38. Goldson AL, Streeter OE Jr, Ashayen E, et al: Intraoperative radiotherapy for intracranial malignancies. Cancer 54:2807–2813, 1984.

39. Gonzalez-Vitale JC, Garcia-Bunuel R: Meningeal carcinomatosis. Cancer 37:2906–2911, 1976.

40. Goodkin R, Carr BI, Perrin RG: Herniated lumbar disc disease in patients with malignancy. J Clin Oncol 5:667–671, 1987.

41. Grisoli F, Vincentelli F, Foa J, et al: Effect of bromocriptine on brain metastasis in breast cancer. Lancet 2:745–746, 1981.

42. Grossman SA, Finkelstein DM, Ruckdeschel JC, et al: Randomized prospective comparison of intraventricular methotrexate and thiotepa in patients with previously untreated neoplastic meningitis. J Clin Oncol 11:561–569, 1993.

43. Grossman SA, Trump DL, Chen DCP, et al: Cerebrospinal fluid flow abnormalities in patients with neoplastic meningitis. Am J Med 73:641–647, 1982.

44. Gutin PH, Levi JA, Wiernik PH, et al: Treatment of malignant meningeal disease with intrathecal thiotepa: A phase II study. Cancer Treat Rep 61:885–887, 1977.

45. Hagenau C, Grosh W, Currie M, et al: Comparison of spinal magnetic resonance imaging and myelography in cancer patients. J Clin Oncol 5:1663–1669, 1987.

46. Harrison KM, Muss HB, Ball MR, et al: Spinal cord compression in breast cancer. Cancer 55:2839–2844, 1985.

47. Hazuka MB, Kinzie JJ: Brain metastases: Results and effects of re-irradiation. Int J Radiat Oncol Biol Phys 15:433–437, 1988.

48. Hendrickson FR: Radiation therapy of metastatic tumors. Semin Oncol 2:43–46, 1975.

49. Hill ME, Richards MA, Gregory WM, et al: Spinal cord compression in breast cancer: A review of 70 cases. Br J Cancer 68:969–973, 1993.

50. Hitchins RN, Bell DR, Woods RL, et al: A prospective randomized trial of single-agent versus combination chemotherapy in meningeal carcinomatosis. J Clin Oncol 5:1655–1662, 1987.

51. Hoskin PJ, Drow J, Ford HT: The influence of extent and local management on the outcome of radiotherapy for brain metastases. Int J Radiat Oncol Biol Phys 19:111–115, 1990.

52. Iaconetta G, Lamaida E, Rossi A, et al: Leptomeningeal carcinomatosis: Review of the literature. Acta Neurol Napoli 16:214–220, 1994.

53. Kamby C, Soerensen PS: Characteristics of patients with short and long survivals after detection of intracranial metastases from breast cancer. J Neuro-Oncol 6:37–45, 1988.

54. Khan FR, Glicksman AS, Chu FCH, et al: Treatment by radiotherapy of spinal cord compression due to extradural metastases. Radiology 89:495–500, 1967.

55. Kim RY, Spencer AS, Meredith RF, et al: Extradural spinal cord compression: Analysis of factors determining functional prognosis—prospective study. Radiology 176:279–282, 1990.

56. Kocher M, Muller R-P, Staar S, et al: Long-term survival after brain metastases in breast cancer. Strahlentherapie Onkologie 171:290–295, 1995.

57. Koehler PJ: Use of corticosteroids in neuro-oncology. Anticancer Drugs 6:19–33, 1995.

58. Krol G, Heier L, Becker R, et al: Value of magnetic resonance imaging in the evaluation of patients with complete and high degree block due to intracanal neoplasm. Acta Radiol 369S:741–743, 1986.

59. Kurup P, Reddy S, Hendrickson FR: Results of re-irradiation for cerebral metastases. Cancer 46:2587–2589, 1980.

60. Lewi HJ, Roberts MM, Donaldson AA, et al: The use of cerebral computed assisted tomography as a staging investigation of patients with carcinoma of the breast and malignant melanoma. Surg Gynecol Obstet 151:385–386, 1980.

61. Lien EA, Wester K, Lonning PE, et al: Distribution of tamoxifen and metabolites into brain tissue and brain metastases in breast cancer patients. Br J Cancer 63:641–645, 1991.

62. Little JR, Dale AJD, Okazaki H, et al: Meningeal carcinomatosis: Clinical manifestation. Arch Neurol 30:138–143, 1974.

63. Loeffler JS, Shrieve DC: What is appropriate therapy for a patient with a single brain metastasis? Int J Radiat Oncol Biol Phys 29:915–917, 1994.

64. Marnazano E, Latini P, Checcaglini F, et al: Radiation therapy of spinal cord compression caused by breast cancer: Report of a prospective trial. Int J Radiat Oncol Biol Phys 24:301–306, 1992.

65. Marcus FS, Dandolos EM, Friedman MA: Meningeal carcinomatosis in breast cancer presenting as central hypoventilation: A case report with a brief review of the literature. Cancer 47:982–984, 1981.

66. Markesbery WR, Brooks WH, Gupta GD, et al: Treatment for patients with cerebral metastases. Arch Neurol 35:754–756, 1978.

67. McKelvey EM: Meningeal involvement with metastatic carcinoma of the breast treated with intrathecal methotrexate. Cancer 22:576–580, 1968.

68. Milburn L, Hibbs GB, Hendrickson FR: Treatment of spinal cord compression from metastatic carcinoma. Cancer 21:447–452, 1968.

69. Murray JJ, Greco FA, Wolff SN, et al: Neoplastic meningitis: Marked variations of cerebrospinal fluid composition in the absence of extradural block. Am J Med 75:289–294, 1983.

70. Noordijk EM, Vecht CJ, Haaxma-Reiche H, et al: The choice of treatment of single brain metastasis should be based on extracranial tumor activity and age. Int J Radiat Oncol Biol Phys 29:711–717, 1994.

71. Olson Me, Chernik NL, Posner JB: Infiltration of the leptomeninges by systemic cancer: A clinical and pathologic study. Arch Neurol 30:122–137, 1974.

72. Ongerboer de Visser BW, van Zanten AP, Twijnstra A, et al: Sensitivity and specificity of cerebrospinal fluid biochemical markers of central nervous system metastases. Prog Exp Tumor Res 29:105–115, 1985.

73. O'Rourke T, George CB, Redmond J III, et al: Spinal computed tomography and computed tomographic metrizamide myelography in the early diagnosis of metastatic disease. J Clin Oncol 4:576–583, 1986.

74. Patchell RA, Tibbs PA, Walch JW, et al: A randomized trial of surgery in the treatment of single metastases to the brain. N Engl J Med 322:494–500, 1990.

75. Peretti-Viton P, Margain D, Murayama N, et al: Les metastases cerebrales: Brain metastases. J Neuroradiol 18:161–172, 1991.

76. Pigott KH, Baddeley H, Maher EJ: Pattern of disease in spinal cord compression on MRI scan and implications for treatment. Clin Oncol 6:7–10, 1994.

77. Pors H, von Eyben FE, Sorensen OS, et al: Longterm remission of multiple brain metastases with tamoxifen. J Neuro-Oncol 10:173–177, 1991.

78. Portenoy RK, Lipton RB, Foley KM: Back pain in the cancer patient: An algorithm for evaluation and management. Neurology 37:134–138, 1987.

79. Posner JB: Management of central nervous system metastases. Semin Oncol 4:81–91, 1977.

80. Posner JB: Surgery for metastases to the brain. N Engl J Med 322:544–545, 1990.

81. Ransohoff J: Surgical management of metastatic tumors. Semin Oncol 2:21–27, 1968.

82. Ratcheson RA, Ommaya AB: Experience with the subcutaneous cerebrospinal fluid reservoir; preliminary report of 60 cases. N Engl J Med 279:1025–1031, 1968.

83. Rodichok LD, Harper GR, Ruckdeschel JC, et al.: Early diagnosis of spinal epidural metastases. Am J Med 70:1181–1188, 1981.

84. Rodichok LD, Ruckdeschel JC, Harper GR, et al: Early detection and treatment of spinal epidural metastases: The role of myelography. Ann Neurol 20:696–702, 1986.

85. Rosner D, Nemoto T, Lane WW: Chemotherapy induces regression of brain metastases in breast carcinoma. Cancer 58:832–839, 1986.

86. Russell EJ, Geremia GK, Johnson CE, et al: Multiple cerebral metastases: Detectability with Gd-DTPA–enhanced MR imaging. Radiology 165:609–617, 1987.

87. Salvati M, Capoccia G, Ramundo E, et al: Single brain metas-

tases from breast cancer: Remarks on clinical pattern and treatment. Tumori 78:115–117, 1992.

88. Salvati M, Cervoni L, Innocenzi G, et al: Prolonged stabilization of multiple and single brain metastases from breast cancer with tamoxifen. Report of three cases. Tumori 79:359–362, 1993.

89. Sarpel S, Sarpel G, Yu E, et al: Early diagnosis of spinal-epidural metastasis by magnetic resonance imaging. Cancer 59:1112–1116, 1987.

90. Sepkowitz KA, Brown AE, Telzak EE, et al: *Pneumocystis carinii* pneumonia among patients without AIDS at a cancer hospital. JAMA 267:832–837, 1992.

91. Shalen PR, Hayman LA, Wallace S, et al: Protocol for delayed contrast enhancement in computed tomography of cerebral neoplasia. Radiology 139:397–402, 1981.

92. Shapiro WR, Young DF, Mehta BM: Methotrexate distribution in cerebrospinal fluid after intravenous ventricular and lumbar injections. N Engl J Med 293:161–166, 1975.

93. Shehata WM, Hendrickson FR, Hindo WA: Rapid fractionation technique and re-treatment of cerebral metastases by irradiation. Cancer 34:257–261, 1974.

94. Siegal T, Lossos A, Pfeffer MR: Leptomeningeal metastases: Analysis of 31 patients with sustained off-therapy response following combined-modality therapy. Neurology 44:1463–1469, 1994.

95. Smalley S, Schray M, Lans E, et al: Adjuvant radiation therapy after surgical resection of solitary brain metastases: Association with pattern of failure and survival. Int J Radiat Oncol Biol Phys 6:1215–1228, 1980.

96. Smith FP, Slavik M, Macdonald JS: Association of breast cancer with meningioma. Cancer 42:1992–1994, 1978.

97. Sorensen PS, Borgesen SE, Rohde D, et al: Metastatic epidural spinal cord compression: Results of treatment and survival. Cancer 65:1502–1508, 1990.

98. Sorensen SC, Eagan RT, Scott M: Meningeal carcinomatosis in patients with primary breast or lung cancer. Mayo Clin Proc 59:91–94, 1984.

99. Stark RJ, Henson RA, Evans SJW: Spinal metastases: A retrospective survey from a general hospital. Brain 105:189–213, 1982.

100. Stein DA, Chamberlain MC: Evaluation and management of seizures in the patient with cancer. Oncology 5:33–39, 1991.

101. Stewart DJ, Dahrouge S: Response of brain metastases from breast cancer to megestrol acetate: A case report. J Neuro-Oncol 24:299–301, 1995.

102. Stewart JF, King RJB, Sexton SA, et al: Oestrogen receptors, sites of metastatic disease and survival in recurrent breast cancer. Eur J Cancer 17:449–453, 1981.

103. Sundaresan N, Galicich JH: Surgical treatment of brain metastases: Clinical and computerized tomography evaluation of the results of treatment. Cancer 55:1382–1388, 1985.

104. Sundaresan N, Sachdev VP, DiGiacinto GV, et al: Reoperation for brain metastases. J Clin Oncol 6:1625–1629, 1988.

105. Sze G, Milano E, Johnson C, et al: Detection of brain metastases: Comparison of contrast-enhanced MR with unenhanced MR and enhanced CT. Am J Neuroradiol 11:785–791, 1990.

106. Sze G, Shin J, Krol G, et al: Intraparenchymal brain metastases: MR imaging versus contrast-enhanced CT. Radiology 168:187–194, 1988.

107. Sze G, Sloetsky S, Bronen R, et al: MR imaging of the cranial meninges with emphasis on contrast enhancement and meningeal carcinomatosis. Am J Neuroradiol 10:965–975, 1989.

108. Tsukada Y, Fouad A, Pickren JW, et al: Central nervous system metastasis from breast carcinoma: Autopsy study. Cancer 52:2349–2354, 1983.

109. Trump DL, Grossman SA, Thompson G, et al: Treatment of neoplastic meningitis with intraventricular thiotepa and methotrexate. Cancer Treat Rev 66:1549–1551, 1982.

110. Van der Gaast A, Alexieva-Figusch J, Vecht C, et al: Complete remission of a brain metastasis to third-line hormonal treatment with megestrol acetate. Am J Clin Oncol 13:507–509, 1990.

111. Vecht CJ, Haaxma-Reiche H, van Putten LF, et al: Initial bolus of conventional versus high-dose dexamethasone in metastatic spinal cord compression. Neurology 39:1255–1257, 1989.

112. Viadana E, Cotter R, Pickren JW, et al: An autopsy study of metastatic sites of breast cancer. Cancer Res 33:179–181, 1973.

113. Wasserstrom WR, Glass JP, Posner JB: Diagnosis and treatment of leptomeningeal metastases from solid tumors. Cancer 49:759–772, 1982.

114. Williams MP, Cherryman GR, Husband JE: Magnetic resonance imaging in suspected metastatic spinal cord compression. Clin Radiol 40:286–290, 1989.

115. Yap BS, Yap HY, Fritsche HA, et al: CSF carcinoembryonic antigen in meningeal carcinomatosis from breast cancer. JAMA 244:1601–1603, 1980.

116. Yap HY, Yap BS, Rasmussen S, et al: Treatment for meningeal carcinomatosis in breast cancer. Cancer 50:219–222, 1982.

117. Yap HY, Yap BS, Tashima CK, et al: Meningeal carcinomatosis in breast cancer. Cancer 42:283–286, 1978.

CHAPTER 77

MANAGEMENT OF PERICARDIAL METASTASES IN BREAST CANCER

Karen A. Johnson, M.D., Ph.D., M.P.H. / Barnett S. Kramer, M.D., M.P.H. / Jeffrey M. Crane, M.D.

In patients known to have metastatic breast cancer, when malignant pericardial disease comes to clinical attention, it usually presents insidiously. An increasing accumulation of fluid within the pericardium containing malignant cells or a constriction of the pericardium by tumor, with or without fluid, has the potential to cause a medical emergency. Cardiac tamponade refers to any degree of cardiac compression caused by increased intrapericardial pressure that results in a functional decompensation of the heart.

The incidence of pericardial effusion and tamponade in breast cancer patients is unknown. Autopsy series with breast cancer patients reveal pericardial metastases in 12 to 35 percent of necropsied patients.[1, 14, 15, 20] However, Thurber and associates[33] noted that the presence of metastatic pericardial disease at autopsy in patients with a variety of tumors was accompanied by effusion in only 16 percent of cases. In one medical center where 307 breast cancer patients were seen between 1977 and 1982, 2 percent developed clinical cardiac tamponade.[3] A similar experience at the Guy's Hospital Breast Unit was reported for 1802 patients with metastatic breast cancer between 1969 and 1985, of whom 2 percent developed pericardial effusions.[37] These results are consistent with the observation that an antemortem diagnosis of cardiac metastases is made in 10 percent or less of autopsy-proved cases.[9, 33] There is other evidence that many pericardial effusions do not come to clinical attention. Buck and associates[4] found that among 30 breast cancer patients routinely given an echocardiogram on entering a phase II protocol for progressive metastatic disease that had been previously treated, 53 percent had small occult effusions. Subsequently, only 1 of these patients had evidence of having frank pericardial disease. In contrast, the presentation of clinically apparent pericardial disease in breast cancer patients with known metastatic disease is ominous. In a group of 38 such patients, 50 percent were documented to have malignant pericardial disease either by positive cytology on examination of pericardial fluid or by histological evidence of carcinoma from surgical specimens.[4]

PATHOPHYSIOLOGY

Many pericardial effusions in breast cancer patients are not malignant. Although some of these nonmalignant effusions may be related to infection or metabolic disease, others will be related to previous treatments for the tumor. Both cyclophosphamide and radiation can induce pericardial injury. In 117 patients with breast cancer who underwent postoperative radiation therapy in the series by Stewart and associates, 4 developed radiation-induced heart disease.[31] In the report by Buck and colleagues[4] there were another 32 breast cancer patients with clinical evidence of pericardial disease, but without any other evidence to suggest metastatic disease. In this particular subset, an associated diagnosis of pre-existing cardiac disease was the most frequent finding and occurred in about 40 percent of patients; but radiation-induced pericardial reaction was suspected in one third and half of this group had histological findings consistent with that diagnosis.[4]

In patients with malignant pericardial effusion, breast cancer metastases from involved mediastinal lymph nodes reach the heart and pericardium by retrograde movement along lymphatic channels.[20] It is thought that the normal flow of lymph from the endocardium and interstitium of the myocardium is via the epicardial lymphatics to the mediastinal collecting system.[21] Kline[20] was able to find only 1 of 61 patients with various malignancies metastatic to the pericardium in whom there was no evidence of mediastinal node involvement. This single case was consistent with pure hematogenous spread of metastases to the pericardium. Six other cases of the 61 were thought to be a result of direct extension to the pericardium from involved mediastinal lymphatics.

The severity of cardiac tamponade is related to the rate of pericardial fluid accumulation, its volume, and the underlying functional status of the patient's myocardium. Gradual accumulation of fluid allows the pericardium to stretch to accommodate the pressure; the myocardium can also adapt to a gradual increase in pericardial pressure. Thus, the pericardium may accommodate several liters of fluid when fluid accumulation is insidious. A critical point occurs when the reflex tachycardia and peripheral vasoconstriction are no longer adequate to compensate for the falling stroke volume. Venous return diminishes as pressures within the vena cava, the pulmonary venous and arterial systems, and the atria rise to the level of ventricular diastolic filling pressures and cardiac output precipitously falls. When the pericardium is thickened by tumor infiltration or radiation fibrosis, compensatory stretching is impossible, and the critical point is reached early. Occasionally, therefore, neoplastic and postirradiation constrictive pericarditis progress rapidly or present as cardiac tamponade. Spodick provides a detailed review of these events.[29]

CLINICAL MANIFESTATIONS

A variety of symptoms can occur in patients with cardiac tamponade. Apprehension or extreme anxiety are likely to accompany the most common symptoms, which include progressive dyspnea, precordial pressure or retrosternal pain, cough, fever and edema. Also observed are orthopnea, hoarseness, singultus (hiccups), and various gastrointestinal symptoms, including dysphagia, nausea, vomiting, and abdominal pain. At the extreme, cardiovascular collapse can occur.

The physical signs of pericardial effusion or cardiac tamponade are primarily related to the effects of decreased cardiac output and compensatory peripheral vasoconstriction. Common signs include diaphoresis, confusion (including coma), tachypnea, and pallor with or without peripheral cyanosis. Peripheral pulses are weak, and jugulovenous distention is evident. The presence of diminished systolic blood pressure as well as decreased pulse pressure should suggest the diagnosis of tamponade. Also useful is the physical finding of pulsus paradoxus. Moreover, a decrease in the magnitude of pulsus paradoxus may accurately reflect the clinical response to therapy of the effusion. Chest examination may disclose pleural effusions, absence of the apical cardiac impulse, and faint heart sounds. The pericardial knock commonly heard in constrictive pericarditis is usually not a component of pericardial effusion with tamponade. The presence of ascites, hepatomegaly, or hepatojugular reflex may be additional clues to pericardial effusion with tamponade in the cancer patient.

Electrocardiographic (ECG) findings may include low-voltage sinus tachycardia and other arrythmias, elevation of ST segments diffusely, and variable T wave abnormalities. Electrical alternans in all segments (P, QRS, and T waves), termed *total electrical alternans*, is unusual but is quite specific for pericardial effusions.[29] In fact, this ECG finding in the patient with metastatic breast cancer should immediately prompt investigation for suspected neoplastic pericardial effusion with incipient tamponade.[22] Partial electrical alternans (QRS complex only) is less specific, being present commonly in other nonmalignant or nontamponade conditions.[4]

The roentgenographic signs of pericardial effusion in metastatic malignancies are variable. A normal chest roentgenogram does not rule out the possibility of neoplastic pericarditis.[25] However, a globose "water bottle heart" shadow is frequently seen in neoplastic pericardial effusions. Even more commonly, simple enlargement of the cardiac silhouette is seen on serial chest x-ray films.[2] Of 55 patients with pericardial metastases, only 4 had a normal chest x-ray film, whereas 50 percent had findings of cardiac enlargement, mediastinal widening, hilar adenopathy or hilar mass.[33]

The echocardiogram is a simple, relatively inexpensive, safe, rapid, and noninvasive test that is very sensitive for the diagnosis of pericardial effusion.[4, 11, 25, 29] Collapse of the right ventricle on echocardiogram is highly diagnostic of tamponade (sensitivity 92 percent, specificity 100 percent, accuracy 94 percent).[27] Right heart catheterization, with pressure-wave tracings of the vena cava, right atrium, right ventricle, and pulmonary artery along with pulmonary capillary wedge pressure measurement, is also a sensitive and specific test for cardiac tamponade. However, this invasive test is rarely indicated except when the diagnosis may be in question after noninvasive testing, particularly where a diagnosis of neoplastic constrictive pericarditis is under consideration.[32]

Once a clinical diagnosis of cardiac tamponade has been made, the pericardial fluid must be removed as quickly as possible. There are few medical oncology emergencies in which as rapid an alleviation of the patient's discomfort may occur. The fluid is nearly always exudative. Approximately one third of pericardial effusions are serous; the remainder are serosanguinous or grossly bloody. However, cytologic reviews of the fluid may not provide pathological confirmation of the clinical diagnosis of a neoplastic pericardial effusion. Approximately 80 percent of specimens are positive for tumor.* False positive results are rare.

TREATMENT

Sudden cardiovascular collapse and death are always possible in cardiac tamponade, whether of neoplastic or benign etiology.[4] Supportive care should be immediately instituted as emergency pericardiocentesis is prepared. Intravascular volume should be expanded with intravenous fluids. Normal saline will usually suffice, but 5 percent serum albumin or its synthetic analogues may be more effective in intravascular volume expansion in tamponade.[30] Blood and other volume expanders may also be used, and if needed, pressor agents may be initiated. In cases of dyspnea or tachypnea, the administration of oxygen will help to partially alleviate some of the patient's distressing symptoms. Positive end-expiratory pressure by mechanical ventilation reduces cardiac output via reduction in central venous return and thus should not be used.[29]

The only immediately effective treatment for pericardial effusion with tamponade is removal of the fluid. To save the patient's life, pericardiocentesis should be performed as soon as possible.[19] Pericardiocentesis is generally indicated when there is (1) cyanosis, dyspnea, a shock-like syndrome, or impairment of consciousness; (2) rising peripheral venous pressure above 130 mm H_2O; or (3) measured pulsus paradoxus exceeding 50 percent of the pulse pressure

---

* References 7, 9, 10, 18, 26, 33, and 39.

or falling pulse pressure below 20 mm Hg.[29] The complications of pericardiocentesis have been reviewed. For patients with malignant pericardial effusion, 2 to 3 percent can expect a serious complication in addition to a mortality rate of about 1 percent from the procedure.[34, 38] Cardiac arrhythmias, bleeding, and myocardial trauma are potentially fatal complications of pericardiocentesis, which can be reduced by conducting the pericardiocentesis under controlled conditions. When it is possible to use two-dimensional echocardiography[5] or real-time ultrasound scanning[8] to guide the procedure, these are recommended. Removal of the first 50 to 100 ml of fluid usually results in an impressive improvement in the patient's symptoms and signs of tamponade, but it is recommended that as much fluid as possible be removed.

Reaccumulation of the pericardial fluid often occurs within 48 to 72 hours of the initial pericardiocentesis. In the past, long-term control of the effusion was accomplished by sclerosis of the pericardial sac with tetracycline.[10, 26, 28] However, since 1991, the injectable tetracycline hydrochloride that was previously used for pericardiocentesis has been unavailable in the United States.[16] Bleomycin is a possible alternative to tetracycline, but reported experience is limited to very small series of patients with malignant effusions.[34, 35] The irritative sclerosing action of bleomycin (20 to 30 mg in 30 ml of sterile saline)[35] is best accomplished after the pericardial sac has been drained completely to allow apposition of the pericardial surfaces. Other agents, including talc, nitrogen mustard, cisplatin or thiotepa have also been used. Although some have noted diminished reaccumulation of fluid using only short-term catheter drainage of the pericardium,[12] the duration of the response to this limited approach is generally short. However, drainage is often used in conjunction with systemic therapy.[34] Woll and associates have reported on a series of breast cancer patients with pericardial effusions including 22 who, as a rule, were started on endocrine or chemotherapy as soon as possible after catheter drainage for tamponade.[37] Only 4 of the 22 required further local treatment for pericardial fluid, and the median survival for this group was about 9 months.

The value of radiation therapy delivered to the pericardium either alone or in conjunction with a pleuropericardial window after failed repetitive attempts at sclerosing therapy is well described.[3, 7, 15, 28, 29, 33] External beam irradiation has replaced instillational therapy with radioactive phosphorous (^{32}P), yttrium (^{90}Y) or gold (^{198}Au). External beam irradiation, 2500 to 3500 rad delivered in 3 to 4 weeks by anterior and posterior ports after pericardiocentesis to tap the effusion dry, controlled pericardial effusion in 11 of 16 breast cancer patients for a period ranging from 2 to 36 months.[7] All these patients had cytologically confirmed malignant pericardial effusions.

If the patient has the potential for long-term survival and sclerosis or radiation fails, the creation of a pleuropericardial window has been reported to provide effective control of pericardial effusions in patients with tamponade resulting from cancer.[13, 17] When in doubt, the neoplastic diagnosis may also be confirmed with this procedure. A compilation of data from three studies estimated the success rate (no further intervention needed to control the effusion) for the pleuropericardial window to be 86 percent.[34] Using a subxyphoid approach, other groups have demonstrated that a pleuropericardial window can be established under local anesthesia, avoiding the drawbacks of general anesthesia in a compromised patient.[6, 24] A percutaneous procedure to create a pericardial window also shows promise as an effective intervention that can be done under local anesthesia.[23, 36, 40] In the series by Buck and colleagues, 10 of 19 patients with histological proof of neoplastic pericarditis were treated either with pericardiectomy or window procedure, and none had recurrence.[4] Median survival was 18.3 months from diagnosis. Postoperative complications from neoplastic pericardial disease are probably less frequent than those described for pleuropericardial windows performed for infectious etiologies.[13] Nevertheless, these complications as well as the inherent problems of submitting a cancer patient to thoracotomy must be weighed against the good results reported for sclerosis therapy. Some authors recommend sclerosis as first-line therapy.[32] As second-line therapy and in patients failing local sclerosing therapy and whose pericardium is not encased with tumor, pleuropericardial windows offer excellent long-term control of the symptoms of neoplastic pericardial effusion. Finally, pericardiectomy is the treatment of choice for radiation-induced pericardial effusion.[32]

Concomitant with local therapy directed toward the malignant effusion, systemic therapy with cytotoxic drugs or hormonal manipulation should be initiated in those patients who are candidates. Given the durable response rates to sclerosis or pericardiectomy in some patients with neoplastic pericardial effusion and the frequency of extrapericardial disease, systemic chemotherapy should be considered in patients who have not exhausted their chemotherapeutic options.

PROGNOSIS

Untreated, neoplastic cardiac tamponade is rapidly fatal. Nevertheless, even if the acute episode is successfully managed, other systemic metastases are nearly always present, and long-term survival is unusual.

In those patients with neoplastic tamponade as the first sign of pericardial metastases (from breast and other carcinoma primaries), the prognosis is grave. An exceptionally grave sign is total electrical alternans, after which most patients have died within a few days despite removal of pericardial fluid.[22] Those patients without frank malignant tamponade have a much better prognosis, with a median survival of 12.8 months and 15 to 16 months for patients with complete response to local therapy.[28]

The range of options available for the treatment of malignant pericardial effusions includes drainage, pericardial sclerosis, systemic antitumor therapy, radiation therapy and surgery. More often than not, it is inappropriate to limit the approach to pericardial disease to a single intervention. The role of the clinician is to individualize therapeutic interventions according to the circumstances so that the best possible outcome is realized.

References

1. Abrams HL, Spiro R, Goldstein N: Metastases in carcinoma; Analysis of 1000 autopsied cases. Cancer 3:74–85, 1950.
2. Abrams HL, Adam DF, Grant JA: The radiology of tumors of the heart. Radiol Clin North Am 9:299–326, 1971.
3. Bitran JD, Evans R, Brown C: The management of cardiac tamponade in patient with breast cancer. J Surg Oncol 27:42–44, 1984.
4. Buck M, Ingle JN, Giuliani ER, et al: Pericardial effusion in women with breast cancer. Cancer 60:263–269, 1987.
5. Callahan JA, Seward JB, Nishimura RA, et al: Two-dimensional echocardiographically guided pericardiocentesis: Experience in 117 consecutive patients. Am J Cardiol 55:476–479, 1985.
6. Campbell PT, Van Trigt P, Wall TC, et al: Subxiphoid pericardiotomy in the diagnosis and management of large pericardial effusions associated with malignancy. Chest 101:938–943, 1992.
7. Cham WC, Freiman AN, Carsteus PHB, et al: Radiation therapy of cardiac and pericardial metastases. Radiology 114:701–704, 1975.
8. Clarke DP, Cosgrove DO: Real-time ultrasound scanning in the planning and guidance of pericardiocentesis. Clin Radiol 38:119–122, 1987.
9. Cohen GU, Peery TM, Evans JM: Neoplastic invasion of the heart and pericardium. Ann Intern Med 42:1238–1245, 1955.
10. Davis SD, Sharma SM, Blumberg ED, et al: Intra pericardial tetracycline for the management of cardiac tamponade secondary to malignant pericardial effusion. N Engl J Med 299:1113–1114, 1978.
11. D'Cruz IA, Cohen HC, Prabhu R, et al: Diagnosis of cardiac tamponade by echocardiography: Changes in initial valve motion and ventricular dimensions with special reference to paradoxical pulse. Circulation 52:460–465, 1975.
12. Flannery EP, Gregoratos G, Corder MP: Pericardial effusions in patients with malignant diseases. Arch Int Med 135:976–977, 1975.
13. Fredriksen RT, Cohen LS, Mullins CV: Pericardial windows or pericardiocentesis for pericardial effusions. Am Heart J 82:158–162, 1971.
14. Hagemeister FB Jr, Buzdar AU, Luna MA, et al: Causes of death in breast cancer: A clinicopathologic study. Cancer 46:162–167, 1980.
15. Hanfling SM: Metastatic cancer to the heart: Review of the literature and report of 127 cases. Circulation 22:474–483, 1960.
16. Heffner JE, Unruh LC: Tetracycline pleurodesis: Adios, farewell, adieu. Chest 101:5–7, 1992.
17. Hill GJ II, Cohen BI: Pleural pericardial window for palliation of cardiac tamponade due to cancer. Cancer 26:81–93, 1970.
18. Johnson WD: The cytological diagnosis of cancer in serous effusions. Acta Cytol 10:161–172, 1966.
19. Kilpatrick ZM, Chapman CB: On pericardiocentesis. Am J Cardiol 16:722–728, 1965.
20. Kline IK: Cardiac lymphatic involvement by metastatic tumor. Cancer 29:799–808, 1972.
21. Lokich JJ: The management of malignant pericardial effusions. JAMA 224:1401–1404, 1973.
22. Niarchos AP: Electrical alternans in cardiac tamponade. Thorax 30:228–233, 1975.
23. Palacios IF, Tuzcu EM, Ziskind AA, et al: Percutaneous balloon pericardial window for patients with malignant pericardial effusion and tamponade. Cathet Cardiovasc Diagnos 22:244–249, 1991.
24. Park JS, Rentschler R, Wilbur D: Surgical management of pericardial effusion in patients with malignancies: Comparison of subxiphoid window versus pericardiectomy. Cancer 67:76–80, 1991.
25. Pories WJ, Guandiani BA: Cardiac tamponade. Surg Clin North Am 55:573–589, 1975.
26. Shepherd FA, Ginsberg JS, Evans WK, et al: Tetracycline sclerosis in the management of malignant pericardial effusion. J Clin Oncol 3:1678–1682, 1985.
27. Singh S, Wann S, Schuchard GH, et al: Right ventricular and right atrial collapse in patients with cardiac tamponade: A combined echocardiographic and hemodynamic study. Circulation 70:966–971, 1984.
28. Smith FE, Lane M, Hidgins PT: Conservative management of malignant pericardial effusion. Cancer 33:47–57, 1974.
29. Spodick DH: Acute cardiac tamponade: Pathologic physiology, diagnosis and management. Prog Cardiovasc Dis 10:64, 1967.
30. Stein L, Shubin H, Weil MH: Recognition and management of pericardial tamponade. JAMA 225:503–506, 1973.
31. Stewart JR, Cohn KE, Fajardo LF, et al: Radiation induced heart disease: A study of twenty-five patients. Radiology 89:302–310, 1976.
32. Theologides A: Neoplastic cardiac tamponade. Semin Oncol 5:181–192, 1978.
33. Thurber DL, Edwards JE, Anchor RWP: Secondary malignant tumors of the pericardium. Circulation 26:228–241, 1962.
34. Vaitkus PT, Herrmann HC, LeWinter MM: Treatment of malignant pericardial effusion. JAMA 272:59–64, 1994.
35. Van Der Gaast A, Kok TC, Van Der Linden NH, et al: Intrapericardial instillation of bleomycin in the management of malignant pericardial effusion. Eur J Cancer Clin Oncol 25:1505–1506, 1989.
36. Vora A, Lokhandwala YY: Echocardiography guided creation of balloon pericardial window. Cathet Cardiovasc Diagn 25:164–165, 1992.
37. Woll PJ, Knight RK, Rubens RD: Pericardial effusion complicating breast cancer. J R Soc Med 80:490–491, 1987.
38. Wong B, Murphy J, Chang J, et al: The risk of pericardiocentesis. Am J Cardiol 44:1110–1114, 1979.
39. Zipf RE, Johnston WW: The role of cytology in the evaluation of pericardial effusions. Chest 62:593–596, 1972.
40. Ziskind AA, Pearce AC, Lemmon CC, et al: Percutaneous balloon pericardiotomy for the treatment of cardiac tamponade and large pericardial effusions: Description of technique and report of the first 50 cases. J Am Coll Cardiol 21:1–5, 1993.

CHAPTER 78
BILATERAL BREAST CANCER

Hiram S. Cody III, M.D. / Patrick I. Borgen, M.D.

Foote and Stewart's[18] assertion that "the most frequent antecedent of cancer of one breast is the history of having had cancer in the opposite breast" is as true now as when written 50 years ago, yet the proper management of the opposite breast remains a subject of both confusion and controversy. Contributing to this uncertainty, both in the medical literature and in clinical practice, are the following considerations:

1. *Is the contralateral cancer a new primary or a metastatic lesion?* Metastasis of a breast cancer to the opposite breast, except in the context of a locally advanced index cancer or widespread metastatic disease, is a rare event. A true second primary breast cancer (as described by Chaudary and coworkers[12]) may be *absolutely identified* by the presence of an *in situ* tumor component, and *relatively identified* by the presence of (a) a different histological pattern, (b) a greater degree of differentiation, and (c) no evidence of local/regional/distant disease from the first cancer. A discrepancy in biomarker studies (such as steroid hormone binding protein status) may be useful as well. *In the absence of other sites of disease, a contralateral breast cancer should always be treated as a new primary.* Metastatic lesions to the breast (from either a previous breast cancer or other sites) will not be further addressed in this chapter.

2. *Is the contralateral cancer synchronous or metachronous?* In the comprehensive review by Wanebo and coworkers,[49] 836 of 22,563 breast cancers (3.7 percent) were bilateral, with one third of these synchronous and two thirds metachronous. The time interval beyond which different authors have defined a contralateral breast cancer as metachronous rather than synchronous has ranged widely, from 6 months to 5 years. Furthermore, the proportion of metachronous cancers varies as a function of patient selection, the method of screening used, the type and stage of the first cancer, and, especially, the length of follow-up. The management of a clinically or mammographically evident contralateral breast cancer is, of course, dictated by standard criteria and will not be discussed further here; management of the apparently normal opposite breast will be the focus of this chapter.

3. *How should the risk of contralateral cancer be reported?* Risk expressed as a total percentage is the least precise and varies widely, subject to the preceding variables and other variables. *Relative risk* (the ratio of observed to expected cases of cancer) is easily calculated but subject to exaggerated risk estimates: "normal lifetime risk" multiplied by relative risk does not equal absolute risk, as anxious patients often assume. *Absolute risk per year* is the most clinically useful measure; in Robbins and Berg's[36] classic study of bilateral breast cancer, the risk of a contralateral breast cancer was 0.7 percent per year of follow-up (Fig. 78–1). The risk of death from a contralateral breast cancer (assuming 70 to 80 percent curability with early diagnosis) is perhaps 0.2 percent per year. All treatment decisions pertaining to the opposite breast must be made in the context of this small level of risk and carefully weighed against the baseline risk imposed by the first cancer.

Over the past decade, widespread mammographic screening has led to earlier diagnosis (often as *in situ* disease), breast conservation with postoperative radiotherapy has become a standard treatment, and postoperative chemotherapy and tamoxifen have been used increasingly often. In the mid-1990s, the potential impact of a contralateral cancer, while small, is perhaps greater than ever. Paradoxically, interest in the contralateral breast has waned, and surveillance alone has become the norm for most physicians and oncological specialists. Should this practice change? If so, for which patients? This chapter will address the following issues:

1. By which parameters can the risk of a contralateral breast cancer be predicted in advance?
2. To what extent have changing patterns in the use of mammography, radiotherapy, chemotherapy, and tamoxifen affected the incidence of contralateral breast cancer?
3. Among the three treatment options for the apparently normal opposite breast—(a) observation alone, (b) contralateral biopsy, and (c) contralateral prophylactic mastectomy—which option is most appropriate for which patients?

RISK FACTORS FOR BILATERAL BREAST CANCER
Age

Young breast cancer patients are substantially more likely to develop contralateral breast cancers. In the

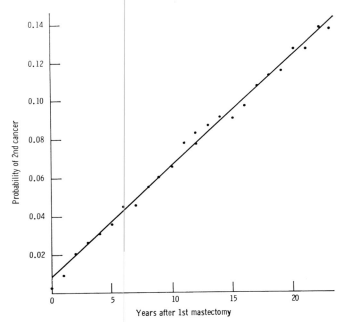

Figure 78–1 *Cumulative net probability of developing a second breast cancer (other causes for removal from series have been corrected). (From Robbins GF, Berg JW: Cancer 17:1501–1527, 1964. Reprinted by permission.)*

study of Robbins and Berg,[36] women under age 50 were 10 to 14 times more likely than the general population to develop contralateral cancers, but patients over age 70 were only twice as likely. The results of large population-based studies from England[35] and Connecticut[23] (as compared with Haagensen's[21] personal series from New York) show striking similarities (Table 78–1), with the greatest contralateral risk existing for the youngest patients. Chaudary and coworkers'[12] series of patients from Guy's Hospital demonstrates a similar result (Fig. 78–2) and again emphasizes the persistence of contralateral cancer risk over time. A careful population-based case-control study by Adami and colleagues[1] confirmed the highest risk of bilaterality in the youngest patients, as well as a greater risk in patients over age 50 than had been suggested by other studies (Table 78–2).

Family History

The interpretation of studies linking family history and bilaterality of breast cancer is difficult. First, there must be a clear distinction between (1) the risk of breast cancer developing in first-degree relatives of patients with bilateral disease (for which the evidence is strong) and (2) the risk of bilateral breast cancer developing in patients whose first-degree relatives had unilateral breast cancer (for which the evidence is less clear). Second, results will be a function of both study design and case selection. For the study of familial breast cancer risk, a large population-based study will have the advantage of eliminating selection biases but may overlook strong associations in small high-risk subsets of patients (a real possibility for the small minority of breast cancers, perhaps 5 percent, that are hereditary).

Since Anderson's[4] initial report in 1971, a number of studies have demonstrated the increased risk of breast cancer associated with a family history of early onset or bilateral disease. Anderson's[4] finding of an increased risk of bilateral breast cancer among patients with positive family histories has been more controversial, with some studies confirming increased bilaterality[11, 17, 25, 46] but others finding no difference.[2, 30, 50] Apparently the only population-based prospective study of the impact of family history on risk of a second breast cancer is by Bernstein and coworkers[6] who found, among 4660 breast cancer patients in the Cancer and Steroid Hormone Study (accrued 1980–1982, with 4 to 6 years' follow-up) that the risk of a contralateral breast cancer was significantly increased with (1) a first-degree family history, (2) an early age of onset in the family member, and (3) bilateral disease in the mother. Interestingly, the same study found that younger age at onset of the first cancer did not predict bilaterality, perhaps because of the relatively short follow-up and a limited age range in the study population.

The discovery of a susceptibility gene for early

TABLE 78–1. RELATIVE RISK OF A SECOND BREAST CANCER ACCORDING TO AGE AT TIME OF DIAGNOSIS OF FIRST CANCER

	Prior and Waterhouse, 1936–1964		Hankey and Coworkers, 1935–1975		Haagensen, 1936–1979	
Age at First Cancer	No. Cases	RR (%) (OBS/EXP)	No. Cases	RR (%) (OBS/EXP)	No. Cases	RR (%) (OBS/EX)
<45	89	5.3	430	5.7	45	5.9
45–54	118	3.4	454	3.6	48	3.2
>54	103	1.3	660	2.4	45	2.3
Total	310	2.4	1544	3.2	138	3.3

RR = Relative risk; OBS = observed cases; EXP = expected cases.
Data from Prior P, Waterhouse JAH: Incidence of bilateral tumours in a population-based series of breast-cancer patients: I. Two approaches to an epidemiological analysis. Br J Cancer 37:620–634, 1978; Hankey BF, Curtis RE, Naughton DN: A retrospective cohort analysis of second breast cancer risk for primary breast cancer patients with an assessment of the effect of radiation therapy. J Natl Cancer Inst 70:797–804, 1983; Haagensen CD: Diseases of the Breast. Philadelphia, WB Saunders, 1986.

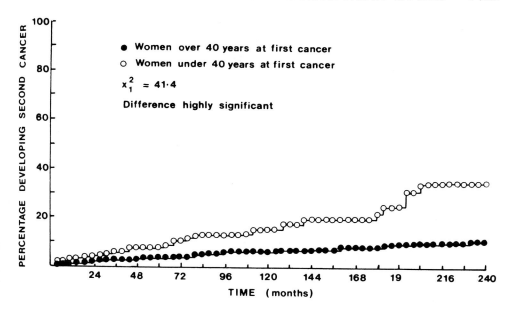

Figure 78–2 *Occurrence of second cancers in relation to age at first cancer. (From Chaudary MA, Millis RR, Bulbrook RD, Hayward JL: Breast Cancer Res Treat 5:201–205, 1985.)*

onset breast cancer (*BRCA1*) has added a new dimension to studies of both familial and bilateral breast cancer risk. In a study by the Breast Cancer Linkage Consortium of 33 families with germline mutations in *BRCA1*,[19] the risk of a first breast cancer by age 70 was 87 percent, and the risk of a contralateral cancer was 64 percent. Whether *BRCA1* mutations predict breast cancer bilaterality independently of family history (or add a predictive value over and above that given by family history alone) is not yet established.

Exposure to Ionizing Radiation

The widespread adoption of conservative surgery and radiotherapy for the treatment of early stage breast cancer has raised concern about the possibility of contralateral cancer being induced by low-dose scatter of radiation to the other breast. Large breast conservation series from Milan (1232 patients),[48] Marseilles (2850 patients),[27] and Boston (1624 patients)[24] all reassuringly demonstrate with long-term follow-up a rate of contralateral breast cancer *no higher than that associated with the first cancer alone*, 0.7 percent (or less) per year. In addition, although one might expect radiation scatter to produce a greater proportion of medial tumors than usual, the Milan group noted instead an identical distribution of contralateral cancer sites between the radiated and nonirradiated groups. These findings are consistent with data from the earlier mastectomy era; both Boice and colleagues[8] (regarding 41,109 breast cancer patients treated in Connecticut between 1935 and 1982), and Storm and colleagues[44] (regarding 56,540 Danish patients treated between 1943 and 1978) found no increased incidence of contralateral cancers in patients given postoperative chest wall radiotherapy.

Radiotherapy given to young women for Hodgkin's disease, on the other hand, dramatically increases the risk of breast cancer, as reports from Stanford and Memorial Sloan-Kettering Cancer Center indicate. In the first report Hancock and coworkers[22] demonstrated relative risks of 136 for women irradiated before age 15, 19 for ages 15 to 24, 7 for ages 24 to 29, and normal risk for age 30 or older. The risk was greatest more than 15 years after treatment. In the latter study, Yahalom and coworkers[51] found that breast cancers occurring after radiotherapy for Hodgkin's disease were significantly more likely to occur at a younger age, to be bilateral (22 percent), and to involve the inner quadrants more than was the case for breast cancer patients generally. Moreover, 95 percent of these breast cancers occurred 10 or more years after irradiation.

Pathological Features of the First Cancer

A second breast cancer can develop only if the patient survives the first. Adverse pathological features in the first cancer may lack a correlation with the devel-

TABLE 78–2. CUMULATIVE RISK OF BILATERAL BREAST CANCER ACCORDING TO AGE AT TIME OF DIAGNOSIS OF FIRST CANCER

Age at First Cancer	Unilateral Incidence (No. Cases)	Bilateral Incidence (No. Cases)	Cumulative Risk (%)*
<40	52	5	9.6
40–49	166	24	14.5
50–59	243	10	4.1
60–69	347	16	4.6
70–79	319	8	2.5
80+	158	3	1.9
Total	1285	66	5.1

*Bilateral/unilateral.
Adapted from Adami H, Bergstrom R, Hansen J: Age at first primary as a determinant of the incidence of bilateral breast cancer. Cumulative and relative risks in a population-based case-control study. Cancer 55:643–647, 1985. Copyright © 1985 American Cancer Society. Reprinted by Wiley-Liss, Inc., a subsidiary of John Wiley & Sons, Inc.

opment of second cancers, simply by reducing the number of survivors. The many contradictory findings in this area may simply reflect variations in mortality from the index cancer rather than a truly independent predictive value for the pathological feature of interest. Among the most consistent pathological correlates of bilaterality are the following:

1. *Stage of disease.* Storm and Jensen,[45] Hankey and coworkers,[23] and Lesser and coworkers[30] have all found increased bilaterality in patients with more advanced tumors. Fisher and coworkers,[17] in a multivariate analysis of 38 pathological and eight clinical features (in the 1578 patients in NSABP Protocol B-04, of whom 66 developed metachronous second cancers), demonstrated increased bilaterality for patients with first cancers greater than 2.0 cm in diameter. By distinction, Robbins and Berg[36] found a higher risk for bilaterality among patients with negative axillary nodes, perhaps reflecting a better survival in this group.

2. *Multicentricity.* Many investigators have associated multicentricity with bilaterality.[17, 25, 30, 36] Both may reflect the same biological phenomenon. As a cautionary note, tumor multicentricity is difficult both to define and to quantitate, and its precise incidence is unknown. As increasing numbers of patients are treated with breast conservation, the impact of occult multicentricity on bilaterality will probably become less clear than it was when most patients were treated by mastectomy (and the entire breast was available for study).

3. *Lobular carcinoma in situ (LCIS, "lobular neoplasia").* The classic studies of Haagensen[21] (Table 78–3) and Rosen and colleagues[39] both document an invasive breast cancer risk in patients with LCIS of about 30 percent at 20 to 25 years' follow-up; about half of this in the ipsilateral and half in the contralateral breast. The cancer risk for patients with LCIS is substantially higher than for the general population, with a relative risk of 7.2 in Haagensen's[21] and 9.0 in Rosen's[39] study. The risk to the opposite breast, however, is about the same as that conferred by a first breast cancer. LCIS is currently regarded as a marker of risk rather than a malignant lesion per se, and in most patients LCIS is managed by close clinical and mammographic follow-up, with equal atten-

TABLE 78–3. CUMULATIVE INCIDENCE OF BREAST CANCER ACCORDING TO TIME INTERVAL FROM TIME OF DIAGNOSIS OF LOBULAR CARCINOMA *IN SITU* ("LOBULAR NEOPLASIA")

Years After Diagnosis	Ipsilateral Breast (N = 280) Cumulative % Cancer	Contralateral Breast (N = 276) Cumulative % Cancer
5	4	6
10	8	7
15	12	8
20	18	12

Adapted from Haagensen CD: Diseases of the Breast. Philadelphia, WB Saunders, 1986.

TABLE 78–4. ROUTINE CONTRALATERAL BREAST BIOPSY: PREDICTORS OF OUTCOME IN 871 PATIENTS

	Positive Biopsy, LCIS Included (%)	Positive Biopsy, LCIS Excluded (%)
Age		
Under 50	4.5	1.0
50 and over	7.1	4.0
	(*p* = .13)	(*p* = .016)
Tumor Size		
T1 (0–2.0 cm)	5.0	2.4
T2 (2.1–5.0 cm)	7.9	3.6
T3 (>5.0 cm)	6.8	2.3
	(*p* = .24)	(*p* = .56)
Axillary Node Status		
Negative	5.5	2.7
1–3 nodes positive	6.1	2.8
>3 nodes positive	9.3	4.3
	(*p* = .24)	(*p* = .61)
Family History		
Negative	5.3	2.2
Positive	9.7	6.3
	(*p* = .03)	(*p* = .004)
Pathology of First Cancer		
Invasive duct	5.9	2.9
Invasive lobular	13.8	5.2
	(*p* = .018)	(*p* = .32)
Invasive versus *in situ* Cancer		
Invasive cancer	6.4	3.0
In situ cancer	3.8	2.5
	(*p* = .31)	(*p* = .76)

Adapted from Cody HS: Routine contralateral breast biopsy: Helpful or irrelevant? Experience in 871 patients, 1979–1993. Ann Surg 225:370–376, 1997.

tion given to each breast. In addition, LCIS is an absolute entry criterion for the current NSABP trial evaluating tamoxifen as a chemopreventive agent.

4. *Invasive lobular carcinoma (ILC).* ILC is associated more with bilaterality[5, 17] than duct carcinoma, although the reported incidence of bilaterality in ILC patients has been biased by the use of (a) clinical follow-up only,[5] (b) routine contralateral biopsy,[47] (c) selective contralateral biopsy,[41] or (d) prophylactic contralateral mastectomy,[28] as well as by the inclusion of LCIS as a "positive" result. In a series of 871 truly random contralateral breast biopsies—defining a positive biopsy as either DCIS or invasive cancer—Cody[14] (Table 78–4) demonstrated that ILC was not significantly more bilateral than invasive duct carcinoma (5.2 percent versus 2.9 percent); thus, the greater contralateral risk from ILC is a metachronous rather than a synchronous cancer.

5. *Atypical hyperplasia.* Atypical proliferative changes in the ipsilateral breast have been associated with an increased risk of contralateral cancer,[17, 25] suggesting (as for multicentricity and LCIS) a field effect of the entire breast epithelium.

PROGNOSIS FOR PATIENTS WITH BILATERAL BREAST CANCER

Opinion is equally divided regarding the prognosis for patients with bilateral breast cancer, supporting either no difference in survival between bilateral and unilateral disease[17, 21] or shorter survival rates for those with bilateral disease.[20, 40] Intuitively, one might postulate that prognosis in cases of bilateral breast cancer reflects the stage of the more advanced lesion (especially when one lesion is *in situ*), and that for two invasive cancers of equal stage the prognosis is in fact worse than for unilateral disease of the same stage. Fracchia and associates,[20] in a report from Memorial Sloan-Kettering Cancer Center, demonstrated exactly this point. The 10-year rate of recurrence for bilateral stage I cancers was 29 percent versus 16 percent for unilateral stage I tumors. As expected, patients with bilateral *in situ* disease had the best survival rate, followed by patients with one invasive and one *in situ* cancer (whose prognosis was identical to that of patients with unilateral disease), followed by patients with bilateral invasive cancers. This prognostic heterogeneity within the group of bilateral breast cancers has not been consistently documented in all studies and may explain the conflicting results reported by other researchers. Second breast cancers unquestionably contribute to breast cancer mortality overall, as shown in the 20-year follow-up studies of Rosen and colleagues.[37, 38] Among patients dying of the disease, 2.6 percent with T1, N0–N1 tumors[38] and 4.6 percent with T2, N0 tumors[37] died of contralateral breast cancers.

IMPACT OF MAMMOGRAPHY AND ADJUVANT THERAPY ON BILATERAL BREAST CANCER

Mammography

Increased use of mammography over the past two decades has been invaluable in diagnosing second breast cancers. Senofsky and coworkers[40] examined the stage of contralateral breast cancer both before (1969–1975) and after (1977–1985) the institution of mammographic monitoring. The proportion of contralateral *in situ* disease increased from 5 to 33 percent while the proportion of stage III–IV disease fell from 35 to 4 percent. Mellink and coworkers[32] compared two populations of breast cancer patients in the Netherlands, one with and one without mammographic follow-up of the opposite breast. With mammography, 35 percent of second cancers were either smaller than 1 cm or *in situ*, versus 7 percent with clinical follow-up alone. Also, with mammography, 75 percent were node-negative versus 57 percent with clinical follow-up alone. These findings, as one would expect, exactly parallel the impact of mammography on the stage at time of diagnosis of a first breast cancer.[13]

Radiotherapy

As noted earlier, radiotherapy given after either mastectomy or breast conservation surgery has not increased the risk of contralateral cancer. Because breast conservation has come into widespread use only during the last decade, longer follow-up will be required, especially in the youngest breast cancer patients, to establish with certainty this apparent lack of risk.

Chemotherapy

Few studies address the impact of adjuvant chemotherapy on the risk of a contralateral breast cancer. In Bernstein and colleagues'[7] prospective cohort study of 4660 patients, treatment with chemotherapy significantly reduced the risk of a second breast cancer (relative risk was 0.56, 95 percent confidence interval [CI] 0.33 to 0.96). A report of 4748 patients from the Institut Curie demonstrated a strikingly similar risk reduction with chemotherapy (relative risk was 0.54, 95 percent CI 0.36 to 0.81).[9] A "world overview" meta-analysis of all randomized adjuvant trials for early stage breast cancer was unable to address the issue of post-chemotherapy contralateral cancer risk, as this information was available for only a very small subset of these patients.[15]

Tamoxifen

The Early Breast Cancer Trialists' meta-analysis found contralateral breast cancers in 184 of 9135 control patients (2.0 percent), and in 122 of 9128 patients treated with adjuvant tamoxifen (1.3 percent), representing a highly significant odds reduction of 39 percent ($p < .00001$), with a trend toward the greatest reduction in risk (53 percent) for patients receiving tamoxifen longer than 2 years. This risk reduction may not be a long-lasting effect; the Cancer Research Campaign (CRC) Adjuvant Breast Trial has demonstrated that the significant contralateral cancer reduction seen in tamoxifen-treated patients at 3 years of follow-up disappeared by 7.8 years.[10] Whereas the CRC trial demonstrated a persisting trend toward benefit from tamoxifen in postmenopausal women, in premenopausal women there were more contralateral cancers among tamoxifen patients than in controls. Further follow-up of existing trials will be required to resolve this issue.

MANAGEMENT OPTIONS FOR THE NORMAL CONTRALATERAL BREAST

Close Observation

Of the available options, most physicians and patients have chosen close observation, with breast examination every 4 to 6 months and mammography annually. Arguments in favor of this approach are the following:

1. The risk of the present cancer will usually far outweigh that of a potential cancer on the other side.
2. Most patients perceive the 0.7 percent per year contralateral cancer risk to be a small one, with

contralateral cancer mortality even smaller. For the two thirds of breast cancer patients older than age 50, this risk may be smaller still.

3. Mammographic screening techniques continue to improve, allowing earlier diagnosis, less radical treatment, and greater likelihood of cure for a contralateral cancer.

4. Adjuvant treatment (either tamoxifen or chemotherapy) may itself reduce the risk of a second breast cancer.

Contralateral Biopsy

Biopsy of the normal contralateral breast remains the subject of controversy. Arguments in favor of routine contralateral biopsy are the following:

1. The procedure is done at the time of the definitive cancer surgery and thus adds little cost or morbidity to the operation.

2. Viewed as a screening test, contralateral biopsy's cancer yield (about 3 percent)[14] exceeds that of a single round of screening mammography (about 0.2 percent)[42] at least tenfold.

3. Patients are reassured by a negative result.

4. A proportion of biopsy-positive patients may benefit from earlier diagnosis of the contralateral cancer.

Despite the preceding arguments, contralateral breast biopsy has never been (and probably never will be) the subject of a randomized trial. Many series of contralateral biopsy are biased by preselection on the basis of clinical suspicion, abnormal results on mammogram, or type of first cancer (with particular emphasis on LCIS and invasive lobular carcinoma). The results of ten contralateral biopsy series in which clinical or mammographic examination of the opposite breast was normal are summarized in Table 78–5. Overall, unsuspected invasive cancers were found in 2.2 percent and *in situ* cancers in 5.2 percent of biopsied patients. Inclusion of LCIS with DCIS (as an *in situ* cancer) inflates the rate of "positive" biopsies. In the series in which LCIS and DCIS are reported separately, 50 of the 69 "positive" *in situ* biopsies (73 percent) were LCIS.[14, 34, 43] Of the studies

that include follow-up information, none convincingly demonstrates that patients with a negative biopsy subsequently have fewer contralateral cancers than would normally be expected. Nevertheless, routine contralateral biopsy will identify conditions (either invasive cancer or DCIS) requiring further treatment in about 3 percent of cases, and, given this information, many patients willingly elect to undergo biopsy if it is offered.

Many surgeons favor a selective approach to contralateral biopsy, with emphasis on known risks for bilaterality, such as age, family history, tumor stage, and tumor type (especially lobular), in an effort to individualize treatment and increase the yield of the procedure. All of these factors are well-correlated with bilaterality, but the largest series (Cody,[14] see Table 78–4) found that only one factor—a first-degree family history—was correlated with *synchronous bilaterality*, as demonstrated by routine contralateral biopsy. *The greater contralateral risk associated with these factors is a metachronous and not a synchronous cancer.* This lack of predictive value would suggest that (except for patients with a strong family history or those with unusual risks such as that posed by previous radiotherapy for Hodgkin's disease) selective contralateral biopsy of the normal breast may offer little advantage over the procedure done on a routine basis.

Contralateral biopsy is best done through a circumareolar incision, removing a small sample of breast tissue from the upper outer quadrant, to ensure the best cosmetic result. It is *not* necessary to excise 25 percent of the contralateral breast tissue, as Urban and coworkers[47] suggested in 1977. A later series from the same practice demonstrated comparable results with a much more conservative sampling of tissue.[14] Similarly, there is no need to perform a "mirror image biopsy." Cancers in the contralateral breast do not "mirror" the site of the first lesion (as the phrase suggests) but have the same frequency distribution by site as any other breast cancer, with most occurring in the upper outer quadrant.

Contralateral Prophylactic Mastectomy

Prophylactic mastectomy is the most controversial and least used of the available options for the other

TABLE 78–5. ROUTINE CONTRALATERAL BREAST BIOPSY: SUMMARY OF RESULTS

Researchers	No. Cases	Positive Biopsy, Invasive No. Cases (%)	Positive Biopsy, *In Situ* No. Cases (%)	Positive Biopsy, Total No. Cases (%)
Fenig[16] 1995	314	11 (3.5)	12 (3.8)	23 (7.3)
King[26] 1976	109	1 (1)	4 (3.7)	5 (4.6)
Urban[47] 1977	301	5 (1.7)	18 (6.0)	23 (7.7)
Leis[29] 1978	321	10 (3.1)	14 (4.4)	24 (7.5)
Pressman[33] 1980	85	0	7 (12)	7 (12)
Andersen & Murchardt[3] 1980	170	7 (4.1)	3 (1.8)	10 (5.9)
Martin[31] 1982	100	2 (2)	0	2 (2)
Wanebo[49] 1985	40	1 (2)	6 (15)	7 (17.5)
Pressman[34] 1986	226	4 (1.8)	28 (12.4)	32 (14.2)
Smith[43] 1992	95	2 (2.1)	3 (3.2)	5 (5.3)
Cody[14] 1997	871	14 (1.6)	40 (4.6)	54 (6.2)
Total	2632	57 (2.2)	135 (5.2)	192 (7.3)

breast. In favor of prophylactic mastectomy are the following arguments:

1. The procedure, properly done, should reduce contralateral breast cancer risk to a minimal level.

2. Patient anxiety associated with follow-up examination and mammography may be lessened.

3. For cases requiring mastectomy with breast reconstruction, contralateral mastectomy (and bilateral reconstruction) may allow the most symmetrical result for some patients. In addition, for patients selecting an immediate tissue transfer reconstruction (such as a TRAM flap, which can be done only once), a single-stage bilateral mastectomy/reconstruction should be considered.

Balanced against the factors favoring contralateral mastectomy is the morbidity of the procedure, which is certainly greater than that of the other options. The benefit appears to be relatively small, although this has not been confirmed by prospective trials. In Leis's[29] series of 101 prophylactic contralateral mastectomies (done selectively in a high-risk group of stage 0–I patients under age 50), only 5 percent were found to have invasive disease, a yield only slightly higher than that of contralateral biopsy. The risk of death from the first cancer is substantially greater than that from a second breast cancer: more than 95 percent of breast cancer deaths in the 20-year studies by Rosen and coworkers[37, 38] were due to the first cancer, and more patients died of second nonmammary malignant tumors than died of second breast cancers.

Prophylactic mastectomy is appropriate treatment for a definite but very small subset of breast cancer patients, primarily those with an extremely high-risk family history or with disabling anxiety about the other breast. For occasional patients having tissue transfer reconstruction, a bilateral procedure may have appeal. Under the stress of a newly diagnosed breast cancer many patients will express a strong interest in prophylactic mastectomy, feeling incorrectly that the opposite breast represents a risk equal to that of the first cancer. The decision to perform prophylactic mastectomy is never an urgent one and is best made (1) after the patient has fully recovered from the first cancer, (2) with the benefit of several different opinions, and (3) after very serious consideration by the patient.

If elected, prophylactic mastectomy is best done as a careful total mastectomy through an adequate incision, removing all breast tissue. "Subcutaneous mastectomy" done blindly through a small inframammary crease incision and preserving the nipple (with immediate reconstruction) is not acceptable treatment. There are many reports (published and anecdotal) of cancer later arising in residual breast tissue left behind during this procedure. A promising new method, "skin-sparing mastectomy" (with reconstruction), represents a cosmetic advantage over conventional total mastectomy while still removing all breast tissue. This technique, performed through a small-diameter circumareolar incision, relies on fiberoptic retractor technology for exposure and may become a more standard approach in the future. See Chapter 41, "General Principles of Mastectomy," for a discussion of skin-sparing mastectomy.

RECOMMENDATIONS AND FUTURE DIRECTIONS

Any decisions regarding the normal contralateral breast must be made considering (1) the prognosis associated with the first cancer (which usually carries a risk far greater than that of the opposite breast), (2) factors predisposing to bilaterality (of which patient age may be the best documented and the least appreciated), (3) the degree to which required adjuvant treatment may reduce this risk, (4) patient anxiety about the opposite breast, (5) the degree of difficulty for physical and mammographic examination, and (6) aesthetic factors relating to breast symmetry after reconstruction.

Close observation of the contralateral breast with physical examination every 4 to 6 months and mammograms annually is suitable for many breast cancer patients, especially those who are older (with fewer potential years at risk), have more advanced disease (stages II–III), have a soft and radiolucent breast, are not anxious regarding the opposite breast, and for whom neither reconstruction nor breast symmetry is an issue.

Contralateral biopsy is reasonable for younger breast cancer patients, especially those with early stage disease (stages 0–I), strong risk factors (such as family history or previous radiotherapy for Hodgkin's disease), a difficult physical and radiographic breast examination, anxiety about the other breast, or the need for a symmetry procedure as part of breast reconstruction. It is precisely this group of patients in whom the relatively small yield of contralateral biopsy may have the greatest impact. With progressively earlier breast cancer diagnoses, the risk posed by a contralateral cancer is greater than ever before, and contralateral screening biopsy deserves wider consideration in this setting.

Contralateral prophylactic mastectomy is reasonable treatment for a very small proportion of breast cancer patients, primarily those with a highly curable first breast cancer, an extremely high-risk family history (including *BRCA1* or *BRCA2* positivity), persistent disabling anxiety regarding the other breast, or the need for symmetry following breast reconstruction. Because of greater morbidity and small marginal benefit, contralateral prophylactic mastectomy will continue to have a definite but very small role in the management of the opposite breast.

The biological heterogeneity of breast cancer ensures that management of the contralateral breast will never become absolutely codified. To what degree will advances in breast imaging such as mammography, ultrasonography, and magnetic resonance imaging as well as newer techniques of biopsy such as stereotaxic or sonographically guided core needle or fine needle aspiration affect management of the opposite breast? Will ever-earlier diagnosis of the first breast cancer lend greater prognostic impact to a cancer on the other side? What will longer follow-up of existing clinical trials demonstrate regarding the effects of radiotherapy, chemotherapy, and tamoxifen on the other breast? Finally, to what degree will the rapidly evolving field of molecular genetics give the individual patient a more precise estimate of breast cancer risk, especially of bilaterality? Only with specific answers to these challenging questions can the oncological surgeon of tomorrow expect to achieve a reasonable adjustment of a means to an end in the management of the contralateral breast.

References

1. Adami H, Bergstrom R. Hansen J: Age at first primary as a determinant of the incidence of bilateral breast cancer. Cumulative and relative risks in a population-based case-control study. Cancer 55:643–647, 1985.
2. Adami H, Hansen J, Jung B, Rumsten A: Characteristics of familial breast cancer in Sweden: Absence of relation to age and unilateral versus bilateral disease. Cancer 48:1688–1695, 1981.
3. Andersen LI, Murchardt O: Simultaneous bilateral cancer of the breast: Evaluation of the use of a contralateral biopsy. Acta Chir Scand 146:407–409, 1980.
4. Anderson DE: Some characteristics of familial breast cancer. Cancer 28:1500–1504, 1971.
5. Ashikari R, Huvos AG, Urban JA, Robbins GF: Infiltrating lobular carcinoma of the breast. Cancer 31:110–116, 1973.
6. Bernstein JL, Thompson WD, Risch N, Holford TR: The genetic epidemiology of second primary breast cancer. Am J Epidemiol 136:937–948, 1992.
7. Bernstein JL, Thompson WD, Risch N, Holford TR: Risk factors predicting the incidence of second primary breast cancer among women diagnosed with a first primary breast cancer. Am J Epidemiol 136:925–936, 1992.
8. Boice JD, Harvey EB, Blettner M, et al: Cancer in the contralateral breast after radiotherapy for breast cancer. N Engl J Med 326:781–785, 1996.
9. Broet P, de la Rochfordiere A, Scholl SM, et al: Contralateral breast cancer: Annual incidence and risk parameters. J Clin Oncol 13:1578–1583, 1995.
10. Cancer Research Campaign Breast Cancer Trials Group: The effect of adjuvant tamoxifen: The latest results from the Cancer Research Campaign Adjuvant Breast Trial. Eur J Cancer 28A:904–907, 1992.
11. Chaudary MA, Millis RR, Bulbrook RD, Hayward JL: Family history and bilateral primary breast cancer. Breast Cancer Res Treat 5:201–205, 1985.
12. Chaudary MA, Millis RR, Hoskins EOL, et al: Bilateral primary breast cancer: A prospective study of disease incidence. Br J Surg 71:711–714, 1984.
13. Cody HS: The impact of mammography in 1096 consecutive patients with breast cancer, 1979–1993. Cancer 76:1579–1584, 1995.
14. Cody HS: Routine contralateral breast biopsy: Helpful or irrelevant? Experience in 871 patients, 1979–1993. Ann Surg 225:370–376, 1997.
15. Early Breast Cancer Trialists' Collaborative Group: Systemic treatment of early breast cancer by hormonal, cytotoxic, or immune therapy: 133 randomised trials involving 31,000 recurrences and 24,000 deaths among 75,000 women. Lancet 339:1–15, 1992.
16. Fenig J, Arlen M, Livingston SF, Levowitz BS: The potential for carcinoma existing synchronously on a microscopic level within the second breast. Surg Gynecol Obstet 141:394–396, 1995.
17. Fisher ER, Fisher B, Sass R, Wickerham L: Pathologic findings from the National Surgical Adjuvant Breast Project (Protocol No. 4). XI. Bilateral Breast Cancer. Cancer 54:3002–3011, 1984.
18. Foote FW, Stewart FW: Comparative studies of cancerous versus noncancerous breasts. Ann Surg 121:197–222, 1945.
19. Ford D, Easton DF, Bishop DT, et al: Risks of cancer in BRCA1-mutation carriers: Breast Cancer Linkage Consortium. Lancet 343:692–695, 1994.
20. Fracchia AA, Robinson D, Legaspi A, et al: Survival in bilateral breast cancer. Cancer 55:1414–1421, 1985.
21. Haagensen CD: Diseases of the Breast. Philadelphia, WB Saunders, 1986.
22. Hancock SL, Tucker MA, Hoppe RT: Breast cancer after treatment of Hodgkin's disease. J Natl Cancer Inst 85:25–31, 1993.
23. Hankey BF, Curtis RE, Naughton DN, et al: A retrospective cohort analysis of second breast cancer risk for primary breast cancer patients with an assessment of the effect of radiation therapy. J Natl Cancer Inst 70:797–804, 1983.
24. Healey E, Cook EF, Orav EJ, et al: Contralateral breast cancer: Clinical characteristics and impact on prognosis. J Clin Oncol 11:1545–1552, 1993.
25. Hislop TG, Elwood JM, Boldman AJ, et al: Second primary cancers of the breast: Incidence and risk factors. Br J Cancer 49:79–85, 1984.
26. King RE, Terz JJ, Lawrence W, et al: Experience with opposite breast biopsy in patients with operable breast cancer. Cancer 37:43–45, 1976.
27. Kurtz JM, Amalric R, Brandone H, et al: Contralateral breast cancer and other second malignancies in patients treated by breast-conserving therapy with radiation. Int J Radiat Oncol Biol Phys 15:277–284, 1988.
28. Lee JSY, Grant CG, Donohue JH: Arguments against routine contralateral mastectomy or undirected biopsy for invasive lobular breast cancer. Surgery 118:640–648, 1995.
29. Leis HP: Bilateral breast cancer. Surg Clin North Am 58:833–842, 1978.
30. Lesser ML, Rosen PP, Kinne DW: Multicentricity and bilaterality in invasive breast cancer. Surgery 91:234–240, 1982.
31. Martin JK, van Heerden JA, Gaffey TA: Synchronous and metachronous carcinoma of the breast. Surgery 91:12–16, 1982.
32. Mellink WAM, Holland R, Hendriks JHCL, et al: The contribution of routine follow-up mammography to an early detection of asynchronous contralateral breast cancer. Cancer 67:1844–1848, 1991.
33. Pressman PI: Bilateral breast cancer: The contralateral biopsy. Breast 5:23–29, 1980.
34. Pressman PI: Selective biopsy of the opposite breast. Cancer 57:577–580, 1986.
35. Prior P, Waterhouse JAH: Incidence of bilateral tumours in a population-based series of breast-cancer patients: I. Two approaches to an epidemiological analysis. Br J Cancer 37:620–634, 1978.
36. Robbins GF, Berg JW: Bilateral primary breast cancers: A prospective clinicopathologic study. Cancer 17:1501–1527, 1964.
37. Rosen PP, Groshen S, Kinne DW: Prognosis in T2N0M0 stage I breast carcinoma: A 20-year follow-up study. J Clin Oncol 9:1650–1661, 1991.
38. Rosen PP, Groshen S, Kinne DW, Hellman S: Contralateral breast carcinoma: An assessment of risk and prognosis in stage I (T1N0M0) and stage II (T1N1M0) patients with 20-year follow-up. Surgery 106:904–910, 1989.
39. Rosen PP, Lieberman P, Bruan D: Lobular carcinoma in situ of the breast: Detailed analysis of 99 patients with an average follow-up of 24 years. Am J Surg Pathol 2:225–251, 1978.
40. Senofsky GM, Wanebo HJ, Wilhelm MC, et al: Has monitoring of the contralateral breast improved the prognosis in patients treated for primary breast cancer? Cancer 57:597–602, 1985.
41. Simkovich AH, Sclafani LM, Masri M, Kinne DW: Role of contralateral breast biopsy in infiltrating lobular cancer. Surgery 114:555–557, 1993.
42. Smart CR: Highlights of the evidence of benefit for women aged 40–49 years from the 14-year follow-up of the Breast Cancer Detection Demonstration Project. Cancer 74:296–300, 1994.

43. Smith BL, Bertagnolli M, Klein BB, et al: Evaluation of the contralateral breast: The role of biopsy at the time of treatment of primary breast cancer. Ann Surg 216:17–21, 1992.
44. Storm HH, Andersson M, Boice JD, et al: Adjuvant radiotherapy and risk of contralateral breast cancer. J Natl Cancer Inst 84:1245–1250, 1992.
45. Storm HH, Jensen OM: Risk of contralateral breast cancer in Denmark 1943–1980. Br J Cancer 54:483–492, 1986.
46. Tulusan R, Ronay G, Egger H, Wilgeroth F: A contribution to the natural history of breast cancer: Bilateral primary breast cancer: Incidence, risks, diagnosis of simultaneous primary cancer in the opposite breast. Arch Gynecol 237:85–91, 1985.
47. Urban JA, Papachristou D, Taylor J: Bilateral breast cancer: Biopsy of the opposite breast. Cancer 40:1968–1973, 1977.
48. Veronesi U, Salvadori B, Luini A, et al: Conservative treatment of early breast cancer: Long-term results of 1232 cases treated with quadrantectomy, axillary dissection, and radiotherapy. Ann Surg 211:250–259, 1990.
49. Wanebo HJ, Senofsky GM, Fechner RE, et al: Bilateral breast cancer: Risk reduction of contralateral biopsy. Ann Surg 201:667–677, 1985.
50. Wobbes T, van der Wiel MP, van der Sluis RF, Theeuves AM: The effect of familiality on clinical presentation and survival in mammary carcinoma. Eur J Surg Oncol 13:119–121, 1987.
51. Yahalom J, Petrek JA, Biddinger PW, et al: Breast cancer in patients irradiated for Hodgkin's disease: A clinical and pathologic analysis of 45 events in 37 patients. J Clin Oncol 10:1674–1681, 1992.

CHAPTER 79
CANCER OF THE MALE BREAST

Morton C. Wilhelm, M.D. / Scott E. Langenburg, M.D. / Harold J. Wanebo, M.D.

Cancer of the male breast is a rare disease, accounting for less than 1 percent of cancers in males as well as less than 1 percent of all breast cancers. Although the first description of male breast cancer was made by an English surgeon, John of Aderne, in 1307 and was subsequently followed by case reports by renowned people such as Ambroise Paré and Fabricus Hildanus in the sixteenth and seventeenth centuries, large series were not reported until well into the twentieth century.[33]

EPIDEMIOLOGY

Male breast cancer accounts for approximately 0.7 percent of all cases of breast cancer in the United States, with an estimated 1400 new cases and 240 deaths occurring in 1995.[4] LaVecchia and coworkers[17] studied male cancer death rates in 25 countries in Europe for 1955–1989. The rates varied from 1.5 to 3 per million, with the highest rates occurring in France, Hungary, Austria, and Scotland. The rates were lower for 1985–1989 compared with 1955–1959. LaVecchia and coworkers[17] concluded that there was no generalized increase in mortality, and thus no new cause of the disease.[17]

Sasco and colleagues[29] reported a meta-analysis of worldwide published, case-controlled studies and found that about 1 percent of all breast cancer cases occurred in males.[29] The male-female ratio was higher in black than in white populations. This ratio was evident in the United States cancer registries and markedly so in African data as well.[1]

Breast cancer appears at an older age in males than in females. The average age of presentation is 63.6 years. It is rarely found before the age of 26, although it has been reported in a boy as young as 5 years of age.[27] Early reports suggested a higher incidence in Jewish males.[31] In about 2 percent of cases, male breast cancer is bilateral.

Testicular hormonal factors appear to play a role in male breast cancer.[6] Klinefelter's syndrome carries a risk of male breast cancer in about 3 percent of cases.[9] Complications of mumps' infections in males 20 years of age and older carry an increased risk of breast cancer, as does infectious orchitis. Other viral infections appear not to cause an increased risk of male breast cancer.[20] Gynecomastia was found in 23 percent of male breast cancer cases reported by Borgen and coworkers[5] and has been reported in as many as 43 percent of male breast cancer cases, but there is no convincing evidence associating gynecomastia with the development of breast cancer.[15] Un-

descended testicles have been associated with an increased risk.[29]

Occupational exposure to heat has been reported in association with an increased incidence of breast cancer in males. It has been suggested that heat exposure has a suppressive effect on testicular function.[20] Exposure to electromagnetic fields was not found to be associated with an increase in male breast cancer in a study by Rosenbaum and associates,[26] but a report by the Office of Epidemiology and Health Surveillance suggested an increased risk in individuals whose jobs exposed them to electromagnetic fields if they were employed before the age of 30 and worked for at least 30 years in this job.[22]

The role of trauma is hard to document, but exposure to ionizing radiation for the treatment of childhood malignancies is a definite risk factor and survivors of such treatment should be observed regularly.[29] Liver disease is associated with an increase in circulating estrogens and has been implicated in male breast cancer.

Familial cancer risks for relatives of males with breast cancer appear to be slight for males, but the risk for female first-degree relatives is significantly higher. Olsson and coworkers[23] reported that data from the Swedish cancer registry showed a significant increase of breast cancer in mothers, sisters, and daughters of male patients with breast cancer. Anderson and Bodzioch[2] found a twofold increased risk of familial cancer as compared with expected rates and a fourfold increase when prostate cancer occurred in the family of a male with breast cancer. Borgen and coworkers[5] found that 12 out of 87 patients (14 percent) had a first-degree relative with a history of breast cancer.

Genetic information regarding male breast cancer suggests little, if any, association between the male breast cancer and breast cancer gene *BRCA1*.[32] There does seem to be an association with *BRCA2*.[30] An androgen receptor gene has been found in male breast cancer with Reifenstein's syndrome, an androgen resistance syndrome.[18] Mutations in p53 for male breast cancers (43 percent) parallel the incidence in females.[3] Predisposing factors are summarized in Table 79–1.

CLINICAL FINDINGS

Male breast cancer is usually detected as a palpable mass. Public awareness is leading to detection at an earlier stage, but skin fixation, chest wall fixation, and ulceration are found more commonly in males than in females. Nipple ulceration and nipple dis-

TABLE 79–1.   MALE BREAST DISEASE: PREDISPOSING FACTORS

Benign Breast Enlargement (Gynecomastia)[a]

Etiology—Disease

Abnormal thyroid function
Adrenal insufficiency
Chronic hepatic disease
Chronic renal failure
Klinefelter's syndrome
Malnutrition
Testicular tumors

Etiology—Medications

Androgens	LSD
Amphetamine	Marijuana
Cimetidine	Methadone
Cyclophosphamide	Methyldopa
Diazepam	Reserpine
Digitalis	Spironolactone
Exogenous estrogens	Thiazides
Heroin	Tricyclic antidepressants
Isoniazid	

Male Breast Cancer

Genetic Associations

BRCA2[b]
Androgen receptor gene found in Reifenstein
    syndrome
p53 mutations (43%)

Familial Association

Incidence of associated breast cancer in female
    relatives, 10–12%

Ethnic-racial

Increased incidence in Jewish and black males

Predisposing Disease

Mumps orchitis
Testicular tumors
Klinefelter's syndrome

Other Predisposing Conditions

Radiation of childhood cancer
Occupational exposure to high environmental
    temperatures
Excess phytoestrogen (soy)

[a]Although there are reports of gynecomastia in association with breast cancer, and there is a 27–42 percent frequency of microscopic gynecomastia in association with male breast cancer, there is no histological or statistical evidence to show gynecomastia as a premalignant lesion.
[b]BRCA1 has a questionable association with male breast cancer.

charge occur in males and requires prompt investigation. Breast enlargement in adolescents is rarely due to carcinoma but may indicate a systemic disorder. In young adults with breast enlargement, the testicles should be carefully examined for the purpose of ruling out a testicular tumor. In some males, breast enlargement can also be caused by systemic disease or medications.

A firm, non-tender mass in the male breast requires investigation. It occurs most commonly in the subareolar location but can occur in adjacent areas. Gynecomastia is more likely to be tender, soft, and more diffuse. The distinction between benign and malignant breast enlargement is usually not difficult to make, but tissue evaluation is necessary if the mass persists or if the examiner has any doubts. Fine needle aspiration or core biopsy can be readily

performed on masses in the male breast, but an open biopsy should be carried out if an adequate sample cannot be obtained.[12]

Mammography has been used in evaluating the male breast, but unless there is significant enlargement, adequate imaging may be difficult. Microcalcifications alone were found in 8 percent of 50 mammograms reported by Borgen and colleagues.[5] Cooper and coworkers[8] reported on 263 mammograms performed in males and found typical gynecomastia in 199, with no cancer on follow-up. Cooper and coworkers[8] recommended confining mammography in males to patients over the age of 50 unless there was strong clinical suspicion of malignancy. Biopsy was not recommended when the mammogram was considered as the diagnostic test for gynecomastia unless the physical examination was highly suspect. False-negative examinations can occur in males, just as in females. Evaluation of the male breast should not require mammography in the majority of cases. Ultrasonography has not been as useful as mammography. Galactograms may have a limited place in identifying abnormal ductal areas in cases with nipple discharge and with no palpable mass.

PATHOLOGY

Male breast cancer is ductal in origin. Lobules are absent in the normal male breast, but cytoarchitectural changes can occur in Klinefelter's syndrome or upon exposure to estrogens. A case of lobular carcinoma has been reported in a male with no known estrogen exposure.[21] The incidence of lobular carcinoma in males varies between zero and 4.7 percent. Infiltrating ductal carcinoma makes up 85–90 percent of the cases and intraductal carcinoma 5–15 percent. Papillary, medullary, and tubular forms, as well as rare forms such as cystosarcoma phyllodes, have been reported. Paget's disease is associated with invasive ductal or intraductal carcinoma. Male breast cancer is staged using the TNM (tumor, node, metastasis) system that is used for staging female breast cancer.

TREATMENT

The treatment of primary breast cancer in males is surgical. Mastectomy is the most common procedure. The proximity of the tumor to the chest wall and the relatively small amount of breast tissue preclude the use of partial mastectomy in the majority of cases. Salvadori and colleagues[28] reported 170 cases from 1961 to 1990 from the National Cancer Institute of Milan. Radical mastectomy was performed in 92 of these cases, modified radical in 58, and total mastectomy in 11.[28] Memorial Sloan-Kettering and the Ochsner Clinic reported 106 cases from 1975 to 1990, with 28 cases treated with radical mastectomy, 71 with modified radical mastectomy, and five with total mastectomy. Modified radical mastectomy is now the surgical treatment of choice unless there is involvement of the pectoral muscle or of Rotter's nodes.[5] Taking exceptions into account, the results are similar for radical mastectomy and modified radical mastectomy.

Levels 1 and 2 axillary dissections are advised for invasive carcinomas. The use of total mastectomy followed by radiation therapy has been reported. The local recurrence rate varies between 4 percent and 26 percent, and adjuvant radiation therapy seems to reduce this occurrence but does not improve overall survival.[32] Camus and associates[7] reported on the treatment of ductal carcinoma *in situ* and recommended total mastectomy in this group. Estrogen and progesterone receptor studies should be carried out for all patients with malignant tumors.

Prognostic factors for breast cancer are being reported with increasing frequency. In males the most important prognostic factors are lymph node status, tumor size, and stage. Guinee and coworkers[11] reported on a multicenter study that evaluated chest wall and skin involvement, tumor diameter, and nodal status. Patients were grouped according to whether they had one to three positive nodes versus four or more. The presence of chest wall and skin fixation did not influence survival. Skin ulceration was associated with a decreased survival, but because of its frequent association with other factors, it was hard to separate as an isolated factor. Tumor size was a definite factor. Patients with tumors 40 mm or more had a significantly lower survival rate. Patients with one to three positive nodes had a survival rate at 5 years of 73 percent compared with 55 percent for patients with four or more positive nodes. Patients with negative nodes had a survival rate of 90 percent at 5 years and 84 percent at 10 years. The risk of death resulting from breast cancer in a patient with four or more positive nodes was 6.75 times that for a patient with negative nodes.[11]

The overall survival rate at 5 years for patients with male breast cancer at Memorial Sloan-Kettering and the Ochsner Clinic was 100 percent for those with negative nodes and 60 percent for those with positive nodes. This unusually high 5-year overall survival rate was attributed primarily to the fact that 17 percent of patients were stage 0 and 27 percent were stage I.[5] Salvadori and coworkers[28] reported 73.1 percent and 45.7 percent overall survival rates at 5 and 10 years, respectively, in 170 cases. The results of representative series show that survival rates at 5 years are 82–100 percent for stage I disease, 63–83 percent for stage II disease, and 74 percent for stage III disease (Table 79–2).

Estrogen and progesterone receptors are positive in 85 percent and 75 percent, respectively, of male breast cancer cases.[5, 14, 10, 24] The influence of receptor positivity on survival is difficult to ascertain, but receptor status does provide valuable information for the decision between cytotoxic and hormonal adjuvant therapy. A Swedish study showed no prognostic significance for DNA ploidy and S-phase fraction in male breast cancer,[13] but Hecht and Winchester's preliminary study suggested that S-phase fraction was a significant predictor of disease-free survival.[14] The significance of the p53 suppressor gene and *ERBB2* oncoprotein in males has not been determined.[16]

ADJUVANT THERAPY

Whereas numerous large and long-term studies exist on the use of adjuvant therapy in women, the small number of cases in each series of male breast cancer patients has resulted in few meaningful conclusions. The use of tamoxifen in the adjuvant setting has been studied by Ribeiro and Swindell[25] since 1976. A total of 39 patients were analyzed, with a median follow-up of 49 months. Tamoxifen was given for 1 year initially, but in 1988 the course of treatment was increased to 2 years. The actuarial survival for the tamoxifen-treated patients was 61 percent at 5 years compared with 44 percent for historical controls. The disease-free survival rate was 56 percent at 5 years compared with 28 percent for historical controls. No serious side effects were recorded.

Anelli and coworkers[4] reported on the side effects of adjuvant tamoxifen treatment in 24 male patients

TABLE 79–2.   SURVIVAL RATES FOR MALE BREAST CANCER CASES

	Heller,[16] 1978	Borgen,[6] 1992	Guinee,[12] 1993	Joshi,[17] 1996
No. Patients	97	106	335	46
Overall Survival (%)				
5-year	72	85	77.5	76
10-year	40			42
Survival for Node-Negative Patients (%)				
5-year	90	100	90	
10-year	79		84	58
Survival for Node-Positive Patients (%)				
5-year	59	60	65	
10-year	11		29	18
5-Year Survival per Stage (%)				
Stage I	100	83		100
Stage II	63	70		83
Stage III	45	74		60

and found that one quarter of them stopped taking the medication because of side effects, in contrast to a noncompliance rate of only 4 percent in women. The most common side effects were decrease in libido (29 percent), weight gain (25 percent), hot flashes (20.8 percent), mood alterations (20.8 percent), and depression (16.6 percent).

Reports on adjuvant cytotoxic chemotherapy are sparse. Borgen and coworkers'[5] report from Memorial Sloan-Kettering and Ochsner Clinic on 13 patients who received cytotoxic chemotherapy showed a distant relapse in 46 percent. In 14 node-positive patients receiving no adjuvant therapy, the relapse rate was 57 percent. In view of the experience in treating female patients, adjuvant hormonal or cytotoxic chemotherapy, or a combination of both, is recommended for node-positive male patients. The use of cytotoxic chemotherapy followed by toilet mastectomy and chest wall radiation for patients with locally advanced disease has been recommended by researchers from several centers.[5]

METASTATIC DISEASE

The high rate of hormone receptor-positive tumors in males (80 percent) makes hormonal manipulation excellent therapy for recurrent disease. Whereas ablation by orchiectomy or adrenalectomy and the use of estrogens or androgens were common in the past, antiestrogen therapy in the form of tamoxifen is the treatment most frequently used at the present time. The response rate in patients with positive estrogen receptors approximates 70 percent and the overall response rate is approximately 50 percent.[14] Lopez and colleagues[19] reported on the combined use of buserelin and cyproterone acetate in treatment of metastatic male breast cancer and found objective responses in seven out of 11 patients, with a median survival of 18.5 months. Cytotoxic chemotherapy should be administered to those who experience relapse after hormonal treatment. Cytotoxic chemotherapy is considered to be the first-line approach in those who are receptor-negative. The response can be expected to be comparable with that in women.

SUMMARY

The incidence of male breast cancer has remained fairly stable throughout the world. There does seem to be a higher incidence in Jewish males and in males with any of the following: Klinefelter's syndrome, mumps orchitis after 20 years of age, positive *BRCA2*, or an androgenic gene. The incidence in black males is higher than in white males in certain parts of the world. Ductal carcinoma is the most frequent cellular type that results in an increased incidence of earlier-stage disease.

Mastectomy is the treatment of choice in the majority of cases, with the tendency being toward less radical procedures. Postoperative radiation therapy is appropriate in high-risk cases and will reduce the rate of local recurrence, which is higher in males than in females. Nodal status is the most important prognostic factor. Overall survival rates for node-negative male patients are comparable with those of node-negative female patients. Overall survival rates for node-positive male patients do not seem to be as good as for node-positive female patients. The development of a treatment strategy that incorporates adjuvant therapy is important. Hormonal manipulation remains an important tool in the management of male breast cancer.

References

1. Ajayi DO, Oseghe DN, Ademiluyi SA: Carcinoma of the male breast in West Africans and a review of world literature. Cancer 50:1664–1667, 1982.
2. Anderson DE, Bodzioch MD: Breast cancer risks in relatives of male breast cancer patients. J Natl Cancer Inst 84(14): 1114–1117, 1992.
3. Anelli A, Anelli TF, Youngson B: Mutations of the p53 gene in male breast cancer. Cancer 75(9):2233–2238, 1995.
4. Anelli TF, Anelli A, Tran KN, et al: Tamoxifen adminstration is associated with a high rate of treatment-limiting symptoms in male breast cancer patients. Cancer 74(1):74–77, 1994.
5. Borgen PI, Wong GY, Vlamis V, et al: Current management of male breast cancer. Ann Surg 215:5, 1992.
6. Brown P, Terez J: Breast cancer associated with Klinefelter's syndrome. J Surg Oncol 10:413–415, 1978.
7. Camus M, Joshe M, Mackarem G, et al: Ductal carcinoma in situ of the male breast. Cancer 74(4):1289–1293.
8. Cooper RA, Gunter BA, Ramamuthy L: Mammography in men. Radiology 191:651–656, 1994.
9. Evans DB, Crichlow RW: Carcinoma of male breast and Klinefelter's syndrome—Is there an association? CA Cancer J Clin 37:246–260, 1987.
10. Friedman MA, Hoffman PG, Dandolos EM, et al: Estrogen receptors in male breast cancer. Cancer 47:134–137, 1981.
11. Guinee VF, Olsson H, Moller T, et al: The prognosis of breast cancer in males. Cancer 71(1):154–161, 1993.
12. Gupta RK, Naran S, Doule CS, et al: The diagnostic impact of needle aspiration cytology of the breast on clinical decision making with emphasis on aspiration cytodiagnosis of male breast masses. Diagn Cytopathol 7(6):637–639, 1991.
13. Hatschek T, Wingren S, Carstensen J, et al: DNA content and S-phase fraction in male breast carcinomas. Acta Oncol 33(6):609–613, 1994.
14. Hecht RJ, Winchester DJ: Male breast cancer: Review. Am J Clin Path 102 (suppl):525–530, 1994.
15. Heller K, Rosen P, Schattenfeld D, Ashihari R, Kinne D: Male breast cancer. Ann Surg 188:60–65, 1978.
16. Joshi MG, Lee AKC, Loda M, et al: Male breast carcinoma: An evaluation of prognostic factors contributing to a poorer outcome. Cancer 77(3):490–498, 1996.
17. LaVecchia C, Levi F, Luccini F: Descriptive epidemiology of male breast cancer in Europe. Int J Cancer 51:62–66, 1992.
18. Lobaccaro JM, Lumbroso S, Belon C, et al: Androgen receptor gene mutation in male breast cancer. Human Mol Genet 2(11):1799–1802, 1993.
19. Lopez M, Natali M, Dilauro L, et al: Combined treatment with buserelin and cyproterone acetate in metastatic male breast cancer. Cancer 72(2):502–505, 1993.
20. Mabuchi A, Bross D, Kessler I: Risk factors in male breast cancer. J Natl Cancer Inst 74:371–375, 1985.
21. Michaels BM, Nunn CR, Roses DF: Lobular carcinoma of the male breast. Surgery 115(3):402–405, 1994.
22. Occupational exposure to electromagnetic fields and male breast cancer. Health Bulletin, U.S. Department of Energy, Washington, DC, Issue 91-4, October 1991.
23. Olsson H, Anderson H, Johansson O, et al: Population-based cohort investigations of the risk for malignant tumors in first-

degree relatives and wives of men with breast cancer. Cancer 71(4):1273–1278, 1993.

24. Ribeiro G: Male breast cancer: Review of 301 cases from Christie Hospital and the Holt Radium Institute, Manchester. Br J Med 51:115–119, 1985.

25. Ribeiro G, Swindell R: Adjuvant tamoxifen for male breast cancer. Br J Cancer 65(2):252–254, 1992.

26. Rosenbaum PF, Vena JE, Zielezmy MA, et al: Occupational exposure associated with male breast cancer. Am J Epidemiol 139(1):30–36, 1994.

27. Saltzstein EC, Tanof M, Latomoca R: Breast carcinoma of a young male. Arch Surg 113:880–881, 1978.

28. Salvadori B, Saccozzi R, Manzari A: Prognosis of breast cancer in males—An analysis of 170 cases. European J of Cancer 30A(7):930–935, 1994.

29. Sasco AJ, Lowenfels AB, Pasker-Dejong P: Review article: Epidemiology of male breast cancer. A meta-analysis of published case control studies and discussion of selected aetiological factors. Int J Cancer 53:538–549, 1993.

30. Sokol H, Bibnon YJ, Eisinger F, et al: Genetics and cancer of the breast. Ann Chir 48(4):303–308, 1994.

31. Steintz R, Katz L, Ben-Hur M: Male breast cancer in Israel: Selected epidemiological aspects. Isr J Med Sci 17:816–821, 1981.

32. Stratton MR, Ford D, Neuhasen S: Familial male breast cancer is not linked to the *BRCA1* locus on chromosome 17q. Nat Genet 7(1):103–107, 1994.

33. Van Geel AN, van Slooten EA, Mavrunac M, Hart AA: A retrospective study of male breast cancer in Holland. Br J Surg 72:724–727, 1985.

34. Wingo PA, Tong T, Bolden S: Cancer statistics, 1995. CA Cancer J Clin 45:8–30, 1995.

CHAPTER 80

LOCAL RECURRENCE, THE AUGMENTED BREAST, AND THE CONTRALATERAL BREAST

D. Scott Lind, M.D. / Edward M. Copeland III, M.D.

The optimal postoperative surveillance strategy for breast cancer patients remains undefined. Few well-designed, prospective, clinical trials have addressed this important question. Therefore, significant physician variation exists in the follow-up of breast cancer patients. Although intuitively one would anticipate that frequent intensive surveillance would lead to earlier detection of recurrences and permit earlier intervention, thereby improving survival, the absence of proven curative therapy for metastatic disease makes it unlikely that early detection of metastatic disease will affect patient outcome.[24] In addition, diagnostic tests to detect metastatic disease, such as computed tomography and radionuclide scans, are expensive. On the other hand, the minimalist approach to follow-up fails to alleviate patient fears and anxiety about the development of recurrent disease. Therefore, the follow-up of breast cancer patients must take into account individual psychosocial issues as well as economic concerns. From the standpoint of detecting local/regional recurrences and contralateral breast cancers, physical examination and mammography are critical.[44] This chapter addresses situations in the care of breast cancer patients that deserve special attention such as recurrence cancer in the operative site following mastectomy, recurrence of cancer in the reconstructed breast, breast cancer after subcutaneous mastectomy, recurrence of cancer in the intact irradiated breast, primary breast cancer in the augmented breast, and risk of cancer in the contralateral breast.

RECURRENCE OF CANCER IN THE OPERATIVE SITE FOLLOWING MASTECTOMY

Local/regional recurrence following mastectomy refers to reappearance of breast cancer in the skin flaps or mastectomy scar on the chest wall or the ipsilateral regional lymphatics (axillary, internal mammary and supraclavicular lymph nodes). Local/regional recurrences are a heterogenous group of lesions ranging from a small, solitary tumor nodule in the surgical scar to diffuse carcinoma en cuirass involving the entire chest wall and regional lymphatics. Local/regional recurrence is directly related to the extent of disease at the time of mastectomy. Factors that influence local/regional recurrence include tumor characteristics (i.e., size, location, skin involvement, and close or positive margins) and lymph node histology (number and percentage of positive lymph nodes, and presence of extracapsular extension). The vast majority of chest wall recurrences are detected by physical examination; therefore, patients must understand the importance of careful evaluation of the chest wall and axilla and bring any changes to a physician's attention.

The incidence of local recurrence following mastectomy varies from 7 to 32 percent[81, 83] and is dependent not only on the initial extent of disease but the type of primary therapy and length of follow-up.[2] Sixty to eighty percent of all chest wall recurrences appear within the first 2 years after mastectomy, but they can occur throughout the lifetime of the patient.[21, 25, 88, 120] There is also a tendency for patients with advanced disease at initial diagnosis to develop local/regional recurrence more rapidly. Unfortunately, most studies examining local/regional recurrence following mastectomy have been retrospective and have employed outdated radiotherapeutic techniques. In addition, the heterogeneity of patients with local/regional recurrences makes the design of prospective randomized trials difficult. Historically, local recurrences following mastectomy have carried a poor prognosis, with the majority of patients ultimately developing distant metastases.[6, 15, 26, 75] Multiple local recurrences that arise after a short disease-free interval probably represent hematogenous spread of tumor cells to the surgical wound and should prompt a metastatic work-up. Therapy in this group of patients tends to be palliative, but efforts toward local/regional control even in patients with metastatic disease should be maximized. Very few studies, however, have evaluated patients who have local recurrence as the first and only site of failure. Some local recurrences may simply represent a solitary focus of tumor incompletely excised or tumor cells deposited in the surgical wound at the time of operation. Rarely, an isolated local recurrence may represent a new primary cancer in residual breast tissue left on the skin flaps at the time of mastectomy. In these instances, cure may be possible with appropriate local therapy. If these local recurrences involve the chest wall (i.e., ribs, intercostal musculature), radical chest wall resection may be indicated. Shah and Urban[103] reported a 43-percent 5-year survival rate using full-thickness chest wall resection for isolated chest wall recurrences. The recent advent of free flaps, made possible by microsurgery, and better prosthetic materials have extended the limits of chest wall resection.

Gilliland and associates[42] reported 60 patients with

TABLE 80–1. TIME INTERVAL BETWEEN TREATMENT OF PRIMARY TUMOR AND DISCOVERY OF CHEST WALL RECURRENCE

Stage (No.)	Mean Disease-free Interval (yrs)	Range (yrs)
I (11)	6.2	2.5–21.0
II (9)	4.3	1.2–6.8
III (31)	2.1	0.2–11.0

Stage I vs. II, $p = 0.26$; stage I vs. III, $p = 0.01$; stage II vs. III, $p = 0.11$.
Adapted from Gilliland MD, et al: Ann Surg 197:284–287, 1983.

ipsilateral chest wall recurrence of breast cancer and no detectable distant metastases. These authors made several interesting observations. More than 50 percent of the nodules were solitary and easily removed. Only 10 percent of patients had more than five nodules. The majority of the recurrences were in the mastectomy scar or immediate vicinity. Mean disease-free interval between treatment of the primary cancer and discovery of the chest wall recurrence, and time interval between local recurrence and death were directly related to stage of initial disease (Tables 80–1 and 80–2). All stage I patients had at least a 2-year disease-free interval, and this interval was as long as 21 years in some patients. Others have also noted a direct correlation between disease-free interval and progression of disease and survival.[6, 15, 26, 42] Surgical resection resulted in the best local control. Even in the most favorable group of patients with no detectable distant metastases at the time of local recurrence, all 60 patients eventually died of metastatic breast cancer. Consequently, this report supports the concept that chest wall recurrence rarely represents a site of isolated disease but is almost always a manifestation of distant metastasis. Mendenhall and coworkers,[81] however, reported a small subset of patients who were aggressively treated for local recurrence and who had 5- and 10-year actuarial survival rates of 50 percent and 34 percent, respectively. Differences in patient follow-up may account for the discrepancy between these two studies.

Prevention of local/regional recurrence at the time of initial treatment is a primary goal. Adjuvant radiation therapy has been shown to decrease the rate of local/regional recurrence after mastectomy.[110] Unfortunately, which subgroups of patients are at sufficient risk for local/regional recurrence to justify

adjuvant postmastectomy radiotherapy has not been precisely defined. In addition, controversy exists concerning the influence of adjuvant radiation therapy on overall survival.[34–36] Although adjuvant chemotherapy improves survival, the effect of chemotherapy on local recurrence has been difficult to establish. If, in the majority of cases, local/regional recurrence is a manifestation of systemic disease and chemotherapy impacts on systemic relapse, then logically, chemotherapy may also impact on local/regional relapse. Without a doubt, chemotherapy given preoperatively to patients with advanced local disease reduces the risk of local recurrence in those patients who respond to treatment. However, these patients are usually treated by mastectomy and chest wall radiation therapy as well, making the impact of chemotherapy on local recurrence difficult to evaluate. The delivery of postoperative chemotherapy is impeded by the interruption of blood supply and scar in the healing wound where residual breast cancer is deposited and thus renders chemotherapy somewhat ineffective locally. Nevertheless, three studies using different cytotoxic chemotherapy protocols in a large number of node-negative patients who received no radiotherapy have been completed.[32, 33, 80] These patients were randomized to treatment with postoperative chemotherapy versus observation only. The group receiving chemotherapy had a prolonged disease-free interval and a reduction in local and regional recurrences at a maximum follow-up of 4 years (Table 80–3). Chemotherapy may only delay the inevitable recurrence and will not replace chest wall radiation therapy as the major deterrent to chest wall relapse following surgery. Future follow-up of these patients may be enlightening.

The optimal sequence of adjuvant radiation and chemotherapy in the overall management of breast cancer remains to be defined. Although radiation oncologists emphasize the importance of adjuvant radiotherapy in achieving optimal local disease control, medical oncologists argue that potential gains in terms of local control may be at the expense of increased distant relapse. The correct integration of these modalities requires individual patient assess-

TABLE 80–2. TIME INTERVAL BETWEEN LOCAL RECURRENCE AND DEATH

Stage (No.)	Average Time Interval (yrs)	Range (yrs)
I (11)	7.2	1.0–23.0
II (9)	6.0	2.1–13.0
III (31)	2.5	0.3–6.3

$p < 0.05$, stage III versus stage I or II.
Adapted from Gilliland MD, et al: Ann Surg 197:284–287, 1983.

TABLE 80–3. LOCAL/REGIONAL RECURRENCE AS FIRST SITE OF TREATMENT FAILURE IN LYMPH NODE-NEGATIVE PATIENTS

Type of Adjuvant Therapy	Surgery Alone (%)	Surgery + Adjuvant (%)
Methotrexate, 5-FU[24] ER negative	8.0	4.0*
Tamoxifen[23] ER positive	3.0	1.0*
Cyclophosphamide, methotrexate 5-FU, leucovorin[62]		
ER positive	3.9	0.9†
ER negative	8.1	1.1†

*$p < 0.05$.
†Significance of values not started.

ment. A delay in the initiation of radiation therapy until completion of chemotherapy in those patients at greatest risk for systemic relapse has little negative impact on local control and therefore seems prudent. Local recurrence should be treated aggressively because short-term prognosis and patient comfort improve markedly if local control of the recurrence can be obtained. Furthermore, the ability to provide local control of recurrent disease is also associated with overall survival. Those lesions amenable to surgical removal (including major chest wall resections) should be treated surgically, and if it has not previously used, radiation therapy is indicated. Our policy is to treat the chest wall and internal mammary nodes to 5000 cGy in 25 fractions with electron beam. The supraclavicular nodes are treated with a combination of photons and electrons to a dose of 5000 cGy in 25 fractions as well. This dose may be boosted through reduced fields to areas of gross disease.[79] The role of chemotherapy in the setting of isolated local/regional recurrence is not clear; however, treatment philosophies developed for other high-risk patients dictate it be used based on the hormone receptor and menopausal status of the patient. Again, no data on sequencing of multimodality treatment exist, but it would be reasonable to deliver appropriate chemotherapy either before or after surgical resection and before radiation therapy.

RECURRENCE OF CANCER IN THE RECONSTRUCTED BREAST

Despite the increasing use of breast-conserving surgery, many women either are not appropriate candidates for lumpectomy or simply prefer mastectomy. This fact, combined with improved reconstructive techniques, has made breast reconstruction increasingly popular. However, there remains some controversy about the appropriate timing of breast reconstruction after mastectomy. The advantages of immediate reconstruction include an immediate breast form on the chest wall, the positive psychological impact of improved self-image, and perhaps a final cosmetic result superior to delayed reconstruction. Immediate reconstruction may also eliminate another operation required with delayed reconstruction, thereby reducing overall cost. Initial concerns that immediate reconstruction might inhibit the detection of local recurrences have not been substantiated. Until several years ago, an empirical interval of 2 years between mastectomy and reconstruction was recommended in order to not mask recurrent disease during this critical time interval. Studies by Gilliland and associates[43] and others[38, 40, 41] demonstrated that almost no patients with stage I disease who experienced recurrence on the chest wall did so in the first 2 years postoperatively. Therefore, waiting a designated time interval is of no practical value in patients with stage I disease. Although immediate reconstruction may offer psychological benefits to patients, other potential problems must be considered.

Significant differences in complication rates associated with immediate reconstruction have been noted. One recent report demonstrated a 15-percent complication rate, with only 9 percent of patients undergoing autologous tissue transfer requiring additional operative procedures.[28] On the other hand, another recent retrospective review of 50 patients reported a 50-percent complication rate, prolonged hospitalization, and frequent use of blood transfusion with immediate breast reconstruction.[59] In addition, more than one operation was frequently required to manage associated complications and to achieve the desired cosmetic result. Wound healing complications after immediate reconstruction may also significantly delay the initiation of adjuvant therapies. However, these delays must be compared with delays associated with wound complications following mastectomy without reconstruction for such a comparison to be meaningful. The possible adverse effect of blood transfusion on tumor recurrence in some cancer patients makes autologous blood donation an important consideration in breast cancer patients undergoing immediate reconstruction with autologous tissue.[20]

In an occasional early report of chest wall recurrence as the first site of treatment failure in a reconstructed breast, the entire capsule surrounding the silicone implant was infiltrated with metastatic breast cancer.[119] Fortunately, subsequent reports of chest wall recurrence after reconstruction have not been of this form of en cuirass disease.[38, 40] For example, with the implant in place subpectorally, Georgiade et al.[40] had no problem with early detection of four local recurrences in 50 patients. Likewise in this series, five patients on final pathological evaluation of the initial specimen had unsuspected evidence of nipple/areolar involvement. Therefore, these authors did not recommend use of autologous nipple/areolar complex for reconstruction.

If a reconstruction procedure were to mask a chest wall recurrence, the best method of reconstruction would be the transverse abdominal island flap, in which a composite graft of autologous muscle and fat from the abdominal wall is transported with its blood supply intact to the chest wall. A recurrence deep to this tissue could go undetected for some period of time. In fact, of the five recurrences reported by Hartrampf and Bennett[54] in their series of 300 patients reconstructed by the transverse abdominal island flap method, only one recurrence was delayed in its discovery (for 3 months). Several other studies have demonstrated no difference in disease-free or overall survival between patients undergoing immediate versus delayed breast reconstruction.[59, 65, 87]

Some reports have demonstrated satisfactory early cosmetic and oncologic results from radiation therapy or chemotherapy with a silicone- or a saline-filled implant in place, but these studies require longer follow-up.[64, 105] Thus, it would appear that immediate reconstruction may be best offered to patients who are anticipated to be at lower risk for postoperative adjuvant therapies.

BREAST CANCER AFTER SUBCUTANEOUS MASTECTOMY

Brief mention should be made of the possibility of developing breast cancer after prophylactic subcutaneous simple mastectomy. The nipple/areolar complex is left intact after this operation, and therefore, breast tissue remains on the chest wall in the nipple because the ducts pass through it to exit on the surface. Also, in an attempt to not devascularize the nipple/areolar complex, a pledget of breast parenchyma may be left beneath the nipple. Subcutaneous mastectomy is often done via an incision in the inframammary crease; consequently breast tissue is not dissected from the skin flaps under direct vision. Likewise, the axillary tail of the breast may be inadequately excised, because it is at the most distant site from the inframammary incision and troublesome bleeding may be encountered in this area. Patients undergoing subcutaneous mastectomy should be made aware of the possibility of some breast tissue remaining on the chest wall, especially if the operation is being performed as prophylaxis against breast cancer. Breast cancer is both a multicentric and multifocal disease, particularly in patients with atypical hyperplasia, a strong family history of breast cancer, and *in situ* disease. Because these are the individuals who are often offered subcutaneous mastectomy as a prophylactic operation, the risk of developing breast cancer in residual ductal tissue after the operation is even higher. It has not been proved whether removal of 95 percent of the breast tissue would reduce the subsequent risk of breast cancer proportionately. There are numerous anecdotal reports in the literature about women developing breast cancer after subcutaneous mastectomy, and these cancers were often detected at an advanced stage, possibly owing to a false sense of security on the part of the women who believed that their risk of developing breast cancer had been eliminated.[9]

Although no operation assures the removal of all breast tissue,[58] the best[56] method of complete extirpation of all breast tissue is via simple mastectomy in which the nipple/areolar complex is excised as part of the specimen and the breast tissue is removed from the skin flaps under direct vision. Some authors have even recommended frozen section analysis to ensure removal of all breast tissue during simple mastectomy.[106]

Researchers have identified specific genes that are responsible for the development of some inherited forms of breast cancer (*BRCA1* and *BRCA2* genes).[51, 117] The development of a simple diagnostic test to identify patients who carry these genes will immediately create a sizeable patient population who may be candidates for prophylactic simple mastectomy and reconstruction. In the absence of any proven chemoprevention, prophylactic mastectomy may be preferable to life-long surveillance with physical examination and mammography because it appears that women who inherit these genes develop breast cancer early in life, at a time when the density of breast tissue impairs mammographic screening.

RECURRENCE OF CANCER IN THE INTACT IRRADIATED BREAST

Several randomized prospective studies have documented that segmental resection (lumpectomy), axillary dissection, and postoperative radiation therapy to the intact breast results in disease-free and overall survival rates equal to those for modified radical mastectomy.[18, 30, 31, 98] Fraudulent data in the National Surgical Adjuvant Breast and Bowel Project Protocol B-06 (NSABP-B06), one of the landmark trials of breast conservation, led some to question the accuracy of results and dampened public perception about clinical trials. Recent publication of the re-analysis of NASBP-B06 excluding all falsified data,[30] and the National Cancer Institute (NCI) audit of the trial,[17] have confirmed the initial interpretation. These findings are also supported by a recent meta-analysis of over 17,000 women involved in randomized trials of surgery and radiotherapy for early breast cancer that demonstrated that the addition of radiotherapy to surgery reduced the risk of local recurrence by approximately one third but had no effect on overall survival.[27] Whether there exists a subset of women who can be treated by surgery alone with an acceptable local recurrence rate awaits the results of carefully designed clinical trials.

Controversy exists regarding the risk factors for and the consequences of local recurrence after lumpectomy and radiation. One fear is that a recurrence in the breast may have the same grave prognostic implications as a chest wall recurrence following mastectomy.[42] It would appear that mammary parenchymal recurrences after lumpectomy[18, 19, 67, 82] are distinctly different entities from chest wall recurrences after mastectomy.[42, 81] Mammary recurrence does not necessarily herald a distant metastasis. Local recurrence after breast-conserving surgery may be a marker of aggressive disease at the time of lumpectomy rather than a failure to remove all local disease with a mastectomy. This concept should not, however, lessen the importance of careful patient selection and meticulous surgical technique to minimize the risk of local recurrence.

In an effort to improve selection criteria and reduce local relapse rates, investigators have sought to identify risk factors for local recurrence after breast-conserving surgery. Factors that may favor recurrence after lumpectomy are positive surgical margins at the time of lumpectomy (inadequate incision),[31, 53, 91, 99] lymphatic invasion,[77] anaplasia,[19, 53, 99] associated *in situ* disease in both the primary cancer and surrounding parenchyma,[53, 91, 99] tumor necrosis,[77] invasive lobular carcinoma,[77] inadequate radiation dose,[19] and a delay of radiation therapy for longer than 7 weeks after lumpectomy.[19] Unfortunately, studies that attempt to identify risk factors for local recurrence are subject to inherent patient heterogeneity and treatment selection biases. For example, not every investigator has found that positive margins,[19] associated *in situ* diseases,[19] or histological subtypes[19] would result in a higher recurrence rate. Although one would assume that tumor cells present at the inked margin of a lumpectomy specimen might lead to an increased risk of local recurrence, there is a lack of consensus among pathologists about what constitutes a positive histological margin.[46] In addition, there is a direct correlation between the number of margins assessed and the frequency of a positive margin.[46] These inconsistencies make it difficult to define precisely the impact of a positive margin on local recurrence after breast-conserving surgery. The relationship between extensive intraductal component and local recurrence is also controversial. The assumption is that if tumor cells may disseminate locally by way of the ducts then a greater intraductal component may increase the risk of local recurrence. The presence of EIC is not, however, a contraindication to breast-conserving surgery, but it may require a more extensive resection to achieve uninvolved margins. The relationship between infiltrating lobular histologic subtype and risk of local recurrence after mastectomy is also unsettled. Lobular cancers tend to be diffusely infiltrative and individual tumor cells are difficult to identify pathologically at the tumor margin. Also, mammography tends to underestimate the pathological extent of disease. Thus, obtaining histologically-free surgical margins may be more difficult with invasive lobular cancer.[116] Several reports have documented, however, that selected patients with invasive lobular cancer can be treated with lumpectomy, axillary dissection, and radiotherapy with an acceptable local recurrence rate.[89, 101, 116, 118] Therefore, lobular histology is not an absolute contraindication to breast-conserving surgery.

An idea of the magnitude of risk for recurrence can be obtained from studies by Harris and associates.[53] Patients who had a combination of the three risk factors of *in situ* disease in the tumor and adjacent tissue and anaplasia had a 37 percent local recurrence rate at 8 years compared with 8 percent for all other patients. Local recurrence was reduced by a radiation boost to the lumpectomy site. The survival rate was 69 percent for patients with all three risk factors compared with 90 percent for the remainder of the patients. These authors have also noted a greater actuarial risk of local recurrence at 5 years for patients who have an incomplete excision (36 percent) compared with those patients in whom excision is complete (8 percent).

Kurtz and colleagues[69] have followed 276 patients with T1 and T2 lesions treated by lumpectomy only for 10 to 21 years. No chemotherapy was employed, and radiation therapy was administered appropriately. The recurrence rate in the treated breast was 15.6 percent. Contralateral breast cancer developed in 7.2 percent of patients. Breast recurrence was rare in the first 2 years postoperatively (data similar to the infrequency of early chest wall recurrence after mastectomy for stage I disease). Only 63 percent of

all eventual failures occurred before 5 years, and 53 percent of failures in patients with T1 lesions occurred 5 or more years postoperatively. The true recurrence rate in the intact irradiated breast may not be known for many years; therefore, results from breast conservation trials must have long-term follow-up.

Somewhat contrary to this concept of late recurrence are data from the NSABP-B06 protocol, which identified the majority of failures following lumpectomy to occur in the first 39 months of the study.[31] Accrual of only a few additional patients with recurrence occurred during the next 4 years of the study. Salvage surgery has been most often accomplished by modified radical mastectomy. In the conservation surgery series by Kurtz and colleagues[69] 49 percent of patients had positive axillary lymph nodes in the salvage mastectomy specimen, a figure much higher than would have been predicted at the initial operation had axillary dissections been performed. Five-year survival after salvage mastectomy was 62 percent, again a lower figure than is expected for patients with T1 or T2NO lesions. Why then was the pathological situation and survival worse for the cohort of patients with recurrent disease? Probably those patients who had local recurrences also had more aggressive cancer. In fact, early recurrences after mastectomy have a distinctly unfavorable prognosis. The type of local failure affects survival as well. An isolated breast parenchymal recurrence without inflammation is much more amenable to cure by mastectomy than is nodal or dermal relapse.[18] The prognosis for dermal relapse appears to be as poor as that for relapse on the chest wall after mastectomy.[18, 31]

It is difficult to know whether an isolated recurrence in the irradiated breast is a true recurrence or a new primary cancer.[74] The ipsilateral mammary tissue is still available for malignant degeneration. Schnitt and coworkers[100] for example, found evidence of multicentricity in 22 percent of patients undergoing salvage mastectomy for solitary mammary recurrences. From the experience of surgeons at the Princess Margaret Hospital in Toronto,[19] however, multicentricity seldom became clinically apparent after radiation therapy. Nevertheless, a new primary malignancy is possible. Kurtz and associates[68] reported 52 patients who were treated for a mammary recurrence by a repeat lumpectomy and axillary dissection rather than by mastectomy. The 5- and 10-year actuarial survival rates calculated from the date of the second operation were 79 percent and 64 percent, respectively. Seventy-three percent of patients were disease-free at a mean of 6 years after salvage surgery. These data compare favorably to previous series reported by these authors[67] and others[18, 19] in which salvage surgery was performed by modified radical mastectomy. In fact, the physician teams at both the Princess Margaret Hospital[18] and the Institute Gustave-Roussy[19] have concluded that a relapse in the breast alone, if appropriately treated, does not adversely affect survival. Haffty and colleagues attempted to differentiate between relapse in the breast and a new primary lesion. The three criteria for determining a new primary lesion were origin in a different breast quadrant, a distinctly different histological pattern, and a different pattern of DNA. Of 82 cancers that developed in the ipsilateral breast after conservative surgery and radiation therapy 47 (57%) were considered a relapse and 35 (43%) were new primary lesions. Time to diagnosis since original treatment was 3.2 years and 5.4 years, respectively, and the survival rates were 36% and 89%, respectively. Determining a second ipsilateral breast cancer to be a relapse or new primary lesion would have significant impact on treatment, especially with the use of adjuvant chemotherapy.[50]

Early detection of local recurrences after breast-conserving surgery is important. A post-treatment mammogram is required to establish a new baseline, because the lumpectomy scar will be visible and radiation fibrosis may distort the image. Otherwise, follow-up is the same after lumpectomy as after modified mastectomy. Any suspicious areas in the breast must be biopsied; therefore, areas of fibrotic tissue are commonly removed, particularly near the scar. After 5 to 7 years, radiation fibrosis usually stabilizes, and a previously firm breast should become compliant. An experienced examiner is required to follow the irradiated breast, and patients should request to be examined by the same individual at each physician visit. The treatment of local recurrence after mastectomy is influenced by the type of recurrence and the treatment of the initial primary tumor. Although there are anecdotal reports of repeat lumpectomy for small local recurrences after breast conserving surgery, the follow-up is relatively short and the relapse rate for conservative salvage surgery appears to be high.[19] Therefore, if the patient has previously undergone lumpectomy and axillary dissection followed by radiotherapy, the appropriate local therapy is simple mastectomy. If the axilla has not been dissected previously, modified radical mastectomy would be indicated. The complication rate is similar to the complication rate for mastectomy in unirradiated patients. If immediate breast reconstruction is being considered after salvage mastectomy, then autogenous tissue transfer (i.e., TRAM flap) may be preferable compared with the placement of an implant in an irradiated field. If the patient had not received adjuvant chemotherapy after the initial lumpectomy, some consideration should be given to administration of chemotherapy following salvage mastectomy, depending on the disease-free interval as well as the type and extent of recurrence.

PRIMARY BREAST CANCER IN THE AUGMENTED BREAST

Safe and effective methods for breast augmentation have been available now for several decades. Estimates are that well over one million women have undergone augmentation,[8, 115] many of these women have reached the prevalent age for the development of breast cancer. Consequently, reports of breast cancer in augmented breasts are now beginning to appear[8, 10, 22, 23, 38, 84] and are stimulating debates on the possibility of the implant material, usually silicone, being causative. Experimental data from subcutaneous implantation of silicone has not shown a causal relationship with malignancy.[12, 14, 45, 56, 60, 73]

Several large retrospective studies in women who have undergone augmentation showed no increase in the risk of breast cancer.[22, 38, 52, 62] Deapen and coworkers[22] reported 3111 women in whom frequency-distribution epidemiological analysis would have predicted 15.7 breast cancers. Only nine breast cancers were actually detected. Of the subpopulation of 447 women in this series who had implants in place for 10 years or more, 3.5 cases of breast cancer were expected and only three were detected. Breast cancers that were identified seemed no more virulent than those in the general population. The conclusion from this study was that breast implants do not appear to increase the risk of breast cancer. The study was performed, however, by 35 plastic surgeons in the Los Angeles County area who submitted their augmentation mammaplasty patients' records for review. Those who developed breast cancer were identified through a population-based cancer registry (The Los Angeles County Cancer Surveillance Program). There is selection bias in any study that retrospectively compares the risk of breast cancer in women who have undergone augmentation mammoplasty with those women who have not undergone the procedure. Women with risk factors for breast cancer are likely to be denied augmentation mammoplasty; therefore, those who undergo the procedure may be a group of women at less risk for the development of breast cancer. Although errors inherent to this method of patient accrual do not invalidate the study, the discovery of the patients with breast cancer relied on accurate record-keeping by a multitude of physicians in the Los Angeles County area. Berkel and coworkers used the Alberta (Canada) Cancer Registry to obtain follow-up on 11,676 augmented patients. Implants were in place for an average of 10.2 years, and similar to the Los Angeles County study, the number of breast cancers predicted for this population was 86, whereas only 41 were observed.[8]

Silverstein and colleagues[104] approached the question from a different perspective. Of the 753 patients treated for primary breast cancer during a 66-month period, 20 had previously undergone a subglandular augmentation mammoplasty with a silicone gel–filled prosthesis. The authors make the point that the augmented group had a worse prognosis than did the general population of nonaugmented patients with breast cancer. None of the cancers in the augmented patients were occult or *in situ*, and 13 patients (65 percent) had positive axillary lymph nodes. All had palpable masses, none of which were discovered mammographically. Although the authors do not suggest that silicone is a causative agent, they do agree with us that women with augmentation have several disadvantages relative to breast cancer detection. The implant, when placed in a retromammary position in a small-breasted woman, compresses the breast parenchyma against the skin and obscures the normal parenchymal pattern (Fig. 80–1). Detection of small clusters of microcalcifications is impaired. Regardless of the plane of the mammogram, the implant will obscure some portion of the breast parenchyma from visualization. When scar and capsule formation occur, stellate masses may occur in the area of the capsule, give a false-positive appearance on physical examination, and present as an indistinct mass on mammogram. If silicone gains access to the breast parenchyma (i.e., from a ruptured implant), granulomas develop that are palpably indistinguishable from carcinoma and may appear as a calcified mass on mammogram. Distortion of the physical examination and the mammographic pattern is not as pronounced when the implant is retromammary in a large-breasted woman or is in the subpectoral position. However, some so-called blind areas still exist on the mammogram. The future use of radiolucent implants and advances in breast imaging techniques will undoubtedly improve our ability to detect breast cancer in women with augmented breasts.

Before augmentation, all women should have a mammogram and have their risk of breast cancer assessed. For those with a strong family history of breast cancer, small dense breasts, atypical hyperplasia on a previous biopsy, or a previous contralateral

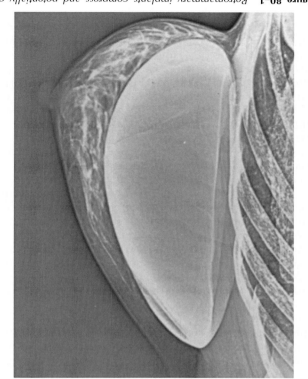

Figure 80–1 Retromammary implants compress and potentially obscure from view several areas of breast parenchyma.

breast cancer, the disadvantages of losing mammography as a potential tool for early detection should be weighed carefully against the cosmetic advantages. Certainly, the woman should be apprised of the problem so that she can actively participate in the decision for augmentation. Following augmentation, annual mammograms using the Eklund push-back technique should be considered when the patient reaches 35 years of age, and all suspicious lesions require biopsy.

The implant does not appear to alter the growth characteristics of the malignancy, although compression of lymphatics and distortion of flow are possibilities, as is the potentiation of neovascularization of the tumor. An initial fear was that a primary breast cancer in an augmented patient with breast augmentation might be first detected as an en cuirass mass surrounding the retromammary implant. To the contrary, in reports to date,[8, 65, 87] the breast cancers have been freely mobile and not attached to the implant capsule (Fig. 80–2). In fact, in large-breasted patients, the lesions are readily visible by mammography (Fig. 80–3).[8]

Treatment regimens for patients developing breast cancer in an augmented breast have not been established. Modified radical mastectomy remains the standard treatment until experience with breast conservation techniques is well established. Previous reports suggested that postoperative radiation in the augmented breast was associated with capsular contracture and poor cosmesis. Recently, however, Geunther and others evaluated the cosmetic outcome and the disease-free survival of 20 women with breast implants who developed breast cancer and were treated with breast-conserving surgery.[47] Good to excellent cosmetic results were achieved in 85% of patients, and there have been no local recurrences with a median follow-up of 4 years. Cosmetic outcome did correlate with the location of the implant; all patients who had retromuscular implants showed excellent results. It is also easier to obtain histologically free margins when the implant is retromuscular because there tends to be more breast parenchyma surrounding the lesion. The effect of cytotoxic chemotherapeutic agents on capsule scar formation is unknown. Doxorubicin does alter wound healing in both human beings and experimental animals.[11] Therefore, long-term follow-up is required before lumpectomy and radiotherapy can be accepted as standard treatment for breast cancer that develops in women with breast implants.

RISK OF CANCER IN THE CONTRALATERAL BREAST

Although the risk of developing breast cancer in the contralateral breast has been discussed in many chapters in this text, a brief summary is provided here. Environmental, genetic, morphological, and biochemical factors affect each breast equally.[16, 74, 76] Because the number of women who have been treated for breast cancer is increasing, more and more women are at risk for developing breast cancer in the opposite breast. The risk of contralateral breast cancer depends on the duration of follow-up and the method of detection. The detection of contralateral breast cancer is lowest when physical examination alone is used as the method of evaluation; identification increases with mammographic surveillance, blind contralateral biopsy, and is highest with prophylactic contralateral mastectomy. Using a combination of physical examination and mammography, 4 percent to 15 percent of surviving breast cancer patients develop a contralateral primary breast cancer, a risk two to six times higher than that for the general population.[13, 70, 72] This risk remains relatively constant throughout the lifetime of the pa-

tient.[55, 57, 70, 93] Horn and Thompson[61] reviewed 292 women with an incident contralateral breast cancer. Factors associated with an increased risk for the opposite breast were lobular histology, a positive progesterone assay in the initial primary cancer, and AB blood type. Interestingly, adjuvant chemotherapy significantly lowered the risk. However, the influence of adjuvant chemotherapy on the development of contralateral breast cancer must be interpreted with caution, because patients receiving chemotherapy are more likely to have more advanced disease in the initially affected breast, and their death from recurrent disease removes the risk of developing contralateral breast cancer. In addition, patients with metastatic disease may not be intensively evaluated for contralateral breast cancer. There is also strong evidence to indicate that adjuvant hormonal therapy (i.e., tamoxifen) significantly reduces the risk of contralateral breast cancer.[32] These clinical data, together with laboratory data, provide the rationale for the NASBP tamoxifen breast cancer prevention trial to evaluate the efficacy of tamoxifen in the prevention of breast cancer in high-risk women. This trial is ongoing, and no clinical results are yet available, but are eagerly awaited.

The need for contralateral breast biopsy in patients with invasive carcinoma is controversial. The work of Urban[107, 108, 109] and Leis[70-72] indicates a potential for detecting a contralateral breast cancer at an early stage; Wanebo and associates[11] have adopted this approach because, in their opinion, the prognosis for patients who develop a contralateral breast cancer is unfavorable. Other investigators, however, have not been able to document any value of a contralateral

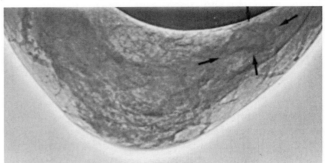

Figure 80-3 Mammogram from the patient whose photomicrograph is depicted in Figure 80-2. The breast cancer was freely mobile from the implant capsule by physical examination and by mammography. (From Bingham H, et al: Ann Plast Surg 20:236-237, 1988. Reprinted by permission.)

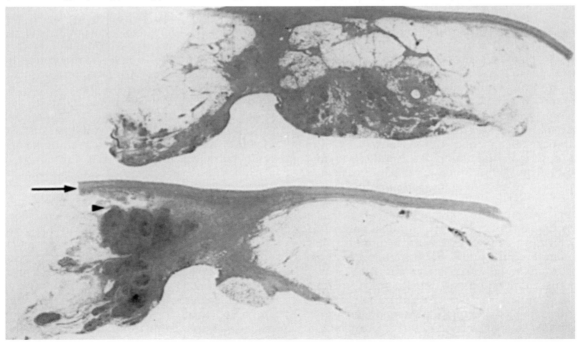

Figure 80-2 Photomicrograph of a breast cancer that developed in a patient with an augmented breast. Note the fibrous capsule around the silicone implant (arrow). The arrowhead points to the advancing border of an adenocarcinoma and demonstrates no attachment to the capsule. (From Bingham H, et al: Ann Plast Surg 20:236-237, 1988. Reprinted by permission.)

report by Haagensen[49] places the incidence of subse-quent invasive breast cancer in either breast at 15 percent. More than half of these invasive lesions develop more than 15 years after the LCIS is diag-nosed.[48,96] Therefore, in those clinical series in which a large percent of patients have LCIS, only a few breast cancers ever develop.

The treatment for the contralateral breast in a patient with LCIS would seem to be careful surveil-lance throughout the remainder of the patient's life. In fact, most investigators now recommend only close follow-up for the ipsilateral breast.[39] Because both breasts are at equal risk for the development of inva-sive cancer, the treatment for both breasts should be the same. Thus, if total mastectomy is the selected surgical therapy, it should be applied bilaterally. However, treating LCIS, a precursor lesion, with mastectomy when breast conservation is used rou-tinely for selected patients with invasive cancer seems paradoxical.

Studies on the bilaterality of intraductal carcinoma are inconclusive. Reports from the Memorial Sloan-Kettering Institute indicate an incidence as high as 26 percent,[5] yet long-term follow-up data on the opposite breast yield an actual breast cancer inci-dence of only 4 to 7 percent.[29,113] Consequently, most investigators recommend close follow-up by physical examination and mammography, just as is done for invasive breast cancer.[63,102]

Prophylactic simple mastectomy for the contralat-eral breast should probably be reserved for those patients who have multiple associated risk factors such as florid LCIS and invasive lobular carcinoma in the ipsilateral breast, multiple first-degree relatives with breast cancer,[4] or a contralateral breast that is difficult to follow clinically because of the density and nodularity of the breast tissue.

References

1. Adami H-O, Hansen J, Jung B, Lindgren A, Rimsten A: Bilateral carcinoma of the breast: Epidemiology and histopa-thology. Acta Radiol Oncol 20:305–309, 1981.
2. Ahlborn TN, Gump FE, Bodian C, Habif DV, Kister S: Tumor to fascia margin as a factor in local recurrence after modified radical mastectomy. Surg Gynecol Obstet 166:523–526, 1988.
3. Anderson LL, Muchardt O: Simultaneous bilateral cancer of the breast—evaluation of the use of a contralateral biopsy. Acta Chir Scand 146:407–409, 1980.
4. Anderson DE: Genetic considerations in breast cancer. In Breast Cancer: Early and Late. 13th Annual Clinical Confer-ence on Cancer, 1968, M.D. Anderson Hospital and Tumor Institute, Houston, 1968. Chicago, Year Book Medical, 1969, pp 27–36.
5. Ashikari R, Hajdu SI, Robbins GF: Intraductal carcinoma of the breast (1960-1969). Cancer 28:1182-1187, 1971.
6. Auchincloss H: The nature of local recurrence following radi-cal mastectomy. Cancer 11:611-619, 1958.
7. Baker RB, Kuhajda F: The incidence of synchronous and metachronous cancers in the contralateral breast of patients with lobular breast cancer. Ann Surg 210:444-448, 1989.
8. Berkel H, Birdsell DC, Jenkins H. Breast augmentation: a risk factor for breast cancer? N Engl J Med 326:1649-1653, 1992.
9. Bilimoria MM, Morrow M. The women at increased risk for breast cancer: evaluation and management strategies. CA Cancer J Clin 45:263-278, 1995.

biopsy in the absence of a detectable physical or radiographic abnormality of the contralateral breast.[3,49,61,70,74,86] Diligent lifelong surveillance of the opposite breast seems most appropriate and avoids overtreatment from data obtained from con-tralateral blind breast biopsy.

A plan for follow-up management of a normal con-tralateral breast in patients with in situ breast can-cer is difficult to obtain from reports in the literature. Data on bilaterality often include patients with a previous or synchronous breast cancer and greatly overestimate the actual risk of cancer developing in a normal contralateral breast. For example, in one of the earliest reports of a large series of patients with minimal breast cancer followed for up to 20 years, 59 percent of patients with lobular carcinoma in situ (LCIS) had bilateral breast cancer,[37] yet none of the patients with a normal contralateral breast at risk developed subsequent breast cancer. Five percent of patients with intraductal carcinoma in situ and the opposite breast at risk developed a subsequent inva-sive breast cancer (Table 80-4). Likewise, in a recent report by Baker and Kuhajda,[7] 6 percent of patients who initially had invasive lobular carcinoma devel-oped a subsequent cancer in the contralateral breast. LCIS was not a reliable marker for predicting the presence of either synchronous or metachronous in-vasive cancer in the opposite breast. The combination of both invasive lobular carcinoma and LCIS, how-ever, may portend a significant increase in the ex-pected incidence of contralateral breast cancer.[39] The actual incidence of invasive carcinoma occurring in either breast at the time of diagnosis of LCIS is about 5 percent (see Table 80-4).[49,95,97]

Estimates of bilateral multicentricity of LCIS range from 25 percent to 69 percent,[66,72,112] and sub-sequent development of breast cancer in either breast ranges from 4 percent[114] to 67 percent.[78] A convincing

TABLE 80-4. BILATERALITY IN MINIMAL BREAST CANCER

Status of Opposite Breast	LCIS	DCIS	MIC
No contralateral disease	7	97	12
Contralateral disease			
Previous invasive carcinoma	3	16	8
Previous noninvasive carcinoma	0	1	0
Simultaneous invasive carcinoma	5	10	1
Simultaneous noninvasive carcinoma	2	4	—
Subsequent invasive carcinoma	0	5	0
Subsequent noninvasive carcinoma	0	3	0
No data	0	1	0
Metastasis from opposite	0	1	0
Total contralateral primary carcinoma	10 (59%)	39 (29%)	9 (42%)

LCIS, lobular carcinoma in situ; DCIS, intraductal carcinoma; MIC, inva-sive ductal carcinoma less than 0.5 cm in size.
Adapted from Frazier TG, et al: Am J Surg 133:697–701, 1977.

10. Bingham H, Copeland EM, Hackett R, Caffee HH: Breast cancer in a patient with silicone breast implants after 13 years. Ann Plast Surg 20:236-237, 1988.

11. Bland KI, Palin WE, von Fraunhofer JA, Morris RR, Adcock RA, Tobin GR: Experimental and clinical observations of the effects of cytotoxic chemotherapeutic drugs on wound healing. Ann Surg 199:782-790, 1984.

12. Bowers DG, Radlauer CB: Breast cancer after prophylactic subcutaneous mastectomies and reconstruction with silastic prostheses. Plast Reconstr Surg 44:541-544, 1969.

13. Broet P, de la Rochefordiere A, Scholl SM, et al: Contralateral breast cancer: Annual incidence and risk parameters. J Clin Oncol 13:1578-1583, 1995.

14. Brown JB, Fryer MP, Ohlwiler DA: Study and use of synthetic materials, such as silicons and Teflon, as subcutaneous prostheses. Plast Reconstr Surg 26:264-279, 1961.

15. Bruce J, Carter DC, Fraser J: Patterns of recurrent disease in breast cancer. Lancet 1:433-435, 1970.

16. Burns PE, Dabbs K, May C, Lees AW, Birkett LR, Jenkins HJ, Hanson J: Bilateral breast cancer in Northern Alberta: Risk factors and survival patterns. Can Med Assoc J 130:881-888, 1984.

17. Christian MC, McCabe MS, Korn EL, Abrams JS, Kaplan RS, Friedman MA: The National Cancer Institute audit of the National Surgical Adjuvant Breast and Bowel Project Protocol B-06. N Engl J Med 333:1469-1474, 1995.

18. Clark RM, Wilkinson RH, Mahoney LJ, Reid JG, MacDonald WD: Breast cancer: A 21-year experience with conservative surgery and radiation. Int J Radiat Oncol Biol Phys 8:967-975, 1982.

19. Clarke DH, Le MG, Sarrazin D, Lacombe M-J, Fontaine F, Travagli J-P, May-Levin F, Contesso G, Arriagada R: Analysis of local-regional relapses in patients with early breast cancers treated by excision and radiotherapy: Experience of the Institut Gustave-Roussy. Int J Radiat Oncol Biol Phys 11:137-145, 1985.

20. Crowe JP, Gordon NH, Fry DE, et al: Breast cancer survival and perioperative blood transfusion. Surgery 106:836-841, 1989.

21. Dao TL, Nemoto T: The clinical significance of skin recurrence after radical mastectomy in women with cancer of the breast. Surg Gynecol Obstet 117:447-453, 1963.

22. Deapen MD, Pike MC, Casagrande JT, Brody GS: The relationship between breast cancer and augmentation mammoplasty: An epidemiologic study. Plast Reconstr Surg 77:361-367, 1986.

23. DeCholnoky T: Augmentation mammoplasty: Study of complications in 10,941 patients by 265 surgeons. Plast Reconstr Surg 45:573-577, 1970.

24. Del Turco MR, Palli D, Cariddi A, Ciatto S, Pacini P, Distante V: Intensive diagnostic follow-up after treatment of primary breast cancer. JAMA 271:1593-1597, 1994.

25. Demaree EW: Local recurrence following surgery for cancer of the breast. Ann Surg 134:863-867, 1951.

26. Donegan WL, Perez-Mesa CM, Watson RF: A biostatistical study of locally recurrent breast carcinoma. Surg Gynecol Obstet 122:529-540, 1966.

27. Early Breast Cancer Trialists' Collaborative Group: The effects of radiotherapy and surgery in early breast cancer—an overview of randomized trials. N Engl J Med 333:1444-1455, 1995.

28. Eberlein TJ, Crespo LD, Smith BL, Hergrueter CA, Douville L, Eriksson E: Prospective evaluation of immediate reconstruction after mastectomy. Ann Surg 218:29-36, 1993.

29. Fechner RE: Ductal carcinoma involving the lobule of the breast: A source of confusion with lobular carcinoma in situ. Cancer 28:274-281, 1971.

30. Fisher B, Anderson CK, Wolmark N, Wickerham DL, Cronin WM: Reanalysis and results after 12 years of follow-up in a randomized clinical trial comparing total mastectomy with lumpectomy with or without irradiation in the treatment of breast cancer. N Engl J Med 333:1456-1461, 1995.

31. Fisher B, Bauer M, Margolese R, Poisson R, Pilch Y, Redmond C, Fisher E, Wolmark N, Deutsch M, Montague E, Saffer E, Wickerham L, Lerner H, Glass A, Shibata A, Deckers P, Ketcham A, Oishi R, Russell I: Five-year results of a randomized clinical trial comparing total mastectomy and segmental mastectomy with or without radiation in the treatment of breast cancer. N Engl J Med 312:665-673, 1985.

32. Fisher B, Constantino J, Redmond C, Poisson R, Bowman D, Couture J, Dimitrov NV, Wolmark N, Wickerham DL, Fisher ER, Feldman MI, Farrar W, Evans J, Lickley HL, Ketner M, et al: A randomized clinical trial evaluating tamoxifen in the treatment of patients with node-negative breast cancer who have estrogen-receptor-positive tumors. N Engl J Med 320:479-484, 1989.

33. Fisher B, Redmond C, Dimitrov NV, Bowman D, Legault-Poisson S, Wickerham L, Wolmark N, Fisher ER, Margolese R, Sutherland C, Glass A, Foster R, Caplan R, et al: A randomized clinical trial evaluating sequential methotrexate and fluorouracil in the treatment of patients with node-negative breast cancer who have estrogen-receptor-negative tumors. N Engl J Med 320:473-478, 1989.

34. Fisher B, Redmond C, Fisher ER, Bauer M, Wolmark N, Wickerham DL, Deutsch M, Montague E, Margolese R, Foster R: Ten-year results of a randomized clinical trial comparing radical mastectomy and total mastectomy with or without radiation. N Engl J Med 312:674-681, 1985.

35. Fisher B, Slack NH, Cavanaugh PJ, Gardner B, Ravdin RG, and cooperating investigators: Postoperative radiotherapy in the treatment of breast cancer. Results of the NSABP clinical trial. Ann Surg 172:711-732, 1970.

36. Fletcher GH, Montague ED: Does adequate irradiation of the internal mammary chain and supraclavicular nodes improve survival rates? Int J Radiat Oncol Biol Phys 4:481-492, 1978.

37. Frazier TG, Copeland EM, Gallager HS, Paulus DD Jr, White EC: Prognosis and treatment in minimal breast cancer. Am J Surg 133:697-701, 1977.

38. Frazier TG, Noone RB: An objective analysis of immediate simultaneous reconstruction in the treatment of primary carcinoma of the breast. Cancer 55:1201-1205, 1985.

39. Frykberg ER, Santiago WL Jr, O'Brien PH: Lobular carcinoma in situ of the breast. Surg Gynecol Obstet 164:1-17, 1987.

40. Georgiade GS, Georgiade NG, McCarty KS, Ferguson BJ, Seigler HF: Modified radical mastectomy with immediate reconstruction for carcinoma of the breast. Trans South Surg Assoc 92:41-49, 1980.

41. Georgiade GS, Riefkohl R, Cox E, et al: Long term clinical outcome of immediate reconstruction after mastectomy. Plast Reconstr Surg 76:415-420, 1985.

42. Gilliland MD, Barton RM, Copeland EM: The implications of local recurrence of breast cancer as the first site of therapeutic failure. Ann Surg 197:284-287, 1983.

43. Gilliland MD, Larson DL, Copeland EM: Appropriate timing for breast reconstruction. Plast Reconstr Surg 72:335-337, 1983.

44. GIVIO (Interdisciplinary Group for Cancer Care Evaluation): Impact of follow-up testing on survival and health-related quality of life in breast cancer patients. JAMA 271:1587-1592, 1994.

45. Gottlieb V, Muench AG, Rich JD, Pagadala S: Carcinoma in augmented breasts. Ann Plast Surg 12:67-69, 1984.

46. Gould EW, Robinson PG: The pathologists examination of the lumpectomy—the pathologists view of surgical margins. Semin Surg Oncol 8:129-135, 1992.

47. Gunther JM, Tokita KM, Giuliano AE. Breast-conserving surgery and radiation after augmentation mammoplasty. Cancer 73:2613-2618, 1994.

48. Gump FE: Personal communication, 1989.

49. Haagensen CD: Lobular neoplasi (lobular carcinoma in situ). In Haagensen CD (ed): Diseases of the Breast. Philadelphia, WB Saunders, 1986, pp 192-241.

50. Haffty BG, Carter D, Flynn SD, et al. Local recurrence versus new primary: Clinical analysis of 82 breast relapses and potential applications for genetic fingerprinting. Int J Radiat Oncol Biol Phys 27:575-583, 1993.

51. Hall JM, Lee MK, Newman B et al. Linkage of early-onset familial breast cancer to chromosome 17q21. Science 250:1684-1689, 1990.

52. Harris HI: Survey of breast implants from the point of view of carcinogenesis. Plast Reconstr Surg 28:81–83, 1961.

53. Harris JR, Connolly JL, Schnitt SJ, Cady B, Love S, Osteen RT, Patterson WB, Shirley R, Hellman S, Cohen RB, Silen W: The use of pathologic features in selecting the extent of surgical resection necessary for breast cancer patients treated by primary radiation therapy. Ann Surg 201:164–169, 1985.

54. Hartrampf CR Jr, Bennett GK: Autogenous tissue reconstruction in the mastectomy patient: a critical review of 300 patients. Trans South Surg Assoc 98:70–81, 1986.

55. Harvey EB, Brinton LA: Second cancer following cancer of the breast in Connecticut, 1935-82. Natl Cancer Inst Monogr 68:99–112, 1985.

56. Hicken NF: Mastectomy: clinical pathologic study demonstrating why most mastectomies result in incomplete removal of mammary gland. Arch Surg 40:6–14, 1940.

57. Hislop TG, Elwood JM, Coldman AJ, Spinelli JJ, Worth AJ, Ellison LG: Second primary cancers of the breast: Incidence and risk factors. Br J Cancer 49:79–85, 1984.

58. Holleb AI, Montgomery R, Farrow JH: The hazard of incomplete simple mastectomy. Surg Gynecol Obstet 121:819–822, 1965.

59. Holley DT, Toursarkissian B, Vasconez HC, et al. The ramifications of immediate reconstruction in the management of breast cancer. Am Surg 61:60–64, 1996.

60. Hoopes JE, Edgerton MT, Shelley W: Organic synthetics for augmentation mammoplasty: Their relation to breast cancer. Plast Reconstr Surg 39:263–270, 1967.

61. Horn PL, Thompson WD: Risk of contralateral breast cancer: associations with histologic, clinical and therapeutic factors. Cancer 62:412–424, 1988.

62. Horn PL, Thompson WD, Schwartz SM: Factors associated with the risk of second primary breast cancer: An analysis of data from the Connecticut Tumor Registry. J Chron Dis 40:1003–1011, 1987.

63. Hutter RVP: The management of patients with lobular carcinoma in situ of the breast. Cancer 53:798–802, 1984.

64. Jacobson GM, Sause WT, Thomson JW, Plenk HP: Breast irradiation following silicone gel implants. Int J Radiat Oncol Biol Phys 12:835–838, 1986.

65. Johnson CH, van Heerden JA, Donohue JH, et al. Oncologic aspects of immediate breast reconstruction following mastectomy for malignancy. Arch Surg 124:819–824, 1989.

66. King RE, Terz JJ, Lawrence W Jr: Experience with opposite breast biopsy in patients with operable breast cancer. Cancer 37:43–45, 1976.

67. Kurtz JM, Amalric R, Brandone H, Ayme Y, Spitalier J-M: Results of wide excision for mammary recurrence after breast-conserving therapy. Cancer 61:1969–1972, 1988.

68. Kurtz JM, Jacquemier J, Torhorst J, et al. Conservative therapy for breast cancers other than infiltrating ductal carcinoma. Cancer 63:1630–1635, 1989.

69. Kurtz JM, Spitalier J-M, Amalric R: Late recurrence after lumpectomy and irradiation. Int J Radiat Oncol Biol Phys 9:1191–1194, 1983.

70. Leis HP Jr: Bilateral breast cancer. Surg Clin North Am 58:833–841, 1978.

71. Leis HP Jr: Managing the remaining breast. Cancer 46:1026–1030, 1980.

72. Leis HP Jr, Urban JA: The other breast. In Gallagher HS, Leis HP Jr, Snyderman RK, Urban JA (eds): The Breast. St Louis, CV Mosby, 1985, pp 487–496.

73. Lilla JA, Vistnes LM: Long-term study of reactions to various silicone breast implants in rabbits. Plast Reconstr Surg 57:637–649, 1976.

74. Lippman ME, Lichter AS, Danforth DN Jr: Diagnosis and Management of Breast Cancer. Philadelphia, WB Saunders, 1988, pp 312–325.

75. Marshall KA, Redfern A, Cady B: Local recurrence of carcinoma of the breast. Surg Gynecol Obstet 139:406–408, 1974.

76. Martin JK Jr, van Heerden JA, Gaffey TA: Synchronous and metachronous carcinoma of the breast. Surgery 91:12–16, 1982.

77. Mate TP, Carter D, Fischer DB, Hartman PV, McKhann C, Merino M, Prosnitz LR, Weissberg JB: A clinical and histopathologic analysis of the results of conservation surgery and radiation therapy in stage I and II breast cancer. Cancer 58:1995–2002, 1986.

78. McDivitt RW, Hutter RVP, Foote FW, Stewart FW: In situ lobular carcinoma: A prospective follow-up study indicating cumulative patient risks. JAMA 201:96–100, 1967.

79. McGrath MH, Burkhardt BR: The safety and efficacy of breast implants for augmentation mammoplasty. Plast Reconstr Surg 74:550–560, 1984.

80. Members of the Ludwig Breast Cancer Study Group: Prolonged disease-free survival after one course of perioperative adjuvant chemotherapy for node-negative breast cancer. N Engl J Med 320:491–496, 1989.

81. Mendenhall NP, Devine JW, Mendenhall WM, Bland KI, Million RR, Copeland EM: Isolated local-regional recurrence following mastectomy for adenocarcinoma of the breast treated with radiation therapy alone or combined with surgery and/or chemotherapy. Radiother Oncol 12:177–185, 1988.

82. Montague ED: Conservation surgery and radiation therapy in the treatment of the operable breast cancer. Cancer 53:700–704, 1984.

83. Montague ED, Fletcher GH: Local regional effectiveness of surgery and radiation therapy in the treatment of breast cancer. Cancer 55:2266–2272, 1985.

84. Morgenstern L, Gleischman SH, Michel SL, Rosenberg JE, Knight I, Goodman D: Relation of free silicone to human breast cancer. Arch Surg 120:573–577, 1985.

85. Newman W: In situ lobular carcinoma of the breast: Report of 26 women with 32 cancers. Ann Surg 157:591–599, 1963.

86. Nielsen M, Christensen L, Andersen JA: Contralateral cancerous breast lesions in women with clinical invasive breast carcinoma. Cancer 57:897–903, 1986.

87. Noone RB, Murphy JB, Spear SL, Little JW III. A six year experience with immediate reconstruction after mastectomy for cancer. Plast Reconstr Surg 76:258–269, 1985.

88. Pawlias KT, Dockerty MB, Ellis FH: Late local recurrent carcinoma of the breast. Ann Surg 148:192–197, 1958.

89. Poen JC, Tran L, Juillard G et al: Conservative therapy for invasive lobular carcinoma. Cancer 69:2789–2795, 1991.

90. Prior P, Waterhouse JAH: Incidence of bilateral tumours in a population-based series of breast cancer patients. I: Two approaches to an epidemiological analysis. Br J Cancer 37:620–634, 1978.

91. Recht A, Silver B, Schnitt S, Connolly J, Hellman S, Harris JR: Breast relapse following primary radiation therapy for early breast cancer. I. Classification, frequency and salvage. Int J Radiat Oncol Biol Phys 11:1271–1276, 1985.

92. Ringberg A, Palmer B, Linell F: The contralateral breast at reconstructive surgery after breast cancer operation—a histological study. Breast Cancer Res Treat 2:151–161, 1982.

93. Robbins GF, Berg JW: Bilateral primary breast cancers: A prospective clinicopathological study. Cancer 17:1501–1527, 1964.

94. Rosen PP: Lobular carcinoma in situ and intraductal carcinoma of the breast. In McDivitt RW, Oberman HA, Ozzello L, et al (eds): The Breast. Baltimore, Williams & Wilkins, 1984 pp 59–105.

95. Rosen PP, Braun DW, Lyngholm B, et al: Lobular carcinoma in situ of the breast: Preliminary results of treatment by ipsilateral mastectomy and contralateral breast biopsy. Cancer 47:813–819, 1981.

96. Rosen PP, Lieberman PH, Braun DW, et al: Lobular carcinoma in situ of the breast: Detailed analysis of 99 patients with average follow-up of 24 years. Am J Surg Pathol 3:225–251, 1978.

97. Rosen PP, Senie R, Schottenfeld D, Ashikari R: Noninvasive breast carcinoma: Frequency of unsuspected invasion and implications for treatment. Ann Surg 189:377–382, 1979.

98. Sarrazin D, Monique LE, Rouesse J, Contesso G, Petit J-Y, Lacour J, Viguier J, Hill C: Conservative treatment versus mastectomy in breast cancer tumors with macroscopic diameter of 20 millimeters or less: The experience of the Institut Gustave-Roussy. Cancer 53:1209–1213, 1984.

99. Schnitt SJ, Connolly JL, Harris JR, Hellman S, Cohen RB: Pathologic predictors of early local recurrence in stage I and II breast cancer treated by primary radiation therapy. Cancer 53:1049–1057, 1984.

100. Schnitt SJ, Connolly JL, Recht A, Silver B, Harris JR: Breast relapse following primary radiation therapy for early breast cancer: Detection, pathologic features and prognostic significance. Int J Radiat Oncol Biol Phys 11:1277–1284, 1985.

101. Schnitt SJ, Connolly JL, Recht A, et al. Influence of infiltrating lobular histology on local tumor control in breast cancer patients treated with conservative surgery and radiotherapy. Cancer 64:448–454, 1989.

102. Schnitt SJ, Silen W, Sadowsky NL, Connolly JL, Harris JR: Current concepts: Ductal carcinoma in situ (intraductal carcinoma) of the breast. N Engl J Med 318:893–903, 1988.

103. Shah JP, Urban JA: Full thickness chest wall resection for recurrent breast cancer involving the bony chest wall. Cancer 35:567–573, 1975.

104. Silverstein MJ, Handel N, Gamagami P, Waisman JR, Gierson ED, Rosser RJ, Steyskal R, Colburn W: Breast cancer in women after augmentation mammaplasty. Arch Surg 123:618–685, 1988.

105. Stabile RJ, Santoto E, Dispaltro F, San Filippo LJ: Reconstructive breast surgery following mastectomy and adjunctive radiation therapy. Cancer 45:2738–2743, 1980.

106. Temple WJ, Lindsay RL, Magi E, Urbanski SJ: Technical considerations for prophylactic mastectomy in patients at high risk for breast cancer. Am J Surg 161:413–415, 1991.

107. Urban JA: Bilaterality of cancer of the breast: Biopsy of the opposite breast. Cancer 20:1867–1870, 1967.

108. Urban JA: Biopsy of the "normal" breast in treating breast cancer. Surg Clin North Am 49:291–301, 1969.

109. Urban JA, Papachristou D, Taylor J: Bilateral breast cancer: Biopsy of the opposite breast. Cancer 40:1968–1973, 1977.

110. Wallgren A, Arner O, Bergstrom J, Blomstedt B, Granberg P-O, Raf L, Silfversward C, Einhorn J: Radiation therapy in operable breast cancer: Results from the Stockholm trial on adjuvant radiotherapy. Int J Radiat Oncol Biol Phys 12:533–537, 1986.

111. Wanebo HJ, Senofsky GM, Fechner RE, Kaiser D, Lynn S, Paradies J: Bilateral breast cancer: Risk reduction by contralateral biopsy. Trans South Surg Assoc 96:131–141, 1984.

112. Warner NE: Lobular carcinoma of the breast. Cancer 23:840–946, 1969.

113. Webber BL, Heise H, Neifeld JP, Costa J: Risk of subsequent contralateral breast carcinoma in a population of patients with in situ breast carcinoma. Cancer 47:2928–2932, 1981.

114. Wheeler E, Enterline JT, Roseman JM, Tomasulo JP, McIlvaine CH, Fitts WT Jr, Kirshenbaum J: Lobular carcinoma in situ of the breast: Long-term follow-up. Cancer 34:544–563, 1974.

115. Whidden P: Augmentation mammaplasty. Transplant Implant Today 3:43–51, 1986.

116. White JR, Gustafson GS, Wimbash K et al. Conservative surgery and radiation therapy for infiltrating lobular carcinoma of the breast: The role of preoperative mammograms in guiding treatment. Cancer 74:640–647, 1994.

117. Wooster R, Neuhausen S, Mangion J et al. Localization of a breast cancer susceptibility gene, BRCA-2 to chromosome 13q 12-13. Science 265:2088–2090, 1994.

118. Yeatman TJ, Canctor AB, Smith TJ et al. Tumor biology of infiltrating lobular carcinoma: Implications for management. Ann Surg 222:549–561, 1995.

119. Zaworski RE, DerHagopian RP: Locally recurrent carcinoma after breast reconstruction. Ann Plast Surg 3:326–329, 1979.

120. Zimmerman KW, Montague ED, Fletcher GH: Frequency, anatomical distribution and management of local recurrences after definitive therapy for breast cancer. Cancer 19:67–74, 1966.

CHAPTER 81
CARCINOMA OF THE BREAST IN PREGNANCY AND LACTATION

David S. Robinson, M.D. / Magesh Sundaram, M.D. / Gregory E. Lakin

Approximately one fourth of all women diagnosed with breast cancer are premenopausal, making breast cancer the second most common cause of death in women in the United States younger than 35 years of age.[1] Although breast carcinoma is generally considered to be a disease of older women, the risk of its discovery is 1 in 213 for those of 40 years of age and younger, increasing to 1 in 26 women during the next decade.[2]

The average age of a patient diagnosed with breast cancer during pregnancy is between 28 and 32 years.[3] The accepted definition of this synchronous condition, pregnancy-associated breast carcinoma (PABC), is a breast cancer diagnosed during the gestational or lactational period or in the year following birth.[4] As the second most common malignancy associated with pregnancy, following carcinoma of the cervix (Table 81–1), breast carcinoma is found in one of every 3000 pregnancies.[5]

Family practitioners and obstetricians, who are vital to both routine breast cancer screening and the management of pregnancy, are often the first to make the diagnosis of PABC. Of concern is the unique dilemma facing the clinician who considers both the well-being of the fetus and the timely, appropriate treatment of the mother's cancer. For the pregnant patient newly diagnosed with breast cancer, a joyous time of her life is drastically altered to one of turbulent desperation, leading to a perceived contest between the mother's life and the well-being of the child. With that understanding, the role of a psycho-oncologist should be considered vital as well. Management of PABC is often controlled by a multispecialty team, including a surgeon, a medical oncologist, and an obstetrician. Issues to be reckoned with include the diagnosis and staging of the cancer, the consideration of terminating the pregnancy, the risks of surgery and anesthesia during pregnancy, the risks and timing of local and systemic adjuvant therapy, and the question of future pregnancies.

HISTORICAL PERSPECTIVE AND POPULAR MISCONCEPTIONS

Traditionally, PABC was considered a postpartum death knell for the mother and a state of antepartum risk for the fetus. The earliest anecdotal literature established widely held misconceptions. Kilgore found a 5-year survival rate of only 17 percent in 1929.[6] Harrington in 1937 reported a mere 5.7 percent 5-year survival[7]; of greater significance was his finding of 61 percent 5-year survival for node negative patients. A better understanding of the condition subsequently has led to greater optimism. This shift is exemplified in the progression of Christian Haagensen's philosophy over two and a half decades. In 1943, Haagensen and Stout declared that pregnant patients who developed breast cancer should not undergo mastectomy because the cancer was uniformly incurable in the 20 patients they identified.[8] By 1967, Haagensen stated that "carcinoma of the breast developing during pregnancy or lactation is a dread disease," but he elaborated that ". . . in a patient with early stage carcinoma of a favorable histologic type and in whom no axillary metastases are found and ultimate cure is likely, it would seem reasonable not to interrupt the pregnancy if the child is much desired."[9]

Although early reports stated that a woman with PABC had a shorter survival period,[10, 11] studies over the past 30 years have established that PABC patients demonstrate a length of survival similar to that of nonpregnant patients.[12, 13] Often a poorer prognosis is due to a significant delay in diagnosis and treatment. For many, the stage of PABC at diagnosis is often advanced; an estimated 70 to 75 percent of patients present with axillary lymph node metastasis.[10, 11, 14, 15] Cohort-matched analyses of PABC patients and nonpregnant patients by stage reveal no significant differences in overall survival.[12, 13]

In identifying myths and misconceptions surrounding this disease, Saunders and Baum[16] surveyed surgeons, obstetricians, and general practitioners. Misconceptions included the belief that pregnancy confers a worse prognosis due to an in-

TABLE 81–1. INCIDENCE OF CANCER DIAGNOSED IN PREGNANCY

Site	Incidence (per 1000 Pregnancies)
Cervix	1.3
Breast	0.33
Melanoma	0.14
Ovary	0.10
Colorectal	0.02
Leukemia	0.01

From Allen HH, Nisker JA: Cancer in pregnancy therapeutic guidelines. *In* Allen HH, Nisker JA (eds): Cancer and Therapy. Therapeutic Guidelines. Mount Kisco, NY, Futura Publishing, 1986, p 4.

creased incidence of inflammatory breast carcinoma, that the hormonal milieu of pregnancy accelerated tumor growth, and that cancer in young patients was inherently more aggressive than cancer in older patients. Of note was their finding that none of the clinicians thought diagnostic delay contributed to an overall poorer prognosis of PABC. These practitioners held the misconceptions that the increased vascularity and lymphatic engorgement of the pregnant breast promote tumor dissemination, and that any diagnostic surgical procedure on the breast commonly leads to a milk fistula.

PREGNANCY AND THE PHYSIOLOGY OF THE BREAST

A woman who completes a full-term pregnancy by her 30th[17] (or in another series, her 35th[18]) birthday statistically reduces her risk of developing breast cancer. Pregnancy may confer protection against cancer by bringing the breast to a state of physiologic and teleologic maturation. Russo and Russo[19] propose that a full-term pregnancy induces maturation of the breast's cellular elements from the immature prepubertal state to one of highly organized ductules and lobules. This differentiation to a more quiescent, adult mitotic state may afford a degree of protection from carcinogenic influences that eventuate in cancer.

During pregnancy, the breast undergoes physiological hypertrophy as mesenchymal elements decline while stromal elements increase in the metamorphosis to milk-bearing ductules and organized lobules. This hypertrophic state is supported by engorgement of vascular and lymphatic channels with increased permeability. Clinically, the gravid breast is tense and multinodular against a background of thickened or edematous parenchyma. The changes that take place during the course of a pregnancy mandate careful, serial examinations at each prenatal visit. That should facilitate the discovery of any new, suspicious, or rapidly growing mass against an altered but less rapidly changing parenchyma. Circulating levels of estrogen, human chorionic gonadotropin, and corticosteroids, which are markedly increased during pregnancy, stimulate the breast toward differentiation and lactation.[17] The maturation of the milk-producing cells also requires prolactin and insulin. At parturition, the estrogen and progesterone levels quickly fall while prolactin remains high, lending to lactation.

After more than 2 decades of investigation, there is little evidence that human breast cancer is immunogenic.[20] Still, the decreased recognition of non-self during pregnancy could, in theory, be permissive to subtle antigenic manifestations of breast cancer cells. Immunologically, gestation demonstrates survival of antigenic foreign tissue—the fetus—within the immunocompetent host mother. This reduction in maternal immunity is a consequence of both the placental barrier to fetal tissue, decreasing an opportunity for recognition, and of fetal-antibody blocking factors that decrease the effectiveness of maternal cytotoxic T cells.[21] Additional nonspecific cell-mediated immune suppression is brought about by the two- to threefold increase in corticosteroid levels during pregnancy.[22] Still, documented enhancement of breast carcinoma's growth or aggressiveness during the course of pregnancy remains unproven.[23]

A tumor's estrogen receptor (ER) and progesterone receptor (PR) status plays a role in determining the course of adjuvant therapy. Quantitative levels of tumor hormonal receptors can be determined through standard cytosolic competitive ligand-binding assays (LBA). During pregnancy, estrogen levels are 10 times greater than those found during menses, and progesterone levels are threefold greater during late pregnancy.[3] Consequently, a routine cytosolic assay may produce false-negative results because the receptor sites are already saturated by high hormone levels that prohibit binding of the test ligands. In addition, elevated estrogen and progesterone concentrations may downregulate receptor levels, possibly below that detectable by the LBA threshold.[24] This is of secondary importance. In most circumstances with correction, the incidence of receptor-positive breast cancer is the same in pregnant patients as it is in nonpregnant premenopausal patients. DeSombre and colleagues[25] have previously shown that quantitative hormone levels reflect the overall response rate of ER-positive cancers to hormonal therapy. Qualitative determination of ER/PR status, through tumor receptor immunohistochemical staining techniques, may more accurately present the ER status in this circumstance. Immunohistochemical positivity of receptor markers reflects that some part of a PABC tumor's estrogen response system may still be intact, despite a negative ER finding by routine LBA.[24] The antibody to the receptor (largely nuclear) binds at a separate locus from estrogen. Consequently, circulating and receptor-bound levels of estrogen do not interfere. As with the general premenopausal population, women with PABC appear more likely to have ER-negative tumors. Nugent and O'Connell[26] found that 10 of 14 (71 percent) of PABC tumors were ER negative. Similarly, Elledge and associates found that the percentage of ER-positive tumors was not significantly different between pregnant and nonpregnant groups. Of note in this study was the finding that there was no difference in outcome regardless of receptor status—4 of 10 patients with hormone-positive tumors died, whereas 3 of 5 patients with hormone negative tumors died.[24]

DIAGNOSIS OF PABC

Patient procrastination in bringing attention to a breast mass, as well as the physician's tendency to discount the possibility of malignancy, are significant factors in delaying the diagnosis of PABC. With regard to tumor size, as might be expected from a delay in treatment, Petrek and coworkers[4] found that only

31 percent of pregnant women had T1 carcinomas (size <2 cm) versus 50 percent of the control group. Nonrecognition and delay in the diagnosis of breast cancer during pregnancy or the postpartum period remain the primary reasons for the poor prognosis associated with this disease.[27] Several series have shown an interval from 2 to 15 months between the initial recognition of a breast mass and confirmation of cancer through breast biopsy.[26, 28, 29] In fear of bad news, a pregnant patient may let several months pass before seeking medical attention for a new breast mass she has discovered. Physicians harbor denial as well. In women younger than 35, Treves and Holleb[30] found that a physician identifying an abnormal breast mass during pregnancy or lactation tended to observe the mass without suspecting cancer for an average of 2 months. It is imperative that the clinician carry out a timely evaluation of any suspicious breast mass, regardless of pregnancy, including a history and a physical examination as well as standard diagnostic studies.

In taking the patient's medical history, specific attention should be directed to any family history of breast cancer, a previous contralateral breast cancer, and to the current assessment. In the postpartum period, a nursing history is also important. An infant's failure to nurse from a lactating breast, possibly indicative of an occult malignancy, was termed the milk-rejection sign by Goldsmith in 1974.[31]

Physical examination of the breasts should take note of symmetry and mobility, fixation or retraction, skin thickening or dimpling, discharge, and nipple inversion, as well as axillary or supraclavicular adenopathy. Any of these findings warrant further diagnostic evaluation and surgical consultation. If the clinician identifies a vaguely prominent breast mass amidst the surrounding multinodularity with no other suspicious findings, serial examinations over a short period of time (2 to 4 weeks) can clarify the suspicion of cancer and diagnostic evaluation may then proceed.

Although the value of screening mammography lies in the early diagnosis of nonpalpable breast cancer, both radiologists and patients avoid diagnostic x-ray studies during pregnancy for fear of harming the fetus. In women younger than 35 mammography is generally not performed because breast density is often prohibitive. Moreover, the physiological alterations of pregnancy further reduce the sensitivity of mammography.[32] An increase in breast density due to hyperemia and increased water content, along with a loss of contrasting fatty tissue surrounding a tumor, makes a mammographic diagnosis of cancer more difficult in the gravid breast. If it is truly indicated, mammography can be performed safely on the pregnant patient, using lead shielding of the abdomen, with a radiation dose of less than 1 cGy per breast and minimal exposure to the fetus.

Ultrasonography of the breast may be a useful diagnostic alternative to mammography in this setting. Real-time ultrasound provides a noninvasive evaluation of the breast during pregnancy without exposure to radiation. Ultrasound can differentiate discrete solid from cystic lesions against an increased background density and multinodularity altered by pregnancy. In selected groups of patients, including pregnant women who refused mammography, Frazier and associates[33] were able to identify solid lesions by breast ultrasound leading to an eventual diagnosis of breast cancer. Although only an incisional biopsy can truly differentiate inflammatory breast carcinoma from an acute inflammatory mastitis, breast ultrasonography can identify small fluid collections or dilated ducts harboring abscesses indicating an infectious process in the pregnant or lactating breast.[34]

If cancer is suspected, a microscopic analysis of cells or tissue must be undertaken. A straightforward cost-effective approach is fine needle aspiration performed in the outpatient office setting. Disappearance of the mass on aspiration usually differentiates a benign cyst or galactocele from a solid tumor. Cystic degeneration of a carcinoma, often masquerading as a simple cyst, may refill rapidly after aspiration. If a cyst refills rapidly or if an aspirate contains blood, a biopsy should be performed. It is reported that fine needle aspiration is as effective in establishing a diagnosis in the pregnant patient as in the nonpregnant patient for the experienced cytologist who is made aware of the history; Kline and his colleagues[35] suggest that if a diagnosis of malignancy is made by cytologic examination, treatment of the PABC may be instituted because a greater than 95 percent specificity is recognized with fine needle aspiration. Before initiating therapy, the authors believe that a TruCut or incisional biopsy should confirm that diagnosis. The sensitivity of fine needle aspiration cytology in identifying malignancy depends on both the sampling technique and the experience of the cytopathologist. PABC is rare enough that even an experienced cytologist will encounter this problem infrequently. The issue of false-positive cytology arises with the hypercellular breast tissue of gravidity, showing active nuclear elements and prominent nucleoli, misinterpreted for malignancy by the inexperienced or uninformed cytopathologist who is unaware of the pregnancy.[36] A negative cytologic result should not deter further investigation of a suspicious lesion; if he or she is concerned, the surgeon should proceed with an open biopsy. In addition to fine needle aspiration, core biopsy (TruCut) can be readily performed with minimal local anesthesia to establish the diagnosis of PABC. A breast biopsy under local anesthesia can be performed with minimal risk to the fetus. Both needle localization and stereotactic biopsy are limited to nonpalpable mammographically suspicious lesions; because mammograms are not taken, they have no role in establishing the diagnosis of breast carcinoma during pregnancy.

A diagnostic operative procedure on the gestational breast requires meticulous attention to technique with special regard to hemostasis. The risk of intraoperative bleeding and postoperative hematoma is elevated because of an increase in vascularity and increased capillary microcirculation. Fear of creating a milk fistula is the most common reason, historically stated, for avoiding an operation on the pregnant or lactating breast. Engorged lactating glands and ducts present ready sources of milk that may drain from the surgical wound. When a biopsy is planned, the patient should discontinue breast feeding for a minimum of 1 to 2 weeks before the surgery. Although breast binding and postoperative ice packs are anecdotally suggested, bromocriptine given 48 hours before biopsy is more likely to reduce the risk of a milk fistula. The location of the surgical incision and depth of the wound play a role in formation of a milk fistula. Petrek[14] points out that the risk of milk fistula is low following a peripheral biopsy and that it increases to a high risk with a central biopsy.

Although antibiotic prophylaxis is not considered mandatory for a routine breast biopsy, it may be more important for an operation on the pregnant breast. Because of vascular and lymphatic alterations during pregnancy, infection and secondary sepsis are of concern. In the lactating breast, milk may be a ready culture medium for infection. The antibiotics usually selected for the pregnant patient are the penicillins and cephalosporins because these agents have few known adverse fetal effects.[37] In patients with penicillin allergies, erythromycin is an alternative that is said to carry a low fetal risk.[37] Tetracyclines, aminoglycosides, and sulfa drugs should be avoided because of their established fetal sequelae including, respectively, the permanent discoloration of teeth, renal and oto-toxicity, and hepatic dysfunction.[38]

PATHOLOGY

The histopathologic spectrum of breast masses during pregnancy is the same as that for nonpregnant patients. Of 134 biopsies performed during pregnancy and lactation, Byrd and colleagues[39] found 29 patients had malignant disease, whereas 105 patients had benign findings. In addition, 39 patients (37 percent) had common, benign tumors, including fibroadenomas, lipomas, papillomas, and cystosarcoma phyllodes, while 36 patients (34 percent) had fibrocystic changes. Twenty-three patients (22 percent) had findings unique to gestation and lactation, such as galactocele, lobular hyperplasia, and lactating adenoma. Seven patients (7 percent) were diagnosed with breast abscesses or inflammatory mastitis.[39] If incision and drainage is required for such inflammatory or infectious breast processes, tissue should always be sent for pathological examination to exclude breast carcinoma. Another benign process mimicking gestational breast carcinoma is the rapid expansion and eventual infarction of a fibroadenoma of a focus hyperplastic breast tissue that is responsive to the exaggerated endocrine change of pregnancy. Clinically, these masses appear as rapidly growing, painful tumors; only a surgical biopsy differentiates these fibroadenomatous infarctions from malignancy.

Byrd and colleagues[39] identified malignancy in 22 percent of pregnant patients biopsied compared with 19 percent in a comparable control group. In addressing the histology, they observed no difference in the subtype of breast malignancy associated with pregnancy. In an analysis presented by Petrek and coworkers,[4] a study of 56 pregnant and 166 nonpregnant patients reported that the respective incidences of invasive ductal cancer were 78 percent and 75 percent and the incidences of medullary cancer were 10 percent and 11 percent, respectively.[4] The misconception that inflammatory carcinoma is more common during pregnancy is unfounded, despite an early report by White.[2] The incidence of inflammatory breast carcinoma in the general population is 1.5 to 4 percent; various studies of PABC patients report an incidence of 1.8 to 4.3 percent.[3, 11, 14] Beyond this, rare malignancies of the breast, such as lymphoma, leukemia, and sarcoma, are not found with any greater frequency during pregnancy.[3]

EVALUATION FOR STAGING AND METASTATIC DISEASE

Once the diagnosis of breast cancer has been made in the pregnant patient, an appropriate evaluation to stage the cancer and identify distant metastases should be undertaken. Recognition of distant metastases alters the treatment plan of a patient with PABC. In the same way that a nonpregnant patient is evaluated, radiological imaging is important in determining the presence of distant disease; however, minimizing fetal exposure to ionizing radiation is important. Although they are old standards, a comprehensive history and physical examination are still the primary and most important parts of the workup. Attention to signs and symptoms suggestive of metastases to the brain, lungs, liver, and bones will tailor and direct hematological studies and radiological procedures needed to accurately stage the patient (Table 81–2). Routine blood testing, including a complete blood count, liver function tests, and evaluation of tumor markers, should be taken as a baseline study with the understanding that pregnancy itself will cause an elevation of some of these tests, such as alkaline phosphatase and carcinoembryonic antigen (CEA).[40] Any patient with breast cancer exhibiting neurological symptoms should undergo a neurological evaluation and a computed tomography (CT) or magnetic resonance imaging (MRI) scan of the brain. With abdominal shielding, a head CT may be performed on the pregnant patient with limited fetal exposure. MRI brain scanning, although virtually unstudied in PABC, is an excellent approach if cerebral staging is to be performed during early pregnancy. MRI has been used in fetal imaging for prenatal diagnosis of congenital malformations with no apparent adverse fetal effect,[41] although the long-term consequences of exposing the fetus to a high magnetic field are unknown.

A chest x-ray study should be obtained to exclude pulmonary metastases for all stages of breast cancer. Pregnancy is not a contraindication to a chest x-ray study (exposure to the fetus is less than 0.01 cGy with abdominal shielding); however, lead shielding during late pregnancy, when the uterus reaches the xyphoid, may obscure the lower lung fields.

Patients with abdominal complaints or with abnormal liver function tests should be evaluated for hepatic metastases. Although a CT scan of the abdomen is routinely performed for the nonpregnant patient, the dosage of fetal radiation from this technique is prohibitive. Hepatic ultrasonography is preferred in this situation.[42]

The incidence of bony metastases in this setting is estimated to be less than 3 percent in Stage I breast cancer and less than 8 percent in Stage II breast cancer, increasing to 20 percent to 40 percent for Stage III and IV breast cancer, respectively.[3] Therefore, asymptomatic bone scans are appropriate only for advanced breast cancer. Routine gestational elevation of serum alkaline phosphatase levels preclude the use of this marker to evaluate the presence of bony metastases.[3] The estimated fetal dose of radiation with a bone scan is 0.02 cGy.[43] The maternal blood pool, urinary tract, and skeleton are the primary sources of fetal exposure to radioactivity during bone scanning.[43] Reduction of the fetal radioactive dose may be accomplished through brisk hydration and placement of an indwelling urinary catheter.[44]

Malignancy may metastasize to the placenta or the fetus, but only 54 such cases have been reported in the world's literature.[45] Given its propensity for early hematogenous dissemination, it is not surprising that melanoma is the most common malignancy to metastasize to the placenta and to the fetus (9 of the 14 reported cases of fetal metastases).[45] Placental metastases of breast cancer have been recognized, however, and Eltorky and associates[45] recommend careful pathological examination of the placenta and intervillous spaces for cancer when maternal malignancy has been identified.

THERAPY

Multiple treatment options render decision-making for the nongravid breast cancer patient difficult enough. Compound these options with the addition of a pregnancy, and the complexity more than doubles; it becomes exponential. Many questions regarding the impact of therapy on the fetus and, reciprocally, the consequence of treatment modifications on the mother's outcome raise concern. Therapy aside, will the pregnancy and the cancer have adverse biological effects on one another? Does the pregnancy need to be terminated to preserve the mother's life? Moreover, if treatment were delayed to allow the pregnancy to progress until a viable child could be delivered, would that time interval have an adverse outcome for the mother? Does any treatment performed during pregnancy carry significant sequelae for the child? What impact does successful treatment have on fertility, and will a future pregnancy produce recurrence? These are a few of the many issues colored by the expected anxiety of the patient and her family. Clearly, the management of breast cancer during pregnancy poses a real clinical challenge.

The best approach to accomplish resolution of these presentations is to examine each of the issues separately in the development of a treatment plan. This requires a working knowledge of the potential effects on both the mother and her yet-to-be-born child. In this section of the chapter, the authors examine the impact of radiation therapy, surgery, and antineoplastic agents on the future of both the mother and the child. A more comprehensive discussion of each of these, aside from pregnancy, is presented in other chapters of this text.

Radiation Therapy

At present, radiation therapy for breast cancer is most often given as an adjuvant treatment following partial mastectomy. Postoperative treatment of the chest wall after a complete mastectomy, which was at one time routine, is now reserved following the removal of large, aggressive breast cancers. Anatomically, breast treatment fields to the upper torso are at some distance from the embryo during early pregnancy, but as the fetus enlarges and assumes full abdominal domain, the fundus in the epigastrium lies closer to the site of radiation in the later stages of gestation. Because the developing fetus does not lie directly in the path of the beam, any radiation received is indirect. The sources of significant indirect radiation exposure to the fetus are photons that are discharged from the machine hood, scatter within the mother, and scatter from collimators and beam modifiers.[46, 47] The well-described contributions of each are roughly equivalent.[48–52]

The most significant factor in determining a pe-

TABLE 81–2. STAGING EVALUATION FOR PREGNANCY ASSOCIATED BREAST CARCINOMA

Site	Procedures of Choice	Fetal Risk
Stage I and II (Asymptomatic)		
CNS*	Not indicated	N/a
Bone	Not indicated	N/a
Pulmonary	Chest x-ray study	<0.01 cGy*
Liver	Serum LFTs	N/a
Stage I and II (Symptomatic) or Stage III & IV		
CNS	MRI, CT brain	Minimal*
Bone	Tc-99m DP bone scan	<0.02 cGy†
Pulmonary	Chest x-ray study, bronchoscopy	<0.01 cGy
Liver	Ultrasound abdomen	N/a

*With fetal shielding.
†With hydration techniques, as per Baker et al.[43]
CNS = Central nervous system; LFT = liver function test; N/a = not applicable.

ripheral dose to the fetus is the distance of the site from the radiation field edge. Here, the dose increases directly with the field size[46] and is more pronounced closer to the beam edge because of scatter within the patient.[51] The contribution of incidental neutrons (a product of linear accelerators in the generation of photons by electrons with energies of greater than 10 MeV) is believed to be negligible.[53] In aggregate, the amount of radiation that the fetus might receive is a consequence of the field size, the distance from the beam edge, and the magnitude of the primary energy delivered. Within 10 cm of the beam edge, the major sources are collimator scatter and scatter within the patient.[46]

The biological effects of radiation on the pregnancy depend both on the gestational age as well as the dose of radiation (Table 81–3). Although the effects of radiation on pregnancy and offspring are derived in part from retrospective clinical analyses of therapy given in standard treatment fractions to pregnant women, more information has been gathered from prospective, small animal trials (largely murine)[54] and from analyses of a single large dose and its fallout upon atomic bomb survivors of Hiroshima and Nagasaki.[55–57] Each approach with its strengths and limitations emphasizes the impact on the fetus and the developmental outcome. The most frequently reported problems are developmental anomalies, severe mental retardation, and a subsequent development of cancer.

Congenital anomalies or malformations have an accepted global incidence in live-born children of 6 percent.[46] Ionizing radiation increases this risk. Current evidence suggests that a minimal threshold dose exists for most defects,[55] and the severity of the defect is directly proportional to dose.[56] Small head size has received the most attention; its incidence among atomic bomb survivors who were in utero at Hiroshima and Nagasaki is 28 percent for those between 4 and 12 weeks' gestation when exposed and 7 percent for those of greater gestational age.[57] The threshold risk of small head size seems low at dose levels between 0.10 and 0.19 Gy. As might be expected, severe mental retardation was reported in the same population,[58] and although there was significant overlap with small head size, there was not

a complete correlation between the two. Otake, Yoshimaru, and Schull, in identifying 30 people who were found to be severely retarded from a cohort of 1544, noted that the risk was higher with increased dose and greater exposure in the first trimester than in the second trimester.[58] In another study, Schull and Otake reported a loss of 30 IQ points per Gy in this group.[56]

Although investigations of single-dose atom bomb exposure are enlightening with regard to malformations and mental retardation, to evaluate the carcinogenic risk of fetal radiation, retrospective epidemiological case-controlled studies may provide a more correlative model. In the Oxford survey, Stuart[59] notes a higher probability of cancer in children whose mothers underwent pelvimetry in the 3rd trimester (0.01 Gy), but these data bear little resemblance to the risk of a fetus whose mother is receiving fractionated treatment doses over a 4- to 6-week period. Still, such low levels of radiation strongly suggest that even a small amount directed to the fetus can cause cancer, and the data on atom bomb victims suggest that this may be a lifetime risk.[60]

Other problems that may occur as a consequence of in utero radiation include loss of the pregnancy (lethal radiation to the fetus), hereditary (genetic) damage, sterility, and general growth retardation. In the preimplantation period (days 0 to 8 after conception) or the early days of the embryonic period (the period of organogenesis; days 8 to 56), little is known both because of the natural frequency of expected loss in the normal population (23 percent of conceptions are thought to abort spontaneously[61]) and the difficulty in determining the course, and even the presence of pregnancy, before implantation. Consequently, the loss of a pregnancy due to radiation is the only untoward event reported at this early stage. Still in animal studies, as little as 0.1 Gy may be lethal[62]; human investigations report that 3.6 Gy can cause abortion in the first trimester.[63]

Several other problems have also been described. Genetic or inheritable risks to children of the fetus are not certain, but it is agreed that 1 Gy will double the spontaneous incidence of mammalian abnormalities.[46, 64] Decreased human fertility in those irradiated during the organogenesis and fetal phases[65]

TABLE 81–3. ESTIMATION OF MINIMAL MALFORMING DOSES, CELL-DEPLETING DOSE, AND LETHAL DOSES FOR THE HUMAN EMBRYO

Age	Approximate Minimum Lethal Dose (Rads)	Minimum Dose for Recuperable Growth Retardation in Adult (Rads)	Minimum Dose for Recognizable Gross Malformation (Rads)	Minimum Dose for Induction of Genetic, Carcinogenic, and Minimal Cell Depletion Phenomena
Day 1	10	No effect	No effect	Unknown
Day 14	25	25	—	Unknown
Day 18	50	25–30	25	Unknown
Day 28	>50	50	25	Unknown
Day 50	>100	50	50	Unknown
Late fetus to term		50	>50	Unknown

From Brent RL: The effects of embryonic and fetal exposure to x-ray, microwaves and ultrasound. Clin Obstet 26:484–510, 1983.

may occur after an exposure of less than 1 Gy.[46] Several reports of growth retardation[65–67] in humans and other mammals have been attributed to cell death during organogenesis in doses exceeding 0.5 Gy. Blatt and Bleyer[68] postulate that long-term growth retardation may be due to damage to the hypothalamic-pituitary axis. No threshold dose is known.

The stage of pregnancy is important in assessing the risk associated with gestational age (Fig. 81–1). Gestation is usually divided into three parts: preimplantation (week 1), organogenesis (weeks 2 to 7), and fetal period here divided into early (weeks 8 to 15), middle (weeks 16 to 25), and late (weeks after 25). The consequences of radiation therapy are far greater in the first trimester. As stated earlier, the only well-defined problem in the preimplantation period is embryonic death. During the embryonic period, the major problems are malformations of specific organs, which are largely neuropathic with small head size discussed earlier, and growth retardation from a threshold dose as low as 0.1 Gy.

During the early fetal period (weeks 8 to 15), small head size and mental retardation remain the principal problems, with the risk for the latter reported to be 40 percent per Gy and a threshold of 0.12 Gy. In the middle fetal period (weeks 16 to 25), severe phenotypic malformations are seen less frequently; small head size and growth retardation have been reported in doses of 0.5 Gy or greater.[66, 69] In the late fetal period (weeks 25 to 40), the major risk is that of cancer development derived largely from scatter, with a fetal incidence of 14 percent per Gy.[70] Reducing this risk by shielding and by dose fractionation should minimize the risk to the pregnancy. In brief, the major risk to the fetus occurs in the first trimester, diminishes in the second trimester, and is negligible in the third trimester; still, radiation should be kept to a minimum because of the risks of functional disorders such as sterility and future malignancy.[28, 57, 65]

Despite the large volume written about fetal hazard from therapeutic radiation, little is written about the impact and efficacy of radiation treatment to the pregnant breast itself. Three reasons account for this paucity of information: (1) The impact to the fetus even from a small dose is so profound that on consideration of either partial mastectomy (lumpectomy) followed by radiation or complete mastectomy as equally efficacious, the former is often not chosen because of the fetal risk. (2) Because it is not known if a delay in the initiation of radiation after lumpectomy will render this a less effective treatment, a patient diagnosed with breast cancer in the 2nd or 3rd trimester may decide to undergo partial mastectomy with axillary dissection and wait until weeks 32 to 35 of pregnancy to induce delivery before beginning adjuvant radiation therapy to the postpartum breast. (3) A breast cancer, often masked by breast enlargement consequent to pregnancy, may be discovered so late that the tumor will be too large for a partial mastectomy; the patient, undergoing a modified radical mastectomy, will obviate the need for radiation therapy.

Despite our current understanding of the physiological and anatomical changes that occur in the pregnant and lactating breast, we do not know whether the standard radiation treatment plan should be altered to account for those differences. The increased water content, increased vascular flow, and increase of glandular elements may not significantly change the way treatment in that setting is approached.

One issue that has been studied is the effect of breast-conserving surgery and radiation on lactation. The extent to which lactation is diminished is proportionate to the radiation dose to the breast, especially to glandular and ductal elements. A standard dose of 4600 Gy to the whole breast can cause lobular atrophy, periductal and perilobular fibrosis with ductal shrinking, and cytoplasmic loss with a subsequent significant reduction in the ability to lactate. Dow and colleagues[71] note that 34 percent of 52 patients studied by Trolius reported lactation from the irradiated

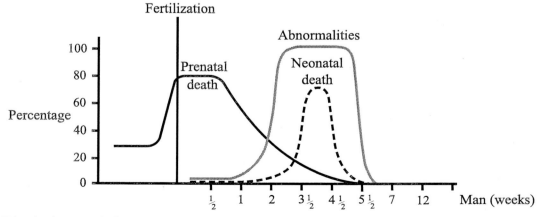

Figure 81–1   *Risks of radiation to the human embryo and fetus. The percentage of risk is plotted against the age in weeks. The risk of embryonic death is highest for radiation received at fertilization and for the first week. Neonatal abnormalities have a peak incidence between weeks 2 and 5. (From Brill AB, Forgotson EH: Radiation and congenital malformations. Am J Obstet Gynecol 90:1149–1168, 1964.)*

breast, and 24 percent were successful at breast feeding after radiation therapy. Still, many women are advised not to breast feed from the irradiated breast because it is feared that mastitis, should it occur, would be more difficult to resolve, especially if these women had also undergone an axillary dissection.

In summary, even at low doses, radiation therapy appears to have profound consequences in the first trimester of pregnancy, but it may be less significant later in the pregnancy. The risks are high enough in the first trimester that when radiation therapy is essential, consideration should be given to termination of the pregnancy because of the high probability of poor outcome for the fetus. For a patient discovered to have breast cancer later in the course of her pregnancy there are several options: (1) shielding of the abdomen in the treatment of a pregnant patient, or (2) partial mastectomy with deferral of adjuvant radiation to the post partum period may be considered after weighing the risks both to the mother and the yet-to-be-born-child. This may be moved forward by early induction of labor. Each of these decisions should be made with the mother, educated by her doctors as to the consequences, taking into full account the impact both on the mother and her baby.

Surgery

The literature defining the surgical management of the pregnant breast cancer patient has focused largely on either diagnostic concerns,[72, 73] or on the anesthetic risk to the fetus.[74–77] Very little has been written from a technical perspective about any operative aspect unique to this situation because there is little from that perspective that is different about the pregnant patient. In reporting on 11 patients who attempted postpartum breast feeding sometime after breast-conserving therapy (surgery and radiation) for cancer, Higgins and Haffty[78] observed that a circumareolar incision (and presumably a deeper interruption of some of the subareolar ducts) was associated with an absence of lactation in that breast. The physiological changes of vascular engorgement and the presence of milk late in the pregnancy and in the postpartum state require very careful hemostasis to prevent surgically iatrogenic galactoceles and fistulas from forming.

The decision to perform a complete or partial mastectomy (lumpectomy) for the patient whose cancer makes her eligible for either operation initiates a therapeutic decision process predicated on the technique, dosage, and requirements for radiation therapy. Because of the profound problems encountered after even a small amount of fetal radiation, a *mastectomy* should be the operation of choice in the *first two trimesters*. In the *third trimester* consideration may be given to *lumpectomy* for a small cancer in a patient with appropriate breast size if some distance between the cancer and the resection margin can be obtained with deferral of radiation to the postpartum period. In the patient who is eligible for conservation surgery, radiation should not begin during the third

trimester itself. The question of a delay in the initiation of radiation therapy after breast-conserving surgery for the nonpartum patient has been considered by Leonard and colleagues[79]; these authors suggest that there is no increase in local recurrence when the radiation was delayed. In this circumstance, the administration of any adjuvant therapy, designed to decrease the risk of recurrence to a patient who has been surgically cleared of all known cancer, should be deferred until completion of the pregnancy. If there is great urgency to begin treatment, the delivery may be induced at the 34th week of gestation (and perhaps even earlier) with a small risk to the baby. The decision regarding the performance of an axillary dissection is based on the histological finding of invasive cancer from the biopsy, just as it is in the nonpregnant state.

The fetal risk of anesthesia delivered to the pregnant woman requiring an operation for a problem unrelated to her pregnancy has been investigated.[75–77] An increased rate of spontaneous abortion does occur,[76, 77] especially in the first and early second trimester, as well as an increase in the number of babies who die within 1 week after delivery.[75] Apparently there is no increase in the number of stillbirths in the third trimester.[75] Mazze also reports an increase in the number of infants with low (less than 2500 g) and very low (less than 1500 g) birth weights both due to premature delivery and to intrauterine growth retardation.[75] None of the reports show an increase in congenital anomalies in any trimester for patients receiving general anesthesia. The choice of anesthetic agents does not seem to make a difference, and most of the standard anesthetic approaches have been investigated. In discussing the literature regarding teratogenic effects of nitrous oxide, Mazze notes that extreme conditions—way beyond any clinical norm—were required to produce teratogenic changes in rats.[75]

Little information is conveyed in the current literature about the anesthetic impact on the mother with breast cancer. Several authors point out that it is difficult to separate the illness from the operation and the anesthetic in evaluating an adverse outcome. Fortunately, the instance of adverse outcomes remains rare.

Antineoplastic Agents and Chemotherapy

The administration of chemotherapy to a pregnant breast cancer patient raises its own concerns (Table 81–4). Although the consequences of chemotherapy to the cancer patient, both in the treatment of metastatic disease as well as in the adjuvant setting, are well documented, the impact on the fetus is less adequately defined. In comparison with the dramatic and well-described impact of radiation therapy on the fetus, chemotherapeutic effects on the progeny of patients being treated for solid tissue tumors are less well documented. Garber[80] notes that the teratogenic effects of approximately 20 cytotoxic agents must be

TABLE 81–4.   ADVERSE EFFECTS OF ANTINEOPLASTIC AGENTS ON THE FETUS AND NEONATE

Immediate
  Spontaneous abortion
  Teratogenesis
  Organ toxicity
  Premature birth
  Low birth weight
Delayed*
  Carcinogenesis
  Sterility
  Retarded physical or mental growth
    and development, or both
  Mutation
  Teratogenic in second generations

*Potential long-term complications of *in utero* exposure to antineoplastic agents.
From Doll DC, Ringenberg QS, Yarbro JW: Antineoplastic agents and pregnancy. Sem Oncol 16:337–346, 1989.

TABLE 81–5.   FETAL OUTCOME IN MOTHERS WHO RECEIVED CHEMOTHERAPY DURING PREGNANCY VERSUS OUTCOME IN MATCHED CONTROL GROUP

	Study Group (n = 11)	Matched Control Group (n = 11)
Mean (± SD) gestational age, wk	36.4 ± 4.2*	40.8 ± 1.3*
No. of preterm births (<37 wk)	5	0
Mean (± SD) birth weight, g	2227 ± 558†‡	3519 ± 272†
Delivery method, No.		
Spontaneous	6	10
Cesarean	5	1

*P < .0056.
†P < .001.
‡N = 9.
From Zemlickis D, Lishner M, Degendorfer P, et al: Fetal outcome after *in utero* exposure to cancer chemotherapy. Arch Intern Med 152:573–576, 1992. Copyright 1992, American Medical Association.

extracted from more than 300 anecdotal reports and reviews. In her 1989 review, she presents a long-term follow-up of all children she could find described in the literature who had been exposed in utero to antineoplastic agents; she cites 64 cases in which children were followed for at least 12 months. Sixty of these children were treated with chemotherapy for lymphoma or leukemia, and of the remaining four, only two had mothers who were treated for breast carcinoma, both in the first trimester. One of the children who received in utero cyclophosphamide and doxorubicin was born with low birth weight, imperforate anus, and a rectovaginal fistula,[81] whereas the other who received those same drugs as well as methotrexate and fluorouracil was described as normal.[82] This description, albeit an opportunity to look at long-term follow-up, contains a surprisingly small cohort of breast cancer patients. The reason for the paucity of patients under study may be due in part to a clinical decision to undergo therapeutic abortion if breast cancer is discovered relatively early in the pregnancy and to an increased instance of spontaneous abortion to patients who received therapeutic doses of chemotherapy within the first trimester of pregnancy. In support of this concept, Zemlickis and coworkers[83] in 1992 reported an analysis of the impact of chemotherapy on 21 pregnant women who were treated over 3 decades at the University of Toronto. Five of them were treated for breast cancer. Of the 13 first-trimester pregnancies, four came to therapeutic abortion and four terminated in spontaneous abortion; two of the remaining five that continued to term had major malformations. Of four women evaluated during the second trimester of pregnancy, one underwent therapeutic abortion and one had a stillbirth; two had normal live births. Four patients were treated with chemotherapy during the third trimester, and all gave birth to healthy live babies.[83] With regard to the breast cancer patients in this analysis, three underwent spontaneous abortions in the first trimester and the third gave birth to a healthy live baby at term. No second-trimester breast

cancer patients were treated. In the third trimester, two patients both had uneventful live births, whereas one demonstrated intrauterine growth retardation. A preponderance of both therapeutic and spontaneous abortions would explain why there are so few reports on the impact of chemotherapy on the infant.

A summary of information regarding fetal outcome is depicted in Table 81–5. Moreover, these authors assessed whether lower birth weights in infants of patients with cancer were due to the increased frequency of premature births or to intrauterine growth retardation. Zemlickis and associates determined the distribution of birth weight percentiles (compensated for gestational age) and compared this factor between the study and control groups. This analysis confirmed that infants born to women receiving chemotherapy during pregnancy were significantly more likely to have birth weights below the 50th percentile ($p < .01$) (Table 81–6).

In consequence of the low numbers of breast cancer patients reported to have received chemotherapy while pregnant, consideration of the impact of antineoplastic drugs on pregnancy and children exposed in utero must be based on the leukemia-lymphoma literature. Reports of spontaneous abortions and

TABLE 81–6.   DISTRIBUTION OF BIRTH WEIGHT PERCENTILES IN THE STUDY AND CONTROL GROUPS

		Birth Weight Percentile for Gestational Age at Delivery				
	n	<25th	25th–50th	50th–75th	75th–90th	>90th
Cases*	9	5	2	1	1	0
Matched controls*	11	0	2	5	4	0

*P < .01.
From Zemlickis D, Lishner M, Degendorfer P, et al: Fetal outcome after *in utero* exposure to cancer chemotherapy. Arch Intern Med 152:573–576, 1992.

birth malformations have appeared over the last 40 years in the several comprehensive reviews.[84–88] In a 1968 analysis of 185 pregnant women who received cytotoxic drugs, Nicholson notes a significant instance of fetal malformation often leading to death in the first trimester, whereas exposure during the second and third trimester carried an increased risk of abnormality similar to that found in the general population.[85] In evaluating fetal malformations from both single agents and multiple drugs administered to pregnant women, Doll observed a 25 percent rate of fetal malformations for mothers who received multiple agents versus a 6 percent rate for those who received single agents in the first trimester of pregnancy.[89] Exposure again during the second and third trimesters yields an instance (1.3%) not unlike that found in the general population.[90] In evaluating the reports of placental transportation of drugs administered to the mother, Pacifici and Nottoli[91] offer discussion only of doxorubicin and cyclophosphamide in a comprehensive review in 1995. They discuss three conflicting reports about transplacental crossing of doxorubicin. No other reports of any antineoplastic agents are offered.

The long-term, functional consequences of chemotherapy are not unlike those of radiation therapy but are less dramatic and largely anecdotal. With regard to intellectual function, the consequences are unknown; there is one case report of gestational exposure to cyclophosphamide and prednisone resulting in mental retardation and multiple congenital anomalies.[92] In two other reports that evaluate psychometric standardized testing, children of mothers treated with chemotherapy during the time of pregnancy are considered to be otherwise unremarkable.[93, 94]

With regard to gonadal dysfunction and infertility of children who received chemotherapeutic agents in utero, the results are unavailable. Most reports evaluate the consequences of adult germ cell function from children with cancer who were treated with multiple chemotherapeutic agents. Boys treated with alkylating agents before puberty have been reported to have normal gonadal function[95] or small testes and elevated follicle-stimulating hormone levels.[96, 97] Because adverse effects on both ovarian and testicular dysfunction have been seen later in life in children exposed to cytotoxic agents, the possibility of sensitivity to the same effects in utero should be considered.[80]

The literature regarding other functional and phenotypic alterations is sparse. The impact on growth, while less dramatic than that seen in radiation therapy, has been reported.[68, 98] Small stature may be due to pituitary-hypothalamic deficits, but a causal relationship is difficult to establish. Genetic defects that can be passed from one generation to another have been variably found.[99–102] The long-term mutagenic impact on germ cells of children treated in utero is not known. With regard to the carcinogenic potential of chemotherapeutic agents delivered to children in utero, the literature shows only one reported case of neoplasia.[92]

In summary, regarding chemotherapy, the administration of combinations of antineoplastic agents to pregnant breast cancer patients carries a significant risk in the first trimester, specifically that of spontaneous abortion and clinically apparent birth defects. The impact is significantly lower in the second and third trimesters. All of this information is based on a very small number of patients. Consequently, our clinical decisions are based on data extrapolated both from a larger cohort of children of mothers who were treated with chemotherapy for leukemia and lymphoma and from long-term results of children treated for childhood cancer. If a woman's disease is metastatic, requiring systemic cytotoxic therapy within the first trimester of pregnancy, she would be well advised to undergo therapeutic abortion because of the high incidence of spontaneous abortions and fetal abnormalities that occur. In the second and third trimesters of pregnancy, this risk of spontaneous abortion apparently is not as significant and patients may proceed to receive cytotoxic treatment with caution.

The question of delaying adjuvant therapy is one to consider seriously. In evaluating an 8-year, relapse-free survival rate, Brufman and colleagues reported a decrease from 77 to 44 percent when adjuvant chemotherapy was delayed for more than 3 months from the time of diagnosis; moreover, they noted that the rate of distal treatment failures rose from 13 to 44 percent in the delayed treatment group.[103] In contrast, Leonard and colleagues[79] were unable to identify any interval that resulted in an increased local recurrence if radiotherapy was delayed because of adjuvant therapy, but they point out that because of the heterogeneous population of breast cancer patients, the results need to be further investigated. Consequently, if there is concern about treatment consequences on the outcome of the pregnancy in the third trimester, early induction with a plan to initiate a course of adjuvant chemotherapy earlier might be an appropriate approach. Because of remarkably small numbers of breast cancer patients reported, the impact of in utero chemotherapy on the outcome of children from patients treated for breast cancer remains to be defined.

LONG-TERM PROGNOSIS AND FUTURE PREGNANCIES

The prognostic implications of breast cancer discovered during pregnancy are inconsistent. Several authorities have suggested that concurrence carries a poor prognosis,[15, 104–107] others have suggested that it makes little difference,[4, 26, 108, 109] and there is one report that shows a survival advantage.[110] The reason for these discrepancies may be that pregnant women present with more advanced disease than their nonpregnant cohorts, but even when adjustments are made for stage, Guinee and coworkers suggest that the relative risk of dying is higher than it is for the nonpregnant cancer patient but that the difference decreases 15 percent per year.[104]

Because many of the patients who die will do so within the first 2 years, especially with axillary nodal involvement, it is recommended—not because of any risk conferred by the pregnancy—but because of the actuarial risk of death in the first 18 months that additional childbearing be deferred until the greatest opportunity for recurrence has passed.[111] A subsequent pregnancy does not affect long-term outcome.[111–113] Many women may be unable to become pregnant after receiving chemotherapy. The risk of premature ovarian failure consequent to cytotoxic chemotherapy may be between 63 and 85 percent in all breast cancer patients; the incidence of permanent failure (30 to 50 percent) may be slightly lower in women younger than 40 years of age.[114] When ovarian failure occurs, the opportunity for pregnancy is unlikely.

SUMMARY

The occurrence of breast cancer in pregnancy is a relatively rare event (1 in 3000 pregnancies) that may be masked by physiological events, allowing the patient to present with more advanced disease. The principal treatment is surgical. The use of adjuvant radiation therapy should be avoided during the pregnancy itself but may be given to the breast after induction of early delivery. The administration of chemotherapy, whether in the adjuvant setting or in the treatment of recognized metastasis, should be avoided in the first trimester but may be given with less risk during the second and third trimesters. If chemotherapy is necessary during the first trimester, consideration should be given to terminating the pregnancy. The long-term impact of the pregnancy and breast cancer on one another is not certain.

References

1. Parker SL, Tong T, Bolden S, et al: Cancer statistics, 1996. CA Cancer J Clin 46:1–28, 1996.
2. White TT, White WC: Breast cancer and pregnancy: Report of 49 cases followed 5 years. Ann Surg 1956; 144:384.
3. Wallack MK, Wolf JA, Bedwinek J, et al: Gestational carcinoma of the female breast. Curr Probl Cancer 7:1–58, 1983.
4. Petrek JA, Dukoff R, Rogatko A: Prognosis of pregnancy-associated breast cancer. Cancer 67:869, 1991.
5. Allen HH, Nisker JA: Cancer in pregnancy therapeutic guidelines. In Allen HH, Nisker JA (eds): Cancer and Therapy. Therapeutic Guidelines. Mount Kisco, NY, Futura Publishing, 1986, p 4.
6. Kilgore AR: Tumors and tumor-like lesions of the breast in association with pregnancy and lactation. Arch Surg 18:2079–2098, 1929.
7. Harrington SW: Carcinoma of the breast. Results of surgical treatment when the carcinoma occurred in the course of pregnancy or lactation and when pregnancy occurred subsequent to operation (1910–1933). Ann Surg 106:690–700, 1937.
8. Haagensen CD, Stout AP: Carcinoma of breast; criteria of operability. Ann Surg 118:859–870, 1943.
9. Haagensen CD: Cancer of the breast in pregnancy and during lactation. Current Developments. Am J Obstet Gynecol 98:141–149, 1967.
10. Applewhite RR, Smith LR, DiVincenti F: Carcinoma of the breast associated with pregnancy and lactation. Am Surg 39:101, 1973.
11. Montgomery TL: Detection and disposal of breast cancer in pregnancy. Am J Obstet Gynecol 81:926, 1961.
12. Petrek JA: Breast cancer during pregnancy. Cancer 74S:518, 1994.
13. Zemlickis D, Lishner M, Degendorfer P, et al: Maternal and fetal outcome after breast cancer in pregnancy. Am J Obstet Gynecol 166:781–787, 1992.
14. Graber EA: Breast disease in pregnancy. In Barber HRK, Graber EA (eds): Surgical disease in pregnancy. Philadelphia, PA, WB Saunders, 1974, pp 303–307.
15. Holleb AJ, Farrow JH: The relation of carcinoma of the breast and pregnancy in 283 patients. Surg Gynecol Obstet 115:65, 1962.
16. Saunders CM, Baum M: Breast cancer and pregnancy: A review. J Royal Soc Med 86:162–165, 1993.
17. Kelsey JL, Gammon MD, John EM: Reproductive factors and breast cancer. Epidemiol Rev 15:36, 1993.
18. Kalache A, Maguire A, Thompson SG: Age at last full-term pregnancy and risk of breast cancer. Lancet 341:33–36, 1993.
19. Russo J, Russo IH: The etiopathogenesis of breast cancer prevention. Cancer Lett 90:81–89, 1995.
20. Higuchi M, Robinson DS, Cailleau R, et al: A serologic study for cultured breast carcinoma lines: Lack of antibody response to tumor specific membrane antigens in patients. Clin Exp Immunol 39:90–96, 1980.
21. Hellstrom KE, Hellstrom I: Lymphocyte mediated cytotoxicity and blocking serum activity to tumor antigens. Adv Immunol 18:209, 1974.
22. Fiorica JV: Special problems: breast cancer and pregnancy. Obstet Gynecol Clin North Am 21:721–731, 1994.
23. Vange NVD, Dongen JAV: Breast cancer and pregnancy. Eur J Surg Oncol 17:1, 1991.
24. Elledge RM, Ciocca DR, Langone G, et al: Estrogen receptor, progesterone receptor, and HER-2/neu protein in breast cancers from pregnant patients. Cancer 71:2499, 1993.
25. DeSombre ER, Carbone PP, Jensen EV, et al: Steroid receptors in breast cancer. Report of a consensus-development meeting. N Engl J Med 301:1011, 1979.
26. Nugent P, O'Connell TX: Breast cancer and pregnancy. Arch Surg 120:1221–1224, 1985.
27. Zinns JS: The association of pregnancy and breast cancer. J Reprod Med 22:297, 1979.
28. Gallenberg MM, Loprinzi CL: Breast cancer and pregnancy. Semin Oncol 16:369–376, 1989.
29. Nicholson RI, Wilson DW, Colin P, et al: Influence of pregnancy on the time of presentation of primary breast cancer. Ann NY Acad Sci 464:463–465, 1986.
30. Treves N, Holleb AI: A report of 549 cases of breast cancer in women 35 years of age or younger. Surg Gynecol Obstet 107:271, 1958.
31. Goldsmith HS: Milk-rejection sign of breast cancer. Am J Surg 127:280, 1974.
32. Hoeffken W, Lanyi M: Normal and abnormal development, hormonal influences. In Hoeffken W, Lanyi M (eds): Mammography, Philadelphia, WB Saunders, 1977, p 76.
33. Frazier TG, Murphy JT, Furlong A: The selected use of ultrasound mammography to improve diagnostic accuracy in carcinoma of the breast. J Surg Oncol 29:231, 1985.
34. Hayes R, Mitchell M, Nunnerley HB: Acute inflammation of the breast—the role of breast ultrasound in diagnosis and management. Clin Radiol 44:253, 1991.
35. Kline TS, Josh LP, Neal HS: Fine needle aspiration in the diagnostic evaluation of the breast: diagnosis and pitfalls—a review of 3545 cases. Cancer 44:1458, 1979.
36. Finley JL, Silverman JC, Lannin DR: Fine needle aspiration cytology of breast masses in pregnancy and lactating women. Diagn Cytopathol 5:255, 1989.
37. Gianopoulos JG: Establishing the criteria for anesthesia and other precautions for surgery during pregnancy. Surg Clin North Am 75:33, 1995.
38. Briggs GG, Freeman RK, Yaffe SJ: Drugs in Pregnancy and Lactation. A Reference Guide to Fetal and Neonatal Risk.

Baltimore, MD, Williams & Wilkins, 1994, pp 65–74, 418, 424.

39. Byrd BF Jr, Bayer DS, Robertson JC, et al: Treatment of breast tumors associated with pregnancy and lactation. Ann Surg 155:940, 1962.

40. Surgova TM, Vinnitsky VB, Sidorenko MV: Cancer in pregnancy. Characterization of common markers. Int J Biol Markers 6:203, 1991.

41. Mattison DR, Angtuaco T: Magnetic resonance imaging in prenatal diagnosis. Clin Obstet Gynecol 31:353, 1988.

42. Sugarbaker JH, Drum DE, Beard JO: Detection of hepatic metastases from cancer of the breast. Am J Surg 133:531, 1977.

43. Baker J, Ali A, Groch MW, et al: Bone scanning in pregnant patients with breast carcinoma. Clin Nucl Med 12:519, 1987.

44. McKenzie AF, Budd RS, Yang C, et al: Technetium-99m-methylene diphosphonate uptake in the fetal skeleton at 30 weeks' gestation. J Nucl Med 35:1338, 1994.

45. Eltorky M, Khare VK, Osborne P, et al: Placental metastasis from maternal carcinoma. A report of three cases. J Reprod Med 40:399–403, 1995.

46. Stovall M, Blackwell CR, Cundiff J: Fetal dose from radiotherapy with photon beams: report of AAPM radiation therapy committee task group No. 36. Med Phys 22:63–82, 1995.

47. Van der Giessen P-H, Hurkmans CW: Calculation and measurement of the dose to points outside the primary beam for CO-60 gamma radiation. Int J Radiat Oncol Biol Phys 27:717–724, 1993.

48. Fraass BA, Van de Geijn J: Peripheral dose from megavolt beams. Med Phys 10:809–818, 1983.

49. Greene D, Chu G-L, Thomas DW: Dose levels outside radiotherapy beams. Br J Radiol 56:543–550, 1983.

50. Greene D, Karup PGG, Sims C, et al: Dose levels outside radiotherapy beams. Br J Radiol 58:453–456, 1985.

51. Kase KR, Svensson GK, Wolbarst AB, et al: Measurements of dose from secondary radiation outside a treatment field. Int J Radiat Oncol Biol Phys 9:1177–1183, 1983.

52. Keller B, Mathewson C, Rubin P: Scattered radiation doses as a function of x-ray energy. Radiology 111:447–449, 1974.

53. National Council on Radiation Protection and Measurements: Influence of dose and its distribution in time on dose-response relationships for low-LET radiations. Report No. 64. Bethesda, MD, National Council on Radiation Protection and Measurements, 1980.

54. United Nations Scientific Committee on the Effects of Atomic Radiation: Genetic and Somatic Effects of Ionizing Radiation. Report to the General Assembly, Vol Annex C, New York, United Nations, 1986, pp 263–341.

55. Brent RL: Response of the 9-1/2 day-old rat embryo to variations in exposure rate of 150 R x-irradiation. Radiat Res 45:127–136, 1971.

56. Schull WJ, Otake M: Effects on intelligence of prenatal exposure to ionizing radiation. Tech Report. Hiroshima, Radiation Effects Research Foundation, 1986, pp 7–86.

57. Miller RW, Mulvihill JJ: Small head size after atomic irradiation. Teratology 14:355–357, 1976.

58. Otake M, Yoshimaru H, Schull WJ: Severe mental retardation among the prenatally exposed survivors of the atomic bombing of Hiroshima and Nagasaki: A comparison of the T65DR and DS 86 dosimetry system. Tech Report. Hiroshima, Radiation Effects Research Foundation, 1987, pp 16–87.

59. Stewart A, Webb J, Hewitt D: A survey of childhood malignancies. BMJ 1:1495–1508, 1958.

60. Jablon S, Kato H: Childhood cancer in relation to prenatal exposure to A-bomb radiation. Lancet 2:1000–1003, 1970.

61. Ford JH, MacCormac L: Pregnancy and lifestyle study: The long-term use of the contraceptive pill and the risk of age-related miscarriage. Hum Reprod 10:1397–1402, 1995.

62. Domon M: Cell cycle dependent radiosensitivity in two-cell mouse embryos in culture. Radiat Res 81:236–245, 1980.

63. Mayer M, Harris W, Winpfheimer S: Therapeutic abortion by means of x-ray. Am J Obstet Gynecol 32:945–957, 1936.

64. International Commission on Radiological Protection: Recommendations of the Commission. Publication 60. New York, Pergamon, 1991.

65. Brent RL: The effects of embryonic and fetal exposure to x-ray, microwaves and ultrasound. Clin Obstet 26:484–510, 1983.

66. Dekaban AS: Abnormalities in children exposed to X-radiation during various stages of gestation. I. Tentative timetable of radiation injury to the human fetus. J Nucl Med 9:471–477, 1968.

67. National Research Council, Committee on the Biological Effects of Ionizing Radiations: The Effects on Populations of Exposure to Low Levels of Ionizing Radiation, BEIR III Report. Washington, DC, National Academy, 1980, pp 441–452, 479, 483.

68. Blatt J, Bleyer WA: Late effects of childhood cancer and its treatment. In Pizzo PA, Poplack DG (eds): Principles and Practice of Pediatric Oncology, Philadelphia, JB Lippincott, 1989, pp 1003–1025.

69. Otake M, Schull WJ: Radiation-related small head sizes among prenatally exposed survivors. Int J Radiat Biol 63:255–270, 1992.

70. National Research Council, Committee on the Biological Effects of Ionizing Radiations: Health Effects of Exposure to Low Levels of Ionizing Radiation. BEIR V Report. Washington, DC, National Academy, 1990, pp 175, 359–360.

71. Dow KH, Harris JR, Roy C: Pregnancy after breast-conserving surgery and radiation therapy for breast cancer. Monogr Natl Cancer Inst 16:131–137, 1994.

72. Canter JW, Oliver GC, Zaloudek CJ: Surgical diseases of the breast during pregnancy. Clin Obstet Gynecol 26:853–864, 1983.

73. Collins JC, Liao S, Wile AG: Surgical management of breast masses in pregnant women. J Reprod Med 40:785–788, 1995.

74. Kim Y, Pomper J, Goldberg ME: Anesthetic management of the pregnant patient with carcinoma of the breast. J Clin Anesth 5:76–78, 1993.

75. Mazze RI, Källén B: Reproductive outcome after anesthesia and operation during pregnancy: A registry study of 5405 cases. Am J Obstet Gynecol 161:1178–1185, 1989.

76. Duncan PG, Pope WDB, Cohen MM, et al: Fetal risk of anesthesia and surgery during pregnancy. Anesthesiology 64:790–794, 1986.

77. Brodsky JB, Cohen EN, Brown BB Jr, et al: Surgery during pregnancy and fetal outcome. Am J Obstet Gynecol 138:1165–1167, 1980.

78. Higgins S, Haffty BG: Pregnancy and lactation after breast-conserving therapy for early stage breast cancer. Cancer 73:2175–2180, 1994.

79. Leonard CE, Wood ME, Zhen B, et al: Does administration of chemotherapy before radiotherapy in breast cancer patients treated with conservative surgery negatively impact local control? J Clin Oncol 13:2906–2915, 1995.

80. Garber JE: Long-term follow-up of children exposed in utero to antineoplastic agents. Semin Oncol 16:437–444, 1989.

81. Murray CL, Reichert JA, Anderson J, et al: Multimodal cancer therapy for breast cancer in the first trimester of pregnancy. A case report. JAMA 252:2607–2608, 1984.

82. Blatt J, Mulvihill JJ, Ziegler JL, et al: Pregnancy outcome following cancer chemotherapy. Am J Med 69:828–832, 1980.

83. Zemlickis D, Lishner M, Degendorfer P, et al: Fetal outcome after in utero exposure to cancer chemotherapy. Arch Intern Med 152:573–576, 1992.

84. Sokal JE, Lessmann EM: Effects of cancer chemotherapeutic agents on the human fetus. JAMA 172:151–157, 1960.

85. Nicholson HO: Cytotoxic drugs in pregnancy. J Obstet Gynaec Brit Comm 75:307–312, 1968.

86. Sweet DL, Kinzie J: Consequences of radiotherapy and antineoplastic therapy for the fetus. J Reprod Med 17:241–246, 1976.

87. Sieber SM, Adamson RH: Toxicity of antineoplastic agents in man: Chromosomal aberrations, antifertility effects, congenital malformations, and carcinogenic potential. Adv Cancer Res 22:57–155, 1975.

88. Gililland J, Weinstein L: The effects of cancer chemotherapeutic agents on the developing fetus. Obstet Gynecol 38:6–13, 1983.

89. Doll DC, Ringenberg QS, Yarbro JW: Management of cancer during pregnancy. Arch Intern Med 148:2058–2064, 1988.

90. Doll DC, Ringenberg QS, Yarbro JW: Antineoplastic agents and pregnancy. Semin Oncol 16:337–346, 1989.
91. Pacifici GM, Nottoli R: Placental transfer of drugs administered to the mother. Clin Pharmacokinet 28:235–256, 1995.
92. Reynoso EE, Shepherd FA, Messner HA, et al: Acute leukemia during pregnancy: The Toronto leukemia study group experience with long-term follow-up of children exposed *in utero* to chemotherapeutic agents. J Clin Oncol 5:1098–1106, 1987.
93. Aviles A, Niz J: Long-term follow-up of children born to mothers with acute leukemia during pregnancy. Med Pediatr Oncol 16:3–6, 1988.
94. Doney KC, Draemer KG, Shepard TH: Combination chemotherapy for acute myelocytic leukemia during pregnancy: Three case reports. Cancer Treat Rep 63:369–371, 1979.
95. Pennisi AJ, Grushkin CM, Lieberman E: Gonadal function in children with nephrosis treated with cyclophosphamide therapy before and during puberty. Am J Dis Child 129:315–318, 1975.
96. Lentz RD, Bergstein J, Steffes MW, et al: Postpubertal evaluation of gonadal function following cyclophosphamide therapy before and during puberty. J Pediatr 91:385–394, 1977.
97. Guesry P, Lenoir G, Broyer M: Gonadal effects of chlorambucil given to prepubertal and pubertal boys for nephrotic syndrome. J Pediatr 92:299–303, 1978.
98. Nesbit M, Krivit W, Heyn R, et al: Acute and chronic effects of methotrexate on hepatic, biliary and skeletal systems. Cancer 37:1048–1054, 1976.
99. Li FP, Fine W, Jaffe N, et al: Offspring of patients treated for cancer in childhood. J Natl Cancer Inst 62:1193–1197, 1979.
100. Mulvihill JJ, McKeen EA, Rosner F, et al: Offspring of patients treated for cancer in childhood. Cancer 60:1143–1150, 1987.
101. Holmes G, Holmes FF: Pregnancy outcome of patients treated for Hodgkin's disease. Cancer 41:1317–1322, 1978.
102. Mulvihill JJ, Byrne J, Steinhorn SA, et al: Genetic disease in offspring of survivors of cancer in the young. (Abstract.) Am J Hum Genet 39:A72, 1986.
103. Brufman G, Sulkes A, Biran S: Adjuvant chemotherapy with and without radiotherapy in stage II breast cancer. Biomed Pharmacother 42:351–355, 1988.
104. Guinee VF, Olsson H, Möller T, et al: Effect of pregnancy on prognosis for young women with breast cancer. Lancet 343:1587–1589, 1994.
105. Tretli S, Kvalheim G, Thoresen S, et al: Survival of breast cancer diagnosed during pregnancy or lactation. Br J Cancer 58:382–384, 1988.
106. Clark RM, Chua T: Breast cancer and pregnancy: The ultimate challenge. Clin Oncol 1:11–18, 1989.
107. Noyes RD, Spanos WJ, Montague ED: Breast cancer in women aged 30 and under. Cancer 49:1302–1307, 1982.
108. Cooper DR, Butterfield J: Pregnancy subsequent to mastectomy for cancer of the breast. Ann Surg 171:429–433, 1970.
109. Danforth DN Jr: How subsequent pregnancy affects outcome in women with a prior breast cancer. Oncol 5:23–30, 1991.
110. Sankila R, Heinävaara S, Hakulinen T: Survival of breast cancer patients after subsequent term pregnancy: "Healthy mother effect." Am J Obstet Gynecol 170:818–823, 1994.
111. Mignot L, Morvan F, Sarrazin D, et al: Breast carcinoma and subsequent pregnancy. Proceedings of American Society of Clinical Oncology 5:219, 1986.
112. Von Schoultz E, Johansson H, Wilking N, et al: Influence of prior and subsequent pregnancy on breast cancer prognosis. J Clin Oncol 13:430–434, 1995.
113. Harvey JC, Rosen PP, Ashkikari R, et al: The effect of pregnancy on the prognosis of carcinoma of the breast following radical mastectomy. Surg Gynecol Obstet 153:723–725, 1981.
114. Shapiro CL, Recht A: Late effects of adjuvant therapy for breast cancer. Monogr Natl Cancer Inst 16:101–112, 1994.

CHAPTER 82

THE UNKNOWN PRIMARY PRESENTING WITH AXILLARY LYMPHADENOPATHY

Daniel W. Tench, M.D. / David L. Page, M.D.

Carcinoma presenting as regional metastatic disease in lymph nodes is uncommon, but well studied. Location of the lymph nodes and histological features of the metastatic tumor guide the search for the primary lesion. The rare presentation of adenocarcinoma compatible with breast primary in an axillary lymph node without an identifiable primary lesion poses special considerations in diagnosis and therapeutic decision making. This problem and its natural history was first outlined by Halsted[7] in 1907:

> I have twice seen extensive carcinomatous involvement of the axilla due to mammary cancer, which later in neither instance became palpable or demonstrable for a considerable period after the axillary glands had attained conspicuous dimensions. In each case the "axillary tumors" had been removed, in one of them a year before, and in the other perhaps two years prior to my first examination which, though made in the most careful manner, failed to find the slightest evidence of cancer of either breast. In the course of a few months thereafter the mammary disease manifested itself in both patients.

In 1909, Cameron[3] recommended ipsilateral mastectomy in the face of axillary adenocarcinoma and a clinically benign breast. This course of action has been the usual mode of therapy in reported series and is predicated on the assumption that a solitary axillary metastasis of adenocarcinoma is likely to represent breast carcinoma in female patients with no other obvious malignancy after a limited workup in search of another primary tumor. Despite the introduction of sensitive modern mammographic and other diagnostic modalities that have redefined the "occult primary," there remain cases in which the breast fails to reveal its tumor, and therapy must be undertaken on the basis of relative certainty.

INCIDENCE AND CLINICAL PRESENTATION

The three largest reported series of breast cancer patients in the premammographic era had a range of 0.3 to 1 percent of women presenting with axillary metastases and inapparent primary tumors within the breast. Vilcoq and colleagues[20] reported a similar incidence of 0.9 percent from the Institute Curie in Paris in women with mammographically benign breasts. In other studies where mammographic results were reported, abnormalities in the ipsilateral breast were noted in 12 to 35 percent of cases.[1, 8, 12, 16, 18, 21] Perhaps surprisingly, in few of these cases did

the mammographic abnormality lead to identification of the primary carcinoma. Thus, the addition of mammography has not permitted a marked decrease in the number of clinically undetected primary tumors (Table 82–1). It is likely that numbers of occult primary tumors are slightly magnified as a result of the practice of referring patients with unusual manifestations of disease to the larger centers from which these reports arise. The median age and age range of these patients do not differ significantly from those of breast carcinoma patients in general. In the majority of such cases, the axillary swelling is discovered by the patient and has been present for several months or less.[1, 13]

GROSS AND MICROSCOPIC ANATOMY

The size of the axillary node on clinical examination has been usually in the range of 2 to 5 cm. Among those patients who underwent formal axillary node dissection, histological examination revealed that one third had only the presenting solitary metastasis as the only involved node. Many studies have not described the histological appearance of the intranodal carcinoma other than to document compatibility with a primary breast tumor. However, when histological pattern is reported, a distinctive pattern of solid sheets of tumor without gland formation and large cells with apocrine cytologic features is often reported (Fig. 82–1). This tumor pattern was noted in 65 percent of cases reported by Rosen and Kimmel,[16] and neoplastic glandular structures alone or in combination with solid patterns were present in the remainder of cases.

Differential diagnosis may include metastases from distant sites, primarily melanoma. As many as one quarter of patients presenting with lymph nodal metastases and inapparent primary melanomas will present with tumor in the axilla.[19] Immunohistologi-

TABLE 82–1. PRESENTATION OF BREAST CARCINOMA AS AXILLARY ADENOPATHY

Investigator	Number	%
Fitts et al.[6]	13/1300	1.00
Haagensen et al.[6a]	18/6000	0.30
Owen et al.[13]	25/5451	0.45
Vilcoq et al.[20]	11/1250	0.90

1447

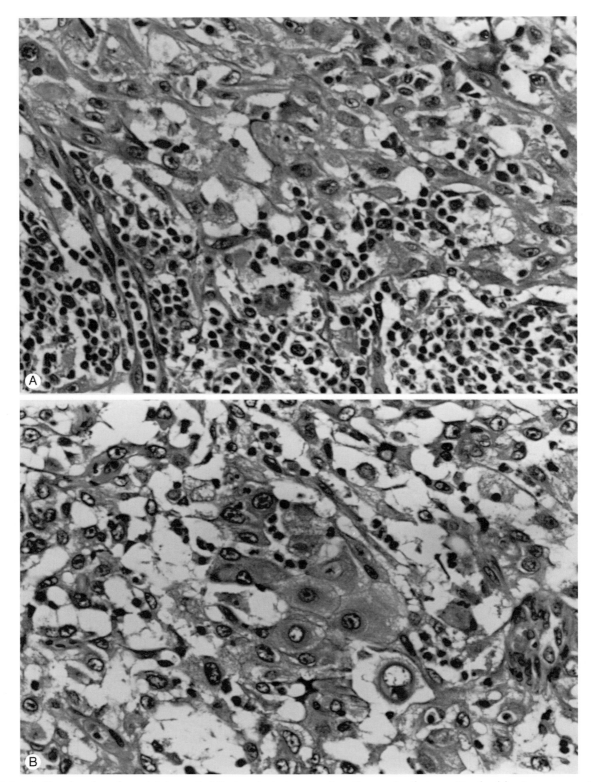

Figure 82–1. *Axillary lymph node containing metastatic breast carcinoma cells with apocrine features. No gland lumina are seen. Large tumor cells have abundant granular, eosinophilic-to-clear cytoplasm and large single nucleoli.* × *650.*

cal methods and stains for mucin will be helpful in this setting.

The possibility that the axillary carcinoma may represent a local primary breast cancer in the axil-

lary tail of Spence must be considered. Careful study to confirm the presence of lymph nodal tissue, primarily by extensive sampling, may be necessary. At-tention to identification of architectural features including capsule, sinuses, and cortical germinal centers will usually distinguish such a lesion from an axillary tail primary with a dense lymphoid reaction. The presence of extensive adjacent benign breast tissue supports a primary breast tumor. Primary breast tumors may locally invade lymph nodes from the axillary breast tissue, presenting special problems in interpretation and explaining some of the cases in which a primary within the breast is never detected. An exceptionally rare carcinoma may develop from heterotopic mammary epithelial inclusions in a lymph node.[17]

Of the 282 cases reported in which the result of mastectomy or biopsy are available, 72 percent contained carcinoma in the resected breast tissue (Table 82–2). Slightly more than half were located in the upper outer quadrant. As the mode of presentation and the difficulty in finding tumor in surgically removed tissue suggest, these tend to be smaller tumors. Ten of 16 cases reported by Patel and associates[14] were microscopically detected only. In most series, the majority of cases have primaries of 1 to 2 cm or smaller. The median size reported by Rosen and Kimmel was 1.5 cm.[16] However, in at least four cases in the literature, the primary tumor was 5 cm or greater and had a diffuse pattern of growth accounting for the nonpalpable nature of the tumor.[6, 10, 14, 18]

The histology of the tumor identified in the breast is similar to that found in the lymph node. Owen and associates[13] report a high incidence of medullary carcinomas, but these cases may well represent usual-type carcinomas with a heavy lymphocytic infiltrate and apocrine cytology rather than pure medullary carcinomas, because the required gross circumscription of medullary carcinoma is not reported in these cases. Tumor is found in the breast tissue by gross examination after mastectomy in the majority of cases, but some tiny primary infiltrating tumors and diffusely infiltrative lobular-type carcinoma may be grossly undetectable. Occasionally, only

in situ carcinoma is found in the specimen.[1, 2, 10, 21] In these series, lobular carcinoma *in situ* (LCIS) accounts for only slightly fewer cases than ductal carcinoma *in situ* (DCIS). Together LCIS and DCIS make up 8 to 10 percent of the tumors found in clinically benign breasts with axillary metastases.[12, 13, 15] It is likely that the failure to demonstrate invasive tumor in this situation is largely a sampling problem deriving from the difficulty of sampling an entire breast for a lesion that may be discovered only microscopically.

CLINICAL WORK-UP

Most unilateral lymphadenopathy does not represent metastatic carcinoma. The rationale involved in the decision to perform a biopsy on an enlarged lymph node is commonplace, yet so complex, that it need not be discussed in detail here. However, we wish to emphasize that the usual main concern is to exclude metastatic carcinoma, and fine-needle aspiration of a superficial node should be considered. With requisite operator and interpreter experience, this procedure is simple, accurate, requires no special equipment, and is associated with essentially no morbidity (see Chapter 37). If the aspiration yields malignant cells, cytologic clues may lead to a focused evaluation of potential primary neoplasms other than the breast. Sites other than the breast most commonly metastatic to the axillary nodes include melanoma prominently and also include thyroid, kidney, lung, stomach, and liver. A limited immunohistochemical study, particularly if the cytologic results or clinical suspicion include melanama, can be performed on cytologic material. After fine-needle aspiration, a lymph node biopsy can be undertaken with a more focused differential diagnosis.

The extent of the work-up of a woman with axillary carcinoma and benign breasts has been addressed,[10, 14] with the consensus of opinion being that studies need

TABLE 82–2. RESULTS OF TISSUE EXAMINATION AND MAMMOGRAPHY

Investigator	No. of Patients	% Tumor in Breast*	Quadrant If Known (%) Upper Outer	Other	Abnormal Mammogram
Ashikari et al.[1]	42	65	71	29	3/25
Feuerman et al.[5]	10	70			
Fitts et al.[6]	13	85	55	45	
Haagensen[6b]	28	84	42	58	
Haupt et al.[8]	43	72			11/43
Kemeny et al.[10]	20	45			1/20
Merson et al.[12]	60	82	60	40	21/32
Owen et al.[13]	25	60	42	58	
Patel et al.[14]	29	55	55	45	10/17
Rosen and Kimmel[16]	48	75			9/37
Weinberger and Stetten[20a]	5	100	50	50	
Westbrook and Gallagher[21]	18	75			6/17
Total	341	72			

*Percent of those examined histologically, totalling 282 cases.

1450 SECTION XXII: SPECIAL PRESENTATIONS OF BREAST CANCER

not be exhaustive. Physical examination should include careful thyroid, pelvic, and rectal exams as well as a search for other palpable lymph nodes and pigmented skin lesions. Other mandatory studies include chest radiographs, measurement of liver enzymes, and, of course, mammography. Bone scans are recommended by some and may be performed to establish a baseline. The efficacy of mammography in identifying or suggesting a mammary carcinoma in the setting of a solitary axillary metastasis has varied widely in reported series, ranging from 5 to 59 percent and averaging 25 percent (see Table 82-2). This variation probably is a reflection of differences in methodology and interpretation as well as case definition.

In any case, the major determinant of further work-up after detection of palpable axillary lymph nodes is the mammogram. In the event that a suspicious mammographic lesion is detected, the immediate course of action is evident. If the axillary lymph node is not greatly enlarged, the breast biopsy may be performed first, in the routine manner. If this breast biopsy finds evidence of invasive carcinoma, then the usual pathways of clinical practice will be followed. These patients will be properly regarded as having preoperative palpable axillary adenopathy.

When the surgical biopsy of a mammographically detected lesion is negative in the presence of a palpable axillary node, then one returns to the clinical setting of this chapter and the clinical algorithm as outlined in Figure 82–2.

If the axillary tumor shows solid sheets of malignant cells, mucin stains demonstrating intracellular positivity can be helpful in determining that the tumor is an adenocarcinoma rather than other types of tumor such as melanoma and lymphoma, which may share this pattern of growth. Immunoperoxidase studies performed on paraffin-embedded tissue are quite reliable in classifying a poorly differentiated malignant neoplasm as epithelial, melanocytic, or lymphoid, but they are of limited help in pointing toward breast as the primary once it has been determined that the tumor is an adenocarcinoma. Electron microscopy demonstration of intracellular canaliculi, apical desmosomes, and secretory vesicles has been shown to be helpful in cases that appear undifferentiated by light microscopy.[9] Positive estrogen and progesterone receptors in a poorly differentiated adenocarcinoma are suggestive but not themselves diagnostic of a breast primary. Performance of tests for these hormone receptors should be considered at the time of lymph node biopsy for the purpose of determining therapy. Awareness of the need for estrogen receptor studies at the time of initial node biopsy is especially important, because this may be the only tumor-containing tissue that will be available for study.

MANAGEMENT

The majority of women reported in these studies have been treated with ipsilateral mastectomies. However, Kemeny and colleagues[10] retrospectively reported on 20 women with axillary presentation of breast carcinoma, of whom 11 received mastectomies and 7 had only axillary dissection or biopsy alone or in combination with radiation or chemotherapy. They showed no difference in survival between those treated by mastectomy and those treated without mastectomy, and they concluded that mastectomy is unnecessary. Vilcoq and associates[20] recommend removal of the axillary mass followed by radiotherapy to the breast and axilla. Eleven patients were thus treated during a 13-year period, with a 91 percent 5-year survival. Feigenberg and co-workers[4] recommend upper outer quadrant sector mastectomy based on the statistical likelihood that this quadrant harbors the tumor. Only three of the eight women in their series were treated in this fashion; these three demonstrated tumor in the upper outer quadrant.

Because axillary presentation of breast carcinoma is rare, questions of appropriate therapy are not likely to be answered on the basis of randomized prospective trials. However, we can tell a woman who has an axillary metastasis "consistent with breast primary" and who has a negative "other primary" work-up that there is a greater than 90 percent chance that the ipsilateral breast contains invasive tumor. Even if that breast is removed and no tumor is demonstrated, still the odds are that the breast does contain tumor that has not been located.

Based on the pathological findings of mastectomy specimens from the largest series (see Table 82–2),

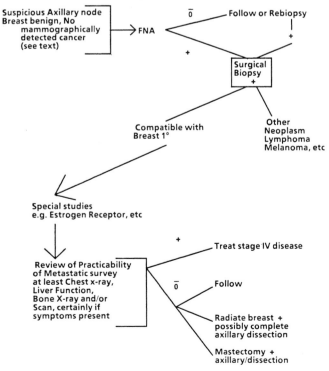

Figure 82–2. *Flow chart outlining approach to female patient with suspected metastatic axillary carcinoma. FNA = Fine needle aspiration.*

the sector mastectomy approach would be expected to leave as many as one half of the tumors behind in other quadrants. Upper outer quadrantectomy is an unproved approach but may be acceptable if the tumor is located within the resected tissue, is not multifocal, and does not have an extensive diffuse *in situ* component, and surgical margins are free. Should the tumor not be found in this quadrant, then consideration of further therapy may be appropriate. Axillary dissection should be performed in all surgically treated cases for adequate staging, prevention of axillary recurrence, and for further determining the need of adjuvant chemotherapy.

PROGNOSIS

The prognosis of women with axillary metastases from occult breast carcinomas has been shown to be no worse and perhaps slightly better than that of stage-matched patients with palpable breast cancer. The reported equivalent or somewhat better prognosis after mastectomy for this form of breast carcinoma as compared with historical controls argues in favor of considering the same breast conservation approaches that have become routine for the treatment of smaller tumors in the breast. The larger series of studies report "a better prognosis than is observed for the average carcinoma of the breast with nodal metastases,"[13] survival rates "higher than that for any group of our patients with carcinoma of the breast except for those without axillary metastases,"[6] and "prognosis is as good or better than it is for palpable breast cancer with axillary metastases."[21] An important study from Memorial Sloan-Kettering[16] compares 22 patients with occult breast carcinoma and axillary metastases whose mastectomy specimens contained measurable invasive tumor and matched them on the basis of tumor size, number of involved lymph nodes, tumor type, and age at diagnosis with patients presenting with palpable tumors (Fig. 82–3). Those with occult lesions demonstrated a more favorable, although not statistically different, prognosis.

The advent of mammography has changed some aspects of this topic of breast cancer presenting with disease in the axilla as it has changed most other aspects of breast cancer detection and treatment. Certainly, the basic definition of "occult" has changed because some lesions undetectable by palpation alone will be detectable by mammography, but many remain undetected.[11] What has remained consistent is that the prognosis, in general, is that of low-stage regional metastatic breast cancer, that is to say, better than the majority of women with axillary metastases at diagnosis.

Reported series of patients treated in a consistent fashion are relatively small but consistent in their message that survival is in the favorable range of stage II patients, and, that mastectomy is thought unnecessary. In one series from Edinburgh,[22] 20 such patients seen between 1977 and 1989 were generally

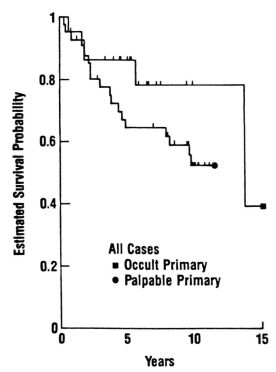

Figure 82–3. *Survival of women (N = 22) with occult primary breast cancers of measurable size compared with similar patients presenting with palpable primary tumors. (From Rosen PP, Kimmel M: Hum Pathol 21:518–523, 1990.)*

treated by radical radiotherapy to the breast and peripheral lymphatics. Local control was achieved in the axilla in 17 of 20 patients (85 percent). No primary tumors appeared in the breast, with average follow-up of about 5 years. The 5-year actuarial survival of the group was 66 percent, similar to stage II breast carcinoma patients.

VanOoijen and colleagues[18] reviewed 15 women presenting with axillary nodal metastases from an occult primary consistent with breast carcinoma. Nine patients underwent complete axillary clearance, and in 6 the clinical mass only was excised. Radiotherapy to the axilla was given to 8 patients. One woman underwent mastectomy at the time of axillary surgery, but no tumor was found in the excised breast; in the remaining 14 patients, the breast was left untreated. One premenopausal woman received adjuvant systemic chemotherapy and 1 postmenopausal patient was given tamoxifen. Three patients died of recurrent disease at 16, 50, and 56 months after treatment of the axillary mass; 1 is alive at 42 months with systemic recurrence. In 2 of these patients, the tumor in the breast became apparent before other metastases. Eleven patients survived, for a median of 92 (range, 18–144) months without evidence of disease. The prognosis of this patient group is better than that generally reported for stage II breast carcinoma, and treatment of the breast appears to be unnecessary. As noted by Rosen and Kimmel,[16] vanOoijen and colleagues,[18] and Whillis and associates,[22] this may well be because of the small size of the primary tumors as well as the fact that few nodes are usually involved.

References

1. Ashikari R, Rosen PP, Urban JA: Breast cancer presenting as an axillary mass. Ann Surg 183:415–417, 1976.
2. Breslow A: Occult carcinoma of second breast following mastectomy. JAMA 226:1000–1001, 1973.
3. Cameron HC: Some clinical facts regarding mammary cancer. Br Med J 1:577–582, 1909.
4. Feigenberg Z, Zer M, Dintsman M: Axillary metastases from an unknown primary source: A diagnostic and therapeutic approach. Isr J Med Sci 12:1151–1158, 1976.
5. Feuerman L, Attie JN, Rosenberg B: Carcinoma in axillary lymph nodes as an indicator of breast cancer. Surg Gynecol Obstet 114:5–8, 1962.
6. Fitts WT, Steiner GC, Enterline HT: Prognosis of occult carcinoma of the breast. Am J Surg 106:460–463, 1963.
6a. Haagensen CD, Bodian CD, Haagensen DE: Breast carcinoma, risk and detection. *In* Haagensen CD (ed): Diseases of the Breast. Philadelphia, WB Saunders, 1971, p 441.
6b. Haagensen CD: Physicians' role in the detection and diagnosis of breast disease. *In* Haagensen CD (ed): Diseases of the Breast. 3rd ed. Philadelphia, WB Saunders, 1986, p 550.
7. Halsted W: The results of radical operations for the cure of carcinoma of the breast. Ann Surg 46:1–19, 1907.
8. Haupt HM, Rosen PP, Kinne DW: Breast carcinoma presenting with axillary lymph node metastases: An analysis of specific histopathologic features. Am J Surg Pathol 9:165–175, 1985.
9. Iglehart JD, Ferguson BJ, Shingleton WW, et al: An ultrastructural analysis of breast carcinoma presenting as isolated axillary adenopathy. Ann Surg 196:8–13, 1982.
10. Kemeny MM, Rivera DE, Tarz JJ, Benfield JR: Occult primary adenocarcinoma with axillary metastases. Am J Surg 152:43–47, 1986.
11. Leibman AJ, Kossoff MB: Mammography in women with axillary lymphadenopathy and normal breasts on physical examination: Value in detecting occult breast carcinoma. AJR 159:493–495, 1992.
12. Merson M, Anderola S, Galimberti V, Bufalino R, Marchini S, Veronesi U: Breast carcinoma presenting as axillary metastases without evidence of a primary tumor. Cancer 70:504–508, 1992.
13. Owen HW, Dockerty MB, Gray HK: Occult carcinoma of the breast. Surg Gynecol Obstet 98:302–308, 1954.
14. Patel J, Nemoto T, Rosner D, et al: Axillary node metastasis from an occult breast cancer. Cancer 47:2923–2927, 1981.
15. Rosen PP: Axillary lymph node metastases in patients with occult noninvasive breast carcinoma. Cancer 46:1298–1306, 1980.
16. Rosen PP, Kimmel M: Occult breast carcinoma presenting with axillary lymph node metastases: A follow-up of 48 patients. Hum Pathol 21:518–523, 1990.
17. Sawicki MP, Howard TJ, Passaro EJ: Heterotopic tissue in lymph nodes. An unrecognized problem. Arch Surg 25:1394–1398, 1990. Review.
18. vanOoijen B, Bontenbal M, Henzen-Logmans SC: Axillary nodal metastases from an occult primary consistent with breast carcinomas. Br J Surg 80:1299–1300, 1993.
19. Velez A, Walsh D, Karakousis CP: Treatment of unknown primary melanoma. Cancer 68:2579–2581, 1991.
20. Vilcoq JR, Calle R, Ferme F, et al: Conservative treatment of axillary adenopathy due to probable subclinical breast cancer. Arch Surg 117:1136–1138, 1982.
20a. Weinberger HA, Stetten D: Extensive secondary axillary lymph node carcinoma without clinical evidence of primary breast lesion. Surgery 29:217–222, 1951.
21. Westbrook KC, Gallagher HS: Breast carcinoma presenting as an axillary mass. Am J Surg 122:607–611, 1971.
22. Whillis D, Brown PW, Rodger A: Adenocarcinoma from an unknown primary presenting in women with an axillary mass. Clin Oncol 2:189–192, 1990.

CHAPTER 83

MANAGEMENT OF THE PATIENT AT HIGH RISK

David L. Page, M.D. / Susan W. Caro, M.S.N., R.N.C. /
William D. Dupont, Ph.D.

This chapter concerns women identified to be at increased cancer risk because of histological determinants from breast biopsy. Nonanatomical factors such as nodularity or painful breast disease have no consistently known risk correlates or implication.[17] Mammographic patterns may be associated with cancer risk,[16, 33] but they are not known to be sufficiently reliable to form the basis for clinical judgments. Epidemiological as opposed to clinical associations and other nonanatomical factors such as familial associations are covered more completely elsewhere (see Chapters 17 and 19). We present a summary of approaches to risk counseling, first summarizing the relevant background material of Chapters 8, 12, and 23 and then proceeding with clinical management recommendations for women at heightened risk for breast cancer.

We consider patients at clinically meaningful elevated risk for the development of carcinoma only if the risk is reliably determined to approach double that of the general population.[9, 35, 36] Note that use of the word "patients" rather than "women" in this operational definition denotes a clinical setting. Lesser degrees of risk may be important in nonclinical settings but are not fully considered here. Elevated risk is of unquestioned clinical importance when its magnitude approaches five times the general population. From epidemiological studies we may derive such information, comparing risk, but to derive useful information for individual women, absolute risk figures that require a time definition are used, e.g., 10 percent risk in 10 years. Note that comments on magnitude of relative risks (RR) are inherently confusing without an immediate reference group, because the term indicates and requires a comparison (see next section). This reference group is usually a population of women without the risk factor or the general population. The age of a patient as well as the number of years at risk are directly relevant and must be comparable. Usually, RR figures should be understood to have been derived while controlling the two comparison groups for age and number of years at risk. Application and derivation of risk statements are discussed in detail in the section on slightly increased risk lesions.

By elevated risk, not otherwise specified, we mean any risk of breast cancer that is reliably identified and is of a magnitude that at least approaches twice that of the general population. When making more specific reference to the implications and magnitude of elevated risk, it is stratified as follows derived from experience with histological markers:

Slight or mild risk elevation	1.5–2 times
Moderate elevation	4–5 times
High elevation	9–11 times

In this borderland between invasive carcinoma and nonproliferative breast tissue lies a group of histological lesions whose association with cancer and cancer risk varies. The levels are further discussed in Chapter 23 and were the focus of a consensus conference organized by the College of American Pathologists and the American Cancer Society in 1985.[21] We and many others[30] prefer that the term *fibrocystic disease* be avoided[40, 47] and replaced with less negative or pejorative terms such as *fibrocystic change* or, simply and descriptively, *dense* or *lumpy breasts*.

BREAST CANCER RISK COUNSELING

Women are often told by well-meaning health care providers that, because of a family history, pathological finding, or other circumstance, they are at "high risk" for breast cancer. But then little else is explained and much is left to the woman's imagination as to how high her risk is and what she is supposed to do with this information. Breast cancer risk is an incredibly complex issue that is difficult for anyone to comprehend. It is even more difficult for the individual woman to make sense of the vast information reported in the media concerning breast cancer. Thus, the major challenge is to relate risk estimates for groups and even the entire society to an individual woman.

Medical information is sometimes reported in the news in short sensational sound bites that leave the viewer or reader confused as to the relevance of the information in the context of the body of medical literature behind the headline. A memorable example of this occurred in the summer of 1995. The June 15, 1995, *New England Journal of Medicine* reported on results of the Nurses' Health Study[7] showing a relative risk for women taking hormone replacement therapy to be 1.32 for women on estrogen and 1.41 for women on estrogen and progestin therapy. This was reported on the news as a 40 percent increase in risk for women on hormone therapy. Only a few weeks later, a report in *JAMA*[49] stated that neither long-term use of estrogen alone nor combined estrogen/progestin therapy was associated with an increased risk of breast cancer. This was also reported in the news, but received less attention. The result is that the American woman has bits of information, but not the whole picture. This can produce significant anxiety, as is evidenced by the phone calls and questions health care providers receive in the wake of such news stories. The past decade has seen an explosion of information and an increase in awareness about breast cancer. A possible consequence of this increase in awareness and information is increased anxiety and fear for women concerned about their risk for breast cancer.[50]

"Only in the past few years have high-risk but healthy relatives emerged as a group with distinct problems, issues, and reactions." This statement was published in 1992 in *Challenging the Breast Cancer Legacy*,[42] a book on the emotional impact and coping strategies for dealing with a family history of breast cancer. With the isolation of breast cancer genes and the availability of testing for a genetic predisposition to breast cancer as a clinical service, the need is even greater to recognize these *and similar* "high-risk but healthy women" as unique and in need of special services. Perception of risk has been evaluated in several studies, and women consistently and inaccurately overestimate their risk for breast cancer.[8, 12, 26, 28, 51, 52] Other research has found an association between increased anxiety and poor compliance with screening.[19, 22, 28]

Risk counseling is not a new concept. Some aspect of risk counseling goes into almost any health care encounter. Most health care decisions are based on some assessment of risk versus benefit. Specific counseling, education, and assessment of risk in relation to breast cancer is a service that may be provided to women who believe themselves to be at increased risk. The goal of the counseling is to provide an understanding of general information about breast cancer risk, to address specific risks as they relate to the individual woman, and to develop a plan of breast health care.

Individualized counseling is a time-consuming process, and it is likely that this will fall to nonphysician providers. Any health care professional that can develop an understanding of the complex issues surrounding breast cancer risk and develop a comfortable therapeutic relationship with the client is appropriate to counsel about risk.[14, 24] A team approach may be ideal, combining the genetic background and counseling skills of the genetic counselor with the clinical knowledge of a specialized nurse clinician. Patient education and emotional support are integral parts of nursing and genetic counseling. A multidisciplinary center is the ideal setting for risk consultation. Available consultative services may include a pathologist, medical geneticist, epidemiologist, medical oncologist, surgical oncologist, plastic surgeon, and psychologist or family therapist.

Breast cancer risk consultation is appropriate for any woman who perceives herself to be at increased risk for breast cancer and wants assistance in understanding and dealing with this risk. Appropriate concerns include pathological indicators of increased risk, family history of breast cancer, and questions concerning other health care decisions such as hormone replacement therapy, screening practices, or prophylactic measures.

Breast cancer risk counseling begins by explaining the counseling process to the patient and collecting relevant information. Initial contact is usually by phone. It is most efficient if the patient is responsible for obtaining medical records or pathology slides when indicated. A sample pedigree is provided and the patient is asked to gather as much information as possible about family history. Of special importance is type of cancers in the family, age at diagnosis, unilateral or bilateral disease, and deaths related to breast cancer. To aid in documentation, the patient is asked to obtain medical records, pathology reports, and pathological slides of previous breast biopsies or family members' cancers. Understandably, this can be an emotionally trying experience if the woman has lost loved ones to breast cancer. The counseling process is outlined for the patient, and she is asked to call back when she is ready to proceed.

The length of the counseling process is dependent on the issues of concern. In most cases, a minimum of two visits is indicated. The initial session is to collect information for review, history taking, and providing general information about breast cancer risk. Follow-up sessions are scheduled as appropriate to discuss review of records, possible histopathological re-review of biopsies and to provide personal risk information.

The impact of the woman's personal experience must be taken into consideration in the counseling process. A woman who has a breast biopsy and has learned that she has a pathological finding that increases her risk of breast cancer carries with her the experience of finding out she has an abnormal mammogram or finding a change on breast self-examination, the experience of the surgery, and the waiting for results. This is particularly disturbing if she has been through this repeatedly or recently. For a woman with a family history of breast cancer, she carries her individual experience of her relative's suffering with breast cancer. Although every woman's experience is unique, some general assessments have been made about family experience of breast cancer.[42] The initial reaction to the diagnosis of breast cancer in a family member is often one of concern for the affected family member. It may be some time later that the impact of the diagnosis on one's own life is realized. Relationships influence the reaction. A mother's illness has a very different impact on a young child or adolescent than it does on an adult woman.[42] Diagnosis in a sister may increase the woman's sense of vulnerability to the disease as it touches her own generation.[42] The diagnosis of additional cancers in the family is less likely to be perceived as bad luck or chance and becomes more of a "personal threat."[42] It should also be considered that the experience of cancer in a close personal friend or even non–blood relative may increase a woman's anxiety and fear of the disease. Also, the experience of cancers other than breast in the family may contribute to the woman's concerns. Clearly, when a relative or friend dies the impact is different than when they survive.

At the first interview, the woman is allowed time to describe her experience with breast cancer. This often occurs during the drawing of the pedigree for those with a family history. A mental or written checklist[23–25, 41] may aid the counselor in the counseling process to ensure that appropriate points are addressed. Such a checklist might include (1) reason for consultation; (2) personal experience with breast cancer; (3) current screening practices; (4) communication: who does the woman talk to about fears and concerns; (5) support systems and coping strategies; and (6) does the patient need additional psychological counseling or support?

The history obtained in the counseling session should include personal medical history, family history, and social history. Specific information related to breast cancer risk factors and current medications should be documented. Concerns about breast disease, past history of breast problems, procedures, and results should be documented. Family history is documented by pedigree as discussed earlier, and written documentation and pathological samples may be collected if relevant.

Basic concepts of risk are taught, along with a review of breast cancer risk factors. This is achieved with the use of visual aids. The educational session begins with a definition of cancer, discussion of prevalence of cancer in this country, and definitions of terms relating to risk, including lifetime risk, relative risk, and absolute risk. Many women are aware that the lifetime risk of breast cancer in this country is 1 in 8.[1, 13] However, it is unclear what this means to the individual because it seeks to relate societal, aggregate risk and not cancer risk for one woman, particularly not in the next 10 to 15 years. Concepts of familial and inheritance are addressed. For example, when one family member is affected with breast cancer, this is more likely a sporadic breast cancer with a minimal implication for increase in risk or a familial basis for the rest of the family. The concepts of risk in relation to time are explained, as well as

the fact that risk may change over time. Breast cancer risk counseling in conjunction with genetic testing is rapidly evolving. Important considerations and psychological implications of testing are described in Chapter 19 and elsewhere.[15, 27, 43, 44] If genetic testing is not desired, not appropriate, or not possible for an individual woman, a risk "estimate" may be obtained by applying data from the literature to the patient's situation. There are many available studies* evaluating breast cancer risk and family history to provide empirical risk estimates. Care must be taken to inform the patient of the limitations of this technique of applying information from research to the individual, and it should be stressed that this is a wide risk "estimate" made with our assessment from the data available at the current time.

Most information in the medical literature is reported as relative risk, usually with the general population as the reference population. This is not directly helpful to the individual woman in understanding her personal risk.[10, 23, 24] Absolute risk estimation for the individual in the next few decades is more helpful. Figure 83–1 shows the relationship between absolute and relative risk of breast cancer.[10] This graph shows a woman's risk of developing breast cancer in the next 15 years given her current age and current relative risk of breast cancer. For example, this graph shows that a 50-year-old woman with a relative risk of 4 will have a 15 percent chance of developing breast cancer by age 65. A computer program is now available on the Internet for performing such calculations for breast and other cancers (see *ftp://ftp.vanderbilt.edu/pub/biostat/absrisk/.txt* at web page *http://www.mc.Vanderbilt.edu/prevmed/brisk.htm* and Dupont and Plummer[10]). The outcome of risk counseling should be an understanding of what is known (and what is not known) about breast cancer risk to date and how this applies to the individual woman. The counselor must consider the individual woman's perspective in receiving the risk information. For a woman who believes herself to have a

---

* References 2, 4–6, 20, 31, 32, 43, 45, 48.

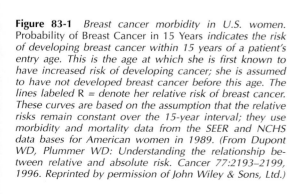

Figure 83-1 *Breast cancer morbidity in U.S. women.* Probability of Breast Cancer in 15 Years *indicates the risk of developing breast cancer within 15 years of a patient's entry age. This is the age at which she is first known to have increased risk of developing cancer; she is assumed to have not developed breast cancer before this age. The lines labeled* R = *denote her relative risk of breast cancer. These curves are based on the assumption that the relative risks remain constant over the 15-year interval; they use morbidity and mortality data from the SEER and NCHS data bases for American women in 1989. (From Dupont WD, Plummer WD: Understanding the relationship between relative and absolute risk.* Cancer 77:2193–2199, 1996. Reprinted by permission of John Wiley & Sons, Ltd.)

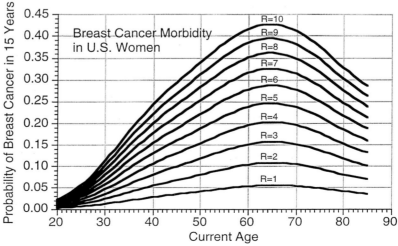

100 percent likelihood of developing breast cancer to learn that she has a 50 percent risk may seem a great relief, whereas the same numbers for another woman may be very distressing. Kelly[23, 24] aptly describes the role of the risk counselor as a "conduit between the growing body of information and the concerned patients." The counselor can serve as an ongoing resource for information and appropriate referral source to her clients.

HIGH-RISK LESIONS

The high-risk lesions (some *in situ* carcinomas) are discussed here primarily to give a backdrop or template for the understanding of the moderate-risk lesions (the atypical hyperplasias). Both the magnitude of risk and variety of accepted approaches to clinical management should be considered. The high level of risk is understood to approximate the magnitude of that associated with lobular carcinoma *in situ*. Women with lobular carcinoma *in situ* (LCIS) are understood to have a risk of subsequent carcinoma development that in relative terms is approximately 10 times that of the general population. The absolute risk of invasive breast cancer after LCIS is as high as 20 percent at 15 years (adjusted for withdrawals). Subsequent invasive cancer is almost equally likely to occur in either breast[29] (see Chapter 23). There may be some differences associated with extensiveness of disease or age at presentation that are currently not well understood. This restriction derives largely from our lack of experience with women in the younger and older age groups.[21] Thus, the great majority of women who undergo biopsy for benign breast disease other than fibroadenoma are in the premenopausal and perimenopausal group from 35 to about 55 years of age.[9, 29, 38] This uncertainty with younger and older women extends to those groups discussed in the sections that follow.

Clinical management of LCIS as a practical matter involves a decision between extremes. The original diagnoses were made by only a few institutions in the 1940s and occasioned no action clinically. As the diagnosis of LCIS was accepted in the 1960s and early 1970s, a simple mastectomy on the side involved with a large biopsy on the other side became a frequent clinical practice. However, at other institutions this was not done, and these women were put under careful clinical surveillance.[3, 18] The study by Haagensen and co-workers[18] found no deaths from metastatic carcinoma after treatment of the carcinomas that developed. This experience led many to believe that careful clinical follow-up is appropriate for this disease. It is important to note that this experience was in the premammographic era. We can only assume that detection of smaller invasive carcinomas will be greatly facilitated by close surveillance with mammography.

Undoubtedly, some physicians will continue to extirpate breast tissue, an option that must be conceded to be appropriate in some clinical settings. The historical and management perspectives are comprehensively reviewed in Chapter 52, as is the treatment of ductal carcinoma *in situ* (DCIS), which may be considered a high-risk lesion because microscopic, noncomedo DCIS lesions are associated with a tenfold increase in risk of invasive cancer after treatment by surgical biopsy only extending at least 25 years.[34, 37, 39] They were found in approximately 0.25 percent of biopsy specimens originally diagnosed as benign in the premammographic era and are seen currently in greatly increased numbers because of their greater incidence in women undergoing open biopsy as a result of mammographically detected, nonpalpable lesions.[11, 39]

NO-ELEVATED-RISK CONDITIONS

In the category of no elevated risk may be placed approximately 70 percent of women who undergo biopsy on the basis of nodules or nodularity seen by a surgeon in the era before mammography. With the different selectivity associated with mammographic evaluation, it is likely that this balance in the different histological findings will change somewhat. We have no reason to believe that the hyperplastic lesions themselves should have different indications but rather that their relative incidence and prevalence will be different. Recent evaluation of breast biopsies performed on the indication of mammography supports this contention and documents an increased prevalence of the atypical hyperplasias.[2, 30]

SLIGHTLY INCREASED-RISK LESIONS

The term *slightly increased risk* is assigned to those conditions that have a statistically significant elevation in cancer risk of a magnitude that approaches twice that of the general population controlled for age and number of years at risk. We will consistently highlight the variable of years at risk. It is important not to extrapolate such risks to time intervals that are much longer than those documented in the literature. In particular, we believe that projecting risk over the entire lifetime of an individual patient is misleading and usually overstates the magnitude of the patient's absolute risk.

The various methods of stating magnitude and relevance of increased risk should be understood by anyone counseling women thought to have increased risk. Most of our discussions are presented in terms of relative risk, which is a complex statement of a fraction divided by a fraction. Thus, the statement that women with atypical hyperplasia (AH) have a four times increased risk of cancer (CA) is derived as follows: incidence of CA in women with AH divided by incidence of CA in general equals RR (incidence of CA in AH equals women with AH developing CA divided by all women with AH), or relative risk equals

women with HH developing CA/All women with AH
÷ Women in reference population developing CA/All women in reference population

Note that the choice of the reference population is a major influence on the credibility and magnitude of the end result. The variables of age at biopsy and number of years followed are critical and are carefully accounted for in credible studies, making the study and reference groups comparable. The RR is a construct designed for the comparison of groups to determine the credibility of the effect of one factor on another. By its nature, it groups different sorts of persons in one statement. Thus, it should only be used in application to a single patient after careful thought to comparability. This comparability is derived from a consideration of age and number of years at risk. These are just the factors amalgamated in the RR statement, which must be dissected out when a statement of risk is individualized. A clinically relevant statement is made in terms of absolute risk (AR), which states the percentage likelihood of an event occurring in a certain period of time. Absolute risk is stated as 10 percent in 10 to 15 years. In general terms, we do not believe that risk should be interpreted beyond that length of time. Moreover, we have also recently shown that RR is not constant with time. Thus, the all-too common practice of taking presumed lifetime risk of breast cancer in North America (about 10 percent) and multiplying it by an RR figure is incorrect. Such a prediction can be shown to be false even when the RR remains constant for the remainder of the patient's life. Studies have been performed that approach 20 years of follow-up but have observed few events after 15 years. Thus, prediction should be confined to the next 10 to 15 or 20 years maximally; AR should be used preferentially in the clinical setting with an individual patient but should be carefully sculpted to the setting. AR may be derived from RR as seen in Figure 83–1. However, the RR is assumed to be constant for the full 20 years, and for proliferative disease, RR falls when observed 10 years after biopsy (see Chapter 23). This latter observation emphasizes the tenuous nature of prediction beyond 10 to 15 years.

Conditions associated with slightly increased risk connote a risk of breast cancer similar to that associated with a weak (few or distant relatives only) family history of breast carcinoma (see Chapters 17 and 19). These histological changes, collectively termed *proliferative disease without atypia* (PDWA) (see Chapter 8), are quite frequent and were long thought to be part of the spectrum of such broadly embracing terms as *mammary dysplasia* and *fibrocystic disease*. The reported magnitudes of risks are statistically significant, but whether they are medically significant is somewhat doubtful. Thus, the risk for breast cancer of the general female population of North America is approximately 0.15 percent per year, or 15 per 1000 women between the ages of 40 and 50 years.[10, 31] The average incidence in the decade between the ages of 40 and 50 years for women with a slight risk elevation would be about 25 per 1000.

We believe that the best way to relay this information to a patient is in terms of the next 10 to 15 years. The reliable knowledge of what will happen

after that time is not available. Events separated by more than a decade in the future become clouded, particularly by the possibility of different associations with carcinoma development in different age groups, and become greatly altered by competing causes of death, which go up very quickly after the age of 65.[10, 31]

The current suggestion followed by most practitioners at this time is that women falling in this slightly elevated risk group should be encouraged to follow the recommendation for a yearly mammogram commencing at approximately the age of 40. There seems to be no other indication to do anything else except to also encourage self-examination in these women. The greatest importance of this group is to delineate and define the majority of women who have had a breast biopsy and have no elevation of risk or the same breast cancer risk as that in the general population.

Despite the lack of certainty as to the cancer preventive effect of increased clinical surveillance on women with elevated risk, it is the only known alternative to denial. The approach to patients with these lesions should be made with humility, because we do not know if the anxiety we may cause could outweigh any therapeutic benefit that we may provide. We recommend no additional surveillance for women with slight risk elevation. This should include, however, a somewhat stronger encouragement of yearly mammography than might be done for the general population.

MODERATELY INCREASED-RISK LESIONS

For women with a moderately elevated risk of subsequent carcinoma development, careful surveillance is probably or certainly mandatory. They should be told that this surveillance by mammography will, in all probability, reduce their risk of death from breast carcinoma to that experienced by the general population. This concept and promise is not made with the proof of specific experience but is certainly strongly supported by the experience of Haagensen and co-workers.[18] Women with lobular neoplasia and related lesions who were followed by Haagensen and co-workers using only clinical exams had no deaths from breast carcinoma, despite a moderate to high level of risk of developing carcinomas. Occasionally, particularly if they have a positive family history, women with specifically defined atypia lesions will approach a relative risk of ten times. This risk is similar to that associated with LCIS, a lesion long known to be associated with high risk of breast cancer (see previous discussion of LCIS).

In addition to women with *in situ* carcinomas, women treated for primary carcinoma in one breast may also be considered in this category. The subsequent risk for the contralateral breast is well accepted to be 0.7 percent to 1 percent per year, at least for the first 10 years (see Chapters 14 and 78).

Again, several clinical management possibilities are available, but breast removal is only occasionally performed.[32, 46, 53] The magnitude of risk for these patients is comparable to that for women with AH at biopsy.

Of greatest concern here is the problem of the length of time at which this elevated risk persists. Although many prefer to be concerned with cumulative risk, which purports to deal with a lifetime risk, we are strongly in favor of the idea that clinical decision-making should be based on knowledge of events in the ensuing 10 to 15 years and not beyond.[34, 40] These are the limits of certainty that may be derived from follow-up studies. It is our experience (see Chapters 14 and 23), particularly with older women, that these elevated risks will fall 10 to 15 years after detection (see Chapter 23).

Our fervent belief is that once a high-risk lesion is determined, no decision should be rushed. It is not a medical emergency or an emergent situation of any type. Even the carcinomas *in situ* of greatest magnitude and extent have not been demonstrated to threaten life within several months after biopsy. Indeed, the "latent" period between detection of the microscopic DCIS and LCIS and the appearance of invasive carcinoma averages 10 years or more (see Chapters 8 and 52). Thus, no harm is likely to result if several months pass between the detection of a high-risk or moderately high-risk lesion and formalizing a clinical decision; the decision should be made without the overlay of immediate drama and stress. It should also be made in the full knowledge of the impact of this diagnosis and risk assessment on the individual woman's quality of life. However difficult it might be to understand risk elevation in the sense of a group or defined population, it is certainly even more difficult to do so in the case of an individual. Thus, if the individual's level of concern is extremely high (impairing sleep, etc.), the patient and her physicians should seriously consider the removal of breast tissue in the hope of reducing risk.[32, 46, 53]

As noted, mammographic surveillance is widely accepted as a clinical alternative over extirpative surgery for most women. The logic of this decision rests largely in the following knowledge:

1. Mastectomy would remove many more breasts than ever would develop cancer.
2. The patient's breast cancer risk will more closely approximate that of slightly elevated risk if she remains free of cancer for 10 years after biopsy, indicating moderate risk, i.e., relative risk often falls with time.[8]
3. The current era of mammography should only improve the good prognosis after treatment of later developing breast cancer in women with moderate and high risk followed closely by palpation.[18]

There is no generally accepted program for clinical surveillance of women with moderate risk. However, yearly mammography with clinical examination once or twice yearly should be considered almost mandatory along with a recommendation for breast self-examination. Whether more frequent mammographic examinations would have practical utility is questionable. The reason for this is based on the intrinsic rate of growth to detectability of many breast cancers. However, there is no specific reason to refuse twice yearly mammography for these women if it brings a calmer acceptance of the situation. A repeat mammogram at 5 to 6 months after initial diagnosis is useful for slightly different reasons (e.g., the possible effect of scarring at the biopsy site may be assessed and the early evaluation of a possible coexisting carcinoma may be accomplished). This suggestion is analogous to the guidelines made after radiation therapy (see Chapters 60 to 65).

It is abundantly clear that many factors will impinge on the clinical management of the woman with moderate- and high-risk lesions. Although indications for biopsy (surgical or needle) will remain the same as for other women, it is also clear that biopsies will be performed more frequently in this group on less certain indications. When frequent biopsies are necessary, then preventive surgical strategies will become more seriously considered.[32] However, with the passage of time and the advance of age, the cancer risk for those women not developing carcinoma at 10 years after biopsy approximates that of women with lesions denoting slightly elevated risk (see Chapter 23).

NONANATOMICAL RISK FACTORS

Family history of breast cancer, mammographic patterns of increased density, nulliparity, delayed parity, and other nonanatomical indicators of elevated breast cancer risk are not further discussed here. However, we would like to highlight the interaction of positive family history (FH) with the moderate risk anatomical indicators of AH. Not only are the risks of later carcinoma for women with AH and FH synergistically interactive (see Chapter 23), but the emotional set of a woman with memories of ill family members will have great impact on decisions made for clinical management. It is in these women that the strategies with greatest physical impact such as total glandular ("subcutaneous") mastectomy will be most likely considered. Even for these women, we believe that several months should pass before undertaking a final decision. It should be certain the woman knows that the anxiety and hindrance of lifestyle is and will be personally relentless.

Other nonsurgical interventional strategies are being tested, mostly those that affect diet or the endocrine milieu. These are discussed elsewhere as a matter of prevention strategies (see Chapter 18).

References

1. American Cancer Society: Cancer Facts and Figures. Atlanta, American Cancer Society, 1996.
2. Anderson DE, Badzioch MD: Risk of familial breast cancer. Cancer 56:383–387, 1985.

3. Bodian CA, Perzin KH, Lattes R: Lobular neoplasia: Long term risk of breast cancer in relation to other factors. Cancer 78:1024–1034, 1996.
4. Claus EB, Risch N, Thompson WD: Age at onset as an indication of familial risk of breast cancer. Am J Epidemiol 131: 961–972, 1990.
5. Claus EB, Risch N, Thompson WD: Genetic analysis of breast cancer in the Cancer and Steroid Hormone Study. Am J Hum Genet 48:232–242, 1991.
6. Claus EB, Risch N, Thompson WD: Autosomal dominant inheritance of early-onset breast cancer. Cancer 73:643–651, 1994.
7. Colditz GA, Hankinson SE, Hunter DJ, et al: The use of estrogens and progestins and the risk of breast cancer in postmenopausal women. N Engl J Med 332:1589–1639, 1995.
8. Daly M, Lerman C, Sands C, Boyce A, Engstrom P: Impact of coping styles on risk perception and health behavior in women genetically predisposed to breast cancer. Am J Hum Genet 49 (suppl):314, 1991.
9. Dupont WD, Page DL: Risk factors for breast cancer in women with proliferative breast disease. N Engl J Med 312:146–151, 1985.
10. Dupont WD, Plummer WD: Understanding the relationship between relative and absolute risk. Cancer 77:2193–2199, 1996.
11. Ernster VL, Barclay J, Kerlikowske K, Grady D, Henderson IC: Incidence of and treatment for ductal carcinoma in situ of the breast. JAMA 275:913–918, 1996.
12. Evans DGR, Burnell LD, Hopwood P, Howell A: Perception of risk in women with a family history of breast cancer. Br J Cancer 67: 612–614, 1993.
13. Feuer EJ, Wun L-M, Boring CC, Flanders WD, Timmel MJ, Tong T: The lifetime risk of developing breast cancer. J Natl Cancer Inst 85:892–897, 1993.
14. Fitzsimmons ML, Conway TA, Madsen N, Lappe JM, Coody D: Hereditary cancer syndromes: Nursing's role in identification and education. Oncol Nurs Forum 16:87–94, 1989.
15. Garber J, Schrag D: Testing for inherited cancer susceptibility. JAMA 275:1928–1929, 1996.
16. Goodwin PJ, Boyd NF: Mammographic parenchymal pattern and breast cancer risk: A critical appraisal of the evidence. Am J Epidemiol 127:1097–1108, 1988.
17. Goodwin PJ, DeBoer G, Clark RM, et al: Cyclical mastopathy and premenopausal breast cancer risk: Results of a case-control study. Breast Cancer Res Treat 33:63–73, 1995.
18. Haagensen CD, Lane N, Lattes R, Bodian C: Lobular neoplasia (so-called lobular carcinoma in situ) of the breast. Cancer 42:737–769, 1978.
19. Halper M, Roush G, Diemer K: Recruitment procedures for a high risk breast cancer detection clinic. Prog Clin Biol Res 293:183–189, 1989.
20. Henderson IC: Risk factors for breast cancer development. Cancer 71(suppl):2127–2140, 1993.
21. Hutter RVP: Consensus meeting: Is fibrocystic disease of the breast precancerous? Arch Pathol Lab Med 110:171–173, 1986.
22. Kash KM, Holland JC, Halper MS, Miller DG: Psychological distress and surveillance behaviors of women with a family history of breast cancer. J Natl Cancer Inst 84:24–30, 1992.
23. Kelly PT: Understanding Breast Cancer Risk. Philadelphia, Temple University Press, 1991.
24. Kelly PT: Breast cancer risk: The role of the nurse practitioner. Nurse Pract Forum 4:91–95, 1993.
25. Kelly PT: Cancer risk counseling for individual and families at increased cancer risk. Cancer Bull 46:275–276, 1994.
26. Lerman C, Daly M, Sands C, et al: Mammography adherence and psychological distress among women at risk for breast cancer. J Natl Cancer Inst 85:1074–1080, 1993.
27. Lerman C, Narod S, Schulman K, et al: BRCA1 testing in families with hereditary breast-ovarian cancer: A prospective study of patient decision making and outcomes. JAMA 275:1885–1892, 1996.
28. Lerman C, Schwartz M: Adherence and psychological adjustment of women at high risk for breast cancer. Breast Cancer Res Treat 28:145–155, 1993.
29. London SJ, Connolly JL, Schnitt SL, Colditz GA: A prospective study of benign breast disease and risk of breast cancer. JAMA 267:941–944, 1992.
30. Love SM, Gelman RS, Silen W: Fibrocystic "disease" of the breast: A nondisease. N Engl J Med 307:1010–1014, 1982.
31. Mettlin C, Croghan I, Natarajan N, Lane W: The association of age and familial risk in a case-control study of breast cancer. Am J Epidemiol 131:973–983, 1990.
32. Ottman R, King M-C, Pike MC, Henderson BE: Practical guide for estimating risk for breast cancer. Lancet Sept 3:556–558, 1983.
33. Oza AM, Boyd NM: Mammographic parenchymal patterns: A marker of breast cancer risk. Epidemiol Rev 15:196–208, 1993.
34. Page DL: The woman at high risk for breast cancer: Importance of hyperplasia. Surg Clin North Am 76:221–230, 1996.
35. Page DL, Dupont WD: Anatomic markers of human premalignancy and risk of breast cancer. Cancer 66:1326–1335, 1990.
36. Page DL, Dupont WD: Anatomic indicators (histologic and cytologic) of increased cancer risk: Breast cancer research and treatment. Breast Cancer Res Treat 28:157–166, 1993.
37. Page DL, Dupont WD, Rogers LW, Jensen RA, Schuyler PA: Continued local recurrence of carcinoma 15–25 years after a diagnosis of low grade ductal carcinoma in situ of the breast treated only by biopsy. Cancer 76:1197–1200, 1995.
38. Page DL, Dupont WD, Rogers LW, Rados MS: Atypical hyperplastic lesions of the female breast: A long-term follow-up study. Cancer 55:2698–2708, 1985.
39. Page DL, Jensen RA: Ductal carcinoma in situ of the breast: Understanding the misunderstood stepchild. JAMA 275:948–949, 1996.
40. Page DL, Steel CM, Dixon JM: Carcinoma in situ and patients at high risk of breast cancer. Br Med J 310:39–42, 1995.
41. Peters J: Breast cancer risk counseling. Genet Res 8:20–25, 1994.
42. Royak-Schaler R, Benderly BL: Challenging the Breast Cancer Legacy: A Program of Emotional Support and Medical Care for Women at Risk. New York, Harper Perennial, 1992.
43. Schneider KA: Counseling About Cancer: Strategies for Genetic Counselors. Dennisport, MA, Graphic Illusions, 1994.
44. Schneider KA, Diller LR, Garber JA: Overview of familial cancers. Genet Res 8:12–19, 1994.
45. Schwartz G, King M-C, Belle SH: Risk of breast cancer to relatives of young breast cancer patients. J Natl Cancer Inst 75:665–668, 1985.
46. Shack RB, Page DL: The patient at risk for breast cancer: Pathologic and surgical considerations. Perspect Plast Surg 2:43–62, 1988.
47. Simpson JF, Page DL: Pathology of preinvasive and excellent-prognosis breast cancer. Curr Opin Oncol 7:501–505, 1995.
48. Slattery ML, Kerber RA: A comprehensive evaluation of family history and breast cancer risk: The Utah population data base. JAMA 270:1563-1568, 1993.
49. Stanford JL, Weiss NS, Voight LF, Daling JR, Habel LA, Rossing MA: Combined estrogen and progestin hormone replacement therapy in relation to risk of breast cancer in middle-aged women. JAMA 274:137–142, 1995.
50. Swanson GM: Breast cancer risk estimation: A translational statistic for communication to the public. J Natl Cancer Inst 85:848–849, 1993.
51. Vernon SW, Vogel VG, Halabi S, Bondy ML: Factors associated with perceived risk of breast cancer among women attending a screening program. Breast Cancer Res Treat 28:137–144, 1993.
52. Vogel VG, Graves DS, Vernon SW, Lord JA, Winn R, Peters GN: Mammographic screening of women with increased risk of breast cancer. Cancer 66:1613–1620, 1990.
53. Vogel VG, Yeomans A, Higginbotham E: Clinical management of women at increased risk for breast cancer. Breast Cancer Res Treat 28:195–210, 1993.

FOLLOW-UP CARE AND REHABILITATION OF THE BREAST CANCER PATIENT

CHAPTER 84
GENERAL CONSIDERATIONS FOR FOLLOW-UP

Kelly K. Hunt, M.D. / Kirby I. Bland, M.D. / Lee M. Ellis, M.D.

Despite advances in the treatment of breast cancer, up to 70 percent of patients will develop recurrent disease.[47] Early identification of recurrent cancer, whether it is local, regional, or disseminated, aids in control of the disease, thus allowing a greater probability for palliation or improved survival. The patterns of recurrence and overall prognosis strongly correlate with the stage of disease at the time of initial treatment.[77] However, because of the diverse biological nature of breast cancer, predicting the patterns of recurrence remains a diagnostic problem. Further compounding the difficulty in diagnosing recurrent cancer is the ability of this heterogeneous tumor to remain dormant for years, only to recur as late as 20 years following treatment of the primary tumor. Recurrences are generally classified as local, regional, or disseminated. *Local recurrence* is defined as the reappearance of cancer in remaining breast tissue, scar, skin, chest wall, soft tissues, or the underlying muscles. *Regional recurrence* is defined as the presence of tumor in the regional lymph node basins, including internal mammary, axillary, supraclavicular, and Rotter's nodes. *Disseminated disease* is defined as metastatic disease at distant sites. The most common sites of distant metastases are bone, lung, pleura, soft tissues, and liver.

It is the responsibility of the physician following the patient after treatment of the primary breast cancer to recognize patterns and sites of recurrence and to be able to detect these recurrences at an early (and potentially treatable) stage. This chapter addresses the efficacy of follow-up for patients with breast cancer. Both the timing of follow-up visits and the use of radiographic and laboratory studies for the detection of recurrences are discussed. Although significant controversy exists regarding the use of radiographic and biochemical studies, suggested guidelines are proposed for the use of such studies in the management of patients during follow-up. With the infiltration of managed care plans and capitation contracts into clinical medicine, costs resulting from long-term follow-up of breast cancer patients must be supported by outcome benefit.

CHARACTERISTICS OF RECURRENT DISEASE

The vast majority of relapses in patients with breast cancer are either local/regional or confined to the skeletal system or chest (Table 84–1).[34] Local/regional recurrences are best detected clinically, whereas osseous or thoracic metastases are more easily detected using radiologic studies, with symptoms guiding the radiologic evaluation. As is discussed later in this chapter, it is difficult to demonstrate that *routine* radiologic surveillance significantly alters the natural history in the patient with recurrent breast cancer. Several factors contribute to the incidence of recurrent disease, and these are addressed in detail in other chapters of this text. Overall, large (T2-T4), node-positive tumors that are poorly differentiated and estrogen receptor negative are more likely to recur than are tumors without those characteristics.

Kamby and associates[40] attempted to demonstrate the importance of the initial stage of disease as a predictor for the site of recurrence in 863 patients with stage I and II breast cancer. These investigators evaluated patients with a single site of recurrence and showed a relative increased incidence of local/regional recurrence in the stage I (62 percent) versus stage II patients (16 percent). Stage II patients were more likely to develop distant metastatic disease, but the anatomical distribution of metastases was the same in both groups (Fig. 84–1). The only notable difference was that stage II patients were more likely to have lymph node metastases outside the regional nodal basins. However, all stage II patients had postoperative radiotherapy and 67 percent had adjuvant chemotherapy, which may have altered the pattern of recurrence. These investigators concluded that

TABLE 84–1. SITE OF FIRST RELAPSE

Site	Number of Relapses	Percent
Bone	171	21
Chest wall	150	19
Lung	153	19
Homolateral axilla	131	16
Liver	75	9
Opposite breast	51	6
Homolateral supraclavicular fossa	26	3
Brain	19	2
Other	33	4
Total	809	~100

From Heitanen P, et al: Ann Clin Res 18:143, 1986. Reprinted by permission.

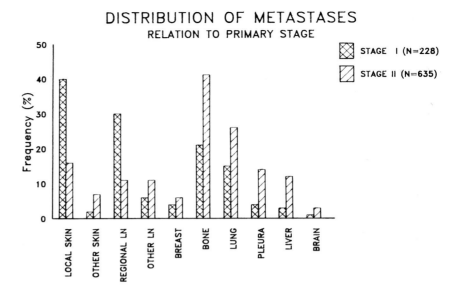

Figure 84-1 *Distribution of patients according to primary stage and anatomical location of first recurrence. (From Kamby C, et al: Eur J Cancer Clin Oncol 23:1925–1934, 1987. Reprinted by permission.)*

screening for recurrent disease should *not* be directed toward any specific site on the basis of the initial stage of disease.

The most important prognostic indicator for recurrent disease and survival is nodal status (Fig. 84–2).[9, 77] Node-negative patients have a 20- to 25-percent incidence of relapse, whereas node-positive patients have a 50- to 75-percent incidence of relapse (Tables 84–2 and 84–3). When more than three nodes are involved, the incidence of recurrence increases significantly. Node-positive patients also tend to develop recurrences at distant sites in addition to a higher rate of local/regional relapses. The most common sites of distant metastases include bone (49 to 60 percent),

lung (15 to 22 percent), pleura (10 to 18 percent), soft tissue (7 to 15 percent), and liver (5 to 15 percent).[47] Overall, 10 to 30 percent of recurrences are local, 60 to 70 percent are detected at distant sites, and 10 to 30 percent are both local and distant.[34, 47, 77] In patients treated with mastectomy, postoperative radiation therapy may decrease the local/regional recurrence rate but has little effect on overall survival.[38] A recent meta-analysis of randomized trials in early breast cancer confirmed that the rate of local recurrence was lower with postoperative radiation but that there was no significant difference in 10-year survival.[24] Adjuvant systemic therapy, on the other hand, has been shown to improve both disease-free

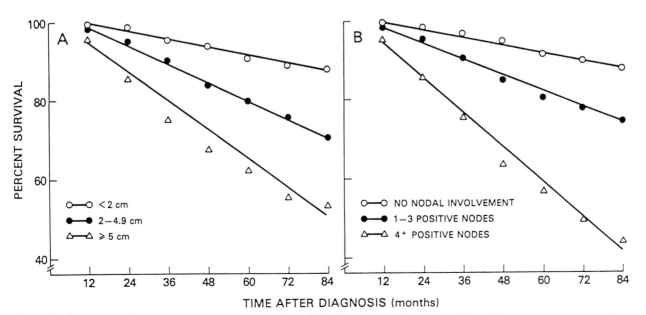

Figure 84-2 *Relative survival of breast cancer patients as a function of (A) primary tumor diameter and (B) axillary lymph node status. (From Carter CL, et al: Cancer 63:181–187, 1989. Reprinted by permission.)*

TABLE 84–2. CUMULATIVE FAILURE PERCENT RELATED TO THE SITE OF FIRST RELAPSE IN AXILLARY NODE–POSITIVE PATIENTS (ACTUARIAL ANALYSIS)

Site of First Relapse	3 Yr	5 Yr	10 Yr
Local/regional* only	14.5	16.6	17.8
Distant	16.7	22.3	28.2
Bone	8.9	11.2	14.4
Viscera	6.8	8.8	10.9
Soft tissue	1.0	2.3	2.9
Multiple sites	17.3	19.6	23.3
Local/regional + distant	6.8	7.6	9.1
Multiple distant	10.5	12.0	14.2
Contralateral breast	3.2	5.1	6.2
Total	51.7	63.6	75.5

*Chest wall and/or ipsilateral supraclavicular region.
From Valagussa P, et al: Cancer 41:1170–1178, 1978. Reprinted by permission.

and overall survival in selected women with breast cancer.[4] Thus, the overall frequency of metastatic relapse is significantly affected by postoperative adjuvant systemic treatment.

To determine the appropriate frequency of follow-up visits and overall duration of follow-up, it is necessary to be aware of the period over which recurrences appear. Although the majority of recurrences occur within the first 36 months of treatment, breast cancer commonly remains occult and indolent for many years, necessitating prolonged follow-up. Romsdahl and associates[65] studied 177 patients with recurrent or metastatic breast cancer and found that 29 percent of their recurrences occurred during the first year, 30 percent during the second year, 13 percent during the third year, 27 percent during the fourth through eleventh years, and 5 percent at 12 years or later. Donegan determined that the peak incidence of local/regional recurrences was observed in the second year following treatment.[23] Others[5, 75] have observed similar recurrence patterns and report 75 to 80 percent of recurrences being detected within 3 years of treatment. It is important to note, however, that as many as 20 percent of patients with breast cancer

TABLE 84–3. CUMULATIVE FAILURE PERCENT RELATED TO THE SITE OF FIRST RELAPSE IN AXILLARY NODE–NEGATIVE PATIENTS (ACTUARIAL ANALYSIS)

Site of First Relapse	3 Yr	5 Yr	10 Yr
Local/regional* only	3.8	4.5	6.0
Distant	6.4	9.0	10.0
Bone	2.9	5.2	6.2
Viscera	2.6	2.6	2.6
Soft tissue	0.9	1.2	1.2
Multiple sites	3.0	4.4	7.2
Local/regional + distant	0.7	1.2	2.0
Multiple distant	2.3	3.2	5.2
Contralateral breast	1.8	3.1	4.7
Total	15.0	21.0	27.9

*Chest wall and/or ipsilateral supraclavicular region.
From Valagussa P, et al: Cancer 41:1170–1178, 1978. Reprinted by permission.

may suffer a recurrence more than 5 years after treatment of the primary tumor.

CLINICAL EVALUATION

The most important mode of detecting recurrent disease is clinical evaluation and physical examination. In a study by Pandya and coworkers[61] of 175 patients with node-positive breast cancer who had a relapse, the first indicator of relapse was symptoms in 38 percent of patients, physical findings at self-examination in 18.3 percent, physical examination by a clinician in 19.4 percent, abnormal blood chemistry findings in 12 percent, abnormal bone scans in 8 percent, abnormal chest radiographs in 5.1 percent, and abnormal mammograms in 1.1 percent. Therefore, 75 percent of recurrent cancers were detected clinically.

Similarly, Scanlon and colleagues[68] studied 194 patients with stage II or III breast cancer treated with chemoimmunotherapy. Patients were examined before each 6-week course of chemotherapy for the first year and at 6-month intervals thereafter. Of the 38 (19.6 percent) patients who had recurrent disease, 33 (86.8 percent) had their recurrence detected by routine history and physical examination. Of the 33, 29 were symptomatic and four were asymptomatic. A second group of 60 patients who developed recurrent breast cancer were evaluated off protocol. This group had postoperative follow-up visits monthly for the first 6 months, bimonthly for the next 6 months, quarterly for 6 months, and then semiannually for life. In this group, 43 patients had symptoms related to their recurrence, and 14 recurrences were discovered by routine history and physical examination. When combined, 90 of 98 recurrences (91.8 percent) were detected by routine history and physical examination. Scanlon and coworkers concluded that history and physical examination, with careful monitoring of symptoms, identify most recurrences at an early stage, diminishing the necessity for routine laboratory or radiologic testing.

Valagussa and colleagues[78] reviewed the records of 278 patients who had a relapse following mastectomy, or mastectomy and systemic chemotherapy. History and physical examination during routine follow-up visits were successful in detecting 78 percent of the recurrences in this series. Sites of recurrence were soft tissue (38 percent), bone (37 percent), and viscera (34 percent). In symptomatic patients, additional sites of occult metastatic disease were detected in only 8 percent of patients. Twenty-two percent of patients who had a relapse were asymptomatic and had recurrent disease detected by routine radiographic examinations. Intrathoracic and bone recurrences were more likely to be asymptomatic when they were solitary sites of metastases. When bone and intrathoracic disease were detected simultaneously, only 2 (20 percent) of 10 patients were asymptomatic. The authors concluded that 6-month intervals were appropriate for follow-up of breast cancer patients in the absence of symptoms.

Other investigators have confirmed the overwhelming importance of the history and physical examination for the detection of recurrent breast cancer. Cantwell and associates[8] observed that 86.5 percent of recurrences in patients with breast cancer were detected by history and physical examination, whereas only 11.9 percent were detected by bone scans and 2.3 percent by chest radiograph. Winchester[87] studied 87 patients with recurrent breast cancer after mastectomy and reported that 79 recurrences (90.8 percent) were accompanied by clinical symptoms. Of those patients with recurrent disease, 38 percent developed osseous metastases, 16 percent had a local recurrence, 10 percent had local and systemic disease, and 10 percent had pulmonary metastasis. Five recurrences were found on physical examination in asymptomatic patients. Only 3 of 87 recurrences (3.4 percent) were discovered by radiologic examinations in the absence of symptoms.

With the knowledge that the majority of recurrences are detected by history and physical examination, two important questions arise. First, are routine follow-up visits after primary treatment for breast cancer efficacious (i.e., are recurrences detected earlier at routine, scheduled visits than with nonscheduled, interval visits)? Second, if a recurrence is detected in an asymptomatic patient, does early detection alter the natural course of the disease? The majority of studies that address these issues have demonstrated that routine screening is *not* superior to interval evaluation of the patient with breast cancer and that early detection of recurrent disease does *not* affect survival, thus minimizing the importance of detecting asymptomatic recurrences.

Holli and Hakama[36] suggested that routine follow-up visits were not efficacious in a Finnish study of 551 breast cancer patients with 5-year follow-up. These investigators observed that recurrent disease was detected five times as often in patients who presented with symptoms at spontaneous visits as it was in patients who were examined at routine visits. However, a false-positive clinical diagnosis of recurrent disease was more commonly made at spontaneous visits. Marrazzo and coworkers[51] retrospectively reviewed 85 patients with breast cancer treated by radical mastectomy and evaluated follow-up parameters. All of the node-positive patients (41) had postoperative chemotherapy (cyclophosphamide, methotrexate, and 5-fluorouracil). Thirty-two patients developed recurrent disease, and 28.1 percent of these recurrences were discovered in asymptomatic patients. Seventy-five percent of the recurrences were detected within 2 years of treatment. These authors acknowledged the lack of evidence demonstrating improved survival with early detection of recurrences in asymptomatic patients. They concluded that asymptomatic patients should have follow-up visits every 3 months for the first 5 years after treatment and that specific examinations (roentgenography and biochemical tests) could be done annually or at 6-month intervals. Brøyn and Frøyen[5] evaluated 81 women with recurrent breast cancer and determined

that the majority of recurrences were diagnosed at nonroutine visits. In addition, 75 percent of these recurrences were detected within the first 3 years after treatment. These investigators concluded that commonly used parameters for follow-up were *not* of value in allowing early detection of recurrent cancer and that routine follow-up did *not* prolong survival. In summary, these studies demonstrated no benefit from early detection of recurrent breast cancer in the asymptomatic patient.

In contrast, others have reported improved survival in asymptomatic patients with early detection of recurrences. Tomin and Donegan[75] evaluated patterns of recurrence and overall prognosis in 1230 women treated for breast cancer. Of the 248 recurrences identified, 36 percent were diagnosed in asymptomatic patients, and this group of patients had survival rates superior to those of patients with symptomatic recurrences (Fig. 84-3). However, the investigators concluded that few recurrences are detectable in asymptomatic patients and that improved survival rates in asymptomatic patients may be a result of so-called lead time bias. When follow-up interval was examined, there was no difference in survival after recurrence between compliant (regular follow-up) and noncompliant (irregular follow-up) patients (Fig. 84-4). These results suggest that detection of recurrences in the asymptomatic patient may afford an enhanced survival, but the appropriate follow-up interval and necessary tests were not well defined.

Bedwinek and colleagues[3] found that when local/regional recurrences were detected when tumor volume was minimal, nearly 50 percent 5-year survival could be achieved. Specifically, the detection of asymptomatic local recurrences afforded a 5-year survival rate of 50 percent, compared with 10.8 percent for symptomatic recurrences. The difference in survival for osseous metastases in symptomatic versus asymptomatic patients approached statistical significance ($p = 0.06$). Dewar and Kerr[22] studied

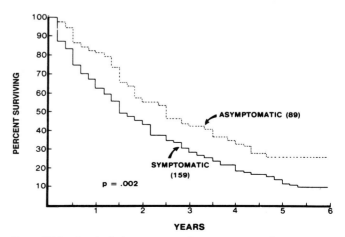

Figure 84-3 *Survival after symptomatic vs. asymptomatic recurrences. Survival is significantly longer in patients with recurrent disease discovered in the asymptomatic state. (From Tomin R, Donegan WL: J Clin Oncol 5:62–67, 1987. Reprinted by permission.)*

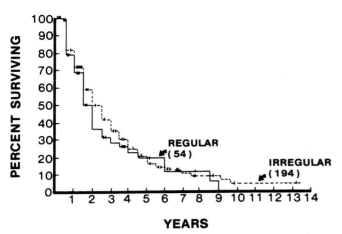

Figure 84-4 *Survival after recurrence of breast cancer according to regular or irregular follow-up examinations. There is no difference in overall survival. (From Tomin R, Donegan WL: J Clin Oncol 5:62–67, 1987. Reprinted by permission.)*

546 patients treated for early breast cancer with mastectomy with or without radiation therapy. One hundred ninety-two relapses were detected over 8 years; 93 were noted at routine visits, and 99 were found at unscheduled (interval) visits. These investigators reported that 74 percent of recurrences detected at routine follow-up visits were in the treated area or contralateral breast, whereas only 26 percent were at distant sites. This study further revealed that for locally recurrent disease, patients whose relapse was detected at a routine visit had a significantly better survival rate than patients whose relapse was detected at an interval visit. Overall, however, a potentially curable relapse (local disease or disease in the contralateral breast) was detected in only 66 patients (1 percent of 6764 routine visits), and only 26 (39 percent) of these 66 patients were free of disease at the completion of the study.

Controversy persists regarding the value of routine follow-up visits for patients with breast cancer. This has special significance in light of the need to establish cost-effective means of surveillance for patients after primary treatment. Routine office visits may increase the lead time in detection of recurrences before they are symptomatic or evident on self-examination; however, it has been difficult to establish that this translates into a survival benefit.[89] With improvements in systemic therapy programs, however, this lead time may result in improvement in survival rates and quality of life for patients with recurrent breast cancer.

RADIOGRAPHIC EVALUATION

Bone Scanning

Many clinical studies have documented that the most common site of recurrent metastatic breast cancer is bone. Osseous metastases are most often osteolytic; mixed osteolytic and osteoblastic metastases are less

common. The lesion must be greater than 1.5 cm in diameter with greater than 50-percent demineralization to allow adequate radiologic visualization and detection.[27] Therefore, routine skeletal surveys may not detect osseous metastases until advanced stages of growth. Lesions often remain asymptomatic until the disease involves the periosteum, initiating intense skeletal pain (see Chapter 74, by Dempsey Springfield, "Management of Osseous Metastases and Impending Pathological Fractures").

Bone scans performed using technetium 99m–labeled phosphate are more sensitive than skeletal roentgenograms and may increase the probability of detection of asymptomatic osseous metastases. Bone scans should be correlated, however, with radiographs and clinical symptoms to rule out abnormalities caused by other disease processes.[27] The incidence of positive bone scans (i.e., presumed osseous metastases) directly correlates with the stage of disease. With symptoms of bone tenderness or pain, more than 35 percent of patients are observed to have an abnormal bone scan.[43] When these symptoms are associated with abnormal skeletal roentgenograms, more than 80 percent of patients have an abnormal bone scan.[43] However, the value of routine bone scanning in asymptomatic patients has not been proved.[7] Bone scans may aid in detecting unsuspected osseous disease in patients with documented recurrences at other sites. Kunkler and Merrick[43] found that with documented local/regional recurrences, 37 percent of patients had positive bone scans. When nonosseous metastases were identified, bone scans were positive in 54 percent of patients.

Pedrazzini and colleagues[62] studied 1601 patients with node-positive breast cancer and determined that radionuclide scans would have detected first recurrences in only 2.4 percent of those studied. Thus, this series suggests that bone scans are not indicated when the patient does not present with clinical evidence of osseous pathology (e.g., symptoms of bone pain or fractures). In addition to yielding a small number of positive results, the routine use of bone scanning to detect asymptomatic recurrence in patients with breast cancer is not cost effective.

In the National Surgical Adjuvant Breast and Bowel Project's trial B-09, Wickerham and colleagues[85] prospectively evaluated 2697 patients with stage II (node-positive) breast cancer. Bone scans were performed every 6 months for the first 3 years and yearly thereafter. Only 0.6 percent of these scans detected lesions in asymptomatic patients. In light of the lack of evidence that the early diagnosis and treatment of osseous metastases improves survival, the investigators suggested that bone scans should be performed only in symptomatic patients. Pandya and associates[61] reviewed 175 patients with recurrent breast cancer from Eastern Cooperative Oncology Group adjuvant chemotherapy studies. Bone scans were obtained every 3 months for the first year and every 6 months thereafter. These studies confirmed metastatic disease in symptomatic patients and identified osseous metastases in asymptomatic patients (18.2 percent of all osseous recurrences). Chaudary and coworkers[14] evaluated the utility of serial bone scans in 241 breast cancer patients treated with postoperative chemotherapy. A total of 832 bone scans in the 241 patients detected only 25 patients with bone metastases (10.4 percent), and only 13 of these patients (5 percent) were asymptomatic. These investigators concluded that routine bone scanning is not indicated in the follow-up of the asymptomatic breast cancer patient.

Advocates of routine bone scanning report higher rates of detection of recurrences in asymptomatic patients.[28] Citrin and colleagues[16] evaluated 75 patients with early breast cancer (stage I or II) who underwent routine preoperative bone scans and subsequent scanning at 6-month intervals. Eleven patients (14.7 percent) had abnormal bone scans at presentation, and 13 patients (17.3 percent) with a normal bone scan at presentation had an abnormal bone scan at subsequent follow-up. The authors concluded that almost one third of their patients (all with stage I or II disease) had evidence of occult bone metastases by bone scan. There was no correlation of bone scan results with symptoms, but the investigators showed that there was a statistically significantly higher death rate in the group with abnormal scans. There was no summary of lymph node status or other prognosticators between the two groups. Probably the most valuable information from this study is that a small number of patients will have abnormal bone scans at presentation, and thus baseline bone scans may be useful in patients who are at high risk for metastatic disease.

Selective bone scanning in patients at high risk for developing osseous metastases may prove more rewarding. McNeil and associates[52] have shown that the rate of conversion from negative bone scans to positive bone scans strongly correlates with stage of disease. These investigators reported a conversion rate for stage I disease of 7 percent; for stage II, 45 percent; and for stage III, 58 percent. Most of these conversions occurred within the first 2 years after surgery. Coker and colleagues[17] likewise demonstrated that the conversion rates from negative to positive bone scans correlate with stage of disease, with conversion rates for stage I, II, and III disease being 6 percent, 26 percent, and 60 percent, respectively. Whether earlier detection of bone metastases translated into improved survival was not addressed in this study.

The results of a randomized trial of intensive diagnostic follow-up with bone scans and chest roentgenograms versus clinical follow-up were reported by the Italian National Research Council Project on Breast Cancer Follow-up.[67] These investigators followed 1243 patients with breast cancer for 5 years after surgical treatment. Both groups had annual mammography and physical examination every 3 months for the first 2 years and every 6 months for the following 3 years. In addition, the intensive follow-up group had chest roentgengrams and bone scans every 6 months. The rate of detection of isolated intrathoracic and bone metastases was higher in the intensive follow-up group (112 versus 71 cases), but local/regional recurrences and metastatic disease at other sites were identified at an equal rate in both groups. The investigators reported a statistically significant difference in 5-year relapse-free survival; patients in the intensive follow-up group had earlier detection of recurrences ($p = 0.01$). At 5 years, 64.8 percent of the intensive follow-up group were free of relapse versus 72 percent of the clinical follow-up group. However, most importantly, there was no difference in the overall 5-year survival between the two groups. The authors concluded that intensive follow-up with chest roentgengrams and bone scans should not be recommended as routine policy.

Chest Roentgenography

Chest roentgenography (CXR) as a routine follow-up study may identify occult disease, but early detection of intrathoracic disease has not been proved to influence survival. Ciatto and Herd-Smith[15] followed 1697 breast cancer patients, performing clinical examination and CXR every 6 months for the first 3 years and yearly thereafter. With a mean follow-up of 4.2 years, 523 patients (31 percent) had a relapse. Twenty-six percent of first recurrences were intrathoracic metastases; however, only 13 percent of first recurrences were isolated intrathoracic metastases. Pleural recurrences were the most likely to be symptomatic (89 percent), followed by multiple (35 percent) and single pulmonary nodules (5 percent). The sensitivity of CXR in detecting metastases was 86 percent. In this study, half of the patients with intrathoracic metastases had metastatic disease detected concurrently at other sites. A trend toward prolonged survival was noted when intrathoracic metastases were detected in asymptomatic patients as opposed to symptomatic patients, but this trend did not reach statistical significance (20.2 months versus 17 months). Thus, this study does not support the use of routine CXR in the follow-up of breast cancer patients. The previously noted study by Chaudary and associates[14] likewise supports the conclusion that routine chest radiographs are not indicated. In their analysis of 241 patients who had 1091 serial CXR, only 5 percent of patients were found to have metastatic disease on CXR, and of those 12 patients, only 8 were asymptomatic. Thus only 3 percent of patients had intrathoracic metastases detected by CXR during an asymptomatic stage.

Metastatic disease is detected in the thorax in up to 40 percent of patients who develop recurrent disease.[47] Thus, CXR identifies a significant number of patients with metastatic breast cancer. However, at the present time, there is no evidence that early detection of intrathoracic metastases affects survival. Therefore, follow-up chest roentgenograms are not routinely recommended in the asymptomatic patient.

Computerized Tomography Scanning of the Chest and Abdomen

At present, data do not support the use of routine computerized tomography (CT) scanning of the chest for the follow-up of asymptomatic breast cancer patients. However, patients with local/regional recurrence may harbor unsuspected disease in bone or soft tissues of the chest or upper abdomen that would not be diagnosed by routine CXR.[55, 80] Rosenman and coworkers[66] found that 22 of 33 patients (67 percent) with locally recurrent breast cancer after mastectomy had unsuspected disease noted on chest and upper abdominal CT scans. Findings on CT prompted changes in the treatment protocol in 10 patients (30 percent). Other investigators have also reported that CT scanning of the chest detects unsuspected disease in a high percentage of patients with local/regional recurrences, prompting alterations in therapy.[55, 80] The CT findings of internal mammary node involvement or unsuspected axillary disease were the most common reasons that CT scanning altered treatment planning in the Rosenman study. CT scanning is not recommended for follow-up of asymptomatic patients but may be helpful in treatment planning for patients with locally recurrent breast cancer.

Radiographic and Diagnostic Studies for Liver Metastases

Routine liver evaluation using CT scanning or radionuclide studies has not been found to be efficacious in detecting hepatic metastases in the asymptomatic patient following treatment of primary breast cancer.[10, 70, 86] Kauczor and colleagues[41] reviewed their experience with abdominal sonography in the follow-up of 414 patients with a diagnosis of breast cancer. During the study period, 2657 examinations were performed and only 28 (1 percent) revealed metastases. The vast majority of these metastases were in the liver (26 patients). The investigators used CT scan or biopsy, or both, to confirm the ultrasound findings in most cases. Kauczor and colleagues concluded that abdominal ultrasound is not indicated for routine screening in the regular follow-up of breast cancer patients. Because the CT scan will most likely be used to confirm suspicion of hepatic metastases, it would appear that the most cost-effective approach is to use the CT scan as the first examination when hepatic metastases are suspected because of symptoms or abnormal biochemical studies.

DeSouza and Shinde[21] reported a remarkably high incidence of asymptomatic liver metastases (up to 23 percent) in patients with breast cancer undergoing screening laparoscopic liver examination. Although laparoscopy may be a sensitive method of identifying metastases, there is risk associated with the procedure and general anesthesia; therefore, laparoscopy is not recommended over available noninvasive methods. In addition, until further studies substantiate the efficacy of early detection of asymptomatic hepatic metastases, hepatic imaging is not indicated as a routine screening modality.

Brain Scanning

Brain metastases following treatment of primary breast cancer are relatively rare; it has been esti-

mated that less than 10 percent of all patients with breast cancer will develop metastatic disease involving the central nervous system. There is no role for CT scans of the brain in breast cancer patients *without* central nervous system symptoms. However, CT scans demonstrate metastases in nearly half of patients *with* central nervous system symptoms, providing important prognostic information. CT scanning is superior to radionuclide scanning for investigation of central nervous system symptoms in patients with breast cancer.[20, 59]

Mammography

Women with a diagnosis of breast cancer have an increased risk of developing a second primary breast cancer. This risk has been estimated to be three to five times higher than that of a woman in the general population developing breast cancer.[53] In addition, women who have undergone breast-conserving therapy are at risk for local recurrence in the treated breast. For these reasons, annual mammography should be performed as part of the routine follow-up of breast cancer patients.

Mellink and associates[53] compared physical examination alone with physical examination and mammography in the follow-up program of breast cancer patients in two different cities in the Netherlands. There were 24 (3 percent) new breast cancers detected in 880 patients followed with mammography and physical examination and 14 (3 percent) new breast cancers found in the 411 patients followed by physical examination alone. Eight (35 percent) of the tumors detected in the group undergoing annual mammography were less than 10 mm in size or were *in situ* carcinomas, compared with only one (7 percent) detected in the group evaluated with physical examination alone. In addition, 18 (75 percent) of the 24 new breast cancers in the mammography group were node negative, whereas only eight (57 percent) of the 14 new breast cancers in the group evaluated with physical examination alone were node negative. These findings parallel the results seen with mammographic screening programs where breast cancers can be detected at an earlier stage with the potential for improved survival.

Women are generally advised to begin routine annual mammographic screening at age 50. Women who have been diagnosed with breast cancer should have annual mammography even if they are younger than 50, although interpretation is more difficult in the dense breasts of younger women. Evaluation after breast-conserving surgery and radiation therapy may be even more difficult depending on the degree of postoperative scarring. The placement of surgical clips at the lumpectomy site can be extremely helpful to the radiotherapist in treatment planning and also to the mammographer who can then focus carefully on the surgical bed.[54] Breast ultrasound is a useful adjunct to mammography in the treated breast because it can distinguish the margins of the surgical bed and can distinguish fluid from soft tissue density seen on mammogram. Magnetic resonance imaging has been shown to help differentiate between postsurgical scarring and recurrent tumor in the treated breast.[83] The use of other imaging modalities such as positron emission tomography scanning and sestamibi scanning to image the postoperative breast remains investigational at this time.

SERUM BIOCHEMICAL STUDIES

Biochemical analysis of serum is commonly used to follow patients with malignancy. Serum is easily obtained, and routine liver chemistry tests are relatively inexpensive. However, specificity and sensitivity are lost when individual parameters are assessed. Sensitivity increases with the number of parameters studied, but specificity is virtually unaffected. Alkaline phosphatase is the most sensitive serum marker for liver metastases; levels are elevated in 58 percent of patients with hepatic metastases.[10] Although there are other causes of elevated alkaline phosphatase levels (e.g., osseous disease), an increase of this isoenzyme in patients with breast cancer signifies liver metastases 85 percent of the time.[10] Serum glutamate oxaloacetate transaminase is also a sensitive biochemical parameter to aid in the detection of liver metastases; levels are increased in 60 percent of patients with liver metastases.[10] Serum glutamate pyruvate transaminase is less sensitive than serum glutamate oxaloacetate transaminase as an indicator of hepatic involvement.[10] Hypoproteinemia with a decrease in serum albumin levels may also be evident in patients with liver metastases; however, a significant number of breast cancer patients without liver metastases also have decreased serum albumin levels that are related to other causes. Combining liver chemistries with radiographic imaging increases the diagnostic sensitivity for liver metastases but has not proved to be cost effective at this time.[86]

Tumor markers, along with physical and radiologic examinations, may help detect a large percentage of patients with recurrent cancer in an early stage. Coombes and associates[18, 19] studied 141 patients with primary breast cancer with no evidence of metastases at diagnosis. One third of these patients subsequently had a relapse during follow-up.[18] Serial markers were obtained every 3 months; clinical examination, CXR, bone scan, liver scan, bone marrow aspiration, and skeletal radiography were performed every 6 months. Carcinoembryonic antigen (CEA), gamma glutamyl transpeptidase, and alkaline phosphatase were found to be the most useful biochemical markers for detecting metastatic disease. These tests, in combination with the chest radiograph and clinical examination, allowed the identification of 98 percent of patients with metastases, with only a 3.5-percent risk of false-positive tests. These authors found that the aforementioned studies provided a lead time of approximately 3 months before detection of overt metastasis, but a survival benefit was not evaluated.

Waalkes and colleagues[81, 82] studied multiple urine and serum markers in patients undergoing chemotherapy for node-positive breast cancer. These authors reported that overall, a higher proportion of elevated values in multiple markers was found in patients diagnosed with recurrent disease than in patients without recurrent disease. The investigators also evaluated biochemical markers for metastases to specific organs and determined that gamma glutamyl transpeptidase and alkaline phosphatase were the best indicators of hepatic disease and urinary hydroxyproline was the best biochemical marker for bone disease. CEA was not site specific, but levels were elevated in a high proportion of patients with hepatic or osseous involvement.

Lee[48] studied biochemical and hematological testing in 500 patients who had undergone mastectomy for breast cancer. Blood was obtained for studies every 2 to 4 months in the first year of follow-up and every 4 to 6 months thereafter. Patients with disseminated soft tissue or lung metastases had blood test results similar to those of patients without metastases. Patients with metastases to bone or other viscera were noted to have decreased albumin and total serum protein levels. In addition, gamma globulin and CEA levels were higher in patients with distant metastases than in patients without metastatic disease.

Although determination of biochemical or hematological parameters is common, there is no objective evidence to support the use of such studies in the routine surveillance of the breast cancer patient. However, if the clinician suspects recurrent disease, these tests may support the clinical findings and even help determine the organ system involved.

Tumor Markers

Several biological markers specific for breast tumors are under investigation for their effectiveness in detecting recurrent breast cancer in the asymptomatic patient (Table 84–4). For a tumor marker to be efficacious, it must fulfill the following criteria:

1. It must be produced by the primary tumor and its metastases.
2. It must be specific to the tumor and not be present in benign conditions.

TABLE 84–4. POTENTIAL SERUM BREAST CANCER TUMOR MARKERS

CA 15-3
CA 27.29
CA 549
Carcinoembryonic antigen (CEA)
ERBB2
MAM-6
Mammary serum antigen (MSA)
Mucin-like carcinoma–associated antigen (MCA)
Tissue polypeptide–specific antigen

3. It must be detected early in tumor growth.

4. It must reflect changes in cell growth and correlate with therapy.

5. It must be measureable by reproducible methods.

6. It must be cost effective.

Carcinoembryonic Antigen

CEA is an oncofetal glycoprotein discovered by Gold and Freedman[29] in 1965 in patients with adenocarcinoma of the colon. CEA is present on the cell surface membrane and is easily released into surrounding fluids. CEA is found in normal embryonic and fetal gut as well as certain malignant cells. This serum glycoprotein is commonly used as a tumor marker for colorectal cancer, but levels have also been found to be elevated in other malignancies. In addition, elevated serum CEA levels are found in some patients with various benign disease states such as colorectal polyps, pancreatitis, liver disease, and pulmonary infections. Heavy cigarette smokers may also have elevated serum CEA levels.

Several prospective studies have shown that serum CEA levels correlate with the stage of disease at the time of diagnosis of breast cancer.[49] Furthermore, serum CEA has been found to be an indicator of prognosis and a predictor of response to therapy.[49] Many investigators have examined the efficacy of monitoring serial serum CEA levels following potentially curative therapy for breast cancer in an attempt to identify patients with recurrent disease at an early stage. The conclusions of multiple studies have led to a wide spectrum of recommendations. At one end of the spectrum are those investigators who propose obtaining serial serum CEA levels as frequently as every 3 months after treatment[1, 2, 13, 26, 32, 44, 49, 57]; at the other extreme are those who insist that CEA monitoring has no role whatsoever in the follow-up of the patient with breast cancer.[31, 42, 45, 50]

Several studies have demonstrated that routine serial serum CEA determinations can identify a subset of patients with subclinical recurrence of breast cancer. Proponents of serial CEA testing have suggested that early detection of recurrences may allow more effective treatment. Elevations of CEA before clinical evidence of disease may lead the clinician to obtain the appropriate studies in the search for recurrent disease. Thus the discovery of an elevated CEA level before overt clinical disease may help identify the site of recurrence and afford earlier and potentially more effective eradication of recurrent disease. Several investigators have reported lead times of 2 to 8 months before clinical manifestations of recurrent disease.[1, 13, 49] Although a few studies have shown that early discovery of recurrence results in improved survival, the majority of studies do not show that survival is affected by lead time.[1, 13, 19, 26, 49, 79]

The major drawback to monitoring serial serum CEA levels is the low sensitivity and specificity of the assay. As previously stated, other malignant and nonmalignant states are associated with elevated serum CEA levels. In one study of 2095 patients following mastectomy for breast cancer, 41 percent of patients *with* verified metastases had a normal CEA level.[44] Thus false-negative results are obtained in greater than 40 percent of patients. In another study, 67 percent of patients with an increased serum CEA developed evidence of recurrent disease.[60] However, there was no difference between the percentage of patients who suffered a recurrence without an increase in CEA and those without recurrent disease who did have an increased CEA level.

In the majority of studies, half of the patients with recurrent breast cancer also have elevated serum CEA levels.[2, 13, 26, 36] Beard and Haskell reviewed several series studying the use of serial serum CEA monitoring in the early detection of recurrent breast cancer and found an overall false-positive rate of 53 percent (patients with an elevated serum CEA without recurrent disease) (Table 84–5).[2] Another subgroup of patients with consistently low serum CEA levels developed metastatic disease.[42] Obviously, a low serum CEA is not useful when patients have documented metastases, and a false-positive CEA result can be worrisome and lead to extensive unnecessary testing.

Others have identified specific instances in which serial monitoring of serum CEA may be useful.[26, 57, 60, 79] Van Der Linden and colleagues[79] found that serial serum CEA monitoring for the first 2 years after treatment may be helpful in screening for distant metastasis in patients with primary tumors 2 cm or greater in diameter and with positive axillary nodes and positive estrogen receptor status. However, even these authors concluded that serial CEA determination is probably not cost effective.

An elevated serum CEA level (>5 ng/ml) is, in part, organ specific. Patients with an elevated serum CEA level are more likely to have visceral or osseous metastases than local or local/regional recurrent disease.[32, 45, 46, 50] If higher serum CEA levels (10 ng/ml)

TABLE 84–5.   CEA AND EARLY DETECTION OF RECURRENT BREAST CANCER

No. of Patients at Risk for Recurrence	Patients with Recurrence	No. of Patients with an Elevated CEA	Elevated or Rising CEA Level Preceding Documented Recurrence (True-Positive)	Elevated or Rising CEA Level *Without* Recurrence During Study (False-Positive)
1626	312 (19%)	227	107 (47%)	120 (53%)

From Beard DB, Haskell CM: Am J Med 80:241–245, 1986. Reprinted by permission.

are used as the cut-off point, then the only patients with elevated serum CEA levels and recurrent disease are those with disseminated metastases.[46]

Overall, it does *not* appear that CEA monitoring is a useful or cost-effective test for detecting recurrent breast cancer.[30, 31] If CEA levels are elevated, however, recurrence is more likely to be present in distant organs rather than on the chest wall or in regional lymph node basins.

Other Serum Tumor Markers

Other tumor-associated antigens have been studied with regard to their usefulness as tumor markers. Almost all of the markers studied thus far in patients with breast cancer have been found to be more sensitive and specific than serum CEA.

CA 15-3. CA 15-3 is a high-molecular-weight, carbohydrate breast cancer–associated antigen. Increases in serum CA 15-3 levels greater than 25 percent above baseline strongly correlate with disease progression.[33, 76] Higher levels are found in patients with multiple sites of metastases and osseous metastases.[39, 63] CA 15-3 has been found to be a sensitive and specific marker for breast cancer and is superior to serum CEA determinations in its sensitivity.[33, 63, 76] Increased serum CA 15-3 levels have been found to precede clinical evidence of recurrent breast cancer by up to 13 months.[39] The high sensitivity and specificity of CA 15-3 make this antigen a potentially efficacious marker for early detection of recurrent breast cancer.

The cut-off point for a positive CA 15-3 level varies depending on the laboratory. In a study of 659 patients, Busetto and colleagues[6] showed a positive predictive value of 99.4 percent for CA 15-3 when a cut-off of 40 U/ml was used. Most other investigators have used a value of 32 U/ml to 35 U/ml for the upper limit of normal. Hölzel and associates[37] proposed the use of individual patient reference ranges calculated on the basis of average intraindividual variation. In this series, 22 recurrences were detected in 55 patients during the follow-up period. Using measurements of CEA and CA 15-3 in combination, Hölzel and colleagues detected all 14 cases of distant metastases with a mean lead time of 12 months and 7 of the 8 cases of local recurrence with a mean lead time of 7 months.

CA 27.29. CA 27.29 is a breast cancer–associated antigen that is structurally similar to CA 15-3 and is defined by reactivity with the B27.29 monoclonal antibody. A recent study comparing CEA, CA 15-3, and CA 27.29 showed that CA 27.29 was more sensitive than CA 15-3 (62 percent versus 57 percent) but was less specific (83 percent versus 87 percent).[64] In addition, the investigators in this study found that CA 27.29 was a better predictor of osseous and visceral metastases, but that CA 15-3 was the most efficacious marker overall.

CA 549. CA 549 is a glycoprotein breast cancer–associated antigen. Elevated CA 549 serum levels correlate more closely with systemic disease than with local recurrence. In addition, changes in serum CA 549 levels correlate with clinical response to therapy.[12] Sölétormos and associates[72] used measurements of CA 549 to monitor patients with metastatic breast cancer during chemotherapy. They concluded that serum CA 549 combined with physical examination identified or predicted clinical progression and could be of benefit over other investigative procedures. Other studies have corroborated these findings and suggested that CA 549 is best used for therapeutic monitoring.[11]

MAM-6. MAM-6 is another tumor-associated glycoprotein that has been found to be increased in the serum of patients with breast cancer. Serum MAM-6 levels correlate with the progression of metastatic disease and are more sensitive than serum CEA levels in detecting recurrent disease.[35] Rising levels may precede clinical evidence of metastases.

Mammary Serum Antigen. Mammary serum antigen (MSA) is a breast tumor–associated glycoprotein discovered in the early 1980s. Changes in MSA have been found to correlate with the clinical course of patients with breast cancer in nearly 90 percent of cases. MSA monitoring is more sensitive than serum CEA in detecting recurrent disease but does not appear as promising as other previously mentioned tumor markers overall.[73, 74] False-positive results are common.

Tissue Polypeptide–Specific Antigen. Tissue polypeptide–specific antigen is a marker of tumor proliferative rate. It is not specific for breast cancer but may be useful in monitoring response to treatment.[25]

Mucin-Like Carcinoma-Associated Antigen. Mucin-like carcinoma-associated antigen MCA is a tumor antigen with a long protein backbone and many carbohydrate side-chains.[56] Zenklusen and colleagues[88] studied breast carcinoma specimens for evidence of MCA and reported that MCA was detected in all of 122 tumors tested using a monoclonal antibody to intracytoplasmic MCA. These investigators also found MCA-positive cells in lymph nodes containing metastatic breast cancer. Subsequently, Miserez and coworkers[56] compared the usefulness of MCA with that of CA 15-3 and found that MCA levels were significantly higher in patients with metastatic disease than in patients who did not suffer relapse. Measured values of MCA were low after treatment of the primary tumor and increased with time during follow-up in the patients who developed metastatic disease. In this study, the negative predictive value of MCA was significantly higher than that of CA 15-3. There was no attempt to correlate symptoms with CA 15-3 or MCA levels in this study; therefore, the usefulness of MCA in the follow-up of asymptomatic patients cannot be determined from this report.

ERBB2 Proto-Oncogene. Amplification of the *ERBB2* proto-oncogene (also called *HER2/Neu*) has been found in 20 to 30 percent of human breast cancers.[71] Several studies have shown that amplification of *ERBB2* is associated with decreased survival in both node-negative and node-positive breast cancer patients. Isola and colleagues[38] recently studied serum levels of a soluble fragment of the *ERBB2* oncogene product in 225 patients both before surgery and during follow-up. Ten of the 11 patients who had preoperative elevation of serum *ERBB2* levels had evidence of *ERBB2* protein expression when the tumor tissues were tested by immunohistochemistry. During postoperative follow-up, elevated ERBB2 serum levels were associated with the development of metastatic disease within the next 6 months in 10 of 27 patients (37%) who had a relapse. This lead time could be important in *ERBB2* overexpressors because there are several ongoing clinical trials with new therapeutic modalities directed at *ERBB2*.

Future Use of Serum Tumor Markers

The clinical usefulness of the available tumor markers in human breast cancer is not well defined. The physiologic function of the majority of these markers is unknown, and none are detected in all breast cancers tested. When the measurement of combinations of several markers is necessary to detect relapse during routine follow-up, it is difficult to demonstrate cost effectiveness. If patients become eligible for new treatment protocols on the basis of elevation of a specific marker (e.g., *ERBB2*), then interval measurements may be justified for high-risk patients.

SUGGESTED GUIDELINES FOR FOLLOW-UP

Follow-up of the patient with breast cancer depends on facilities available to the clinician as well as patient compliance and the stage of disease. Follow-up must be tailored to the individual patient and that patient's associated risk factors. Patients with multiple risk factors for recurrent disease, such as nodal involvement, estrogen receptor–negative tumors, or chest wall involvement, may need more frequent follow-up than patients with small, node-negative, hormone receptor-positive tumors.

Our recommendations (Table 84–6) for follow-up are based on the clinical studies previously referenced, clinical experience, and cost effectiveness. For reference, Table 84–7 outlines follow-up schedules used by other investigators. It should be noted that data are not available to support specific follow-up intervals. Frequent follow-up may allow for early detection of local-regional failures. Early identification of local-regional disease will aid in the ability to achieve eventual local-regional control. More frequent follow-up intervals may also provide a longer lead time before clinical manifestations of distant disease are evident. Although numerous studies have

TABLE 84–6. RECOMMENDED FOLLOW-UP OF THE PATIENT WITH BREAST CANCER FOLLOWING CURATIVE THERAPY*

	Preoperative	Follow-up (Interval)
History and physical	Yes	4-month intervals for 2 years; 6-month intervals for years 2–5; annually after 5 years
Mammography	Yes	Annually†
Serum liver chemistry tests	Yes	As indicated
Chest roentgenography	Yes	As indicated
Bone scan	No‡	As indicated
Computerized tomography, abdomen and chest	No	As indicated
Brain scan	No	As indicated

*Recommended follow-up for patients with stages I to III breast cancer.
†Patients undergoing breast conservation therapy should have a baseline mammogram 6 months after completion of their radiotherapy.
‡Preoperative bone scan should be considered in stage II and III patients.

failed to show a survival benefit with routine follow-up, quality of life has not been evaluated. Patients with metastatic disease detected in the asymptomatic state may have a better quality of life than those who are not treated until their disease becomes symptomatic. The goal of the oncologist is to convert this lead time into an improvement in overall and disease-free survival. Based on these premises, our recommendations are as follows:

All patients should have routine serum liver chemistry tests, CXR, and mammography performed *before* primary treatment. A baseline bone scan should be considered in patients with stage II or III disease. Patients should be evaluated clinically every 4 months for the first 2 years and every 6 months for the next 3 years. After 5 years of follow-up, patients can be evaluated on an annual basis with history and physical examination and mammograms. Patients should be instructed in breast self-examination of the chest wall or conserved breast as well as the opposite breast. CXRs and bone scans should be obtained only when physical examination or symptoms warrant further investigation. Routine biochemical or biological marker studies are not indicated at routine follow-up visits unless examination or symptoms warrant further investigation. CT scans of the brain, chest, and abdomen are also not indicated on a routine basis.

If local recurrence is detected, radiographic studies may be helpful in detecting asymptomatic distant metastases. Bone scanning has been found to show evidence of metastatic disease in one third of patients who harbor local-regional recurrent disease without symptoms of osseous metastases. Likewise, occult intrathoracic disease may be detected by CT scanning of the chest in 67 percent of patients.[66] We recommend both bone scanning and CXR or CT scan of the chest in patients with local-regional recurrent disease.

TABLE 84–7. FOLLOW-UP SCHEDULES UTILIZED BY OTHER INVESTIGATORS

Author	History and Physical Examination	Serum Chemistry Tests	Chest Roentgenogram	Bone Scan	Skeletal Survey	Liver Scan
Marrazzo[51]	3-mo intervals	3-mo intervals	3-mo intervals	6-mo intervals	Annually	Annually
Muss[59]	6-mo intervals	Annually	Annually	Annually	—	—
Pandya[61]	3-mo intervals	3-mo intervals	3-mo intervals	3-mo intervals for 1 yr, 6-mo intervals yr 2–5	3-mo intervals	—
Tomin and Donegan[75]	3-mo intervals for 2 yr, annually after 5 yr	6-mo intervals for 5 yr	6-mo intervals for 5 yr	—	As indicated	—
Valagussa[78]	3-mo intervals for 1 yr, then every 4 mo	6-mo intervals for 3 yr, annually after 3 yr	4-mo intervals for 3 yr, biannually after 3 yr	—	6-mo intervals	Annually
Winchester[87]	6-mo intervals for 3–5 yr, annually after 5 yr	3- to 4-mo intervals for 3 yr	Annually	As indicated	—	—

It must be emphasized that the vast majority of recurrences are recognized by a detailed history and physical examination, along with careful attention to symptoms.[58] This has proved to be the case in other disease sites as well.[84] Therefore, the clinician should not rely solely on radiologic or laboratory studies to detect recurrent or metastatic disease because it is best recognized by a thorough history and physical.

As new tumor markers are developed and assessed, these studies may play an important role in detecting recurrent or metastatic breast cancer during follow-up. However, at present, none of these markers have sufficient sensitivity or specificity to recommend their use on a routine basis during follow-up. Furthermore, the cost of routine application of these tests cannot be justified at present. Schapira and Urban[69] evaluated the cost of routine surveillance for patients with breast cancer to determine the impact of reducing surveillance visits and testing. They estimated that a cost savings of $636 million in 1990 could have been achieved if follow-up was minimized to annual history, physical examination, and mammograms. This issue becomes pivotal as we enter the age of managed care plans and capitation contracts.

The early detection of recurrent breast cancer has not been shown to have a significant impact on survival. However, new advances in systemic therapy may eventually lead to improvements in survival for patients who develop recurrent disease. Early diagnosis of a second primary breast cancer in the conserved breast or in the contralateral breast has the greatest potential to impact survival of women with breast cancer at this time.

References

1. Ahlemann LM, Staab HJ, Anderer FA: Serial CEA determinations as an aid in postoperative therapy management of patients with early breast cancer. Biomedicine 32:194, 1980.
2. Beard D, Haskell CM: Carcinoembryonic antigen in breast cancer: Clinical review. Am J Med 80:241, 1986.
3. Bedwinek JM, Lee J, Fineberg B, et al: Prognostic medicators in patients with isolated local-regional recurrence of breast cancer. Cancer 47:2232, 1981.
4. Bonadonna G, Brusamolino E, Valagussa P, et al: Combination chemotherapy as an adjuvant treatment in operable breast cancer. N Engl J Med 294:405, 1976.
5. Brøyn T, Frøyen J: Evaluation of routine follow-up after surgery for breast carcinoma. Acta Chir Scand 148:401, 1982.
6. Busetto M, Vianello L, Franceschi R, et al: CA 15-3 value and neoplastic disease predictivity in the follow-up for breast cancer. Tumor Biol 16:243, 1995.
7. Butzelaar RM, Van Dongen JA, De Graaf PW, et al: Bone scintigraphy in patients with operable breast cancer stages I and II. Final conclusion after five-year follow-up. Eur J Cancer Clin Oncol 20:877, 1984.
8. Cantwell B, Fennelly JJ, Jones M: Evaluation of follow-up methods to detect relapse after mastectomy in breast cancer patients. Ir J Med Sci 151:1, 1982.
9. Carter CL, Allen C, Henson DE: Relation of tumor size, lymph node status, and survival in 24,740 breast cancer cases. Cancer 63:181, 1989.
10. Castagna J, Benfield JR, Yamada H, et al: The reliability of liver scans and function tests in detecting metastases. Surg Gynecol Obstet 134:463, 1972.
11. Cazin JL, Gosselin P, Boniface B, et al: An evaluation of CA 549, a circulating marker of breast cancer using a procedure for comparison with CA 15.3. Anticancer Res 12:719, 1992.
12. Chan DW, Beveridge RA, Bruzek DJ, et al: Monitoring breast cancer with CA-549. Clin Chem 34:2000, 1988.
13. Chatal JF, Chupin F, Ricolleau G, et al: Use of serial carcinoembryonic antigen assays in detecting relapses in breast cancer involving high risk of metastasis. Eur J Cancer 17:233, 1981.
14. Chaudary MM, Maisey MN, Shaw PJ, et al: Sequential bone scans and chest radiographs in the postoperative management of early breast cancer. Br J Surg 70:517, 1983.
15. Ciatto S, Herd-Smith A: The role of chest x-ray in the follow-up of primary breast cancer. Tumori 69:151, 1983.
16. Citrin DL, Furnival CM, Bessent RG, et al: Radioactive technetium phosphate bone scanning in preoperative assessment and follow-up study of patients with primary cancer of the breast. Surg Gynecol Obstet 143:360, 1976.
17. Coker DD, Lambrecht RW, Kehn BD: The value of initial and follow-up bone scans in patients with operable breast cancer. Mil Med 145:492, 1980.
18. Coombes RC, Gazet JC, Ford HT, et al: Treatment of malignant disease. Assessment of biochemical tests to screen for metastases in patients with breast cancer. Lancet 1:296, 1980.
19. Coombes RC, Powles TJ, Gazet JC, et al: Screening for metastases in breast cancer: An assessment of biochemical and physical methods. Cancer 48:310, 1981.
20. Dearnaley DP, Kingsley DPE, Husband JE, et al: The role of computed tomography of the brain in the investigation of breast cancer patients with suspected intracranial metastases. Clin Radiol 32:375, 1981.
21. DeSouza LJ, Shinde SR: The value of laparoscopic liver examination in the management of breast cancer. J Surg Oncol 14:97, 1980.
22. Dewar JA, Kerr GR: Value of routine follow up of women treated for early carcinoma of the breast. BMJ 291:1464, 1985.
23. Donegan WL: Local and regional recurrence. In Donegan WL, Spratt JA (eds): Cancer of the Breast, 3rd ed. Philadelphia, WB Saunders, 1988, p 648.
24. Early Breast Cancer Trialists' Collaborative Group: Effects of radiotherapy and surgery in early breast cancer. An overview of the randomized trials. N Engl J Med 333:1444, 1995.
25. Einarsson R: TPS—A cytokeratin marker for therapy control in breast cancer. Scand J Clin Lab Invest Suppl 221:113, 1995.
26. Falkson HC, Falson G, Portugal MA, et al: Carcinoembryonic antigen as a marker in patients with breast cancer receiving postsurgical adjuvant chemotherapy. Cancer 49:1859, 1982.
27. Feig SA: The role of new imaging modalities in staging and follow-up of breast cancer. Semin Oncol 13:402, 1986.
28. Gerber FH, Goodreau JJ, Kirchner PT, et al: Efficacy of preoperative and postoperative bone scanning in the management of breast carcinoma. N Engl J Med 297:300, 1977.
29. Gold P, Freedman SO. Demonstration of tumor-specific antigens in human colonic carcinomata by immunological tolerance and absorption techniques. J Exp Med 121:439, 1965.
30. Gray BN: Value of CEA in breast cancer. Aust N Z J Surg 54:1, 1984.
31. Gray BN, Walker C, Barnard R: Value of serial carcinoembryonic antigen determinations for early detection of recurrent cancer. Med J Aust 1:177, 1981.
32. Haagensen DW, Kister SJ, Vandevoorde JP, et al: Evaluation of carcinoembryonic antigen as a plasma monitor for human breast carcinoma. Cancer 42:1512, 1978.
33. Hayes DF, Zurawski VR Jr, Kufe DW: Comparison of circulating CA 15-3 and carcinoembryonic antigen levels in patients with breast cancer. J Clin Oncol 4:1542, 1986.
34. Hietanen P: Relapse pattern and follow-up of breast cancer. Ann Clin Res 18:134, 1986.
35. Hilkens J, Bonfrer JMG, Kroezen V, et al: Comparison of circulating MAM-6 and CEA levels and correlation with the estrogen receptor in patients with breast cancer. Int J Cancer 39:431, 1987.
36. Holli K, Hakama M: Effectiveness of routine and spontaneous follow-up visits for breast cancer. Eur J Cancer Clin Oncol 25:251, 1989.
37. Hölzel WGE, Beer R, Deschner W, et al: Individual reference

ranges of CA 15-3, MCA, and CEA in recurrence of breast cancer. Scand J Clin Lab Invest 221(Suppl):93, 1995.

38. Isola JJ, Holli K, Oksa H, et al: Elevated *ERB*B-2 oncoprotein levels in preoperative and follow-up serum samples define an aggressive disease course in patients with breast cancer. Cancer 73:652, 1994.

39. Kallioniemi O-P, Oksa H, Aaran R-K, et al: Serum CA 15-3 assay in the diagnosis and follow-up of breast cancer. Br J Cancer 58:213, 1988.

40. Kamby C, Rose C, Ejlertsen B, et al: Stage and pattern of metastases in patients with breast cancer. Eur J Cancer Clin Oncol 23:1925, 1987.

41. Kauczor H-U, Voges EM, Wieland-Schneider C, et al: Value of routine abdominal and lymph node sonography in the follow-up of breast cancer patients. Eur J Radiol 18:104, 1994.

42. Krieger G, Wander HE, Kneba M, et al: Metastatic breast cancer with constantly low CEA blood levels. J Cancer Res Clin Oncol 108:341, 1984.

43. Kunkler IH, Merrick MV: The value of non-staging skeletal scintigraphy in breast cancer. Clin Radiol 37:561, 1986.

44. Lamerz R, Leonhardt A, Ehrhart H, et al: Serial carcinoembryonic antigen (CEA) determinations in the management of metastatic breast cancer. Oncodevelopmental Biology and Medicine 1:123, 1980.

45. Lee YTN: Carcinoembryonic antigen as a monitor of recurrent breast cancer. J Surg Oncol 20:109, 1982.

46. Lee YTN: Serial tests of carcinoembryonic antigen in patients with breast cancer. Am J Clin Oncol 6:287, 1983.

47. Lee YTN: Breast carcinoma: Pattern of recurrence and metastasis after mastectomy. Am J Clin Oncol 7:443, 1984.

48. Lee YTN: Biochemical and hematological tests in patients with breast carcinoma: Correlations with extent of disease, sites of relapse, and prognosis. J Surg Oncol 29:242, 1985.

49. Lokich JJ, Zamcheck N, Lowenstein M: Sequential carcinoembryonic antigen levels in the therapy of metastatic breast cancer. Ann Intern Med 89:902, 1978.

50. Loprinzi CL, Tormey DC, Rasmussen P, et al: Prospective evaluation of carcinoembryonic antigen levels and alternating chemotherapeutic regimens in metastatic breast cancer. J Clin Oncol 4:46, 1986.

51. Marrazzo A, Solina G, Pocosa V, et al: Evaluation of routine follow-up after surgery for breast carcinoma. J Surg Oncol 32:179–181, 1986.

52. McNeil BJ, Pace PD, Gray EB, et al: Preoperative and follow-up bone scans in patients with primary carcinoma of the breast. Surg Gynecol Obstet 147:745, 1978.

53. Mellink WAM, Holland R, Hendriks JHCL, et al: The contribution of routine follow-up mammography to an early detection of asynchronous contralateral breast cancer. Cancer 67:1844, 1991.

54. Mendelson EB: Evaluation of the postoperative breast. Radiol Clin North Am 30:107, 1992.

55. Meyer JE, Munzenrider JE: Computed tomographic demonstration of internal mammary lymph-node metastasis in patients with locally recurrent breast carcinoma. Radiology 139:661, 1981.

56. Miserez AR, Günes I, Müller-Brand J, et al: Clinical value of a mucin-like carcinoma-associated antigen in monitoring breast cancer patients in comparison with CA 15-3. Eur J Cancer 27:126, 1991.

57. Mughal AW, Hortobagyi GN, Fritsche HA, et al: Serial plasma carcinoembryonic antigen measurements during treatment of metastatic breast cancer. JAMA 249:1881, 1983.

58. Muss HB, McNamara MCJ, Connelly RA: Follow-up after stage II breast cancer: A comparative study of relapsed versus non-relapsed patients. Am J Clin Oncol 11:451, 1988.

59. Muss HB, White DR, Cowan RJ: Brain scanning in patients with recurrent breast cancer. Cancer 38:1574, 1976.

60. Palazzo S, Liguori V, Molinari B, et al: The role of carcinoembryonic antigen in the postmastectomy follow-up of primary breast cancer and in the prognostic evaluation of disseminated breast cancer. Tumori 70:57, 1984.

61. Pandya KJ, McFadden ET, Kalish LA, et al: A retrospective study of earliest indicators of recurrence in patients on Eastern Cooperative Oncology Group adjuvant chemotherapy trials for breast cancer. Cancer 55:202, 1985.

62. Pedrazzini A, Gelber R, Isley M, et al: First repeated bone scan in the observation of patients with operable breast cancer. J Clin Oncol 4:389, 1986.

63. Pons-Anicet DMF, Krebs BP, Mira R, et al: Value of CA 15-3 in the follow-up of breast cancer patients. Br J Cancer 55:567, 1987.

64. Rodríguez de Paterna L, Arnaiz F, Estenoz J, et al: Study of serum tumor markers CEA, CA 15.3, and CA 27.29 as diagnostic parameters in patients with breast carcinoma. Int J Biol Markers 10:24, 1995.

65. Romsdahl MM, Sears ME, Eckles NE: Posttreatment evaluation of breast cancer. *In* The University of Texas M. D. Anderson Hospital and Tumor Institute: Breast Cancer: Early and Late. Chicago, Year Book Medical Publishers, Inc., 1970, p 291.

66. Rosenman J, Churchill CA, Mauro MA, et al: The role of computed tomography in the evaluation of postmastectomy locally recurrent breast cancer. Int J Radiat Oncol Biol Phys 14:57, 1988.

67. Rosselli Del Turco M, Palli D, Cariddi A, et al: Intensive diagnostic follow-up after treatment of primary breast cancer. A randomized trial. JAMA 271:1593, 1994.

68. Scanlon EF, Oviedo MA, Cunningham MP, et al: Preoperative and follow-up procedures on patients with breast cancer. Cancer 46:977, 1980.

69. Schapira DV, Urban N: A minimalist policy for breast cancer surveillance. JAMA 265:380, 1991.

70. Sears HF, Gerber FH, Sturts DL, et al: Liver scan and carcinoma of the breast. Surg Gynecol Obstet 140:409, 1975.

71. Slamon DJ, Godolphin W, Jones LA, et al: Studies of the HER-2/*neu* proto-oncogene in human breast and ovarian cancer. Science 244:707, 1989.

72. Sölétormos G, Nielsen D, Schiøler V, et al: Carbohydrate antigen 549 in metastatic breast cancer during cytostatic treatment and follow-up. Eur J Cancer 28A:845, 1992.

73. Stacker SA, Sacks NPM, Golder J, et al: Evaluation of MSA as a serum marker in breast cancer: A comparison with CEA. Br J Cancer 57:298, 1988.

74. Tjandra JJ, Russell IS, Collins JP, et al: Application of mammary serum antigen assay in the management of breast cancer: A preliminary report. Br J Surg 75:811, 1988.

75. Tomin R, Donegan WL: Screening for recurrent breast cancer—its effectiveness and prognostic value. J Clin Oncol 5:62, 1987.

76. Tondini C, Hayes DF, Gelman R, et al: Comparison of CA15-3 and carcinoembryonic antigen in monitoring the clinical course of patients with metastatic breast cancer. Cancer Res 48:4107, 1988.

77. Valagussa P, Bonadonna G, Veronesi U: Patterns of relapse and survival following radical mastectomy. Analysis of 716 consecutive patients. Cancer 41:1170, 1978.

78. Valagussa P, Tess T, Rossi A, et al: Adjuvant CMF effect on site of first recurrence, and appropriate follow-up intervals, in operable breast cancer with positive axillary nodes. Breast Cancer Res Treat 1:349, 1981.

79. Van Der Linden JC, Baak JPA, Postma T, et al: Monitoring serum CEA in women with primary breast tumours positive for oestrogen receptor and with spread to lymph nodes. J Clin Pathol 38:1229, 1985.

80. Villari N, Fargnoli R, Mungai R: CT evaluation of chest wall recurrences of breast cancer. Eur J Radiol 5:206, 1983.

81. Waalkes TP, Abeloff MD, Ettinger DS, et al: Multiple biological markers and breast carcinoma: A preliminary study in the detection of recurrent disease after primary therapy. J Surg Oncol 18:9, 1981.

82. Waalkes TP, Enterline JP, Shaper JH, et al: Biological markers for breast carcinoma. Cancer 53:644, 1984.

83. Weinreb JC, Newstead G: MR Imaging of the breast. Radiology 196:593, 1995.

84. Weiss M, Loprinzi CL, Creagan ET, et al: Utility of follow-up tests for detecting recurrent disease in patients with malignant melanomas. JAMA 274:1703, 1995.

85. Wickerham L, Fisher B, Cronin W, et al: The efficacy of bone scanning in the follow-up of patients with operable breast cancer. Breast Cancer Res Treat 4:303, 1984.

86. Wiener SN, Sachs SH: An assessment of routine liver scanning in patients with breast cancer. Arch Surg 113:126, 1978.

87. Winchester DP, Sener SF, Khandekar JD, et al: Symptomatology as an indicator of recurrent or metastatic breast cancer. Cancer 43:956, 1979.

88. Zenklusen H-R, Stähli C, Gudat F, et al: The immunohistochemical reactivity of a new anti-epithelial monoclonal antibody (MAb b-12) against breast carcinoma and other normal and neoplastic human tissues. Virchows Arch A Pathol Anat 413:3, 1988.

89. Zwaveling A, Albers GHR, Felthuis W, et al: An evaluation of routine follow-up for detection of breast cancer recurrences. J Surg Oncol 34:194, 1987.

CHAPTER 85

HORMONE REPLACEMENT THERAPY AND THE RISK OF BREAST CANCER

Michele G. Cyr, M.D. / Anne W. Moulton, M.D.

HORMONE REPLACEMENT THERAPY AND THE RISK OF BREAST CANCER

Background

In 1985 there were 40.5 million women older than 45 years in the United States. This number is predicted to rise to 52.5 million by the year 2000.[46] As a consequence, many more women will be facing decisions regarding the use of hormone replacement therapy at menopause. In spite of the attention menopausal hormone replacement therapy has received in the medical literature and lay press, relatively few postmenopausal women are taking hormone therapy. The number of women on hormone therapy varies widely even within the United States, with 15% of women on treatment in the Northeast versus 30% of women on the West Coast.[49]

The single best determinant for hormone use is hysterectomy.[3] Most women who have not had hysterectomies begin estrogen use because of symptoms.[3] Comparatively fewer women initiate hormone therapy for prevention of heart disease and osteoporosis.

Many reasons have been proposed to explain why women do not start hormone therapy. In the Massachusetts Women's Health Survey of 2500 women, 1 in 5 women never had their prescription filled.[62] More than half of the women who stopped or never started estrogen in the Massachusetts study cited fear of cancer as the reason.[54] When women are queried about their biggest health concern, they are much more likely to cite breast cancer than heart disease, even though cardiovascular disease is the leading cause of death for women.[1] Therefore, it is no surprise that the fear of breast cancer is a major deterrent to hormone therapy.

To assess women's knowledge and attitudes about hormone therapy, a postal survey was conducted in Iowa.[24] The majority of women in the study who were taking estrogen therapy had undergone a hysterectomy. Of the 125 postmenopausal women who were not taking estrogen, 80 (64 percent) had never discussed estrogen use with their physician. When these women were asked whether their physicians' recommendation would convince them to take estrogen, 75 percent agreed. It is also noteworthy that only 27 percent of the women not taking hormone replacement therapy (HRT) knew that estrogen was important in reducing the risk of osteoporosis, versus 89 percent of those taking estrogen.[24] These results were replicated in another survey conducted by mail in Scotland.[75] Only 11.9 percent of the 411 postmenopausal women who had never taken HRT had ever discussed it with their doctor. The majority of women did not know that estrogen could reduce the risk of heart disease or osteoporosis.

These studies point to the importance of shared decision-making between patients and physicians, particularly with regard to the long-term risks and benefits of hormone therapy. Most women still view hormone therapy as treatment rather than prevention. In the next decade, many more postmenopausal women will consider hormone replacement therapy and will discuss with their physicians the benefits (treatment of symptoms and prevention of coronary disease and osteoporosis) versus the major risk (potential for development of breast cancer). As more data become available documenting the benefits of HRT in the prevention of various conditions, it is more critical that patients and physicians engage in discussion about the risks and benefits.

This chapter presents what is known at present of the association between hormones and breast cancer. The hormonally mediated risk factors for breast cancer and hormonal effects on breast tissue are reviewed. The indications, benefits and risks of postmenopausal hormone therapy are presented. For women at average, additional, and high risk of breast cancer, the literature linking breast cancer to HRT is explored in detail. Finally, the alternatives to HRT are reviewed.

Risk Factors for Breast Cancer: The Role of Hormonally Mediated Risk Factors

Several known risk factors for breast cancer, including age at menarche, age of first pregnancy, number of pregnancies, age at menopause, postmenopausal obesity and estrogen use, offer evidence that ovarian hormones (primarily estrogens) play a major role in the development of breast cancer.[39] Unlike other cancers for which rates continue to climb with age, breast cancer incidence slows substantially after menopause with the concurrent reduction of endogenous estrogen levels.[78] Estrogens are established carcinogens in experimental settings, increasing the incidence of breast tumors in several animal models.[67] There is some evidence from epidemiologic studies that populations at higher risk for breast cancer have higher levels of circulating estrogens.[82]

Duration of Menstruation

A reduced risk of breast cancer is associated with shorter durations of menstruation. Earlier age of menarche is associated with the earlier onset of regular menstrual cycles and thus earlier exposure to normal endogenous estrogen and progesterone levels. Breast cancer risk is reduced by approximately 10 percent for each year the menarche is delayed. Similarly, breast cancer risk is increased by a comparable amount for each year the menopause is delayed. Early menopause, whether natural or related to bilateral oophorectomy, reduces breast cancer risk.

Pregnancy and Age at First Pregnancy

Nulliparity or older maternal age at first pregnancy are both risk factors that increase the lifetime incidence of breast cancer. The risk of breast cancer in women who have their first pregnancy after the age of 30 is approximately two times that of women who have their first pregnancy before the age of 20.[35] Women who delay pregnancy beyond the age of 35 actually have a slightly higher risk than nulliparous women.[39] The absolute number of pregnancies has only a small effect on breast cancer risk, after controlling for age at the time of pregnancy.

An early pregnancy is not only associated with extensive proliferation of breast tissue (ductal, lobular, and alveolar) under the stimulus of high levels of estrogen and progesterone, but it also results in stem cell differentiation in the terminal ducts and lobules.[39] This conversion of omnipotent stem cells to more differentiated forms is thought to leave the breast permanently less susceptible to genotoxic insults. Late age of first pregnancy and nulliparity both increase breast cancer risk. However, after controlling for age at first pregnancy, women who have a first birth at a late age show a short-term increase of breast cancer followed by a long-term reduction in risk, relative to nulliparous women.

Obesity

Postmenopausal obesity is an important risk factor for breast cancer.[16] This association is thought to be mediated predominantly by increased estrogenic stimulation of the breast. Androstenedione derived from the adrenal gland is the major endogenous source of estrogen precursors in postmenopausal women, and adipose cells are the major sites of aromatization of androstenedione to estrone (the major form of postmenopausal estrogen). Estrone is subsequently converted to the more biologically potent estradiol. It has been shown that serum levels of estrogen are higher in postmenopausal obese women than in thin women.[39] In contrast to postmenopausal obesity, premenopausal obesity decreases breast cancer risk, but the mechanism for this is unknown.[51, 88]

Hormone Use

Oral contraceptive use appears to increase the risk of breast cancer by approximately 50 percent; this risk declines rapidly after the drug is stopped.[35] However, there is some concern that longer duration of use (for more than a few years) may be associated with increased risk. Women who start oral contraceptive use at an early age (i.e., teenagers or before first full-term pregnancies) may be at increased risk of developing early onset (less than age 45) breast cancer. Furthermore, because oral contraceptives became available to U.S. women in the 1960s, it is only now that the long-term effects of oral contraceptives (albeit with larger doses of estrogen and progesterone than currently used) can be identified. There is at least one ongoing study to address this.[39]

Use of postmenopausal estrogen replacement therapy (ERT) may cause a modest increase in the risk of breast cancer, with a drop in risk after discontinuation of ERT.[39] The greatest risk is seen in patients who have used estrogen for more than 15 years. This issue is discussed in more detail later.

ESTROGEN EFFECTS ON BREAST TISSUE

Hormone Activity in Normal Breast Tissue

Steroid hormones play a significant role in promoting proliferation and cell differentiation in normal breast epithelium. The biological effects of estrogen and progesterone, two steroid hormones, are thought to be mediated through transcriptional activation of particular sets of genes recognized by specific receptor proteins.[15] The estrogen-receptor (ER) gene is located on the long arm of chromosome 6 (band q24-27)[44] and the progesterone receptor (PR) on the long arm of chromosome 11 (band q13).[47] Estrogen induces the formation of both ER and PR, whereas progesterone downregulates the formation of both receptors.[39] ER and PR are located mostly in the nucleus of the cell. Studies have suggested that there are four major functional regions in the ER and PR. These regions consist of a ligand-binding domain, a hinge region, a DNA-binding domain, and a variable or regulatory domain.[15] Certain amino acids in the hormone-binding domains of the ER and PR are essential for hormone recognition. Binding of the ligand to the receptors is thought to result in an allosteric change that allows the receptor-hormone complex to bind to its DNA response element in the promoter region of a target gene. In the absence of the hormone, the hormone-binding domain prevents the receptor from binding.

There is limited information on the pattern of ER and PR expression in normal breast tissue during the menstrual cycle. In normal breast tissue, ER and PR appear to be heterogeneous. Both are located in the nuclei of ductal and lobular epithelial cells but not in the myoepithelial or stromal cells. The percentage of epithelial cells in normal breast tissue expressing either ER or PR is actually low compared with observations made in breast cancer: Studies average less than 5 percent of epithelial cells expressing ER and less than 20 percent expressing PR. ER concentrations are highest in the follicular phase of the menstrual cycle, with ER levels in the luteal cell phase only 60 percent of the follicular phase levels.[15] In contrast, PR has been found to be relatively stable during both phases of the menstrual cycle. Studies show no effect of age or parity on percentage of ER or PR among premenopausal women.

The ratio of epithelial cells expressing ER to those expressing PR is reversed in postmenopausal tissue compared with premenopausal tissue. In one study, 26 percent of epithelial cells in postmenopausal breast were immunostained for ER and 2 percent for PR.[41]

Proliferative Activity of Normal Breast Tissue

The exact relationship between steroid–hormone receptor levels and breast cell proliferation is unclear. With the onset of menses, ductal growth is stimulated by estrogen. In the luteal phase of the menstrual cycle, terminal ducts per lobule are greatly increased, with an increase in the number of cells per terminal duct lobular unit. In the late luteal and early follicular phase, there is substantial loss of terminal duct lobular unit cells. Final proliferative development of the terminal region of the mammary tree occurs during pregnancy, when both estrogen and progesterone are present.

Hormonal effects on the terminal duct lobular unit are important because the majority of breast carcinomas arise in this area. There is great individual variation in breast tissue proliferation and no studies to date relate the observed cell division rates with serum hormone concentrations. Studies performed with tritiated thymidine labeling suggest that most proliferative activity occurs during the luteal phase of the cycle, with peak activity between postovulation days 9 and 12. Overall, the percentage of cells incorporating thymidine is 2 to 2½ times higher in the luteal phase than in the follicular phase.[15]

Mechanism of Hormonal Effect on the Development of Breast Cancer

ER content in malignant breast tissue is significantly higher than in normal breast tissue. Increased ER content has also been noted in dysplasias and adenomas.[39] It has been suggested that the reason for the high ER content of malignant breast tissue from postmenopausal women is the absence of circulating progesterone to downregulate the ER. However, in breast tumor tissue from premenopausal women, the ER content is stable throughout the menstrual cycle despite fluctuations in serum estrogen and progesterone.[39]

It is still not clear what role ovarian hormones play in the initiation, promotion, or dissemination of breast cancer. In cell lines, in vitro studies suggest that estrogen increases levels of transforming growth factor-α, an activator of growth, and decreases levels of transforming growth factor-β, which normally de-

presses cell proliferation activity. These effects are reversed by estrogen withdrawal. Estrogen also appears to stimulate expression of insulin-like growth factor, or somatomedin-C. Generally, estrogen appears to control breast cancer cell proliferation with upregulation of positive growth factors and receptors and downregulation of negative growth factors.[39] The potential risks associated with HRT could vary in specific clinical situations depending on the exact mechanism of hormonal action.

The ER and PR content of breast cancers has been shown to be important in predicting a patient's response to endocrine therapy, presumably by influencing mitotic activity. Women with ER-positive and PR-positive breast cancers who develop recurrent disease are more likely to respond to endocrine therapy (60 percent) with a regression or growth arrest of the tumor. Women with ER-negative and PR-negative breast cancers seldom (less than 10 percent) respond to endocrine therapy.[15] In general, use of ERT is not differentially associated with ER-positive versus ER-negative tumors. Interestingly, studies that have evaluated more specific use patterns, such as long-term use, recent versus remote use, or high dose, are more likely to show a positive association between ERT and ER-negative tumors.[39]

Several studies report growth stimulatory effects of progestins in animal models and in human cells. During the menstrual cycle, the mitotic activity of breast cells is higher during the luteal phase than the follicular phase, suggesting that estrogen and progesterone in combination may increase the risk of breast cancer over that of estrogen alone.[91] The exact role of progesterone in controlling the rate of mitosis in breast tissue and in the development of breast cancer remains unclear. Some authors suggest that increased mitosis in the luteal phase may be a reflection of increased estrogen levels in the previous follicular phase, as well as the short-lived surge in mitotic activity that occurs at the onset of the luteal phase.

Although estrogens and progestins appear to play important roles in breast cell proliferation, as noted earlier, there are other hormones and growth factors that regulate proliferative activity in breast cells. Insulin and estrogen exert synergistic effects on breast cancer cell proliferation. Numerous growth factors and hormones, including insulin, growth hormone, thyroid hormone, glucocorticoids, somatostatin, and prolactin may play important roles in breast cell development and differentiation.[15]

INDICATIONS FOR HORMONE REPLACEMENT THERAPY: SYMPTOMATIC TREATMENT VERSUS PREVENTION

At the time of menopause, ERT is prescribed to treat hot flashes and genitourinary symptoms. Another indication for prescribing estrogen is the prevention of osteoporosis and heart disease. This decision is based in part on knowledge of a woman's lifetime risk of breast cancer versus heart disease, osteoporosis, and hip fractures (Table 85–1) and the projected benefit of HRT.[13] Most of the available data is derived from observational studies. In fact, to date there are no prospective, randomized, double-blind, placebo-controlled clinical trials that show a clear benefit in morbidity or mortality of women at average risk for heart disease or osteoporosis.

Treatment of Symptoms

The median age at menopause is 51.3, with a range of 48 to 55.[77] The majority of women (58 to 93 percent) in the perimenopausal transition experience symptoms of vasomotor instability, although there is considerable individual variation in the frequency and intensity of these episodes. Most patients describe a hot flash as the sensation of heat across the upper thorax, neck, and head, typically accompanied by flushing and perspiration in the same distribution and followed by a chill. Associated symptoms may include palpitations, chest pain, and anxiety. Hot flashes that occur during the night may cause substantial impairment of the normal sleep pattern. Much of the mood disturbance that has been attributed to menopause in the past is now known to be related to disrupted sleep. Hot flashes are thought to be caused by the decreasing estrogen levels. It is known that estrogen influences thermoregulatory, neural, and vascular functioning, but the specific role of estrogen in the etiology of hot flashes is not fully understood.[43]

Estrogen therapy effectively controls hot flashes in more than 95 percent of perimenopausal women. Most women are treated with 0.625 mg of conjugated equine estrogen or its equivalent; however, some may require higher doses, whereas others may be treated with less. For symptom control, the lowest effective dose of estrogen should be used. The duration of therapy varies with the duration of symptoms, but it usually ranges from 1 to 3 years. Although most patients experience hot flashes for 1 to 3 years after the cessation of menses, some may have them for up to 10 years. In women with an intact uterus, a progestin must be added to the regimen to eliminate the

added risk of endometrial cancer. Other therapies are discussed in the section on alternatives to HRT at the end of the chapter.

Genitourinary symptoms usually begin 3 to 5 years after the cessation of menses. As estrogen levels decline, the vulva loses most of its collagen, adipose, and water-retaining ability, becoming flattened and thin. The vagina shortens and narrows, and the vaginal walls become thinner, less elastic, and less able to produce lubricating secretions during intercourse. Symptoms include vaginal dryness, dyspareunia, vaginal bleeding, increased vaginal infections, urinary incontinence, and urinary tract infections. Treatment with estrogen (oral medication or vaginal cream) is effective in most cases, and alternative therapies are discussed later.

Hormone Replacement Therapy for Prevention

Cardiovascular Disease

Cardiovascular disease is the leading cause of death for women in the United States, accounting for 50 percent of deaths in women older than age 50.[84] A 50-year-old woman has a 31-percent lifetime chance of dying from ischemic heart disease in contrast to a 2.8-percent risk from breast cancer, a 2.8-percent risk from an osteoporotic hip fracture, and a 0.7-percent risk from endometrial cancer (see Table 85–1).[13] Women lag 10 to 15 years behind men in the development of heart disease, which is presumed to be secondary to early protection by estrogen, with rates of coronary disease increasing in postmenopausal women as they age. It was originally thought that this effect was mediated entirely via lipids. A recent randomized double-blind, placebo-controlled trial confirms a short-term beneficial effect of estrogen on lipids, with an increase in high-density lipoproteins and a decrease in total cholesterol.[91] However, estrogen's indirect effect on cholesterol metabolism accounts for only part of its beneficial effect on the heart.[85] Estrogen appears to retard atherosclerotic processes directly by inhibiting intimal hyperplasia and other steps in the development of atherosclerosis. It acts as an antioxidant and may protect the endothelial cell from injury. It inhibits platelet aggregation and decreases fibrinogen levels. Finally, it has a direct effect on vasomotor tone by stimulation of the release of endothelium-derived relaxing factor. ERs have been identified in the smooth muscle cells of human coronary arteries.[85]

Most women placed on HRT for prevention have an intact uterus and thus are placed on a progestin therapy as well. There has been ongoing concern that progestins might attenuate or eliminate the cardiovascular benefit of estrogen. This should become less of an issue with the findings of the Postmenopausal Estrogen/Progestin Interventions (PEPI) trial that support the beneficial effects of estrogen and progesterone on lipid profiles. In this study, the greatest benefit was derived from unopposed estrogen, but

TABLE 85–1. LIFETIME RISKS OF DEATH DUE TO SELECTED CONDITIONS FOR 50-YEAR-OLD WHITE POSTMENOPAUSAL WOMEN

Condition	Lifetime Risk (%)
Coronary heart disease	31.0
Hip fracture	2.8
Breast cancer	2.8
Endometrial cancer	0.7

From Cummings SR, Black DM, Rubin SM: Lifetime risks of hip, Colles' or vertebral fracture and coronary heart disease among white postmenopausal women. Arch Intern Med 149:2445–2448, 1989. Copyright 1989, American Medical Association.

estrogen in combination with micronized progesterone showed similar but somewhat less substantial changes.[92] Even as the benefits of estrogen become more obvious, the role of progesterone remains uncertain with respect to heart disease. HRT for the prevention of coronary disease should continue for 20 to 25 years after menopause.

Osteoporosis

Osteoporosis is a leading cause of morbidity in women as they age. In the United States, there are at least 250,000 hip fractures each year; the majority of these fractures occur in women. However, these fractures represent only a small fraction of the fractures attributable to osteoporosis. The lifetime risk of a 50-year-old woman for a hip fracture is 16 percent; for a wrist fracture, 15 percent; and for vertebral fracture, 32 percent.[13] Osteoporosis is a disease characterized by low bone mass with microarchitectural deterioration of bone tissue, leading to enhanced bone fragility and an increase in fracture risk. Bone mass increases rapidly in young women, reaching a peak between the second and third decades. After age 35 to 40, bone mass begins to decline in both men and women, but in women, the rate of bone loss accelerates dramatically after menopause.[64] Calcium metabolism changes as estrogen levels decline, but the mechanism by which estrogen influences this change is not clear. The withdrawal of estrogen results in increased bone turnover and, in particular, increased bone resorption.[64] Multiple observational studies document reduced hip fracture rates with ERT. The pooled estimate for relative risk of hip fracture is 0.75 for estrogen users versus nonusers.[34] The addition of progestin has not been shown to influence the beneficial effects of estrogen on osteoporotic fractures. As with the prevention of coronary disease, HRT for osteoporosis is presumed to be a lifelong commitment.

Other Potential Benefits of Hormone Replacement Therapy

The list of potential benefits of HRT grows longer as the results of more observational studies are analyzed (Table 85–2). Included among the recent additions are HRT's effects on dental health, colon cancer, and Alzheimer's disease.

The Leisure World Cohort Study has demonstrated a beneficial effect of estrogen on tooth loss. Denture wearing was less common among estrogen users than nonusers, and rates of dental loss were lower among women treated with estrogen.[57]

An association between colon cancer and estrogen has been suggested in several epidemiological studies. Recently, women selected for the Cancer Prevention Study II were studied to assess this association.[6] Women who had ever used ERT had a significantly decreased risk of fatal colon cancer (relative risk [RR] = 0.71, confidence interval [CI] 0.61–0.83). Current users of estrogen experienced the greatest risk reduction (RR = 0.55, CI 0.40–0.76) with a trend toward decreased risk with increased duration of estrogen use. The authors concluded that exogenous estrogens exert a protective effect against the development of colorectal cancer.

Based on several observational studies, it appears that estrogen may have a protective effect against Alzheimer's disease. Women treated with estrogen were less likely to carry a diagnosis of Alzheimer's disease and related dementias.[36, 58] Additionally, two clinical trials have suggested that estrogen treatment may improve cognition in postmenopausal women with established Alzheimer's disease.[25, 37] These results need to be confirmed because neither of the studies were controlled. Nonetheless, there does appear to be an association between cognitive function and estrogen use.

RISKS OF HORMONE REPLACEMENT THERAPY

Endometrial Cancer

Endometrial cancer is the most common malignant disease of the female genital tract. There were 32,000 new cases of endometrial cancer, resulting in 5600 deaths in 1992. A woman's lifetime risk of developing endometrial cancer is 2 to 3 percent. This risk is increased by a history of early menarche, late menopause, nulliparity, obesity, anovulation, liver disease, and the use of unopposed exogenous estrogens. Chronic unopposed estrogen, either from endogenous or exogenous sources, is associated with endometrial cancer. The endometrium can be stimulated by the increased estrogen levels related to obesity (increased production), liver disease (decreased degradation), or exogenous sources (postmenopausal estrogen). Conditions associated with anovulation also favor a high estrogen environment because the ovarian thecal cells are no longer stimulated to produce progesterone. Since the mid-1970s, several retrospective studies have implicated ERT as a risk factor for the development of endometrial cancer in postmenopausal women.[29]

The recently published results of the PEPI Trial not only reinforced this association but also accentu-

TABLE 85–2. BENEFITS AND RISKS OF HORMONE REPLACEMENT THERAPY

Benefits	Risks
Treatment	
• Treats genitourinary atrophy	• Breast cancer
• Treats hot flashes	• Endometrial cancer
	• Gallbladder disease
Prevention	
• Reduces cardiovascular disease	
• Reduces risk of osteoporosis	
• Decreases dental loss	
• Prevents Alzheimer's disease	
• Prevents colon cancer	

ated it.[92] The addition of a progestin eliminates the observed excess risk from estrogen use. Consequently, progesterone has become a near-mandatory addition to postmenopausal HRT for nonhysterectomized women and, therefore, ERT must be considered in the context of progesterone treatment.

Gallbladder Disease

Exogenous estrogen has been associated with the development of gallbladder disease. Estrogen administration decreases bile acid concentration, increases biliary cholesterol, and raises the cholesterol concentration in bile. Epidemiological studies have shown conflicting results comparing gallstone development in users versus nonusers of estrogen. A recent report from the Nurses' Health Study indicates that current hormone users are at increased risk for cholecystectomy compared with women who had never used hormones. The risk of gallbladder surgery increased with increasing duration and dose of hormones.[32]

Breast Cancer

The potential for increased risk of breast cancer with HRT represents the major concern for patients and their physicians. This subject is addressed with considerations of individual baseline risk for breast cancer (see later).

Risks and Benefits for Women at Average Risk of Breast Cancer

Based on the results of approximately 35 observational studies, hormonal replacement therapy does not appear to increase substantially the risk of breast cancer in the general population.[34] Most of these studies suggest that the overall risk of breast cancer in hormone users (without regard to type, amount and duration of use) is not substantially different from that of nonusers. Relative risks of 1.3 to 2 are reported in special populations of hormone users depending on the duration of use, recency of use, and chronological age.[39] In addition, several U.S. and European studies have shown an interaction between age at menopause and hormone use.[39] Hormone users with late age at natural menopause exhibit an increased breast cancer risk. Recent studies have also shown an interaction between alcohol consumption and estrogen risk (see later). In all of these associations, the high-risk subgroups exhibit relative risk estimates of 2 or less.

Of six meta-analyses reported in the literature (Table 85-3), none has shown a statistically significant effect for lifetime use of hormone replacement therapy on breast cancer risk.[2, 8, 19, 33, 74, 80] However, two of the six meta-analyses show a 25- to 30-percent increase in breast cancer risk with prolonged use (10 to 15 years) compared with controls.

In the mid- to late 1980s, there were some suggestions in the literature that progestins exerted a protective effect on the risk of breast cancer. However,

TABLE 85–3. META-ANALYSES OF BREAST CANCER RISK AMONG USERS OF HORMONE REPLACEMENT THERAPY VERSUS NONUSERS

Reference	Effects of Use (RR [95% CI]*)	Chronic Use (# yrs) (RR [95% CI])
Armstrong (1988)[2]	0.96 (0.98–1.05)	1.04 (15 yr) (0.88–1.24)
Dupont and Page (1991)[19]	1.08 (0.96–1.2)	No conclusion
Steinberg et al (1991)[80]	1.0	1.3 (15 yr) (1.2–1.6)
Grady and Ernster (1991)[33]	1.02 (0.98–1.06)	1.25 (15 yr) (1.04–1.51)
Sillero-Arenas et al (1992)[74]	1.06 (1.00–1.12)	1.23 (12 yr) (1.07–1.42)
Colditz et al (1993)[8]	1.02 (0.93–1.12)	1.23 (10 yr) (1.08–1.4)

*RR = relative risk, CI = confidence interval.

careful review of the available data refuted this conclusion.[23] The results from subsequent studies evaluating breast cancer risk from estrogen and progestin have been conflicting.[34] This variability in the published results to date prevents any firm conclusion from being reached.

Two studies published in 1995 underscore the continuing controversy about HRT and the risk of breast cancer. Both studies assessed the risk of breast cancer for women taking both estrogen and progesterone but arrived at very different conclusions. The Nurses' Health Study, a prospective cohort study, demonstrated an increase in the relative risk for breast cancer in postmenopausal women taking HRT. The risk was greatest in older women and in those who had used hormones for more than 5 years (Fig. 85–1).[9] In contrast, a case-controlled study by Stanford and colleagues suggested that women who had used combination therapy for more than 8 years had a reduced risk of breast cancer (RR = 0.4, CI = 0.2–1.0) compared with users of estrogen and progesterone.[79] Both studies raise the concern that observational studies cannot truly assess the association between HRT and breast cancer. Randomized trials are clearly needed to answer the question.

Grady and associates presented a thorough and cogent analysis of the available data on risks and benefits of HRT, and applied the calculated relative risks of associated conditions to specific case scenarios.[34] The authors summarized the current literature as of 1992 and generated lifetime probabilities for the four specific conditions that would be affected either positively or negatively by the addition of HRT. They found that in non-hysterectomized women (approximately 60 percent) who are at no increased risk (i.e., average risk) for these conditions, estrogen use could reduce the risk of coronary heart disease by 35 percent and the risk of a hip fracture by 25 percent.

However, unopposed estrogen could be expected to increase the risk of endometrial cancer eight-fold and to increase the risk of breast cancer by 25 percent. The addition of progestin to the regimen alters the probabilities substantially, effectively removing any added risk of endometrial cancer. However, the effect of progestin on heart disease is unclear; it could reduce the beneficial effect of estrogen by as much as 50 percent. The role of progestins in the development of breast cancer is similarly uncertain (see later), and some studies suggest a potential increase in the risk of breast cancer. Overall, the expected gain in life expectancy with HRT for 50-year-old women with no increased risk of heart disease, osteoporosis, or breast cancer was 1 month to 1 year. This range is based on calculations from the most conservative to the most generous estimates of progesterone's influence on the conditions considered.

Based on existing evidence for HRT in women at average risk, the authors concluded that "the best course of action is unclear."[34]

Women with Additional Breast Cancer Risks

The literature on the relationship between estrogen and breast cancer suffers from numerous methodological problems. Among them is the relatively small sample size of most studies. This problem is accentuated when one looks at specific subsets of women who may be at increased risk based on estrogen exposure. At the present time, most of the data available are those from meta-analyses, which systematically combine data sets to generate numbers adequate enough to identify specific additional risks for breast cancer.

Family History

Five to twenty percent of women have a family history of breast cancer, depending on the population studied.[38] There is great concern that these women will have an increased risk of breast cancer with postmenopausal HRT. There is no clear consensus to advise patients with a family history of breast cancer against HRT. The literature raises the possibility of a slightly increased risk of breast cancer for women with a family history of breast cancer compared with those without a family history.

In a meta-analysis, Steinberg and associates reported an increased risk of breast cancer among estrogen using women with a family history of breast cancer.[80] The relative risk was 3.4 (CI = 2.0–6.0) for women with a family history, compared with those without a family history of breast cancer. However, other meta-analyses have not found this degree of increased risk with estrogen use in patients with a family history of breast cancer.

Grady and colleagues used meta-analytic methods to determine summary relative risks for breast cancer with and without HRT.[34] They applied these calculations to lifetables to estimate changes in life expectancy (Table 85–4).

The authors assume that for a 50-year-old woman with a family history of breast cancer, the risk of breast cancer is twice that of an individual without a family history (Table 85–5). This, in turn, confers a 19.3 percent lifetime risk of breast cancer, which reduces life expectancy by 0.5 years compared to an average risk woman (see Tables 85–4 and 85–5). If this 50-year-old woman were to take estrogen at menopause, her lifetime probability of breast cancer would increase from 19.3 to 24.1 percent. These numbers are based on their assumptions from meta-analyses estimating the risk of breast cancer related to estrogen. Without the addition of progestin, the risk of endometrial cancer rises even more dramatically. Nonetheless, the woman's life expectancy is increased by 0.7 years, based on the benefits of estrogen related to coronary artery disease and hip fracture. In this situation, even though the risk of breast cancer rises significantly, the long-term benefits of estrogen outweigh the risks when life expectancy is the outcome considered.

When progestins are added, the added risk of endometrial cancer is completely eliminated. It is still unknown what the effects of adding progestin are on breast cancer risk. The authors calculate a worst-case scenario based on the literature that assumes a twofold increased risk of breast cancer with estrogen and progestin. In the patient with a family history,

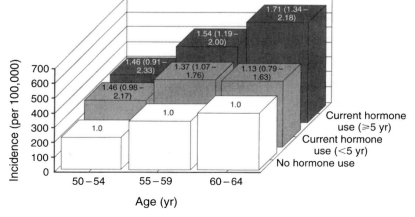

Figure 85–1 *Incidence and relative risk of breast cancer according to age and the duration of current postmenopausal hormone therapy. Relative risks and 95 percent confidence intervals are shown on the top of the bars; relative risks are expressed in comparison with the risk among women in each age group who never received hormone therapy. Data have been adjusted for age at menopause, type of menopause, and family history of breast cancer in a proportional-hazards analysis. (From Colditz GA, Hankinson SE, Hunter DJ, et al: The use of estrogens and progestins and the risk of breast cancer in postmenopausal women. N Engl J Med 332:1589–1593, 1995.)*

TABLE 85–4.   LIFETIME PROBABILITIES OF SELECTED CONDITIONS FOR A 50-YEAR-OLD WHITE WOMAN TREATED WITH LONG-TERM HORMONE REPLACEMENT

Variable	Lifetime Probability*			
	No Treatment	*Estrogen*	*E + P†*	*E + P‡*
Coronary heart disease, %	46.1	34.2	34.4	39.0
Stroke, %	19.8	20.2	20.3	19.3
Hip fracture, %	15.3	12.7	12.8	12.0
Breast cancer, %	10.2	13.0	13.0	19.7
Endometrial cancer, %	2.6	19.7	2.6	2.6
Life expectancy, yr	82.8	83.7	83.8	82.9

*Estimated lifetime probability of developing the condition.

†Assuming that the addition of a progestin to the estrogen regimen does not alter any of the relative risks for disease from estrogen therapy, except to prevent the increased risk due to endometrial cancer (relative risk for endometrial cancer estimated to be 1.0).

‡Assuming that the addition of a progestin to the estrogen regimen provides only two thirds of the coronary heart disease risk reduction afforded by estrogen therapy (relative risk for coronary heart disease estimated to be 0.8) and relative risk for breast cancer in treated women is 2.0.

E + P = estrogen plus progestin.

From Grady D, Rubin SM, Petitti DB, et al: Hormone therapy to prevent and prolong life in postmenopausal women. Ann Intern Med 117:1016–1037, 1992.

the lifetime probability increased from 19.3 to 35.1 percent and resulted in a loss of life expectancy of 0.5 years.

Based on these calculations and the degree of uncertainty that exists at present, many clinicians advise women with a family history of breast cancer against HRT. The authors of a recent review of this topic commented, "We recommend that all women at increased risk of breast cancer avoid use of exogenous estrogens when possible . . . In the absence of data, we have chosen to abide by the Hippocratic principle of 'First do no harm.' "[38]

The isolation of the *BRCA1* gene and localization of the *BRCA2* gene have made it clear that individuals with a family history of breast cancer are not a homogeneous group. Yet the studies relating HRT and breast cancer were done before these advances, and they characterize all family history as equivalent. It is likely that future research will make these distinctions in order that the specific group at high-

est risk of HRT-related breast cancer can be counseled accordingly.

Benign Breast Disease

Several studies have been published that address the risk of breast cancer in estrogen users with benign breast disease.[5, 20, 65, 68, 89] Of five studies published, only one has demonstrated an increased risk of estrogen use in women with benign breast disease.[68] In a meta-analysis, Dupont and Page calculated the relative risk of breast cancer with HRT in the setting of benign breast disease to be 1.16 (CI = 0.89–1.5). They concluded that there was no extra risk conferred based on a history of benign breast disease with ERT, and that benign breast disease should not be a contraindication to HRT.[19]

Some studies suggest that oral contraceptives or progestational agents can reverse intraductal hyperplasia and atypical hyperplasia in nearly half of the

TABLE 85–5.   LIFETIME PROBABILITIES OF SELECTED CONDITIONS FOR A 50-YEAR-OLD WHITE WOMAN AT RISK FOR BREAST CANCER TREATED WITH LONG-TERM HORMONE REPLACEMENT*

Variable	Lifetime Probability†			
	No Treatment	*Estrogen*	*E + P‡*	*E + P§*
Coronary heart disease, %	44.9	33.1	33.3	37.1
Stroke, %	19.2	19.5	19.6	18.2
Hip fracture, %	14.8	12.2	12.3	11.2
Breast cancer, %	19.3	24.1	24.2	35.1
Endometrial cancer, %	2.5	19.3	2.6	2.5
Life expectancy, yr	82.3	83.0	83.1	81.8

*Relative risk for developing or dying of breast cancer was estimated as 2.0, as for a woman with a mother or sister who has had breast cancer.

†Estimated lifetime probability of developing the condition.

‡Assuming that the addition of a progestin to the estrogen regimen does not alter any of the relative risks for disease seen with estrogen therapy, except to prevent the increased risk due to endometrial cancer (relative risk for endometrial cancer estimated to be 1.0).

§Assuming that the addition of a progestin to the estrogen regimen provides only two thirds of the coronary heart disease risk reduction afforded by estrogen therapy (relative risk for coronary heart disease estimated to be 0.8) and relative risk for breast cancer in treated women is 2.0.

E + P = estrogen plus progestin.

From Grady D, Rubin SM, Petitti DB, et al: Hormone therapy to prevent and prolong life in postmenopausal women. Ann Intern Med 117:1016–1037, 1992.

patients treated for between 1 and 3 years.[83] Clearly, more studies are needed to determine the effects of progestins on postmenopausal breast disease.

Alcohol Use

Alcohol consumption, estrogen use, and breast cancer have been linked in several epidemiological studies.[27, 72, 88] There have also been some data suggesting a synergistic effect between alcohol and estrogen on the risk of breast cancer. Based on Nurses' Health Study data, the relative risk of breast cancer among alcohol consumers who concurrently used estrogen was 1.56 (CI = 1.2 − 2.0).[10] There was no increased risk of breast cancer among nondrinkers who took hormones. The authors described this difference in risk of breast cancer due to estrogen according to level of alcohol intake to be "unexpected and intriguing," and called for further study of this association. Similarly, Iowa's Women's Health Study demonstrated a relationship between alcohol and breast cancer in estrogen users versus nonusers.[31]

Investigators reported a synergistic interaction between alcohol and other risk factors for breast cancer based on ER and PR status. The results suggested an increased risk of ER-negative and PR-negative related breast cancers in estrogen users who drank alcohol. Specifically, women drinking more than 4 gm of ethanol per day who had ever used estrogen had a relative risk for ER-negative and PR-negative related breast cancers of 2.6 when compared with abstainers who had ever used estrogen. Of interest, the authors also demonstrated an increased risk of ER-negative and PR-negative related breast cancers in women who drank and had a family history of breast cancer.[30]

Other Cancers

There is growing evidence that ERT may be safe in patients treated for endometrial cancer.[40] Although a definitive study has not been conducted, many patients with treated endometrial cancer are receiving estrogen. The question of initiating other estrogen-sensitive primary tumors has not been addressed. This is an area that warrants increased attention. Nonetheless, a history of endometrial cancer is still listed among the absolute contraindications for hormone therapy.

Women with Breast Cancer (High Risk)

Approximately 175,000 women are diagnosed with breast cancer in the United States each year, and of these 67 percent will survive. Between 75 and 90 percent of these patients are postmenopausal and 10 to 25 percent are still in their reproductive years.[33] Of those younger women treated for breast cancer, many will have menopause induced by treatment with chemotherapy.[7] For these women, the vasomotor and genitourinary symptoms of menopause are likely to be particularly severe because of the precipitous

drop in estrogen levels. In addition, their earlier menopause will put them at increased risk for osteoporosis and heart disease as compared with women who experience natural menopause later in life.

For all women who have survived breast cancer, and particularly for those who have had menopause prematurely induced by treatment, it is crucial to know the risk of ERT because the benefits from both symptom control and prevention of long-term consequences of menopause could be great.

Use of Estrogen by Breast Cancer Patients

Listed among the absolute contraindications to estrogen use is a personal history of breast cancer. In fact, until recently there would be little if any reason to approach this topic with anything more than a very clear warning that estrogen should not be used in breast cancer survivors under any circumstances. This dogma has been challenged recently. Several reviews of the literature have been published and reflect the growing concern that a large number of women are being denied access to the potential benefits of HRT based on their past history of breast cancer.[7, 12, 14, 17, 40, 52, 61, 70] The major argument is that in the absence of clearly established increased risks of treatment, many women are being excluded unnecessarily from the symptomatic and preventive benefits of HRT.

To date, there have been few trials of ERT in breast cancer patients. Many who advocate the use of estrogen in such patients point to the natural experiments of estrogen exposure in patients with breast cancer. One such natural experiment is in patients who have become pregnant after treatment for breast cancer. For these patients, there has been no demonstrably adverse effect of pregnancy on their breast cancer.[42, 63] Additionally, there is evidence from cohort studies that estrogen treatment before breast cancer diagnosis may improve the prognosis.[4] This is similar to the observation that women who develop breast cancer while taking oral contraceptives have no worse prognosis and in some studies have had better-differentiated tumors than women not taking birth control pills.[53, 76]

There have been only five published studies on estrogen use in breast cancer survivors to date.[18, 22, 60, 81, 87] The results of these studies are summarized in Table 85–6. Stoll treated breast cancer survivors with estrogen for hot flashes and reported that there were no relapses after 2 years.[81] Wile and colleagues studied 25 breast cancer survivors treated with HRT for menopausal symptoms. After an average of nearly 3 years of treatment, three patients had relapsed. The overall survival of the high-risk patients was 94 percent. Although their study did not have sufficient power to establish safety of hormonal therapy in breast cancer patients, the authors used their results to justify further investigation.[86]

Eden and associates conducted a case-controlled study of combined continuous estrogen-progestin re-

TABLE 85–6.   HORMONE REPLACEMENT THERAPY IN WOMEN WITH A HISTORY OF BREAST CANCER

Study	Hormone Replacement Therapy	Number	Median Age	Stage					Follow-Up (months)	Outcome† %
				In Situ	1	2	3	4		
Wile et al[87]	Varied	25	51	2	13	7	1	2	35	88 NED 12 REL
DiSaia et al[18]	Varied	77	50	6	43	17	5	6	59	92 NED 8 REL
Stoll[81]	Combined continuous‡	50	?	—					24	100 NED
Powles et al[60]	Varied	35	51		12	14	9		43	94 NED 6 REL
Eden et al[22]	Varied	90	47	—					>72	93 NED 7 REL

†NED, no evidence of disease; REL, relapse.
‡Three to six months of 0.625 mg conjugated estrogen and 0.15 mg norgestrel.
From Sands R, Boshoff C, Jones A, et al: Current opinion: Hormone replacement therapy after a diagnosis of breast cancer. Menopause: The Journal of the North American Menopause Society 2:77, 1995.

placement in women with a breast cancer history.[22] Of 901 women with breast cancer, 90 had taken estrogen for menopausal symptoms. Most of these women were taking combined continuous estrogen and progestin. Controls were matched from the same data base and had not taken hormones after their breast cancer diagnosis.

Among the 90 estrogen users, there were no deaths and only 7 percent had a recurrence. Conversely, among the nonusers of estrogen, 17 percent experienced a recurrence. This corresponded with a relative risk of 0.4 (Cl = 0.17–0.93) for estrogen users versus nonusers. The authors concluded that short-term use (median treatment of 1.5 years) of HRT could be safe for women with breast cancer and might reduce the recurrence rate. Interestingly, their findings are compatible with other evidence that continuous moderate progestins reduce breast cell activity in vitro and in vivo, whereas cyclic progestins increase mitotic activity.[28]

Powles and colleagues reported their experience with 35 patients who received hormone therapy with conjugated equine estrogen (0.625 mg to 1.25 mg) and tamoxifen (20 mg per day) after a diagnosis of breast cancer.[60] These women were treated for menopausal hot flashes for a mean duration of 14.6 months (range = 1 to 44 months). The mean follow-up was 43 months (range = 1 to 238 months). During follow-up, only two patients experienced a relapse. The majority of treated patients had partial or complete relief of their menopausal symptoms. Based on their findings, the authors conclude that it may be possible to design HRT regimens that control menopausal symptoms while protecting the patient from breast cancer.

In a report in the *Lancet*, DiSaia and coworkers described their experience with HRT breast cancer survivors.[18] The authors routinely counsel all patients about the benefits and risks of HRT in the setting of breast cancer. Of the women counseled, 77 accepted HRT after treatment for breast cancer and were followed for 15 years. The median duration of therapy was 27 months (range = 1 to 233 months). Most of the women used conjugated estrogen, with fewer using estradiol patches. The median follow-up from diagnosis was 59 months (range = 10 to 425 months). Among the 77 patients treated with hormone therapy, 7 had recurrent breast cancer. At the time of the report, 71 patients (91 percent) had no evidence of disease, 3 (4 percent) were alive with disease, and 3 died. Among the 70 patients with no recurrences, only 3 had stopped their HRT.

Other trials are in progress, and data should be available in the near future. There is nothing yet to substantiate the harmful effects of short-term ERT in breast cancer survivors. Yet there are still no randomized trials that can definitively answer the question.

In assessing the risk of estrogen treatment in breast cancer survivors, it should also be acknowledged that other related cancers could be initiated or stimulated by ERT. Of particular concern are cancers of the ovaries, endometrium, and possibly, the cervix. At the annual meeting of the Society of Gynecologic Oncologists, researchers presented evidence for a link between breast cancer and gynecological cancers of the ovary, cervix, and endometrium.[72] This preliminary data might suggest the possibility of yet another risk of ERT in survivors of breast cancer.

If shorter term, lower dose estrogen were established to be safe in breast cancer patients, menopausal symptom treatment with estrogen would be possible. The safety of treating with estrogen to prevent osteoporosis and heart disease needs to be addressed separately because there is insufficient evidence that lower dose, shorter term ERT is effective.

Tamoxifen

Much interest has been generated in tamoxifen as an alternative to estrogen in the prevention of postmenopausal osteoporosis and cardiovascular disease. For women at high risk for primary or secondary estrogen-related cancer in particular, tamoxifen could be a safer choice.

Tamoxifen has been shown to be effective in controlling breast cancer. In fact, tamoxifen's classification as antiestrogenic has been invoked to argue that if it is beneficial for breast cancer, then estrogen must be detrimental. This argument is far too simplistic, however, because tamoxifen has complex actions that are not uniformly antiestrogenic. Tamoxifen has been shown to act like estrogen in increasing the risk of endometrial cancer, improving lipid profile (decreased total and low-density lipoprotein cholesterol) and maintaining bone mass.[26] It is plausible that tamoxifen's effect on breast cancer is not solely related to its antiestrogenic actions. Premenopausal women treated with tamoxifen are hyperestrogenemic, yet they have been shown to benefit from treatment.[71]

There is growing interest in the possibility of concomitant use of tamoxifen and estrogen in patients who have had breast cancer. This combination is particularly appealing for patients who have symptoms of estrogen deficiency with tamoxifen use. To date, there have been no well-controlled trials substantiating the benefit and safety of such regimens, although there are suggestive reports from Great Britain.[59] Because both tamoxifen and estrogen increase the risk of endometrial cancer, progestins must be given concomitantly in patients with intact uteri.

Tamoxifen has successfully reduced the recurrence of contralateral breast cancer among breast cancer patients. One study has investigated the risks of second primary cancers of the ovary, endometrium, and contralateral breast among breast cancer survivors treated for short periods with tamoxifen.[11] The study was designed as a nested case-control within a cohort study of breast cancer patients. Ovarian, endometrial, and contralateral breast cancer cases were less likely to have received tamoxifen than were the cancer-free controls, although the differences achieved statistical significance only for breast cancer. The authors concluded that short duration of tamoxifen (mean of 2 years) was not associated with an increased risk of endometrial or ovarian cancer and was associated with reduced risk of contralateral breast cancer in breast cancer patients. However, more studies are needed to determine the risks of long-term tamoxifen use.

In a meta-analysis of 133 randomized adjuvant therapy trials, 30,000 women with breast cancer treated with tamoxifen experienced significantly reduced recurrence and mortality rates. The finding that spurred interest in tamoxifen as a preventive agent was that the incidence of contralateral breast cancer was reduced 39 percent in tamoxifen-treated patients.[21]

In 1992, the National Cancer Institute and the National Surgical Adjuvant Breast and Bowel Project began a randomized, placebo-controlled, double-blinded clinical trial of 16,000 healthy women. All subjects are older than 35 and at high risk for breast cancer. Subjects will receive 5 years of treatment with placebo or tamoxifen. The major outcome studied will be that of breast cancer, but tamoxifen's effect on cardiovascular disease and bone density will also be studied.[26]

The Breast Cancer Prevention Trial has sparked controversy in the medical community. Many contend that the potential benefits of tamoxifen in reducing breast cancer outweigh the potential risks of endometrial cancer and thromboembolic disease.[55] Nonetheless, the trial continues and is likely to add to our knowledge of tamoxifen's effects. Certainly, this is an area where further study is desperately needed.

Alternative Treatment for Menopause

Although some of the literature would imply otherwise, there are alternatives to ERT for both the treatment of menopausal symptoms and the prevention of associated long-term conditions. Although it is true that estrogen is highly effective for the treatment of hot flashes and vaginal dryness, it is by no means the only effective treatment. Similarly, there are alternatives to estrogen for the prevention of osteoporosis and heart disease. Particularly for patients with breast cancer, these alternative therapies may be the only choices for symptom relief and the prevention of associated conditions.

Because there are relatively few controlled trials of treatment for hot flashes, much of the information that is available is anecdotal. However, there is evidence that suggests that clonidine, lofexidine, veralipride, and sotalol can decrease hot flashes.[92] Although none of these drugs completely eliminate hot flashes and their use may be limited by side effects, many women who choose not to take estrogen may find them effective.

The safety of vitamin E in low doses (100-400 IU per day) makes it a reasonable first-line treatment for hot flashes. Although the data on vitamin E and hot flashes is mostly anecdotal, there are claims that up to two thirds of women experience relief from hot flashes with it. Ginseng has been promoted as a "natural" treatment for menopausal symptoms. Ginseng is an herbal source of estrogen and, as such, should be used only in circumstances in which estrogen would be prescribed. Although it is likely that the amount of estrogen ingested in the form of ginseng is less than that which would be prescribed, this is by no means guaranteed. Other herbs have been touted as effective in the treatment of menopausal symptoms, but clear evidence is lacking.

Preventive strategies may also be effective for women who can identify triggers of hot flashes. Also, paced breathing and relaxation techniques can be used to abort a hot flash at its outset. Unfortunately, these techniques may be less helpful for nighttime hot flashes that can cause night sweats and severe sleep disturbances.

Low doses of megestrol acetate have been shown to reduce hot flashes by 85 percent versus an observed 25 percent reduction in the placebo group.

This treatment could have great promise for women with breast cancer if its long-term safety is established.[50] As yet, it is not known whether megestrol affects hormonally sensitive cancers such as breast cancer and, therefore, cannot be recommended with complete confidence as an alternative to ERT for hot flashes in breast cancer patients.

Postmenopausal genitourinary atrophy can cause symptoms of vaginal dryness, dyspareunia, dysuria, and urinary incontinence. Although estrogen is highly effective in reversing the atrophic changes, there are other means of prevention and treatment. Continued sexual activity prevents some of the postmenopausal changes by mucosal stimulation. For women who have established symptoms of vaginal atrophy, a short course of estrogen (topically or systemically) may be necessary so that they can resume sexual activity to prevent ongoing and progressive problems. There are now topical treatments that contain polycarbophil, a mucoadherent compound, that are superior to conventional lubricants and are effective for several days after a single application.[93] These can be very effective for women who cannot use estrogen.

Estrogen is certainly not the only effective means of preventing osteoporosis and heart disease. Weight-bearing exercise and calcium both have important roles in osteoporosis prevention. Newer agents to treat osteoporosis include nasal calcitonin, slow-release fluoride, and bisphosphonates.[56] The bisphosphonates, which inhibit osteoclastic activity, are particularly promising in the treatment of osteoporosis.[48] Diet, exercise, and smoking cessation are effective in reducing the risk of heart disease. These strategies should all be employed whether estrogen is or is not recommended. For most women, these life style changes will have additional health benefits.

SUMMARY

There has been a concern on the part of many that HRT is being prescribed without a clear assessment of individual risks and benefits.[66] The Women's Health Initiative has been designed to provide data that will distinguish real from potential benefits in subsets of women.[69]

At the present time, estrogen is still contraindicated for use in women who have had breast cancer. However, it must be made absolutely clear to the patient that this exclusion is based largely in theory.

It is ultimately the patient who must decide whether the potential benefits of HRT outweigh the potential risks. As health care providers, it is our responsibility to educate patients to the extent that the information is available so that they can make the most informed decision in the context of their individual beliefs and values. Fortunately, there is an ever-expanding list of resources available to help patients in the decision-making process.[45]

References

1. Andrews WC: The transitional years and beyond. Obstet Gynecol 85:1–5, 1995.
2. Armstrong BK: Oestrogen therapy after the menopause—boon or bane? Med J Aust 148:213–214, 1988.
3. Barrett-Connor E: Prevalence, initiation and continuation of hormone replacement therapy. J Women's Health 4:143–148, 1995.
4. Bergkvist L, Adami HO, Persson I, et al: Prognosis after breast cancer diagnosis in women exposed to estrogen and estrogen-progesterone replacement therapy. Am J Epidemiol 130:221–228, 1992.
5. Brinton LA, Hoover R, Fraumeni JR Jr: Menopausal oestrogens and breast cancer risk: An expanded case-control study. Br J Cancer 54:825–832, 1986.
6. Calle EE, Miracle-McMahill HL, Thun MJ, Health CW Jr: Estrogen replacement therapy and risk of fatal colon cancer. J Natl Cancer Inst 87:517–523, 1995.
7. Cobleigh, MA, Berris RF, Bush T, et al: Estrogen replacement therapy in breast cancer survivors. JAMA 272:540–545, 1994.
8. Colditz GA, Egan KM, Stampfer MJ: Hormone replacement therapy and risk of breast cancer: Results from epidemiologic studies. Am J Obstet Gynecol 168:1473–1480, 1993.
9. Colditz GA, Hankinson SE, Hunter DJ, et al: The use of estrogens and progestins and the risk of breast cancer in postmenopausal women. N Engl J Med 332:1589–1593, 1995.
10. Colditz GA, Stampfer MJ, Willett WC, et al: Prospective study of estrogen replacement therapy and risk of breast cancer in postmenopausal women. JAMA 264:2648–2653, 1990.
11. Cook LS, Weiss NS, Schwartz SM, et al: Population-based study of tamoxifen therapy and subsequent ovarian, endometrial and breast cancers. J Natl Cancer Inst 87:1359–1364, 1995.
12. Creasman WT: Estrogen replacement therapy: Is previously treated cancer a contraindication? Obstet Gynecol 77:308–312, 1991.
13. Cummings SR, Black DM, Rubin SM: Lifetime risks of hip, Colles' or vertebral fracture and coronary heart disease among white postmenopausal women. Arch Intern Med 149:2445–2448, 1989.
14. Cyr MG: Postmenopausal estrogen replacement therapy in the patient with breast carcinoma. Rhode Island Medicine 78:261–263, 1995.
15. Dahmoush L, Pike MC, Press MF: Hormones and breast cell proliferation. *In* Lobo RA (ed): Treatment of the Postmenopausal Woman: Basic and Clinical Aspects. New York, Raven Press, 1994, pp 325–337.
16. deWaard F, Nornelis JP, Aoki K, et al: Breast cancer incidence according to weight and height in two cities of the Netherlands and in Aichi Prefecture, Japan. Cancer 40:1269–1275, 1977.
17. DiSaia PJ. Hormone replacement therapy in patients with breast cancer. Cancer 71(Suppl):1490–1500, 1993.
18. DiSaia PJ, Odicino F, Grosen EA: Hormone replacement therapy in breast cancer. [Letter.] Lancet 342:1232, 1993.
19. Dupont WD, Page DL: Menopausal estrogen replacement therapy and breast cancer. Arch Intern Med 151:67–71, 1991.
20. Dupont WD, Page DL, Roger LW, et al: Influence of exogenous estrogens, proliferative breast disease, and other variables on breast cancer risks. Cancer 63:948–957, 1989.
21. Early Breast Cancer Trialists' Collaborative Group: Systemic treatment of early breast cancer by hormonal, cytotoxic, or immune therapy: 133 randomized trials involving 31,000 recurrences and 24,000 deaths among 75,000 women. Lancet 339:1–15, 1992.
22. Eden JA, Bush T, Nand S, et al: A case-controlled study of combined continuous estrogen-progestin replacement therapy among women with a personal history of breast cancer. Menopause: The Journal of the North American Menopause Society 2:67–72, 1995.
23. Ernster VL, Cummings SR: Progesterone and breast cancer. Cancer 68:715–717, 1986.
24. Ferguson KJ, Hoegh C, Johnson S, et al: Estrogen replacement therapy: A survey of women's knowledge and attitudes. Arch Intern Med 149:133–136, 1989.

25. Filit H, Weinreb H, Cholst I, et al: Observations in a preliminary open trial of estradiol therapy for senile dementia—Alzheimer's type. Psychoneuroendocrinology 11:337–345, 1986.
26. Ford LG, Brawley OW, Perlman JA, Nayfield SG, et al: The potential for hormonal prevention trials. Cancer 74(Supp):2726–2733, 1994.
27. Friedenraich CM, Howe GR, Miller AB: A cohort study of alcohol consumption and the risk of breast cancer. Am J Epidemiol 137:512–520, 1993.
28. Gambrell RD: Hormone replacement therapy in patients with previous breast cancer. Menopause: The Journal of the North American Menopause Society 2:55–57, 1995.
29. Gambrell RD: Pathophysiology and epidemiology of endometrial cancer. In Lobo RA (ed): Treatment of the Postmenopausal Woman: Basic and Clinical Aspects. New York, Raven Press, 1994, pp 355–362.
30. Gapstur SM, Potter JD, Drinkard C, et al: Synergistic effect between alcohol and estrogen replacement therapy on breast cancer differs by estrogen progestin receptor states in Iowa's Women's Health Study. Cancer Epidemiol Biomarkers Prev 4:313–318, 1995.
31. Gapstur SM, Potter JD, Folsom AR: Increased risk of breast cancer with alcohol consumption in postmenopausal women. Am J Epidemiol 136:1221–1231, 1993.
32. Goldstein F, Colditz G, Stampfer M: Postmenopausal hormone use and cholecystectomy in a large propsective study. Obstet Gynecol 83:5–11, 1994.
33. Grady D, Ernster V: Invited commentary: Does postmenopausal hormone therapy cause breast cancer? Am J Epidemiol 134:1396–1400, 1991.
34. Grady D, Rubin SM, Petitti DB, et al: Hormone therapy to prevent disease and prolong life in postmenopausal women. Ann Intern Med 117:1016–1037, 1992.
35. Harris JR, Lippman ME, Veronesi U, et al: Medical Progress, Breast Cancer. N Engl J Med 327:319–328, 1992.
36. Henderson VW, Paganini-Hill A, Emanuel CK, et al: Estrogen replacement therapy in older women. Arch Neurol 51:896–900, 1994.
37. Honjo H, Ogino Y, Naithoh K, et al: In vivo effects by estrone sulfate on the central nervous system—senile dementia (Alzheimer's type). J Steroid Biochem 34:521–525, 1986.
38. Hoskins KF, Stopfer JE, Calzone KA, et al: Assessment and counselling for women with a family history of breast cancer: A guide for clinicians. JAMA 273:577–585, 1995.
39. Hulka BS, Liu ET, Lininger RA: Steroid hormones and risk of breast cancer. Cancer suppl 74(Suppl):111–124, 1994.
40. Hutchinson-Williams KA, Gutmann JN: Estrogen replacement therapy (ERT) in high risk cancer patients. Yale J Biol Med 64:607–626, 1991.
41. Jacquemier JD, Hassoun J, Torrente M, et al: Distribution of estrogen and progesterone receptors in healthy tissue adjacent to breast lesions at various stages—immunohistochemical study of 107 cases. Breast Cancer Res Treat 15:109–117, 1990.
42. King RM, Welch JS, Martin JK Jr, et al: Carcinoma of the breast associated with pregnancy. Surg Gynecol Obstet 150:119–128, 1985.
43. Kronenberg F: Hot flashes. In Lobo RA (ed): Treatment of the Postmenopausal Woman: Basic and Clinical Aspects. New York, Raven Press, 1994, pp 97–117.
44. Kumar V, Green S, Stack G: Functional domains of the human estrogen receptor. Cell 51:941–951, 1987.
45. Landau CL, Cyr MG, Moulton AW: The Complete Book of Menopause: Every Woman's Guide to Good Health. New York, GP Putnam's & Sons, 1994.
46. Lane HU: The World Almanac and Book of Facts: 1987. New York, Pharos Books, 1987.
47. Law ML, Kao FT, Wei Q, et al: The progesterone receptor maps to chromosome band 11q13, the site of mammary oncogene int-2. Proc Natl Acad Sci USA 84:2877–2881, 1987.
48. Liberman UA, Weiss SR, Broll J, et al: Effect of oral alendronate on bone mineral density and the incidence of fractures in postmenopausal osteoporosis. N Engl J Med 333:1437–1443, 1995.
49. Lobo RA: Benefits and risks of estrogen replacement therapy. Am J Obstet Gynecol 173:982–989, 1995.
50. Loprinzi CL, Michalar JC, Quella SK, et al: Megestrol acetate for the prevention of hot flashes. N Engl J Med 331:347–352, 1994.
51. Lubin F, Ruder AM, Wax Y, et al: Overweight and changes in weight throughout adult life in breast cancer etiology. Am J Epidemiol 122:579–588, 1985.
52. Marchant DJ: Estrogen replacement therapy after breast cancer. Cancer 55:2169–2176, 1993.
53. Matthews PN, Millis RR, Hayward JL: Breast cancer in women who have taken contraceptive steroids. BMJ 282:774–776, 1981.
54. Nachtigall LE: Enhancing patient compliance with hormone replacement therapy at menopause. Obstet Gynecol 75:77S–80S, 1990.
55. Nease RF, Ross JM: The decision to enter a randomized trial of tamoxifen for the prevention of breast cancer in healthy women: An analysis of the tradeoffs. Am J Med 99:180–189, 1995.
56. New drugs for osteoporosis. Med Lett Drugs Ther 38:1–3, 1996.
57. Paganini-Hill A: The benefits of estrogen replacement therapy on oral health: The Leisure World Cohort. Arch Intern Med 155:2325–2329, 1995.
58. Paganini-Hill A, Henderson VW: Estrogen deficiency and risk of Alzheimer's disease in women. Am J Epidemiol 140:256–261, 1994.
59. Powles TJ: Tamoxifen and oestrogen replacement. Lancet 336:48, 1990.
60. Powles TJ, Hickish T, Casey S, et al: Hormone replacement after breast cancer. Lancet 342:60–61, 1993.
61. Pritchard KI, Sawka CA: Menopausal estrogen replacement therapy in women with breast cancer. Cancer 75:1–3, 1995.
62. Ravnikar VA: Compliance with hormone therapy. Am J Obstet Gynecol 156:1332–1334, 1987.
63. Riberio G, Jones DA, Jones M: Carcinoma of the breast associated with pregnancy. Br J Surg, 73:607–609, 1986.
64. Riggs BL, Melton LJ III: The prevention and treatment of osteoporosis. N Engl J Med 327:620–627, 1992.
65. Rohan TE, McMichael AJ: Non-contraceptive exogenous oestrogen therapy and breast cancer. Med J Aust 148:217–221, 1988.
66. Rosenberg L: Hormone replacement therapy: The need for reconsideration. Am J Public Health 85:1670–1673, 1993.
67. Ross RK, Bernstein L: Influence of sex hormones on breast cancer risk and mortality. In Lobo RA (ed): Treatment of the Postmenopausal Woman: Basic and Clinical Aspects. New York, Raven Press, 1994, pp 339–347.
68. Ross RK, Paginini-Hill A, Gerkins VR, et al: A case-controlled study of menopausal estrogen therapy and breast cancer. JAMA 243:1635–1639, 1980.
69. Rossouw JE, Finnegan LP, Harlan WR, et al: The evolution of the Women's Health Initiative: Prospectives from the NIH. J Am Med Women's Assoc 50:50–55, 1995.
70. Sands R, Boshoff C, Jones A, et al: Current opinion: Hormone replacement therapy after a diagnosis of breast cancer. Menopause: The Journal of the North American Menopause Society 2:73–80, 1995.
71. Sawka CA, Prtichard KR, Paterson AHG, et al: Role and mechanism of action of tamoxifen in premenopausal women with metastatic breast carcinoma. Cancer Res 46:3152–3156, 1986.
72. Schatzkin A, Jones DY, Hoover RN et al: Alcohol consumption and breast cancer in the epidemiologic follow-up study of the First National Health and Nutrition Examination Survey. N Engl J Med 316:1169–1173, 1987.
73. Shaffer M: Breast cancer linked to other gynecologic tumors. Medical Tribune March 23:10, 1995.
74. Sillero-Arenas M, Delgado-Rodriguez M, Rodrigues-Canteras R, et al: Menopausal hormone replacement therapy and breast cancer: A meta-analysis. Obstet Gynecol 78:286–294, 1992.
75. Sinclair HK, Bond CM, Taylor RJ: Hormone replacement therapy: A study of women's knowledge and attitudes. Br J Gen Prac 43:365–370, 1993.
76. Spencer JD, Millis RR, Hayward JL: Contraceptive steroids and breast cancer. BMJ 1:1024–1026, 1978.

77. Speroff L: The menopause: A signal for the future. *In* Lobo RA (ed): Treatment of the Postmenopausal Women: Basic and Clinical Aspects. New York, Raven Press, 1994, pp 1–8.

78. Spicer DV, Pike MC: Sex steroids and breast cancer prevention. Monogr Natl Cancer Inst 16:139–147, 1994.

79. Stanford JL, Weiss NS, Voigt LF, et al: Combined estrogen and progestin hormone replacement therapy in relation to risk of breast cancer in middle-aged women. JAMA 274:137–142, 1995.

80. Steinberg KK, Thacker SB, Smith SJ, et al: A meta-analysis of the effect of estrogen replacement therapy on the risk of breast cancer. JAMA 265:1885–1890, 1991.

81. Stoll BA: Hormone replacement in women treated for breast cancer. Eur J Clin Oncol 25:1909, 1989.

82. Toniolo PG, Levitz M, Zeleniuch-Jacquotte A, et al: A prospective study of endogenous estrogens and breast cancer in postmenopausal women. J Natl Cancer Inst 87:190–197, 1995.

83. Voherr H: Oral contraceptives and hormone replacement therapy: Are progestogens and progestins breast mitogens? Am J Obstet Gynecol 155:1140–1142, 1986.

84. Wenger NK: Introduction to Cardiovascular Health and Disease in Women. *In* Wenger NK, Speroff L, Packard B (eds): Proceedings of an N.H.L.B.I. Conference. Greenwich, LeJacq Communications, Inc., 1993, pp 1–2.

85. Wild RA: Estrogen effects on the vascular tree. Obstet Gynecol 87:27S–35S, 1996.

86. Wile AG, Opfellt RW, Margileth DA: Hormone replacement therapy in previously treated breast cancer patients. Am J Surg 165:372–375, 1993.

87. Willett WC, Browne ML, Bain C, et al: Relative weight and risk of breast cancer among premenopausal women. Am J Epidemiol 122:579–588, 1985.

88. Willett WC, Stampfer JM, Colditz GA, et al: Moderate alcohol consumption and the risk of breast cancer. N Engl J Med 316:1174–1179, 1987.

89. Wingo PA, Layde PM, Lee NC, et al: The risk of breast cancer in postmenopausal women who have used estrogen replacement therapy. JAMA 257:209–215, 1987.

90. Wren BG, Eden JA: Do progestogens reduce the risk of breast cancer? A review of the evidence. Menopause 3:4–12, 1996.

91. Writing Group for the PEPI Trial: The effects of estrogen or estrogen/progestin regimens on heart disease risk factors in postmenopausal women. JAMA 273:199–208, 1995.

92. Young RL, Kumar NS, Goldzicher JW: Management of menopause when estrogen cannot be used. Drugs 40:220–230, 1990.

CHAPTER 86
BREAST CANCER: NURSING MANAGEMENT ISSUES

Carol Reed Ash, Ed.D., R.N. /
Carmen S. Rodriguez, R.N., M.S.N., A.R.N.P., O.C.N.

The role of the nurse in the management of patients with breast cancer encompasses the provision of care to address specific needs that may arise during the process of diagnosis, treatment, or rehabilitation. This chapter includes an overview of breast cancer screening and early detection issues, nursing implications in association with breast cancer treatment options, and psychosocial issues commonly affecting the breast cancer patient.

SCREENING AND EARLY DETECTION ISSUES

Breast cancer remains the most common cancer among women in the United States and the second major cause of cancer death in women. It is estimated that 184,300 new cases of invasive breast cancer will be diagnosed in 1996, which may in part be related to an increased use of breast cancer screening methods, but may also be associated with the prevalence of breast cancer risk factors.[1] Established risk factors associated with the development of breast cancer[1] include increasing age, family history of breast cancer, a personal history of breast cancer, history of benign breast disease, and hormonal factors leading to prolonged exposure to endogenous estrogen (e.g., early age at menarche, late age at menopause, late age at first live birth) (see Chapter 17).

Early detection of breast cancer continues to be the goal of current screening methods. The major components of current screening recommendations include a breast self-examination (BSE) (Fig. 86–1), a clinical breast examination (CBE) performed by a trained health care professional, and a mammogram. Existing screening guidelines incorporate specifications by age group, including a monthly BSE and a CBE every 3 years for women 20 to 39 years; a monthly BSE, annual CBE, and a baseline mammogram by age 40 for women 40 to 49 years; and a monthly BSE, annual CBE, and annual mammography for women 50 years or older.[1]

Findings associated with the continuous development of molecular genetics have resulted in the ability to identify genetic mechanisms associated with the development of breast cancer. Cancer genes BRCA1 and BRCA2 have been identified in a small number of patients with breast cancers, offering hope for the development of a screening test for women who have high rates of breast cancer in their families.[2, 3] The role of other genetic conditions that may be associated with increased breast cancer risk for

specific individuals (e.g., Li-Fraumeni syndrome, Cowden's disease, Muir-Torre syndrome, Peutz-Jeghers syndrome, ataxia-telangiectasia) also continues to be evaluated[4] (see Chapter 19). As a result, these findings not only impact the medical approach used to identify breast cancer risk, diagnosis, and treatment, but also emphasize the need for health care practitioners to keep abreast of advances that may affect the traditional medical and nursing management for the breast cancer patient. As findings associated with breast cancer molecular genetics develop, they may result in new responsibilities associated with cancer risk assessment "counseling" and in the emergence of ethical issues associated with the provision of information and decision making about treatment alternatives.

Special Populations

Elderly

The lack of direct evidence associated with the efficacy of the screening mammography and the CBE or BSE in women 70 years or older has resulted in limited screening and prevention efforts for the elderly. Despite the association among breast cancer risk, increasing age, and rising breast cancer cases for women 60 to 79 years, with a slight decline in women 80 years or older, breast cancer screening efforts remain limited in this population.[1] Barriers to breast cancer screening include issues associated with the client, the health care provider, and the health care system (Fig. 86–2).[5] These barriers also contribute to the elderly woman's lack of access to breast cancer prevention, early detection, and treatment.

To provide some direction to health care practice associated with the needs of the elderly woman, the Forum on Breast Screening in Older Women made the following recommendations (also supported by the Surviving and Prevention Editorial Board of the National Cancer Institute).[6]

- Women 65 to 74 years: annual CBE, mammography at regular intervals of approximately 2 years
- Women 75 years and older with good general health and life expectancy: annual CBE, mammography at regular intervals of approximately 2 years
- Women 65 years and older: monthly BSE to identify clinical lesions

❧ LOOK FOR CHANGES

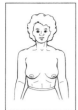

Hands at side.

Compare for symmetry.
Look for changes in:
- ❧ shape
- ❧ color

Check for:
- ❧ puckering
- ❧ dimpling
- ❧ skin changes
- ❧ nipple discharge

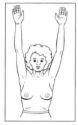

Hands over head.

Check front and side
view for:
- ❧ symmetry
- ❧ puckering
- ❧ dimpling

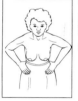

Hands on hips,
press down,
bend forward.

Check for:
- ❧ symmetry
- ❧ nipple direction
- ❧ general appearance

❧ FEEL FOR CHANGES

Lie down with a
towel under right
shoulder; raise
right arm above
the head.

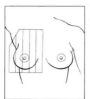

Examine area
from:
- ❧ underarm to
  lower bra line
- ❧ across to breast
  bone
- ❧ up to collar
  bone
- ❧ back to armpit

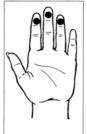

Use the pads of the
three middle fin-
gers of the left
hand.

Hold hand in
bowed position.

Move fingers in
dime-size circles.

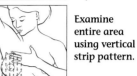

Use three levels
of pressure:
- ❧ light
- ❧ medium
- ❧ firm

Examine
entire area
using vertical
strip pattern.

Now check your left breast with your right
hand in the same way. If there are any
lumps, knots or changes, tell your doctor
right away.

> ❧ **AMERICAN CANCER SOCIETY**
> **GUIDELINES FOR EARLY DETECTION**
> **Breast Self-Exam:**
> • Once a month
> • Age 20 and over
> **Clinical Exam:**
> • See a doctor or nurse for a physical breast
>   exam
> • Age 20-40, every 3 years
> • Over 40, every year
> **Mammography:**
> • Have your first mammogram by age 40
> • Age 40-49, have a mammogram every 1
>   to 2 years
> • Age 50 and over, have a mammogram
>   every year

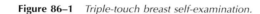

Figure 86–1   *Triple-touch breast self-examination.*

Male Population

Male breast cancer accounts for less than 1 percent
of the overall incidence and mortality for all cancers.[7]
Statistical evidence associated with breast cancer incidence indicates that men are at a lower risk of
developing breast cancer (approximately 1400 cases
in 1996).[6] The lower risk for the development of
breast cancer in males should not deter health care
practitioners in the provision of available information associated with breast cancer prevention to this
population.

Multicultural

Cultural values and beliefs may affect the
individual's perceived susceptibility to a disease.[8]
Health from the viewpoint of the individual must be
understood by the health care practitioner to prevent
misunderstandings and to facilitate the individual's
participation in health-related interventions. The development of culturally sensitive breast cancer
screening and educational programs may facilitate
the participation of those individuals who in many
instances are unable to benefit from or access resources directed to meet the needs of the general
population.

TREATMENT OPTIONS

Nursing Implications

The continuous development of research efforts that
influence treatment choices challenges breast cancer
patients to understand the information and their role
in the decision-making process. Advances in breast
cancer management have given patients the opportunity to take an active role in decision making associated with treatment options that have the potential
to eradicate the disease and result in less disfigurement. The nurse also has been challenged to remain
abreast of new approaches in the treatment of breast
cancer to facilitate the patient's understanding of
treatment options.

Diagnosis

Additional diagnostic evaluation may be recommended after the detection of a breast lump by
means of BSE, clinical examination, or a mammogram. Patients must understand that despite the
use of other diagnostic techniques (i.e., ultrasound)
histological confirmation to detect the presence of a
malignancy and establish a definitive diagnosis is

Client
lack of perception of breast cancer as a major
    health concern
association of cancer symptoms with the aging
    process
delays in seeking medical treatment or care
limited education about breast cancer screening
    tests
fears of findings/the effect of cumulative
    radioactivity/pain associated with procedure
embarrassment/modesty

Health Care System
cost associated with CBE and mammograms
inconsistency between practitioners about CBE
general lack of availability of promotional
    information regarding breast cancer screening
practitioners set an upper age limit for screening
    procedures based on biologic years and not
    on individual developmental status
limited outreach to the elderly woman

Health Care Provider
tendency to spend less time with the elderly
busy practices leading to not conducting
    clinical breast exam
provider's perception of projected life span
    and quality of life of the elderly

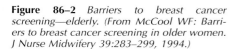

Figure 86–2 *Barriers to breast cancer screening—elderly. (From McCool WF: Barriers to breast cancer screening in older women. J Nurse Midwifery 39:283–299, 1994.)*

necessary. Available alternatives to determine such information must be explained as they apply to the individual's specific situation (e.g., fine needle aspiration, percutaneous needle biopsy, or incisional or excisional biopsy) (Table 86–1). Patients must also be educated about specific aspects associated with selected procedures, such as potential complications, anesthesia requirements, follow-up care after the

TABLE 86–1   DIAGNOSTIC PROCEDURES

Procedure	Description	Test Results
Fine needle aspiration	Simple and quick office procedure, used when an abnormality is known to be solid or to determine if the lump is a cyst.	Experienced cytopathologist to interpret smears; a risk for false negative results of up to 10 percent.
Stereotactic fine needle aspiration (SFNA); stereotactic core needle biopsy (SCNB)	Procedure takes place in a specially equipped room that contains breast-imaging equipment to assist with radiologic guidance while obtaining biopsy sample.	SFNA drawbacks: lack of widespread cytologic expertise, inability to diagnose invasion, low capacity to give benign diagnoses. SCNB drawbacks: problems in sampling women with small breasts, superficial lesions, and microcalcifications. Experienced cytopathologist required.
Incisional biopsy	Surgical procedure that involves the removal of a core of tissue for diagnostic examination.	May be used for metastatic disease, locally advanced breast cancer; provides information limited to core of tissue obtained; experienced cytopathologist required.
Excisional biopsy	Lump is removed along with a small amount of surrounding normal tissue.	Allows for complete evaluation of the tumor size and its histological characteristics; experienced cytopathologist required.

Data from Harris JR, Morrow M, Bonadionna G: Cancer of the breast. *In* DeVita VT, Hellman S, Rosenberg SA (eds): Cancer Principles and Practice of Oncology. Philadelphia, JB Lippincott, 1993, pp 1264–1332; and Schmidt RA: Stereotactic breast biopsy. CA Cancer J Clin 44:172–191, 1994.

procedure, and how to obtain information about test results.

Individuals facing a breast cancer diagnosis not only need to cope with the stress of a new diagnosis, but also need to make critical decisions about treatment options within a limited time frame. Patients may experience difficulties with attention capacity at a time in which their ability to direct attention or concentrate to learn about their diagnosis and treatment choices are crucial.[11]

Luker and colleagues,[12] in a study that examined the information needs of 150 women newly diagnosed with breast cancer in a large university teaching hospital, demonstrated that patients are able to identify their own information needs around the time of diagnosis. Topics such as the likelihood of cure, the spread of the disease, and treatment options were perceived as the most important areas to be addressed at the time of diagnosis. Other information, in order of descending priority, included information about the risk to the family, side effects of treatment, impact on family, self-care, effect on social life, and sexual attractiveness. These findings support the role of assessing the educational needs of patients and the need to tailor educational efforts to the individual's needs. The nurse may also assist in decreasing the risk of overloading the patient with more information than needed at a time in which multiple sources of information may be accessible.

Surgery

Regardless of the surgical treatment option selected, all breast cancer patients must be informed about the surgical procedure, expected cosmetic results, duration of hospital stay, postoperative care, potential complications, and psychosocial and rehabilitative issues as applicable.

Procedure

Candidates who meet criteria for local treatment options should be informed about the rationale associated with recommending breast-preserving surgery and adjuvant radiation therapy versus a modified radical mastectomy. Information that supports recommended treatment choices, such as factors considered and prognostic information associated with each surgical intervention, may help to clarify and facilitate the decision-making process. Criteria that lead to recommendation of a mastectomy include tumor- and breast-size ratios, an extensive intraductal carcinoma at margins, multiple tumors in different areas of the breast, local recurrence in a previously irradiated breast, and specific situations in which radiation therapy would be contraindicated (e.g., asthma, emphysema).[13] Patients should also be made aware of the survival rates associated with each breast treatment alternative. Local control interventions can provide the survival equivalent to total mastectomy and axillary dissection while preserving the breast.[14]

Wound Management

The patient's responsibility in wound management may incorporate monitoring of the surgical site and dressings for the presence of drainage or signs of infection or actually performing dressing changes. It is important to remember that the responsibility for managing wound care may vary between institutions and that wound management during the early postoperative period may be limited to the surgeon or nurse until the patient returns for a follow-up visit. Clear instructions related to the patient's role in performing dressing changes, frequency of change, technique, and signs and symptoms of infection should be discussed with the patient before discharge.

Other topics to be discussed in association with wound management requirements include pain control, level of activity for affected extremity, potential complications, and the need for medical follow-up. Nurses must take into consideration the time restrictions that may result from shorter hospital stays or changes in health care settings (i.e., surgery performed as an ambulatory service). The average hospital stay after breast cancer surgery is reported to be from 1 to 4.7 days, which consequently may result in less time to assist patients with their educational needs.[15–18]

Seroma Formation

Seroma formation is a common complication associated with breast cancer surgery. The use of flap tacking to the underlying chest wall and a closed suction drainage system have been reported as effective methods to minimize seroma formation.[19–21] The function of a closed continuous suction drain in the control of postoperative fluid accumulation should be explained to patients as applicable. The drain is inserted while in surgery and usually remains in place until a volume of drainage less than 30 ml is produced during a 24-hour period.[20, 21] Information regarding the frequency and how to empty the reservoir, how to measure and record the volume of drainage, and reportable signs and symptoms (e.g., fever, color of drainage) should be discussed with the patient. It is expected that the drainage will decrease as time evolves. Patients should be aware of the need to notify the nurse if fluid volume increases rather than decreases. Early discharge of patients with a closed continuous suction drain has been documented as an effective strategy in multiple studies.[15–18]

Lymphedema

Patients who have undergone a surgical resection of lymph nodes and those who have received radiation therapy to the lymphatic channels are at risk of developing lymphedema (see Chapter 51).[22] Lymphedema as a complication of breast cancer treatment has been reported from days to 30 years after surgery.[23] Patients should be made aware of clinical characteristics associated with the development of lymphedema and preventive measures to be followed as a lifelong practice. Clinical characteristics associated with the development of lymphedema include edema of affected limb, sensory changes, pain, discomfort and heaviness, mobility impairment, and skin changes, such as cellulitis, weeping, or hardening of skin.[24] Preventive measures that should be discussed with patients at risk include avoidance of physical, chemical, or thermal trauma; the need to assess skin for breakdown or changes on a daily basis; the importance of protecting the affected extremity by wearing appropriate clothing; and adherence to mobility and exercise guidelines as recommended.[24] Patients should also be instructed about the need to avoid blood pressure measurements or venipuncture on affected extremity. Written information related to the prevention and management of lymphedema should be made available to patients as applicable. Information booklets for professionals and consumers have been developed by various agencies, including the National Lymphedema Network and the American Cancer Society.

Pain Control

Information related to pharmacological and nonpharmacological pain control alternatives should be described to patients undergoing breast cancer surgery. While in the hospital setting, patients should be reassessed at frequent intervals (every 2 to 4 hours during the first 24-hour period) to determine if the pain management interventions are effective in controlling pain.[26] The nurse must also be cognizant of the need to discuss pain management strategies before the patient's discharge. Those experiencing pain upon discharge should be reassured that acute pain associated with the surgical intervention should improve as the healing process occurs.

Postmastectomy pain as a result of injury to the cutaneous branch of the intercostobrachial nerve may appear any time after surgery, but appears more commonly several weeks after surgery.[27] This type of pain is characterized by a burning numbness and dysesthetic squeezing sensation along the anterior chest wall, axilla, and medial upper arm. Therapies regularly used for the management of neuropathic pain have a role in the management of postmastectomy pain (e.g., tricyclic antidepressants, anticonvulsants, oral local anesthetics, transcutaneous electrical nerve stimulation units, and physical therapy). Lack of control of postmastectomy pain may lead to guarding of the affected extremity, which results in development of frozen shoulder, contractures, and reflex sympathetic dystrophy (RSD) syndrome.[27]

Motion Limitation

Patients may experience limited or painful shoulder motion as a result of breast cancer surgery. An exercise program directed to restore and maintain function of the involved extremity should be implemented as part of the rehabilitation process of these patients.

Recommendations for beginning exercise vary from 1 day after surgery to 1 week after surgery.[24, 25]

Lotze and colleagues[28] and Petrek and associates[29] evaluated the influence of early versus delayed initiation of shoulder mobilization on postoperative drainage in 57 women with a clinical stage I or II breast cancer. Patients were randomized to either early (postoperative day 2) or delayed (postoperative day 5) shoulder motion. Early versus delayed time of exercise initiation had no effect on total amount or duration of drainage. Based on the findings of Petrek and associates, some institutions begin their exercise program on the second postoperative day and continue it daily for the remaining hospitalization time.[29] A study of 144 patients who had axillary lymph node dissection explored the role of delayed shoulder exercises on wound drainage and shoulder function. Patients in Group 1 started active shoulder exercises 1 day postoperatively and patients in Group 2 started on the eighth postoperative day after 1 week of arm immobilization.[25] Although results of the study revealed less wound drainage volume (14 percent) in Group 2, this was not considered significant. The authors recommended a change in postoperative instructions to allow patients to mobilize the affected arm and shoulder as much as desired during the first week after surgery, and they recommended providing follow-up physiotherapy when a marked reduction in function was found 1 week after surgery.

Time schedules associated with the initiation of an exercise program after breast cancer surgery may vary between institutions. Clear instructions regarding appropriate timing, frequency, and type of exercises should be provided in verbal and written form. Common rehabilitative exercises recommended after breast cancer surgery are presented in Figures 86–3 to 86–6.

Breast Reconstruction

Women who have chosen a mastectomy as their primary cancer treatment have the option of breast reconstruction immediately after surgery or a delayed reconstruction. The progress associated with new techniques and the availability of well-trained experts have enhanced the opportunities for breast cancer patients in dealing with body image and the emotional sequelae resulting from breast surgery.

The selection and timing of breast reconstruction should be based on a careful evaluation of the patient's situation, incorporating factors such as stage of disease (early stage versus locally advanced disease), access to a reconstructive surgeon, the patient's motivation and desire for breast restoration, and type of procedure.[30–32]

The discussion of breast reconstruction options should be considered as an integral part of the education that breast cancer patients should receive. Patients should become aware of the most common procedures and techniques used for breast reconstruction (Table 86–2).

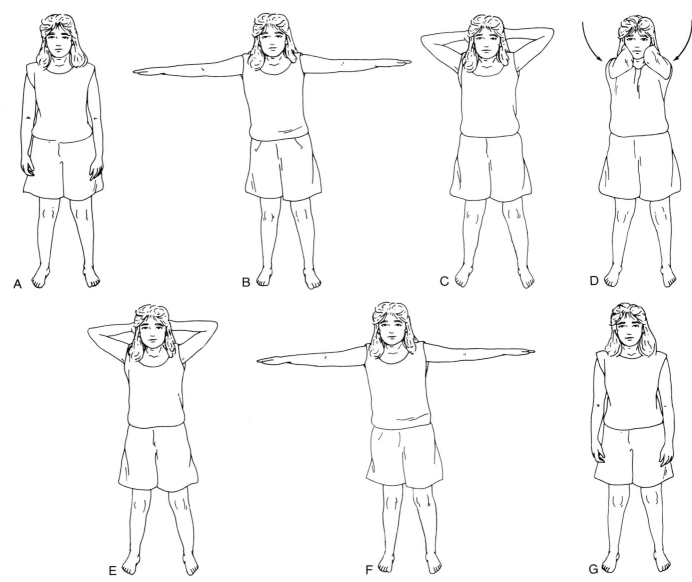

Figure 86–3 *Exercise 1: Elbow pull-in.* **A,** Stand facing straight ahead with feet 6 to 12 inches apart. **B,** Extend arms sideways to shoulder level. **C,** Bend elbows and clasp fingers at the back of neck. **D,** Pull elbows in toward each other until they touch. **E,** Return to position *C* with elbows bent. **F,** Unclasp fingers and extend arms sideways at shoulder level. *G,* Return to original position; rest and repeat.

Radiation Therapy

Radiation therapy (RT) after breast-preserving surgery is a significant component of breast cancer treatment to promote an increased rate of local control of cancer (see Chapters 60–65, 68, and 71). Patients undergoing RT as an adjuvant treatment after breast-preserving surgery should be educated about the process preceding the actual implementation of the treatment, including simulation and planning appointment, location of treatment area and permanent marks, and specifics of daily schedule. Information related to the type of RT, schedule guidelines, and necessary arrangements while undergoing RT (e.g., work schedule, housing arrangements) should be provided to patients before beginning of RT.

The patient should be informed about acute and long-term complications that may occur as a result of radiation treatments. Early complications that may be experienced by the patient include erythema, hyperpigmentation, dry and moist desquamation, and epilation.[32] Other acute complications may include intermittent pain in the treated area, chest wall, or axilla; breast edema; fatigue; and bone marrow suppression.[33] Although the management of irradiated skin may vary from one institution to another, general guidelines to be followed include avoidance of chemical, physical, or thermal skin irritation or further breakdown; infection prevention; and adherence to prescribed topical measures for the management of the skin (e.g., hydrocortisone, compresses with antibacterial agents).

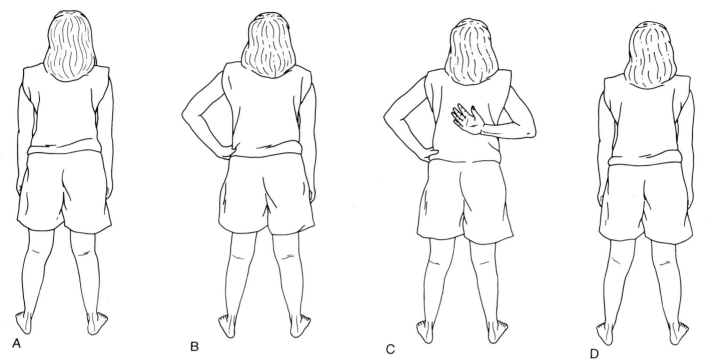

Figure 86–4 *Exercise 2: Scratcher.*   **A,** Stand facing straight ahead with feet 6 to 12 inches apart.   **B,** Place hand of unoperated side on your hip.   **C,** Bend elbow at operated arm, placing back of hand in the middle of back. Gradually work the hand up your back until your fingers reach the opposite shoulder blade.   **D,** Slowly lower your arm; rest and repeat.

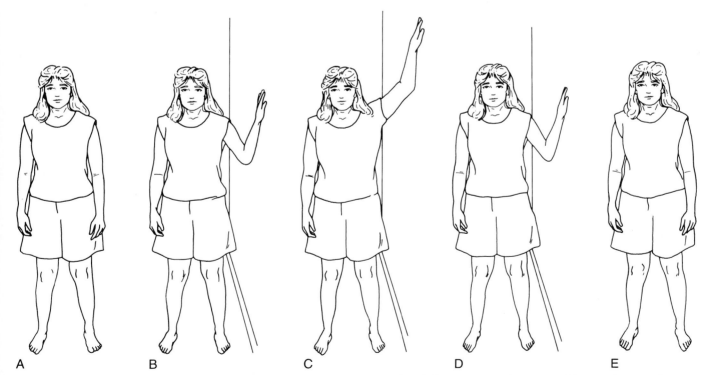

Figure 86–5 *Exercise 3: Hand wall climbing.*   **A,** Stand facing straight ahead with feet 6 to 12 inches apart with operative arm closest to wall.   **B,** Bend elbow and place palm against wall at shoulder level.   **C,** Walk hand up wall until incisional pulling or pain occurs. Mark the level so progress can be checked.   **D,** Slowly work hand down to shoulder level.   **E,** Return to original position; rest and repeat.

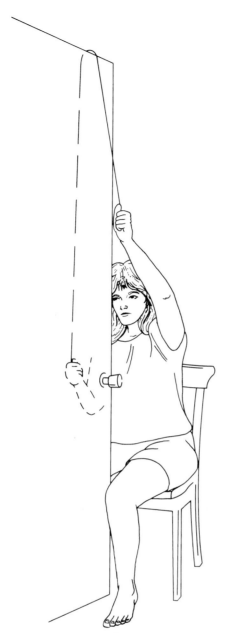

Figure 86–6   *Exercise 4: Door pulley. Equipment*: A 6-foot rope or 6 feet of bandage; a door and chair. *Procedure*: Place knots in the rope at each end and toss it over the door with the unaffected arm. Sit on armless chair with soles placed firmly on floor and door held closely between the legs. Hold the ends of the rope between the third and fourth fingers. Slowly pull the rope down with the unaffected arm, and raise the operative arm. Keep the raised arm close to the head and raise as far as is comfortable. Reverse the motion and raise the unaffected arm; rest and repeat.

Patients should also become aware of potential long-term complications that may arise as a result of RT and the need for ongoing monitoring after treatment completion. Long-term complications associated with RT for breast cancer may include rib fractures; radiation pneumonitis; swelling, firmness, or shrinkage of the breast; brachial plexopathy; secondary sarcomas; and soft tissue fibrosis.[34, 35] Although

modern RT techniques expose smaller volumes of the heart to radiation doses, the potential for cardiac toxicity exists, and it may be compounded by the interaction of certain chemotherapy agents (i.e., anthracyclines) when used concurrently.[36]

Systemic Treatment

Patients for whom adjuvant systemic therapy is integrated in the treatment plan should be clear about its role in the eradication of microscopic disease, treatment options, rationale for treatment selection and duration, and potential acute and long-term effects. The nurse must keep abreast of information associated with systemic treatment options, such as conventional-dose adjuvant chemotherapy, dose-intensive chemotherapy with hematopoietic support, and hormonal therapy.

Conventional Chemotherapy

Chemotherapy used for breast cancer is based on the combination of alkylating agents, antimetabolites, and anthracycline antibiotics (see Chapters 66 and 72).[37] Chemotherapy regimens commonly used as adjuvant therapy for breast cancer include cyclophosphamide, methotrexate, and fluorouracil (CMF); cyclophosphamide, doxorubicin, and fluorouracil (CAF); and cyclophosphamide, mitoxantrone, and fluorouracil (CNF). The development of drugs such as the taxanes and ongoing studies to determine their role and efficacy in the management of breast cancer have resulted in additional treatment alternatives for the patient with advanced disease. The side effects and nursing management issues associated with the use of specific cytotoxic agents incorporated in breast cancer regimens are outlined on Table 86–3.

Despite advances in the management of symptomatology associated with the administration of chemotherapeutic agents, patients still experience significant distress as a result of treatment side effects. Common symptoms experienced by breast cancer patients undergoing chemotherapy include nausea and vomiting, mucositis, alopecia, menopausal symptoms, weight gain and fatigue.[33]

Nausea and Vomiting. Nausea, vomiting, and retching are described as three of the most disruptive and distressing side effects of antineoplastic therapy.[38] The incidence and severity of chemotherapy-induced emesis is affected by the following factors: emetogenic potential of the drug, dose administered, route of administration, schedule, infusion rate, patient characteristics, and combination of drugs.[39] Nausea and vomiting may be characterized by an acute (within 24 hours of administration), delayed (after 24 hours of chemotherapy administration), or anticipatory (prior to receiving the treatment) pattern. Chemotherapy agents commonly used to treat breast cancer have emetogenic potential at various levels and diverse patterns. Agents such as cyclophosphamide and doxorubicin are associated with

TABLE 86–2   BREAST RECONSTRUCTION OPTIONS

Procedure	Type	Common Problems	Implications for Nursing Practice and Patient Education
Implants	Silicone gel–filled; saline-filled	Capsular contracture (fibrous scar that forms around implant). May interfere with mammograms. Potential to rupture, leak or displace.	Surgical intervention to release or remove scar tissue may be necessary for minor contractures. Patient should be educated about the importance of notifying mammographer of the presence of implants; special views may be ordered. Saline leak is harmlessly absorbed by the body; can be exchanged for another implant. Silicone leak has the potential for long-term sequelae associated with the development of autoimmune diseases and cancer.
Musculocutaneous flaps (autologous)	Transverse rectus abdominis musculocutaneous (TRAM) flap	Associated with more blood loss than reconstruction with implants.	Transfusion may be necessary.
	Latissimus dorsi musculocutaneous flap	Operation is complex and requires the skill of a reconstructive surgeon experienced in the technique.	Patient should be educated about the magnitude of the surgery and their role in the rehabilitative process.
	Gluteus maximus musculocutaneous flap with microsurgical transfer	Potential for delayed healing, partial or total flap failure, infection, venous clots, fluid accumulation, and hematoma. Hospitalization of 4 to 7 days.	Patient should be educated about possible complications and reportable signs and symptoms. May require a lengthier hospital stay and recovery time.

Data from Bostwick J III: Breast reconstruction following mastectomy. CA J Nurs Clin 45:289–304, 1995.

a high emetic potential and a delayed emetogenic pattern.[39]

Antiemetic drugs commonly used in the management of chemotherapy-induced nausea and vomiting include serotonin antagonists (5HT$_3$), phenothiazines, butyrophenones, benzamides, benzodiazepines, corticosteroids, cannabinoids, and antihistamines.[38] These drugs may be used as single agents or in combination regimens that have been proved effective in the control of nausea and vomiting. Drug combination regimens are available that take into consideration factors such as the antiemetic potential of the chemotherapy regimen used, physiological mechanism associated with the development of nausea and vomiting, and the drug's properties in the prevention and control of nausea and vomiting. The use of serotonin antagonists (i.e., granisetron and ondansetron) is associated with the absence of side effects such as sedation and extrapyramidal symptoms. As a result, the serotonin antagonists have become first-line agents for the control of chemotherapy-associated nausea and vomiting.

Preparing the breast cancer patient to effectively manage nausea and vomiting while at home or when returning to the demands of daily living (e.g., return to work or school) must not be underestimated. Preparation should also incorporate an assessment re-

garding financial limitations that may hinder the patient's ability to obtain the prescribed antiemetic regimen. The importance in understanding potential complications that may emerge as a result of uncontrolled nausea and vomiting must also be discussed with the patient.

The clinical expertise of other health care team members, such as the pharmacist and the dietitian, should be incorporated in the management of chemotherapy-associated nausea and vomiting before or early in the treatment phase. The incorporation of nonpharmacological interventions, such as relaxation techniques, music therapy, and distraction, in addition to prescribed pharmacological interventions may also assist to control the stress associated with emesis-inducive cancer treatment.

Mucositis. Cytotoxic drugs incorporated in the treatment of breast cancer, such as methotrexate, the antibiotic tumor agents, and fluorouracil, are associated with the development of mucositis.[39] Factors that may influence the severity of stomatitis include dose and schedule of drugs, combination drug therapy, and the presence of renal or hepatic dysfunction.

The development of mucositis may result in the inability to eat and swallow, difficulty to communicate, a higher risk of developing oral mucosa infec-

TABLE 86–3 COMMON CYTOTOXIC AGENTS FOR BREAST CANCER TREATMENT

Agent	Common Side Effects	Nursing Management Issues
Doxorubicin (Adriamycin)	Alopecia, n&v, bone marrow suppression, stomatitis, cardiac toxicity (acute and long term), potential for extravasation skin injury, radiation recall reaction	Implement educational efforts associated with acute signs and symptoms, cytotoxic safety guidelines, prevention of infection as a result of bone marrow suppression, n&v management, oral care protocol, alternatives to manage hair loss, potential long-term complications and the need for ongoing monitoring. Avoid extravasation. Monitor IV/CV access patency and for signs of extravasation. Monitor cumulative dose.
Cyclophosphamide	N&V; alopecia, bone marrow suppression, gonadal failure, hemorrhagic cystitis, secondary malignancies, high dose has potential for cardiac toxicity	Encourage schedule of oral cyclophosphamide early in the morning with adequate hydration during the day. Avoid fast IV administration to control symptoms of nasal congestion. Promote adequate hydration (IV/PO). Instruct patient regarding the risk for delayed n&v and measures to be implemented, signs and symptoms associated with hemorrhagic cystitis, infection prevention measures, review potential long-term complications and provide reinforcement as necessary.
5-Fluorouracil	Bone marrow suppression, GI mucosa effects (stomatitis, diarrhea), dermatological toxicity (dermatitis, hyperpigmentation, nail changes)	Provide information related to oral care protocol, importance in maintaining adequate hydration, reportable signs and symptoms, long-term effects as a result of dermatological toxicity, need to avoid sun exposure and to practice sun protective behaviors.
Methotrexate	Dose-related bone marrow suppression, mild GI mucosa effects, renal/hepatic dysfunction, dermatological toxicity	Assess oral mucosa and implement oral care protocol as per institutional guidelines. Instruct patient to avoid sun exposure and to practice sun protective behaviors. High dose: assess for signs and symptoms of renal/liver dysfunction, follow guidelines for urine alkalinization and hydration, administer leucovorin rescue as ordered
Mitoxantrone	Bone marrow suppression, GI symptoms (n&v, anorexia), phlebitis, discoloration of the vein and urine	Implement educational interventions, including infection prevention measures, urine and vein discoloration, GI symptoms management, signs and symptoms associated with phlebitis or extravasation. Avoid drug extravasation. Monitor for presence of phlebitis.
Paclitaxel	Hypersensitivity reactions, bone marrow suppression, cardiovascular side effects, peripheral neuropathy, alopecia	Implement protocol for the prevention and management of hypersensitivity reactions. Monitor for the development of syncope, rhythm abnormalities, blood pressure changes. Follow administration guidelines as per institutional standards.
Vinblastine	Bone marrow suppression, GI mucosa effects (mucositis, n&v), neurotoxicities, acute respiratory complications (bronchospasm, interstitial pulmonary infiltrates), dermatological toxicity (alopecia, photosensitivity), potential for extravasation skin injury	Implement educational efforts associated with acute signs and symptoms, prevention of infection as a result of bone marrow suppression, n&v management, oral care protocol, alternatives to manage hair loss. Assess for the presence of neurotoxicities: bowel function, peripheral nerves dysfunction. Avoid extravasation. Monitor IV/CV access patency and for signs of extravasation.

N&V = Nausea and vomiting; IV = intravenous; CV = central venous; PO = by mouth; GI = gastrointestinal.
Data from Kardinal CG: Chemotherapy of breast cancer. *In* Perry MC (ed): The Chemotherapy Sourcebook. Batimore, Williams & Wilkins, 1993, pp 289, 305, 307, 324–328, 349, 366, 948–988.

tion, bleeding, and pain. Severe mucositis may also result in interruption of the chemotherapy schedule. Management and prevention of chemotherapy-associated mucositis may vary between institutions, but they are generally directed to maintain a clean mucosa, prevent/control the development of complications such as infection and bleeding, and promote optimal oral intake to prevent nutritional imbalances. Recommendations related to oral complica-

tions associated with cancer therapy emphasize the need for an oral examination before the initiation of cancer treatment, treating pre-existing oral disease before therapy initiation, diagnosing and treating infections of the oral mucosa, and maintaining appropriate oral care.[40]

The nursing assessment of the oral mucosa should be performed before, during, and after the initiation of chemotherapy treatments. The assessment of the oral mucosa should be focused on the identification of changes in the oral cavity, ability to speak, swallow and eat, and the presence of pain or infection. Ambulatory care patients or those treated at home should be instructed about signs and symptoms indicative of mucositis, oral care guidelines to be followed during and after the administration of chemotherapy, how to maintain appropriate nutrition, and reportable signs and symptoms.

Fatigue. Fatigue resulting from cancer treatment has been described based on the disease and cancer treatment effects on the patient. Subjective reports associated with the presence of fatigue may incorporate multiple descriptions, including signs and symptoms such as tiredness, weakness, lack of energy, exhaustion, lethargy, depression, inability to concentrate, malaise, asthenia, boredom, sleepiness, lack of motivation, and decreased mental status.[41] Variations in fatigue pattern have been found in association with factors such as the presence of pathophysiological changes as a result of treatment (e.g., electrolyte imbalances and pancytopenia), the effects of antiemetics, and the psychological impact of the diagnosis and treatment.[42] In a study of 86 breast cancer patients receiving chemotherapy treatment with three commonly used regimens (CMF, CAF, and CNF), fatigue was one of the most frequently reported side effects of all three treatment regimens at four data collection times.[42]

Research associated with nursing interventions to manage cancer-related fatigue, although limited, has demonstrated the potential roles of education, exercise, and attention-restoring activities.[43, 44]

Alopecia. Hair loss as a result of chemotherapy administration may be characterized by partial or total absence of hair or thinning of hair (scalp, pubic area, axillary, or facial). Chemotherapy-induced hair loss is temporary, usually occurring within 2 to 3 weeks after treatment with multiple agents. The agents commonly used in the treatment of breast cancer patients are associated with the development of alopecia.

Patients at risk of experiencing alopecia should be instructed about alternative methods to deal with this symptom while hair regrowth occurs. Information related to options such as the use of a wig, hat, or scarf should be made available before the initiation of chemotherapy. Assisting patients to anticipate the hair loss experience offers them the option of exploring available alternatives before experiencing the problem.

Information related to the controversies surrounding the use of hair preservation techniques (i.e., scalp hypothermia) should also be discussed with the patient. A referral to community groups such as the "Look Good Feel Good" program (American Cancer Society) should be considered for those patients who may benefit from group dynamics. As patients progress through their treatment schedule, their ability to cope with appearance and self-esteem changes should be assessed.

Dose-Intensive Chemotherapy

Oncology nurses may be faced with the challenge of managing patients with metastatic disease or high-risk primary breast cancer undergoing the administration of high-dose chemotherapy with hematocellular support (e.g., autologous bone marrow transplant or peripheral blood progenitor cell transplant) (see Chapter 72). These patients will not only demand high levels of skill and knowledge associated with symptom management but will also require intense efforts to minimize the potential for complications in comparison with the patient undergoing standard therapy.

Similar to what other nurses are experiencing as a result of changes in the health care environment, oncology nurses caring for breast cancer patients undergoing high-dose chemotherapy with hematocellular support are faced with the need to provide the same quality of care in an environment surrounded by limited admission days, cost containment, and the need to provide expeditious, efficient, and safe care. Innovative methods such as the development of nursing care guidelines (i.e., clinical pathways) have the potential to facilitate the management of these patients taking into consideration the factors listed above. The use of a clinical pathway facilitates the incorporation of critical elements to be considered in the management of a specific population with a certain level of structure by which necessary health care interventions should be accomplished within a reasonable time frame. Figures 86–7 and 86–8 illustrate a clinical pathway developed for a breast cancer patient undergoing a bone marrow transplant for uncomplicated breast cancer. General guidelines related to the most critical elements to be considered in the management of this population, including proposed time frames, are outlined.

Hormonal Therapy

The use of hormonal therapy (i.e., tamoxifen) as a systemic option for the adjuvant treatment of breast cancer as well as a chemopreventive agent has offered a new set of challenges for those involved in the management of the breast cancer patient (see Chapters 18 and 73). Toxicities associated with the use of tamoxifen and its potential to promote the development of complications such as endometrial carcinoma are some of the issues faced by the breast cancer patient.

Patients who may benefit from tamoxifen treatment should be made aware of side effects associated with its use and the importance in adhering to follow-up guidelines established by health care members involved in their management. The most common side effects associated with the use of tamoxifen include hot flashes, mild nausea, vaginal bleeding or discharge, fluid retention, and irregular menses.[45] Other toxicities that have been reported in association with tamoxifen therapy include thromboembolic disease and ocular effects.

Patients undergoing treatment with tamoxifen

SHANDS HOSPITAL
at the University of Florida

ADDRESSOGRAPH

The Clinical Pathway is a general guideline. Patient care continues to require individualization based on patient needs and response.

Patient's Name: MR#

CLINICAL PATHWAY

TITLE: BONE MARROW TRANSPLANT FOR UNCOMPLICATED BREAST CANCER (Pre-Admission through Day 6)
SERVICE: MEDICINE HEMATOLOGY/ONCOLOGY

ALLERGIES:____

CARE ELEMENT	Pre-admission with BMTU Coordinators	Day 1 Admission (-8)	Day 2 to Day 6 (-7 to -3)	Day 7 (-2)
CARE UNIT	BMTU	BMTU	BMTU	BMTU
CONSULTS	• Psychology • Social services	• PT • Social services • +/- Pastoral care	• PT • Social services • +/- Pastoral care	• PT • Social services • +/- Pastoral care
TESTS/LABS	• 24 hr urine • Spirometry only • MUGA scan • CBC with diff, renal battery, liver battery, hepatitis panel, HSV, EBV, VZV, HIV • Bone marrow biopsy • Bone marrow harvest • Stem cell collection • Bone Scan • Chest, Abdominal CT • Head MRI • UA	• Chemo catheter placement • EKG • CXR • CBC, renal battery, liver battery, PT/PTT	• CBC/diff, Renal qd • liver MWF • Initial fever spike: pan culture and CXR • Blood cultures qd for temp ≥38.5 or 38.0 x 3 in 24 hrs.	• CBC/diff, Renal qd • liver MWF • Initial fever spike: pan culture and CXR • Blood cultures qd for temp ≥38.5 or 38.0 x 3 in 24 hrs.
ACTIVITY		• LAF room • Up ad lib • Strict handwashing • Compromised host precautions • Chemo precautions	• LAF room • Up ad lib • Strict handwashing • Compromised host precautions • Chemo precautions • Thrombocytopenia precautions if platelets < 50,000	• LAF room • Up ad lib • Strict handwashing • Compromised host precautions • Chemo precautions • Thrombocytopenia precautions if platelets < 50,000
ASSESSMENTS		• Physical exam with special attention to: skin, mucous membranes, perirectal area, IV puncture sites, surgical wounds, respiratory system, GI/GU, neuro status, hydration status • VS qs • Routine nursing assessment q shift • Weight/height/m² • Check urine void for heme after CTX started • ABT	• Physical exam with special attention to: skin, mucous membranes, perirectal area, IV puncture sites, surgical wounds, respiratory system, GI/GU, neuro status, hydration status, po intake • VS qs • Routine nursing assessment q shift • Weight bid • Check urine and stool for heme	• Physical exam with special attention to: skin, mucous membranes, perirectal area, IV puncture sites, surgical wounds, respiratory system, GI/GU, neuro status, hydration status, po intake • VS qs • Routine nursing assessment q shift • Weight bid • Check urine and stool for heme
TREATMENTS		• Mouth care protocol • Peri care • CVL dressing change • Change adapter caps to click lock system • Label chemo catheter lines	• Mouth care protocol • Peri care • Strict I&O • Blood product support prn • CVL dressing change qd if bleeding or q 72/ adapter change q 72	• Mouth care protocol • Peri care • Strict I&O • Blood product support prn • CVL dressing/adapter change q 72

Figure 86–7 *Clinical pathway. Bone marrow transplant for complicated breast cancer (preadmission through day 6). Day 2. ANC, absolute neutrophil count; bid, twice per day; BMTU, bone marrow transplant unit; CBC, complete blood count; CT, computed tomography; CTX, cytoxan; CVL, central venous line; CXR, chest x-ray study; EBV, Epstein-Barr virus; EKG, electrocardiogram; GCSF, granulocyte colony–stimulating factor; GI/GU, gastrointestinal/genitourinary; HIV, human immunodeficiency virus; HSV, herpes simplex virus; I & O, intake and output; IV, intravenous; LAF, laminar air flow; MRI, magnetic resonance imaging; MUGA, multiple-gated acquisition; MWF, Monday, Wednesday and Friday; n/v, nausea and vomiting; prn, as necessary; PT, physical therapist; PT/PTT, prothrombin time and partial prothrombin time; qs, every shift; q, every; UA, urinalysis; vs, vital signs; VZV, varicella zoster virus.*

CARE ELEMENT	Pre-admission with BMTU Coordinators	Day 1 Admission (-8)	Day 2 to Day 6 (-7 to -3)	Day 7 (-2)
MEDICATION		• CTX 750 mg/m² q 12 hr • Thiotepa 62.5 mg/m² q 12 hr • Carboplatin 100mg/m² q 12 hr • Kytril 2mg/kg IV qd • Decadron 8 mg iv qd	• CTX 750 mg/m² q 12 hr • Thiotepa 62.5 mg/m² q 12 hr • Carboplatin 100mg/m² q 12 hr • Hyperhydration * • Kytril 2 mg/kg IV qd • Decadron 8 mg iv qd	• Kytril 2 mg/kg IV qd • Decadron 8 mg iv qd
PAIN/SYMPTOM CONTROL		• Tylenol 650 mg/po prn pain d/c with neutropenia • Tylenol 650 mg/po prn temp ≥38.5	• Tylenol 650 mg/po prn pain d/c with neutropenia • Tylenol 650 mg/po prn temp ≥38.5 • Urokinase lines prn • Phenergan 25 mg iv for n/v prn or Compazine 10 mg IV q4h prn • Ativan 1-2 mg iv (n/v mgmt prn) • Fluid mgmt with Lasix prn	• Tylenol 650 mg/po prn pain d/c with neutropenia • Tylenol 650 mg/po prn temp ≥38.5 • Urokinase lines prn • Phenergan 25 mg iv for n/v prn or Compazine 10 mg IV q4h prn • Ativan 1-2 mg iv (n/v mgmt prn) • Fluid mgmt with Lasix prn
NUTRITION		•Regular diet except for raw shell fish and sushi	•Regular diet except for raw shell fish and sushi • Oral dietary supplements	•Regular diet except for raw shell fish and sushi • Oral dietary supplements
D/C PLANNING/ TEACHING	• Orientation to BMTU by Transplant Coordinators	• BMTU teaching and orientation (patient/family) • Chemo precautions (patient/family)	• BMTU teaching (patient/family) • Chemo precautions (patient/family)	• BMTU teaching (patient/family) • Chemo precautions (patient/family)

*12 hr prior to chemo and 24 hr p̄ chemo

Anita Stephen, RN, BSN
Nurse Practice Coordinator-BMTU

Kathy Conner, RN, MN, OCN
Coordinated Care Manager

Department of Nursing and Patient Services
Shands Hospital at the University of Florida

Figure 86–7   *See legend on opposite page*

The Clinical Pathway is a general guideline.   Patient care continues to require individualization based on patient needs and response.

ADDRESSOGRAPH

CLINICAL PATHWAY
TITLE: **BONE MARROW TRANSPLANT FOR UNCOMPLICATED**
         BREAST CANCER (Day 6 through Day 21)
SERVICE: MEDICINE HEMATOLOGY/ONCOLOGY

ALLERGIES:_____

Patient's Name: MR#:

CARE ELEMENT	Day 8 (-1)	Day 9 (0) Transplant Day	Day 10 to Day 21 (+1 to + 12)	Day 22 (+13) Anticipated discharge date from unit
CARE UNIT	BMTU	BMTU	BMTU	BMTU
CONSULTS	• PT • Social services • +/- Pastoral care	• PT • Social services • +/- Pastoral care	• PT • Social services • +/- Pastoral care	• Social services
TESTS/LABS	• CBC/diff, Renal qd • liver MWF • Initial fever spike: pan culture and CXR • Blood cultures qd for temp ≥38.5 or 38.0 x 3 in 24 hrs	• CBC/diff, Renal qd • liver MWF • Initial fever spike: pan culture and CXR • Blood cultures qd for temp ≥38.5 or 38.0 x 3 in 24 hrs	• CBC/diff, Renal qd • liver MWF • Initial fever spike: pan culture and CXR • Blood cultures qd for temp ≥38.5 or 38.0 x 3 in 24 hrs	• CBC/diff, Renal qd • liver MWF
ACTIVITY	• LAF room • Up ad lib • Strict handwashing • Compromised host precautions • Thrombocytopenia precautions if platelets < 50,000	• LAF room • Up ad lib • Strict handwashing • Compromised host precautions • Thrombocytopenia precautions if platelets < 50,000	• LAF room • Up ad lib • Strict handwashing • Compromised host precautions • Thrombocytopenia precautions if platelets < 50,000	• LAF room • Up ad lib • Strict handwashing • Compromised host precautions • Thrombocytopenia precautions if platelets < 50,000
ASSESSMENTS	• Physical exam with special attention to: skin, mucous membranes, perirectal area, IV puncture sites, surgical wounds, respiratory system, GI/GU, neuro status, hydration status, po intake • VS qs • Routine nursing assessment q shift • Weight bid • Check urine and stool for heme	• Physical exam with special attention to: skin, mucous membranes, perirectal area, IV puncture sites, surgical wounds, respiratory system, GI/GU, neuro status, hydration status, po intake • VS q4 • Routine nursing assessment q shift • Weight bid • Check urine and stool for heme	• Physical exam with special attention to: skin, mucous membranes, perirectal area, IV puncture sites, surgical wounds, respiratory system, GI/GU, neuro status, hydration status, po intake • VS q4 • Routine nursing assessment q shift • Weight bid • Check urine and stool for heme	• Physical exam with special attention to: skin, mucous membranes, perirectal area, IV puncture sites, surgical wounds, respiratory system, GI/GU, neuro status, hydration status, po intake • VS q4 • Routine nursing assessment q shift • Weight qd • Check urine and stool for heme
TREATMENTS	• Mouth care protocol • Peri care • Strict I&O • Blood product support prn • CVL dressing/adapter change q 72	• Mouth care protocol • Peri care • Strict I&O • Blood product support prn • CVL dressing/adaptor change q 72 • Bone marrow transplant: Transplant orders written MD/PA on BMTU Emergency transplant pack in room Place patient on heart monitor and pulse oximetry VS q5 x 4, then q15 till end of transplant	• Mouth care protocol • Peri care • Strict I&O • Blood product support prn • CVL dressing/adapter change q 72	• Mouth care protocol • Peri care • Strict I&O • Blood product support prn • CVL dressing/adapter change q 72

Figure 86–8   *Bone marrow transplant for uncomplicated breast cancer (Day 6 through Day 21). ANC, absolute neutrophil count; bid, twice per day; BMTU, bone marrow transplant unit; CBC, complete blood count; CT, computed tomography; CTX, cytoxan; CVL, central venous line; CXR, chest x-ray study; EBV, Epstein-Barr virus; EKG, electrocardiogram; GCSF, granulocyte colony–stimulating factor; GI/GU, gastrointestinal/genitourinary; HIV, human immunodeficiency virus; HSV, herpes simplex virus; I & O, intake and output; IV, intravenous; LAF, laminar air flow; MRI, magnetic resonance imaging; MUGA, multiple-gated acquisition; MWF, Monday, Wednesday and Friday; n/v, nausea and vomiting; prn, as necessary; PT, physical therapist; PT/PTT, prothrombin time and partial prothrombin time; qs, every shift; q, every; UA, urinalysis; vs, vital signs; VZV, varicella zoster virus.*

CARE ELEMENT	Day 8 (-1)	Day 9 (0) Transplant Day	Day 10 to Day 21 (+1 to + 12)	Day 22 (+13) Anticipated discharge date from unit
MEDICATION	• Acyclovir if HSV+ -400 mg po tid or -125 mg/m² IV q8	• Fluconzole 100 mg qd po/iv • Acyclovir if HSV+ -400 mg po tid or -125 mg/m² IV q8 • Transplant pre-med: -Benadryl 25 mg iv -Tylenol 650 mg po	• Fluconzole 100 mg qd po/iv • Acyclovir if HSV+ -400 mg po tid or -125 mg/m² IV q8 • GCSF 5 mg/kg SQ iv qd unless weight >75 kg on day +1 • If temp > 38.5 or 38 x3 in 24 hours, then initiate antibiotics within one hour of fever spike If culture is positive consider narrowing antibiotic coverage	• GCSF 5 mg/kg SQ iv qd unless weight >75 kg on day +1 and until ANC ≥1500 X 2 days then D/C
PAIN/SYMPTOM CONTROL	• Tylenol 650 mg/po prn pain d/c with neutropenia • Tylenol 650 mg/po prn temp ≥38.5 • Urokinase lines prn • Phenergan 25 mg iv for n/v prn or Compazine 10 mg IV q4h prn • Ativan 1-2 mg iv (n/v mgmt prn) • Fluid mgmt with Lasix prn	• Urokinase lines prn • Phenergan 25 mg iv for n/v prn or Compazine 10 mg IV q4h prn • Ativan 1-2 mg iv (n/v mgmt prn) • Fluid mgmt with Lasix prn •Give Tylenol 650 mg po prn temp ≥ 38.5, ONLY if on antibiotics	• Pain management prn • Urokinase lines prn • Phenergan 25 mg iv for n/v prn or Compazine 10 mg IV q4h prn • Ativan 1-2 mg iv (n/v mgmt prn) • Fluid mgmt with Lasix prn •Give Tylenol 650 mg po prn temp ≥ 38.5, ONLY if on antibiotics	• Pain management prn
NUTRITION	• Regular diet except for raw shell fish and sushi • Oral dietary supplements	• Regular diet except for raw shell fish and sushi • Oral dietary supplements	• Regular diet except for raw shell fish and sushi •Neutropenic diet when ANC <500 • Oral dietary supplements • +/- Calorie count	• Regular diet except for raw shell fish and sushi
D/C PLANNING/ TEACHING	• BMTU teaching (patient/family) • Reinforce neutropenia precautions (patient/family)	• BMTU teaching (patient/family) • Reinforce neutropenia precautions (patient/family)	• Continue BMTU teaching and initiate discharge teaching (patient/primary caregiver) • Reinforce neutropenia precautions (patient/family)	• Discharge teaching complete (patient/primary caregiver) • Reinforce neutropenia precautions (patient/family) • BMTU discharge sheet complete • Discharge supplies and medications ready • Clinic visit scheduled

Anita Stephen, RN, BSN
Nurse Practice Coordinator-BMTU

Kathy Conner, RN, MN, OCN
Coordinated Care Manager

Department of Nursing and Patient Services
Shands Hospital at the University of Florida

Figure 86–8 *See legend on opposite page*

must be educated about its effectiveness and its toxicities. Assistance should be provided to balance available information that will ensure an informed decision regarding the use of this agent for cancer control. Patients who may benefit from tamoxifen as a cancer treatment alternative or as a chemopreventive approach should be educated about the potential benefits and complications associated with its use. They should be made aware of the risk for endometrial cancers as a result of its use and the importance of following cancer screening guidelines as indicated. A baseline endometrial sampling followed by a yearly sampling is recommended by the American College of Obstetrics and Gynecology.[46]

Yearly endometrial biopsies or transvaginal ultrasound with biopsy in patients with thickened endometrial linings were recommended by the National Cancer Institute Advisory Meeting in 1994.[46] Nurses working with patients undergoing tamoxifen treatment must keep abreast of ongoing research associated with its role in chemoprevention and long-term complications associated with its use. The oncology nurse is instrumental in assessing the level of understanding of patients regarding risk factors associated with the development of endometrial cancer and signs and symptoms associated with uterine abnormalities.

PSYCHOSOCIAL ISSUES

The impact of a breast cancer diagnosis not only imposes significant physical, physiological, and psychological demands on the patient, but may also result in psychological distress that may extend to family members or their support system. Northhouse studied the impact of breast cancer on 50 mastectomy patients and their husbands and identified the following adjustment issues: concerns about the extent of their disease, potential for cancer's recurrence, family matters, and the need to return to previous lifestyle.[47] The majority of the women and husbands included in the study identified the preoperative period as the most stressful because of uncertainty associated with the situation, delays with surgery/scheduling problems, insufficient information about their condition, and the need to make treatment choices with minimal guidance from health professionals. Hilton studied 35 families coping with breast cancer and also identified similar themes and issues, including uncertainty during initial diagnostic stage; difficulties associated with making treatment decisions, being informed, and making informed decisions; and issues regarding the functional patterns of the family.[48]

Welch-McCaffrey and associates in a review of the literature (1979 to 1988) categorized the following psychosocial variables as issues with the potential to affect long-term cancer survivors: fear of recurrence and death, relationships with the health care team, adjustment to physical compromise, alterations in customary social support, isolationism, psychosocial reorientation, and employability and insurability problems.[49] Recent studies on cancer survivorship had revealed the impact of a breast cancer diagnosis in the quality of life of those affected. The following themes have been identified as needs or concerns by breast cancer survivors: the need to continue integrating the disease process into current life (e.g., information seeking, problem solving); changes in relationships with friends, family, and others; restructuring of life perspective (i.e., to be of service to others); and unresolved issues such as patient's relationships with health care providers and fears of susceptibility to cancer.[50]

The impact of breast cancer and its treatment on sexuality and body image has also been associated with adaptation issues and high levels of stress. Cancer treatments such as chemotherapy may result in physical deficits that may impair the functioning of the gonads; patients may experience sexual difficulties and marital problems as a result of the emotional consequences associated with a mastectomy or other body image changes associated with cancer treatment (e.g., alopecia, weight changes).[51] The sexual effects of breast cancer and its treatment are poorly addressed by health care professionals.

A diagnosis of cancer is also accompanied by financial and economic adjustments in association with treatment and rehabilitation needs. The treatment phase may be accompanied by difficulties in adjusting and managing cancer treatment–related symptoms that may deter the patient from work-related activities and eventually impact the patient's financial status. Interventions to assist patients with cosmetic changes associated with surgical cancer treatment (e.g., breast implants, wigs) may also create a financial burden on the patient as well as on the family.

A diagnosis of breast cancer has the potential to impact the psychosocial stability of patients, family members, and those involved in providing support to the patient at different intervals during the treatment phase. The struggle to maintain psychosocial adjustment may continue as a lifelong issue for breast cancer survivors. Nurses play a significant role in the early identification of issues that may be affecting the patient's ability to adjust to demands associated with a new diagnosis. Oncology nurses are also instrumental in facilitating necessary understanding to assist patients during the decision-making process at different intervals during the diagnosis, treatment, or rehabilitative phase. The need to coordinate services with other health care practitioners (e.g., social workers, clinical psychologists) must be assessed on an ongoing basis given the diversity of psychosocial issues that may be affecting the patient and her or his support system. Nursing interventions or strategies to promote psychosocial adjustment should also incorporate family members and the patient's support system.

Nursing management of the patient with breast cancer requires knowledge of the disease process, understanding of the complexity of the treatment options, and skill in providing physical and psychosocial support. Understanding the continuum of care, communicating accurate information so that the patient can make informed decisions, and facilitating treatment and rehabilitation interventions will provide the supportive and caring environment the patient requires and deserves.

References

1. American Cancer Society. Breast Cancer Facts and Figures. ACS 1–6, 1996.
2. Wooster R, Neuhausen SL, Mangion J, et al: Localization of a breast cancer susceptibility gene, BRCA2, to chromosome 13 q 12-13. Science 265:2088–2090, 1994.
3. Miki Y, et al: A strong candidate for the breast and ovarian cancer susceptibility gene BRCA1. Science 266:66–71, 1994.
4. Hoskins KF, Stopfer JE, Calzone K, et al: Assessment and counseling for women with a family history of breast cancer: A guide for clinicians. JAMA 273:577–585, 1993.
5. McCool WF: Barriers to breast cancer screening in older women. J Nurse Midwifery 39:283–299, 1994.
6. Constanza M: Issues in breast cancer screening in older women. Cancer Supplement 74:2009–2015, 1994.
7. American Cancer Society. ACS Facts and Figures. ACS 11–13, 1996.
8. Spector RE: Cultural Diversity in Health and Illness. Stamford, Connecticut, Appleton & Lange. 1996, p 24.
9. Harris JR, Morrow M, Bonadionna G: Cancer of the breast. *In* DeVita VT, Hellman S, Rosenberg SA (eds): Cancer Principles and Practice of Oncology. Philadelphia, JB Lippincott, 1993, pp 1264–1332.
10. Schmidt RA: Stereotactic breast biopsy. CA Cancer J Clin 44:172–191, 1994.
11. Cimprich B: Development of an intervention to restore attention in cancer patients. Cancer Nurs 16:83–92, 1993.
12. Luker KA, Beaver K, Leinster SJ, et al: The information needs of women newly diagnosed with breast cancer. J Adv Nurs 22:134–141, 1995.
13. Kalinowski BH: Local therapy for breast cancer: Treatment choices and decision making. Semin Oncol Nurs 7:187–193, 1993.
14. NIH Consensus Conference: Treatment of early stage breast cancer. JAMA 265:391–394, 1991.
15. Clark A, Kent RB: One day hospitalization following modified radical mastectomy. Am Surg 58:239–242, 1992.
16. Edwards MJ, Broodwater RJ, Bill JL, et al: Economic impact of reducing hospitalization for mastectomy patients. Ann Surg 208:330–336, 1988.
17. Cohen AM, Schaeffer N, Chen Z, et al: Early discharge after modified radical mastectomy. Am J Surg 151:465–466, 1986.
18. Orr RK, Ketcham AS, Robinson DS, et al: Early discharge after mastectomy: A safe way of diminishing hospital costs. Am Surg 53:161–63, 1987.
19. Chilson TR, Chan F, Lonsen R, et al: Seroma prevention after modified radical mastectomy. Surg Clin North Am 63:1331–1351, 1983.
20. Somers RG, Jablon LK, Kaplan MJ, et al: The use of closed suction drainage after lumpectomy and axillary node dissection for breast cancer. Ann Surg 215:146–149, 1992.
21. Aitken R, Hunsaker R, James AG: Prevention of seromas following mastectomy and axillary node dissection. Surg Gynecol Obstet 158:327–330, 1984.
22. Humble CA: Lymphedema: Incidence, pathophysiology, management, and nursing care. Oncol Nurs Forum 22:1503–1509, 1995.
23. Brennan MJ, Weitz J: Lymphedema 30 years after radical mastectomy. Am J Phys Med Rehabil 71:12–14, 1992.
24. Farncombe M, Daniels G, Cross L: Lymphedema: The seemingly forgotten complication. J Pain Symptom Manage 9:269–276, 1994.
25. Jansen RFM, Van Geel AN, De Groot HGW, et al: Immediate

versus delayed shoulder exercises after axillary lymph node dissection. Am J Surg 160:481–484, 1990.
26. U.S. Department of Health and Human Service: Acute Pain Management: Operative or Medical Procedures and Trauma Clinical Practice Guidelines. U.S. Department of Health and Human Services, Agency for Health Care Policy and Research, 1992, p 26.
27. Campa JA III, Payne R: Pain syndromes due to cancer treatment. *In* Patt RB (ed): Cancer Pain. Philadelphia, JB Lippincott, 1993, pp 52–53.
28. Lotze MT, Duncar MA, Guber LH, et al: Early vs delayed shoulder motion following axillary dissection. Ann Surg 193:288–295, 1981.
29. Petrek J, Peters M, Nori S, et al: Axillary lymphadenopathy. Arch Surg 125:378–382, 1990.
30. Bostwick J III: Breast reconstruction following mastectomy. CA J Nurs Clin 45:289–304, 1995.
31. Knobf MT, Stahl R: Reconstructive surgery in primary breast cancer treatment. Semin Oncol Nurs 7:200–206, 1991.
32. Sitton E: Early and late radiation-induced skin alterations. Part I: Mechanisms of skin changes. Oncol Nurs Forum 19:801–807, 1992.
33. Barnicle MM: Managing symptoms related to chemotherapy. *In* Dow KH (ed): Contemporary Issues in Breast Cancer. Boston, Jones and Bartlett, 1996, pp 27–42.
34. Pierce SM, Harris JR: Radiation therapy to the breast: Practical aspects. J Am Med Wom Assoc 47:174–177, 1992.
35. O'Rourke N, Robinson LMP: Breast cancer and the role of radiation therapy. *In* Dow KH (ed): Contemporary Issues in Breast Cancer. Boston, Jones and Bartlett, 1996, pp 43–58.
36. Shapiro CL, Recht A: Late effects of adjuvant therapy for breast cancer. J NCI Monogr 16:101–109, 1994.
37. Kardinal CG: Chemotherapy of breast cancer. *In* Perry MC (ed): The Chemotherapy Sourcebook. Baltimore, Williams & Wilkins, 1993, pp 948–988.
38. Rhodes VA, Johnson MH, McDaniel RW: Nausea, vomiting, and retching: The management of the symptom experienced. Semin Oncol Nurs 11(4):256–265, 1995.
39. Mitchell EP, Schein PS: Gastrointestinal toxicity of chemotherapeutic agents. *In* Perry MC (ed): The Chemotherapy Sourcebook. Baltimore, Williams and Wilkins, 1993, pp 620–634.
40. National Institutes of Health: Oral complications of cancer therapies: Prevention and treatment. NIH Consensus Development Conference Statement 7:7–19, 1989.
41. Winningham ML, Nail LM, Burke MB, et al: Fatigue and the cancer experience: The state of the knowledge. Oncol Nurs Forum 21:23–36, 1994.
42. Greene D, Nail LM, Fieler VK, Dudgeon D, Jones LS: A comparison of patient-reported side effects among three chemotherapy regimens for breast cancer. Cancer Pract 2:57–62, 1994.
43. MacVicar M, Winningham M, Nickel J: Effects of aerobic interval training on cancer patient's functional capacity. Nurs Res 38:348–351, 1989.
44. Cimprich B: Development of an intervention to restore attention in cancer patients. Cancer Nurs 16:83–92, 1993.
45. Jaiyesimi IA, Buzdar AU, Decker DA, Hortobagyi GN: Use of tamoxifen for breast cancer: Twenty eight years later. J Clin Oncol 13:513–529, 1995.
46. Crabbe WW: The tamoxifen controversy. Oncol Nurs Forum 23:761–766, 1996.
47. Northhouse LL: The impact of breast cancer on patients and husbands. Cancer Nurs 12:276–284, 1989.
48. Hilton BA: Issues, problems and challenges for families coping with breast cancer. Semin Oncol Nurs 9:88–100, 1993.
49. Welch-McCaffrey D, Hoffman B, Leigh SA, et al: Surviving adult cancers. Part 2: Psychosocial implications. Ann Intern Med 11:517–523, 1989.
50. Wyatt G, Kurtz ME, Liken M: Breast cancer survivors: An exploration of quality of life issues after breast cancer. Cancer Nurs 16:440–447, 1993.
51. Kaplan HS: A neglected issue: The sexual side effects of current treatments for breast cancer. J Sex Marital Ther 18:3–17, 1992.

CHAPTER 87
REHABILITATION

Thomas A. Gaskin III, M.D. / Lindsey A. Trammell, R.N., M.S.N.

"The cancer patient who is cured of his malignancy but is left a physical or emotional cripple represents a sort of tawdry triumph of our therapeutic skills."[25] Rehabilitation is the process for minimizing physical, psychological, and vocational dysfunction that may result from the disease or its treatment. Although these disabilities or dysfunctions are not exclusively found in patients with breast cancer, breast cancer is an appropriate model because of its prevalence, its demography, and the presence of essentially all categories of disability. The tragedy of curing a woman of breast cancer but having her life devastated by the physical or emotional effects of the cancer or its treatment occurs far too commonly. Society has made the breast a focus of aesthetics and affection. Nevertheless, it is a fallacy that maladjustment to the cosmetic deformity of mastectomy constitutes the principal disability that a woman faces. The woman with breast cancer also faces physical, sexual, psychosocial, and vocational disabilities.[25] The impact of these disabilities spreads far beyond the individual and involves her family, friends, and workplace.[13] This places an additional burden on the patient, her family, and those who treat her.

Correction of these disabilities follows the same general principles and approaches as the treatment of the disease itself. The following items are essential:

1. Knowledge of the disabilities
2. Prospective action to prevent or minimize disabilities
3. An organized system of assessment
4. Interventions of varying complexity that may involve a variety of individuals with varying degrees and types of expertise (team approach) (Table 87–1)[14]
5. Surveillance and reassessment to monitor effectiveness

Recognition of the interrelationships between the categories of disability is an essential step in understanding, preventing, and ameliorating these conditions. This chapter addresses physical, sexual, and vocational disabilities; Chapter 89 addresses the psychosocial disabilities. Of necessity, the chapter addresses many of the interrelationships that mutually contribute to recovery.

Approaching breast cancer–related disabilities is little different from the approach to managing illness. Table 87–1 categorizes services likely to be available at various levels of health care facilities. This table has changed minimally since 1981 and continues to be a useful format for illustrative purposes. Although the vast majority of women will be managed in the physician's office, advanced or complicated situations may require specialized or uncommon services.[14]

Medicine has moved, organizationally, from cottage industry to industrial revolution. The fragmentation of diagnosis, primary treatment, and surveillance has had a detrimental effect on the prevention, detection, and management of disability. Psychosocial support should begin with the diagnostic procedures and continue through the spectrum of primary surgical care, adjuvant treatment, and surveillance. This assembly-line process often involves diagnostic radiologists, the radiation oncologist, the oncologic surgeon, the reconstructive surgeon, the medical oncologist, and the primary care physician. It is understandable with this system that efforts to address disabilities may be absent, uncoordinated, and ineffective and that women will not know to whom to turn to discuss problems. Managed care is often a confounding rather than a constructive ingredient. Our format will enumerate dysfunctions and discuss their causes, opportunities for prevention, practical detection instruments appropriate to an office-based practice, and interventions consonant with the degree of dysfunction.

PHYSICAL REHABILITATION

The fear of death, loss of control, uncertainty of outcome, and alteration of body image so characteristic of women with breast cancer are profoundly affected by and affect physical problems such as lymphedema, restriction of range of motion, strength and conditioning, pain, sexual function and desire, and circumstances of employment and insurability.

Occupational and physical therapy have important roles in helping women with breast cancer overcome their most obvious disability. The physical disabilities are related primarily to mastectomy but are also found in women who have had partial mastectomy and axillary dissection.[16] A variety of factors play a part in determining the type and extent of disabilities encountered, including decreased range of motion in the shoulder on the operated side, lymphedema, scar tissue, decreased strength in the arm and shoulder girdle, changes in sensation, and pain. Contributing factors are pre-existing problems, major and minor nerve injury, extent of lymphatic dissection, removal or denervation of muscles, postoperative wound problems including seroma and infection, type of incision, and even such details as type of surgical dressing.[18, 19]

Physical disabilities are commonly present and un-

TABLE 87-1. REHABILITATION TEAM MEMBERS FOR INTERVENTIONAL APPROACH

Rehabilitation Team Member	Cancer Center	500-Bed Hospital	200–300-Bed Hospital	Small Community Hospital	Physician's Office	Ambulatory Health Service
Physician (M.D.)	Psychiatrist or specially trained	Interested or specially trained	Interested and/or attending	Interested and/or attending	M.D.	M.D.
Nurse	Nurse coordinator	Nurse coordinator	Nurse	Nurse	Nurse	Nurse
Chaplain	Chaplain	Chaplain	Chaplain	Chaplain	Refer	Refer
Physical therapist (P.T.)	P.T.	P.T.	P.T., part-time	P.T., part-time	Refer P.T. center or visiting nurse (V.N.)	Refer P.T. center or V.N.
Occupational therapist (O.T.)	O.T.	O.T.	O.T., part-time or consultant	O.T. consultant or center	Refer O.T. center or V.N.	Refer O.T. center or V.N.
Social worker	Social worker	Social worker	Possible social worker or refer	Refer or V.N.	Refer community agency or V.N.	Refer community agency or V.N.
Psychiatrist or clinical psychologist	Psychiatrist	Psychiatrist or clinical psychologist	Consultant	Consultant	Refer	Refer
Speech and hearing specialist	Speech pathologist	Speech pathologist or consultant	Refer	Refer	Refer	Refer
Prosthodontist	Prosthodontist	Prosthodontist consultant	Consultant	Refer	Refer	Refer
Prosthetist or orthotist	Prosthetist orthotist consultant	Prosthetist orthotist consultant	Consultant	Consultant or refer	Refer	Refer
Vocational counselor	Counselor on call	On call	Refer	Refer	Refer	Refer

*Adapted from Dietz JH: Rehabilitation Oncology. New York, John Wiley & Sons, 1981.

commonly treated in an organized way in breast cancer. Physical disabilities are a constant reminder of the malignancy and adversely affect coping skills, which in turn contributes to psychosocial dysfunction. Petrek and Blackwood observe that many of the recommendations of the American Cancer Society, the National Cancer Institute Cancer Information Service, and the National Lymphedema network serve to perpetuate the sense of illness. "The long term survivor is reminded that she is not or will never be 'normal.'"[28] The admonitions against heavy lifting and carrying purses with the ipsilateral arm serve to promote the one-sidedness that many women develop. These admonitions stem from anecdotal observations that some women who have been lymphedema free for years after their surgery suddenly developed lymphedema after a precipitating event that strains the arm. Thus, efforts intended to lessen the chance of lymphedema, even when the risk is quite small, paradoxically contribute to psychological disability. There has been neither quantification of the protective benefit of many of the recommended precautions nor quantification of an adverse psychological effect.[11]

Fitness

Lack of fitness is extremely common—almost to the point of universality. Lack of fitness results in a decreased sense of well-being and, frequently, weight gain. Weight gain contributes to the sense of altered body image, especially when hair loss or loss of a breast is part of the picture. Lack of fitness with attendant decrease in sense of well-being is more than additive in the demands placed on a woman's coping skills.

Causes. The decrease in fitness is primarily caused by abandonment of physical activity. This initially results from preoccupation with the cancer and its treatment. Side effects of chemotherapy or radiation therapy often make exercise uncomfortable or especially demanding. Later on, however, women are frequently concerned that exercise will have an adverse impact on the surgery or will, in some way, reactivate the cancer. The authors identified an almost universal sense of self-consciousness about physical appearance that inhibited women from participating in exercise groups.[16]

Prevention. Prevention is best accomplished by anticipatory counseling and by encouragement to participate in a group exercise program such as STRETCH (Strength Through Recreation Exercise Togetherness Care Help) (see Appendix).[16] In discussions with women as they enter treatment, it is useful to encourage them to maintain an exercise and fitness program and to caution them against inordinate weight gain. STRETCH, a group exercise–based rehabilitation program for women with breast cancer, is discussed in more detail in the Appendix at the end of the chapter.

Detection. The most obvious detection instrument is the scale. An increase in weight should prompt questions specific to exercise and the woman's daily routine.

Interventions. When lack of fitness and weight gain do not respond to encouragement and if "informational" counseling has been ineffective, then more specific counseling using peers (women with breast cancer) and professional counselors may be needed. Group exercise and specific exercise prescriptions are additional tools that have been found to be effective.

Lymphedema

Lymphedema occurs in 15 to 20 percent of women with axillary dissection. It is estimated that 210,000 axillary dissections are performed annually and that 400,000 long-term survivors suffer from lymphedema.[28] The attention paid to the appearance of the breast far outweighs that paid to the appearance of the arm, yet, lymphedema cannot easily be disguised by clothing. Its very presence calls attention to the breast cancer by the patient and those she encounters. Repeated episodes of cellulitis and lymphangitis are painful, frightening, and often confusing because of an absence of consistent explanations of etiology and lack of a systematical, organized approach to treatment.

Causes. Lymphedema is a sequelum of axillary node dissection and is often exacerbated by radiation or infection. It is profound, disturbing, and unfortunate that a partial mastectomy and radiation, performed to preserve breast cosmesis, can result in lymphedema and is worsened by radiation scattered to the axilla. Paradoxically, the more complete and elegant the axillary dissection is, the greater the likelihood of lymphedema. Axillary wound infection and prolonged seroma formation are additional factors that increase the risk of lymphedema.

Prevention. The prime determinant of the risk of lymphedema is axillary dissection. For patients in whom axillary dissection can be avoided and still be consistent with good oncological care, it seems reasonable to omit axillary dissection.[23] The extent of axillary dissection necessary to be consistent with sound oncological principles also varies from patient to patient. If the sentinel node technique proves reliable in identifying patients in whom axillary dissection can be omitted, a substantial number of women treated for breast cancer can be spared the risk of lymphedema without compromise to their survival. Avoidance of overenthusiastic dissection of the tissue around and superior to the axillary vein is a technical detail that may prove to be useful. The combination of radiation therapy and axillary dissection is especially likely to result in lymphedema. It seems prudent, therefore, for the dissected axilla not to be subjected to routine radiation. The avoidance of infection can be assisted by the performance of a one-stage rather than a two-stage operation. Preoperative needle biopsy often makes the one-stage technique appropriate. Antibiotic prophylaxis has been established to be effective in a randomized prospective trial.[31] Seroma formation does not seem to be dependent on timing of arm mobilization, an increase in the number of drains, or the use of compression dressings.[29, 30]

Detection. The simplest instrument to detect early lymphedema is information from the patient. Observation may identify a visible difference in the size of the arms and hands. Tightness of rings is an early sign of swelling. Measurement of the arm and forearm circumference is a reasonable, quantitative way to detect and follow lymphedema. Volumetric studies using liquid displacement are more accurate but are not practical in most circumstances.

Interventions. Interventions for lymphedema must be made in a timely fashion. Long-standing lymphedema seems to result in chronic dilation of lymph vessels that do not recoil but provide a chamber waiting to be filled. Avoidance of injury or infection, elevation, centripetal massage, fitted external elastic sleeves, lymphedema pumps, and "decongestive" therapy all play a role in intervention.[15]

Surveillance. Lymphedema may occur years after axillary dissection for reasons not yet clear. Anecdotal accounts of women who have been free of lymphedema for a number of years sustaining a single physical event to that arm with subsequent development of lymphedema are not uncommon.[11]

Range of Motion

A significant number of women have limitation in the range of motion of the ipsilateral shoulder, although the "frozen shoulder" is seldom encountered today.

Causes. The causes of restricted range of motion are immobility by dressing, instruction, pain, fear, or scarring.

Prevention. Prevention of loss of range of motion is accomplished by early mobilization and by instruction in postoperative range of motion exercises. The range-of-motion exercises in pamphlets provided by the American Cancer Society are useful.[2] An exercise-based rehabilitation program such as STRETCH is effective in the prevention and treatment of restricted range of motion (see Appendix).[16]

Detection. The simplest instrument for early detection of loss of range of motion is the use of the checklist described in Table 87–2.[45] Goniometric measurements are seldom needed.

Interventions. Range-of-motion exercises, deep friction massage, use of moisturizers, and prolonged

TABLE 87–2.   ASSESSING RANGE OF MOTION

Using the arm on your operated side are you able to
1. Brush and comb your hair?
2. Get a T-shirt, blouse that does not unbutton, or tight-necked sweater over your head?
3. Pull on a pair of pants or pantyhose and pull them up?
4. Close a back-fastening bra?
5. Completely zip up a dress with a back-fastening zipper?
6. Wash the upper part of your back, i.e., shoulder-blade area, on the same side as the operation?
7. Wash the upper part of your back, i.e., the shoulder-blade area, on the opposite side from the operation?
8. Reach into a cupboard over your head?
9. Make a double bed?
10. Carry a grocery bag containing three 1-pound cans, a 3-pound roast, a 3-pound bag of apples, and one or two other items so that the bag weighs approximately 10 pounds?

Adapted from Wingate L: Efficacy of physical therapy for patients who have undergone mastectomies. Phys Ther, June, 1985.

stretching of fibrous bands can help preserve and restore range of motion. Operative release of wound contracture or frozen shoulder is seldom required.

Surveillance. Quantitative surveillance is not necessary in the asymptomatic patient. Questions regarding shoulder mobility at surveillance visits is usually sufficient to identify late problems and allow for intervention at that time.

Posture

Changes in posture occur in about 90 percent of women, and the types of changes are not consistent. The authors' evaluation of 114 women examined from 2 months to 22 years postoperatively, with the average postoperative time being 2 years, subjectively identified only 14 women who were thought to have "normal" posture.[16]

Causes. Changes in posture have a variety of causes, including subconscious or conscious protection of the affected side, physical and mental awareness of the scar, reconstructive surgery, or the weight and presence of a prosthesis.

Prevention. Emphasis on restoration of shoulder and arm use often avoids the physical factors (strength, flexibility, range of motion) that affect posture. Proper prosthetic fitting and clothing selection can reduce the compensatory changes in posture caused by these two factors.

Detection. Detection of posture changes is among the most difficult of all the features of physical disability. Subtle changes in posture may not be apparent to the patient, her family, or the physician. Changes in posture occur commonly with age in women without breast cancer. The signs that characteristically are associated with breast cancer treatment are folding the arms across the chest or upper abdomen, lack of symmetry in shoulder elevation, and forward rotation of the affected shoulder with resultant reluctance to use the ipsilateral arm.

Interventions. The primary intervention is education. Physical therapy, exercise, and clothing consultation are useful once education has provided the awareness of the condition.

Surveillance. Surveillance is qualitative rather than quantitative and is even more subtle than early detection.

Pain

Tightness from the scar and paresthesias in the intercostal brachial nerve distribution cause discomfort in a significant proportion of women after breast surgery.[7, 48] Less common (4 to 6 percent) is more severe pain that may be disabling.[28]

Cause. Symptomatic cicatrix formation most commonly follows skin flap necrosis or infection. Division of the intercostal brachial nerve is a direct cause of paresthesias or pain.

Prevention. Prevention is accomplished by preservation of the intercostal brachial nerve and techniques designed to minimize skin edge necrosis and wound infection.

Detection. Detection of pain from cicatrix or nerve injury is usually readily accomplished by the postoperative interview and physical examination. In women with increasing pain and paresthesias, it may be useful to search for a trigger point.

Interventions. Pain from cicatrix formation is, thankfully, usually of limited duration and responds to moisturizers, skin lubrication, and massage. The treatment of mild paresthesias is frequently expectant, because the severity of these is also often self-limited. In the minority of patients who develop a disabling pain syndrome, excision of neuromas or therapeutic injection have limited utility.

Muscle Weakness

Cause. Ipsilateral muscle weakness may result from removal of muscle, prolonged immobilization, or nerve injury. A kinesiological study by Nikkanen and colleagues reports a 25 percent decrease in muscle strength on the operated side compared with the muscle strength on the control side.[27] Although there are physical causes for much of the muscle weakness seen after breast surgery, it is not uncommon for women to become "one armed" after a mastectomy or axillary dissection. The resultant favoring of the affected extremity is a prominent cause of loss of muscle strength and reduced range of motion.

Interventions. The primary interventions are muscle strengthening and education to dispel the myth that muscular activity will reactivate the malignancy.[32, 34]

Summary

Physical disabilities are constant reminders of the cancer and, therefore, affect psychosocial health, sexuality, and employment. Because of these interactions, physical disabilities that may seem relatively minor assume an emphasized role against the background of breast cancer.

Physical and occupational therapies provide education and techniques for minimizing a variety of physical disabilities that, if not corrected, could result in significant change in appearance and in modification of activities of daily living. Physical and educational techniques can promote a sense of control and wellness correlated with improved function and cosmesis. The value of this should not be underestimated as a factor in the overall recovery and adjustment of the woman with breast cancer.[45]

SEXUAL REHABILITATION

Sexuality is more than the union of an erect penis with a lubricated vagina. For a woman, it is the expression of her gender on her personality, her view of "self," and her relationship with others.[9] Changes in sexuality accompany many malignancies; breast cancer has no monopoly on this phenomenon (Table 87–3).[33, 40] Breast cancer, however, has an especially pronounced impact as a public health issue because of its commonness and because of the status of the breast in Western sexual culture. The concept of breast removal as mutilation is not a twentieth century invention; Decius punished St. Agatha (the patron saint of breast cancer) in 251 A.D. by amputating her breasts.[17] The effect of breast removal has almost universal effects on a woman's expression of her gender.[39] The basic underlying factor is a change in self-image that manifests itself by difficulty in expressing intimacy, in selecting clothing, and in avoidance of participation in many sports and activities that involve brief clothing.

The threat to sexuality is a major source of distress for the recovering breast cancer patient. Issues of sexuality are often neglected in oncology, leaving the woman to confront alone the loss of sexual desire, a decrease in the range of sexual activities, the impaired feeling of attractiveness, and, commonly, the absence of the ability to reproduce. Sexual rehabilitation should be an integral component of treatment planning and after care, because feeling sexually desirable and attractive and being able to receive and make love are critical components of quality of life. The incidence of sexual dysfunction is reported to be between 25 and 40 percent, but it is seldom addressed in the routine clinical situation.[4, 26, 35]

TABLE 87–3. FEMALE SEXUAL PROBLEMS CAUSED BY CANCER TREATMENT

Treatment	Low Sexual Desire	Less Vaginal Moisture	Reduced Vaginal Size	Painful Intercourse	Trouble Reaching Orgasm	Infertility
Chemotherapy	Sometimes	Often	Sometimes	Often	Rarely	Often
Pelvic radiation therapy	Rarely	Often	Often	Often	Rarely	Often
Radical hysterectomy	Rarely	Often*	Always	Rarely	Rarely	Always
Radical cystectomy	Rarely	Often*	Sometimes	Sometimes	Rarely	Always
Abdominoperineal resection	Rarely	Often*	Sometimes	Sometimes	Rarely	Sometimes
Total pelvic exenteration with vaginal reconstruction	Sometimes	Always	Sometimes	Sometimes	Sometimes	Always
Radical vulvectomy	Rarely	Never	Sometimes	Often	Sometimes	Never
Conization of the cervix	Never	Never	Never	Rarely	Never	Rarely
Oophorectomy (removal of one tube and ovary)	Rarely	Never*	Never*	Rarely	Never	Rarely
Oophorectomy (removal of both tubes and ovaries)	Rarely	Often*	Sometimes*	Sometimes*	Rarely	Always
Mastectomy or radiation to the breast	Rarely	Never	Never	Never	Rarely	Never
Antiestrogen therapy for breast or uterine cancer	Sometimes	Often	Sometimes	Sometimes	Rarely	Always
Androgen therapy	Never	Never	Never	Never	Never	Uncertain

*Vaginal dryness and size changes should not occur if one ovary is left in or if hormone replacement therapy is given.
Adapted from Schover LR: Sexuality & Cancer: For the Woman Who Has Cancer, and Her Partner. Randers-Pehrson M (ed). Rev. ed. No. 4657-PS. New York, American Cancer Society, 1995.

Etiology. Sexuality is such a fragile, multifaceted component of human life that any listing of etiologies is automatically incomplete. The common etiologies in women with breast cancer are:

1. Physical deformity
2. Change in the hormone milieu
3. Pharmacological effects and side effects
6. Decrease in energy level
7. Local discomfort from surgery or radiation
8. Psychological problems in the patient or her partner related to inadequate or mythical information
9. Pre-existing psychological problems in the patient or her partner or pre-existing difficulties in their relationship

Loss of the Breast. The psychological impact of breast cancer has been widely studied because of the disease's effects on an organ associated with self-esteem, self-image, femininity, sexuality, and reproduction.[22] Any visual or perceived alteration in the breast may affect a woman's perception of herself in terms of gender, physical well-being, and attractiveness. Most local therapy involving the breast is viewed as disfiguring, and body image disturbance has been suggested as central to the sexual disruption that occurs in breast cancer patients.[4] The impact of body image disturbance hinges on the woman's and her partner's value of the breast. The patient's partner is also vulnerable to psychological factors that may impede normal sexual expression.[20, 42, 43] The partner may believe that the woman with breast cancer is too sick for sexual activity and may feel guilty about making sexual overtures to her while she is experiencing the trauma of cancer and its treatment. Partners may falsely believe that the cancer is contagious or that the treatment will somehow affect them.[20, 42, 43] Other partners have difficulty adjusting to the altered appearance of the breast. Wellisch described five variables that determine the impact of breast cancer on a relationship:

1. The status of the relationship before the cancer developed
2. The longevity of the marriage
3. The stage of the breast cancer
4. The point in the course of the illness
5. The interpersonal skills available to the partner[43]

According to Schover, "A woman's overall psychological health, relationship satisfaction, and premorbid sexual life appear to be far stronger predictors of post cancer sexual satisfaction than is the extent of the damage to the breast."[39]

Breast conservation and reconstruction have as their *raison d'être* a diminution in the physical disfigurement of the breast. Studies of the impact of breast conservation on the quality of life demonstrate an advantage, albeit not as great as would be intuitively expected, for breast conservation. Two comprehensive reviews describe studies comparing quality of life, including sexuality, of patients undergoing mastectomy versus breast conservation.[21, 36, 39, 41] For the majority of patients, the studies reflected no difference in the outcomes of quality of life and of sexual functioning.[21, 41]

When the studies demonstrated a difference in the quality of life and in the sexual functioning outcomes, the benefit favored breast conservation. Breast conservation patients had more positive feelings about their bodies, particularly their appearance nude.[39] Breast conservation seems to produce less psychological hardship, although it does not eliminate all the psychosocial morbidity associated with mastectomy.[36] Although the fundamental objective of breast conservation is to preserve the integrity of the woman's body image, it should not be assumed that body image changes will not occur. Radiation effects on the breast include changes in the texture of breast tissue, contour and size of the breast, thickening of the skin, and discoloration of the skin. This information should dampen the sometimes overenthusiastic assertions regarding breast conservation, just as unfounded claims of improved survival should not be made in favor of mastectomy.

Techniques of breast reconstruction are improving year by year, with some truly spectacular results. Restoration of body image is accomplished in many undergoing reconstructions, and yet, only a fraction of women eligible for reconstruction choose this option. Overall, women who choose reconstruction generally report satisfaction. No benefit has been consistently reported between immediate and delayed reconstruction on sexuality.[39] Detailed studies of the effects of reconstruction on sexuality and the impact on the partner have not been forthcoming.[41] Because there is evidence that local treatment for breast cancer is the major factor in a minority of women, studies directed toward that subset deserve special consideration regarding the effect of local therapy on sexual functioning.[39]

Systemic Therapy. Chemotherapy can cause sexual disruption directly and indirectly.[5, 20, 37, 44] It can produce nausea, fatigue, malaise, and decrease in sense of well-being as well as sleep and appetite disturbances. All of these interfere with libido. Changes in physical appearance such as alopecia, weight gain or loss, and pallor present significant challenges to a woman's self-esteem and self-perception.[39] In premenopausal and perimenopausal women, chemotherapy often results in ovarian failure with resultant menopausal symptoms, alteration in sexual function, and infertility.[20] Hot flashes, loss of vaginal lubrication, and eventual vulvar and vaginal atrophy create a loss of desire, decreased arousal, and orgasmic difficulties.[39]

Tamoxifen is the most common form of hormonal treatment among a variety of surgical and pharmacological options.[20, 39] Hormonal manipulation may not only affect estrogen, but androgens as well. Tamoxifen has been associated with vasomotor changes, weight gain, and depression symptoms, which are hard to separate causally from other aspects of breast cancer treatment. Symptoms of hot flashes, irregular menses, vaginal discharge, and vaginal atrophy are more directly associated with tamoxifen and other agents or interventions that interfere with estrogen and have a more direct effect on sexual dysfunction. Sexual expression after breast cancer is largely affected by the quality of sexual expression before breast cancer, including existing self-esteem, quality of the relationship, and degree of sexual functioning. Schover states, "The most common culprit in causing sexual dysfunction may prove to be not loss of a breast, but the premature and severe menopausal impact of systemic therapy."[39]

Treatment. Characteristically, women who experience sexual difficulty are hesitant to initiate communication with their caregivers or their partners. It is incumbent, therefore, on the treatment team to establish an open line of communication on the subject early in the course of treatment planning and therapy. The absence of a discussion of sexual issues conveys the message that these critical concerns are unimportant, inappropriate, or uncommon. Using Annon's PLISSIT (Permission, Limited Information, Specific Suggestions, and Intensive Therapy) model is a useful scheme for approaching sexual issues with breast cancer patients.[6]

Permission. The breast cancer patient is given permission to discuss sexual concerns with the health care team. The health care professional communicates an attitude of acceptance and encouragement so that the patient feels comfortable as a sexual being to discuss sexual issues. Any discussion of treatment options involves local therapy, mastectomy with and without reconstruction, and breast conservation. Talking about the value placed on the breast by the woman and her partner is an introduction to discussions of sexuality. Although issues of survival are usually foremost, the consideration of potential sexual consequences serves the additional purpose of introducing sexual concerns as a permissible topic. It also provides the physician and other members of the treatment team with some insight into the quality of the relationship. At any time in the course of therapy, the simple question "Are you having trouble with your sex life?" is often sufficient to indicate that sexual activity and thoughts are okay and that problems in this area are appropriate topics of concern to the treatment team.[39]

Limited Information. Factual information about the effects that breast cancer and its treatment have on sexuality and fertility is communicated to the patient and her partner by the health care team. During treatment planning, women at risk for premature menopause should be counseled about infertility. Explaining to a couple the importance of open communication between them about their sexual relationship and its difficulties is extremely valuable in minimizing the sexual disruption that they experi-

ence.[39] A general discussion of the effects of hormonal manipulation or chemotherapy on sexual functioning is the sort of limited information appropriate to almost every woman. Identification of merchants who are knowledgeable, helpful, and sensitive about prostheses and fashions can be automatically provided. The American Cancer Society's publication *Sexuality and Cancer: For the Woman and Her Partner* is useful for a detailed discussion of specific suggestions, but identification or provision of this booklet is an example of limited information.[40] That is, the information provided in this book includes specific suggestions, but simply directing the patient to the booklet is "limited information."

Specific Suggestions. Specific strategies to enable a woman to overcome her individual problems are sometimes necessary. This level of therapy may require expertise not available to the usual health care team. Although it may be worthwhile for someone on the team to develop this expertise, it is usually sufficient to be able to identify a community resource. *Sexuality and Cancer* is a valuable guide for the health care professional and for the patient.[40] Women or their partners often are faced with feelings of discomfort with nudity in sexual situations. Communication with the partner and imagination usually serve to solve this problem inherently, but the health professional (the choice usually depends on rapport rather than expertise) may be called on for help. Communication is the first suggestion to determine if nudity is a problem to either. If it is, then appropriate lingerie and lifelike prostheses may ease the discomfort. Vaginal dryness may be alleviated by nonestrogenic lubricants, and vaginal dilation may relieve another cause of dyspareunia. Alternative activities to express physical intimacy other than intercourse such as massage or embrace may prove to be helpful. Dryness or hypersensitivity resulting from irradiation can be addressed by skin lubricants or modification of the firmness of the stimulation.[40]

Intensive Therapy. Intensive treatment of a couple's sexual dysfunction warrants referral to a sex therapist or a psychotherapist. Intensive therapy often goes beyond practical suggestions to help with specific problems and delves into the relationship and what each partner contributes. For couples with preexisting marital problems or sexual dysfunction, breast cancer may precipitate divorce, worsening of the sexual dysfunction, or major psychological disturbance. This degree of disability cannot be left unaddressed.

Witkin concluded:

1. Sexual self-concept supersedes mortality as a primary concern of most recovering mastectomy patients.

2. The attitude of the partner—husband or lover—is crucial to that self-concept.

3. Most partners are eager to help.

4. Psychosexual counseling is helpful and found to be appropriate.[47]

Women often have difficulty finding health professionals who are knowledgeable about the sexual effects of their treatment and who are willing to talk to them about these issues. Every woman with breast cancer should be asked about her current sexual functioning and concerns by a member of her oncology team. Restoration of sexual functioning carries benefits far beyond private sexual behavior of a couple by enabling the woman's femininity to express herself in all of her relationships, including her very important relationship with herself.[47]

VOCATIONAL REHABILITATION

Historically, employment discrimination against people with a history of cancer was a serious and well-documented problem.[8] The cause of the discrimination arose from myths regarding communicability of the disease but also was based on economic prejudice. Our society increasingly places emphasis on what we do as a measure of who we are. Aside from a source of income, a job provides an identity and a sense of self-worth.[24]

Health insurance is a benefit of employment, and loss of employment often means loss of health insurance. Individual policies for a person with a history of cancer are either unavailable or carry extraordinary premiums beyond the reach of even an employed person. Suitability for employment often means more than suitability for the position—it means insurability. By and large, employers are not obligated to provide employment for anyone, and yet, there are certain legal safeguards and remedies to protect certain classes of employees from discrimination.

The fifth and fourteenth amendments of the United States Constitution provide some general protection against actions of government; actions of government can be widely interpreted to include actions of those who do substantial business with the government. The Rehabilitation Act of 1973 is most often cited as the source of relief for cancer patients. This act, however, applies to "disabled" persons, and several courts have ruled that recovered cancer patients are not disabled. The Americans with Disabilities Act (ADA) provides legal protection for cancer patients against employment discrimination. As of July 26, 1994, the ADA applies to any private employer with 15 or more employees. The American Cancer Society's pamphlet 4571 details examples of the Act's provisions (Table 87–4).[1]

The main enforcement agency for the ADA is the United States Equal Employment Opportunity Commission. Under the ADA, employers are prohibited from asking about a history of cancer or requiring a medical examination before making a job offer. If a job offer is accepted, the employer is required to provide the same insurance coverage available to other employees. For persons already employed who are under treatment for cancer, "reasonable accommodations must be made by the employer to allow the person to continue to perform his or her job."

TABLE 87–4.   PRINCIPAL PROVISIONS OF THE AMERICANS WITH DISABILITIES ACT (ADA)

1. An employer cannot refuse to hire or continue employing a person with a disability, as long as that person is otherwise able and qualified to do the job.
2. An employee cannot be demoted or fired because of disability or because the employer thinks there is or will be a disability.
3. An employer cannot refuse insurance or other benefits to an employer with a disability, when the same insurance or other benefits are provided to other employees.
4. Employers must provide reasonable accommodations to persons with disabilities, if they need the help to perform their job, as long as the reasonable accommodations do not cause undue hardship to the employer.
5. The ADA covers individuals who had or have cancer.
6. Persons disabled by cancer are protected against discrimination by people who have misunderstandings about cancer.
7. Persons with disabilities are guaranteed equal access to any public facilities that are available to persons without disabilities.
8. Persons with disabilities must have access to any public transit that is available to persons without disabilities in the same city or town including bus, rail, or any other method of travel, except aircraft.
9. Persons with disabilities will have equal access to communication services that are available to persons without disabilities.

Adapted from American Cancer Society: Americans with Disabilities Act: Legal protection for cancer patients against employment discrimination. No. 4571. Atlanta, American Cancer Society, 1993.

Those reasonable accommodations may include schedule changes to allow rest or time for treatment, borrowing sick days from future years, working from home when appropriate, or job sharing. It can now be said that legal safeguards exist to protect people with cancer from the type of employment discrimination so prevalent in the past.[1]

PRACTICAL ASPECTS OF CARE

The authors' strategy for the office-based practice includes a hospital-provided "package" that includes an abbreviated length of stay combined with preoperative and postoperative education regarding disability.* "The healing begins before the treatment starts. . . " is a motto appropriate to this approach. Psychosocial assessment and support begins informally with the initial visit to evaluate a palpable or mammographic abnormality. Survival and preservation of choice are emphasized, recognizing that these are the two primary concerns of women when a breast abnormality is discovered. Needle biopsy—free hand or guided—preserves choice, lowers risk of infection, is less threatening, and avoids an operating room encounter with its attendant anxieties and loss

---

*Life After Cancer. Marie Garner, Director of Surgical Services. Videotape. Baptist Health System–Princeton, December 1994. Contact Person: Angela Collins, Surgical CNA, Baptist Health System–Princeton, 701 Princeton Ave., Birmingham, AL 35211.

of control. After a diagnosis of malignancy is rendered, there is opportunity to assess coping skills, personal support network, the employment and insurance environment, and the attitude of the spouse. Directed counseling is made easier by avoiding an atmosphere of urgency. The liberal use of second opinions—surgical, reconstructive, medical, medical oncology, radiation oncology—can facilitate an informed decision and at the same time provide the patient a sense of control and confidence. A hospital-based surgical interdisciplinary team developed a videotape that is given to women undergoing surgery for breast cancer at the preoperative visit, the morning postoperatively, or at discharge depending on the individual circumstances.* The tape provides specific verbal, written, and visual instruction on wound and drain care and on convalescence. It also contains interviews with a number of women who have "experienced just what you're going through," which helps lessen the sense of isolation, frankly introduces issues of sexuality, and encourages assertive communication. Our operative strategy includes many of Petrek's principles[28]:

1. Avoid axillary dissection when reasonable.
2. Limit axillary dissection consonant with reasonable oncological principles.
3. Preserve intercostal brachial nerve and lateral pectoral nerves.
4. Use short axillary drains.
5. Use preoperative antibiotics.
6. Avoid dressings that constrict shoulder movement.

Postoperative stay is usually 24 hours and, after discharge, a visiting nurse monitors drain care. Patients are instructed in the videotape to bring an analgesic for the first postoperative visit to help relieve any pain caused by drain removal. The Reach to Recovery visit is made in the surgeon's office at this visit or a subsequent one or, alternatively, at the American Cancer Society's office.[2] Instructions for arm care and shoulder exercises are given verbally and in written form (Table 87–5).[3] The tape includes visual demonstration of simple shoulder exercises. One month postoperatively, shoulder motion is assessed by physical examination and by a checklist questionnaire (see Table 87–2).[45] STRETCH is suggested and prosthetic recommendations are made at this time. At 3 months, the "permissive" step in sexual rehabilitation is initiated by a simple question about problems with intimate relations. Depending on the relative rapport, this question is asked by either the surgeon or the office nurse. The arms are examined for signs of lymphedema, and shoulder motion and strength are assessed. If the STRETCH program has not been used, exercise is encouraged. Patients at high risk for lymphedema may require

*Life After Cancer. Marie Garner, Director of Surgical Services. Videotape. Baptist Health System–Princeton, December 1994. Contact Person: Angela Collins, Surgical CNA, Baptist Health System–Princeton, 701 Princeton Ave., Birmingham, AL 35211.

TABLE 87–5. ARM CARE

1. Have blood drawn, blood pressure taken, and injections given in the opposite arm.
2. Pay early and careful attention to cuts, bites, or burns.
3. Wear gloves for gardening and other hazardous activities.
4. Use thimbles when sewing.
5. Push cuticles back rather than cutting.
6. Be careful with underarm shaving.
7. Avoid heavy lifting.
8. Avoid tight constriction.
9. Avoid sunburn.
10. Use deodorant rather than antiperspirant.

Adapted from American Cancer Society: Mastectomy: A Patient Guide. Rev. ed. No. 4600. Atlanta, American Cancer Society, 1994.

some modification of the instructions. Job and insurance caveats are provided. If surveillance visits are allowed, specific examinations to detect recurrence, new primaries, or indications of disability are addressed. If surveillance visits are not permitted, the discharge letter to the primary physician outlines recommended oncological surveillance as well as surveillance for early detection of disabilities, along with an invitation for re-referral should any signs of recurrence, a new primary, or disability occur.

THE TEAM APPROACH

Rehabilitation is important in the treatment of women with breast cancer and is applicable to all women who have it.[12] As in any treatment, accurate assessment of the problems and competent interventions are needed. Cancer care is a prototype of multidisciplinary care with the team approach. Rehabilitation fits well into this concept.[46] The team composition will vary in different environments and must often be extended beyond the primary treatment group (see Table 87–1).[34, 38] The concept of an extended team is useful because it allows a treatment unit of any size to avail itself of community or regional resources or to use a specially organized group such as STRETCH to expand its expertise and effectiveness.[14]

A satisfactory assessment instrument is an astute and sensitive physician or nurse involved in treatment. A questionnaire is followed by an interview with a nurse clinician, counselor, or other trained professional as a thorough and efficient means, although not without bias, of identifying psychosocial problems.[10] Physical restrictions can be quantitated by physical and occupational therapists.

Interventions, in the same way, may require little more than the immediate treatment group, family, and friends. Beyond these, there are many resources of professionals and volunteers who can become part of the extended team.

Professionals. These include those in physical therapy, occupational therapy, psychological care, pastoral care, sexual therapy, and vocational rehabilitation counseling.

Volunteer. The American Cancer Society has long been in the forefront of rehabilitation activities.[12] Reach to Recovery has been an extremely successful program. A specially trained volunteer who has had breast cancer visits the woman in the postoperative, or occasionally, the preoperative period to provide an information list, a temporary prosthesis, and first-hand experience with encouragement. The program has been expanded to include a group for husbands of married patients.[2]

The American Cancer Society also has information and referral services, transportation services, loan and gift items, and financial assistance. Additionally, it sponsors or supports community programs such as TOUCH, STRETCH, Bosom Buddies, and others that provide a variety of services.

For the optimal functioning of the team—especially the extended team—the involvement, leadership, and direction of the physician is desirable, if not essential.

Stretch*

STRETCH (Strength Through Recreation Exercise Togetherness Care Help) is an exercise-based rehabilitation program for women that began in February 1985 (Fig. 87–1). Inspired by a number of women with breast cancer who left group exercise programs and requested private instruction, a local instructor broached the problem with the Lurleen B. Wallace Cancer Center, the National Cancer Institute–designated Comprehensive Cancer Center at the University of Alabama in Birmingham.[16]

A pilot project was begun in collaboration with the community's surgeons, physical and occupational therapists, oncology counselors, and others. The women were studied for physical and psychosocial disabilities before, during, and after completion of an 8-week exercise program. Using that information and help from the Alabama Division of the American Cancer Society, a standardized regimen of exercise and education was established.

Specifically designed for postsurgery patients, the exercise routines consist of five major segments:

*STRETCH: A program of the American Cancer Society, Mid-South Division. Address: 504 Brookwood Boulevard, Birmingham, AL 35209. Contact person: Lori Langer.

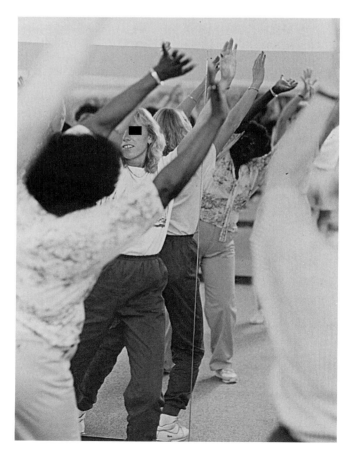

Figure 87–1 *Stretch program.*

1. *Warm-up* (10 to 15 minutes). Slow rhythmic head-neck exercises; gentle stretching and flexibility routines; arm-leg and arm-shoulder motions; all done slowly and deliberately.

2. *Floor Routine* (10 minutes). Abdominal exercises, including curls and sit-backs (no sit-ups); back, leg, and static stretches; all at a smooth rhythmic pace.

3. *Upper Body Concentration* (10 minutes). Mobility improvements; exercises require use of a dowel to position arm, hand, and shoulder correctly.

4. *Cool Down* (10 to 15 minutes). Relaxation routines.

5. *Group Discussion* (30 minutes). Speakers are periodically invited to address the group on educational, service, and social topics relating to the group's needs or requests.[16]

What began as an exercise program became a support group. The need for exercise is consistently reported as the reason for entering the program and physical improvement as the most important benefit. However, emotional support, which is seldom listed as a reason for entering the program, is cited as the second most important benefit.[16]

The physical benefits are improvement in flexibility and strength, reduction of arm swelling, endurance, becoming "two-handed" again, and the sense of well-being that comes with fitness. The exercises are designed for this purpose. The psychosocial benefits first come from seeing that other women do not look "funny" in exercise clothing. The education sessions are directed at basic information about the disease, but also at reconstruction, clothing styles, sexual adjustment, assertiveness, and a number of optional topics. The sessions involving reconstruction evolved quickly into a personal demonstration of results by women who had undergone a variety of operations. The camaraderie that permeates the group fosters intense personal interaction monitored and directed by professionals. These shared experiences and discussions in a loosely controlled environment among women ostensibly brought together for the purpose of exercise has enabled the program to function as a support group. The support, however, is not crisis intervention, but rather is directed at the common problems experienced by most women with breast cancer. The value of this program lies in its simplicity, reproducibility, attention to both physical and psychosocial disabilities, and applicability to most women with breast cancer.

Acknowledgment

The authors acknowledge the invaluable help of Sandy Edwards and Natalie Taylor in the preparation of this chapter.

References

1. American Cancer Society: Americans with disabilities act: Legal protection for cancer patients against employment discrimination. No. 4571. Atlanta, American Cancer Society, 1993.
2. American Cancer Society: Exercises after breast surgery: Reach to recovery. Rev. ed. No. 4668. Atlanta, American Cancer Society, 1994.
3. American Cancer Society: Mastectomy: A patient guide. Rev. ed. No. 4600. Atlanta, American Cancer Society, 1994.
4. Anderson BL: Sexual functioning morbidity among cancer survivors. Cancer 55:1835-1842, 1985.
5. Anderson BL, Jochimsen PR: Sexual functioning among breast cancer, gynecologic cancer, and healthy women. J Consult Clin Psychol 53:25-32, 1985.
6. Annon JS: A proposed conceptual scheme for the behavioral treatment of sexual problems. *In* Behavioral Treatment of Sexual Problems. Honolulu, Enabling Systems, Inc., 1975.
7. Assa J: The intercostobrachial nerve in radial mastectomy. J Surg Oncol 6:123-126, 1974.
8. Barofsky I: Job discrimination: A measure of the social death of the cancer patient. Western States Conference on Cancer Rehabilitation. Palo Alto, Bull Publishing, 1982.
9. Barton A: Sexual rehabilitation of the cancer patient. Syllabus of rehabilitation of the cancer patient in the community hospital. Princeton, AL, Baptist Medical Center, 1984.
10. Bloom JR, Ross RD: Measurements of the psychosocial aspects of cancer: Sources of bias. *In* Cohen J, Cullen JW, Martin LR (eds): Psychosocial Aspects of Cancer. New York, Raven Press, 1982.
11. Brennan MJ: Lymphedema following the surgical treatment of breast cancer: A review of pathophysiology and treatment. J Pain Symptom Manage 7:110-116, 1992.
12. Cerra FB: A Manual for Practitioners. Atlanta, American Cancer Society, 1982.
13. Cohen MM: Psychosocial morbidity in cancer: A clinical perspective. *In* Cohen J, Cullen JW, Martin LR (eds): Psychosocial Aspects of Cancer. New York, Raven Press, 1982.
14. Dietz JH: Rehabilitation Oncology. New York, John Wiley and Sons, 1981.
15. Foldi E, Foldi M, Clodius L: The lymphedema chaos: A lancet. Ann Plast Surg 22:505-515, 1989.
16. Gaskin TA, Lo Buglio A, Kelly D, et al: STRETCH: A rehabilitation program for breast cancer. South Med J 82:467-469, 1989.
17. Holweck FG: A Biographical Dictionary of the Saints With a General Introduction to Hagiology. St. Louis, Herder Book Company, 1924.
18. Ivens D, Hoe AL, Podd CR, et al: Assessment of morbidity from complete axillary dissection. Br J Cancer 66:136-138, 1992.
19. Jansen RFM, van Geel AN, de Groot HGW, et al: Immediate versus delayed shoulder exercises after axillary lymph node dissection. Am J Surg 160:481-484, 1990.
20. Kaplan HS: A neglected issue: The sexual side effects of current treatments for breast cancer. J Sex Marital Ther 18:3-19, 1992.
21. Kiebert GM, de Haes JCJM, van de Velde CJH: The impact of breast conserving treatment and mastectomy on quality of life of early-stage breast cancer patients: A review. J Clin Oncol 9:1059-1070, 1991.
22. Knobf MKT: Primary breast cancer: Physical consequences and rehabilitation. Semin Oncol Nurs 1:214-224, 1985.
23. Lin PP, Allison DC, Wainstock J, et al: Impact of axillary lymph node dissection on the therapy of breast cancer patients. J Clin Oncol 11:1536-1544, 1993.
24. Mellette SJ: The cancer patient at work. Cancer 35:360-373, 1985.
25. Mellette SJ: Comprehensive cancer rehabilitation. Syllabus of rehabilitation of the cancer patient in the community hospital. Princeton, AL, Baptist Medical Center, 1984.
26. Miller PJ: Mastectomy: A review of psychosocial research. Health Social Work 4:60-65, 1980.
27. Nikkanen TAV, Vanharanta H, Helenius-Reunanen H: Swelling of the upper extremity, function and muscle strength of

shoulder joint following mastectomy combined with radiotherapy. Ann Clin Res 10:273-279, 1978.

28. Petrek JA, Blackwood MM: Axillary dissection: Current practice and technique. Curr Probl Surg 32:257-323, 1995.

29. Petrek JA, Peters MM, Cirrincione C, et al: A prospective randomized trial of single versus multiple drains in the axilla after lymphadenectomy. Surg Gynecol Obstet 175:405-409, 1992.

30. Petrek JA, Peters MM, Nori S, et al: Axillary lymphadenectomy: A prospective, randomized trial of thirteen factors influencing drainage, including early or delayed arm mobilization. Arch Surg 125:378-382, 1990.

31. Platt R, Zaleznik DF, Hopkins CC, et al: Perioperative antibiotic prophylaxis for herniorrhaphy and breast surgery. N Engl J Med 332:153-160, 1990.

32. Pollard R, Callum KG, Altman DG, et al: Shoulder movement following mastectomy. Clin Oncol 2:343-349, 1976.

33. Rosenbaum EH, Rosenbaum IR, Bullard JS, et al: How you can help cancer patients solve their sexual concern. Your Patient and Cancer 3:45-54, 1983.

34. Sachs SH, Davis JM, Reynolds SA, et al: Postmastectomy rehabilitation in a community hospital. J Fam Pract 11:395-401, 1980.

35. Schain WS: Breast cancer surgeries and psychosexual sequelae: Implications for remediation. Semin Oncol Nurs 1:200-205, 1985.

36. Schain WS, Edwards BK, Gorell CR, et al: Psychosocial and physical outcomes of primary breast cancer therapy: Mastectomy versus excisional biopsy and irradiation. Breast Cancer Res Treat 3:377-382, 1983.

37. Schain WS, Wellisch DK, Pasnau RO, et al: The sooner the better: A study of psychological factors in women undergoing immediate versus delayed breast reconstruction. Am J Psychiatry 142:40-46, 1985.

38. Schmid WL, Kiss M, Hibert L: The team approach to rehabilitation after mastectomy. AORN J 19:821-836, 1974.

39. Schover LR: The impact of breast cancer on sexuality, body image, and intimate relationships. CA Cancer J Clin 41:112-120, 1991.

40. Schover LR: Sexuality and Cancer: For the Woman Who Has Cancer, and Her Partner. Randers-Pehrson M (ed). Rev. ed. No. 4657-PS. New York, American Cancer Society, 1995.

41. Schover LR, Yetman RJ, Tuason LJ, et al: Partial mastectomy and breast reconstruction: A comparison of their effects on psychosocial adjustment, body image, and sexuality. Cancer 75:54-64, 1995.

42. Small EC: Psychosocial sexual issues. Obstet Gynecol North Am 21:773-780, 1994.

43. Wellisch DK: The psychologic impact of breast cancer on relationships. Semin Oncol Nurs 1:195-199, 1985.

44. Wilmoth MC, Townsend J: A comparison of the effects of lumpectomy versus mastectomy on sexual behaviors. Cancer Pract 3:279-285, 1995.

45. Wingate L: Efficacy of physical therapy for patients who have undergone mastectomies. Phys Ther 65:896-900, 1985.

46. Winick L, Robbins GF: The post-mastectomy rehabilitation group program. Am J Surg 132:599-602, 1976.

47. Witkin MH: Psychosexual counseling of the mastectomy patient. J Sex Marital Ther 4:20–28, 1978.

48. Wood KM: Intercostobrachial nerve entrapment syndrome. South Med J 71:662-666, 1978.

CHAPTER 88
DIETARY MANAGEMENT IN BREAST DISEASE

Barbara L. Winters, Ph.D., R.D., M.Ed. / Ernst L. Wynder, M.D.

OVERVIEW

In this chapter, we review the relationship between nutrition and breast cancer, with an emphasis on dietary fat intake. We also provide recommendations and guidelines to help patients optimize nutritional status. Recommendations on dietary practices are based on the role of diet in both the incidence and progression of breast cancer and on the recently promoted health recommendations for the general population[260, 261]: achieve and maintain ideal body weight, reduce fat and increase fiber intake with fruits, vegetables and grains, limit or eliminate alcohol consumption, and incorporate exercise as a life style practice. In more specific, measurable terms, the optimal diet should contain 25 percent or less calories from fat and 25 gm of fiber per day.[295] Dietary patterns to reduce the risk of breast cancer should be promoted in childhood as well as when a breast cancer patient reaches a surgeon or an oncologist. The challenge lies in translating our clinical and epidemiological knowledge on diet and breast disease into optimal dietary practices that will be adopted and maintained.

DIETARY FAT AND BREAST CANCER

In 1981, Doll and Peto[56] estimated that 35 percent of all cancer mortality in the United States was related to diet, and previously, Wynder and Gori[291] estimated that nearly 40 percent of cases of cancer among women is related to diet. A key element relative to dietary intake and cancer is a condition known as metabolic overload, a condition of excess consumption, particularly excess fat intake.[294] The international variation in breast cancer incidence rates and the changes in incidence among migrant populations[214] have pointed to a high fat intake, or metabolic overload, as a significant factor influencing risk of and mortality from this disease. A marked number of ongoing animal studies and striking evidence compiled over the last 50 years[28, 73] supports the concept that high-fat diets promote tumor development and progression, and that dietary fat also influences the metastatic dissemination of breast tumor cells.[156, 216, 217] These studies are backed by data showing a variety of mechanisms by which fat exerts its effect.

Animal Studies and Fat

In the early 1940s, using a mouse model, Tannenbaum and Silverstone[248] demonstrated that a high-fat diet stimulated mammary tumor development when compared to a low-fat diet (12 percent versus 3 percent fat). In further studies, the effect was demonstrated to be independent of caloric intake, and the response to fat was nonlinear, with a plateau at around 16 percent fat (wt/wt). Later, in the 1960s, studies[29, 69] showed that the tumor-enhancing effect of fat was exerted during the promotional phase of mammary carcinogenesis in rats and mice. Similar findings in transplanted mammary tumor models[1] also support the idea that fat acts after the initiating event because transplantable tumors have progressed through all but the metastatic stage of carcinogenesis. These studies have been extended to include the last and most lethal stage in carcinogenesis, the metastatic stage. Katz and Boylan,[134] using a metastatic rat mammary tumor model, and Rose and colleagues,[213, 216, 217] using human breast cancer cells inoculated into nude mice, demonstrated that high-fat intake significantly increased the size and the number of pulmonary metastases compared with mice fed low-fat diets.

Mechanistic Studies

A variety of mechanisms have been proposed to explain the tumor-promoting effects of dietary fat, adding additional weight for a causal effect.[274] These mechanisms can be categorized as having either indirect or direct effects. Indirect effects include the effects of fat on (1) the hypothalamus-pituitary axis, which influences hormone levels as well as regulators of plasma hormones*; (2) membrane-bound enzymes such as mixed function oxidases, which regulate estrogen catabolism;[165] (3) structural and functional changes in cell membranes resulting in alterations of hormone growth factors and other cellular receptors;[274] and (4) immune functions including T and B cells and natural killer cell recognition activities.[97, 129, 130, 192] Direct effects of fat include the (1) conversion of essential fatty acids to eicosanoids (short-lived hormones) that are related to breast cancer promotion (primarily eicosanoids derived from linoleic acid from the omega-6 family of fatty acids);[38, 43, 104, 156, 214] (2) reactions between oxygen and the conjugated double bonds in polyunsaturated fatty acids, leading to reactive oxygen species, which, in turn, induce DNA damage;[54–56, 62, 81, 164, 190] and (3) interaction between fatty acids and genomic DNA, leading to alterations in gene expression.†

---

*See references 13, 24, 78, 90, 124, 187, 193, 211, and 215.
†See references 34, 36, 64, 66, 211, 216, 249, and 253.

HUMAN STUDIES AND BREAST CANCER

Ecologic and Descriptive Epidemiological Studies

The animal work and the supporting mechanistic studies on the link between fat intake and breast cancer incidence and mortality are consistent with intercountry comparisons correlating the effect of fat over wide ranges of intake.[86] Breast cancer incidence varies widely between those countries with the highest and lowest fat intakes.[214] The age-adjusted incidence of breast cancer varies from 22 per 100,000 in Japan to 68 per 100,000 in the Netherlands.[5] Similarly, survival rates of breast cancer are greater in Japan than in Western countries.[290] The ratio of premenopausal and postmenopausal breast cancer mortality between the United States and Japan is 3:1 and 8:1, respectively,[180, 191] and cannot be explained by known prognostic factors, except perhaps by a low-fat diet[290] and leanness.[33] The international correlations between per-capita fat intake and age-adjusted mortality rates from breast cancer are approximately 0.8.[27, 205, 293]

Evidence from descriptive epidemiology also supports the international correlations, suggesting that cultural factors or life styles, especially diet, are important etiological factors in the development of breast cancer. In general, breast cancer rates shift toward those prevalent in the country to which the women migrate.[197, 198, 303] Japanese migrant women living in Hawaii have a higher incidence of breast cancer than Japanese women living in Japan consuming traditional foods.[140] Genetic differences do not account for ethnic variation in breast cancer mortality rates. The age-standardized incidence ratio of breast cancer in Chinese-American women is 2.3 relative to native Chinese women, but 0.55 relative to the white American population.[300] These differences are not due to menstrual and reproductive factors,[303] but are believed to reflect the adoption of Western diets among the Chinese migrants.[296]

Although this evidence is strong, it has been suggested that there may exist confounding environmental and reporting factors associated with dietary fat intake.[203, 276] International correlations between fat disappearance data and breast cancer incidence do not indicate whether those individuals with high fat intakes within the country are the ones who get the disease. That is, relations at the group level or aggregate data might not accurately reflect relationships among individuals. Further, it has been suggested that epidemiological evidence may be confounded by known risk factors associated with breast cancer. Women who live in more Westernized, affluent countries generally eat more fat, have an earlier age of menarche, deliver their first child later in life, have lower parity, and have minimal levels of physical activity compared with women in Eastern countries. All of these factors are associated with increased risk. However, none of them, either alone or in combination, explain all the global variations in breast cancer.[102, 185, 198]

Dietary Fat and Breast Cancer Recurrence

From a clinical perspective, the data supporting an association between dietary fat intake and clinical outcome for patients with established breast cancer also comes from epidemiological studies comparing survival of breast cancer patients in the United States and Japan.[163, 186, 222, 290] In these studies, stage-for-stage survival rates of patients with resected breast cancer was consistently and significantly greater in Japan, where dietary fat consumption is low, compared with those of the United States, where fat consumption is twice as high. At the time of this initial observation, dietary fat intake as a percent of calories was approximately three times higher in the United States compared with that of Japan: 37 percent versus 11 percent, respectively.[163] Recent observations of the natural history of breast cancer in Japanese and American women confirm the earlier observations.[185] The survival difference reported in epidemiological studies comparing fat intake with breast cancer survival are of the same magnitude as the benefit currently identified for systemic adjuvant tamoxifen or chemotherapy use in these patient groups.[58] Although little difference in survival rates was seen in premenopausal patients, Sakamoto and associates[222] identified a 93 percent greater 10-year survival rate for postmenopausal patients with localized disease in Japan compared with that of the United States. These differences cannot be explained by known prognostic factors.[290] In fact, prognostic studies of women with postmenopausal breast cancer show increased recurrence with increasing intake of fat.[88, 103, 272] Such provocative epidemiological results do not establish a causal relationship between dietary fat intake and survival of breast cancer patients but suggest a potential magnitude of effect worth prospective evaluation.

Case-Control and Cohort Studies

Although not all studies are supportive,[145] there are a number of case-control studies that demonstrate a strong association between dietary fat intake and breast cancer risk in both premenopausal and postmenopausal women[161, 176, 200] Kushi and associates[144] reported a modest positive association of total fat intake with risk of breast cancer in a study of 34,388 postmenopausal women from Iowa. A number of smaller case-control studies, summarized in a meta-analysis by Howe and coworkers,[109] have demonstrated a weak positive association. Four of the 12 studies in the meta-analysis showed positive associations between fat intake and breast cancer risk, and the pooled data from all studies showed a significant but weak association for both total and saturated fat in postmenopausal women. In contrast to the supportive case-control studies, Graham and associates[84] compared the fat intake of 2024 breast cancer cases with 1463 controls and found that both animal fat and total fat intake were nearly identical in the two groups.

Conflicting results have also been reported in prospective studies.[11, 112, 278, 286] The Nurses Health Study by Willett and colleagues[278, 286] has not supported the inverse relationship of fat intake with breast cancer. Also, a pooled analysis (which included the Nurses Health Study) of seven prospective studies reported by Hunter and coworkers[119, 120, 123] found no evidence of a positive association between total dietary fat intake and the risk of breast cancer. The authors of this study suggested that lowering the total intake of fat in midlife is unlikely to substantially reduce the risk of breast cancer. However, "lowering" implies that we know what the optimally or ideally low level is. The definition of low fat often differs among research groups. Researchers have defined low fat ranging from 30 percent to 20 percent calories from fat. It is uncertain whether a lower fat intake than has been reported in most studies to date could be protective. Further conclusions on the effect of lower fat diets have been made on few cases. Only 1.7 percent of the cases in Hunter and associates' pooled analysis consumed less than 20 percent fat calories.[119]

Another reason for the inconsistent findings in cohort and case-control studies is that many studies examine fat intake in smaller, higher level ranges (25–30 percent of calories from fat).[162, 266, 275] Insufficient variation in fat intake within countries like the United States makes it nearly impossible to establish potential differences even if they do exist. Within a defined population such as exists in the United States, virtually everyone may be "over exposed" in terms of calorie and especially fat intake.[289, 292] Therefore, the so-called overexposed control group phenomenon appears to be responsible in part for the inconsistent results. Another difficulty with these studies is that the research populations may be underreporting fat intake because of a "social desirability" bias.[96] There is a tendency for individuals to report intakes consistent with acceptable social norms, such as eating a low-fat diet, as conveyed by the media and the popular press.

The inconsistent results in case and cohort studies may also result from a threshold effect of fat intake, which suggests that a threshold may exist above which risk is no longer enhanced by increasing fat consumption. Using the animal models, Cohen and colleagues[39] and others[298] provide evidence suggesting a threshold point between 20 percent and 30 percent fat calories. Recently Tang and coworkers[247] reported results consistent with the threshold hypothesis. No difference in mammary tumor incidence was reported in animals fed 5 percent to 25 percent or in those fed 30 percent to 40 percent energy from fat. However, when they combined the data from both groups, it clearly showed that mammary tumor incidence was significantly higher in the 30 percent to 40 percent fat intake groups compared with the 5

percent to 25 percent fat intake group. These results suggest that one reason for the null effect may be that the lowest percent of intake in the population lies above the hypothetical threshold. Human studies support the likelihood of a threshold effect, reporting no relationship between dietary fat and breast cancer risk over a range of fat intake between 44 percent and 28 percent of total energy.* Another unresolved question is whether fat intake earlier in life may influence the incidence of breast cancer.[45] Prospective studies of fat intake and breast cancer have involved only middle-aged women.

EXCESS CALORIES AND SPECIFIC FATTY ACIDS AND OILS

Excess Calories

Some experiments have been interpreted to suggest that the effect of a high-fat diet in breast cancer is entirely attributable to increased caloric intake.[142, 143] However, analysis of the collective animal literature reveals a specific enhancing effect of dietary fat, with a separate enhancing effect of calories.[73] The type and the amount of fat appears to be an important determinant of the effect on disease.[29] In animal model studies, specific types of fat exert different effects under high-fat conditions, arguing against the possibility that the tumor-promoting effects of fat are due simply to its high caloric content.[143] Nonetheless, as distinct from fat, excess caloric intake may be of importance in humans, especially when overnutrition leads to obesity. Interestingly, in animal models, the only modulation of diet that consistently maintains maximal longevity is caloric restriction.[168]

Specific Fatty Acids and Oils

Although all fats provide identical caloric loads, there are distinctive effects of different fats on mammary carcinogenesis. In rodent models, omega-6 polyunsaturated fats (e.g., corn, sunflower, and safflower oil) are strong cancer promoters, particularly the omega-6 fatty acid, linoleic acid.[126, 149] In contrast, the omega-9–rich monounsaturated oils (e.g., olive, peanut, and canola oil) appear neutral.[38] Data also suggest that omega-3–rich polyunsaturated fats (marine-based/fish oils) are protective.[42, 241] The relationship between specific fats and cancer also holds true for the metastatic process. The growth and metastasis of transplantable human breast tumors is suppressed by high levels of omega-3 fatty acids but is enhanced by omega-6 fatty acids.[216]

Human studies corroborate the animal research on the effect of different fats. Recent dietary studies support the observation that consumption of omega-9–rich, monounsaturated fat does not increase the risk of breast cancer. Women in southern Europe who

---

*See references 101, 127, 133, 146, 161, 176, 178, 209, 254, and 275.

consume more monounsaturated fat (olive oil) than their northern neighbors have a lower incidence of breast cancer.[63, 79, 166, 258, 259] The high intake of marine mammals and fish in the Eskimo and Japanese diets and the associated high blood levels of the omega-3 fatty acid, eicosapentanoic acid, is linked with the low breast cancer rates in these populations.[131, 153] In contrast, several studies suggest that the high consumption of animal fat from red meat rich in saturated fat increases the incidence of cancer. Meat and whole milk, which contribute approximately 40 percent and 20 percent of fat, respectively, in the adult American diet, are positively associated with hormone-related cancers.[171, 179, 235] Red meat is not only an important source of saturated fat in the diet, it is also a major contributor to dietary cholesterol, thus having negative effects on both carcinogenesis and cardiovascular incidence. It has been suggested that red meat consumption may be excessive in Western cultures.[279]

SUMMARY: BREAST CANCER AND DIETARY FAT

Before any conclusions are drawn from case-control and cohort studies, the composite of research on the relationship of fat intake to breast cancer must be weighed. The extensive evidence from animal and ecological studies demonstrates the strength of association between fat intake and breast cancer. Furthermore, this relationship is supported by a substantial amount of data on the plausible biological effects of fat on breast tissue biomechanisms such as hormone metabolism, oxidative damage, and immune function. There is no question that rates of breast cancer are higher in countries with a higher per capita consumption of fat. It is unclear whether a lower intake of fat than has been studied to date could be protective. Data from animal studies suggest that there is a threshold effect that may be at or below 25 percent of calories from fat. Another unresolved question is whether fat intake earlier in life may influence the incidence of breast cancer.

OTHER NUTRITIONALLY RELATED FACTORS: OBESITY/EXCESS WEIGHT, BODY MASS INDEX, BODY FAT DISTRIBUTION, AND HEIGHT AND AGE AT MENARCHE

Obesity/Excess Weight and Body Mass Index

A number of studies* but not all[65, 87, 95, 236, 283] have suggested that obesity or excess weight may be associated with poor prognosis and greater breast cancer recurrence or mortality. A study of 8427 women with

---

*See references 12, 19, 23, 26, 48, 53, 229, 256, 270, and 299.

breast cancer identified a death rate 1.7 times higher for women with initially localized cancer who were in the highest percentile of body mass compared to those in the lowest percentile.[257] The association has been reported more consistently in postmenopausal than premenopausal women and in women with less advanced than in those with more advanced disease.[82] Possible explanations for poorer prognosis among overweight women have been hypothesized, including (1) it may be harder to detect early stage breast cancer in the obese, making advanced diagnosis more common; (2) the increased endogenous estrogen level of obese women may accelerate metastasis; and (3) obesity is a marker of another adverse dietary contributor, such as excess fat intake. Relative to these hypotheses, Zhang and associates[299] reported that obesity was associated with more advanced disease at diagnosis and that obesity was a statistically significant predictor of mortality in age-adjusted but not multivariately adjusted results. This finding supports the first hypothesis that breast cancer is more advanced in the obese patient at diagnosis because it is harder to detect, although this finding does not rule out other hypotheses.

The association of breast cancer incidence to body mass index (BMI, weight in kilograms g/height in m^2), a means to measure obesity, appears to vary according to menopausal status. Most studies support an inverse association with BMI among premenopausal women and a positive association in postmenopausal women.[114, 117]

Body Fat Distribution

Differences in body fat distribution have also been related to breast cancer risk[25, 224, 228] survivorship.[51, 52] Schapiro and colleagues[224] examined the extent of breast cancer at diagnosis in premenopausal and postmenopausal women in relation to fat distribution and found a positive association with upper body fat distribution, expressed as an increased abdomen-to-thigh skin-fold ratios. It has been suggested that the poor outcome associated with an increase in waist-hip ratio (WHR) may be related to factors associated with insulin resistance or lower serum sex hormone–binding globulin and higher free testosterone and elevated estrogen levels.[243] On the other hand Zhang and coworkers[299] reported results from a prospective study of postmenopausal women that showed that WHR was unrelated to survival after breast cancer. They concluded that overall adiposity, not its distribution, appears to be the link between obesity and higher breast cancer mortality rates.

Weight Gain Associated with Adjuvant Therapy

Against these background observations on body weight, it is recognized that there is a tendency for breast cancer patients receiving adjuvant chemotherapy to gain weight.[17, 26, 31, 48, 53, 71, 94] Weight gains of between 2.5 and 6.2 kg have been associated with chemotherapy regimens, both with and without prednisone. In a population of 646 breast cancer patients, Camoriano and coworkers[26] showed that adjuvant therapy–associated weight increase adversely influences breast cancer patient survival. After 7 years of follow-up, premenopausal women gaining more than the median weight at 1 year after being on chemotherapy were 1.5 times more likely to have relapsed and 1.7 times more likely to have died than women gaining less than the median weight. Similar trends are reported for postmenopausal women.

Weight gains have also been reported in patients receiving hormonal therapy including tamoxifen, megestrol acetate, aminoglutethimide, and fluoxymesterone.[47, 107, 108, 122, 123] Each of these agents has a differential effect on weight status, an effect that may be modified by the patient's disease. In a study of early-stage patients, Hoskin and associates[107] reported significantly greater gains in weight in patients taking tamoxifen than in patients receiving local therapy alone. Weight gains were most pronounced in premenopausal women. Ingle and coworkers[122] reported a 5 to 10 percent increase in body weight in patients with metastatic disease receiving tamoxifen. In contrast, appreciable weight gain was not reported in the tamoxifen arm (10 mg bid) of Protocol B-14 of the National Breast Cancer and Bowel Project (NSABP) when compared with patients randomized to the placebo regimen (n = 2644).[68] Given the widespread use of tamoxifen, including its potential use as a preventive agent, further research investigating its use is needed.

There are few accounts of weight gain in women who receive only localized treatment (i.e., surgery alone or surgery plus radiation).[50] In one of the few studies that addressed weight gain in women randomized to surgery alone versus those who received surgery plus CMF (cyclophosphamide, methotrexate, and fluorouracil) therapy, Goodwin and associates[83] reported that weight gain may be due to the cancer itself or resulting psychosocial problems.

Although weight gain in breast cancer patients is clinically well appreciated, little research has been done to investigate the underlying mechanisms. Plausible mechanisms include changes in the rate of metabolism (i.e., resting metabolic rate, thermogenesis), physical activity, and dietary intake.[50] This area requires continued investigation because weight gain during therapy may increase the risk of recurrence. Disease-free survival and psychological research point to the profound negative impact of weight gain on the quality of life in breast cancer patients.[144, 160]

Height and Age at Menarche

There is some evidence that height,[23, 86, 302] possibly an indicator of early childhood nutrition,[241] is related to breast cancer. Most case-control studies suggest a modest positive association between attained height and risk of breast cancer.[117] Data from women in Europe who were infants during World War II and who experienced famine show that the shorter women, presumably those who experienced more deprivation, have a lower incidence of breast cancer.[269, 270] In the National Health and Nutrition Examination Survey I (NHANES I), Swanson and associates[245] observed a significant increased risk with increased height. However, height is not consistently related to breast cancer in other studies.[158, 301] For example, height was not associated with breast cancer risk in premenopausal women and was only weakly associated in postmenopausal women in the Nurses Health Cohort Study.[158]

Ecological studies[87] indicate a correlation between age at menarche and adult height with breast cancer rates. It has been suggested that more advanced age at menarche in Japan may account for as much as 40 percent of the differences between rates in the United States. However, an analysis by Prentice and colleagues[204] showed no significant effect of age at menarche after controlling for per capita fat disappearance.

VITAMINS, MINERALS, AND BREAST CANCER

Antioxidant Vitamins A, C, and E

Vitamin A

Experimental studies provide data on the beneficial effects of vitamin A with breast cancer.[237] Retinol inhibits the growth of human breast carcinoma cells in vitro,[72] and retinyl acetate reduces breast cancer incidence in rodent models.[163, 183, 184] Data from human studies, with both preformed vitamin A as retinol and retinyl esters, as well as the carotenoids, are not conclusive, but suggest a possible protective effect.[116, 201, 279] Howe and colleagues' meta-analysis results from 12 studies[109] showed that total vitamin A (preformed vitamin and carotenoids) had a significant apparent protective effect against breast cancer. However, when they distinguished between both forms of vitamin A, they found a significant effect for beta-carotene in eight studies but no associations for preformed vitamin A. Prospective studies on vitamin A intake and breast cancer from New York[132] and California[196] found nonsignificant inverse associations, and a Canadian study[209] found a marginally significant association. The Nurses' Health Study[121] found a modest but significant association with preformed vitamin A that was slightly more strongly associated with lower risk of breast cancer than was intake of carotenoids. The Nurses' Health Study also examined the effect of vitamin A supplements and the risk of breast cancer. This study indicated that supplement intake may be beneficial for those with low dietary intake but was unlikely to reduce risk of breast cancer in women who already consume sufficient vitamin A in their diet.[121] Another recent study with premenopausal women also does not demonstrate a beneficial effect of vitamin A supplementation; these authors suggest that vitamin A may just be a marker for other anticarcinogenic factors in vitamin A–rich foods.[74]

Vitamins C and E

The weight of evidence to date from human studies cannot determine whether there is a protective effect of vitamins C and E against breast cancer. Two case-control studies on vitamin C by the same group reached conflicting results.[84, 85] The Nurses' Health Study found no evidence of a lower risk when comparing women in the highest quintile, who were generally taking vitamin C doses of more than 500 mg/d, with those in the lowest quintile.[116] In contrast, other studies suggest a beneficial role for vitamin C. Howe and coworkers[109] reported that each 300 mg/d increase in vitamin C reduced the risk of breast cancer. A recent study by Freudenheim and colleagues[74] on the effects of fruit and vegetable intake reported a reduction in risk for breast cancer associated with vitamin C intake (odds ratio [OR] 0.53) but suggested that risk reduction may be due in part to non-nutrient components associated with vitamin C–rich foods.

Similar to studies with vitamin C, further research into vitamin E intake is required. Vitamin E has an inhibitory effect on mammary tumor incidence in rodents in some[92, 152] but not all experiments. Vitamin E blood levels correlated moderately with vitamin E intake after controlling for blood lipid livels.[284] Three case-control studies suggest a negative association between vitamin E intake and an increased risk of breast cancer, whereas other studies do not.[114] Reduced risk in premenopausal women has been recently linked with vitamin E intake with an odds ratio of 0.55.[74] London and associates[157] reported a weak inverse association with breast cancer and vitamin E intake from food sources but not with supplement intake. However, no evidence of a protective effect of vitamin E was noted in the Nurses' Health Study[121] or the European Community Multicenter Study on Antioxidants.[7] It may be that the beneficial effects of vitamin E are linked with a synergistic effect with selenium intake in the context of a low-fat diet. It has also been suggested that vitamin E could exert an effect by its impact with selenium as an antioxidant[106] or by an effect on oncogene expression.[240]

Vitamin D

Data from animal studies suggest that vitamin D deficiency may be a risk factor for mammary carcinogenesis.[128] In its active form, the vitamin has demonstrated protective effects in experimental models.[46, 188] Human studies have shown that women with vitamin D receptor–positive tumors have longer disease-free survival than those with vitamin D receptor–negative tumors,[46] and vitamin D receptor status has been proposed as a potential prognostic indicator.[14] However, a human case-control study investigating the hypothesis of vitamin D deficiency

and cancer of the breast showed no differences between patients and controls in their mean intake of the vitamin.[231] There are ongoing studies investigating the therapeutic effects of vitamin D alone as well as with other nutrients such as vitamin A.

Selenium

There is an extensive body of literature describing the protective effect of selenium on mammary carcinogenesis.[61, 125] Ecological studies have also demonstrated strong inverse associations between selenium exposure and international breast cancer rates.[35, 237] A recent case control study in Sweden[91] showed a preventive effect in breast cancer with increasing plasma selenium levels in women over the age of 50. Data from a prospective study conducted in Finland by Knekt and associates[137] showed evidence of increased risk among women with low dietary intake of selenium. Because Finland is among the countries with the lowest dietary selenium levels in the world, this is consistent with the possibility that a threshold exists below which low selenium intake does increase breast cancer risk. However, not all types of human studies support this finding.[262, 267] In a prospective study by Hunter and colleagues[115, 118] the relative risk for selenium for concentrations from highest to lowest quintiles was not different. They concluded that selenium intake later in life is not likely to be an important factor in the etiology of breast cancer. Others have also proposed that evidence appears to indicate a lack of appreciable effect of selenium intake on breast cancer risk within the range of human diets.[77] Unfortunately, selenium intake cannot be measured accurately by means of dietary assessment in geographically dispersed populations, because the selenium content of individual foods is highly variable depending on the geographical area in which the foods were grown.[154] This has made prospective studies difficult to evaluate. Also the effect of organic selenium in the context of a low-fat diet has been inadequately evaluated.

BREAST CANCER AND DIET-RELATED CONSIDERATIONS

Fruits and Vegetables

Low or inadequate intakes of fruits and vegetables in the Western diet has been linked epidemiologically to an increased risk of several cancers[15, 238–240] including breast cancer.[84, 148] People who eat greater amounts of fruits and vegetables have approximately one-half the risk and, if cancer is diagnosed, lower mortality rates from many cancers.[306] In 82 percent of 156 recently reviewed studies, it was found that fruit and vegetable consumption provides significant protection against cancer.[15] The Nurses' Health Study[121] showed that low intake of vegetables was associated with a 25 percent increase in the risk of breast cancer. The benefits associated with a diet containing fruits and vegetables are likely derived in part from adequate levels of antioxidant and other potentially beneficial nutrients. In addition, consuming a diet rich in fruits and vegetables provides a milieu of non-nutrient components called phytochemicals that appear to possess health-protective qualities.[16, 74]

Non-nutrient Food Components— Phytochemicals/Phytoestrogens

Experimental evidence demonstrates that a number of phytochemicals (non-nutrient food components produced in plants) have anticarcinogenic properties as well as estrogenic properties.[4] Non-nutrient components (e.g., allyl sulfides, phytates, isoflavones, lignans, isothiocyanates, indoles, and ellagic acid) have been linked with various metabolic pathways as well as various hormonal actions associated with the development of cancer. Dietary phytoestrogens present in foods such as legumes and grains may provide potential prevention of estrogen-dependent cancers such as breast cancer.[16, 105, 138]

Epidemiological and other human studies support the experimental evidence that the risk-reduction properties of fruits and vegetables may relate to their roles as dietary sources of phytochemicals. Human studies[3, 80, 138] have demonstrated that compounds in the diet (lignans, isoflavonoids, and plant heterocyclic phenols similar in structure to estrogens) may affect uptake and metabolism of sex hormones and thus may inhibit cancer cell growth by competing for estrogen binding sites[9, 172] or by altering the balance of estrogen metabolites. The intake of soy, a major source of isoflavonoid phytoestrogens, is associated with lower risk of breast cancer,[30, 151, 172, 288] although not all studies are conclusive.[199] Typically, Western diets are low in isoflavones. The lower incidence of and mortality rates from breast cancer in Eastern populations has been linked to this population's intake of soy.[151]

Other phytochemicals have also been associated with the incidence of breast cancer in humans. High consumption of indole-3-carbinol found in cruciferous vegetables (cabbage, brussels sprouts, broccoli, cauliflower) appears to alter the balance of estrogen metabolism toward less potent forms[20, 21, 175] and has been shown to reduce the incidence of mammary cancer in mice.[22] Research, including human studies, on indole-3-carbinol and other non-nutritive factors is ongoing and expansive.

Fiber

The increased cancer risks associated with low intake of fruits and vegetables also relate to fiber intake.[209, 212, 218, 242, 272] This is because many fruits and vegetables are excellent sources of fiber, as are cereals and grains. The protective role for dietary fiber from grains, vegetables, and fruits relative to hormone-related cancers is likely due to two actions of fiber. One action is fiber's ability to bind to estrogen, thereby reducing intestinal reabsorption. A second action is fiber's ability to change bowel microflora through promoting bacteria with low beta-glucuronidase activity, which may also lower plasma estrogens through decreasing the re-entry of estrogens into the circulation.[37]

Although there is substantial support for the anticarcinogenic effect of fiber in the diet, some studies have reported a lack of effect. The conflicting reports have been attributed to disagreements by experts on the best way to measure levels of different fibers in epidemiological studies[279, 281] and on the relative significance of the effects of different types of fibers. Both the physical form and the chemical compositions of fiber are probably biologically important. Dietary fiber is composed of crude insoluble fiber that is excreted unchanged and many soluble fiber fractions that may have different biological effects. A recent animal study by Cohen and colleagues[40] compared the inhibitory effect of different ratios of fibers, insoluble (wheat bran) and soluble (psyllium), and observed a maximum and significant reduction in mammary tumors with an equal combination of soluble and insoluble fibers. More detailed dietary data in epidemiological studies, including information on the intake of different amounts and types of fiber, is needed to accurately assess the role of fiber in human breast cancer.

Other Diet-Related Considerations

Caffeine

Caffeine consumption has been examined as a risk factor for breast cancer because elimination of caffeine from the diet has been proposed as a treatment for benign breast disease.[181, 182] However, the epidemiologic evidence does not suggest substantial increase in breast cancer risk associated with drinking coffee. Snowdon and Phillips[234] observed no increase in breast cancer risk among a cohort of Seventh-Day Adventist women who consumed coffee. Further, no association of caffeine with breast cancer incidence was observed in the Iowa Women's Study.[70] On the other hand, Hunter and coworkers[118] observed a weak but significant inverse association between caffeine consumption and breast cancer risk. Although most case-control studies show no positive association with the disease,[170, 223] a link between caffeine consumption and breast cancer cannot be ruled out.[273]

Alcohol

Reports of a possible association between alcohol intake and an increased risk of breast cancer have led to considerable epidemiological debate.[220] Most studies of this issue have suggested an association,* yet several have not.[2, 181, 219, 221] Among the studies that have found alcohol intake to be a risk factor,

---

*76, 93, 159, 160, 189, 226, and 268.

there is considerable variability in the intake required to produce a measurable increase in risk. Some studies have suggested that even low intake can have an impact,[67, 147, 150, 225, 278] whereas others have implicated the impact of only heavier drinking.[98, 255] In various studies, younger women[93, 195, 208] or older women[67, 99] seem to display the association more strongly. Although recent studies favor the association between increased risk of breast cancer and alcohol, the degree of increased risk is still uncertain. The mode of action is also unresolved, although alcohol intake has been associated with statistically significant increased rise in several estrogenic hormones.[206]

Pesticides

Although a diet high in fat may increase exposure to pesticides, this is not specifically a dietary exposure route. But, given the widespread dissemination of organochlorines in the environment and the food chain, and their association with an estrogenic effect, organochlorines have been implicated as dietary etiological agents for human breast cancer.[6] There is some evidence, although it is not consistent, to implicate polychlorinated biphenyls (PCBs) and 2,2-bis(p-chlorophenyl)-1,1,1,-trichloroethane (DDT) in increased risk of breast cancer.[141, 286] Wolff and associates[286] reported that blood levels of organochlorines such as DDT and PCBs were higher in breast cancer patients than in controls. On the other hand, other studies[141] do not support this finding. Additional research studies such as the Long Island Breast Cancer Project[75] are needed before drawing conclusions in this area.

NUTRITIONAL STRATEGIES FOR BREAST CANCER

General Dietary Recommendations

Those working in the public health sector are looked to for making recommendations as to the type and amount of foods to consume for optimal health. Tables 88–1 and 88–2 summarize general guidelines for

TABLE 88–1. DIETARY GUIDELINES FOR AMERICANS 1995

- Eat a variety of foods.
- Balance the food you eat with physical activity. Maintain or improve your weight.
- Choose a diet with plenty of grain products, vegetables, and fruits.
- Choose a diet low in total fat, saturated fat, and cholesterol.
- Choose a diet moderate in sugars.
- Choose a diet moderate in salt and sodium.
- If you drink alcoholic beverages, do so in moderation.

United States Department of Agriculture, United States Department of Health and Human Services: Nutrition and Your Health: Dietary Guidelines for Americans, 3rd ed. Washington, DC: US Government Printing Office, 1990.

TABLE 88–2. UNITED STATES DEPARTMENT OF AGRICULTURE FOOD GUIDE PYRAMID 1992

Food Categories and Recommended Servings per Day
Bread, cereal, rice, and pasta group: 6 to 11 servings
Fruit group: 2 to 4 servings
Vegetable group: 3 to 5 servings
Milk, yogurt, and cheese group: 2 to 3 servings
Fats, oils, and sweets: use sparingly

United States Department of Agriculture (USDA): USDA's Food Guide Pyramid: Home and Garden Bulletin no. 249. Hyattsville, MD; Human Nutrition Information Services, 1992.

the prevention of disease, and include the most recent dietary recommendations of several groups. The recent recommendations of the Committee on Diet and Health of the National Academy of Sciences (NAS), the *Dietary Guidelines for Americans*,[260] and the *Food Guide Pyramid*,[261] published by the U.S. Department of Agriculture (USDA), are universal recommendations for chronic disease reduction and are pertinent to breast cancer management. These recommendations focus on decreasing risks of a variety of chronic diseases and conditions, and aim to provide sufficient intake of essential nutrients.

The American Cancer Society (ACS) Guidelines for Adults[250] (Table 88–3) address a total dietary pattern

TABLE 88–3. CANCER-SPECIFIC GUIDELINES, AMERICAN CANCER SOCIETY 1996

- Choose most of the foods you eat from plant sources.
  Eat five or more servings of fruits and vegetables each day.
  Choose fruits and vegetables for snacks.

- Eat other foods from plant sources, such as breads, cereal products, rice, pasta, or beans several times each day.
  Include grain products in every meal.
  Choose whole grains in preference to processed (refined) grains.
  Choose beans as an alternative to meats.

- Limit your intake of high-fat foods, particularly from animal sources.
  Choose foods low in fat.
  Replace fat-rich foods with fruits, vegetables, grains, and beans.
  Eat smaller portions of high-fat foods.
  Choose baked and broiled foods instead of fried foods.
  Select nonfat and low-fat milk and dairy products.
  When you eat packaged snack, convenience, and restaurant foods, choose those low in fat.

- Limit your consumption of meats, especially high-fat meats.
  When you eat meat, select lean cuts.
  Eat smaller portions of meats.
  Choose beans, seafood, and poultry as an alternative to beef, pork, and lamb.
  Select baked and broiled meats, seafood, and poultry, rather than fried.

- Be physically active: achieve and maintain a healthy weight.
  Be at least moderately active for 30 minutes or more on most days.
  Stay within your healthy weight range.

- Limit consumption of alcoholic beverages, if you drink at all.

**TABLE 88–4. AMERICAN HEALTH FOUNDATION
25:25 DIETARY PLAN**

- To eat no more than 25% of calories from fat
  *A typical adult woman eating 1800 calories should eat no
  more than 50 gm of fat per day*
  *A typical adult man eating 2200 calories should eat no
  more than 60 gm of fat per day*
- Adults should eat 25 gm of fiber daily

for lowering cancer risk. The ACS Guidelines are very similar to the general recommendations (see Tables 88–3 and 88–4) but with more detailed specifications. There is also a nationwide campaign to promote increased consumption of fruits and vegetables. The National Cancer Institute–sponsored *5-a-Day for Better Health* program is designed to encourage the consumption of at least five servings of fruits and vegetables per day.[244] Unfortunately, at present, the average American is not meeting this goal.

Breast Cancer: An Optimal Diet and Guidelines; The 25:25 Diet Plan

The wealth of animal and human data supporting the potential to reduce the risk of primary or secondary breast cancer through diet is of little use unless we adopt healthy eating behaviors. We need means to translate research on an optimal diet into realistic dietary practices. As a general guide, the American Health Foundation's recommendation for an optimal diet is the *25:25 Diet*.[284, 289, 295] This diet is in line with the above general recommendations from the American Cancer Society and the National Cancer Institute's Five-a-Day program, as well as the recommendations found in the *Dietary Guidelines for Americans*, and the *Food Guide Pyramid*. For adults, the 25:25 Diet comprises 25 percent or fewer calories from fat and 25 gm of fiber per day (see Table 88–4, The American Health Foundation 25:25 Dietary Plan). Simplified food choices make it possible for individuals to follow the 25:25 plan (Tables 88–5 and 88–6, Fat and Fiber Choices).

Definitive recommendations for including more profound fat reduction (i.e., 15 percent of calories from fat) await results from the Women's Intervention Nutrition Study (WINS) and a Canadian study with high-risk women.[18] The WINS trial is a National Cancer Institute–funded dietary trial that is enrolling 2500 women from over 30 clinical sites nationwide. The objective of WINS is to determine whether dietary fat intake reduction, together with adjuvant therapy, would reduce the incidence of recurrence of early-stage breast cancer.[32, 33, 44] A similar dietary study is the Women's Health Initiative (WHI).[194, 203] The WHI, a larger study, recruiting 163,000 healthy postmenopausal women, is conducted with women for their clinical trial and observational study. As part of the WHI, they will investigate the effect of a low-fat diet on the incidence of breast disease. Findings from these and other trials will further define

our fat recommendations. Until these studies are completed, it is recommended that the public and women with newly diagnosed cancer follow a diet consisting of 25 percent or less calories from fat and 25 grams of fiber, along with the detailed recommendations of other agencies and organizations as found in Tables 88–2 and 88–3.

Childhood: Nutrition and Breast Cancer

Because cancer is a chronic condition that develops over time, with certain cancers having their inceptions during childhood, guidelines are needed for a cancer-preventive life style beginning in childhood. Studies have suggested the potential for a significant effect of diet in early life on breast cancer incidence,[45, 263] perhaps even in utero.[59, 60, 100, 113, 174, 263] It has also been suggested that at menarche, during the time of breast development, dietary factors such as a high-fat diet are influential in the later development of breast cancer.[45] This has led to the suggestion that dietary intervention programs to reduce the incidence of breast cancer should be targeted at early adolescent girls.[45]

Whereas the current level of fat intake for children is around 35 percent,[252] the dietary recommendation for children older than age 2 years is that no more than 30 percent of their total calories should come from fat,[8, 136] with suggestions that children should quickly move in the direction of adult recommendations of 25 percent or less calories from fat.[282] The average dietary fiber intake of children and adolescents, like that of adults, is probably only about half the optimal intake. The optimal fiber intake (in grams) for children is "age plus 5."[285] Therefore the recommended fiber intake for a 3 year old is 8 gm per day (3 + 5), whereas an 11 year old should consume 16 gm per day.

Guidelines for Dietary Management of Breast Cancer

Nutritional messages for breast cancer risk reduction and treatment practices must be reinforced by the medical community, both verbally and by example. The following eight guidelines are designed to be used by health professionals to help individuals adopt and maintain life style dietary practices that maximize nutritional quality.

1. *Place diet in the context of overall risk reduction strategies*: When it comes to health promotion and risk reduction, guidelines cannot focus on diet alone. Dietary recommendations for breast cancer must be in the context of recommendations for appropriate exercise levels, smoking cessation, stress reduction, and moderation in alcohol consumption.

2. *Support modifications in dietary patterns as opposed to megadoses of supplements*: Our knowledge of the risks and benefits associated with megadoses of supplements and the cancer-prevention properties of many nutrients is still evolving. Consuming a less

TABLE 88–5. FAT SUBSTITUTIONS*

Amount	Food	Fat Grams
1 tbsp	Nonfat mayonnaise, nonfat yogurt	0
1 tbsp	Mayonnaise	11
1 tbsp	Oil-free dressing	0
1 tbsp	Oil/creamy dressing	8
1 tbsp	Lemon juice, wine	0
Coated 9″ skillet with cooking spray		1
1 tbsp	Cooking oil	14
1 tbsp	Butter buds	0
1 tbsp	"Light" butter	6
1 tbsp	Butter	12
1 tbsp	Fruit preserves, jam, jelly	0
1 tbsp	Diet margarine	2
1 tbsp	Margarine	11
3 oz	1/2 whole grain bagel or 2 slices toast	1
3 oz–1 small	Bran muffin	11
3 oz–1 small	Doughnut	18
1 oz	Fat-free mozzarella	0
1 oz	Part skim mozzarella	5
1 oz	Whole milk mozzarella	6
1 oz	Fat-free cheddar cheese	0
1 oz	Reduced fat (low-fat) cheddar cheese	5
1 oz	Cheddar cheese	9
1 tbsp	Fat-free cream cheese	0
1 tbsp	Cream cheese	5
2 tbsp	Fat-free sour cream or nonfat yogurt	0
2 tbsp	Sour cream	5
1/2 cup	Fat-free cottage cheese	0
1/2 cup	1% cottage cheese	2
1/2 cup	Creamed (4%) cottage cheese	5
1 cup	Nonfat yogurt	0
1 cup	Plain low-fat yogurt	4
1 cup	Whole milk yogurt	7
1 cup	Skim milk	0
1 cup	1% low-fat milk	3
1 cup	Whole milk	8
2 oz–1/2 cup	Pasta	1
2 oz–1/2 cup	Cheese or beef ravioli	6
2″ × 2″	Lasagna	13
2 oz–1/4 cup	Tomato sauce (no oil added)	0
2 oz–1/4 cup	Alfredo sauce	16
2 oz–1/4 cup	Pesto sauce	30

than optimal diet and hoping to correct it by a magic pill or supplement are not supported by current scientific data.[202] In fact, excess intake of a single nutrient may increase risk.[7, 49, 251] Further, it has been suggested that the synergistic effects of nutrients may be more important than single nutrients.[74, 202, 239] Until more data are obtained and clinical trials are conducted, changes in total dietary patterns are preferable over modifications in specific nutrients.

3. *Keep an open mind and listen when individuals talk about their alternative practices (yet unproven or questionable remedies) related to nutrition*: Individuals and the public should be provided with strategies to deal with questionable remedies.[233] Questionable remedies can decrease the quality of life, can cause financial burden, and may be harmful. On the other hand, they may also be harmless and provide psychological benefit to an individual. There is also the potential that alternative practices may have beneficial effects that have not yet been proved via the conventional rigors of scientific inquiry.[10] Organizations such as the American Cancer Society and the Food and Drug Administration Office of Consumer Affairs can provide objective reviews of alternative treatments and help identify situations of outright fraud. We need to encourage patients to thoroughly investigate all claims.

4. *Individuals—even those with breast cancer or those trying to reduce their risk of breast cancer—still eat primarily for taste, not for nutritional or health reasons*: When the focus is on nutrition, we must consider the palatability of the food. Long-term dietary change is very closely linked to the individual's food preferences and the overall palatability of foods. All health professionals as well as food scientists and those in the food industry should be part of an interdisciplinary approach to changing what we serve and how we eat.[57]

5. *Discourage individuals from "blaming the cook" or blaming themselves for breast cancer*: Individuals with cancer, or those aiming at preventing cancer, often believe that what they eat or what they have eaten is solely responsible for causing disease. People need to be informed that diet is only one of many of the genetic and environmental factors related to the development and recurrence of cancer.[57]

TABLE 88–5. FAT SUBSTITUTIONS* *Continued*

Amount	Food	Fat Grams
1 medium	Baked potato	0
3 oz	French fries	██████████12
2 oz	Tuna packed in water	█1
2 oz	Tuna packed in oil	█████████10
3 oz	Shrimp (peel & eat)	█1
3 oz	Fried shrimp	█████████10
1 oz–1 slice	Canadian bacon	██2
1 oz–2 link	Sausage	████████8
1 oz–5 slices	Bacon	███████████12
3 oz	Turkey breast, no skin	██2
3 oz	Turkey (dark) without skin	█████5
3 oz	Turkey (dark meat) with skin	█████████10
3 oz	Chicken (light or breast) no skin	███3
3 oz	Chicken (dark) no skin	███████7
3 oz	Chicken thigh, fried with skin	█████████████14
3 oz	Beef, round tip select	████4
3 oz	Filet mignon or pot roast	████████8
3 oz	London broil or minute steak	█████5
3 oz	Hamburger, lean	█████████████14
4 oz–1/2 cup	Sorbet, frozen nonfat yogurt, or 1 fruit pop	0
4 oz–1/2 cup	Ice cream	███████7
1 oz	Fortune cookie	█1
1 oz	Fig bar	██2
	Chocolate chip cookie, graham crackers, granola bar, brownie	█████5
1 medium	Baked apple	0
3 oz–1 small slice	Apple pie	████████9
1 oz	Popcorn (air-popped), pretzels, baked chips	█1
1 oz	Potato chips	█████████10
1 oz	Salsa	0
1 oz	Guacamole	█████5
1.5 oz	Gum drops, jelly beans, licorice, marshmallows	0
1.5 oz	M & Ms	████████9
1.5 oz	Chocolate bar	█████████████14
1 oz	Chestnuts	█1
1 oz	Almonds, peanuts, walnuts	█████████████14
3 oz	Angel food cake	0
3 oz	Cheesecake	███████████████16
3 oz	Devil's food cake with icing	█████████████████18

* From the American Health Foundation 25:25 Dietary Plan.

6. *Avoid so-called good food/bad food terminology for individuals of all ages*: In considering individual foods, good food/bad food terminology does not encourage healthful food consumption practices.[57] There are dietary practices that are good or better than others in the sense that some patterns are more likely to foster good health than others. Distributing lists of bad or forbidden foods often promotes a sense of guilt. This can result in cancer patients' using diet as a means to express defiance or anger. It is important to emphasize positive choices and the social desirability of eating and drinking in healthy ways.

7. *Supports and barriers to dietary changes—do not assume that dietary change is always easy*: For a variety of reasons, including physical, social, and psychological, an individual may have difficulty achieving dietary modifications. Intentions to change do not automatically lead to the corresponding behavior.[57] Likewise, nutrition knowledge does not always translate into healthy behavior. A nutritional regimen that does not fit into the individual's cul-tural or age-related needs may be ignored or followed inconsistently.[89] For long-term life style modifications, dietary risk reduction plans should be tailored to fit the individual's favored foods and cultural preferences.[89] Effective strategies for shaping eating behavior and healthy lifelong eating habits recognize that occasional lapses are inevitable and are unlikely to be critical in the long term. Several factors contribute to a diminished adherence or the lack of commitment to changing or maintaining dietary patterns including a history of defeats, a negative attitude, and self-doubt.[232] Most times, these barriers to change can be overcome. The best source of information on disease and individualized dietary plans and dietary relapse prevention is a nutritionist with an expertise in oncology.

8. *Research is ongoing, and recommendations change as new data are generated*: There are ongoing trials investigating how various nutritive (e.g., vitamin A, ascorbic acid, fiber sources) and non-nutritive substances (e.g., lignans, phytoestrogens) may inhibit or promote carcinogenesis. As results become

TABLE 88–6. FIBER CONTENT OF VARIOUS FOODS

	Food	Fiber (g)
1/2 cup	Wheat bran cereal	13
1 cup	Whole grain/wheat cereal or oatmeal	4–7
1 cup	Dried beans	6–9
1/2 cup	Dried apricots	6
1/4 cup	Wheat germ	4
1 whole	Whole wheat English muffin	4
1/2 cup	Dried apples	4
1 cup	Blueberries	4
1/2 cup	Sweet potato	4
1 cup	Brown rice	3
2 slices	Whole wheat bread	3
1 cup	Applesauce	3
1 medium	Apple, banana, or orange	3
1/2 cup	Raisins	3
1 cup	Strawberries	3
2	Dried figs	3
1/2 cup	Brussels sprouts	3
1 medium	Baked potato	2
1/2 cup	Cooked broccoli, cabbage, corn, or spinach	2
1/2 cup	Cooked carrots, parsnips, or green peas	2
1 cup	Vegetable juice	2
1 cup	Fruit nectar	2
2 slices	Raisin bread	2

available, revisions of recommendations may be made. Radical changes in recommendations are unlikely.

SUMMARY AND CONCLUSIONS

The predominant message that emerges from the data on nutrition and breast cancer points to the supporting role of dietary fat as well as a variety of biologically plausible mechanisms by which the promoting effect of fat could occur. There are few other nutrients that demonstrate so compelling a role in the development or the progression of breast cancer. The data on antioxidant vitamins seem to demonstrate the potential protective effect of vitamin A and a weakly positive protective effect of vitamin C with not enough evidence for evaluating vitamin E. The role of selenium as an inhibitory agent of breast cancer is inconclusive, as are the synergistic effects of vitamin E and selenium. Overall, more work needs to be undertaken to investigate the mechanisms of the antioxidant vitamins as a form of protection against human breast cancer. Data on the relationship of alcohol intake to breast cancer incidence is accumulating, but the degree of the risk and exposure is unresolved. Data is not conclusive about the breast cancer–preventing properties of a number of specific micronutrients because the optimal levels are yet to be defined. Further, there are no recommendations on dietary phytochemicals because our knowledge of the associated risks and benefits from phytochemicals is far from complete. Thus, the recommendation is for an overall modification of total dietary patterns rather than the administration of individual agents, the exception being the case of

very high risk populations in whom potent chemopreventive agents are being tested.

One effective means to address breast cancer risk reduction appears to be through dietary prevention in childhood, although much more work is needed on the relationship of nutrition in early life to breast cancer. At the other end of the spectrum, it is clear that secondary prevention is worth preaching at the point when a breast cancer patient reaches a surgeon or an oncologist, as demonstrated by epidemiological and animal studies that support a beneficial role for diet after cancer has occurred. Human studies supporting the benefits of dietary modifications to prevent disease recurrence, such as the Women's Intervention Nutrition Study,[32, 33] are ongoing. As more research into the genetics of breast cancer emerges, it will become more important to understand the nutritional factors in this disease in the context of genetic risk factors.

The conclusions and implications for women in terms of what type of diet could be beneficial to them are the same as those that have been promoted by all health groups in recent years: maintain ideal body weight; reduce fat and increase fiber intake (25:25 plan); eat plenty of fruits, vegetables, and grains; limit alcohol consumption; and increase exercise as a life style practice. The challenge lies in translating our clinical and epidemiological knowledge about diet and breast disease into optimal dietary practices that will be adopted and successfully maintained through life.

References

1. Abraham S, Hillyard LA: Effect of dietary 18 carbon fatty acids on growth of transplantable mammary adenocarcinoma in mice. J Natl Cancer Inst 71:601–608, 1983.

2. Adami HO, Lund E, Bergstrom R, Meirik O: Cigarette smoking, alcohol consumption and risk of breast cancer in young women. Br J Cancer 58:832–837, 1988.

3. Adlercreutz H, Hockerstedt K, Bannerwart C, Hamalainen E, Fotsis T, Bloigu S: Association between dietary fiber level, urinary excretion of lignans and isoflavonic phytoestrogens, and plasma nonprotein bound sex hormones in relation to breast cancer. Prog Cancer Ther 35:409–412, 1988.

4. Adlercreutz H, Moousavi Y, Clark J, Hockerstedt K, Hamalainen E, Wahala K, Makela T, Hases T: Dietary phytoestrogens and cancer: In vitro and in vivo studies. J Steroid Biochem Mol Biol 41:331, 1992.

5. Age-standardized incidence rates, four-digit rubrics, and age-standardized and cumulative incidence rates, three-digit rubrics. Cancer incidence in five continents. IARC Scientific Publications 120:871–1011, 1992.

6. Ahlborg UG, Lipworth L, Titus-Ernstoff L, Hsieh CC, Hanberg A, Baron J, Trichopoulos D, Adami HO: Organochlorine compounds in relation to breast cancer, endometrial cancer, and endometriosis: An assessment of the biological and epidemiological evidence. Review. Crit Rev Toxicol 25:463–531, 1995.

7. Albanes D, Heinonen, OP, Taylor PR, et al: α-Tocopherol and β-carotene supplements and lung cancer incidence in the Alpha-tocopherol, Beta-carotene Cancer Prevention Study: Effects of base-line characteristics and study compliance. J Natl Cancer Inst 88: 21:1560–1570, 1996.

8. American Academy of Pediatrics Committee on Nutrition: Statement on cholesterol. Pediatrics 90:469, 1992.

9. Barnes S: Effect of genistein on in vitro and in vivo models of cancer. Review. J Nutr 125 (3 Suppl):777S–783S, 1995.

10. Barrett S: Health schemes, scams, and frauds. New York: Consumer Reports Books, 1990.

11. Barrett-Connor E, Friedlander NJ: Dietary fat, calories, and the risk of breast cancer in postmenopausal women: A prospective population-based study. J Am Coll Nutr 12:390, 1993.

12. Basarrachea Jorge, Hortobagyi GN, Smith TL, Shu-Wan CK, Buzdar AU: Obesity as an adverse prognostic factor for patients receiving adjuvant chemotherapy for breast cancer. Ann Intern Med 119:18–25, 1993.

13. Bennett FC, Ingram DM: Diet and female sex hormone concentrations: An intervention study for the type of fat consumed. Am J Clin Nutr 52:808–812, 1990.

14. Berger U, McClelland RA, Wilson P, Greene GL, Haussler MR, Pike JW, Colson K, Easton D, Coombes RD: Immunocytochemical determination of estrogen receptor and 1,2-dihydroxyviatimin D₃ receptor in breast cancer and relationship to prognosis. Cancer Res 51:239, 1991.

15. Block G, Patterson B, Subar A: Fruit, vegetables and cancer prevention: A review of the epidemiological evidence. Nutr Cancer 18:1–29, 1992.

16. Block A, Thomson CA: Position of the American Dietetic Association: phytochemicals and functional foods. J Am Diet Assoc 95:493–496, 1995.

17. Bonadonna G, Valagussa P, Rossi A: Ten-year experience with CMF-based adjuvant chemotherapy in resectable breast cancer. Breast Cancer Res Treat 5:95–115, 1986.

18. Boyd NF, Greenberg C, Lockwood G, Little L, Martin L, Byng M, et al: The effects at 2 years of a low-fat high-carbohydrate diet on radiological features of the breast: Results from a randomized trial. Dietary fat and cancer: Genetic and molecular interactions. American Institute for Cancer Research Poster Abstract Booklet August 29 & 30, 1996.

19. Boyd NF: Nutrition and breast cancer. J Natl Cancer Inst 85:6–7, 1993.

20. Bradlow HL, Michnovicy JJ, Teleang NT, Osborne MP: Effect of dietary indole-3-carabinol or estradiol metabolism and spontaneous mammary tumors in mice. Carcinogenesis 12:1571–1574, 1991.

21. Bradlow HL, Hershcopf RJ, Martucci CP et al: 16α-hydroxylation of estradiol: A possible risk marker for breast cancer. Ann NY Acad Sci 464:138–151, 1989.

22. Bradlow HL, Michnovicz JJ, Telang NT, Osborne MD, Goldin BR: Diet, oncogenes and tumor viruses as modulators of estrogen metabolism in vivo and in vitro. Cancer Prev Detect 516:35–42, 1991.

23. Brinton LA, Swanson CA: Height and weight at various ages and risk of breast cancer. Ann Epidemiol 2:597–609, 1992.

24. Bruning PF, Bonfrèr JMG: Free fatty acid concentrations correlated with the available fraction of estradiol in human plasma. Cancer Res 16:2606–2609, 1986.

25. Bruning PF, Bonfrèr JMG, Hart AAM, van Noord PAH, van der Hoeven H, Collette HJA, et al: Body measurements, estrogen availability and the risk of human breast cancer: A case-control study. Int J Cancer 51:14–19, 1992.

26. Camoriano JK, Loprinzi CL, Ingle JN: Weight change in women treated with adjuvant therapy or observed following mastectomy for node-positive breast cancer. J Clin Oncol 8:1327–1334, 1990.

27. Carroll KK, Gammal EB, Plunkett ER: Dietary fat and mammary cancer. Can Med Assoc J 98:590–594, 1968.

28. Carroll KK, Khor HT: Dietary fat in relation to tumorigenesis. Prog Biochem Pharmacol 10:308, 1975.

29. Carroll KK, Khor HT: Effect of level and the type of dietary fat on incidence of mammary tumors induced in female Sprague-Dawley rats by 7,12-dimethylbenz(a)anthracene. Lipids 6:415–420, 1971.

30. Cassidy A, Bingham S, Carlson J, Setchell KD: Biological effects of plant estrogens in premenopausal women. (Abstract). FASEB J 7:A866, 1993.

31. Chlebowski RT, Weiner JM, Reynold R, et al: Long-term survival following relapse after 5-FU but not CMF adjuvant breast cancer therapy. Breast Cancer Res Treat 7:23–29, 1986.

32. Chlebowski RT, Rose D, Buzzard IM, et al: Adherence to a dietary fat intake reduction program in postmenopausal women receiving therapy for early breast cancer. J Clin Oncol 11:2072–2080, 1993.

33. Chlebowski RT, Rose D, Buzzard M, Blackburn GL, Insull W Jr, Grosvenor M et al: Adjuvant dietary fat intake reduction in postmenopausal breast cancer patient management. Breast Cancer Res Treat 20:73–84, 1991.

34. Clark S, Jump D: Dietary polyunsaturated fatty acid regulation of gene expression. Ann Rev Nutr 14:83–88, 1994.

35. Clark LC: The epidemiology of selenium and cancer. Fed Proc 44:2584–2589, 1985.

36. Clarke SD, Armstrong MK: Cellular lipid binding proteins: Expression, function and nutritional regulation. FASEB J 3:2480–2487, 1989.

37. Cohen LA, Kendall ME, Zang E, Meschter C, Rost DP: Modulation of N-nitrosomethylurea-induced mammary tumor promotion by dietary fiber and fat. J Natl Cancer Inst 83:496–501, 1991.

38. Cohen LA, Thompson DO, Masura Y, Choi K, Blank ME, Rose DP: Dietary fat and mammary cancer. II. Modulation of serum and tumor lipid composition and tumor prostaglandins by different dietary fats. Association with tumor incidence patterns. J Natl Cancer Inst 77:43–51, 1986.

39. Cohen LA, Choi K, Weisburger JH, Rose DP: Effect of varying proportions of dietary fat on the development of N-nitrosomethylurea-induced rat mammary tumors. Anticancer Res 6:215–218, 1986.

40. Cohen LA, Zhao Z, Zang EA, Wynn TT, Simi B, Rivenson A: Wheat bran and psyllium diets: Effects on N-methylnitrosourea–induced mammary tumorigenesis in F344 rats. J Natl Cancer Inst 88:899–907, 1996.

41. Cohen LA, Thompson DO, Masura Y, Choi K, Blank ME, Rose DP: Dietary fat and mammary cancer. I. Promoting effect of dietary fats on N-nitrosomethylurea–induced rat mammary tumorigenesis. J Natl Cancer Inst 77:33–42, 1986.

42. Cohen LA, Chen-Backlund J-Y, Sepkovic D, Sugie S: Effect of varying proportions of dietary menhaden and corn oil on experimental rat mammary tumor promotion. Lipids 28:449–456, 1993.

43. Cohen LA, Karmali RA: Endogenous prostaglandin production by established cultures of neoplastic rat mammary epithelial cells. In Vitro 20:119–126, 1984.

44. Cohen LA, Rose DP, Wynder EL: A rationale for dietary intervention in postmenopausal breast cancer patients: An update. Nutr Cancer 19:1–10, 1993.

45. Colditz GA, Fazier AL: Models of breast cancer show that risk is set by events of early life: Prevention efforts must shift focus. Cancer Epidemiol Biomarkers Prev 4:567–571, 1995.

46. Colston KW, Berger U, Coombes RC: Possible role for vitamin D in controlling breast cancer cell proliferation. Lancet 28:188, 1989.

47. Cruz JM, Muss HB, Brockschmidt JK, Eans G: Weight changes in women with metastatic breast cancer treated with megastrol acetate: A comparison of standard versus high-dose therapy. Semin Oncol 17:63–67, 1990.

48. DeConti R: Weight gain in the adjuvant chemotherapy of breast cancer. Proc Am Soc Clin Oncol 1:73, 1982.

49. DeLuca LM, Ross S: Beta-carotene increases in lung cancer incidence in cigarette smokers. Nutr Rev 54:178–180, 1996.

50. Demark-Wahnefried W, Winer EP, Rimer BK: Why women gain weight with adjuvant chemotherapy for breast cancer. J Clin Oncol 11:1418–1429, 1993.

51. Den Tonkelaar I, Seidell JC, Collett HJ: Body fat distribution in relation to breast cancer in women participating in the DOM-project. Breast Cancer Res Treat 34:55–61, 1995.

52. Den Tonkelaar I, Seidell JC, Collette HJ, de Waard F: Obesity and subcutaneous fat patterning in relation to breast cancer in postmenopausal women in the Diagnostic Investigation of Mammary Cancer Project. Cancer 69:2663–2667, 1992.

53. Dixon J, Moritz DA, Baker FL: Breast cancer and weight gain: An unexpected finding. Oncol Nurs Forum 5:5–7, 1978.

54. Djuric Z, Heilbrun LK, Reading B, Boome A, et al: Effects of a low fat diet on levels of oxidative stress to DNA in human peripheral nucleated blood cells. J Natl Cancer Inst 83:766–769, 1992.

55. Djuric Z, Lu MH, Lewis SM, Luongo DA, Chen XW, Heibrun LK et al: Oxidative damage levels in rats fed low-fat, high-fat and calorie-restricted diets. Toxicol Appl Pharmacol 115:156–160, 1992.

56. Doll R, Peto R: The causes of cancer: Quantitative estimates of avoidable risks in the United States today. J Natl Cancer Inst 66:1191, 1981.

57. Dwyer JT. Diet and nutritional strategies for cancer risk reduction. Cancer 72(Suppl):1024–1031, 1993.

58. Early Breast Cancer Trialists' Collaborative Group: Effects of adjuvant tamoxifen and of cytotoxic therapy on mortality in early breast cancer. An overview of 61 randomized trials among 28,396 women. N Engl J Med 319:1681–1692, 1988.

59. Ekbom A, Trichopoulos D, Adami HO, Hsieh CC, Lan SJ: Evidence of prenatal influences on breast cancer risk. Lancet 340:1015–1018, 1992.

60. Ekbom A, Chung-Cheng H, Lipworth L, Adami HO, Trichopoulas D: Intrauterine environment and breast cancer risk in women: A population based study. J Natl Cancer Inst 88:71–76, 1997.

61. El Bayoumy K: Evaluation of chemopreventive agents against breast cancer and proposed strategies for future clinical intervention trials. Review. Carcinogenesis 15:2395–2420, 1994.

62. Esterbauer H, Zollner H, Schaur RJ: Aldehydes formed by lipid peroxidation: mechanisms of formation, occurrence and determination. In Vigo-Pelfrey C (ed): Membrane Lipid Oxidation. Boca Raton, FL, CRC Press, 1990, pp 239–263.

63. Esteve J, Kriker A, Ferlay J, Parkin DM: Facts and figures of cancer in the European Community. Lyon: International Agency for Research on Cancer, 1993.

64. Etkind PR: Dietary effects on gene expression in mammary tumorigenesis. Adv Exp Biol 375:75–84, 1995.

65. Ewertz M, Gillanders S, Meyer L, Zedeler K: Survival of breast cancer patients in relation to factors which affect the risk of developing breast cancer. Int J Cancer 49:526–530, 1991.

66. Fernandez G, Chandresekar B, Troyer DA, Ventutraman JT, Good RA: Dietary lipids and calorie restriction affect mammary tumor incidence and gene expression in mouse mammary tumor virus/v-Ha-ras transgenic mice. Proc Natl Acad Sci (USA) 92:6494–6498, 1995.

67. Ferraroni M, Decarli A, Willett WC, Marubini E: Alcohol and breast cancer risk: A case-control study from northern Italy. Int J Epidemiol 20:859–864, 1991.

68. Fisher B, Costantino J, Redmond C: A randomized trial evaluating tamoxifen in the treatment of patients with node-negative breast cancer who have estrogen receptor–positive tumors. N Engl J Med 320:479–484, 1989.

69. Fisher SM, Conti CJ, Lochniskar M, Belury MA, Maldve RE, Lee ML et al: The effect of dietary fat on the rapid development of mammary tumors induced by 7,12-dimethylbenz(a) anthracene in SENCAR mice. Cancer Res 52:662–666, 1992.

70. Folsom AR, McKenzie DR, Bisgard KM, Kushi LH, Sellers TA: No association between caffeine intake and postmenopausal breast cancer incidence in the Iowa Women's Health Study. Am J Public Health 74:820–823, 1984.

71. Foltz AT: Weight gain among stage II breast cancer patients: A study of five factors. Oncol Nurs Forum 12:21–26, 1985.

72. Fraker LD, Halter SA, Forbes JT: Growth inhibition by retinol of a human breast carcinoma cell line in vitro and in athymic mice. Cancer Res 5757–5763, 1984.

73. Freedman LS, Clifford C, Messina M et al: Analysis of dietary fat, calories, body weight, and the development of mammary tumors in rats and mice: A review. Cancer Res 50:5710–5719, 1990.

74. Freudenheim JL, Marshall JR, Vena JE, Laughlin R, Brasure JR, Swanson MK, Nemoto T, Graham S: Premenopausal breast cancer risk and intake of vegetables, fruits and related nutrients. J Natl Cancer Inst 88:340–348, 1996.

75. Gammon MD, Wolff MS, Neugut AI, Terry MB, et al: Treatment for breast cancer and blood levels of chlorinated hydrocarbons. Cancer Epidemiol Biomarkers Prev 5:467–472, 1996.

76. Gapstur SM, Potter JD, Sellers TA, Folsom AR: Increased risk of breast cancer with alcohol consumption in postmenopausal women. Am J Epidemiol 136:1221–1231, 1992.

77. Garland M, Willett WC, Manson JE, Hunter DJ: Antioxidant micronutrients and breast cancer. J Am Coll Nutr 12:400, 1993.

78. Gates JR, Parpia B, Campbell TC, Junshi C: Association of dietary factors and selected plasma variables with sex hormone binding globulin in rural Chinese women. Am Soc Clin Nutr 63:22–31, 1996.

79. Gerber M: Olive oil and cancer. In Giacosa A, Hill MJ (eds): The Mediterranean diet and cancer prevention. Proceedings of a workshop organized by the European Cancer Prevention Organization (ECP) and the Italian League against Cancer, Cosenza, Italy, June 28–30, 1991. Andover, England, European Cancer Prevention Organization 1991, pp 127–139.

80. Goldin BR, Adlercreutz H, Gorbach SL, et al: Estrogen excretion patterns and plasma levels in vegetarian and omnivorian women. N Engl J Med 307:1542–1547, 1982.

81. Gonzales MJ, Schemmel RA, Gray JI, Dugan JL, Sheffield LG, Welsch CW: Effect of dietary fat on growth of MCF-7 and MDA-MB-231 human breast carcinomas in athymic nude mice: Relationship between carcinoma growth and lipid peroxidation product levels. Carcinogenesis 17:1231–1235, 1991.

82. Goodwin PJ, Panzarella T, Boyd NF: Weight gain in women with localized breast cancer—a descriptive study. Breast Cancer Res Treat 11:59–66, 1988.

83. Goodwin PJ, Boyd NF: Body size and breast cancer prognosis: A critical review of the evidence. Breast Cancer Res Treat 16:205–214, 1990.

84. Graham S, Hellmann R, Marshall J, Freudenheim J, Vena J, Swanson M, et al: Nutritional epidemiology of postmenopausal breast cancer in western New York. Am J Epidemiol 134:552–566, 1991.

85. Graham S, Marshall J, Mettlin C, Rzepka T, Nemoto T, Byers T: Diet in the epidemiology of breast cancer. Am J Epidemiol 116:68, 1982.

86. Gray GE, Pike MC, Henderson BE: Breast cancer incidence and mortality rates in different countries in relation to known risk factors and dietary practices. Br J Cancer 39:1–7, 1979.

87. Greenberg ER, Vessey MP, McPherson K, Doll R, Yeates D: Body size and survival in premenopausal breast cancer. Br J Cancer 51:691–697, 1985.

88. Gregorio DI, Emrich LJ, Graham S, et al: Dietary fat con-

sumption and survival among women with breast cancer. J Natl Cancer Inst 75:37–41, 1985.

89. Gritz ER, Bastani R: Cancer prevention—behavior changes: The short and the long of it. Prev Med 22:676–688, 1993.

90. Hagerty MA, Howie BJ, Tan S, Schultz TD: Effect of low- and high-fat intakes on the hormonal milieu of premenopausal women. Am J Clin Nutr 47:653–659, 1988.

91. Hardell L, Danell M, Angqvist CA, Marklund SL, Fredriksson M, Azkari AL, Kjellgren A: Levels of selenium in plasma and glutathione peroxidase in erythrocytes and the risk of breast cancer: A case-control study. Biol Trace Elem Res 36:99, 1993.

92. Harman D: Dimethylbenzanthracene-induced cancer; inhibitory effect of dietary vitamin E. (Abstract.) Clin Res 17:125, 1969.

93. Harvey EB, Schairer C, Brinton LA, Hoover RN, Fraumeni JF Jr: Alcohol consumption and breast cancer. J Natl Cancer Inst 78:657–661, 1987.

94. Heasman KZ, Sutherland HJ, Campbell JA, Elhaken T, Boyd N: Weight gain during adjuvant chemotherapy for breast cancer. Breast Cancer Res Treat 5:195–200, 1985.

95. Hebert JR, Augustine A, Barone J, Kabat GC, Kinne DW, Wynder EL: Weight, height and body mass index in the prognosis of breast cancer: Early results of a prospective study. Int J Cancer 42:315–318, 1988.

96. Hebert JR, Clemow L, Pbert L, Ockene IS, Ockene JK: Social desirability bias in dietary self-report may compromise the validity of dietary intake measures. Int J Epidemiol 24:389–398, 1995.

97. Hebert JR, Barone J, Reddy MM, Backlund JY: Natural killer cell activity in a longitudinal dietary fat intervention trial. Clin Immunol Immunopathol 54:103–107, 1989.

98. Hiatt RA, Bawol RD: Alcoholic beverage consumption and breast cancer incidence. Am J Epidemiol 120:676–683, 1984.

99. Hiatt RA, Klatsky AL, Armstrong MA: Alcohol and breast cancer: A cohort study. Prev Med 17:686–693, 1988.

100. Hilakivi-Clarke L, Onojafe I, Raygda M, Cho E, Clarke R, Lippman ME: Breast cancer risk in rats fed a diet high in n-6 polyunsaturated fatty acids during pregnancy. J Natl Cancer Inst 88:1821–1827, 1996.

101. Hirohata T, Nomura AMY, Hankin JH, Kolonel LN, Lee J: An epidemiologic study on the associations between diet and breast cancer. JNCI 78:595–600, 1987.

102. Hoel DG, Wakabayashi T, Pike MC: Secular trends in the distributions of the breast cancer risk factors—menarche, first birth, menopause, and weight—in Hiroshima and Nagasaki, Japan. Am J Epidemiol 118:78–89, 1983.

103. Holm L-E, Nordevang E, Hjalmar M-L, Lidbrink E, Callmer E, Nilsson B: Treatment failure and dietary habits in women with breast cancer. J Natl Cancer Inst 85:32–36, 1993.

104. Honn KV, Bockman RS, Marnett LJ: Prostaglandins and cancer: A review of tumor initiation through tumor metastasis. Prostaglandins 21:833–864, 1981.

105. Horn-Ross PL: Phytoestrogens, body composition, and breast cancer. Review. Cancer Causes Control 6:567–573, 1995.

106. Horvath P, Ip C: Synergistic effect of vitamin E and selenium in the chemoprevention of mammary carcinogenesis in rats. Cancer Res 43:5335–5341, 1983.

107. Hoskin PJ, Ashley S, Yarnold JR: Weight gain after primary surgery for breast cancer—effect of tamoxifen. Breast Cancer Res Treat 22:129–132, 1992.

108. Hoskin PJ, Ashley S, Yarnold JR: Changes in body weight after treatment for breast cancer and effect of tamoxifen. Br J Cancer 62(supp XI):26, 1990.

109. Howe GR, Hirohata T, Hislop TG, Iscovich JM, Yuan JM, Katsouyanni K, Lubin F, Marubini E, Modan B, Rohan T: Dietary factors and risk of breast cancer: Combined analysis of 12 case-control studies. J Natl Cancer Inst 82:561, 1990.

110. Howe GR: Dietary fat and cancer. Cancer Causes Control 1:99–100, 1990.

111. Howe GR, Hirohata R, Hislop TG, et al: Dietary factors and the risk of breast cancer: Combined analysis of 12 case-control studies. J Natl Cancer Inst 82:565–569, 1990.

112. Howe GR, Friedenreich CM, Jain M, Miller AB: A cohort study of fat intake and risk of breast cancer. J Natl Cancer Inst 83:336–340, 1991.

113. Hsieh CC, Lan SJ, Ekbom A, Petridou E, Adami HO, Trichopoulos D: Twin membership and breast cancer risk. Am J Epidemiol 136:1321–1326, 1992.

114. Hunter DJ, Willett WC: Diet, body build, and breast cancer. Ann Rev Nutr 14:393–418, 1994.

115. Hunter DJ, Morris JS, Stampfer MJ, Colditz GA, Speizer FE, Willett WC: A prospective study of selenium status and breast cancer risk. JAMA 264:1128–1131, 1990.

116. Hunter DJ, Stamfer MJ, Colditz GA, Manson J, Rosner B, Hennekens CH, Speizer FE, Willett WC: A prospective study of consumption of vitamins A, C and E and breast cancer risk. Am J Epidemiol 134:715, 1991.

117. Hunter DJ, Willett WC: Diet, body size, and breast cancer. Epidemiol Rev 15:110–132, 1993.

118. Hunter DJ, Manson JE, Stampfer MJ, et al: A prospective study of caffeine, coffee, tea and breast cancer. Am J Epidemiol 136:1000–1001, 1992.

119. Hunter DJ, Spiegelman D, Adami H-O, Beeson L, Van Den Brandt P, Folsom AR, et al: Cohort studies of fat intake and the risk of breast cancer—a pooled analysis. New Engl J Med 334:356–361, 1996.

120. Hunter DJ, Speigelman D, Willett WC: Dietary fat and the risk of breast cancer. (Letter.) New Engl J Med 334:1607, 1996.

121. Hunter DJ, Manson JE, Colditz GA, et al: A prospective study of the intake of vitamins C, E and A and the risk of breast cancer. N Engl J Med 329:234–240, 1993.

122. Ingle JN, Twito DI, Schaid DDJ, Cullinan SA, Krrok JE, Maillard JA, Tschetter LK, Long HJ, Gerstner JG, Windschitl HE: Combination hormonal therapy with tamoxifen plus fluoxymestrone versus tamoxifen alone in postmenopausal women with metastatic breast cancer. Cancer 67:886–891, 1991.

123. Ingle JN, Everson LK, Wieand HS: Randomized trial of observation versus adjuvant therapy with cyclophosphamide, flourouracil, prednisone with or without tamoxifen following mastectomy in postmenopausal women with node positive breast cancer. J Clin Oncol 6:1388–1396, 1988.

124. Ingram DM, Benett FC, Willcox D, de Klerk N: Effect of low-fat diet on female sex hormone levels. J Natl Cancer Inst 79:1225–1229, 1987.

125. Ip C, Lisk DJ: Efficacy of cancer prevention by high-selenium garlic is primarily dependent on the action of selenium. Carcinongenesis 16:2649–2652, 1995.

126. Ip C: Fat and essential fatty acids in mammary carcinogenesis. Am J Clin Nutr 45:218–224, 1987.

127. Iscovich JM, Iscovich RB, Howe G, Shiboski S, Kaldar JM: A case-control study of diet and breast cancer in Argentina. Int J Cancer 44:770–776, 1989.

128. Jacobson EA, James KA, Newmark HL, Carroll KK: Effects of dietary fat, calcium and vitamin D on growth and mammary tumorigenesis induced by 7,12-dime-thylbenz(a)-anthracene in female Sprague-Dawley rats. Cancer Res, 49:6300, 1989.

129. Johnson PO: Dietary fats, eicosanoids and immunity. Adv Lipid Res 21:103–123, 1985.

130. Jonnalagadda SS, Mustad VA, Yu S, Etherton TD, Kris-Etherton PM: Effects of individual fatty acids on chronic diseases. Nutr Today 31:90–106, 1996.

131. Kaizer L, Boyd NF, Krivkov U: Fish consumption and breast cancer risk: An ecologic study. Nutr Cancer 12:61–68, 1989.

132. Kalish LA: Relationships of body size with breast cancer. J Clin Oncol 2:287–293, 1984.

133. Katsouyanni K, Trichopoulos D, Boyle P, Xirouchaki E, Trichopolou A: Diet and breast cancer: A case-control study in Greece. Int J Cancer 38:815–820, 1986.

134. Katz EB, Boylan ES: Stimulatory effect of high polyunsaturated fat diet on lung metastasis from the 13762 mammary adenocarcinoma in female retired breeder rats. J Natl Cancer Inst 79:351–358, 1987.

135. Key TJA, Chen J, Wang DY, Pike MC, Boreham J: Sex hormones in women in rural China and in Britain. Br J Cancer 62:631–636, 1990.

136. Kleinman RD, Finberg LF, Kersh WJ, Laver RV: Dietary guidelines for children: U.S. recommendations. J Nutr 125:10285–10305, 1995.

137. Knekt P, Aromma A, Maatela J, et al: Selenium in human mammary carcinogenesis: A case cohort study. Eur J Cancer 27:900–902, 1991.

138. Knight DC, Eden JA: Phyoestrogens—a short review. Maturitas 22:167–175, 1995.

139. Knobf MK, Mullen JC, Xistris D, Mortiz PA: Weight gain in women with breast cancer receiving adjuvant chemotherapy. Oncol Nurs Forum 10:28–34, 1983.

140. Kolonel LN: Cancer patterns of four ethnic groups in Hawaii. J Natl Cancer Inst 65:1127, 1980.

141. Kreiger N, Wolff MS, Hiatt RA, Vogelman J, Orentreich N: Breast cancer and serum organochlorines: a prospective study among white, black and Asian women. J Natl Cancer Inst 86:589–599, 1994.

142. Kritchevsky D: The effect of over- and undernutrition on cancer. Review. Eur J Cancer Prev 4:445–451, 1995.

143. Kritchevsky D: Caloric restriction and experimental carcinogenesis. Adv Exp Med Biol 322:131–141, 1992.

144. Kushi LH, Sellers TA, Potter JD, et al: Dietary fat and postmenopausal breast cancer. J Natl Cancer Inst 84:1092–1099, 1992.

145. Kyogoku S, Hirohata T, Nomura Y, Shigematsu T, Takeshita S, Hirohata I: Diet and prognosis of breast cancer. Nutr Cancer 17:271–277, 1992.

146. La Vecchia C, Decarli A, Franceschi S, Gentile A, Negri, et al: Dietary Factors and the risk of breast cancer. Nutr Cancer 10:205–214, 1987.

147. La Vecchia C, Negri E, Parazzini F, Boyle P, Fasoli M, Gentile A, Franceschi S: Alcohol and breast cancer: Update from an Italian case-control study. Eur J Cancer Clin Oncol 25:1711–1717, 1989.

148. Landa MC, Frago N, Tres A: Diet and the risk of breast cancer in Spain. Eur J Cancer Prev 3:313–320, 1994.

149. Lasekan JB, Clayton MK, Gendron-Fitzpatrick A, Ney DM: Dietary olive and safflower oils in promotion of DMBA-induced mammary tumorigenesis in rats. Nutr Cancer 13:153–163, 1990.

150. Lê MG, Hill C, Kramar A, Flamant R: Alcoholic beverage consumption and breast cancer in a French case-control study. Am J Epidemiol 120:350–357, 1984.

151. Lee HP, Gourley L, Duffy SW, Estève J, Lee J, Day NE: Dietary effects on breast cancer risk in Singapore. Lancet 337:1197–1200, 1991.

152. Lee C, Chen C: Enhancement of mammary tumorigenesis in rats by vitamin E deficiency. (Abstract.) Proc Am Assoc Cancer Res 20:132, 1979.

153. Lenfant C, Ernst N: Daily dietary fat and total food-energy intakes. Third National Health and Nutrition Examination Survey, Phase I, 1988–1991. MMWR 43:116–117, 1994.

154. Levander OA: The need for a measure of selenium status. J Am Coll Toxicol 5:37–44, 1986.

155. Levine EG, Raczynski JM, Carpenter JT: Weight gain with breast cancer adjuvant treatment. Cancer 67:1954–1959, 1991.

156. Liu X-H, Rose DP: Stimulation of type IV collagenase expression by linoleic acid in a metastatic human breast cancer cell line. Cancer Lett 76:71–77, 1994.

157. London SJ, Stein EA, Henderson IC, et al: Carotenoids, retinol, and vitamin E and risk of proliferative benign breast disease and breast cancer. Cancer Causes Control 3:503–512, 1992.

158. London SJ, Colditz GA, Stampfer MJ, Willett WC, Rosner B, Speizer FE: Prospective study of relative weight, height, and risk of breast cancer. JAMA 262:2853–2858, 1989.

159. Longnecker M, Berlin JA, Orza MJ, Chalmers TC: A meta-analysis of alcohol consumption in relation to risk of breast cancer. JAMA 260:652, 1988.

160. Longnecker M: Alcoholic beverage consumption in relation to risk of breast cancer: Meta-analysis and review. Cancer Causes Control 5:73–82, 1994.

161. Lubin JH, Blot WJ, Burns PE: Breast cancer following high dietary fat and protein consumption. Am J Epidemiol 116:68, 1982.

162. Lubin JH, Burns PE, Bot WJ, Ziegler RG, Lees AW, et al: Dietary factors and breast cancer risk. Int J Cancer 28:685–689, 1981.

163. Makita M, Sakamoto G, et al: Natural history of breast cancer among Japanese and Caucasian females. Gan To Kagaku Ryoho 17:1239–1243, 1990.

164. Malins D, Polissar NL, Gunselman SJ: Progression of human breast cancers to the metastatic state is linked to hydroxyl radical-induced DNA damage. Proc Natl Acad Sci (USA) 93:2557–2563, 1996.

165. Marshall WJ, McClean REM: A requirement for dietary lipids for induction of cytochrome P450 by phorbarbitone in rat liver microsomal drug metabolism. Biochem Pharmacol 21:2887–2897, 1992.

166. Martin-Moreno JM, Willett WC, Corgojo L, et al: Dietary fat, olive oil intake and breast cancer risk. Int J Cancer 54:774–780, 1994.

167. Marubini E, Decarli A, Costa A, et al: The relationship of dietary intake and serum levels of retinol and β-carotene with breast cancer. Cancer 61:173–180, 1988.

168. Masoro EJ: Caloric restriction and aging in rats. *In* Ingram DK, Baker GT III, Shock NW, Trumbull CN (eds): The Potential for Nutritional Modulation of Aging Processes. Trumbull, CT, Food & Nutrition Press, 1991, p 123.

169. McCormick DL, Burns PJ, Albert RE: Growth inhibition by retinol of a human breast carcinoma cell line in vitro and in athymic mice. Cancer Res 44:5757–5763, 1984.

170. McLaughlin CC, Mahoney MC, Nasca PC, Metzger BB, Baptiste MS, Field NA: Breast cancer and methylxanthine consumption. Cancer Causes Control 3:175–178, 1992.

171. Meara J, McPherson K, Roberts M, Jones L, Vessey M: Alcohol, cigarette smoking and breast cancer. Br J Cancer 60:70–73, 1989.

172. Messina MJ, Persky V, Setchell K: Soy intake and cancer risk: A review of the in vitro and in vivo data. Nutr Cancer 21:113–131, 1994.

173. Mettlin JC, Selenskas S, Natarajan N, Huben R: Beta-Carotene and animal fats and their relationship to prostate cancer risk. Cancer 64:605–612, 1989.

174. Micheles KB, Trichopoulos D, Robins JM, et al: Birth weight as a risk factor for breast cancer. Lancet 348:1542–1546, 1996.

175. Michnovicz JJ, Bradlow HL: Induction of estradiol metabolism by dietary indole-3-carbinol in humans. J Natl Cancer Inst 82:947–949, 1990.

176. Miller AB, Kelly A, Choi NW, Matthews V, Morgan RW, Munan L, Burch JD, Feather J, Howe GR, Jain M: A study of diet and breast cancer. Am J Epidemiol 107:499, 1978.

177. Miller AB: An overview of hormone-associated cancers. Cancer Res 38:3985, 1978.

178. Mills PK, Beeson WL, Phillips RL, Fraser GE: Dietary habits and breast cancer incidence among Seventh Day Adventists. Cancer 64:582–590, 1989.

179. Mills PK, Beeson WL, Phillips RL, et al: Cohort study of diet, lifestyle, and prostate cancer in Adventist men. Cancer 64:598–604, 1989.

180. Ministry of Health and Welfare of Japan: Vital Statistics, 1985. Tokyo, Ministry of Health and Welfare, 1986.

181. Minton, JP, Foeking MK, Webster DJ, Matthews RH: Response of fibrocystic disease to caffeine withdrawal and correlation of cyclic nucleotides with breast disease. Am J Obstet Gynecol 135:157, 1979.

182. Minton JP, Foecking MK, Wevster DJ, Matthews RH: Response of fibrocystic disease to caffeine withdrawal and correlation of cyclic nucleotides with breast disease. Am J Obstet Gynecol 135:157–158, 1979.

183. Moon RC, McCormick DL, Mehta RG: Inhibition of carcinogenesis by retinoids. Cancer Res 43:2469S–2475S, 1983.

184. Moon RC, Grubbs CJ, Sporn MB, Goodman DG: Retinal acetate inhibits mammary carcinogenesis induced by *N*-methyl-*N*-nitrosourea. Nature 267:620–621, 1977.

185. Morabia A, Wynder EL: Epidemiology and breast cancer. Implications for the body weight–breast cancer controversy. Surg Clin North Am 70:739–752, 1990.

186. Morrison AS, Lowe CCR, MacMahon B, et al: Some international differences in treatment and survival in breast cancer. Int J Cancer 18:269–273, 1976.

187. Nandi S, Guzman RC, Yang J: Hormones and mammary

carcinogenesis in mice, rats and humans: A unifying hypothesis. Proc Natl Acad Sci (USA) 92:3650–3657, 1995.
188. Narraez CJ, Vanweelden K, Bryne I, Welsh J: Characterization of a vitamin D$_3$–resistant MCF-7 cell line. Endocrinology 137:400–409, 1996.
189. Nasca PC, Baptiste MS, Field NA, Metzger BB, Black M, Kwon CS, Jacobson H: An epidemiological case-control study of breast cancer and alcohol consumption. Int J Epidemiol 19:532–538, 1990.
190. Nath RG, Ocando JE, Chung F-L: Detection of 1,N2-propano-deoxyguanosine adducts as potential endogenous DNA lesions in rodent and human tissues. Cancer Res 56:452–456, 1996.
191. National Cancer Institute: Annual Cancer Statistics Review including Cancer Trends: 1950–1985. Bethesda, MD, U.S. Department of Health and Human Services, 1988.
192. Newberne PM: Dietary fat, immunological response and cancer in rats. Cancer Res 41:3783–3786, 1981.
193. Nunez EA: Nonesterified fatty acids: Role in the molecular events linking endocrinology and oncology via nutrition. Tumor Biol 8:273–280, 1987.
194. Office of Research on Women's Health: Women's Health Initiative: Overview Statement. Bethesda, MD, National Institutes of Health, 1994, p 1.
195. O'Connell DL, Hulka BS, Chamless LE, Wilkinson WE, Deubner DC: Cigarette smoking, alcohol consumption, and breast cancer risk. J Natl Cancer Inst 78:229–234, 1987.
196. Paganini-Hill A, Chao A, Ross RK, et al: Vitamin A, beta-carotene and the risk of cancer: A prospective study. J Natl Cancer Inst 79:443–448, 1987.
197. Parkin DM: Studies of cancer in migrant populations. IARC Scientific Publications 123:1–10, 1993.
198. Parkin DM: Cancers of the breast, endometrium and ovary: geographic correlations. European J Cancer Clin Oncol 25:1917–1925, 1989.
199. Petrakis NL, Barnes S, King EB, Lowenstein J, Wiencke J, Lee MM, Miike R, Kirk M, Coward L: Stimulatory influence of soy protein isolate on breast secretion in pre- and post-menopausal women. Cancer Epidemiol Biomarkers Prev 5:785–794, 1996.
200. Phillips RL: Role of life-style and dietary habits in risk of cancer among Seventh-Day Adventists. Cancer Res 35:3513, 1975.
201. Potischman N, McCullock CF, Byers T, et al: Breast cancer and plasma concentrations of carotenoids and vitamin A. Am J Clin Nutr 52:909–915, 1990.
202. Potter JD: Food and phytochemicals, magic bullets and measurement error: A commentary. Am J Epidemiol 144:1026–1027, 1996.
203. Prentice RL, Sheppard L: Dietary fat and cancer: Rejoinder and discussion of research strategies. Cancer Causes Control 2:53–58, 1990.
204. Prentice RL, Sheppard L: Dietary fat and cancer: Consistency of the epidemiologic data, and disease prevention that may follow from a practical reduction in fat consumption. Cancer Causes Control 1:81–97, 1990.
205. Prentice RL, Kakar F, Hursing S, Sheppard L, Klein R, Kushi L: Aspects of the rationale for the Women's Health Trial. J Natl Cancer Inst 11:802–814, 1988.
206. Reichman ME, Judd JT, Longcope C, Schatzkin A, Clevidence BA, Nair PP, Campbell WS, Taylor PR: Effects of alcohol consumption on plasma and urinary hormone concentrations in premenopausal women. J Natl Cancer Inst 85:722, 1993.
207. Rohan TE, McMichael AJ, Baghurst PA: A population-based case-control study of diet and breast cancer in Australia. Am J Epidemiol 128:478–489, 1988.
208. Rohan TE, McMichael AJ: Alcohol consumption and risk of breast cancer. Int J Cancer 41:695–699, 1988.
209. Rohan TE, Howe GR, Friedenreich CM, Jain M, Miller AM: Dietary fiber, vitamins A, C, and E, and risk of breast cancer: A cohort study. Cancer Causes Control 4:29–37, 1993.
210. Ronai Z, Tillotson J, Cohen L: Effect of dietary fatty acids on gene expression in breast cells. Adv Exp Med Biol 375:85–96, 1995.
211. Rose DP, Boyar AP, Cohen C, Strong LE: Effect of a low-fat diet on hormone levels in women with cystic breast disease. I. Serum steroids and gonadotropins. J Natl Cancer Inst 78:623–626, 1987.
212. Rose DP, Goldman M. Connolly JM, Strong LE: High-fiber diet reduces serum estrogen concentrations in premenopausal women. Am J Clin Nutr 54:520–525, 1991.
213. Rose DP, Connolly JM, Liu X-H: Dietary fatty acids and human breast cancer cell growth invasion and metastasis. Adv Exp Med Bio 364:83–91, 1994.
214. Rose DP, Boyar AP, Wynder EL: International comparison of mortality rates for cancer of the breast, ovary, prostate, and colon, and per capita food consumption. Cancer 58:2363–2371, 1986.
215. Rose DP: Diet, hormones and cancer. Ann Rev Public Health 14:1–17, 1993.
216. Rose DP, Connolly JM, Liu X-H: Effects of linoleic acid on the growth and metastasis of two human breast cell lines in nude mice, and the invasive capacity of these cell lines in vitro. Cancer Res 54:6557–6562, 1994.
217. Rose DP, Connolly JM, Meschter CL: Effect of dietary fat on human breast cancer growth and lung metastases in nude mice. J Natl Cancer Inst 83:1491–1493, 1991.
218. Rose DP: Dietary fiber and breast cancer. Nutr Cancer 13:1–8, 1990.
219. Rosenberg L, Palmer JR, Miller DR, Clarke EA, Shapiro S: A case-control study of alcoholic beverage consumption and breast cancer. Am J Epidemiol 13:6–14, 1990.
220. Rosenberg L, Metzger LS. Palmer JR: Alcohol consumption and risk of breast cancer: A review of the epidemiologic evidence. Epidemiol Rev 15:133–144, 1993.
221. Rothman KJ: Modern Epidemiology. Boston, Little, Brown and Co, 1986, pp 63–64.
222. Sakamoto G, Sugano H, Hartman WH: Stage-by-stage survival from breast cancer in the U.S. and Japan. Jpn J Cancer 25:161–170, 1979.
223. Schairer C, Brinton LA, Hoover RN: Methylxanthines and breast cancer. Int J Cancer 40:469–473, 1987.
224. Schapiro DV, Kumar NB, Lyman GH, Cox CE: Abdominal obesity and breast cancer risk. Ann Intern Med 112:182–186, 1990.
225. Schatzkin A, Carter CL, Green SB, Kreger BE, Splansky GL, Anderson KM, Jelsel EW, Kannel WB: Is alcohol consumption related to breast cancer? Results from the Framingham Heart Study. J Natl Cancer Inst 81:31–35, 1989.
226. Schatzkin A, Jones Y, Hoover RN, Taylor PR, Brinton LA, Ziegler RG, Harvey EB, Carter CL, Licitra LM, Dufour MC, Larson DB: Alcohol consumption and breast cancer in the epidemiologic follow-up study of the First National Health and Nutrition Examination Survey. N Engl J Med 316:1169–1173, 1987.
227. Schrauzer GN, White DA, Scheider CJ: Cancer mortality correlation studies, III: Statistical associations with dietary selenium intakes. Bioinorg Chem 7:23–34, 1977.
228. Sellers TA, Kushi LH, Potter JD, Kaye SA, Nelson CL, McGovern PG, et al: Effect of family history, body fat distribution, and reproductive factors on risk of postmenopausal breast cancer. N Engl J Med 326:1323–1329, 1992.
229. Senie RT, Rosen PP, Rhodes P, Leser ML, Kinne DW: Obesity at diagnosis of breast carcinoma influences duration of disease-free survival. Ann Intern Med 116:26–32, 1992.
230. Shamberger RJ, Tytko SA, Willis CE: Antioxidants and cancer, VI: Selenium and age-adjusted human cancer mortality. Arch Environ Health 31:231–235, 1976.
231. Simard A, Vobecky J, Vobecky JS: Vitamin D deficiency and cancer of the breast: An unprovocative ecological hypothesis. Can J Public Health 82:300, 1991.
232. Snetselaar L: Nutrition Counseling Skills: Assessment, Treatment and Evaluation, 2nd ed. Rockville, MD, Aspen Publishers, 1989.
233. Snow L: Folk medical beliefs and their implications for care of patients. Ann Internal Med 72:1024–1031, 1993.
234. Snowdon DA, Phillips RL: Coffee consumption and risk of fatal cancers. Am J Public Health 74:820–823, 1984.
235. Snowdon DA, Phillips RL, Choi W: Diet, obesity, and risk of fatal prostate cancer. Am J Epidemiol 120:244–250, 1984.

236. Sohrabi A, Sandoz J, Spratt JS, Polk HC Jr: Recurrence of breast cancer: obesity, tumor size, and auxiliary lymph node metastases. JAMA 244:264–265, 1980.

237. Sporn MB, Roberts AB: Role of retinoids in differentiation and carcinogenesis. Cancer Res 43:3034–3040, 1983.

238. Steinmetz K, Potter J: Vegetables, fruit and cancer. I. Epidemiology. Cancer Causes Control 2(Suppl):325–357, 1991.

239. Steinmetz K, Potter JD: A review of vegetables, fruit, and cancer. I. Epidemiology. Cancer Causes Control 2:325–357, 1991.

240. Steinmetz KA, Potter JD: Vegetables, fruits and cancer. II. Mechanisms. Cancer Causes Control 2:427–442, 1991.

241. Stoll BA, Vatten LJ, Kvinnsland S: Does early physical maturity influence breast cancer risk? Review. Acta Oncol 33:171–176, 1994.

242. Stoll BA: Can supplementary dietary fibre suppress breast cancer growth? Br J Cancer 73:557–559, 1996.

243. Stoll BA: Breast cancer risk in Japanese women with special reference to the growth hormone-insulin-like growth factor axis. Review. Jpn J Clin Oncol 22:1–5, 1992.

244. Subar AS, Heimendingeer J, Krebs-Smith SM, et al: 5-a-day for better health: A baseline study of Americans' fruit and vegetable consumption. Rockville, MD, National Cancer Institute, NIH, 1991, p 7.

245. Swanson CA, Jones DY Schatzkin A, Brinton LA, Ziegler RG: Breast cancer risk assessed by anthropometry in NHANES I epidemiological follow-up study. Cancer Res 48:5363–5367, 1988.

246. Takata T, Minara T, Takuda H, Sagauchi M, Yamamura M, Hioki K, Yamamato M: Specific inhibitory effect of dietary eicosapentaenoic acid on N-nitroso-N-methylurea–induced mammary carcinogenesis in female Sprague-Dawley rats. Carcinogenesis 11:2015–2019, 1990.

247. Tang ZC, Shivapurkar N, Frost A, Alabaster O: The effect of dietary fat on the promotion of mammary and colon cancer in a dual-organ rat carcinogenesis model. Nutr Cancer 25:151–159, 1996.

248. Tannenbaum A, Silverstone H: Nutrition in relation to cancer. Adv Cancer Res 1:451–465, 1953.

249. Telang NT, Basu A, Kurihara H, Osborne MD, Modak MJ: Modulation in the expression of murine mammary tumor virus, ras proto-oncogene, and of alveolar hyperplasia by fatty acids in mouse mammary explant cultures. Anticancer Res 8:971–976, 1988.

250. The American Cancer Society 1996 Advisory Committee on Diet, Nutrition, and Cancer Prevention: American Cancer Society Guidelines on diet, nutrition, and cancer prevention: Reducing the risk of cancer with healthy food choices and physical activity. CA Cancer J Clin 46:325–342, 1996.

251. The Alpha-Tocopherol, Beta Carotene Cancer Prevention Study Group: The effects of vitamin E and beta carotene on the incidence of lung cancer and other cancers in male smokers. N Engl J Med 330:1029–1035, 1994.

252. Third National Health and Nutrition Examination Survey, Phase 1, 1988–1991. Daily dietary fat and total food-energy intake. MMWR 43:116–125, 1994.

253. Tiwari RK, Mukhopadhyay B, Telang NT, Osborne MD: Modulation of gene expression by selected fatty acids in human breast cancer cells. Anticancer Res 11:1383–1388, 1991.

254. Toniolo P, Riboli E, Protta F, Charrel M, Cappa APM: Calorie-providing nutrients and risk of breast cancer. J Natl Cancer Inst 81:278–286, 1989.

255. Toniolo P, Riboli E, Protta F, Charrel M, Cappa APM: Breast cancer and alcohol consumption: A case-control study in northern Italy. Cancer Res 49:5203–5206, 1989.

256. Tretli S: Height and weight in relation to breast cancer morbidity and mortality. A prospective study of 570,000 women in Norway. Cancer 44:23–30, 1989.

257. Tretli S, Haldorsen T, Ottestad L: The effect of pre-morbid height and weight on the survival of breast cancer patients. Br J Cancer 62:299–304, 1990.

258. Trichopoulou A, Katsouyanni K, Stuver S, et al: Consumption of olive oil and specific food groups in relation to breast cancer risk in Greece. J Natl Cancer Inst 87:110–116, 1995.

259. Trichopoulou A, Toupadaki N, Tzonou A, Katsouyani K, Manousos O, Kadi E, et al: The macronutrient composition of the Greek diet: Estimates derived from six case-control studies. Eur J Clin Nutr 47:549–558, 1993.

260. United States Department of Agriculture, United States Department of Health and Human Services: Nutrition and your health: Dietary guidelines for Americans. 3rd ed. Washington, DC: US Government Printing Office, 1990.

261. United States Department of Agriculture (USDA): USDA's food guide pyramid: Home and garden bulletin no. 249. Hyattsville, MD, Human Nutrition Information Services, 1992.

262. Van Noord PA, Collette HJ, Maas MJ, De Waard F: Selenium levels in nails of premenopausal breast cancer patients assessed prediagnostically in a cohort-nested case-referent study among women screened in the DOM project. Int J Epidemiol 16(Suppl):318–322, 1987.

263. Van't Veer P: Diet and breast cancer: Trial and error? Ann Med 26:453–460, 1994.

264. Van't Veer P, van Leer EM, Rietdijk A, Kok FJ, Schouten EG, Hermus RJ, et al: Combination of dietary factors in relation to breast-cancer occurrence. Int J Cancer 47:649–653, 1991.

265. Van't Veer P, Kalb CM, Verhoef P, et al: Dietary fiber, β-carotene and breast cancer: Results from a case-control study. Int J Cancer 45:825–828, 1990.

266. Van't Veer P, Kok FJ, Brants HA, Ockhuizen T, Sturmans F, et al: Dietary fat and the risk of breast cancer. Int J Epidemiol 19:12–18, 1990.

267. Van't Veer P, Strain JJ, Fernandez-Crehuet J, Martin BC, Thamm M, Kardinall AFM, Kohlmeier L, Huttunen JK, Martin-Moreno JM, Kok FJ: Tissue antioxidants and postmenopausal breast cancer: The European community multicentre study on antioxidants, myocardial infarction, and cancer of the breast (EURAMIC). Cancer Epi Biom & Prev, 5:441–447, 1996.

268. Van't Veer P, Kok FJ, Hermus RJJ, Sturmans F: Alcohol dose, frequency and age at first exposure in relation to the risk of breast cancer. Int J Epidemiol 18:511–517, 1989.

269. Vatten LJ, Kvinnsland S: Body height and risk of breast cancer. Br J Cancer 61:881–885, 1990.

270. Vatten LJ, Kvinnsland S. Prospective study of height, body mass index and risk of breast cancer. Acta Oncol 31:195–200, 1992.

271. Verreault R, Brisson J, Deschenes L, et al: Dietary fat in relation to prognostic factors in breast cancer. J Natl Cancer Inst 80:819–825, 1988.

272. Weisburger JH, Reddy BS, Rose DP, Cohen LA, Kendall ME, Wynder EL: Protective mechanisms of dietary fibers in nutritional carcinogenesis. Review. Basic Life Sci 61:45–63, 1993.

273. Welsch CW: Caffeine and the development of the normal and neoplastic mammary gland. Proc Soc Exp Biol Med 207:1:1–12, 1994.

274. Welsch CW: Enhancement of mammary tumorigenesis by dietary fat: Review of potential mechanisms. Am J Clin Nutr 45:192–202, 1987.

275. Willett WC, Stampfer MJ, Colditz GA, Rosner BA, Hennekens CH, et al: Dietary fat and the risk of breast cancer. N Engl J Med 316:22–28, 1987.

276. Willett WC, Stampfer MJ: Dietary fat and cancer: Another view. Cancer Causes Control 1:103–109, 1990.

277. Willett WC: Dietary fat reduction among women with early breast cancer. J Clin Oncol 11:2061–2062, 1993.

278. Willett WC, Stampfer MJ, Colditz GA, Rosner BA, Hennekens CH, Speizer FE: Moderate alcohol consumption and the risk of breast cancer. N Engl J Med 316:1174–1180, 1987.

279. Willett WC: Diet and cancer: what do we know now? Adv Oncol 11:3–8, 1995.

280. Willett WC, Stampfer MJ, Underwood BA, Speizer FE, Rosner B, Hennekens CH: Validation of a dietary questionnaire with plasma carotenoid and alpha-tocopherol levels. Am J Clin Nutr 38:631–639, 1983.

281. Willett WC, Hunter DJ, Stampfer MJ, et al: Dietary fat and fiber in relation to risk of breast cancer. An 8-year follow up. JAMA 268:2037–2044, 1992.

282. William CL: Nutrition in childhood: A key component of

primary cancer prevention. *In* Watson RR, Mufti SI (eds): Nutrition and Cancer Prevention. Boca Raton, FL, CRC Press, 1996, pp 25–50.

283. Williams G, Howell A, Jones M: The relationship of body weight to response to endocrine therapy, steroid hormone receptors and survival of patients with advanced cancer of the breast. Br J Cancer 58:631–634, 1988.

284. Williams GM, Wynder EL: Diet and cancer: A synopsis of causes and preventive strategies. *In* Watson RR, Mufti SI (eds): Nutrition and Cancer Prevention. Boca Raton, FL, CRC Press, 1996, pp 1–12.

285. Williams C, Bolella M, Williams GM: Cancer prevention beginning in childhood. *In* De Vita VT Jr, Hollman S, Rosenberg SA (eds): Cancer Prevention. Philadelphia, JB Lippincot, 1993, p 1.

286. Wolff MS, Toniolo PG, Lee EW, Rivera M, Dubin N: Blood levels of organochlorine residues and risk of breast cancer. J Natl Cancer Inst 85:648–652, 1993.

287. Wu AH, Ziegler RG, Horn-Ross PL, Nomura AMY, West DW, Kolonel LN, Rosenthal JF, Hoover RN, Pike MC: Tofu and risk of breast cancer in Asian-Americans. Cancer Epidemiol Biomarkers Prev 5:901–906, 1996.

288. Wu AH, Ziegler RG, Pike MC, Nomura AMY, West DW, Kolonel LN, et al: Menstrual and reproductive factors and risk of breast cancer in Asian-Americans. Br J Cancer 73:680–686, 1996.

289. Wynder EL, Hebert JR: Homogeneity in nutritional exposure: An impediment in cancer epidemiology. (Letter.) J Natl Cancer Inst 79:605–607, 1987.

290. Wynder EL, Kajitani T, Kuno J, Lucas JC, et al: A comparison of survival rates between American and Japanese patients with breast cancer. Gynecol Obstet 111:196–200, 1963.

291. Wynder EL, Gori GB: Contributions of the environment to cancer incidence: An epidemiological exercise. J Natl Cancer Inst 58:825, 1977.

292. Wynder EL, Stellman SD. The "over-exposed" control group. Am J Epi 135:459–461, 1992.

293. Wynder EL, Rose DP, Cohen LA: Diet and breast cancer in causation and therapy. Cancer 58:1804–1813, 1986.

294. Wynder EL, Williams GM: Metabolic overload and carcinogenesis form the viewpoint of epidemiology. *In* Somosyi A, Appel KE, Katenkamp A (eds): Chemical Carcinogenesis: The Relevance of Mechanistic Understanding in Toxicological Evaluations. Munich, MMV Medizin Verlag, 1993, p 17.

295. Wynder EL, Weisburger JH, Ng SK: Nutrition: The need to define "optimal intake" as a basis for public policy decisions. Am J Public Health 82:34, 1992.

296. Yu H, Harris RE, Gao YT, Wynder EL: Comparative epidemiology of cancers of the colon, rectum, prostate and breast in Shanghai, China versus the United States. Int J Epidemiol 20:76–78, 1991.

297. Zeigler RG: Vegetables, fruits, and carotenoids and the risk of cancer. Am J Clin Nutr 53(suppl):251S–259S, 1991.

298. Zevenberger JL, Verschuren PM, Zaalberg J: Effect of the amount of dietary fat on the development of mammary tumors in BALB/c-MTV mice. Cancer 17:9–18, 1992.

299. Zhang S, Folsom AR, Sellers TA, Kushi LH, Potter JD: Better breast cancer survival for postmenopausal women who are less overweight and eat less fat. Cancer 76:275–283, 1995.

300. Zhang J, Sukuki S, Sasaki R: Cancer incidence among native Chinese and Chinese residing in Hong Kong, Singapore and the United States. J Aichi Med Univ Assoc 23:427–436, 1995.

301. Zhang Y, Rosenberg L, Colton, Cupples LA, Palmer JR, Strom BL, Zauber AG, Warshauer ME, Harlap S, Shapiro S: Adult height and risk of breast cancer among white women in a case-control study. Am J Epidemiol 143:1123–1128, 1996.

302. Ziegler RG, Hoover RN, Nomura Am, et al: Relative weight, weight change, height, and breast cancer risk in Asian-American women. J Natl Cancer Inst 88:650–660, 1996.

303. Ziegler RG, Hoover RN, Pike MC, Hildsheim A, Nomura AMY, West DW, et al: Migration patterns and breast cancer risk in Asian-American women. J Natl Cancer Inst 85:1819–1827, 1993.

CHAPTER 89
THE PSYCHOSOCIAL CONSEQUENCES OF BREAST CANCER

James R. Zabora, Ph.D., M.S.W.

OVERVIEW

Despite improved overall survival, the diagnosis of breast cancer continues to generate fear and turmoil in the lives of women and their families. All phases related to diagnosis, treatment, and recovery create challenges and problems that patients and survivors must face. Clearly, at the time of diagnosis patients experience uncertainty, confusion, and distress. Psychological distress can be exacerbated by inadequate information, complex treatment decisions, and scheduling difficulties with various specialists such as surgeons, medical oncologists, radiotherapists, and plastic surgeons.[1] As treatment begins, concerns related to physical functioning, body image, mood, sexuality, family, and vocational pursuits quickly emerge. Surgical options—which include lumpectomy, mastectomy, and reconstruction—present unique issues as patients contemplate the advantages and disadvantages of each procedure. Following postsurgical care, little time is available for a full psychological recovery, since adjuvant chemotherapy and radiotherapy must also be considered and discussed. Adjuvant treatments generate additional physiological assaults that further affect body image, sexuality, and family. As women move beyond treatment, their role of patient transforms to that of survivor, and the fear of recurrence arises. Breast cancer survivors require rehabilitative assistance beyond the physical domain. Major rehabilitation problem areas include physical, psychological, social, sexual, nutritional, financial, and vocational ones.[2] Each of these domains contributes to each patient's sense of overall well-being or quality of life; however, rehabilitation efforts frequently ignore the spiritual domain, which also figures into any such measurement.

While breast cancer treatments present significant challenges and distress, the majority of patients learn to live with the disease and to incorporate it into day-to-day living.[3] In essence, the majority of patients possess problem-solving skills that effectively resolve the many difficulties associated with treatment and rehabilitation. Since patients vary in their ability to respond to these challenges and problems, careful consideration must be given to understanding the individual variations in psychological reactions. Each adverse reaction and symptom requires the patient to appraise the event to determine the level of potential harm or threat.[4] In this way, patients determine the significance of each side effect or symptom and the impact on well-being and survival. These appraisals related to the diagnosis, treatments, and adverse events are directly influenced by factors such as psychological status, level of optimism, spirituality, and support from sources such as family, friends, employers, and the health care team. Evidence suggests that one of the best predictors of positive adaptation to breast cancer is the psychological state of the patient before the diagnosis.[5] Prevalence studies of psychological distress indicate that one of every three newly diagnosed patients experiences significant difficulty in adjustment.[6-8] Further evidence suggests that the diagnosis of breast cancer generates more anxiety than any other cancer diagnosis.[9] In addition, this prevalence rate of psychological distress remains constant over the disease continuum, as patients move from diagnosis and treatment to recovery and survivorship.[10] These factors present unique challenges to the health care team since undetected and untreated psychological distress can jeopardize treatment outcomes and actually increase health care costs.[11]

IMPACT OF SPECIFIC TREATMENTS

Mastectomy. Initial treatment decisions focus on mastectomy versus lumpectomy, and if mastectomy is chosen, reconstruction requires examination. Clearly, mastectomy is a radical approach to an aggressive disease and a significant assault on overall body image and self-esteem. Without question, the breast is a cultural symbol that is closely intertwined with a definition of femininity.[12] The loss of self-esteem associated with mastectomy causes anger, anxiety, fear, and sadness. While these emotions and symptoms are appropriate, the duration of these reactions may be prolonged. In these cases, the health care team may consider a referral for psychosocial services.

Lumpectomy. Breast conservation provides an alternative to mastectomy that lessens the effect on body image and self-esteem. Lumpectomy is a viable option for early-stage cancers; however, women may still opt for the more radical mastectomy, in an effort to achieve a maximum level of comfort with the removal of the entire breast being linked to elimination of all of the disease. Even when breast conservation provides equal survival statistics, mastectomy is the choice of some women.

Reconstruction. Immediate or delayed reconstruction offers an opportunity to restore a positive body image and to increase self-esteem.[13] An intact body enhances sexual functioning and satisfaction; however, pretreatment levels of sexual satisfaction may be the best predictor of overall post-treatment sexual functioning.

Adjuvant Chemotherapy. As with other solid tumors, distant metastases may develop months to years after the initial surgery. Consequently, while the value of a systemic therapy is apparent, the rigors of most chemotherapeutic protocols can further debilitate the patient. Regardless of the classification of these agents, adverse reactions and symptoms significantly challenge all breast cancer patients. Alopecia, fatigue, hemorrhagic cystitis, myelosuppression, and nausea and vomiting consistently affect the psychological well-being of every patient. While dramatic improvements have occurred in the management of nausea and vomiting, symptoms such as alopecia and fatigue exacerbate the assault on body image, sexual satisfaction, and overall quality of life.[14]

Radiation Therapy. Radiation therapy with conservation surgery or in combination with alternating chemotherapy treatments can enhance overall survival, but treatment does not come without a price. The degree of organ injury due to radiation therapy depends on the dose of radiation absorbed and the volume of the particular organ that is irradiated. Despite the use of molds and shields, the precision of the system to deliver the radiation dose must be closely monitored. Damage to the esophagus, heart, and lungs is possible, but effective treatment planning and the close co-operation among radiation specialists reduces the chance of any significant damage. Often, the most frequently cited side effect of radiation therapy is fatigue, which inhibits day-to-day functioning, disrupts activities, and decreases quality of life. Patients also possess significant concerns related to pain and the duration of treatments.

Autologous Bone Marrow Transplantation (ABMT). The intensity of treatment associated with ABMT is well-established; however, improvements in the overall procedure with the use of agents such as hematopoietic growth factors have reduced the length of hospital stays and complications due to prolonged aplasia. Evidence suggests that despite the intensity, many patients adapt favorably and recover psychologically. In many respects, the patient's psychological status before transplant may be the best predictor of adjustment after the procedure and discharge from the hospital.

PSYCHOSOCIAL VULNERABILITY

Cancer is more than the initial diagnosis. As patients move through their early reactions, they gain experience as cancer survivors. For many breast cancer patients, survivorship begins on the day of diagnosis as women begin to redefine all aspects of their lives.[15]

Four primary points exist in the psychosocial care of cancer patients. First, patients experience an "existential plight"[16] during the first 3 months after their diagnosis. While many patients strive to regain a sense of normalcy, many experience intense distress and are forced to acknowledge that their lives will never be the same. Second, if a remission occurs, patients begin to live with their cancer. They incorporate disruptions of daily life into their routines. Third, the fear of recurrence or the actual event further complicates the psychosocial course for each patient. While many health care providers assume patients may experience recurrence as the point of highest distress, this is often not the case. Patients gain critical information and knowledge concerning their disease and treatments, while forming supportive relationships with members of the health care team and with other patients. Knowledge and support from the team enable patients to anticipate and understand their course after recurrence. While absent at diagnosis, this critical knowledge often lessens distress at recurrence.[17] Finally, if treatment fails, terminal illness and the potential threat of abandonment confronts patients with the greatest challenge to adaptation. Some patients possess the capability to adapt to a terminal illness, but many will never accept death.[18]

Since patients vary significantly in their ability to adapt to their cancer diagnosis and treatment, the essential task is to define those variables which promote adaptation. Table 89–1 summarizes the critical variables that promote or inhibit psychosocial adap-

TABLE 89–1.   VARIABLES ASSOCIATED WITH PSYCHOSOCIAL ADAPTATION

Social Support
Marital Status
Living arrangements
Number of family members and relatives in vicinity
Church attendance

History
Substance abuse
Depression
Mental health
Major illness
Past regrets
Optimism versus pessimism

Current Concerns
Health
Religion
Work-finance
Family
Friends
Existential
Self-Appraisal

Other
Education
Employment
Physical symptoms
Anatomical staging

From Weisman AD, Worden JW, Sobel HJ: Psychosocial Screening and Intervention With Cancer Patients: Research Report. Boston, Harvard Medical School and Massachusetts General Hospital, 1980.

TABLE 89–2. COPING STRATEGIES AND THEIR LEVEL OF EFFECTIVENESS

Most Effective
Confrontation
Redefinition
Compliance with authority

Intermediate Effective
Seek information
Share concern
Humor
Distraction

Least Effective
Suppression
Stoic submission
Acting out
Repetition compulsion
Tension reduction
Withdrawal
Blame others
Self-blame

Data from Weisman AD, Worden JW, Sobel HJ: Psychosocial Screening and Intervention With Cancer Patients: Research Report. Boston, Harvard Medical School and Massachusetts General Hospital, 1980.

tation. While single variables do not determine successful adaptation, patient profiles can be constructed to describe who will experience higher levels of difficulty. For example, a widow who lives alone and has only a few relatives in her immediate area may experience greater difficulty. If this same individual possesses a history of depression and a pessimistic life orientation, her difficulty will be even greater and she will probably require psychosocial intervention to enable her to move from ineffective strategies to behaviors that will resolve illness-related problems (Table 89–2).

Psychosocial Screening

Methods exist that can effectively identify patients who are more likely to experience higher levels of distress. Psychosocial screening provides the opportunity to identify and predict which patients are more distressed and, consequently, are unlikely to adapt to the many stressors associated with a cancer diagnosis and its treatments.[19] Traditional psychosocial services are available on a referral basis from the health care team. Often, referrals occur when a patient reaches a crisis. Such a reactive approach allows the patient to experience a crisis that may jeopardize her relationship with the health care team as well as effective participation in her treatment. In some cases, patients withdraw from treatment or exhibit a lack of compliance with health directives.[20, 21] Estimates of low compliance with chemotherapy regimens range from 20 to 75 percent.[22] Given the difficulties that very distressed patients experience and their greater likelihood not to fully participate in treatment, psychosocial screening to prospectively identify these patients becomes imperative. Identification of "high-distress patients" results in the offer of psychosocial services early in the treatment course and creates the opportunity for a more effective alliance between the patient and the health care team. Techniques for psychosocial screening of newly diagnosed patients range from structured interviews to self-report psychological instruments. Brief and efficient methods that utilize self-report measures may also be cost-effective.[19, 23] In some cases, a brief psychological instrument can be incorporated into an outpatient clinic registration process and require only 5 to 7 minutes of patient time. Such a process also maximizes the utilization of psychosocial resources, since these providers can identify patients with the highest level of distress.

CANCER AND THE FAMILY

Since social support is a critical variable in the patient's adaptation, the family most often fulfills this role. Weisman, Worden, and Sobel[24] attempt to quantify social support (see Table 89–1) by an objective examination of pertinent variables such as marital status, living arrangements, and availability of family members and other relatives, but a quantitative description does not equate with the ability of any family system to actually provide the support a patient needs. In some instances, families may attempt to provide too much support, which can also disrupt a patient's attempt to adapt successfully to the illness.[25] For example, family members may attempt to protect the patient through encouragement to delay participation in physical therapy or a return to eating after dietary restrictions.

Critical Family Constructs

Family literature provides a range of theories to describe how families function. Family unity,[26] enmeshment,[27] and cross-generational alliances[28] are concepts that describe certain aspects of family behavior. Olson and colleagues[29] developed the Circumplex Model of Family Functioning, which focuses on two of the most salient family constructs—adaptability and cohesion. This model can be helpful in the medical setting to assess the resources and limitations of a family system. Methods exist that actually measure these critical variables and possess highly acceptable levels of reliability and validity.[30] If possible, psychosocial screening can also be undertaken to prospectively identify families that might present difficulties for the health care team.[31]

Adaptability and Cohesion

Adaptability can be defined as the capability of any family to reorganize or restructure itself when confronted by a stressful event. Under significant stress, families need to reassign internal roles, modify rules for daily living, or revise its decision-making process. While many families accept this challenge, approximately 30 percent of them cannot adapt and may be lost to or disrupt the health care team.[31] *Cohesion*

TABLE 89–3.   EARLY INDICATORS OF POSITIVE FAMILY ADJUSTMENT

Seek information appropriately
Provide support to the patient
Visit regularly
Assist with activities of daily living
Facilitate medical treatment plans
Possess a positive attitude
Demonstrate support to one another
Focus on patient rather than family needs

is the amount of emotional bonding between family members. Cohesion can be high, moderate, or low. High cohesion tends to suggest enmeshment: each individual member has little autonomy. Low cohesion or minimal emotional bonding expresses a lack of commitment to other members, and such families may be unavailable to medical staff for support of the patient or decision-making.[32]

Often, in the care of the patient and family, early indicators suggest which families may be an asset or a liability to care (Table 89–3). Early identification, combined with a comprehensive family assessment, maximizes the health care team's ability to respond to a wide range of behaviors exhibited by diverse family types. Interactions between the team and family members during the diagnostic and initial treatment phases set the stage for ongoing contact. Specific interventions of the team—information giving, emotional support, availability, and the instilling of a sense of hope and interest—provide the opportunity to build an effective alliance with the family on behalf of the patient.

Family Life Cycle

A final consideration of Olson's Circumplex Model is the concept of the family life cycle. While patients are often broadly characterized by their developmental stage (i.e., middle age, elderly), families also follow a life cycle. Within the Circumplex Model, the age of the oldest child determines movement through the family life cycle. At each of the seven stages, families confront normal developmental tasks and these dynamic changes over time create natural stressors. Table 89–4 contains Olson's Family Life Cycle and defines each of the seven stages. Critical to this con-

TABLE 89–4.   OLSON'S FAMILY LIFE CYCLE

Stage	
1	Young couples without children
2	Families with preschoolers (age 0 to 5)
3	Families with school-age children (age 6 to 12)
4	Families with adolescents (age 13 to 18)
5	Launching families (age 19 or older)
6	Empty nest families (all children gone)
7	Families in retirement (over age 65)

From Olson DH, McCubbin HI, Barnes HL, et al: Families: What Makes Them Work. London, Sage, 1989.

cept of the family life cycle is its dynamic nature. Daily living generates normal stressors within families. As a result, overall marital satisfaction, family satisfaction, and quality of life are constantly in flux. Normal changes or stressors may intensify if the family cannot respond to tasks at each developmental stage. Adaptability and cohesion levels are critical to how successfully families move through the life cycle. Within this framework, unanticipated stressful events such as a cancer diagnosis can occur and disrupt a family's natural transition from one stage to the next.

The diagnosis of breast cancer severely disrupts the normal course of events in a family. A range of variables determine the family's response. For example, the response of a family at Stage 1 (young couples, no children) may be quite different from a family at Stage 5 (launching stage, children leaving home). Families may be more vulnerable at stages when normal stressors reach their maximum. Given that most women will be diagnosed at a later age, most families may be approaching or experiencing Stage 5. Consequently, most families may experience breast cancer at a time when normal stressors in the family may be at the highest point.

In summary, factors such as a family's level of adaptability and cohesion in conjunction with the stage in the life cycle greatly influence a family's response to the diagnosis of cancer. Families may be temporarily impaired, or if their functioning is already in an extreme category their behavior may be problematic to the health care team.

SEXUALITY

Advances in cancer treatments continue to increase and extend survival. As a result, cancer patients need help in normalizing their daily lives to achieve optimal physical, psychological, and social functioning.[33] Sexual functioning is a critical factor in the physical, psychological, and social rehabilitation, given that breast cancer can affect body image and self-esteem. Thus, decreased sexual functioning and perceptions of sexual attractiveness can diminish a patient's overall sense of well-being.[34]

Timely recognition of patients' sexual needs and dysfunctions is essential to comprehensive cancer care. Unfortunately, health professionals often stress survival and control of the disease and ignore sexuality as an essential aspect of the cancer patient's quality of life. Physicians and nurses may refrain from providing information that addresses sexuality because they assume that sexual desires and the need for intimacy fade in the face of life-threatening illness. Patients may also be reluctant to raise sexual issues as a concern because they are embarrassed to discuss this intimate topic.[33] Reluctance may be due to the fact that myths about cancer and sexuality are still prevalent today. Fears that cancer is contagious through sexual activity, that having sex may cause a recurrence, that cancer is a punishment for past sexual misconduct, or that a sexual partner may be exposed to radiation if the patient is receiving external-beam radiation therapy are but a few of the common misunderstandings.[35]

To address these misconceptions and to engage in a total psychosocial rehabilitation of the breast cancer patient, health care personnel need to conduct a sexual assessment as part of their routine care. A health review of the vital systems of the body with routine questions about eating, smoking, drinking, and sleeping habits ought to include specific inquiries about sexual functioning and relationships.[36]

A comprehensive clinical assessment must take an orderly approach to systematically ascertain the role of sexuality for each patient.[37] A large proportion of sexual dysfunctions have psychological as well as physiological origins, and it is thus important to differentiate between the anatomic changes and the emotional effects of the disease.[33] Even when sexual functioning is negatively affected by physiological processes, however, psychological support and guidance is no less important. According to Wise,[37] there are a number of possible psychological effects: regression due to the sick role; lowered self-esteem; fears of appearance (scars, odors); comfort minimized by pain; and agility and mobility limited by disease or treatment. Organic limitations, on the other hand, are easily divided into two categories: endogenous ones attributable to the disease effects, and exogenous ones that are drug or treatment induced.

SPIRITUALITY

One salient aspect of the distress of life-threatening or terminal illness is spirituality or one's spiritual self-awareness. Studies concerned with the spiritual well-being,[38] spiritual coping strategies,[39] and the relationship of spiritual well-being to hope,[18] indicate that an awareness of spirituality should be fundamental to the study of psychosocial distress related to any life-threatening or terminal illness. Many traditional psychological approaches fail to recognize spirituality and transcendency as intrinsic aspects of human needs.[40, 41] Therefore, medical and psychosocial providers may not meet the needs of those facing a life-threatening or terminal illness. An essential principle for meaningful intervention with these populations is the fundamental perspective that as human beings we are far more than either the sum of our biological parts or the effects of our environment. Acknowledgment of the spiritual aspect of the person is based on the principle that there are powerful forces within the psyche that propel us toward greater wholeness and integration. Bodian describes this journey as a potential psychospiritual transformation beyond the ego.[42] However, traditional theories of psychology, upon which many psychosocial interventions are based, are very dependent on ego psychology and as a result lack a theoretical framework for an ego-transcending phenomenon such as death. Therefore, terminally ill patients or those fac-

ing a life-threatening illness often approach illness, dying, and death from a fearful and reactive stance. People can be helped to accept their own mortality within a framework which normalizes death.

Whether or not a poor prognosis is ever indicated, clinicians observe that breast cancer patients, at the time of diagnosis and throughout their illness, enter a process of exploring what life and death mean to them. As this exploration begins, traditional values and spiritual belief systems are questioned and challenged. A redefinition of one's attitude toward death may be necessary in order to formulate a personal death perspective that serves as a comfort rather than a threat. If the patient is able to move beyond commonly held beliefs, this developmental task can be accomplished; however, the interactive process of formulating a personal death perspective and a heightened spiritual awareness can generate elevated levels of distress for cancer patients and their families. If a patient is unable to find a comforting death perspective, or if the level of spiritual orientation is inadequate, the patient may experience significant psychosocial distress.

Smith and colleagues[43] found that a higher level of spirituality is associated with an increase in the patient's ability to normalize death. As a result, patients experienced lower levels of psychosocial distress. In this study of 116 adult medical oncology outpatients, a significant negative relationship was found between the interaction of spiritual awareness with the patient's personal death perspective and psychosocial distress. The findings of this study empirically support the suppositions of others working in the field of spiritual well-being[44] and spiritual distress.[45] Patients accrue spiritual perspectives over the life span, and as a result they can maintain a sense of well-being in the face of perceptual losses associated with a life-threatening illness and death.

Smith[46] has also proposed a model of intervention in the transpersonal realm to facilitate and normalize death and to heighten spiritual awareness.

QUALITY OF LIFE

The concept of quality of life continues to create struggles for clinicians and researchers in that it is difficult to reach consensus on its definition and on techniques to measure it. Despite a consensus that the goal of medical care is the preservation of life and well-being,[47, 48] the clear majority of clinical trials fail to include any qualitative assessments of the subjective experience of the patient as an outcome.

It must be acknowledged that any quality of life assessment requires value judgments. In many respects, patients can judge their own values and their losses. The most commonly studied domains are physical, psychological, social, economic, and global well-being.[49] Self-report provides patients the opportunity to describe their quality of life from their perspective rather than relying on evaluations by physicians, family members, or other caregivers. Repeat measurements of quality of life over time enable providers to examine this concept within short time frames. Consequently, recall bias is avoided and the effect of personality traits can be ascertained. Quality of life can be measured globally through such instruments as the Functional Living Index—Cancer[50] or the Functional Assessment of Cancer Therapy,[51] the Satisfaction with Life Domains Scale,[52] or through the use of multiple instruments to assess the specific domains that comprise quality of life. Given that life can be defined from both a quantitative and a qualitative perspective, quality of life in relation to cancer therapies and rehabilitation provides an additional measure that can be utilized to substantiate treatment outcomes.

SURVIVORSHIP

Owing to recent technological advances in the detection and treatment of cancer, nearly half of the people diagnosed with these life-threatening diseases are expected to be alive after 5 years.[53] As an increasing number of breast cancer patients are now either cured of their disease or live for many years with it, they face the complex process of adjusting to life after cancer treatment. This has created a growing population of cancer survivors who have successfully completed their cancer treatment, but have a number of special needs. A number of studies[54, 55] indicate that, while cancer survival may be achieved, it is still a disease that can substantially affect several physical and psychological aspects of a survivor's life. These physical and psychological "late effects" that plague survivors appear to result from the physical complications of aggressive cancer treatments, the stress of being near death, and the stigma of being a cancer patient.[56, 57] Survivors have to deal with problems related to being in a dependent patient role, which generates difficulty in a return to preillness roles. Cancer survivors and their family members seldom shake the fear of recurrence. Hypervigilance and hypochondriasis are common reactions that should be addressed at every opportunity.

According to Zampini and Ostroff,[58] cancer survivors generally experience challenges in four critical life domains: (1) physical health; (2) psychological and social well-being; (3) maintaining adequate health insurance; and (4) employment. Physical health challenges for breast cancer survivors include fear of recurrence, the possibility of a secondary malignancy, and other late medical effects of aggressive treatments. Many survivors actively strive to meet these challenges by maintaining their physical health through preventive regimes of diet, exercise, stress reduction, and smoking cessation. These activities restore some sense of control to the cancer survivor in the realm of physical health.

Psychological and social well-being of cancer survivors are challenged on a number of fronts. While no two breast cancer survivors respond identically, emotions confronted include elation to be finishing treatment, residual shock, anger, grief, sadness, and existential questioning. In general, most breast cancer survivors report mild to moderate psychological distress. Those patients who lack social support, have a psychiatric history, have severe physical limitations, or have a pattern of maladaptive coping may experience even higher levels of distress and will be impeded in their adjustment.

The maintenance of adequate health coverage is extremely important to breast cancer survivors; however, cancer survivors often may be threatened with policy cancellations or reductions in coverage. Furthermore, the link between job and insurance creates difficulties for survivors who feel compelled to retain their current employment rather than risk the possibility of losing their health care coverage. Finally, employment issues that concern cancer survivors center around failure to be promoted, negative attitudes toward cancer, and undue criticism from supervisors or coworkers. Few cancer patients actually encounter dismissal from their place of employment, but a larger number experience more subtle difficulties.[58]

Because the bulk of the survivorship literature tends to cluster around the four domains set forth above, a number of programs are being established to address the specialized needs of this population. The National Cancer Institute has developed a booklet as a guide for cancer survivors entitled *Facing Forward*,[59] which addresses these four domains. Major cancer centers have also developed patient programs such as Memorial Sloan-Kettering's Post-Treatment Resource Program and The Johns Hopkins Oncology Center's Cancer Survivors' Program.

COPING WITH LOSS

To maintain a sense of hope and optimism and a positive definition of quality of life, the losses breast cancer patients experience must be acknowledged. While loss is a universal experience, breast cancer represents multiple losses. Partial or complete loss of a breast in conjunction with the actual cancer diagnosis generates a series of losses that every patient confronts. Given the symbolic nature of the breast in our culture,[13] definitions of femininity are challenged. Many spouses and partners attempt to provide support through statements that diminish the importance of the breast. Often, health and survival are emphasized, and the loss of the breast may be discounted; however, spouses and partners also experience a loss. If the emotions associated with these losses remain hidden, relationships can be severely disrupted. Acknowledgment and open communication foster awareness of the meaning of the loss for both the patient and her partner. In many respects, involvement of the spouse or partner prior to surgery in medical discussions and education programs provides opportunities for them to prepare for these issues.

A secondary loss that is also significant relates to

overall health. For many women, breast cancer is the first serious illness of their lives. Life before breast cancer proceeded with health as a given as women moved along a developmental line toward middle age, and eventually retirement. Women lose a life that was free of any serious health concern or illness. These losses, in conjunction with others in areas of career, financial security, and family, require attention and direction from the health care team and psychosocial providers.

To provide direct assistance, patients can be encouraged to consider how they have managed other losses. For example, a newly diagnosed 51-year-old married woman with two teenage daughters sought assistance for her emotional reactions following surgery. In examining past losses, the patient clearly identified the death of her father as the most traumatic event in her life. In exploring her response to her father's death, she described how she experienced the pain of this loss, how her family provided comfort, and how her spiritual beliefs created relief. In many respects, her response can be characterized as the use of positive coping skills to gain control and an understanding of her father's death. Through this exploration, the patient realized that these same approaches would be helpful to her as she attempts to respond to the meaning of her surgery and prepares for potential adjuvant treatments.

Finally, loss generates fear, anguish, sadness, and grief. Each is a normal reaction to the diagnosis of breast cancer and surgery. Acknowledgment of emotional reactions facilitates movement through treatment, rehabilitation, and recovery. If these reactions persist or increase in intensity, counseling through a masters-prepared social worker or a psychologist may be indicated. A support group may be helpful for open discussion, clarification of emotions, and problem-solving suggestions. If the reactions are severe, psychotherapy may be appropriate to address persistent symptoms such as anxiety or depression. Given that breast cancer patients experience more anxiety,[9] cognitive-behavioral interventions should also be considered.

COGNITIVE-BEHAVIORAL INTERVENTIONS

Breast cancer patients frequently manifest a variety of symptoms as direct effects of the cancer and its treatments. Most commonly identified symptoms include acute and chronic pain, anxiety, insomnia, hypochondriasis, anticipatory nausea and vomiting, and depression. To varying degrees, cognitive-behavioral interventions can ameliorate symptoms that challenge the integrity of patients and families.

Anxiety, pain, and nausea and vomiting represent some of the most common noxious symptoms experienced by breast cancer patients. Affectual, behavioral, motivational, and perceptual variables significantly influence these symptoms. Consequently,

cognitive-behavioral techniques emerge as the focal approach for the treatment of these symptoms.[60-64]

Cognitive-behavioral approaches originate with the laws of learning and conditioning. With an adequate appreciation for the importance of the interaction between the patient's thoughts, feeling, and behaviors (especially the unexamined automatic responses), a variety of cognitive and behavioral interventions can be systematically employed.[65] Specifically, the synergy of reinforcers from the internal and external domains of the patient and the immediate environment serve to determine both the frequency and degree of effectiveness of patient responses. Patient activities, whether they are thoughts, feelings, or behavior, can be socially rewarded or encouraged and as a result, physical tension, distress, or pain can be reduced.

Usually, interactions between patients and families produce the vast majority of reinforcing, inhibiting, or extinguishing responses. Consequently, a cognitive-behavioral treatment plan actively engages and integrates key family members into the implementation of strategies to resolve the problematic symptom. Exclusion of the patient's primary caregiver or significant other often results in family resistance. As previously discussed, the family may be lost as allies or resources in the implementation of the treatment plan. This loss is even more significant if the patient is significantly impaired, has advanced disease, or is terminally ill. For the health care provider it should be emphasized that cognitive-behavioral approaches enable cancer patients and their families to maximize their sense of control and hope, which are often the first and second casualties after a cancer diagnosis.

Since breast cancer patients and families pass through different phases following the diagnosis, this dynamic process necessitates revisions of goals and treatment plans so that specific needs can be met. Over the course of their illness, the most common needs are maintenance of quality of life, attention to mood, acquisition of coping skills, and reduction of suffering.[66]

EMPLOYMENT AND FINANCES

Return to work after surgery and adjuvant treatments provides relief as well as potential stress. On the positive side, work represents the beginning of a return to normalcy, and in many ways work serves as a distraction from the rigors associated with a breast cancer and related treatments. However, the lack of physical endurance related to fatigue may persist, which in turn can hinder work performance. While case reports exist concerning highly supportive work environments, negative responses clearly outnumber the positive ones. Cancer in the workplace can be equated with a social stigma as colleagues and coworkers are unprepared to respond to dramatic physiological changes. Openness is simply not encouraged. As a result, breast cancer patients must

TABLE 89–5. FACTORS FOR RISK ASSESSMENT OF BREAST CANCER

Age
Family history in first- or second-degree relatives
History of biopsy for benign breast disease
Nulliparity or first live birth after age 30
Menarche before age 12

From Vogel VG: Assessing women's potential risk of developing breast cancer. Oncology 10:1451, 1996.

attempt to conceal treatment effects. Discomfort in the work environment can result in social isolation and significant fears of termination from the job, which in turn may create the most significant fear, loss of health care benefits.

DAUGHTERS OF BREAST CANCER PATIENTS

Given the significant advances in cancer genetics, concerns continue to increase related to the increased risks of breast cancer for first-degree relatives. For daughters of premenopausal breast cancer patients, the risk can increase sixfold.[67] Given the media attention in this area, the general public possesses an awareness of the genetic link of breast cancer from generation to generation. The major issue is how to manage the anxiety of these daughters as they gradually approach the age when their mothers were diagnosed. Clearly, risk-related information must focus on the probability of developing breast cancer rather than of dying from the disease.[68] Identification of risk without an effective management plan can only exacerbate pre-existing psychological distress. Furthermore, distress may cause a woman to dramatically overestimate her cancer risk. Table 89–5 details factors for risk assessment.

Increased risk of breast cancer can generate significant anxiety and fear. Exploration of this issue should result in a detailed understanding of women's fears and worries of developing breast cancer. If consistent reassurance and support do not reduce distress, appropriate referrals for psychological assessment and counseling are warranted.[67]

CONCLUSIONS

Patients and families have very personal perceptions of breast cancer and treatments that are influenced and developed over time as a result of many factors. A clear understanding of how patients and family members perceive supportive care significantly enhances the health care team's ability to provide care and anticipate potential problems. Information and education must be consistently available as patients and families move across the disease continuum from diagnosis to treatment to recovery.

Comprehensive psychosocial assessment of the pa-

tient must move beyond traditional considerations and include intimacy, sexuality, and spirituality and a realistic appraisal of the capabilities and limitations of each family. Health care providers tend to assume, erroneously, that all patients are capable of withstanding the multiple and complex demands of a prolonged illness. Because of the ongoing trend to reduce inpatient length of stay, families must be carefully assessed to determine if the level of care and support for the patient is adequate. If indications of marginal or inadequate care exist, the patient may require additional support services.

Health care professionals practice in an extremely demanding environment. Although prepared to function well in the context of multiple technical and instrumental tasks, staff are seldom prepared for the psychological and emotional demands of patients and families and of their own idiosyncratic responses. For the patient and family, loss is at the center of the breast cancer experience. For the health care professional with a commitment to comprehensive care, facilitation of the patient's adjustment through adequate support for the family can lead to a sense of control and satisfaction. Undetected and untreated psychological distress can jeopardize treatment outcomes,[21] stimulate dissatisfaction with care,[69] and increase overall health care costs.[11]

References

1. Wainstock JM: Breast cancer: Psychosocial consequences for the patient. Semin Oncol Nursing 7:207, 1991.
2. Ganz PA: Advocating for the women with breast cancer. CA Cancer J Clin 45:114, 1995.
3. Weisman AD: Early diagnosis of vulnerability in cancer patients. Am J Med Sci 271:187, 1976.
4. Lazarus RS: Coping with the stress of illness. WHO Reg Publ Eur Ser 44:11, 1992.
5. Carlsson M, Hamrin E: Psychological and psychosocial aspects of breast cancer and breast cancer treatments. Cancer Nursing 17:418, 1994.
6. Derogatis LR, Morrow GR, Fetting J: The prevalence of psychiatric disorders among cancer patients. JAMA 249:751, 1983.
7. Farber JM, Weinerman BH, Kuypers JA: Psychosocial distress in oncology outpatients. J Psychosocial Oncol 2:109, 1984.
8. Stefanek M, Derogatis L, Shaw A: Psychological distress among oncology outpatients. Psychosomatics 28:530, 1987.
9. Zabora JR, Smith ED, Brintzenhofe Szoc K: Prevalence of psychological distress by cancer site. Proc Am Soc Clin Oncol 15:507, 1996.
10. Zabora J, Blanchard C, Smith E, et al: Prevalence of psychological distress across the disease continuum. J Psychosocial Oncol 15:21, 1997.
11. Allison TG, Williams DE, Miller TD, et al: Medical and economic costs of psychologic distress in patients with coronary artery disease. Mayo Clin Proc 70:734, 1995.
12. Williams TR, O'Sullivan M, Snodgrass SE, Love N: Psychosocial issues in breast cancer: Helping patients get the support they need. Postgrad Med 98:97, 1995.
13. Elberg JJ, Blichert-Toft M, Drzewiecki KT: Primary breast reconstruction after mastectomy for breast cancer. Ugeskr Laeger 157:1013, 1995.
14. Levine MN, Guyatt GH, Gent M, et al: Quality of life in stage II breast cancer. J Clin Oncol 6:1978, 1988.
15. Mullan F: The cancer consort: Making cancer survivors a positive political force. J Psychosocial Oncol 5:81, 1987.
16. Weisman AD, Worden JW: The existential plight in cancer:

Significance of the first hundred days. Psychiatry Med 7:1, 1976.

17. Weisman AD, Worden JW: The emotional impact of recurrent cancer. J Psychosocial Oncol 3:5, 1985.

18. Carson V, Soeken K, Grimm P: Hope and its relationship to spiritual well-being. J Psychol Theol 6:159, 1988.

19. Rainey LC, Wellisch DK, Fawzy FI: Training health professionals in psychosocial aspects of cancer: A continuing education model. J Psychosocial Oncol 1:41, 1983.

20. Weisman AD: A model of psychosocial phasing in cancer. Gen Hosp Psychiatry 1:187, 1979.

21. Hyland JM, Travis JW, Pruyser H, et al: Problems of compliance with treatment among patients receiving radiotherapy. J Psychosocial Oncol 1:65, 1983.

22. Richardson JL, Mark G, Levine A: The influence of symptoms and side effects of treatment on compliance with cancer therapy. J Clin Oncol 6:1746, 1988.

23. Zabora JR, Smith-Wilson R, Fetting JH, et al: An efficient method for the psychosocial screening of cancer patients. Psychosomatics 3:192, 1990.

24. Weisman AD, Worden JW, Sobel HJ: Psychosocial Screening and Intervention With Cancer Patients: Research Report. Boston, Harvard Medical School and Massachusetts General Hospital, 1980.

25. Berkman L, Leo-Summers L, Horwitz RI: Emotional support and survival after myocardial infarction. Ann Intern Med 117:1003, 1992.

26. Geismar LL, La Sorte MA: Understanding the Multi-Problem Family. New York, Associated Press, 1964.

27. Minuchin S: Families and Family Therapy. Cambridge, Harvard University Press, 1974.

28. Haley J: Strategies of Psychotherapy. Orlando, Grune & Stratton, 1963.

29. Olson DH, McCubbin HI, Barnes HL, et al: Families: What Makes Them Work. London, Sage, 1989.

30. Olson DH, Sprenkle RH (eds): Circumplex Model: Systemic Assessment and Treatment of Families. New York, Haworth, 1988.

31. Zabora JR, Fetting JH, Shanley VB, et al: Predicting conflict with staff among families of cancer patients during prolonged hospitalizations. J Psychosocial Oncol 7(3):103, 1989.

32. Zabora JR, Smith ED: Early assessment and intervention with dysfunctional family systems. Oncology 5:31, 1992.

33. Mantell JE: Sexuality and Cancer: Psychosocial Aspects of Cancer. New York, Raven Press, 1982.

34. Burbie GE, Polinsky ML: Intimacy and sexuality after cancer treatment: Restoring a sense of wholeness. J Psychosocial Oncol 10(1):19, 1992.

35. Schover L, Johnson S: Sexuality and Chronic Illness: A Comprehensive Approach. New York, Guilford, 1988.

36. Wasow M: Sexuality assessment as a tool for sexual rehabilitation in cancer patients. Sexuality Disability 5:28, 1982.

37. Wise T: Sexuality in the aging and incapacitated: Disabilities and treatment. Psychiatr Clin North Am 3:1873, 1980.

38. Reed P: Spirituality and well-being in terminally ill hospitalized adults. Res Nursing Health 10:335, 1987.

39. Sodestrom L, Martinson I: Patients' spiritual coping strategies: A study of nurse and patient perspectives. Oncol Nursing Forum 14:41, 1987.

40. Walsh R, Vaughn F (eds): Beyond Ego. Los Angeles, Jeremy P. Tarcher, 1980.

41. Welwood J: Awakening the Heart. Boulder, CO, Shambhala Publications, 1983.

42. Bodian S: If Buddha had been a shrink. Yoga J 88:43, 1989.

43. Smith E, Stefanek ME, Joseph MV: Spiritual awareness, personal death perspective and psychosocial distress among cancer patients: An initial investigation. J Psychosocial Oncol 11:89, 1993.

44. Reed P: Death perspectives and temporal variables in terminally ill and healthy adults. Death Stud 10:467, 1968.

45. Ellerhorst-Ryan J: Selecting an instrument to measure spiritual distress. Oncol Nursing Forum 12:93, 1985.

46. Smith E: The Relationship of Transpersonal Development to Psychosocial Distress of Cancer Patients. The Catholic University of America, Doctoral dissertation, 1990.

47. Zittoun R (ed): Quality of life of cancer patients. In International Congress of Psychosocial Oncology, Beaune, France, October 12–14, 1992.

48. Cella DF, Tulsky DS: Measuring quality of life today: Methodological aspects. Oncology 4:29, 1990.

49. De Haes CJM, van Knippenberg FCE: The quality of life of cancer patients: A review of the literature. Social Sci Med 20:809, 1985.

50. Schipper H, Clinch A, McMurray A, et al: Measuring the quality of life of cancer patients: The functional living index-cancer: Development and validation. J Clin Oncol 2:472, 1984.

51. Cella DF, Lee-Riordan D, Silberman M, et al: Quality of life in advanced cancer: Three new disease-specific measures, abstracted (1225). Proc Am Soc Clin Oncol, May 21–23, 1989.

52. Baker F, Curbow B, Wingard J: Development of the satisfaction with life domains scale for cancer. J Psychosocial Oncol 10:75, 1992.

53. Cancer Facts and Figures-1994. Atlanta, American Cancer Society, 1994.

54. Ganz PA, Rofessart J, Polinsky ML, et al: A comprehensive approach to cancer patients' needs assessment: The cancer inventory of problem situation (CIPS) and a companion interview. J Psychosocial Oncol 4:75, 1986.

55. Andrykowski MA, Curren SL, Cunningham L, et al: Psychosocial adjustment and quality of life in women with breast cancer and benign breast problems. J Clin Epidemiol 48:827, 1996.

56. Hoffman B: Employment discrimination: Another hurdle for cancer survivors. Cancer Invest 9:589, 1991.

57. Nessim S, Ellis J: Cancervive: The Challenge of Life After Cancer. Boston, Houghton-Mifflin, 1991.

58. Zampini K, Ostroff JS: The post-treatment resource program: Portrait of a program for cancer survivors. Psycho-oncology 2:1, 1993.

59. National Cancer Institute: Facing Forward: A Guide for Cancer Survivors. Washington, DC, U.S. Department of Health and Human Services, Public Health Service, National Institutes of Health, 1990.

60. Chapman CR: Psychologic and behavioral aspects of cancer pain. In Bonica JJ, Ventafridda V (eds): Advances in Pain Research and Therapy. Vol. 2. New York, Raven Press, 1979, p 655.

61. Morrow GR, Dobkin PL: Anticipatory nausea and vomiting in cancer patients undergoing chemotherapy treatment: Prevalence, etiology, and behavioral interventions. Clin Psychol Rev 8:517, 1988.

62. Loscalzo M, Jacobsen PB: Practical behavioral approaches to the effective management of pain and distress. J Psychosocial Oncol 8:139, 1990.

63. Turk DC, Rennert K: Pain and the terminally ill cancer patient: A cognitive-social learning perspective. In Sobel H (ed): Behavior Therapy in Terminal Care. Cambridge, MA, Ballinger, 1981, p 95.

64. Morrow GR, Morrell BS: Behavioral treatment for the anticipatory nausea and vomiting induced by cancer chemotherapy. N Engl J Med 307:1476, 1982.

65. Turk D, Meichenbaum D, Genest M: Pain and Behavioral Medicine. New York, Guilford, 1983.

66. Bandura A: Self-efficacy: Toward a unifying theory of behavioral change. Psychol Rev 84:191, 1977.

67. Vogel VG: Assessing women's potential risk of developing breast cancer. Oncology 10:1451, 1996.

68. Hoskins RF, Stopfer JE, Calzone KA, et al: Assessment and counseling for women with a family history of breast cancer. JAMA 273:577, 1995.

69. Greenley JR, et al: Psychological distress and patient satisfaction. Med Care 20:373, 1982.

CHAPTER 90

PSYCHOSOCIAL RESOURCES FOR BREAST CANCER PATIENTS AND THEIR FAMILIES

Susan Stillman, M.S.W.

BACKGROUND

Each year, more than 180,000 women in the United States learn they have breast cancer.[1] Most women possess the emotional strength to tolerate the challenges associated with the rigors of diagnosis and treatment; however, cancer disrupts all aspects of daily life, including family, work, fiancees, friends, as well as the woman's psychological status.[2] Previous studies have shown that two out of every three newly diagnosed people with cancer complete a successful adaptation 2 to 6 months after the initial diagnosis.[3, 4] These patients have positive sources of emotional support, greater social connectedness, and higher levels of adaptability in resolving problems and crisis events. The third of patients who fail to adapt have weaker social support, a greater likelihood of past psychosocial problems such as alcoholism or a psychiatric history, and a pessimistic orientation to life events.[5] When considering what types of resources women with breast cancer need, health care providers must focus on the needs of all patients, not assuming that people who successfully adapt have no psychosocial needs. Psychoeducational services, such as the provision of information concerning treatment options and decision making, insurance dilemmas, employment discrimination, or sexual difficulties, facilitate a successful adaptation for any person with cancer.[6] Even after women adapt successfully, patients may need to pursue more intensive services such as psychotherapy to gain additional support, control, and insight. A variety of national organizations exist that address many of the psychosocial needs of women with breast cancer.[7]

In addition, a variety of health care professionals can provide key clinical interventions or educational programs for women and their families. Clinical interventions focus on teaching effective problem-solving skills. Clinical social workers often provide crisis intervention as a means of identifying problems amenable to problem-solving techniques. While social workers frequently detect levels of distress associated with psychiatric diagnoses and provide psychotherapy, psychologists and psychiatrists provide consultation and evaluation for more severe disorders that may require psychotropic medications. At times, a clinical nurse specialist with psychiatric training may also fulfill this role. Table 90–1 presents a comprehensive psychosocial model of care that is appropriate for the management of psychosocial problems experienced by breast cancer patients and survivors.[8]

NATIONAL ORGANIZATIONS

A number of national organizations have emerged over the years to help women with information and resources about breast cancer. A description of the most prominent ones follows.

National Alliance of Breast Cancer Organizations (NABCO). Founded in 1986, NABCO is a network of over 300 breast cancer organizations, including comprehensive cancer centers, breast centers, private and government agencies, research centers, professional organizations, and support services. NABCO provides information, assistance, and referral to anyone with questions about breast cancer and acts as a voice for the interests and concerns of breast cancer survivors and women at risk. In addition, members receive the following benefits:

- *Information Services*: Up-to-date information on all aspects of breast cancer—risk factors, early detection, treatment options, support services, recurrence, hospice care, financial assistance/reimbursement, and free or low-cost services—is available. An individualized package is mailed in response to a member's queries that addresses both medical and emotional needs.
- *NABCO News*: This quarterly newsletter covers the latest developments in medical and scientific research. It covers the policies and politics that affect women with breast cancer and shares information about what women are doing to help themselves.
- *Breast Cancer Resource List*: A comprehensive listing of more than 1500 resources nationally—books and other printed materials—covers every aspect of breast cancer and breast health: videos, hotlines, and a database of over 300 local support organizations; detailed information about medical services, advocacy efforts and more. This list of resources is updated and published annually.
- *Advocacy Efforts*: Through testimony and expertise, NABCO addresses a range of important issues, regulations, and policies on the local, state, and national level.

National Breast Cancer Coalition (NBCC). NBCC is a grassroots advocacy effort conceived in January 1991. Since that time, the Coalition has grown to more than 350 organizations, representing several million patients, professionals, women, their

TABLE 90–1. INTERDISCIPLINARY MODEL FOR A COMPREHENSIVE PSYCHOSOCIAL PROGRAM

Social Work	Psychiatry	Nursing	Cancer Counseling Center
Psychosocial Screening Phase			
Coordinates screening to identify high-distress patients	Provides consultation for high-distress patients (suicidal ideation, major depressive episodes, medication evaluations)	Provides education and counseling on disease and treatment	Receives referrals for high-distress patients and families in need of psychotherapy
Diagnostic Phase			
Provides crisis intervention or short-term therapy to moderate- to high-distress patients Provides linkages to community resources	Assesses patients for major psychiatric problems on a consulting basis Provides evaluation for need for psychotropic medications	Provides education (early treatment issues) Provides support to facilitate decision-making and normalize emotions	Provides long-term counseling or psychotherapy to patients and families with severe psychosocial histories
Treatment Phase			
Provides short-term therapy, relaxation techniques, and support to facilitate adaptation to the diagnosis and treatments Teaches specific coping skills to relieve anxiety and physical discomfort Assists with referrals to community resources for specific needs Provides discharge planning for patients with complex needs	Acts as a consultant to psychosocial team concerning high-distress patients Prescribes psychotropic medications when indicated Facilitates psychiatric hospitalization, when appropriate	Provides treatment, education, and follow-up of rehabilitation needs Focuses on treatment side effects, such as nausea, vomiting, pain, and weight loss Facilitates referrals to social work, nutrition, physical therapy, as indicated Explores specific rehabilitation needs, such as concerns related to body image or sexuality	Provides ongoing long-term psychotherapy to patients and families Addresses severe psychosocial problems such as substance abuse and sexual abuse
Follow-Up Evaluation			
Provides short-term therapy, or crisis intervention as needed Develops, coordinates, and facilitates patient and family support groups with appropriate team members Acts as a liaison between patient and resources, as needed Provides additional information concerning the American Cancer Society's program and other community resources	Monitors patients on psychotropic medications Refers patients to the community for psychiatric follow-up evaluation	Reinforces information concerning report of new symptoms and how to access assistance Provides telephone consultation to patients with specific disease- or treatment-related problems Facilitates referrals for appropriate follow-up, such as social work and nutrition	Continues long-term psychotherapy or counseling to resolve significant problem areas Counsels families (long-term issues exacerbated by the patient's cancer diagnosis)

From Zabora JR, Smith ED, Loscalzo MJ: Psychosocial rehabilitation. *In* Abeloff MD, et al. (eds): Clinical Oncology. New York, Churchill Livingstone, 1995.

families, and friends. Coalition members include cancer support, information, and service groups, as well as women's, consumer health, and provider organizations. Since its inception, the NBCC has had significant impact on general awareness about the breast cancer epidemic, and has had major influence on public policy.

The mission of the NBCC is to eradicate breast cancer by focusing national attention on it and by involving patients and caring others as advocates for action and change. The Coalition informs, supports, and directs patients and concerned others in knowledgeable and effective advocacy efforts. Nationwide, women and men are bringing about meaningful prog-

ress in breast cancer policy through legislative and regulatory input, promotion of media coverage, and participation in activities such as marches and campaigns.

The goals of the NBCC are

- To promote research into the cause of, optimal treatments, and cure for breast cancer through increased funding, recruitment, and training of scientists and improved co-ordination and distribution of research funds;
- To improve access to high-quality breast cancer screening, diagnosis, treatment, and care for all women, particularly the underserved and unin-

sured, through legislation and change in the regulation and delivery of breast health care;

- To increase the involvement and influence of those living with breast cancer in the areas of legislation, regulatory process, and all aspects of clinical trial design, including access to clinical trials.

American Cancer Society (ACS). In 1913, 10 physicians and 5 laymen founded the American Society for the Control of Cancer. Its stated purpose was to "disseminate knowledge concerning the symptoms, treatment, and prevention of cancer; to investigate conditions under which cancer is found, and to compile statistics in regard thereto." Later renamed the *American Cancer Society, Inc.*, the organization now consists of over 2 million Americans working to conquer cancer. While there are many Patient Service Programs to help people in their rehabilitation from cancer treatment, those most relevant to women with breast cancer are these:

- *Community Connection: Resources, Information, and Guidance (RIG)*: Community Connection: RIG is a woman's connection to the local services of the American Cancer Society. RIG provides the most current information about cancer and guidance to the Society's programs and to other resources in a particular community. Volunteers speak with callers about their fears and concerns, and provide help in finding solutions for the varied problems surrounding the illness and its treatment.
- *Reach to Recovery*: Reach to Recovery is a visitation program for women and families who have a personal concern about breast cancer. It addresses breast cancer patients' needs preoperatively and postoperatively. It answers cosmetic, physical, and emotional questions. It gives one-on-one support at this critical time. All volunteers have been treated for breast cancer. Gift kits with information are given to all patients. Terese Lasser, who herself had breast cancer, started Reach to Recovery in 1952. In 1969, it became a program of the American Cancer Society.
- *Look Good, Feel Better*: This service teaches women with cancer about beauty techniques to enhance their appearance and self-image during chemotherapy and radiation treatments. The program is co-sponsored by the Cosmetic, Toiletry and Fragrance Association Foundation and the National Cosmetology Association.
- *Self-Help and Support Groups*: These programs, which vary according to local needs and resources, are offered to patients, families, and friends.
- *Transportation*: Trained volunteer drivers provide transportation for patients to and from treatment (called *Road to Recovery* in some areas).
- *Home Care Items*: The local American Cancer

Society may have a variety of medical equipment such as hospital beds, walkers, wheelchairs, or other supplies available for loan to cancer patients. Insurance or Medicare benefits will be utilized when appropriate. Limited financial assistance for services such as housekeeping may be available in some areas.

- *CanSurmount*: This short-term program connects cancer patients and their families to trained volunteers who have experienced the same type of cancer and who offer support through one-on-one visits.
- *Patient and Family Education*: The ACS provides a number of pamphlets and brochures to help patients understand and cope with their disease. Topics include caring for the cancer patient at home, sexuality and cancer, talking with your doctor, pain control, and many others. The local ACS office should be contacted for these free materials.

Y-ME. Because of their own experiences with breast cancer, Ann Marcou and Mimi Kaplan founded Y-ME in 1978. Y-ME is a not-for-profit organization that provides information, hotline counseling, educational programs, and self-help meetings for breast cancer patients, their families, and friends. Y-ME is the largest and most comprehensive breast cancer support program in the country. All of Y-ME's trained hotline volunteers have had a breast cancer experience. They share concerns, feelings, and information with new patients and each other. Y-ME does not give medical opinions or provide any treatments; however, all programs are carefully monitored by well-known breast cancer specialists who serve on Y-ME's Medical Advisory Board.

Activities:
- *Hotline Services*: Trained peer counselors who have experienced breast cancer answer questions and lend support via the Y-ME hotline. Callers can be matched as closely as possible to a volunteer by age, lifestyle, and diagnosis. Y-ME hotline volunteers have had a wide range of treatments, including lumpectomies, mastectomies, chemotherapy, reconstruction, and bone marrow transplants. Though it is rare, men can get breast cancer too, and several men survivors are available to lend support through the hotline. Y-ME has a dedicated phone line for Spanish-speaking callers. Y-ME recognizes that breast cancer affects the entire family and has formed a group for men whose partners have been treated for breast cancer. Men are encouraged to call the Y-ME hotline and ask to speak to a man who understands the special concerns of a partner.
- *Open-Door Educational Meetings*: Y-ME offers regular meetings for individuals who have had breast cancer or are concerned about it. These volunteer-co-ordinated programs provide information from experts on topics such as chemo-

therapy, radiation, reconstruction, sexuality, nutrition, and stress. Meetings are free and open to the general public. Family members, friends, and health professionals are welcome. Meetings often conclude with an informal discussion session.

- *Presurgical Counseling and Referral Service*: Information on where to go and what to expect if a symptom is detected is available from the Y-ME staff and hotline volunteers. Reading material selected to meet personal needs is sent to each caller. An extensive list of physicians and clinics that specialize in breast care is maintained in the Y-ME headquarters and updated continuously. Resource material on treatment options and prosthesis and wig information is also available. A lending library of current readings on breast cancer is housed in the Y-ME office.

- *Educational Workshops and Newsletter*: Trained volunteers and staff are available to present workshops to organizations and businesses using excellent audiovisuals on all the importance of early detection, the correct method of breast self-examination, and options for diagnosis and treatment. Y-ME sends its contributing members an award-winning newsletter six times a year.

- *In-service Programs for Health Professionals*: Special workshops on the psychosocial needs of breast cancer patients are offered to nurses, technologists, social workers, and other health professionals. From time to time, Y-ME sponsors special full-day conferences designed to share ideas, insights, and experience in the care and counseling of breast cancer patients.

- *Technical Assistance*: Support groups and other self-help programs are encouraged to learn from the Y-ME experience. Y-ME has several handbooks available for purchase, including a 150-page workbook, *Guidelines for Breast Cancer Support Programs*, and a workshop manual, *Just for Teens*, focusing on their successful high school project. Y-ME has also published several booklets targeted to special audiences including husbands and single women.

- *Wig and Prosthesis Bank*: A selection of donated wigs and prostheses is available to women with limited financial resources.

- *Advocacy*: As a founding member of the National Breast Cancer Coalition, Y-ME provides information on public policy and legislative activities related to breast cancer. Y-ME participates in national advocacy efforts to increase federal funding for breast cancer research.

- *Volunteer Opportunities*: Y-ME attributes its success to the help of volunteers. Breast cancer affects everyone in some way, and volunteers—survivors, friends, health professionals—are needed for a variety of projects and special events. Y-ME requires hotline counselors to be breast cancer survivors, but there are many other opportunities that need volunteer support.

The Susan G. Komen Breast Cancer Foundation. The Komen Foundation is a national organization with a network of volunteers working through local chapters and the Race for the Cure events in 56 cities in 32 states and the District of Columbia. Thanks to its volunteers and supporters, the Komen Foundation has raised more than $27.5 million dollars and has become the largest private funder of research, dedicated solely to breast cancer in the United States. Its mission is to eradicate breast cancer as a life-threatening disease by advancing research, education, screening, and treatment.

The purpose of the foundation is threefold:

- To provide funding for breast cancer research, education, screening, and treatment.
- To make mammography available to the medically underserved women in America who should be screened according to the American Cancer Society Guidelines.
- To promote positive awareness, education, and early detection of breast cancer among women of all ages.

CONCLUSIONS

Psychosocial resources exist in hospitals and communities and on a national level to facilitate the adjustment to breast cancer and related treatments. Although resources in specific hospitals can vary significantly, patients and families should be encouraged to explore programs and services in the hospital and local community. Psychosocial screening affords the ability to quickly identify high-risk patients who may experience significant distress as they move through the diagnostic phase into treatment and on to recovery. Screening for psychological distress also enables the team to link patients to psychosocial services from which they may derive the greatest benefit.[9, 10] Patients who experience significantly elevated levels of distress that goes untreated are less likely to follow treatment regimens[11] and to be satisfied with their medical care[12] and more likely to generate higher health care costs.[13]

References

1. Cancer Facts and Figures—1997. Atlanta, American Cancer Society. 1997.
2. Ganz PA: Advocating for women with breast cancer. CA Cancer J Clin 45:114–126, 1995.
3. Farber JM, Weinerman BH, Kuypers JA: Psychosocial distress in oncology outpatients. J Psychol Oncol 2:109–118, 1984.
4. Stefanek M, Derogatis L, Shaw A: Psychological distress among oncology outpatients. Psychosomatics 28:530–535, 1987.
5. Weisman AD, Worden JW, Sobel HS: Psychosocial Screening and Interventions with Cancer Patients: A Research Report. Boston, Massachusetts General Hospital, 1980.
6. Zampini KA, Ostroff JS: The post-treatment resource pro-

gram: Portrait of a program for cancer survivors. Psychooncology 2:1–9, 1993.

7. Maryland Affiliate of The Susan G. Komen Breast Cancer Foundation: Opening Doors to Breast Health and Healing: A Resource Guide. Baltimore, The Foundation, 1995.

8. Zabora JR, Smith ED, Loscalzo MJ: Psychosocial rehabilitation. *In* Abeloff MD, et al. (eds): Clinical Oncology. New York, Churchill Livingstone, 1995.

9. Zabora JR, Smith-Wilson R, Fetting JH, Enterline JP: An efficient method for the psychosocial screening of cancer patients. Psychosomatics 31:192–196, 1990.

10. Zabora JR, Loscalzo MJ: Comprehensive psychosocial programs: A prospective model of care. Oncol Issues 11:14–18, 1996.

11. Richardson JL, Mark G, Levine A: The influence of symptoms and side effects of treatment on compliance with cancer therapy. J Clin Oncol 6:1746–1749, 1988.

12. Greenley JR, et al: Psychological distress and patient satisfaction. Med Care 20:373–385, 1982.

13. Allison TG, Williams DG, Miller TD, et al: Medical and economic costs of psychologic distress in patients with coronary artery disease. Mayo Clin Proc 70:734–742, 1995.

CHAPTER 91
PATIENT AND FAMILY RESOURCES

Marlene McCarthy

When a woman is suspected of having breast cancer or it is actually diagnosed, she most often feels immediately vulnerable, overwhelmed by impending mortality, and profoundly alone. Statistics such as, "One in eight women may develop breast cancer in their lifetime" or "Some 2.6 million women have breast cancer today in the United States" are not comforting. These details, offered to counter a sense of isolation, may only add to the emotional drama of the diagnosis.

There is no way for a woman to prepare herself to hear, "There is something on your mammogram. We have to look further," or "There's a lump in your breast. We have to do a biopsy." Instant fear, and oftentimes panic, seem to take over her entire being. The mind goes blank, voices she knows she should be listening to intently become muffled, and she envisions the worst-case scenario. Her heart may pound so loudly that she is unable to concentrate and ask appropriate questions. She feels afraid, utterly alone, and in the dark. The same sequence often repeats itself when the woman's worst fears are confirmed and she is told her biopsy is positive: *She has breast cancer.*

The following suggestions and resources are offered to surgeons and medical staff, who have a chance to offer the patient assistance. It is essential that the breast cancer patient and her significant supporters (family, friends, and others) regard their relationship with the health caregivers as *the patient's team,* who are focused on helping her to make the best-informed decisions on treatment.

When the patient is offered the opportunity and encouragement to learn about her disease and understand that she has options to consider for her treatment that are presented in an atmosphere where her questions and opinions are respected, she is much more trusting of her medical treatment team and confident in the choices identified. As a participant in the healing process, the patient becomes a general in the war with her breast cancer. Armed with appropriate resources, she can effect a more positive outcome from her treatment. Knowing that no cure for breast cancer is known but that treatments and clinical trials with good results are available to her, is encouraging. Also, knowing that breast cancer advocates, women like her who have been treated for breast cancer, are lobbying the U.S. Congress to dedicate more money to find the causes and cure for this disease will help her to feel she has an army of supporters for her personal fight.

The surgeon is also on the front line of the battle, calling the charge, the first to invade the battlefield, the leader of her medical team. It is the surgeon's responsibility to provide her with the tools she will need to make her experience as positive as possible:

Encourage the patient to keep a notebook where she can write her questions, concerns, names and telephone numbers of contacts, resources, and her physicians' comments.

Encourage her to review books and educational pamphlets about breast cancer to help her prepare for the choices she will make during this experience.

Encourage her to contact a support group that focuses on the issues of women with breast cancer for peer support and shared strength.

Validate her feelings of sadness. Encourage her to practice deep-breathing exercises and meditation. Remind her that physical activity such as walking and swimming is very important to her well-being.

Every patient is a medical consumer who has selected caregivers for their expertise, their reputations, and their communication skills. It is their responsibility to provide her with the necessary comforts that will secure her ongoing confidence. Surgeons would do well to consider the following measures:

- Prepare preprinted fact sheets about themselves and facts about their practice, including information on board certification and the percentage of practice accorded to breast care.
- List hospital affiliations, insurances accepted, and if they are willing to adjust fees if the patient does not have adequate insurance coverage.
- Set forth hours when they are available to take telephone calls, and the days of the week and hours they see patients.
- Provide instructions for emergencies.
- If the practice involves medical residents or interns, describe their roles on the patient's medical team.
- Identify a member of the staff who will be accessible to the patient when the surgeon is not available. Make certain that staff member understands the critical potential of a patient's need for emotional support.
- Schedule her postoperative appointment *before* she undergoes surgery.
- If there is an ACS Reach to Recovery program in the area, encourage a volunteer to visit the patient.

Visual aids work wonders when the patient is trying to understand her choices for the operative procedure and what she will look like after surgery. A sketch of a breast is useful for demonstrating where tissue will be cut and what the scar may look like.

Surgeons should obviously be prepared to answer the patient's questions about the benefits and drawbacks of mastectomy and lumpectomy and why they are recommending the particular surgery. The patient should be urged to consider her options carefully by reviewing her reasoning and the doctor's recommendation before choosing a procedure.

The patient will want to know the latest research data on the success rate of certain procedures and to be clear about the recovery period. She should be provided a printed sheet on how she must care for her incision, how long it will take to heal, and what problems might occur. If drains are to be inserted, she will want to know how long they will be needed.

The potential for numbness in her arm that will last for some time after the surgery should be explained, as should possible lymphedema and physical limitations. In talking about pain management, the surgeon should assure the patient that she will be provided medication for any discomfort after the surgical procedure. The staging of the disease should be presented in a clear and concise manner, and copies of her pathology, blood, and scan reports should be provided.

After surgery, patients who need to see an oncologist or radiotherapist often ask the surgeon for a recommendation. If the practice and personal time permit, the surgeon may consider participating in a consultation with the patient and the new members of her medical team. After all breast surgery, there is a chance of recurrence; so it is important to remain involved in the patient's care.

A patient enrolling in a clinical trial must give informed consent after the information is clearly presented to her, and fact sheets should be available for her personal use. Every effort must be made to share new information about treatment of her breast cancer.

Future encounters may find the patient still fearful and apprehensive, even after her surgeries and additional treatments are completed. It is important to continue to encourage her to remain informed about her disease, asking questions and searching for answers. Most women continue to feel a shadow of uncertainty after treatment, and that is perfectly normal. Caregivers should validate this feeling for her. Breast cancer is a challenge. No one can explain how it happened *to her*, and no one can assure her that it is no longer in her body. The patient should be encouraged to contact the surgeon when she is worried that something may be wrong. Oftentimes, women identify an imbalance in their body—that "something is wrong"—before a recurrence can be determined by a medical workup.

The patient could stagger her follow-up medical appointments rather than seeing each specialist in the same month. Thus, she might feel more secure because she is being examined and followed closely over a longer period of time. The surgeon should explain that blood tests will be done that can alert the physician to early signs of recurring cancer and, that if the cancer does come back, other treatment options are available to her.

When patients need counseling, the surgeon should be prepared to suggest the appropriate professional. Breast cancer is a chronic illness, and when coping strategies can be established, most once-fragile patients can do very well emotionally. Finally, the surgeon should encourage a hopeful attitude and suggest that the patient might want to become involved in joining with other women as advocates to increase research funding to find a cure for breast cancer.

PRINTED RESOURCES

General Information

The Breast Cancer Handbook: Taking Control After You've Found a Lump
by Joan Swirsky and Barbara Balaban (New York, Harper Collins, 1994, $11).
This user-friendly guide in workbook format is full of practical information that will be helpful to any woman.
Available through bookstores.

Dr. Susan Love's Breast Book
by Susan M. Love, MD, with Karen Lindsey (Reading, MA, Addison Wesley, 1995 edition, paperback, $17).
A breast surgeon and feminist discusses all conditions of the breast, from benign to malignant. A balanced view of treatment options and controversies is clearly presented in a friendly, accessible style.
Available through bookstores.

Your Breast Cancer Treatment Handbook
by Judy C. Kneece, RN, OCN (Columbia, SC, Edu Care Publishing, 1995, $19.95 plus $3.50 shipping and handling).
This easy-to-use book contains useful information about managing treatment decisions and addresses sensitive emotional issues in an insightful manner.
Available from Edu Care Publishing, P.O. Box 280305, Columbia, SC 29228. (800) 849–9271, http://www.cancerhelp.com/ed.

Examining Myself: One Woman's Story of Breast Cancer Treatment and Recovery
by Musa Mayer (Winchester, MA, Faber and Faber, 1993, $19.95/paperback edition 1994, $10.95).
A sensitive exploration of the emotional aspects of disease and recovery. Faber and Faber is donating a portion of the proceeds from this book to the National Breast Cancer Coalition.
Available through bookstores.

The Race Is Run One Step at a Time: My Personal Struggle and Every Woman's Guide to Taking Charge of Breast Cancer
by Nancy Brinker with Catherine McEvily Harris (Dallas, Summit Publishing Group, 1995, paperback $13.95 plus shipping and handling).
Nancy Brinker's updated edition is a guide to taking charge of breast cancer. Ms. Brinker is founder of the

Susan G. Komen Breast Cancer Foundation, to which all royalties are donated for breast cancer research.
Available through The Komen Foundation, 5005 LBJ Freeway, Suite 370, Dallas, TX 75244. Order from (800) I'M AWARE/462–9273.

Cancer in Two Voices
by Sandra Butler and Barbara Rosenblum (MN, Spinsters Book Company, 1991, paperback, $12.95).
This is a particularly moving and honest account of the authors' identities as Jewish women and as lesbians, and of living with advanced breast cancer. Based on excerpts from their diaries.
Available through bookstores.

Handbook for Mothers Supporting Daughters with Breast Cancer
(1995)
This book gives practical advice and sources of information to the mothers of women with breast cancer.
Order from Mothers Supporting Daughters with Breast Cancer, 21710 Bayshore Road, Chestertown, MD 21620–4401, (410) 778–1982.

Helping Your Mate Face Breast Cancer
by Judy C. Kneece, RN, OCN (Columbia, SC, Edu Care Publishing, 1995, $12.95 plus $3.50 shipping and handling).
A support partner's guide to understanding the emotional responses of mates and other family members. Provides helpful suggestions on coping strategies and how to support the physical and emotional recovery of a partner.
Available from Edu Care Publishing, P.O. Box 280305, Columbia, SC 29228, (800) 849–9271.

For Single Women with Breast Cancer
(1994)
Y-ME has created this booklet to offer practical guidance and emotional support for women without partners or women who live alone. Single copies are available free. Bulk orders available on request.
Call (800) 221–2141.

Kemoshark
by H. Elizabeth King and illustrated by Diane Willford Steele (1995).
A colorfully illustrated booklet to help children understand chemotherapy when a parent is undergoing treatment.
Order from KIDSCOPE, Inc., Charles N. Center, 3400 Peachtree Road, N.E., Suite 703, Atlanta, GA 30326, (404) 233–0001.

Man to Man: When the Woman You Love Has Breast Cancer
by Andy Murcia and Bob Stewart (New York, St. Martin's Press, 1990, paperback, $10.95).
This book is written for the male partner of the woman with breast cancer. It addresses the emotional issues and encourages partners to "participate."
Available through bookstores.

Sammy's Mommy Has Cancer
by Sherry Kohlenberg (New York, Magination Press, 1993, $8.95).
The author, diagnosed with breast cancer when she was

34 and her son was 18 months old, offers parents a thoughtful and sensitive way to explain breast cancer to a child. Ms. Kohlenberg, a co-founder of the Virginia Breast Cancer Foundation, died in 1993.
Available through bookstores or (800) 825–3089; in New York, (212) 924–3344.

Sexuality and Cancer: For the Woman Who Has Cancer and Her Partner
(1991 edition)
Gives information about cancer and sexuality and areas of concern to the patient and her partner. Resource list included.
Call ACS (800) ACS–2345.

When the Woman You Love Has Breast Cancer
by Larry T. Eiler (Ann Arbor, MI, Queen Bee Publishing, 1994, $9.95 plus $4 shipping).
Based on the personal experiences of the author, this book addresses issues faced by a man whose wife or friend has the disease and what steps he can take to be supportive of her.
Order from Queen Bee Publishing, 900 Victors Way, Suite 180, Ann Arbor, MI 48108, (313) 761–3399.

Waking Up, Fighting Back: The Politics of Breast Cancer
by Roberta Altman (Boston, Little, Brown, 1996, $24.95).
An award-winning journalist's provocative survey of the issues and controversies relating to breast cancer advocacy.
Available through bookstores.

Resources for Treatment and Choices

"Breast Cancer"
(Time Life Medical, 1996, $19.95)
Produced under the guidance of C. Everett Koop, MD, and hosted by journalist Linda Ellerbee, this 30-minute videotape offers patients and their families information and education to better understand their diagnosis and determine how best to manage their disease with their physicians. A 22-page workbook is included.
Available at retail pharmacies nationwide.

Cancerfax
This service allows access to NCI's Physician Data Query (PDQ) system (see entry below) via fax machine, 24 hours a day, 7 days a week, at no charge other than the fax call charge. Information is also available in Spanish.
For information and codes, call the Cancer Information Service, (800) 4–CANCER or on the Internet, http://wwwicic.nci.nih.gov.

PDQ (Physician Data Query)
The cancer information data base of the NCI, providing prognostic, stage, and treatment information and a listing of more than 1500 clinical trials that are open to patient accrual. Access by computer equipped with a modem and by fax.
Additional information available through NCI at (800) 4–CANCER or via the Internet, http://wwwicic. nci.nih.gov.

Ten Questions (and Answers) If You Are Diagnosed with Breast Cancer
(1995)
This free brochure from the American Society for Therapeutic Radiology and Oncology (ASTRO) answers questions about breast cancer treatment.
Order from ASTRO, (800) 96–ASTRO.

Resources for Reconstruction

Breast Implants: Everything You Need to Know
by Nancy Bruning (Alameda, CA, Hunter House, 1995, paperback, $11.95).
This newly revised edition is a valuable resource for any woman considering breast implants. Includes details of potential health risks, alternatives to implants, and advice on whether or not to remove them. A resource list is included.
Available through bookstores, or call (800) 266–5592.

Breast Reconstruction After Mastectomy
(1991)
Describes types of surgery with photographs and drawings and gives answers to commonly asked questions and a glossary of terms.
Available through ACS (800) ACS–2345.

FDA (Food and Drug Administration) Breast Implant Information Line
Answers consumer and professional inquiries about breast implants; assists in registering complaints and accessing implant registries. Established in 1992.
Call (800) 532–4440.

A Woman's Decision, Breast Care, Treatment, and Reconstruction
by Karen Berger and John Bostwick III, MD (Quality Medical Publishing, MO, 1995, $18.50 plus shipping and handling).
This book provides a comprehensive discussion of the subject.
Order from Quality Medical Publishing, (800) 348–7808.

COMPUTER RESOURCES

Computer Programs

Compuserve: toll-free 1–800–848–8199
Medline: toll-free 1–800–478–1126
GratefulMed: toll-free 1–800–638–8480

Important Breast Cancer Web Sites

Avon's Breast Cancer Awareness Crusade
   http://www.pmedia.com/Avon/avon.html
The Breast Cancer Information Clearinghouse
   http://nyscrnet.org/breast/Default.html
CANSearch
   http://access.digex.net/~mkragen/cansearch.html
The National Cancer Institute
   http://wwwicic.nci.nih.gov
Oncolink
   http://cancer.med.upenn.edu
National Breast Cancer Coalition
   http://www.natlbcc.org

Computer Bulletin Boards

Commercial on-line services have added a new dimension to the availability of support and information through computer bulletin boards for people with cancer. *America Online, Compuserve,* and *Prodigy* all have bulletin boards where cancer survivors provide support and information to each other.
America Online: **(800) 827–6364**
Look in *America Online*'s Health and Medical Forum as well as Keyword: Avon, for a bulletin board dedicated solely to breast cancer support and information.
Compuserve: **(800) 848–8199**
Go to the Cancer Forum in the Health Professional section, or GO CANCER.
Prodigy: **(800) 776–3449**
Go to the Medical Support Board under the Cancer topic.

Journal Searches

The largest data base, with 3600 contributing medical journals, is *Medline*, which has a separate cancer data base called *Cancerlit*. Some major libraries and medical libraries (if open to the public) subscribe and will permit searches, sometimes for a fee.

Medline is available at no cost on the Internet through **HealthGate** at **http://www.healthgate.com.** You can also use special software such as *Grateful Med*; for a free demo disk and brochure, call **(301) 496–6308** or E-mail **gmhelp@gmedserv.nlm.nih.gov.**

Compuserve and *America Online* also provide access to *Medline*.

CD-ROM

Be a Survivor: Your Interactive Guide to Breast Cancer
Available from Lange Productions.
Call for pricing information: **(213) 874–0132**

Understanding Breast Cancer ($49.90)
Available from Tiger Software: **(800) 238–4437**

Breast Self-Examination ($49.95)
Available from CMC ReSearch: **(800) 854–9126**

Combined Health Information Database (CHID)
An on-line computerized data base from the U.S. Public Health Service.
Call for information: (800) 950–2035 x400

INFORMATION AND SUPPORT

Organizations and Programs

National Alliance of Breast Cancer Organizations (NABCO)
This is the leading nonprofit national central resource for breast cancer information.
NABCO, 9 East 37th Street, 10th Floor, New York, NY 10016. (800) 719–9154, http://www.nabco.org.

AMC Cancer Research Center's Cancer Information and Counseling Line
Professional cancer counselors offer easy-to-understand answers to questions about cancer, and mail instructive, free publications upon request. Equipped for deaf and hearing-impaired callers.
(800) 525–3777.

American Cancer Society
The society's nationwide toll-free hot line provides information on all forms of cancer, and referrals for the ACS-sponsored "Reach to Recovery" program.
(800) ACS–2345, http://www.cancer.org.

The Cancer Information Service of the National Cancer Institute
The service furnishes information and direction on all aspects of cancer through its regional network, provides informational brochures, and refers callers to medical centers and clinical trial programs. Spanish-speaking staff members available.
(800) 4–CANCER, http://wwwicic.nci.nih.gov.

The Susan G. Komen Breast Cancer Foundation
This national volunteer organization seeks to eradicate breast cancer as a life-threatening disease, working through local chapters and Race for the Cure events in 60 cities. The Foundation is the largest private funder of breast cancer research in the United States.
Information: (800) I'M AWARE or The Susan G. Komen Breast Cancer Foundation, Occidental Tower, 5005 LBJ Freeway, Suite 370, Dallas, TX 75244, (972) 855–1600, http://www.komen.com.

The National Coalition for Cancer Survivorship (NCCS)
The coalition raises awareness of cancer survivorship through its publications and advocacy for insurance, employment, and legal rights for people with cancer.
NCCS, 1010 Wayne Avenue, 5th Floor, Silver Spring, MD 20910, (301) 650–8868. Use a search engine to locate NCCS on the World Wide Web via CANSEARCH.

Y-ME National Breast Cancer Organization
Y-ME provides support and counseling through its national toll-free 24-hour hot line, **(800) 222–2141. Call or write to 212 W. Van Buren Street, Chicago, IL 60607, http://www.Y-ME.org.**

The YWCA of the U.S.A.'s Encore Plus Program
Located throughout the United States, this program provides early detection outreach, education, postdiagnostic support, and exercise to all women.
To locate the program nearest you, **call (202) 628–3636.**

The National Breast Cancer Coalition
The mission of the National Breast Cancer Coalition is to work to eradicate breast cancer, the most common form of cancer among women in the United States, through focusing national attention on breast cancer and by involving all who are concerned about this disease as advocates for action, advances, and change.
NATIONAL BREAST CANCER COALITION, 1701 L Street, NW, Suite 1060, Washington, DC 20036, (202) 296–7477, http://www.natlbcc.org.

REGIONAL SUPPORT GROUPS
(Arranged by State, Includes Canada)

Alabama	Gadsden	Women to Women	(205) 543-8896
	Montgomery	SISTAs CanSurvive	(334) 277-5224
	Tuscaloosa	UPFRONT Support Group	(205) 759-7000
Alaska	Anchorage	The Anchorage Women's Breast Cancer Support Group	(907) 261-3607
Arizona	Phoenix	Good Samaritan Medical Center	(602) 239-3250
		Bosom Buddies	(602) 231-6648
		New Beginnings/Maryvale Samaritan Hospital	(602) 848-5588
	Scottsdale	Y-ME Breast Cancer Network of Arizona	(602) 231-6666
	Tucson	Arizona Cancer Center	(520) 626-6044
Arkansas	Fayetteville	Northwest Arkansas Cancer Support Home	(501) 521-8024
	Fort Smith	Phillips Cancer Support House	(501) 782-6302
	Little Rock	CARTI CancerAnswers	(800) 482-8561
California	Anaheim	Anaheim Memorial Hospital	(714) 999-3880
	Berkeley	Alta Bates Hospital	(510) 204-1591
		Women's Cancer Resource Center	(510) 548-9272
	Chico	Beyond Breast Cancer Support Group	(916) 892-6888
	Covina	WIN Against Breast Cancer	(818) 332-2255
	Encino	Vital Options and "The Group Room" Cancer Radio Talk Show	(818) 508-5657
	Escondido	Pallmar Pomerado Health System	(619) 737-3960
	Fresno	St. Agnes Medical Center	(209) 449-5222
	La Habra	Bloomers-Y-ME of Orange County	(714) 447-6975
	La Jolla	Scripps Memorial Hospital	(619) 626-6756
		UCSD Cancer Center	(619) 543-6650

	Lancaster	Ladies of Courage/Y-ME	(805) 266-4811
	Long Beach	Long Beach Memorial Breast Center	(310) 933-7880
		Y-ME South Bay/Long Beach	(310) 984-8456
	Los Angeles	Rhonda Flemming Mann Resource Center for Women with Cancer	(310) 794-6644
	Lynwood	Sisters Network for African-American Women	(310) 639-6511
	Monterey	Breast Self-Help Group	(408) 649-1772
	Napa	Bosom Buddies	(707) 257-4047
	Orange	The Breast Care Center	(714) 541-0101
	Palm Springs	The Desert Comprehensive Breast Center	(619) 323-6676
	Palo Alto	Community Breast Health Project	(415) 725-1788
		Discovery Breast Cancer Support Group/YWCA	(415) 494-0972
	Pasadena	Breast Cancer Networking Group	(818) 796-1083
	Sacramento	Save Ourselves/Y-ME of Sacramento	(916) 921-9747
	San Diego	WIN Against Breast Cancer	(619) 488-6300
		Women's Cancer Task Force/Y-ME San Diego Chapter	(619) 239-9283
	San Francisco	Bay Area Lymphedema Support Group	(415) 921-2911
		Breast Cancer Action	(415) 243-9301
		The Breast Care Center	(415) 476-5555
		The Cancer Support Community	(415) 648-9400
	San Jose	Bay Area Breast Cancer Network	(408) 261-1425
	Santa Monica	Wellness Community	(310) 314-2555
	Sausalito	Center for Attitudinal Healing	(415) 331-6161
	Van Nuys	The Breast Center	(818) 787-9911
	Walnut Creek	John Muir Medical Center	(510) 933-4107
	West Covina	Queen of the Valley	(818) 814-2464
Canada	Burlington, Ont.	Burlington Breast Cancer Support Services	(905) 634-2333
	Montreal	Breast Cancer Action	(514) 483-1846
	Ottawa, Ont.	Breast Cancer Action	(613) 736-5921
	St. Cath., Ont.	Niagara Breast Cancer Support Group	(905) 687-3333
Colorado	Colorado Springs	Penrose Cancer Center	(719) 776-5273
	Denver	AMC Cancer Research Center	(303) 239-3424
		Rose Medical Center	(303) 320-7142
		Rose Medical Center: Discussion Group for Male Partners	(303) 320-7142
Connecticut	Branford	Y-ME of New England	(203) 483-8200
	Danbury	I Can	(203) 830-4621
	Hartford	St. Francis Hospital and Medical Center	(203) 548-4366
	Norwalk	Cancer Care, Inc.	(203) 854-9911
	Ridgefield	The Revivers	(203) 438-5555
	Stamford	Building Bridges	(203) 325-7447
Delaware	Wilmington	Looking Ahead Support Group	(302) 421-4161
District of Columbia		National Capital/Y-ME	(800) 970-4411
		George Washington University	(202) 994-4589
		Georgetown University	(202) 784-4000
		The Mary-Helen Mautner Project for Lesbians with Cancer	(202) 332-5536
Florida	Coral Springs	Y-ME of Florida	(305) 752-2101
	Daytona Beach	Halifax Medical Center Women's Services	(904) 254-4211
	Jacksonville	Bosom Buddies	(904) 633-8246
		Evenings and weekends	(904) 396-5973
	Orlando	Bosom Buddies	(407) 281-8663
		Florida Hospital	(407) 897-1617
	Pensacola	Ann L. Baroco Center for Women's Health	(904) 474-7878
	Sarasota	Sarasota Memorial Hospital	(941) 917-1375
	Tampa	FACTORS/H. Lee Moffit Cancer Center	(813) 972-8407
Georgia	Atlanta	Northside Hospital	(404) 851-8635
	Tucker	Bosom Buddies—Also, bone marrow transplant support group	(404) 493-7517
		Bosom Buddies—men's bereavement support group	(404) 493-7517
Hawaii	Honolulu	Queens Medical Center	(808) 547-4243

Idaho	Boise	Women's Life Center	(208) 381-2764
	Ketchum	The Wellness Group	(208) 726-8464
Illinois	Alton	CARE-Alton Memorial Hospital	(618) 463-7150
	Barrington	Good Shepherd Hospital	(847) 381-9600 Ext. 5336
	Belleville	St. Elizabeth Hospital	(618) 234-2120 Ext. 1260
	Chicago	Lesbian Community Cancer Project	(312) 561-4662
		Moving Towards Recovery	(312) 205-2017
		Y-ME National Breast Cancer Organization	(312) 986-8338
	Decatur	Decatur Memorial Hospital	(217) 876-2380
	Elmhurst	Elmhurst Memorial Hospital	(708) 782-7900
	Joliet	St. Joseph Medical Center	(815) 741-7560
	Macomb	McDonough District Hospital	(309) 836-1584
	Moline	Quad City's Breast Cancer Survivors	(309) 764-2888
	Pekin	Pekin Hospital—Mastectomy Support Group	(309) 353-0807
	Peoria	Susan G. Komen Breast Center	(309) 689-6622
	Rockford	Breast Cancer Support Group for Younger Women	(815) 961-6215
	Springfield	Sangamon Breast Cancer Support Group	(217) 787-7187
Indiana	Bluffton	Women's Cancer Support Group	(219) 824-6493
	Gary	Methodist Hospital, Northlake Campus	(800) 952-7337
	Indianapolis	Uplifter's Breast Cancer Support Group	(317) 355-1411
		Y-ME of Central Indiana	(317) 240-3331
	South Bend	St. Joseph's Medical Center	(219) 234-4097
	Terre Haute	Y-ME of Wabash Valley	(812) 877-3025
	Warsaw	Women Winning Against Cancer	(219) 269-9911
Iowa	Cedar Rapids	"ESPECIALLY FOR YOU" After Breast Cancer	(319) 398-6265
	Marshalltown	Marshalltown Support Group	(515) 752-6486
	Sioux City	ABC—After Breast Cancer Support Group	(712) 279-2989
	Waterloo	Breast Cancer Support Group	(319) 292-2100
Kansas	Wichita	Breast Cancer Care Group	(316) 262-7559
Kentucky	Ashland	Breast Cancer Support Group	(606) 327-4535
	Edgewood	St. Elizabeth Women's Center	(606) 344-3939
	Lexington	The Thursday Group	(606) 269-4836
	Louisville	After Breast Cancer	(502) 589-6000
	Owensboro	Women of Owensboro Mastectomy Association c/o the American Cancer Society	(502) 584-6782
	Prestonsburg	Breast Cancer Support Group	(606) 886-8511 Ext. 7575
Louisiana	Marrero	West Jefferson Medical Center	(504) 349-1640
	Metairie	Center For Living With Cancer	(504) 454-4500
	New Orleans	Breast Cancer Support Group	(504) 897-4223
		Ochsner Breast Cancer Support Group	(504) 842-4251
		Tulane Medical Center	(504) 587-2120
	Slidell	North Shore Regional Medical Center	(800) 749-6363
Maine	Bangor	Breast Cancer Support Group	(207) 581-3433
	Lewiston	Breast Cancer Support Group	(207) 784-3591
	Portland	Breast Cancer Support Group	(207) 773-1919
Maryland	Hagerstown	Y-ME of the Cumberland Valley	(301) 791-5843
	Pasadena	Cancer Resource and Support Center	(410) 760-CARE
	Timonium	Arm in Arm	(410) 494-0083
Massachusetts	Amherst	Margaret Gozlin Counseling Center	(413) 256-4600
	Boston	Beth Israel Hospital Support Program	(617) 667-2900
		Dana Farber Cancer Institute	(617) 632-3459
		Faulkner Breast Centre Support Group	(617) 983-7967
		New England Medical Center	(617) 636-9227
	Burlington	Lahey Clinic Breast Cancer Treatment Center	(617) 273-8989
	Cambridge	Harvard University	(617) 495-2936

	Framingham	Metro West Medical Center	(508) 383-1378
	Marion	Strength for Tomorrow	(508) 748-0561
	Pittsfield	Y-ME of the Berkshires	(413) 499-2486
	Springfield	Baystate Medical Center	(413) 784-8010
	Worcester	University of Massachusetts	(508) 856-3112
Michigan	Ada	"EXPRESSIONS" for Women	(616) 752-8124
	Ann Arbor	University Hospital	(313) 936-9425
	Detroit	Barbara Anne Karmanos Cancer Institute for Caring Partners	(313) 745-8618
		Barbara Anne Karmanos Cancer Institute Unique Breast Cancer Support Group	(313) 966-0761
		Breast Cancer Support Group	(313) 343-3684
	Farmington Hills	Berry Health Center	(313) 493-6507
	Flint	McLaren Mastectomy Support Group	(810) 342-2375
	Grand Rapids	St. Mary's Breast Center	(616) 774-6756
	Lansing	Sparrow Regional Cancer Center	(517) 483-2689
	Marquette	Marquette General Hospital	(906) 225-3500
	Midland	Midland Community Cancer Services	(517) 835-4841
	Petoskey	Just for Us	(616) 347-8443
Minnesota	Duluth	Duluth Clinic—Breast Diagnostic Center	(218) 725-3195
	Fridley	Mercy Unity Oncology Services	(612) 780-7780
	Minneapolis	Medformation Support Group Referral	(612) 863-3333
	St. Louis Park	Methodist Hospital	(612) 932-6086
	St. Paul	Medformation Support Group Referral	(612) 863-3333
Mississippi	Biloxi	Biloxi Regional Medical Center	(601) 436-1694
Missouri	Jefferson City	St. Mary's Hospital	(573) 634-5423
	Kansas City	Bloch Cancer Support Center	(816) 363-6969
		Menorah Medical Park	(816) 276-8848
		The Cancer Institute of Health Midwest	(816) 751-2929
	Springfield	Reach Together	(417) 866-LADY
		St. John's Breast Center	(417) 885-2385
	St. Charles	St. Joseph Health Center—Hospital West	(314) 947-5000
	St. Louis	Barnes Jewish Hospital	(314) 362-5574
		FOCUS—St. Luke's Hospital	(314) 205-6055
		Missouri Baptist Medical Center	(314) 569-5263
		SHARE Breast Cancer Education & Support Center	(314) 991-4424
		St. John's Mercy Cancer Center	(314) 569-6400
Montana	Billings	The Women's Center	(406) 657-8730
	Missoula	Breast Cancer Support Group	(406) 251-3995
	Sidney	Bosom Buddies	(406) 482-2423
Nebraska	Lincoln	St. Elizabeth Community Health Center	(402) 486-7567
Nevada	Reno	St. Mary's Regional Medical Center	(702) 789-3232
New Hampshire	Concord	Breast Cancer Support Group	(603) 224-2051
		Concord Hospital	(603) 225-2711
	Lebanon	Norris Cotton Cancer Center	(603) 650-5789
	Manchester	Catholic Medical Center	(603) 626-2049
		Elliot Hospital	(603) 628-2338
New Jersey	Bayonne	Bayonne Hospital	(201) 339-7573
	Bergen County	After Breast Cancer	(201) 487-2224
	Brick	Brick Hospital	(908) 295-6427
	Camden	Cooper Hospital University Medical Center	(609) 342-2000 Ext. 3572
	Dover	Northwest Covenant Health Care System	(201) 989-3106
	Flemington	Breast Cancer Support Group	(908) 782-6112
	Freehold	Women's Health Center	(908) 308-0292
	Hackensack	Hackensack Medical Center	(201) 996-5800
	Little Silver	Mid–Monmouth County Recurrence Support Group	(908) 933-1333
	Livingston	St. Barnabas Medical Center	(201) 533-8414
	Long Branch	Monmouth Medical Center	(908) 870-5360

	Millburn	Cancer Care, Inc.	(201) 379-7500
	Neptune	Jersey Shore Cancer Center	(908) 776-4240
	New Brunswick	Cancer Institute of New Jersey	(908) 235-6790
	Pomona	Atlantic City Medical Center	(609) 652-3500
	Princeton	Beyond Cancer	(609) 683-0692
		Breast Cancer Resource Center (for men and women), Princeton YWCA	(609) 497-2126
	Randolf	Women at Risk (for women considering prophylactic mastectomy)	(800) 82-BREAST
	Red Bank	Riverview Regional Cancer Center	(908) 530-2382
	Ridgewood	Cancer Care, Inc.	(201) 444-6630
		Valley Hospital	(201) 447-8656
	Somerville	Somerset Medical Center	(908) 685-2953
	South River	WISE-Women's International Support Environment	(908) 257-6611
	Summit	Pathways	(908) 273-4242
	Toms River	Community Medical Center	(908) 240-8148
	Wash. Township	After Breast-Cancer Surgery	(201) 666-6610
	Westfield	CHEMOcare	(800) 55-CHEMO
			(908) 233-1103
New Mexico	Albuquerque	People Living Through Cancer	(505) 242-3263
	Farmington	The Four Corners Breast Cancer Support Group	(505) 326-0743
New York	Binghamton	Brass Ears—Breast Cancer Support Group	(607) 693-1759
		Southern Tier Y-ME	(607) 722-5839
	Brooklyn	Cancer Institute of Brooklyn	(718) 283-6599
		Long Island College Hospital	(718) 780-2947
	Buffalo	Breast Cancer Network of Western New York	(716) 631-8665
	Cold Spring Harbor	Maurer Foundation for Breast Health Education	(800) 853-LEARN
	Elmhurst	St. John's Queens Hospital	(718) 558-1000 Ext. 2250
	Flushing	Flushing Hospital Medical Center	(718) 670-5640
	Garden City	Adelphi New York Statewide Breast Cancer HOTLINE and Support Program	(516) 877-4444
		Sisters Network for African-American Women	(516) 538-8086
	Glens Falls	Glens Falls Hospital	(518) 696-2000
	Huntington	Huntington Hospital	(516) 351-2568
	Ithaca	Cayuga Medical Center	(607) 274-4011
		Ithaca Breast Cancer Alliance	(607) 277-9410
	Johnson City	Women's Health Connection, United Health Services	(607) 763-6546
	Kingston	Benedictine Hospital	(914) 338-2500 Ext. 4453
	Manhasset	North Shore University Hospital	(516) 926-HELP
	New Hyde Park	Long Island Jewish Medical Center Post-Lumpectomy Support Group	(718) 470-7188
	New York	Beth Israel Medical Center	(212) 420-5688
		Beth Israel Medical Center, North Division	(212) 870-9502
		Breast Examination Center of Harlem	(212) 864-0600
		Cancer Care, Inc.	(212) 302-2400
		Creative Center for Women With Cancer	(212) 868-4766
		Gilda's Club	(212) 647-9700
		Memorial Sloan-Kettering Cancer Center	(212) 717-3527
		Mount Sinai Medical Center	(212) 987-3063
		SHARE: Support Service for Women with	(212) 719-0364
		Breast or Ovarian Cancer Spanish	(212) 719-4454
	No. Tarrytown	Side by Side	(914) 347-2649
	Pt. Jefferson	John T. Mather Memorial Hospital	(516) 476-2723
	Putnam Valley	Breast Cancer Support Group	(914) 528-8213
	Rochester	Cancer Action, Inc.	(716) 423-9700
	Rye Brook	Cancer Support Team, Inc.	(914) 253-5334
	Syosset	FEGS/Jewish Community Services	(516) 364-8040
	Valley Stream	Franklin Hospital	(516) 256-6012
	Woodbury	Cancer Care, Inc.	(516) 364-8130
No. Carolina	Asheville	Life After Cancer/Pathways, Inc.	(704) 252-4106
	Chapel Hill	Chapel Hill Support Group	(919) 929-7022
	Charlotte	Charlotte Organization for Breast Cancer Education	(704) 846-2190
		Presbyterian Hospital	(704) 384-4750

		Women Living with Cancer	(704) 355-2884
	Durham	Duke Comprehensive Cancer Center	(919) 684-4497
	New Bern	Breast Cancer Support Group	(919) 636-0186
	Raleigh	Triangle Breast Cancer Support Group	(919) 787-2637
	Rocky Mount	Boice Willis Clinic	(919) 937-0200
		Nash Day Hospital	(919) 443-8607
	Wilson	Kathy Farris Memorial Mastectomy Group	(919) 237-0439
	Winston-Salem	Pink Broomstick—Cancer Services, Inc.	(910) 725-7421
No. Dakota	Bismarck	Great Plains Rehabilitation Services Mastectomy Support Group	(701) 224-7988
Ohio	Cincinnati	Bethesda Oak Breast Center	(513) 731-3346
		Cancer Family Care, Inc.	(513) 569-5152
		University of Cincinnati Hospital	(513) 558-8567
	Cleveland	Cleveland Clinic Foundation	(216) 444-3770
	Columbus	Arthur G. James Cancer Hospital	(614) 293-3237
		Riverside Cancer Institute	(614) 566-4321
	Dayton	St. Elizabeth Breast Center	(513) 229-7474
		Y-ME of the Greater Dayton Area	(513) 274-9151
	Hamilton	Fort Hamilton Hughes Hospital	(513) 867-2700
	Kettering	SOAR/Strength, Optimism and Recovery	(513) 296-7231
	Marietta	Marietta Memorial Hospital	(614) 374-1450
	Springfield	Mercy Medical Center	(513) 390-5030
	Youngstown	Cancer Care Center	(216) 740-4176
Oklahoma	Oklahoma City	Central Oklahoma Cancer Center	(405) 636-7104
		University of Oklahoma	(405) 271-4514
Oregon	Portland	St. Vincent Hospital and Medical Center	(503) 215-4673
	Springfield	McKenzie-Willamette Hospital	(503) 726-4452
	Tualatin	Meridian Park Hospital	(503) 692-2113
Pennsylvania	Allentown	John and Dorothy Morgan Cancer Center	(610) 402-0500
	Bristol	Lower Bucks Hospital	(215) 785-9056
	Bryn Mawr	Bryn Mawr Hospital	(610) 526-3073
	Coatesville	Brandywine Hospital and Trauma Center	(610) 383-8549
	Dresher	Abington Memorial Hospital	(215) 646-4954
	Ft. Washington	Advanced Care Associates	(800) 289-8001
	Hershey	Milton S. Hershey Medical Center	(717) 531-5867
	Kingston	Wyoming Valley Health Care System	(717) 283-7851
	Lancaster	Lancaster Breast Cancer Network	(717) 393-7477
	Norristown	Montgomery Breast Cancer Support Program	(610) 270-2703
	Philadelphia	Fox Chase Cancer Center	(215) 728-2668
		Linda Creed Breast Cancer Foundation	(215) 545-0800
		Thomas Jefferson University Hospital	(215) 955-8370
	Pittsburgh	Burger King Cancer Caring Center	(412) 622-1212
		Magee-Women's Hospital	(412) 641-4255
	Ridley Park	Taylor Hospital	(610) 522-0203
	West Reading	Breast Cancer Support Services of Berks County	(610) 478-1447
	York	York Cancer Center	(717) 741-8100
Rhode Island	Providence	Hope Center for Life Enhancement	(401) 454-0404
	Providence	Rhode Island Hospital	(401) 444-5013
	Providence	Women & Infants Hospital	(401) 453-7540
	Narragansett	Kathy's Group for Lesbians	(401) 783-1601
	Warwick	Toll Gate Surgical	(401) 739-8010
	(Statewide)	Rhode Island Breast Cancer Coalition	(800) 216-1040
So. Carolina	Columbia	Bosom Buddies and Man to Man	(803) 771-5244
		Breast Cancer Support Group	(803) 434-3378
	Florence	McLeod Resource Center	(803) 667-2888
	Greenville	Breast Cancer Support Group	(803) 455-7591
	Lexington	Supporting Sisters	(803) 796-6009
So. Dakota	Sioux Falls	After Breast Cancer Survivors' Program	(605) 333-5244
Tennessee	Chattanooga	Y-ME of Chattanooga	(423) 886-4171
	Knoxville	Breast Cancer Networker	(423) 546-4661

	Memphis	EMBRACE—Memphis Cancer Center	(901) 763-0446
		Memphis Area Mastectomy/Lumpectomy Assoc.	(901) 382-9500
	Nashville	Mastectomy Support Group	(615) 665-0628
Texas	Arlington	Together We Will	(817) 277-7434
	Dallas	Between US	(214) 521-5225
		Common Cares	(214) 692-8893
		Medical City Hospital	(214) 661-4997
		Patient to Patient	(214) 821-2962
		Presbyterian Hospital of Dallas	(214) 345-2600
		Sammons Cancer Center	(214) 820-2608
		Sisters Network for African-American Women	(214) 637-7451
	Forth Worth	Breast Reconstruction Educational Support Group	(817) 335-6363
		Doris Kupferle Breast Center	(817) 882-3650
	Houston	Sisters Network for African-American Women	(713) 781-0255
		The Rose Garden	(713) 484-4708
		The Rosebuds	(713) 665-2729
	Lake Jackson	Sisters Network for African-American Women	(409) 297-4419
	Plano	North Texas Cancer Center	(214) 867-3577
	Richardson	Bosom Buddies	(214) 238-9516
	Woodlands	Coping With Breast Cancer	(800) 450-0026
Utah	Salt Lake City	Salt Lake Regional Breast Care Center	(801) 350-4973
	Vernal	Ashley Valley Medical Center	(801) 789-3342
Vermont	Burlington	Breast Care Center	(802) 656-2262
Virginia	Alexandria	National Capital/Y-ME	(703) 462-9616
	Charlottesville	Martha Jefferson Hospital	(804) 982-8407
		University of Virginia Cancer Center	(804) 924-2477
	Falls Church	Fairfax Hospital	(703) 698-3201
	Harrisonburg	Rockingham Memorial Hospital	(540) 433-4100
	Norfolk	Sentara Leigh Hospital	(804) 466-5738
		Sentara Norfolk General	(804) 668-4268
	Richmond	Massey Cancer Center	(804) 828-0450
	Salem	Lewis-Gale Regional Cancer Center	(800) 543-5660
Washington	Bellevue	Overlake Hospital	(206) 688-5261
	Bremerton	Breast Cancer Support Group of Kitsap County	(360) 373-1057
	Edmonds	Puget Sound Tumor Institute	(206) 640-4300
	Everett	Providence General Medical Center	(206) 258-7255
	Gig Harbor	Gig Harbor Breast Cancer Support Group	(206) 857-5802
	Kirkland	Evergreen Hospital	(206) 899-2265
	Olympia	St. Peter Hospital Regional Cancer Center	(360) 493-4111
	Seattle	Highline Community Hospital	(206) 439-5577
		Northwest Hospital	(206) 368-1457
		Providence	(206) 320-2100
		Swedish Hospital Tumor Institute	(206) 386-2323
W. Virginia	Charleston	Women and Children's Hospital	(304) 348-2545
Wisconsin	Madison	Meriter Hospital Women's Center	(608) 258-3750
	Sheboygan	Sheboygan Memorial Medical Center	(414) 451-5536
Wyoming	Cheyenne	United Medical Center	(307) 634-2273

AMERICAN CANCER SOCIETY CHARTERED DIVISIONS

The American Cancer Society is the nationwide, community-based, voluntary health organization dedicated to eliminating cancer as a major health problem by preventing cancer, saving lives from cancer, and diminishing suffering from cancer through research, education, and service. National Headquarters: American Cancer Society, Inc., 1599 Clifton Road, N.E., Atlanta, GA 30329–4251, (404) 320–3333.

Alabama Division, Inc.
504 Brookwood Boulevard
Homewood, Alabama 35209
(205) 879–2242

Alaska Division, Inc.
1057 West Fireweed Lane, Suite 204
Anchorage, Alaska 99503
(907) 277–8696

Arizona Division, Inc.
2929 East Thomas Road
Phoenix, Arizona 85016
(602) 224–0524

Arkansas Division, Inc.
901 North University
Little Rock, Arkansas 72207
(501) 664–3480

California Division, Inc.
1710 Webster Street
Oakland, California 94604
(510) 893–7900

Colorado Division, Inc.
2255 South Oneida
Denver, Colorado 80224
(303) 758–2030

Connecticut Division, Inc.
Barnes Park South
14 Village Lane
Wallingford, Connecticut 06492
(203) 265–7161

Delaware Division, Inc.
92 Read's Way, Suite 205
New Castle, Delaware 19720
(302) 324–4227

District of Columbia Division, Inc.
1875 Connecticut Avenue, NW
Suite 730
Washington, DC 20009
(202) 483–2600

Florida Division, Inc.
3709 West Jetton Avenue
Tampa, Florida 33629–5146
(813) 253–0541

Georgia Division, Inc.
2200 Lake Boulevard
Atlanta, Georgia 30319
(404) 816–7800

Idaho Division, Inc.
2676 Vista Avenue
Boise, Idaho 83705–0386
(208) 343–4609

Illinois Division, Inc.
77 East Monroe
Chicago, Illinois 60603–5795
(312) 641–6150

Indiana Division, Inc.
8730 Commerce Park Place
Indianapolis, Indiana 46268
(317) 872–4432

Iowa Division, Inc.
8364 Hickman Road, Suite D
Des Moines, Iowa 50325
(515) 253–0147

Kansas Division, Inc.
1315 SW Arrowhead Road
Topeka, Kansas 66604
(913) 273–4114

Kentucky Division, Inc.
701 West Muhammad Ali Boulevard
Louisville, Kentucky 40201–1807
(502) 584–6782

Louisiana Division, Inc.
2200 Veterans Memorial Boulevard
Suite 214
Kenner, Louisiana 70062
(504) 469–0021

Maine Division, Inc.
52 Federal Street
Brunswick, Maine 04011
(207) 729–3339

Maryland Division, Inc.
8219 Town Center Drive
Baltimore, Maryland 21236–0026
(410) 931–6850

Massachusetts Division, Inc.
30 Speen Street
Framingham, Massachusetts 01701
(508) 270–4600

Michigan Division, Inc.
1205 East Saginaw Street
Lansing, Michigan 48906
(517) 371–2920

Minnesota Division, Inc.
3316 West 66th Street
Minneapolis, Minnesota 55435
(612) 925–2772

Mississippi Division, Inc.
1380 Livingston Lane
Lakeover Office Park
Jackson, Mississippi 39213
(601) 362–8874

Missouri Division, Inc.
3322 American Avenue
Jefferson City, Missouri 65102
(573) 893–4800

Montana Division, Inc.
17 North 26th Street
Billings, Montana 59101
(406) 252–7111

Nebraska Division, Inc.
8502 West Center Road
Omaha, Nebraska 68124–5255
(402) 393–5800

Nevada Division, Inc.
1325 East Harmon
Las Vegas, Nevada 89119
(702) 798–6857

New Hampshire Division, Inc.
Gail Singer Memorial Building
360 Route 101, Unit 501
Bedford, New Hampshire 03110
(603) 472–8899

New Jersey Division, Inc.
2600 US Highway 1
North Brunswick, New Jersey 08902–0803
(908) 297–8000

New Mexico Division, Inc.
5800 Lomas Boulevard, NE
Albuquerque, New Mexico 87110
(505) 260–2105

New York State Division, Inc.
6725 Lyons Street
East Syracuse, New York 13057
(315) 437–7025

Long Island Division, Inc.
75 Davids Drive
Hauppauge, New York 11788
(516) 436–7070

New York City Division, Inc.
19 West 56th Street
New York, New York 10019
(212) 586–8700

Queens Division, Inc.
112–25 Queens Boulevard
Forest Hills, New York 11375
(718) 263–2224

Westchester Division, Inc.
2 Lyon Place
White Plains, New York 10601
(914) 949–4800

North Carolina Division, Inc.
11 South Boylan Avenue, Suite 221
Raleigh, North Carolina 27603
(919) 834–8463

North Dakota Division, Inc.
123 Roberts Street
Fargo, North Dakota 58102
(701) 232–1385

Ohio Division, Inc.
5555 Frantz Road
Dublin, Ohio 43017
(614) 889–9565

Oklahoma Division, Inc.
4323 63rd, Suite 110
Oklahoma City, Oklahoma 73116
(405) 843–9888

Oregon Division, Inc.
0330 SW Curry
Portland, Oregon 97201
(503) 295–6422

Pennsylvania Division, Inc.
Route 422 & Sipe Avenue
Hershey, Pennsylvania 17033–0897
(717) 533–6144

Philadelphia Division, Inc.
1626 Locust Street
Philadelphia, Pennsylvania 19103
(215) 985–5400

Puerto Rico Division, Inc.
Calle Alverio #577
Esquina Sargento Medina
Hato Rey, Puerto Rico 00918
(787) 764–2295

Rhode Island Division, Inc.
400 Main Street
Pawtucket, Rhode Island 02860
(401) 722–8480

South Carolina Division, Inc.
128 Stonemark Lane
Westpark Plaza
Columbia, South Carolina 29210–3855
(803) 750–1693

South Dakota Division, Inc.
4101 Carnegie Place
Sioux Falls, South Dakota 57106
(605) 361–8277

Tennessee Division, Inc.
1315 Eighth Avenue, South
Nashville, Tennessee 37203
(615) 255–1227

Texas Division, Inc.
2433 Ridgepoint Drive
Austin, Texas 78754
(512) 928–2262

Utah Division, Inc.
941 East 3300 South
Salt Lake City, Utah 84106
(801) 483–1500

Vermont Division, Inc.
13 Loomis Street
Drawer C
Montpelier, Vermont 05602
(802) 223–2348

Virginia Division, Inc.
4240 Park Place Court
Glen Allen, Virginia 23060
(804) 527–3700

Washington Division, Inc.
2120 First Avenue, North
Seattle, Washington 98109–1140
(206) 283–1152

West Virginia Division, Inc.
2428 Kanawha Boulevard, East
Charleston, West Virginia 25311
(304) 344–3611

Wisconsin Division, Inc.
PO Box 902
Pewaukee, Wisconsin 53072-0902
(414) 523–5500

Wyoming Division, Inc.
4202 Ridge Road
Cheyenne, Wyoming 82001
(307) 638–3331

ADVOCACY ORGANIZATIONS

If the contact in your state listed below cannot be reached, call the National Breast Cancer Coalition office at **(202) 296–7477**.

U.S. Territories
American Samoa
Amata Coleman Radewagen
Box 26142
Alexandria, Virginia 22313–6142
(703) 548–2244

Alabama
Caroline T. Noogin, RN
Huntsville Hospital Women's Center
1963 Memorial Parkway
Huntsville, Alabama 35801
(205) 517–6614
Fax: (205) 517–6611

Alaska
Sharon Yerbich
Alaska Breast Cancer Coalition
329 F Street, Suite 210
Anchorage, Alaska 99501–2217
(907) 274–5631

Arizona
Vanette Hickey
Arizona Women's Cancer Network
HC 30 Box 1225
Prescott, Arizona 86301
(520) 776–4935

Arkansas
Maureen Colvert
Arkansas Cancer Research Center
4301 W. Markham, Slot 725
Little Rock, Arkansas 72205
(501) 686–6503

California
Arlyne Draper
California Breast Cancer Organizations
8755 Aero Drive, #302
San Diego, California 92123
(619) 569–9283

Colorado
Anne Wylie Weiher
Colorado Breast Cancer Coalition
3486 16th Circle
Boulder, Colorado 80304
(303) 415–1883

Connecticut
Barbara Stillman
Connecticut Breast Cancer Coalition
158 Main Street
Thomaston, Connecticut 06787
(860) 283–1155

Delaware
Maureen Lauterbach
Delaware Breast Cancer Coalition
2300 Riddle Avenue #303
Wilmington, Delaware 19806
(302) 658–4589

District of Columbia
Jean M. Lynn, RN
Breast Care Center
George Washington University Medical Center
Washington, DC 20037
(202) 994–4589

Florida
Jane Torres
Florida Breast Cancer Coalition
600 Grapetree Drive, Apt. 10BS
Key Biscayne, Florida 33149
(305) 371–2773

Georgia
Ruth Eldredge
Georgia Breast Cancer Coalition
3639 Shallowford Road
Doraville, Georgia 30040
(770) 889–8950

Hawaii
Ginnie Coggins
American Cancer Society
Hawaii Pacific Division
2370 Nuuanu Avenue
Honolulu, Hawaii 96817
(808) 595–7500
Fax: (808) 595–7502

Idaho
Cordelia (Percy) Persigehl
Mountain States Tumor Institute
151 East Bannock
Boise, Idaho 83712
(208) 386–2764

Illinois
Carol White
Y-ME National Office
212 West Van Buren, 4th Floor
Chicago, Illinois 60607
(312) 986–8338

Indiana
Michele Wood
St. Francis Hospital
8111 South Emerson Avenue
Indianapolis, Indiana 46237
(317) 865–5864

Iowa
Suki Cell, Co-Coordinator
Iowa Breast Cancer Action
424 First Avenue NE
Cedar Rapids, Iowa 52401
(319) 398–5317
Fax: (319) 398–5228

Kentucky
Doris Rosenbaum
Kentucky Breast Cancer Coalition
3605 Gloucester Drive
Lexington, Kentucky 40510
(606) 233–3601

Louisiana
Lorre Lei Jackson
Louisiana Breast Cancer Task Force
9605 Red Gate Drive
New Orleans, Louisiana 70123
(504) 737–0992
Fax: (504) 738–3794

Maine
Laurel Bezanson
Maine Breast Cancer Coalition
51 Sandy Hill Road
South Portland, Maine 04106
(207) 874–0943

Maryland
Marsha Oakley
Arm-in-Arm
302 Presway Road
Timonium, Maryland 21093
(410) 368–2962

Massachusetts
Judi Hirshfield-Bartek, RN
Beth Israel Hospital
330 Brookline Avenue
Boston, Massachusetts 02215
(617) 667–4491

Michigan
Deanna Makela
4852 Marseilles
Detroit, Michigan 48224
(313) 885–2105

Minnesota
Chris Norton
Minnesota Breast Cancer Coalition
8601 Indian Boulevard
Cottage Grove, Minnesota 55016–2147
(612) 459–7923

Missouri
Ileane Kanter Fagin
St. Louis Breast Cancer Coalition
7 Beaver Drive
St. Louis, Missouri 63141
(314) 994–3346
Fax: (314) 692–8022

Montana
Kim Alexandre Powell
205 Evans Avenue
Missoula, Montana 59801
(406) 728–1949
Fax: (406) 728–5772

Nebraska
Kathy Zeitz
423 S. 160th Street
Omaha, Nebraska 68118
(712) 328–6084

Nevada
Gail Allen
Breast Cancer Coalition of Nevada
P.O. Box 97084
Las Vegas, Nevada 89193
(702) 361–5393
Fax: (702) 361–5453

New Hampshire
Nancy Ryan
New Hampshire Breast Cancer Coalition
18 Belle Lane
Lee, New Hampshire 03824
(603) 659–3482

New Jersey
Jane Rodney
Breast Cancer Resource Center
Princeton YWCA
Paul Robeson Place
Princeton, New Jersey 08540
(609) 497–2126

New Mexico
Joann Huff
New Mexico Breast Cancer Coalition
1705 Singletary NE
Albuquerque, New Mexico 87112
(505) 822–9922
Fax: (505) 822–0801

New York
Hillary Rutter
Adelphi NY Statewide Breast Cancer Hotline & Support
    Program
Adelphi University School of Social Work
Garden City, New York 11530
(516) 877–4313
Fax: (516) 877–4336

North Carolina
Emma Lu Bullard
1505 Kenan Street
Wilson, North Carolina 27893–2252
(919) 237–0439

North Dakota
Jan Buckner
1512 34th Street SW
Fargo, North Dakota 58103
(218) 299–6337

Ohio
Janie Ehrman
Women's Health Information Network, Inc.
7144 Youngstown-Salem Road
Canfield, Ohio 44406–9434
(330) 533–1750

Oklahoma
Debbie Clark
Breast Care Center
13509 North Meridian, Suite 6
Oklahoma City, Oklahoma 73120
(405) 755–2273

Oregon
Lee Smith
Oregon Breast Cancer Coalition Fund
1430 Willamette, Suite 193
Eugene, Oregon 97401
(541) 744–5630

Pennsylvania
Barbara DeLuca
Linda Creed Breast Cancer Foundation
255 17th Street, #905
Philadelphia, Pennsylvania 19103
(215) 545–0800

Rhode Island
Marlene McCarthy
Rhode Island Breast Cancer Coalition
300 Quaker Lane, Suite 7
Warwick, Rhode Island 02886
(401) 822–0095
Fax: (401) 823–4945
email: RIBCC@aol.com

South Carolina
Anita Throw
3720 Palmer Drive
Florence, South Carolina 29506
(803) 661–1692

Tennessee
Marianne Sartin Bouldin
Vanderbilt Cancer Center
649 Medical Research Building II
Nashville, Tennessee 37323
(615) 936–1782

Texas
Dale Eastman
Alamo Breast Cancer Foundation & Coalition
3715 Hunters Point
San Antonio, Texas 78230
(210) 344–3364
Fax: (210) 344–4611

Utah
Judy Smith
Breast Cancer Coalition of Utah
3510 West 2460 South
West Valley, Utah 84119
(801) 943–6500

Vermont
Pat Barr
Vermont Breast Cancer Coalition
507 Main Street
Bennington, Vermont 05201
(802) 442–6341

Virginia
Patricia Goodall
Virginia Breast Cancer Foundation
P.O. Box 17884
Richmond, Virginia 23226
(804) 285–1200
Fax: (804) 285–7735
email: 14775.3233@compuserve.com

Wisconsin
Kathleen Harris
Wisconsin Breast Cancer Coalition
P.O. Box 17031
Milwaukee, Wisconsin 53217
(414) 962–7180
Fax: (414) 962–7180
email: MedVC@aol.com

MEDICAL AND LEGAL ISSUES SPECIFIC TO THE CARE OF BREAST CANCER

CHAPTER 92

BREAST CANCER: A MODEL FOR CANCER EDUCATION

Stephen N. Birrell, M.D., Ph.D. / David A. Sloan, M.D. / Richard W. Schwartz, M.D.

BREAST CANCER EDUCATION: THE NEED FOR IMPROVEMENT

The treatment of patients with breast cancer is complex; patients are increasingly treated in a multimodal fashion that requires the input of several cancer specialists.[1] The care of breast cancer patients may include oncologic surgeons, medical oncologists, radiotherapists, radiologists, pathologists, medical social workers, and nurse oncologists. Furthermore, it is unusual for a patient with a breast tumor to have only a single treatment option; generally, several options and several timetables are possible. The side effects, risks, and potential benefits of the available options must be carefully explained to each patient, individually, in terms that she can clearly understand.

Analysis of current practice patterns reveals that many general practitioners continue to screen patients inadequately and that many surgeons continue to treat breast cancer with mastectomy. These findings suggest that these practitioners have inadequate knowledge of screening guidelines and treatment options.[2–5] Despite incontrovertible evidence for the efficacy of breast conservation surgery (BCS) from the National Surgical Adjuvant Breast and Bowel Project (NSABP) and other trials, most women with early breast cancer undergo mastectomy rather than BCS.[6–8] Margolis and colleagues reported that women who underwent mastectomy felt less attractive than did women treated with BCS, and half regretted their choice.[9] Since the widespread publicity of the BCS trials, disturbing data have suggested that the rate of modified radical mastectomies is returning to pre-1985 levels, especially in remote areas of the country.[3, 10] The issues that have led to these findings are complex, and research is urgently needed to see how individual breast cancer patients and their physicians decide what type of treatment is most appropriate. The solution does not lie in the Breast Cancer Disclosure Acts that since 1979 have been enacted in many states, because these acts vary much with respect to what treatment alternatives physicians are required to disclose to patients, what responsibilities are placed on physicians, and how the written summaries of treatment alternatives are constructed.[11]

The multitude of options and the burgeoning body of oncological knowledge make education in breast cancer (undergraduate and graduate) difficult. Many medical schools lack an integrated oncology curriculum, and reviews of undergraduate medical curricula have documented many weaknesses in the presentation of the oncology curriculum.[12–15] An overview of undergraduate education in 142 medical schools showed that educational activity in general oncology was distinctly lacking.[15] This lack of a structured oncology curriculum may explain the poor performance of medical students in oncology-related areas. Bleyer and coworkers noted that medical students' performance on oncology-related questions was significantly poorer than their performance on other subjects.[14] Jewell and Deslauriers at the University of Kansas Medical Center found that it was possible for students to graduate from medical school without having any appreciable insight into the care of cancer patients.[16] A recent survey of fourth-year medical students at three institutions revealed that most of the students had never palpated a breast involved by cancer.[17] Furthermore, in a recent survey of oncology education in Australian medical schools, Smith and colleagues were alarmed at the many important deficits in oncology skills and knowledge among medical undergraduates.[18] Knowledge of common cancers, including recommendations for screening, was very poor, and experience with important components of cancer treatment such as radiotherapy and palliative care was virtually nonexistent. The authors identified "worrying levels of incorrect knowledge" about cancer and lamented that there was no valid instrument in the literature with which to evaluate cancer instruction.[18]

Physicians clearly need to learn more than simply how to perform a breast examination and when to order a mammogram, although such basic education is needed.[2–5, 19–23] Additional components of clinical assessment include patient counseling, risk assessment, and instruction in breast self-examination.[24–26] Stefanek has summarized the future of breast cancer intervention as follows: "The focus of the intervention should center upon the benefits of early detection, assessment of breast self-examination skills, individualized breast cancer screening, recommendations such as mammography and physical examinations, and recommendations for life-style changes for possible prevention."[27]

It is assumed that such clinical skills are acquired in medical school. Unfortunately, a growing body of evidence indicates that assuming that students have acquired such clinical skills may be misleading.[28–32] Only recently, with the development of the Objective Structured Clinical Examination (OSCE), has a true appreciation of the failure of medical schools to teach clinical skills become apparent.[29–33] In this examination format, students or residents encounter patients individually and are asked to take a history or perform a focused physical examination. The use of both actual and simulated patients in the OSCE creates real-life settings for students and residents. In addition, these patients can very effectively evaluate the trainees for both their clinical skills and their ability to interact with patients.[34–37] Use of the OSCE has revealed substantial deficits in students' and residents' understanding of breast cancer and other oncology problems.[29, 30, 33, 38, 39]

Mean OSCE performance scores in an initial pilot study at the University of Kentucky (UK) were very poor: most students and interns failed almost all of the problems.[30] For example, when presented with a patient with breast pain who was worried about cancer, students and residents performed poorly (Fig. 92–1). To our knowledge, this pilot study was the first to use performance-based testing to evaluate the ability of residents and students to treat cancer patients. Subsequent OSCE studies that examined the entire group of surgery residents at UK found their understanding of common breast cancer problems disappointing.[38, 39]

Most recently, 16 primary care trainees at UK were tested on a 12-station breast cancer OSCE (Fig. 92–2). The trainees were presented with several standardized patients, some of whom were breast cancer survivors. The problems were basic ones—breast pain, nipple discharge, explanation of treatment options, among others. The mean OSCE score was very low (41.1 percent). The mean score at the station in which the trainee presented options to a "standardized patient" (a breast cancer survivor) with newly diagnosed breast cancer was 29.6 percent.

The ability of physicians to communicate with cancer patients is paramount. We have demonstrated that interpersonal skills can be measured with good reliability by both patients and faculty members during the OSCE.[35–37] Patients' evaluations correlated very well with those given by faculty members ($r = 0.87$, $P < .001$) in one study.[36] The ability of patients to evaluate residents' interpersonal skills was underscored by the observation that the ratings of both faculty members ($P < .0001$) and patients ($P < .001$) differentiated levels of training (the more senior residents received higher ratings). Breast cancer survivors have recently been involved as standardized OSCE patients at UK, and feedback from these patients has been very helpful.

Despite this evidence, very little in the way of innovative, structured education has been applied to the problem of breast cancer. This is in marked con-

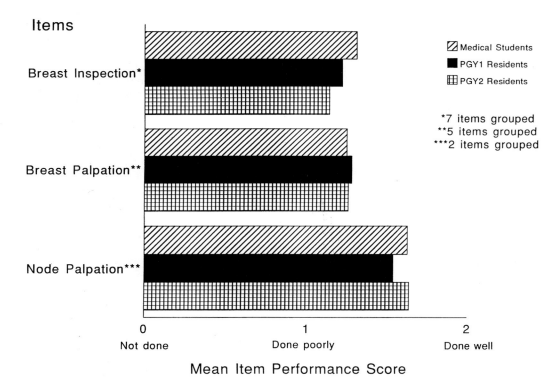

Figure 92–1 *Mean performance scores for medical students, postgraduate year (PGY)-1 residents, and PGY-2 residents for selected data-gathering items concerning a patient with breast pain who is worried about cancer.*

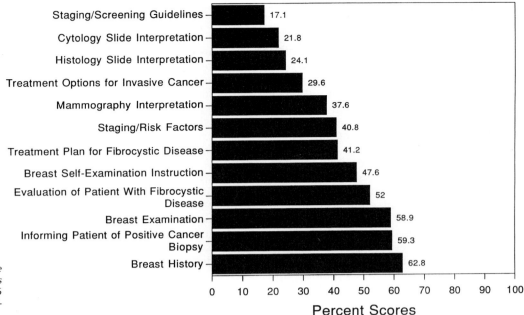

Figure 92–2 *Mean performance scores for the various components of an OSCE given to a group of 16 primary care trainees at the University of Kentucky.*

trast to education in acute trauma or cardiac disease, for which groups of specialists have laid out and encoded competent behavior (e.g., the Advanced Cardiac Life Support [ACLS] and Advanced Trauma Life Support [ATLS] programs).[40–43] Both the ACLS program and the ATLS program use packaged standardized instruction formats and have been successfully administered to hundreds of thousands of physicians, residents, and students. Both programs are associated with improved physician performance and improved patient survival.[44–46] Similar educational strategies must be applied to the task of reducing breast cancer morbidity and mortality.

NOVEL STRATEGIES FOR IMPROVING BREAST CANCER EDUCATION

Development of the Structured Clinical Instruction Module for Breast Cancer Education

In an effort to improve the quality of breast cancer education, a multidisciplinary group at UK developed a clinical workshop specifically to address breast cancer skills. This workshop, called the Structured Clinical Instruction Module (SCIM), was then presented as a pilot effort to 30 medical students.[47] The SCIM consisted of twelve 10-minute stations, each covering a different aspect of breast disease. The students rotated through the various stations in groups of three. Nine patients and fourteen faculty members participated. At the patient stations, a designated student conducted the interview or examination. The other students in the group were given the opportunity to ask additional questions, after which the students were given feedback evaluation; faculty members then took the opportunity to emphasize key points. A checklist of key items was used to guide instructional feedback. At nonpatient stations, students were asked, for example, to identify the important features of several mammograms and then to make an interpretation. The faculty member then provided instructional feedback, again on the basis of predetermined objective criteria. All ratings of the SCIM by faculty members, patients, and students were very positive.[47]

As this pilot study demonstrated, the SCIM concept has several distinct advantages over conventional clinical teaching: (1) a detailed curriculum containing all essential elements for competent performance as defined by experts; (2) comprehensive and consistent teaching of skills that generally are not learned from textbooks, the usual source of information for students and residents; (3) instruction in an environment isolated from external disruptions such as hectic clinics; (4) the opportunity for trainees to show what they do not know, a powerful stimulus for receiving instruction; (5) important feedback from the patients participating in the SCIM; and (6) reproducible teaching.

On the basis of the success of the SCIM as a format for clinical instruction, an NIH-funded multi-institutional consortium of five institutions (UK, University of Louisville, Harvard University, Brown University, and the University of Texas M.D. Anderson Cancer Center [UTMDACC]) was created, first to determine content and then to implement a breast cancer SCIM for general surgery residents at the five institutions. This Breast Cancer Education Working Group (BCEWG) consisted of professionals from the following disciplines: surgical oncology, medical oncology, radiation oncology, pathology, radiology, plastic and reconstructive surgery, nursing oncology, and behavioral science. Representative breast cancer survivors were also members of the BCEWG.

The curriculum developed by the BCEWG encompassed all aspects of the assessment of a breast cancer patient, including history and physical examination, risk factor assessment, attention to psychosocial and interpersonal factors, explanation of treatment options and patient counseling, basic tumor imaging studies, key cytologic and pathological techniques, and assessment for protocol enrollment.

The SCIM was piloted with a group of 25 residents at UK and was very well received by cancer patients, residents, and faculty members.[48, 49] For the patients, the three most positive aspects of the SCIM were as follows: (1) the patient enjoyed participating in the workshop; (2) the SCIM was a valuable educational experience for the residents; and (3) the faculty members appeared to enjoy the SCIM. The residents judged their own clinical competence on 16 specific breast cancer–related skills before and after the SCIM (Fig. 92–3). For every skill the post-SCIM ratings were significantly higher than the pre-SCIM ones. "Less than competent" mean ratings were observed for 10 of the 16 skills on the pre-SCIM evaluation; in contrast, only one skill (interpreting breast cytology and histology slides) was rated "less than competent" on the post-SCIM evaluation. The SCIM was then given to surgical residents at the remaining BCEWG institutions, with similar results. Table 92–1 shows the course content.

A pilot SCIM has also been developed for primary care trainees. Input was obtained from professionals in family medicine, general internal medicine, and gynecology, as well as from the nurse practitioner and physician's assistant schools. The primary care SCIM consisted of eight 15-minute stations. The 20 primary care trainees at UK agreed (on a 5-point Likert scale; 1 = strongly disagree and 5 = strongly agree) that the SCIM faculty members were well-prepared (mean 4.9), that the SCIM was well-organized (mean 4.9), and that the SCIM was a valuable educational experience (mean 4.8). The faculty members enjoyed participating (mean 4.9) and believed that the SCIM was a unique method for teaching clinical skills (mean 4.8). The patients believed that feedback from faculty members to trainees was excellent (mean 5.0), and they rated the SCIM very highly overall (mean 5.0).

Breast cancer survivors play an integral role in the SCIM. Although the use of standardized patients in evaluating and instructing students and residents is increasingly common, there is no prior experience with the participation of actual cancer patients as standardized patients and as instructors of physicians.[34, 50–54] Thirty-one breast cancer survivors have participated in the SCIM to date (Fig. 92–4). All survivors from whom data have been collected evaluated the SCIM as either outstanding or above average, and 73 percent were willing to participate as often as needed; none said that they would not participate again. There were significant differences in the levels of agreement for the various SCIM characteris-

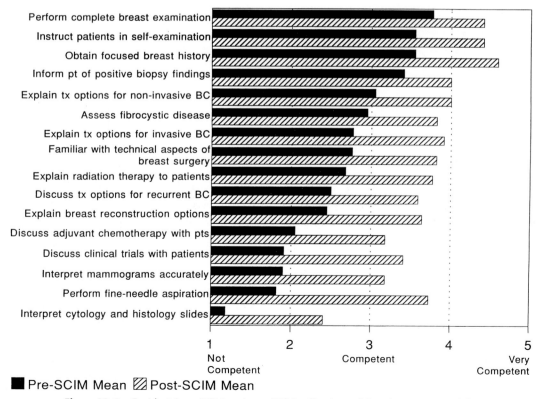

Figure 92–3 *Residents' pre-SCIM and post-SCIM self-ratings of their breast cancer skills.*

TABLE 92–1.   STATIONS OF THE STRUCTURED CLINICAL INSTRUCTION MODULE

Station Number	Station Name	Station Tasks
1	Focused breast history; breast self-examination instruction	Obtain a focused history from a patient with a complaint of a breast lump; then instruct patient in breast self-examination technique. (AP)
2	Mammogram interpretation	Interpret seven mammograms with diagnoses including spiculated mass, simple cyst, and fibroadenoma.
3	Breast cytology; fine needle aspiration biopsy technique	Practice fine needle aspiration biopsy technique on artificial tissue (oranges).
4	Breast cytology/histology; slide interpretation	View and interpret cytologic and histological slides with diagnoses of fibroadenoma, ductal carcinoma, fibrocystic changes, and proliferative fibrocystic disease without atypia.
5	Explanation of treatment options	Explain treatment options to a patient with a newly diagnosed breast cancer. (AP)
6	Radiation therapy treatment planning	Discuss radiation therapy treatment plans with a patient contemplating breast conservation treatment. (AP)
7	Reconstruction options	Discuss options for breast reconstruction with a patient planning to undergo modified radical mastectomy. (AP)
8	Informing patient of positive cancer biopsy	Explain to a patient that she has cancer. (SP or AP)
9	Surgical anatomy and breast biopsy	Review of surgical anatomy of the breast and axilla; review of open biopsy techniques.
10	Medical oncology evaluation	Discuss with a patient the possibility of adjuvant treatment and its benefits. (AP)
11	Evaluation and examination of patient with fibrocystic disease or nipple discharge	After being given history results, perform a breast physical examination on a patient; then provide diagnosis and treatment plan. (SP)
12	Consent for protocol enrollment	Discuss the Breast Cancer Prevention Trial with a patient at high risk for developing breast cancer. (SP)

AP, actual cancer patient; SP, simulated patient.

tics ($P<.0001$ from a repeated-measures analysis of variance). Patients agreed most that (1) they enjoyed participating in the workshop (mean 4.90 on a 5-point Likert scale); (2) it was beneficial to use real cancer patients (mean 4.87); (3) the SCIM is a valu-able educational experience for the residents (mean 4.90); (4) the patients' participation in the workshop was important and effective (mean 4.74); and (5) the faculty members gave useful feedback at the end of the station (mean 4.84). From these data we can conclude that the patients viewed the SCIM as a valuable educational experience and believed strongly that their participation contributed to its effectiveness.

The efficacy of both the primary care and the surgery resident versions of the SCIM has been tested. Forty-two primary care trainees at UK were randomized to one of four groups; training background (e.g., family practice versus internal medicine) and level of training (e.g., post graduate year level) were used as stratification variables. The groups were as follows: (1) SCIM plus immediate post-SCIM OSCE; (2) untreated control plus immediate OSCE; (3) SCIM plus OSCE administered after 6 months; and (4) untreated control plus OSCE administered after 6 months. The SCIM group (mean OSCE score 62 percent) performed much better than the untreated control group (mean score 43 percent) on the OSCE immediately after the SCIM ($P<.001$). This difference between groups was maintained over a 6-month period, as evidenced by performance on the OSCE administered 6 months after the SCIM (Fig. 92–5). There was no significant decline in skills ($P=.645$). This same pattern of performance was found for judged competence, interpersonal skills judged by faculty members and patients, and organizational skills exhibited during the patient interactions.

In a similar fashion, 48 general surgery residents were randomized to the same four experimental groups. The only difference was that the second OSCE was given 8 months after the SCIM. The pattern of results was similar. Residents assigned to the SCIM group (mean OSCE score 63 percent) performed significantly better ($P=.001$) than an untreated control group (mean 49 percent). This differ-

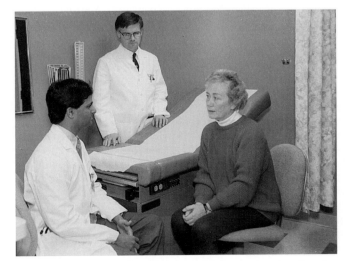

Figure 92–4 *A surgical resident is explaining treatment options to a breast cancer survivor participating in the SCIM.*

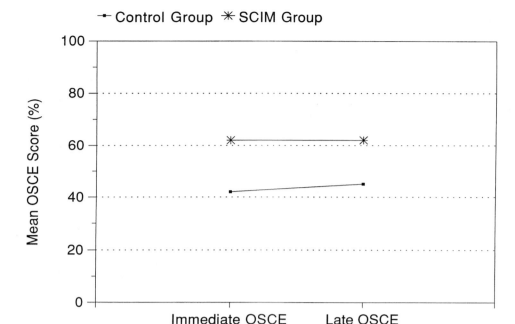

Figure 92–5 *Impact of the primary care breast cancer SCIM on immediate and late OSCEs measuring breast cancer skills.*

ence was sustained at the end of 8 months, although there was a small but significant decline ($P = .0104$) in the performance of the SCIM group (mean 55 percent). The nonsignificant ($P = .286$) interaction between testing and group indicates that the SCIM and control groups had parallel decreases in performance. This same pattern of results was observed for judged competence; however, in the cases of organizational skills and of interpersonal skills judged by faculty members and by patients, the SCIM group performed better than the control group with no decrease over time.

Computer-Based Instruction

Medical schools around the world are using problem-based learning (PBL) as a didactic tool to improve students' ability to solve complex medical problems.[55–58] Recently, this educational platform has been incorporated into computerized educational packages. The Technology in Medical Education (TIME) group at the University of Liverpool has developed Liverpool's Electronic Study Guide for Oncology (LETSGO). This computerized breast cancer education program for undergraduate medical students is based on the principles of problem-based learning, and, to the best of our knowledge, the description of this program in *Medical Education* contains the only published data about this innovative and exciting combination of PBL and computerized learning.[59] Unlike many bland computerized education and assessment tools, which are little more than electronic textbooks, LETSGO presents a dynamic user interface combining tools such as brainstorming and mindmap pads, a comprehensive personal information manager, and interactive educational self-assessment and quiz games. The learner is provided

with feedback on both personal and peer-referenced levels. The short- and long-term effectiveness of the LETSGO program has not yet been determined.

CONCLUSIONS

Conventional medical education has failed to prepare students and physicians to effectively manage problems related to breast cancer. Medical educators must re-evaluate the methods of cancer education. The continued development and implementation of novel educational packages such as the SCIM and LETSGO programs should enhance problem-solving and clinical skills in the management of breast cancer. It is hoped that such educational strategies will lead to a reduction in breast cancer morbidity and mortality rates. Such programs are not only appropriate for students and residents but can also be modified for practicing physicians.

References

1. Balch CM, Singletary SE, Bland KI: Clinical decision-making in early breast cancer. Ann Surg 217:207–225, 1993.
2. Albanes D, Weinberg GB, Boss L, Taylor PR: A survey of physicians' breast cancer early detection practices. Prev Med 17:643–652, 1988.
3. Lazovich DA, White E, Thomas DB, Moe RE: Underutilization of breast-conserving surgery and radiation therapy among women with stage I or II breast cancer. JAMA 266:3433–3438, 1991.
4. Survey of physicians' attitudes and practices in early cancer detection. CA Cancer J Clin 35:197–213, 1985.
5. Nattinger AB, Gottlieb MS, Veum J, Yahnke D, Goodwin JS: Geographic variation in the use of breast-conserving treatment for breast cancer. N Engl J Med 326:1102–1107, 1992.
6. Fisher B, Redmond C, Poisson R, et al: Eight-year results of a randomized clinical trial comparing total mastectomy and

lumpectomy with or without irradiation in the treatment of breast cancer. N Engl J Med 320:822–828, 1989.

7. Veronesi U, Banfi A, Salvadori B, et al: Breast conservation is the treatment of choice in small breast cancer: Long-term results of a randomized trial. Eur J Cancer 26:668–670, 1990.

8. Farrow DC, Hunt WC, Samet JM: Geographic variation in the treatment of localized breast cancer. N Engl J Med 326:1097–1101, 1992.

9. Margolis G, Goodman RL, Rubin A: Psychological effects of breast-conserving cancer treatment and mastectomy. Psychosomatics 31:33–39, 1990.

10. Samet JM, Hunt WC, Farrow DC: Determinants of receiving breast-conserving surgery. The Surveillance, Epidemiology, and End Results Program, 1983–1986. Cancer 73:2344–2351, 1994.

11. Nayfield SG, Bongiovanni GC, Alciati MH, Fischer RA, Bergner L: Statutory requirements for disclosure of breast cancer treatment alternatives. J Natl Cancer Inst 86:1202–1208, 1994.

12. Brincker H: Undergraduate oncology education in Scandinavia. J Cancer Educ 3:97–101, 1988.

13. Robert KH, Einhorn J, Kornhuber B, Peckham M, Zittoun R: European undergraduate education in oncology. A report of the EORTC Education Branch. Acta Oncol 27:423–425, 1988.

14. Bleyer WA, Hunt DD, Carline JD, Trevisan M, Johnson S, Phillips TJ: Improvement of oncology education at the University of Washington School of Medicine, 1984–1988. Acad Med 65:114–119, 1990.

15. Bernard LJ, Carter RA: Surgical oncology education in US and Canadian medical schools. J Cancer Educ 3:239–242, 1988.

16. Jewell WR, Deslauriers MP: Teaching surgical oncology to medical students. J Surg Oncol 24:218–220, 1983.

17. Kennedy BJ, Foley JF, Yarbro JW, Ringenberg QS: Breast cancer examination experience of medical students and residents. J Cancer Educ 3:243–245, 1988.

18. Smith WT, Tattersall MH, Irwig LM, Langlands AO: Undergraduate education about cancer. Eur J Cancer 27:1448–1453, 1991.

19. Thomas DC, Spitzer WO, MacFarlane JK: Inter-observer error among surgeons and nurses in presymptomatic detection of breast disease. J Chronic Dis 34:617–626, 1981.

20. Fletcher SW, O'Malley MS, Bunce LA: Physicians' abilities to detect lumps in silicone breast models. JAMA 253:2224–2228, 1985.

21. Observer variation in recording clinical data from women presenting with breast lesions. Report from the Yorkshire Breast Cancer Group. Br Med J 2:1196–1199, 1977.

22. Boyd NF, Sutherland HJ, Fish EB, Hiraki GY, Lickley HL, Maurer VE: Prospective evaluation of physical examination of the breast. Am J Surg 142:331–334, 1981.

23. Rudolph A, McDermott RJ: The breast physical examination. Its value in early cancer detection. Cancer Nurs 10:100–106, 1987.

24. Huguley CM Jr, Brown RL, Greenberg RS, Clark WS: Breast self-examination and survival from breast cancer. Cancer 62:1389–1396, 1988.

25. Mettlin CJ, Bard M, Boyd FJ, Kushner HD, McKenney SJ, Mellette SJ, Saltzstein SL, Schain WS, Shover LR, Wellisch DK: Patient/psychosocial issues. Patient and family education. Cancer 68(5 Suppl):1184–1185, 1991.

26. Maguire P, Faulkner A: Improve the counselling skills of doctors and nurses in cancer care. Br Med J 297:847–849, 1988.

27. Stefanek ME: Counselling women at high risk for breast cancer. Oncology (Huntingt) 4:27–33, 1990.

28. Gleeson F: Defects in postgraduate clinical skills as revealed by the objective structured long examination record (OSLER). Ir Med J 85:11–14, 1992.

29. Sloan DA, Donnelly MB, Johnson SB, Schwartz RW, Strodel WE: The use of an Objective Structured Clinical Examination (OSCE) to measure improvement in clinical competence during the surgical internship. Surgery 114:343–351, 1993.

30. Sloan DA, Donnelly MB, Schwartz RW, Munch LC, Wells MD, Johnson SB, Strodel WE: Assessing medical students' and surgery residents' clinical competence in problem solving in surgical oncology. Ann Surg Oncol 1:204–212, 1994.

31. Endean ED, Sloan DA, Veldenz HC, Donnelly MB, Schwarcz TH: Performance of the vascular physical examination by residents and medical students. J Vasc Surg 19:149–156, 1994.

32. Reisner E, Dunnington G, Beard J, Witzke D, Fulginiti J, Rappaport W: A model for the assessment of students' physician-patient interaction skills on the surgical clerkship. Am J Surg 162:271–273, 1991.

33. Sloan DA, Donnelly MB, Schwartz RW, Strodel WE: The Objective Structured Clinical Examination (OSCE). The new gold standard for evaluating postgraduate clinical performance. Ann Surg 222:735–742, 1995.

34. Stillman PL, Swanson DB, Smee S, et al: Assessing clinical skills of residents with standardized patients. Ann Intern Med 105:762–771, 1986.

35. Strodel WE, Donnelly M, Schwartz R, Sloan D: Faculty and patient ratings of residents' interpersonal skills. Clin Invest Med 17 (suppl 4):B84, 1994.

36. Sloan PA, Donnelly MB, Schwartz RW, Sloan DA: Cancer pain assessment and management by housestaff. Pain 67:475–481, 1996.

37. Sloan DA, Donnelly MB, Johnson SB, Schwartz RW, Strodel WE: Assessing surgical residents' and medical students' interpersonal skills. J Surg Res 57:613–618, 1994.

38. Sloan D, Donnelly M, Schwartz, Strodel W: Measuring the ability of residents to manage oncologic problems. J Surg Oncol 64:135–142, 1997.

39. Sloan D, Donnelly M, Schwartz R, Strodel WE, Kenady DE, McGrath PC: How well do medical students and residents understand ductal carcinoma in situ (DCIS)? Presented at the Society of Surgical Oncology, Boston, Massachusetts, March, 1995.

40. Carveth SW, Burnap TK, Bechtel J, McIntyre K, Donegan J, Buchman RJ, Reese HE: Training in advanced cardiac life support. JAMA 235:2311–2315, 1976.

41. Kaye W, Mancini ME, Rallis SF: Advanced cardiac life support refresher course using standardized objective-based Mega Code testing. Crit Care Med 15:55–60, 1987.

42. Collicott PE: Advanced trauma life support course, an improvement in rural trauma care. Nebr Med J 64:279–280, 1979.

43. Collicott PE: Advanced trauma life support (ATLS): Past, present, future; 16th Stone Lecture, American Trauma Society. J Trauma 33:749–753, 1992.

44. Ali J, Adam R, Butler AK, Chang H, Howard M, Gonsalves D, Pitt-Miller P, Stedman M, Winn J, Williams JI: Trauma outcome improves following the advanced trauma life support program in a developing country. J Trauma 34:890–899, 1993.

45. Lowenstein SR, Sabyan EM, Lassen CF, Kern DC: Benefits of training physicians in advanced cardiac life support. Chest 89:512–516, 1986.

46. Townsend RN, Clark R, Ramenofsky ML, Diamond DL: ATLS-based videotape trauma resuscitation review: Education and outcome. J Trauma 34:133–138, 1993.

47. Sloan DA, Donnelly MB, Plymale M, McGrath PC, Kenady DE, Schwartz RW: The structured clinical instruction module as a tool for improving students' understanding of breast cancer. American Surgeon 63:255–260, 1997.

48. Sloan DA, Donnelly MB, Schwartz RW, Plymale MA, Kenady DE, McGrath PC, Edwards MJ, Singletary SE, Evans DB, Souba WW, Bland KI, and the Breast Cancer Education Working Group: The Multidisciplinary Structured Clinical Instruction Module (SCIM) as a Vehicle for Cancer Education. Am J Surg 173:220–225, 1997.

49. Rosenbaum ME, Wilson JF, Sloan DA: Clinical instruction for delivering bad news. Acad Med 71:529, 1996.

50. Norman GR, Tugwell P, Feightner JW: A comparison of resident performance on real and simulated patients. J Med Educ 57:708–715, 1982.

51. Sanson-Fisher RW, Poole AD: Simulated patients and the assessment of medical students' interpersonal skills. Med Educ 14:249–253, 1980.

52. Burdick WP, Escovitz ES: Use of standardized patients in a freshman emergency medicine course. J Emerg Med 10:627–629, 1992.

53. Burchard KW, Rowland-Morin PA: A new method of assessing the interpersonal skills of surgeons. Acad Med 65:274–276, 1990.
54. Plymale M, Donnelly M, Scholes S, Schwartz R, Sloan D: Participation of breast cancer survivors in structured clinical teaching. Abstract presented at the Annual Meeting of the Association for Surgical Education, Lexington, Kentucky, April 10–13, 1996.
55. Schwartz RW, Nash PP, Middleton JL, Witte FM, Weeks LE, Young B: Problem-based learning in the surgery clerkship: A change in philosophy. Clin Anat 5:69–77, 1992.
56. Schwartz RW, Middleton JL, Nash PP, Witte FM, Young B: The history of developing a student-centered, problem-based surgery clerkship. Teach Learn Med 3:38–44, 1991.
57. Schwartz RW, Donnelly MB, Sloan DA, Young B: Knowledge gain in a problem-based surgery clerkship. Acad Med 69:148–151, 1994.
58. Schwartz RW, Donnelly MB, Nash PP, Johnson SB, Young B, Griffen WO Jr: Problem-based learning: An effective educational method for a surgery clerkship. J Surg Res 53:326–330, 1992.
59. Mooney GA, Bligh JG, leinster SJ, Warenius HM: An electronic study guide for problem-based learning. Med Educ 29:397–402, 1995.

CHAPTER 93
LEGAL ISSUES IN BREAST DISEASE

Marvin A. Dewar, M.D., J.D.

It is no surprise that women report that diseases of the breast are their most significant health concern. The fact that breast cancer is the most common major cancer among women, and ranks second only to lung cancer as a cause of cancer death in women, provides a sufficient basis for the importance of breast disease in women's health care. In addition, recent projections that the lifetime prevalence of breast cancer in women may be as high as 1 in 9 underscore the importance of providing expert medical care for breast disease.

Emphasis on the medical aspects of breast disease should be accompanied by an awareness of the importance of legal issues that may arise when managing breast disease.[1] Health care providers encounter a wide variety of legal issues while caring for patients with breast disorders, including professional liability for alleged misdiagnosis, delayed diagnosis of breast cancer, and improper treatment of breast disease. Legal issues other than medical malpractice also impact the care of breast disorders. For example, many state legislatures have established statutory informed consent requirements for treating patients with breast cancer. Finally, legislation and litigation regarding insurance coverage for mammography screening and new breast cancer treatments, such as high-dose chemotherapy and autologous bone marrow transplantation, are increasingly common.[2]

The most publicized legal issue facing those who care for women with breast disease is the malpractice risk that attends the diagnosis and treatment of breast cancer. Malpractice cases involving allegations of delay in the diagnosis of breast cancer are among the most expensive categories of claims and are very difficult to defend and settle for liability insurers.[3] At least in part, the special challenge of these cases derives from the emotionally charged nature of the cancer diagnosis, combined with what some suggest are unbridled high public expectations as to the current capability of breast cancer detection techniques and treatment results.[4–6]

The trend toward an increasing number of liability cases related to breast cancer was identified as early as the 1970s.[7] Currently, breast cancer–related cases are among the leading causes of physician malpractice claims, both in frequency and in cost.[8] Furthermore, a number of factors point toward continued growth and prominence of breast cancer cases. The increasing incidence of breast cancer with resulting increased malpractice exposure to clinicians, developments in malpractice law that favor the filing of cancer-related claims, and continued public emphasis on breast cancer detection and treatment all create an environment that is favorable for even greater breast cancer–related liability risk in the future.[9] An understanding of the legal issues encountered when managing breast disease, therefore, is important for all health providers caring for patients with breast disorders.

MEDICAL MALPRACTICE: GENERAL PRINCIPLES

During the past two decades, the impact of the medical liability system on health care delivery has increased substantially. A major portion of this impact is the direct financial cost of supporting the medical liability system. Throughout the early 1980s, the average dollar amount paid for medical malpractice claims rose almost 30 percent per year.[10] As a result, medical malpractice liability insurance premiums rose dramatically during the same time period. In addition to this direct financial impact of the medical liability system, there are also substantial indirect effects on health care delivery, such as the practice of defensive medicine, in which physicians alter medical practice patterns in response to the risk of medical malpractice liability, adding additional costs to the health care system.[11] Because of the importance of medical liability issues in the care of breast disorders, it is important that health care providers have a good general understanding of medical malpractice law.

The law of medical malpractice is a subset of the law of torts, which is the branch of civil law that provides a private remedy for certain individual actions that cause an injury to another individual. An important concept in tort law is the idea of "negligence," in which a tortfeasor fails to adhere to a standard of care or responsibility established for the protection of others. As it applies to health care, medical negligence is the failure of a health care provider to adhere to a standard of health care delivery established to protect patients.

To successfully recover on a claim of medical malpractice, a plaintiff must demonstrate that actual harm or damage is legally caused by the negligent actions of the defendant physician or other health care provider.[1] To be a legally sufficient claim, a plaintiff seeking to prove a case of medical malpractice must show that the health care provider had a legal responsibility to the patient (duty), and that the health care provider failed to adhere to, or breached, that legal duty, causing legally recognizable injury or harm to the patient.[1] In an early American case, *Pike v. Honsinger*,[12] a New York court articulated the principles of medical malpractice, which are largely still in place to this day. In *Pike v. Honsinger*, which involved an allegation of negligent medical treatment of an injured knee, the court stated: "[a physician] represents that he possesses the reasonable degree of learning and skill ordinarily possessed by physicians... [it is the physician's] duty to use reasonable care and diligence in the exercise of his skill and his learning. He is bound to keep abreast of the times, and departure from approved methods, if it injures the patient, will render him liable."

DUTY

Physicians have a legal responsibility, or duty, to provide reasonable and appropriate medical care in every professional interaction with a patient. Although the rules of tort law do not affirmatively require a physician to become involved in any particular patient's care, once the physician embarks upon a professional relationship with the patient, a duty of reasonable care attaches to the relationship. The scope of a physician's duty to a particular patient is largely determined by the explicit and implicit understanding between the physician and patient about the extent of care that is to be delivered. It is possible for physicians to limit the scope of their responsibility to a patient (for example, embarking on the care of a patient's breast disease, but not assuming responsibility for the care of other health problems), but this should be done cautiously and with the clear understanding and acknowledgment of both patient and provider.[13]

Because most malpractice cases involve circumstances where the physician-patient relationship is clearly established, whether a physician owes a legal duty of reasonable medical care to a patient is not usually a hotly contested item in medical malpractice lawsuits. There are circumstances, however, where the physician-patient relationship is not immediately apparent, but liability may still ensue. For example, if a physician speaks to a woman about breast complaints over the telephone while on-call for another physician, or in a social setting outside the office or hospital, a legally recognizable physician-patient relationship may be established, even if the physician has no prior or subsequent contact with the patient.

Furthermore, when more than one physician is involved in the care of a patient with breast disease, each physician has a duty to provide reasonable professional care for the patient within the scope of their respective specialty expertise. The practical danger in such situations is that each physician may rely upon the other to perform some necessary diagnostic or therapeutic service, with the patient actually receiving the necessary care from neither physician.[1, 14]

Finally, breast radiography raises several interesting legal duty issues. In general, professional liability considerations in radiology have always accounted for the fact that radiologists typically perform a specific and episodic patient service, at the request of another health provider who has primary responsibility for the patient's care. Breast imaging, and particularly screening mammography, provides a variation on this theme. For women who are referred for mammography by another health care provider with primary responsibility for the woman's care, the traditional paradigm is largely unchanged. The duty of the radiographer in this setting is to perform a satisfactory imaging study and issue a reasonable interpretive report. For women who initiate the request for breast imaging themselves (D'Orsi and Debor[15] refer to these women as "self-requesting" when they also have a personal physician, and "self-referred" when they have no personal health care provider), the radiographer may be held to have the additional legal duty of performing or arranging for a clinical breast examination, and potentially even a derivative duty to provide follow-up and referral services for women with abnormal examinations. The extent of the radiographer's duty in such cases is largely determined by the explicit and the reasonable implicit understanding between the radiologist and patient at the time services are rendered.[15, 16]

BREACH OF THE STANDARD OF CARE

After establishing a duty of care between the physician and patient, the next essential legal element of a medical malpractice case is proving that the physician breached, or failed to adhere to, an acceptable standard of care. As early as the eighteenth century and according to English common law, the practice of medicine was considered a public calling, which required that the practitioner display that level of care and expertise that would be followed by a reasonably prudent provider practicing in the same or similar circumstances. For the most part, definitions of the appropriate standard of care for medical practice are derived from the common law, which represents the sum total of prior case law preserved as written appellate court decisions and which serves as precedent for deciding future cases.[17] In some cases, state legislatures have attempted to remove the ambiguity inherent in determining the standard of care by looking to common law by codifying the definition of medical negligence into statutes. For example, the Florida legislature codified the appropriate standard of care as "... that level of care, skill and treatment which, in light of all relevant surrounding circumstances, is recognized as acceptable and appropriate by reasonably prudent similar health care providers."[18] Other states' statutes have similar language.

Many physicians refer to the standard of care as if it has an independent existence and can be empirically determined. The medical care that meets the standard of care in any particular case, however, is actually established by the jury (or judge, in some circumstances) after evaluating all the legally admissible evidence. Jury determinations of what the applicable standard of care required in a particular circumstance are highly dependent on the facts of the specific case; therefore, physicians and others should be very cautious about attempting to derive a general rule of medical practice from the legal result in any particular case.[1, 17]

A simple error in medical judgment is not necessarily medical malpractice.[13] When determining whether a physician's actions in a particular case breached the applicable standard of care, juries primarily consider medical evidence presented as testimony by medical experts. Historically, most jurisdictions followed the locality rule, which required that testifying medical experts reside in and practice in the same community as the defendant physician. More recently, many jurisdictions have modified the locality rule to allow testimonial evidence from medical experts who practice in medical communities that are sufficiently similar to that of the defendant, even though the expert may not live or practice in the community. Some jurisdictions have taken the additional step of abolishing the locality requirement altogether, thereby further expanding the number of medical experts qualified to testify in a particular case and effectively establishing what amounts to a national standard of care.[19]

Qualification of a medical expert at trials usually requires a showing that the expert is a "similar health care provider" to the defendant. This does not necessarily mean, however, that the expert physician and the defendant must practice in identical medical specialties. For example, in *Green v. Goldberg*,[20] a breast surgeon challenged the admissibility of testimony from a medical oncologist about the applicable standard of care concerning whether a breast biopsy should have been performed. In finding the medical oncologist's testimony admissible, the court stated, "in this case, the given field of medicine is breast cancer, not surgery in general. [The oncologist] is a specialist in cancer; the defendant doctor is a general surgeon." Even though he did not actually perform breast biopsies, the oncologist was considered to have a sufficient level of expertise to testify regarding the need for a biopsy in a specific case.

Finally, juries may also consider other types of evidence when determining the applicable standard of care. For example, medical literature and practice guidelines are increasingly used to help establish the standard of medical care in particular cases.[21] In some jurisdictions, including federal courts, generally accepted and authoritative literature may be admitted directly into evidence. In many state courts, such evidence can be admitted only through the testimony of a qualified medical expert.

Recently, many medical organizations and specialty societies have promulgated guidelines and recommendations to guide medical practice. Examples include the screening mammography guidelines published by the American Cancer Society and consensus statements on adjuvant chemotherapy for breast cancer published by the National Cancer Institute. Of note is the possibility that practice parameters and clinical guidelines might be used as evidence in malpractice cases. When clearly written and promulgated by a physician's own medical specialty organization, such guidelines may provide compelling evidence when used as evidence in malpractice litigation. On the other hand, clinical guidelines will not be admitted into evidence in every case. For example, in *Quigley v. Jobe*,[22] the physician defendant's liability insurance carrier promulgated risk management guidelines that recommended follow-up examination within 6 weeks after the discovery of a palpable breast lesion. As part of obtaining insurance coverage, the physician signed a form acknowledging that he was aware of the company guidelines. During a malpractice case against the surgeon for delayed diagnosis of breast cancer, the plaintiff sought to introduce evidence that the physician failed to follow the insurance company's guideline. Refusing to admit the guidelines into evidence, the court noted that the materials were created as part of an insurance company's risk management effort and did not necessarily reflect a generally recognized standard of care within the medical profession. The whole issue of practice guidelines and their applicability to medical malpractice litigation will continue to evolve with time.

CAUSATION

Medical malpractice liability exists only when negligent conduct is the legal cause of patient's injury. To be recognized as the legal cause of an injury, the tortfeasor's negligence must have a nexus, or association, with the resulting injury that is sufficiently close to hold the tortfeasor liable for damages.

Historically, U.S. jurisdictions used a "but for" test to establish legal, or proximate, causation. Under the but for test, an injured patient is not awarded malpractice damages for the injury unless a better outcome was probable, better than even, or more likely than not, absent the negligent actions. Under the but for test, negligent acts that only possibly, or with a likelihood of 50 percent or less, result in injury are deemed too speculative and insufficient to make the tortfeasor liable for damages.

Previously the major test in the United States, the but for standard has now been replaced in most states by legal causation theories that allow recovery in circumstances where the probability that the negligent action led to patient injury is less than 50 percent.[9] The first of these alternative causation theories is the "substantial factor" test, which permits recovery when the negligent behavior is a substantial factor in producing injury, even if the plaintiff's chance at a better outcome absent the negligent behavior was less than 50-50. A distinct, but related, alternative causation standard is the "loss of a chance" theory. In jurisdictions that allow recovery for loss of a chance, a physician may be held liable for actions that deny the patient some chance or prospect of a better outcome. For example, in *Herskovitz v. Group Health Co-op of Puget Sound*,[23] a patient won a malpractice award after the physician's negligent delay in the diagnosis of lung cancer, which, according to expert medical testimony, produced a reduction in the patient's chance of survival from 39 percent to 24 percent. Recovery for a less than probable impact on outcome such as this would not be possible in a jurisdiction that followed the traditional but for causation analysis. Table 93–1 lists those states which have adopted a loss of a chance standard for causation.

The causation standard a particular jurisdiction follows can have a tremendous impact on the outcome of medical malpractice liability cases in general, particularly so for malpractice cases related to the diagnosis and treatment of cancer.[24] The heightened importance of causation analysis in these cases results from the fact that patients with cancer already have a diagnosis that may substantially impact the quality and length of their life, with or without treatment. Negligent diagnosis or treatment by a physician in cancer cases may have a negative impact on the anticipated outcome, but must be considered in context of the expected prognosis with appropriate care. In this setting, whether the malpractice causation standard is but for, substantial factor, or loss of a chance can be the determining factor in the outcome of litigation.

A number of cases demonstrate the impact of causation analysis on breast cancer malpractice litigation. In *Kilpatrick v. Bryant*,[25] a patient alleged that a misinterpreted mammogram resulted in a 4-month delay in the diagnosis of her breast cancer. Rejecting the claim for recovery on the basis that the delayed diagnosis caused the patient to lose some chance for a better outcome, the Tennessee Supreme Court stated that a patient must demonstrate a better than even chance (*probability*) of improved outcome absent the negligent care to recover damages in a malpractice suit. The court went on to comment that the mere *possibility* that medical negligence produced a worse outcome in a particular case does not establish the requisite degree of medical certainty required to establish legal causality. On the other hand, the

plaintiff successfully met the but for causation standard in *Mezrah v. Bevis*,[26] a malpractice claim against a gynecologist in Florida for delayed diagnosis of breast cancer. In *Mezrah v. Bevis*, the plaintiff introduced evidence that, without the negligent diagnostic delay, the patient's breast cancer "more likely than not" would have been completely cured. The court held that this testimonial evidence was sufficient to establish legal causation.

An Alabama case, *Pope v. Elder*,[27] provides an interesting application of but for causation analysis in a case involving the diagnosis and treatment of breast cancer. In *Pope v. Elder*, the initial pathology review identified no cancer in 46 lymph nodes removed during a mastectomy done for primary breast cancer treatment. Two years later, the patient developed metastatic breast cancer, and eventually died after undergoing chemotherapy and autologous bone marrow transplantation. After breast cancer recurrence, a review of the pathology slides from the initial mastectomy showed a single micrometastasis in a single lymph node. In a malpractice action against the pathologist who performed the initial review, the plaintiff's estate introduced testimony from the treating oncologist that the misread pathology slides resulted in a delay in chemotherapy that "might possibly have caused some small statistical chance for longer survival." Upholding a summary judgment in favor of the defendant pathologist, the court held that the mere showing of a statistically diminished chance of cure does not meet the plaintiff's burden of proving that the alleged negligence probably caused the injuries sustained.

Courts that reject the but for test in favor of substantial factor or loss of a chance analysis usually do so, at least in part, on the basis that a rule that gives zero recovery for a reduction in survival from 49 percent to 0 percent as a result of negligence, while giving full recovery for a reduction in survival from 51 percent to 49 percent, is arbitrary and capricious.[28] For example, a malpractice case in New Jersey involving an alleged 7-month delay in diagnosing infiltrating ductal carcinoma in a 38-year-old woman was dismissed by the trial judge because of a lack of probable cause. The plaintiff's expert could not state that, "in all medical probability," the patient experienced a worse outcome as a result of the delay. The New Jersey Supreme Court subsequently reversed the trial judge's decision, using substantial factor analysis, and held that evidence within a reasonable degree of medical probability that the delayed diagnosis increased the patient's risk, and that the increased risk was a substantial factor in the medical outcome and was sufficient to establish legal causation.[29] Similarly, in *Werner v. Blankfort*,[30] a delay in the diagnosis and treatment of recurrent melanoma decreased the patient's chance of 5-year survival from 40 percent to 13 percent. Using a variation of loss of chance analysis, a California Court found this level of injury sufficient to justify a malpractice award.

Whether a particular act of medical negligence

TABLE 93–1. LEGAL CAUSATION: STATES ADOPTING LOSS OF CHANCE STANDARD

Arizona	Missouri
Arkansas	Montana
Colorado	Nevada
Connecticut	New York
District of Columbia	Oklahoma
Georgia	Pennsylvania
Hawaii	South Dakota
Iowa	Virginia
Kansas	Washington
Louisiana	West Virginia
Michigan	Wisconsin

Data from Frickleton JC, Bartimus J: Applying the loss-of-chance doctrine in cancer litigation. Cancer Litigation 1:1–4, 1995.

rises to a sufficient level to pass the substantial factor test is basically a question for the jury. This is demonstrated in the case of *Clayton v. Sabeth*,[31] in which the estate of a patient who died of breast cancer brought a malpractice action against the patient's physician for failing to order screening mammography, which allegedly would have resulted in an earlier diagnosis of the cancer and prevented the patient's death. Although the case was heard in a jurisdiction that followed the substantial factor test, the jury determined that any increased risk the patient experienced as a result of not undergoing screening mammography did not constitute a substantial factor causing her subsequent demise.

Under the best of circumstances, determining the specific impact of a health care provider's diagnostic or therapeutic actions on any particular patient's clinical outcome is difficult. Regardless which legal causation standard a court chooses, making the same determination in the context of adversarial malpractice litigation and a cancer diagnosis is all the more difficult still.

DAMAGES

In addition to proving duty, breach, and causation, plaintiffs must demonstrate that medical negligence resulted in an *actual patient injury* to recover on a claim for medical malpractice. Medical malpractice damages can be classified as economic, noneconomic, and punitive. Economic damages represent the actual out-of-pocket losses incurred as a result of the negligent actions, such as medical and rehabilitation costs, lost wages, lost earning capacity, etc. Economic damages make up approximately two thirds of the damage amount awarded in most malpractice cases. Noneconomic damages provide compensation for injury to noneconomic interests, such as the experience of pain and suffering and loss of consortium (injury to a relationship, usually with a close family member). Punitive damages are designed to punish a tortfeasor for negligent behavior that is particularly wanton or reckless. Punitive damages are only very rarely awarded in medical malpractice cases. Damage awards in malpractice cases involving the diagnosis of cancer in general, and breast cancer in particular, tend to be higher than those in other types of cases.[1]

MALPRACTICE CLAIMS REVIEW

A number of studies have examined trends and characteristics of malpractice cases that involve the diagnosis of breast cancer. Among the first of these studies was an analysis of closed malpractice claims from the Aetna Life & Casualty Insurance Company.[32] Between 1962 and 1974, 36 closed claims at Aetna involved a cancer diagnosis, with breast cancer the most common cancer involved. Delayed diagnosis was the most common allegation in these cases, and

obstetricians/gynecologists the most common defendants. In 1980, Mittlemann and Scholhamer[6] expanded this review of Aetna claims to include a total of 67 closed claims. The findings were largely the same. Failure to diagnose breast cancer was again the most common type of claim found in the follow-up study.

A number of published studies analyzed malpractice claims involving a cancer diagnosis and arising out of a single jurisdiction. For example, Dewar and Love[1] completed a retrospective review of a Florida Department of Insurance data base that included all medical malpractice cases in Florida involving an indemnity payment. Analyzing all cases that involved a primary care physician defendant during 1991, failure to diagnose cancer was the single most common and most expensive category of claim. Among cases involving failure to diagnose cancer, cases involving breast cancer were reported most often, followed by lung, colon and prostate cancer. A review of claims from the leading medical malpractice insurance carrier in North Carolina in the early 1990s produced similar findings.[33]

Kern[34] analyzed a computerized legal data base to identify written court decisions between 1972 and 1990 from malpractice cases involving the diagnosis of breast cancer. He identified 45 cases, all involving the allegation of delay in the diagnosis of breast cancer. Kern noted that the patients involved in these claims tended to be relatively young for breast cancer patients (mean age, 40 years) and experienced a mean delay of 15 months in the diagnosis of breast cancer. Other findings included a patient-identified mass in more than 80 percent of cases, and a high false negative mammography rate of 80 percent. The highest malpractice awards went to younger patients, pregnant patients, patients residing in the northeastern United States, and those who experienced longer diagnostic delays.

Mitnick and associates,[35] in a review of voluntary malpractice case reports to the New York Jury Verdict Reporter between 1985 through 1991, found 34 cases involving breast cancer, with 32 cases involving an allegation of diagnostic delay. The average delay from the time of presentation to definitive diagnosis was 11.6 months. Like Kern's study, Mitnick and associates also found a relatively young patient age (76 percent of patients younger than 50 years) and a high portion of cases involving a palpable mass (49 percent). The medical specialty most frequently involved as defendant was obstetrician/gynecologist (41 percent), followed by internal medicine (30.7 percent), general or breast surgery (12.8 percent) and radiology (7.7 percent).

Zylstra and colleagues[36] reviewed the Massachusetts Medical Professional Insurance Association claims data base to identify malpractice cases involving the diagnosis or treatment of breast cancer filed between 1989 and 1993. The study found 26 total cases and used multivariate analysis techniques to establish a mathematical model for predicting litigation outcome and total financial cost. The model identified smaller tumor size at diagnosis and patient age younger than 40 years as predictors of a litigation outcome favorable to defendants. Failure of the clinician to perform a biopsy on a identifiable mass predicted a litigation outcome in favor of the plaintiffs. Younger patient age, longer periods of diagnostic delay, and failure to biopsy a palpable mass lesion were all factors associated with higher indemnity amounts.

In a study that underscores the increasing number of malpractice cases involving breast cancer, Berlin and Berlin[37] performed a retrospective analysis of all medical malpractice suits involving a radiologist as defendant and filed in Cook County, Illinois, between 1975 and 1994. Allegations of missed diagnosis represented the claim category with the greatest increase in frequency during the study period, with cases related to breast cancer demonstrating the most substantial increase within the category. From 1975 through 1979, the study found only 4 cases alleging misdiagnosis of breast cancer. This increased to 9 claims for 1980 through 1984, 24 claims for 1985 through 1989, and 53 claims for 1990 to 1994.

PIAA BREAST CANCER STUDIES

The most comprehensive analyses of malpractice cases involving the diagnosis or treatment of breast cancer come from the Physician Insurers Association of America (PIAA). The PIAA is a professional association of insurance companies that provide medical malpractice liability insurance to physicians. The PIAA Data Sharing Project was established in 1985 to assist member companies collect and analyze data on medical malpractice claims. From the outset, one of the PIAA projects focused on malpractice cases involving breast cancer. The first PIAA breast cancer study was released in March 1990[38] and reported data on 273 paid breast cancer malpractice claims from 21 member PIAA companies, which collectively insured almost 96,000 U.S. physicians. The study found that cases involving malignant neoplasms of the breast were the most expensive and second most common category of malpractice claim against physicians. Women younger than 50 years represented almost 70 percent of all breast cancer–related mal-

practice claims and more than 80 percent of the total paid indemnity. Similar to the findings from other studies, a breast lesion was most commonly first identified by the patient (69 percent of all claims), with physicians frequently not impressed by the physical findings on clinical breast examination. Thirty percent of all claims in the 1990 study involved cases with a negative mammography report, and another 14 percent involved equivocal mammography results. The average period of diagnostic delay was 12.7 months, with the most common cause of delay that the physical findings on clinical breast examination failed to impress the physician. The average indemnity payment for the 273 cases was $221,524, ranging from $1,000 to $2 million. The specialties involved as defendants in the claims are shown in Table 93–2.

The second PIAA Breast Cancer Study was published in June 1995[8] and analyzed 487 paid malpractice claims reported by 33 PIAA member companies. Consistent with the 1990 study, claims involving malignant neoplasms of the breast were again the most common and second most expensive condition resulting in physician malpractice claim payments. Analysis again revealed women who were relatively young for the diagnosis of breast cancer (60 percent of study patients were younger than 50 years) and a high occurrence of false negative mammogram results (nearly 80 percent of claims with either negative or equivocal mammogram results). The average length of diagnostic delay was 14 months, with the average malpractice award or settlement increasing with longer periods of delay. The reasons underlying the diagnostic delay are listed in Table 93–3.

Compared to the 1990 results, the 1995 PIAA Breast Cancer Study found that radiologists rather than obstetricians/gynecologists were the most frequently sued physicians (see Table 93–2) and the average indemnity payment increased 36 percent, from $221,524 in 1990 to $301,460 in 1995.

IMPACT AND CAUSE OF DIAGNOSTIC DELAY

The outcome of medical malpractice litigation involving breast cancer often hinges on the impact, if any,

TABLE 93–2. SPECIALTIES INVOLVED AS PIAA DEFENDANTS

PIAA Breast Cancer Study 1990 (350 Claims)	Percent	PIAA Breast Cancer Study 1995 (675 Claims)	Percent
Obstetrics/gynecology	39	Radiology	24
Family practice/general practice	17	Obstetrics/gynecology	23
Surgical specialty	16	Family practice/general practice	17
Internal medicine	12	Surgical specialty	14
Radiology	11	Internal medicine	9
Pathology	2	Pathology	2

PIAA: Physician Insurers Association of America

TABLE 93–3. REASONS UNDERLYING DIAGNOSTIC DELAY (PERCENT)

Physical findings fail to impress physician	35
Failure to follow-up in a timely fashion	31
Negative mammogram report	26
Misread mammogram	23
Failure to do a proper biopsy	23
Delayed or failure to consult	16
Failure to react to mammogram	12
Other health problems	11
Repeat exams failed to impress clinician	11
Failure to order mammogram	11
Communication failure	11
Poor clinical examination	10

of diagnostic delay on the subsequent clinical outcome. The legal basis for the importance of this determination derives from the requirement that the plaintiff prove causation, as already described in the previous section.

A fundamental tenet of cancer care is that early diagnosis is better than a late diagnosis. The wide media attention given to early breast cancer detection leads to a public perception that improved outcome invariably follows earlier diagnosis.[36] Epidemiological studies demonstrate that women with breast cancer diagnosed in early stages have improved survival rates and a wider range of therapeutic options than do women with breast cancer diagnosed in later stages.[39, 40] Wilkinson and colleagues[41] performed a retrospective study using tumor registry data for 1784 women with histologically confirmed breast cancer to evaluate the effect on disease stage and survival of delay between first recognition of symptoms and diagnosis. Patient delay greater than 2 months between the onset of symptoms and diagnosis was associated with a significant negative impact on survival rates and an increase in the stage of disease at diagnosis. The negative impact of patient delay on survival rates in this study occurred through the impact of delay on disease stage at the time of diagnosis.

Elwood and Moorehead[42] performed a retrospective review of the records of 1591 women with primary breast cancer to determine the effect of diagnostic delay after the presentation of the first symptom of breast cancer on stage and survival. The study found better patient survival rates when the delay from the first symptom to definitive diagnosis was less than 1 month when compared to delays greater than 12 months. Within a given breast cancer clinical stage, Elwood and Moorehead found no significant impact of diagnostic delay on survival.

Statistical evidence of "cure" after primary breast cancer treatment for a particular patient is problematic because death from breast cancer recurrence has been noted up to 40 years after initial diagnosis and treatment. Nevertheless, Rosen and associates[43] attempted to estimate breast cancer cure rates in a longitudinal survival study of 644 patients with T1 breast cancer. By comparing the survival of breast cancer patients with standard expected survival curves, an estimated 80% cure rate was found for T1N0M0 tumors less than 1 cm in size, and a cure rate of approximately 70 percent for T1N0M0 tumors 1.1 to 2.0 cm in diameter. The study found no evidence of cure among T1N1M0 patients.

Although these studies support clinical efforts at early diagnosis, the importance of diagnostic or therapeutic delay in any given patient is far less clear. Many experts point to the complex relationship which exists between the time of diagnosis and clinical outcome.[34, 35, 44–46] The inherent biological characteristics of a particular tumor and host-tumor relationships may be more important in determining patient outcome than the timing of clinical diagnosis.[35, 46] Furthermore, by the time a patient's breast cancer is clinically palpable, the label of early diagnosis may be misapplied. In malpractice litigation, these issues are raised in the context of testimony about tumor biology, cancer cell doubling time, and the tendency of breast cancer to undergo early metastatic spread.[34, 35] Unfortunately, these principles are often arcane and counterintuitive and may be difficult to explain to patients and jurors.[14]

Cytokinetic tumor data may provide critical information when deciding causation issues in medical negligence lawsuits. About 20 cell doublings are required to generate a breast cancer that is 1 mm in diameter, weighing 1 mg and containing approximately 10^6 malignant cells. Ten more doublings produce a clinically palpable tumor with a mass of 1 gm and 10^9 malignant cells. Another four doublings is required to produce a tumor 3.3 cm in diameter (the average size of a clinically diagnosed tumor), weighing 10 gm and containing 10^{10} malignant cells. Although mammography can detect breast cancer six or seven doublings before it is detectable by clinical examination, Plotkin and Blakenship[24] note that axillary metastasis usually occurs within the first 20 doublings of a primary tumor's life span, before it is detectable by either mammography or clinical palpation. Tumor biology considerations such as this suggest that, except for occult breast cancer detected mammographically, current clinical diagnostic tools and physical examination may be insufficient to detect breast cancer early enough in the cancer life cycle to make a significant difference in long-term survival.[14]

Doubling-time analysis is also sometimes used to work backward from a known tumor mass and establish whether a patient's tumor should have been clinically palpable at a given prior point in time. This type of tumor sizing analysis uses information from breast imaging studies or pathology analysis combined with known average cell-doubling times to make sizing projections. Size analysis is complicated by the fact that tumor growth tends to undergo significant deceleration late in the course of the cancer life cycle. Also, interval cancers in the Breast Cancer Demonstration and Detection Project tended to be aggressive tumors, with more rapid predetection growth than would have been predicted from sizing analysis.[35, 48] Conclusions from retrospective tumor sizing using doubling-time analysis should therefore be approached cautiously. Some authorities even question the usefulness of this type of information in the context of medical malpractice litigation.[49]

Results of studies of the impact of diagnostic delay on survival in patients with breast cancer have been inconsistent. Fisher and associates[50] studied 1539 women with clinical stage I and II invasive breast cancer entered in the National Surgical Adjuvant Breast and Bowel Project. Although the study found an association between longer symptom duration and increased tumor size, no statistically significant increase in monthly treatment failure rates were found when comparing symptom duration of 0 and more than 9 months. Another study of 237 women undergoing radical mastectomy for treatment of breast cancer[45] found no significant relationship between patient survival and diagnostic delay of up to 12 months.

Porta and coworkers[51] used a hospital-based tumor registry to perform a retrospective follow-up study on 1247 patients with lung, breast, stomach, colon, and rectal cancer to assess the relationship between survival and the interval from first disease symptom to diagnosis. The mean interval from first symptom to diagnosis for breast cancer was 7.44 months. Mean time to diagnosis was not a significant predictor of long-term survival.

The explanation for this ambiguous relationship between diagnostic delay and patient survival may be the tendency of breast cancer to become a systemic disease relatively early in the course of the cancer life cycle.[52–54] Reintgen and colleagues[55] recently compared clinical delectability of breast lesions by palpation, tumor size, and axillary lymph node status in 435 women consecutively registered for treatment of invasive breast cancer at a university cancer center. The threshold of palpation by an experienced breast surgeon performing clinical breast examination was a tumor more than 5 mm in diameter, with most tumors not identified by palpation until they were greater than 15 mm in diameter on histological examination. By the time tumor size was such that most lesions were clinically palpable, more than one third of patients already had positive axillary nodes.

Other researchers have reported positive axillary metastasis in up to 26 percent of nonpalpable breast cancers 0.6 to 1 cm in diameter.[56] Another study found positive axillary nodes in 7.7 percent of women with primary breast cancers less than 5 mm in diameter, and 17.5 percent in women with a primary tumor 6 to 10 mm in diameter.[57] Although studies on the impact of diagnosis delay on clinical outcome are inconsistent, and it is possible that axillary micrometastasis and tumor biology have a greater impact on survival than does diagnostic delay, it nonetheless behooves clinicians to diagnose breast cancer as early as possible in the natural history of the disease.[36]

INFORMED CONSENT

The informed consent doctrine promotes patient self-determination and privacy as well as autonomy in medical decision making. Informed consent facilitates a voluntary decision made by a competent patient after consideration of adequate descriptions of diagnostic or therapeutic options.[1] The failure to obtain informed consent before an invasive procedure exposes the physician to liability for battery regardless of whether the outcome of the procedure is good or bad. In contrast to liability for battery, which occurs when the physician fails to obtain *any* level of consent from the patient, a claim of negligent consent implies that the consent that was obtained was *insufficient* to promote an informed decision by the patient. Physicians must disclose the information that reasonable individuals would consider material and necessary to make a decision to obtain legally sufficient informed consent from patients. The concept of information materiality takes into account both the severity and frequency or likelihood of a particular side effect or other outcome.[58]

It is important to remember that the key component in informed consent is the *communication of sufficient information* to the patient in a way that empowers an informed choice. Although it is tempting for physicians to focus on the format of the written informed consent documents that patients are asked to read and sign, these documents serve only as evidence of the more important informed consent discussion that occurs between a patient and physician. The prudent degree of documentation of informed consent varies with the medical procedure involved. As the medical risk attendant to a procedure increases, or the appropriate medical course or decision is less clear, documentation of the detail of the informed consent discussion should likewise increase. On the other hand, in many ambulatory settings, extensive documentation of the informed consent discussion may not be practical. In this setting, the chart notation "GAR informed consent obtained" indicates that the physician reviewed the following important facts with the patient:

- G General information about the medical condition
- A Alternatives for diagnosis or therapy
- R Risks of proposed diagnostic or therapeutic alternatives

In general, the task of obtaining informed consent should not be delegated, but should be performed by the physician or provider who is making a medical recommendation or planning to do a particular test or procedure. Also, informed consent is specific to a particular procedure or clinical decision. Brenner[58] emphasizes this point by noting that informed consent for a breast cyst aspiration is not likely to be sufficient to cover a subsequent core needle biopsy attempt.

Adequate informed consent regarding treatment options for women with breast cancer includes discussing the relative benefits and risks of extensive surgery, conservative surgery, radiation therapy, and adjuvant chemotherapy. Although the general law of informed consent also applies to breast cancer, sev-

TABLE 93-4.   SPECIFIC INFORMED CONSENT LAWS FOR TREATMENT OF BREAST CANCER IN VARIOUS STATES

State	State Law	Information Required	Specific Signed Informed Consent
California	Cal. Health & Safety Code 1704.5	Treatment alternatives	Required
Florida	Fla. Stat. 458.324	Treatment alternatives	Required
Georgia	Ga. Code 43-34-21	Treatment alternatives	Recommended
Hawaii	Haw. Rev. Stat. 671-3	Treatment alternatives	Required
Illinois	Ill. Rev. Stat. Ch. 127, 55.49	Treatment alternatives	Required
Kansas	Kan. Stat. Ann. 65-2836	Treatment alternatives	Required
Kentucky	Ky. Stat. 311.935	Treatment alternatives	Required
Maine	Me. Stat. 24.2905-A	Treatment alternatives	Required
Maryland	Md. Health Gen 20.113	Treatment alternatives	Required
Massachusetts	Mass. Stat. 111.70E	Treatment alternatives	Required
Michigan	Mich. Stat. 333.17013	Treatment alternatives	Required
Minnesota	Minn. Stat. 144.651	Treatment alternatives	Required
New Jersey	NJ Stat. Ann. 45.9-22.2	Treatment alternatives	Required
New Mexico	NM IIj Mem 4. 36th Leg. 2d Sess	Treatment alternatives	Required
New York	N.Y. Pub. Health Law 2404	Treatment alternatives	Required
Pennsylvania	Pa. Cons. Stat. 5641	Treatment alternatives	Required
Texas	Tex. Health & Safety Code 86.002	Treatment alternatives	Recommended
Virginia	Va. Code Ann. 54.1-2971	Treatment alternatives	Required

eral states have passed specific laws detailing the informed consent requirements for breast cancer treatment (Table 93–4). Physicians should become familiar with the specific requirements of their state law.

RISK MANAGEMENT CONSIDERATIONS

Because of the medical and medical legal importance of breast disorders and breast cancer, much has been written about risk management techniques for physicians caring for women with breast disorders as a way of reducing malpractice liability risk.* Although many of these recommendations are appropriate and likely to lead to improved overall care for women with breast disease, it is important to note that these are guidelines only, susceptible to modification as appropriate by qualified clinicians who must evaluate the specific circumstances of each particular case.[44] An old adage from the field of medical law is worth repeating here, "Good medicine is good law." The guiding principles for care of women with breast disease must be grounded in medical science and sound clinical judgment. Good medicine is also good risk management.

Patient education and effective communication are key components of good clinical care and effective risk management. Significant diagnostic or therapeutic uncertainty should be explained to the patient so that informed consent may be obtained for all critical clinical decisions.[1, 15, 17] Although it is important to maintain a positive and optimistic tenor in the doctor/patient relationship, physicians should guard against minimizing clinical concerns to the extent that patients may not be aware of the importance or

true implications of returning for follow-up examinations, repeat diagnostic tests, or other procedures.[13]

Another sound risk management technique is good documentation. For women with breast symptoms, the medical record should include a description of findings from the history and physical examination that is sufficient to allow effective comparison of findings during follow-up examinations. The chart notation "breasts okay" or "breasts normal" is not adequate chart documentation for a woman who presents with breast symptoms. The use of a specific breast encounter form may help facilitate sufficient chart documentation. Clinicians should also record the rationale for their important clinical decisions in the medical record. If the subsequent clinical course is unfavorable, documentation that includes clinical reasoning may demonstrate that the decision made was appropriate in the light of the information available at the time.[1]

Practice guidelines for the care of women with common breast disorders help promote good clinical care and may reduce liability risk. A number of guidelines for the care of breast disorders have been published.[4, 8, 14] Office reminder systems, such as tickler or recall files, are particularly helpful to identify patients who should undergo breast cancer screening as well as to ensure that appropriate follow-up is maintained for patients being evaluated for breast abnormalities.

Women with a dominant breast mass found on examination or breast imaging should be evaluated thoroughly. Mammography, breast ultrasonography, fine needle aspiration, needle core biopsy, and open biopsy should be used as necessary to rule out cancer.[33, 44] Breast ultrasonography may be particularly useful to evaluate for the presence of an underlying mass lesion in patients with asymmetric nodularity.[34] Primary care physicians should consider obtaining second opinions from a colleague experienced in breast disease when patients have persistent focal

*References 1, 3, 6, 8, 9, 13–15, 17, 22, 33–35, 44, 55, 59

breast symptoms, even when the results of clinical and radiological examinations are normal.[1]

Follow-up of women with breast symptoms should be explicit and clear. Appointments at predetermined dates are preferable to patient-initiated ("PRN") follow-up. Continuity of care for breast complaints must be carefully ensured, even when other medical problems become interposed. Reminder telephone calls and letters are appropriate for patients with particularly suspicious clinical presentations who miss follow-up appointments.

In general, breast abnormalities of uncertain significance should be followed through no more than one or two menstrual cycles before arriving at a diagnosis. No currently available data suggest that diagnostic delay of less than 2 months between the onset of symptoms and diagnosis of treatment adversely influences outcome in breast cancer care.[1] For certain nonpalpable and probably benign mammographic abnormalities with a less than 1 percent chance of representing cancer, mammography follow-up at 6 month intervals may be appropriate.[55, 60]

References

1. Dewar MA, Love N: Legal issues in managing breast disease. Postgrad Med 92:137-154, 1992.
2. Wynstre NA: Breast cancer: Selected legal issues. Cancer 74(Suppl):491-511, 1994.
3. Cancer-related claims: High in frequency, higher in cost. Focus 2:1-4, 1990.
4. Trombly ST: The breast cancer "epidemic." Forum 13:2-5, 1992.
5. Brenner RJ: Evolving medical-legal concepts for clinicians and imagers in evaluation of breast cancer. Cancer 69(Suppl): 1950-1953, 1992.
6. Mittlemann M, Scholhamer CG: What are the chances when malignancy leads to a malpractice suit? Leg Aspects Med Pract, February 1980, pp 40-47.
7. Curran WJ: Malpractice claims: New data and new trends. N Engl J Med 300:26-27, 1979.
8. Physician Insurers Association of America: Breast Cancer Study, June 1995. Washington, DC, Physician Insurers Association of American, 1995.
9. Heland KV, Rutledge P: Medicolegal issues. Obstet Gynecol Clin North Am 21:781-788, 1994.
10. Nye DJ, Gifford DG, Dewar MA, et al: The causes of the medical malpractice crisis: An analysis of claims data and insurance company finances. Georgetown Law J 76:1495-1561, 1988.
11. Dewar MA: Defensive medicine: It may not be what you think. Fam Med 26:36-38, 1994
12. Pike v. Honsinger, 49 N.E. 716 (1898).
13. Henderson IC, Danner D: Legal pitfalls in the diagnosis and management of breast cancer. Hematol Oncol Clin North Am 3:823-842, 1989.
14. Osuch JR, Bonham VC: The timely diagnosis of breast cancer: Principles of risk management for primary care providers and surgeons. Cancer 74:271-278, 1994
15. D'Orsi CJ, Debor MD: Communication issues in breast imaging. Radiol Clin North Am 33:1230-1245, 1995.
16. Brenner RJ: Screening mammography: Medical legal considerations. Cancer 66:1348-1350, 1990.
17. Brenner RJ: Breast cancer evaluation: Medical-legal and risk management considerations for the clinician. Cancer 74:486-490, 1994.
18. Florida Statutes 766.101(1) (1995).
19. Flamm MB: Cases of failure to diagnose cancer. Trial, Sept. 1986, pp 82-87.
20. Green v. Goldberg, 630 So.2d 606 (Fla. App. 4 Dist. 1993).
21. Hirshfeld EB: Should practice parameters be the standard of care in malpractice litigation? JAMA 266:2886-2891, 1991.
22. Quigley v. Jobe, 851 P.2d 1992 (Colo. App. 5 1992).
23. Herskovitz v. Group Health Co-op of Puget Sound, 663 P.2d 474 (1983).
24. Plotkin D, Blakenship F: Breast cancer: Biology and malpractice. Am J Clin Oncol 14:254-266, 1991.
25. Kilpatrick v. Bryant, 868 S.W.2d 594 (Tenn. 1993).
26. Mezrah v. Bevis, 593 So.2d 1214 (Fla. 2d DCA 1992).
27. Pope v. Elder, 671 So.2d 730 (Ala. Civ. App. 1995).
28. Frickleton JC, Bartimus J: Applying the loss-of-chance doctrine in cancer litigation. Cancer Litigation 1:1, 3–4, 1995.
29. Gabin JH: The Evers Care: 1984 decision has lasting impact. New Jersey Med 90:563-537, 1993.
30. Werner v. Blankfort, 36 Cal. App. 4th 298 (1995).
31. Clayton v. Sabeth, 594 A.2d 365 (Pa. Super. 1991).
32. Mittelman M, Scholhamer CF: Cancer and malpractice claims. Cancer 39:2573-2378, 1977.
33. Yarborough MF: Breast cancer malpractice litigation in North Carolina, 1984 - 1992. North Carolina Med J 54:202-205, 1993.
34. Kern K: Causes of breast cancer malpractice litigation: A 20-year civil court review. Arch Surg 127:542-547, 1992.
35. Mitnick JS, Vazquez MF, Plesser KP, Roses DF: Breast cancer malpractice litigation in New York state. Radiology 189:673-676, 1993.
36. Zylstra S, Bors-Koefoed R, Mendor M, Anti D, Giordano K, Ressequie LJ: A statistical model for predicting the outcome in breast cancer malpractice lawsuit. Obstet Gynecol 84:392-398. 1994.
37. Berlin L, Berlin JW: Malpractice and radiologists in Cook County, IL: Trends in 20 years of litigation. AJR Am J Roentgenol 165:781-788, 1995.
38. Physician Insurers Association of America: Breast Cancer Study March 1990. Physician Insurers Association of America, Lawrenceville, NJ, 1990.
39. Dodd GD: American Cancer Society guidelines on screening for breast cancer: An overview. CA Cancer J Clin 42:177-180, 1992.
40. Miller W, Dorr FA: Treatment of early stage breast cancer: January 1985 through May 1990. Current bibliographies in medicine No. 90-6. Bethesda, US Dept of Health and Human Services, 1990.
41. Wilkinson GS, Edgerton F, Wallace HJ, Reese P, Patterson J, Priore R: Delay, stage of disease and survival from breast cancer. J Chron Dis 32:365-373, 1979.
42. Elwood JM, Moorehead WP: Delay in diagnosis and long-term survival in breast cancer. Bri Med J 1291-1294, 1980.
43. Rosen PP, Groshen S, Saig PE, Kinne DW, Hellman S: A long-term follow-up study of survival in stage I (T.N.M.) and stage II (T.N.M.) breast carcinoma. J Clin Oncol 17:355-366, 1989.
44. Gump FE: Medicolegal pitfalls in the diagnosis of breast cancer. Compr Ther 21:3-6, 1995.
45. Dennis CR, Gardner B, Lim B: Analysis of survival and recurrence vs patient and doctor delay in treatment of breast cancer. Cancer 35:714-720, 1975.
46. Rubin D: The effect of delay in treatment of prognosis. JAMA 200:136-138, 1967.
47. Spratt JS, Spratt SW: Medical and legal implication of screening and follow-up procedures for breast cancer. Cancer 66:1351-1362, 1990.
48. Spratt JS, Meyer JS, Spratt JA: Rates of growth of human neoplasms: Part III. J Surg Oncol 61:68-83, 1996.
49. Citron R: Faulty reasoning guides doubling time defense. Med Malpract Law Strategy 9:1-5, 1991.
50. Fisher ER, Redmond C, Fisher B: A perspective concerning the relation of duration of symptoms to treatment failure in patients with breast cancer. Cancer 40:3160-3167, 1977.
51. Porta M, Gallen M, Malats N, Planes J: Influence of "diagnostic delay" upon cancer survival: An analysis of five tumor sites. J Epidemiol Community Health 45:225–230, 1991.
52. Spratt JS, Greenberg RA, Henser LS: Geometry, growth rates, and duration of cancer and carcinoma in sites of the breast before detection by screening. Cancer Res 46:970-974, 1986.
53. Redding WH, Monaghan P, Imrie SF: Detection of micrometastases in patients with primary breast cancer. Lancet 2:1271-1273, 1983.

54. Fisher ER, Redmond C, Fisher B: A perspective concerning the relation of duration of symptoms to treatment failure in patients with breast cancer. Am J Clin Pathol 88:123-131, 1987.
55. Reintgen D, Cox C, Greenberg H, Baekey P, Nicosia S, Berman C, Clark R, Lyman G: The medical legal implications of following mammographic breast masses. Ann Surg 59:99-105, 1993.
56. Wilhelm MC, Edge SB, Cole DD: Nonpalpable invasive breast cancer. Ann Surg 213:600-603, 1991.
57. Tinnemans JGM, Webbes T, Holland R: Treatment and sur-
vival of female patients with nonpalpable breast carcinoma. Ann Surg 209:249-253, 1989.
58. Brenner RJ: Interventional procedures of the breast: Medicolegal considerations. Radiology 195:611-615, 1995.
59. Brenner RJ, Berlin L: Evaluation of the mammographic abnormality. AJR Am J Roentgenol 167:17-19, 1996.
60. Brenner RJ, Sickles EA. Acceptability of periodic follow-up as an alternative to biopsy for mammographically detected lesions interpreted as probably benign. Radiology 171:645-646, 1989.

CHAPTER 94

THE DELAYED DIAGNOSIS OF SYMPTOMATIC BREAST CANCER

Kenneth A. Kern, M.D.

The delayed diagnosis of symptomatic breast cancer is a leading source of error in clinical practice. Delays in diagnosis of symptomatic breast cancer, by definition, result from the failure to diagnose breast lesions (either by biopsy or other methods) that later prove to be malignant. Given the limited number of diagnostic elements used to evaluate breast symptoms—in essence, only the physician's physical findings, the reports of mammograms or sonograms, and a decision regarding biopsy—one might presume that errors in diagnosis should occur infrequently. Yet, historically, even long-established authorities in the field, such as Haagensen, recognized the difficulties inherent in preventing the delayed diagnosis of breast cancer.[94] Reflecting on his own 1-percent rate of diagnostic errors in breast cancer examinations over a 30-year interval, Haagensen's writings emphasized that diagnostic errors occurred chiefly because many of the symptoms of breast cancer closely mimicked benign conditions, including masses, infections, and skin rashes. "The price of skill in the diagnosis of breast carcinoma is a kind of eternal vigilance," Haagensen wrote, "based upon an awareness that any indication of disease in the breast may be due to carcinoma."[94]

Although inaccurate diagnosis of breast cancer may be viewed simply as the result of substandard medical care by a "bad physician," the events that lead to misdiagnosis are far more complex. It is important for practitioners to recognize that delayed diagnosis of breast cancer is not simply the inverse of diagnosing breast cancer by prompt recognition of its symptoms. Indeed, underlying these misdiagnoses rest the unique features of breast cancer that make delays in diagnosis not only possible but under certain conditions highly probable. In fact, delayed diagnosis of breast cancer almost always falls within a specific category of patients, an identifiable class of physicians, and a reproducible set of clinical circumstances. These three factors interact to produce delays in diagnosis that are frequent and often lengthy. This chapter attempts to clarify many of the scenarios for diagnostic error.

Because delays in diagnosis occur repeatedly under certain clinical conditions, it follows that (1) the circumstances producing diagnostic failures should be predictable, and (2) theoretically, diagnostic delays should be largely avoidable. A thorough understanding of the causes and consequences of the delayed diagnosis of breast cancer is central to risk management for clinicians managing breast disease. Ultimately, an analysis of the determinants of delayed diagnosis of breast cancer is an important and useful tool in defining the limits of the perceptual and cognitive detection and understanding of breast cancer, by patients and clinicians alike.

MAGNITUDE OF THE PROBLEM

In terms of all diagnostic errors among providers of primary health care to women, the delayed diagnosis of breast cancer ranks among the top three misdiagnoses, as illustrated in Table 94–1. This table was created from data compiled in 1995 by the Physician Insurers Association of America (PIAA).[191, 192] The PIAA is an insurance trade association of 36 domestic insurance companies, providing malpractice insurance to over 90,000 physicians in the United States. The data represent indemnity claims over the ten-year interval from December 1984 to 1994. In a more detailed analysis of the same data, Tables 94–2 and 94–3 demonstrate the magnitude of the problem surrounding the delayed diagnosis of breast cancer according to two points of view: (1) in terms of all errors in diagnosis within the specialties most frequently involved in the management of breast disease; and (2) in terms of the frequency of lawsuits caused by these same specialties.

Overall, the delayed diagnosis of breast cancer is the most frequent medicolegal claim against physicians. It is also the second-most expensive area of claims to indemnify by liability carriers. Tables 94–4 and 94–5 demonstrate these findings and compare

---

TABLE 94–1.   TOP THREE ERRORS IN DIAGNOSIS RESULTING IN CLAIMS FOR MEDICAL MALPRACTICE BY PHYSICIAN SPECIALTY

General Surgery
Breast cancer, appendicitis, spinal fracture

Family Practice
Myocardial infarct, *breast cancer*, appendicitis

Internal Medicine
Lung cancer, myocardial infarct, *breast cancer*

Obstetrics/Gynecology
Breast cancer, ectopic pregnancy, pregnancy

Radiology
Breast cancer, lung cancer, spinal fracture

Table created from data compiled in the Physician Insurers Association of America (PIAA) Data Sharing Reports, Executive Summary (1995). Washington, DC, PIAA, 1995. The report documents malpractice claims indemnified by the 36-member companies of the PIAA over the 10-year interval December, 1984 to December, 1994. The full report analyzes information on 126,000 claims for medical malpractice.

TABLE 94–2.   DELAYED DIAGNOSIS OF BREAST CANCER—MAGNITUDE OF PROBLEM WITHIN EACH SPECIALTY

	General Surgery	Family Practice	Internal Medicine	Obstetrics/ Gynecology	Radiology
Of all errors in diagnosis:					
Rank order–frequency	No. 1	No. 2	No. 3	No. 1	No. 1
Rank order–expense	No. 1	No. 2	No. 3	No. 1	No. 1

Table created from data compiled in the Physician Insurers Association of America (PIAA) Data Sharing Reports, Executive Summary (1995). Washington, DC, PIAA, 1995. The report documents malpractice claims indemnified by the 36 member companies of the PIAA over the 10-year interval December, 1984 to December, 1994. The full report analyzes information on 126,000 claims for medical malpractice.

TABLE 94–3.   DELAYED DIAGNOSIS OF BREAST CANCER—MAGNITUDE OF PROBLEM CAUSED BY EACH SPECIALTY

	No. 1	No. 2	No. 3	No. 4	No. 5
Of all physicians sued:					
Rank order—frequency	Radiology	Obstetrics/gynecology	Family practice	General surgery	Internal medicine
Rank order—expense	Obstetrics/gynecology	Radiology	General surgery	Family practice	Internal medicine

Data from Physician Insurers Association of America (PIAA) Data Sharing Reports, Executive Summary (1995). Washington, DC, PIAA, 1995. The report documents malpractice claims indemnified by the 36 member companies of the PIAA over the 10-year interval December, 1984 to December, 1994. The full report analyzes information on 126,000 claims for medical malpractice.

TABLE 94–4.   MOST PREVALENT CONDITIONS RESULTING IN CLAIMS OF MEDICAL MALPRACTICE

Condition	N	Percent*	Total Paid	Average Cost
Breast cancer	2986	8	212,408,523	204,436
Brain-damaged infant	2613	7	419,819,766	449,486
Pregnancy	1953	5	68,358,114	128,978
Acute myocardial infarction	1770	5	107,165,159	190,347

*The data in this table reflect only claims which were closed with payment, representing 37,935 claims, or 30% of the total data base of 126,000 claims for medical malpractice tabulated by the PIAA. Percentiles are calculated by dividing the number of claims for each diagnosis, listed under "N", by the total number of paid claims (37,935).
Data from Physician Insurers Association of America (PIAA) Data Sharing Reports, Executive Summary (1995). Washington, DC, PIAA, 1995. The report documents malpractice claims indemnified by the 36 member companies of the PIAA over the 10-year interval December, 1984 to December, 1994.

TABLE 94–5.   MOST EXPENSIVE CONDITIONS TO INDEMNIFY FOR MEDICAL MALPRACTICE

Condition	N	Percent*	Total Paid	Average Cost
Brain-damaged infant	2613	8	419,819,766	449,486
Breast cancer	2986	9	212,408,523	204,436
Acute myocardial infarction	1770	5	107,165,159	190,347
Lung cancer	1639	5	75,510,568	149,823

*The data in this table reflect only claims which were closed with payment, representing 37,935 claims, or 30% of the total data base of 126,000 claims for medical malpractice tabulated by the PIAA. Percentiles are calculated by dividing the number of claims for each diagnosis, listed under "N", by the total number of paid claims (37,935). Table created from data compiled in the Physician Insurers Association of America (PIAA) Data Sharing Reports, Executive Summary (1995). Washington, DC, PIAA, 1995. The report documents malpractice claims indemnified by the 36 member companies of the PIAA over the 10-year interval December, 1984 to December, 1994.

TABLE 94–6. DISTRIBUTION OF MALPRACTICE CASES BY ORGAN SITE (N = 711)

Organ Site	N	Percent	References
Breast	172	24	122, 123, 126–131, 132, 134, 136, 137
Colorectum and gastrointestinal	148	21	124, 134, 127
Bile duct	86	12	122a, 135a, 135b
Head and neck	76	11	127
Other cancer sites	74	10	127
Endocrine	62	9	125, 127
Lung	49	7	127
Melanoma	44	6	127
Total	711	100	

From Kern KA: The anatomy of surgical malpractice claims. Bull Amer Coll Surg 80:34–49, 1995.

TABLE 94–7. MOST FREQUENT DIAGNOSES RESULTING IN NEGLIGENCE LITIGATION AGAINST GENERAL SURGEONS

Most Frequent Diagnosis	N	Percent	Cost per Claim (Average Cost)
Female breast cancer	288	3	183,349
Inguinal hernia	283	3	57,894
Appendicitis	270	3	66,491
Calculus of gallbladder	185	2	98,544
Cholecystitis	160	2	69,133
Obesity operations	151	2	91,442
Postoperative infections	131	1	114,581
Arterial embolus and thrombosis	117	1	158,977
Colorectal cancer	115	1	152,410
Foreign body left in patient	99	1	49,190
Total	1649	17	94,728

Total number of malpractice claims against general surgeons = 9515. Not all categories shown. Table created from data compiled in the Physician Insurers Association of America (PIAA) Data Sharing Reports, Executive Summary (1995). PIAA, Washington, DC, 1995. From Kern KA: The anatomy of surgical malpractice claims. Bull Am Coll Surg 80:34–49, 1995.

the delayed diagnosis of breast cancer with four other frequent and expensive conditions resulting in malpractice actions. Delayed breast cancer diagnosis is but one element making up the problems of delayed cancer diagnosis overall, which accounts for 20 percent of all diagnostic errors. For example, in 1990, the PIAA noted that the delayed diagnosis of cancer in general accounted for 2956 claims out of a total of 15,356 claims for diagnostic errors.[189, 190] Indemnity payments for misdiagnosed cancer approached $200 million annually, or approximately 30 percent ($194 million out of $698 million) of paid-out liability claims for medical misadventures. Indemnification of

misdiagnosed cancer, therefore, represents almost 8 percent of the total yearly liability payout by insurers ($2.6 billion).[191, 192]

We corroborated the frequency and expense of misdiagnosed breast cancer using data derived from our own nationwide medicolegal study of 338 cases of misdiagnosed cancer occurring in 13 major organ

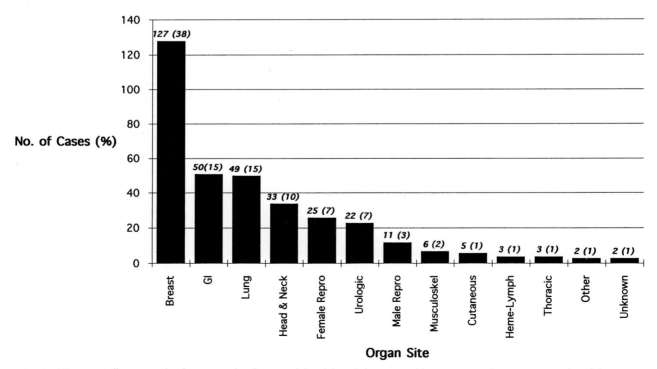

Figure 94–1 *Histogram illustrating the frequency distribution of the delayed diagnosis of breast cancer, by organ site, plotted for 338 cases of malpractice litigation nationwide. The data represent 338 jury verdicts surrounding misdiagnosed cancer from 42 states, covering the years 1985 to 1990. The 338 cases are divided into 13 principal organ sites. Four cancer sites accounted for nearly 80% (259/338, 77%) of the claims frequency against physicians: breast (38%, n = 127), gastrointestinal (15%, n = 51), lung (15%, n = 50), and head and neck cancers (10%, n = 33). (Data from Kern KA: Medicolegal analysis of the delayed diagnosis of cancer in 338 cases in the United States. Arch Surg 129:397–404, 1994.)*

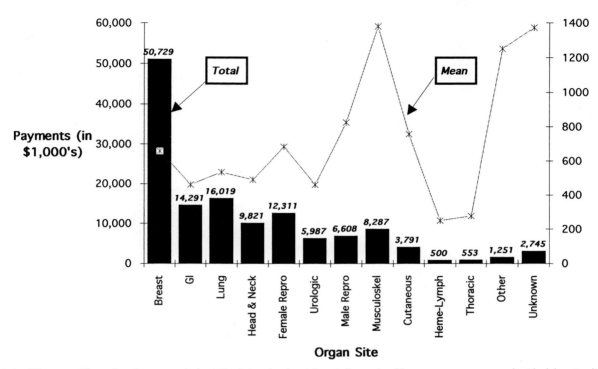

Figure 94–2   *Histogram illustrating the cost to indemnify claims for the delayed diagnosis of breast cancer, compared with delays in diagnosis for 12 other organ sites. The solid bars indicate the total expense for each organ site; the dashed line represents the average payment for each organ site. The graph demonstrates that the average cost to indemnify a breast cancer claim is lower than that for six other organ sites. However, the high frequency of claims for the delayed diagnosis of breast cancer results in a significant increase in total liability costs, compared with other organ sites. (Data from Kern KA: Medicolegal analysis of the delayed diagnosis of cancer in 338 cases in the United States. Arch Surg 129:397–404, 1994.)*

sites, as shown in Figure 94–1.[127] This histogram illustrates that breast cancer ranked first in misdiagnosed cancer, accounting for 127 out of 338 cases. The delayed diagnosis of breast cancer exceeded the next most common organ site involved in diagnostic delays, colon cancer, by over twofold (38 versus 15 percent). The author's study demonstrated that the expense of liability claims for misdiagnosed breast cancer totaled over $50 million, or 38 percent of the combined total for all 13 organ sites of $133 million. A comparison of the expense of delayed diagnosis of breast cancer to delayed diagnosis of other cancer sites is illustrated in Figure 94–2. Table 94–6 is taken from our recent article reviewing 711 negligence claims in the field of general surgery. Breast cancer claims again ranked first on this list, with 172 cases (24 percent) out of the total caseload of 711 liability claims.[136] Despite the frequency with which general surgeons evaluate and treat breast cancer, misdiagnosis of this condition ranks first in diagnoses resulting in negligence litigation against general surgeons, as shown in Table 94–7.[136]

Other studies have supported these findings. In 1988, The St. Paul Fire and Marine Insurance Company, a large medical liability carrier, reported that failure to diagnose cancer was the third most frequent allegation against physicians. Of these diagnostic delays, one third focused on breast cancer.[222] In 1963, Harper reviewed 1000 cases of litigation while serving as a medicolegal defense consultant to California insurers. The delayed diagnosis of cancer was reported in 1.4 percent of negligence cases (42 of 1005 cases), equally divided among cancers of the rectum, breast, and cervix.[102] In a study of 1371 malpractice claims from an insurance survey in New Jersey, Kravitz and colleagues noted that breast operations accounted for 9 percent (26 of 304) of general surgery operations resulting in negligence claims.[138]

The frequency of delayed diagnosis of breast cancer is not a direct result of the high incidence of breast cancer in the population. Figure 94–3, derived from data tabulated in the author's 1994 study of delayed diagnosis of cancer nationwide,[127] illustrates that the frequency for delayed diagnosis of breast cancer is twice as great, on a proportionate basis, as the frequency of breast cancer in the U.S. population. Interestingly, the mortality rate of breast cancer patients from this medicolegal study was no different from that of breast cancer patients in the 1973–1987 Surveillance, Epidemiology, and End Results (SEER) Program of the National Cancer Institute. As illustrated in Figure 94–4, the mortality rate of breast cancer patients who experienced a delayed diagnosis was equal to that of patients in the SEER database,

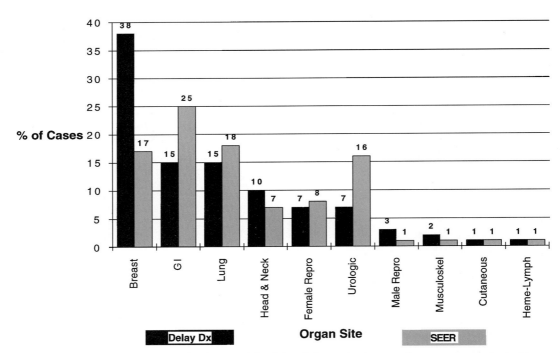

Figure 94–3 *Histogram comparing the frequency distribution of the delayed diagnosis of cancer, by organ site, to the incidence of cancer in the SEER database of the National Cancer Institute (Surveillance, Epidemiology, and End-Results Program of the National Institutes of Health). Each column represents the proportionate representation of each organ site in either the series of delayed diagnoses resulting in malpractice litigation (black bars), or in the SEER population (gray bars). The percentage figures represented by the black bars were calculated by dividing the total number of cases in our medicolegal study, by organ site on a yearly basis, by the number of litigated cases per year. The percentage figures represented by the gray bars were calculated by dividing the yearly incidence by organ site per 100,000 population by the total number of cases per year per 100,000 population in the SEER program. Breast cancer, the most frequently litigated condition, has proportionately twice as many lawsuits as its incidence in the general population. Thus, the frequency distribution of diagnostic delays for breast cancer, on a proportionate basis, is not the same as the incidence of breast cancer in the general population. (Data from Kern KA: Medicolegal analysis of the delayed diagnosis of cancer in 338 cases in the United States. Arch Surg 129:397–404, 1994.)*

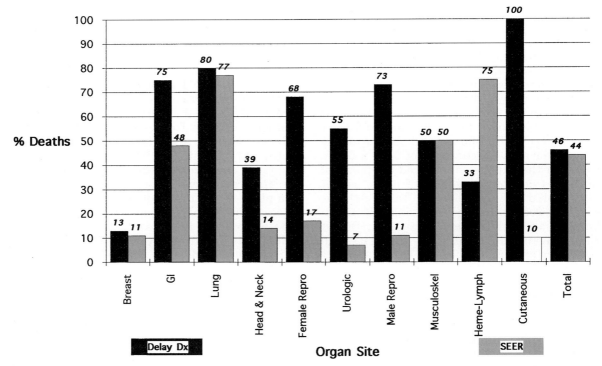

Figure 94–4 *Histogram comparing the death rate of cases in our medicolegal study population to that of the SEER data base. The mortality rates are calculated on a proportionate basis, in a similar fashion to the method described in Figure 94–2. Data from Kern KA: Medicolegal analysis of the delayed diagnosis of cancer in 338 cases in the United States. Arch Surg 129:397–404, 1994.)*

when calculated on a proportionate basis (the difference in mortality rates was 1.2 between delayed diagnosis cases and SEER cases). The proportionate mortality rate of breast cancer patients with delayed diagnosis was 13 percent (17 deaths in 127 cases of delayed diagnoses), compared with a mortality rate of 11 percent for the SEER breast cases (24 deaths from breast cancer per 10^5 population/212 breast cancer events per 10^5 population). Taken together, the data illustrated in Figures 94–1 through 94–4 define diagnostic delays for breast cancer as a unique but relatively frequent clinical problem in the field of oncology.

Understanding the mechanism of diagnostic delays is important to clinicians for several reasons. First, this information can serve as an effective educational tool to improve the diagnostic capabilities of physicians. In essence, early diagnosis by physicians can only succeed when physicians are truly aware of the possibility of breast cancer, particularly in groups of women thought unlikely to harbor breast malignancy (such as women under age 45). Second, an understanding of the delayed diagnosis of breast cancer highlights limitations imposed by modern imaging technology and routine physical diagnosis. Lastly, understanding the causes and consequences of delayed diagnosis provides a deeper understanding of our scientific knowledge regarding the biological behavior, predictability, and curability of breast cancer. This information is vital to the physician-patient relationship, because many patients believe that any delay in the diagnosis and treatment of breast cancer decreases their chances for survival, regardless of the length of time involved, the biology of the breast tumor, or the clinical circumstances surrounding the delay.

Unfortunately, there is strong evidence that many clinicians do not fully understand the problem of the delayed diagnosis of breast cancer. This evidence is derived from medical malpractice claims for failure to diagnose breast cancer, as described in the preceding discussion. When stratified by which actions on the part of physicians are most costly to malpractice carriers, manual examination of the female breast ranks 9 out of 20, accounting for $38 million (162 claims out of 8234 total malpractice cases, or 2 percent).[189–192] An approximate calculation of the numbers of misdiagnosed breast cancer resulting in litigation may be derived from findings accrued by the PIAA. This group defends approximately 300 cases of misdiagnosed breast cancer each year among its 100,000 insured physicians (encompassing a wide range of specialties). Because there are about 1 million physicians in the United States, with roughly one third caring for adult women, it can be estimated that there may be as many as 1000 cases per year of misdiagnosed breast cancer undergoing evaluation for medical negligence (on average 20 cases per state). This represents 0.5% of the new cases of breast cancer (180,000) diagnosed each year.

Several factors contribute to persistence of errors in the delayed diagnosis of breast cancer. First,

breast cancer and benign breast disease are common, and both may adopt similar signs and symptoms. Over 180,000 cases of breast cancer, or 100 cases per 100,000 females, were diagnosed in 1993.[121, 225] Estimates of the number of breast biopsies performed in the United States are reflective of the volume of benign breast disease, which includes 250,000 open surgical procedures and 37,000 needle biopsies of palpable breast lesions.[70] Second, clinically occult, undetectable breast cancer is present in up to 10 percent of women. Holford and associates showed that the percentage of women with breast cancer at autopsy in whom the diagnosis was overlooked antemortem ranged between 3 and 11 percent.[108] Both contralateral biopsy and prophylactic contralateral mastectomy have revealed an incidence of occult breast cancer of 5 to 10 percent.[144, 233, 234] Thus, some fraction of women presenting with breast symptoms who are not biopsied initially (for defensibly correct reasons) will later be diagnosed with breast cancer that was detected incidentally. Finally, many physicians evaluate breast complaints. In the absence of specialists in the field or well-defined, clinical practice guidelines, errors in diagnosis are bound to occur.

DEFINITION OF DELAYED DIAGNOSIS OF BREAST CANCER

Delayed diagnosis of breast cancer may be classified in several ways. In terms of a general definition, delayed diagnosis of breast cancer is the failure to recognize the signs and symptoms of breast cancer, by either a patient or a physician, resulting in a prolonged interval between the appearance of breast cancer symptoms and its diagnosis and treatment. The terminology applied to diagnostic delays is not standardized. More specific classifications of delayed diagnosis of breast cancer are based on who is primarily responsible for the delay: the doctor, the patient, or the medical system itself. Terms that define these specific delays reflect the source of responsibility for the delay, and include patient-associated delays, doctor-associated delays, symptom-to-hospital time, symptom-to-doctor consultation time, and symptom-to-completion of therapy interval.[1] For example, Katz[119] placed emphasis on the terms symptom-delay time, diagnosis-delay time, and surgery-delay time. Similarly, Sheriden[215] defined patient-delay as the interval between the patient's noticing an abnormality and the time when she first sought medical advice. Doctor-delay was defined as the interval from first consultation to the commencement of definitive treatment. Total delay time was defined as the sum of the two types of delay. Some have given quantitative definitions to these terms. Harms[100] defined a patient-associated delay as having persistent symptoms for one month or longer before seeing a doctor. Delay by the physician was defined as waiting for any period longer than three weeks.

In this chapter we will discuss the general categories of patient-associated and doctor-associated delays in the diagnosis of breast cancer.

PATIENT-ASSOCIATED DELAYS IN DIAGNOSIS

Studies of Patient-Associated Delays in Diagnosis

Regardless of the type of cancer under review, studies of the delayed diagnosis of cancer have shown that most delays occur before medical consultation.[34] This finding has been noted for over 50 years. For example, in 1943 Harms[100] studied 158 cancer patients and reported that the median interval between the onset of symptoms and treatment was 8.5 months. Breast cancer had the second longest delay time, with cancer of the skin having the longest time of delay in presentation to a physician.

While studying a wide range of cancers, Mor[170] showed that 25 percent of cancer patients delayed seeking medical consultation for more than 3 months. Other studies have shown similar results, with 35 to 50 percent of cancer patients delaying more than three months before seeking medical attention.[9] Hackett,[95] in a study of 563 cancer cases from the Massachusetts General Hospital with a wide range of diagnoses, showed that 15.6 percent of cancer patients delayed their presentation to a doctor for over 1 year. Hackett reported that between the years 1917 and 1970, only modest decreases in the length of delayed diagnosis of cancer of all types were appreciated. In the years 1917 to 1918, delays averaged 5.4 months; between 1921 and 1922, the average delay was 4.6 months; and by 1930, the delay interval remained at 4.8 months. The median time to presentation was 3 months.

By creation of a kinetic curve describing the rate of presentation for medical evaluation versus time, Hackett demonstrated that the half-time curve of delay in diagnosis for a variety of cancer types was slightly over 2 months. Based on this kinetic analysis, it can be predicted that 10 to 20 percent of cancer patients will never consult their physician about their symptoms. In essence, this kinetic analysis is a mathematical predictor that a group of patients will demonstrate extraordinarily long symptomatic intervals before presenting to a doctor for diagnosis. Clinical studies have confirmed this mathematical prediction. For example, Aitken-Swann[3] reported on a series of patient interviews with British cancer patients. In this study, approximately 50 percent of cancer patients overall delayed seeking advice for 3 months or more, and 25 percent of cancer patients with a wide variety of tumors delayed seeking treatment for a year or more after first noticing symptoms. In a subset of women with breast cancer, Wool[246] confirmed that symptomatic delays could reach extraordinarily lengthy intervals, with some patient-associated delays approaching 2 to 3 years.

Historically, studies specific to the delayed diagnosis of breast cancer have shown that diagnostic delays were usually long. Nonetheless, a chronological analysis demonstrates that delays have been steadily decreasing over time. In 1892, Dietrich (as reported in reference 19) reported that only 23 percent of breast cancer patients presented within 6 months of discovering their breast tumor. Over the next 50 years the proportion of patients sustaining lengthy delays continued to decrease.[21] By 1910 to 1914, Harrington[103] at the Mayo Clinic reported that 33 percent of breast cancer patients were treated within 6 months of discovery of a breast tumor, and 54 percent were treated in less than 1 year; by the late 1930s, these proportions had increased to 50 and 70 percent, indicating earlier diagnosis of these cases. Lewis and Reinhoff[145] in the late 1930s, and later, Eggers and de Cholnoky[64] in the 1940s, reported less optimistic findings, with only 34 percent of cases seeking medical advice within 6 months, and 55 percent within 1 year. By the 1950s, Bloom[19, 22] reported a series of 406 cases and showed that 65 percent of patients came for treatment within 6 months of the first symptom and 85 percent of patients presented for evaluation within 1 year. Hultborn[112] reported on 517 cases from the years 1930 to 1955. Patients presented for treatment in less than 1 month in 30 percent of patients; in less than 6 months in 37 percent of patients; and in less than 1 year in 22 percent of patients. Between 1930 and 1955, there was no change in the rate at which cases presented for diagnosis on a proportionate basis.

In 1959, Waxman[241] reported on 740 patients with breast cancer and showed that the number of patients reporting their symptoms to a physician within 1 month of discovery increased 10 percent between the years 1940 and 1951. He attributed this effect to increased publicity about breast cancer. Robbins[202] compared the range of pretreatment symptom delays among 3802 patients treated by radical mastectomy between 1940 and 1955. Patients were divided into two groups: Those treated between 1940 and 1943, and those treated between 1950 and 1955. In the patients from the 1940s, delays of less than 2 months were present in 42.9 percent of patients, compared with patients in the 1950s, of whom 47.5 percent presented with delays of less than 2 months. Delays exceeding 6 months were present in 30.8 percent of the 1940s group, and 27.7 percent of the 1950s group. Between the two time periods, the median delay for delayed presentation of symptoms dropped by only 0.8 months. Tumor sizes at presentation in these same time periods showed a shift downward in tumor size at diagnosis in 2 to 10 percent of patients. For patients in the 1940s (1281 patients), T1 tumors (smaller than 2 cm) were present in 20 percent; T2 tumors (smaller than 4 cm), 46.7 percent; and T2 tumors (larger than 4 cm), 33.3 percent. In the 1950s (2168 patients), these same figures were T1, 28.4 percent; small T2, 48.7 percent; and larger T2, 22.9 percent.

More recent studies have shown a continued decline in the time to presentation for medical evaluation after the appearance of the first symptom of breast cancer. In 1971, Sheriden[215] reported that among 1860 women in Western Australia, 24 percent had patient delays of 1 to 4 weeks, 32 percent had delays of 1 to 3 months, 18 percent had delays of 3 to 6 months, and 6 percent had delays of over 6 months. A small fraction of patients (2 percent) sustained lengthy delays in presentation of 4 years or more: Only 5 percent of patients visited a doctor within 1 week of symptoms. Nichols and coworkers[178] confirmed that 23 percent of women delayed consultation for more than 3 months. Gould-Martin and associates[87] reported that in a study of 275 women with breast cancer aged 40 to 65, 7 percent of patients delayed for more than 6 months before seeking medical attention. Waters and colleagues[239] and Cameron and Henton[34] noted that between 20 to 30 percent of patients delayed presentation to a physician for over 3 months. Pilipshen and Robbins[193] reported in 1984 that 63 percent of breast cancer patients treated at Memorial Hospital in New York delayed for less than 2 months. Robinson and associates[203] studied 523 women with breast cancer and noted a mean delay from symptoms to diagnosis of 5.5 months (median 4 months). Mor and colleagues[170] studied nearly 500 breast cancer patients and showed that one third of patients delayed presentation to a physician for over 3 months after the onset of symptoms. Rossi and colleagues[206] demonstrated that the median symptom-delay time was 2 months, with 35 percent of women waiting more than 3 months before presenting to a physician.

Keinan and coworkers[120] noted that typical delays for American and Canadian women from symptoms to diagnosis were 3 to 6 months. Katz and associates[119] noted that in a study of women in Washington State and British Columbia, 16 to 17 percent of patients had a symptom-delay time of 3 months and 13 percent had a symptom-delay time of 6 months. Diagnosis-delay times of 3 months were present in 4.6 percent of Canadian patients and 13.1 percent of American patients; patient-associated diagnostic delays exceeding 6 months were present in 3.5 percent of Canadian and American patients. Most recently, in 1995, Andersen[6] confirmed that the mean delay time from first noticing a symptom in breast patients to clinical evaluation is 3 months. In a subset of women, delays can be extreme, approaching 2 to 3 years.[246] Given the large number of new cases of breast cancer expected to be diagnosed in American women in 1996 (180,000), it has been estimated that over 60,000 American women will sustain patient-associated diagnostic delays exceeding 3 months.[69]

Delays approximating 3 months from the onset of symptoms to presentation by the patient appear to be universal throughout the world. In a study of Australian women, Margarey and coworkers[157] confirmed that 25 percent of patients delayed presentation to a physician for over 4 months. In a study of 48,000 women from Sweden, Mansson and Bengtsson[160] noted that the average delay to visiting a doc-

tor was 5 months and that only 40 percent of women visited a doctor within 1 month of symptoms. In third-world countries delays may extend over a far greater period of time. Goel and associates[85] noted that in India the average patient delay time was 6.7 months. Ajekigbe[4] noted similar results in Nigeria, and Chie and Chang[42] confirmed lengthy patient-associated diagnostic delays in Taiwan.

Theories of Patient-Associated Delay in Diagnosis

Various theories have been proposed to explain patient-associated delay in diagnosis. These theories have included: (1) psychological factors; (2) socioeconomic level; (3) race; (4) age; (5) parity; and (6) anatomical factors. These factors are listed in Table 94–8.

Psychological Factors

Many attempts have been made to define the personality traits that lead to prolonged delays in seeking medical attention for symptomatic breast disease. Attempts to define the psychological profile of the patient who delays presentation is of more than academic interest. The price to pay for psychological processes that inhibit early evaluation of breast symptoms may be progression of disease. For example, Wool[246] compared patients presenting quickly to a physician, within 1 month of discovering breast symptoms, with a group of patients exhibiting extreme denial of breast symptoms, in which delays in presenting to a physician exceeded 20 months. He found a 30-percent increase in regional or metastatic disease in patients exhibiting extreme denial (85 percent nondeniers versus 54 percent deniers, $p < .01$).

Studies of how a woman's personality characteristics may influence behavior patterns leading to potential delays in diagnosis have revealed a complex interaction between many levels of mental processes. Margarey and Todd[155] applied psychological testing to a group of women with the delayed diagnosis of breast cancer who were facing surgical therapy. Personality inventories revealed that conscious fear, for example, the consciously expressed fear of mastectomy, was not a central factor in causing lengthy diagnostic delays. Rather these investigators found that subconscious defense mechanisms, not recognized by the patients themselves, were responsible for the delay in presenting to a physician. In further detailed studies, the defense mechanisms of denial and suppression of reality became the dominant psychological behaviors responsible for delays.[156, 157] An-

TABLE 94–8. THEORIES OF PATIENT-ASSOCIATED DELAYS IN DIAGNOSIS OF BREAST CANCER

Psychological factors	Age
Socioeconomic status	Parity
Ethnic background	Anatomical factors

dersen and Cacioppo[6] recently showed that two thirds (77 days) of the typical 3-month delay by a patient are spent in appraisal of the illness; the decision to seek help is rapidly carried out thereafter. Those who suppress this need for help go on to exhibit prolonged delays.

A reproducible finding in patients who delay presentation to a physician is a significantly lower level of conscious anxiety than would be expected with a possible diagnosis of cancer.[156, 157] Others have also confirmed that conscious anxiety is an important psychological element in bringing patients with newly discovered breast symptoms to medical attention. Thus, although some have assumed that conscious fear prevents women from presenting to their physicians for diagnosis,[169] the opposite dynamic appears to function in patients who delay. Cameron and Hinton[34] found that delays in diagnosis occurred in patients who exhibited little or no anxiety over the presence of a breast tumor. Cameron labeled this behavior as "conscious indifference" to the potential presence of cancer. Introverts also exhibit long delays in seeking help for breast symptoms.[34] Hackett and colleagues[95] suggested that delays in diagnosis were a conscious and deliberate act performed by patients in full awareness of their condition. Based on a kinetic analysis of time to presentation in a wide group of patients, he suggested, "It is as though motivation to seek medical help for this group is a negatively accelerated function that rapidly reaches an asymptote of complete indifference."[95]

These studies have led to the important conclusion that attempts to motivate the public to seek early diagnosis of breast symptoms by invoking fear of a delayed diagnosis of cancer is unlikely to work in many patients. Beginning in the late 1940s, public health campaigns designed to decrease delays in diagnosis have been predicated on the premise that increased information, particularly focused on the fear of late cancer, would motivate the public to seek early medical attention for symptoms of breast cancer.[100] Yet, such campaigns may not be successful or may have the opposite effect. Wool[246] confirmed this hypothesis through an attempted 3-year health educational campaign in England, designed to test the hypothesis that public education regarding the importance of an early diagnosis of breast cancer would reduce delays in diagnosis. The result of the campaign, which appealed to people's rational, conscious mind, was a failure: No significant decrease in time to diagnosis of breast cancer occurred. In particular, the proportion of women with long delay times did not change throughout the 3-year interval of the study.

Buttlar and Templeton[31] also confirmed the inability of public educational campaigns to decrease the size of tumors detected by breast self-examination. These investigators analyzed a 12-year public education campaign through a community hospital foundation. In this study, the percent of tumors smaller than 2 cm remained constant at 33 percent over the 12-year study interval. Surprisingly, health profes-sionals had a worse record for early diagnosis compared with the general population. The percentage of tumors larger than 5 cm was greatest in professionals with prior health training (doctors, nurses, hospital workers), and the fraction of women with delays in diagnosis of 6 months or more, was 7 percent greater in health professionals than in the population at large.

In similar studies, Sheriden and associates[215] reported no decrease in patient-associated delays in diagnosis in Western Australia between the years 1954 and 1957 and 1961 and 1965, despite an extensive public campaign geared toward early recognition by patients of breast cancer symptoms. In a study by Harms and colleagues,[100] 57 percent of patients did nothing about a breast lump because they believed the symptom was "not serious enough" to warrant a medical evaluation, despite patient education to the contrary. Hackett and coworkers[95] used interview techniques to demonstrate that the speed of response to breast cancer symptoms is related to the degree of conscious awareness and depth of specific knowledge about breast cancer. During patient interviews, rapid responders to symptoms referred to their condition using the specific word "cancer," instead of the non-specific term "tumor." Interestingly, those with a family history of breast cancer tended to have a longer delay in presentation to a physician.

In contrast to some of the previous findings, several investigators have shown no relationship between personality traits and delays in diagnosis. Watson and associates[240] found that the length of diagnostic delay was not related to psychological denial. In this study, denial appeared to have a short-term beneficial effect by relieving anxiety, without the detrimental effect of increasing the delay in diagnosis. In a follow-up study, Wool[246] found that immature ego development or affective disorders could not explain the behavior pattern of extreme denial. Keinan and colleagues[120] also found personality traits, such as the ability to handle responsibility or chronic level of anxiety, were not related to diagnostic delays. Rather longer diagnostic delays occurred in women with little body awareness, a feature defined as those women who did not examine themselves in a mirror frequently, did not exercise, and did not touch their bodies frequently. This theory lends itself well to the somewhat surprising finding by Gould-Martin and colleagues[87] that 38 percent of 274 women diagnosed with breast cancer found their tumors solely by accidental touching, and not by a planned program of breast self-examination.

Socioeconomic Status

A consistent finding throughout many studies has been the correlation between socioeconomic status and length of diagnostic delay. While no single socioeconomic category accounts for all reasons for diagnostic delays,[188] certain broad conclusions can be drawn from sociological studies. Those of lower socioeconomic class consistently show greater delays in presentation to physicians.[170] In one of the earliest studies documenting this effect, Haagensen[93] compared the length of delay in diagnosis between privately insured patients and uninsured charity patients at Columbia-Presbyterian Hospital admitted in the years 1915 to 1934. He noted the percentage of patients who presented to a doctor within 1 month of discovering a breast mass was twofold greater in private patients compared with uninsured charity patients. Cameron and Hinton[34] also found that patients with fewer years of education exhibited longer delays.

In terms of economic status, Mor and associates[170] found that women below the poverty line exhibited greater delays in presentation to a physician compared with more affluent women, a finding also confirmed by Cameron and Hinton.[34] Facione[69] noted those patients with no health insurance had longer delays in diagnosis. Polednak[194] noted an effect of income distribution on stage of breast cancer at diagnosis. In a group of black and white women, the income differential was 39 percent higher in whites, or $3000 yearly. This difference correlated with the increased numbers of late cases (stage III) in blacks presenting for diagnosis. In a study of the effect of marital status on time to presentation of breast cancer in 1261 women (910 married, 351 widowed), Neale and colleagues[176] noted that white women have the lowest incidence of late-presenting tumors, compared with widowed or single women. They also lived longer than widowed women. This effect was thought to represent an economic disparity between the marital status of these groups of women. Gould-Martin and coworkers[87] noted that women most likely to present for a breast examination were young, premenopausal, married at the time of diagnosis, and held a high socioeconomic status, as measured by four factors: site of residence, income level, husband's occupation, and educational level achieved by the patient. Hackett and colleagues[95] confirmed a significant relationship between social class and length of diagnostic delays. Those patients with the highest index of social position had the shortest diagnostic delays, confirmed at a statistical level of significance of $p = .001$.

Lower socioeconomic status also has an impact on the frequency with which women sustaining a physician-associated delay in diagnosis of breast cancer bring a lawsuit against their physicians. Recently, Burstin and associates[30] studied liability claim rates for medical malpractice of all types among the poor and elderly, and reported indigent and elderly patients sue at rates one fifth to one tenth that of higher socioeconomic groups. This low rate of lawsuits among the poor and elderly stands in contrast to what many physicians believe to be true, because these indigent groups are perceived to sue more often than higher socioeconomic classes. While preparing a recent study on risk prevention related to medical malpractice in breast cancer, we noted that the poor and elderly rarely sue for the delayed diagnosis of breast cancer.[135] We derived the data from three surveys of the professional liability claims experience of the American College of Obstetricians and Gynecologists (ACOG) during the years 1987, 1990, and 1992.[129] Tabulating the results from all three surveys, members reported 104 total claims for breast cancer malpractice (largely failure to diagnose breast cancer) out of a total of 1542 overall obstetric-gynecological claims (7 percent). Importantly, patients with indemnity insurance plans (private insurance, Blue Cross/Blue Shield, or HMO) accounted for 92 percent (96/104) of these claims, whereas Medicaid and Medicare patients accounted for less than 2 percent (2/104) of total breast cancer malpractice claims (1/104 for each category). A breakdown of claims by these three payor categories, for each year surveyed, is as follows (the category "other" not included): (1) 1987: indemnity 92 percent (60/66); Medicaid 2.2 percent (1/66), Medicare n/a; (2) 1990: indemnity 96 percent (25/26), Medicaid 0 percent (0/26); Medicare 0 percent (0/26); (3) 1992: indemnity 95 percent (11/12); Medicaid 0 percent (0/12); Medicare 1 percent (1/12); (4) all years: indemnity 92 percent (96/104), Medicaid 1 percent (1/104), Medicare 1 percent (1/104). These data are illustrated in Figure 94–5. Based on the three professional liability surveys of the ACOG, higher socioeconomic groups possessing indemnity insurance account for over 90 percent of the malpractice cases, confirming that the indigent and elderly rarely sue for breast cancer malpractice.

The influence of socioeconomic status on time to presentation of breast cancer is a worldwide phenomenon, particularly evident in rural countries of the developing world. In Taiwan, Chie and Chang[42] noted that tumors smaller than 2 cm were more common if patients were employed or were part of families with higher overall income. In a study of rural patients in India with the delayed diagnosis of breast cancer, patients listed financial concerns as the second most common reason for late presentation to a health clinics.[85]

Ethnic Background

Richardson and colleagues[199] found that greater delays in diagnosis occurred among blacks and Hispanics. Facione[69] confirmed that race adversely influences delay time. Hunter and coworkers[114] confirmed that long delays occurred among blacks of low socioeconomic status, but the same held true for economically-disadvantaged white women. No firm conclusions could be drawn on the mechanism of the delay related to racial differences, which might include any of the following factors: (1) differences in health care access, (2) prior medical experiences that might inhibit the patient from presenting to physicians for treatment, or (3) differences in life style patterns, making an early presentation to a physician unlikely because of financial or social difficulties.

Age and Parity

The influence of age on patient-associated time to presentation with breast symptoms remains contro-

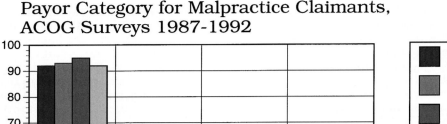

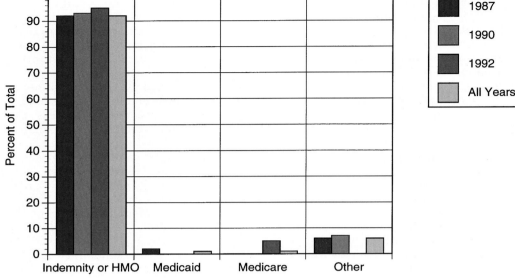

Figure 94–5 *Histogram demonstrating the percentage distribution of patients (claimants) who sue for misdiagnosed breast cancer, based on the type of insurance coverage held by each patient. The data were derived from surveys performed by the American College of Obstetrics and Gynecology, during the years 1987, 1990, and 1992. The bars represent the results from these years individually, and from all years combined. The graph demonstrates that patients holding private or HMO-type insurance account for nearly all liability claims stemming from the delayed diagnosis of breast cancer. (Data from Kern KA: Do the poor sue more? JAMA 271:504, 1994.)*

versial. Finley and Francis[73] noted that older women presented sooner with symptoms, whereas Facione[69] and Kaae[118] demonstrated that older women delayed their presentation. Nichols and coworkers[178] reported that women over age 65 were likely to significantly delay their presentation to a doctor. Robinson and coworkers[203] demonstrated that in a study of women over age 70, 15 percent more women delayed presenting for evaluation compared with those under age 50 (a statistically significant finding). In an evaluation of patients with extreme denial syndromes (average time to presentation, 20.9 months), Wool[246] confirmed that the elderly were more likely to fall into this category.

The effect of age on time to patient presentation has also been studied in the subset of women under age 35. Treaves and colleagues[231] evaluated 549 patients with breast cancer who were under age 35. The median delay was 2 months from self-discovery of symptoms (range 1 day to 1 year). Williams and associates[244] demonstrated that women younger than age 35 had a 50 percent decrease in time to presentation with serious breast symptoms (only 17 percent waiting more than 3 months to seek help) compared with women over age 35 (28 percent waiting more than 3 months to seek medical evaluation). Max and Klamer[162] noted in a study of 120 women with an average age of 31 years that 34 percent of patients waited more than 6 weeks to present to a doctor. Backhouse and coworkers[11] showed that in a study of 54 patients with a mean age of 31 years, 45 percent delayed more than 3 months before presenting for

evaluation. Of these 24 patients, 22 had an obvious breast mass. Three patients (12.5 percent) had a known family history of breast cancer. Brightmore and colleagues[26] studied 101 women under age 35 and reported that 15 percent had delays of less than 1 month, 18 percent had delays of less than 2 months, and 10 percent had delays of less than 3 months. Bennett and associates[17] noted that Australian women with breast cancer younger than age of 35 had an average duration of symptoms of 6.5 months. However, Sheridan and coworkers[215] reported that among women in Western Australia, younger patients presented more quickly for medical consultation.

In an investigation of the effect of parity on time to delay with malignant breast symptoms, Williams and coworkers[244] noted that nulliparous women presented within 1 month in 75 percent of patients and only 8.5 percent delayed for more than 3 months. In contrast, parous women presented within 1 month in only 45 percent of cases and delayed more than 3 months in 28.80 percent of cases (a factor of three compared with nulliparous women). Apparently, those women with previous pregnancies showed less concern about breast symptoms, believing these changes represented fibrocystic tissue, which frequently develops on return of the lactating breast to the non-pregnant state.

Anatomical Factors

Anatomical factors may also influence the time interval of patient-associated delays in diagnosis of breast cancer. It is widely documented that the first sign of breast cancer in 60 to 80 percent of women is a painless mass. For those patients with symptoms other than a mass (such as pain, discharge, or skin changes), diagnostic delays may ensue. Williams and coworkers[244] noted that over half of women thought breast lumps were "nothing to worry about," particularly because they were not painful. Nichols and colleagues[178] noted that women with painless lumps presented to physicians with a median delay of 16 days. Those women presenting with breast symptoms other than a lump sustained significant delays in diagnosis. In Nichols' study, those women with malignant breast symptoms involving indistinct findings, such as asymmetrical nodularity, tenderness, or skin puckering, sustained median delays ranging from 126 to 250 days. In a different study, Mor and associates[170] demonstrated that women with shorter delays in diagnosis were aware that a lump may be cancerous twice as often as those who delayed seeking medical advice. However, in women with breast pain as their only symptom of cancer, over 40 percent did not recognize this symptom as a possible sign of malignant disease. Gould-Martin and colleagues[87] demonstrated that in patients who did not have lumps as their first symptom of breast cancer, patient-associated diagnostic delays were four times longer than in women with isolated breast masses (7 days with a lump versus 31 days without a lump). Facione[69] demonstrated that prior fibrocystic disease or symptoms other than a breast mass led to longer delays in patient presentation for consultation.

The lack of pain in most breast cancers is one reason for delayed patient presentation to a doctor. Hein and coworkers[105] showed that a painful breast process, such as a breast abscess, brings the patient to a doctor within 2 weeks. In contrast, painless breast processes, such as fibroadenomas, are accompanied by a much longer delay in patient presentation. In Hein's study, patients with fibroadenomas delayed their presentation to a physician for an average of 7.1 months, whereas those patients with breast cysts waited on average over 15 months before seeking medical attention. Paradoxically, patients with painful masses may seek medical attention rapidly and yet be misled by physicians into believing painful breast masses are benign. Because breast cancers are associated with breast pain in about 10 percent of patients, doctors may cause diagnostic delays by falsely reassuring patients that painful breast masses are benign.

In 1989, Ingram and associates[115] studied breast size in mastectomy specimens to determine if larger breasts obscure breast cancer diagnosis. Ingram measured the weight and thickness of mastectomy specimens, and found that those with heavier and thicker breasts (over 800 gm, and over 5 cm thick) more often had tumors greater than 2.25 cm, and more often demonstrated positive lymph nodes. Ingram could not determine, however, if the more advanced tumors were a result of simple anatomical masking, or if local breast hormones were accelerating tumor growth (for example, breast lipocytes produce estrogen). Hormone receptors did not vary in these two groups.

Lanin and coworkers[141] reported that women younger than age 50 had more visits to a dedicated breast clinic (1567 versus 838) to diagnose breast cancer but had fewer breast cancers detected rapidly (38 versus 100). These workers ascribed this effect to anatomical factors masking tumor detection by physical examination and mammography. The sensitivity of mammography was 91 percent in women older than age 50 but only 68 percent in younger women. The tumors in younger women (under age 50) were more ill defined and were less easily palpated (45 versus 72 percent). Lanin proposed that anatomical differences in either the breast itself (for example, increased breast inelasticity) or in the tumor stroma (for example, a diffusing-type cancer) accounted for the difficulty in physical diagnosis of breast cancer in women under age 50. In contrast, in women over age 50, tumors were nonpalpable simply because they were small (1.0 cm versus 4.1 cm in younger women). In younger women, the tumors were large, yet they could not be palpated because they could not be differentiated easily from the background mammary tissue, which was typically dense and inelastic. Reintgen and coworkers[196, 197] in a study of 435 patients with an average age in the mid-50s reported that no tumor smaller than 5 mm in size could be palpated, 26 percent of tumors 6 to 10 mm could be palpated, and 48 percent of tumors 11 to 15 mm could be palpated. Ninety-six percent of tumors larger than 2 cm could be detected by palpation.

The histological type of breast cancer also contributes to delay in diagnosis. Joensuu and colleagues[117] found that 65 percent of cases with delayed diagnosis of breast cancer were of the lobular invasive type. This is in contrast to the usually reported proportion of lobular carcinoma, which generally does not exceed 10 percent.[117] Yeatman and associates[247] recently confirmed that the sizes of infiltrating lobular carcinomas are underestimated by mammographic examination by at least 1 cm, compared with their final pathological size. Both mammograms and fine needle aspiration biopsies are frequently false negative with infiltrating lobular carcinoma, leading to delays in diagnosis.[247] In Yeatman's series, the histology of patients sustaining delays in diagnosis was infiltrating lobular carcinoma in 76 percent of cases and infiltrating ductal carcinoma in 24 percent of cases. This ratio of histological types is a reversal of the usual ratio in breast cancer patients. Hollingsworth and coworkers[109] confirmed that diffuse malignant histology, such as invasive lobular carcinoma or multifocal, widely invasive ductal carcinoma, is an important cause of misdiagnosed breast cancer. In six patients with diffuse tumors measuring 1.0 to 1.9 cm, Hollingsworth documented that no significant mammographic density was created by the tumor to allow for radiographic diagnosis, regardless of its size.

DOCTOR-ASSOCIATED DELAYS IN DIAGNOSIS

Compared with patient-associated delays, many factors accounting for doctor-associated delays in diagnosis are less well-studied. Facione[69] noted that the true extent of provider delay is underresearched and underestimated. However, since the 1930s, it has been recognized that doctors are responsible for many delays in diagnosis of breast cancer. Lane-Claypon[139] reported in 1926 that in a series of 670 breast cancer cases, the average interval from first medical consultation to treatment averaged 6 months. Pack and Gallo[181] stated that physicians were solely responsible for 17 percent of delays in diagnosis in a series of 1000 patients and proposed that an equal number of delays resulted from the combination of patient and doctor delays. Rimstein and colleagues,[200] confirming earlier reports of Leach and Robbins,[142] noted that physicians were responsible for diagnostic delays in 28 percent of patients and contributed to the combination of patent-doctor responsibility in another 11 percent. In a series of 400 patients, Kaae[118] noted that doctors were responsible for delays in 12 percent. As is discussed later, these delays were often related to the age of the patient: Those women under age 40 were twice as likely to sustain delays in diagnoses as those over age 50.

The relationship between young patients and delay in diagnosis of breast cancer has been noted since the 1940s. Harnett[101] found that in a series of 2000 patients with breast cancer, 7 percent of patients sustained a delayed biopsy because of a physician's missed diagnosis. Over one quarter of these delays were sustained in patients younger than age 50. Rimstein and associates[200] noted that 25 percent of women younger than age 50 had a delay in diagnosis ranging from 4 months to 2 years and that doctors were solely responsible for these delays in nearly one quarter of patients. Nichols and colleagues[178] noted

that 10 percent of malignant breast diseases were delayed in their diagnosis by physicians for more than 1 month. Robinson and coworkers[203] noted that physician-associated delay in diagnosis occurs in 8 to 30 percent of patients.

Physician Factors in Delayed Diagnosis of Breast Cancer

Interval of Diagnostic Delay

Doctor-associated errors in diagnosis tend to follow reproducible and predictable patterns. From the author's medicolegal studies, it was found that the average length of a delay in diagnosis of breast cancer is 15 months, with a median length of diagnostic delay of 11 months (90th percentile, 24 months).[122, 127] Others have confirmed this average length of diagnostic delay in breast cancer.[59, 167, 168, 189, 191, 249] In the author's 1992 study,[122] it was found that the range of diagnostic delay in 37 cases was 1 to 60 months from the time of the patient's presentation to the biopsy-proven diagnosis of breast cancer. Broken down on a yearly basis, 67 percent (25/37) of patients were diagnosed as having breast cancer within 1 year; 78 percent (29/37) of patients, within 2 years; and 95 percent (35/37) of patients, within 3 years.

A comparison of intervals of diagnostic delay in breast cancer and other cancers is given in Table 94–9. The mean length of diagnostic delay for 212 cases was 17 months, with a median of 12 months (90th percentile, 33.5 months). This comparison shows surprisingly similar lengths of median diagnostic delay among the 13 types of cancers, including cancer of the colon (11 months),[124, 133] thyroid cancer (12 months),[125] and cancer of the lung (15 months).[127] Figure 94–4 is a statistical chart of the median and 90th percentile for diagnostic delays in these anatomical sites, constructed from the data in Table 94–9.[127] Figure 94–6 graphically illustrates the remarkable similarity between the breast and 12 other

TABLE 94–9.   LENGTH OF KNOWN DELAYS IN DIAGNOSIS BY ORGAN SITE (IN MONTHS)

Organ Site	N	Mean*	SE	Median	SD	90th Percentile	5th Percentile	Range
Breast	86	15.3	2	10	19	24	2.5	2–120
Gastrointestinal	16	21	3.3	14	17	44.5	5.5	5–70
Lung	34	15	1.6	12	9.4	25	2.5	1–42
Head and neck	16	14.1	2.0	12	7.7	20	5	5–36
Female reproductive	17	15	2.4	12	9.8	21.5	2	2–45
Urologic	14	31	7.1	24	26	59	3	3–97
Male reproductive	5	9.2	2	10	4.7	13.5	n/a	4–15
Musculoskeletal	6	6.2	2.5	4	6	13.5	n/a	1–14
Cutaneous	2	66	18	66	2.5	n/a	n/a	48–84
Heme-lymph	2	4.5	1.5	4.5	2.1	n/a	n/a	3–6
Thoracic	1	36	n/a	n/a	n/a	n/a	n/a	n/a
Other	1	24	n/a	n/a	n/a	n/a	n/a	n/a
All sites	212	17	1.2	12	17.6	33.5	2.5	1–120

*N.S. by Student's t-test for comparison of mean diagnostic delays between groups.

Modified from Kern KA: Medicolegal analysis of the delayed diagnosis of cancer in 338 cases in the United States. Arch Surg 129:397–404, 1994. Copyright 1992–1994, American Medical Association.

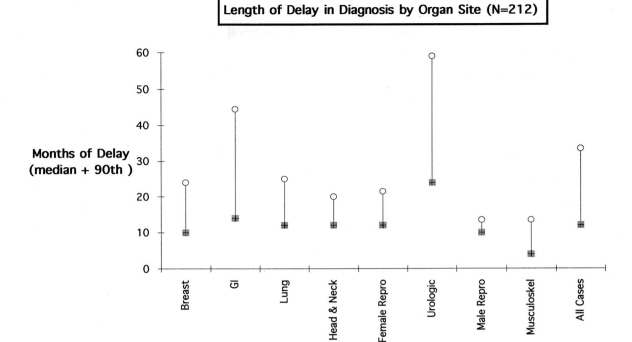

Figure 94–6   *A statistical plot of the median length of diagnostic delay, by organ site, for delayed diagnosis of cancer resulting in malpractice litigation. The hatched box and cross represents the median length of diagnostic delay; the open circle indicates the 90th percentile. Note the striking similarity in diagnostic delays for these nine different organ sites. This figure is a visual representation of the data in Table 94–9. (Data from Kern KA: Medicolegal analysis of the delayed diagnosis of cancer in 338 cases in the United States. Arch Surg 129:397–404, 1994.)*

anatomical sites for the typical length of diagnostic delay (median 12 months).

In the author's study of 338 misdiagnosed cancers nationwide, 156 cases were recorded with a death or terminal condition (46 percent, or 156/338). These cases were not all breast cancers. In 88 of the fatal cases, the length of diagnostic delay was known and averaged 16 months, with a median length of delay of 12 months (90th percentile, 25 months). This length of delay was not different statistically from the 17-month average delay of the entire group of 212 cases. The author also analyzed the lengths of diagnostic delays for 296 cancers overall in relation to the outcome of subsequent malpractice litigation. No statistical difference was found in the average lengths of diagnostic delays between defense verdicts (14 months, n = 64), plaintiff verdicts (19 months, n = 61), settlements out of court (17 months, n = 83), and all deaths (16 months, n = 88). A histogram of this data is shown in Figure 94–7, which demonstrates the similarity in lengths of diagnostic delay between patients who died, patients who succeeded in their lawsuit, patients who lost their lawsuit, and patients who settled their negligence lawsuits out of court.

A frequency distribution by 3-month intervals of the delayed diagnosis of breast cancer, derived from the author's previous civil court study[122] is shown in Figure 94–8. There is a bi-modal distribution of diagnostic delays, with the first peak at 7 to 9 months, and a second later peak at 31 to 33 months of delay. We analyzed the diagnostic delays in 273 cases from the PIAA 1990 study of misdiagnosed breast cancer, grouping delays in 5-month intervals, as shown in Figure 94–9.[189] Here a single peak at 6-to-11 months of delay was found, with a long tail to the frequency distribution curve, extending out to 72 to 77 months. Based on these data, it appears that most cancers make their presence known after misdiagnosis within a 1-year interval of time; however, a smaller fraction continue to go undiagnosed for lengthy periods of time.

Using data from the author's nationwide study of 338 cases, the outcomes of litigation were correlated versus the lengths of diagnostic delay, categorized by 3-month intervals, as shown in Figure 94–10. The 205 verdicts were divided into 65 defense verdicts (40 percent), 59 plaintiff verdicts (29 percent), and 81 settlements out of court (40 percent). At less than 3 months, the 11 jury verdicts largely favored the defense, in the following proportion: 64 percent defense verdicts (7/11), 9 percent plaintiff verdicts (1/11), and 27 percent settlements out of court (3/13). At 4 to 6 months, the proportion of defense verdicts decreased to 42 percent (13/31), plaintiff verdicts rose to 29 percent (9/31), and settlements also rose to 29 percent (9/31). By 7 to 9 months, defense verdicts decreased further still but stabilized at the level of 26 percent (7/27), plaintiff verdicts remained roughly the same at 22 percent (6/27), and settlements stabi-

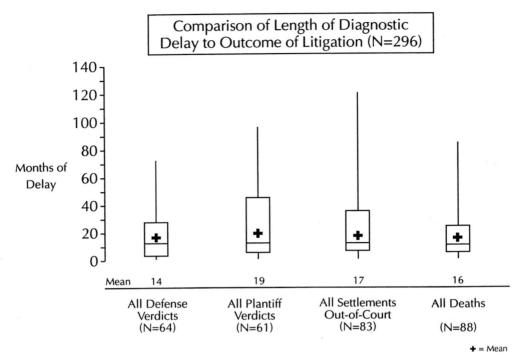

Figure 94–7 *Box-and-whisker plots of the months of diagnostic delay versus the outcome of litigation in 296 cases of delayed diagnosis of cancer. The dark cross in the center of the box indicates the mean length of diagnostic delay. The line through the center of the box represents the median length of diagnostic delay. The edges of the box represent the interquartile ranges. The ends of the whiskers represent the 95th percentile (upper end) and 5th percentile (lower end) of the range in diagnostic delay. There is no statistical difference in the length of diagnostic delay between any of the categories represented. (Data from Kern KA: Medicolegal analysis of the delayed diagnosis of cancer in 338 cases in the United States. Arch Surg 129:397–404, 1994.)*

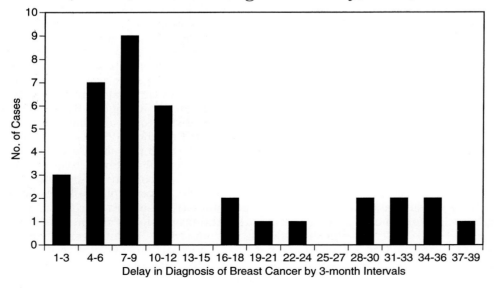

Figure 94–8 *Histogram displaying a frequency distribution for the length of diagnostic delay in breast cancer, grouped into 3-month intervals. The histogram demonstrates a bimodal distribution of diagnostic delay intervals. (Data from Kern KA: Causes of breast cancer malpractice litigation: A 20-year civil court review. Arch Surg 127:542–545, 1992.)*

Frequency Distribution of Delayed Diagnosis of Breast Cancer, By 5-Month Intervals (N = 273, PIAA, 1990)

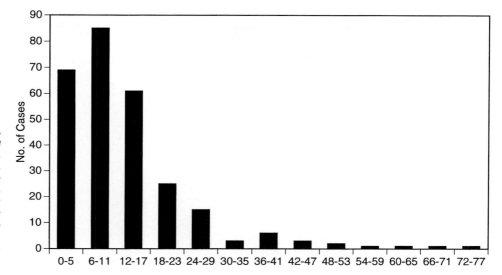

Figure 94–9 *Histogram displaying the frequency of delays in misdiagnosed breast cancer, grouped into 5-month intervals, derived from the Physician Insurers Association of America (PIAA) Breast Cancer Study (1990). The chart demonstrates an initial peak delay interval of 12 months, with a long tail extending out as far as 5 years. (Data derived from the Physician Insurers Association of America, Breast Cancer Study (1990). PIAA, Washington, DC, 1990.)*

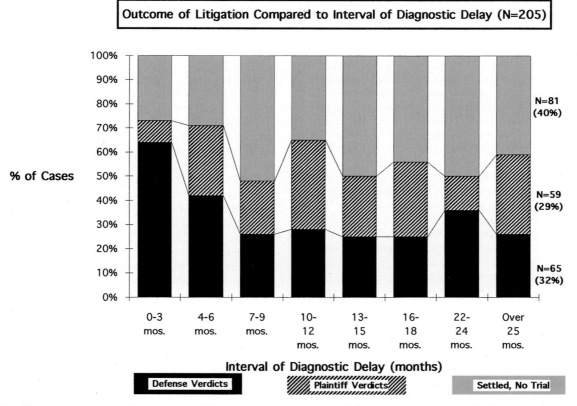

Figure 94–10 *Histogram comparing the outcomes of litigation versus the lengths of diagnostic delay, categorized by 3-month intervals, for 205 cancer cases of different types. Breast cancer accounted for over 100 cases. The dark bars represent jury verdicts in favor of the physician being sued for negligent delay in diagnosis. The hatched bars indicate jury verdicts in favor of the patient. The gray bars indicate a settlement before trial, where no blame is assigned to the physician. When the length of diagnostic delay exceeds three months, verdicts in favor of the physician decline rapidly and plaintiff verdicts and settlements increase in number. After 6 months of diagnostic delay in cancer, the combination of settlements out of court and jury verdicts against the physician account for two thirds of the case decisions. (Data from Kern KA: Medicolegal analysis of the delayed diagnosis of cancer in 338 cases in the United States. Arch Surg 129:397-404, 1994. Copyright 1992–94, American Medical Association. With permission.)*

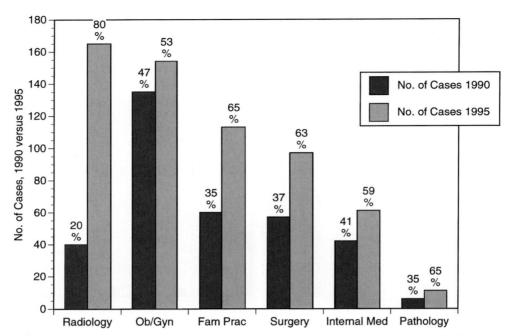

Figure 94–11 *Comparative distribution of specialty training of physicians involved in the delayed diagnosis of breast cancer, derived from PIAA reports in 1990 compared with those of 1995. The black bars represent the distribution of specialties in the PIAA 1990 study; the gray bars represent the distribution in 1995. There is a marked increase in the number of radiologists named in lawsuits in the 5-year interval between studies. (Data derived from Physician Insurers Association of America. Breast Cancer Study 1990, 1995. PIAA, Washington, DC, 1990, 1995).*

lized at 52 percent (14/27). Grouped by 3-month intervals thereafter (10 to 12 months, 13 to 15 months, 16 to 18 months, 22 to 24 months, and over 25 months), the proportion of verdicts remained roughly the same. At greater than 25 months of diagnostic delay, the verdicts were 26 percent (7/27) for the defense, 33 percent (9/27) for the plaintiff, and 41 percent (11/27) for settlements out of court.

How juries view delays in diagnosis as negligent is a complex and incompletely understood process. Experimental research on jury decision-making has focused on criminal cases, and little is known about how juries in civil trials of medical negligence allocate liability among parties, or assess compensatory and punitive damages.[150] One theory, derived from basic research on human judgment, suggests that juries reach decisions through an information-integration model, in which evidence is mentally averaged until a decision threshold is reached.[7, 209] Thereafter, exact statistics are disregarded in favor of the mentally weighted average. This model best explains the decline in number of defense verdicts at 3 months and the stabilization of these verdicts after 6 months. Apparently, juries view 6 months of diagnostic delay as the threshold for negligent delay in diagnosis. Beyond this point, the length of diagnostic delay, or survival of the patient, appears to be irrelevant to the jury's final deliberation.

Specialty Training of Physicians

The specialty distribution of doctors involved in diagnostic delay from our 1992 study was obstetricians and gynecologists in 21 (50 percent) of 42 cases, fam-

ily practitioners in 15 (36 percent) of 42 cases, general surgeons in 12 (29 percent) of 42 cases, radiologists in four (10 percent) of 42 cases, and internists in two (5 percent) of 42 cases. The numbers of physicians involved in these 42 cases ranged from one through four in each case. The distribution of physicians involved in these cases was one physician in 27 cases, two physicians in 10 cases, three physicians in three cases, and four physicians in two cases.

A frequency distribution of the specialty training of physicians, created from data from two PIAA studies of the delayed diagnosis of breast cancer, is shown in Figure 94–11.[189, 191] This histogram compares two time periods, demonstrating a change in the specialty distribution of physicians involved in delayed diagnosis. In 1990, the three most frequently implicated physician specialties in the delayed diagnosis of breast cancer, in rank order, were obstetricians and gynecologists, family practitioners, and general surgeons. This distribution in 1990 was consistent with the author's findings, published in 1992. A re-assessment of data reported by the PIAA in 1995 showed that radiologists had increased in frequency of misdiagnosis from 20 percent of the total cases, to involvement in 80 percent of the cases. In 487 cases reported by the PIAA in 1995, 917 physicians were involved in delayed diagnosis. There was an average of two physicians involved in each case. The increase in radiologists involved in diagnostic delays between 1990 and 1995 suggests that more emphasis is being placed on mammographic interpretation of breast findings suggestive of cancer. When the diagnosis of detectable breast cancer is delayed, both the radiologist and other primary care providers to the patient might be named in any negligence lawsuit.

Diagnostic Work-ups Requested by Physicians

From the author's medicolegal studies in 1992 and 1994,[122, 127] it was determined that the diagnostic work-up of patients sustaining misdiagnosis was largely inadequate, reflecting the mistaken idea that these young women with breast masses could not have breast cancer. For example, 51 percent (23/45) of patients in our 1992 study had no work-up of breast masses beyond visual observation and physical examination alone. Forty-four percent (20/45) of patients underwent mammography. Of the 20 mammograms performed, 80 percent (16/20) of the results were read as normal, despite the presence of a malignant breast mass. Only one patient (2 percent) underwent fine needle aspiration biopsy, but this patient sustained a false-negative result, leading to a diagnostic delay. No patients underwent ultrasonographic evaluation.

In the following section, the clinical scenarios leading to these inadequate work-ups of symptomatic breast disease are presented.

Clinical Scenarios Leading to the Delayed Diagnosis of Breast Cancer by Physicians

There are several well-recognized clinical scenarios that lead to delays in diagnosis on the part of physicians. Table 94–10 lists these factors leading to a delay in diagnosis on the part of a physician.

Triad of Error for Delay in Diagnosis of Breast Cancer

In several previous publications the author has proposed that women are at highest risk to sustain a delayed diagnosis of breast cancer when they fulfill these three criteria: (1) they are age 45 or younger,

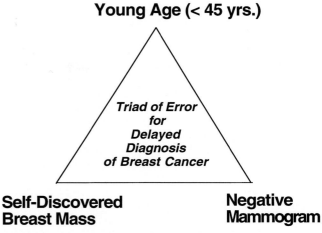

Figure 94–12 *The "triad of error" for misdiagnosed breast cancer describes women at the highest risk for a delayed diagnosis of breast cancer. The three legs of the triad are (1) women under age 45, with (2) a self-discovered breast mass, and (3) a negative mammogram. Women who fulfill these criteria account for over two thirds of patients sustaining the delayed diagnosis of breast cancer.*

(2) they present to their doctor with a self-discovered breast mass, and (3) they undergo diagnostic mammography, resulting in a false-negative study because it will not image their breast mass.[122, 123, 126–132, 134, 137] To help clinicians remember these elements, the author named them the Triad of Error for misdiagnosed breast cancer, succinctly stated as young age, self-discovered breast mass, and negative mammogram (illustrated in Fig. 94–12).[129] Patients who harbor the triad are the subjects of misdiagnosis in over three quarters of cases. These patients are believed to be too young to develop breast cancer, and their mammograms, if obtained, are frequently read as negative, despite the presence of a breast mass. An analysis of actual medical malpractice litigation reveals that physicians are lulled into the misdiagnosis of breast cancer by the young age of patients, not by vague findings or difficult diagnostic situations. Data from medicolegal studies show that in over 80 percent of misdiagnosed breast cancers, a physical finding clearly compatible with breast cancer is present. Because of the relative youth of these patients, physicians are not aggressive in pursuing a diagnosis, often believing a negative mammogram is sufficient proof of benign disease, even in the presence of a breast lump. This is the clinical situation leading to the delayed diagnosis of breast cancer and subsequent cases of medical malpractice. Much of the evidence for this triad of error comes from the author's own studies of the delayed diagnosis of breast cancer and its attendant malpractice litigation. Medicolegal data were analyzed from several perspectives, including a clinical,[122, 127] historical,[128] and risk prevention viewpoint.[129, 132] The following paragraphs evaluate each of the legs of the triad individually.

Young Age

Most patients with the delayed diagnosis of breast cancer are young, with a median age of 42 years.[59, 122, 127]

TABLE 94–10.   CLINICAL SCENARIOS LEADING TO PHYSICIAN-ASSOCIATED DELAYS IN DIAGNOSIS OF BREAST CANCER

"Triad of error" for misdiagnosis
  Young age
  Self-discovered breast mass
  Negative mammogram
Pregnancy-associated breast cancer
Male breast cancer
Fine needle aspiration biopsies
Miscellaneous
  Paget's disease of breast
  Carcinomas arising near old surgical scar
  Lobular invasive cancer
  Post-augmentation mammoplasty with silicone gel
    breast implants
  Surgical biopsy errors during needle-localization
    excisional biopsy

In the author's previous 20-year review of the delayed diagnosis of breast cancer,[122] 45 cases of breast cancer malpractice litigation tried in the U.S. Federal and state civil court system between 1971 and 1990 were critically analyzed. In 21 cases in which a patient's age could be identified, the patients were young, with a mean age of 40 years (age range, 22 through 59 years). When cases were grouped by 10-year intervals, the ages of these patients were as follows: four (19 percent) were aged 20 to 29 years; eight (39 percent), 30 to 39 years; five (30 percent), 40 to 49 years; and four (19 percent) were aged 50 to 59 years. Of the patients with known ages, four (19 percent) were younger than age 29; 11 (52 percent), younger than age 39; 16 (76 percent), younger than age 49; and all patients were younger than age 59. The menopausal status of the patients was identified in 25 (55.5 percent) of cases. These results confirmed the youthfulness of the group. Of these 25 women, 68 percent were hormonally active, 15 (60 percent) were known to be premenopausal, and 2 (8 percent) were pregnant. Postmenopausal women made up five (11.1 percent) members of the group. The PIAA 1995 Breast Cancer Study[191] noted the average age of misdiagnosed patients was 46 years, an increase of 2 years over the average age of 44 years reported in their previous 5-year study.[189] A comparison of the frequency distribution of the ages of the patients in the two studies is shown in Figure 94–13, demonstrating a shift toward slightly older patients sustaining misdiagnosed breast cancer.

Perhaps the most important finding from the author's study was that the misdiagnosed breast cancer patient is 20 years younger than the median age of 63 years for breast cancer patients in the SEER data base of the National Cancer Institute.[127] The same finding holds true for other types of misdiagnosed cancer as well. Figure 94–14 illustrates the age differential in misdiagnosed cancer patients from our study of delayed diagnosis in 13 different organ sites. For all organ sites, a delayed diagnosis occurred in patients at a younger age than the typical age of presentation in the SEER population. The difference in median ages between diagnostic delays and the SEER data base ranged from 8 to 27 years. On average, patients with diagnostic delays were younger than SEER patients by 16.2 years (S.E., 2 years).

The author refers to the age differential in misdiagnosed cancer as a "litigation gap" rather than an age gap, because the young age of cancer patients, in general, leads to delays in biopsy and radiographic diagnosis, leading to malpractice litigation. Other studies have confirmed the author's findings of young ages in misdiagnosed cancer patients. Diercks and Cady also confirmed a median age of 42 years for 57 patients in Massachusetts sustaining delays in diagnosis of breast cancer.[59] Max and Klamer[162] studied 120 women with breast cancer younger than age 35. In this group of women with a mean age of 31 years, 9.1 percent were pregnant or lactating. Delays in diagnosis were common: In 7 percent of patients, physicians delayed more than 2 months before recommending a biopsy. In this study, 61 percent presented with a painless lump; mammography was done in 61 percent of patients, and in 52 percent of this group, mammography was negative; in 11 percent it was equivocal and did not lead to biopsy. Pregnancy-associated delays in diagnosis are discussed more completely later but are mentioned here to emphasize the importance of young age as a cause of misdiagnosis. The average age of pregnant patients with breast cancer is 32 to 38 years, but such patients can be extremely young and have been described as young as 16 to 18 years of age.[82] This is in contrast to nonpregnant patients, in whom breast cancer under age 20 to 25 is extremely rare. Hein and associates[105] in a series of 95 adolescent females showed no breast cancers in these women with an average age of 15.9 years (range 12 to 20 years).

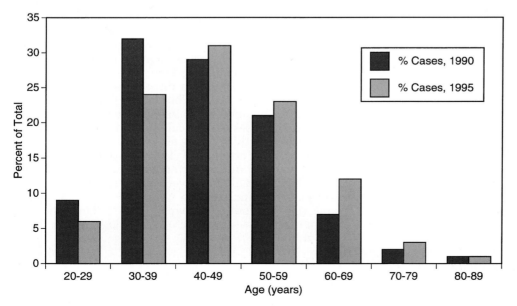

Figure 94–13 *Histogram comparing the ages of patients, by 10-year intervals, who sustained the delayed diagnosis of breast cancer in studies by the PIAA in 1990 (black bars) compared with ages of patients in 1995 (gray bars). The average age of patients in 1990 was 44 years, whereas in 1995, the average age of a misdiagnosed patient was 46 years. (Data derived from (Physician Insurers Association of America: Breast Cancer Study 1990, 1995. PIAA, Washington, DC, 1990, 1995).*

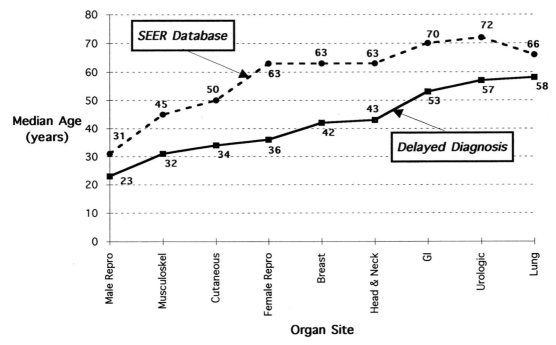

Figure 94–14 *Line chart comparing the ages of patients with misdiagnosed cancer in nine organ sites with the median age of patients presenting with cancer derived from the SEER (Surveillance, Epidemiology, and End-Results Reporting Program of the National Cancer Institute) data base. Patients receiving a delayed diagnosis of cancer are younger than the median age for cancer in the SEER population, by intervals ranging from a minimum of 8 years (male reproductive cancer) to a maximum of 27 years (female reproductive cancer). For the delayed diagnosis of breast cancer, the difference in age between those misdiagnosed and the SEER population is 21 years. This age differential is called a litigation gap because it is the most common cause of misdiagnosis leading to malpractice litigation. (From Kern KA: The anatomy of surgical malpractice claims. Bulletin American College of Surgeons 80:34–49, 1995. With permission.)*

However, two cases of cystosarcoma phylloides were noted.

The young age of patients with the delayed diagnosis of cancer is a unique aspect of misdiagnosis and negligence litigation in malignant disease. Generally, it is the elderly who are more likely to sustain negligence-related, adverse events. In one study, patients over age 64 were twice as likely to experience legally compensible complications during hospitalization as patients younger than age 45.[143] Many physicians are unaware that nearly one quarter of all breast cancer deaths occur in women whose age is not usually associated with the presence of breast cancer. Two percent of breast cancers occur in women between the ages of 15 and 34; 10 percent occur under age 40, and 21 percent of breast cancers occur in women between the ages of 35 and 54 years.[26, 35, 47] A recent study of rates of breast cancer in women 30 years of age or younger with breast masses found the incidence of cancer was 2.5 percent.[183] McWhirter[165] calculated that each general practitioner in England is likely to see a case of breast cancer in women under age 40 only once in every 15 years of his working life.

Self-Discovered Breast Mass

Palpable masses are frequently present in misdiagnosed younger women with breast cancer. As outlined in Table 94–11, in the author's civil court analysis of 45 cases of misdiagnosed breast cancer,[122] definite

physical findings were present in 82 percent (37/45) and included the following: painless mass, 64 percent (29/39); painful mass, 9 percent (4/45); nipple discharge (bloody or green) or rash, 6 percent (3/45).

TABLE 94–11. **PRESENTATION OF 45 PATIENTS WITH DELAY IN DIAGNOSIS OF BREAST CANCER (U.S. CIVIL LITIGATION SURVEY)**

	Number of Cases	Percent
Person who discovered lesion		
Patient	37	82.2
Physician	6	13.3
Incidental discovery	2	4.4
Total	45	100
Signs and symptoms		
Painless mass	29	64
Painful mass	4	9
Asymmetrical nodularity	6	13
Total	39	100
Other		
Bloody nipple discharge	1	2.2
Green-tinged nipple discharge	1	2.2
Eczematous nipple rash	1	2.2
Mastalgia	1	2.2
Incidental mammographic finding	1	2.2
Incidental chest radiographic finding	1	2.2
Total	45	100

From Kern KA. Causes of breast cancer malpractice litigation. A 20-year civil court review. Arch Surg 127:542–547, 1992. Copyright 1992–1994, American Medical Association. Reprinted with permission.

Thus, 73 percent of misdiagnosed breast cancer patients presented with a self-discovered breast mass.[122] The author confirmed this finding in a larger series of 127 breast cancer cases, in which 61 percent of patients presented with a breast mass.[127] In the 1990 PIAA study of misdiagnosed breast cancer,[189] the findings at physical diagnosis were reported. In 273 cases, 62.1 percent (159/273) presented with a mass without palpable axillary nodes and 9.8 percent (25/273) presented with a mass and palpable nodes. Thus, 72 percent of patients with delayed diagnosis of breast cancer originally presented to a physician with a self-discovered breast mass. Abnormal physical findings exclusive of breast masses were present in a smaller percentage of patients: 5.9 percent (15/273) presented with bleeding or nipple discharge, 3.5 percent (9/273) presented with palpable axillary nodes only, and only 16 percent (41/273) presented with no physical findings. Summing these figures, 81.3 percent (208/273) of patients presented with a physical finding compatible with breast cancer. In these litigated cases, only 72.9 percent (199/273) of patients received a mammogram, only 19.8 percent (54/273) underwent a fine needle biopsy or aspiration, and only 2.9 percent (8/273) received an ultrasound examination. These studies show that a physical abnormality was detected and was documented by physicians on initial presentation in over three quarters of patients sustaining the delayed diagnosis of breast cancer.

Unfortunately, the physical abnormalities detected initially in patients with misdiagnosed breast cancer are misinterpreted as benign disease, largely because further work-ups of these breast abnormalities are either inadequate (relying solely on mammography) or not performed at all. In this author's opinion, the standard of care in breast diagnosis dictates that isolated, dominant, and solid masses of the breast in women older than age 25 receive a cytologic or histological diagnosis (by fine needle aspiration biopsy, or open excisional biopsy). Such lesions cannot be accurately diagnosed by visual observation, physical examination, or even mammography alone. Unfortunately, before the definitive diagnosis of breast cancer is made in misdiagnosed patients, a benign label is applied to their breast condition, without attempts to obtain a histological diagnosis. In 1992, we reported the pre-diagnostic labels for 29 cases of misdiagnosed breast cancer.[122] The benign labels were as follows: Fibrocystic disease was diagnosed in nine cases, a simple or premenstrual cyst was diagnosed in four cases, abnormal milk gland or galactocele was diagnosed in four cases, mastitis was diagnosed in four cases, a "hormonal" mass was diagnosed in four cases, and an intraductal papilloma was diagnosed in four cases. None of these diagnoses were confirmed by the results of biopsy. These conditions and their percentage distributions are listed in tabular form in Table 94–12.

Other studies have confirmed that palpable breast lesions presenting as isolated breast lumps are misdiagnosed frequently. Nichols and colleagues,[178] in a

TABLE 94–12. INITIAL MISDIAGNOSIS IN 29 CASES OF MISDIAGNOSED BREAST CANCER (U.S. CIVIL LITIGATION SURVEY)

Misdiagnosis	Number (%) of Cases
Fibrocystic disease	9 (30)
Simple or premenstrual cyst	4 (14)
Galactocele or abnormal milk gland	4 (14)
Mastitis	4 (14)
Hormonal mass	4 (14)
Intraductal papilloma	4 (14)
Total	29 (100)

Table created from data compiled in Kern KA: Causes of breast cancer malpractice litigation. A 20-year civil court review. Arch Surg 127:542–547, 1992.

study of the National Health Service and breast cancer evaluation, reported that 25 out of 57 women with discrete lumps were not referred immediately for evaluation. Many errors are due to the initial inability of a physician to palpate a mass detected by the patient. Deschenes and coworkers[56] reported the high frequency of mislabeling of breast cancers in middle-aged women as benign fibroadenomas. Reintgen and associates studied the threshold of physical detection of breast cancers.[196] From a study of 509 breast cancers at a university breast clinic, they determined the following: (1) the threshold of clinically detected breast cancer is 5 mm, (2) the median detection limit (50 percent of cancers detected) occurs at 11 mm, and (3) experienced clinicians do not detect the majority (i.e., over 80 percent) of breast cancers until the cancer is larger than 16 mm. Because the absolute threshold of detection of breast cancer by patients has never been specifically evaluated, one explanation for physician error in physical examination is simply that patients can detect breast masses at smaller sizes than physicians can.[37]

False-Negative Mammogram

The role of diagnostic mammography in women with symptomatic breast disease is a subject of controversy because it has been linked to the creation of diagnostic delays by physicians. This chapter does not address the issue of screening mammography in asymptomatic women, which has been shown through seven clinical studies (three randomized, three case-control, and one quasiexperimental study) to improve survival in women older than age 50 and perhaps those younger as well.[36, 166, 228] Instead, this section addresses the question of failure to image symptomatic or palpable breast cancers.

Errors in reading mammograms include technical errors in 5 percent, observer errors in 30 percent, and nonimaging of breast tumors because of dense or dysplastic breast parenchyma.[28] Nonimaging because of dense or dysplastic breast parenchyma is an age-related phenomenon and the greatest cause of mammographically associated delays in diagnosis.[59, 122, 127, 189, 191] In the majority of cases, diagnostic delays in women with symptomatic breast cancer are a result of false reassurance to physicians that the mammogram does not show breast cancer (i.e., false-negative mammography). Although the threshold size for detection of breast cancer (the minimum size required to consistently see the lesion) is thought to be approximately 2.3 to 2.6 mm,[28, 224] this applies to women with optimal breast tissue for imaging, which occurs in women generally older than age 50. For those women younger than age 50, the threshold size of tumor visualization may be considerably greater; it may not be reached until 2 cm or greater, particularly in the youngest of women. Thus, despite the presence of an obvious breast mass, the mammogram may show nothing suspicious. In such women, the cancer may have grown to a size allowing metastasis long before it can be imaged by modern mammography. By the time a tumor has reached only 2 mm in size, it contains 4 million cells and has undergone 22 net cell doublings. Tumor angiogenesis, a mandatory process before metastases can reach the systemic circulation, is thought to occur much earlier, at 13 net cell doublings or 0.3 mm in size.[221, 223] Tumor size alone, however, is not the sole determinant of metastases. The role of histological determinants of prognosis and the future role of molecular genetic determinants of metastases remain central to any discussion regarding the timing of metastatic spread of disease.[182] As yet, our understanding of the interaction between tumor growth, local nodal spread, and systemic spread of metastases is incomplete.

The high frequency of false-negative mammograms in middle-aged women with breast masses is unappreciated by many physicians. Although the false-negative rate for mammography is generally reported as being 7 to 20 percent,[122, 127] this figure applies to women older than age 50; the actual false-negative rate increases greatly in younger women. For example, the false-negative rate of mammography approaches 80 percent in the author's studies[122, 127] and other studies of the delayed diagnosis of breast cancer, in which the average age of women is 42 to 45 years.[59] In the 1995 PIAA study of breast cancer lawsuits, 407 patients underwent diagnostic mammography to evaluate a palpable breast lesion. In 70 percent of cases, the results of diagnostic mammography were false negative and did not incite further diagnostic efforts: Mammograms were negative in 49.2 percent (96/273) and equivocal in 19 percent (37/273). Thus, a breast mass was documented by physicians on initial presentation in almost three quarters of patients. However, evaluation by physicians rarely proceeded beyond a negative mammogram, resulting in the delayed diagnosis of breast cancer.[191]

In another study of women younger than age 30 with an isolated breast mass, 74 percent of these masses did not produce an image on mammography.[123] In the Breast Cancer Detection and Demonstration Project involving 280,000 women, patients aged 40 with breast cancer sustained false-negative

mammography in 36 percent of cases, compared with 9 percent of cases in women 75 years old.[128, 129] Woods reported the average age of those with palpable breast lesions and false-negative mammograms was 44 years. This was significantly less than the average age of those with positive mammograms of 57 years.[245] Mann and associates[159] reported on 36 women with palpable breast cancer and false-negative mammography. The average age of patients was 45 years. The subsequent delays in diagnosis ranged from 3 to 24 months. Mann noted that 52 percent of women less than 45 years of age had normal mammograms despite a malignant breast mass. Bennett[17] reported a false-negative mammography rate in 227 women with symptomatic breast cancer of 24 percent (8/33 cancers). The reported delay caused by false-negative mammography was 8 months. Max and Klamer[162] noted that 52 percent of mammograms were false negative in women younger than age 35 with palpable breast cancers. Walker[236, 237] noted a false-negative rate of 30.7 percent in a group of 230 women with a median age of 50 years. The false-negative report led to a mean treatment delay of 12.7 months, ranging between 3 and 60 months. Joensuu[117] reported that the false-negative rate in women under 50 was 35 percent in a study of 306 women with invasive cancer. This was significantly different than the rate of 13 percent in women over age 50 ($p < .0001$). In those with a false-negative mammogram, 30 percent had delays of 6 months or more. For those with true-positive mammograms, no patients were delayed 6 months.

Others have reported that false-negative mammography is frequent in middle-aged women.[167, 168] Thus, the woman with a breast mass who is 45 years old or younger faces two perils in the diagnostic process: First, physicians assume she is too young to have breast cancer, and second, mammograms may not provide useful diagnostic information about the mass. Kern reported that of the 44 percent of patients (20/45) who underwent mammography, studies were negative in 80 percent (16/20). Only one patient (2 percent) underwent fine needle aspiration of a breast mass, which proved to be false negative.[122] As in palpable masses, the reason for false-negative mammography related to the increased breast density of younger women, which makes x-ray penetration more difficult.[44]

The impact of false-negative mammograms on delay in diagnosis was studied by Burns and colleagues.[29] In a group of 80 women with negative mammograms, 63 percent (50) presented with palpable breast masses. The negative mammogram resulted in a delay in diagnosis in this group of 1 month to 5.4 years; it averaged 11 months. Burns and associates pointed out the irony that although women were being urged to learn breast self-examination and that over 80% of breast cancers are found on palpation by the patient herself, false-negative mammography was creating delays in diagnosis after patients presented to a physician with a breast mass. Others have also noted the curious anomaly that the introduction of mammography into clinical practice as a technique for the early detection of asymptomatic breast cancer has resulted in delayed diagnosis because of its widespread use as a diagnostic tool in symptomatic women. Max and Klamer[162] noted in a study of 120 women with breast cancer with an average age of 31 years (range 22 to 35 years), that in 7 percent of women who contacted a physician immediately after the onset of symptoms, the physician delayed for more than 2 months before recommending biopsy. Locklear and Langlands[146] noted that in a study of 735 women with breast cancer, 13 percent had false-negative mammograms, resulting a diagnostic delay of 11.2 months, ranging from 2.5 to 48 months. Age played a significant role in the rate of false-negative mammography: Seventy-three percent of women with false-negative mammograms were premenopausal, compared with 38% premenopausal women in the no-delay group.

Others have reported that delays in diagnosis occur in almost 50 percent of premenopausal women because of false-negative mammography.[159] Although some authors have argued that it would take 80 biopsies of benign palpable lesions in this age group to detect four misdiagnosed breast cancers,[146] this author believes it unlikely that patients will accept these probabilistic arguments as a reason not to seek a timely diagnosis of mammographic abnormalities. Katz and coworkers[119] reported that in a series of women in British Columbia and Washington State, the preponderance of diagnostic delays was due to nonsuspicious, false-negative mammograms. Tennvall and colleagues[230] demonstrated that women with both negative or inconclusive mammograms and negative fine needle aspiration cytology of palpable breast masses were found to be 11 years younger that the group with combined positive findings. In these young patients, negative cytology and negative mammography led to extended diagnostic delays. Delays in diagnosis, even when the end result is benign, can have significant adverse psychological impact on patients.[72]

The high rate of false-negative mammograms in young women have led some to recommend that it not be used in symptomatic women.[137, 158] Mahoney and Csima[158] studied 302 women with breast cancer and found 87 or 29 percent had false-negative mammograms. Mahoney noted that mammography is most productive when used as a routine screening study in women older than age 50 with clinically normal breasts. These workers noted that 53 percent of palpable breast cancers did not image in women younger than age 45. The mean age for a false-negative mammogram with a palpable breast cancer was 49.3 years; for a positive mammogram with a palpable cancer, it was 58 years. The mean size for a negative mammogram was 2.1 cm, and for a positive mammogram, it was 3.3 cm. Mahoney recommended three rules related to mammography and breast cancer: (1) use mammography as a screening study in older women with normal breasts, (2) never delay biopsy of a breast lump that is solid on aspiration

because of a negative mammogram, and (3) mammography in symptomatic women younger than age 35 is unrewarding and should not be used.

Woods and coworkers[245] reviewed 1433 consecutive patients undergoing mammography and found a false-negative rate in those with palpable abnormalities of 30 percent. In 16 percent of these patients, the false reassurance of mammography directly contributed to diagnostic delays ranging from 2 to 24 months. Langlands and Tiver[140] used a statistical argument to show that the use of diagnostic mammography in women with a palpable breast lesion of any age is inappropriate for two reasons: (1) the low probability of imaging the lesion in the young, and (2) and the inability to make definitive statements about a cancer diagnosis without a confirmatory biopsy, even in older women. In this series, diagnostic delays due to false-negative mammography ranged from 2 months to 3 years.

Some authors have disputed the rate of false-negative mammography. Cregan and coworkers[50] studied the extent of delay in 219 women and found that only 11 percent of women had false-negative mammography. This led to a delay in diagnosis of 1 to 3 months in 10 percent of women (3/32 cases). These authors pointed to the value of mammography in women as young as 25 (in whom early signs of familial cancer may be detected, such as irregular, clustered microcalcifications), especially in those with a family history of breast cancer in which early onset is the rule. Bassett and associates[15] argued for a tailored mammographic examination in women younger than age 35 with localized breast symptoms, particularly those without a palpable lump. In a study of 1016 women younger than age 35 with breast cancer, Bassett evaluated a group of 454 women with palpable breast masses. He noted that two women sustained delays of 4 months and 10 months because mammograms did not image palpable lesions of 2 cm and 1.5 cm, and these lesions were labeled as fibroadenomas without biopsy confirmation. In terms of nonlump symptoms in a group of 53 patients, one 34-year-old patient with localized breast tenderness was diagnosed with architectural distortion on tailored mammogram, leading to an immediate breast biopsy and cancer diagnosis. One 26-year-old patient with unilateral discharge had a negative mammogram and sustained a delay of 6 weeks before biopsy. Based on these results, Bassett reminded readers that a negative mammogram should not preclude biopsy of a palpable, solid mass. Blichert-Toft and coworkers,[18] in a series of 167 patients in a Danish breast clinic, showed that immediate work-up of vague symptoms or unilateral palpable findings by needle aspiration biopsy or open biopsy prevented delayed diagnosis, despite false-negative mammograms in eight patients (5 percent).

Screening mammograms that show highly suspicious lesions in younger women with no palpable breast abnormalities may diagnose breast cancer with great accuracy, and with a detection rate as high as 40 percent.[96] However, when mammograms are read as nondiagnostic, indeterminate, or not suspicious, the rate of missed cancers approaches 5 percent (6/127).[96] Erickson and colleagues[68] showed that 2 percent of patients observed because of an indeterminate mammogram, without the presence of symptoms, were later diagnosed with cancer. Three patients out of the study group of 114 women sustained delays of 3, 12, and 15 months. Nonetheless, with an average delay of 10 months, patients had no progression in stage, as measured by the rate of positive axillary nodes.

Delays Related to Pregnancy-Associated (Gestational) Breast Cancer

Although only 1 to 2 percent of cases of breast cancer overall are diagnosed during pregnancy,[61, 62, 111] the number of pregnancies that are complicated by breast cancer ranges from 0.03 percent[111] to 3.1 percent for women in the childbearing age group of 15 to 45 years.[61, 62] Others have estimated the rate of gestational breast cancer to be between 1 case per 1360 deliveries[54] and 1 case per 6200 deliveries.[23] Donegan has provided a table of age-specific frequency[61, 62] that demonstrates a rate for women in the United States during 1970 as having gestational breast cancer ranging between 0.25 to 2.0 cases per 100,000. As cited by Scott-Connor,[213] other reviewers have placed this rate at 10 to 39 gestational breast cancers per 100,000 women. Because there are approximately 3.4 million live births in the United States annually,[229] the author estimates the number of gestational breast cancers to range between 350 to 1400 cases yearly. Because the average obstetrician manages between 150 to 250 pregnant women yearly, the frequency of an obstetrician seeing gestational breast cancer in any one practice will be extremely low. A large multiphysician group that delivers over 3000 babies yearly might expect to see one to three cases of gestational breast cancer each year. Because of its rarity, it is important for clinicians managing pregnant women to understand the potential for pregnancy and breast cancer. Special attention should be given to high-risk groups, such as women in breast cancer–prone families, who may develop gestational breast cancer.

Because the incidence of gestational breast cancer in clinical practice is low, diagnostic delays are the rule. In the 1950s, McWhirter[165] pointed out that pregnant patients were frequently given wrong advice when presenting with a breast mass. Instead of being advised to undergo diagnostic biopsy, they were often asked to do what McWhirter believed were potentially harmful maneuvers such as massaging the lump or applying a poultice. As noted by Bottles and Taylor,[23] delayed diagnosis in gestational pregnancy presents a paradox, because pregnant patients are seen many more times than usual by physicians compared with nonpregnant patients. In 1958, Treaves and Holleb[231] reported from a study of 108 patients with gestational breast cancer that the median delay in diagnosis in pregnant woman was 4 months, which was twice as long as nonpregnant women. In one report, 50 percent of gestational breast cancers were not diagnosed until 3 weeks after delivery.[229] Petrek has shown that less than 20 percent of patients with gestational breast cancer were diagnosed during pregnancy.[186, 187] Others have shown that the duration of symptomatic breast cancer before diagnosis in pregnant women ranges between 2 and 15 months.* Byrd and coworkers noted that two thirds of women with a breast cancer first detected during pregnancy were advised to defer biopsy until after delivery, on the incorrect assumption that their breast masses were benign.[32] Supporting this finding, Donegan has shown that only one third of pregnant women are admitted to the hospital for definite treatment of breast cancer within 6 months of discovery of a breast mass.[61] Donegan also determined that the delay in diagnosis of breast cancer in pregnant women averages 13 months. Deemarsky and associates confirmed that the delay in diagnosis of breast cancer in pregnant women ranges between 11 and 15 months.[54] Gallenberg and Loprinzi[82] noted that delays in diagnosis of breast cancer generally exceed 5 months. Treves and Holleb[231] reported that physicians watched an abnormal breast mass for an average of 2 months longer than they normally would in nonpregnant patients.

Advanced, late stage breast tumors are often finally diagnosed in gestational breast cancer. This finding of late disease has been attributed to delay in diagnosis, largely by physicians.[186, 187, 238, 242, 246] Zinns[248] concluded that delay in diagnosis is "the most significant, controllable factor in the patient's prognosis." Westberg[242] stated that "it would seem thus that pregnancy has no very great effect on prognosis of breast cancer, apart from the fact that patients delay in consulting a doctor, and the doctor is inclined to postpone surgery." Many other authors believe delay in diagnosis is the sole factor accounting for the diminished survival of pregnant patients with breast cancer,[246] because stage-for-stage, survival is equivalent in the two groups.[116, 161, 185–187, 213, 235] Opposing the idea that delay is solely responsible for late-stage tumors, other authors cite the unfavorable biological factors favoring rapid tumor growth and early dissemination in gestational breast cancer, such as the high nutrient hormone levels and relatively low host immunity during pregnancy.[186, 187, 238]

Barnavon and Wallack[13] used a comprehensive review of the world literature to demonstrate that, regardless of diagnostic delay, pregnant patients with breast cancer fare worse overall than their nonpregnant, premenopausal counterparts. Typically, gestational breast cancers are large, with the median size in one study of 3.5 cm.[186, 187, 229] Gestational breast cancers are often associated with positive axillary nodes; up to 70% to 89% of patients are node positive.[89, 111, 198] Byrd and colleagues[32] reported that pregnant patients with involved axillary lymph nodes had a longer delay from first symptom to definite

---

*See references 10, 13, 23, 54, 111, 186, 187, and 242.

diagnosis nearly twice that of nonpregnant patients (7.4 months versus 3.1 months). Guinee and coworkers[89] have shown that the odds ratio of a pregnant patient dying of breast cancer is threefold that of a woman with breast cancer who has never been pregnant.

Given the high risk for misdiagnosis of gestational breast cancer, the use of fine needle biopsy has been advocated to diagnose any dominant or suspicious breast abnormality in the pregnant or lactating woman,[23, 213] particularly when it is believed to be different than usual by the patient. Cytologic atypia should be followed by open breast biopsy, because such features suggest breast cancer and are not caused by pregnancy.[179] Open breast biopsy is safe when performed under local anesthesia and should not be delayed in the pregnant woman with an isolated, dominant mass that has either clinically suspicious characteristics or has been needle aspirated and found to contain cytologic atypia, an indeterminate diagnosis, or frank cancer.

Delays in Diagnosis Related to Male Breast Cancer

Delays in the diagnosis of male breast cancer are common.[165, 219, 226] In males, more advanced stages of disease are present at final diagnosis,[24, 44, 45, 219, 226] and this is hypothesized to be due to a combination of delay in diagnosis and anatomical factors. In males, there is less intervening tissue between breast, skin, and chest wall. Bounds and colleagues[24] noted that only 1 percent of cases of breast cancer is due to male breast cancer. Of all male cancers, only 0.2 percent are due to breast cancer.[219] The incidence of male breast carcinoma in the United States is 1 per 100,000, nearly 150 to 200 times less frequent than breast cancer in females. The median age of patients has been reported to vary between 63 years[226] and 70 years. Because of its infrequent nature and presentation in elderly patients who often exhibit typical senile gynecomastia, delays in diagnosis by doctors (and delayed recognition of symptoms by patients) are common.[45, 226] This is believed to be one factor accounting for the percentage of patients with positive axillary nodes on diagnosis (50 percent) and metastatic disease (80 percent). Stierer and associates documented that the delay in diagnosis from first onset of symptoms and onset of therapy ranged from 1 week to 84 months, with a median delay of 3 months. Tumor size correlated with the median delay: Small T1 tumors had a median delay of 2 months, whereas large T3 and T4 tumors had a median delay of 10 months. Stierer and colleagues[226] believe that diagnostic delays are so common as to establish proof that early diagnosis is virtually never reached in male breast cancer.

Delays in Diagnosis Related to False-Negative Fine Needle Aspiration Biopsy

Fine needle aspiration (FNA) biopsy plays an important role in the rapid diagnosis of palpable breast masses and other palpable abnormalities of the breast. Although the test is operator dependent and may lead to false-positive interpretations if it is performed before ultrasonography,[227] it is still an indispensable tool for diagnosis. Svensson and associates[227] demonstrated the ability of FNA biopsy to diagnose malignant tumors in women as young as 20 years old, an age generally not recognized as prone to breast cancer development. In a series of over 3000 FNA biopsies, Gupta evaluated 691 women under age 30. The false-negative FNA rate was 0.4 percent (3/691).[89–91]

The introduction of FNA has been shown to decrease the rate of excisional biopsies in dedicated breast clinics.[16] However, FNA biopsy may be accompanied by false-negative studies. Giard and Hermans[83] reviewed 29 articles containing information on over 31,000 aspiration biopsies and could not determine a reproducible accuracy rate for FNA biopsy. Bates and colleagues[16] showed that a delay in diagnosis of more than 50 days occurred in 6.9 percent of a series of over 1000 women evaluated in a dedicated breast clinic in Great Britain. Although the rate of excisional biopsies fell by over 50 percent (from 238 to 110 annually), the rate of delayed diagnosis did not change over a 2-year interval. However, the group of patients affected by delay did change. In the interval before the initiation of FNA, the median age of delay was 47 years; after the introduction of FNA, the age of patients misdiagnosed dropped to a median of 40. The type of symptom changed from isolated breast mass to an area of asymmetrical thickening, which frequently resulted in nondiagnostic FNA biopsies. Thus, FNA biopsy has its best role in the diagnosis of isolated, dominant breast masses. The young patient with indefinite thickening of nodularity may need open biopsy despite negative FNA findings.

We believe that FNA biopsy should always be followed by total excisional biopsy to confirm the diagnosis before initiating therapy. In our 1992 study of 45 malpractice cases related to the delayed diagnosis of breast cancer, one patient who underwent FNA biopsy had a false-negative result. More recently, a jury trial in New York resulted in a $1.5 million verdict against a surgeon, pathologist, and internist for failure to diagnose breast cancer, based on an erroneous FNA biopsy. In this instance a 37-year-old homemaker with a breast mass underwent FNA biopsy, read incorrectly by a pathologist as benign. Because of this falsely negative report, the mass was not excised. Sixteen months later, the mass grew larger and excisional biopsy revealed invasive breast cancer. Despite mastectomy and chemotherapy, the patient died 33 months after initial misdiagnosis (*Smith v. Dutkewych*, No. 88-1980 [Madison Cty. Sup. Ct. N.Y. June 8, 1992]).

Miscellaneous Factors Leading to the Delayed Diagnosis of Breast Cancer

Several other conditions are typically associated with the delayed diagnosis of breast cancer. Paget's dis-

TABLE 94–13.   EXAMPLES OF CLINICAL SITUATIONS LEADING TO DELAYED DIAGNOSIS OF BREAST CANCER (U.S. CIVIL LITIGATION SURVEY)

Case Number	Clinical Factors	Patient Age (yr)	Length Delay (mo)
1	Hospital lost biopsy specimen on transport from operating room to pathology department	38	3
2	Breast mass palpated and documented by doctor, but subsequently overlooked during work-up of rectal bleeding	n/a	5
3	Breast mass noted on chest x-ray film, but no comment made, no follow-up requested	58	n/a
4	Bloody nipple drainage; no biopsy	n/a	7
5	Mass during pregnancy; patient died	n/a	3
6	Paget's disease of nipple; no biopsy	27	6
7	Breast mass grew while receiving estrogen replacement therapy; no biopsy	49	n/a
8	Breast thickening diagnosed as "normal"; no biopsy	22	18
9	Mass grew during pregnancy; patient died	30	6
10	Final diagnosis lobular carcinoma-in-situ and ductal carcinoma-in-situ, treated by mastectomy	47	18
11	Misread mammogram with lengthy delay	58	36

Modified from Kern KA: Causes of breast cancer malpractice litigation: A 20-year civil court review. Arch Surg 127:542–547, 1992. Copyright 1992–94, American Medical Association. With permission.

ease of nipple is frequently misdiagnosed as eczema, breast infection, or psoriasis.[94, 180, 210] Surgical biopsy errors, particularly needle localization biopsy in which the actual tumor mass is not identified on the follow-up mammogram, are potential risks for the surgeons. The failure to follow-up yearly and thereby detect metachronous breast cancer many years after initial therapy is also an error. In one study, delays in diagnosis of second metachronous breast cancers contributed to larger tumor sizes and more lymph node involvement.[205] Scar-associated breast cancer may present many years after a breast biopsy, and the surgeon mistakes the thickening of the tumor for the presumed thickening of the scar. FNA biopsy would prevent this dilemma. The potential problem for masking of breast cancers after silicone implant breast augmentation is a phenomenon being evaluated and prevented by displacement of the prosthesis on a screening mammogram,[65, 212, 216, 217] or by use of magnetic resonance imaging (MRI).[175]

A variety of additional situations leading to the delayed diagnosis of breast cancer, taken from actual civil litigation proceedings, is shown in Table 94–13.

INFLUENCE OF DELAYED DIAGNOSIS OF BREAST CANCER ON SURVIVAL

Medical liability in breast cancer diagnosis has its origin in the workers' compensation system begun in the early 1900s.[128] At that time, because of a limited understanding of cancer epidemiology based largely on anecdotes, trauma was thought to initiate cancer de novo. Based on this incorrect biological concept, the random association of workplace trauma with subsequent breast cancer was thought to be causally linked, a situation calling for compensible legal remedies. Later, with the maturation of scientific knowledge and the acceptance that breast cancer was a spontaneous cellular aberration and not associated with single episodes of acute, limited trauma, workers' compensation cases disappeared from the civil justice system. However, in their place arose cases alleging that a delayed diagnosis of breast cancer breached the standard of medical care because it led directly to injury through diagnostic delay itself; therefore, delayed diagnosis cases were equivalent to legally compensible injuries. Here, the biological basis of litigation rests on a theoretical but critically dependent relationship between the timing of diagnosis, cancer progression, and cancer metastases. Although much debate surrounds the workings and details of this theory, it lies at the core of the medicolegal controversy surrounding all liability in the delayed diagnosis of cancer.

The influence of a delayed diagnosis of breast cancer on prognosis, including staging and patient survival, has been the subject of study for over 60 years. The following section traces chronologically the influence of a delay in diagnosis on the prognosis and survival from breast cancer.

Historical Background to Importance of Early Diagnosis

The importance of rapidly diagnosing and treating breast cancer, once symptoms or signs are present (or preferably sooner), has long held an important role in the minds of clinicians. In the absence of a truly effective cure for breast cancer and in the presence of an unpredictable disease, contemporary medical philosophy holds that physicians must rely on an early diagnosis to deliver a better prognosis and better chance for cure. From this philosophy has arisen the public health basis for widespread mammographic screening for breast cancer.

Problems in achieving an early diagnosis of breast cancer have been debated for over 100 years. Halsted, presenting a paper before the American Surgical Association in 1907,[97, 98] noted that the diagnosis of breast cancer was a field considered to be a trite subject, with little of importance to be discussed. Halsted believed, however, that much could be contributed by the astute clinician. He proposed that the examiner spend up to an hour on the examination of difficult breast cases. He noted that women were presenting themselves more promptly, realizing that a cure of breast cancer was possible if they were operated upon early. Halsted emphasized that "the slightest delay [in diagnosis and treatment] is dangerous," noting that "the prognosis is quite good in the early stage of breast cancer, two in three being cured; and bad, three in four succumbing, when the axillary glands are demonstrably involved." Paradoxically, Halsted also noted that despite radical surgery and microscopically negative axillary lymph nodes, 23.4 percent of his patients died of metastatic breast cancer.

Halsted drew much of his philosophy and inspiration for understanding breast cancer from the British surgeon Handley. Handley published his treatise on cancer of the breast in 1906[63, 99] and argued that breast cancer was a local, diffusing disease of lymphatic tissue, advancing through tissues at different rates of spread. Rapid removal of this advancing front (much like the advancing front of a bacterial infection) would result in cure. Based on this reasoning, early diagnosis and treatment should provide the best chance for cure.

The role of early diagnosis and treatment was later questioned, however, by several investigators who proposed that breast cancer spreads by multiple pathways, and does so early in its course. Through the work of Gray,[88] Engell,[67] and the Fishers,[74, 75] the early embolic spread of breast cancer via blood-borne metastases became defined and experimentally proved as one of the most important routes of tumor spread.[63] Given the evidence for early occult tumor growth with rapid dissemination by tumor emboli from the time of angiogenic vascularization, some have proposed that breast cancer can no longer be thought of as strictly a local disease like skin cancer, permeating by local lymphatic spread to the rest of the body. Thus, many believe the aim of current breast cancer surgery should be essentially cytoreductive, reducing the primary tumor burden to allow host immunology,[79] systemically administered anticancer agents, or both, to destroy the breast cancer.[76, 77] The controversy surrounding the role of temporal delays in decreasing survival from breast cancer stems from this basic controversy of how mammary carcinoma grows and metastasizes: either (1) as a process that occurs late, mostly locally, and in a tissue-diffusing fashion; or (2) as a process that occurs early, acts systemically, and occurs through blood-borne tumor emboli. Further complicating the discussion is a third possibility, that different breast cancers may adopt partially or completely either of these two processes, or may switch between them during their cycle of growth.

Because of this persistent scientific controversy, contemporary thinking on the influence of delay on survival itself remains controversial. Numerous studies on the impact of diagnostic delay on survival may be cited to support the three positions on the effect of diagnostic delay on survival: (1) delays adversely effect survival, (2) delays have no effect on survival, or (3) delays result in an improvement in survival.

The basic premise of breast cancer treatment, as is the case for all types of cancer treatment, is that intervention and removal of the disease process prolongs survival. Bloom and colleagues[22] attempted to validate this hypothesis for breast cancer by comparing treatment outcomes to the survival of 356 untreated breast cancer patients, identified in hospital archives in England from 1805 to 1933. He found that treatment by radical or modified radical mastectomy, with or without radiotherapy, did indeed influence the length of survival for each of three grades of cancer (low, intermediate, and high grade). The median duration of life for untreated breast cancer patients, in his and other comparable studies, varied between 2.5 years for high-grade lesions, and 3.5 years for low-grade lesions. In contrast, treatment of primary breast cancer increased the median survival rate to 4.5 years for high-grade lesions, and to 11.5 years for low-grade lesions. The most striking difference between untreated breast cancer patients versus those who received mastectomy was noted in the highly malignant grade III tumors. Without therapy, no patients with high-grade tumors lived beyond 4.25 years. With therapy, some patients with high-grade lesions (approximately 10 percent) lived to 15 years.

For grade I tumors, Bloom and coworkers found that there was a marked increase in survival (300 percent) between the treated and untreated series. An interesting side note to these studies relates to the length of survival of a small proportion of the untreated patients with low-grade tumors. Despite the absence of any treatment, approximately 4 percent of the untreated patients with grade I lesions, or 14 patients, demonstrated survival surpassing 10 years. The longest survival of an untreated breast cancer patient with a low-grade lesion was 18 years and 3 months. In the 1920s, Daland[53] noted a similar long-term survival in untreated, low-grade breast cancer patients. From this standpoint, if untreated breast cancer is considered to be the ultimate example of the delayed diagnosis of breast cancer, then a small segment of breast cancer patients seem to withstand these delays with a limited (albeit negative) impact on surgery.

The question left incompletely answered, however, by studies that confirm that intervention in breast cancer improves survival, is the quantitative effect of the timing of intervention on prognosis. In other words, does intervening early in the disease process quantitatively improve length of survival? If so, by what quantity? And are all types of breast cancer equally affected? This is the central focus of any investigation into the delayed diagnosis of symptomatic breast cancer.

Unfortunately, the impact of delayed diagnosis on survival from cancer in general has remained controversial for over 60 years. The remaining discussion defines, in chronological order, studies on the impact of a delayed diagnosis of breast cancer. The first section reviews those studies that show an adverse effect of diagnostic delay on survival.

Studies Showing an Adverse Effect of Diagnostic Delay on Survival

In the 1930s, Luff[147] noted a progressive increase in mortality in a group of 1500 cases with delayed diagnosis of breast cancer derived from case files of the British Medical Association. Those cases with a delay of 1 to 3 months had a 4-year survival rate of 31 percent, compared with patients with delays of greater than 12 months, who had a survival rate of only 16 percent. Referring to this analysis, in 1950, Cade[33] stated that "the mortality of cancer of the breast in England and Wales could be reduced from 7000 yearly to 1000, if all cases were adequately treated in the first month of the appearance of the disease." Other investigators in the 1930s to 1940s confirmed the detrimental effect of a delayed diagnosis of breast cancer. Haagensen and Stout[92] reported on a series of patients from 1915 to 1934 and showed a 12 percent difference between those presenting within less than 1 month from discovery of symptoms compared with patients with a symptomatic intervals exceeding 6 months. Those presenting within 1 month had positive axillary metastases in 56.5 percent of cases compared with those with lengthier delays in which 68.8 percent of cases had positive axillary nodes. Hoopes and McGraw,[110] in the 1940s, found that the percentage of 5-year survivors after radical mastectomy decreased slightly with increased duration of symptoms before treatment. In a series of 240 patients undergoing the Halsted radical mastectomy, patients with negative axillary nodes and symptoms of 1 month or less had 5-year survival rates of 71.4 percent compared with a survival rate of 65.6 percent in those with delays exceeding 6 months. When axillary metastases were present, 5-year survival with delays of 1 month or less were 34.6 percent and dropped to 25.8 percent when delays exceeded 6 months. The number of patients with positive axillary nodes increased when delays in symptoms increased from less than 1 month (55 percent) to more than 6 months (63 percent).

During this same era, MacDonald (1942)[151] demonstrated that the highest rate of survival in a large series of breast cancer patients was found in those treated within 2 months of discovery of the tumor. Paradoxically, as delays exceeded 1 year, survivals began to increase. Eggers, de Cholnoky, and Jessup (1941)[64] confirmed these findings. They noted a 5-year survival rate of 76 percent for patients operated on within 1 month of symptoms compared with a 20 percent 5-year survival rate for delays of 1 to 2 years.

Yet, as delays increased beyond 2 to 3 years, survivals rose to 41 percent. In the 1950s, Smithers and associates[218] analyzed 846 English breast cancer patients and demonstrated a shift in anatomical staging dependent on the length of diagnostic delay. When patients had symptomatic intervals of less than 6 months, 64 percent were stage I or II, whereas when delays exceeded 12 months, only 32 percent were stage I or II; at more than 18 months, the percentage of early tumors dropped to 18 percent. The percentage of advanced stage III and IV tumors doubled as delays exceeded 12 months, from 31 percent (for delays less than 6 months) to 65 percent.

Robbins (1957) and Bross[202] evaluated the significance of diagnostic delay in 1281 patients undergoing radical mastectomy between 1940 and 1943. Later, Robbins and coworkers[201] compared results of the initial study with those of 2168 patients treated between 1950 and 1955. In the initial series, as delays in diagnosis increased from less than 1 month to more than 12 months in node-positive women, 5-year survival rates decreased from 55 percent to 30 percent. In node-negative patients, as delays increased to over 12 months, survival decreased from 88 percent to 70 percent. An analysis of variance was undertaken in patients who delayed more than 6 months, in an effort to determine the relative importance of several factors influencing survival. Three factors were found to account for 89 percent of the variance in the results between patients without diagnostic delay, and those delaying for more than 1 year: (1) spread to lymph nodes (62 percent of variance), (2) tumor size (23 percent of variance), and (3) delay in presentation (4 percent of variance).

Based on these data, Robbins reasoned that delay in diagnosis contributed to decreased survival but at a very low level of importance on a hierarchy of prognostic factors, as demonstrated by its minimal contribution to the variance in results. Using this same analysis of variance, Robbins demonstrated a correlation between delay in treatment and node involvement but at a nonstatistical level of significance. In patients who stated they delayed 1 month or less before surgery, 45.2 percent had negative nodes compared with patients who delayed one year or more, in which only 25 percent had negative nodes. This effect was only noted for level I and II nodes; there was no correlation between level III nodes and duration of symptoms. Robbins concluded that "We have not found any report offering any data on a preoperative clinical or laboratory procedure that will predict the growth rate of any specific breast cancer. Until such testing is available, it is important and imperative to institute definitive therapy with a minimum delay in all cases of proved operable cancer."

In 1959, Robbins and Bross[201] compared results of a similar study in women treated between 1950 and 1955. Patients in both groups reporting long delays had a 50 percent increase in the number of large cancers compared with those patients with shorter delays. However, based on an analysis of variance,

95 percent of the changes in stage appeared to be independent of the duration of pretreatment symptoms. At most, Robbins hypothesized that delay in presentation for treatment of cancer accounted for 5 percent of changes in clinical stage and survival. Robbins concluded that more could be gained from a search for asymptomatic lesions than by a drive for less delay in treatment. He believed that it would be easier to persuade patients and doctors alike to search for asymptomatic lesions through radiographic screening studies, because of reticence to change practice patterns, and because of emotional factors induced by cancer-related fears in patients.

In 1959, Waxman and Fitts[241] demonstrated a direct correlation between survival and length of diagnostic delays in a group of 740 patients. The 5-year survival rates of patients according to length of diagnostic delay were (1) delays of less than 1 month, 67 percent; (2) 1 to 2 months, 60 percent; (3) 3 to 5 months, 55.8 percent; (4) 6 to 9 months, 44.8 percent; and (5) more than a 10-month delay, 37.1 percent. Waxman and Fitts concluded that patients who reported cancer symptoms early had a better chance of survival. In a study of 549 patients younger than age 35, Treaves and Holleb (1958)[231] demonstrated that there was a loss of 7 percent in 5-year survival rate and an increase of 12 percent in axillary node positivity rate when delays in diagnosis increased from less than 1 month to more than 12 months. In a subset analysis of 116 patients seen within 6 months, the clinical 5-year cure rate was 42 percent and the positive axillary node rate was 58.3 percent. In 65 patients seen after 6 months of symptoms, the 5-year cure rate was 33.8 percent, and the incidence of metastatic disease to the axilla was 64 percent. Treaves and Holleb concluded that delays in diagnosis had an adverse impact on survival but only at a modest level of significance (5 to 10 percent).

In several important studies of the influence of delay in diagnosis on the natural history and prognosis of breast cancer, Bloom (1965)[20] demonstrated that delays decreased survival in grade I breast cancers and, to a lesser extent, in grade II tumors. High-grade breast cancers were not affected by delays in diagnosis of up to 3 years. In his study of 1411 cases from the Middlesex Hospital in London, England, 1200 cases were treated by radical mastectomy and followed for over 20 years. Overall, for all grades combined, Bloom demonstrated no difference in survival over 20 years for any length of diagnostic delay. Here, the distribution of tumor grades counterbalanced the influence of delay on survival. However, when Bloom categorized tumors by their degree of cellular differentiation, he demonstrated that patients with tumors of intermediate and low-grade histology may lose years of life because of diagnostic delay. Bloom was the first to demonstrate that the effect of delay on survival can be understood only when the degree of tumor differentiation is taken into account.[21] He therefore concluded that "early treatment must be the undoubted principle for all cases."

In 1970, Brightmore and associates[26] demonstrated that in a series of 101 women younger than age 35, 5-year overall survival rates were correlated with length of diagnostic delays. If delays were less than 1 month, the survival was 43 percent; for 3 to 7 months of delay, the survival was 26 percent, and for more than a 1 year delay, the survival was 22 percent. Delays in diagnosis may not completely explain the poorer survival of young women with breast cancer. Chung and coworkers[43] reported that women younger than age 40 have more advanced anatomical stages than their older counterparts. In an analysis of 3000 women with carcinoma of the breast in Rhode Island, the majority of women younger than age 40 had stage II lesions; this is in contrast to the usual finding that approximately one third of women overall present with stage II disease.*

In 1971, Anglem and Leber[8] studied a group of 47 patients treated by radical mastectomy, who had an extremely short duration of preoperative symptoms of 1 week or less. The 10-year survival rate for this group was 79 percent compared with a poorer survival rate for patients with a duration of symptoms of more than 1 week. Of patients dying within 5 years of diagnosis, only 6 percent had a short duration of symptoms of 1 week or less; 96 percent of those patients dying within 5 years had longer delays in diagnosis. Anglem and Leber concluded that these findings were a "natural argument" in support of the great importance of an early diagnosis of breast cancer.

Sheriden (1971) and colleagues[215] demonstrated that the effect of delayed diagnosis was stage dependent. Patients with stage I breast cancer had no effect on 5-year survival despite delays ranging from 1 week to over 6 months. Paradoxically, in stage I patients, survival was 74 percent for those with less than 4 weeks of delay but rose to 85 percent for patients with 6 to 9 months of delay. This improvement with increasing delay suggests that stage I tumors form a unique classification of tumor types, characterized by indolent and nonaggressive biological behavior. In contrast, the stage II tumors demonstrated a decreased 5-year survival rate with increasing intervals of diagnostic delay. When the treatment was less than 4 weeks from the first symptoms, the survival rate was 65.8 percent; at 5 to 12 weeks, it was 55.9 percent; at 3 to 6 months, it was 59.5 percent; and more than 9 months, it was 46.8 percent.

In 1973, Balachandra and associates[12] analyzed 5549 cases of radical mastectomy treated at Memorial Hospital between the years 1940 and 1965. These investigators determined delay in diagnosis from symptoms to treatment, and correlated these findings with the tumor size and degree of node positivity in several groups of patients (the groups of patients were divided into 15- to 20-year time intervals). In the 25-year interval between 1940 and 1943 and 1960 and 1965, the distribution of tumor sizes

---

*Personal communication, Connecticut Tumor Registry.

shifted to a greater proportion of smaller tumors: Of 1281 patients treated in 1940 to 1943, 20 percent had tumors less than 2 cm, whereas in 1960 to 1965, 38 percent of the 2100 patients treated had tumors less than 2 cm in diameter. These investigators found a similar effect regarding the distribution of positive axillary nodes, although the magnitude of the effect did not approach the nearly twofold difference regarding tumor size. In the 20-year study interval, the percentage of patients with positive axillary nodes decreased from 55.5 to 46.4 percent. Balachandra and coworkers believed decreases in time to presentation were responsible for this improved anatomical staging in patients from the 1960s. In 1940 to 1943, 42.9 percent of patients had delays of less than 2 months and 30.8 percent of patients had delays of more than 6 months. Twenty years later, 60.5 percent of patients were treated in less than 2 months and 25.6 percent of patients were treated in less than 6 months. During this same time interval, the 10-year overall survival from breast cancer treated by radical mastectomy increased from 51.6 to 74.2 percent. Although these differences in tumor size, node involvement, and survival only ranged between 5 and 23 percent, these investigators concluded that earlier detection of breast cancer results in improved anatomical staging; they linked this improved anatomical staging to improved overall survival. The difference in delay in diagnosis between those operable and inoperable was threefold. Differences in operative technique, postoperative radiotherapy, and chemotherapy were not discussed.

In 1974, Say and Donegan[211] reported on 1344 patients from the Ellis Fishel State Cancer Hospital treated by radical mastectomy between 1940 and 1965. The data showed that smaller tumors had less frequent node metastases. Because these investigators believed that tumor size on presentation was decreasing over the years of the study as a result of public health campaigns regarding breast cancer, they concluded that decreased delay in diagnosis led to smaller tumor size at presentation. From this reasoning they extrapolated that node metastases would be less frequent; therefore, survival would increase. This indirect argument begs the question of how delay in diagnosis and outcome are related, because the entire argument is based upon an untested, indirect chain of reasoning.

Wilkinson and associates (1979)[243] evaluated 1784 cases from Roswell Park Memorial Institute and confirmed a significant relationship between length of delay and extent of disease, length of survival, and age. Delay by patients was found to affect survival through the influence on extent of disease at diagnosis. Wilkinson proposed that a 2-month symptom delay time should be a standard time in which patients should recognize their symptoms, and doctors should act upon these findings through referral for definitive treatment. Patients with less than a two-month symptom delay time demonstrated a better survival rate ($p < .001$) compared with those sustaining delays of more than 3 months. The extent of disease was directly related to the length of delay: For delays of less than 2 months, local disease was seen 53 percent of the time, but only 27 percent of the time when the delay was more than 6 months. Regional disease increased from 41 to 50 percent when delays increased to more than 6 months. Distant metastatic disease also increased from 6 to 24 percent as delays increased to more than 6 months. Even when controlling for the stage of disease, delays of more than 3 months resulted in greater numbers of patients with regional and metastatic disease. This effect was not seen in patients with stage I disease. Wilkinson emphasized that the problem of delayed diagnosis is not an "either/or" phenomenon. Both delay and the biological nature of breast cancer are important in determining survival.

Others have also shown an adverse effect on prognosis by delays in diagnosis of breast cancer. In an attempt to answer the question of whether prompt diagnosis of breast cancer improves survival as assessed from the date of the first symptom, Elwood and Moorehead (1980)[66] studied 1059 women in British Columbia with histologically confirmed primary breast cancer. Patients with long delays in diagnosis had a poor average survival from the date of diagnosis, with an overall average relative survival rate at 5 years of 57 percent compared with 70 percent in those with short delays. For patients with delays in diagnosis of 1 month or less, survival at 5, 10, 15, and 20 years was 65, 55, 50, and 45 percent, respectively. However, for patients with delays of more than 12 months, overall survival decreased by 15 to 20 percent for each length of follow-up. Barr and Bailey (1980)[14] showed that tumors with short delays had an average diameter of 1.6 cm, whereas those with longer delays had an average size of 3.1 cm.

Gould-Martin and coworkers (1982)[87] confirmed that increased intervals of symptom delay from self-discovery of a breast cancer were associated with more frequent instances of positive axillary lymph nodes. In a group of 2299 cancer patients, Robinson[204] demonstrated delays of more than 6 weeks from onset of symptoms to diagnosis were associated with decreased survival in carcinoma of the breast but not in other tumor types. Porta and colleagues (1991)[195] analyzed 1247 cases of cancer from five sites: lung, breast, stomach, colon, and rectum. Porta found that only breast cancer showed a distinct pattern of increasing anatomical stage of disease with increasing delays between symptoms and diagnosis. Overall, the average symptom-to-diagnosis interval in this study was 7.4 months. Correlating stage and delay in diagnosis demonstrated significant differences in extent of disease versus length of delay: For localized breast cancer, the symptom-to-diagnosis interval was 2.5 months; for regional disease, it was 3.4 months; and for disseminated disease, it was 4.2 months. The difference in the symptom-to-diagnosis interval between localized disease and more advanced stages was significant at the $p < .01$ level. The probability of survival decreased linearly with increasing stage of breast cancer.

Dohrmann and colleagues (1982)[60] studied 435 breast cancer patients and compared staging when symptom duration increased from 1 week to over 6 months. Dohrmann found that there was a significant difference in the distribution of advanced tumors in those patients with lengthy symptom duration. In this study, 12 percent of patients had delays of less than 1 week; 26 percent of 1 week to 1 month; 33 percent of 1 month to 6 months; and 21 percent of 6 months or more. Compared with patients with symptom durations of less than 1 week, those with symptoms of more than 6 months had increased numbers of stage III lesions, 8 versus 19 percent. During the same time period, the number of stage I lesions decreased from 39 to 26 percent. The differences in the number of stage IV tumors also increased with delays of more than 6 months, with a significance level of $p < .003$. Survival rates were greater by 18 percent for patients with symptoms of less than 1 week, as compared with those with symptoms of 6 months or more (82 versus 64 percent, $p < .007$).

Feldman and coworker (1983)[71] studied 664 patients in 15 hospitals in New York and were able to demonstrate the biological heterogeneity of breast cancer and associated diagnostic delays. These investigators categorized tumors as relatively small, nonmetastatic tumors (5 cm or less with negative lymph nodes, termed class I) and large, aggressive tumors associated with cancers over 5 cm in diameters and positive axillary lymph nodes (termed class III). Whereas class I tumors had 4-year survival rates that increased from 83 to 91 percent after 12 months delay in diagnosis, the Class III tumors had a 50 percent decrease in survival rate after a 12-month diagnostic delay. In class III tumors, ominous changes in breast symptoms occurred more frequently after lengthy delays. For example, skin changes doubled from 4.2 to 7.8 percent; nipple discharge rose from 3.3 to 7.8 percent; nipple changes, from 3.3 to 6.9 percent; and two or more grave signs, from 9.4 to 18.6 percent. These findings were interpreted to demonstrate that breast cancer patients can be divided into two biological subgroups. One group (Feldman's class I) are slow-growing, nonmetastasizing tumors that remain in Class I even after a period of delay of 12 months. According to this study, in another subgroup of relatively fast-growing, metastatic tumors, delay in treatment appears to be harmful, leading to reduced survival rates. By the time grave symptoms began to show during the delay, the prognosis is reduced further still.

Pilipshen and colleagues (1984)[193] reviewed a large series of patients from Memorial Hospital and determined that patients delaying more than 6 months before presentation with breast symptoms had twice the chance of having tumors of at least 4 cm compared with those with symptom delays of less than 6 months. Patients with delays of less than 2 months had T1 tumors (less than 2 cm) in 35 percent of cases, whereas those patients with delays of more than 6 months were diagnosed with T1 tumors in

only 17 percent of cases. Patients with long diagnostic delays were 40 percent more likely to have positive axillary nodes than those with short delays. Yet, if tumor size were held constant, delay in diagnosis had no impact on the presence of positive axillary nodes. For example, T1 lesions were accompanied by positive axillary nodes in 21 percent of cases in which the delay was less than 2 months, and in 24 percent of cases in which the delay was more than 6 months. T2 tumors (greater than 4 cm) had 65 percent positive axillary nodes for delays of less than 2 months and 69 percent positive axillary nodes for delays greater than 6 months.

Charlson and Feinstein (1985)[38–41] studied 685 women treated between 1962 and 1969. They noted that patients with less than 3 months' duration from symptoms to treatment had better survival rate than those with longer delays. At 10 years of survival, those patients with less than 3 months delay had a 60 percent survival rate, compared with a 50 percent survival rate in those with greater than a 6-month delay. The patients with the shorter delays fared better than those with longer delays because they had a more favorable distribution of clinical stages. With increasing delay, there was a stepwise increase in the proportion of patients in more advanced stages III or IV. In patients with less than a 3-month delay, 76 percent were stage I or II, compared with only 46 percent with more than six months of delay.

Charlson identified a subset of patients who demonstrated adverse changes during the diagnostic delay (termed a "change in clinical state"), and demonstrated a poorer prognosis than the group that remained clinically stable during the delay. Despite breaking delays into 3-month intervals, those without changes in clinical state had a 10-year survival of 61 percent. Despite longer delays, in those patients without a change in clinical state of breast symptoms, the survival rates were as good or better than those with short delays. However, those patients developing adverse clinical signs during the delay—for example, skin and nipple retraction, ulceration, axillary adenopathy, pain, or edema—demonstrated a significantly worse outcome in overall and stage-specific survival. Nonetheless, only a limited number of patients were ultimately affected by delays in diagnosis, because most patients remained clinically stable during the interval of delay. Charlson estimated that 5.5 percent of patients (37 of 685) were adversely affected by diagnostic delays. This number was estimated to be the maximum amount of potentially preventable deaths that would result from prevention of the delayed diagnosis of breast cancer. Charlson concluded that decreased survival resulting from the delayed diagnosis of breast cancer is related to an increase in the stage of the disease; however, the impact of delay is limited to a subset of patients who had biologically active and aggressive disease during the interval of diagnostic delay.

In a study of 179 patients, Robinson (1984),[203] demonstrated those patients with delays exceeding six weeks from the onset of symptoms had 43% stage I tumors, compared with 66% stage I tumors in a group without diagnostic delay. Stage III tumors increased from 44% to 80% as delays increased past six weeks. In another study, Robinson and coworkers (1986)[203, 204] evaluated 523 patients with delays in diagnosis of breast cancer. She determined that patients who delayed presentation past 6 weeks incurred upstaging to a more advanced stage of cancer in 10 to 15 percent of cases. Stage III disease was more frequently found in those with delays, whereas stage I disease was found most commonly in those patients without diagnostic delays.

Neale and colleagues (1986)[176] studied 1261 women at MD Anderson Hospital between 1949 and 1968, and correlated the duration of symptoms with the relative risk of surviving 10 years from diagnosis. Those women with less than 3 months of symptom delay had a relative risk of dying within 10 years of 0.8 (indicating a slightly improved survival rate compared with a group with intermediate delays); when the delay was 3 to 6 months, the relative risk of dying within 10 years was 1.1 (virtually the same as a standard population); and when the delay was greater than 6 months, the relative risk of dying within 10 years was increased by 50 percent, to an odds ratio of 1.5. In this pairwise analysis of the relative risk of dying in relation to diagnostic delays, the inverse relationship was statistically significant at $p = .001$. In addition, the three categories of delays were statistically different from each other. Nearly 50 percent of those with little or no delay in seeking treatment were living after 10 years. Only about half as many patients who waited more than 6 months to seek medical attention survived 10 years. Neale proposed that diagnostic delay decreased survival by leading to more advanced clinical stages of disease.

The Italian Group for Cancer Care (GIVIO, 1986)[84] conducted a study at 63 Italian general hospitals to determine the impact of diagnostic delays in 1110 women. They noted a doubling of the stage III and IV cases in women with more than a 3-month delay in diagnosis (34 versus 17 percent). At 6 months of diagnostic delay, the size of the tumors increased, as demonstrated by the odds ratio for a T3 or T4 tumor of 3 to 4 times those with no delay. The relative risk of node positivity in those patients with a delay of greater than 6 months was twice that of patients without diagnostic delay.

In a study of 596 breast cancer patients, Machiavelli and associates (1989)[154] demonstrated that a larger proportion of patients with delays in diagnosis of more than 3 months had advanced stage III and IV disease. At 10 years of survival, there was a 10 percent difference in survival, for the group as a whole, between patients with less than 3 months versus those with more than 6 months of delay (33 versus 22 percent). In patients with stage I or II lesions, survival was 68 percent at 10 years for those with less than 3 months' delay versus 50 percent for those with longer delays. Machiavelli and colleagues calculated that 51 patients, or roughly 10% of the group, were affected by diagnostic delays through

upstaging to stage III or IV disease. These stage shifts resulted in 30 excess deaths. Interestingly, the negative influence of delay was almost exclusively demonstrated in the patients over age 50. This is the same age group of patients demonstrated by mammographic studies, such as the HIP study (Health Insurance Plan of New York) to benefit from early diagnosis from mammographic screening.[171, 172, 214]

Rossi and associates (1990)[206] studied 189 women and correlated symptoms, age, tumor grade, and diagnostic delay with prognosis. Delays were divided into groups of less than 1 month, 1 to 3 months, 3 to 6 months, and 6 months to 1 year. A consistent and direct relationship was found between delay and tumor size, nodal involvement, and the presence of metastases. As delays increased from 1 month to 1 year, there was a 46-percent increase in the number of T4 tumors and a 50-percent decrease in the number of T1 tumors. Lymph node metastases were present in 37 percent of patients with delays of less than 1 month, in 62 percent of patients with delays of at least 3 months, and in 100% (12/12) of patients with delays of greater than 1 year. Systemic organ metastases increased from 5 percent of cases to 25 percent of cases as delays increased from 1 month to 1 year. Survival rates decreased with longer delays: Those with less than 1 month of delay had a 90% survival at 3 years, whereas those with over a 3-month delay had a 66 percent survival at 3 years; for patients with over 1 year of delay, the survival was only 56 percent.

Tennvall and coworkers (1990)[230] also recently showed that patient delay and age adversely affected survival through a shift in anatomical staging. For 273 patients studied, the mean age was 56 years. Stage I tumors had an average delay of 1 month or less, and patients averaged 49 years of age. Stage II tumors also had a delay averaging 1 month with an average patient age of 56 years. Stage III tumors had an average delay time of 2 months with an average patient age of 63 years. Stage IV tumors had an average delay time of 6 months, with an average patient age of 70 years.

Afzelius and colleagues (1994)[2] studied the prognostic implications of patient and doctor delay in primary operable breast cancer in 7068 patients in Copenhagen, Denmark. A long patient delay was associated with an unfavorable stage and poor survival as compared with a short delay. If the patient delay was more than 60 days, the mortality rate was 24 percent higher than for a shorter delay. A long patient delay of more than 60 days was associated with larger tumors, more positive lymph nodes, and rate of survival. For example, only 8 percent of patients with short delays had tumors larger than 5 cm compared with 19 percent in long patient delays (more than 60 days). The number of node-negative patients dropped from 62 to 51 percent as the delay increased. Those with more than four positive lymph nodes increased from 12 to 20 percent with long delays. Afzelius hypothesized that delay times reflect biological characteristics of breast cancer and its presentation.

One unusual aspect of this study was that long doctor delay times were associated with better survival because tumors were smaller and less anaplastic. This factor suggests that doctors recognized aggressive and rapidly growing tumors, and diagnosed them promptly. In comparison, smaller, more indolent tumors may have presented in a more subtle fashion, and were more difficult to diagnose. Although the delays in recognizing these tumors were longer, a negative impact on stage brought about by a delayed diagnosis could not be demonstrated.

Studies Showing No Effect of Diagnostic Delay on Survival

Several series of patients treated by radical mastectomies in the 1940s to 1950s have shown that delay in diagnosis does not increase mortality from breast cancer; indeed, in some series, those with longer delays exhibit improved survival.

In 1944, Hawkins[104] evaluated the duration of disease before treatment in white and black females. For white females, the mean duration of disease before treatment was 15.2 months, and for black females, it was 22.6 months. The duration of disease was not correlated with survival rates when corrections were made for stage of disease. Hawkins explained this finding by noting that the biology of breast cancer is highly variable; some tumors may grow slowly and metastasize rarely, whereas others may grow rapidly and metastasize early. In order to understand the true impact of a delayed diagnosis of breast cancer on survival, it would be necessary to understand more precisely these three factors: (1) the actual time of onset of the disease, (2) the rate of growth of the disease, and (3) the inherent tendency of breast tumors to metastasize.

In 1941, Eggers and colleagues[64] reported 5-year survival rates in 235 patients with surgically treated breast cancer. Although delays in treatment of up to 2 years were associated with decreases in survival rates from 76 to 20 percent, the survival rate increased to 41 percent for a subgroup of 22 patients with diagnostic delays exceeding 3 years. Beginning in the 1940s, MacDonald[151–153] developed his theory of biological predeterminism to explain the variability and unpredictability of breast cancer prognosis. To explain the difficulty of diagnosing and curing breast cancer, MacDonald postulated that the events that determine survival occur in the very early preclinical phase of the tumor, long before the tumor itself is detectable. This theory of biological predeterminism, constructed in the 1940s, is the forerunner of the modern day alternative theory of breast cancer pathophysiology, which emphasizes that breast cancer is often a systemic disease from its inception. During the preclinical phase, the predetermined biological aggressiveness of the cancer directs the timing and extent of occult metastases, which will later overwhelm the host. In this regard, MacDonald believed that it was the influence of natural selection of aggressive clones of malignant cells rather than the timing of treatment that determined the end results of breast cancer therapy.

The evidence for the theory of biological predeterminism rested largely on the finding from MacDonald's 1951 study[152] that 56 percent of tumors studied by him that were 1 cm or less had metastasized to the nodes of the axilla, whereas 23 percent of tumors more than 5 cm had not metastasized. Thus, MacDonald argued that although there was broad conformance to the spatial size of the tumor increasing with longer duration of symptoms (tumors 1 cm or less decreased in number from 19 to 5 percent when duration of symptoms increased from 1 month to more than 12 months), there was no direct relationship between metastatic spread of disease to the axilla and tumor size. MacDonald demonstrated that as tumors increased in size from 1 to 5 cm, there was no increase in the rate of regional node disease.

MacDonald was one of the first investigators to posit that the average breast cancer is invisible to detection by radiological studies from the time of its inception to its eighth year of growth, at which time it would appear to be 1 cm in size. The remainder of a breast cancer's clinical phase would last about 4 years. The calculations for these tumor dimensions were based on tumor doubling times averaging 100 days. The variability in life cycle of breast tumors would depend on the wide range in tumor doubling times, which others have shown ranges between 42 to 944 days.* Heuser and coworkers (1979)[10] analyzed serial mammograms from 23 women selected from the Breast Cancer Detection Demonstration Project of 10,120 women undergoing screening mammography. He reported that the average tumor volume doubling time in 23 breast cancers was 325 days, with several tumors either growing too fast between mammogram intervals to be measured or, in 9 of 23 cases, not growing at all. Fast-growing tumors had an incidence of positive nodes at surgery of 34 percent, and slow-growing tumors were accompanied by positive nodes at surgery in 15 percent of cases.[107] Thus, those tumors that metastasize in the preclinical, nondetectable phase would lead to an ultimately fatal outcome, despite the apparent efficacy of an early diagnosis. Spratt has emphasized the importance of recognizing the silent interval of potential tumor spread and of recognizing the limitations of anatomical staging without taking into account the malignant potential of tumors.[221, 223]

Interestingly, as early as 1942, Haagensen and Stoutz[92] also noted from retrospective clinical reviews two groups of women who responded differently to diagnostic delays. In a group of 623 women who underwent radical mastectomies for breast cancer, Haagensen noted that one group had an adverse effect on survival with up to 35 months of delay. Thereafter, those women with diagnostic delays exceeding 36 months had increased survival compared with the group as a whole. For example, those women with delays of 2 weeks or less had 5-year survival

---

*See references 28, 48, 49, 86, 106, 107, 148, and 149.

rates of 54 percent; at 1 year of delay, the 5-year survival rate was 28 percent; and at 24 to 35 months of delay, the 5-year survival rate was 22 percent. However, after 36 months of delay, no further decline in survival rate was noted; instead, the overall survival increased to 42 percent. Axillary node metastases increased 18 percent (from 50 to 68 percent) in patients with diagnostic delays that increased from 1 month to more than 6 months. Explaining the paradox in these survival figures for patients with very long delays, Haagensen concluded that this represented a subgroup of women who manifested indolent, nonmetastatic breast cancer. This provided an explanation for the paradox of why early diagnosis and treatment seemed to be an important factor increasing the survival of some women, whereas other women had poor survival rates despite entering treatment soon after diagnosis.

In 1951, Park and Lees[184] summarized current knowledge about diagnosis and survival from breast cancer. They concluded that the difference in survival between those operated on without diagnostic delay and those with lengthy diagnostic delays exceeding 3 years was only 7.5 percent. Commenting on the fact that the difference between treated and untreated patients at the time (when adjuvant chemotherapy was rarely used) was only 20 percent, these investigators believed early treatment was simply selecting out slow-growing, smaller (and therefore favorable) tumors for treatment. In 1953, Harnett[101] evaluated 2880 cancer patients overall for relationship between length of delay, stage, and survival. In a group of 660 breast cancer patients divided into those with delays in diagnosis ranging between 0 and 12 months, there was no difference in survival among the groups when all stages I through III were combined. In 53 patients with untreated breast cancer, the actual duration of survival averaged 35.9 months, with a decrease in the percentage of normal life expectancy of only 27 percent (a somewhat surprising finding in the absence of any therapy).

In the 1950s Bloom reported on a series of 406 breast cancer patients and noted that regardless of the duration of symptoms (from less than 6 weeks to more than 12 months), diagnostic delays held no influence on survival.[19] Five-year survival rates at 6 weeks of delay were 50 percent, whereas survival rates at 12 months or more of delay were 52 percent. In a more detailed analysis, Bloom demonstrated that as the duration of symptoms increased, the clinical stage of the patients progressed: for patients with delays of 3 months or less, 37 percent were stage I, whereas with delays of 1 year or more, only 25 percent were stage I. Those patients with advanced stage III breast cancer increased from 19 percent with short delays to 44 percent with delays longer than 1 year. Paradoxically, longer duration of symptoms was also correlated with increasing numbers of grade I tumors: 24 percent with grade I with a 6-week delay versus 38 percent Grade I with a 1-year delay. In addition, longer delays correlated with decreasing numbers of grade II tumors (45 percent

for 6-week delay versus 34 percent for a 1-year delay) and grade III tumors (31 percent for a 6-week delay versus 28 percent for a 1-year delay). From an analysis of grade and survival, Bloom concluded that grade III tumors presented earliest, had the shortest mean duration of symptoms (7.1 months), and were not influenced in terms of 5-year survival rates by delays in diagnosis of any time interval (29 percent with a 6-week delay versus 21 percent with a 1-year delay). In contrast, grade I tumors had the latest presentation, the longest duration of symptoms (mean 10.1 months), and were affected by delays in diagnosis (92 percent with a 6-week delay versus 78 percent with a 1-year delay). Ultimately, Bloom concluded that outcome in mammary carcinoma was largely a function of histology and growth rate rather than of the promptness of treatment.

In 1952, Smithers and colleagues[218] determined that prognosis in a group of 846 British breast cancer patients was related to a clinically determined rate of tumor growth. The rate of growth was said to be slow when the tumor changed less than a centimeter in 6 months, and these patients had 5-year survival rates of 84 percent. When the tumor changed no more than 1 cm in 6 months, growth was said to be moderate and survival rates decreased to 64 percent. Tumor growth was said to be fast when the tumor changed more than 1 cm in 6 months, in which the survival rate was 18%. Smithers[218] also documented a paradoxical increase in survival in patients with duration of symptoms exceeding 18 months. In a study of 846 British patients with breast cancer, those with a duration of symptoms of less than 6 months (364 cases) demonstrated a 5-year absolute survival of 43 percent. When the duration of symptoms was less than 12 months, the survival rate dropped to 26 percent but rose again to 41 percent when the duration of symptoms exceeded 18 months.

In 1955, McKinnon[163, 164] raised the important issue that stage I breast cancer is not synonymous with short-duration or earlier diagnosed breast cancer. Rather, stage I breast cancer is more reflective of a unique type of breast cancer biology, one that holds low metastatic potential and low lethality for the patient. McKinnon made the prescient point that the wide variations in survival of patients with cancers of other stages also reflects the wide variations in malignancy in these stages that are not accurately revealed by histopathology. Only advances in the newer fields of molecular oncology, which will reveal the genetic determinants of malignancy, will be truly predictive of tumor behavior.

McWhirter, in 1957,[165] in a study of 1000 patients in England, noted that there was no correlation between the size of primary breast cancer and the duration of symptoms as stated by the patient. Indeed, comparing patients with delays of more than 1 year with those with delays of 1 month, the number of tumors smaller than 1 cm was roughly the same as the number of tumors larger than 6 cm in size. The 5-year survival rate of those patients who delayed for more than 1 year was slightly higher than that of patients who delayed for less than 3 months (a 1-year delay resulted in a 61-percent survival rate versus a 58-percent survival rate in less than 3 months' delay). Yet, when all groups of patients were combined, including the inoperable group and the group of patients with locally advanced carcinoma, the survival rate declined from 49 to 40 percent with delays of more than 1 year compared with those of less than 3 months. McWhirter explained this effect as resulting from the additive effect of poor prognosis in patients with metastatic disease, because these patients increase in number if delays are greater than 1 year. In 1960, Hultborn and Tornberg[112] reported that the duration of symptoms in 517 patients with breast cancer gave no significant information of prognostic value. Postoperative survival curves showed no difference for patients with pretreatment delays of less than 1 month versus delays of increasing intervals up to 2 years.

In one of the first kinetic analyses of breast cancer growth related to survival, Humphrey constructed a "coefficient of growth rate" from a large group of breast cancer patients, and correlated this number to their overall 5-year survival rate. Initially, Humphrey and Severdlow (1963)[113] reported that the overall survival rate at 5 years for a group of breast cancer patients was decreased by 10% when delays exceeded 30 days from diagnostic biopsy to radical mastectomy (47 versus 36.8 percent). Despite this finding, the duration of tumor symptoms had no effect upon the 5-year survival rate, except for those with symptomatic delays between 7 to 9 months, in whom the survival was 36.4 percent. This is in comparison to the other groups of patients with delays ranging up to 1 year, in whom the 5-year survival rate was 50 percent. To clarify this issue, Humphrey used the coefficient of growth rate, defined as the ratio of tumor size in centimeters to duration of symptoms in months. When the coefficient was 0.1 to 0.5 (indicating either a very small tumor, or a tumor whose delay far exceeds its size), the 5-year survival rate was 62 percent. When the coefficient of growth was 0.6 to 1 (indicating a larger tumor, or a tumor whose growth rate is beginning to exceed its duration of symptoms), the 5-year survival rate fell to 38.5 percent. This finding suggests that the duration of symptoms can only be interpreted prognostically when the biology of tumor growth is integrated into the analysis.

In 1967, Devitt[57, 58] challenged the idea that advanced stages of breast cancer are due to the disease having been present and untreated for increased periods of time. Devitt studied 1440 patients from the Ottawa Clinic in Ontario, Canada from 1946 to 1961. Correlating the stage of breast cancer with the length of pretreatment symptoms, he found that the distribution of patients with stages I and II lesions, in terms of the symptomatic interval, was identical. Although the distribution of patients with stage III and IV lesions was increased with longer pretreatment symptomatic intervals, he believed this finding was not enough to account for the vastly different 5-

and 10-year survival rates. For example, those with 1 month or less of delay made up 31 percent of stage I; 26 percent of stage II; 18 percent of stage III; and 13 percent of stage IV. With delays of 4 to 6 months, 17 percent were stage I; 16 percent were stage II; 17 percent were stage III; and 8 percent were stage IV. At symptomatic intervals before treatment of greater than 1 year, 12 percent were stage I; 16 percent were stage II; 35 percent were stage III; and 49 percent were stage IV. However, survival rates did not change with increasing intervals of treatment delay. For delays of 1 month or less, 5-year survival rate for those with stage I lesions was 75 percent, stage II, 56 percent, and stage III, 20 percent. For delays of 1 year or more, survival for patients with stage I lesions at 5 years was 80 percent, 54% stage II, and 21% stage III.

Devitt's study showed that survival rates were independent of the time before treatment, regardless of the clinical stage. The shapes of the survival curves for each clinical stage described the rate of dying from systemic disease; each of the curves was different for the three stages described. The yearly death rate for stage I breast cancer was 6 percent; for stage II breast cancer, 12 percent; and for stage III, 21 percent. Based on these different behaviors, Devitt proposed that tumor biology, and not diagnostic delay, was the central determinant of the tumor stage and its prognosis. Using a simplified mathematical formula, Devitt proposed that the tumor stage at the time of definitive diagnosis was not simply defined by growth rate × time. Instead, tumor size and spread was more closely approximated by an equation which adjusts for tumor biology and the tumor-host interaction, which Devitt proposed could be schematically stated as tumor stage at diagnosis = tumor growth potential ÷ host resistance × time.

Further support for the importance of the tumor-host interaction and tumor biology comes from a study by Devitt of the survival times for patients diagnosed with metastatic disease after primary treatment for breast cancer. Those who originally had stage I primary cancers lived longer after their metastases than those who had presented initially with primary tumors of more advanced clinical stage. For example, if the patient had an osseous recurrence, and her primary cancer stage was stage I, then her median time to death was 10 months. This is twofold greater than the median time to death (5 months) of a patient whose primary tumor was stage III at the time of diagnosis. These data support the idea that presenting clinical stage was a measure of the tumor-host interaction as much as a measure of the chronological age or physical extent of the tumor.

In 1968, Brinkley and Haybittle[27] reported on a 15-year follow-up study of patients treated for breast cancer in England. He reported that for a given clinical stage and age group, the length of pretreatment history did not significantly affect survival rates. This finding suggested that the growth rate of the tumor was not of primary importance in determining prognosis. However, Brinkley noted that longer clinical histories of breast cancers were associated with later clinical stages and poorer survival rates.

In 1971, Alderson and associates[5] performed a multivariate analysis of 21 prognostic factors in 272 cases of breast cancer treated by radical mastectomy. The duration of symptoms in the months preceding initial hospital treatment was evaluated for its predictive power in estimating 5-year survival both as an independent and dependent predictor of local and systemic recurrence. The correlation coefficient between duration of symptoms and survival was 0.09, not a statistically significant relationship. Indeed, the total contribution of the factor "duration of symptoms" to the variance in survival determined by 22 prognostic factors was only 0.4 percent. Thus, delay in diagnosis, or length of pretreatment symptoms, had no predictive power or statistical significance as an independent prognostic factor of survival. In contrast, the three factors of axillary node metastases, clinical stage, and pathological size of the primary tumor were highly predictive of future survival. All of these factors are critical elements defining the inherent biology of a breast cancer.

Dennis and coworkers (1975)[55] studied 237 patient with breast cancer treated by mastectomy. The average symptom delay was 4.8 months and was not correlated with race, age, or socioeconomic group. When plotting the length of survival versus the length of delay, no correlation was noted between the two. The average time to recurrence throughout the group ranged between 20 and 24 months, and there was no difference between less than 1 month of delay, 3 months of delay, or more than 12 months of delay. Patients free of disease at 5 years and those with recurrent disease, had similar symptom delay times (5.8 ± 1.4 mo) and doctor delay times (0.56 ± 0.15 mo). There was no correlation between delay in diagnosis and the number or presence of positive axillary lymph nodes.

Fisher and coworkers (1977)[78, 80] noted that delays in diagnosis were correlated with a significant increase in grave signs of breast cancer, including skin changes, nipple irregularities and discharge, and nodal disease. As the duration of symptoms increased from 1 month to more than 9 months, tumor sizes and grave signs increased: the number of tumors larger than 1 cm increased from 63 to 78 percent; the frequency of clinically positive nodes increased from 31 to 41 percent; nipple involvement was present more commonly, increasing from 9.8 to 17.5 percent; and skin involvement was found more often, increasing from 2.3 to 11.4 percent. The number of positive axillary nodes did not correlate strongly with length of delay: at 9 months of delay, those patients with more than four positive nodes increased slightly from 30.1 to 32.9 percent, and those with no positive nodes decreased from 48 to 43 percent. Consistent with the findings from several studies reviewed earlier, Fisher showed that the number of treatment failures decreased as symptoms increased beyond 9 months of diagnostic delay.

In 1979, Fox[81] reported a similar analysis of survival in women with breast cancer. Fox identified two populations of cancer patients with different kinetic rates of death from breast cancer. One population died at a yearly rate exceeding 2.5 percent. A second population died at a much slower rate, more closely akin to the rate of death in the normal population. Fox raised the possibility that what has been labeled as a single disease under the heading of breast cancer should be considered as representing two or more distinct populations with different biological behaviors.

Further studies on the relationship between the clinical history of breast cancer as an estimate of its growth rate are derived from Boyd and coworkers (1981).[25] Boyd studied 756 patients from 1965 to 1972 at the Princess Margaret Hospital. These investigators characterized by clinical means transition events during the diagnostic delay interval of patients. Transition events were defined as changes in the symptoms in the breast reflecting structural or anatomical progression of disease. These events included a change in size of the breast mass, a change in consistency of the mass, the development of other masses, skin changes, contracture or a change in the size or shape of the breast itself, retraction of the skin, pain, or edema. Those patients with transition events and a delay in diagnosis measured in months were categorized as having fast-growing tumors. Such patients had a relative death rate twice that of those with slow-growing tumors, defined as those with no transition events and a lengthy symptomatic interval. Boyd concluded that differences in the clinical history of a breast cancer's growth rate correspond to true biological differences, which can be classified by clinical characteristics. For example, in Boyd's study, the relative risk of having more than four positive lymph nodes was nearly 10 times greater in those with fast-growing tumors (1.87 relative risk) compared with slow-growing tumors (0.2 relative risk). In separate investigations, Cummings and associates (1983)[51] also noted the importance of the relationship of tumor growth rate to survival. In 160 breast cancer patients with a variety of pretreatment delays, fast-growing tumors appeared to be unaffected by diagnostic delays. For the group as a whole, the overall survival was better in those patients with shorter diagnostic delays.

Heuser and coworkers (1984)[106] noted two groups of breast cancer growth rates during an evaluation of 10,120 women in the Breast Cancer Detection Demonstration Project over a 5-year interval. These investigators noted fast-growing cancers that surfaced between yearly mammographic screenings. These tumors were characterized by aggressive biological characteristics, including higher mitotic index, poor cellular differentiation, and larger tumor size. These tumors tended to occur in young women, demonstrating lymphatic invasion around the tumor and accompanied by a higher proportion of axillary metastases. Patients with fast-growing tumors had a cumulative 5-year survival rate of 74 percent compared with a 94-percent survival rate in patients with cancers found on screening that developed over a period of time longer than 1 year.

Mueller[173, 174] brought attention to the different mortality kinetics in breast cancer, described by the half-time death rate and annual death rate. These two mortality figures were not the same in stage I and stage II disease. Studying the kinetics of breast cancer mortality in the National Surgical Adjuvant Breast Project and from the Tumor Registry of Connecticut, Mueller identified a small but statistically different result between stages I and II for both half-time death rates and annual death rates. This differential mortality for stages I and II ranged between 3 and 5 percent. For example, stage I breast cancer had a half-time death rate of 11.8 to 12 years, with an annual death rate of 4.7 to 5 percent. In contrast, stage II disease has a half-time death rate of 7.4 to 8.5 years and an annual death rate of 8 to 9 percent. These data suggest that stage I and II breast cancers are not the same disease as reflected by a direct progression from early to intermediate stages. Instead, these data appear to reflect three populations of breast malignancies: stage I; an overlap between stages I and II; and a separate stage II population. Mueller proposed that "women with stage II breast cancer are not those who seek medical care later but are instead those who have a tumor that is more aggressive, whose axillary lymph node metastases are more obvious, whose distant metastases show themselves sooner, whose local recurrences are more frequent, and whose death is therefore likely to occur earlier." In essence, those patients who are going to die of breast cancer after surgical treatment and local radiation already have micrometastases at the time of treatment. One hypothesis to link the factors of tumor size and poor prognosis is related to an increase in metastatic cell clones as tumors increase in size. Larger tumors may become multiclonal and thereby have an increased potential to metastasize. Small tumors are likely to be monoclonal and will likely behave in an indolent and controllable fashion. With an increase in tumor size, a breast cancer may lose its monoclonal features, and its behavior becomes more erratic, leading to greater chances for metastases.

Neave (1990)[177] studied 1675 women in New Zealand who sustained delays in diagnosis of 6 weeks or more. There was no difference in survival based on diagnostic delay, although variables in tumor size, skin attachment, and nipple retraction were worse in the group with longer delays. A 5- to 10-percent difference in tumor size and grave signs of malignancy accompanied delays of more than 6 weeks. For example, tumors larger than 5 cm were present in 17 percent of those who delayed compared with 12 percent of nondelayers; nipple retraction was present in 87 percent of delayers and 81 percent of nondelayers. However, the number of positive axillary nodes was no different between the two groups. Interestingly, Neave found an adverse prognostic significance to a group with short delay. This included a group of women whose tumors had grade III histology and

negative estrogen receptors. If patients with these tumors presented quickly for diagnosis, prognosis was decreased compared with other groups. Neave ascribed this finding to a particularly aggressive biology in these tumors. Clayton[46] supported the prognostic implications of biological aggressiveness as determined by high mitotic count in breast cancer.

In a different approach to the problem using an analysis of lawsuits for failure to diagnose breast cancer in Massachusetts, Diercks and Cady[59] demonstrated biological differences indicating a more benign clinical course in a subpopulation of patients sustaining long diagnostic delays. These investigators compared patients with delays in diagnosis of 18 months with those patients with less than 6 months of delay. The tumor sizes in the long-delay group were smaller (average 3 cm in 8 cases) compared with patients with shorter delay (average 5 cm in 18 cases). Furthermore, compared with patients with an 18-month delay, patients with a less than 6-month delay had a 10-percent increase in positive axillary nodes (72 versus 62 percent). Patients were found to have more than five positive axillary nodes 50 percent of the time in less than 6 months of delay, but only 40 percent of the time with more than 18 months of delay. Thus, the data from lawsuits in Massachusetts suggest that there are two groups of patients with breast cancers of different degrees of biological aggressiveness.

Rudan and colleagues[207] (1994) studied node-posi-

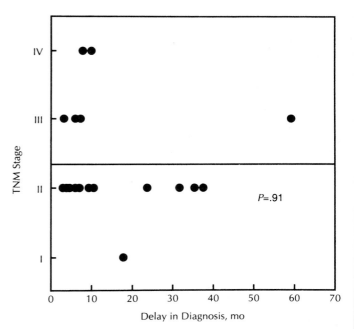

Figure 94–15 *Regression analysis between TNM stage of breast cancer and the length of the diagnostic delay in 24 cases that had data sufficient for study (from a total of 45 cases of breast cancer malpractice litigation). Six points in the scattergram are hidden by overlap. No correlation was noted between the increasing length of diagnostic delay and the advancing stage of disease by TNM classification (p = .91). (From Kern KA: Causes of breast cancer malpractice litigation: A 20-year civil court review. Arch Surg 127:542–547, 1992. Copyright 1992-94, American Medical Association. With permission.)*

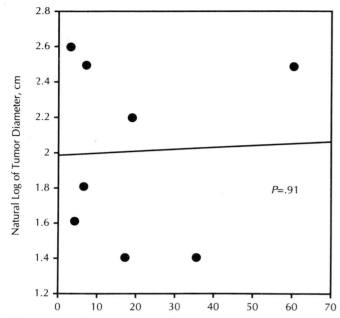

Figure 94–16   *Regression analysis between natural log of tumor diameter and the length of diagnostic delay in eight cases that had data sufficient for study (from a total of 45 cases of breast cancer malpractice litigation). No correlation was noted between the increasing length of diagnostic delay and enlarging tumor size. (From Kern KA: Causes of breast cancer malpractice litigation: A 20-year civil court review. Arch Surg 127:542–547, 1992. Copyright 1992–94, American Medical Association. With permission.)*

tive patients and correlated delay with survival at less than 1 month, 1 to 3 months, 3 to 6 months, and more than 6 month of delay. The average delay was 4.6 months. The influence of delay on 5-year survival was not significant, even in patients with less than 6 months of delay, compared with those with more than 24 months of delay. A similar study[208] in patients with metastatic disease showed no influence of delay on survival.

Kern[122, 127] addressed the issue of the impact of a delayed diagnosis of breast cancer on prognosis by using data derived from U.S. civil trials. Actual tumor sizes and data on lymph node status was extracted from legal data bases of completed malpractice trials. By plotting data on tumor stage and size versus diagnostic delay, the relationship between delay and tumor behavior was determined in this select group of patients. No correlation was found between TNM stage or tumor size and the length of diagnostic delay (illustrated in Figs. 94–15 and 94–16). Linear regression analysis was nonsignificant ($p = .91$) for the relationship between months of delay and tumor stage and for the relationship between months of delay and tumor size (plotted as natural log of tumor diameter). Importantly, virtually all cases were stage II or greater. It is possible that once a tumor is stage II, delay has a limited impact on survival. At what point these tumors became stage II during the interval of delay is unknown.

The lack of correlation between diagnostic delays and survival time reported by the studies reviewed earlier probably reflects the fact that other factors such as cell kinetics, rate of growth, immune response, hormone factors, and patient age, may also play a role in survival.[52, 182, 220, 232] Spratt[221] has argued that the duration of symptoms represents only a small fraction of the life span of the tumor; therefore, events influencing survival are occurring in a time at which the tumor is occult and nondiagnosable by present technology.

CONCLUSION: HOW TO PREVENT THE DELAYED DIAGNOSIS OF BREAST CANCER: SYNOPSIS OF CLINICAL RISK PREVENTION

Limited attempts to prevent errors in breast cancer diagnosis by codifying clinical pitfalls have been undertaken previously. Over 20 years ago, Haagensen gave an excellent account of problems related to breast diagnosis.[94] In his textbook, he noted that, since 1926, the percent of carcinomas of the breast discovered by physicians on routine breast examination had increased nearly 20-fold to 17 percent. However, errors in the diagnosis of breast cancer remained common. In his personal series of 1433 patients with breast cancer, 19 percent (270) sustained misdiagnoses before referral to him, resulting in an average diagnostic delay of 14 months. In 19 percent of these cases, two or more physicians had examined the breast and missed the diagnosis of breast cancer. Based on the experience with these patients, Haagensen classified diagnostic errors in breast disease into nine types, all related to a failure to biopsy a breast lesion in a timely fashion:

1. Failure to examine a breast containing an obvious tumor while treating the patient for an unrelated disease.
2. Failure of the physician, in his palpation of the breast, to feel the tumor that the patient had discovered and for which she came for consultation.
3. Mistaking a carcinomatous tumor of the breast for a breast infection.
4. Wrongly diagnosing a carcinomatous tumor of the breast as a benign lesion, and failing to advise biopsy or excision.
5. Disregarding a history of acute and sharp pain in the breast.
6. Disregarding a definite retraction sign.
7. Failure to determine the cause of a nipple discharge.
8. Relying upon negative aspiration biopsy.
9. Relying on mammography rather than palpation.

In the same text, Haagensen analyzed his own diagnostic errors, which occurred at a rate of 1 percent (17 misdiagnosed breast cancers in 1669 women studied between 1935 and 1967). He highlighted pitfalls in diagnosis based on his errors, and presented solutions to these problems, as follows:

1. Ignoring the patient's statements that a mass is present, even if the physician cannot initially palpate

it. Ask for the location of the mass, and search again for it.

2. Ignoring the statements of referring physicians that a mass was present. If not detected initially, ask for a re-visit soon thereafter.

3. Failing to ask patients with a nipple discharge, but no obvious cause, for re-visits and frequent examinations until the cause is found. Monthly re-visits may be necessary.

4. Rushing and examining patients under inadequate conditions, with less than optimal time spent in the examination.

5. Failure to biopsy benign-appearing masses in women over age 25, even if they appear to be fibroadenomas on clinical evaluation.

6. Assuming new masses in the breast of patients with previously biopsied benign lesions are also benign. For women 25 years or older, aspiration and biopsy of solid breast masses is mandatory.

7. Allowing patients with nodularity to go without re-examination for 6 months or more. Every 2 months is mandatory.

8. Failing to impress upon patients the need to keep follow-up appointments, even at frequent intervals, until a definite diagnosis is determined.

Haagensen's analysis of diagnostic errors in breast disease provides a valuable contribution and excellent clinical guide to preventing errors in the diagnosis of breast cancer. Perhaps Haagensen's greatest contribution, however, was something not stated explicitly in his solutions to diagnostic dilemmas: Personal commitment provides the key to the early diagnosis of breast cancer. Haagensen stated

> It is a heavy responsibility that we, as physicians, bear in the diagnosis of lesions of the breast. Each one of us must set for [ourselves] the highest standard of exactitude in the diagnosis of lesions of the breast, always seeking to improve our personal clinical skill and to discipline it by the pathologic diagnoses in our patients. We must also improve our medical education in regard to the diagnosis of breast lesions.[94]

Risk Prevention Profile in Delayed Diagnosis of Breast Cancer

A risk prevention profile constructed from the findings of this chapter can be condensed into a scenario of high risk for the delayed diagnosis of breast cancer.[129] The patient most likely to sustain a delayed diagnosis of breast cancer meets the following criteria: (1) a woman of upper socioeconomic means, with private health insurance, under age 45, who presents with a self-discovered, painless mass; (2) a work-up includes a physical examination in which the mass is discovered and thought to be benign because of the patient's age; (3) a mammogram is ordered and returned negative for abnormalities or malignancy, despite the presence of the palpable mass; (4) the patient is diagnosed with fibrocystic disease and told she does not have cancer, based on the physical examination and negative mammogram; (5) a biopsy or referral for consultation is not recommended; (6) a delay averaging 13 to 15 months precedes the diagnosis of breast cancer; (7) the TNM stage will be at least stage II at final operation and pathological staging.

The primary physician most likely involved in the delayed diagnosis of breast cancer meets the following criteria: (1) an obstetrician-gynecologist evaluates a woman under age 45; (2) despite the presence of a mass, the physician is unimpressed with the potential for breast cancer; (3) a needle aspiration, needle biopsy, or ultrasound is not performed; (4) a mammogram is ordered and returns negative, and is accepted as providing a benign diagnosis, despite the presence of the breast mass; (5) no consultation regarding the mass is obtained; (6) the mass is labeled as fibrocystic disease or as another benign breast condition; (7) the physician supports a settlement if a lawsuit is filed; (8) the radiologist responsible for any mammograms is likely to be named in the lawsuit; (9) the physician believes that some action could have prevented the lawsuit, the most likely being referral for consultation regarding evaluation of an apparently benign breast mass or abnormality.

Potential solutions to reduce the risk of misdiagnosed breast cancer may be derived directly from these high-risk profiles. These solutions tie in directly with the goals of good communication about risk management: identify incorrect ideas leading to errors, and tailor communication to these beliefs. Because women younger than age 40 are consistently found to be the focus of the misdiagnosed breast cancer, one belief of physicians leading to errors must relate to the incidence of breast cancer in young women.

Correction of other errors requires physicians to accept a sequence of steps tailored to evaluate breast abnormalities that are noted only by patients and not by physicians. This includes the following: (1) understanding that a small mass may indeed be present, even when undetected by the physician's initial physical examination; (2) evaluating the breast by imaging studies, including ultrasound (looking for occult cysts and solid masses), in addition to mammography; (3) biopsying by FNA (or other minimally invasive methods) any area believed by the patient to be new and abnormal; (4) following the patient closely and repeating examinations monthly for several visits; and (5) explaining to the patient that the only way to detect some breast cancers is by careful, sequential, and repeated breast examinations, added to the imaging techniques and other diagnostic methods discussed earlier.

References

1. Adam SA, Horner JK, Vessey MP: Delay in treatment for breast cancer. Community Med 2:195–201, 1980.
2. Afzelius P, Zedeler K, Sommer H, et al: Patient's and doctor's delay in primary breast cancer. Acta Oncol 33:345–351, 1994.
3. Aitken-Swan J, Paterson R: The cancer patient: Delay in seeking advice. BMJ 1:623–627, 1955.
4. Ajekigbe AT: Fear of mastectomy: The most common factor responsible for late presentation of carcinoma of the breast in Nigeria. Clin Oncol 3:78–80, 1991.

5. Alderson MR, Hamlin I, Staunton MD: The relative significance of prognostic factors in breast carcinoma. Br J Cancer 25:646–656, 1971.
6. Andersen BL, Cacioppo JT: Delay in seeking a cancer diagnosis: Delay stages and psychophysiological comparison processes. Br J Social Psychol 34:33–52, 1995.
7. Anderson NH: Foundations of Information Integration Theory. New York, Academic Press, 1981.
8. Anglem TJ, Leber RE: Characteristics of ten year survivors after radical mastectomy for cancer of the breast. Am J Surg 121:363–367, 1971.
9. Antonovsky A, Hartman H: Delay in the detection of cancer: A review of the literature. Health Education Monograph 2:98–128, 1974.
10. Applewhite RR, Smith LR, DiVincenti F: Carcinoma of the breast associated with pregnancy and lactation. Am Surg 39:101–105, 1973.
11. Backhouse CM, Lloyd-Davies ERV, Shousha S, Burn JI: Carcinoma of the breast in women aged 35 or less. Br J Surg 74:591–593, 1987.
12. Balachandra VK, Schottenfeld D, Berg JW, et al: Patterns of delay and extent of disease in radical mastectomy patients. Clin Bull (Memorial Sloan-Kettering Cancer Center) 3:10–13, 1973.
13. Barnavon Y, Wallack MK: Management of the pregnant patient with carcinoma of the breast. Surg Gynecol Obstet 171:347–352, 1990.
14. Barr L, Bailey M: Delay in diagnosis of breast cancer. BMJ 281:146–147, 1980.
15. Bassett LW, Ysrael M, Gold RH, Ysrael C: Usefulness of mammography and sonography in women less than 35 years of age. Radiology 180:831–835, 1991.
16. Bates AT, Bates T, Hastrich, et al: Delay in the diagnosis of breast cancer: The effect of the introduction of fine needle aspiration cytology to a breast clinic. Eur J Surg Oncol 18:433–437, 1992.
17. Bennett IC, Freitas R, Fentiman IS: Diagnosis of breast cancer in young women. Aust NZ Surg 61:284–289, 1991.
18. Blichert-Toft M, Dyreborg U, Andersen J: Diagnostic strategy in the management of patients with breast symptoms. Acta Oncol 27:597–600, 1988.
19. Bloom HJG: Further studies on prognosis of breast carcinoma. Br J Cancer 4: 347–367, 1950.
20. Bloom HJG: The influence of delay on the natural history and prognosis of breast cancer. Br J Cancer 19:228–262, 1965.
21. Bloom HJG, Richardson WW: Histologic grading and prognosis in breast cancer. Br J Cancer 11:359–377, 1957.
22. Bloom HJG, Richardson WW, Harries EJ: Natural history of untreated breast cancer (1805–1933). Comparison of untreated and treated cases according to histological grade of malignancy. BMJ 2:213–221, 1962.
23. Bottles K, Taylor RN: Diagnosis of breast masses in pregnant and lactating women by aspiration cytology. Obstet Gynecol 66:76S–78S, 1985.
24. Bounds WE, Burton GV, Schwalke MA: Male breast cancer. J Louisiana State Med Soc 145:353–355, 1993.
25. Boyd NF, Meakin JW, Haywood JL, et al: Clinical estimation of the growth rate of breast cancer. Cancer 48:1037–1042, 1981.
26. Brightmore TG, Greening WP, Hamlin I: An analysis of clinical and histopathical features in 101 cases of carcinoma of breast in women under 35 years of age. Br J Cancer 24:644–669, 1970.
27. Brinkley D, Haybittle JL: A 15-year follow-up study of patients treated for carcinoma of the breast. Br J Radiol 41:215–221, 1968.
28. Buchanan JB, Spratt JS, Heuser LS: Tumor growth, doubling times, and the inability of the radiologist to diagnose certain cancers. Radiol Clin North Am 21:115–126, 1983.
29. Burns PE, Grace MGA, Lees AW, May C: False negative mammograms causing delay in breast cancer diagnosis. J Can Assoc Radiol 30:74–76, 1979.
30. Burstin HR, Johnson WG, Lipsitz ST, Brennan TA: Do the poor sue more? JAMA 270:1697–1701, 1993.
31. Buttlar CA, Templeton AC: The size of breast masses at presentation. The impact of prior medical training. Cancer 51:1750–1753, 1983.
32. Byrd BF Jr, Bayer DS, Robertson JS, et al: Treatment of breast tumors associated with pregnancy and lactation. Ann Surg 155:940–945, 1962.
33. Cade S: Malignant Disease and Its Treatment by Radium, 2nd ed. Bristol, England, Wright, 1948–1952.
34. Cameron A, Hinton J: Delay in seeking treatment for mammary tumors. Cancer 21:1121–1126, 1968.
35. Cancer statistics. Cancer 39:31, 1989.
36. Caplan LS, Helzlsouer KJ: Delay in breast cancer: A review of the literature. Public Health Rev 20:187–214, 1992.
37. Cardona G, Cataliotti L, Ciatto S, Del Turco MR: Reasons for failure of physical examination in breast cancer detection (analysis of 232 false-negative cases). Tumori 69:531–537, 1983.
38. Charlson ME: Delay in the treatment of carcinoma of the breast. Surg Gynecol Obstet 160:393–399, 1985.
39. Charlson ME, Feinstein AR: The auxometric dimension. A new method for using rate of growth in prognostic staging of breast cancer. JAMA 228:180–185, 1974.
40. Charlson ME, Feinstein AR: A new clinical index of growth rate in staging of breast cancer. Am J Med 69:527–536, 1980.
41. Charlson ME, Feinstein AR: Rapid growth rate in breast cancer: A confounding variable in adjuvant-chemotherapy trials. Lancet 1:1343–1345, 1982.
42. Chie W-C, Chang K-J: Factors related to tumor size of breast cancer at treatment in Taiwan. Prev Med 23:91–97, 1994.
43. Chung M, Chang H, Bland KI, Wanebo HJ: Younger women with breast carcinoma have a poorer prognosis than older women. Cancer 77:97–103, 1996.
44. Ciatto S, Iossa A, Bonardi R, Pacini P: Male breast carcinoma: Review of a multicenter series of 150 cases. Tumori 76:555–558, 1990.
45. Ciatto S, Zappa M: A prospective study of the value of mammographic patterns as indicators of breast cancer risk in a screening experience. Eur J Radiol 17:122–125, 1993.
46. Clayton F: Pathologic correlates of survival in 378 lymph node–negative infiltrating ductal breast carcinomas. Mitotic count is the best single predictor. Cancer 68:1309–1317, 1991.
47. Cohen MI, Mintzer RA, Matthies HJ, Bernstein JR: Mammography in women less than 40 years of age. Surg Gynecol Obstet 160:220–222, 1985.
48. Collins VP: Time of occurrence of pulmonary metastasis from carcinoma of the colon and rectum. Cancer 15:387–395, 1962.
49. Collins VP, Loeffler K, Tivey H: Observation on growth rates of human tumors. Am J Radiol 76:988–1000, 1956.
50. Cregan PC, Parer JG, Power AR: Accuracy of mammography in an Australian community setting. Med J Aust 149:408–409, 1988.
51. Cummings KM, Michalek AM, Gregoria D, Walsh D: Effects of behavioral and biological factors on survival from breast cancer. Cancer Detect Prev 6:485–494, 1983.
52. Cutler SJ, Myers MH, White PL: Who are we missing and why? Cancer 37:421–425, 1976.
53. Daland EM. Untreated cancer of the breast. Surg Gynecol Obstet 44:264–268, 1927.
54. Deemarsky LJ, Semiglzov VF: Cancer of the breast and pregnancy. In Ariel IM, Cleary JB (eds): Breast Cancer: Diagnosis and Treatment. New York, McGraw-Hill, 1987, p 475.
55. Dennis CR, Gardner B, Lim B: Analysis of survival and recurrence vs patient and doctor delay in treatment of breast cancer. Cancer 35:714–720, 1975.
56. Deschenes L, Jacob S, Fabia J, Christen A: Beware of breast fibroadenomas in middle-aged women. Can J Surg 28:372–374, 1985.
57. Devitt JE: The clinical stages of breast cancer. What do they mean? Can Med Assoc J 97:1257–1262, 1967.
58. Devitt JE: The enigmatic behavior of breast cancer. Cancer 27:12–17, 1971.
59. Diercks DB, Cady B: Lawsuits for failure to diagnose breast cancer. Tumor biology in causation and risk management strategies. Surg Oncol Clin North Am 3:125–139, 1994.

60. Dohrmann PJ, Hughes ES, McDermott F: Symptom duration, tumor staging, and survival in patients with carcinoma of the breast. Surg Gynecol Obstet 154:707–710, 1982.

61. Donegan WL: Management of pregnancy and lactation. In Stoll B (ed): Breast Cancer Management, Early and Late. London, Heinemann, 1977, p 195.

62. Donegan WL: Breast carcinoma and pregnancy. In Donegan WL, Spratt JS (eds): Cancer of the Breast, 4th ed. Philadelphia, WB Saunders, 1995, pp 732–733.

63. Donegan WL: Introduction to the history of breast cancer. In Donegan WL, Spratt JS (eds): Cancer of the Breast, 4th ed. Philadelphia, WB Saunders, 1995, pp 4–10.

64. Eggers C, deCholnoky T, Jessup DSD: Cancer of the breast. Ann Surg 113:321–340, 1941.

65. Eklund GW, Busby RC, Miller SH, Job JS: Improved imaging of the augmented breast. AJR Am J Roentgenol 151:469–473, 1988.

66. Elwood JM, Moorehead WP: Delay in diagnosis and longterm survival in breast cancer. BMJ 280:1291–1294, 1980.

67. Engell HC: Cancer cells in the circulating blood. Acta Chir Scand 201(Suppl):1–70, 1955.

68. Erickson EJ, McGreevy JM, Muskett A: Selective nonoperative management of patients referred with abnormal mammograms. Am J Surg 160:659–663, 1990.

69. Facione NC: Delay versus help seeking for breast cancer symptoms: A critical review of the literature on patient and provider delay. Soc Sci Med 36:1521–1534, 1993.

70. Fajardo LL, Davis JR, Wiens JL, et al: Mammography-guided stereotactic fine-needle aspiration cytology of nonpalpable breast lesions: Prospective comparison with surgical biopsy results. AJR Am J Roentgenol 155:977–981, 1990.

71. Feldman JG, Saunders M, Carter AC, Gardner B: The effects of patient delay and symptoms other than a lump on survival in breast cancer. Cancer 51:1226–1229, 1983.

72. Fentiman IS: Pensive women, painful vigils: Consequences of delay in assessment of mammographic abnormalities. Lancet 1:1041–1042, 1988.

73. Finley ML, Francis A: Risk factors and physician delay in the diagnosis of breast cancer. Prog Clin Biol Res 130:351–360, 1983.

74. Fisher B, Fisher ER: The interrelationship of hematogenous and lymphatic tumor cell dissemination. Surg Gynecol Obstet 122:791–796, 1966.

75. Fisher B, Fisher ER: Barrier function of lymph node to tumor cells and erythrocytes: I. Normal nodes. Cancer 20:1907–1913, 1967.

76. Fisher B: A commentary on the role of the surgeon in primary breast cancer. Breast Cancer Res Treat 1:17–26, 1981.

77. Fisher B, Gebhardt MC: The evolution of breast cancer surgery. Past, present, future. Semin Oncol 5:385–394, 1978.

78. Fisher B, Slack NH, Bross IDJ, et al: Cancer of the breast: Size of neoplasm and prognosis. Cancer 24:1071–1080, 1969.

79. Fisher ER, Gregorio RM, Redmond C, et al: Pathologic findings from the National Surgical Adjuvant Breast Project (protocol no. 4). The significance of regional node histology other than sinus histiocytosis in invasive mammary cancer. Am J Clin Pathol 197:21–30, 1976.

80. Fisher ER, Redmond C, Fisher B: A perspective concerning the relation of duration of symptoms to treatment failure in patients with breast cancer. Cancer 40:3160–3167, 1977.

81. Fox MS: On the diagnosis and treatment of breast cancer. JAMA 241:489–494, 1979.

82. Gallenberg MM, Loprinzi CL: Breast cancer and pregnancy. Semin Oncol 16:369–376, 1989.

83. Giard RW, Hermans J: The value of aspiration cytologic examination of the breast. A statistical review of the medical literature. Cancer 69:2104–2110, 1992.

84. GIVIO (Interdisciplinary Group for Cancer Care Evaluation) Italy: Reducing diagnostic delay in breast cancer: Possible therapeutic implications. Cancer 58:1756–1761, 1986.

85. Goel AK, Seenu V, Shukla NK, Raina V: Breast cancer presentation at a regional cancer centre. Natl Med J India 8:6–9, 1995.

86. Goodsen WH, Ljung BM, Waldman F, et al: In vivo measurement of breast cancer growth rate. Arch Surg 126:1220–1224, 1991.

87. Gould-Martin K, Paganini-Hill A, Casagrande C, et al: Behavioral and biological determinants of surgical stage of breast cancer. Prev Med 11:429–440, 1982.

88. Gray JH: The relation of lymphatic vessels to the spread of cancer. Br J Surg 26:462–472, 1938.

89. Guinee VF, Olsson H, Moller T, Hess KR, et al: Effect of pregnancy on prognosis for young women with breast cancer. Lancet 343:1587–1589, 1994.

90. Gupta RK, Dowle CS, Simpson JS: The value of needle aspiration cytology of the breast, with an emphasis on the diagnosis of breast disease in young women below the age of 30. Acta Cytol 34:165–168, 1990.

91. Gupta RK, Naran S, Buchanan A, Fauck R, Simpson J: Fine-needle aspiration cytology of breast: Its impact on surgical practice with an emphasis on the diagnosis of breast abnormalities in young women. Diagn Cytopathol 4:206–209, 1988.

92. Haagensen CD, Stout AP: Carcinoma of the breast. I—Results of treatment. Ann Surg 116:801–815, 1942.

93. Haagensen CD, Stout AP: Carcinoma of the breast. III. Results of treatment, 1935–1942. Ann Surg 134:151–172, 1951.

94. Haagensen CD: Diseases of the Breast. Philadelphia, WB Saunders, 1971, pp 478–502.

95. Hackett TP, Cassem NH, Raker JW: Patient delay in cancer. N Engl J Med 289:14–20, 1973.

96. Hall FM, Storella JM, Silverstone DZ, Wyshak G: Nonpalpable breast lesions: Recommendations for biopsy based on suspicion of carcinoma at mammography. Radiology 167:353–358, 1988.

97. Halsted WS: The results of operations for the cure of cancer of the breast at Johns Hopkins Hospital from 1889 to 1894. Johns Hopkins Hospital Rep 4:297–350, 1894–1895.

98. Halsted WS: The results of radical operations for the cure of carcinoma of the breast. Trans Am Surg Assoc 25:61–79, 1907.

99. Handley WS: Cancer of the Breast and Its Operative Treatment. London, John Murray Publishers, 1906.

100. Harms CR, Plaut JA, Oughterson AW: Delay in the treatment of cancer. JAMA 121:335–338, 1943.

101. Harnett WL: The relationship between delay in treatment of cancer and survival rate. Br J Cancer 7:19–26, 1953.

102. Harper D: Medical lessons from malpractice cases. JAMA 183:1073–1077, 1963.

103. Harrington WW: Survival rates of radical mastectomy for unilateral and bilateral carcinoma of the breast. Surgery 19:154–166, 1946.

104. Hawkins JW: Evaluation of breast cancer therapy as a guide to control programs. J Natl Cancer Inst 4:445–460, 1944.

105. Hein K, Dell R, Cohen MI: Self-detection of a breast mass in adolescent females. J Adolesc Health 3:15–17, 1982.

106. Heuser LS, Spratt JS, Kuhns JG, et al: The association of pathologic and mammographic characteristics of primary human breast cancers with "slow" and "fast" growth rates and with axillary lymph node metastases. Cancer 53:96–98, 1984.

107. Heuser L, Spratt JS, Polk HC: Growth rates of primary breast cancers. Cancer 43:1888–1894, 1979.

108. Holford TR, Roush GC, McKay LA: Trends in female breast cancer in Connecticut and the United States. J Clin Epidemiol 44:29–33, 1991.

109. Hollingsworth AB, Taylor LD, Rhodes DC: Establishing a histologic basis for false-negative mammograms. Am J Surg 166:643–647, 1993.

110. Hoopes BJ, McGraw AB: The Halsted radical mastectomy—five-year results in 246 consecutive operations at the same clinic. Surgery 12:892–905, 1942.

111. Hoover HC: Breast cancer during pregnancy and lactation. Surg Clin North Am 70:1151–1163, 1990.

112. Hultborn KA, Tornberg B: Mammary carcinoma—the biologic character of mammary cancer studied in 517 cases by a new form of malignancy grading. Acta Radiol Suppl 196:1–143, 1960.

113. Humphrey LJ, Swerdlow M: Factors influencing the survival of patients with carcinoma of the breast. Am J Surg 106:440–444, 1963.

114. Hunter CP, Redmond CK, Chen VW, et al: Breast cancer:

Factors associated with stage at diagnosis in black and white women. J Natl Cancer Inst 85:1129–1137, 1993.

115. Ingram DM, Huang H-Y, Catchpole BN, Roberts A: Do big breasts disadvantage women with breast cancer? Aust NZ J Surg 59:115–117, 1989.

116. Isaacs JH: Cancer of the breast in pregnancy. Surg Clin North Am 75:47–51, 1995.

117. Joensuu H, Asola R, Holli K, et al: Delayed diagnosis and large size of breast cancer after a false negative mammogram. Eur J Cancer 30A:1299–1302, 1994.

118. Kaae S: The prognostic significance of early diagnosis in breast cancer. Acta Radiol 29:475–479, 1948.

119. Katz SJ, Hislop G, Thomas DB, Larson EB: Delay from symptom to diagnosis and treatment of breast cancer in Washington State and British Columbia. Med Care 31:264–268, 1993.

120. Keinan G, Carmil D, Rieck M: Predicting women's delay in seeking medical care after discovery of a lump in the breast: The role of personality and behavior patterns. Behav Med 177–183, Winter 1991/1992.

121. Kelsey JL, Gammon MD: The epidemiology of breast cancer Cancer 41:146, 1991.

122. Kern KA: Causes of breast cancer malpractice litigation. A 20-year civil court review. Arch Surg 127:542–547, 1992.

122a. Kern KA: Risk management goals involving injury to the common bile duct during laparoscopic cholecystectomy. Am J Surg 163:551–552, 1992.

123. Kern KA: Breast biopsy in young women. Am J Surg 166:776–777, 1993.

124. Kern KA: Medical malpractice involving colon and rectal disease: A twenty-year review of United States civil court litigation. Dis Colon Rectum 36:531–539, 1993.

125. Kern KA: Medicolegal analysis of errors in the diagnosis and treatment of surgical endocrine disease. Surgery 114:1167–1174, 1993.

126. Kern KA: Medical liability and breast cancer diagnosis: Breast Surgery: Index and Reviews, Vol 1, No. 4. Cedar Knolls, NJ, World Medical Communications Organization, 1993.

127. Kern KA: Medicolegal analysis of the delayed diagnosis of cancer in 338 cases in the United States. Arch Surg 129:397–404, 1994.

128. Kern KA: Historical trends in breast cancer litigation: A clinician's perspective. Surg Oncol Clin North Am 3:1–24, 1994.

129. Kern KA: Preventing the delayed diagnosis of breast cancer through medical litigation analysis. Surg Oncol Clin North Am 3:101–123, 1994.

130. Kern KA, Cady B: The delayed diagnosis of breast cancer and health care reform (editorial). Breast Dis Q 6:14–15, 1994.

131. Kern KA, Cady B: Breast cancer: Selected legal issues (annotated bibliographic note). Breast Dis Q 6:120–121, 1994.

132. Kern KA: The delayed diagnosis of breast cancer. Biologic, technologic, or sociologic failure? Contemp Surg 45:286–289, 1994.

133. Kern KA: Medical malpractice in colon and rectal disease. Dis Colon Rectum 37:95–96, 1994.

134. Kern KA: Causes of breast cancer malpractice litigation. J Am Coll Surg 179:505–506, 1994.

135. Kern KA: Do the poor sue more? JAMA 271:504, 1994.

135a. Kern KA: Medicolegal analysis of bile duct injury during open cholecystectomy and abdominal surgery. Am J Surg 168:217–222, 1994.

135b. Kern KA: Medicolegal perspectives on laparoscopic bile duct injury. Surg Clin North Am 74:979–984, 1994.

136. Kern KA: The anatomy of surgical malpractice claims. Bull Am Coll Surg 80:34–49, 1995.

137. Kern KA: Unnecessary mammograms in women with palpable breast masses. J Am Coll Surg 182:462–463, 1996..

138. Kravitz RL, Rolph JE, McGuigan K: Malpractice claims data as a quality improvement tool. I. Epidemiology of error in four specialties. JAMA 266:2087–2091, 1991.

139. Lane-Claypon JE: Report of Public Health. London, British Ministry of Public Health, 1924–1928.

140. Langlands AO, Tiver KW: Significance of a negative mammogram in patients with a palpable breast tumour. Med J Aust 1:30–31, 1982.

141. Lannin DR, Harris RP, Swanson FH, Pories WJ: Difficulties in diagnosis of carcinoma of the breast in patients less than fifty years of age. Surg Gynecol Obstet 177:457–462, 1993.

142. Leach JE, Robbins GF: Delay in the diagnosis of cancer. JAMA 135:5–9, 1947.

143. Leape LL, Brennan TA, Nan Laird MPH, et al: The nature of adverse events in hospitalized patients. Results of the Harvard Medical Practice Study II. N Engl J Med 324:377–384, 1991.

144. Leis HP: Selective elective prophylactic contralateral mastectomy. Cancer 28:956–961, 1971.

145. Lewis D, Reinhoff WF: A study of the results of operations for the cure of cancer of the breast. Ann Surg 95:336–400, 1931.

146. Locklear QJ, Langlands AO: The misuse of mammography in the management of breast cancer. Med J Aust 145:185–187, 1986.

147. Luff AP: The incidence of cancer of the breast, and its history after treatment. BMJ 1:897–903, 1932.

148. Lundgren B: Diagnosis and screening in breast cancer; a review. Eur J Cancer Clin Oncol 19:1709–1710, 1983.

149. Lundgren B: Observations on growth rate of breast carcinomas and its possible implications for lead time. Cancer 40:1722–1725, 1977.

150. MacCoun RJ: Experimental research on jury decision-making. Science 244:1046–1050, 1989.

151. MacDonald I: Mammary carcinoma—a review of 2636 cases. Surg Gynecol Obstet 74:75–82, 1942.

152. MacDonald I: Biological predeterminism in human cancer. Surg Gynecol Obstet 92:443–452, 1951.

153. MacDonald I: The natural history of mammary carcinoma. Am J Surg 111:435–442, 1966.

154. Machiavelli M, Leione B, Romero A, et al: Relation between delay and survival in 596 patients with breast cancer. Oncology 46:78–82, 1989.

155. Magarey CJ, Todd PB: Breast loss and delay in breast cancer diagnosis: Behavioural science in surgical research. Aust NZ J Surg 40:391–393, 1976.

156. Magarey CJ, Todd PB: The doctor and the patient in early breast cancer diagnosis. Aust Fam Physician 6:243–247, 1977.

157. Magarey CJ, Todd PB, Blizard PJ: Psychosocial factors influencing delay and breast self examination in women with symptoms of breast cancer. Soc Science Med 11:229–232, 1977.

158. Mahoney L, Csima A: Use and abuse of mammography in the early diagnosis of breast cancer. Can J Surg 26:262–265, 1983.

159. Mann BD, Giuliano AE, Bassett LW, et al: Delayed diagnosis of breast cancer as a result of normal mammograms. Arch Surg 118:23–24, 1983.

160. Mansson J, Bengtsson C: The diagnosis of breast cancer—experiences from the community of Kungsbacka, Sweden. Neoplasma 39:305–308, 1992.

161. Marchant DJ: Breast cancer in pregnancy. Clin Obstet Gynecol 37:993–997, 1994.

162. Max MH, Klamer TW: Breast cancer in 120 women under 35 years old. A 10-year community-wide survey. Am Surg 50:23–25, 1984.

163. McKinnon NE: Limitations in diagnosis and treatment of breast and other cancers. Can Med Assoc J 73:614–625, 1955.

164. McKinnon NE: Control for cancer mortality. Lancet 1:251–254, 1954.

165. McWhirter R: Some factors influencing prognosis in breast cancer. J Fac Radiol 8:220–234, 1957.

166. Miller AB: Mammography: A critical evaluation of its role in breast cancer screening, especially in developing countries. J Public Health Policy 10:486–498, 1989.

167. Mitnick JS, Vazquez MF, Kronovet SZ, Roses DF: Malpractice litigation involving patients with carcinoma of the breast. J Am Coll Surg 181:315–321, 1995.

168. Mitnick JS, Vazquez MF, Plesser KP, Roses DF: Breast cancer malpractice litigation in New York State. Radiology 189:673–676, 1993.

169. Mittelmann M, Scholhamer CF: Cancer and malpractice claims. Cancer 39:2573–2578, 1977.

170. Mor V, Masterson-Allen S, Goldberg R, et al: Prediagnostic symptom recognition and help seeking among cancer patients. J Community Health 15:253–266, 1990.

171. Moskowitz M: Breast cancer: Age-specific growth rates and screening strategies. Radiology 1:3741–3746, 1986.

172. Moskowitz M: Guidelines for screening for breast cancer. Is a revision in order? Radiol Clin North Am 30:221–233, 1992.

173. Mueller CB: Surgery for breast cancer: Less may be as good as more. N Engl J Med 312:712–714, 1985.

174. Mueller CB: Stage II breast cancer is not simply a late stage I. Surgery 104:631–638, 1988.

175. Mund DF, Farria DM, Gorczyca DP, et al: MR imaging of the breast in patients with silicone-gel implants: Spectrum of findings. AJR Am J Roentgenol 161:773–778, 1993,

176. Neale AV, Tilley BC, Vernon SW: Marital status, delay in seeking treatment and survival from breast cancer. Soc Sci Med 23:305–312, 1986.

177. Neave LM, Mason BH, Kay RG: Does delay in diagnosis of breast cancer affect survival? Breast Cancer Res Treat 15:103–108, 1990.

178. Nichols S, Waters WE, Fraser JD, et al: Delay in the presentation of breast symptoms for consultant investigation. Community Med 3:217–225, 1981.

179. Novotny DB, Maygarden SJ, Shermer RW, Frable WJ: Fine needle aspiration of benign and malignant breast masses associated with pregnancy. Acta Cytol 35:676–686, 1991.

180. Osther PJ, Balslev E, Blichert-Toft M: Paget's disease of the nipple. A continuing enigma. Acta Chir Scand 156:343–352, 1990.

181. Pack GT, Gallo JS: The culpability for delay in the treatment of cancer. Am J Cancer 33:443–447, 1938.

182. Page DL: Prognosis and breast cancer. Recognition of lethal and favorable prognostic types. Am J Surg Pathol 15:334–349, 1991.

183. Palmer ML, Tsangaris TN: Breast biopsy in women 30 years old or less. Am J Surg 165:708–712, 1993.

184. Park WW, Lees JC: The absolute curability of cancer of the breast. Surg Gynecol Obstet 93:129–152, 1951.

185. Petrek JA: Pregnancy-associated breast cancer. Semin Surg Oncol 7:306–310, 1991.

186. Petrek JA: Breast cancer during pregnancy. Cancer 74:518–527, 1994.

187. Petrek JA: Breast cancer and pregnancy. Natl Cancer Inst Monogr 16:113–121, 1994.

188. Phelan M, Dobbs J, David AS: 'I thought it would go away': Patient denial in breast cancer. J R Soc Med 141:768–769, 1992.

189. Physician Insurers Association of America: Breast Cancer Study 1990. Washington, DC, PIAA, 1990.

190. Physician Insurers Association of America: Data Sharing Reports, Executive Summary. Washington, DC, PIAA, 1990.

191. Physician Insurers Association of America. Breast Cancer Study 1995. Washington, DC, PIAA, 1995.

192. Physician Insurers Association of America. Data Sharing Reports: Executive Summary (1995). Washington, DC, PIAA, 1995.

193. Pilipshen SJ, Gerardi J, Bretsky S, Robbins GF: The significance of delay in treating patients with potentially curable breast cancer. Breast 10:16–23, 1984.

194. Polednak AP: Breast cancer in black and white women in New York State. Case distribution and incidence rates by clinical stage at diagnosis. Cancer 58:807–815, 1986.

195. Porta M, Gallen M, Malats N, Planas J: Influence of diagnostic delay upon cancer survival: An analysis of five tumour sites. J Epidemiol Community Health 45:225–230, 1991.

196. Reintgen D, Berman C, Cox C, et al: The anatomy of missed breast cancers. Surg Oncol 2:65–71, 1993

197. Reintgen D, Cox C, Greenberg H, et al: The medical legal implications of following mammographic breast masses. Am Surg 59:99–105, 1993.

198. Ribeiro G, Jones DA, Jones M: Carcinoma of the breast associated with pregnancy. Br J Surg 73:607–609, 1986.

199. Richardson JL, Langholz B, Bernstein L, et al: Stage and delay in breast cancer diagnosis by race, socioeconomic status, age, and year. Br J Cancer 65:922–926, 1992.

200. Rimsten A, Stenkvist B: Diagnostic delay in cancer of the breast. Ann Chir Gynaecol 64:353–358, 1975.

201. Robbins GF, Berg JW, Bross IDJ, et al: The significance of early treatment of breast cancer. Cancer 12:688–692, 1959.

202. Robbins GF, Bross I: The significance of delay in relation to prognosis of patients with primary operable breast cancer. Cancer 10:338–344, 1957.

203. Robinson E, Mohelever J, Borovik R: Factors affecting delay in diagnosis of breast cancer: Relationship of delay to stage of disease. Isr J Med Sci 22:333–338, 1986.

204. Robinson E, Sapir D, Zeiden G, Mohelever J: Delay in diagnosis of cancer. Possible effects on the stage of disease and survival. Cancer 54:454–60, 1984.

205. Robinson E, Rennert G, Bar-Deroma R, et al: The pattern of diagnosis of a second primary tumor in the breast. Breast Cancer Res Treat 25:211–215, 1993.

206. Rossi S, Cinini C, Di Pietro C, et al: Diagnostic delay in breast cancer: Correlation with disease stage and prognosis. Tumori 76:559–562, 1990.

207. Rudan I, Skoric T, Rudan N: Breast cancer prognosis. II. Prognostic factors in patients with node-positive (N1-3) breast cancer. Acta Med Croatica 48:165–170, 1994.

208. Rudan I, Skoric T, Rudan N: Breast cancer prognosis. III. Prognostic factors in patients with distant metastases (M1) at the time of diagnosis. Acta Med Croatica 48:171–174, 1994.

209. Saks MJ, Kidd RF: Human information processing and adjudication: Trial by heuristics. Law and Society Review 15:123–160, 1980.

210. Sanchez JA, Feller WF: Paget's disease of the breast. Am Fam Physician 36:145–147, 1987.

211. Say CC, Donegan WL: Invasive carcinoma of the breast: Prognostic significance of tumor size and involved axillary lymph nodes. Cancer 34:468–471, 1974.

212. Schirber S, Thomas WO, Finley JM, et al: Breast cancer after mammary augmentation. South Med J 86:263–268, 1993.

213. Scott-Connor CE, Carol EH, Schorr SJ: The diagnosis and management of breast problems during pregnancy and lactation. Am J Surg 170:401–405, 1995.

214. Shapiro S, Venet W, Strax P, et al: Ten- to fourteen-year effect of screening on breast cancer mortality. J Natl Cancer Inst 69:349–355, 1982.

215. Sheridan B, Fleming J, Atkinson L, Scott G: The effects of delay in treatment on survival rates in carcinoma of the breast. Med J Aust 1:262–7, 1971.

216. Silverstein MJ, Gierson ED, Gamagami P, et al: Breast cancer diagnosis and prognosis in women with silicone gel–filled implants. Cancer 66:97–101, 1990.

217. Silverstein MJ, Handel N, Gamagami P, et al: Mammographic measurements before and after augmentation mammaplasty. Plast Reconstr Surg 86:1126–1130, 1990.

218. Smithers DW, Rigby-Jones P, Galton DA, Payne PM: Cancer of the breast—review. Br J Radiol (Suppl) 4:1–13, 1–90, 1952.

219. Spatz MW: Breast cancer in men. Am Fam Physician 38:187–189, 1988.

220. Spratt JS Jr, Ackerman LV: Relationship of the size of colonic tumors to their cellular composition and biological behavior. Surg Forum 10:56–61, 1960.

221. Spratt JS, Spratt JA: What is breast cancer doing before we can detect it? J Surg Oncol 30:156–160, 1985.

222. Spratt JS, Spratt SW: Medical and legal implications of screening and follow-up procedures for breast cancer. Cancer 66:1351–1362, 1990.

223. Spratt JS: Anatomic staging systems for cancer. Fixed end-point survival rates and tort claims. J Pelvic Surg 1:8–11, 1995.

224. Spratt JS, Spratt JA: Growth rates. In Donegan WL, Spratt JS (eds): Cancer of the Breast, 4th ed. Philadelphia, WB Saunders, 1995, pp 317–345.

225. Spratt JS, Donegan WL, Sigdestad CP: Epidemiology and etiology. In Donegan WL, Spratt JS: Cancer of the Breast, 4th ed. Philadelphia, WB Saunders, 1995, p 118.

226. Stierer M, Rosen H, Weitensfelder W, et al: Male breast cancer: Austrian experience. World J Surg 19:687–693, 1995.

227. Svensson WE, Tohno E, Cosgrove DO, et al: Effects of fine-

needle aspiration on the US appearance of the breast. Radiology 185:709–711, 1992.
228. Tabar L, Gad A: Screening for breast cancer—the Swedish trial. Radiology 138:219–222, 1981.
229. Tabbarah HJ: Cancer and pregnancy. *In* Haskell CM (ed): Cancer Treatment, 4th ed. Philadelphia, WB Saunders, 1995.
230. Tennvall J, Moller T, Attewell R: Delaying factors in primary treatment of breast cancer. Acta Chir Scand 156:591–596, 1990.
231. Treves N, Holleb AI: A report of 549 cases of breast cancer in women 35 years of age or young. Surg Gynecol Obstet 107:271–283, 1958.
232. Tubiana M, Koscielny S: Natural history of human breast cancer: Recent data and clinical implications. Breast Cancer Res Treat 18:125–40, 1991.
233. Urban JA: Early diagnosis of breast cancer Cancer 9:1173–1176, 1956.
234. Urban JA: Bilateral breast cancer Cancer 24:1310–1316, 1969.
235. Waalen J: Pregnancy poses tough questions for cancer treatment. J Natl Cancer Inst 83:900–902, 1991.
236. Walker QJ, Langlands AO: The misuse of mammography in the management of breast cancer. Med J Aust 145:185–187, 1986.
237. Walker QJ, Gebski V, Langlands AO: The misuse of mammography in the management of breast cancer revisited. Med J Aust 151:509–511, 1989.
238. Wallack MK, Wolf JA, Bedwinek J, et al: Gestational carcinoma of the female breast. Curr Probl Cancer 7:1–58, 1983.
239. Waters WE, Nichols S, Wheeller MJ, et al: Evaluation of a health education campaign to reduce the delay in women presenting with breast symptoms. Community Medicine 5:104–108, 1983.
240. Watson M, Greer S, Blake S, Shrapnell K: Reaction to a diagnosis of breast cancer. Relationship between denial, delay and rates of psychological morbidity. Cancer 53:2008–2012, 1984.
241. Waxman BD, Fitts WT: Survival of female patients with cancer of the breast. Am. J Surg 97:31–35, 1959.
242. Westberg SV: Prognosis of breast cancer for pregnancy and nursing women. A clinical-statistical study. Acta Obstet Gynecol 25:1–5, 1946.
243. Wilkinson GS, Edgerton F, Wallace HJ, et al: Delay, stage of disease and survival from breast cancer. J Chronic Dis 32:365–373, 1979.
244. Williams EM, Baum M, Hughes LE: Delay in presentation of women with breast disease. Clin Oncol 2:327–331, 1976.
245. Woods WGA, Earlam RJ, Turner MJ: Mammography in hospital patients: Use and misuse. J R Coll Surg Edinb 37:16–18, 1992.
246. Wool MS: Extreme denial in breast cancer patients and capacity for object relations. Psychother Psychosom 46:196–204, 1986.
247. Yeatman TJ, Cantor AB, Smith TJ, et al: Tumor biology of infiltrating lobular carcinoma. Implications for management. Ann Surg Onc 222:549–561, 1995.
248. Zinns JS: The association of pregnancy and breast cancer. J Reprod Med 22:297–301, 1979.
249. Zylstra S, Bors-Koefoed R, Mondor M, et al: A statistical model for predicting the outcome in breast cancer malpractice lawsuits. Obstet Gynecol 84:392–398, 1994.

INDEX

Note: Page numbers in *italics* refer to illustrations; page numbers followed by t refer to tables.

Cyclosporine, gynecomastia with, 173
Cyproterone acetate, gynecomastia with, 173
Cyst(s), 192–195, 234
  apocrine, 193–194, *193, 194*
  apocrine-like epithelium of, 193, *193,* 235–236, 236t
  breast cancer risk and, 194–195, 431
  fine needle aspiration of, 714, *714*
  fluid aspiration from, 808–809, *809*
  GCDFP-15 marker in, 194
  histopathology of, 192–195, *193, 194*
  mammography of, 658, *660*
  palpability of, 193
  papillary apocrine change of, 193–194, *194*
    breast cancer risk and, 195
  pathology of, 234–236
  pigment-laden macrophages and, 195
  ultrasonography of, *660*
  vellus hair, 329, *329*
Cystic fibrosis, gynecomastia in, 176
Cystosarcoma phyllodes, 206–208, 315–318. See also *Phyllodes tumor.*
  border of, 317, *317*
  clinical features of, 315–316
  diagnosis of, 318
  fine needle aspiration of, 727
  histopathology of, 207–208, *207, 208,* 316, *316*
  pathological features of, 316, *316*
  prognosis for, 316–318, *317*
  recurrence of, 317
  stromal overgrowth in, 317
  treatment of, 318
Cytokines, in breast cancer, 607, 609
Czerny, Vincenz, 13

Dahl-Iversen, E., 785
Danazol, in drug-related breast gigantism, 223–224
  in gynecomastia, 177, 178t
  in mastalgia, 251t, 253, 257
Danocrine, for mastalgia, 241
Darier's disease (keratosis follicularis), 325, *325*
DDT (dichlorodiphenyltrichloroethane), breast cancer risk and, 349, 1526
Dehydroepiandrosterone sulfate, serum, breast cancer risk and, 353
Dementia, hormone replacement therapy and, 1479
Deoxyribonucleic acid (DNA), estrogen receptor interaction with, 520
Depression, *BRCA1* gene testing and, 387, *387*
Dermatitis, contact, 324–325
  radiation, 326
    vs. inflammatory breast cancer, 1282
  seborrheic, 324
Dermatofibrosarcoma protuberans, fine needle aspiration of, 728
Dermatomyofibroma, 336
Dermatoses, inflammatory, 324–328, 324t, *325–328*
Desmoid tumor (fibromatosis), 309, *310*
  vs. fibroadenoma, 206
D'Etiolles, Jean-Jacques-Joseph Leroy, 9
Dexrazoxane, cardioprotective effects of, 1292
  in stage IV breast cancer, 1341
DF3 antigen, in breast carcinoma *in situ,* 1017

Diabetes mellitus, breast abscess in, 146
  hypogonadotropism in, 43
Diabetic fibrous mastopathy, vs. granulomatous mastitis, 88
Diagnostic delay, 1582–1584, 1583t, 1626. See also *Breast cancer, delayed diagnosis of; Interval breast cancer.*
Diana of Ephesus, *2*
Diazepam, gynecomastia with, 172
Dicumarol, tissue necrosis with, 97–98, *98*
Diet, 1519–1530. See also specific dietary components.
  25:25 Diet for, 1527, 1528t–1529t, 1530t
  alcohol in, 349, 357t, 362, 616, 1525–1526
  caffeine in, 241, 250–252, 357t, 362, 1525
  caloric value of, 1521
  childhood, breast cancer and, 1527
  fat in, 1519–1522
    animal studies of, 1519, 1521
    breast cancer and, 348–349, 354, 1520–1521
    mastalgia and, 250–251, 252
    mechanistic studies of, 1519
    types of, 1521–1522
  fiber in, 1525
  fruits in, 1524–1525
  guidelines for, 1527–1530
  in breast cancer prevention, 354–355, 357t, 365, 1527–1530
  in mastalgia, 251–253
  pesticides in, 1526
  phytochemicals in, 1525
  phytoestrogens in, 1525
  recommendations for, 1526–1527, 1526t, 1527t, 1528t–1529t, 1530t
  selenium in, 1524
  vegetables in, 1524–1525
  vitamin A in, 354, 1523–1524
  vitamin C in, 357t, 362, 1524
  vitamin D in, 355, 357t, 362, 1524
  vitamin E in, 354–355, 357t, 362, 1524
25:25 Diet, 1527, 1528t–1529t, 1530t
Diethylstilbestrol (DES), carcinogenic effects of, 523–524
  gynecomastia with, 171, 172
  in estrogen receptor assay, 466, *466*
  in hormonal therapy, 1361
  in stages I and II breast cancer, 1224
Difluoromethylornithine, in breast cancer prevention, 361
Digitalis, gynecomastia with, 171
Dihydrotestosterone heptanoate, for gynecomastia, 177
7,12-Dimethylbenz[*a*] anthracene (DMBA)–induced carcinogenesis, 353–354
  hormone effects on, 524–525
  limonene effect on, 362
  tamoxifen effect on, 353–354, 357–358
Diphenylhydantoin, in metastases-induced seizures, 1392
Diuretics, in benign breast disease, 241
  in mastalgia, 256
  in postmastectomy lymphedema, 1008
Docetaxel, in stage IV breast cancer, 1331–1332, 1332t
Domperidone, gynecomastia with, 175
Dopamine, serum, in mastalgia, 250
Dormancy, tumor, 593
Doxorubicin (Adriamycin), antiangiogenic effects of, 597
  cardiotoxicity of, 1217, 1330

Doxorubicin (Adriamycin) *(Continued)*
  in stage IV breast cancer, 1328, 1329–1330, 1334–1336, 1334t, 1336t, 1337t
  in stages I and II breast cancer, 1207–1208, 1208t
  liposomal, in stage IV breast cancer, 1333
  MCF-7 breast cancer cell line resistance to, 543–544
  side effects of, 1292, 1498
  with CMF, 1211
Doxycycline pleurodesis, in malignant pleural effusion, 1385
Dracunculiasis, 89
Dressing, postmastectomy, 995
Droloxifene, 1356
Drugs. See also specific drugs.
  galactorrhea with, 49, 68
  gynecomastia with, 46
Ductal carcinoma, 285. See also *Breast cancer* and specific stages of breast cancer at *Stage* entries.
  after ductal carcinoma *in situ,* 1023–1024, 1023t
  after lobular carcinoma *in situ,* 1021–1022
  cytologic features of, 64–65, *65*
  nipple discharge in, 66, *66,* 67, *67*
Ductal carcinoma, not otherwise specified (carcinoma, no special type), 285, 288–289, *289*
  familial, 380, *381*
  fine needle aspiration of, 721, 723, *724*
  histopathology of, 288–289, *289*
  mammography of, 666, *666–668*
  mitotic grade of, *381*
  multicentricity of, 303
    case study of, 298, *299, 300,* 301, *301*
Ductal carcinoma *in situ,* 1020t, 1044–1068
  angiogenic switch in, 586, *587, 588*
  axillary lymph node dissection in, 957
  bilateral disease and, 1025–1026, 1429t
  calcifications in, *264,* 272, 273, 1026–1027, *1027*
  cancerization of lobules in, *270*
  cathepsin D in, 440
  classification of, 271–272, 271t, 272t, 1046–1048, *1046,* 1046t, *1047*
  comedo, 271, 271t
    definition of, 1046–1048, 1046t
    fine needle aspiration of, 720, *720*
    histopathology of, *269,* 270, *270,* 1018–1019, 1046–1047, 1046t
    historical studies of, 1013–1014
    invasive potential of, 1019
    mammography of, *674,* 675, *675*
    necrosis in, 1018, 1019
    NM23 protein in, 276
    prognosis for, 1019, 1134
  cribriform, *264,* 1018, *1046*
  cytometry in, 275–276
  diagnosis of, 1026–1027, *1027*
    biopsy in, 1027–1028, 1049–1054, *1050–1054,* 1054t
      coordinated team for, 1050, 1053
      dressing after, 1053, *1054*
      mammography after, 1053, *1054*
      specimen mammography after, 1027, *1027,* 1050
      tissue processing for, 1049–1050, *1053*
    fine needle aspiration biopsy in, 1027, 1049